The Practice
of Clinical
Echocardiography

Catherine M. Otto, MD

J. Ward Kennedy-Hamilton Endowed Professor of Cardiology
Department of Medicine
Director, Training Programs in Cardiovascular Disease
Associate Director, Echocardiography Laboratory
University of Washington School of Medicine
Seattle, Washington

The Practice of Clinical Echocardiography

THIRD EDITION

SAUNDERS

ELSEVIER

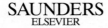

1600 John F. Kennedy Blvd.
Ste 1800
Philadelphia, PA 19103-2899

THE PRACTICE OF CLINICAL ECHOCARDIOGRAPHY, THIRD EDITION   ISBN: 978-1-4160-3640-1

Copyright © 2007, 2002, 1997 by Saunders, an imprint of Elsevier Inc.

Notice

Knowledge and best practice in this field are constantly changing. As new research and experience broaden our knowledge, changes in practice, treatment and drug therapy may become necessary or appropriate. Readers are advised to check the most current information provided (i) on procedures featured or (ii) by the manufacturer of each product to be administered, to verify the recommended dose or formula, the method and duration of administration, and contraindications. It is the responsibility of the practitioner, relying on their own experience and knowledge of the patient, to make diagnoses, to determine dosages and the best treatment for each individual patient, and to take all appropriate safety precautions. To the fullest extent of the law, neither the Publisher nor the Editor assumes any liability for any injury and/or damage to persons or property arising out of or related to any use of the material contained in this book.

The Publisher

Library of Congress Cataloging-in-Publication Data

The practice of clinical echocardiography / [edited by] Catherine M. Otto ; Starr Kaplan, illustrator. -- 3rd ed.
    p. ; cm.
  Includes bibliographical references.
  ISBN 978-1-4160-3640-1
  1. Echocardiography. I. Otto, Catherine M. II. Title: Clinical echocardiography.
  [DNLM: 1. Echocardiography. 2. Cardiovascular Diseases--diagnosis. WG 141.5.E2 P8942 2007]

RC683.5.U5C57 2002
616.1′207543--dc22

                             2007026986

Executive Publisher: Natasha Andjelkovic
Developmental Editor: Pamela Hetherington
Project Manager: Mary Stermel
Design Direction: Ellen Zanole
Marketing Manager: Paul Leese

Printed in China

Last digit is the print number: 9 8 7 6 5 4 3 2 1

Contributors

Gerard P. Aurigemma, MD
Professor of Medicine and Radiology
Director, Noninvasive Cardiology
Director, Cardiology Fellowship Program
Department of Medicine, Division of Cardiology
University of Massachusetts Memorial Medical School
Worcester, Massachusetts

Thomas Bartel, MD
Professor of Medicine
Division of Cardiology
Department of Internal Medicine
Medical University Innsbruck
Innsbruck, Austria

Ann F. Bolger, MD
William Watt Kerr Professor of Clinical Medicine
Division of Cardiology
University of California, San Francisco
Director, Echocardiography
San Francisco General Hospital
San Francisco, California

Johan G. Bosch, PhD
Assistant Professor
Laboratory for Experimental Echocardiography
Department Thoraxcenter Biomedical Engineering
Erasmus Medical Center
Rotterdam, The Netherlands

Charles J. Bruce, MD, MBChB
Associate Professor of Medicine
Division of Cardiovascular Diseases and Internal
  Medicine
Mayo Clinic and Mayo Foundation
Rochester, Minnesota

Ian G. Burwash, MD
Associate Professor of Medicine
Division of Cardiology
University of Ottawa Heart Institute
Ottawa, Ontario, Canada

Christopher H. Cabell, MD, MHS
Assistant Professor of Medicine
Division of Cardiology
Duke Clinical Research Institute
Duke University Medical Center
Durham, North Carolina

Kwan-Leung Chan, MD
Professor of Medicine
Department of Cardiology
University of Ottawa Heart Institute
Ottawa, Ontario, Canada

Edmond W. Chen, MD
Assistant Clinical Professor of Medicine
Department of Medicine, Division of Cardiology
University of California, San Francisco
San Francisco, California

Michael A. Chen, MD, PhD
Assistant Professor of Medicine
University of Washington
Department of Medicine, Division of Cardiology
Attending Physician
Harborview Medical Center
Seattle, Washington

John S. Child, MD
Streisand-American Heart Association Professor of
  Medicine and Cardiology
Director, Ahmanson-UCLA Adult Congenital Heart
  Disease Center
David Geffen School of Medicine at University of
  California, Los Angeles
Los Angeles, California

Lori B. Croft, MD
Assistant Professor of Medicine
Zena and Michael A. Wiener Cardiovascular Institute
Marie-Josée and Henry R. Kravis Center for
  Cardiovascular Health
Mt. Sinai Medical Center
New York, New York

Milind Y. Desai, MD
Physician
Department of Cardiovascular Medicine
The Cleveland Clinic Foundation
Cleveland, Ohio

Thor Edvardsen, MD, PhD
Associate Professor
Director, Cardiovascular Imaging Research
Consultant Cardiologist
Department of Cardiology
Rikshospitalet University Hospital
Oslo, Norway

Raimund Erbel, MD
Professor of Medicine/Cardiology
European Cardiologist
Department of Cardiology
West-German Heart Center
University Duisburg-Essen
Essen, Germany

Husam H. Farah, MD
Assistant Clinical Professor of Medicine
University of California, San Francisco
San Francisco, California

Kirsten E. Fleischmann, MD, MPH
Associate Professor of Medicine
Department of Medicine, Division of Cardiology
University of California, San Francisco
San Francisco, California

Paul R. Forfia, MD
Assistant Professor of Medicine
Department of Medicine, Cardiovascular Division
University of Pennsylvania School of Medicine
Philadelphia, Pennsylvania

Elyse Foster, MD
Professor of Clinical Medicine
Araxe Vilensky Endowed Chair in Medicine
Department of Medicine, Division of Cardiology
University of California, San Francisco School of
   Medicine
Director, Echocardiography Laboratory
University of California, San Francisco
San Francisco, California

Rosario V. Freeman, MD, MS
Assistant Professor of Medicine
Acting Director, Echocardiography Laboratory
University of Washington School of Medicine
Seattle, Washington

William H. Gaasch, MD
Professor of Medicine
Department of Cardiovascular Medicine
University of Massachusetts Medical School
Worcester, Massachusetts
Senior Consultant in Cardiology
Department of Cardiovascular Medicine
Lahey Clinic
Burlington, Massachusetts

Ivor L. Gerber, MD, MBChB
Consultant Cardiologist
Green Lane Cardiovascular Service
Auckland City Hospital
Auckland, New Zealand

Martin E. Goldman, MD
Dr. Arthur and Hilda Master Professor of Medicine
Director, Echocardiography Laboratory
Zena and Michael A. Wiener Cardiovascular Institute
Marie-Josée and Henry R. Kravis Center for
   Cardiovascular Health
Mt. Sinai Medical Center
New York, New York

John S. Gottdiener, MD
Professor of Medicine
University of Maryland School of Medicine
Director, Adult Echocardiography Laboratory
University of Maryland Hospital
Baltimore, Maryland

Brian P. Griffin, MD
Director, Cardiovascular Disease Training Program
John and Rosemary Brown Chair of Cardiovascular
   Medicine
Cleveland Clinic
Cleveland, Ohio

Michelle Gurvitz, MD
Assistant Professor of Pediatrics
Division of Pediatric Oncology
University of Washington
Seattle, Washington

Achim Gutersohn, MD
Assistant Physician
Division of Cardiology and Division of Pharmacology
West-German Heart Center
University Duisburg-Essen
Essen, Germany

Judy Hung, MD
Assistant Professor of Medicine
Harvard University
Associate Director, Clinical Echocardiography
Massachusetts General Hospital
Boston, Massachusetts

Bernard Iung, MD
Professor
Department of Cardiology
Paris VII University, Denis Diderot
Paris, France

Mary Etta E. King, MD
Associate Professor
Department of Pediatrics
Harvard University
Pediatrician and Director, Pediatric Echocardiography
Massachusetts General Hospital
Boston, Massachusetts

Allan L. Klein, MD
Professor of Medicine
Cleveland Clinic Lerner College of Medicine of Case
    Western Reserve University
Director, Cardiovascular Imaging Research
Department of Cardiovascular Medicine
Cleveland Clinic
Cleveland, Ohio

Thomas Konorza, MD
Assistant Physician
Division of Cardiology
West-German Heart Center
University Duisburg-Essen
Essen, Germany

Mark Lewin, MD
Associate Professor of Pediatrics
University of Washington School of Medicine
Interim Chief of Cardiology
Co-Director, Noninvasive Imaging
Children's Hospital and Regional Medical Center
Seattle, Washington

Warren J. Manning, MD
Assistant Professor of Medicine
Professor of Radiology
Harvard Medical School
Chief, Noninvasive Cardiac Imaging
Co-Director, Cardiac MR Center
Beth Israel Deaconess Medical Center
Boston, Massachusetts

Thomas H. Marwick, MBBS, PhD
Professor of Medicine
University of Queensland
Queensland, Australia
Director, Cardiac Imaging Group
Princess Alexandra Hospital
Brisbane, Australia

Gary S. Mintz, MD
Chief Medical Officer
Cardiovascular Research Foundation
Washington, DC

Robert R. Moss, MD
Clinical Assistant Professor
Internal Medicine (Cardiology)
University of British Columbia
Attending Cardiologist
St. Paul's Hospital
Vancouver, British Columbia, Canada

Silvana Müller, MD
Division of Cardiology
Department of Internal Medicine
Medical University Innsbruck
Innsbruck, Austria

Brad I. Munt, MD
Clinical Instructor
University of British Columbia School of Medicine
Attending Cardiologist
St. Paul's Hospital
Vancouver, British Columbia, Canada

Tasneem Z. Naqvi, MD
Associate Professor of Clinical Medicine
UCLA School of Medicine
Associate Director, Cardiac Noninvasive Lab
Cedars-Sinai Medical Center
Los Angeles, California

Catherine M. Otto, MD
J. Ward Kennedy-Hamilton Endowed Professor of
    Cardiology
Department of Medicine
Director, Training Programs in Cardiovascular Disease
Associate Director, Echocardiography Laboratory
University of Washington School of Medicine
Seattle, Washington

Donald C. Oxorn, MD
Professor
Department of Anesthesia
University of Washington School of Medicine
Seattle, Washington

Michael H. Picard, MD
Associate Professor of Medicine
Harvard Medical School
Director, Echocardiography
Massachusetts General Hospital
Boston, Massachusetts

Thomas R. Porter, MD
Assistant Professor
Section of Cardiology
University of Nebraska Medical Center
Omaha, Nebraska

Harry Rakowski, MD
Professor of Medicine
Division of Cardiology
University of Toronto
Toronto, Ontario, Canada

Rita F. Redberg, MD, MSc
Robert Wood Johnson Foundation Health Policy
    Fellow
Professor of Medicine
Director, Women's Cardiovascular Services
Division of Cardiology
University of California, San Francisco
San Francisco, California

Carlos A. Roldan, MD
Professor of Medicine
Division of Cardiology
University of New Mexico School of Medicine
Director, Echocardiography Laboratory
Veterans Affairs Medical Center
Albuquerque, New Mexico

Raphael Rosenhek, MD
Associate Professor of Medicine
Department of Cardiology
Medical University Vienna
Vienna, Austria

Florence H. Sheehan, MD
Research Professor
Department of Medicine
Division of Cardiology
University of Washington School of Medicine
Seattle, Washington

Otto A. Smiseth, MD, PhD
Professor of Medicine
Chief, Department of Cardiology
University of Oslo
Oslo, Norway

William J. Stewart, MD
Associate Professor of Medicine
Cleveland Clinic Lerner College of Medicine of Case
    Western Reserve University
Staff Cardiologist
Department of Cardiovascular Medicine
Section of Cardiovascular Imaging
The Cleveland Clinic Foundation
Cleveland, Ohio

Marcus F. Stoddard, MD
Professor of Medicine
Director, Noninvasive Cardiology
Division of Cardiology
University of Louisville
Director, Echocardiography
Veterans Administration Medical Center
Louisville, Kentucky

Karen K. Stout, MD
Assistant Professor of Medicine
Division of Cardiology
Adjunct Assistant Professor of Pediatrics
Director, Adult Congenital Heart Disease Program
University of Washington School of Medicine
Seattle, Washington

Martin St. John Sutton, MD
John W. Bryfogle Professor of Medicine
Division of Cardiovascular Medicine
Director, Cardiac Imaging
University of Pennsylvania Medical Center
Director, Cardiology Fellowship Program
Hospital of the University of Pennsylvania
Philadelphia, Pennsylvania

Christopher R. Thompson, MD
Director, Echocardiography Laboratory
St. Paul's Hospital
Vancouver, British Columbia, Canada

Brandon R. Travis, PhD
Research Fellow
Department of Thoracic and Cardiovascular Surgery
Skejby Sygehus
Arhus, Denmark

Alec Vahanian, MD
Professor
Department of Cardiology
Paris Universite VII, Denis Diderot
Head, Cardiology Department
Hopital Bichat
Paris, France

Nozomi Watanabe, MD
Assistant Professor of Medicine
Department of Cardiology
Director, Echocardiographic Laboratory
Kawasaki Medical School
Okayama, Japan

Sarah Weeks, MD
Echocardiography Fellow
Department of Cardiology
University of California, San Francisco
San Francisco, California

Neil J. Weissman, MD
Associate Professor of Medicine
Georgetown University
Director, Cardiac Ultrasound and Ultrasound Core Labs
Cardiovascular Research Institute/Washington
   Hospital Center
Washington, DC

Susan E. Wiegers, MD
Associate Professor of Medicine
Department of Medicine/Cardiovascular Division
University of Pennsylvania School of Medicine
Philadelphia, Pennsylvania

E. Douglas Wigle, MD
Professor of Medicine
University of Toronto
Toronto, Ontario, Canada

Anna Woo, MD
Assistant Professor of Medicine
University of Toronto
Toronto, Ontario, Canada

Audrey H. Wu, MD, MPH
Lecturer
Department of Internal Medicine
Division of Cardiovascular Medicine
University of Michigan Health System
Ann Arbor, Michigan

Feng Xie, MD
Assistant Professor, Internal Medicine
Division of Cardiology
University of Nebraska Medical Center
Omaha, Nebraska

Ajit P. Yoganathan, PhD
Wallace H. Coulter Distinguished Faculty Chair in
   Biomedical Engineering
Regents Professor
Associate Chair for Research
Georgia Institute of Technology and Emory University
Atlanta, Georgia

Miguel Zabalgoitia, MD
Professor of Medicine
University of Texas Health Center at San Antonio
Staff Cardiologist
University Hospital
South Texas Veterans Health Care System
San Antonio, Texas

William A. Zoghbi, MD
Professor of Medicine
William L. Winters Chair in Cardiovascular Imaging
Director, Cardiovascular Imaging Center
The Methodist DeBakey Heart Center
Houston, Texas

Preface

This book has two underlying goals: to serve as an advanced reference text on the clinical applications of echocardiography and to provide an introduction to newer echocardiographic modalities and research methods. As an advanced reference text, this book reflects our role as clinicians caring for patients with cardiovascular disease. The clinical information in this book will be of value to all cardiovascular specialists, not just those focused on cardiovascular imaging. This book also will be of interest to cardiology fellows, cardiovascular anesthesiologists, and other health care providers using echocardiographic approaches in the clinical setting, including radiologists, interventional cardiologists, electrophysiologists, emergency medicine physicians, and internists with an active interest in cardiovascular disease. Cardiac sonographers, cardiovascular technologists, physician assistants, nurse practitioners, and nursing professionals who wish to go beyond the basics in echocardiographic imaging will also find this book useful. For the researcher using echocardiography, there are 12 chapters focused on instrument, methodology, validation, and future prospects for newer advanced echocardiographic modalities.

Echocardiography is a vital component in the evaluation of patients with suspected or known cardiovascular disease. As this technique has evolved and matured, the role of the echocardiographer has shifted from simply providing a description of the images to providing an integrated assessment of the echocardiographic data in conjunction with the other clinical data in each patient. Often, echocardiography provides all the data needed for clinical decision making. When additional information is needed, the echocardiographic findings help define which other imaging modalities might be helpful. In effect, echocardiography has become a specialized type of cardiology consultation.

The information now requested by the referring physician includes not only the qualitative and quantitative interpretation of the echocardiographic images and Doppler flow data, but also a discussion of how this information might affect clinical decision making. Specific examples include decisions regarding interventional procedures (e.g., detection of coronary ischemia), medical or surgical therapy (e.g., treatment of endocarditis, surgery for aortic dissection), optimal timing of intervention in patients with chronic cardiac diseases (e.g., valvular regurgitation, mitral stenosis), prognostic implications (e.g., heart disease in pregnancy, patients with heart failure), and the possible need for and frequency of periodic diagnostic evaluation (e.g., congenital heart disease, the postoperative patient). In addition, echocardiography is critical in choosing the optimal therapy for each patient (e.g., selection of patients with heart failure for biventricular pacing) and in monitoring the effects of medical, percutaneous, or surgical intervention.

The clinical practice of echocardiography no longer is restricted to the full diagnostic examination performed in an imaging laboratory. Instead echocardiography has become so integrated into cardiovascular care that specialized instruments are now used in the intensive care unit, in the emergency department, in the interventional laboratory, during electrophysiology procedures, and in the operating room. As instruments become easier to use, smaller, and less expensive, it is likely that the clinical applications of this imaging modality will continue to expand.

Each chapter provides an advanced level of discussion, written by an expert in the field, building upon the basic material in the *Textbook of Clinical Echocardiography*, third edition, by Catherine M. Otto. The primary focus of each chapter is the role of echocardiography in clinical decision making and the impact on clinical outcomes. Emphasis is also placed on the principles of optimal data acquisition, quantitative approaches to data analysis, potential technical limitations, and areas of active research. In addition, the strengths and limitations of alternative diagnostic approaches are reviewed to put the role of echocardiography into the context of clinical practice. Detailed tables, color illustrations, echocardiographic images and Doppler tracings, and figures with important data from published outcome studies are used to provide clarity and depth.

In this edition, all the chapters have been updated to reflect recent advances, including revision of the text, references, figures, and tables. Key points that provide a quick overview or review of the most important concepts have been added to each chapter. There are over 40, full-color artist-drawn anatomic illustrations oriented to match echocardiographic image planes that demonstrate cardiac anatomy in different disease states. A new feature is the inclusion of a DVD that complements the material presented in the text. For each chapter, there are clinical cases (80 total), with echocardiographic images and cine loops, that demonstrate the clinical applications of the material discussed in the chapter. Multiple choice questions (over 210 total) provide an opportunity for readers to test their knowledge or quickly review the core material. The detailed explanation of the correct answer that is included with each question also provides an opportunity for additional learning.

The first two parts of the book are dedicated to advances in echocardiographic imaging. The chapters in these parts provide a detailed description of advanced imaging modalities, which includes basic principles, instrumentation, technical aspects of data acquisition, measurement of data, any limitations of the approach, and interpretation of results. Chapters are included on transesophageal echocardiography, intraoperative echocardiography, contrast echocardiography, three-dimensional echocardiography, and intravascular ultrasound. In addition, three new chapters have been added on intracardiac echocardiography, tissue-Doppler echocardiography, and handheld echocardiography to reflect the increasing use of these approaches in clinical practice. The next section focuses on methods to evaluate the left ventricle, with chapters spanning the spectrum from critical appraisals of quantitative techniques for evaluation of ventricular size, shape, and global and regional systolic function to chapters on edge detection and assessment of diastolic function.

The greater portion of the book is organized into parts based on major diagnostic categories. These chapters expand from a concise summary of data acquisition to focus on the clinical application of basic and advanced echocardiographic techniques in each disease state. The part on ischemic heart disease includes chapters on the role of echocardiography in the emergency department and coronary care unit, stress echocardiography (exercise and nonexercise), and a new chapter on echocardiographic imaging of coronary blood flow. The central role of echocardiography in management of patients with valvular heart disease is evident with chapters on quantitation of regurgitant severity, the optimal timing of surgery in patients with chronic valvular regurgitation, management of patients undergoing balloon mitral commissurotomy, clinical decision making in patients with endocarditis, evaluation of disease severity and progression in valvular aortic stenosis, and evaluation of prosthetic valves.

The following parts discuss the role of echocardiography in patients with cardiomyopathies (the patient with heart failure, hypertrophic cardiomyopathy, and restrictive cardiomyopathy and the posttransplant patient) and pericardial disease. Cardiac resynchronization therapy is addressed in the chapter on heart failure. There is a separate chapter on heart disease in pregnant women. In a part on other vascular and systemic diseases that lead to cardiac dysfunction (hypertension, aortic dissection, pulmonary disease, systemic immune-mediated diseases, renal disease, aging, systemic embolic events, and cardiac arrhythmias), a new chapter on connective tissue disorders now is included.

The part on congenital heart disease will be of value to clinicians caring for the increasing number of patients being seen with this diagnosis, as more children with corrective or palliative surgical procedures now survive to adulthood. The first chapter is entirely new and focuses on the general echocardiographic approach to the patient with congenital heart disease. The next chapter discusses congenital heart disease in adults without prior surgical procedures, and the third chapter discusses the often complex echocardiographic findings in adults with prior intervention for congenital heart disease. Finally, a new chapter on cardiac tumors has been added.

It is hoped that this book will provide the needed background to support and supplement clinical experience and expertise. Of course, competency in the acquisition and interpretation of echocardiographic and Doppler data depends on appropriate clinical education and training as detailed in accreditation requirements for both physicians and technologists and as recommended by professional societies, including the American Society of Echocardiography, the American College of Cardiology, and the American Heart Association. I strongly support these educational requirements and training recommendations; readers of this book are urged to review the relevant documents.

In addition, there continue to be advances both in the technical aspects of image and flow data acquisition and in our understanding of the clinical implications of specific echocardiographic findings. This book represents our knowledge base at one point in time; readers will wish to consult the current literature for the most up-to-date information. Although an extensive list of carefully selected references is provided with each chapter, the echocardiographic literature is so robust that it is impractical to include all relevant references; the reader can use an online medical literature search if an all-inclusive listing is desired.

Acknowledgments

Sincere thanks are due to the many individuals who made this book possible. Primary recognition goes to the chapter contributors who provided scholarly, thoughtful, and insightful discussions and integrated the clinical and echocardiographic information into a format that will benefit our readers. The support staff at each of our institutions deserves our appreciation for manuscript preparation and providing effective communication, with special thanks to Sharon Kemp and Angie Frederickson. The many research subjects who contributed to the data on which our current understanding is based certainly are worthy of our appreciation. The cardiac sonographers at all our institutions are due thanks as our partners in the clinical practice of echocardiography and as the individuals who acquired most of the images shown in this book. I also wish to express my appreciation to Starr Kaplan for her outstanding illustrations of cardiac anatomy and pathology. In addition, gratitude is due to Natasha Andjelkovic, Pamela Hetherington, Leah Bross, and the production team at Elsevier/Saunders. Finally, I thank my family for their constant encouragement and support.

Contents

Abbreviations

ABD	automatic border detection
ABG	arterial blood gas
ACE	angiotensin-converting enzyme
aCL	anticardiolipin antibodies
ACS	acute coronary syndrome
AFib	atrial fibrillation
AFl	atrial flutter
AIH	aortic intramural hematoma
AMI	acute myocardial infarction
aPL	antiphospholipid antibodies
APTT	activated partial thromboplastin time
AQ	acoustic quantification
AR	aortic regurgitation
ARB	angiotensin receptor blocker
ARVD	arrhythmogenic right ventricular dysplasia
AS	aortic stenosis
ASD	atrial septal defect
ASH	asymmetric septal hypertrophy
ASO	arterial switch operation
ATP	adenosine triphosphate
AV	atrioventricular
AVSD	atrioventricular septal defect
BNP	B-type natriuretic peptide
BP	blood pressure
BSA	body surface area
CABG	coronary artery bypass graft
CAD	coronary artery disease
CCTGA	congenitally corrected transposition of the great arteries
CCU	coronary care unit
CHD	coronary heart disease
CHF	congestive heart failure
CNS	central nervous system
CO	cardiac output
COPD	chronic obstructive pulmonary disease
CPAP	continuous positive airway pressure
CPB	cardiopulmonary bypass
CRT	cardiac resynchronization therapy
CSA	cross-sectional area
CT	computed tomography
CTEPH	chronic thromboembolic pulmonary hypertension
CW	continuous wave
CXR	chest x-ray
DCM	dilated cardiomyopathy
DES	drug-eluting stent
DHF	diastolic heart failure
DICOM	digital imaging and communications in medicine
DORV	double-outlet right ventricle
DSE	dobutamine stress echocardiography
DST	disproportionate septal thickening
DT	deceleration time
d-TGA	d-transposition of the great arteries
ECG	electrocardiogram
ED	end-diastolic
EDP	end-diastolic pressure
EDV	end-diastolic volume
EEM	external elastic membrane
EF	ejection fraction
EOA	effective orifice area
EROA	effective regurgitant orifice area
ES	end-systolic
ESV	end-systolic volume
FDA	Food and Drug Administration
FPV	flow propagation velocity
HCM	hypertrophic cardiomyopathy
HCU	hand-carried ultrasound
HF	heart failure
HLA	human leukocyte antigen
HR	heart rate
IABP	intraaortic balloon pump
IAS	interatrial septum
ICD	internal cardiac defibrillator
ICE	intracardiac echocardiography
ICU	intensive care unit
INR	international normalized ratio
IPAI	intraluminal phased-array imaging
IV	intravenous; intravenously
IVMD	interventricular mechanical delay
IVPG	intraventricular pressure gradient

IVR	isovolumic relaxation
IVRT	isovolumic relaxation time
IVUS	intravascular ultrasound
LA	left atrium; left atrial
LAD	left anterior descending
LBBB	left bundle branch block
LDH	lactate dehydrogenase
LDL	low-density lipoprotein
LMCA	left main coronary artery
l-TGA	l-transposition of the great arteries
LV	left ventricular; left ventricle
LVAD	left ventricular assist device
LVEDP	left ventricular end-diastolic pressure
LVOT	left ventricular outflow tract
MAIVF	mitral-aortic intervalvular fibrosa
MAP	mean arterial pressure
MCE	myocardial contrast echocardiography
MI	myocardial infarction; mechanical index
MLD	minimum lumen diameter
MMPs	myocardial matrix metalloproteinases
MPI	myocardial performance index
MR	mitral regurgitation
MRI	magnetic resonance imaging
MS	mitral stenosis
MVP	mitral valve prolapse
NPO	nothing by mouth
NSAIDs	nonsteroidal antiinflammatory drugs
OR	operating room
PA	pulmonary artery
PACS	picture archiving and communications systems
PAH	pulmonary arterial hypertension
PAPS	primary antiphospholipid syndrome
PAPVR	partial anomalous pulmonary venous return
PASP	pulmonary arterial systolic pressure
PCWP	pulmonary capillary wedge pressure
PDA	patent ductus arteriosus
PE	pericardial effusion
PEEP	positive end-expiratory pressure
PH	pulmonary hypertension
PHT	pressure half-time
PISA	proximal isovelocity surface area
PLAATO	percutaneous left atrial appendage transluminal occlusion
PR	pulmonary regurgitation
PTCA	percutaneous transluminal coronary angiography
PTSMA	percutaneous transluminal septal myocardial ablation
P-V	pressure-volume

PVE	prosthetic valve endocarditis
PVOD	pulmonary veno-occlusive disease
PVR	pulmonary venous resistance
PW	pulsed wave
QCA	quantitative coronary angiographic
RBC	red blood cell
RCA	right coronary artery
RNA	ribonucleic acid
ROA	regurgitant orifice area
ROC	receiver operated characteristic
RV	right ventricular; right ventricle
RVAD	right ventricular assist device
RVOT	right ventricular outflow tract
RVUs	relative value units
RWT	relative wall thickness
SAM	systolic anterior motion
SBP	systolic blood pressure
SD	standard deviation
SEC	spontaneous echocardiographic contrast
SLE	systemic lupus erythematosus
SPECT	single photon emission computed tomography
SR	strain rate
STE	speckle tracking echocardiography
SV	stroke volume
SVC	superior vena cava
SVR	systemic vascular resistance
TAAD	thoracic aortic aneurysm and dissection
TAPSE	tricuspid annular plane systolic excursion
TAPVC	total anomalous pulmonary venous connection
TAPVR	total anomalous pulmonary venous return
TCPC	total cavopulmonary connection
TDI	tissue-Doppler imaging
TEE	transesophageal echocardiography
3D	three-dimensional
TIA	transient ischemic attack
TIMI	thrombolysis in myocardial infarction
TIMPs	tissue inhibitors of metalloproteinases
TLR	target lesion revascularization
TMR	transmyocardial laser revascularization
TNF	tumor necrosis factor
TOF	tetralogy of Fallot
TR	tricuspid regurgitation
TTE	transthoracic echocardiography
TVI	time velocity integral
2D	two-dimensional
US	ultrasound
VC	vena contracta
VSD	ventricular septal defects

Part One

Advanced Echocardiographic Techniques

Chapter 1

Transesophageal Echocardiography

IAN G. BURWASH, MD • KWAN-LEUNG CHAN, MD

Since the initial description of transesophageal echocardiography (TEE) in 1976,[1] TEE has become a valuable diagnostic imaging modality for the dynamic assessment of cardiac anatomy and function in the evaluation of diseases of the heart and great vessels. The close proximity of the esophagus to the heart and great vessels provide the echocardiographer with an easily accessible window with the potential for excellent visualization of cardiac structures, avoiding the intervening lung and chest wall tissues that limit transthoracic imaging. The potential of TEE to provide a valuable imaging tool became widely recognized in the 1980s with advancements in TEE probe technology, including the availability of single-plane phased array transducers and the addition of color flow and continuous wave Doppler imaging technology. TEE does not supplant transthoracic echocardiography (TTE), however; it is a complementary imaging modality with its own strengths and weaknesses. The introduction of biplane TEE transducers in the late 1980s and multiplane transducers in the 1990s has resulted in a further expansion of potential diagnostic applications.

Perhaps the best evidence of the diagnostic utility and value in patient management of TEE is the widespread use of this technology. TEE is found in the inpatient and outpatient ambulatory setting, in the operating room (OR), in the intensive care unit (ICU), and in the emergency department (ED). Currently, TEE accounts for approximately 5% to 10% of all echocardiography studies performed. The indications and utility of TEE will likely expand in the future with new technologic advancements, such as three-dimensional (3D) echocardiography.

Performance of Transesophageal Echocardiography

TEE is a semi-invasive procedure that should be performed only by a properly trained physician who understands the indications for and potential complications of the procedure. Both technical and cognitive skills are required for the competent performance and interpretation of TEE studies (Table 1-1), and guidelines on training have been published.[2] The physician should be assisted by an experienced sonographer whose tasks are to ensure that optimal images are obtained by adjusting the controls of the echocardiographic system and to ensure safety by monitoring the responses of the patient during the procedure. Although family members or friends are usually not allowed in the room when the procedure is being performed, there are situations in which their presence can be helpful. The presence of a parent can have a calming effect when one is dealing

TABLE 1-1. Cognitive and Technical Skills Required for the Performance of Transesophageal Echocardiography

Cognitive Skills

Knowledge of appropriate indications, contraindications, and risks of TEE
Understanding of differential diagnostic considerations in each clinical case
Knowledge of physical principles of echocardiographic image formation and blood flow velocity measurement
Familiarity with the operation of the ultrasonographic instrument, including the function of all controls affecting the quality of the data displayed
Knowledge of normal cardiovascular anatomy as visualized tomographically
Knowledge of alterations in cardiovascular anatomy resulting from acquired heart disease and CHD
Knowledge of normal cardiovascular hemodynamics and fluid dynamics
Knowledge of alterations in cardiovascular hemodynamics and blood flow resulting from acquired heart disease and CHD
Understanding of component techniques for general echocardiography and TEE, including when to use these methods to investigate specific clinical questions
Ability to distinguish adequate from inadequate echocardiographic data and to distinguish an adequate from an inadequate TEE examination
Knowledge of other cardiovascular diagnostic methods for correlation with TEE findings
Ability to communicate examination results to patient, other health care professionals, and in the medical record

Technical Skills

Proficiency in performing a complete standard echocardiographic examination, using all echocardiographic modalities relevant to the case
Proficiency in safely passing the TEE transducer into the esophagus and stomach and in adjusting probe position to obtain the necessary tomographic images and Doppler data
Proficiency in correctly operating the ultrasonographic instrument, including all controls affecting the quality of the data displayed
Proficiency in recognizing abnormalities of cardiac structure and function as detected from the transesophageal and transgastric windows, in distinguishing normal from abnormal findings and in recognizing artifacts
Proficiency in performing qualitative and quantitative analysis of the echocardiographic data

CHD, congenital heart disease; TEE, transesophageal echocardiography.
From Pearlman AS, Gardin JM, Martin RP, et al: *J Am Soc Echocardiogr* 5:187-194, 1992.

with an apprehensive teenager. A friend or a relative who speaks the same language can relieve much of the anxiety when dealing with an anxious patient who is not fluent in English.

TEE should be performed in a spacious room that can comfortably accommodate a stretcher. The room should be equipped with an oxygen outlet and suction facilities. A pulse oximeter should be available, for use mainly in cyanotic patients and patients with severe lung disease. The TEE probe should be carefully examined before each use. In addition to visual inspection, it is important to palpate the probe, particularly the flexion portion, to ensure that there is no unusual wear and tear of the probe.[3] Stretching of the steering cables may result in increased flexibility and mobility of the probe tip with buckling of the probe tip within the esophagus.[4] This phenomenon is associated with a poor TEE image and resistance to probe withdrawal. The probe should be advanced into the stomach and straightened by retro-flexion of the extreme antiflexed probe tip. A perforation of the TEE probe sheath by a ruptured steering cable can occur and inspection of the casing for any protruding wires before probe insertion is recommended.[3] The flexion controls need to be tested on a regular basis. Anterior flexion should exceed 90 degrees, and right and left flexion should approach 90 degrees.

Preparation of Patient

Patients should be contacted at least 12 hours before the procedure and instructed to fast for at least 4 hours before the procedure. They should be informed that they should be accompanied because they will not be able to drive or return to work for several hours owing to the lingering effect of sedation. On the day of the study, a health care provider explains the procedure in greater detail and obtains informed consent. A health care provider tells the patient to expect mild abdominal discomfort and gagging following the insertion of the probe and reassures them that these responses are transient. A 20-gauge intravenous (IV) cannula is then inserted for administration of medications and contrast agents, if necessary. Lidocaine hydrochloride spray is routinely used for topical anesthesia, which should cover the posterior pharynx and the tongue. For sedation, 2 to 10 mg of IV diazepam is used.[5] Midazolam at 0.05 mg/kg, with a total dose between 1 and 5 mg, can also be used.

Sedation is used in about 85% of patients and should be more sparingly used in elderly patients, because they tend to be more stoic and the effect of sedation is more likely prolonged. On the other hand, sedation is essential in young, anxious patients and when the study is expected to be protracted. The aim is for light sedation so that at the end of the procedure the patients are awake and can leave with an escort. Heavy sedation is needed in situations in which blunting the hemodynamic responses to the procedure is desirable. One obvious example is a patient undergoing TEE for suspected aortic dissection.[6]

Anticholinergic agents, such as glycopyrrolate, to decrease salivation are rarely used. In the rare circumstances in which there is excessive salivation, it is usually adequate to simply instruct the patient to let the saliva dribble onto a towel placed under the chin, or the saliva can be removed by intermittent suction. Bacteremia is not a significant risk in TEE, and we do not use antibiotic prophylaxis to prevent endocarditis even in patients with prosthetic heart valves.[7,8]

Esophageal Intubation

The TEE study is performed with the patient in the left decubitus position. The physician, the sonographer, and the echocardiographic system are all positioned on the left-hand side of the patient.[5] Artificial teeth or dentures are routinely removed. The flexion controls should be unlocked to allow for maximum flexibility of the probe when it is being inserted. The patient's head should be in a flexed position. The tip of the probe is kept relatively straight and gently advanced to the back of the throat. It should be maintained in a central position because deviation to either side increases the likelihood that it may become lodged in the piriform fossa. The operator can facilitate this process by inserting one or two fingers into the patient's oropharynx to direct the path of the probe. Gentle pressure is exerted, and the patient is instructed to swallow. The swallowing mechanism helps guide the probe into the esophagus. In older patients, cervical spondylosis with prominent protrusion into the posterior pharynx can create difficulty with passage of the probe.[5] Manually depressing the back of the tongue provides more room, allowing the TEE probe to assume a less acute angle and facilitating the intubation of the esophagus. If significant resistance is encountered when the probe is advanced, it is prudent to withdraw the probe and then initiate a new attempt. Esophageal intubation is more difficult with the multiplane probe than with the smaller monoplane and biplane probes.[9,10] The latter can be used, if available, when esophageal intubation cannot be achieved with a multiplane probe. In experienced hands, the rate of failure of esophageal intubation should be less than two percent.[5,9,11]

A bite guard should always be used, except in edentulous patients. Putting it between the patient's teeth before the TEE probe is passed into the oropharynx and esophagus is useful because patients with a sensitive pharynx may close their mouths involuntarily during esophageal intubation. The patient is instructed to keep the guard between the teeth throughout the procedure, and regular checks are made to ensure that it is in the proper position to prevent damage to the probe or injury to the patient.

Even when the probe is inserted without difficulties, it is not uncommon for the patient to develop nausea with or without mild retrosternal or abdominal discomfort. Pausing for 10 to 15 seconds allows these symptoms to subside before proceeding with echocardiographic imaging. Start with images acquired from the esophagus before advancing the probe into the stomach for the gastric views. The gastroesophageal sphincter is usually reached when the probe is advanced 40 cm from the teeth. Gentle pressure is all that is required to advance the probe through the gastroesophageal sphincter. The patient may again experience nausea and mild discomfort, and it may be advisable to pause momentarily for these symptoms to subside. Imaging of the proximal descending thoracic aorta and aortic arch is generally reserved for the end of the study because the probe needs to be positioned in the upper esophagus and the patient is generally more aware of the probe at this position and tends to have more discomfort and gagging.

Inadvertent passage of the probe into the trachea can occur, particularly in deeply sedated patients. The development of stridor and incessant cough should alert the operator of this possibility. Furthermore, it would be difficult to advance the probe beyond 30 cm from the teeth, and the image quality is usually poor.[5]

In patients on mechanical ventilation, esophageal intubation is more difficult. In these cases the probe can be introduced with the patient lying supine because the airway is protected, and aspiration is unlikely. The probe is positioned behind the endotracheal tube and gently advanced. It is helpful to have the patient's mandible pulled forward when the probe is being advanced. If there is undue resistance at about 25 to 30 cm from the teeth, slight deflation of the cuff of the endotracheal tube can be considered to ease the passage of the probe. The gastric tube can be used as a guide to help in the proper positioning and passage of the TEE probe and may not need to be removed. In a minority of intubated patients, successful esophageal intubation may be achieved only with direct laryngoscopy.

Image Format

There is no general agreement on how the imaging planes should be displayed. Our preference is to orient the images such that the right-sided structures are on the left side of the screen and the left-sided on the right. The apex of the imaging plane with the electronic artifact is at the top of the screen. Thus, in the longitudinal views, superior structures are to the right of the screen and the inferior to the left.[12]

Standard Imaging Planes

Advances in TEE transducer technology have culminated in the development of the multiplane probe capable of two-dimensional (2D) and color flow imaging in multiple planes. The imaging plane can be steered electronically from 0 to 180 degrees by means of a pressure-sensitive switch, providing views unattainable by monoplane and biplane probes. This discussion focuses only on standard imaging views routinely performed at the University of Ottawa Heart Institute using multiplane TEE (Table 1–2). These views are considered "standard" because they have important clinical

TABLE 1–2. **Standard Imaging Planes with Multiplane Transesophageal Echocardiography**

Imaging View	Standard Imaging Plane	Angle of Imaging Array (Degrees)	Main Cardiac Structures
Basal	Aortic valve	0-60	Aortic valve, coronary arteries, left atrial appendage, pulmonary veins
	Atrial septum	90-120	Fossa ovalis, SVC, inferior vena cava
	Pulmonary bifurcation	0-30	Pulmonic valve, main and right PAs, proximal left PA
Four-chamber	Left ventricle	0-180	Left ventricle (regional and global function), right ventricle, tricuspid valve
	Mitral valve	0-180	Anterior and posterior mitral leaflets, papillary muscles, chords
	Left ventricular outflow tract	120-160	Aortic valve, ascending aorta, left and right ventricular outflow tracts, pulmonic valve, main PA
Transgastric	Left ventricle	0-150	Left ventricle, right ventricle, tricuspid valve
	Mitral valve	0-150	Anterior and posterior mitral leaflets, papillary muscles, chords
	Coronary sinus	0	CS, tricuspid valve
Aortic	Descending thoracic aorta	0	Entire descending thoracic aorta
	Aortic arch	90	Aortic arch, arch vessels, left PA

CS, coronary sinus; PA, pulmonary artery; SVC, superior vena cava.

relevance and can be obtained in most patients with specific imaging planes.

Four basic maneuvers are used to obtain specific tomographic views with TEE.[13] The first relates to the positioning of the transducer by advancement or withdrawal of the probe. Although this is a simple maneuver, it is the most crucial, and the imaging views can be conveniently categorized according to the location of the TEE probe within the esophagus or stomach into four groups: basal, four-chamber, transgastric, and aortic views (Fig. 1–1). The second maneuver involves rotation of the probe from side to side. This is particularly useful when using longitudinal imaging planes, which provide a better demonstration of the continuity between vertically aligned structures, such as the superior vena cava and the arch vessels[12,13] (Fig. 1–2). Steering the imaging plane using the pressure-sensitive switch is the third maneuver to obtain different tomographic views (Fig. 1–3). The ability to image cardiac structures from 0 to 180 degrees not only enhances understanding of cardiac anatomy but also provides a ready means for 3D reconstruction.[14,15] The accompanying images in Figures 1–1, 1–2, and 1–3 represent the typical images obtained with one of the basic maneuvers and provide the starting points for further adjustment of the imaging plane to obtain optimal long- or short-axis views of specific structures. This may be achieved using the fourth maneuver, which involves manipulation of the anterior-posterior and right-left flexion control knobs. The availability of a steerable imaging plane has drastically reduced the need to use the flexion knobs, but there are situations in which these knobs play a crucial role in obtaining proper tomographic views.[10,13] These maneuvers provide an almost infinite number of imaging planes. Table 1–2 summarizes the standard imaging planes and the cardiac structures evaluated in these four groups of views.

Basal Views

The basal group of views is obtained with the TEE probe located in the midesophagus. The base of the heart, particularly the aortic valve, is well seen. The relationship of the two great arteries can be well defined and followed cephalad to at least the level of the pulmonary bifurcation. Beyond this level, the interposing trachea makes imaging impossible. Three basal tomographic planes are routinely performed: short axis aortic valve, atrial septum, and pulmonary bifurcation.

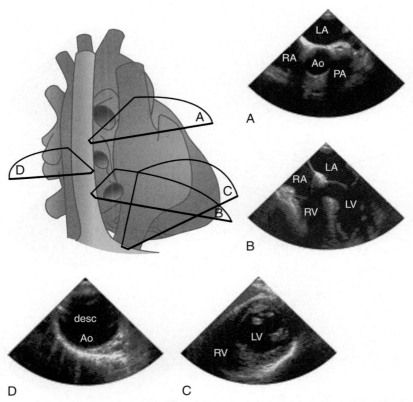

Figure 1–1. Diagram showing the transesophageal echocardiography transducer locations for the four standard imaging positions: basal (A), four-chamber (B), transgastric (C), and aortic (D). Ao, aorta; desc Ao, descending aorta; LA, left atrium; LV, left ventricle; PA, pulmonary artery; RA, right atrium; RV, right ventricle.

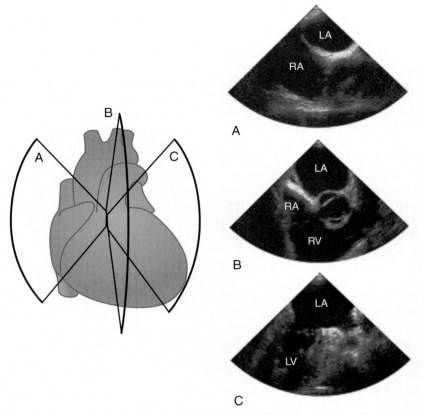

Figure 1–2. *Diagram showing the transesophageal echocardiography longitudinal imaging planes obtained by rotation of probe: atrial septum (A), right ventricular outflow tract (B), and two-chamber view (C). LA, left atrium; LV, left ventricle; RA, right atrium; RV, right ventricle.*

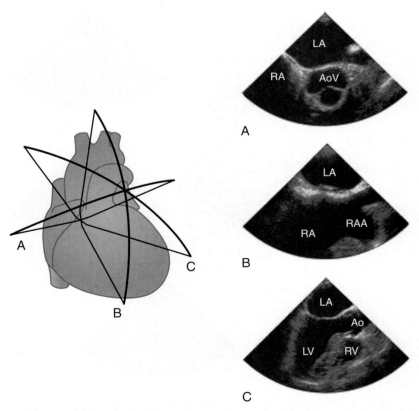

Figure 1–3. *Diagram showing the transesophageal echocardiography rotational imaging planes (0 to 180 degrees): aortic valve (A, 40 degrees), SVC (B, 100 degrees), and left ventricular outflow tract (C, 140 degrees). Ao, aorta; AoV, aortic valve; LA, left atrium; LV, left ventricle; RA, right atrium; RAA, right atrial appendage; RV, right ventricle.*

Aortic Valve

A short-axis view of the aortic valve can be obtained with the probe at about 30 to 35 cm from the teeth. The left coronary cusp often appears to have nodular thickening if the aortic valve is cut obliquely, which is often the case at 0 degrees.[12] Steering the imaging plane to 30 to 60 degrees should eliminate this artifact by providing an optimal short-axis view of the aortic valve[13] (see Fig. 1–3A). Pulling the transducer slightly back should allow visualization of both the left and right coronary arteries. The left coronary artery can be followed to its bifurcation into the left anterior descending and circumflex arteries (Fig. 1–4). The right coronary artery is more difficult to display, and usually only the proximal 2 to 3 cm is seen (Fig. 1–5). Other structures seen well in this view are the left atrial appendage and the left pulmonary veins. The partition between these structures can be quite bulbous and should not be confused

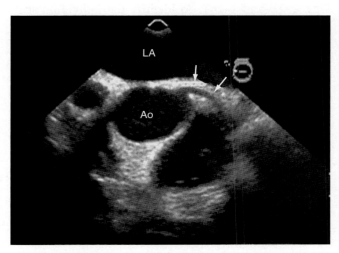

Figure 1–4. The left coronary artery (arrows) *was imaged at 0 degrees. Ao, aorta; LA, left atrium.*

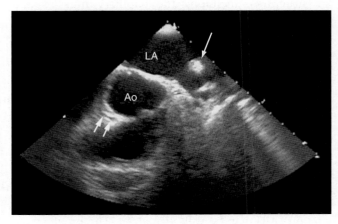

Figure 1–5. The proximal right coronary artery (small arrows) *and the bulbous partition between the left atrial appendage and the left upper pulmonary vein* (large arrow) *are demonstrated. Ao, aorta; LA, left atrium.*

with an abnormal intracardiac mass[16] (see Fig. 1–5). Rotating the probe to the right should reveal the right pulmonary veins.

The horizontal plane is useful in imaging the four pulmonary veins. The left and right pulmonary veins are imaged separately. It is difficult to image the upper and lower pulmonary veins, left or right, in the same view because the veins are not located in the same plane with the lower pulmonary veins posterior and inferior to the upper pulmonary veins.[17] When one pulmonary vein is identified, a slight translational movement of the probe should bring out the other because the orifices of the upper and lower pulmonary veins are in close proximity. The lower pulmonary veins run horizontal to the imaging plane, whereas the upper veins are more anterior and at an obtuse angle, making them more suitable for Doppler assessment. The right and left atrial appendages wrap around the great arteries anteriorly. The left atrial appendage is more prominent and can consist of multiple lobes.[18]

A comprehensive interrogation using multiple imaging planes should be performed to exclude left atrial appendage thrombus in the appropriate clinical setting. The right atrial appendage is smaller and triangular in shape (see Fig. 1–3B). The endocardial surfaces of both appendages are corrugated and should not be confused with small thrombi.[16] A long-axis view of the aorta can be achieved with the imaging plane at about 120 degrees. A more rightward imaging plane, such as 150 degrees, may be needed if the ascending aorta is dilated and tortuous. This view allows the visualization of a longer length of the ascending aorta and thus significantly reduces the blind spot caused by the interposing trachea.

Atrial Septum

We prefer to image the atrial septum using the longitudinal plane at 90 to 120 degrees. The fossa ovalis, which is the thinnest part of the atrial septum, and the continuity of the superior vena cava (SVC) with the right atrium are well demonstrated in this view (see Fig. 1–3B). This view is particularly valuable in demonstrating the sinus venosus atrial septal defect, which is usually located just inferior to the entrance of the SVC.[19,20] The foramen ovale, if present, is located at the superior aspect of the fossa ovalis and is readily seen in this view. It is important to advance the probe to the level of the inferior vena cava so as not to neglect the inferior aspect of the atrial septum.[21] Careful sweep of the atrial septum with left-right rotation is needed to visualize the entire atrial septum. Continuous rotation from right to left will sequentially demonstrate the left ventricular outflow tract and the right ventricular outflow tract (see Fig. 1–2B). Rotating the probe to the right shows the right upper pulmonary vein and provides parallel alignment for Doppler assessment.

Pulmonary Bifurcation

The pulmonary bifurcation view is achieved by withdrawal of the probe with the imaging plane at 0 degrees. The pulmonic valve and main pulmonary artery are best seen slightly superior to the aortic valve (Fig. 1–6). The pulmonic valve is thinner than the aortic valve and is usually difficult to image in a true cross section. Further slight withdrawal allows imaging the pulmonary bifurcation. The entire length of the right pulmonary artery but only the proximal portion of the left pulmonary artery can be seen. The right pulmonary artery can usually be followed to its first bifurcation by rotation of the probe rightward, but this maneuver is better performed with the longitudinal plane at 90 degrees. Gradual rotation from left to right provides good visualization in cross section of the entire right pulmonary artery and its first bifurcation. This is an important view in the detection of proximal pulmonary emboli.[22,23]

Four-Chamber Views

Four-chamber views are obtained with the transducer within the middle to lower esophagus. It is difficult to image the left ventricle in its true long axis. Excessive anterior flexion should be avoided to prevent foreshortening of the ventricles. Indeed, to optimize visualization of the left ventricle, it is advisable to withdraw the probe slightly and at the same time attempt gentle retroflexion while maintaining adequate contact between the imaging surface and the esophagus. In the setting of a dilated and unfolded aorta, rotating the imaging plane to about 20 to 30 degrees may be necessary to obtain the four-chamber view without the aorta obscuring the tricuspid valve and part of the right ventricle.

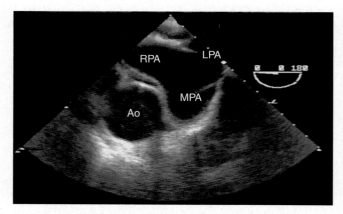

Figure 1–6. *The bifurcation of the main pulmonary artery into the right and left pulmonary arteries was imaged using the transverse plane. Ao, aorta; LPA, left pulmonary artery; MPA, main pulmonary artery; RPA, right pulmonary artery.*

Left Ventricle

The inferior septum and anterolateral wall are usually seen in the four-chamber view (see Fig. 1–1B). The left ventricular apex is difficult to visualize, particularly in patients with a dilated left ventricle. In addition to retroflexion, rightward flexion can often be helpful to minimize foreshortening of the left ventricle. Far-field imaging can be improved by decreasing the transmission frequency or by using harmonic imaging. A continuous sweep from 0 to 180 degrees should be performed to examine the different left ventricular segments so as to have a comprehensive assessment of left ventricular global and regional function (see Fig. 1–2C).

Mitral Valve

The mitral valve is well seen using the four-chamber view, but the depth of the imaging plane should be reduced to enhance the resolution of the image (see Figs. 1–1B and 1–2C). To identify the individual scallops of the anterior and posterior mitral leaflets, a careful sweep from 0 to 180 degrees should be made. The technique of visualizing specific scallops of the mitral leaflets have been published,[24] but patient-to-patient variation should be kept in mind. The presence of a good long-axis view of the aortic valve and proximal ascending aorta, usually at 120 degrees, is a good indication that the middle scallops of both the anterior and the posterior mitral leaflets are imaged and provides the internal reference for the analysis of the other imaging planes. Both papillary muscles can be imaged but usually not in the same plane. The subvalvular chords are seldom completely imaged because they are frequently obscured by the mitral leaflets. The morphologic information obtained from this view should be corroborated by the short-axis view of the mitral valve obtained from the transgastric view, which also allows a better assessment of the subvalvular structures, including the papillary muscles and chords. Four-chamber views are ideal for the assessment of mitral regurgitation (MR) in relation to the number of regurgitant jets, the direction of the regurgitant jets, and the severity of regurgitation.[25,26]

Left Ventricular Outflow Tract

We like to image the left ventricular outflow tract at 120 to 160 degrees because the outflow tract has a horizontal alignment in this plane that may allow optimal imaging even in the setting of a prosthetic aortic valve (see Fig. 1–3C). The opening and closing of the aortic valve, as well as the presence or absence of aortic regurgitation (AR), can be well visualized. The proximal ascending aorta is present in this view. A slight withdrawal of the probe will allow more of the ascending aorta to be visualized (Fig. 1–7). A slight rotation to the

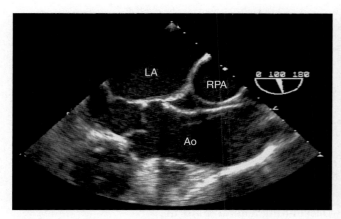

Figure 1-7. *Slight withdrawal of the probe relative to the probe position used to acquire the image shown in Figure 1-3C, which showed the right pulmonary artery in short axis and more of the ascending aorta. Ao, ascending aorta; LA, left atrium; RPA, right pulmonary artery.*

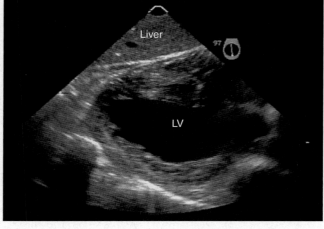

Figure 1-8. *Transgastric long-axis view of the left ventricle with visualization of the apex. LV, left ventricle.*

left will show the right ventricular outflow tract with the thin pulmonic valve. Both the motion of the pulmonic valve and the presence or absence of pulmonic regurgitation can be adequately assessed using this view.

Transgastric Views

There is slight resistance during the passage of the TEE probe through the gastroesophageal junction; the appearance of the liver is a clear indication that the probe is in the stomach. Anterior flexion, often with leftward rotation and flexion, is required to achieve good contact between the imaging surface and the gastric wall. Extreme anterior flexion with further advancement of the probe can sometimes produce images similar to the five-chamber views obtained from the subxiphoid surface approach.

Left Ventricle

Multiple cross sections of the left ventricle can usually be obtained using the transgastric approach (see Figs. 1–1C and 1–8). These are the views commonly used in the intraoperative assessment of left ventricular function.[24] Optimization of the short-axis views of the left ventricle can be achieved with leftward rotation accompanied by leftward flexion. To visualize the left ventricular apex, gentle advancement of the probe is required together with slight retroflexion. In our experience, the short-axis view of the left ventricular apex can be obtained in about 60% of cases. Another way to visualize the left ventricular apex is to use the longitudinal plane at about 90 degrees (see Fig. 1–8). Careful lateral rotation can be used to obtain comprehensive regional assessment of the left ventricle. Leftward rotation of this imaging plane can yield a good alignment with the left ventricular outflow tract and aortic valve to allow accurate measurement of

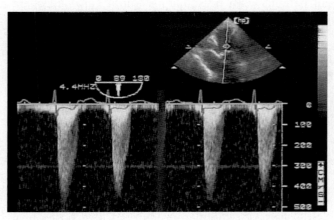

Figure 1-9. *Transgastric transesophageal echocardiography approach to assess the severity of aortic stenosis using continuous wave Doppler echocardiography.*

the transaortic pressure gradients in the setting of aortic stenosis (AS)[27] (Fig. 1–9). The right ventricle can be seen with rightward rotation of the probe. Both short- and long-axis views of the tricuspid valve are achievable, although the tricuspid valve and its papillary muscles are better assessed with the long-axis plane.

Mitral Valve

The mitral valve can be best assessed using the horizontal imaging plane with the transducer brought up to near the gastroesophageal junction (Fig. 1–10). Anterior flexion and leftward flexion are usually required to optimize this view. Adjusting the imaging plane to about 20 degrees will help to bring out the lateral commissure. This view provides unambiguous assessment of the individual scallops of both the anterior and pos-

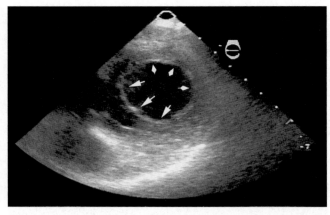

Figure 1–10. *The mitral valve was demonstrated in the short axis showing the anterior* (arrows) *and posterior* (arrowheads) *mitral leaflets.*

terior mitral leaflets and thus should be attempted in all patients with myxomatous mitral valve degeneration. In our experience, this view is achievable in about 70% of patients. Both the papillary muscle and chords can be demonstrated, and the continuity between these structures and the mitral leaflets is best seen in the long-axis plane.

Coronary Sinus

The coronary sinus (CS) comes into view when the probe is withdrawn to be near the gastroesophageal junction, and the flexion knobs are in relatively neutral positions (Fig. 1–11). This view can also be achieved by retroflexion with the probe in the lower esophagus. The CS is seen as a vascular structure located posterior to the left ventricle at the atrioventricular (AV) groove draining into the right atrium. The tricuspid valve can be visualized to the right and anterior. A dilated CS should raise the possibility of the presence of a persis-

tent left SVC, which is the most common cause. Leftward rotation while following the CS may sometimes demonstrate this anomalous vein. In the esophageal views, the left SVC is usually sandwiched between the left atrial appendage and the left upper pulmonary vein.[28]

Aortic Views

The thoracic aorta is well assessed by TEE because of its close proximity to the esophagus.

Descending Thoracic Aorta

The best way to assess the descending thoracic aorta is to use the horizontal imaging plane with the transducer rotated leftward and posterior, followed by slow withdrawal from the level of the diaphragm to the aortic arch[16] (see Fig. 1–1D). Because of the relationship between the esophagus and the aorta, slight rotational adjustment is required to visualize the entire circumference of the aortic wall as the probe is slowly withdrawn.[29] If the aorta is dilated or tortuous, proper short-axis views of the descending aorta will require adjustment of the imaging plane by 0 to 90 degrees.

Aortic Arch

The longitudinal imaging plane at 90 degrees is preferred in imaging the aortic arch because it allows visualization of the entire circumference of the aorta[29] (Fig. 1–12). Anterior rotation of the longitudinal plane should visualize the entire aortic arch, but the proximal aortic arch may not be visualized when the aortic arch is unfolded. The transducer will need to be withdrawn slightly to image the arch vessels, which

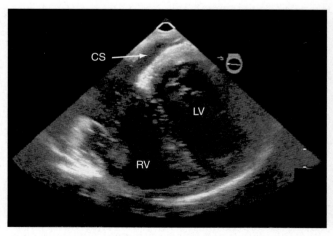

Figure 1–11. *The coronary sinus was demonstrated with the probe at the gastroesophageal junction. CS, coronary sinus; LV, left ventricle; RV, right ventricle.*

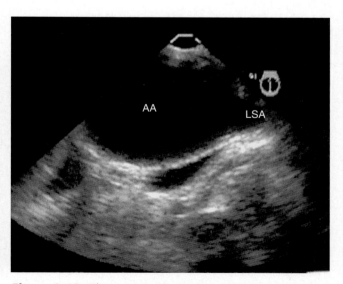

Figure 1–12. *The aortic arch was imaged using the longitudinal plane, showing the origin of the left subclavian artery. AA, aortic arch; LSA, left subclavian artery.*

course superiorly. In one third of patients, all three arch vessels can be imaged, but in the other two thirds of patients, only the two distal arch vessels can be imaged. It is rare not to be able to image at least one arch vessel. As a rule, the brachiocephalic artery, which is anterior and more rightward, is the most difficult to image because of the interposing trachea. The transverse plane in a more superior location may sometimes show the three arch vessels in their short axis. Advancing the probe by 1 to 2 cm so that the imaging plane is just inferior to the aortic arch can frequently image the proximal left pulmonary artery (PA). It is sometimes possible to follow it to the first bifurcation. This view should be sought in the assessment of patients suspected of having pulmonary embolism.

Doppler Examination

TEE can be used to assess the flow patterns across the four cardiac valves, but it does not provide additional information to TTE. Furthermore, good ultrasound (US) beam alignment with the transvalvular flow may not be feasible because of the anatomic confines of the esophagus. On the other hand, some intracardiac flows, such as pulmonary vein flow and left atrial appendage flow, are better and more consistently obtained by TEE and provide important insight into intracardiac hemodynamics.

Transmitral and Transtricuspid Flow

The pulsed-Doppler ultrasound beam can be aligned parallel to transmitral flow in the midesophageal four-chamber view or long-axis view to accurately measure transmitral filling velocities. The pulsed-Doppler sample volume should be kept small (2 to 5 mm) and positioned at the mitral valve leaflet tips for the evaluation of diastolic function and filling pressures.[30,31] In contrast, transmitral stroke volume is measured by placing the sample volume at the mitral valve annulus, so that velocity and annular dimensions are measured at the same location.[32,33]

Transtricuspid filling can be assessed by pulsed Doppler measurements obtained in the midesophageal four-chamber view. However, it is frequently not possible to align the Doppler US beam parallel to blood flow. The transtricuspid filling pattern is similar to the transmitral filling pattern, although lower velocities are present.

Transaortic and Transpulmonary Flow

Transaortic flow can be assessed by imaging the left ventricular outflow tract and aortic valve in either the transgastric long-axis view (100 to 135 degrees) or the deep transgastric long-axis view (0 degrees), in which the probe is advanced deep into the stomach adjacent

to the left ventricular apex and anteflexed until the imaging plane is directed superiorly toward the base of the heart. In these views, the pulsed-Doppler or continuous wave Doppler beam can be aligned parallel to blood flow to measure transaortic velocity. Stroke volume can then be derived by measuring the midesophagus left ventricular outflow tract diameter or the short-axis aortic valve orifice area at valve leaflet level.[34,35] In patients with AS or left ventricular outflow tract obstruction, transaortic pressure gradient can be derived using the continuous wave Doppler signal from the transgastric long-axis or deep transgastric long-axis view and the simplified Bernoulli equation.[27]

Transpulmonary flow has been measured by combining pulsed Doppler or continuous wave Doppler velocity measurements of pulmonary artery flow from the midesophagus short-axis view of the main PA and the main PA diameter.[36,37]

Left Atrial Appendage Flow

The left atrial appendage can be imaged from the midesophagus aortic valve short-axis view (30 to 60 degrees) or the midesophagus two-chamber view (80 to 100 degrees). Left atrial appendage flow should be recorded by positioning the color flow sector over the left atrial appendage and placing the pulsed-Doppler sample volume at the site of maximal flow velocity. This usually occurs in the proximal or middle third of the left atrial appendage. Velocity recordings from the distal third of the left atrial appendage frequently have wall motion artifacts and are usually unsatisfactory. Wall filters should be set low because low-velocity flow may be present.

The pattern of left atrial appendage flow is dependent on cardiac rhythm.[38,39] In patients with sinus rhythm, four left atrial appendage flow waves have been described (Fig. 1–13): (1) a large positive wave after the electrocardiographic P-wave representing left atrial appendage contraction and emptying; (2) a large

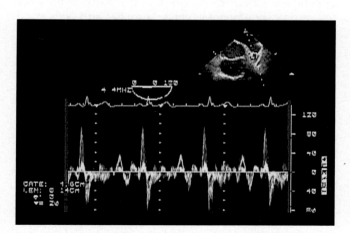

Figure 1–13. Normal left atrial appendage flow pattern in sinus rhythm, showing prominent atrial emptying and filling velocities.

negative early systolic wave immediately following the QRS complex representing left atrial appendage filling; (3) alternating positive and negative waves of decreasing velocity throughout the remainder of systole representing passive flow in and out of the appendage; and (4) a low-velocity positive emptying wave in early diastole coinciding with rapid left ventricular filling. In addition, a low-velocity mid-diastolic negative filling wave representing appendage filling from the pulmonary veins may follow the early diastolic atrial appendage emptying wave. The normal left atrial appendage velocities are as follows: contraction, 60 ± 14 cm/s; filling, 52 ± 13 cm/s; and early diastolic filling, 20 ± 11 cm/s.[38,40]

In atrial fibrillation, a regular atrial contraction wave is absent. However, the left atrial appendage continues to contract, resulting in irregular oscillating positive and negative emptying and filling waves with variable velocities. The velocities are usually larger during ventricular diastole when the mitral valve is open, and smaller during systole when the valve is closed. Mean left atrial appendage velocity tends to be lower at higher heart rates because of the smaller proportion of time spent during diastole. The early diastolic emptying wave, which coincides with early rapid left ventricular filling, may still be seen in atrial fibrillation (AFib). In atrial flutter (AFl), the velocity waves are more regular and tend to be of greater velocity resulting from the slower atrial rate.

Other factors affecting left atrial appendage velocities include age, gender, heart rate, left atrial contractility, left atrial pressure, left ventricular systolic and diastolic function, mitral stenosis (MS), and MR.[38,39] Increases in heart rate during sinus rhythm can result in higher emptying velocities due to fusion of the early diastolic emptying and atrial contraction velocities. Increasing age is associated with a decrease in early diastolic emptying and atrial contraction velocities. Women also have lower atrial contraction velocities.

The potential clinical utility of measuring left atrial appendage velocities relates to their association with left atrial spontaneous echo contrast and left atrial thrombus.[38,39,41,42] Patients with AFib and a left atrial appendage emptying velocity less than 20 cm/s are more likely to have left atrial thrombus and a 2.6-fold greater risk of ischemic stroke compared to patients with a velocity greater than 20 cm/s.[41,42] Lower left atrial appendage velocities have also been observed in stroke patients in normal sinus rhythm.[43] Left atrial appendage velocities may predict successful cardioversion of AFib,[44] and the maintenance of sinus rhythm at one year.[38,39,45]

Pulmonary Vein Flow

Pulmonary venous flow patterns provide unique and ancillary information for evaluating left ventricular diastolic function, measuring left ventricular filling pressure, assessing MR severity, differentiating constrictive pericarditis from restrictive cardiomyopathies, and identifying pulmonary vein stenosis after radiofrequency ablation of AFib.[46] TTE can obtain pulmonary vein flow in up to 90% of patients,[47] however TEE allows a more consistent and reliable acquisition of high quality laminar Doppler signals.[46]

The pulmonary veins are imaged from the midesophagus level. Pulmonary vein flow can be evaluated by placing the pulsed-Doppler sample volume 1 to 2 cm into the pulmonary veins. The anterior to posterior direction of the left and right upper pulmonary veins allows the Doppler ultrasound beam to be aligned parallel to blood flow. This often cannot be achieved when interrogating the lower pulmonary veins.

The normal pulmonary venous flow pattern can be divided into three phases: (1) antegrade systolic flow, (2) antegrade diastolic flow, and (3) retrograde atrial contraction flow reversal (Fig. 1–14). Biphasic antegrade systolic flow can usually be appreciated on TEE. Systolic flow is dependent on apical displacement of the annulus, which is predominantly determined by left ventricular function, atrial relaxation, and atrial compliance.[30,46] Antegrade systolic flow is also affected by left atrial pressure and decreases with increasing left atrial pressure.[30,46] MR increases left atrial pressure during systole and may result in systolic flow reversal in one or all pulmonary veins.[30,46] Diastolic antegrade flow occurs as the mitral valve opens and left atrial pressure falls. The diastolic flow profile is dependent on left atrial pressure, left ventricular relaxation, and ventricular compliance.[30,46] Late diastolic atrial contraction flow reversal is dependent on atrial contractility, atrial systolic pressure, and left ventricular compliance. The normal pulmonary venous flow pattern is dependent on age, heart rate, and AV conduction, with older individuals having higher pulmonary venous systolic and atrial reversal velocities and smaller diastolic flow velocities.[46,48]

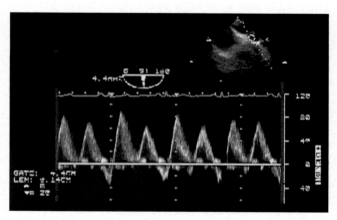

Figure 1–14. Normal pulmonary venous flow showing two antegrade flows in ventricular systole and diastole, with a diminutive retrograde flow caused by atrial contraction.

Coronary Artery Flow

The evaluation of coronary artery flow may be limited by motion of the heart during the cardiac and respiratory cycle and difficulties aligning the Doppler US beam parallel to blood flow. Coronary artery blood flow is best measured in the distal left main or proximal left anterior descending artery by imaging the aortic valve in short-axis from the midesophagus and then withdrawing the probe 1 to 2 cm such that the pulsed-Doppler US beam can be aligned parallel to coronary blood flow. Color flow imaging can assist in the proper positioning of the pulsed-Doppler sample volume. The US beam can only rarely be aligned parallel to flow in the left circumflex artery, and the right coronary artery cannot be imaged in up to half of patients. Identification of the right coronary artery is often best achieved using the high-esophagus long-axis view, in which the ostium of the coronary artery is visualized arising from the right sinus of Valsalva. The normal Doppler flow signal is characterized by a large diastolic velocity and small systolic velocity moving away from the transducer. In general, diastolic velocities are less than or equal to 60 cm/s, with velocities greater than 100 cm/s suggestive of a significant stenosis.[49-51] Coronary artery flow reserve can be evaluated using TEE by measuring peak or mean diastolic velocities at rest and following dipyridamole or adenosine infusion.[50,52-54] In normal subjects, coronary artery flow reserve tends to be greater than 3, with a flow reserve greater than 2.1 having a high negative predictive value for a critical stenosis in the left anterior descending artery.[52,54]

Tissue Doppler Imaging

Tissue Doppler imaging using TEE is feasible and allows the measurement of transverse and longitudinal myocardial velocities, strain, and strain rate to evaluate ventricular function and detect myocardial ischemia.[31,55,56] Longitudinal motion and deformation of individual wall segments can be assessed using the midesophageal four-chamber, two-chamber, and long-axis views, whereas transverse motion of the inferior and anterior walls can be assessed from the transgastric midpapillary muscle short-axis view.[31,55,56] Tricuspid annular velocities can be measured from a transgastric right ventricular inflow view to assess right ventricular function.[57]

Indications for Transesophageal Echocardiography

The utility of TEE in the assessment and management of patients with suspected and overt cardiac disease encompasses the spectrum of cardiac problems encountered in clinical cardiology. TEE can be performed in the ambulatory setting, intensive care unit, coronary care unit (CCU), or operating room. In general, TTE should be employed as the initial diagnostic investigation because this technique is noninvasive and entails no risk to the patient. However, obesity, emphysema, or chest deformities frequently limit ultrasound penetration and result in a nondiagnostic TTE study. Surgical bandages may limit the number of available acoustic windows, whereas mechanical ventilation and surgical devices, such as traction and intra-aortic balloon pumps (IABPs), may limit the ability to properly position the patient. Subcutaneous emphysema may result in the complete inability of TTE to visualize cardiac structures. TEE should be considered in these patients to obtain the necessary diagnostic information.

Despite an adequate TTE, TEE may be indicated to visualize cardiac structures not usually seen by TTE (i.e., SVC, pulmonary veins, and the descending thoracic aorta), or to provide improved anatomic details, such as the detection of a flail mitral valve scallop or the presence of a valvular vegetation, which are not consistently detected by TTE. Finally, TEE has important applications in the OR, which are discussed in Chapter 2. The common clinical indications for TEE are listed in Table 1–3.

Native Valve Disease

The presence, etiology, and severity of native valve disease can usually be determined by TTE. TEE is usually reserved for the clinical situations in which TTE findings are inconclusive or a more precise characterization of the valve morphology or lesion severity will alter patient management. Excellent visualization of the mitral valve anatomy is possible by TEE because of the close proxim-

TABLE 1–3. **Common Indications for Transesophageal Echocardiography**

Nondiagnostic TTE
Evaluation of native valve disease
Evaluation of prosthetic valves
Evaluation of suspected and definite infective endocarditis
Evaluation of a suspected cardioembolic event
Evaluation of cardiac tumors
Evaluation of an atrial septal abnormality
Evaluation of aortic disease
AFib (TEE-guided strategy for "early" cardioversion)
Evaluation of CHD
Detection of CAD
Evaluation of pericardial disease
Evaluation of the critically ill patient
Intraoperative monitoring
Monitoring during interventional procedures

CAD, coronary artery disease; CHD, congenital heard disease; TEE, transesophageal echocardiography; TTE, transthoracic echocardiogram.

ity of the mitral valve to the posteriorly positioned TEE transducer and the ability to image with a high-frequency transducer. The mitral annulus, leaflets, chordal structures, and papillary muscles can all be visualized and evaluated. A multiplane transducer allows a comprehensive, detailed examination of the valve to determine the location and mechanism of mitral regurgitation.[25,58] Ruptured chordae tendineae can be visualized, and precise anatomic localization of prolapsing or flail scallops is possible, which allows prediction of the likelihood of successful mitral valve repair (Chapter 20).[25,58-61] Abnormalities of the papillary muscles, such as a partial or complete rupture, are better visualized by TEE than TTE.[62]

The severity of MR can be quantified using the same methods employed for TTE (Chapter 18),[63] however color Doppler regurgitant jet areas tend to be larger on TEE than TTE.[64] Pulmonary vein flow can be assessed in nearly all patients and provides a valuable measure of MR severity.[46,65-68] The vena contracta width, regurgitant volume, and regurgitant orifice area derived using the proximal flow convergence zone can be obtained using TEE and provide prognostic information in asymptomatic patients with MR.[69-72]

In MS, TTE is usually satisfactory in evaluating the valve morphology and stenosis severity (see Chapter 21). TEE appears equivalent to TTE in assessing valve mobility and leaflet thickening, but subvalvular disease and calcification may be underestimated in the esophageal views resulting from the shadowing effect from mitral leaflet and annular thickening and calcification.[73] Transvalvular pressure gradients can be measured by aligning the continuous wave Doppler beam through the mitral valve parallel to left ventricular inflow in the midesophageal views.[74] Effective orifice area can be derived by the pressure half-time method,[74] proximal flow convergence method, or orifice planimetry.[75] Orifice planimetry requires a tomographic cut of the distal or most narrowed portion of the mitral orifice, however, this is technically difficult to obtain by TEE and frequently not possible. The suitability of a patient for percutaneous balloon mitral valvuloplasty usually incorporates a detailed TEE assessment of the left atrial chamber and appendage to identify thrombus,[76] in addition to an evaluation of the mitral valve morphology score and MR severity.[77] Mitral valve morphology on TEE can predict the prognosis of patients following percutaneous balloon mitral valvuloplasty, however TTE is preferred to evaluate valve morphology because of the preceding described limitations.[73,78] TEE can also be employed during the procedure to guide the transeptal puncture, balloon placement, and identify potential procedural complications, including severe MR, cardiac tamponade, or a significant atrial septal defect.[79]

TTE can adequately visualize most aortic valve abnormalities, and only rarely is TEE required. However, subvalvular abnormalities, such as subaortic membranes, frequently require TEE for definitive diagnosis.[80] The severity of AS is best quantified using transvalvular pressure gradients or valve area derived by TTE (see Chapter 23). Continuous wave Doppler interrogation of the aortic valve is possible by TEE using the transgastric long-axis view (100 to 135 degrees) or deep transgastric long-axis view (0 degrees) (see Fig. 1–13). Good correlations between TTE and TEE gradients have been reported despite a limited number of accessible TEE windows.[27] Anatomic aortic valve area can be measured on TEE by planimetry of the maximum systolic orifice area in the esophageal short-axis (30 to 60 degree) view. Proper transducer position should be confirmed by rotating to the longitudinal plane and verifying that the leaflet tips are being imaged. Aortic valve areas derived by orifice planimetry correlate well with valve areas derived by TTE using the continuity equation and Gorlin equation valve areas.[27,81,82] However, valve calcification may affect the accuracy of orifice areas measured by TEE.[83] TEE may also provide additional information on the presence and extent of aortic dilation, calcification, and ascending aorta atheroma, which may alter the surgical approach.

The evaluation of AR severity only rarely necessitates TEE (see Chapter 18). Standard Doppler methods employed with TTE may be used with TEE.[63,84] However, color jet areas on TEE tend to be larger than those obtained with TTE.[64] The ratio of color jet area to left ventricular outflow tract area can be obtained from the esophageal short-axis view of the outflow tract immediately inferior to the aortic valve. The ratio of jet height to outflow tract height can be obtained from the esophageal long-axis view. Vena contracta width on TEE correlates well with the regurgitant fraction and regurgitant volume.[85] AR severity may also be quantified using proximal flow convergence methods.[86,87] Holo-diastolic flow reversal in the descending aorta can be detected by TEE using pulsed Doppler.[88]

Prosthetic Valves

TEE is a valuable technique for evaluating prosthetic valve function because TTE visualization of the prosthetic valve components and function is often limited by the echogenicity of the prosthetic components (Chapter 25). Reverberation artifacts, attenuation artifacts, and acoustic shadowing obscure visualization of the prosthetic components and limit visualization beyond the prosthesis. TEE has increased sensitivity for detecting abnormalities of bioprosthetic and mechanical prostheses when compared to TTE.[89,90] Small abnormalities, such as leaflet thickening and calcification, flail leaflets, vegetations, thrombi, and filamentous strands, are better appreciated on TEE.[90-96] The structure and motion of the occluding device may also be better evaluated by TEE.[97] TEE can be used to distinguish pannus from thrombus formation[98-100] and guide the use of thrombolytic therapy in the latter condition.[101-103] TEE is especially valuable in assessing mitral prostheses because the transducer's posterior position provides excellent visualization of vegetations and thrombi usually located on the left atrial aspect of the prosthesis.[89,92] However, the ventricular aspect of a mitral prosthesis may not be adequately seen, and TTE should be performed to complement the TEE assessment.[104]

TEE can differentiate normal from pathologic prosthetic valve regurgitation.[90-94,105] Prosthetic MR is frequently better evaluated by TEE than TTE[90,91,93] because the left atrial cavity can be visualized without any intervening prosthetic material. TEE should be performed in patients in whom significant MR is a clinical concern but not seen on TTE.[106] Importantly, TEE allows characterization of MR jets as paravalvular or transvalvular in origin, which may modify the surgical procedure.[91,93,107] The incremental benefit of TEE in the assessment of AR severity is less clear for aortic prostheses because the regurgitation jet is usually well seen on TTE, and TEE visualization may be compromised by partial obstruction of the regurgitation jet by either the aortic or mitral prosthesis when imaged in the esophageal views.[94]

All bioprostheses and mechanical prostheses are inherently stenotic. The degree of stenosis is dependent on the prosthesis type and size and the presence of an associated pathologic condition, such as leaflet calcification, pannus formation, or valve thrombosis.[108] In general, TTE is sufficient to assess the severity of prosthetic AS or MS, but only TEE has sufficient resolution to distinguish these pathologic conditions.[98,99] In patients with an inadequate TTE, TEE can quantify prosthetic MS by measuring the diastolic pressure gradient, pressure half-time, and effective orifice area using the proximal flow convergence method, as described for native mitral stenosis.[75,109] Prosthetic AS can be quantified by measuring the transvalvular pressure gradient, as described for native AS.[27,110]

Infective Endocarditis

The presence of a vegetation is a hallmark finding of infective endocarditis, and its identification in the clinical setting of suspected endocarditis confirms the diagnosis (Chapter 22).[111] In native valve endocarditis, the sensitivity of TTE for the detection of a vegetation has ranged from 28% to 70%, inferior to the 86% to 98% sensitivity observed with TEE.[112-117] Smaller vegetations are more likely to be detected by TEE than TTE because of improved spatial resolution.[113] The specificity of TTE and TEE for detecting vegetations is similar and greater than 90% when strict criteria are used for diagnosis.[112,113,115] Pulmonic valve vegetations may also be better seen by TEE.[118] However, TEE does not appear to have an improved sensitivity for the detection of tricuspid valve vegetations or the assessment of re-

gurgitation severity.[119] Prosthetic valve endocarditis is more difficult to diagnose using either TTE or TEE. The sensitivity of TTE for detecting prosthetic valve vegetations has ranged from 0% to 43%, and increases to 33% to 86% using TEE.[89,114,120,121] Thus, TEE is warranted in patients with suspected prosthetic valve endocarditis if the TTE does not identify a vegetation.

Although TEE has a higher sensitivity for detecting vegetations than TTE, the impact of TEE is greatest in patients with suspected endocarditis and an intermediate clinical probability of endocarditis, especially patients with prosthetic valves.[122] The absence of a vegetation on TEE makes the diagnosis of endocarditis unlikely (<10%), and alternative diagnoses should be considered.[121,123] However, false-negative TEE studies have been reported and a negative TEE should not supplant a clinical and microbiological diagnosis. Patients with a high index of suspicion of endocarditis, prosthetic valves, or a persistent bacteremia may benefit from a follow-up TEE in 7 to 10 days if the initial study was negative.[121,123] TEE has a low diagnostic yield in patients with a low clinical probability of endocarditis and is likely not warranted.[122]

Complications of infective endocarditis, including abscess formation, leaflet diverticula, leaflet perforation, fistula tracts, mycotic aneurysms, and pseudoaneurysm formation, are better detected by TEE than TTE.[114,124-129] In one large series, only 28% of surgical or autopsy confirmed abscess cavities were identified by TTE, compared to 87% using TEE.[124] The specificity of both techniques for detecting abscess formation exceeded 90%. Thus, patients with a suspected abscess based on clinical grounds or persistent bacteremia should undergo TEE.

The potential utility of TEE in patients with uncomplicated confirmed endocarditis remains to be determined. However, TEE may provide the clinician with prognostic information on the clinical course of infective endocarditis. Larger (>10 mm), severely mobile vegetations on TEE are associated with systemic embolization,[116,130,131] and vegetation size on TEE has been shown to be an independent predictor of survival.[131] Complications including embolism, abscess formation, need for valve replacement, and death may be more likely to occur in patients in whom a vegetation fails to decrease in size with therapy.[132] However at this time, we do not perform routine follow-up TEE for cases of uncomplicated confirmed endocarditis.

Suspected Cardioembolic Event

A potential cardioembolic event should be considered in patients suffering cerebral ischemia or a peripheral artery embolus, especially in those patients without significant cerebrovascular disease. The Cerebral Embolism Task Force has suggested that cardiac emboli account for 15% to 20% of cerebral ischemic events.[133]

Potential cardioembolic sources are conditions that have a propensity for thrombus formation, intracardiac or intra-aortic masses, or potential passageways for paradoxical emboli. Several cardiac abnormalities have a strong association with cardioembolic events and are considered major risk sources (Chapter 40). These abnormalities include AFib, left atrial or left ventricular thrombi, vegetations, intracardiac tumor, MS, mechanical valves, recent myocardial infarction (MI), dilated cardiomyopathy, ischemic left ventricular dysfunction (EF < 28%) and intra-aortic debris.[134,135] Minor risk sources with weaker associations include atrial septal aneurysms, patent foramen ovale, spontaneous echo contrast, mitral annular calcification, and mitral valve prolapse (MVP).[134-136] Many of these conditions can be diagnosed clinically, but echocardiography is frequently required to diagnosis anatomic abnormalities. Although TTE can detect these potential cardioembolic sources, in general, TEE is superior at identifying major and minor risk sources.

Left atrial thrombus is frequently located in the left atrial appendage, a region poorly visualized on TTE. The sensitivity of TTE in detecting left atrial thrombi has been reported to be 0% to 53%, whereas TEE has a sensitivity of 93% to 100% and a specificity exceeding 95%.[137,138] Care must be taken not to confuse the pectinate muscles of the appendage for thrombus. Left ventricular thrombi can be detected by TTE with a sensitivity and specificity approaching or exceeding 90%[139] and may be better appreciated by TTE than TEE because of the close proximity of the left ventricular apex to the TTE transducer, and the far-field position and frequent apical foreshortening on TEE.[140] However, TEE may be helpful if the TTE is inconclusive.[141] Left atrial spontaneous echocardiographic contrast is rarely appreciated on TTE but well seen on TEE.[142] TEE may better detect small myxomas.[143,144] Similarly, TEE is superior for detecting patent foramen ovale and atrial septal aneurysms.[145,146] The cardioembolic risk of a patent foramen ovale is related to the defect size and can be better appreciated by TEE.[147-149] A comprehensive evaluation of aortic arch atheroma is rarely possible by TTE alone. TEE is required to adequately assess the extent, degree of lumen protrusion, and morphological features (i.e., mobility, ulceration) that characterize the potential embolic risk.[41,150-154]

The indication for performing a TEE in a patient with a suspected cardioembolic event is controversial.[134,155,156] Although TEE has a better sensitivity than TTE for detecting potential cardioembolic abnormalities (TEE abnormalities have been documented in over 50% of patients with cryptogenic stroke or transient ischemic attack [TIA]),[157-159] the yield for identifying a major risk source is limited. An analysis of pooled data suggested an overall detection rate for intracardiac masses of 4% for TTE and 11% for TEE.[134] However, the yield was greater in patients with cardiac disease.

TTE and TEE identified an intracardiac mass in 13% and 19% of patients with cardiac disease and only 0.7% and 1.6% in patients without cardiac disease. In addition, the information obtained by TEE, which may include the identification of minor risk sources, may not significantly alter patient management.[134,159] Many management decisions will be predetermined by the clinical setting (e.g., a patient with AFib requires anticoagulation), and the management of patients with minor-risk cardiac abnormalities is frequently controversial. Thus, TEE should only be performed if the results have a reasonable chance of altering patient management or therapy. In this regard, TEE may have the greatest impact on patient management in the clinical setting of patients younger than 55 years of age with unexplained cerebral ischemia, in patients having recurrent events or events in multiple cerebrovascular territories, in patients with occlusion of a large peripheral vessel (i.e., femoral or renal artery), or in patients with suspected endocarditis and in who the TTE fails to identify a cardioembolic source.

Atrial Septal Abnormalities

TEE provides excellent visualization of the atrial septum because of the close proximity of the transducer and perpendicular orientation to the US beam. Atrial septal defects, atrial septal aneurysms, and patent foramen ovale, are identified more frequently by TEE than TTE.[19,144,146,160-162] TTE with harmonic imaging can improve the detection rate of a patent foramen ovale[162] but may lead to decreased specificity.[163] Sinus venosus defects and associated anomalous pulmonary venous drainage are frequently not identified on TTE but can be easily detected on TEE.[19,20] TEE can delineate the morphological details of an atrial septal defect, assess the severity of left-to-right shunting, measure the size of a patent foramen ovale, determine the potential for percutaneous closure, and assist in proper device placement during percutaneous closure.[148,164-166] TEE can also detect thrombus formation within an atrial septal aneurysm or an impending paradoxical embolus.[147,161,167]

Cardiac Tumors

TEE appears superior to TTE, computed tomography (CT), angiography, and magnetic resonance imaging (MRI) for detecting intracardiac tumors.[144,168] The sensitivity of TTE and TEE for the detection of atrial myxomas has been reported to be 95% and 100%, respectively.[168] Nonmyxomatous intracardiac tumors are identified by TTE and TEE in 91% and 100% of patients, respectively.[168] However, the sensitivity of TTE and TEE is dependent on tumor size and may be as low as 62% and 77%, respectively, for cardiac papillary fibroelastomas less than or equal to 2 mm in size.[169] Pericardial or paracardial tumors are detected in only 67% of patients using TTE and 97% by TEE.[168] TEE appears especially valuable for detecting tumors located at the base of the heart, adjacent to the great vessels, or adjacent to the right heart.[144,168] In addition, TEE is superior to TTE in characterizing the features of a cardiac tumor that may assist in the diagnosis and management, such as the involvement of multiple chambers, site of tumor attachment, presence of multiple tumors, infiltration of adjacent structures, tumor calcification, or cyst formation.[144,168] TEE has been used to guide the percutaneous biopsy of intracardiac tumors.[170] Importantly, the size and extent of paracardial involvement is not well assessed by TTE or TEE. In this setting, tomographic imaging with a wider field of view (MRI or CT) is required. In addition, intracardiac tumor can be missed when there are associated cardiac lesions confounding visualization, the tumor is small, or when the operator has an insufficient level of suspicion. Thus, care should be taken to consider the potential presence of an intracardiac tumor when performing the examination.

Aortic Dissection, Intramural Hematoma, and Rupture

Aortic dissection can be detected by TEE with a high degree of accuracy and is the diagnostic investigation of choice for suspected aortic dissection in many institutions (see Chapter 33).[171,172] The ascending aorta, aortic arch, and descending thoracic aorta can be visualized with excellent resolution resulting from the close proximity of the transducer to the aorta. The presence of an intimal flap is diagnostic of aortic dissection and can be distinguished from reverberation artifacts commonly occurring in the ascending aorta by using M-mode echocardiography.[173,174] However, a small segment of the superior ascending aorta may not be visualized by TEE resulting from the interposition of the air-filled trachea and bronchus, and TTE should be performed to visualize this region before ruling out a dissection. The sensitivity of monoplane and biplane TEE for the detection of aortic dissection has been reported to be 97% to 100%, with a specificity of 77% to 100%.[171,175-177] The specificity was greater than 95% in all but one study.[175] Multiplane TEE has been associated with a sensitivity and specificity of 98% to 100% and 94% to 95%.[178,179] Thus, TEE compares favorably with other technologies, such as aortography, CT, and MRI, but has several advantages related to its portability, rapid diagnostic potential, and ability to be performed in hemodynamically unstable patients.[172,175-177]

In addition to diagnosis, TEE can determine the extent of the dissection, differentiate true and false lumens, identify thrombus within the false lumen, locate the site of the intimal tear, evaluate for aortic valve involvement, and the potential for valve repair.[171,175,180] Arch vessel and coronary artery involvement can also

be determined by TEE.[171] Importantly, TEE can detect findings suggestive of aortic rupture, such as a pericardial effusion, pleural effusion, or mediastinal hematoma, which may significantly alter surgical therapy.[171] An algorithm using TEE has been proposed to guide stent graft implantation for descending thoracic aorta dissections.[181] Aortic complications following surgical repair can also be detected with TEE.[182]

Intramural hematoma and penetrating aortic ulcers can have a presentation similar to aortic dissection and can be diagnosed using TEE.[177,178,183-185] TEE appears to have a high sensitivity and specificity (100% and 91%, respectively) for detecting intramural hematoma, diagnosed by a crescentric or circular local aortic wall thickening (>5 to 7 mm) that may have associated echolucent areas, in the absence of an intimal flap or tear, and with displacement of intimal calcification.[178,186-188] TEE can serially evaluate patients with intramural hematoma to assess for hematoma regression, progression, or the development of classic dissection.[189,190] The diagnostic accuracy of TEE for detecting penetrating aortic ulcers is unclear, however a sensitivity of 83% has been reported.[183] The presence, depth, and diameter of a penetrating ulcer are predictive of disease progression and prognosis in patients with intramural hematoma.[191]

TEE has been used in the setting of chest trauma for the diagnosis and grading of blunt aortic trauma and traumatic aortic rupture.[151,192] The reported sensitivity and specificity of TEE for the detection of traumatic aortic rupture has ranged from 63% to 100% and 84% to 100%, respectively.[151,192,193] However, TEE cannot consistently visualize the superior ascending aorta and aortic arch branch vessels, a frequent site of traumatic injury.[194] The role of TEE in the diagnostic evaluation of chest trauma patients remains undefined. However, limited data suggests that the TEE findings can be used to guide acute management and select patients for conservative therapy, immediate surgery, or postponed surgical repair.[195]

Atrial Fibrillation

AFib predisposes the left atrium to contractile dysfunction, chamber dilation, and thrombus formation. TEE is clearly superior to TTE for detecting left atrial thrombus and has a sensitivity ranging from 93% to 100% and a specificity exceeding 95%.[137,138] However, TEE can also stratify atrial fibrillation patients into their risk of thromboembolism. The prevalence of left atrial thrombus, spontaneous echo contrast, left atrial appendage velocity less than 20 cm/s, and complex aortic atheroma on TEE are associated with a patient's clinical risk of thromboembolism,[196] and a left atrial abnormality (thrombus, dense spontaneous echo contrast, left atrial appendage velocity less than 20 cm/s) or complex aortic atheroma on TEE are predictive of thromboembolic events in high-risk patients based on clinical criteria.[197]

A TEE-guided strategy has been proposed to allow "early" cardioversion of AFib that is greater than 2 days in duration. In the ACUTE trial, a TEE-guided strategy of "early" electrical cardioversion in patients without left atrial thrombus was compared to a conventional strategy of 3 to 4 weeks of anticoagulation before and after electrical cardioversion.[198] The TEE-guided strategy had an incidence of embolic events, stroke, and TIA similar to the conventional strategy at 8 weeks follow-up but fewer hemorrhagic events. This data suggests that a TEE-guided strategy may be an acceptable alternative in patients at increased risk for hemorrhagic complications or who are not tolerating their AFib despite rate control. However, a TEE-guided approach does not obviate the need for anticoagulation postcardioversion.[199] An economic analysis has demonstrated that the cost of the TEE-guided strategy and conservative strategy are similar.[200]

Congenital Heart Disease

TTE is the primary modality for evaluating patients with congenital heart disease (CHD). However, previous surgery or chest deformities may result in an inadequate examination. TEE frequently adds information to the diagnostic evaluation and management of patients with CHD, whether in the preoperative, interventional, intraoperative, or postoperative setting (see Chapters 42 to 44).[166,201-206] However, a detailed systematic segmental approach is of the utmost importance during these studies.[205,206] The indications for TEE in patients with CHD are extensive,[205,206] and in 2005, the American Society of Echocardiography published recommendations for the performance of TEE in patients with pediatric acquired heart disease or CHD.[204] TEE better appreciates abnormalities of the atrial septum and pulmonary veins, and can be used to guide the percutaneous closure of atrial and ventricular septal defects.[19,20,160,164-166,205,207,208] In patients with AV canal defects, the AV valves and site of chordal insertion can be visualized to determine the potential for surgical valvuloplasty.[209] Intracardiac and extracardiac baffles may not be well seen on TTE. TEE provides good visualization of an atrial baffle and can detect stenoses or leaks.[210] Complications of a Fontan procedure, such as obstruction or thrombosis, can be detected.[211] TEE can characterize outflow tract obstructions,[80,201,205,209] and abnormalities of the aorta, such as aortic coarctation and patent ductus arteriosus, are better appreciated by TEE.[212,213]

Coronary Artery Disease

TEE can be used to diagnosis coronary artery disease (CAD) by (1) visualizing coronary stenoses in the proximal vessels[54,214] or (2) detecting stress-induced regional wall motion abnormalities. Thus, TEE is uniquely positioned to evaluate the anatomic and physiologic significance of a coronary stenosis.

The left main coronary artery can be visualized by TEE in more than 85% of patients.[49,215-218] The proximal left anterior descending artery and left circumflex artery can also be visualized in most patients.[215-217] The proximal right coronary artery is more difficult to visualize but may still be seen in greater than 50% of patients.[215,217] In patients with visualized vessels, the sensitivity of TEE for identifying a significant left main coronary stenosis has been reported to be 91% to 100%, with a specificity greater than 90%.[49,215-218] The sensitivity for detecting significant proximal left anterior descending artery disease, left circumflex artery disease, or right coronary artery disease has been reported to be 78% to 100%, 50% to 89%, and 82% to 100%, respectively but significantly decreases if nonvisualized segments are included in the analysis.[215-217] Left anterior descending artery stenoses have been quantified by TEE using the continuity equation, however the severity tends to be underestimated.[51] Coronary artery flow reserve can be measured using TEE, and a flow reserve greater than 2.1 is highly predictive of the absence of a critical stenosis in the left anterior descending artery.[50,52-54,214,219] Abnormal flow reserve in the CS may also be useful in detecting left coronary artery stenoses.[220] However, TEE should not replace coronary angiography in the diagnosis of proximal coronary artery stenoses but rather, may be useful in assessing angiographically questionable stenoses of the left main or left anterior descending artery in centers where intravascular US is unavailable.[221]

Stress echocardiography with TEE imaging has been used to evaluate patients with suspected or confirmed CAD.[222-227] Transesophageal atrial pacing and pharmacologic stimulation using either dobutamine or dipyridamole have been shown to be highly accurate in detecting CAD, to provide information for risk stratification, and can evaluate myocardial viability in patients with left ventricular dysfunction.[222-230] However, TEE is an invasive procedure with potential risks and therefore, should be reserved for patients with poor TTE images. The widespread use of contrast agents during TTE stress echocardiography has reduced the need to perform TEE stress echocardiography.

Additional applications of TEE include the detection of anomalous coronary arteries, coronary artery aneurysms, and coronary artery fistulas.[54,231]

Pericardial Disease

Pericardial effusions and cardiac tamponade are usually easily diagnosed on TTE (Chapter 30). However, cardiac tamponade after cardiac surgery can be difficult to diagnose by TTE. Local compression of the right atrium by extracardiac thrombus may not be apparent on TTE because of the posterior position of the thrombus and poor image quality related to suboptimal patient position, surgical bandages, and drainage tubes. TEE circumvents these problems and can better detect extracardiac compression.[232] Constrictive pericarditis and restrictive cardiomyopathies can usually be differentiated by TTE using a combination of Doppler echocardiography, respiratory monitoring, and tissue Doppler imaging. However, TEE with respiratory monitoring may be useful in patients with a nondiagnostic TTE.[233] TEE is superior to TTE in assessing pericardial thickening, intrapericardial metastases, intrapericardial thrombus, and pericardial cysts.[232,234] However, CT and MRI have unique advantages over TEE by better localizing pericardial abnormalities, characterizing pericardial masses, or detecting pericardial calcification and are the preferred techniques for assessing pericardial thickness.[235]

Critically Ill Patient in the Intensive Care Unit

The TTE images obtained in the ICU are frequently inadequate resulting from surgical bandages, drains, mechanical ventilation, and an inability to properly position the patient. In this setting, TEE can provide rapid access to essential diagnostic information that alters patient management.[236,237] TEE provides information on myocardial function, valve function, volume status, and hemodynamics critical in the evaluation and management of patients with unexplained hypotension or pulmonary edema.[236-239] In patients with unexplained hypoxia, TEE can detect right-to-left intracardiac shunting through a patent foramen ovale, which may occur in ventilated patients requiring high levels of pressure support or right ventricular infarction.[240,241] The presence of massive or proximal pulmonary emboli can be diagnosed by TEE.[22,23] Potential complications of MI, including left ventricular dysfunction, papillary muscle rupture, and myocardial rupture, may be detected.

Intraoperative Monitoring

Intraoperative TEE can provide detailed information on cardiac anatomy and function without disrupting the surgical procedure.[242-244] TEE can evaluate global and segmental left ventricular function, detect intraoperative myocardial ischemia, and monitor hemodynamics, including cardiac output, left ventricular filling pressures, and volume status.[236,244] The cause of hemodynamic disturbances can be determined and intraoperative complications identified. Importantly, the adequacy of valve repairs or replacements and surgical reconstructions for congenital and acquired diseases can be evaluated before leaving the OR.[203,244-246] The value of intraoperative TEE is well established in patients undergoing mitral valve reconstructive surgery and predictive of both early and late mitral valve dysfunction.[247-249] Practice guidelines for perioperative TEE have been published by the American Society of Anesthesiologists and the Society of Cardiovascular Anesthesiologists based on the strength of supporting evidence and expert opinion that TEE improves clinical outcome.[242] In 1999, the American Society of Echocardiography and Society of Cardiovascular Anesthesiologists published guidelines for the performance of a comprehensive intraoperative multiplane TEE examination.[250] The complete list of potential indications for TEE in the intraoperative period is extensive and is discussed in more detail in Chapters 2 and 20.

Monitoring during Interventional Procedures

TEE is a valuable adjunct to percutaneous interventional procedures in patients with both congenital and acquired diseases. For percutaneous mitral valvuloplasty, TEE can guide catheter positioning during the transseptal puncture, assist in proper balloon placement, evaluate the result, identify complications, and shorten procedure and fluoroscopy times.[164,251] TEE can also guide catheter positioning for radiofrequency ablation.[252] During percutaneous closure of an atrial septal defect or patent foramen ovale, TEE can detect the defect, exclude multiple defects, identify the location in relation to the pulmonary veins or mitral valve, size the defect during balloon inflation, guide proper positioning of the occluder device, and assess for residual shunting.[165,166,208] TEE has also been used to guide catheter positioning during percutaneous closure of a patent ductus arteriosus, ventricular septal defect, or coronary artery fistula.[166,207,253-255] Biopsies of the right ventricle or intracardiac masses can be guided by TEE, as can alcohol septal ablation procedures for hypertrophic cardiomyopathy (HCM).[170,256] TEE has been useful in the pediatric population during creation or enlargement of an interatrial communication or balloon dilation of obstructive left-sided heart lesions.[166,257]

Contraindications to Transesophageal Echocardiography

See Table 1–4 for common contraindications to TEE. Patients undergoing TEE should be kept at nothing by mouth (NPO) status for 4 to 6 hours before the procedure because of the potential for vomiting and aspiration. However, urgent procedures can likely be performed earlier with minimal risk of vomiting and aspiration if there has been only clear fluid intake up to 2 hours before the procedure.[258] TEE should not be performed on the uncooperative patient. Patients who are uncooperative should either have the study deferred or be sedated and paralyzed, if necessary. Patients with a tenuous cardiorespiratory status should be intubated and ventilated to avoid

TABLE 1-4. Contraindications for Transesophageal Echocardiography

Absolute
Uncooperative patient
Severe respiratory depression
Tenuous cardiorespiratory status
Esophageal obstruction (stricture, mass)
Tracheoesophageal fistula
Perforated viscous
Active GI bleed

Relative
Esophageal diverticulum
Esophageal varices
Previous esophageal surgery
Severe cervical arthritis
Dislocation of the atlanto axial joint
Severe coagulopathy

GI, gastrointestinal.

TABLE 1-5. Procedural Complications with Transesophageal Echocardiography

Major Complications
Death
Esophageal rupture
Laryngospasm or bronchospasm
CHF or pulmonary edema
Sustained ventricular tachycardia

Minor Complications
Excessive retching or vomiting
Sore throat
Hoarseness
Minor pharyngeal bleeding
Blood-tinged sputum
Nonsustained or sustained supraventricular tachycardia
AFib
Nonsustained ventricular tachycardia
Bradycardia or heart block
Transient hypotension
Transient hypertension
Angina
Transient hypoxia
Parotid swelling
Tracheal intubation

Afib, atrial fibrillation; CHF, congestive heart failure.

decompensation during the procedure. To avoid esophageal rupture, TEE should not be attempted in a patient with an esophageal obstruction caused by a stricture or mass. An esophageal diverticulum should also be considered a relative contraindication because of the possibility of the probe entering and perforating the diverticulum. Techniques have been proposed to successfully perform a TEE in a patient with a Zenker's diverticulum by using fluoroscopic balloon guidance or a fiberoptic endoscope and overtube.[259] TEE is contraindicated in the patient with an unrepaired tracheoesophageal fistula, perforated viscus, or active gastrointestinal (GI) bleed. Esophageal varices are not an absolute contraindication to TEE. However, the potential additive information should be weighed against the small risk of major bleeding. Severe cervical arthritis or dislocation of the atlantoaxial joint, where flexion of the neck is severely limited, should be considered a relative contraindication to TEE. TEE can be performed safely in patients on anticoagulation therapy, although a severe coagulopathy should be considered a relative contraindication.

Complications of Transesophageal Echocardiography

TEE is a relatively safe procedure with a low complication rate. Procedural complications have been observed in 0.47% to 2.8% of patients with successful esophageal intubation, however the vast majority of complications are minor[5,9,11,260] (Table 1-5). Major complications, defined in one study as death, laryngospasm, sustained ventricular tachycardia, or congestive heart failure (CHF), occur in approximately 0.3% of patients.[260] In the Multicenter European Survey of 10,419 examinations, the TEE examination had to be interrupted before completion in 0.88% of studies.[11] Patient intolerance of the probe, including excessive retching or vomiting, was the most common complication resulting in premature termination of the procedure.[11] In the largest patient series, deaths have been reported in 0% to 0.03% of patients.[5,9,11,260] Reported cardiac complications have included nonsustained and sustained supraventricular tachycardias or AFib, nonsustained and sustained ventricular tachycardia, bradycardia, transient hypotension or hypertension, angina pectoris, CHF, and pulmonary edema. Pulmonary complications have included transient hypoxia and laryngospasm. Bleeding complications have included minor pharyngeal bleeding or blood-tinged sputum, Mallory-Weiss tear, and severe hematemesis in a patient with a malignant tumor invading the esophagus. A minor sore throat may be present for 24 hours after the procedure.

Complication rates during intraoperative TEE may be higher resulting from the patient's inability to comply with the examination or signal procedural discomfort. However, a complication rate of only 0.2% was observed in 7200 patients undergoing cardiac surgery.[261] Odynophagia warranting further investigations with either endoscopy or Gastrografin swallow was the most common complication (0.1%). Dental injury and significant upper GI bleeding occurred in 0.03% of patients, respectively. Esophageal perforation occurred in only one patient (0.01%). There were no deaths.

The complication rate has been reported to be 2.4% (excluding failed intubations) in 1650 pediatric patients undergoing TEE, predominantly in the intraoperative setting. Most complications related to airway obstruction and occurred predominantly in smaller subjects.[262]

Adverse reactions may occur as a result of IV sedation, topical anesthesia, or drying agents, such glycopyrrolate. IV sedation may result in respiratory depression, hypoxia, hypotension, or paradoxical reactions. Topical anesthesia with benzocaine or lidocaine may result in acute toxic methemoglobinemia, a rare but potentially lethal condition in which hemoglobin is oxidized by the topical anesthesia agent and unable to deliver oxygen to the tissues.[263-265] In this condition, the partial pressure of oxygen in the blood is normal, but oxyhemoglobin levels are decreased. Patients usually develop cyanosis and may have lethargy, tachycardia, or dyspnea. Oxygen saturation by pulse oximetry is often only mildly reduced because pulse oximetry is unable to distinguish methemoglobin and reduced hemoglobin. The diagnosis can be confirmed with an arterial blood gas (ABG) sample and measurement of the methemoglobin level. The incidence of overt clinical methemoglobinemia associated with TEE in clinical practice has been estimated at 0.115%.[265] Rapid recognition is essential to prevent serious cardiopulmonary compromise and a potential fatal reaction.[263] Methylene blue (1 to 2 mg/kg) given as a 1% solution over 5 minutes will result in prompt resolution of the cyanosis, and is indicated when the methemoglobin levels are greater than or equal to 30%, or if the patient has cyanosis, central nervous system (CNS) depression or cardiopulmonary compromise.[265]

Future Developments

At present, 3D TEE relies on the sequential acquisition of multiple 2D TEE images at predefined imaging plane locations every 3 to 5 degrees over a 180-degree range, gated to the electrocardiogram (ECG) and respiration.[266] These images are stored for offline 3D reconstruction, which is time consuming and laborious, limiting the utility of 3D TEE in clinical practice. Recent introduction of a 3000-element matrix transducer has allowed real-time 3D TTE with high-quality images. Miniaturization of the matrix transducer as a result of ongoing advances in microprocessor technology will likely make real-time 3D TEE a reality in the near future.

Summary

TEE is a powerful diagnostic tool that can evaluate cardiac structure and function in a wide range of clinical situations. A comprehensive study should include the standard views discussed in this chapter with additional views obtained as necessary depending on the clinical problem and diagnostic information required. In critically ill patients, the initial views acquired should be those that are most pertinent to the clinical question. Adequate diagnostic information would then have been obtained even if the study needs to be terminated prematurely. Finally, we need to be mindful that TEE is a semi-invasive procedure and not free of risk. Clear and convincing indications should be present before a TEE is performed.

KEY POINTS

- TTE and TEE have unique and different advantages and limitations in the evaluation of the patient with suspected cardiac disease.

- TEE is a semi-invasive procedure with a small but definite risk of complications.

- Performance of the TEE study requires knowledge of cardiac anatomy and pathology, as well as proficiency in manipulating the transducer imaging plane and ultrasound machine image controls.

- TEE is an essential component of the pre- and intraoperative evaluation of the patient being considered for mitral valve repair.

- TEE is a valuable modality to detect the presence and severity of suspected prosthetic mitral valve dysfunction.

- The impact of TEE in suspected endocarditis is greatest in patients at intermediate risk for disease. Alternate diagnoses should be considered in suspected native valve endocarditis if the TEE study is negative.

- TEE should only be performed in a patient with potential cardioembolic event if the results will alter patient management. The greatest impact of TEE on patient management resides in the young patient with unexplained cerebral ischemia, recurrent events, or events in multiple vascular distributions.

- TEE may be considered the diagnostic investigation of choice for the diagnosis of aortic dissection of the thoracic aorta.

- TEE can provide essential and rapid diagnostic information for the management of the critically ill patient in the ICU in whom TTE images are often suboptimal.

- TEE is a valuable adjunctive imaging modality to monitor device placement and detect potential complications during percutaneous interventional cardiology procedures.

REFERENCES

1. Frazin L, Talano JV, Stephanides L, et al: Esophageal echocardiography. *Circulation* 54:102-108, 1976.
2. Pearlman AS, Gardin JM, Martin RP, et al: Guidelines for physician training in transesophageal echocardiography: Recommendations of the American Society of Echocardiography Committee for physician training in echocardiography. *J Am Soc Echocardiogr* 5:187-194, 1992.
3. Chan K, Burwash I: Unusual structural abnormality in a biplane transesophageal transducer with normal imaging function. *J Am Soc Echocardiogr* 11:310-312, 1998.
4. Kronzon I, Cziner DG, Katz ES, et al: Buckling of the tip of the transesophageal echocardiography probe: A potentially dangerous technical malfunction. *J Am Soc Echocardiogr* 5:176-177, 1992.
5. Chan KL, Cohen GI, Sochowski RA, et al: Complications of transesophageal echocardiography in ambulatory adult patients: Analysis of 1500 consecutive examinations. *J Am Soc Echocardiogr* 4:577-582, 1991.
6. Chan K: Impact of transesophageal echocardiography on the management of patients with aortic dissection. *Chest* 101:406-410, 1991.
7. Steckelberg JM, Khandheria BK, Anhalt JP, et al: Prospective evaluation of the risk of bacteremia associated with transesophageal echocardiography. *Circulation* 84:177-180, 1991.
8. Melendez L, Chan K, Cheung P, et al: Incidence of bacteremia in transesophageal echocardiography: A prospective study of 140 consecutive patients. *J Am Coll Cardiol* 18:1650-1654, 1991.
9. Tam JW, Burwash IG, Ascah KJ, et al: Feasibility and complications of single-plane and biplane versus multiplane transesophageal imaging: A review of 2947 consecutive studies. *Can J Cardiol* 13:81-84, 1997.
10. Yvorchuk K, Sochowski R, Chan K: A prospective comparison of the multiplane probe with the biplane probe in structure visualization and Doppler examination during transesophageal echocardiography. *J Am Soc Echocardiog* 8:111-120, 1995.
11. Daniel WG, Erbel R, Kasper W, et al: Safety by transesophageal echocardiography: A multicenter survey of 10,419 examinations. *Circulation* 83:817-821, 1991.
12. Cohen G, Chan K: Biplane transesophageal echocardiography: Clinical applications of the long-axis plane. *J Am Soc Echocardiogr* 4:155-163, 1991.
13. Seward JB, Khandheria BK, Freeman WK, et al: Multiplane transesophageal echocardiography: Image orientation, examination technique, anatomic correlations, and clinical applications. *Mayo Clin Proc* 68:523-551, 1993.
14. Marx GR, Fulton DR, Pandian NG, et al: Delineation of site, relative size and dynamic geometry of atrial septal defects by real-time three dimensional echocardiography. *J Am Coll Cardiol* 25:482-490, 1995.
15. Flachskampf FA, Chandra S, Gaddipatti A, et al: Analysis of shape and motion of the mitral annulus in subjects with and without cardiomyopathy by echocardiographic 3-dimensional reconstruction. *J Am Soc Echocardiogr* 13:277-287, 2000.
16. Seward JB, Khandheria BK, Oh JK, et al: Transesophageal echocardiography: technique, anatomic correlations, implementation, and clinical applications. *Mayo Clin Proc* 63:649-680, 1988.
17. Anderson R, Dussek J, Evans S, et al: Cardiovascular. In Williams PL (ed): *Gray's Anatomy*, 38th ed. New York, Churchill Livingstone, 1995, pp 1482-1483.
18. Veinot JP, Harrity PJ, Gentile F, et al: Anatomy of the normal left atrial appendage: A quantitative study of age-related changes in 500 autopsy hearts-implications for echocardiographic examination. *Circulation* 96:3112-3115, 1997.
19. Kronzon I, Tunick PA, Freedberg RS, et al: Transesophageal echocardiography is superior to transthoracic echocardiography in the diagnosis of sinus venosus atrial septal defect. *J Am Coll Cardiol* 17:537-542, 1991.
20. Pascoe RD, Oh JK, Warnes CA, et al: Diagnosis of sinus venosus atrial septal defect with transesophageal echocardiography. *Circulation* 94:1049-1055, 1996.
21. Fagan S, Veinot JP, Chan KL: Residual sinus venosus atrial septal defect following surgical closure of atrial septal defect. *J Am Soc Echocardiogr* 14(7):738-741, 2001.
22. Wittlich N, Erbel R, Eichler A, et al: Detection of central pulmonary artery thromboemboli by transesophageal echocardiography in patients with severe pulmonary embolism. *J Am Soc Echocardiogr* 5:515-524, 1992.
23. Pruszczyk P, Torbicki A, Pacho R, et al: Noninvasive diagnosis of suspected severe pulmonary embolism: Transesophageal echocardiography vs spiral CT. *Chest* 112:722-728, 1997.
24. Shanewise JS, Cheung AT, Aronson S, et al: ASE/SCA guidelines for performing a comprehensive intraoperative multiplane transesophageal echocardiography examination: Recommendations of the American Society of Echocardiography Council for Intra-operative Echocardiography and the Society of Cardiovascular Anesthesiologists Task Force for Certification in Perioperative Transesophageal Echocardiography. *J Am Soc Echocardiogr* 12:884-900, 1999.
25. Enriquez-Sarano M, Freeman WK, Tribouilloy CM, et al: Functional anatomy of mitral regurgitation: Accuracy and outcome implications of transesophageal echocardiography. *J Am Coll Cardiol* 34:1129-1136, 1999.
26. Pieper EP, Hellemans IM, Hamer HP, et al: Additional value of biplane transesophageal echocardiography in assessing the genesis of mitral regurgitation and the feasibility of valve repair. *Am J Cardiol* 75:489-493, 1995.
27. Blumberg FC, Pfeifer M, Holmer SR, et al: Transgastric Doppler echocardiographic assessment of the severity of aortic stenosis using multiplane transesophageal echocardiography. *Am J Cardiol* 79:1273-1275, 1997.
28. Catoire P, Beydon L, Delaunay L, et al: Persistent left superior vena cava diagnosed by transesophageal echocardiography. *J Cardiothorac Vasc Anesth* 7:375-379, 1993.
29. Seward JB, Khandheria BK, Edwards WD, et al: Biplanar transesophageal echocardiography: Anatomic correlations, image orientation, and clinical applications. *Mayo Clin Proc* 65:1193-1213, 1990.
30. Nishimura RA, Tajik AJ: Evaluation of diastolic filling of left ventricle in health and disease: Doppler echocardiography is the clinician's Rosetta stone. *J Am Coll Cardiol* 30:8-18, 1997.
31. Groban L, Dolinski SY: Transesophageal echocardiographic evaluation of diastolic function. *Chest* 128:3652-3663, 2005.
32. Hozumi T, Shakudo M, Applegate R, et al: Accuracy of cardiac output estimation with biplane transesophageal echocardiography. *J Am Soc Echocardiogr* 6:62-68, 1993.
33. Pu M, Griffin BP, Vandervoort PM, et al: Intraoperative validation of mitral inflow determination by transesophageal echocardiography: Comparison of single-plane, biplane and thermodilution techniques. *J Am Coll Cardiol* 26:1047-1053, 1995.
34. Feinberg MS, Hopkins WE, Davila-Roman VG, et al: Multiplane transesophageal echocardiographic Doppler imaging accurately determines cardiac output measurement in critically ill patients. *Chest* 107:679-673, 1995.
35. Katz WE, Gasior TA, Quinlan JJ, et al: Transgastric continuous-wave Doppler to determine cardiac output. *Am J Cardiol* 71:853-857, 1993.
36. Gorscan J III, Diana P, Ball BA, et al: Intraoperative determination of cardiac output by transesophageal continuous wave Doppler. *Am Heart J* 123:171-176, 1992.
37. Muhiudeen IA, Kuecherer HF, Lee E, et al: Intraoperative estimation of cardiac output by transesophageal pulsed Doppler echocardiography. *Anesthesiology* 74:9-14, 1991.
38. Agmon Y, Khandheria BK, Gentile F, et al: Echocardiographic assessment of the left atrial appendage. *J Am Coll Cardiol* 34:1867-1877, 1999.

39. Donal E, Yamada H, Leclercq C, et al: The left atrial appendage, a small, blind-ended structure: a review of its echocardiographic evaluation and its clinical role. *Chest* 128:1853-1862, 2005.

40. Tabata T, Oki T, Fukuda N, et al: Influence of aging on left atrial appendage flow velocity patterns in normal subjects. *J Am Soc Echocardiogr* 9:274-280, 1996.

41. The Stroke Prevention in Atrial Fibrillation Investigators Committee on Echocardiography: Transesophageal echocardiographic correlates of thromboembolism in high-risk patients with nonvalvular atrial fibrillation. *Ann Intern Med* 128:639-647, 1998.

42. Goldman ME, Pearce LA, Hart RG, et al: Pathophysiologic correlates of thromboembolism in nonvalvular atrial fibrillation: I. Reduced flow velocity in the left atrial appendage (The Stroke Prevention in Atrial Fibrillation [SPAFF-III] study). *J Am Soc Echocardiogr* 12:1080-1087, 1999.

43. Kamalesh M, Copeland TB, Sawada S: Severely reduced left atrial appendage function: A cause of embolic stroke in patients in sinus rhythm? *J Am Soc Echocardiogr* 11:902-904, 1998.

44. Palinkas A, Antonielli E, Picano E, et al: Clinical value of left atrial appendage flow velocity for predicting of cardioversion success in patients with non-valvular atrial fibrillation. *Eur Heart J* 22:2201-2208, 2001.

45. Antonielli E, Pizzuti A, Palinkas A, et al: Clinical value of left atrial appendage flow for prediction of long-term sinus rhythm maintenance in patients with nonvalvular atrial fibrillation. *J Am Coll Cardiol* 39:1443-1449, 2002.

46. Tabata T, Thomas JD, Klein AL: Pulmonary venous flow by doppler echocardiography: revisited 12 years later. *J Am Coll Cardiol* 41:1243-1250, 2003.

47. Jensen JL, Williams FE, Beilby BJ, et al: Feasibility of obtaining pulmonary venous flow velocity in cardiac patients using transthoracic pulsed wave Doppler technique. *J Am Soc Echocardiogr* 10:60-66, 1997.

48. Klein AL, Burstow DJ, Tajik AJ, et al: Effects of age on left ventricular dimensions and filling dynamics in 117 normal persons. *Mayo Clin Proc* 69:212-224, 1994.

49. Yamagishi M, Yasu T, Ohara K, et al: Detection of coronary blood flow associated with left main coronary artery stenosis by transesophageal Doppler color flow echocardiography. *J Am Coll Cardiol* 17:87-93, 1991.

50. Kozakova M, Palombo C, Pratali L, et al: Assessment of coronary reserve by transoesophageal Doppler echocardiography: Direct comparison between different modalities of dipyridamole and adenosine administration. *Eur Heart J* 18:514-523, 1997.

51. Isaaz K, da Costa A, de Pasquale JP, et al: Use of the continuity equation for transesophageal Doppler assessment of severity of proximal left coronary artery stenosis: A quantitative coronary angiography validation study. *J Am Coll Cardiol* 32:42-48, 1998.

52. Redberg RF, Sobol Y, Chou TM, et al: Adenosine-induced coronary vasodilation during transesophageal Doppler echocardiography: Rapid and safe measurement of coronary flow reserve ratio can predict significant left anterior descending coronary stenosis. *Circulation* 92:190-196, 1995.

53. Chaudhry FA, Ren JF, Ramani K, et al: Validation of transesophageal echocardiography to determine physiologic coronary flow. *Echocardiography* 18:553-557, 2001.

54. Youn HJ, Foster E: Transesophageal echocardiography (TEE) in the evaluation of the coronary arteries. *Cardiol Clin* 18:833-848, 2000.

55. Simmons LA, Weidemann F, Sutherland GR, et al: Doppler tissue velocity, strain, and strain rate imaging with transesophageal echocardiography in the operating room: a feasibility study. *J Am Soc Echocardiogr* 15:768-776, 2002.

56. Skulstad H, Andersen K, Edvardsen T, et al: Detection of ischemia and new insight into left ventricular physiology by strain Doppler and tissue velocity imaging: assessment during coronary bypass operation of the beating heart. *J Am Soc Echocardiogr* 17:1225-1233, 2004.

57. David JS, Tousignant CP, Bowry R: Tricuspid annular velocity in patients undergoing cardiac operation using transesophageal echocardiography. *J Am Soc Echocardiogr* 19:329-334, 2006.

58. Agricola E, Oppizzi M, De Bonis M, et al: Multiplane transesophageal echocardiography performed according to the guidelines of the American Society of Echocardiography in patients with mitral valve prolapse, flail, and endocarditis: diagnostic accuracy in the identification of mitral regurgitant defects by correlation with surgical findings. *J Am Soc Echocardiogr* 16:61-66, 2003.

59. Foster GP, Iselbacher EM, Rose GA, et al: Accurate localization of mitral regurgitation defects using multiplane transesophageal echocardiography. *Ann Thorac Surg* 65:1025-1031, 1998.

60. Grewal KS, Malkowski MJ, Kramer CM, et al: Multiplane transesophageal echocardiographic identification of the involved scallop in patients with flail mitral valve leaflet: Intraoperative correlation. *J Am Soc Echocardiogr* 11:966-971, 1998.

61. Omran AS, Woo A, David TE, et al: Intraoperative transesophageal echocardiography accurately predicts mitral valve anatomy and suitability for repair. *J Am Soc Echocardiogr* 15:950-957, 2002.

62. Moursi MH, Bhatnagar SK, Vilacosta I, et al: Transesophageal echocardiographic assessment of papillary muscle rupture. *Circulation* 94:1003-1009, 1996.

63. Zoghbi WA, Enriquez-Sarano M, Foster E, et al: Recommendations for evaluation of the severity of native valvular regurgitation with two-dimensional and Doppler echocardiography. *J Am Soc Echocardiogr* 16:777-802, 2003.

64. Smith MD, Harrison MR, Pinton R, et al: Regurgitant jet size by transesophageal compared with transthoracic Doppler color flow imaging. *Circulation* 83:79-86, 1991.

65. Klein AL, Obarski TP, Stewart WJ, et al: Transesophageal Doppler echocardiography of pulmonary venous flow: A new marker of mitral regurgitation severity. *J Am Coll Cardiol* 18:518-526, 1991.

66. Hynes MS, Tam JL, Burwash IG, et al: Predictive value of pulmonary venous flow patterns in detecting mitral regurgitation and left ventricular abnormalities. *Can J Cardiol* 15:665-670, 1999.

67. Klein AL, Bailey AS, Cohen GI, et al: Importance of sampling both pulmonary veins in grading mitral regurgitation by transesophageal echocardiography. *J Am Soc Echocardiogr* 6:115-123, 1993.

68. Roach JM, Stajduhar KC, Torrington KG. Right upper lobe pulmonary edema caused by acute mitral regurgitation. Diagnosis by transesophageal echocardiography. *Chest* 103:1286-1288, 1993.

69. Grayburn PA, Fehske W, Omran H, et al: Multiplane transesophageal echocardiographic assessment of mitral regurgitation by Doppler color flow mapping of the vena contracta. *Am J Cardiol* 74:912-917, 1994.

70. Pu M, Vandervoort PM, Griffin BP, et al: Quantification of mitral regurgitation by the proximal convergence method using transesophageal echocardiography: Clinical validation of a geometric correction for proximal flow constraint. *Circulation* 92:2169-2177, 1995.

71. Enriquez-Sarano M, Avierinos JF, Messika-Zeitoun D, et al: Quantitative determinants of the outcome of asymptomatic mitral regurgitation. *N Engl J Med* 352:875-883, 2005.

72. Tribouilloy C, Shen WF, Quere JP, et al: Assessment of severity of mitral regurgitation by measuring regurgitant jet width at its origin with transesophageal Doppler color flow imaging. *Circulation* 85:1248-1253, 1992.

73. Marwick TH, Torelli J, Obarski T, et al: Assessment of the mitral valve splitability score by transthoracic and transesophageal echocardiography. *Am J Cardiol* 68:1106-1107, 1991.

74. Stoddard MF, Prince CR, Tuman WL, et al: Angle of incidence does not affect accuracy of mitral stenosis area calculation by

pressure half-time: Application to Doppler transesophageal echocardiography. *Am Heart J* 127:1562-1572, 1994.

75. Degertekin M, Basaran Y, Gencbay M, et al: Validation of flow convergence region method in assessing mitral valve area in the course of transthoracic and transesophageal echocardiographic studies. *Am Heart J* 135:207-214, 1998.

76. Manning WJ, Reis GJ, Douglas PS: Use of transoesophageal echocardiography to detect left atrial thrombi before percutaneous balloon dilatation of the mitral valve: a prospective study. *Br Heart J* 67:170-173, 1992.

77. Cormier B, Vahanian A, Michel PL, et al: Transesophageal echocardiography in the assessment of percutaneous mitral commissurotomy. *Eur Heart J* 12(suppl B):61-65, 1991.

78. Levin TN, Feldman T, Bednarz J, et al: Transesophageal echocardiographic evaluation of mitral valve morphology to predict outcome after balloon mitral valvotomy. *Am J Cardiol* 73:707-710, 1994.

79. Park SH, Kim MA, Hyon MS: The advantages of on-line transesophageal echocardiography guide during percutaneous balloon mitral valvuloplasty. *J Am Soc Echocardiogr* 13:26-34, 2000.

80. Essop MR, Skudicky D, Sareli P: Diagnostic value of transesophageal versus transthoracic echocardiography in discrete subaortic stenosis. *Am J Cardiol* 70:962-963, 1992.

81. Kim KS, Maxted W, Nanda NC, et al: Comparison of multiplane and biplane transesophageal echocardiography in the assessment of aortic stenosis. *Am J Cardiol* 79:436-441, 1997.

82. Hoffmann R, Flachskampf FA, Hanrath P: Planimetry of orifice area in aortic stenosis using multiplane transesophageal echocardiography. *J Am Coll Cardiol* 22:529-534, 1993.

83. Cormier B, Iung B, Porte JM, et al: Value of multiplane transesophageal echocardiography in determining aortic valve area in aortic stenosis. *Am J Cardiol* 77:882-885, 1996.

84. Meyerowitz CB, Jacobs LE, Kotler MN, et al: Assessment of aortic regurgitation by transesophageal echocardiography: Correlation with angiographic determination. *Echocardiography* 10:269-278, 1993.

85. Willett DL, Hall SA, Jessen ME, et al: Assessment of aortic regurgitation by transesophageal color Doppler imaging of the vena contracta: validation against an intraoperative aortic flow probe. *J Am Coll Cardiol* 37:1450-1455, 2001.

86. Sato Y, Kawazoe K, Nasu M, et al: Clinical usefulness of the proximal isovelocity surface area method using echocardiography in patients with eccentric aortic regurgitation. *J Heart Valve Dis* 8:104-111, 1999.

87. Sato Y, Kawazoe K, Kamata J, et al: Clinical usefulness of the effective regurgitant orifice area determined by transesophageal echocardiography in patients with eccentric aortic regurgitation. *J Heart Valve Dis* 6:580-586, 1997.

88. Sutton DC, Kluger R, Ahmed SU, et al: Flow reversal in the descending aorta: A guide to intraoperative assessment of aortic regurgitation with transesophageal echocardiography. *J Thorac Cardiovasc Surg* 108:576-582, 1994.

89. Daniel WG, Mugge A, Grote J, et al: Comparison of transthoracic and transesophageal echocardiography for detection of abnormalities of prosthetic and bioprosthetic valves in the mitral and aortic positions. *Am J Cardiol* 71:210-215, 1993.

90. Alton ME, Pasierski TJ, Orsinelli DA, et al: Comparison of transthoracic and transesophageal echocardiography in evaluation of 47 Starr-Edwards prosthetic valves. *J Am Coll Cardiol* 20:1503-1511, 1992.

91. Daniel LB, Grigg LE, Weisel RD, et al: Comparison of transthoracic and transesophageal assessment of prosthetic valve dysfunction. *Echocardiography* 7:83-95, 1990.

92. Khandheria BK, Seward JB, Oh JK, et al: Value and limitations of transesophageal echocardiography in the assessment of mitral valve prosthesis. *Circulation* 83:1956-1968, 1991.

93. Chaudhry FA, Herrera C, DeFrino PF, et al: Pathologic and angiographic correlations of transesophageal echocardiography in the prosthetic heart valve dysfunction. *Am Heart J* 122:1057-1064, 1991.

94. Karalis DG, Chandrasekaran K, Ross JJ Jr, et al: Single-plane transesophageal echocardiography for assessing function of mechanical or bioprosthetic valves in the aortic valve position. *Am J Cardiol* 69:1310-1315, 1992.

95. Gueret P, Vignon P, Fournier P, et al: Transesophageal echocardiography for the diagnosis and management of nonobstructive thrombosis of mechanical mitral prosthesis. *Circulation* 91:103-110, 1995.

96. Orsinelli DA, Pearson AC: Detection of prosthetic valve strands by transesophageal echocardiography: Clinical significance in patients with suspected cardiac source of embolism. *J Am Coll Cardiol* 26:1713-1718, 1995.

97. Muratori M, Montorsi P, Teruzzi G, et al: Feasibility and diagnostic accuracy of quantitative assessment of mechanical prostheses leaflet motion by transthoracic and transesophageal echocardiography in suspected prosthetic valve dysfunction. *Am J Cardiol* 97:94-100, 2006.

98. Barbetseas J, Nagueh SF, Pitsavos C, et al: Differentiating thrombus from pannus formation in obstructed mechanical prosthetic valves: An evaluation of clinical, transthoracic and transesophageal echocardiographic parameters. *J Am Coll Cardiol* 32:1410-1417, 1998.

99. Girard SE, Miller FA, Orszulak TA, et al: Reoperation for prosthetic aortic valve obstruction in the era of echocardiography: trends in diagnostic testing and comparison with surgical findings. *J Am Coll Cardiol* 37:579-584, 2001.

100. Montorsi P, De Bernardi F, Muratori M, et al: Role of cine-fluoroscopy, transthoracic, and transesophageal echocardiography in patients with suspected prosthetic heart valve thrombosis. *Am J Cardiol* 85:58-64, 2000.

101. Ozkan M, Kaymaz C, Kirma C, et al: Intravenous thrombolytic treatment of mechanical prosthetic valve thrombosis: A study using serial transesophageal echocardiography. *J Am Coll Cardiol* 35:1881-1889, 2000.

102. Lengyl M: Management of prosthetic valve thrombosis. *J Heart Valve Dis* 13:329-334, 2004.

103. Tong AT, Roudaut R, Ozkan M, et al: Transesophageal echocardiography improves risk assessment of thrombolysis of prosthetic valve thrombosis: results of the international PRO-TEE registry. *J Am Coll Cardiol* 43:77-84, 2004.

104. Tenenbaum A, Fisman EZ, Vered Z, et al: Failure of transesophageal echocardiography to visualize a large mitral prosthesis vegetation detected solely by transthoracic echocardiography. *J Am Soc Echocardiogr* 8:944-946, 1995.

105. Flachskampf FA, O'Shea JP, Griffin BP, et al: Patterns of transvalvular regurgitation in normal mechanical prosthetic valves. *J Am Coll Cardiol* 18:1493-1498, 1991.

106. Fernandes V, Olmos L, Nagueh SF, et al: Peak early diastolic velocity rather than pressure half-time is the best index of mechanical prosthetic mitral valve function. *Am J Cardiol* 89:704-710, 2002.

107. Flachskampf FA, Hoffmann R, Franke A, et al: Does multiplane transesophageal echocardiography improve the assessment of prosthetic valve regurgitation? *J Am Soc Echocardiogr* 8:70-78, 1995.

108. Reisner SA, Meltzer RS: Normal values of prosthetic valve Doppler echocardiographic parameters: A review. *J Am Soc Echocardiogr* 11:201-210, 1998.

109. Gorscan J III, Kenny WM, Diana P, et al: Transesophageal continuous-wave Doppler to evaluate mitral prosthetic stenosis. *Am Heart J* 121:911-914, 1991.

110. Baumgartner H, Khan S, DeRobertis M, et al: Effect of prosthetic aortic design on the Doppler-catheter gradient correlation: An in vitro study of normal St. Jude, Medtronic-Hall, Starr-Edwards, and Hancock valves. *J Am Coll Cardiol* 19:324-332, 1992.

111. Durack DT, Lukes AS, Bright DK: New criteria for diagnosis of infective endocarditis: Utilization of specific echocardiographic findings. *Am J Med* 96:200-209, 1994.

112. Birmingham GD, Rahko PS, Ballantyne F: Improved detection of infective endocarditis with transesophageal echocardiography. *Am Heart J* 123:774-781, 1992.

113. Erbel R, Rohmann S, Drexler M, et al: Improved diagnostic value of echocardiography in patients with infective endocarditis by transesophageal approach: A prospective study. *Eur Heart J* 9:43-53, 1988.

114. Taams MA, Gussenhoven EJ, Bos E, et al: Enhanced morphologic diagnosis in infective endocarditis by transoesphageal echocardiography. *Br Heart J* 63:109-113, 1990.

115. Shively BK, Gurule FT, Roldan CA, et al: Diagnostic value of transesophageal compared with transthoracic echocardiography in infective endocarditis. *J Am Coll Cardiol* 18:391-397, 1991.

116. Mügge A, Daniel WG, Frank G, et al: Echocardiography in infective endocarditis: Reassessment of prognostic implications of vegetation size determined by the transthoracic and the transesophageal approach. *J Am Coll Cardiol* 14:631-638, 1989.

117. Shapiro SM, Young E, De Guzman S, et al: Transesophageal echocardiography in diagnosis of infective endocarditis. *Chest* 105:377-382, 1994.

118. Ramadan FB, Beanlands DS, Burwash IG: Isolated pulmonic valve endocarditis in healthy hearts: a case report and review of the literature. *Can J Cardiol* 16:1282-1288, 2000.

119. San Roman JA, Vilacosta I, Zamorano JL, et al: Transesophageal echocardiography in right-sided endocarditis. *J Am Coll Cardiol* 21:1226-1230, 1993.

120. Zabalgoitia M, Herrera CJ, Chaudhry FA, et al: Improvement in the diagnosis of bioprosthetic valve dysfunction by transesophageal echocardiography. *J Heart Valve Dis* 2:595-603, 1993.

121. Lowry RW, Zoghbi WA, Baker WB, et al: Clinical impact of transesophageal echocardiography in the diagnosis and management of infective endocarditis. *Am J Cardiol* 73:1089-1091, 1994.

122. Lindner JR, Case RA, Dent JM, et al: Diagnostic value of echocardiography in suspected endocarditis: An evaluation based on the pretest probability of disease. *Circulation* 93:730-736, 1996.

123. Sochowski RA, Chan K-L: Implication of negative results on a monoplane transesophageal echocardiographic study in patients with suspected infective endocarditis. *J Am Coll Cardiol* 21:216-221, 1994.

124. Daniel WG, Mugge A, Martin RP, et al: Improvement in the diagnosis of abscesses associated with endocarditis by transesophageal echocardiography. *N Engl J Med* 324:795-800, 1991.

125. Massey WM, Samdarshi TE, Nanda NC, et al: Serial documentation of changes in a mitral valve vegetation progressing to abscess rupture and fistula formation by transesophageal echocardiography. *Am Heart J* 124:241-248, 1992.

126. Castro SD, Cartoni D, d'Amati G, et al: Diagnostic accuracy of transthoracic and multiplane transesophageal echocardiography for valvular perforation in acute infective endocarditis: Correlation with anatomic findings. *Clin Infect Dis* 30:825-826, 2000.

127. Vilacosta I, San Roman JA, Sarria C, et al: Clinical, anatomic, and echocardiographic characteristics of aneurysms of the mitral valve. *Am J Cardiol* 84:110-113, 1999.

128. Tingleff J, Egeblad H, Gotzsche CO, et al: Perivalvular cavities in endocarditis: Abscesses versus pseudoaneurysms? A transesophageal Doppler echocardiographic study in 118 patients with endocarditis. *Am Heart J* 130:93-100, 1995.

129. Piper C, Hetzer R, Korfer R, et al: The importance of secondary mitral valve involvement in primary aortic valve endocarditis. The mitral kissing vegetation. *Eur Heart J* 23:79-86, 2002.

130. Di Salvo G, Habib G, Pergola V, et al: Echocardiography predicts embolic events in infective endocarditis. *J Am Coll Cardiol* 37:1069-1076, 2001.

131. Thuny F, Di Salvo G, Belliard O, et al: Risk of embolism and death in infective endocarditis: prognostic value of echocardiog-

132. Rohmann S, Erhel R, Darius H, et al: Effect of antibiotic treatment on vegetation size and complication rate in infective endocarditis. *Clin Cardiol* 20:132-140, 1997.

133. Cerebral Embolism Task Force: Cardiogenic brain embolism: The second report of the Cerebral Embolism Task Force. *Arch Neurol* 46:727-743, 1989.

134. Kapral MK, Silver FL, with the Canadian Task Force on Preventive Health Care: Preventive health care, 1999 update: 2. Echocardiography for the detection of a cardiac source of embolus in patients with stroke. *CMAJ* 161:989-996, 1999.

135. Ay H, Furie KL, Singhal A, et al. An evidence-based causative classification system for acute ischemic stroke. *Ann Neurol* 58:688-697, 2005.

136. Overell JR, Bone I, Lees KR: Interatrial septal abnormalities and stroke: a meta-analysis of case-control studies. *Neurology* 55:1172-1179, 2000.

137. Hwang JJ, Chen JJ, Lin SC, et al: Diagnostic accuracy of transesophageal echocardiography for detecting left atrial thrombi in patients with rheumatic heart disease having undergone mitral valve operations. *Am J Cardiol* 72:677-681, 1993.

138. Manning WJ, Weintraub RM, Wakomonski CA, et al: Accuracy of transesophageal echocardiography for identifying left atrial thrombi. A prospective intraoperative study. *Ann Intern Med* 123:817-822, 1995.

139. Stratton JR, Lighty GW Jr, Pearlman AS, et al. Detection of left ventricular thrombus by two-dimensional echocardiography: Sensitivity, specificity, and causes of uncertainty. *Circulation* 66:156-166, 1982.

140. Mugge A, Daniel WG, Haverich A, et al: Diagnosis of noninfective cardiac mass lesions by two-dimensional echocardiography: Comparison of the transthoracic and transesophageal approaches. *Circulation* 83:70-78, 1991.

141. Chen C, Koschyk D, Hamm C, et al: Usefulness of transesophageal echocardiography in identifying small left ventricular apical thrombus. *J Am Coll Cardiol* 21:208-215, 1993.

142. Black IW, Hopkins AP, Lee LCL, et al: Left atrial spontaneous echo contrast: A clinical transesophageal echocardiographic analysis. *J Am Coll Cardiol* 18:398-404, 1991.

143. Rittoo D, Cotter L: Detection of a small left atrial myxoma: Value and limitations of four imaging modalities. *J Am Soc Echocardiogr* 10:874-876, 1997.

144. Mügge A, Daniel WG, Haverich A, et al: Diagnoses of noninfective cardiac mass lesions by two-dimensional echocardiography: Comparison of the transthoracic and transesophageal approaches. *Circulation* 83:70-78, 1991.

145. Siostrzonek P, Zangeneh M, Gössinger H, et al: Comparison of transesophageal and transthoracic contrast echocardiography for detection of a patent foramen ovale. *Am J Cardiol* 68:1247-1249, 1991.

146. Pearson AC, Nagelhout D, Castello R, et al: Atrial septal aneurysm and stroke: A transesophageal echocardiographic study. *J Am Coll Cardiol* 18:1223-1229, 1991.

147. Hausmann D, Mügge A, Daniel WG: Identification of patent foramen ovale permitting paradoxical embolism. *J Am Coll Cardiol* 26:1030-1038, 1995.

148. Schuchlenz HW, Weihs W, Beitzke A, et al: Transesophageal echocardiography for quantifying size of patent foramen ovale in patients with cryptogenic cerebrovascular events. *Stroke* 33:293-296, 2002.

149. Schuchlenz HW, Weihs W, Horner S, et al: The association between the diameter of a patent foramen ovale and the risk of embolic cerebrovascular events. *Am J Med* 109:456-462, 2000.

150. Tunick PA, Kronzon I: Atheromas of the thoracic aorta: Clinical and therapeutic update. *J Am Coll Cardiol* 35:545-554, 2000.

151. Willens HJ, Kessler KM: Transesophageal echocardiography in the diagnosis of diseases of the thoracic aorta: Part II-

raphy: a prospective multicenter study. *Circulation* 112:69-75, 2005.

atherosclerotic and traumatic diseases of the aorta. *Chest* 117:233-243, 2000.

152. Guo Y, Jiang X, Zhang S, et al: Application of transesophageal echocardiography to aortic embolic stroke. *Chin Med J (Engl)* 115:525-528, 2002.

153. Di Tullio MR, Sacco RL, Savoia MT, et al: Aortic atheroma morphology and the risk of ischemic stroke in a multiethnic population. *Am Heart J* 139:329-336, 2000.

154. Montgomery DH, Ververis JJ, McGorisk G, et al: Natural history of severe atheromatous disease of the thoracic aorta: a transesophageal echocardiographic study. *J Am Coll Cardiol* 27:95-101, 1996.

155. Warner MF, Momah KI: Routine transesophageal echocardiography for cerebral ischemia: Is it really necessary? *Arch Intern Med* 156:1719-1723, 1996.

156. McNamara RL, Lima JA, Whelton PK, et al: Echocardiographic identification of cardiovascular sources of emboli to guide clinical management of stroke: A cost-effective analysis. *Ann Intern Med* 127:775-787, 1997.

157. Pearson AC, Labovitz AJ, Tatineni S, et al: Superiority of transesophageal echocardiography in detecting cardiac source of embolism in patients with cerebral ischemia of uncertain etiology. *J Am Coll Cardiol* 17:66-72, 1991.

158. Labovitz AJ for the STEPS Investigators: Transesophageal echocardiography and unexplained cerebral ischemia: A multicenter follow-up study. *Am Heart J* 137:1082-1087, 1999.

159. Rauh G, Fischereder M, Spengel FA: Transesophageal echocardiography in patients with focal cerebral ischemia of unknown cause. *Stroke* 27:691-694, 1996.

160. Mehta RH, Helmcke F, Nanda NC, et al: Transesophageal Doppler color flow mapping assessment of atrial septal defect. *J Am Coll Cardiol* 16:1010-1016, 1990.

161. Mugge A, Daniel WG, Angermann C, et al: Atrial septal aneurysm in adult patients: A multicenter study using transthoracic and transesophageal echocardiography. *Circulation* 91:2785-2792, 1995.

162. Ha JW, Shin MS, Kang S, et al: Enhanced detection of right-to-left shunt through patent foramen ovale by transthoracic contrast echocardiography using harmonic imaging. *Am J Cardiol* 87:669-671, 2001.

163. Madala D, Zaroff JG, Hourigan L, et al: Harmonic imaging improves sensitivity at the expense of specificity in the detection of patent foramen ovale. *Echocardiography* 21:33-36, 2004.

164. Rittoo D, Sutherland GR, Shaw TR: Quantification of left-to-right shunting and defect size after balloon mitral commissurotomy using biplane transesophageal echocardiography, color flow Doppler mapping, and the principle of proximal flow convergence. *Circulation* 87:1591-1603, 1993.

165. Ewert P, Berger F, Daehnert I, et al: Transcatheter closure of atrial septal defects without fluoroscopy: Feasibility of a new method. *Circulation* 101:847-849, 2000.

166. Rigby ML: Transoesophageal echocardiography during interventional cardiac catheterisation in congenital heart disease. *Heart* 86(Suppl 2):II23-II29, 2001.

167. Chow BJ, Johnson CB, Turek M, et al: Impending paradoxical embolus: a case report and review of the literature. *Can J Cardiol* 19:1426-1432, 2003.

168. Engberding R, Daniel WG, Erbel R, et al: Diagnosis of heart tumours by transoesophageal echocardiography: A multicentre study in 154 patients. *Eur Heart J* 1993;14:1223-1228.

169. Sun JP, Asher CR, Yang XS, et al: Clinical and echocardiographic characteristics of papillary fibroelastomas. A retrospective and prospective study in 162 patients. *Circulation* 103:2687-2693, 2001.

170. Beaver TA, Robb JF, Teufel EJ, et al: Right ventricular outflow tract obstruction in an older woman: Facilitated diagnosis with transesophageal echocardiography-guided biopsy. *J Am Soc Echocardiogr* 13:622-625, 2000.

171. Cigarrao JE, Isselbacher EM, DeSanctis RW, et al: Diagnostic imaging in the evaluation of suspected aortic dissection: Old standards and new directions. *N Engl J Med* 328:35-43, 1993.

172. Nienaber CA, Eagle KA: Aortic dissection: new frontiers in diagnosis and management: Part I: from etiology to diagnostic strategies. *Circulation* 108:628-635, 2003.

173. Evangelista A, Garcia-del-Castillo H, Gonzalez-Alujas T, et al: Diagnosis of ascending aortic dissection by transesophageal echocardiography: utility of M-mode in recognizing artifacts. *J Am Coll Cardiol* 27:102-107, 1996.

174. Vignon P, Spencer KT, Rambaud G, et al: Differential transesophageal echocardiographic diagnosis between linear artifacts and intraluminal flap of aortic dissection or disruption. *Chest* 119:1778-1790, 2001.

175. Nienaber CA, von Kodolitsch Y, Nicolas V, et al: The diagnosis of thoracic aortic dissection by noninvasive imaging procedures. *N Engl J Med* 328:1-9, 1993.

176. Bansal RC, Chandrasekaran K, Ayala K, et al: Frequency and explanation of false negative diagnosis of aortic dissection by aortography and transesophageal echocardiography. *J Am Coll Cardiol* 25:1393-1401, 1995.

177. Willens HJ, Kessler KM: Transesophageal echocardiography in the diagnosis of diseases of the thoracic aorta: Part I-aortic dissection, aortic intramural hematoma, and penetrating atherosclerotic ulcer of the aorta. *Chest* 116:1772-1779, 2000.

178. Keren A, Kim CB, Hu BS, et al: Accuracy of biplane and multiplane transesophageal echocardiography in diagnosis of typical acute aortic dissection and intramural hematoma. *J Am Coll Cardiol* 28:627-636, 1996.

179. Sommer T, Fehske W, Holzkuecht N, et al: Aortic dissection: A comparative study of diagnosis with spiral CT, multiplanar transesophageal echocardiography and MR imaging. *Radiology* 199:347-352, 1996.

180. Movsowitz HD, Levine RA, Hilgenberg AD, et al: Transesophageal echocardiographic description of the mechanisms of aortic regurgitation in acute type A aortic dissection: Implications for aortic valve repair. *J Am Coll Cardiol* 36:884-890, 2000.

181. Rocchi G, Lofiego C, Biagini E, et al: Transesophageal echocardiography-guided algorithm for stent-graft implantation in aortic dissection. *J Vasc Surg* 40:880-885, 2004.

182. Masani ND, Banning AP, Jones RA, et al: Follow-up of chronic thoracic aortic dissection: Comparison of transesophageal echocardiography and magnetic resonance imaging. *Am Heart J* 131:1156-1163, 1996.

183. Vilacosta I, San Roman JA, Aragoncillo P, et al: Penetrating atherosclerotic aortic ulcer: Documentation by transesophageal echocardiography. *J Am Coll Cardiol* 32:83-89, 1998.

184. Evangelista A, Mukherjee D, Mehta RH, et al: Acute intramural hematoma of the aorta: a mystery in evolution. *Circulation* 111:1063-1070, 2005.

185. Maraj R, Rerkpattanapipat P, Jacobs LE, et al: Meta-analysis of 143 reported cases of aortic intramural hematoma. *Am J Cardiol* 86:664-668, 2000.

186. Kang DH, Song JK, Song MG, et al: Clinical and echocardiographic outcomes of aortic intramural hemorrhage compared with acute aortic dissection. *Am J Cardiol* 81:202-206, 1998.

187. Vilacosta I, San Roman JA, Ferreiros J, et al: Natural history and serial morphology of aortic intramural hematoma: A novel variant of aortic dissection. *Am Heart J* 134:495-507 1997.

188. Song JM, Kang DH, Song JK, et al: Clinical significance of echo-free space detected by transesophageal echocardiography in patients with type B aortic intramural hematoma. *Am J Cardiol* 89:548-551, 2002.

189. Song JK, Kim HS, Song JM, et al: Outcomes of medically treated patients with aortic intramural hematoma. *Am J Med* 113:181-187, 2002.

190. Kaji S, Akasaka T, Katayama M, et al: Long-term prognosis of patients with type B aortic intramural hematoma. *Circulation* 108(Suppl 1):II307-II311, 2003.

191. Ganaha F, Miller DC, Sugimoto K, et al: Prognosis of aortic intramural hematoma with and without penetrating atheroscle-

rotic ulcer: a clinical and radiological analysis. *Circulation* 106:342-348, 2002.

192. Goarin JP, Cluzel P, Gosgnach M, et al: Evaluation of transesophageal echocardiography for diagnosis of traumatic aortic injury. *Anesthesiology* 93:1373-1377, 2000.

193. Smith MD, Cassidy JM, Souther S, et al: Transesophageal echocardiography in the diagnosis of traumatic rupture of the aorta. *N Engl J Med* 332:356-362, 1995.

194. Ahrar K, Smith DC, Bansal RC, et al: Angiography in blunt thoracic aortic injury. *J Trauma* 42:665-669, 1997.

195. Vignon P, Martaille JF, Francois B, et al: Transesophageal echocardiography and therapeutic management of patients sustaining blunt aortic injuries. *J Trauma* 58:1150-1158, 2005.

196. Zabalgoitia M, Halperin JL, Pearce LA, et al: Transesophageal echocardiographic correlates of clinical risk of thromboembolism in nonvalvular atrial fibrillation. Stroke Prevention in Atrial Fibrillation III Investigators. *J Am Coll Cardiol* 31:1622-1626, 1998.

197. Transesophageal echocardiographic correlates of thromboembolism in high-risk patients with nonvalvular atrial fibrillation. The Stroke Prevention in Atrial Fibrillation Investigators Committee on Echocardiography. *Ann Intern Med* 128:639-647, 1998.

198. Klein AL, Grimm RA, Murray RD, et al: Use of transesophageal echocardiography to guide cardioversion in patients with atrial fibrillation. *N Engl J Med* 344:1411-1420, 2001.

199. Moreyra E, Finkelhor RS, Cebul RD, et al: Limitations of transesophageal echocardiography in the risk assessment of patients before nonanticoagulated cardioversion from atrial fibrillation and flutter: an analysis of pooled trials. *Am Heart J* 129:71-75, 1995.

200. Klein AL, Murray RD, Becker ER, et al: Economic analysis of a transesophageal echocardiography-guided approach to cardioversion of patients with atrial fibrillation: The ACUTE economic data at eight weeks. *J Am Coll Cardiol* 43:1217-1224, 2004.

201. Ritter SB: Transesophageal real-time echocardiography in infants and children with congenital heart disease. *J Am Coll Cardiol* 18:569-580, 1991.

202. Weintraub R, Shiota T, Elkadi T, et al: Transesophageal echocardiography in infants and children with congenital heart disease. *Circulation* 86:711-722, 1992.

203. Randolph GR, Hagler DJ, Connolly HM, et al: Intraoperative transesophageal echocardiography during surgery for congenital heart defects. *J Thorac Cardiovasc Surg* 124:1176-1182, 2002.

204. Ayres NA, Miller-Hance W, Fyfe DA, et al: Indications and guidelines for performance of transesophageal echocardiography in the patient with pediatric acquired or congenital heart disease: report from the task force of the Pediatric Council of the American Society of Echocardiography. *J Am Soc Echocardiogr* 18:91-98, 2005.

205. Masani ND: Transoesophageal echocardiography in adult congenital heart disease. *Heart* 86(Suppl 2):II30-II40, 2001.

206. Miller-Hance WC, Silverman NH: Transesophageal echocardiography (TEE) in congenital heart disease with focus on the adult. *Cardiol Clin* 18:861-892, 2000.

207. Fu YC, Bass J, Amin Z, et al: Transcatheter closure of perimembranous ventricular septal defects using the new Amplatzer membranous VSD occluder: results of the U.S. phase I trial. *J Am Coll Cardiol* 47:319-325, 2006.

208. Figueroa MI, Balaguru D, McClure C, et al: Experience with use of multiplane transesophageal echocardiography to guide closure of atrial septal defects using the amplatzer device. *Pediatr Cardiol* 23:430-436, 2002.

209. Sreeram N, Stumper OF, Kaulitz R, et al: Comparative value of transthoracic and transesophageal echocardiography in the assessment of congenital abnormalities of the atrioventricular junction. *J Am Coll Cardiol* 16:1205-1214, 1990.

210. Kaulitz R, Stümper OFW, Geuskens R, et al: Comparative values of the precordial and transesophageal approaches in the echocar-

diographic evaluation of atrial baffle function after an atrial correction procedure. *J Am Coll Cardiol* 16:686-694, 1990.

211. Stümper O, Sutherland GR, Geuskens R, et al: Transesophageal echocardiography in evaluation and management after a Fontan procedure. *J Am Coll Cardiol* 17:1152-1160, 1991.

212. Engvall J, Sjoqvist L, Nylander E, et al: Biplane transoesophageal echocardiography, transthoracic Doppler, and magnetic resonance imaging in the assessment of coarctation of the aorta. *Eur Heart J* 10:1399-1409, 1995.

213. Andrade A, Vargas-Barron J, Rijlaarsdam M, et al: Utility of transesophageal echocardiography in the examination of adult patients with patent ductus arteriosus. *Am Heart J* 130:543-546, 1995.

214. Biederman RW, Sorrell VL, Nanda NC, et al: Transesophageal echocardiographic assessment of coronary stenosis: a decade of experience. *Echocardiography* 18:49-57, 2001.

215. Tardif JC, Vannon MA, Taylor K, et al: Delineation of extended lengths of coronary arteries by multiplane transesophageal echocardiography. *J Am Coll Cardiol* 24:909-919, 1994.

216. Reichert SL, Visser CA, Koolen JJ, et al: Transesophageal examination of the left coronary artery with a 7.5 MHz annular array two-dimensional color flow Doppler transducer. *J Am Soc Echocardiogr* 3:118-124, 1990.

217. Samdarshi TE, Nanda NC, Gatewood RP Jr, et al: Usefulness and limitations of transesophageal echocardiography in the assessment of proximal coronary artery stenosis. *J Am Coll Cardiol* 19:572-580, 1992.

218. Yoshida K, Yoshikawa J, Hozumi T, et al: Detection of left main coronary artery stenosis by transesophageal color Doppler and two-dimensional echocardiography. *Circulation* 81:1271-1276, 1990.

219. Gadallah S, Thaker KB, Kawanishi D, et al: Comparison of intracoronary Doppler guide wire and transesophageal echocardiography in measurement of flow velocity and coronary flow reserve in the left anterior descending coronary artery. *Am Heart J* 135;38-42, 1998.

220. Vrublevsky AV, Boshchenko AA, Karpov RS: Reduced coronary flow reserve in the coronary sinus is a predictor of hemodynamically significant stenoses of the left coronary artery territory. *Eur J Echocardiogr* 5:294-303, 2004.

221. Firstenberg MS, Greenberg NL, Lin SS, et al: Transesophageal echocardiography assessment of severe ostial left main coronary stenosis. *J Am Soc Echocardiogr* 13:696-698, 2000.

222. Panza JA: Transesophageal echocardiography with stress for the evaluation of patients with coronary artery disease. *Cardiol Clin* 17:501-520, 1999.

223. Madu EC: Transesophageal dobutamine stress echocardiography in the evaluation of myocardial ischemia in morbidly obese subjects. *Chest* 117;657-661, 2000.

224. Noguchi Y, Nagata-Kobayashi S, Stahl JE, et al: A meta-analytic comparison of echocardiographic stressors. *Int J Cardiovasc Imaging* 21:189-207, 2005.

225. Anselmi M, Golia G, Rossi A, et al: Feasibility and safety of transesophageal atrial pacing stress echocardiography in patients with known or suspected coronary artery disease. *Am J Cardiol* 92:1384-1388, 2003.

226. Vitarelli A, Dagianti A, Conde Y, et al: Value of transesophageal dobutamine stress echocardiography in assessing coronary artery disease. *Am J Cardiol* 86:57G-60G, 2000.

227. Rainbird AJ, Pellikka PA, Stussy VL, et al: A rapid stress-testing protocol for the detection of coronary artery disease: comparison of two-stage transesophageal atrial pacing stress echocardiography with dobutamine stress echocardiography. *J Am Coll Cardiol* 36:1659-1663, 2000.

228. Chaudhry FA, Tauke JT, Alessandrini RS, et al: Enhanced detection of ischemic myocardium by transesophageal dobutamine stress echocardiography: Comparison with simultaneous transthoracic echocardiography. *Echocardiography* 17:241-253, 2000.

229. Kamalesh M, Matorin R, Sawada S, et al: Comparative prognostic significance of transesophageal versus transthoracic stress echocardiography. *Echocardiography* 19:313-318, 2002.

230. Kamalesh M, Sawada S, Humphreys A, et al: Prognostic value of negative transesophageal dobutamine stress echocardiography in men at high risk for coronary artery disease. *Am J Cardiol* 85:41-44, 2000.

231. Vitarelli A, De Curtis G, Conde Y, et al: Assessment of congenital coronary artery fistulas by transesophageal color Doppler echocardiography. *Am J Med* 113:127-133, 2002.

232. Hutchison SJ, Smalling RG, Albornoz M, et al: Comparison of transthoracic and transesophageal echocardiography in clinically overt or suspected pericardial heart disease. *Am J Cardiol* 74:962-965, 1994.

233. Klein AL, Cohen GI, Pietrolungo JF, et al: Differentiation of constrictive pericarditis from restrictive cardiomyopathy by Doppler transesophageal echocardiographic measurements of respiratory variations in pulmonary venous flow. *J Am Coll Cardiol* 22:1935-1943, 1993.

234. Ling LH, Oh JK, Tei C, et al: Pericardial thickness measured with transesophageal echocardiography: Feasibility and potential clinical usefulness. *J Am Coll Cardiol* 29:1317-1323, 1997.

235. Wang ZJ, Reddy GP, Gotway MB, et al: CT and MR imaging of pericardial disease. *Radiographics* 23:S167-S180, 2003.

236. Poelaert JI, Schupfer G: Hemodynamic monitoring utilizing transesophageal echocardiography: the relationships among pressure, flow, and function. *Chest* 127:379-390, 2005.

237. Vignon P: Hemodynamic assessment of critically ill patients using echocardiography Doppler. *Curr Opin Crit Care* 11:227-234, 2005.

238. Heidenreich PA, Stainback RF, Redberg RF, et al: Transesophageal echocardiography predicts mortality in critically ill patients with unexplained hypotension. *J Am Coll Cardiol* 26:152-158, 1995.

239. Vignon P, Mentec H, Terre S, et al: Diagnostic accuracy and therapeutic impact of transthoracic and transesophageal echocardiography in mechanically ventilated patients in the ICU. *Chest* 106;1829-1834, 1994.

240. Dewan NA, Gayasaddin M, Angelillo VA, et al: Persistent hypoxemia due to patent foramen ovale in a patient with adult respiratory distress syndrome. *Chest* 89:611-613, 1986.

241. Bansal RC, Marsa RJ, Holland D, et al: Severe hypoxemia due to shunting through a patent foramen ovale: A correctable complication of right ventricular infarction. *J Am Coll Cardiol* 15:499-504, 1985.

242. American Society of Anesthesiologists and the Society of Cardiovascular Anesthesiologists Task Force on Transesophageal Echocardiography: Practice guidelines for perioperative transesophageal echocardiography. *Anesthesiology* 84:986-1006, 1996.

243. Kolev N, Brase R, Swanevelder J, et al: The influence of transesophageal echocardiography on intra-operative decision making: A European multicentre study. European Perioperative TOE Research Group. *Anaesthesia* 53:767-773, 1998.

244. Katsnelson Y, Raman J, Katsnelson F, et al: Current state of intraoperative echocardiography. *Echocardiography* 20:771-780, 2003.

245. Shapira Y, Vaturi M, Weisenberg DE, et al: Impact of intraoperative transesophageal echocardiography in patients undergoing valve replacement. *Ann Thorac Surg* 78:579-583, 2004.

246. Ommen SR, Park SH, Click RL, et al: Impact of intraoperative transesophageal echocardiography in the surgical management of hypertrophic cardiomyopathy. *Am J Cardiol* 90:1022-1024, 2002.

247. Saiki Y, Kasegawa H, Kawase M, et al: Intraoperative TEE during mitral valve repair: Does it predict early and late postoperative mitral valve dysfunction? *Ann Thorac Surg* 66:1277-1281, 1998.

248. Freeman WK, Schaff HV, Khandheria BK, et al: Intraoperative evaluation of mitral valve regurgitation and repair by trans-

esophageal echocardiography: incidence and significance of systolic anterior motion. *J Am Coll Cardiol* 20:599-609, 1992.

249. Agricola E, Oppizzi M, Maisano F, et al: Detection of mechanisms of immediate failure by transesophageal echocardiography in quadrangular resection mitral valve repair technique for severe mitral regurgitation. *Am J Cardiol* 91:175-179, 2003.

250. Shanewise JS, Cheung AT, Aronson S, et al: ASE/SCA guidelines for performing a comprehensive intraoperative multiplane transesophageal echocardiography examination: Recommendations of the American Society of Echocardiography Council for Intraoperative Echocardiography and the Society of Cardiovascular Anesthesiologists Task Force for Certification in Perioperative Transesophageal Echocardiography. *J Am Soc Echocardiogr* 12:884-900, 1999.

251. Park SH, Kim MA, Hyon MS: The advantages of on-line transesophageal echocardiography guide during percutaneous balloon mitral valvuloplasty. *J Am Soc Echocardiogr* 13:26-34, 2000.

252. Kantoch MJ, Frost GF, Robertson MA: Use of transesophageal echocardiography in radiofrequency catheter ablation in children and adolescents. *Can J Cardiol* 14:519-523, 1998.

253. Tumbarello R, Sanna A, Cardu G, et al: Usefulness of transesophageal echocardiography in the pediatric catheterization laboratory. *Am J Cardiol* 71:1321-1325, 1993.

254. van der Velde ME, Sanders SP, Keane JF, et al: Transesophageal echocardiographic guidance of transcatheter ventricular septal defect closure. *J Am Coll Cardiol* 23:1660-1665, 1994.

255. McElhinney DB, Burch GH, Kung GC, et al: Echocardiographic guidance for transcatheter coil embolization of congenital coronary arterial fistulas in children. *Pediatr Cardiol* 21:253-258, 2000.

256. Pytlewski G, Georgeson S, Burke J, et al: Endomyocardial biopsy under transesophageal echocardiographic guidance can be safely performed in the critically ill cardiac transplant recipient. *Am J Cardiol* 73:1019-1020, 1994.

257. Cheung YF, Leung MP, Lee J, et al: An evolving role of transesophageal echocardiography for the monitoring of interventional catheterization in children. *Clin Cardiol* 22:804-810, 1999.

258. Greenfield SM, Webster GJ, Brar AS, et al: Assessment of residual gastric volume and thirst in patients who drink before gastroscopy. *Gut* 39:360-362, 1996.

259. Fergus I, Bennett ES, Rogers DM, et al: Fluoroscopic balloon-guided transesophageal echocardiography in a patient with Zenker's diverticulum. *J Am Soc Echocardiogr* 17:483-486, 2004.

260. Khandheria BK, Seward JB, Tajik AJ: Concise review for primary-care physicians: Transesophageal echocardiography. *Mayo Clin Proc* 69:856-863, 1994.

261. Kallmeyer IJ, Collard CD, Fox JA, et al: The safety of intraoperative transesophageal echocardiography: a case series of 7200 cardiac surgical patients. *Anesth Analg* 92:1126-1130, 2001.

262. Stevenson JG: Incidence of complications in pediatric transesophageal echocardiography: Experience in 1650 cases. *J Am Soc Echocardiogr* 12:527-532, 1999.

263. Moore TJ, Walsh CS, Cohen MR, et al: Reported adverse event cases of methemoglobinemia associated with benzocaine products. *Arch Intern Med* 164:1192-1196, 2004.

264. Tsigrelis C, Weiner L: Methemoglobinemia revisited: An important complication after transesophageal echocardiography. *Eur J Echocardiogr* 7:470-472, 2006.

265. Novaro GM, Aronow HD, Militello MA, et al: Benzocaine-induced methemoglobinemia: experience from a high-volume transesophageal echocardiography laboratory. *J Am Soc Echocardiogr* 16:170-175, 2003.

266. Salehian O, Chan KL: Impact of three-dimensional echocardiography in valvular heart disease. *Curr Opin Cardiol* 20:122-126, 2005.

Chapter 2

Monitoring Ventricular Function in the Operating Room: Impact on Clinical Outcome

DONALD C. OXORN, MD

- Standard of Practice
- Evaluation of Intraoperative Ventricular Function
    - *Left Ventricular Filling*
    - *Global Systolic Function*
    - *Regional Wall Motion*
    - *Intraoperative Assessment of Coronary Reserve*
- Use of Transesophageal Echocardiography to Monitor Intraoperative Cardiac Function in Specific Clinical Entities
    - *Separation from Cardiopulmonary Bypass*
    - *Off-Pump Coronary Bypass Surgery*
    - *Cardiac Function in Noncardiac Surgery*
    - *Positioning of Intravascular Devices*
    - *Transplant Surgery*
    - *Laparoscopic Surgery*
- New Technology
    - *Epicardial Echocardiography*
    - *Three-Dimensional Transesophageal Echocardiography*
    - *Transmyocardial Laser Revascularization*

- Transesophageal Echocardiography as a Monitor of Intraoperative Ventricular Function: Impact on Postoperative Outcomes and Cost-Effectiveness
- Summary

Since being introduced into anesthetic practice in the late 1980s, transesophageal echocardiography (TEE) for intraoperative monitoring during cardiac surgery has gained wide acceptance.[1-5] TEE is relatively noninvasive, can be used in most patients, and does not interfere physically with most surgical procedures. In some centers, TEE is used routinely for all cases involving cardiopulmonary bypass (CPB), whereas it is used more selectively at others.

The usefulness of TEE in the diagnosis and management of hemodynamically unstable patients in the intensive care unit (ICU) has long been appreciated,[6] and there has been recent evidence that hemodynamic instability in noncardiac surgical patients is equally well managed by the early implementation of TEE.[7,8]

In this chapter, the focus will be on the use of TEE in the assessment of cardiac function in the setting of both cardiac and noncardiac surgery. In addition, the impact intraoperative TEE has had on the quality of perioperative care is discussed. Intraoperative assessment of valvular function, chamber size, masses, and great vessels are covered in other sections of the book.

Standard of Practice

Intraoperative TEE has become inextricably linked with cardiac anesthesiology. Over the past decade, guidelines for physician training in TEE have been directed primarily at cardiologists and have stressed a background in transthoracic echocardiography (TTE), the acquisition of both cognitive and technical skills, and an ongoing program of maintenance of competence.

Practice guidelines for perioperative TEE were published by the American Society of Anesthesiologists and the Society of Cardiovascular Anesthesiologists in 1996[9]; more recent publications have focused on guidelines for training,[10-12] certification,[13] and maintenance of competence with emphasis on emerging ultrasound (US) modalities.[14] Practitioners approach intraoperative TEE with varying degrees of skill; for that reason, two levels of training—basic and advanced—are generally recognized. Essential to the development of expertise in intraoperative TEE is exposure to varieties of diagnostic techniques, cardiovascular pathology, and an understanding of the complex environment that is the cardiovascular operating room (OR). Educational opportunities abound, and anesthesiologists trained in TEE interpret comprehensive intraoperative examinations at a level comparable to physicians from other disciplines whose primary practice is echocardiography.[15]

A working group of the American Society of Echocardiography and the Society of Cardiovascular Anesthesiologists developed guidelines for performing a comprehensive intraoperative TEE examination.[16] It is the committee's contention that if the practitioner performs a careful and systematized examination every time the probe is inserted, the chance of missing important findings is minimized, and the potential for teaching is enhanced.

Evaluation of Intraoperative Ventricular Function

Left Ventricular Filling

In the OR, rapidity is needed in the assessment of preload during periods of hemodynamic instability. Since the introduction of the pulmonary artery (PA) catheter in the 1970s, use of pulmonary capillary wedge pressure (PCWP) as a surrogate of left atrial pressure and by inference ventricular end-diastolic volume (EDV) has been the intraoperative practice standard. It is recognized, however, that the PCWP may overestimate left atrial pressure resulting from the contributions of pulmonary venous resistance (PVR) and the right ventricular (RV) systolic pressure wave[17] and thus may overestimate preload. TEE has the potential to refine this measurement by allowing Doppler estimation of left atrial pressure, two-dimensional (2D) measurement of left ventricular (LV) cross-sectional area, calculation of LV volume, and assessment of diastolic function.

Left Atrial Pressure

Left atrial pressure can be estimated with Doppler TEE by several methods. If mitral regurgitation (MR) is present, measurement of the peak velocity of the regurgitant jet and application of the modified Bernoulli equation allows calculation of the left ventriculatrial pressure gradient; in the absence of aortic stenosis, subtraction of this number from the peak systolic blood pressure (BP) yields left atrial pressure. Certain mitral inflow and pulmonary venous variables also correlate with left atrial pressure; in patients undergoing cardiovascular surgery, Kuecherer and colleagues[18] found that changes in the systolic fraction of the pulmonary venous tracing correlated inversely and strongly with PCWP and theorized that this related to decreased atrial compliance. Nomura and colleagues[19] found that in patients with ejection fractions (EFs) less than 35% the deceleration time of the early velocity of mitral inflow correlated with PCWP and that a deceleration time greater than 150 msec was strongly predictive of a PCWP pressure of less than 10 mm Hg. Arguing that the aforementioned Doppler parameters were overly influenced by loading conditions, Kinnaird and colleagues[17] proposed that examining the deceleration slope of the diastolic component of pulmonary venous flow allowed the left atrium to be treated as a receiving chamber in its own right and showed that this deceleration time was inversely correlated with left atrial pressure. The ratio of early to atrial LV diastolic filling velocity (E/A ratio) has also been used to predict fluid responsiveness in cardiac surgical patients. Patients with higher E/A ratios tended to have a more rightward position on the diastolic pressure volume curve (Fig. 2–1) and thereby were less likely to increase their cardiac output (CO) with an infusion of colloid.[20]

There are a number of caveats related to the intraoperative estimation of left atrial pressure with TEE. Patients with a rhythm other than sinus or with valvular regurgitation were excluded in most studies; these are the patients in whom preload estimates are often crucial. In suitable patients, correlations but not absolute values of left atrial pressure are usually yielded. Use of the MR jet to calculate left atrial pressure dictates that MR must be present. Finally, an estimate of left atrial pressure, whether obtained by Doppler echocardiography or by PA catheter, may still yield inaccurate estimates of preload

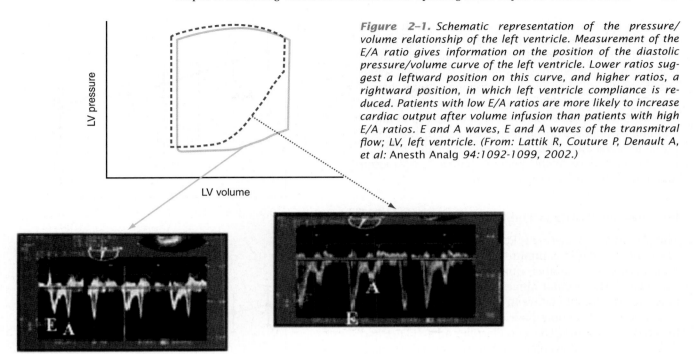

Figure 2–1. Schematic representation of the pressure/volume relationship of the left ventricle. Measurement of the E/A ratio gives information on the position of the diastolic pressure/volume curve of the left ventricle. Lower ratios suggest a leftward position on this curve, and higher ratios, a rightward position, in which left ventricle compliance is reduced. Patients with low E/A ratios are more likely to increase cardiac output after volume infusion than patients with high E/A ratios. E and A waves, E and A waves of the transmitral flow; LV, left ventricle. (From: Lattik R, Couture P, Denault A, et al: Anesth Analg 94:1092-1099, 2002.)

in patients with decreased ventricular compliance[21]; this is the case in many patients following CPB.[22]

Tissue Doppler imaging (TDI) of the mitral annulus (Fig. 2–2) has been proposed as a descriptor of LV relaxation that is less affected by changes in loading conditions and ventricular function than more traditional Doppler parameters.[23,24] In essence, the velocity of movement of the mitral annulus away from the LV apex during diastole (E′) relates directly to LV relaxation; thus this parameter has been used to correct for LV relaxation and render the E wave of mitral inflow more accurate in the estimation of LV filling pressure (E/E′ ratio).

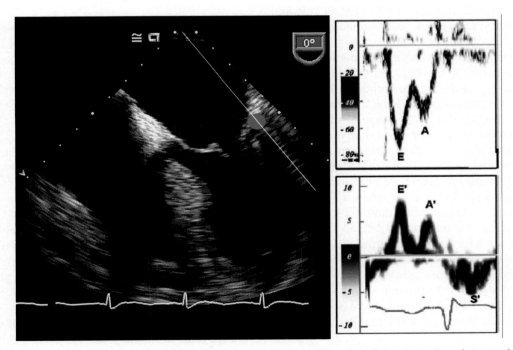

Figure 2–2. In this four-chamber view (left), the correct positioning of the tissue Doppler sample volume is shown by the red circle. Angulation between the sampling cursor and mitral annulus was minimal. On the right, representative Doppler tracing of mitral inflow (above) and mitral annular velocity (below) are shown. E and A represent early diastolic and atrial contraction velocities respectively; E′, A′, and S′ represent early diastolic contraction, atrial contraction, and systolic motions of the mitral annulus respectively. (From Combes A, Arnolt F, Trouillet J-L: Intensive Care Med 30:75-81, 2004. With kind permission of Springer Science and Business Media.)

Although it has shown a strong correlation with PA occlusion pressure when obtained by TEE in a mixed group of patients in the ICU,[25] it has yet to be rigorously tested in the intraoperative setting. The lateral and septal mitral annuli are often used interchangeably in measuring TDI; however, as Malouf and colleagues[26] point out, there is decreased diastolic excursion of the septal mitral annulus as opposed to normal excursion of the lateral mitral annulus after CPB; the authors conclude that this may be secondary to the known change in postpump function of the interventricular septum.

End-Diastolic Area and End-Systolic Area

The American Society of Echocardiography's guidelines and standards committee have published recommendations for chamber quantification in both TTE and TEE.[27] The normal ranges for dimension and volume are comparable between the two techniques.[28]

A number of authors have examined the intraoperative relationship between end-diastolic area (EDA) and end-systolic area (ESA) measured at the transgastric mid-papillary level and cardiac volume status. Cheung and colleagues[29] performed an elegant study examining the effect of graded hypovolemia produced by autologous blood collection on hemodynamic- and TEE-derived indices of LV preload in patients undergoing coronary artery bypass surgery. Patients with valvular insufficiency, rhythms other than sinus, and overt congestive heart failure (CHF) were excluded. Patients were stratified on the basis of resting LV function. EDA, ESA, PCWP, and measures of end-diastolic and end-systolic wall stress decreased linearly as blood volume was reduced by 0% to 15% in all patients; however, in patients with impaired LV function, only the TEE-derived indices maintained linearity (Fig. 2–3). As the authors acknowledge, estimation of ventricular volume in the patient with asymmetric ventricular dysfunction may be problematic, because hypokinetic or akinetic areas may not be represented in the area of the two-dimensional cut.

Other studies have also demonstrated that single plane areas, although not predictive of absolute LV volumes,[30] can generally be used to monitor for a trend toward increased or decreased volume.[31,32] It must also be remembered that the presence of a small EDA or ESA does not always reflect decreased intravascular volume. Small LV volumes can be seen with restrictions to filling, as in pericardial disease, or decreased right-sided heart function (Fig. 2–4), as in RV infarction or large pulmonary embolus. Other causes include increased inotropy or redistribution of blood out of the thoracic cavity.[33]

Left Ventricular Volumes

The most common and generally accepted method for volume measurement is the biplane method of disks (Simpson's rule). Smith and colleagues[34] found that

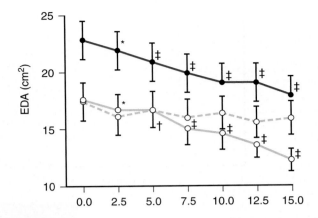

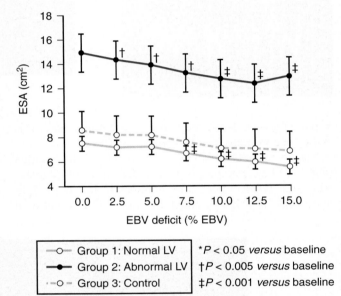

—○— Group 1: Normal LV	*$P < 0.05$ *versus* baseline	
—●— Group 2: Abnormal LV	†$P < 0.005$ *versus* baseline	
⋯○⋯ Group 3: Control	‡$P < 0.001$ *versus* baseline	

Figure 2–3. End-diastolic area and end-systolic area in response to graded hypovolemia, estimated blood volume deficits of 0% to 15%. Patients had either normal left ventricular function or deficient left ventricular function. Control patients were not subjected to hypovolemia. EBV, estimated blood volume; EDA, end-diastolic area; ESA, end-systolic area; LV, left ventricular. (Reproduced with permission from Cheung AT, Savino JS, Weiss SJ, et al: Anesthesiology 81:376-387, 1994.)

measurement of LV volume was underestimated by TEE when compared to ventriculography and attributed this to underestimation of ventricular length; more recent studies using multiplane probes[28] have shown that volumetric data obtained by TTE and TEE show minor or no differences.

In summary, the assessment of preload with intraoperative TEE is in most cases a semi-quantitative estimate based on visual inspection of EDA and ESA and on temporal comparison with the use of videotape or stored cine loops. Confounding conditions, such as RV failure or the administration of inotropic agents, must be considered.

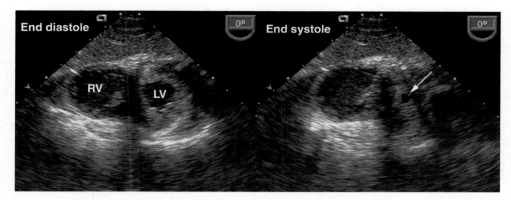

Figure 2–4. Transgastric image of a transesophageal echocardiography scan obtained in a patient with pulmonary hypertension secondary to cystic fibrosis. Although the end-systolic area of the left ventricle is exceedingly small (arrow), this was secondary to right-sided heart failure and not absolute hypovolemia. LV, left ventricle; RV, right ventricle.

Global Systolic Function

Cardiac Output

Ventricular filling, contractility, wall stress, and heart rate (HR) all influence CO. Thus, CO is the measurement most often used in anesthetic and critical care practice as a guide to therapeutic manipulations of cardiac function. Despite its limitations, thermodilution CO measurement with a PA catheter has been considered the gold standard since being popularized in the early 1970s. Recognition of potentially fatal complications related to its use[35] have led to the increasing use of alternative methods of hemodynamic monitoring.

Doppler TEE has the potential to be used in the intraoperative setting for the continuous measurement of CO.

These methods use the concept that the cross-sectional area of a conduit within the cardiovascular system multiplied by the Doppler-derived time-velocity integral yields the stroke volume through that conduit. When the result is multiplied by HR, the product is CO.

Several important assumptions are inherent to this approach. Valid area formulas must be applicable to the anatomic site being analyzed. The velocity profile across the valve must be flat and devoid of skew.[36,37] Whichever anatomic area is chosen, the ability to consistently obtain the image and to interrogate parallel to flow is mandatory.

Pulmonary Artery. With the probe at 0 degrees and retroflexed, the main PA and pulmonic valve can be imaged at the base of the heart (Fig. 2–5). This site has

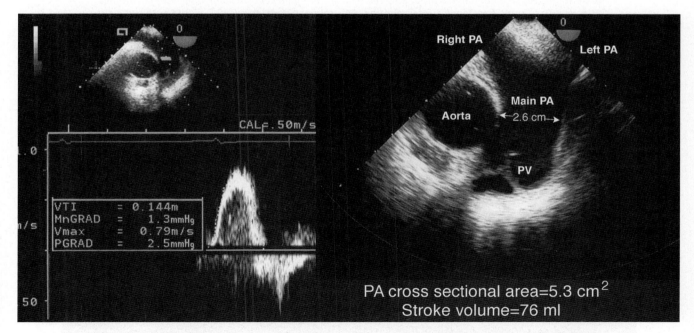

Figure 2–5. Imaging at the base of the heart of the main pulmonary artery and its branches. Pulsed-Doppler velocity time integral and diameter measurement are used to calculate stroke volume. MnGRAD, mean gradient; PA, pulmonary artery; PGRAD, peak gradient; PV, pulmonary valve; Vmax, maximum velocity; VTI, velocity time integral.

been examined with pulsed wave (PW) Doppler[36,38] and in a study by Gorcsan and colleagues[39] using both PW and continuous wave (CW) methodologies. PA diameter was measured just distal to the pulmonic valve. Interobserver variability was low in all studies, and correlation with thermodilution was strong in all but the study by Muhiudeen and colleagues[38] in which patients with inaccurate thermodilution measurements may have been included. Alternatively, the main PA may be imaged at 60 to 90 degrees using the aortic arch as a window (Fig. 2–6).

Right Ventricular Outflow Tract. From the transgastric approach, the probe is turned rightward and flexed to image the RV outflow tract at a rotation angle between 0 and 120 degrees (Fig. 2–7). Imaging frequency must usually be reduced to ensure optimal penetration. Maslow and colleagues[40] found excellent correlation between CO calculated with PW Doppler and thermodilution. Patients with pulmonary hypertension, significant tricuspid regurgitation, and nonsinus rhythms were excluded. In a significant percentage (16%) of patients, the two-dimensional image was not suitable.

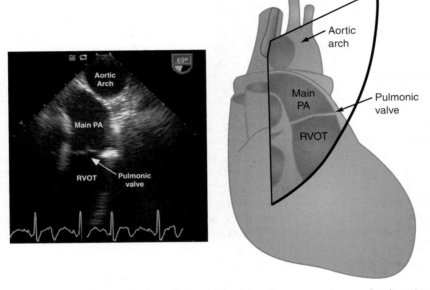

Figure 2–6. *Using the aortic arch as a window, the main pulmonary artery and pulmonic valve are seen. On the left is the high esophageal transesophageal echocardiography image; on the right is an anatomic reproduction illustrating how the transesophageal echocardiography view is obtained. This view is suitable for Doppler interrogation. PA, pulmonary artery; RVOT, right ventricular outflow tract.*

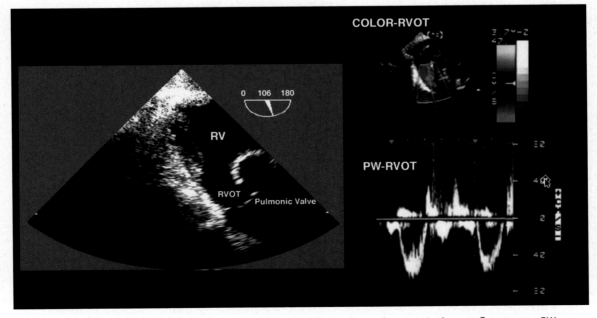

Figure 2–7. *Pulsed wave Doppler measurement from the right ventricular outflow tract. PW, pulsed wave; RV, right ventricle; RVOT, right ventricular outflow tract.*

Left Ventricular Outflow Tract. With the probe in the stomach, turned leftward, in the flexed position, and at low imaging frequency, the aortic valve and LV outflow tract can usually be imaged between 0 and 140 degrees (Fig. 2–8). Imaging from the stomach allows parallel pulsed-Doppler interrogation of the LV outflow tract; its diameter can be obtained from either the stomach or the midesophageal long-axis view. Calculation of the cross-sectional area and CO follow standard formula (Fig. 2–9). Strong correlation with thermodilution and low interobserver variability have been described.[41,42]

To avoid contamination of the Doppler signal by the region of flow acceleration adjacent to the aortic valve orifice, the sample volume must be placed precisely in the LV outflow tract.

Mitral Valve. Using the mitral valve for calculation of CO has the advantages of consistent imaging and parallel Doppler alignment. However, the saddle shape of the mitral annulus makes the area measurement unpredictable, and the cross-sectional velocity skew is of concern when using PW Doppler.

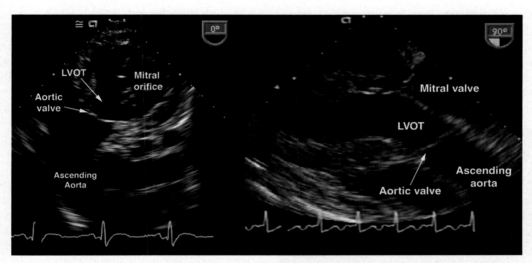

Figure 2–8. *Transesophageal echocardiography imaging from the stomach allows parallel alignment with the ascending aorta.* Left-hand panel *is the deep transgastric long axis view,* right-hand panel *is the transgastric long axis view. LVOT, left ventricular outflow tract.*

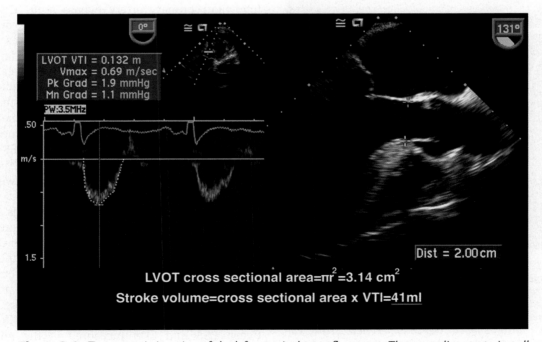

Figure 2–9. *Transgastric imaging of the left ventricular outflow tract. The ascending aorta is well visualized, and the Doppler intercept angle is small. Pulsed-Doppler velocity time integral and diameter measurement are used to calculate stroke volume. LVOT, left ventricular outflow tract; Mn GRAD, mean gradient; Pk GRAD, peak gradient; Vmax, maximum velocity; VTI, velocity time integral.*

The use of color Doppler as a means of obtaining automated CO has been described with TEE and validated against thermodilution CO.[43] The edge of the color profile is detected as the width of the flow tract in each frame. The flow volume is automatically calculated by double integration of Doppler signals in space (across the full width of the flow tract) and in time. This frame-by-frame tracking function of the velocity profile enables the measurement of CO accurately, especially at the mitral valve (Fig. 2-10). This technique has not yet been validated in the intraoperative setting.

Practical Considerations. For intraoperative transesophageal Doppler calculation of CO, the LV outflow tract method is the most reproducible. Adjustments in the degree of probe flexion and imaging angle should be made to ensure that the aortic valve and ascending aorta are clearly visualized and that the Doppler intercept angle is small (see Fig. 2-9). Several measurements should be made and averaged, this being especially important when dealing with rhythms other than sinus. In practical terms, Doppler measurement of CO is used when a PA catheter is not in place or when conditions, such as severe tricuspid regurgitation, render thermodilution inaccurate. There is a need for further validation of this approach in patients with a spectrum of cardiovascular diseases.

Ejection Fraction and Stroke Volume

Although it is somewhat load dependent and therefore not a pure index of "LV function,"[44] EF is often assumed to reflect ventricular contractility. During intraoperative TEE, the fractional area of change measured at the transgastric midpapillary level is often used interchangeably with EF, although gauging volume in a potentially asymmetric chamber based on a measure of area has obvious limitations.[45,46] As mentioned previously, the most common and generally accepted method for volume measurement is the biplane method of disks, Simpson's rule (Fig. 2-11).

A number of studies report the relationship between TEE-derived fractional area of change and radionuclide-derived EF. Clements and colleagues[47] examined the relationship in 12 patients having abdominal aortic aneurysm surgery. There was excellent correlation in patients with both normal and abnormal LV function. In patients with ventricular dyssynergy, fractional area of change led to a slight overestimate of EF. Urbanowicz and colleagues[48] found strong correlation in 10 patients following coronary artery bypass graft (CABG). In a series of 15 patients following CABG, Ryan and colleagues[30] measured TEE EF using volumes calculated from the modified Simpson's rule and area-length methods in addition to TEE-derived fractional area of change and radionuclide-derived EF. Unlike previous studies, variability was calculated and found to be small and not significantly different among the three measurement techniques. Not surprisingly, the TEE volumetric results were more representative of radionuclide EF than fractional area of change. Smith and colleagues[34] also found that EF based on TEE volumetric methods were comparable to those obtained with angiography.

In an attempt to develop online methods of intraoperative functional assessment, the technique of automated border detection has been used (see Chapter 7). Automated border detection is based on the principle of acoustic quantification of ultrasonic back scatter signals to detect the blood-tissue interface and thereby define the endocardial edge.[49] Gorcsan and colleagues[50] examined stroke area, defined as the difference between ESA and EDA measured at the midpapillary level, and compared the results to stroke volume measured in the ascending aorta by an electromagnetic flow probe in nine patients undergoing coronary artery

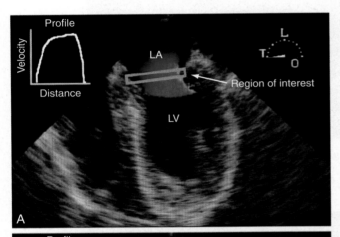

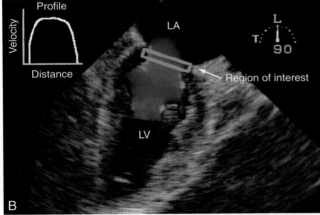

Figure 2-10. (A) *Blood flow through the mitral annulus in the transesophageal four-chamber view. Stroke volume is calculated by integrating velocity in space and time throughout diastole. Cardiac output is calculated by multiplying stroke volume by heart rate.* (B) *Blood flow through the mitral annulus in the transesophageal two-chamber view. Stroke volume is calculated by integrating velocity in space and time throughout diastole. The scale is set at 610 cm s±1. LA, left atrium; LV, left ventricle. (From: Akamatsu S, Oda A, Terazawa T, et al: Anesth Analg 98:1232-1238, 2004.)*

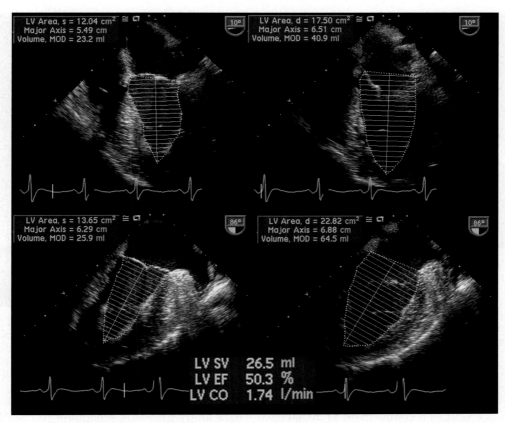

Figure 2–11. Measurements of systolic and diastolic area made in the four-chamber (upper panels) and two-chamber (lower panels) views are used to obtain volumetric data by the method of disks. From these measurements, stroke volume, ejection fraction, and cardiac output can be calculated. CO, cardiac output; D, diastolic; EF, ejection fraction; LV, left ventricle; MOD, method of disks; SV, stroke volume.

bypass. Preoperative LV function was largely preserved. Measurements were made before and after CPB. There was a strong correlation between the measurements at all periods of the study. In a number of other studies using automated border detection, prediction of stroke volume as measured by thermodilution was poor.[51,52]

It would appear that fractional area of change more closely estimates EF in patients with normal ventricular function. The use of TEE-derived volumetric data to estimate EF is more accurate, though manual tracing is tedious; however, software that comes with many TEE machines allows rapid calculation. The use of automated border detection algorithms and programmed volume calculations may prove superior but are largely untested in clinical practice.

Contractility

The end-systolic pressure-volume relationship and resultant end-systolic elastance defines contractility in a load-independent fashion[53] and therefore would be of potential use in the estimation of intraoperative left ventricle contractility and in the quantification of changes resulting from manipulations, such as CPB.

A number of surrogates of this relationship have been described to facilitate the practical acquisition of this information in an OR setting. The substitution of femoral arterial pressure[54] or tonometry[55] for LV end-systolic pressure, ESA for end-systolic volume,[56-58] and end-systolic wall stress for end-systolic pressure[56] have been made. Although these substituted measurements are not construed as replacements for traditional measures of pressure and volume, their directional change suggests that in cardiac surgical patients undergoing CPB, they may be used as an alternative way of assessing load-independent LV function. At present, however, the methods for intraoperative data analysis are prohibitively complex.

Other Indices of Left Ventricular Function

Tissue Doppler Imaging. The use of TDI in the assessment of diastolic function has already been described. Systolic myocardial velocity at the lateral mitral annulus (S′; see Fig. 2–2) is a measure of longitudinal systolic function that correlates with EF.[59] Simmons and colleagues[60] showed the feasibility of using TEE to obtain radial and longitudinal LV wall velocities; there

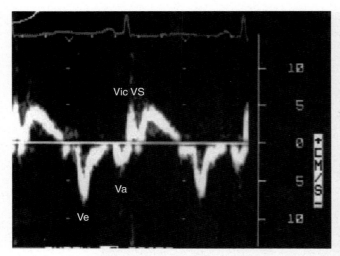

Figure 2-12. *Pulsed-wave tissue Doppler recording of myocardial velocities in the left ventricle anterior midwall. Systolic velocities are directed upward (positive), and diastolic velocities are directed downward (negative). Va, atrial contraction velocity; Ve, early diastolic velocity; Vic, velocity of isovolumic contraction; Vs, systolic thickening velocity. (From: Skarvan K, Filipovic M, Wang J, et al: Br J Anaesth 91:473-480, 2003.)*

was consistency between TTE and TEE measurements, and regional reduction in S′ correlated with decreased regional wall motion. Skarvan and colleagues[61] used TDI of the anterior wall as a complement to visual assessment of systolic wall thickening (Fig. 2-12). Although more work is needed to define what constitutes normal and abnormal velocities, this technique shows promise in intraoperative ischemia detection.

dP/dt. dP/dt is a load-dependent index of systolic performance. Its measurement using CW Doppler of the MR jet has been validated against measurements in the cardiac catheterization laboratory.[62] The time required for an increase of the pressure gradient from 4 to 36 mm Hg (or an increase of velocity from 1 to 3 m/sec) is recorded. Normal values are 800 to 1200 mm Hg/sec[63] (Fig. 2-13). The presence of mitral stenosis (MS) contraindicates the technique. It has not been adequately tested in the intraoperative environment.

Myocardial Performance Index. Also known as the Tei index, the myocardial performance index has been proposed as a combined index of ventricular systolic and diastolic function.[64,65] Because decrements in either systolic or diastolic function require different treatments, its use in the rapidly changing milieu of the OR is limited.[66]

Right Ventricular Function

In the setting of CPB, the evaluation of RV function is important. RV dysfunction often occurs secondary to the inadequate delivery of cardioplegia[67] and to the embolization of intracardiac air down the right coro-

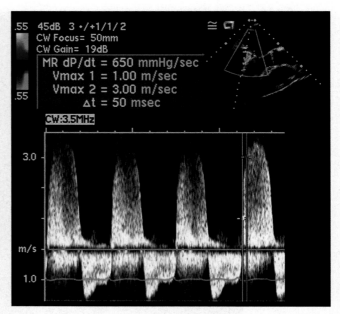

Figure 2-13. *Measurement of dP/dt is taken from the mitral regurgitation jet obtained by continuous wave Doppler. The duration of time required for the velocity to increase from 1 to 3 m/sec (or the pressure to rise from 4 to 36 mm Hg) is recorded. CW, continuous wave; MR, mitral regurgitation; Vmax, maximum velocity.*

nary artery following separation from CPB (Fig. 2-14). The triangular shape of the right ventricle makes its global function hard to quantitate with TEE, although the modified method of disks has been used in offline analysis in the setting of coronary bypass grafting.[68] The abnormal septal motion often seen following CPB[69] makes analysis more difficult. Standards for the measurement of RV volumes with TEE have been published.[27]

Tricuspid annular velocity measurement by TDI has been used to quantitate RV function, with excursions less than 1.5 cm associated with poor prognosis in a variety of cardiovascular diseases.[70] The technique is feasible during cardiac surgery using modified transgastric imaging[71]

At present, TEE assessment of intraoperative RV function is best accomplished by visual inspection and semi-quantitative assessment in both the transgastric and the four-chamber views.

Regional Wall Motion

The suggestion of a link between perioperative myocardial ischemia and cardiac morbidity[72,73] has led to an intensive search for accurate methods of its intraoperative detection (Fig. 2-15). Visual inspection of the electrocardiogram for ST segment changes has been the foundation on which the newer technologies of automated ST analysis and TEE detection of regional wall motion abnormalities have been added. There are several points on which to judge the merits of TEE: ap-

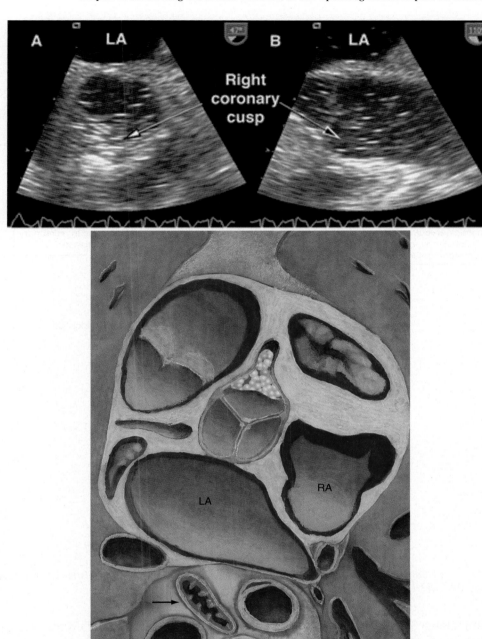

Figure 2-14. *Short-axis (A) and long-axis (B) views of the aortic valve during separation from cardiopulmonary bypass. The cross-sectional figure (C), with the patient supine, shows that the right coronary cusp is most superior so that bubbles collect in the right coronary sinus of Valsalva and may embolize down the right coronary artery. LA, left atrium; RA, right atrium.*

plicability, accuracy, reproducibility, cost, expertise required for interpretation, and prognostic importance.

Segmental analysis is most frequently undertaken using the 16-segment model first proposed by Schiller and colleagues[74] and later modified for TEE by Shanewise and colleagues.[16] In 2002, a seventeenth segment, the apical cap, was added.[75]

The recognition that coronary occlusion leads to the immediate development of regional wall motion abnor-

malities[76] and their frequent regression following revascularization[77] has prompted investigators to examine the usefulness of intraoperative TEE as a monitor of ischemia. The paucity of contraindications to TEE means that it can be used in most patients undergoing general anesthesia. The midpapillary view is generally easy to obtain and demonstrates areas of myocardium subtended by the three major coronary arteries. Interpretation is rarely confounded by rhythm disturbances,

INTRAOPERATIVE MONITORS FOR ISCHEMIA

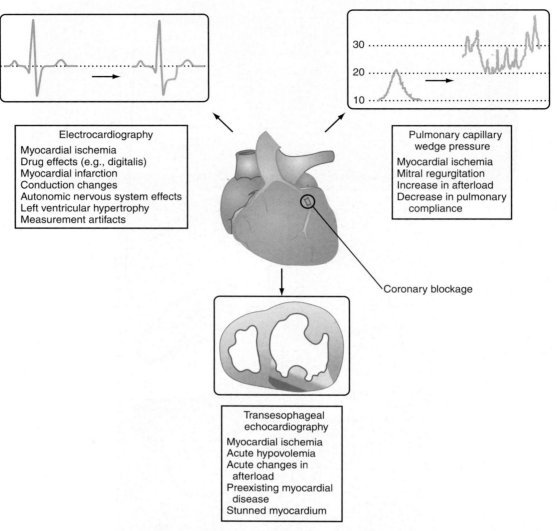

Figure 2–15. Causes of ischemic changes on intraoperative monitors. (From Fleisher LA: Anesthesiology *92:1183-1188, 2000.)*

as is the case for automated ST analysis. TEE cannot be used, however, in patients receiving regional anesthesia, and because the probe is not inserted until after anesthetic induction, it cannot detect changes during this vulnerable period.

Assessment of the accuracy of TEE in the detection of myocardial ischemia has been limited somewhat by the lack of a reliable reference standard. Smith and colleagues[78] found that wall motion changes could be detected more quickly and commonly than ST segment changes in patients at high risk of myocardial ischemia who were analyzed offline.

Conflicting studies[79,80] regarding the prognostic importance of regional wall motion abnormalities were subsequently published. In a study by London and colleagues,[80] 156 patients undergoing noncardiac surgery who were at high risk for coronary artery disease (CAD) were studied. Specific clinical, electrocardio-

graphic, or hemodynamic events prompted analysis of stored images. The number of new wall motion abnormalities detected was low, and discordance with electrocardiographic findings was significant (Table 2–1). The number of postoperative cardiac complications was low. In the study by Leung and colleagues,[79] patients undergoing coronary artery bypass were examined with electrocardiography and TEE. Although prebypass ischemia was rare, postbypass ischemia was more common and postoperative cardiovascular complications were associated more closely with TEE findings than with electrocardiography alone.

It is now accepted that regional wall motion abnormalities, although often the result of myocardial ischemia, may result from hypovolemia, tethering of nonischemic myocardium, and myocardial stunning after CPB.[81,82] Abnormal interventricular septum abnormalities are seen after CPB, with right-sided chamber over-

TABLE 2–1. Comparison of Transesophageal Echocardiography and Intraoperative Electrocardiography Monitoring for Myocardial Ischemia[*]

	TEE+	TEE−
ECG+	8 (1 MI)	11
ECG−	24	2 MI, 1 UA

[*]$P < 0.05$.
ECG, electrocardiography; MI, myocardial infarction; TEE, transesophageal echocardiography; UA, unstable angina.
From London MJ, Tubau JF, Wong MG, et al: *Anesthesiology* 73(4):644-655, 1990.

load, ventricular pacing, and bundle branch blocks. Off-line analysis has been employed in most of the large-scale studies involving comparison of TEE with other methods of ischemia detection, but extrapolation to the accuracy of real-time TEE analysis should not be assumed. Regional wall motion abnormalities that subtend the anatomic distribution of coronary artery flow are more often a result of ischemia than those that do not.

Comunale and colleagues[83] also documented the poor concordance between the TEE and electrocardiography and attributed this finding to the lack of standard definitions of significant regional wall motion abnormalities and ischemic ST changes, the exclusion of longitudinal TEE views, and the use of different models of segment nomenclature.

TEE is the most sensitive test for intraoperative myocardial ischemia and has therefore been adapted by many practitioners as cutting edge technology in this regard. Conditions, which lead to its lack of specificity as mentioned, must be taken into account. The ability to monitor additional tomographic planes[84,85]; the use of cine loops for comparison; and the advent of new technologies, such as automated border detection, color kinesis[86] and TDI,[61] should improve accuracy. Regional wall motion abnormalities precede electrocardiographic changes,[87] and once ischemia is diagnosed, TEE can be used to directly monitor the effects of intervention.

Intraoperative Assessment of Coronary Reserve

Dobutamine stress echocardiography (DSE) is a well-established technique for diagnosing CAD and predicting the improvement of dysfunctional myocardium postoperatively (see Chapter 14).[88,89] The ability to predict the reversibility of LV dysfunction with the use of intraoperative low-dose dobutamine stress TEE (DSTEE) was examined by Aronson and colleagues[90] in the setting of CABG. The odds ratios for early and late improvement in myocardial function were 20.7 and 34.6

times higher if preoperative low-dose dobutamine produced improved function than if it did not. In a subsequent paper, however,[91] low dose DSTEE could not be used to predict which segments would not recover at one year. Leung and colleagues[92] found that in patients undergoing myocardial revascularization, improved myocardial function in response to intraoperative DSTEE was highly specific for viable myocardium; however, worsened myocardial function in response to DSTEE had low sensitivity in predicting nonviable myocardium.

The authors concluded that although DSE has been demonstrated to be a sensitive test in predicting myocardium at risk in patients with CAD, its usefulness in predicting nonviable myocardium in the reperfusion period is relatively small, because a substantial proportion of myocardium may not demonstrate immediate contractile improvement in this early reperfusion period. Williams and colleagues[93] found that systolic velocities obtained with perioperative TDI with TEE in patients undergoing revascularization could not be used to predict late recovery of systolic function. In conclusion, the ability to predict late recovery of systolic function with either DSTEE or TDI appears limited.

Use of Transesophageal Echocardiography to Monitor Intraoperative Cardiac Function in Specific Clinical Entities

The use of TEE has improved our ability to intelligently manage post-CPB instability. It has allowed us to understand the intraoperative changes that occur during some of the newer techniques in coronary revascularization and can guide us in placement of numerous intracardiac and intravascular devices. Its use in monitoring cardiac function during noncardiac surgery is most advantageous in the diagnosis of sudden and unexplained hemodynamic instability.

Separation from Cardiopulmonary Bypass

At the time of separation of the patient from CPB, the use of TEE may guide the anesthesiologist in the use of pharmacologic and nonpharmacologic therapies and can maximize the likelihood of a smooth transition.

Intracardiac Air

Left-sided intracardiac air is ubiquitous following procedures in which left-sided chambers have been open to atmosphere and is identified by its characteristic "firefly" appearance. Air is often seen entering the left

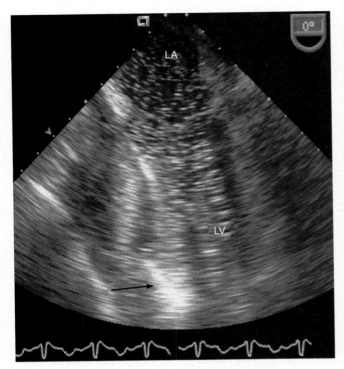

Figure 2-16. Four-chamber midesophageal view. As the patient is being separated from cardiopulmonary bypass, a pocket of air enmeshed in the left ventricular subvalvular apparatus is noted (arrow), with numerous bubbles emanating from it. LA, left atrium; LV, left ventricle.

atrium from the pulmonary veins or enmeshed in the mitral subvalvular apparatus (Fig. 2–16). Echocardiographic inspection is carried out in the four-chamber and transgastric long-axis views. Careful evacuation by the surgeon is important and involves suctioning on the aortic root vent or needle aspiration of the LV apex to evacuate trapped pockets. In addition to guiding evacuation, TEE is useful in diagnosing the consequences of embolization through the right coronary ostium, which results in ventricular dysfunction in a right coronary distribution.

Cardiac Output

There are a number of potential causes of low CO immediately following CPB: perioperative infarction, coronary air emboli, metabolic abnormalities, hypovolemia, LV outflow tract obstruction, and inadequate myocardial protection. It seems intuitive that the yield of TEE when it is used during hemodynamic instability during and after cardiac surgery would be high. Two published series have demonstrated the myriad diagnoses that have been made and the ability to intervene on many patients[94,95] (Table 2–2). No attempt was made to compare TEE with other diagnostic modalities, although the speed with which information is made available appears hard to supersede. The prebypass

TABLE 2-2. Relevant Intraoperative Transesophageal Echocardiographic Findings Categorized by Indication

Finding	Indication, *n*				
	Hemodynamic Instability	Surgical Planning	Trauma	Hypoxemia	Total Number of Patients
Severe left ventricular dysfunction ± regional wall motion abnormality	15	2	—	—	17
Aortic dissection ± aortic regurgitation	1	13	—	—	14
Significant mitral regurgitation	4	2	—	—	6
Intracardiac/great vessel shunt	1	1	—	2	4
Hyperdynamic left ventricular function	2	—	1	—	3
Severe right ventricular dysfunction	2	—	1	—	3
Extracardiac clot	2	—	—	—	2
Significant aortic regurgitation	2	—	—	—	2
Significant tricuspid regurgitation	1	—	—	—	1
Pericardial tamponade	1	—	—	—	1
No relevant findings	5	1	4	3	13

From Brandt RR, Oh JK, Abel MD, et al: *J Am Soc Echocardiogr* 11(10):972-977, 1998.

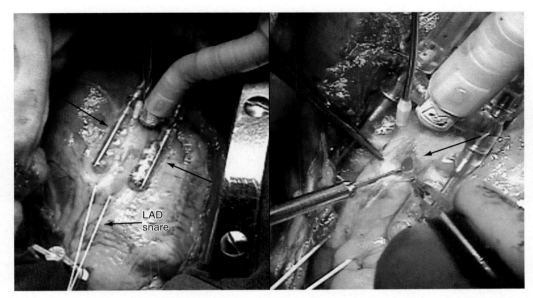

Figure 2–17. *In the* left-hand panel, *the two* arrows *indicate the stabilizing device, which through suction, lifts and immobilizes a portion of the anterior cardiac wall. The two limbs of the device straddle the left anterior descending artery, which has a snare around it. In the* right-hand panel, *an arteriotomy has been made in the left anterior descending artery* (arrow). *LAD, left anterior descending artery.*

TEE-derived wall motion score index was found to independently predict the need for postbypass inotropic support.[96]

Myocardial contrast echocardiography, although not commonly used in the OR, may have a role in determining the adequacy of cardioplegia distribution.[97,98]

Off-Pump Coronary Bypass Surgery

The off-pump bypass surgical approach to coronary revascularization involves bypassing coronary arteries without CPB, otherwise known as the "beating heart" operation. Hemodynamic instability can occur both from intraoperative ischemia and from cardiovascular deformation by the device used to stabilize the heart during coronary anastomoses (Figs. 2–17 and 2–18).[99] Although the number of readable myocardial segment decreases during cardiac displacement, TEE can adequately detect regional wall motion abnormalities in most patients.[100]

Cardiac Function in Noncardiac Surgery

In their comprehensive review of cardiovascular care during noncardiac surgery, Eagle and colleagues[101] concluded that the incremental value of TEE in the diagnosis of intraoperative ischemia is limited.

However, when sudden and unexplained hypotension occurs, TEE may be extremely helpful in establishing the diagnosis. Memtsoudis and colleagues[102] examined the use of TEE in cardiac arrest during noncardiac surgery. In 18 of 22 patients, the etiology was detected

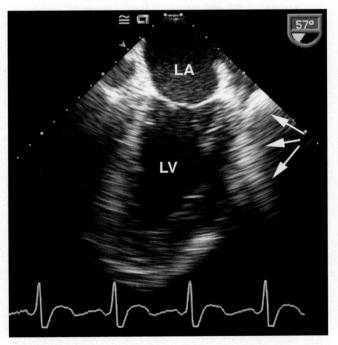

Figure 2–18. *In this two-chamber view, the stabilizer* (arrows) *deforms the anterior wall of the left ventricle. LA, left atrium; LV, left ventricle.*

by TEE and helped guide subsequent management. Much of the remaining literature is in anecdotal form. Diagnoses have included massive pulmonary embolism (PE),[103] intracardiac tumor extension,[104] cardiac tamponade,[105] main PA obstruction by an expanding aortic aneurysm[106] (Fig. 2–19), traumatic cardiac injury,[107-109]

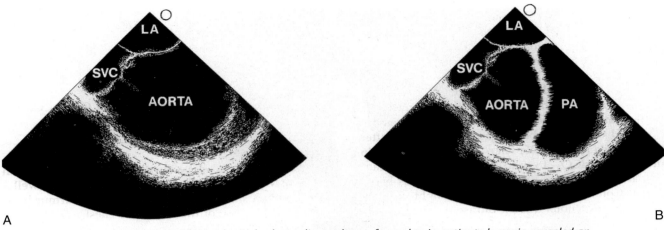

A

B

Figure 2-19. A, *Transesophageal echocardiography performed to investigate hypoxia revealed an expanding ascending aortic aneurysm with main pulmonary artery compression. B, Normal image for comparison. LA, left atrium; PA, pulmonary artery; SVC, superior vena cava. (From Jacka M, Oxorn DC: Anesth Analg 80:185-187, 1995.)*

ventilator-induced systemic air embolism,[110,111] and a case of venous air embolism during pelvic surgery, which resulted in pulseless electrical activity until open cardiac aspiration was undertaken (Fig. 2-20).

Positioning of Intravascular Devices

Intraoperative TEE can be used to guide the positioning of a number of intravascular devices.

Central Venous Pressure Air Aspiration Catheters

These are often used during sitting craniotomies to aspirate air that has gained access to the venous circulation. Correct positioning is at the right atrial–superior

vena caval junction, and imaging is best in the mid-esophagus with rightward rotation and a transducer angle of approximately 90 to 100 degrees (Fig. 2-21).

Intra-Aortic Balloon Pump

The benefits of intra-aortic balloon pump (IABP) have been demonstrated with TEE and include improved LV function and decreased wall stress.[112] The balloon pump is best imaged in the descending aorta in a vertical plane. Correct positioning is at the inferior border of the transverse aortic arch.[113] Once the tip of the balloon is visualized at a transducer angle of approximately 90 degrees, the probe marking at the teeth is noted. The probe is slowly withdrawn until the left subclavian artery orifice is seen; the marking is again noted. The distance between the balloon and the subclavian orifice should be approximately 5 cm (Fig. 2-22).

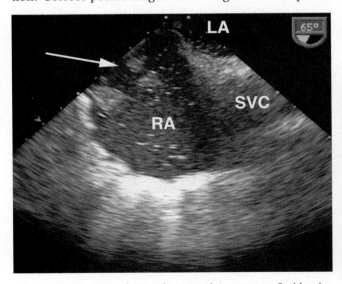

Figure 2-20. *Bicaval view during pelvic surgery. Sudden hypotension and hypoxemia prompted TEE, which revealed massive amounts of air and tissue (likely fat) entering the right atrium via the inferior vena cava (arrow). Air gained access to the left atrium through a patent foramen ovale. LA, left atrium; RA, right atrium; SVC, superior vena cava.*

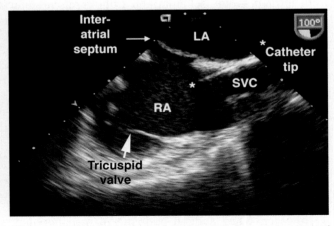

Figure 2-21. *A catheter inserted from the arm is positioned at the junction of the right atrium and superior vena cava to evacuate any air that gains access to the venous circulation during sitting craniotomy. LA, left atrium; RA, right atrium; SVC, superior vena cava.*

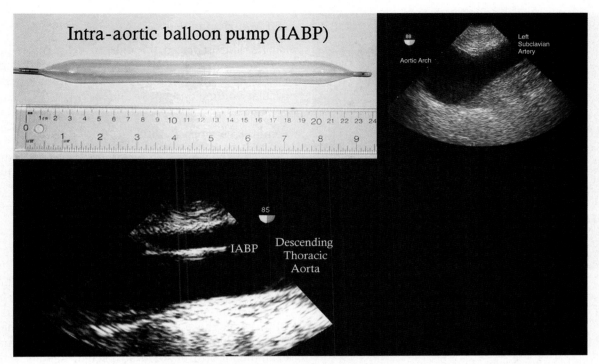

Figure 2–22. *Intra-aortic balloon pump positioned in the descending thoracic aorta. The left sub-clavian artery is visualized and not encroached on. IABP, intra-aortic balloon pump.*

Left Ventricular Assist Device

As the left ventricular assist device (LVAD) withdraws blood from the left ventricle, left atrial pressure falls below right atrial pressure. It is important to determine whether a patent foramen ovale (PFO) is present, because right-to-left shunting will invariably occur. The orifice of the ventricular apical cannula should be imaged in the four-chamber view, and the lack of obstruction by adjacent walls should be ascertained (Fig. 2–23). Because the outflow cannula terminates in the ascending aorta (Fig. 2–24), it is important to rule out significant aortic regurgitation, because this would lead to LV distension during aortic flow.

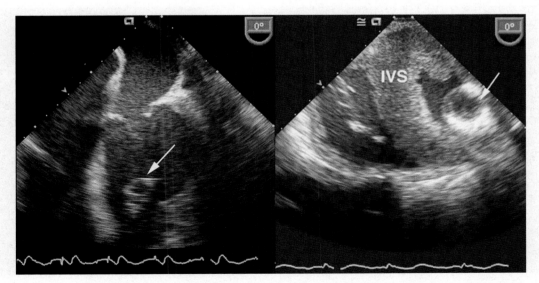

Figure 2–23. *The inflow cannula of the left ventricular assist device (arrow) is seen to freely enter the apical region of the left ventricle and not abut the IVS. Left panel, four-chamber view; right panel, transgastric short-axis view. IVS, interventricular septum.*

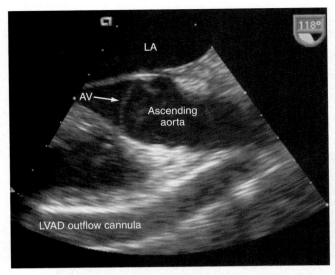

Figure 2–24. The outflow cannula of the left ventricular assist device terminates in the ascending aorta. AV, aortic valve; LA, left atrium; LVAD, left ventricular assist device.

Right Ventricular Assist Device

In positioning the right ventricular assist device (RVAD), it is preferable to avoid impingement on the tricuspid valve (Fig. 2–25).

Coronary Sinus Cannulation

The coronary sinus (CS) is cannulated through blind right atrial puncture for the purposes of administering retrograde cardioplegia. Occasionally, TEE guidance is required (Fig. 2–26).

Left Ventricular Vent

An LV vent is placed through the right upper pulmonary vein into the left atrium and advanced through the mitral valve into the left ventricle to drain excess ventricular volume on bypass (Fig. 2–27).

Femoral Venous Cannula

Occasionally venous drainage on bypass is achieved through femoral venous cannulation with advancement into the right atrium (Fig. 2–28).

Transplant Surgery

Heart Transplantation

TEE is used to examine the native heart for LV thrombi and to assess the function of the donor heart before procurement and after the recipient is separated from CPB, when the effects of the ischemic time may become evident. In addition, the anastomoses may be examined if obstruction is suspected, such as in the PA anastomosis (Fig. 2–29).

Lung Transplantation

During lung transplantation, the use of TEE has been described in the evaluation of vascular anastomoses. The pulmonary venous anastomoses are generally well seen, and velocities are usually less than 1 m/sec in the absence of significant obstruction[114,115] (Fig. 2–30).

The right PA anastomoses (and less likely the left) may be visualized in the midesophageal ascending aor-

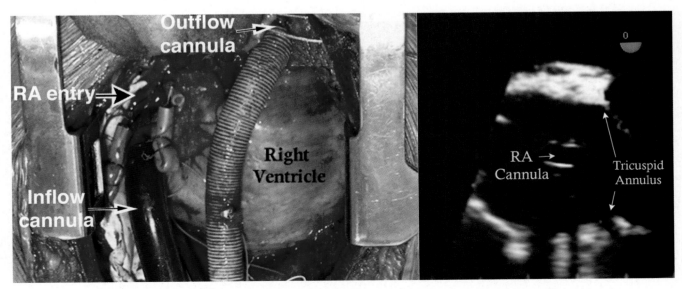

Figure 2–25. The inflow cannula to the right ventricular assist device enters the right atrium through the appendage (left, arrow). The tip is seen in the right atrium and free of the tricuspid valve on TEE (right). RA, right atrium.

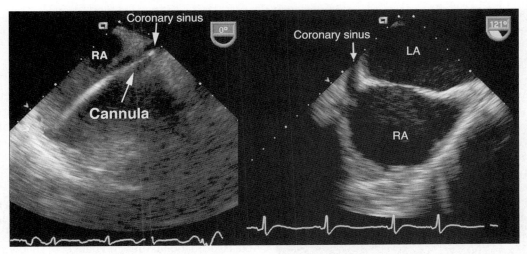

Figure 2–26. *The coronary sinus, visualized in a low esophageal view* (left) *and a bicaval view* (right). *In the* left-hand panel, *the catheter is seen traversing the right atrium and entering the coronary sinus orifice. LA, left atrium; RA, right atrium.*

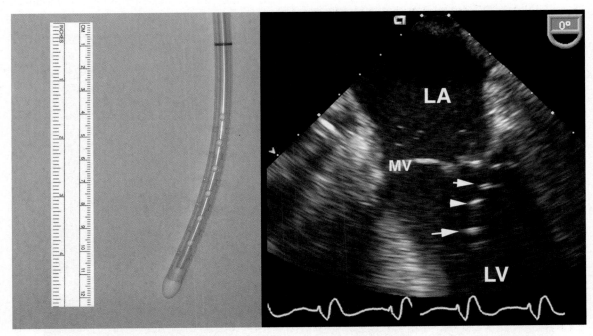

Figure 2–27. *Left ventricular vent. The distal end of the cannula is seen on the* left, *with its multiple orifices. The four-chamber TEE on the* right *demonstrates the correct position of the cannula; the* arrows *represent the orifices. LA, left atrium; LV, left ventricular; MV, mitral valve.*

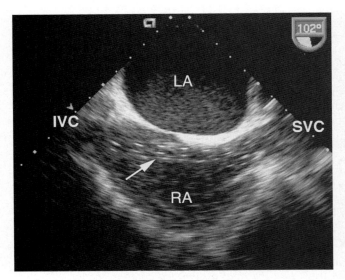

Figure 2–28. The multiorifice femoral venous cannula is seen entering the right atrium from the inferior vena cava. IVC, inferior vena cava; LA, left atrium; RA, right atrium, SVC, superior vena cava.

tic short-axis view, although the angle of flow precludes Doppler interrogation of the anastomosis (Fig. 2–31).

Liver Transplantation

During reperfusion of the transplanted liver, significant right-sided embolization can occur, with resultant hemodynamic instability. TEE can aid in this diagnosis and guide treatment.

Laparoscopic Surgery

As laparoscopic surgery has grown in its application, so has the realization that the associated pneumoperitoneum leads to increased LV wall stress[116,117] and decreased fractional area of change.[118] Following release of the pneumoperitoneum, higher than baseline fractional area of change has been described.[118] These hemodynamic alterations have been attributed to the physical effect of increased intra-abdominal pressure and to the associated neurohumoral changes. TEE has also been used to monitor for intraoperative gas embolization.

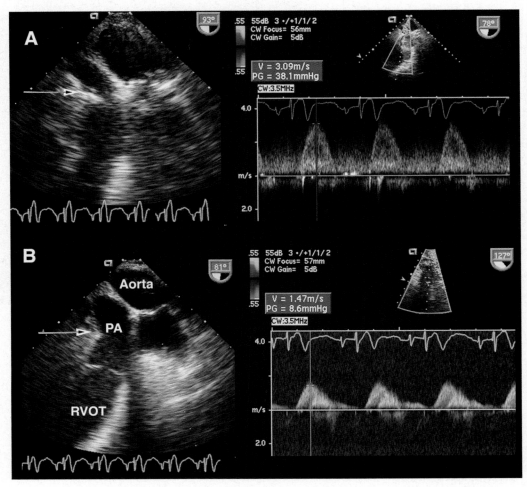

Figure 2–29. Images obtained from a high esophageal window. A, A pressure gradient (PG) of 38 mm Hg across the pulmonary artery led to the diagnosis of an anastomotic obstruction (arrow). B, The anastomosis was revised with resolution of the gradient. CW, continuous wave; PA, pulmonary artery; RVOT, right ventricular outflow tract; V, velocity.

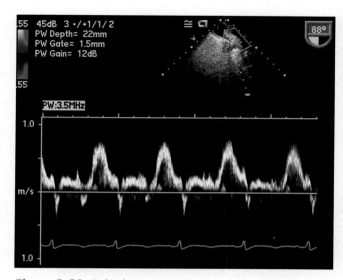

Figure 2–30. *Pulsed wave Doppler across the left pulmonary venous anastomosis shows a normal velocity of <1 m/s. PW, pulsed wave.*

New Technology

Epicardial Echocardiography

On occasion there may be contraindications to TEE, or the images obtained may be suboptimal. Using a high-frequency US probe in a sterile sheath, the cardiac surgeon can image the heart by placing it on the epicardial surface and obtain standard surface echocardiographic images[119] (Fig. 2–32).

Three-Dimensional Transesophageal Echocardiography

Three-dimensional (3D) TEE produces striking images of cardiac pathology. Although now commercially available, reconstruction of images may be time consuming[120] and not well suited to the dynamic environment of the OR.

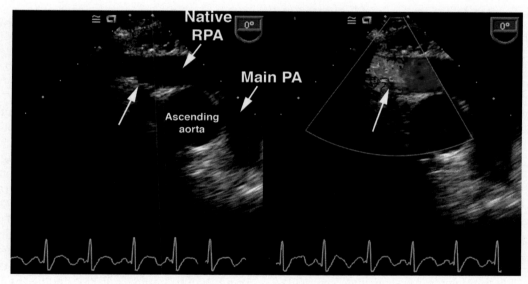

Figure 2–31. *Midesophageal ascending aortic short-axis view in a patient who received a right-sided lung transplant. In the* left-hand panel, *the arrow indicates the slight narrowing of the anastomic site. In the* right-hand panel, *aliasing in the color Doppler signal is seen at the anastomosis. PA, pulmonary artery; RPA, right pulmonary artery.*

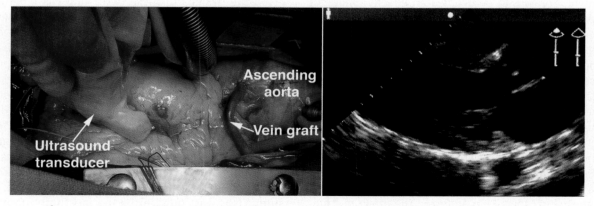

Figure 2–32. *In the* left-hand panel, *the surgeon places an ultrasound probe directly on the epicardial surface after protecting it with a sterile sheath. In the* right-hand panel, *a parasternal long-axis view is obtained.*

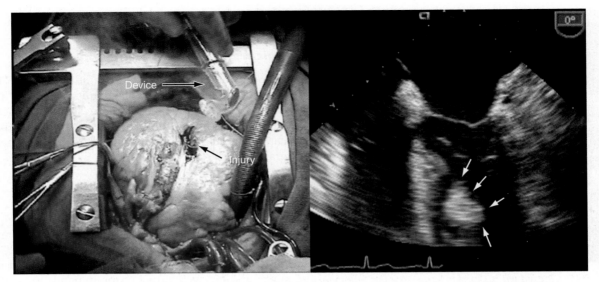

Figure 2–33. In the left-hand panel, *the laser device is seen after producing a small area of epicardial injury. In the* right-hand panel, *the TEE shows air entrained* (arrows) *into the left ventricle.*

Transmyocardial Laser Revascularization

Transmyocardial laser revascularization (TMR) involves penetrating the myocardium with laser and is an accepted mode of symptom control in selected patients with refractory angina.[121] During the procedure, transmyocardial penetration is confirmed by the visualization of small amounts of air entrained into the left ventricle (Fig. 2–33).

Transesophageal Echocardiography as a Monitor of Intraoperative Ventricular Function: Impact on Postoperative Outcomes and Cost-Effectiveness

The use of TEE to monitor intraoperative ventricular function varies significantly between institutions and relates in part to the experience of the operator, the type of surgical procedure, and the cardiopulmonary reserve of the patient. For TEE to be deemed an effective mode of intraoperative monitoring, it must have acceptable risk, impact patient outcome positively, and be cost effective and reproducible. In the position paper of 1996,[9] the Society of Cardiovascular Anesthesiologists listed the routine use of TEE in CABG as category II (possibly beneficial), largely because of the lack of outcome data.

Several studies have addressed the impact of intraoperative TEE monitoring of ventricular function during coronary bypass surgery. In all instances, benefits must be weighed against the reported complication rate of TEE of approximately 0.2%.[122]

In a study conducted at the Mayo Clinic, Click and colleagues[123] prospectively analyzed the effect of intraoperative TEE on surgical management. TEE use (and thus inclusion in the study) was determined by the treating physicians. Of the 292 patients having CABG surgery, there were 97 new TEE findings (33% of all cases) pre-bypass and 24 new TEE findings (8% of all cases) post-bypass. This large number probably reflects a selection bias, because more complex cases were more apt to be selected for TEE.

In a series of unselected and consecutive cardiac surgical patients having exclusively CABG with TEE monitoring, Qaddoura and colleagues[124], also at the Mayo Clinic, noted new prebypass findings in 52 patients, resulting in alterations of the surgical procedure in 21 of them; the most common occurrence was a previously undiagnosed PFO (Table 2–3). Post-bypass there were 19 new findings in 15 patients, resulting in 15 surgical interventions in 10 patients (Table 2–4). In a retrospective review of 2343 unselected patients having cardiac surgery, Forrest and colleagues[125] found a surgical impact of TEE findings of 4.5%. When the data for CABG patients was analyzed, the surgical impact was 6.7% of high-risk patients versus 2.8% of low-risk patients. What would be difficult to determine given the designs of these two studies is whether the additional procedures performed led to improved outcome. Bergquist and colleagues[126,127] studied the concordance between real-time intraoperative TEE interpretation by five cardiac anesthesiologists and offline analysis by two blinded investigators in the assessment of LV filling, EF area, and regional wall motion. Results obtained by the two methods were within 10% of each other 75% of the time with respect to EF and filling. The accuracy of regional assessment was variable: more accurate for normal than for abnormal wall motion and better in anesthesiologists with more advanced echocardiographic training. In the second part of the study, TEE was found to be the most important factor in guiding hemodynamic interventions in 17% of cases examined. What is lacking is a clear demonstration that

TABLE 2–3. New Prebypass Findings in 474 Coronary Artery Bypass Graft Patients and Surgical Impact by Intraoperative Transesophageal Echocardiography

New Findings (46 Patients)	*n*	Surgical Impact (16 Patients)	*n*
PFO	22	PFO closed	7
MVP with MR	3	No surgical impact	—
Significant MR (5), TR (4), AR (3)	12	MV (2), TV (2), AV (1) repair	5
AV disease (Lambl's, mild AS)	2	AV explored (Lambl's excised)	2
Subvalvular AS	1	Myomectomy	1
Improved left VF	4	No IABP	4
Aortic atheroma	5	OPCAB	2
Depressed left and right VF	2	No surgical impact	—
New RWMA	1	No surgical impact	—
Total	52	Total	21

AR, aortic regurgitation; AS, aortic stenosis; AV, aortic valve; IABP, intra-aortic balloon pump; MR, mitral regurgitation; MV, mitral valve; MVP, mitral valve prolapse; OPCAB, off-pump coronary artery bypass; PFO, patent foramen ovale; RWMA, regional wall motion abnormality; TR, tricuspid regurgitation; TV, tricuspid valve; VF, ventricular function.
From Qaddoura FE, Abel MD, Mecklenburg KL, et al: *Ann Thorac Surg* 78:1586-1590, 2004.

TABLE 2–4. New Postbypass Findings in 474 Coronary Artery Bypass Graft Patients and Surgical Impact by Inoperative Transesophageal Echocardiography

New Findings (15 Patients)	*n*	Surgical Impact (10 Patients)	*n*
Significant MR	3	MV Repair	2
Altered cardiac function		Graft flow evaluation	3
Depressed LVF	6	Graft revision	5
New RWMA	7	IABP inserted	5
New RWMA and depressed LV or RV function	2		
Dynamic obstruction	1	Medical treatment	—
Total	19	Total	15

EF, ejection fraction; IABP, intra-aortic balloon pump; LV, left ventricular; LVF, left ventricular function; MR, mitral regurgitation; MV, mitral valve; RV, right ventricular; RWMA, regional wall motion abnormalities.
From Qaddoura FE, Abel MD, Mecklenburg KL, et al: *Ann Thorac Surg* 78:1586-1590, 2004.

the TEE assessments were correct and that the same interventions would not have been undertaken if guided by more traditional monitors. Cost and outcome were not examined. Mathew and colleagues[15] demonstrated that cardiac anesthesiologists interpret TEE examinations at a level comparable to physicians whose practice is echocardiography.

At the Cleveland Clinic, Savage and colleagues[128] examined the use of intraoperative TEE monitoring in a group of high-risk patients undergoing CABG. In addition to documenting numerous management changes related to TEE-derived information (Table 2–5), they documented lower short-term morbidity and mortality rates as compared with a historical group of patients with

similar severity scores[129] who were not monitored with TEE (Table 2–6). An individual not part of the anesthetic or surgical team read the TEE scan; it is uncertain whether someone involved in direct patient management would have as readily garnered the information.

In studies from Australia,[130] Europe,[131] Canada,[1] and India,[132] the real-time accrual of information with TEE was demonstrated to be of value in the management of hemodynamic perturbations and the planning of the surgical procedure in CABG and other cardiac surgical procedures (Tables 2–7, 2–8, and 2–9). No assessment of the effect of intraoperative TEE monitoring on patient outcome was made. These studies and others are summarized in Table 2–10.

TABLE 2-5. Surgical Management Alterations during Coronary Artery Bypass Grafting Based on Transesophageal Echocardiographic Findings

Alteration	Before CPB, *n*	Before CPB Separation, *n*	After CPB Separation, *n*	After CC, *n*	Total Number of Patients
Rush to CPB	2	—	—	—	2
Return to CPB	—	—	3	1	4
Reopen	—	—	—	2	2
LVAD/ECMO	0	0	0	1	1
Additional redo grafts	8	2	3	1	12
IABP	4	3	2	0	9

CC, chest closure; CPB, cardiopulmonary bypass; ECMO, extracorporeal membrane oxygenation; IABP, intra-aortic balloon pump; LVAD, left ventricular assist device.
From Savage RM, Lytle BW, Aronson S, et al: *Ann Thorac Surg* 64(2):368-373, 1997.

TABLE 2-6. Patient Outcomes with and without Intraoperative Transesophageal Echocardiography

Variable	Management with TEE	Management without TEE
Patients, *n*	82	478
Age, y	68.4	64.8
Severity score	6.1	5.9
Hospital deaths, *n* (%)	1 (1.2)	18 (3.8)
Myocardial infarction, *n* (%)	1 (1.2)	14 (3.5)
Cardiac morbidity, *n* (%)	1 (1.2)	7 (1.5)
ICU CNS morbidity, *n* (%)	3 (3.6)	18 (3.8)
Hospital CNS morbidity, *n* (%)	1 (1.2)	16 (3.3)

CNS, central nervous system; ICU, intensive care unit; TEE, transesophageal echocardiography.
From Savage RM, Lytle BW, Aronson S, et al: *Ann Thorac Surg* 64(2):368-373, 1997.

TABLE 2-7. Impact of Routine Transesophageal Echocardiographic Findings on Medical and Surgical Management: Coronary Artery Bypass Grafting after Cardiopulmonary Bypass (*N* = 120)

Clinical Problem/ TEE Finding (Number of Patients)	Consequence (Number of Patients)	Impact
Acute SWMA (8), acute SWMA, and moderate/ severe mitral regurgitation (1)	Graft revision (3), papaverine (1), medical therapy (5)	E (3)*† I (6)
IABP not in optimal position (2)	IABP advanced	V (2)‡
IABP not in descending aorta	IABP reinserted	V (1)
ST depression (II and V5)/no SWMA (3)	De-cannulation—good outcome	I (3)
Pulmonary hypertension 3 minutes post-protamine/widespread SWMA, moderate to severe mitral regurgitation	Medical therapy for ischemia not prot-amine reaction	I (1)

*One patient also classified as valuable for IABP not in descending aorta.
†One patient also classified as informative for ST depression without SWMA.
‡Two patients also classified as informative in problems separating from CPB.
E, essential; I, informative; IABP, intra-aortic balloon pump; SWMA, segmental wall motion abnormality; TEE, transesophageal echocardiography; V, valuable.
From Sutton DC, Kluger R: *Anaesth Intensive Care* 26(3):287-293, 1998.

TABLE 2–8. Influence of Intraoperative Transesophageal Echocardiography as the Driving Force on Interventions Compared with Other Monitors

Intervention, *n* (%)	Monitor					
	TEE	ECG	Arterial Catheter	PA Catheter	Other*	Total
Fluid bolus	275 (28)	0	129 (13)	73 (7)	519	996
Anti-ischemic therapy	207 (56)	114 (31)	11 (3)	31 (8)	9	372
Vasopressor or inotrope therapy	56 (16)	3 (1)	183 (51)	27 (7)	92	361
Change in anesthetic depth	4 (2)	0	164 (78)	2 (1)	41	211
Vasodilator therapy	6 (4)	9 (6)	96 (68)	13 (9)	18	142
Antiarrhythmic therapy	0	55 (89)	0	0	7	62
Surgical intervention	9 (17)	17 (33)	12 (23)	0	14	52
Miscellaneous	3 (8)	2 (6)	27 (75)	3 (8)	1	36
Total	560 (25)	200 (9)	622 (28)	149 (7)	701	2232

*Indicates that the interventions were not based on information from the four monitors studied. More than half of these interventions were transfusion of blood for low hematocrit.
ECG, electrocardiography; PA, pulmonary artery; TEE, transesophageal echocardiography.
From Kolev N, Brase R, Swanevelder J, et al: *Anaesthesia* 53(8):767-773, 1998.

TABLE 2–9. Summary of Surgical Modifications Related to the Intraoperative Use of Transesophageal Echocardiography

Modification	Number
Return on bypass for revision of coronary artery bypass graft	4
Modification of Planned Surgery	
Valvular replacement cancelled	5
Valvular replacement or repair	11
Pleural drainage	3
Detection of air emboli before aortic unclamping	2
Surgical exploration for hemodynamic instability	7
Femoral artery bypass for aortic dissection	2
Others	
Ventricular aneurysm resection	1
Aortoplasty	1
Cancellation of aortic dissection (diagnostic error)	1
Left ventricular assist device	1
Total	38

From Couture P, Denault AY, McKenty S, et al: *Can J Anaesth* 47(1):20-26, 2000.

Cost-effectiveness has been demonstrated by studies of the use of TEE in congenital cardiac surgery,[133] preparation for elective cardioversion,[134] and determination of antibiotic treatment duration in endocarditis.[135] Similar data for routine TEE monitoring in CABG is lacking. Fanshawe and colleagues[3] showed substantial savings with the routine use of TEE in cardiac surgical patients but not specifically CABG. The claim of improved patient outcome must be tempered by the fact that most surgical changes involved closure an asymptomatic PFO.

The impact of monitoring of ventricular function during noncardiac surgery has not been studied as closely. In a retrospective review by Suriani and colleagues,[136] the use of TEE was associated with some alterations in anesthetic and surgical management in most cases. However, the indications for TEE were subjective, and neither the cost-effectiveness nor the effect on outcome was studied. Hofer and colleagues[137] prospectively examined patients at "high risk" for myocardial ischemia who were having major noncardiac surgery. A large number of patients had therapeutic changes based on TEE findings (Table 2–11), but outcome data were lacking. The authors acknowledge that randomized controlled clinical trials to evaluate outcome with intraoperative TEE are difficult to perform and cite the checkered history of the utility of the PA catheter.[138,139]

TABLE 2-10. Summary of Studies Examining the Alterations in Therapy during Cardiac Surgery with the Use of Intraoperative Transesophageal Echocardiography

Study	Population	Surgery	Altered Therapy, n/%	Outcome Reported
Bergquist and colleagues[126,127]	n = 75, 584 interventions	C-revasc	98/17% of all interventions	No
Savage and colleagues[128]	n = 82, "high risk"	C-revasc	Surgical change: 27/33% of patients	Compared to historical controls
Savage and colleagues[128]	n = 82, "high risk"	C-revasc	Hemodynamic change: 42/51% of patients	Compared to historical controls
Sutton and Kluger[130]	n = 120	C-revasc	16/13% of all patients	No
Kolev and colleagues[131]	n = 224, 2232 interventions	C-all NC	560/25% of all interventions	No
Couture and colleagues[1]	n = 851	C-all	125/15% of all patients	No
Mishra and colleagues[132]	n = 5016	C-all	1146/23% of all patients	No
Click and colleagues[123]	n = 3245	C-all	441/14% of all patients pre-bypass 121/4% of all patients post-bypass	No
Qaddoura and colleagues[124]	n = 474	C-revasc	21/4% of all patients pre-bypass	No
Qaddoura and colleagues[124]	n = 474	C-revasc	19/4% of all patients post-bypass	No
Forrest and colleagues[125]	n = 1785 low risk n = 821 medium risk n = 696 high risk n = 268(140)	C-revasc	62/3.5% of all patients 2.8% 2.9% 6.7%	No

C-all, coronary and non-coronary cardiac surgery; C-revasc, coronary revascularizations; NC, noncardiac surgery.

TABLE 2-11. Preoperative Cardiovascular Diagnoses and Intraoperative Transesophageal Echocardiography: Incidence of Therapeutic Consequences

	Total, N	Vasodilator, n (%)	Vasopressor, n (%)	Fluid, n (%)
CAD	61	36(59)	28(46)	11(18)
CAD+ valve	13	7(54)	5(39)	5(39)
Valve	11	4(36)	3(27)	2(18)
SWMA	28	26(93)*	20(71)*	9(32)
EF < 40%	15	8(53)	6(40)	1(7)
LHF	10	8(80)*	3(30)	1(10)
PAH	11	8(73)*	8(73)*	4(36)
RHF	10	7(70)*	5(50)	2(20)
Total	99	54(55)	43(43)	24(24)

*$P < 0.05$.
Vasodilator/vasopressor/fluid, new therapy, or changes of therapy with respect to vasodilator/vasopressor and fluid management.
CAD, coronary artery disease; EF, ejection fraction; LHF, left-sided heart failure; PAH, pulmonary arterial hypertension; RHF, right-sided heart failure; SWMA, systolic wall motion abnormality; Valve, valve diseases.
From Hofer CK, Zollinger A, Rak M, et al: *Anaesthesia* 59:3-9, 2004.

Summary

Although data showing improved outcomes is lacking, intraoperative TEE has become an essential tool in the assessment of ventricular function during cardiac surgery and in the monitoring of specific clinical entities, such as device placement and organ transplantation. It must be emphasized that appropriate physician training and quality assurance are crucial to the correct interpretation of data. Numerous technologic advances are on the horizon and may improve intraoperative applicability.

KEY POINTS

■ TEE is an essential tool for monitoring cardiac function in the OR.

■ TEE allows evaluation of ventricular function and filling pressures.

■ TEE is particularly useful for monitoring ventricular function at the time of separation from CPB and for placement of intracardiac devices.

REFERENCES

1. Couture P, Denault AY, McKenty S, et al: Impact of routine use of intraoperative transesophageal echocardiography during cardiac surgery. *Can J Anaesth* 47:20-26, 2000.
2. Ionescu AA, West RR, Proudman C, et al: Prospective study of routine perioperative transesophageal echocardiography for elective valve replacement: Clinical impact and cost-saving implications. *J Am Soc Echocardiogr* 14:659-667, 2001.
3. Fanshawe M, Ellis C, Habib S, et al: A retrospective analysis of the costs and benefits related to alterations in cardiac surgery from routine intraoperative transesophageal echocardiography. *Anesth Analg* 95:824-827, 2002.
4. Lambert AS, Mazer CD, Duke PC: Survey of the members of the cardiovascular section of the Canadian Anesthesiologists' Society on the use of perioperative transesophageal echocardiography—a brief report. *Can J Anaesth* 49:294-296, 2002.
5. Schmidlin D, Bettex D, Bernard E, et al: Transoesophageal echocardiography in cardiac and vascular surgery: Implications and observer variability. *Br J Anaesth* 86:497-505, 2001.
6. Huttemann E, Schelenz C, Kara F, et al: The use and safety of transoesophageal echocardiography in the general ICU—a mini-review. *Acta Anaesthesiol Scand* 48:827-836, 2004.
7. Denault AY, Couture P, McKenty S, et al: Perioperative use of transesophageal echocardiography by anesthesiologists: Impact in noncardiac surgery and in the intensive care unit. *Can J Anaesth* 49:287-293, 2002.
8. Lin T, Chen Y, Lu C, Wang M: Use of transesophageal echocardiography during cardiac arrest in patients undergoing elective non-cardiac surgery. *Br J Anaesth* 96:167-170, 2006.
9. Practice guidelines for perioperative transesophageal echocardiography. A report by the American Society of Anesthesiologists and the Society of Cardiovascular Anesthesiologists Task Force on Transesophageal Echocardiography. *Anesthesiology* 84:986-1006, 1996.
10. Beique FA, Denault AY, Martineau A, et al: Expert consensus for training in perioperative echocardiography in the province of Quebec. *Can J Anaesth* 50:699-706, 2003.
11. Cahalan MK, Abel M, Goldman M, et al: American Society of Echocardiography and Society of Cardiovascular Anesthesiologists task force guidelines for training in perioperative echocardiography. *Anesth Analg* 94:1384-1388, 2002.
12. Quinones MA, Douglas PS, Foster E, et al: ACC/AHA clinical competence statement on echocardiography: A report of the American College of Cardiology/American Heart Association/American College of Physicians–American Society of Internal Medicine Task Force on Clinical Competence. *J Am Coll Cardiol* 41:687-708, 2003.
13. Aronson S, Butler A, Subhiyah R, et al: Development and analysis of a new certifying examination in perioperative transesophageal echocardiography. *Anesth Analg* 95:1476-1482, 2002.
14. Thys DM: Clinical competence in echocardiography. *Anesth Analg* 97:313-322, 2003.
15. Mathew JP, Fontes ML, Garwood S, et al: Transesophageal echocardiography interpretation: A comparative analysis between cardiac anesthesiologists and primary echocardiographers. *Anesth Analg* 94:302-309, 2002.
16. Shanewise JS, Cheung AT, Aronson S, et al: ASE/SCA guidelines for performing a comprehensive intraoperative multiplane transesophageal echocardiography examination: Recommendations of the American Society of Echocardiography Council for Intraoperative Echocardiography and the Society of Cardiovascular Anesthesiologists Task Force for Certification in Perioperative Transesophageal Echocardiography. *J Am Soc Echocardiogr* 12:884-900, 1999.
17. Kinnaird TD, Thompson CR, Munt BI: The deceleration [correction of declaration] time of pulmonary venous diastolic flow is more accurate than the pulmonary artery occlusion pressure in predicting left atrial pressure. *J Am Coll Cardiol* 37:2025-2030, 2001.
18. Kuecherer HF, Muhiudeen IA, Kusumoto FM, et al: Estimation of mean left atrial pressure from transesophageal pulsed Doppler echocardiography of pulmonary venous flow. *Circulation* 82:1127-1139, 1990.
19. Nomura M, Hillel Z, Shih H, et al: The association between Doppler transmitral flow variables measured by transesophageal echocardiography and pulmonary capillary wedge pressure. *Anesth Analg* 84:491-496, 1997.
20. Lattik R, Couture P, Denault AY, et al: Mitral Doppler indices are superior to two-dimensional echocardiographic and hemodynamic variables in predicting responsiveness of cardiac output to a rapid intravenous infusion of colloid. *Anesth Analg* 94:1092-1099, 2002.
21. Swenson JD, Bull D, Stringham J: Subjective assessment of left ventricular preload using transesophageal echocardiography: Corresponding pulmonary artery occlusion pressures. *J Cardiothorac Vasc Anesth* 15:580-583, 2001.
22. Groban L, Dolinski SY: Transesophageal echocardiographic evaluation of diastolic function. *Chest* 128:3652-3663, 2005.
23. Ho CY, Solomon SD: A clinician's guide to tissue Doppler imaging. *Circulation* 113:e396-e398, 2006.
24. Ommen SR, Nishimura RA, Appleton CP, et al: Clinical utility of Doppler echocardiography and tissue Doppler imaging in the estimation of left ventricular filling pressures: A comparative simultaneous Doppler-catheterization study. *Circulation* 102:1788-1794, 2000.
25. Combes A, Arnoult F, Trouillet JL: Tissue Doppler imaging estimation of pulmonary artery occlusion pressure in ICU patients. *Intensive Care Med* 30:75-81, 2004.
26. Malouf PJ, Madani M, Gurudevan S, et al: Assessment of diastolic function with Doppler tissue imaging after cardiac surgery: Effect of the "postoperative septum" in on-pump and off-pump procedures. *J Am Soc Echocardiogr* 19:464-467, 2006.
27. Lang RM, Bierig M, Devereux RB, et al: Recommendations for chamber quantification: A report from the American Society of

Echocardiography's Guidelines and Standards Committee and the Chamber Quantification Writing Group, developed in conjunction with the European Association of Echocardiography, a branch of the European Society of Cardiology. *J Am Soc Echocardiogr* 18:1440-1463, 2005.

28. Colombo PC, Municino A, Brofferio A, et al: Cross-sectional multiplane transesophageal echocardiographic measurements: Comparison with standard transthoracic values obtained in the same setting. *Echocardiography* 19:383-390, 2002.

29. Cheung AT, Savino JS, Weiss SJ, et al: Echocardiographic and hemodynamic indexes of left ventricular preload in patients with normal and abnormal ventricular function. *Anesthesiology* 81:376-387, 1994.

30. Ryan T, Burwash I, Lu J, et al: The agreement between ventricular volumes and ejection fraction by transesophageal echocardiography or a combined radionuclear and thermodilution technique in patients after coronary artery surgery. *J Cardiothorac Vasc Anesth* 10:323-328, 1996.

31. Hinder F, Poelaert JI, Schmidt C, et al: Assessment of cardiovascular volume status by transoesophageal echocardiography and dye dilution during cardiac surgery. *Eur J Anaesthesiol* 15:633-640, 1998.

32. Tousignant CP, Walsh F, Mazer CD: The use of transesophageal echocardiography for preload assessment in critically ill patients. *Anesth Analg* 90:351-355, 2000.

33. Leung JM, Levine EH: Left ventricular end-systolic cavity obliteration as an estimate of intraoperative hypovolemia. *Anesthesiology* 81:1102-1109, 1994.

34. Smith MD, MacPhail B, Harrison MR, et al: Value and limitations of transesophageal echocardiography in determination of left ventricular volumes and ejection fraction. *J Am Coll Cardiol* 19:1213-1222, 1992.

35. Bowdle TA: Complications of invasive monitoring. *Anesthesiol Clin North America* 20:571-588, 2002.

36. Savino JS, Troianos CA, Aukburg S, et al: Measurement of pulmonary blood flow with transesophageal two-dimensional and Doppler echocardiography. *Anesthesiology* 75:445-451, 1991.

37. Samstad SO, Torp HG, Linker DT, et al: Cross sectional early mitral flow velocity profiles from colour Doppler. *Br Heart J* 62:177-184, 1989.

38. Muhiudeen IA, Kuecherer HF, Lee E, et al: Intraoperative estimation of cardiac output by transesophageal pulsed Doppler echocardiography. *Anesthesiology* 74:9-14, 1991.

39. Gorcsan JD, Diana P, Ball BA, Hattler BG: Intraoperative determination of cardiac output by transesophageal continuous wave Doppler. *Am Heart J* 123:171-176, 1992.

40. Maslow A, Comunale ME, Haering JM, Watkins J: Pulsed wave Doppler measurement of cardiac output from the right ventricular outflow tract. *Anesth Analg* 83:466-471, 1996.

41. Descorps-Declere A, Smail N, Vigue B, et al: Transgastric, pulsed Doppler echocardiographic determination of cardiac output. *Intensive Care Med* 22:34-38, 1996.

42. Stoddard MF, Prince CR, Ammash N, et al: Pulsed Doppler transesophageal echocardiographic determination of cardiac output in human beings: Comparison with thermodilution technique. *Am Heart J* 126:956-962, 1993.

43. Akamatsu S, Oda A, Terazawa E, et al: Automated cardiac output measurement by transesophageal color Doppler echocardiography. *Anesth Analg* 98:1232-1238, 2004.

44. Robotham JL, Takata M, Berman M, Harasawa Y: Ejection fraction revisited. *Anesthesiology* 74:172-183, 1991.

45. Teichholz LE, Kreulen T, Herman MV, Gorlin R: Problems in echocardiographic volume determinations: Echocardiographic-angiographic correlations in the presence of absence of asynergy. *Am J Cardiol* 37:7-11, 1976.

46. Schiller NB, Acquatella H, Ports TA, et al: Left ventricular volume from paired biplane two-dimensional echocardiography. *Circulation* 60:547-555, 1979.

47. Clements FM, Harpole DH, Quill T, et al: Estimation of left ventricular volume and ejection fraction by two-dimensional transoesophageal echocardiography: Comparison of short axis imaging and simultaneous radionuclide angiography. *Br J Anaesth* 64:331-336, 1990.

48. Urbanowicz JH, Shaaban MJ, Cohen NH, et al: Comparison of transesophageal echocardiographic and scintigraphic estimates of left ventricular end-diastolic volume index and ejection fraction in patients following coronary artery bypass grafting. *Anesthesiology* 72:607-612, 1990.

49. Perez JE, Waggoner AD, Barzilai B, et al: On-line assessment of ventricular function by automatic boundary detection and ultrasonic backscatter imaging. *J Am Coll Cardiol* 19:313-320, 1992.

50. Gorcsan JD, Gasior TA, Mandarino WA, et al: On-line estimation of changes in left ventricular stroke volume by transesophageal echocardiographic automated border detection in patients undergoing coronary artery bypass grafting. *Am J Cardiol* 72:721-727, 1993.

51. Greim CA, Roewer N, Laux G, et al: On-line estimation of left ventricular stroke volume using transoesophageal echocardiography and acoustic quantification. *Br J Anaesth* 77:365-369, 1996.

52. Katz WE, Gasior TA, Reddy SC, Gorcsan J, 3rd: Utility and limitations of biplane transesophageal echocardiographic automated border detection for estimation of left ventricular stroke volume and cardiac output. *Am Heart J* 128:389-396, 1994.

53. Sagawa K: The end-systolic pressure-volume relation of the ventricle: Definition, modifications and clinical use. *Circulation* 63:1223-1227, 1981.

54. Gorcsan J 3rd, Denault A, Gasior TA, et al: Rapid estimation of left ventricular contractility from end-systolic relations by echocardiographic automated border detection and femoral arterial pressure. *Anesthesiology* 81:553-562, 1994.

55. Yamaura K, Hoka S, Okamoto H, Takahashi S: Noninvasive assessment of left ventricular pressure-area relationship using transesophageal echocardiography and tonometry during cardiac and abdominal aortic surgery. *J Anesth* 19:106-111, 2005.

56. O'Kelly BF, Tubau JF, Knight AA, et al: Measurement of left ventricular contractility using transesophageal echocardiography in patients undergoing coronary artery bypass grafting. The Study of Perioperative Ischemia (SPI) Research Group. *Am Heart J* 122:1041-1049, 1991.

57. Declerck C, Hillel Z, Shih H, et al: A comparison of left ventricular performance indices measured by transesophageal echocardiography with automated border detection. *Anesthesiology* 89:341-349, 1998.

58. De Hert SG, Rodrigus IE, Haenen LR, et al: Recovery of systolic and diastolic left ventricular function early after cardiopulmonary bypass. *Anesthesiology* 85:1063-1075, 1996.

59. Galiuto L, Ignone G, DeMaria AN: Contraction and relaxation velocities of the normal left ventricle using pulsed-wave tissue Doppler echocardiography. *Am J Cardiol* 81:609-614, 1998.

60. Simmons LA, Weidemann F, Sutherland GR, et al: Doppler tissue velocity, strain, and strain rate imaging with transesophageal echocardiography in the operating room: A feasibility study. *J Am Soc Echocardiogr* 15:768-776, 2002.

61. Skarvan K, Filipovic M, Wang J, et al: Use of myocardial tissue Doppler imaging for intraoperative monitoring of left ventricular function. *Br J Anaesth* 91:473-480, 2003.

62. Bargiggia GS, Bertucci C, Recusani F, et al: A new method for estimating left ventricular dP/dt by continuous wave Doppler-echocardiography. Validation studies at cardiac catheterization. *Circulation* 80:1287-1292, 1989.

63. Poelaert JI, Schupfer G: Hemodynamic monitoring utilizing transesophageal echocardiography: The relationships among pressure, flow, and function. *Chest* 127:379-390, 2005.

64. Tei C, Nishimura RA, Seward JB, Tajik AJ: Noninvasive Doppler-derived myocardial performance index: Correlation

with simultaneous measurements of cardiac catheterization measurements. *J Am Soc Echocardiogr* 10:169-178, 1997.

65. Tei C, Dujardin KS, Hodge DO, et al: Doppler echocardiographic index for assessment of global right ventricular function. *J Am Soc Echocardiogr* 9:838-847, 1996.

66. Lutz JT, Giebler R, Peters J: The 'TEI-index' is preload dependent and can be measured by transoesophageal echocardiography during mechanical ventilation. *Eur J Anaesthesiol* 20:872-877, 2003.

67. Winkelmann J, Aronson S, Young CJ, et al: Retrograde-delivered cardioplegia is not distributed equally to the right ventricular free wall and septum. *J Cardiothorac Vasc Anesth* 9:135-139, 1995.

68. Maslow AD, Regan MM, Panzica P, et al: Precardiopulmonary bypass right ventricular function is associated with poor outcome after coronary artery bypass grafting in patients with severe left ventricular systolic dysfunction. *Anesth Analg* 95:1507-1518, 2002.

69. Wranne B, Pinto FJ, Siegel LC, et al: Abnormal postoperative interventricular motion: New intraoperative transesophageal echocardiographic evidence supports a novel hypothesis. *Am Heart J* 126:161-167, 1993.

70. Samad BA, Alam M, Jensen-Urstad K: Prognostic impact of right ventricular involvement as assessed by tricuspid annular motion in patients with acute myocardial infarction. *Am J Cardiol* 90:778-781, 2002.

71. David JS, Tousignant CP, Bowry R: Tricuspid annular velocity in patients undergoing cardiac operation using transesophageal echocardiography. *J Am Soc Echocardiogr* 19:329-334, 2006.

72. Fleisher LA: Real-time intraoperative monitoring of myocardial ischemia in noncardiac surgery. *Anesthesiology* 92:1183-1188, 2000.

73. Slogoff S, Keats AS: Does perioperative myocardial ischemia lead to postoperative myocardial infarction? *Anesthesiology* 62:107-114, 1985.

74. Schiller NB, Shah PM, Crawford M, et al: Recommendations for quantitation of the left ventricle by two-dimensional echocardiography. American Society of Echocardiography Committee on Standards, Subcommittee on Quantitation of Two-Dimensional Echocardiograms. *J Am Soc Echocardiogr* 2:358-367, 1989.

75. Cerqueira MD, Weissman NJ, Dilsizian V, et al: Standardized myocardial segmentation and nomenclature for tomographic imaging of the heart: A statement for healthcare professionals from the Cardiac Imaging Committee of the Council on Clinical Cardiology of the American Heart Association. *Circulation* 105:539-542, 2002.

76. Tennant R, CJ W: The effect of coronary occlusion on myocardial contraction. *Am J Physiol* 112:351-361, 1935.

77. Koh TW, Pepper JR, Gibson DG: Early changes in left ventricular anterior wall dynamics and coordination after coronary artery surgery. *Heart* 78:291-297, 1997.

78. Smith JS, Cahalan MK, Benefiel DJ, et al: Intraoperative detection of myocardial ischemia in high-risk patients: Electrocardiography versus two-dimensional transesophageal echocardiography. *Circulation* 72:1015-1021, 1985.

79. Leung JM, O'Kelly B, Browner WS, et al: Prognostic importance of postbypass regional wall-motion abnormalities in patients undergoing coronary artery bypass graft surgery. SPI Research Group. *Anesthesiology* 71:16-25, 1989.

80. London MJ, Tubau JF, Wong MG, et al: The "natural history" of segmental wall motion abnormalities in patients undergoing noncardiac surgery. S.P.I. Research Group. *Anesthesiology* 73:644-655, 1990.

81. Seeberger MD, Cahalan MK, Rouine-Rapp K, et al: Acute hypovolemia may cause segmental wall motion abnormalities in the absence of myocardial ischemia. *Anesth Analg* 85:1252-1257, 1997.

82. Leung JM, O'Kelly BF, Mangano DT: Relationship of regional wall motion abnormalities to hemodynamic indices of myocar-

dial oxygen supply and demand in patients undergoing CABG surgery. *Anesthesiology* 73:802-814, 1990.

83. Comunale MEHP, Body SC, Ley C, et al: The concordance of intraoperative left ventricular wall-motion abnormalities and electrocardiographic S-T segment changes: Association with outcome after coronary revascularization. Multicenter Study of Perioperative Ischemia (McSPI) Research Group. *Anesthesiology* 88:945-954, 1998.

84. Rouine-Rapp K, Ionescu P, Balea M, et al: Detection of intraoperative segmental wall-motion abnormalities by transesophageal echocardiography: The incremental value of additional cross sections in the transverse and longitudinal planes. *Anesth Analg* 83:1141-1148, 1996.

85. Koide Y, Keehn L, Nomura T, et al: Relationship of regional wall motion abnormalities detected by biplane transesophageal echocardiography and electrocardiographic changes in patients undergoing coronary artery bypass graft surgery. *J Cardiothorac Vasc Anesth* 10:719-727, 1996.

86. Podgoreanu MV, Djaiani GN, Davis E, et al: Quantitative echocardiographic assessment of regional wall motion and left ventricular asynchrony with color kinesis in cardiac surgery patients. *Anesth Analg* 96:1294-1300, 2003.

87. Hauser AM, Gangadharan V, Ramos RG, et al: Sequence of mechanical, electrocardiographic and clinical effects of repeated coronary artery occlusion in human beings: Echocardiographic observations during coronary angioplasty. *J Am Coll Cardiol* 5:193-197, 1985.

88. Elhendy A, Cornel JH, Roelandt JR, et al: Impact of severity of coronary artery stenosis and the collateral circulation on the functional outcome of dyssynergic myocardium after revascularization in patients with healed myocardial infarction and chronic left ventricular dysfunction. *Am J Cardiol* 79:883-888, 1997.

89. Geleijnse ML, Fioretti PM, Roelandt JR: Methodology, feasibility, safety and diagnostic accuracy of dobutamine stress echocardiography. *J Am Coll Cardiol* 30:595-606, 1997.

90. Aronson S, Dupont F, Savage R, et al: Changes in regional myocardial function after coronary artery bypass graft surgery are predicted by intraoperative low-dose dobutamine echocardiography. *Anesthesiology* 93:685-692, 2000.

91. Dupont FW, Lang RM, Drum ML, Aronson S: Is there a long-term predictive value of intraoperative low-dose dobutamine echocardiography in patients who have coronary artery bypass graft surgery with cardiopulmonary bypass? *Anesth Analg* 95:517-523, 2002.

92. Leung JM, Bellows WH, Pastor D: Does intraoperative evaluation of left ventricular contractile reserve predict myocardial viability? A clinical study using dobutamine stress echocardiography in patients undergoing coronary artery bypass surgery. *Anesth Analg* 99:647-654, 2004.

93. Williams RI, Haaverstad R, Sianos G, et al: Perioperative tissue Doppler echocardiography and bypass graft flowmetry in patients undergoing coronary revascularization: Predictive power for late recovery of regional myocardial function. *J Am Soc Echocardiogr* 15:1202-1210, 2002.

94. Brandt RR, Oh JK, Abel MD, et al: Role of emergency intraoperative transesophageal echocardiography. *J Am Soc Echocardiogr* 11:972-977, 1998.

95. Chan KL: Transesophageal echocardiography for assessing cause of hypotension after cardiac surgery. *Am J Cardiol* 62:1142-1143, 1988.

96. McKinlay KH, Schinderle DB, Swaminathan M, et al: Predictors of inotrope use during separation from cardiopulmonary bypass. *J Cardiothorac Vasc Anesth* 18:404-408, 2004.

97. Aronson S, Savage R, Toledano A, et al: Identifying the cause of left ventricular systolic dysfunction after coronary artery bypass surgery: The role of myocardial contrast echocardiography. *J Cardiothorac Vasc Anesth* 12:512-518, 1998.

98. Borger MA, Wei KS, Weisel RD, et al: Myocardial perfusion during warm antegrade and retrograde cardioplegia: a contrast echo study. *Ann Thorac Surg* 68:955-961, 1999.

99. Couture P, Denault A, Limoges P, et al: Mechanisms of hemodynamic changes during off-pump coronary artery bypass surgery. *Can J Anaesth* 49:835-849, 2002.

100. Wang J, Filipovic M, Rudzitis A, et al: Transesophageal echocardiography for monitoring segmental wall motion during off-pump coronary artery bypass surgery. *Anesth Analg* 99:965-973, 2004.

101. Eagle KA, Berger PB, Calkins H, et al: ACC/AHA guideline update for perioperative cardiovascular evaluation for noncardiac surgery—executive summary: a report of the American College of Cardiology/American Heart Association Task Force on Practice Guidelines. *J Am Coll Cardiol* 39:542-553, 2002. Erratum in *J Am Coll Cardiol* 47:2356, 2006.

102. Memtsoudis SG, Rosenberger P, Loffler M, et al: The usefulness of transesophageal echocardiography during intraoperative cardiac arrest in noncardiac surgery. *Anesth Analg* 102:1653-1657, 2006.

103. Newkirk L, Vater Y, Oxorn D, et al: Intraoperative TEE for the management of pulmonary tumour embolism during chondroblastic osteosarcoma resection. *Can J Anaesth* 50:886-890, 2003.

104. Plowman AN, Bolsin SN, Patrick AJ: Unusual cause of intraoperative hypotension diagnosed with transoesophageal echocardiography in a patient with renal cell carcinoma. *Anaesth Intensive Care* 27:63-65, 1999.

105. Swanton BJ, Keane D, Vlahakes GJ, Streckenbach SC: Intraoperative transesophageal echocardiography in the early detection of acute tamponade after laser extraction of a defibrillator lead. *Anesth Analg* 97:654-656, 2003.

106. Jacka M, Oxorn DC: Pulmonary artery obstruction by aortic aneurysm mimicking pulmonary embolism. *Anesth Analg* 80:185-187, 1995.

107. Tousignant C: Transesophageal echocardiographic assessment in trauma and critical care. *Can J Surg* 42:171-175, 1999.

108. Weiss RL, Brier JA, O'Connor W, et al: The usefulness of transesophageal echocardiography in diagnosing cardiac contusions. *Chest* 109:73-77, 1996.

109. Chavanon O, Dutheil V, Hacini R, et al: Treatment of severe cardiac contusion with a left ventricular assist device in a patient with multiple trauma. *J Thorac Cardiovasc Surg* 118:189-190, 1999.

110. Ho AM, Ling E: Systemic air embolism after lung trauma. *Anesthesiology* 90:564-575, 1990.

111. Ibrahim AE, Stanwood PL, Freund PR: Pneumothorax and systemic air embolism during positive-pressure ventilation. *Anesthesiology* 90:1479-1481, 1990.

112. Cheung AT, Savino JS, Weiss SJ: Beat-to-beat augmentation of left ventricular function by intraaortic counterpulsation. *Anesthesiology* 84:545-554, 1996.

113. Shanewise JS, Sadel SM: Intraoperative transesophageal echocardiography to assist the insertion and positioning of the intraaortic balloon pump. *Anesth Analg* 79:577-580, 1994.

114. Michel-Cherqui M, Brusset A, Liu N, et al: Intraoperative transesophageal echocardiographic assessment of vascular anastomoses in lung transplantation. A report on 18 cases. *Chest* 111:1229-1235, 1997.

115. Huang YC, Cheng YJ, Lin YH, et al: Graft failure caused by pulmonary venous obstruction diagnosed by intraoperative transesophageal echocardiography during lung transplantation. *Anesth Analg* 91:558-560, 2000.

116. Branche PE, Duperret SL, Sagnard PE, et al: Left ventricular loading modifications induced by pneumoperitoneum: A time course echocardiographic study. *Anesth Analg* 86:482-487, 1998.

117. Alfonsi P, Vieillard-Baron A, Coggia M, et al: Cardiac function during intraperitoneal CO2 insufflation for aortic surgery: A transesophageal echocardiographic study. *Anesth Analg* 102:1304-1310, 2006.

118. Harris SN, Ballantyne GH, Luther MA, Perrino AC Jr: Alterations of cardiovascular performance during laparoscopic colectomy: A combined hemodynamic and echocardiographic analysis. *Anesth Analg* 83:482-487, 1996.

119. Eltzschig HK, Kallmeyer IJ, Mihaljevic T, et al: A practical approach to a comprehensive epicardial and epiaortic echocardiographic examination. *J Cardiothorac Vasc Anesth* 17:422-429, 2003.

120. Ahmed S, Nanda NC, Miller AP, et al: Usefulness of transesophageal three-dimensional echocardiography in the identification of individual segment/scallop prolapse of the mitral valve. *Echocardiography* 20:203-209, 2003.

121. Bridges CR, Horvath KA, Nugent WC, et al: The Society of Thoracic Surgeons practice guideline series: Transmyocardial laser revascularization. *Ann Thorac Surg* 77:1494-1502, 2004.

122. Kallmeyer IJ, Collard CD, Fox JA, et al: The safety of intraoperative transesophageal echocardiography: A case series of 7200 cardiac surgical patients. *Anesth Analg* 92:1126-1130, 2001.

123. Click RL, Abel MD, Schaff HV: Intraoperative transesophageal echocardiography: 5-year prospective review of impact on surgical management. *Mayo Clin Proc* 75:241-247, 2000.

124. Qaddoura FE, Abel MD, Mecklenburg KL, et al: Role of intraoperative transesophageal echocardiography in patients having coronary artery bypass graft surgery. *Ann Thorac Surg* 78:1586-1590, 2004.

125. Forrest AP, Lovelock ND, Hu JM, Fletcher SN: The impact of intraoperative transoesophageal echocardiography on an unselected cardiac surgical population: A review of 2343 cases. *Anaesth Intensive Care* 30:734-741, 2002.

126. Bergquist BD, Leung JM, Bellows WH: Transesophageal echocardiography in myocardial revascularization: I. Accuracy of intraoperative real-time interpretation. *Anesth Analg* 82:1132-1138, 1996.

127. Bergquist BD, Bellows WH, Leung JM: Transesophageal echocardiography in myocardial revascularization: II. Influence on intraoperative decision making. *Anesth Analg* 82:1139-1145, 1996.

128. Savage RM, Lytle BW, Aronson S, et al: Intraoperative echocardiography is indicated in high-risk coronary artery bypass grafting. *Ann Thorac Surg* 64:368-373; discussion 373-374, 1997.

129. Higgins TL, Estafanous FG, Loop FD, et al: Stratification of morbidity and mortality outcome by preoperative risk factors in coronary artery bypass patients. A clinical severity score. *JAMA* 267:2344-2348, 1992.

130. Sutton DC, Kluger R: Intraoperative transesophageal echocardiography: Impact on adult cardiac surgery. *Anaesth Intensive Care* 26:287-293, 1998.

131. Kolev N, Brase R, Swanevelder J, et al: The influence of transesophageal echocardiography on intra-operative decision making. A European multicentre study. European Perioperative TOE Research Group. *Anaesthesia* 53:767-773, 1998.

132. Mishra M, Chauhan R, Sharma KKHP, et al: Real-time intraoperative transesophageal echocardiography—how useful? Experience of 5,016 cases. *J Cardiothorac Vasc Anesth* 12:625-632, 1998.

133. Bettex DA, Pretre R, Jenni R, Schmid ER: Cost-effectiveness of routine intraoperative transesophageal echocardiography in pediatric cardiac surgery: A 10-year experience. *Anesth Analg* 100:1271-1275, 2005.

134. Seto TB, Taira DA, Tsevat J, Manning WJ: Cost-effectiveness of transesophageal echocardiographic-guided cardioversion: A decision analytic model for patients admitted to the hospital with atrial fibrillation. *J Am Coll Cardiol* 29:122-130, 1997.

135. Rosen AB, Fowler VG Jr, Corey GR, et al: Cost-effectiveness of transesophageal echocardiography to determine the duration of therapy for intravascular catheter-associated Staphylococcus aureus bacteremia. *Ann Intern Med* 130:810-820, 1999.

136. Suriani RJ, Neustein S, Shore-Lesserson L, Konstadt S: Intraoperative transesophageal echocardiography during noncardiac surgery. *J Cardiothorac Vasc Anesth* 12:274-280, 1998.

137. Hofer CK, Zollinger A, Rak M, et al: Therapeutic impact of intraoperative transoesophageal echocardiography during noncardiac surgery. *Anaesthesia* 59:3-9, 2004.

138. Connors AF Jr, Speroff T, Dawson NV, et al: The effectiveness of right heart catheterization in the initial care of critically ill patients. SUPPORT Investigators. *JAMA* 276:889-897, 1996.

139. Wheeler AP, Bernard GR, Thompson BT, et al: Pulmonary-artery versus central venous catheter to guide treatment of acute lung injury. *N Engl J Med* 354:2213-2224, 2006.

Chapter 3

Contrast Ultrasound Imaging: Methods, Analysis, and Applications

THOMAS R. PORTER, MD • FENG XIE, MD

The discovery of ultrasonographic contrast was first described in 1968 and is based on the concept of hand agitation of saline creating a gas-blood interface for ultrasonic enhancement of blood within the heart.[1] During the following years, bubbles from agitated saline and a variety of other substances were used as echocardiographic contrast agents. Because of the large size of the microbubbles, their use was restricted to right-sided heart contrast when administered via a peripheral vein. Applications included the detection of congenital or acquired intracardiac shunts, assessment of right-sided valvular regurgitation, and diagnosis of complex congenital heart defects and pulmonary arteriovenous fistulas. Although color Doppler echocardiography now provides an easier method of detecting left-to-right shunts, agitated saline has remained helpful in detecting right-to-left shunting through a patent foramen ovale (PFO). In the past, use of ultrasonographic contrast agents for left-sided imaging, however, could be performed only by direct injection of bubbles into the left atrium or left ventricle.

Initial studies aimed at detecting myocardial contrast utilized microbubbles produced by hand agitation or solutions containing carbon dioxide gas. Because of the short duration of the contrast, these agents were given either into the aortic root or directly into the coronary artery.[2-6] Since these studies, however, significant developments have been made in how intravenous (IV) microbubbles can be used to study myocardial perfusion. The stimulus for these developments includes an improved understanding of coronary physiology in patients with coronary artery disease (CAD), advances in ultrasonographic imaging, and the development of microbubbles that consistently reach the coronary microcirculation after IV injection.

The purpose of this chapter is first to illustrate the methods used to create ultrasonographic contrast and second how these methods have been used to detect myocardial perfusion and review the results of clinical trials. Finally, newer clinical applications of ultrasound (US) contrast are reviewed.

Characteristics of Microbubbles

Microbubbles have to meet numerous physical and chemical standards to reach the left ventricular (LV) cavity and myocardium following venous injection. The first requirement is size. Microbubbles greater than 8 μm in diameter are filtered from the pulmonary circulation and will not reach the LV cavity.[7] The scattering cross section of a microbubble is related to the sixth power of its radius, and thus the smaller bubbles that reach the left ventricle are less reflective than the bubbles filtered by the pulmonary circulation. To detect the comparatively weak echoes of the bubbles small enough for transpulmonary passage, imaging modalities have been developed that register the more "microbubble-specific" resonant frequencies. The resonant frequency of a microbubble is inversely related to its diameter.[8]

Another problem arising with the small microbubble size requirement is surface tension. The internal pressure of gases within microbubbles is increased dramatically as the size of a microbubble decreases to fewer than 7 μm. Therefore, the gases within the microbubbles are at high concentrations and rapidly diffuse into blood. This immediately reduces the size and hence the contrast effect, a limitation becoming most evident when attempts are made to obtain myocardial ultrasonographic contrast from an IV injection. The transit time required to reach the LV cavity from an IV injection is greater than 5 seconds and therefore, significant amounts of gas will have escaped from the microbubble at this point.

Therefore, a second requirement for IV microbubbles is to have a method of preventing dissolution after exposure to blood. The gas composition is one of the most important factors for retention of microbubble size in circulation. First-generation contrast agents contained room air, which is 78% nitrogen. Because nitrogen rapidly diffuses, these microbubbles survived only seconds.[9] To overcome this problem, slowly diffusing insoluble gases were incorporated into the microbubbles. This improved the duration of ultrasonographic contrast in blood and even achieved myocardial contrast from an IV injection.[10] As shown in Figure 3–1, by incorporating higher molecular weight gases, such as perfluoropropane (molecular weight 188 g/mol), into microbubbles instead of room air, the same IV dose of dextrose albumin-coated microbubbles can produce a signifi-

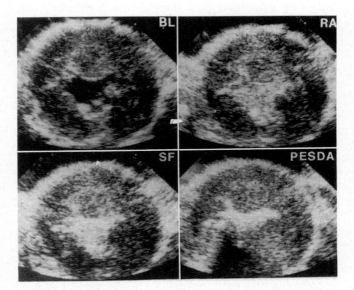

Figure 3–1. Effect of incorporating gases with lower diffusivity and solubility into microbubbles. When microbubbles contain only room air or sulfur hexafluoride, an intravenous injection produces no myocardial contrast compared with baseline. When these microbubbles contain a gas with low diffusivity and solubility, such as perfluorocarbon exposed sonicated dextrose albumin, intravenous injection produces bright myocardial contrast. BL, baseline; RA, room air; PESDA, perfluorocarbon exposed sonicated dextrose albumin; SF, sulfur hexafluoride. (From Porter TR, Xie F, Kilzer K: J Am Soc Echocardiogr 5:710-718, 1995.)

cantly greater amount of myocardial contrast than the same dose of microbubbles containing room air.

Ultrasonographic Contrast Agents

Before the development of sonication, most microbubbles were produced by hand agitation, resulting in bubbles that had both a large size (diameter > 10 μm) and a variable size distribution. The actual concentration of microbubbles in this solution was comparatively low. Various physical and chemical techniques have been developed to create smaller, more stable, and more uniformly sized microbubbles.

Electromechanical Sonication

Electromechanical sonication was first described by Feinstein and colleagues[11] in 1984 as a method to create ultrasonographic contrast. This technique involves a sonicating horn that emits a controlled source of US energy, usually at a frequency of 20 KHz. Application of this energy to a wide variety of liquids produces cavitation waves resulting in bubbles. These bubbles rapidly collapse during sonication to produce stable, smaller microbubbles (4 to 10 μm) that serve as the source of ultrasonographic contrast. Compared with the hand-agitation method to create bubbles, microbubbles produced by sonication pass through the pulmonary and myocardial microcirculation more readily.[12] When this process is applied to 50% to 70% dextrose or iodinated radiographic contrast agents, microbubble concentrations of 1×10^3/mL are produced with a size range of 3 to 5 μm.[13] The half-life of these microbubbles, however, is only minutes. Sonication of serum albumin produces microbubbles of a similar size but with much higher concentrations (1×10^8 microbubbles per mL) that have a shelf life of up to 5 months.[14-16] The mechanism for the improved microbubble stability and concentrations produced by sonication of albumin as compared with sonicating dextrose or iodinated contrast agents is related to both emulsification and cross-linking of sonochemically generated disulfide bonds.[17] Sonicated albumin (Albunex) was the first echocardiographic contrast agent approved by the Food and Drug Administration (FDA) for LV opacification from an IV injection.

Microbubbles produced by electromechanical sonication have been given into the aortic root or directly into the coronary artery to create myocardial contrast. Sonicated iodinated radiographic contrast agents have been used extensively to study regional myocardial blood flow or perfusion territories from either an aortic root[18-20] or intracoronary[21-23] injection. Sonicated albumin microbubbles have also been given into the aortic root[24] or directly into the coronary artery[25-27] to measure coronary flow abnormalities. The stability, small size, and large concentration of microbubbles produced by sonication of albu-

min raised hope that this agent might be able to produce myocardial ultrasonographic contrast from a peripheral IV injection. However, as long as air-filled microbubbles were used, there was no visually evident contrast in the myocardium after IV injection of sonicated albumin and only a variable degree of LV cavity contrast.[28,29]

The high surface tension on the small microbubbles filled with room air results in rapid diffusion of room air gases out of the microbubble.[30] The diffusivity of a gas is inversely proportional to the square root of its molecular weight (Graham's law). By incorporation of less soluble gases with a higher molecular weight inside the microbubble, the microbubbles became more stable so that myocardial contrast could be visualized even when modern imaging techniques, such as second harmonic imaging, were not available. Perfluorocarbons have the added advantage of preferentially remaining a gas instead of becoming a liquid at higher temperatures (low Ostwald coefficient). Several types of microbubble solutions containing perfluorocarbons have been developed for potential clinical use.

Albumin microspheres sonicated (Optison) was the first perfluorocarbon containing IV ultrasonographic contrast agent approved for use in humans. Its indication is enhancement of LV opacification from IV injection. Perfluorocarbon exposed sonicated dextrose albumin (PESDA) is a contrast agent formulated by sonicating 5% dextrose with 5% human serum albumin (3:1 mixture) after hand agitating this mixture with the perfluorocarbon decafluorobutane. Intravenously injected microbubbles with PESDA appear to have a rapid transit through the myocardium and do not affect LV function, coronary and systemic hemodynamics, or pulmonary gas exchange. Both PESDA, which is formulated on-site at institutions throughout the world, and commercially available albumin microspheres sonicated have proven to be capable of creating consistent myocardial contrast enhancement in animal and human studies when utilizing newer imaging techniques.[31-33]

Lipid Encapsulated Microbubbles

Two other microbubbles, perflutren lipid microspheres (Definity) and perfluorooctylbromide (Imagent) have also received FDA approval for endocardial border detection. Perflutren lipid microspheres are lipid-coated microbubbles, which are typically formed from two components: a long-chain lipid and an emulsifier. This is typically a saturated diacyl phosphatidylcholine and a polyethylene glycol (PEG) spacer. To create stable microbubbles, this mixture must be "activated" with a Vialmix device. The perfluorooctylbromide microbubble is a lipid-encapsulated surfactant stabilized microbubble, which is activated by simple agitation. None of these agents are approved as yet for assessing myocardial perfusion, but two synthetic coated microbubbles are nearing their approval for this indication at the time

TABLE 3–1. Currently Clinically Utilized Microbubble Formulations

Name	Manufacturer	Size, μm	Concentration	Shell Composition	Indication	Gas Content	Availability
AI-700	Acusphere	2.9	—	Synthetic polymer	Myocardial perfusion	Perfluoro-carbon	Not yet approved
CARDIOsphere	Point BioMedical	4	—	Polymer bilayer	Myocardial perfusion	Nitrogen	Not yet approved
Definity	Bristol/Myers Squibb	1.1-3.3	1.2×10^{10}	Lipid encapsulated	LVO	Perfluoro-propane	United States
Levovist	Schering	2-4	—	Galactose matrix and palmitic acid	LVO	Air	Europe, Asia
Optison	GE Healthcare	2-4.5	$5-8 \times 10^{8}$	Denatured albumin	LVO	Perfluoro-propane	Not yet approved
SonoVue	Bracco	2.5	$1-5 \times 10^{8}$	Phospholipids	LVO and myocardial perfusion	Sulfur hexa-fluoride	Europe, Asia

LVO, left ventricular opacification.

of this manuscript publication. Table 3–1 demonstrates all active and pending IV microbubble preparations.

Altering microbubble shell thickness is one other method of preventing dissolution within the bloodstream. One of the microbubbles seeking FDA approval for myocardial perfusion imaging is CARDIOspheres. This agent has an albumin and polylactide shell, which is of sufficient thickness that it remains stable in the bloodstream even though the encapsulated gas is nitrogen. Multicenter clinical trials have been performed with this unique microbubble to detect myocardial perfusion abnormalities during dipyridamole stress echocardiography.[34]

Ultrasonographic Imaging Techniques

Although fluorocarbon gases have rendered thin-shelled microbubbles more stable, their detection in the myocardium with echocardiographic equipment is limited with conventional imaging techniques. The development of harmonic imaging, intermittent imaging, harmonic power Doppler, and more recently, low mechanical index (MI) detection techniques has dramatically enhanced the myocardial contrast produced from intravenously injected microbubbles.

Harmonic High Mechanical Index Intermittent Imaging

Microbubbles in an ultrasonic field have the ability to scatter US not only linearly but also non-linearly. At peak incident pressures (above 0.1 megapascals), the microbubbles respond in a nonlinear manner. This physical property is attributable to the fact that gas bubbles are compliant and react to insonification at diagnostic frequencies with compression and rarefaction, thus emitting radial oscillations. The magnitude of compression and rarefaction is not the same with each oscillation, and therefore both linear and nonlinear returning waves occur.[35] The nonlinear responses occur in both the fundamental and harmonic frequencies and can be received and filtered by an appropriate echocardiography system. Because tissue and side lobes exhibit a significantly smaller nonlinear response to US, ultrasonic transducers that selectively receive the nonlinear responses produce a much better signal-to-noise ratio and more sensitive detection of microbubbles than conventional imaging.[36]

Microbubbles are destroyed by real-time US when it is transmitted at diagnostic intensities (MI > 0.3). Destruction can be reduced by selecting one frame out of every one to several cardiac cycles, usually with triggering the frame to the electrocardiogram (ECG). This has been referred to as intermittent imaging.

When the intermittent US impulse is at a high intensity (MI > 0.9), there is a strong and brief nonlinear echo. This transient scattering produces a large contrast signal from the microbubbles.[37,38] Interrupting the high-intensity US for a short period allows replacement of microbubbles, which serve to produce contrast enhancement for the subsequent triggered frame. When microbubbles are administered as a continuous infusion and the US pulsing interval is incrementally varied, the reappearance of bubbles in the myocardium permits the calculation of mean microbubble velocity and plateau (or peak) myocardial signal intensity.[39] Multiplying these two variables together, one can quantify myocardial blood flow changes. Therefore, with a combination of second harmonic and intermittent imaging, it has become possible to non-invasively examine myocardial perfusion in animals and humans using a wide variety of IV higher molecular weight microbubbles.[8,40-43]

(Harmonic) Power Doppler

Power Doppler images are based on the integrated power in the Doppler signal instead of its mean frequency shift, as used in conventional color Doppler.[44] The amplitude of the Doppler signal is related to the concentration of moving scatterers at a particular location. This amplitude is much greater in the presence of microbubbles when compared with the signal of red blood cells (RBCs).[45] This type of Doppler signal is more sensitive, not subject to aliasing, and independent of the angle of insonation. It is, however, subject to flash artifacts, which occur with movement of the heart. Harmonic power Doppler has been successfully employed in animal[46] and human myocardial perfusion studies, showing satisfactory concordance in the comparison between echocardiographic and ^{99m}Tc-sestamibi single photon emission computed tomography (SPECT) stress imaging. [34,47,48]

Low Mechanical Index Imaging Schemes

Pulse Inversion Doppler

Significant achievements have been made in low MI real-time visualization of myocardial function. Pulse inversion Doppler is a multipulse technique that separates linear and nonlinear scattering using the radiofrequency domain. The concept is an extension of pulse inversion, in which alternating positive and negative pulses of identical amplitude are transmitted into the tissue, the sum signal of which is equal to zero (Fig. 3-2). The responses of linear scatterers to these kinds of pulses, therefore, will be canceled. On the other hand, the signal from nonlinear scatterers (which do not react to positive and negative pressures in the same way) will be unequal to zero and can be registered as a bubble-specific response [49] (see Fig. 3-2). Pulse inversion Doppler overcomes motion artifacts by sending multiple pulses of alternating polarity into the myocardium. This allows one to visualize wall thickening and contrast enhancement simultaneously at low MIs (<0.2) while maintaining an excellent signal-to-noise ratio. Because it can receive only even order harmonics, however, there is significant attenuation, especially in basal myocardial segments in apical windows (Table 3-2). Initial studies using this technique in humans have demonstrated bril-

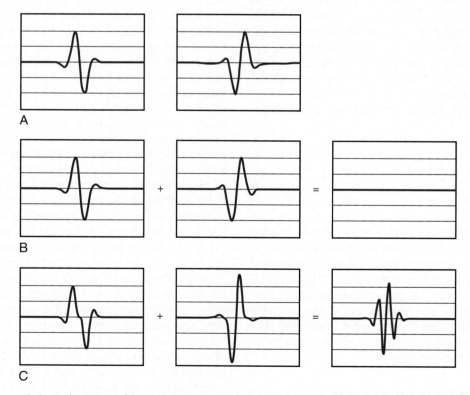

Figure 3–2. A depiction of how pulse inversion is utilized to suppress nonlinear responses from tissue and elicit nonlinear responses from microbubbles. A, Pulses of alternating polarity, when transmitted to tissue will cancel each other out with the summed response shown in B. However, because microbubbles respond non-linearly to these pulses of alternating polarity, there is actually a nonlinear response at twice the transmitted frequency (C). (Taken from Rafter P, Phillips P, Vannan MA: Cardiol Clin 22:181-197, 2004.)

TABLE 3–2. **Different Low Mechanical Index Imaging Techniques***

Name	Company Manufacturer	Tissue Cancellation	Nonlinear Activity	Advantages/Disadvantages
PID	Phillips ATL	Alternating polarity	Even order harmonics	Spatial resolution/attenuation and low sensitivity
PM	Phillips Agilent	Alternating amplitude	Fundamental	Sensitivity/sensitivity Poor resolution
CPS	Siemens Acuson	Alternating amplitude/ polarity	Fundamental and harmonics	Sensitivity and resolution/ sensitivity

*The methods by which the pulse sequence schemes cancel tissue and the frequency in which enhanced nonlinear response is detected is also shown.
CPS, contrast pulse sequencing; PID, pulse inversion Doppler; PM, power modulation.

liant myocardial opacification from small bolus injections of IV albumin microspheres sonicated.[50,51]

Power Modulation and Contrast Pulse Sequencing

Power modulation is another technique that improves the signal-to-noise ratio at low MIs. This technique, developed by Philips, is also a multipulse cancelation technique; only here the power of each pulse is varied. The low-power pulses create a linear response, whereas the slightly higher power pulse results in a linear response from tissue but a nonlinear response from bub-

bles. The linear responses from the two different pulses (the amplified low-power pulse and the slightly higher power pulse) can be subtracted from each other. The transducer then only sees the nonlinear behavior, which emanates exclusively from the microbubbles. Both pulse inversion Doppler and power modulation can be used at low MIs to assess myocardial contrast in real time with excellent spatial resolution at higher bandwidths.

Contrast pulse sequencing extends these multipulse techniques by interpulse phase and amplitude modulation. [52] An example of this technique is displayed in Figure 3–3, in which the second pulse of a sequence scheme has both a 180-degree phase shift and twice the

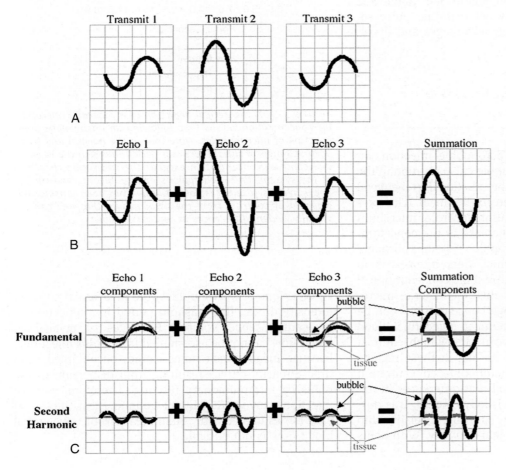

Figure 3–3. *An example of the interpulse phase and amplitude modulation sequence, which involves sending multiple pulses of both alternating polarity and amplitude (A) and stimulating nonlinear responses from microbubbles (B), which have both fundamental and harmonic components (dark arrows; C) and which have marked tissue suppression (lighter arrows). (Reprinted with permission from Rafter P, Phillips P, Vannan MA: Cardiol Clin 22:181-197, 2004.)*

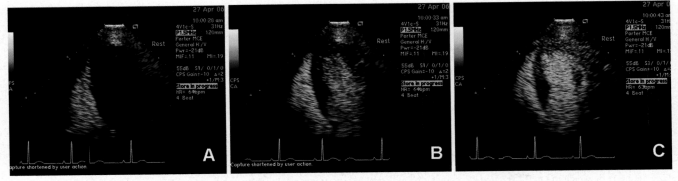

Figure 3–4. *An example of the absence of tissue signal from the left ventricular cavity or muscle apical four-chamber view before contrast in* (A) *and the bright left ventricular cavity* (B) *and myocardial contrast enhancement* (C) *in a patient being imaged with the interpulse phase and amplitude modulation scheme.*

amplitude as the first and third pulses (see Fig. 3–3A). The received echoes (see Fig. 3–3B) from microbubbles reflect the summation of nonlinear responses. Figure 3–3C depicts how this signal can be broken down, such that linear signals (which at this low MI would be from tissue primarily) are canceled, whereas nonlinear signals (primarily from microbubbles) are evident in both the fundamental and harmonic frequencies. An example of the excellent myocardial tissue rejection and increased microbubble signal intensity with contrast pulse sequencing in a normal patient from the apical four-chamber view is displayed in Figure 3–4. Table 3–2 summarizes the different low MI real-time pulse sequence schemes and lists their advantages and disadvantages.

Qualitative and Quantitative Methods of Analysis

Regardless of the route of microbubble injection, an accurate definition of microbubble concentration in the myocardium requires that the relationship between concentration and signal intensity be linear. This precondition is fulfilled at low intramyocardial microbubble concentrations; with an increase of the concentration; however, echocardiographic systems normally reach a saturation point, in which video intensity is no longer proportional to the microbubble concentration.[53] This becomes a factor with bolus injections of microbubbles in which transient high concentrations can be reached even in regions with reduced myocardial blood flow, leading to a brief period during which contrast enhancement falsely appears normal in these regions (Fig. 3–5). It is not until microbubble concentration falls during the washout period that differences in microbubble concentration are visually evident. It is during this time period that there is a linear relationship between concentration and signal intensity. With bolus

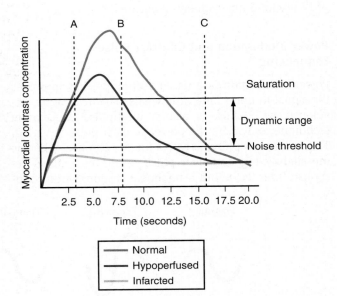

Figure 3–5. *A theoretical depiction of myocardial microbubble concentration versus time following an intravenous bolus injection of microbubbles. Note that in the normal and hypoperfused myocardium, there is a period in which the myocardial contrast concentration exceeds the saturation threshold of the system, and both regions appear bright even though one is hypoperfused. It is not until there has been considerable washout of contrast from the myocardium that one can see visually evident differences in contrast intensity.*

IV injections of microbubbles, the myocardial contrast intensity during this washout period is a reflection of myocardial blood volume. Estimates of myocardial blood flow cannot be ascertained from bolus injections, because mean transit times cannot be obtained from time intensity curves resulting from dispersion of the bolus by intrapulmonary filtering. Therefore, with IV injections, myocardial blood volume (peak intensity) can be estimated but quantification of myocardial blood flow is not possible.

Continuous Infusion Imaging

The difficulties arising with the thresholding effect and saturation point of echocardiography systems can partly be avoided by using a continuous peripheral venous infusion of microbubbles instead of a bolus injection. This method assumes the input of microbubbles into the myocardium is constant. The practical advantage of a continuous infusion is that attenuation artifacts resulting from high contrast intensity in the LV cavity can be reduced.[54,55] Moreover, the contrast dosage administered can easily be adjusted depending on the individual imaging conditions of different patients.[56]

Starting from the presumption that a true continuous venous infusion of a constant number of microbubbles can be achieved, a quantitative assessment of myocardial blood flow is possible. The US beam destroys these microbubbles when a high MI is used, so that insonation at high MIs results in almost complete bubble destruction with every pulse. Triggering US to one frame timed to end-systole in the cardiac cycle at a sequence of incrementally longer cardiac cycles allows a replenishment of contrast agent corresponding to flow to the given region during that time sequence. The longer the triggering intervals are set, the more microbubbles refill the capillaries and the higher the signal intensity to be registered in the tissue until finally a plateau phase is reached. The product of slope of myocardial contrast intensity and plateau intensity is an index of myocardial blood flow. Alternatively, if one is imaging at low MI in real time, brief high MI impulses can be applied to the imaging plane, following which replenishment can be visualized in real time at the low MI (Fig. 3–6). The plateau background subtracted myocardial contrast intensity of a respective myocardial region is related to the capillary cross-sectional area. The rate at which this plateau stage is achieved (slope) is proportional to the blood flow velocity in that region. Because the peak background subtracted myocardial video intensity is directly related to capillary cross-sectional area, the slope times peak or plateau myocardial video intensity represents a measure of myocardial blood flow.[38] Although this methodology holds a good deal of promise, incomplete destruction of microbubbles in the US field could lead to significant underestimation of myocardial blood flow abnormalities.[57] Models have been proposed and validated that correct the plateau myocardial signal intensity (which is subject to regional US beam inhomogeneities) by dividing this value by the adjacent LV cavity intensity (Fig. 3–7). These normalized plateau intensities, when multiplied by the rate of contrast replenishment and divided by tissue density, can be used to compute myocardial blood flow.[58]

Because of the high resolution of echocardiography, subendocardial contrast intensity (in decibels) has been calibrated to adjacent LV cavity contrast intensity with harmonic power Doppler to compute relative

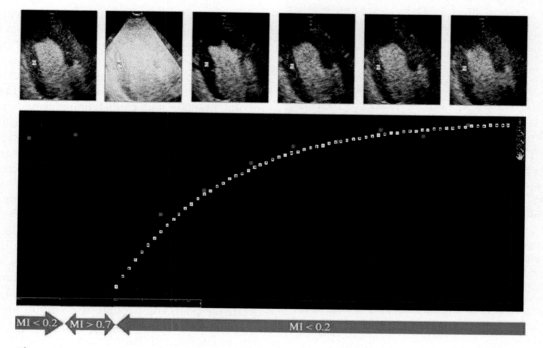

Figure 3–6. An example of myocardial contrast replenishment following a high mechanical index impulse (depicted as the bright flash in the second apical four-chamber image across the top panels) using a typical low mechanical index pulse sequence scheme. Note that after the high mechanical index impulse, there is replenishment of myocardial contrast while imaging at a low mechanical index (0.2). This can be plotted and fitted to the 1-exponential function. MI, mechanical index. (With permission from Rafter P, Phillips P, Vannan MA: Cardiol Clin 22:181-197, 2004).

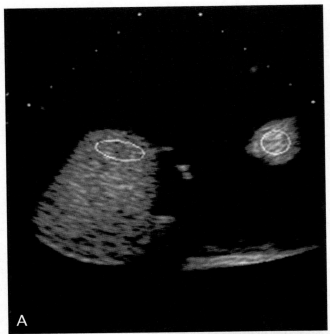

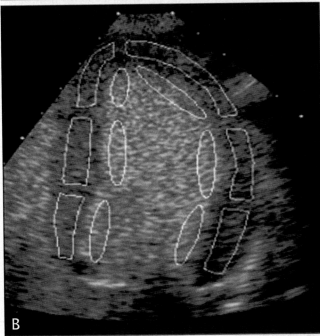

Figure 3-7. The regions of interest deployed in a perfusion phantom (A) and normal human (B) in which quantification of myocardial blood flow is performed by normalizing each myocardial signal intensity with the adjacent left ventricular cavity will compensate for regional beam inhomogeneities and beam attenuation. (With permission from Vogel R, Indermuhle A, Reinhardt J, et al: J Am Coll Cardiol 45:754-762, 2005.)

TABLE 3-3. Specific Clinical Applications of Ultrasound Contrast Agents Based on the Method of Delivery

Route of Injection	Clinical Parameters Measured
Intravenous injection	Doppler enhancement Area at risk infarct size Left ventricular cavity opacification Perfusion defect size Myocardial blood volume
Intravenous infusion	Myocardial blood flow changes Intracardiac mass definition Subendocardial blood flow

Continuous infusion techniques can be done with infusion pumps or handheld infusions. With either of the commercially available contrast agents, one can mix them at the bedside with saline and infuse them either as a continuous drip or as a handheld infusion (Fig. 3-8). Table 3-3 summarizes the different clinical parameters that can be assessed with bolus versus continuous infusion of contrast.

Technical Equipment, Image Processing, and Data Analysis

Processing and analysis play a major role in the quantitative, reproducible assessment of echocardiographic myocardial perfusion. In most cases, myocardial signal intensity in one or more regions of interest per frame is specified. The regions of interest have to be maintained in a constant position, large enough to provide the highest signal-to-noise ratio but without including any parts of the brighter endocardial or epicardial border. The alignment, manually or by a computer algorithm, should be performed before and after contrast at end-systole, to reduce contributions from larger intramyocardial arterioles.[60] Regions of interest should be corrected by using background subtraction,[61] performed by subtracting any background intensity posthigh MI impulses from contrast-enhanced pictures. If the signal intensity in the regions of interest is measured from video data, it can be displayed in a dynamic range of 256 pixels, the different values related to the pixel, which contains the highest signal intensity. Because the ability of the human eye to distinguish between a large amount of gray shades is relatively poor, color-coding is a helpful tool for better detection of perfusion abnormalities.[61,62] To prevent the loss of information that comes from analyzing video images, digital intensity obtained from returning signals before post-processing is more commonly utilized today. This information is unprocessed and not affected by the postprocessing functions of the imaging chain. However, all quantitative analyses to date have been shown to be

blood volume fractions. This quantitative parameter (calibrated contrast intensity) was useful in reducing heterogeneity in myocardial contrast intensity variations and in discriminating viable from nonviable myocardium.[59]

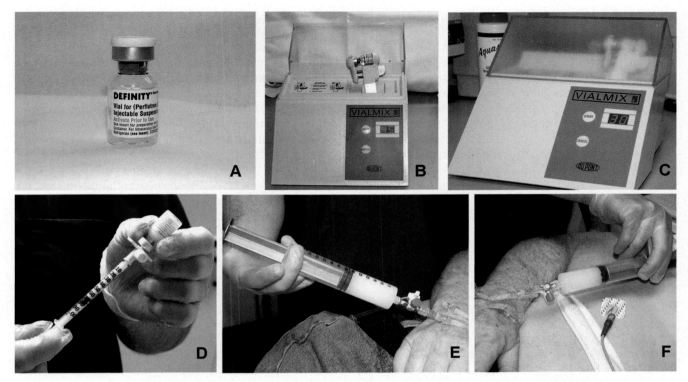

Figure 3–8. One method of administering Definity using a continuous infusion technique during dobutamine stress echocardiography. After agitating the Definity solution with the Vialamix (B and C), half the vial is put into 30 mL of saline and infused for the resting images (D, E, and F). The remaining half is infused during stress image acquisition in the same manner.

time consuming and technically demanding.[63] Nonetheless, there is general agreement that visual analysis of myocardial perfusion data will be inadequate when quantifying myocardial contrast enhancement from venous infusions of contrast.

Commercially available US systems and digital review stations are now equipped with quantitative signal intensity systems, which can measure contrast intensity and myocardial blood flow changes using the 1-exponential function. Quantification of myocardial contrast enhancement will require that we understand which normal variations in contrast enhancement exist within different regions. Animal and human studies have demonstrated that there is a regional heterogeneity in myocardial contrast enhancement from microbubbles.[58,59,64]

Three-dimensional real-time perfusion concepts have been put forth, which attempt to quantify myocardial blood flow changes using volumetric acquisition protocols.[65] The difficulty here is that high MI impulses to destroy microbubbles during continuous infusions of microbubbles in a volume (as opposed to a single imaging plane) of myocardium are probably not going to be feasible. Therefore, background subtracted peak contrast replenishment rates have been measured following brief interruptions in microbubble infusions. The feasibility and accuracy of this approach has yet to be determined.

Clinical Application of Ultrasonographic Contrast

Detecting Acute Ischemia/Risk Area in the Emergency Setting

In several animal and human investigations, intracoronary US contrast injections have successfully delineated the area at risk after acute myocardial infarction (AMI), which is defined as the complete transmural extent of the perfusion bed supplied by an occluded coronary artery.[66-68] These studies have shown that an area at risk measured with intracoronary contrast is superior to clinical, electrocardiographic, hemodynamic, or angiographic data in determining actual risk area. IV microbubbles encapsulating high molecular weight gases in combination with new imaging techniques have made the rapid noninvasive assessment of risk areas possible in an acute setting. In several animal experiments, the spatial distribution of hypoperfusion after coronary artery occlusion and reperfusion has been accurately quantified with IV myocardial contrast echocardiography (MCE).[31,69-71] Perfusion defects delineated by US contrast have correlated with the extent of wall motion abnormality in the corresponding myocardial segment and postmortem measurements of risk area.[69] Continuous infusions of microbubbles have been employed to quantify reductions in myocardial blood flow using the destruction-replenishment techniques described previously.[39]

Resting MCE data has been assessed in the emergency department (ED) in a large number of patients with chest pain and nondiagnostic electrocardiograms. In patients with low or moderate clinical risk scores, myocardial perfusion assessed with intermittent high MI ultraharmonic or harmonic power Doppler imaging provided incremental prognostic information in patients who had resting abnormalities in regional wall motion. Patients with both abnormal regional wall motion and abnormal myocardial perfusion had a significantly worse event-free survival, when compared to patients with abnormal regional function but normal myocardial perfusion.[72]

Assessment of Myocardial Viability in the Acute and Chronic Setting

Identification of patients with the "no-reflow" phenomenon has proven to be an important clinical application for MCE. This phenomenon, described first in an animal setting by Kloner and colleagues[73] in 1974, is characterized by a lack of recovery in microvascular perfusion although the occluded coronary artery is successfully reopened by percutaneous intervention or thrombolysis. Ito and colleagues[74] were the first to systematically examine myocardial microvascular perfusion with intracoronary microbubbles in patients with acute anteroseptal myocardial infarction immediately following restoration of antegrade flow in the left anterior descending artery. Using intracoronary sonicated radiographic contrast, they demonstrated that 23% of the patients had persistent contrast defects (i.e., no reflow) in the area at risk after recanalization. The long-term prognosis of these no-reflow patients was impaired, and there was significant deterioration in regional and global systolic function at follow-up. These findings have been confirmed by other investigators.

Several investigators have recently succeeded in detecting the no-reflow phenomenon from IV administration of microbubbles in patients with acute myocardial infarction following revascularization. Lepper and colleagues[75] studied myocardial contrast enhancement in patients with acute infarction undergoing angioplasty immediately before and 24 hours after recanalization using IV perfluorocarbon-containing microbubbles and intermittent harmonic imaging. An improvement of myocardial perfusion within 24 hours after intervention was predictive of functional recovery verified at 4-week follow-up. These investigators found that myocardial contrast imaging performed within an hour after revascularization is likely to lead to an underestimation of the ultimate infarct size. Actual infarct size in this time frame was best assessed following the use of a coronary vasodilatator.[76] In patients undergoing primary coronary stenting, homogenous myocardial contrast enhancement within the infarct zone by continuous infusion IV MCE was highly predictive of regional recovery of function.[77] Restoration of microvascular perfusion was most likely to occur if patients demonstrated at least partial perfusion to the risk area before primary stenting. MCE performed during dipyridamole infusion 1 week after acute myocardial infarction in patients receiving primary fibrinolytic therapy has been shown to be useful in detecting both a significant residual stenosis within the infarct vessel and predicting when multivessel coronary disease is present.[78]

Visualization of collateral myocardial blood flow before and after revascularization has been demonstrated with intracoronary contrast. In patients with occluded vessels, injection of ultrasonographic contrast material into adjacent coronary arteries can produce myocardial contrast enhancement in the perfusion bed subtended by the occluded vessel.[79,80] This phenomenon is clinically relevant, because it indicates viability of the perfusion bed subtended by the occluded coronary artery.[81] Sabia and colleagues[82] demonstrated that revascularization of an occluded coronary artery after myocardial infarction resulted in improved function only when myocardial contrast enhancement was observed following US contrast injection into the opposite coronary artery.[83] The spatial extent of collateral blood flow as defined by contrast echocardiography correlated closely with improvement in regional function within the infarct zone.

Detection of Coronary Artery Disease

With Vasodilator Stress Perfusion Imaging

Until the last few years, radionuclide scintigraphy has been the diagnostic tool to address myocardial perfusion during stress testing. This method, especially when performed with ^{99m}Tc rather than ^{201}Tl, provides high sensitivity in identifying patients with CAD. It is limited, however, by relatively poor spatial resolution and frequent attenuation artifacts. With IV perfluorocarbon contrast agents and nonlinear ultrasonographic techniques, detection of underperfused myocardial segments during stress echocardiography has become feasible. Initial studies deployed intermittent harmonic or power Doppler imaging techniques to detect coronary stenoses during vasodilator stress. Using IV albumin microspheres sonicated and intermittent harmonic imaging, Kaul and colleagues[84] described a 92% concordance between segmental perfusion scores by MCE and ^{99m}Tc-sestamibi SPECT at rest and during dipyridamole stress. Heinle and colleagues[48] used an IV albumin microspheres sonicated infusion and harmonic power Doppler imaging at long pulsing intervals during adenosine stress testing to compare perfusion with ^{99m}Tc-sestamibi SPECT in 123 patients with suspected CAD. There was an overall concordance between both techniques of 83%; concordance was higher in patients

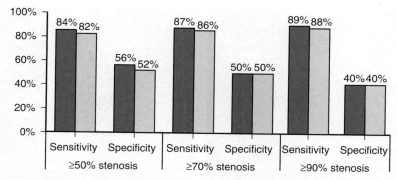

Figure 3–9. *Comparisons of sensitivities and specificities of myocardial contrast echocardiography* (purple bars) *with single-photon computed tomography* (yellow bars) *in detecting coronary stenoses of different severity in a multicenter study using dipyridamole stress and an intermediate mechanical index (0.5) triggered replenishment imaging technique. (From Jeetley P, Hickman M, Kamp O, et al: Am Coll Cardiol 47:141-145, 2006.)*

with no or multivessel CAD. Correlation was also dependent on which coronary territory was involved, with the best agreement occurring in the left anterior descending territory (81%). Agreement was not as good between the two techniques in the left circumflex (72%) or right coronary artery (76%) territories.[48]

Real-time perfusion and other lower MI imaging techniques have been applied to vasodilator stress as well. Recently, the first multicenter studies comparing MCE (triggered replenishment imaging) with radionuclide scintigraphy (SPECT) have taken place. These demonstrated a similar sensitivity and specificity between the two techniques, regardless of stenosis severity (Fig. 3–9).

During Dobutamine or Exercise Stress Echocardiography

Real-time perfusion techniques have been utilized to detect coronary stenoses during exercise and dobutamine stress echocardiography (DSE). Cwajg and colleagues[85] used accelerated intermittent imaging and IV bolus injections of albumin microspheres sonicated and PESDA at rest and during dobutamine stress echocardiography in 45 patients with known or suspected CAD. In this study, the real-time assessment of perfu-

sion improved the sensitivity of the test in detecting angiographically significant stenoses by more than 10%.[85] More recent phase II studies have demonstrated the incremental value of myocardial perfusion assessment using low MI imaging during exercise testing.[86] In predominately single-center studies, real-time perfusion echocardiography has been shown to increase the sensitivity of the dobutamine stress test when compared to wall motion analysis [87] and improve the ability of the test to predict death or nonfatal myocardial infarction.[88] Examples of inducible perfusion defects within single-vessel territories (the left anterior descending and left circumflex) are displayed in Figures 3–10 and 3–11, whereas a multivessel inducible perfusion defect is displayed in Figure 3–12. Table 3–4 demonstrates the clinical studies that have been performed in the previous 5 years examining the sensitivity and specificity of MCE in detecting CAD during different types of stress echocardiography.[34,78,86,89-99]

Artifacts in Myocardial Perfusion Assessments

One must be able to differentiate potential artifacts that create the appearance of perfusion defects. The most common artifact results from attenuation. This typically

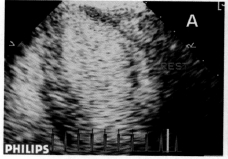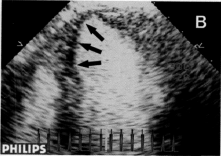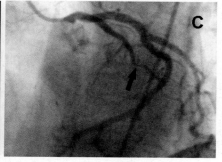

Figure 3–10. *An example of an inducible septal and apical perfusion defect during dobutamine stress echocardiography using real-time contrast echocardiography. The arrows depict the excellent resolution of the subendocardial perfusion defect.*

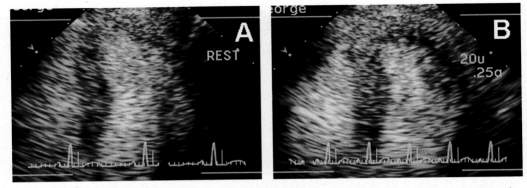

Figure 3–11. *An example of a lateral wall perfusion defect detected with real-time contrast echocardiography during dobutamine stress echocardiography.*

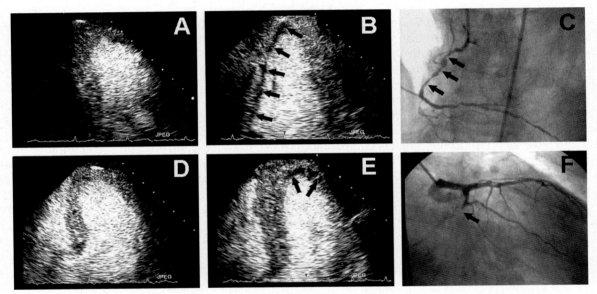

Figure 3–12. *An example of a multivessel pattern of inducible perfusion defect during dobutamine stress echocardiography, in which subendocardial defects are seen with stress (arrows; B and E), compared to resting images (A and B) with the corresponding right coronary (C) and left circumflex (F) lesions shown on coronary angiography.*

occurs in basal segments and is differentiated from true defects by its location. Attenuation typically masks not only the myocardium but adjacent epicardial and endocardial borders as well (Fig. 3–13). Attenuation is usually present both at rest and during stress, whereas inducible defects are present only during stress and typically involve just the subendocardium. Other potential artifacts are lung shadows, which will often mask an entire region (e.g., the anterior wall in the apical two-chamber view). A second location in which artifacts tend to occur is in the apical region. If the near-field gains (time-gain compensation) are set too low, the apex will appear hypoperfused. Unlike true defects, this can be corrected by increasing the near-field potentiometers. Near-field destruction of microbubbles can also cause the false appearance of perfusion defects in the apex. This can be corrected by moving the focus to

the near field, which decreases the scan line density in this region and reduces destruction.

Detection of Coronary Artery Disease with Large Arteriolar Imaging

If a higher MI is used in real time, microbubbles within capillaries are destroyed, but those transiting faster through larger arterioles (>300 microns) can still be visualized. These larger arterioles are not involved with autoregulation, and their contrast intensity exhibits a predominately diastolic component under normal conditions. As the smaller arterioles (150 to 300 microns) involved with autoregulation dilate in response to a coronary stenosis, a correspondingly greater concentration of microbubbles from these arterioles is injected retrograde into the larger arterioles during sys-

TABLE 3-4. Selected Myocardial Perfusion Stress Imaging Studies Performed with Intravenous Ultrasound Contrast during Stress Echocardiography

Reference Number	Test	N	Sensitivity	Specificity	Accuracy	Bolus or Continuous Infusion	Imaging Mode	Reference Standard
89	Dob	40	—	—	83%	Bolus	RT	Angio
86	EX	100	—	—	76%	Bolus	RT	SPECT
90	Dob	44	97%	93%	—	Bolus	RT	Angio
91	Dipy	35	85%	79%	—	CI	RT	Angio
78	Dipy	73	88%	75%	87%	CI	RT	Angio
92	Dipy	46	—	—	83%	—	TRI	SPECT
93	Dipy+Dob	70	91%	70%	—	CI	RT	Angio
94	Dob		—	—	84%	Bolus	RT	Angio
95	Dob	128	89%	53%	81%	Bolus	RT	Angio
96	Dipy or Adeno	36	—	—	TRI 81% RT 85%	Bolus	TRI and RT	SPECT
97	Dob	27	64%-67%	50%-80%	63%-67%	Bolus	RT	Angio
98	Dipy	123	80%	63%	—	CI	TRI	Angio
99	Dipy or Adeno	89	83%	72%	—	CI	RT	Angio
34	Dipy	54	96%	63%	—	CI	TRI	SPECT
*	Dipy	884	63%-75%	48%-60%	—	—	—	Angio

*Data from http://www.pointbio.com/newsroom/release.asp?id5pr32200473615.
Adeno, adenosine; Angio, angiography; CI, continuous infusion; Dipy, dipyridamole; Dob, dobutamine; EX, exercise; RT, real time; SPECT, Single photon emission computed tomography; TRI, triggered.

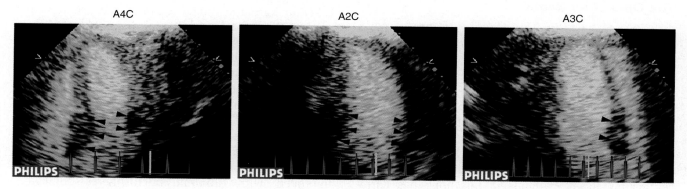

A4C   **A2C**   **A3C**

Figure 3-13. An example of basal segment attenuation (arrowheads) *seen in multiple different apical windows. The attenuation is different from a true defect in that it is not confined to the subendocardium and adjacent structures cannot be visualized as well.*

tole. Recently, Wei and colleagues[60,100] has demonstrated that this increase in systolic contrast intensity (or increase in the systolic-to-diastolic-signal ratio) from these larger arterioles can detect when significant stenoses are present in the left anterior descending artery under resting conditions.

Distribution of Transmural Myocardial Blood Flow

Because of the high spatial resolution of ultrasonographic imaging, several investigators have demonstrated differences in the degree of echocardiographic contrast produced by an intracoronary or aortic root injection between the subendocardial and subepicardial layers of myocardium. Animal studies even demonstrated after an intracoronary injection of a monosaccharide-based contrast agent (SHU-454) that differences in the transmural distribution of contrast could be detected at different times in the cardiac cycle.[86] Lim and colleagues[101] demonstrated with an intracoronary injection of hand-agitated contrast material in humans that there was a lower subendocardial contrast intensity during pacing in regions supplied by a critical coronary stenosis. With IV infusions of microbubbles, the quantitative assessment of myocardial blood flow can also delineate transmural differences.[102] In an open-chest canine study, only the endocardial-to-epicardial ratio of the product of the initial contrast replenishment slope and plateau myocardial signal intensity correlated with radiolabeled microsphere measurements, whereas transmural measurements of myocardial blood volume did not. With real-time pulse sequence schemes, excellent delineation of inducible subendocardial defects during the replenishment phase of contrast are seen during dobutamine stress echocardiography. These defects are observed during the initial 1 to 2 seconds following a high MI impulse during stress imaging and often are not evident at the plateau intensity. An example of such a defect is displayed in Figure 3–9, in which a distal septal and apical subendocardial defect is evident during the replenishment phase of contrast at peak dobutamine stress.

Other Applications of Microbubbles

The Operating Room

When employed in the operating room (OR) during a coronary bypass graft (CABG), intracoronary and aortic root injections of ultrasonographic contrast agent have been useful in several aspects. The effectiveness of saphenous vein grafts has been determined by injection of air-filled microbubbles into the cross-clamped aortic root or directly into the graft.[103-105] Aortic root injections of microbubbles before cardiopulmonary bypass (CPB) have also guided the sequence of bypassing.[106] The peak myocardial video intensity following intra-aortic contrast-enhanced cardioplegia injections has correlated with the eventual improvement in wall motion after bypass grafting.[103,107]

Retrograde (via the coronary sinus [CS]) and antegrade cardioplegic delivery have been compared by using MCE. In these small studies, retrograde delivery was found to be superior in providing myocardial perfusion in certain cases.[108] Keller and colleagues[108] investigated the possibility of quantifying myocardial blood flow in the arrested heart during open-heart surgery and found that the washout of microbubbles was markedly prolonged during antegrade crystalloid cardioplegia, so that it was no longer correlated with tissue flow. The washout delay appeared to result from albumin microbubble adherence to the venules, suggesting that endothelial damage is caused by the cardioplegic solution.[109] This microvasculature damage could be partly avoided when cardioplegia was mixed with blood. The greater the amount of blood in the cardioplegic solution, the higher the observed microbubble transit rate was.[110]

Improved Left Ventricular Cavity Opacification

Several different IV US contrast agents have demonstrated their ability to improve the diagnostic value of echocardiographic examinations in patients with suboptimal imaging conditions. In routine ultrasonographic examinations in patients with poor echocardiographic windows, contrast enhancement of the LV cavity provides better delineation of the endocardial border. Clinically, this could give more information regarding regional and global systolic function that could not be assessed with routine echocardiography. Tissue harmonic imaging by itself has significantly improved endocardial border, often eliminating the need for IV ultrasonographic contrast agents filled with room air.[111] During the past few years, however, studies have shown that because of their consistent left ventricular opacification, IV perfluorocarbon containing micobubbles has improved border definition in the left ventricle of patients with suboptimal tissue harmonic images. Although the use of contrast may increase the costs for routine transthoracic echocardiograms (TTEs), substantial cost savings could still be made in the examination of patients with poor baseline harmonic image quality, because it would prevent the need for additional diagnostic studies in these situations.[112]

Reilly and colleagues[113] recently studied the effect of IV albumin microspheres sonicated injections in harmonic transthoracic echocardiography in the intensive care unit (ICU). Their results indicated a significant increase in interpreter confidence in evaluating myocardial segments that could not be analyzed without contrast application. Furthermore, the ability to estimate LV ejection fraction (EF) was clearly improved with albumin microspheres sonicated. Malhotra and colleagues[114] compared stress echocardiograms performed with both fundamental and harmonic imaging modalities with and without IV albumin microspheres sonicated contrast in 200 patients. They reported that the combination of harmonic ultrasonography with albumin microspheres sonicated resulted in the most consistent endocardial border delineation, which significantly exceeded the quality of either fundamental contrast imaging or tissue harmonic imaging alone. Interobserver agreement with albumin microspheres sonicated and harmonic imaging in this study was 95%. A recent multicenter study compared the reproducibility and accuracy of contrast enhanced cardiac magnetic resonance imaging (MRI), contrast-enhanced and unenhanced echocardiography, and cineventriculography in quantifying ejection fraction using biplane methods. The echocardiographic settings for contrast-enhanced imaging were an MI of 0.3, gain settings of 60%, and compression of 15%. These studies demonstrated that the most reproducible method (lowest intraclass coefficient) for quantifying ejection fraction was contrast enhanced echocardiography.[115] Contrast-enhanced echocardiography also had the highest interobserver agreement for analyzing regional wall motion.[116]

Contrast-induced homogeneous opacification of the LV cavity could also assist physicians in detecting LV thrombi or tumors[117,118] and complications of acute myocardial infarction, such as myocardial rupture and LV pseudoaneurysm.[119] It has also been used during transesophageal echocardiography (TEE) to delineate false and true lumen in patients with aortic dissection.[120] Using a continuous infusion of microbubbles, one can examine the replenishment patterns of contrast within cardiac masses following high MI impulses to differentiate between malignant tumors, stromal tumors, and thrombi.[121] Figure 3–14 demonstrates the excellent delineation of an apical thrombus using real-time perfusion imaging, which was not seen with unenhanced echocardiography or even contrast-enhanced echocardiography with B-mode harmonic imaging at a MI of 0.5. Following high MI impulses, no replenishment of contrast occurred in this mass, confirming that it was a thrombus.

Doppler Enhancement

IV microbubbles affect Doppler recordings, because their scatter is much greater than from red blood cells. Microbubbles therefore can increase the signal strength in a Doppler examination markedly, which may be helpful in patients with suboptimal imaging quality. von Bibra and colleagues[122] described a significant enhancement of spectral and color Doppler and an increase in the signal-to-noise ratio in the quantitative assessment of aortic stenosis (AS), pulmonary venous flow, and mitral regurgitation (MR) by IV injection of galactose (Levovist). Transthoracic pulmonary venous flow velocities have been improved by IV contrast enhancement to the point that they are comparable to those obtained with transesophageal imaging.[123] Moreover, IV microbubble US contrast was successful in providing a clear spectral signal across stenotic aortic valves in cases in which the echocardiogram would have been nondiagnostic without contrast enhancement.[124] The gradients determined using contrast-enhanced Doppler signals correlated well with catheterization calculations.[124] Okura and colleagues[125] studied the effect of albumin (Albunex) in 45 patients with prosthetic aortic valves. They found a significant improvement in transvalvular continuous-wave Doppler signal intensity with IV albumin, increasing the frequency of satisfactory Doppler signals from 64% to 93% of patients. More recently, Jeon and colleagues[126] have demonstrated that a 10% air, 10% blood, 80% saline hand-agitated mixture is more optimal than the traditional agitated air-saline mixture in Doppler enhancement of the tricuspid regurgitant jet. They found that brief premixture of the patient's own blood with air and saline produces greater concentrations of small microbubbles, which improved the accuracy of the pulmonary artery (PA) pressure measurement.

Cerebral, Renal, and Skeletal Muscle Perfusion Imaging

The replenishment curves following microbubble destruction that have been used to detect myocardial blood flow changes can be applied to solid organs as well. The time versus acoustic intensity curve following US-mediated destruction of microbubbles has been validated as a method of measuring blood flow changes within the cerebral microcirculation.[127] This has re-

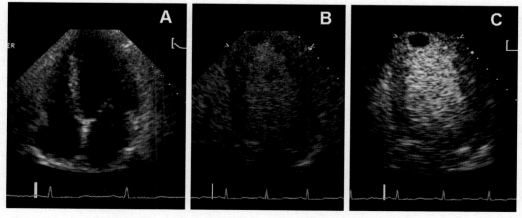

Figure 3–14. An example of how the low mechanical index (0.1) real-time perfusion pulse sequence schemes are even better than low mechanical index (0.5) B-mode harmonic imaging in detecting an apical thrombus. The thrombus was completely missed using noncontrast imaging.

cently been applied in traumatic brain injury (TBI) to documents the beneficial effect of early decompressive surgery on cerebral microvascular blood flow.[128] Quantitative measurements with contrast-enhanced US have also been utilized to demonstrate that physiologic increases in insulin alter microvascular blood volume without altering skeletal muscle blood flow.[129] Contrast-enhanced US has also been shown to accurately quantify renal cortical blood flow changes in response to flow limiting stenoses or during dopamine infusion.[130]

Arteriogenesis and Inflammation Imaging

Several experimental studies have discovered that albumin microbubbles persist in the myocardium in regions undergoing ischemia followed by reperfusion. The reason for this prolonged persistence is not exactly known. There is evidence, however, that endothelial damage and the presence of inflammatory extracellular matrix increase microbubble adherence to vascular endothelium.[131,132]

Lindner and colleagues[133] hypothesized that during the early inflammatory response after reperfusion, activated leukocytes adherent to the venular endothelial surface may bind microbubbles and therefore may be responsible for their prolonged transit. Using tumor necrosis factor-α (TNF-α) injection in an animal setting, they showed that both lipid and albumin microbubbles attach to activated leukocytes. The binding of the albumin microbubbles was mediated by $β_2$-integrins, whereas the interaction between leukocytes and lipid microbubbles involved the complement pathway.[133] In a subsequent investigation, the leukocytes involved were identified to be mostly neutrophils and monocytes. Both lipid and albumin microbubbles were phagocytosed by these cells and remained acoustically active for up to 30 minutes and could be detected in vivo after microbubbles from the blood pool had already vanished.[134]

Microbubbles can be also conjugated with disintegrins. This serves to target the microbubbles to $α_v$ integrins, which are expressed on neovascular endothelium.[135] Unlike unlabeled microbubbles, which pass freely through the microcirculation, these microbubbles are retained within regions of increased arteriogenesis that occur in response to prolonged hind-limb ischemia.[136] The arteriogenic effects of certain agents, such as fibroblast growth factor-2 used to treat ischemic regions, can therefore be assessed non-invasively by measuring signal intensity following IV injections of microbubbles targeted to $α_v$ integrins. Similarly, phosphatidylserine has been incorporated into the shell of microbubbles to increase complement-mediated avidity to activated leukocytes. These microbubbles have been shown to be retained within reperfused myocardium, and the signal intensity derived from these microbubbles correlates closely with the severity and extent of postischemic inflammation.[137] The retained signal intensity from microbubbles targeted to activated leukocytes or up-regulated leukocyte adhesion molecules on the endothelial surface has also been utilized in animal studies to detect rejection following cardiac transplantation.[138,139] Microbubbles targeted to both $α_v$ and $β_3$ integrins and activated leukocytes have been utilized to assess the effects of agents that inhibit endothelial integrin and platelet glycoprotein IIb/IIIa receptors in reducing myocardial infarct size.[140]

Safety of Myocardial Contrast Echocardiography

There have been numerous investigations into the safety of IV microbubbles in humans. The potential concerns related to microbubbles and US are that stabilized gas-containing microbubbles disrupt during insonation. This disruption process (cavitation) could cause endothelial damage or hemorrhage.[141] There is also concern of whether the shell encapsulating the gas-containing microbubble could precipitate allergic reactions. The byproducts of microbubbles are the gas that is emitted from the bubble, which is exhaled via the lungs, and the components of the shell, which are metabolized by liver enzymes. Despite these concerns, microbubble containing perfluorocarbon have been shown to have minimal toxicity in humans. FDA-approved contrast agents include sonicated albumin microspheres and perflutren lipid microspheres. Both of these agents have been used in thousands of patients without toxicity, even in patients with advanced CAD.[94] The reported side effects of sonicated albumin microspheres are headache (5.4%), nausea and vomiting (4.3%), warm sensation or flushing (3.6%), and dizziness (2.5%).[142] Side effects reported with perflutren lipid microspheres are back pain (1.2%), headache (2.3%), flushed sensation in (1.1%), and nausea (1%).[143] No mortalities or prolonged serious adverse effects have been attributed to either of these contrast agents. Postmarket analysis of the contrast agent sulfur hexafluoride (Sonovue) has indicated rare occurrences (0.014%) of severe adverse events that occurred in close association with contrast administration, including three deaths. These deaths, however, were in patients who were considered to have unstable angina at the time of contrast administration. Nonetheless, the use of this agent has had restrictions placed on it when being used in echocardiography.[144,145]

Although diagnostic US MIs do have the potential to disrupt capillaries and induce both hemorrhage and hemolysis, these studies have still only been done in settings in which minimal attenuation of the US beam exists.[146] Much larger human trials using US and contrast during stress echocardiography have confirmed no significant adverse effects occur.[94,145] High MI impulses (up to 1.9) applied during dobutamine stress echocardiography have the potential to elicit isolated ventricular premature depolarizations, but no sustained arrhythmias induced by these transient high MI impulses from diagnostic transducers have been observed.[147]

Therapeutic Applications of Ultrasound and Microbubbles

A number of studies indicate that US-mediated microbubble destruction may also be used for therapeutic purposes. These applications include targeted drug delivery, stimulation of arteriogenesis, and thrombus dissolution.

Drug Delivery

The fact that microbubbles are destroyed by the US beam has led to the study of their potential role in depositing conjugated drugs or genes to an "US-targeted" organ.[148] Skyba and colleagues[149] studied the intravascular destruction of microbubbles containing perfluorocarbon and the bioeffects of this process in the isolated spinotrapezius muscle of rats. With just one sweep of a diagnostic US transducer (2.3 MHz), microbubble destruction was observed that caused local microvessel rupture. When the bubbles were mixed with colloidal particles, these particles were "microinjected" into the interstitial space. The degree of microbubble destruction and resulting "drug delivery" was directly related to the MI used.[150] It has been demonstrated that perfluorocarbon-exposed sonicated dextrose albumin microbubbles bind large quantities of synthetic antisense oligonucleotides.[151] These oligonucleotides are synthetic gene products that can be used to inhibit the translation of messenger ribonucleic acid (RNA) into proteins and enzymes that regulate pathologic processes, such as neointimal hyperplasia following vascular injury. In these studies, external diagnostic US released the synthetic antisense into the insonified kidney if the antisense oligonucleotide was given intravenously already bound to microbubbles. Recombinant adenovirus containing β-galactosidase has been conjugated to the surface of intravenously injected perfluorocarbon-containing albumin microbubbles and successfully targeted to the myocardium of rats by diagnostic US at a high MI (1.5). Postmortem analysis showed β-galactosidase transgene expression in the myocardium after US antigen delivery but no expression of the transgene in the control groups that had received microbubbles alone, virus alone, or virus plus US.[152] Targeted intramyocardial gene delivery has also been reported in vivo with lipid-encapsulated microbubbles.[153] The simultaneous imaging of microbubbles appears to be important in targeted delivery, in that the highest quantity of delivered agent occurs when high MI delivery impulses are applied only when maximal signal intensity from the microbubbles within the region of interest is present[154] (Fig. 3–15). Current diagnostic transducers are equipped with the ability to switch from sensitive low MI pulse sequence schemes, which image the microbubbles, to high MI impulses, which destroy microbubbles carrying drugs. Low frequency, high MI impulses have been shown to create transient, temporary micropores in the endothelial cells.[155] This has led to the observation of microinjections of drugs conjugated to the microbubbles into the subendothelial spaces, even across the blood-brain barrier with transcranial US.[156] Ultrastructural observations following US-mediated destruction of microbubbles in the brain has demonstrated increased numbers of intracytoplasmic vacuoles within the brain capillary endothelium following US-mediated destruction of circulating intracerebral microbubbles.[157] Low MI pulse sequence schemes, therefore, have the advantage of guiding when to apply high MI impulses and thus could significantly reduce unwanted bioeffects of hemorrhage or permanent endothelial injury. Most of these therapeutic effects of diagnostic US transducers are at peak negative pressures and pulse durations that fall within current FDA guidelines.[158]

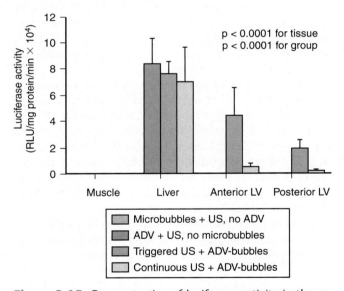

Figure 3–15. *Demonstration of luciferase activity in the anterior and posterior myocardium following intravenous microbubble injections, which are conjugated with the adenovirus encoding the luciferase gene. When diagnostic ultrasound application is in a continuous mode* (yellow bars), *there is minimal deposition of the gene into the myocardium. However, when ultrasound is delivered only when a maximum quantity of microbubbles is present* (triggered ultrasound, green bars), *there is a significant increase in gene transfer. The liver uptake is maximal* (blue bar) *when the adenovirus is administered without microbubbles. Group of microbubbles without ADV* (purple bars) *was not shown due to no activity. ADV, adenovirus encoding the luciferase gene under a cytomegalovirus promoter; LV, left ventricle; RLU, relative light units; US, ultrasound. (From Chen S, Shohet RV, Bekeredjian R, et al: J Am Coll Cardiol 42:301-308, 2003.)*

Thrombolysis

Several investigators have examined the potential use of high-energy US alone to dissolve thrombi in vitro and in an animal setting. Transcatheter US was able to reduce thrombus weight and possibly recanalize occluded femoral arteries.[159] Because this process involves cavitation, more recent investigations have focused on whether microbubbles could potentiate this phenomenon.

When combined with IV perfluorocarbon microbubbles, low-intensity, high-frequency US significantly increased the thrombolytic effect of urokinase in vitro. Even more importantly, US plus microbubbles containing perfluorocarbon alone proved to be equivalent to urokinase in degree of thrombus dissolution. Therefore, it appeared that US and microbubbles could produce a localized clot lysis similar to a fibrinolytic agent without a systemic lytic state.[160] Invasive clot dissolution with therapeutic US and PESDA alone has been successfully tested in animal experiments. In a study involving 10 rabbits, iliofemoral arteries received transcutaneous US treatment on one side and no US treatment on the other after an acute artery thrombotic occlusion. PESDA was given intravenously. After US treatment, all arteries that had received PESDA and US were recanalized by angiography, but none of the arteries treated with PESDA alone were patent. US alone also was unable to recanalize any of the thrombosed vessels.[161]

More recent work has focused on the potential clinical applications of using US and IV microbubbles to recanalize acutely thrombosed arteriovenous grafts and restoring flow in acute intracoronary or intracerebral thrombi.[162-164] Effectiveness may be reduced in the setting of attenuation but may still be feasible if platelet targeted microbubbles are utilized. Although more investigation on this field is required, the combination of US and microbubbles may turn out to be a promising alternative to the established thrombolytic or interventional strategies because of their ability to rapidly localize clot dissolution to just the desired area.

Summary

The use of IV microbubbles for perfusion imaging is now a real-time reality. Multicenter studies are demonstrating whether there is an incremental clinical benefit to examining myocardial perfusion during stress echocardiography and in the evaluation of acute coronary syndromes. IV targeted microbubbles also have a potential role in molecular imaging of arteriogenesis and inflammation. They also may have a significant therapeutic role in the areas of targeted drug delivery, stimulating arteriogenesis, and enhancing thrombolysis.

KEY POINTS

- Ultrasound contrast agents are produced by electromechanical sonification or as lipid encapsulated microbubbles.
- High mechanical index myocardial contrast echocardiography uses intermittent ranging.
- Low mechanical index myocardial contrast echocardiography uses pulse inversion or power modulation.
- Contrast agents may be given as bolus injections or as a continuous infusion.
- Myocardial contrast imaging can be evaluated in a qualitative or quantitative manner.
- Contrast echocardiographic evaluation of myocardial ischemia has been used to detect acute coronary syndromes.
- Myocardial contrast echocardiography can be used to detect myocardial viability.
- Myocardial contrast echocardiography demonstrates areas of inducible ischemia during stress testing.
- Intravenous contrast echocardiography also can be used to detect blood flow in other organs and in tumors.
- Thrombolysis and targeted drug delivery may be possible in the future using microbubbles and ultrasound.

REFERENCES

1. Gramiak R, Shah PM, Kramer DH: Ultrasound cardiography: Contrast studies in anatomy and function. *Radiology* 92:939-948, 1969.
2. Tei C, Sakamaki T, Shah PM, et al: Myocardial contrast echocardiography: A reproducible technique of myocardial opacification for identifying regional perfusion deficits. *Circulation* 67:585-593, 1983.
3. Gross CM, Wann LS, Hurley SE: Evaluation of regional myocardial perfusion by contrast echocardiography using hydrogen peroxide [abstract]. *Circulation* 66 (Suppl II):II-28, 1982.
4. Armstrong WF, West SR, Mueller TM, et al: Assessment of location and size of myocardial infarction with contrast-enhanced echocardiography. *J Am Coll Cardiol* 2:63-69, 1983.
5. Kemper AJ, O'Boyle JE, Sharma S, et al: Hydrogen peroxide contrast-enhanced two-dimensional echocardiography: Real time in vivo delineation of regional myocardial perfusion. *Circulation* 68:603-611, 1983.
6. Armstrong WF, Mueller TM, Kinney EL, et al: Assessment of myocardial perfusion abnormalities with contrast-enhanced two dimensional echocardiography. *Circulation* 66:166-173, 1982.
7. Meltzer RA, Tickner EG, Popp RL: Why do the lungs clear ultrasound contrast? *Ultrasound Med Biol* 6:263-269, 1980.
8. Strauss AL, Beller KD: Persistent opacification of the left ventricle and myocardium with a new echo contrast agent. *Ultrasound Med Biol* 25:763-769, 1999.
9. Porter TR, Xie F: Visually discernible myocardial echocardiographic contrast following intravenous injection of sonicated dextrose albumin microbubbles containing high molecular weight less soluble gases. *J Am Coll Cardiol* 25:509-515, 1995.

10. Xie F, Porter TR: Perfluoropropane enhanced sonicated dextrose albumin produces visually apparent consistent myocardial opacification with physiologic washout and minimal hemodynamic changes following venous injection. *Circulation* 90:I-69, 1994.

11. Feinstein SB, Ten Cate FJ, Zwehl W, et al: Contrast echocardiography. I. In vitro development and quantitative analysis of echo contrast agents. *J Am Coll Cardiol* 3:14-20, 1984.

12. Feinstein SB, Shah PM, Bing RJ, et al: Microbubble dynamics visualized in the intact capillary circulation. *J Am Coll Cardiol* 4:595-600, 1984.

13. Keller MW, Feinstein SB, Briller RA, et al: Automated production and analysis of echo contrast agents. *J Ultrasound Med* 5:493-498, 1986.

14. Barnhart J, Leven H, Villapando E, et al: Characteristics of Albunex: Air-filled albumin microspheres for echocardiography contrast enhancement. *Invest Radiol* 25:S162-S164, 1990.

15. Grinstaff MW, Suslick KS: Air-filled proteinaceous microbubbles: Synthesis of an echo-contrast agent. *Proc Natl Acad Sci U S A* 88:7708-7710, 1991.

16. Christiansen C, Kryvi H, Sontum PC, et al: Physical and biochemical characterization of Albunex, a new ultrasound contrast agent consisting of air-filled albumin microspheres suspended in a solution of human albumin. *Biotechnol Appl Biochem* 19:307-320, 1994.

17. Suslick KS, Grinstaff MW: Protein microencapsulation of nonaqueous liquids. *J Am Chem Soc* 112:7807-7809, 1990.

18. Silverman PR, Feinstein SB, Lang RM, et al: Contrast echocardiography: Effects of microbubbles on coronary blood flow and left ventricular hemodynamics. *Am J Physiol Imaging* 4:158-164, 1989.

19. Vandenberg BF, Kieso R, Fox-Eastham K, et al: Quantitation of myocardial perfusion by contrast echocardiography: Analysis of contrast gray level appearance variables and intracyclic variability. *J Am Coll Cardiol* 13:200-206, 1989.

20. Spotnitz WD, Keller MW, Watson DD, et al: Success of internal mammary bypass grafting can be assessed intraoperatively using myocardial contrast echocardiography. *J Am Coll Cardiol* 12:196-201, 1988.

21. Vandenberg BF, Feinstein SB, Kieso RA, et al: Myocardial risk area and peak gray level measurement by contrast echocardiography: Effect of microbubble size and concentration, injection rate, and coronary vasodilation. *Am Heart J* 115:733-739, 1988.

22. Keller MW, Glasheen W, Smucker ML, et al: Myocardial contrast echocardiography in humans. II. Assessment of coronary blood flow reserve. *J Am Coll Cardiol* 12:925-934, 1988.

23. Monaghan MJ, Quigley PJ, Metcalfe JM, et al: Digital subtraction contrast echocardiography: A new method for the evaluation of regional myocardial perfusion. *Br Heart J* 59:12-19, 1988.

24. Cheirif J, Desir RM, Bolli R, et al: Relation of perfusion defects observed with myocardial contrast echocardiography to the severity of coronary stenosis: Correlation with thallium-201 single-photon emission tomography. *J Am Coll Cardiol* 19:1343-1349, 1992.

25. Reisner SA, Ong LS, Lichtenberg GS, et al: Myocardial perfusion imaging by contrast echocardiography with use of intracoronary sonicated albumin in humans. *J Am Coll Cardiol* 14:660-665, 1989.

26. Rovai D, Ghelardini G, Trivella MG, et al: Intracoronary air-filled albumin microspheres for myocardial blood flow measurement. *J Am Coll Cardiol* 22:2014-2021, 1993.

27. Porter TR, D'Sa A, Turner C, et al: Myocardial contrast echocardiography for the assessment of coronary blood flow reserve: Validation in humans. *J Am Coll Cardiol* 21:349-355, 1993.

28. Feinstein SB, Ten Cate FJ, Cheirif J, et al: Safety and efficacy of a new transpulmonary ultrasound contrast agent: Initial multicenter clinical results. *J Am Coll Cardiol* 16:316-324, 1990.

29. Walker R, Wiencek JF, Aronson S, et al: The influence of intravenous Albunex injection on pulmonary hemodynamics, gas exchange, and left ventricular peak intensity. *J Am Soc Echocardiogr* 5:463-470, 1992.

30. Weyman AE: *Principles and Practice of Echocardiography*. Malvern, PA, Lea & Febiger, 1994, pp 302-326.

31. Meza M, Greener Y, Hunt R, et al: Myocardial contrast echocardiography: Reliable, safe, and efficacious myocardial perfusion assessment after intravenous injection of a new echocardiographic contrast agent. *Am Heart J* 132:871-881, 1996.

32. Colon PJ 3rd, Richards DR, Moreno CA, et al: Benefits of reducing the cardiac cycle-triggering frequency of ultrasound imaging to increase myocardial opacification with FSO69 during fundamental and second harmonic imaging. *J Am Soc Echocardiogr* 10:602-607, 1997.

33. Porter TR, Xie F, Kricsfeld A, et al: Noninvasive identification of acute myocardial ischemia and reperfusion with contrast ultrasound using intravenous perfluoropropane-exposed sonicated dextrose albumin. *J Am Coll Cardiol* 26:33-40, 1995.

34. Wei K, Crouse l, Weiss J, et al: Comparison of usefulness of dipyridamole stress myocardial contrast echocardiography to technetium-99m sestamibi single-photo emission computed tomography for detection of coronary artery disease (PB127 Multicenter Phase 2 Trial Results). *Am J Cardiol* 91:1293-1298, 2003.

35. de Jong N, Ten Cate FJ, Lancee CT: Principles and recent developments in ultrasound contrast agents. *Ultrasonics* 29:324-330, 1991.

36. Chang PH, Shung KK: Second harmonic imaging and harmonic Doppler measurements with Albunex. *IEEE Trans Biomed Eng* 3:1551, 1994.

37. Burns PN, Wilson ST, Muradali D, et al: Microbubble destruction is the origin of harmonic signals from FS069. *Radiology* 201:158, 1996.

38. Burns PN, Wilson SR, Muradali D, et al: Intermittent ultrasound harmonic contrast enhanced imaging and Doppler improves sensitivity and longevity of small vessel detection. *Radiology* 201:159, 1996.

39. Wei K, Jayaweera AR, Firoozan S, et al: Quantification of myocardial blood flow with ultrasound-induced destruction of microbubbles administered as a constant venous infusion. *Circulation* 97:473-483, 1998.

40. Porter TR, Xie F, Kricsfeld D, et al: Improved myocardial contrast with perfluorocarbon-exposed sonicated dextrose albumin. *J Am Coll Cardiol* 27:1497-1501, 1996.

41. Binder T, Assayag P, Baer F, et al: NC100100, a new echo contrast agent for the assessment of myocardial perfusion: Safety and comparison with technetium-99m sestamibi single-photon emission computed tomography in a randomized multicenter study. *Clin Cardiol* 22:273-282, 1999.

42. Main ML, Escobar JF, Hall SA, et al: Detection of myocardial perfusion defects by contrast echocardiography in the setting of acute myocardial ischemia with residual antegrade flow. *J Am Soc Echocard* 11:228-235, 1998.

43. Porter TR, Li S, Kricsfeld D, et al: Detection of myocardial perfusion in multiple echocardiographic windows with one intravenous injection of microbubbles using transient response second harmonic imaging. *J Am Coll Cardiol* 29:791-799, 1997.

44. MacSweeney JE, Cosgrove DO, Arenson J: Colour Doppler energy (power) mode ultrasound. *Clin Radiol* 51:387-390, 1996.

45. Powers JE, Burns PN, Souquet J: Imaging instrumentation for ultrasound contrast agents. In Nanda NC, Schlief R, Goldberg BB (eds): *Advances in Echo Imaging Using Contrast Enhancement*, 2nd ed. Dordrecht, The Netherlands, Kluwer Academic Publishers, 1997, p 139.

46. Broillet A, Puginier J, Ventrone R, et al: Assessment of myocardial perfusion by intermittent harmonic power Doppler using SonoVue: a new ultrasound contrast agent. *Invest Radiol* 33:209-215, 1998.

47. Senior R, Kaul S, Soman P, Lahiri A: Power Doppler harmonic imaging: A feasibility study of a new technique for the assessment of myocardial perfusion. *Am Heart J* 139:245-251, 2000.

48. Heinle SK, Noblin J, Goree-Best P, et al: Assessment of myocardial perfusion by harmonic power Doppler imaging at rest and during adenosine stress: Comparison with (99m) Tc-sestamibi SPECT imaging. *Circulation* 102:55-60, 2000.

49. Simpson DH, Burns PN: Pulse inversion Doppler: A new method for detecting nonlinear echoes from microbubble contrast agents. *Proc IEEE Ultrason Symp* 2:1597, 1997.

50. Burns PN, Wilson SR, Simpson DH: Pulse inversion imaging of liver blood flow: Improved method for characterizing focal masses with microbubble contrast. *Invest Radiol* 35:58-71, 2000.

51. Albrecht T, Hoffmann CW, Schettler S, et al: B-mode enhancement at phase-inversion US with air-based microbubble contrast agent: Initial experience in humans. *Radiology* 216:273-278, 2000.

52. Rafter P, Phillips P, Vannan MA: Imaging technologies and techniques. *Cardiol Clin* 22:181-197, 2004.

53. Skyba DM, Jayaweera AR, Goodman NC, et al: Quantification of myocardial perfusion with myocardial contrast echocardiography during left atrial injection of contrast: Implication for venous injection. *Circulation* 90:1513-1521, 1994.

54. Lindner JR, Villanueva FS, Dent JM, et al: Assessment of resting perfusion with myocardial contrast echocardiography: Theoretical and practical considerations. *Am Heart J* 139:231-240, 2000.

55. Weissman NJ, Mylan CC, Hack TC, et al: Infusion versus bolus contrast echocardiography: A multicenter, open-label, crossover trial. *Am Heart J* 139:399-404, 2000.

56. Wei K, Jayaweera AR, Firoozan S, et al: Basis for detection of stenosis using venous administration of microbubbles during myocardial contrast echocardiography: Bolus or continuous infusion? *Circulation* 32:252-260, 1998.

57. Porter TR, Xie F, Li S, et al: Effect of transducer standoff on the detection, spatial extent, and quantification of myocardial contrast defects caused by coronary stenosis. *J Am Soc Echocardiogr* 12:951-956, 1999.

58. Vogel R, Indermuhle A, Reinhardt J, et al: The quantification of absolute myocardial perfusion in humans by contrast echocardiography. *J Am Coll Cardiol* 45:754-762, 2005.

59. Yano A, Ito H, Iwakura K, et al: Myocardial contrast echocardiography with a new calibration method can estimate myocardial viability in patients with myocardial infarction. *J Am Coll Cardiol* 43:1799-1806, 2004.

60. Wei K, Tong KL, Belcik T, et al: Detection of coronary stenoses at rest with myocardial contrast echocardiography. *Circulation* 112:1154-1160, 2005.

61. Pasquet A, Greenberg N, Brunken R, et al: Effect of color coding and subtraction on the accuracy of contrast echocardiography. *Int J Cardiol* 70:223-231, 1999.

62. Jayaweera AR, Sklenar J, Kaul S: Quantification of images obtained during myocardial contrast echocardiography. *Echocardiography* 11:385-396, 1994.

63. Angermann CE, Kruger TM, Junge R, et al: Intravenous Albunex during transoesophageal echocardiography: Quantitative assessment by videodensitometry and integrated backscatter analysis from unprocessed radiofrequency signals. *J Am Soc Echocardiogr* 8:839-853, 1995.

64. Jiang L, Lu P, Khankirawatana B, et al: Heterogeneity of segmental myocardial video-intensity increments during intermittent harmonic imaging with continuous intravenous infusion of perfluorocarbon microbubbles. *J Am Coll Cardiol* 31:438A:1179, 1998.

65. Toledo E, Lang RM, Collins KA, et al: Imaging and quantification of myocardial perfusion using real-time three-dimensional echocardiography. *J Am Coll Cardiol* 47:146-154, 2006.

66. Ito H, Tomooka T, Sakai N, et al: Time course of functional improvement in stunned myocardium in risk area in patients with reperfused anterior infarction. *Circulation* 87:355-362, 1999.

67. Kaul S, Pandian NG, Okada RD, et al: Contrast echocardiography in acute myocardial ischemia: In-vivo determination of total left ventricular "area at risk." *J Am Coll Cardiol* 4:1272-1282, 1984.

68. Touchstone DA, Nygaard TW, Kaul S: Correlation between left ventricular risk area and clinical, electrocardiographic, hemodynamic, and angiographic variables during acute myocardial infarction. *J Am Soc Echocardiogr* 3:106-117, 1990.

69. Dittrich HC, Bales GL, Kuvelas T, et al: Myocardial contrast echocardiography in experimental coronary artery occlusion with a new intravenously administered contrast agent. *J Am Soc Echocardiogr* 8:465-474, 1995.

70. Grauer SE, Pantely GA, Xu J, et al: Myocardial imaging with a new transpulmonary lipid-fluorocarbon echo contrast agent: Experimental studies in pigs. *Am Heart J* 132:938-945, 1996.

71. Firschke C, Lindner JR, Wei K, et al: Myocardial perfusion imaging in the setting of coronary artery stenosis and acute myocardial infarction using venous injection of a second-generation echocardiographic contrast agent. *Circulation* 96:959-967, 1997.

72. Tong KL, Kaul S, Wang XQ, et al: Myocardial contrast echocardiography versus thrombolysis in myocardial infarction score in patients presenting to the emergency department with chest pain and a nondiagnostic electrocardiogram. *J Am Coll Cardiol* 46:920-927, 2005.

73. Kloner RA, Ganote CE, Jennings RB: The "no-reflow" phenomenon after temporary coronary occlusion in the dog. *J Clin Invest* 54:1496-1508, 1997.

74. Ito H, Tomooka T, Sakaii N, et al: Lack of myocardial perfusion immediately after successful thrombolysis: A predictor of poor recovery of left ventricular function in anterior myocardial infarction. *Circulation* 85:1699-1705, 1992.

75. Lepper W, Hoffmann R, Kamp O, et al: Assessment of myocardial reperfusion by intravenous myocardial contrast echocardiography and coronary flow reserve after primary percutaneous transluminal coronary angiography in patients with acute myocardial infarction. *Circulation* 101:2368-2374, 2000.

76. Firschke C, Lindner JR, Goodman NC, et al: Myocardial contrast echocardiography in acute myocardial infarction using aortic root injections of microbubbles: Potential application in the cardiac catheterization laboratory. *J Am Coll Cardiol* 29:207-216, 1997.

77. Balcells E, Powers ER, Lepper W, et al: Detection of myocardial viability by contrast echocardiography in acute infarction predicts recovery of resting function and contractile reserve. *J Am Coll Cardiol* 41:827-833, 2003.

78. Janardhanan R, Senior R: Accuracy of dipyridamole myocardial contrast echocardiography for the detection of residual stenosis of the infarct-related artery and multivessel disease early after acute myocardial infarction. *J Am Coll Cardiol* 43:2247-2252, 2004.

79. Lim YJ, Nanto S, Masuyama T, et al: Discrepancies between wall motion abnormalities and regional myocardial perfusion in patients with myocardial infarction: Evaluation by myocardial contrast echocardiography. *J Cardiol* 19:343-350, 1989.

80. Lim YJ, Nanto S, Masuyama T, et al: Coronary collaterals assessed with myocardial contrast echocardiography in healed myocardial infarction. *Am J Cardiol* 66:556-561, 1990.

81. Grill HP, Brinker JA, Taube JC, et al: Contrast echocardiographic mapping of collateralized myocardium in humans before and after coronary angioplasty. *J Am Coll Cardiol* 16:1594-1600, 1990.

82. Sabia PJ, Powers ER, Ragosta M, et al: An association between collateral blood flow and myocardial viability in patients with recent myocardial infarction. *N Engl J Med* 327:1825-1831, 1992.

83. Kaul S, Jayaweera AR, Glasheen WP, et al: Myocardial contrast echocardiography and the transmural distribution of flow: A critical appraisal during myocardial ischemia not associated with infarction. *J Am Coll Cardiol* 20:1005-1016, 1992.

84. Kaul S, Senior R, Dittrich H, et al: Detection of coronary artery disease with myocardial contrast echocardiography: Comparison with [99mTc]-sestamibi single-photon emission computed tomography. *Circulation* 96:785-792, 1997.

85. Cwajg J, Xie F, O'Leary E, et al: Detection of angiographically significant coronary artery disease with accelerated intermittent imaging after intravenous administration of ultrasound contrast material. *Am Heart J* 139:675-683, 2000.

86. Shimoni S, Zoghbi WA, Xie F, et al: Real-time assessment of myocardial perfusion and wall motion during bicycle and treadmill exercise echocardiography: comparison with single photon emission computed tomography. *J Am Coll Cardiol* 37:741-747, 2001.

87. Elhendy A, O'Leary EL, Xie F, et al: Comparative accuracy of real-time myocardial contrast perfusion imaging and wall motion analysis during dobutamine stress echocardiography for the diagnosis of coronary artery disease. *J Am Coll Cardiol* 44:2185-2191, 2004.

88. Tsutsui JM, Elhendy A, Anderson JR, et al: Prognostic value of dobutamine stress myocardial contrast perfusion echocardiography. *Circulation* 112:1444-1450, 2005.

89. Porter TR, Xie F, Silver M, et al: Real-time perfusion imaging with low mechanical index pulse inversion Doppler imaging. *J Am Coll Cardiol* 37:748-753, 2001.

90. Olszowska M, Kostkiewicz M, Tracz W, Przewlocki T: Assessment of myocardial perfusion in patients with coronary artery disease. Comparison of myocardial contrast echocardiography and 99mTc MIBI single photon emission computed tomography. *Int J Cardiol* 90:49-55, 2003.

91. Peltier M, Vancraeynest D, Pasquet A, et al: Assessment of the physiologic significance of coronary disease with dipyridamole real-time myocardial contrast echocardiography. Comparison with technetium-99m sestamibi single-photon emission computed tomography and quantitative coronary angiography. *J Am Coll Cardiol* 43:257-264, 2004.

92. Yu EH, Skyba DM, Leong-Poi H, et al: Incremental value of parametric quantitative assessment of myocardial perfusion by triggered Low-Power myocardial contrast echocardiography. *J Am Coll Cardiol* 43:1807-1813, 2004.

93. Moir S, Haluska BA, Jenkins C, et al: Incremental benefit of myocardial contrast to combined dipyridamole-exercise stress echocardiography for the assessment of coronary artery disease. *Circulation* 110:1108-1113, 2004.

94. Tsutsui JM, Elhendy A, Xie F, et al: Safety of dobutamine stress real-time myocardial contrast echocardiography. *J Am Coll Cardiol* 45:1235-1242, 2005.

95. Elhendy A, Tsutsui JM, O'Leary EL, et al: Noninvasive diagnosis of coronary artery disease in patients with diabetes by dobutamine stress real-time myocardial contrast perfusion imaging. *Diabetes Care* 28:1662-1667, 2005.

96. Tsutsui JM, Xie F, McGrain AC, et al: Comparison of low-mechanical index pulse sequence schemes for detecting myocardial perfusion abnormalities during vasodilator stress echocardiography. *Am J Cardiol* 95:565-570, 2005.

97. Xie F, Tsutsui JM, McGrain AC, et al: Comparison of dobutamine stress echocardiography with and without real-time perfusion imaging for detection of coronary artery disease. *Am J Cardiol* 96:506-511, 2005.

98. Jeetley P, Hickman M, Kamp O, et al: Myocardial Contrast Echocardiography for the Detection of Coronary Artery Stenosis. *J Am Coll Cardiol* 47: 141-145, 2005.

99. Korosoglou G, Dubart AE, DaSilva KG Jr, et al: Real-time myocardial perfusion imaging for pharmacologic stress testing: added value to single photon emission computed tomography. *Am Heart J* 151:131-138, 2006.

100. Wei K, Le E, Jayaweera AR, et al: Detection of noncritical coronary stenosis at rest without recourse to exercise or pharmacological stress. *Circulation* 105:218-223, 2002.

101. Lim YJ, Nanto S, Masuyama T, et al: Visualization of subendocardial myocardial ischemia with myocardial contrast echocardiography in humans. *Circulation* 79:233-244, 1989.

102. Linka AZ, Sklenar J, Wei K, et al: Assessment of transmural distribution of myocardial perfusion with contrast echocardiography. *Circulation* 98:1912-1920, 1998.

103. Aronson S, Lee BK, Wiencek JG, et al: Assessment of myocardial perfusion during CABG surgery with two-dimensional transesophageal contrast echocardiography. *Anesthesiology* 75:433-440, 1991.

104. Hirata N, Nakano S, Shimazaki Y, et al: Assessment of the size and distribution of the coronary artery selected for bypass grafting using myocardial contrast echocardiography during coronary artery bypass surgery. *Nippon Kyobu Geka Gakkai Zasshi* 40:13-19, 1992.

105. Mudra H, Zwehl W, Klauss V, et al: Intraoperative myocardial contrast echocardiography for assessment of regional bypass perfusion. *Am J Cardiol* 66:1077-1081, 1990.

106. Goldman ME, Mindich BP: Intraoperative cardioplegic contrast echocardiography for assessing myocardial perfusion during open heart surgery. *J Am Coll Cardiol* 4:1029-1034, 1984.

107. Hirata N, Nakano S, Taniguchi K, et al: Assessment of regional and transmural myocardial perfusion by means of intraoperative myocardial contrast echocardiography during coronary artery bypass grafting. *J Thorac Cardiovasc Surg* 194:1158-1166, 1992.

108. Keller MW, Spotnitz WD, Matthew TL, et al: Intraoperative assessment of regional myocardial perfusion using quantitative myocardial contrast echocardiography: An experimental evaluation. *J Am Coll Cardiol* 16:1267-1279, 1990.

109. Keller MW, Geddes L, Spotnitz WD: Microcirculatory dysfunction following perfusion with hyperkalemic, hypothermic, cardioplegic solutions and blood reperfusion: Effects of adenosine. *Circulation* 84:2485-2494, 1991.

110. Ismail S, Spotnitz WD, Jayaweera AR, et al: Myocardial contrast echocardiography can be used to assess dynamic changes in microvascular function in vivo. *J Am Coll Cardiol* 25:246A, 1995.

111. Main ML, Asher CR, Rubin DN, et al: Comparison of tissue harmonic imaging with contrast (sonicated albumin) echocardiography and Doppler myocardial imaging for enhancing endocardial border resolution. *Am J Cardiol* 83:218-222, 1999.

112. Shaw LJ, Gillam L, Feinstein S, et al: Use of an intravenous contrast agent (Optison) to enhance echocardiography: Efficacy and cost implications. Optison Multicenter Study Group. *Am J Manag Care* 25:SP169-SP176, 1998.

113. Reilly JP, Tunick PA, Timmerman RJ, et al: Contrast echocardiography clarifies uninterpretable wall motion in intensive care unit patients. *J Am Coll Cardiol* 35:485-490, 2000.

114. Malhotra V, Nwogu J, Bondmass MD, et al: Is the technically limited echocardiographic study an endangered species? Endocardial border definition with native tissue harmonic imaging and Optison contrast: A review of 200 cases. *J Am Soc Echocardiogr* 13:771-773, 2000.

115. Hoffmann R, von Bardeleben S, ten Cate F, et al: Assessment of systolic left ventricular function: a multi-centre comparison of cineventriculography, cardiac magnetic resonance imaging, unenhanced and contrast-enhanced echocardiography. *Eur Heart J* 26:607-616, 2005.

116. Hoffmann R, von Bardeleben S, Kasprzak JD, et al: Analysis of regional left ventricular function by cineventriculography, cardiac magnetic resonance imaging, and unenhanced and contrast-enhanced echocardiography. *J Am Coll Cardiol* 47:121-128, 2006.

117. Nagai T, Atar S, Luo H, et al: The usefulness of second generation ultrasound contrast agent to identify intracardiac thrombus [abstract]. *J Am Coll Cardiol* 33:408A, 1999.

118. Thanigaraj S, Schechtman KB, Perez JE: Improved echocardiographic delineation of left ventricular thrombus with the use of intravenous second-generation contrast image enhancement. *J Am Soc Echocardiogr* 12:1022-1026, 1999.

119. Waggoner AD, Williams GA, Gaffron D, et al: Potential utility of left heart contrast agents in diagnosis of myocardial rupture by 2-dimensional echocardiography. *J Am Soc Echocardiogr* 12:272-274, 1999.

120. Kimura BJ, Phan JN, Housman LB: Utility of contrast echocardiography in the diagnosis of aortic dissection. *J Am Soc Echocardiogr* 12:155-159, 1999.

121. Kirkpatrick JN, Wong T, Bednarz JE, et al: Differential diagnosis of cardiac masses using contrast echocardiographic perfusion imaging. *J Am Coll Cardiol* 43:1412-1419, 2004.

122. von Bibra H, Sutherland G, Becher H, et al: Clinical evaluation of left heart Doppler contrast enhancement by a saccharide-based transpulmonary contrast agent. The Levovist Cardiac Working Group. *J Am Coll Cardiol* 25:500-508, 1995.

123. Lambertz H, Schuhmacher R, Tris HP, et al: Improvement of pulmonary venous flow Doppler signal after intravenous injection of Levovist. *J Am Soc Echocardiogr* 10:891-898, 1997.

124. Nakatani S, Imanishi T, Terawawa A, et al: Clinical application of transpulmonary contrast-enhanced Doppler technique in the assessment of severity of aortic stenosis. *J Am Coll Cardiol* 20:973-978, 1992.

125. Okura H, Yoshida K, Akasaka T, et al: Improved transvalvular continuous-wave Doppler signal intensity after intravenous Albunex injection in patients with prosthetic aortic valves. *J Am Soc Echocardiogr* 10:608-612, 1997.

126. Jeon DS, Huai L, Iwami T, et al: The usefulness of a 10% air-10% blood- 80% saline mixture for contrast echocardiography: Doppler measurement of pulmonary artery systolic pressure. *J Am Coll Cardiol* 39:124-129, 2002.

127. Rim SJ, Leong-Poi H, Lindner JR, et al: Quantification of cerebral perfusion with "real-time" contrast-enhanced ultrasound. *Circulation* 104:2582-2587, 2001.

128. Heppner P, Ellegala DB, Durieux M, et al: Contrast ultrasonographic assessment of cerebral perfusion in patients undergoing decompressive craniectomy for traumatic brain injury. *J Neurosurg* 104:738-745, 2006.

129. Coggins M, Linder J, Rattigan S, et al: Physiologic hyperinsulinemia enhances human skeletal muscle perfusion by capillary recruitment. *Diabetes* 50:2682-2690, 2001.

130. Wei K, Le E, Bin JP, et al: Quantification of renal blood flow with contrast-enhanced ultrasound. *J Am Coll Cardiol* 37:1135-1140, 2001.

131. Lindner JR, Ismail S, Spotnitz WD, et al: Albumin microbubble persistence during myocardial contrast echocardiography is associated with microvascular endothelial glycocalyx damage. *Circulation* 98:2187-2194, 1998.

132. Villanueva FS, Jankowski RF, Manaugh C, et al: Albumin microbubble adherence to human coronary endothelium: implications for assessment of endothelial function using myocardial contrast echocardiography. *J Am Coll Cardiol* 30:689-693, 1997.

133. Lindner JR, Coggins MP, Kaul S, et al: Microbubble persistence in the microcirculation during ischemia/reperfusion and inflammation is caused by integrin- and complement-mediated adherence to activated leukocytes. *Circulation* 101:668-675, 2000.

134. Lindner JR, Dayton PA, Coggins MP, et al: Noninvasive imaging of inflammation by ultrasound detection of phagocytosed microbubbles. *Circulation* 102:531-538, 2000.

135. Leong-Poi H, Christiansen J, Klibanov AL, et al: Noninvasive assessment of angiogenesis by ultrasound and microbubbles targeted to alpha (v)-Integrins. *Circulation* 107:455-460, 2003.

136. Leong-Poi H, Christiansen J, Heppner P, et al: Assessment of endogenous and therapeutic arteriogenesis by contrast ultrasound molecular imaging of integrin expression. *Circulation* 111:3248-3254, 2005.

137. Christiansen JP, Leong-Poi H, Klibanov AL, et al: Noninvasive imaging of myocardial reperfusion injury using leukocyte-targeted contrast echocardiography. *Circulation* 105:1764-1767, 2002.

138. Weller GER, Lu E, Csikari MM, et al: Ultrasound imaging of acute cardiac transplant rejection with microbubbles targeted to intercellular adhesion molecule-1. *Circulation* 108:218-224, 2003.

139. Kondo I, Ohmori K, Oshita A, et al: Leukocyte-targeted myocardial contrast echocardiography can assess the degree of acute allograft rejection in a rat cardiac transplantation model. *Circulation* 109:1056-1061, 2004.

140. Sakuma T, Sari I, Goodman CN, et al: Simultaneous integrin $a_v\beta_3$ and glycoprotein IIb/IIIa inhibition causes reduction in infarct size in a model of acute coronary thrombosis and primary angioplasty. *Cardiovasc Res* 66:552-561, 2005.

141. Ay T, Havaux X, Van Camp G, et al: Destruction of contrast microbubbles by ultrasound: Effects on myocardial function, coronary perfusion pressure, and microvascular integrity. *Circulation* 104:461-466, 2001.

142. Optison product information, Mallinckrodt Inc., St. Louis, 1998.

143. Definity product information, Bristol Myers Squibb.

144. Dijkmans PA, Visser CA, Kamp O: Adverse reactions to ultrasound contrast agents: is the risk worth the benefit? *Eur J Echocardiogr* 6(2):363-366, 2005.

145. Timperley J, Mitchell ARJ, Thibault H, et al: Safety of contrast dobutamine stress Echocardiography: A Single Center Experience. *J Am Soc Echocardiogr* 18:163-167, 2005.

146. Miller DL, Driscoll EM, Dou C, et al: Microvascular permeabilization and cardiomyocyte injury provoked by myocardial contrast echocardiography in a canine model. *J Am Coll Cardiol* 47:1464-1468, 2006.

147. Chapman S, Windle J, Xie F, et al: Incidence of cardiac arrhythmias with therapeutic versus diagnostic ultrasound and intravenous microbubbles. *J Ultrasound Med* 24:1099-1107, 2005.

148. Wei K, Skyba DM, Firschke C, et al: Interaction between microbubbles and ultrasound: In vitro and in vivo observations. *J Am Coll Cardiol* 29:1081-1088, 1997.

149. Skyba AM, Price RJ, Linka AZ, et al: Direct in vivo visualization of intravascular destruction of microbubbles by ultrasound and its local effects on tissue. *Circulation* 98:290-293, 1998.

150. Price RJ, Skyba DM, Kaul S, et al: Delivery of colloidal particles and red blood cells to tissue through microvessel ruptures created by targeted microbubble destruction with ultrasound. *Circulation* 98:1264-1267, 1998.

151. Porter TR, Iversen PL, Li S, et al: Interaction of diagnostic ultrasound with synthetic oligonucleotide-labeled perfluorocarbon-exposed sonicated dextrose albumin microbubbles. *J Ultrasound Med* 15:577-584, 1996.

152. Shohet RV, Chen S, Zhou Y-T, et al: Echocardiographic destruction of albumin microbubbles directs gene delivery to the myocardium. *Circulation* 101:2554-2556, 2000.

153. Unger EC, McCreery TP, Sweitzer RH, et al: In vitro studies of a new thrombus-specific ultrasound contrast agent. *Am J Cardiol* 81:58G-61G, 1998.

154. Chen S, Shohet RV, Bekeredjian R, et al: Optimization of ultrasound parameters for cardiac gene delivery of adenoviral or plasmid deoxyribonucleic acid by ultrasound-targeted microbubble destruction. *J Am Coll Cardiol* 42:301-308, 2003.

155. Taniyama Y, Tachibana K, Hiraoka K, et al: Local delivery of plasmid DNA into rat carotid artery using ultrasound. *Circulation* 105:1233-1239, 2002.

156. Kinoshita M, McDannold N, Jolesz FA, Hynynen K: Targeted delivery of antibodies through the blood-brain barrier by MRI-guided focused ultrasound. *Biochem Biophys Res Comm* 340:1085-1090, 2006.

157. Sheikov N, McDannold N, Vykhodtseva N, et al: Cellular mechanisms of the blood-brain barrier opening induced by ultrasound in presence of microbubbles. *Ultrasound Med Biol* 30:979-989, 2004.

158. FDA: *Information for manufacturers seeking marketing clearance of diagnostic ultrasound systems and transducers.* (HHS Publication, FDA, Center for Devices and Radiological Health) Food and Drug Administration, 9200 Corporate Blvd., Rockville MD 20850, 1997.

159. Rosenschein U, Bernstein JJ, DiSegni E, et al: Experimental ultrasonic angioplasty: Disruption of atherosclerotic plaques and thrombi in vitro and arterial recanalization in vivo. *J Am Coll Cardiol* 15:711-717, 1990.

160. Porter TR, LeVeen RF, Fox R, et al: Thrombolytic enhancement with perfluorocarbon-exposed sonicated dextrose albumin microbubbles. *Am Heart J* 132:964-968, 1996.

161. Birnbaum Y, Luo H, Nagai T, et al: Noninvasive in vivo clot dissolution without a thrombolytic drug. *Circulation* 97:130-134, 1998.

162. Xie F, Tsutsui JM, Lof J, et al: Effectiveness of lipid microbubbles and ultrasound in declotting thrombosis. *Ultrasound Med Biol* 31:979-985, 2005.

163. Tsutsui JM, Grayburn PA, Xie F, Porter TR: Drug and gene delivery and enhancement of thrombolysis using ultrasound and microbubbles. *Cardiol Clin* 22:299-312, vii, 2004.

164. Culp WC, Porter TR, Lowery J, et al: Intracranial clot lysis with intravenous microbubbles and transcranial ultrasound in swine. *Stroke* 25:2407-2411, 2004.

Chapter 4

Three-Dimensional Echocardiography

MICHAEL H. PICARD, MD

The author would like to thank MGH sonographers Mary Flaherty, RDCS, and Barbara Jones, RDCS, for their excellent three-dimensional echocardiographic images and Marika Jamacochen, RDCS, and Sarah Fostello, RDCS, for their assistance with three-dimensional image display.

For full use and understanding of two-dimensional (2D) echocardiography, the user must be able to mentally integrate a series of these views into a three-dimensional (3D) image of the heart and its components. For example, when performing 2D echocardiography on a patient with prolapse of a portion of the posterior mitral valve leaflet, the echocardiographer individually examines each portion of the valve from a series of 2D images and mentally reconstructs the entire valve to determine which portion of the valve is prolapsing. To accurately perform this task, one must know the precise relationship of each 2D image to one another. In addition, when quantifying cardiac chamber volumes, mass, or function with 2D echocardiography, one relies on assumptions about the geometry of the chamber to apply specific formulas and calculate these and other parameters. As chambers become distorted in shape, the geometric assumptions about shape become less accurate as do the calculated values using these formulas.

3D echocardiography either via transthoracic or transesophageal approaches eliminates the need for cognitive 3D reconstruction of image planes and the need to use geometric assumptions about shape of structures for cardiac quantitation. This is particularly applicable to complex shapes, such as the right ventricle, an aneurysmal left ventricle, an asymmetrically stenotic or regurgitant valve orifice, eccentric regurgitant jets assessed by color Doppler, valve annulae, and the complex structural relationships observed in congenital heart lesions. The 3D echocardiographic technique has the potential to decrease the time required for complete image acquisition of the heart. Also the 3D echocardiogram can be viewed from various projections by rotation of the images and thus an improved appreciation of the relationships between various cardiac structures can be obtained.

Recently the pace of development and clinical application of 3D echocardiography has increased. Initial development of 3D echocardiography required transducer locating systems. The offline image reconstruction was time- and labor-intensive. As computer hardware and software have matured, these processes have become easier to apply and thus the acquisition and display of 3D ultrasound (US) images has moved from being predominantly a research tool to being used in clinical applications. Transducer technology has also evolved to now enable 3D US imaging in real time. Whereas color Doppler data can also be obtained and displayed in three dimensions, the majority of this chapter will focus on imaging of cardiac structures.

Technical Considerations

The 3D US data set can be acquired either as (1) a series of 2D images and then reconstructed into a 3D image (reconstruction technique) or (2) as a 3D volume of US data (volumetric technique). The reconstruction method requires that the precise location and timing of the each image be known to facilitate the integration of the collection of images. The volumetric approach requires a specialized rectangular (or matrix) array transducer to collect a pyramidal (or 3D) volume of image data. With either method, the image can be displayed in many fashions. The surface of a structure can be displayed as a solid object. Alternatively, the volume can be displayed with varying degrees of transparency and shading to show different depths, thus allowing visualization of various structures within the volume.

Three-Dimensional Echocardiography Using Reconstruction Techniques

The earliest 3D echocardiograms were obtained using the reconstruction technique.[1,2] With this technique, images are obtained from varying transducer locations of known position gated to the cardiac and respiratory cycle. Using various software programs, the 3D coordinates of each image are registered; each image is positioned into its proper three dimensional spatial location at specific times of the cardiac cycle; and then the structure can be reconstructed as a 3D object using image processing techniques, including interpolation and segmentation. The surfaces and volumes are then rendered for display. Objects and their relative positions in this 3D space or coordinate system can be quantified.

For maximum flexibility in obtaining the set of component 2D images, freehand scanning can be performed. With this approach, the position of the transducer and thus the image planes are quantified by one of a variety of spatial locating devices attached to the transducer. Advantages of this method are that nonparallel, intersecting images can be combined and that the transthoracic transducer can be applied to any place on the chest. The spatial locating devices range from mechanical arms to acoustic devices to electromagnetic systems. The spatial resolution of these locating systems is quite precise, and studies have shown that locations computed by these systems differ from true location by <1 mm. A disadvantage of this method is that these locating devices add bulk to the transducer. For the acoustic devices, an unobstructed path from the transmitter to the receiver is required, making some echocardiographic views difficult to obtain. The electromagnetic device requires the absence of metallic objects in a wide area. The process of registering the images in time and space for the reconstruction can be labor intensive and time consuming. Despite these challenges many important studies were performed with this initial approach.[3-9] One example is its role in refining the definition of mitral valve prolapse (MVP).[3] Early 3D echocardiographic reconstructions demonstrated that the mitral valve annulus is saddle-shaped and thus prolapse of the leaflets below the low points of the annulus into the left atrium (LA) can only be observed in 2D echocardiographic views that display the anterior and posterior portions of the annulus (parasternal and apical long-axis views).

A second approach for the reconstruction method is to have the transducer move in preset increments in a known direction ("pull back") and obtain a series of parallel images (Fig. 4–1A). The position of each image relative to the others is known and thus a transducer locating device is not required. Gating to respiration is required to keep the heart in the same position in each image or images are obtained during held respirations. Gating to the cardiac cycle is also necessary. This approach has been used for transesophageal echocardiographic (TEE) 3D reconstructions and for 3D reconstructions of intravascular US images. This technique has proved difficult for transthoracic imaging because optimum acoustic windows across a long enough path of parallel transducer positions is rarely achieved or do not span enough of the cardiac structures of interest.

A third method for 3D reconstruction is to keep the transducer fixed at one position on the chest and for it to be moved in a fan-like motion or rotated around 180 degrees (Fig. 4–1B,C). This is often done with a transthoracic transducer housed within a device that mechanically moves it in known increments or with a multiplane transesophageal transducer (either within the esophagus or applied to the chest wall). Gating to the cardiac and respiratory cycles is still required, but this approach has proven more popular than the free-

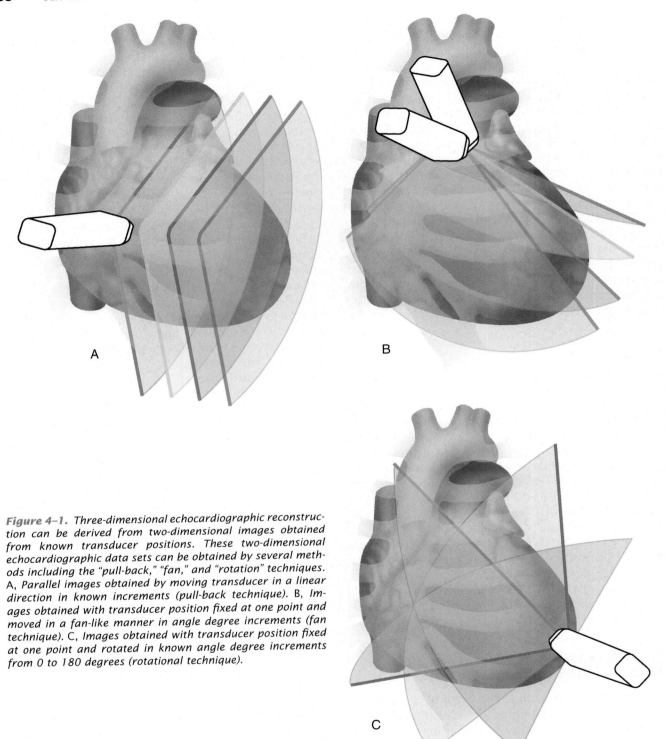

Figure 4-1. *Three-dimensional echocardiographic reconstruction can be derived from two-dimensional images obtained from known transducer positions. These two-dimensional echocardiographic data sets can be obtained by several methods including the "pull-back," "fan," and "rotation" techniques. A, Parallel images obtained by moving transducer in a linear direction in known increments (pull-back technique). B, Images obtained with transducer position fixed at one point and moved in a fan-like manner in angle degree increments (fan technique). C, Images obtained with transducer position fixed at one point and rotated in known angle degree increments from 0 to 180 degrees (rotational technique).*

hand scanning approach that requires transducer locating devices. The reconstruction technique is currently the only method available for transesophageal 3D imaging (Fig. 4-2). The amount of time required to obtain the image set depends on the heart rate, respiratory rate, and the spatial increments of transducer motion.

Whereas the reconstruction method is time consuming because of image acquisition, spatial registration, offline reconstruction, and image rendering and display, this approach has proven accurate and valuable for quantitation of left ventricular (LV) size and function, right ventricular (RV) size and function, pericardial effusions, and valve disease. For 3D echocardiograms obtained by any of the reconstruction methods, the quality of the 3D image depends on the quality of the component 2D images and on the number of com-

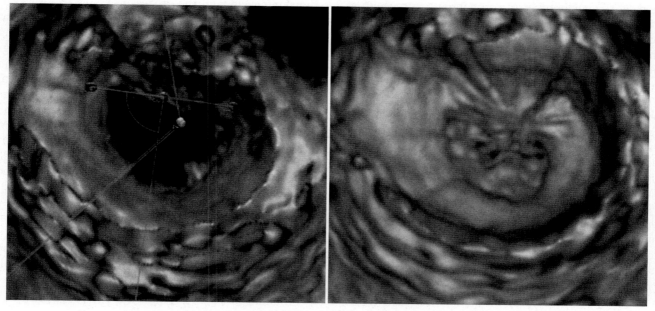

A   B

Figure 4–2. Three-dimensional transesophageal echocardiographic display of the mitral valve in diastole (A) and systole (B) reconstructed from a series of two-dimensional rotational images gated to cardiac and respiratory cycle. (Courtesy of Michael D'Ambra, MD, Brigham and Women's Hospital.)

ponent images used. The more frequent the image sampling, the better the reconstruction. With freehand scanning, quantitation of LV volume has been shown to be accurate with reconstruction from as few as eight intersecting nonparallel 2D images[10]; whereas visualization of focal pathology on smaller or rapidly moving structures, such as the mitral valve, may require a larger number of component images.

3D color flow Doppler can be acquired with reconstruction techniques. With offline processing the volume-rendered 3D color flow jets can be displayed superimposed on gray scale images.[11]

Three-Dimensional Echocardiography Using Volumetric Techniques

The development of a complex transthoracic US transducer enabled acquisition of 3D volume data sets in real time or "near" real time. To achieve this goal, the transducer elements are typically arranged in a rectangular grid or matrix array, and advanced electronics enable beam steering in multiple directions (Fig. 4–3). To scan a volume of adequate size and at a reasonable frame rate, multiple US pulses must be emitted from this matrix array at the same time and processed in parallel. The earliest device utilized a sparse-array matrix transducer with 256 elements and acquired a pyramid-shaped volume of US data within a single cardiac cycle.[12-14] Whereas this provided real-time 3D images, the spatial and temporal resolution were not ideal and volume rendering was not performed on the machine.

Current real-time 3D systems utilize matrix array transducers with 3000 to 4000 elements. A pyramid-shaped 3D US volume of about 30 by 50 degrees can be

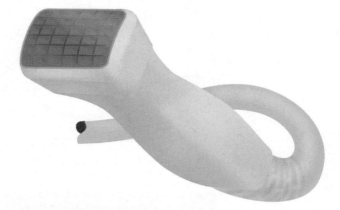

Figure 4–3. Schematic of a matrix array transducer. Over 3000 elements are arranged in a rectangular grid. Multiple ultrasound pulses are transmitted at the same time and processed in parallel to obtain a three-dimensional volume of ultrasound image data. Instead of three-dimensional volumetric acquisition, the firing of the matrix array transducer elements can also be configured to obtain multiple two-dimensional image planes at the same time.

acquired and displayed in real time. With this sized volume, only a portion of the adult heart can typically be displayed in real time and three dimensions. However, this is large enough to display valves, the right ventricle, complex defects, masses, color Doppler jets, the infant left ventricle, or portions of the adult left ventricle. To optimally visualize this real-time 3D US image, one rotates the image to view from all perspectives. Currently, display of a larger volume requires acquisition of at least four smaller 3D US component volumes over a series of cardiac cycles, and these are then combined to yield a 90 by 90 degrees image set. Color Doppler flow mapping is performed with acquisition of a larger number of component volumes. To reduce artifacts that would appear in these fused images resulting from changes in position of the heart during the image acquisition, it is best if the images are acquired with held respiration. Currently these 3D image sets are obtained at a frame rate of 20 to 25 Hz.

Matrix array transducers can also be utilized to obtain multiple image planes of a structure during the same cardiac cycle. Rather than transmit and receive elements from the transducer to obtain a volume of US data, the pattern of firing of the elements can be configured to transmit and receive a series of 2D planes. This real-time multiplane imaging is of particular interest for quantitation. For example, the endocardial borders from a series of simultaneous apical views of the left ventricle can be automatically or manually traced to calculate the LV volume and systolic function. This is similar to the approach with 3D reconstruction methods, except that all images of the heart are obtained in the same cycle, and the processing is faster. This real-time multiplane approach can be used to ensure that 2D images are on axis. For example, while visualizing a parasternal long-axis view as a guide, a second imaging plane can be directed that is perpendicular to the narrowest opening of the leaflet tips of a stenotic mitral valve (Fig. 4–4).

When the 3D US volume is first displayed on the echocardiographic machine or a workstation, only an outer surface of the pyramidal data set is seen and it provides little information. To visualize the cardiac structures within this volume, layers of it must be removed—a process referred to as "cropping" (Fig. 4–5). Multiple cropping planes can be performed to display structures of interest and the relationship of several structures to one another (Fig. 4–6).

3D color flow Doppler can be acquired with the volumetric technique and displayed in real time simultaneously with the gray scale images.[15,16]

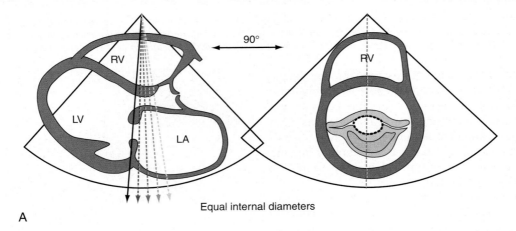

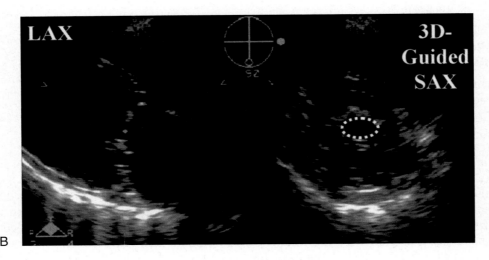

Figure 4–4. *Use of simultaneous transthoracic echocardiographic multiplane images to accurately guide image plane position to quantify mitral stenosis as shown in schematic (A) and real time images (B). Using the parasternal long-axis (LAX) image as a guide, a second scan plane is positioned orthogonally (dotted lines) and then moved until it passes through the smallest orifice at the mitral leaflet tips (solid line). Planimetry of the leaflet tips in the orthogonal short-axis image (SAX) view then yields the mitral valve area. LA, left atrium; LV, left ventricle, RV, right ventricle; 3D, three dimensional. (Reproduced with permission from Sebag I, et al: Am J Cardiol 96:1151-1156, 2005.)*

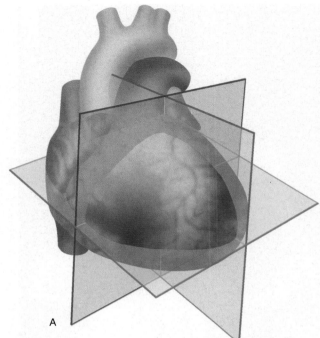

Figure 4–5. *Cropping of a full-volume ultrasound. To visualize structures within the three-dimensional ultrasound volume (B-1), cropping is performed. A, A schematic of standard cropping in transverse, sagittal, and coronal planes is shown with the colors corresponding to the image planes shown below; however, any three-dimensional cropping plane can be created. B, Individual cropping planes through an ultrasound volume collected from the apical transducer position demonstrate cardiac structures from various perspectives. The transverse plane in blue (B-2) yields a short-axis view (B-3) viewed from the left ventricular (LV) apex; the sagittal plane in red (B-4) yields either an apical two-chamber (B-5) view viewed from the right ventricle (RV) or (B-6) viewed from the lateral wall or long-axis view depending on depth and angle of the cropping plane; and the coronal plane in green (B-7) yields an apical four-chamber view viewed from the front (B-8) or from behind (B-9). B-1, full-volume of ultrasound; B-2, transverse crop plane; B-3, transverse plane viewed from LV apex; B-4, sagittal plane; B-5, sagittal viewed from RV; B-6, sagittal viewed from lateral wall; B-7, coronal plane; B-8, coronal viewed from front; B-9, coronal viewed from behind.*

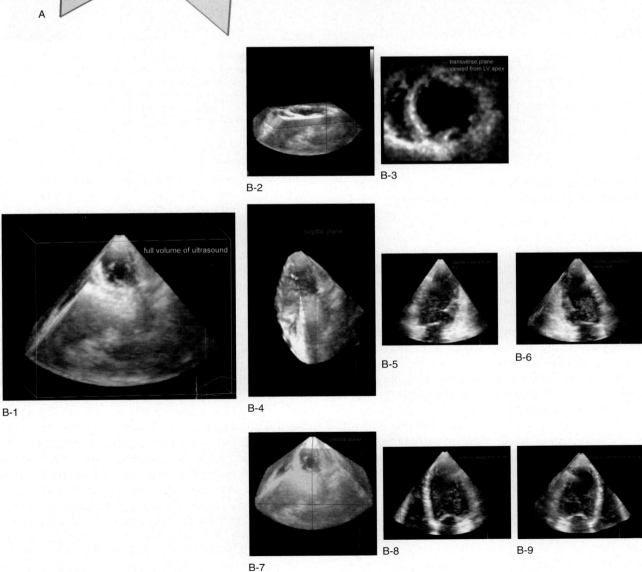

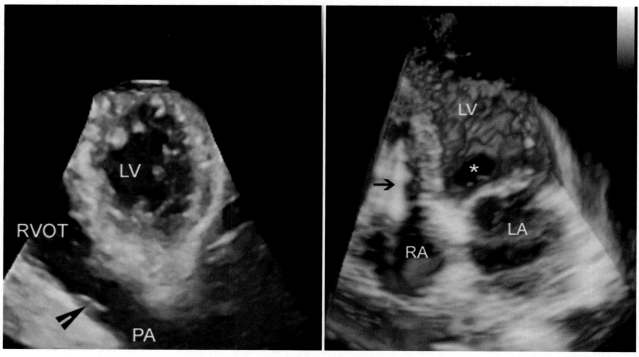

A

B

Figure 4–6. Illustrations of unique transthoracic echocardiographic views obtained by cropping full-volume three-dimensional data sets. A, Cross section of the left ventricle, long axis of right ventricular outflow tract, pulmonic valve (black arrowhead) and main pulmonary artery. B, View of heart from a lateral perspective. The left ventricular outflow tract (*) and open aortic valve are observed along with a pacemaker (arrow) in the right ventricle. LA, left atrium; LV, left ventricle; PA, pulmonary artery; RA, right atrium; RVOT, right ventricular outflow tract. (A, Courtesy of General Electric Healthcare Technologies.)

Advantages and Disadvantages of Three-Dimensional Acquisition Techniques

Compared to the reconstruction technique, image acquisition with the volumetric method is simpler and potentially faster. With the real-time 3D and the real-time multiplane display, there is no time needed for offline reconstruction and display. For the "near real-time, full-volume" method, offline manipulation (cropping) is required but typically the amount of time required compared to reconstruction techniques is short. Whereas for many reconstruction techniques, image rendering, display, and cropping are more complex, these processes with rotational data sets have become simpler. At present, the image quality with the reconstruction techniques and the real-time multiplane display is better compared to the real-time 3D and full-volume 3D images. This results from current limitations of the matrix array transducer—frame rate, number of transducer elements, and so on. For some of the methods, quantitation from the 3D image requires transfer to a special workstation. Because reconstruction techniques and the current full-volume method combine multiple images gated to the cardiac and respiratory cycle, accurate image display can be challenging when the heart rate is irregular, such as during arrhythmias and when the patient is breathing at a rapid rate or

with varying effort. The motion artifacts that may result will be most apparent in the cropped views that include the interfaces of the combined images. For example, if the mitral valve imaging volume is acquired by fusing four sequential volume sets from a parasternal short-axis view (medial commissure to lateral commissure of the valve) during which the patient coughs, when the images are cropped and viewed from the perspective of the LA or the LV apex (i.e., transverse plane or short-axis view of the valve), one will see the motion artifact with the appearance that the images are not stitched together well. However, if one crops and views from the perspective of the ventricular septum to observe a long-axis of the valve (sagittal plane), display of such artifacts would be minimized. Because of the time required for image rendering and display, the reconstruction approach to 3D transthoracic echocardiography (TTE) has not been integrated into clinical practice, but this approach is used with TEE. Because quantitation of cardiac structure and function are accurate with the reconstruction approach, it is used in research applications with both transthoracic and transesophageal modalities. Real-time 3D, full-volume 3D, and real-time 3D multiplane echocardiography have only recently been introduced into clinical practice.

At present depiction of color flow Doppler with both the reconstruction and volumetric methods have limitations. The reconstruction method requires additional offline processing, whereas color flow Doppler jet interrogation with the volumetric method are subject to low frame rates. Lastly, pulse wave and continuous wave Doppler capabilities are not yet available on matrix array transducers.

Three-Dimensional Echocardiographic Work Flow

The images obtained and cropped from a 3D US volume should focus on the goals of the imaging. For example, assessment of ventricular function, aortic valve function, or an atrial septal defect requires reconstructions or volume acquisitions of different parts of the heart. It is likely that in the future, specific imaging protocols will be developed. Ideally this approach will include a rapid acquisition of the 3D US volume and then the majority of image preparation time will be spent cropping the volume to display and quantify cardiac structures, function, and pathology. This cropping may be standardized to demonstrate all cardiac structures in specific orientations. For example, the cardiac volume can be cropped in planes sagittal (apical two-chamber or long axis depending on angle and depth of plane), coronal (apical four-chamber) and transverse (short axis) relative to the heart (see Fig. 4–5). However, because in many cases of cardiac pathology the anatomic relationships may be altered, it is critical to individualize the cropping process to optimize the views of each cardiac structure. This is particularly true for color flow Doppler assessment in which the paths of regurgitant jets do not respect standardized planes.

Evidence-Based Applications of Three-Dimensional Echocardiography

Left Ventricular Volume and Function

Validation studies using a variety of gold standards have demonstrated the improved accuracy of 3D echocardiographic-derived LV volume compared to LV volumes measured from 2D echocardiograms in humans[17] (Table 4–1).

This improvement relates to the fact that a more accurate representation of the LV endocardial surface occurs with the 3D echocardiogram than the 2D echocardiogram. The volume calculation with 2D echocardiograms relies on some assumptions of the symmetry and geometry of the left ventricle, whereas the volume of the left ventricle by the 3D echocardiographic technique is calculated from the reconstructed 3D LV endocardial surface without assumptions of shape. Also, methods used with 2D echocardiography are at risk to yield underestimations if the images used for the quantitation are foreshortened (Fig. 4–7). With 3D echocar-

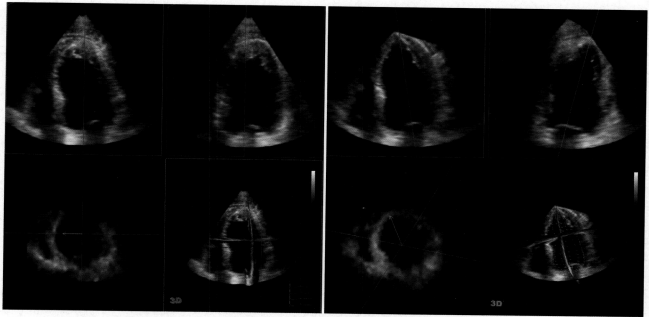

A   B

Figure 4–7. *The full-volume transthoracic ultrasound data set enables positioning of cropping planes so that the true length of the left ventricle is visualized and measured.* A, *Typical two-dimensional imaging planes for the four-chamber (coronal plane, upper left) and two-chamber (sagittal plane, upper right) views fail to include an aneurysm at the anterior apex of the left ventricle.* B, *Coronal (green) and sagittal (red) cropping planes adjusted through the true long axis of the left ventricle in the same full-volume data set. The endocardial borders are then detected and an accurate left ventricular volume quantified. End-diastolic volume (yellow shell) is shown in lower right panel.*

TABLE 4-1. Left Ventricular Volume Quantitation in Humans by Three-Dimensional Echocardiography Compared to a Reference Standard

First Author	3D Technique	Subjects Studied	n	Reference Standard	Pearson Linear Correlation Coefficient (r)	SEE (mL)	Mean Difference ±1 SD of the Difference (Bland-Altman Analysis, mL)	Interobserver Variability (%)
Gopal and colleagues[a]	Reconstruction, freehand scanning, spark gap transducer locator	Normal	15	MRI	EDV 0.92 ESV 0.81	7 4	—	5 8
Sapin and colleagues[b]	Reconstruction, freehand scanning, spark gap transducer locator	Patients evaluated for CAD	35	Ventriculography	EDV 0.97 EDV 0.98	11 10	13±13 -1±13	11 9
Buck and colleagues[c]	Reconstruction, rotational scanning	Patients with CAD and aneurysms	23	MRI	EDV 0.97 ESV 0.97	15 12	-11±15 -3±13	—
Nosir and colleagues[d]	Reconstruction, rotational scanning	Patients with CAD (31) and normal (15)	46	MRI	EDV 0.98 ESV 0.98	—	-1±14 -2±11	—
Lange and colleagues[e]	Reconstruction, rotational scanning	Patients with CAD	16	Ventriculography	Combined EDV+ESV 0.98	7	EDV -13±9 ESV -7±5	10 7
Lange and colleagues[e]	Reconstruction, rotational scanning, tissue Doppler imaging	Patients with CAD	16	Ventriculography	Combined EDV+ESV 0.99	5	EDV -4±5 ESV -2±5	—
Nosir and colleagues[f]	Reconstruction, rotational scanning	Patients with CAD (25) and normal (15)	40	MRI	EDV 0.98 ESV 0.99	—	-1±14 -2±11	—
Schmidt and colleagues[g]	Real-time 3D	Patients with cardiac diseases (21) and normal (4)	25	MRI	EDV 0.88 ESV 0.82 Combined: 0.91	Combined EDV + ESV = 28	Combined EDV + ESV = -17±36	—
Belohlavek and colleagues[h]	Reconstruction, rotational scanning	Patients with several cardiac diseases (10)	11	Electron-beam CT	EDV 0.96 ESV 0.96	21 15	-5±20 -7±16	6 9
Lee and colleagues[i]	Real-time 3D	Patients with "various cardiac disorders"	25	MRI	EDV 0.99 ESV 0.99	11 10	+1±12 +4±10	—
Mannaerts and colleagues[j]	Reconstruction, freehand scanning, electromagnetic locator	Patients with CAD (16), other cardiac diseases and normal (7)	28	MRI	EDV 0.74 ESV 0.88	—	-14±14 -18±24	2 7
Kawai and colleagues[k]	Reconstruction, freehand scanning, electromagnetic locator	Patients with CAD (10) and other cardiac diseases	15	Gated radionuclide ventriculography	EDV 0.94 ESV 0.96	22 15	+7±25 +4±18	7 6

Study	Method	Population (n)	n	Comparison	Correlation (r)		Bias (mean ± SD)	
Kühl and colleagues[l]	Real-time 3D with semi-automated border detection	Patients with cardiomyopathy (14) and normal (10)	24	MRI	EDV 0.98 ESV 0.98	18 18	−14±19 −13±21	—
Arai and colleagues[m]	Real-time 3D	Patients with CAD and wall motion abnormalities	25	SPECT	EDV 0.97 ESV 0.98	—	3±14 2±9	4 6
Jenkins and colleagues[n]	Real-time 3D	Patients referred for echocardiography	50	MRI	—	—	—	—
Corsi and colleagues[o]	Real-time 3D, measurement of LV volume throughout cardiac cycle	Normal and patients with CAD, dilated cardiomyopathy and other cardiac diseases	16	MRI	EDV 0.99 ESV 0.99	—	3±6 3±4	—
Jacobs and colleagues[p]	Real-time 3D with semi-automated border detection	Patients referred for cardiac MRI	50	MRI	EDV 0.96 ESV 0.97	—	−14±17 −7±16	10 11

[a]Gopal AS, Keller AM, Rigling R, et al: Left ventricular volume and endocardial surface area by three-dimensional echocardiography: Comparison with two-dimensional echocardiography and nuclear magnetic resonance imaging in normal subjects. *J Am Coll Cardiol* 22(1):258-270, 1993.

[b]Sapin PM, Schroder KM, Gopal AS: Comparison of two- and three-dimensional echocardiography with cineventriculography for measurement of left ventricular volume in patients. *J Am Coll Cardiol* 24(4):1054-1063, 1994.

[c]Buck T, Hunold P, Wentz KU, et al: Tomographic three-dimensional echocardiographic determination of chamber size and systolic function in patients with left ventricular aneurysm: Comparison to magnetic resonance imaging, cineventriculography, and two-dimensional echocardiography. *Circulation* 96(12):4286-4297, 1997.

[d]Nosir YF, Lequin MH, Kasprzak JD, et al: Measurements and day-to-day variabilities of left ventricular volumes and ejection fraction by three-dimensional echocardiography and comparison with magnetic resonance imaging. *Am J Cardiol* 82(2):209-214, 1998.

[e]Lange A, Palka P, Nowicki A, et al: Three-dimensional echocardiographic evaluation of left ventricular volume: comparison of Doppler myocardial imaging and standard gray-scale imaging with cineventriculography—an in vitro and in vivo study. *Am Heart J* 135(6 Pt 1):970-979, 1998.

[f]Nosir YF, Stoker J, Kasprzak JD, et al: Paraplane analysis from precordial three-dimensional echocardiographic data sets for rapid and accurate quantification of left ventricular volume and function: A comparison with magnetic resonance imaging. *Am Heart J* 137(1):134-143, 1999.

[g]Schmidt MA, Ohazama CJ, Agyeman KO, et al: Real-time three-dimensional echocardiography for measurement of left ventricular volumes. *Am J Cardiol* 84(12):1434-1439, 1999.

[h]Belohlavek M, Tanabe K, Jakrapanichakul D, et al: Rapid three-dimensional echocardiography: Clinically feasible alternative for precise and accurate measurement of left ventricular volumes. *Circulation* 103(24):2882-2884, 2001.

[i]Lee D, Fuisz AR, Fan PH, et al: Real-time 3-dimensional echocardiographic evaluation of left ventricular volume: Correlation with magnetic resonance imaging—a validation study. *J Am Soc Echocardiogr* 14(10):1001-1009, 2001.

[j]Mannaerts HF, Van Der Heide JA, Kamp O, et al: Quantification of left ventricular volumes and ejection fraction using freehand transthoracic three-dimensional echocardiography: Comparison with magnetic resonance imaging. *J Am Soc Echocardiogr* 16(2):101-109, 2003.

[k]Kawai J, Tanabe K, Morioka S, Shiotani H: Rapid freehand scanning three-dimensional echocardiography: Accurate measurement of left ventricular volumes and ejection fraction compared with quantitative gated scintigraphy. *J Am Soc Echocardiogr* 16(2):110-115, 2003.

[l]Kühl HP, Schreckenberg M, Rulands D, et al: High-resolution transthoracic real-time three-dimensional echocardiography: Quantitation of cardiac volumes and function using semi-automatic border detection and comparison with cardiac magnetic resonance imaging. *J Am Coll Cardiol* 43(11):2083-2090, 2004.

[m]Arai K, Hozumi T, Matsumura Y, et al: Accuracy of measurement of left ventricular volume and ejection fraction by new real-time three-dimensional echocardiography in patients with wall motion abnormalities secondary to myocardial infarction. *Am J Cardiol* 94(5):552-558, 2004.

[n]Jenkins C, Bricknell K, Hanekom L, Marwick TH: Reproducibility and accuracy of echocardiographic measurements of left ventricular parameters using real-time three-dimensional echocardiography. *J Am Coll Cardiol* 44(4):878-886, 2004.

[o]Corsi C, Lang RM, Veronesi F, et al: Volumetric quantification of global and regional left ventricular function from real-time three-dimensional echocardiographic images. *Circulation* 112(8):1161-1170, 2005.

[p]Jacobs LD, Salgo IS, Goonewardena S, et al: Rapid online quantification of left ventricular volume from real-time three-dimensional echocardiographic data. *Eur Heart J* 27(4):460-468, 2006.

CAD, coronary artery disease; CT, computed tomography; EDV, end-diastolic left ventricular volume; ESV, end-systolic left ventricular volume; mL, milliliters; MRI, magnetic resonance imaging; SD, standard deviation; SEE, standard error of the estimate; 3D, three dimensional.

Adapted from Hung J, Lang R, Flachskampf F, et al: *J Am Soc Echocardiogr* 20(3):213-233, 2007.

Continued

TABLE 4-1. Left Ventricular Volume Quantitation in Humans by Three-Dimensional Echocardiography Compared to a Reference Standard—cont'd

First Author	3D Technique	Subjects Studied	n	Reference Standard	Pearson Linear Correlation Coefficient (r)	SEE (mL)	Mean Difference ±1 SD of the Difference (Bland-Altman Analysis, mL)	Interobserver Variability (%)
Bu and colleagues[q]	Real-time 3D	Children	19	MRI	EDV 0.97 ESV 0.97	9 3	−7±10 −2±3	3 0
Caiani and colleagues[r]	Real-time 3D	Patients referred for MRI: normal (7), cardiomyopathy (9), CAD (15), other (15)	46	MRI	EDV 0.97 ESV 0.97	17 16	−4±15 −4±17	8 13
Hibberd and colleagues[s]	Reconstruction, freehand scanning, magnetic locator	Normal (12), cardiomyopathy (13)	25	MRI	EDV 0.99 ESV 0.99	9 6	—	6 7
Krenning and colleagues[t]	Reconstruction, rotational scanning	Patients with MI	17	MRI	EDV 0.99 ESV 0.96	7 7	−10±13 −3±15	—
van den Bosch and colleagues[u]	Real-time 3D	Patients with CHD, referred for MRI	29	MRI	EDV 0.97 ESV 0.98	9 5	−3±12 1±10	—
Fukuda and colleagues[v]	Reconstruction, rotational scanning	Patients scheduled for SPECT	25	SPECT	EDV 0.97 ESV 0.99	—	0±5 0±3	5 6
Gutierrez-Chico and colleagues[w]	Real-time 3D	Patients with cardiomyopathy	35	MRI	EDV 0.99 ESV 0.99	—	−13±11 −10±8	—

[q]Bu L, Munns S, Zhang H, et al: Rapid full volume data acquisition by real-time 3-dimensional echocardiography for assessment of left ventricular indexes in children: A validation study compared with magnetic resonance imaging. *J Am Soc Echocardiogr* 18(4):299-305, 2005.

[r]Caiani EG, Corsi C, Zamorano J, et al: Improved semiautomated quantification of left ventricular volumes and ejection fraction using 3-dimensional echocardiography with a full matrix-array transducer: Comparison with magnetic resonance imaging. *J Am Soc Echocardiogr* 18(8):779-788, 2005.

[s]Hibberd MG, Chuang ML, Beaudin RA, et al: Accuracy of three-dimensional echocardiography with unrestricted selection of imaging planes for measurement of left ventricular volumes and ejection fraction. *Am Heart J* 140(3):469-475, 2000.

[t]Krenning BJ, Voormolen MM, van Geuns RJ, et al: Rapid and accurate measurement of left ventricular function with a new second-harmonic fast-rotating transducer and semi-automated border detection. *Echocardiography* 23(6):447-454, 2006.

[u]van den Bosch AE, Robbers-Visser D, Krenning BJ, et al: Real-time transthoracic three-dimensional echocardiographic assessment of left ventricular volume and ejection fraction in congenital heart disease. *J Am Soc Echocardiogr* 19(1):1-6, 2006.

[v]Fukuda S, Hozumi T, Watanabe H, et al: Freehand three-dimensional echocardiography with rotational scanning for measurements of left ventricular volume and ejection fraction in patients with coronary artery disease. *Echocardiography* 22(2):111-119, 2005.

[w]Gutierrez-Chico JL, Zamorano JL, Perez de Isla L, et al: Comparison of left ventricular volumes and ejection fractions measured by three-dimensional echocardiography versus by two-dimensional echocardiography and cardiac magnetic resonance in patients with various cardiomyopathies. *Am J Cardiol* 95(6):809-813, 2005.

CHD, congenital heart disease; MI, myocardial infarction; SPECT, single photon emission computed tomography.

diographic data sets transferred to an offline workstation, the volume can be calculated by several methods. First is a method of discs, in which multiple short-axis planes are derived to create a series of component volumes of the left ventricle, that are summed from base to apex, and this measurement will increase in accuracy as the number of short-axis planes used increases. A second method is to directly sum the voxels enclosed by the endocardial borders of the 3D structure (Fig. 4–7B). Compared to reference standards, the accuracy of 3D echocardiographic LV volume by the reconstruction method will be a function of the number of component images used because this will determine how much interpolation of the endocardial surface between images has occurred.[10] The accuracy of the 3D echocardiographic LV volume by the volumetric method will be a function of the number of elements in the matrix array transducer, the voxel size, and the spatial resolution of the image.

Compared to cardiac magnetic resonance imaging (MRI), both end-diastolic and end-systolic LV volumes of normal subjects and patients with cardiac disease are slightly smaller when calculated from 3D echocardiography regardless of the 3D echocardiographic acquisition technique. Images obtained from the apical transducer position may underestimate the LV cavity slightly because the US point-spread function and beam width.[18-20] In many of the validation studies, the volume of the 3D echocardiogram was calculated from apical (or long-axis) images, whereas the cardiac MRI used short-axis images and this may account for some differences. Another explanation for the discrepancy between 3D echocardiography and cardiac MRI is the difference in definition of the endocardial border. For echocardiography, the inner border of the endocardial trabeculations is traced, whereas on MRI the trabeculations are commonly excluded and so a larger volume will result in the same patient.[21]

Because the LV volumes calculated from 3D echocardiograms are accurate, it follows that the derivation of LV stroke volume and ejection fraction (EF) from these volumes is also accurate.[22] The advantages of this technique for assessment of LV function is most noticeable in subjects with distorted ventricles or wall motion abnormalities such as occurs in coronary artery disease (CAD). LV volume can be calculated throughout the cardiac cycle with real-time 3D echocardiography by generation of volume-time curves as a measure of systolic and diastolic function from either manual or automated border tracing.[23,24] Observer variability is low and change in LV volume, stroke volume and ejection fraction are also more precisely determined with 3D echocardiography compared to other echocardiographic techniques. Thus, one would expect that the 3D echocardiographic technique will be a valuable outcome tool

in clinical trials in which accurate characterization of changes of these parameters is critical.

Left Ventricular Mass

LV mass is an important predictor of prognosis. It is calculated as the product of the volume of the LV myocardium and the myocardial density (gm/cm^3). The specific gravity of cardiac muscle, a ratio of its density relative to water, is often substituted for density. The myocardial volume is calculated with 3D echocardiography as the space between the epicardial and endocardial borders of the left ventricle. This can be calculated directly as a sum of the voxels in this enclosed space or derived from the difference of the epicardial and endocardial volumes.

LV mass measurements by 3D echocardiography are slightly larger than direct LV weight (in vitro studies) or cardiac MIR (in vivo, human studies) (Table 4–2). Again, this difference is best explained by the fact that typically on echocardiographic images the inner border of the endocardium is traced and includes the many spaces between the fine trabeculations. In one human study, however, the 3D echocardiographic LV mass was slightly smaller than cardiac MRI.[25] In that study, the patients had LV hypertrophy and the mean LV mass of this population was much larger than that of the other human validation studies. In all of the studies, however, the 95% confidence intervals of the difference between the 3D echocardiographic measure and the reference method overlap zero or no difference. Potential sources of error with the echocardiographic measures include the need to include the entire epicardial surface of the left ventricle within the image sector and exact tracing of endocardial trabeculations. Regression of 3D echocardiographically measured LV mass with pharmacologic therapy has been demonstrated in a small study of hypertensive patients.[26] Because LV mass derived from 3D echocardiography is more accurate, precise, and less variable than that from 2D echocardiography, it is expected that fewer number of subjects will be required in clinical trials of LV mass regression using this technique compared to trials that have used 2D echocardiography to measure LV mass change.

Right Ventricular Volume

Because the RV inflow, outflow, and apex do not all align within a single 2D plane, calculation of total RV area or volume is challenging by 2D echocardiography, and this is an area in which there is clear value of 3D echocardiographic techniques. As with 3D techniques for LV volume, the need for geometric assumptions or standardized planes is eliminated. The methods for calculating volume from the 3D image are the same as described previously for LV volume. Because

TABLE 4-2. Left Ventricular Mass Quantitation by Three-Dimensional Echocardiography Compared to a Reference Standard

First Author	3D Technique	Subjects or Objects Studied	n	Reference Standard	Pearson Linear Correlation Coefficient (r)	SEE (g)	Mean Difference ± 1 SD (Bland-Altman Analysis, g)	Interobserver Variability (%)
Gopal and colleagues[a]	Reconstruction, free-hand scanning, spark gap locator	In vitro, autopsy hearts	11	Myocardial volume (displacement) × specific gravity	0.99	3	—	—
Gopal and colleagues[a]	Reconstruction, free-hand scanning, spark gap locator	In vivo, patients	15	MRI	EDV 0.90	11	—	13
Kühl and colleagues[b]	Reconstruction, rotational scanning	In vitro, autopsy hearts	14	Myocardial volume (displacement) × specific gravity	0.98	10	+5±10	4
Lee and colleagues[c]	Real-time 3D	Patients with "various cardiac disorders"	25	MRI	0.95	6	+5±26	—
Schmidt and colleagues[d]	Real-time 3D	In vivo, sheep hearts	21	Measurement of weight	0.94	9	+7±5	—
Mor-Avi and colleagues[e]	Real-time 3D	Patients referred for echocardiography	21	MRI	0.90	—	4±14	0-23
Caiani and colleagues[f]	Real-time 3D with automated detection of surfaces/borders	Patients referred for echocardiography	21	MRI	0.96	11	−2±12	12
Oe and colleagues[g]	Real-time 3D	Patients referred for MRI for LV hypertrophy	21	MRI	0.95	20	−14±29	11
van den Bosch and colleagues[h]	Real-time 3D	Patients with CHD	20	MRI	0.94	19	10±19	—
Hubka and colleagues[i]	Reconstruction, free-hand scanning, magnetic locator	In vitro, animal hearts	15	Measurement of weight	0.99	10	8±10	—

Study	Method	Population	N	Reference	Correlation			
Teupe and colleagues[j]	Reconstruction, rotational scanning	In vitro, porcine hearts	10	Measurement of weight	0.92	22	—	6
Bu and colleagues[k]	Real-time 3D	Children	19	MRI	0.97	9	2±10	5
Jenkins and colleagues[l]	Real-time 3D	Patients referred for echocardiography	50	MRI	—	—	0±38	—
Qin and colleagues[m]	Real-time 3D	Patients with cardiomyopathy (25) or AR (2)	27	MRI	0.92	29	−9±33	—

aGopal AS, Keller AM, Shen Z, et al: Three-dimensional echocardiography: In vitro and in vivo validation of left ventricular mass and comparison with conventional echocardiographic methods. *J Am Coll Cardiol* 24(2):504-513, 1994.

bKühl HP, Franke A, Frielingsdorf J, et al: Determination of left ventricular mass and circumferential wall thickness by three-dimensional reconstruction: In vitro validation of a new method that uses a multiplane transesophageal transducer. *J Am Soc Echocardiogr* 10(2):107-119, 1997.

cLee D, Fuisz AR, Fan PH, et al: Real-time 3-dimensional echocardiographic evaluation of left ventricular volume: Correlation with magnetic resonance imaging—a validation study. *J Am Soc Echocardiogr* 14(10):1001-1009.

dSchmidt MA, Freidlin RZ, Ohazama CJ, et al: Anatomic validation of a novel method for left ventricular volume and mass measurements with use of real-time 3-dimensional echocardiography. *J Am Soc Echocardiogr* 14(1):1-10, 2001.

eMor-Avi V, Sugeng L, Weinert L, et al: Fast measurement of left ventricular mass with real-time three-dimensional echocardiography: Comparison with magnetic resonance imaging. *Circulation* 110(13):1814-1818, 2004.

fCaiani EG, Corsi C, Zamorano J, et al: Improved semiautomated quantification of left ventricular volumes and ejection fraction using 3-dimensional echocardiography with a full matrix-array transducer: Comparison with magnetic resonance imaging. *J Am Soc Echocardiogr* 18(8):779-788, 2005.

gOe H, Hozumi T, Arai K, et al: Comparison of accurate measurement of left ventricular mass in patients with hypertrophied hearts by real-time three-dimensional echocardiography versus magnetic resonance imaging. *Am J Cardiol* 95(10):1263-1267, 2005.

hvan den Bosch AE, Robbers-Visser D, Krenning BJ, et al: Comparison of real-time three-dimensional echocardiography to magnetic resonance imaging for assessment of left ventricular mass. *Am J Cardiol* 97(1):113-117, 2006.

iHubka M, Bolson EL, McDonald JA, et al: Three-dimensional echocardiographic measurement of left and right ventricular mass and volume: In vitro validation. *Int J Cardiovasc Imaging* 18(2):111-118, 2002.

jTeupe C, Takeuchi M, Yao J, Pandian N: Determination of left ventricular mass by three-dimensional echocardiography: In vitro validation of a novel quantification method using multiple equi-angular rotational planes for rapid measurements. *Int J Cardiovasc Imaging* 18(3):161-167, 2002.

kBu L, Munns S, Zhang H, et al: Rapid full volume data acquisition by real-time 3-dimensional echocardiography for assessment of left ventricular indexes in children: A validation study compared with magnetic resonance imaging. *J Am Soc Echocardiogr* 18(4):299-305, 2005.

lJenkins C, Bricknell K, Hanekom L, Marwick TH: Reproducibility and accuracy of echocardiographic measurements of left ventricular parameters using real-time three-dimensional echocardiography. *J Am Coll Cardiol* 44(4):878-886, 2004.

mQin JX, Jones M, Travaglini A, et al: The accuracy of left ventricular mass determined by real-time three-dimensional echocardiography in chronic animal and clinical studies: A comparison with postmortem examination and magnetic resonance imaging. *J Am Soc Echocardiogr* 18(10):1037-1043, 2005.

AR, aortic regurgitation; CHD, congenital heart disease; EDV end-diastolic left ventricular volume; LV, left ventricular; MRI magnetic resonance imaging; SD, standard deviation; SEE, standard error of the estimate; 3D, three dimensional.

Adapted from Hung J, Lang R, Flachskampf F, et al: *J Am Soc Echocardiogr* 20(3):213-233, 2007.

the right ventricle is typically smaller and more heavily trabeculated than the LV surface, one might expect lower accuracy of volume quantitation compared to the left ventricle. However, numerous 3D echocardiographic validation studies of RV volume show correlation coefficients, standard errors, biases, precision, and percent interobserver variability that are similar to LV volume quantitation (Table 4–3). In vivo studies tend to show a slight underestimation with the 3D technique compared to other standards, and this may result from the tracing of the trabeculations and exclusion of some of the interstices of the RV cavity. However, in nearly all studies, the 95% confidence intervals show no significant difference with the reference standard.

Most of the validation studies for RV volume and function have used normal right ventricles. Recently, 3D echocardiographic quantification of RV volume and function has been applied to a small number of patients with arrhythmogenic RV dysplasia/cardiomyopathy.[27] Whereas the correlations with cardiac MRI are lower than noted in other validation studies, pathologic right ventricles could be discriminated from normal controls and unaffected family members. Additional validation studies in this and other right ventricular pathologies will be of value to determine if accuracies are lower when the right ventricle is enlarged and if so, why. 3D echocardiographic quantitation of RV volume has been used to assess RV remodeling in secondary pulmonary hypertension.[28] Initial findings suggest that segments closest to the RV outflow are most affected by pressure overload.

Atrial Volume

Left atrial size is not only a marker of diastolic function but has also been shown to be a predictor of risk for atrial fibrillation (AFib), stroke, and cardiac events. In these assessments, left atrial volume has been shown to be a stronger marker than area or linear dimension.[29] Because of the lack of symmetry of the atria, 3D echocardiography is ideally suited for accurate quantitation of left and right atrial volumes. The methods are similar to that for calculation of ventricular volume by 3D echocardiography and accuracy is comparable to MRI.[30-32]

Valvular Heart Disease

3D echocardiography is especially suited for assessments of valve disease with its ability to image nonplanar valve leaflets, demonstrate the spatial relationships of all components of the valve and surrounding structures, and depict color Doppler flow in three dimensions. This technique should be of particular value in the preoperative and intraoperative US evaluation of patients being considered for or undergoing repair and replacement of valves.[33]

Mitral Valve

As previously discussed, since its early development, 3D echocardiographic approaches have been used to understand the complex geometry of the mitral valve and improve the echocardiographic diagnosis of MVP.[3] The delineation of the nonplanar shape of the mitral annulus has led to identification of imaging planes and 2D echocardiographic views from which it can be seen that the mitral leaflets truly prolapse below the annulus into the LA. Recent studies suggest that with real-time 3D TEE, the anterior mitral leaflet is visualized better than the posterior mitral leaflet.[34]

Mitral Stenosis. Characterization of mitral stenosis is a strength of 2D echocardiography. Whereas planimetry and pressure half-time methods with 2D echocardiography and Doppler typically provide equivalent assessments of the mitral valve area, there are some situations particularly immediately after percutaneous mitral valvuloplasty in which only planimetry provides an accurate measure. This accurate planimetry of mitral valve area requires a parasternal image plane that is perpendicular to the long axis of the smallest mitral orifice. This is a time-consuming task especially when the valve orifice is asymmetrically narrowed. Deviations from the ideal image plane positioning will lead to significant overestimations of the valve area.[35] With 3D echocardiographic reconstruction techniques, a series of parallel short-axis planes through the mitral valve are used to identify the smallest mitral valve area for direct planimetry.[36] With the real-time 3D volumetric technique, the best image of the valve can be cropped and rotated to display the best plane for planimetry[37] (Figs. 4–8, 4–9). Because multiple US planes can be created simultaneously with a matrix array probe, another method to planimeter the mitral valve area is to obtain a long-axis view of the mitral valve and then position a second intersecting imaging plane that is perpendicular to the limiting orifice[38] (see Fig. 4–4). Investigations have shown mitral valve area by real-time 3D echocardiography to be more precise than 2D measures and comparable to that of the pressure half-time technique when compared to invasive measures of valve area.[37] In such comparisons, the 3D measurement frequently changed the classification of mitral stenosis severity. For experienced sonographers, there may not be a significant difference in valve area calculation compared with 2D echocardiography, however, the time required to acquire the view of the mitral valve for planimetry is reduced. The benefits will be observed by less experienced personnel. The Wilkins morphology valve score by the 3D approach demonstrates less interobserver variability than the 2D echocardiographic technique.[37] Initial studies also suggest that 3D echocardiography may better quantify the degree of commissural fusion before percutaneous balloon mitral valvotomy and leaflet morphology after the procedure.[39] The presence of atrial fibrillation, especially when the ventricular response is variable, poses a challenge for the application of 3D echocardiography in mitral stenosis.

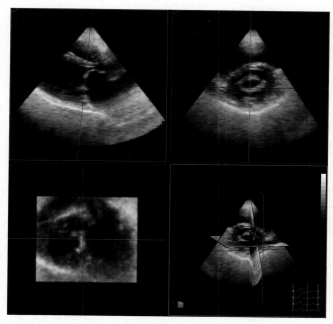

Figure 4–8. *Full-volume three-dimensional transthoracic echocardiogram and various image planes of mitral stenosis obtained from the parasternal transducer position. The* upper left *image is the sagittal (long axis) plane through the middle of the left ventricle and mitral valve viewed from a lateral position. The* upper right *image is the transverse (short axis) plane through the mitral valve viewed from the left ventricle. The* lower left *panel is the coronal image through the posterior leaflet of the mitral valve (looking at the heart from above).*

Mitral Regurgitation. 3D echocardiography has been used for several different aspect of mitral regurgitation (MR). First, it can quantify the severity of MR. Second, it can delineate specific anatomic lesions responsible for MR resulting from degenerative disease, myxomatous valve disease, congenital lesions, or endocarditis. Third, it can provide insights into the mechanisms responsible for functional and ischemic MR. Lastly by better understanding the mechanisms of the regurgitation and the shape and anatomical relationships of surrounding supporting structures, such as annulus and papillary muscles, 3D echocardiography can assist in the design of valve repair techniques and prosthetic supports, such as annular rings.

3D echocardiographic quantification of MR can be performed either by the proximal isovelocity surface area (PISA) method or the vena contracta area method.[16,40,41] For the PISA method, the 3D color Doppler image of the flow convergence zone is examined to find the true shape of this region. The true radius and the convergence angle correction factor are then measured and used in the equations for mitral regurgitant volume and regurgitant orifice area. Alternatively, the true flow convergence area can be quantified free of assumptions of geometry and used in the calculations (Fig. 4–10). This approach is of particular value for quantitation of regurgitation from MVP in which the jet may be eccentrically directed in the LA and the shape of the flow convergence zone may not be a symmetric hemiellipse.[42] For the calculation of vena contracta area, the best image of the vena contracta is obtained, the full-volume color Doppler image set is then cropped in a plane parallel to the leaflets, the image is then rotated to view the vena contracta enface, and then the previously cropped portion of the image is

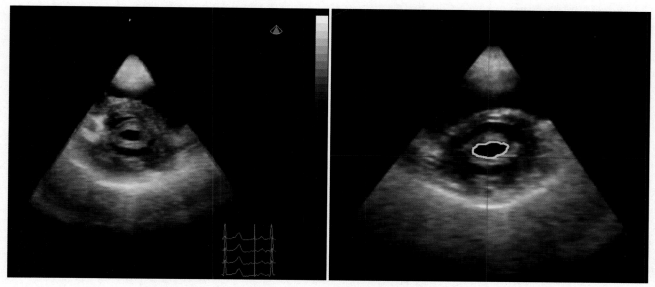

A   B

Figure 4–9. *Full-volume three-dimensional transthoracic echocardiography of mitral stenosis. A,* Transverse (short axis) plane through a stenotic mitral valve viewed from the left atrial perspective. B, Same plane viewed from the left ventricular perspective with planimetry of the orifice in yellow (1.5 cm²).

TABLE 4-3. Right Ventricular Volume Quantitation by Three-Dimensional Echocardiography Compared to a Reference Standard

First Author	3D Technique	Subjects or Objects Studied	n	Reference Standard	Pearson Linear Correlation Coefficient (r)	SEE (mL)	Mean Difference ± 1 SD (Bland-Altman Analysis, mL)	Interobserver Variability (%)
Jiang and colleagues[a]	Reconstruction, freehand scanning, spark gap locator	In vitro, autopsy hearts	12	Volume of casts of RV	0.99	3	2±3	5
Jiang and colleagues[b]	Reconstruction, freehand scanning, spark gap locator	In vivo, canine hearts	5 animals, 20 hemodynamic stages	Intracavitary volume	EDV 0.99 ESV 0.98	2 3	−2±3 −2±2	4
Vogel and colleagues[c]	Reconstruction, rotational and fan scanning	In vivo, patients	16	MRI	EDV 0.95 ESV 0.75	—	5±4 6±5	4 5
Pini and colleagues[d]	Reconstruction, rotational scanning	In vitro, sheep hearts	14	Volume of casts of RV	0.95	4	0±4	5
Shiota and colleagues[e]	Real-time 3D	In vivo, sheep with pulmonary insufficiency	6 animals, 14 hemodynamic stages	Stroke volume by electromagnetic flow probe	0.8	—	−3±6	—
Ota and colleagues[f]	Real-time 3D	In vitro, canine hearts	8	Direct volume measurement	0.97	3	0±4	4
Ota and colleagues[f]	Real-time 3D (with saline echocardiographic contrast)	In vivo, human volunteers	14	3-D echocardiogram calculated right ventricular stroke volume compared to 2-D echocardiogram calculated left ventricular stroke volume	0.88	2	4±4	8

Study	Population	N	Reference standard	Correlation			
Hubka and colleagues[g]	Reconstruction, freehand scanning, magnetic locator — In vitro, bovine hearts	10	Direct volume measurement	0.99	3	6±4	—
Fujimoto and colleagues[h]	Reconstruction, rotational scanning — In vivo, human volunteers	15	MRI	EDV 0.94 ESV 0.97	—	0±10 0±6	8 7
Chen and colleagues[i]	Real-time 3D — In vitro, porcine hearts	10	Volume of casts of RV	0.94	—	—	—
Prakasa and colleagues[j]	Real-time 3D — Patients with ARVD/C, idiopathic ventricular tachycardia and controls	36	MRI	EDV 0.50 ESV 0.72	—	−16±18 −7±9	—

[a]Jiang L, Handschumacher MD, Hibberd MG, et al: Three-dimensional echocardiographic reconstruction of right ventricular volume: in vitro comparison with two-dimensional methods. *J Am Soc Echocardiogr* 7(2):150-158, 1994.

[b]Jiang L, Siu SC, Handschumacher MD, et al: Three-dimensional echocardiography. In vivo validation for right ventricular volume and function. *Circulation* 89(5):2342-2350, 1994.

[c]Vogel M, Gutberlet M, Dittrich S, et al: Comparison of transthoracic three dimensional echocardiography with magnetic resonance imaging in the assessment of right ventricular volume and mass. *Heart* 78(2):127-130, 1997.

[d]Pini R, Giannazzo G, Di Bari M, et al: Transthoracic three-dimensional echocardiographic reconstruction of left and right ventricles: in vitro validation and comparison with magnetic resonance imaging. *Am Heart J* 133(2):221-229, 1997.

[e]Shiota T, Jones M, Chikada M, et al: Real-time three-dimensional echocardiography for determining right ventricular stroke volume in an animal model of chronic right ventricular volume overload. *Circulation* 97(19):1897-1900, 1998.

[f]Ota T, Fleishman CE, Strub M, et al: Real-time, three-dimensional echocardiography: feasibility of dynamic right ventricular volume measurement with saline contrast. *Am Heart J* 137(5):958-966, 1999.

[g]Hubka M, Bolson EL, McDonald JA, et al: Three-dimensional echocardiographic measurement of left and right ventricular mass and volume: In vitro validation. *Int J Cardiovasc Imaging* 18(2):111-118, 2002.

[h]Fujimoto S, Mizuno R, Nakagawa Y, et al: Estimation of the right ventricular volume and ejection fraction by transthoracic three-dimensional echocardiography. A validation study using magnetic resonance imaging. *Int J Cardiovasc Imaging* 14(6):385-390, 1998.

[i]Chen G, Sun K, Huang G: In vitro validation of right ventricular volume and mass measurement by real-time three-dimensional echocardiography. *Echocardiography* 23(5):395-399, 2006.

[j]Prakasa KR, Dalal D, Wang J, et al: Feasibility and variability of three dimensional echocardiography in arrhythmogenic right ventricular dysplasia/cardiomyopathy. *Am J Cardiol* 97(5):703-709, 2006.

ARVD/C, arrhythmogenic right ventricular dysplasia/cardiomyopathy; EDV, end-diastolic left ventricular volume; ESV, end-systolic left ventricular volume; MRI, magnetic resonance imaging; RV, right ventricle; SEE, standard error of the estimate; 3D, three dimensional; 2D, two dimensional.
Adapted from Hung J, Lang R, Flachskampf F, et al: *J Am Soc Echocardiogr* 20(3):213-233, 2007.

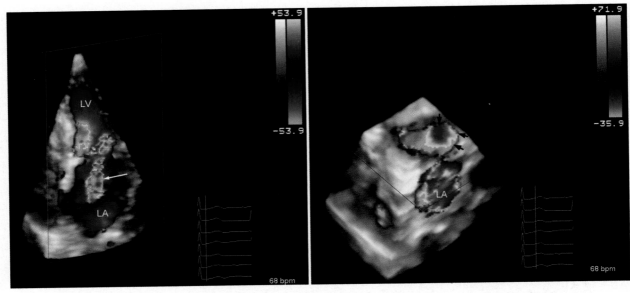

Figure 4-10. Full-volume three-dimensional transthoracic echocardiogram of mitral regurgitation. A, Cropping of the full-volume image set to display the full extent of an eccentrically directed jet of mitral regurgitation (white arrow) as viewed from the anterior aspect of the right ventricle and similar to an apical five-chamber view but with the right heart cut away. B, A transverse plane above the mitral valve viewed from the perspective of the left ventricle to display the proximal isovelocity surface area (orange-blue interface, black arrows). LA, left atrium; LV, left ventricle.

added back until the largest vena contracta area is depicted. Because a better quantification of the complex geometry of the vena contracta and flow convergence areas is possible with the 3D technique, it is not unexpected that these methods have shown better correlations with invasive measurements of MR than the same methods by 2D echocardiography (3D vena contracta versus angiography r = 0.88; 3D PISA versus flow probe r = 0.87).[16,40] The direct measurement of the regurgitant orifice area by 3D echocardiography is feasible and may overcome some of the limitations of the calculation of this area by the PISA method.[15]

As noted previously, one of the initial applications of 3D echocardiography was to understand the relationship between mitral valve leaflets and annulus, thus improving the echocardiographic diagnosis of MVP. Another early application has been the direct visualization and localization of prolapsed segments of leaflets before surgical repair[43,44] (Fig. 4–11). When compared to surgical findings, intraoperative 3D TEE identified the correct location of prolapse in 94% of patients. Differences in the extent of prolapse were noted in 17% of the cases.[45] Typically, enface views of the mitral valve or views that are parallel to the closed valve leaflets from the left atrial perspective have been utilized. However, one study has demonstrated that longitudinal reconstructions (i.e., perpendicular to the enface view) provide additive and perhaps more accurate depiction of regurgitant mitral valve abnormalities with 3D transesophageal reconstructions.[46] These

longitudinal views through specific segments of the anterior and posterior leaflets may yield improvements because they take advantage of the axial resolution of the system and are less subject to artifacts in the LA. Few studies have quantitatively compared 3D TEE to surgical findings in patients with MVP undergoing repair. The ability to visualize all aspects of the mitral valve with real-time 3D TTE is lower than that reported for 3D TEE reconstructions. In a study of consecutive patients with the transthoracic technique, complete visualization of the anterior mitral leaflet was noted in 58% and posterior leaflet in 51% of the time, whereas this improved to 84% for the anterior and 77% for the posterior leaflet if patients were selected on the basis of image quality.[34] For 3D transthoracic imaging with current matrix array transducers, the parasternal transducer position provides better visualization of the leaflets most of the time compared to the apical window because the structure of interest will be closer to the transducer and thus scan line density will be greater and beam spread artifact will be less. Regardless of the 3D imaging approach used, a complete visualization of all leaflet segments from all planes is recommended to define the pathology. Display of this pathology in an enface view may then be the best way to display the valve for those not familiar with the component echocardiographic views. It remains to be demonstrated whether either a 3D TTE or 3D TEE for evaluation of mitral valve morphology is superior to a well-performed 2D TEE.

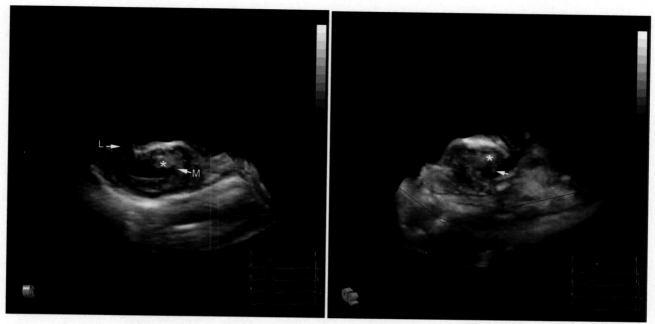

A   B

Figure 4–11. *Three-dimensional transthoracic echocardiogram of mitral valve prolapse. A, Mitral valve viewed from the left atrium demonstrating prolapse (*) of the midportion of the anterior leaflet of the mitral valve. B, Same valve viewed from the left ventricular cavity. The left ventricular perspective allows visualization of a ruptured chord to the prolapsed segment (white arrow). L, lateral commissure; M, medial commissure.*

Whereas limitations may exist in the morphologic evaluation, observations from quantitative 3D echocardiography have provided important insights into mechanisms responsible for both functional and ischemic MR.[47-50] 3D echocardiography has shown that as the left ventricle dilates, it leads to displacement of normal papillary muscle position such that the mitral leaflets are apically tethered (increased mitral valve tenting area) and the resulting *functional* MR occurs through incompletely closing leaflets. 3D echocardiography has shown that, in contrast, regional distortion of wall motion and/or distortion of the wall shape, such as aneurysm formation, adjacent to a papillary muscle will lead to a disruption of the normal spatial relationships between a papillary muscle and mitral valve resulting in disruption of normal coaptation and *ischemic* MR. Clinical studies with 3D echocardiography have confirmed prior experimental studies and demonstrated that with ischemia and infarction, as the mitral annulus flattens, it enlarges predominantly in the anterior-posterior direction, and annular motion during the cardiac cycle is reduced, especially compared to that of the posterior segments.[51,52] Based on these observations, repair techniques that reduce anterior-posterior annular diameter,[53] decrease tenting area,[54] restore normal ventricular geometry,[49,55] and reposition papillary muscles[56] have each been proposed for treatment of ischemic MR, whereas those that reduce global dilation and enhance reverse LV remodeling are being tested for functional MR.[57]

Aortic Valve

3D echocardiography may have value in the assessment of aortic valve disease because all aspects of the three leaflets of the aortic valve cannot be visualized in a single 2D plane and the 2D US imaging plane often is oblique through the stenotic or regurgitant aortic orifice. Direct planimetry of the aortic valve in aortic stenosis, description of valve morphology (i.e., number of leaflets) (Fig. 4–12), localization and description of subvalvular obstruction (both discrete membranes and hypertrophic septum/left ventricular outflow tract [LVOT] obstruction), quantification of aortic regurgitation, and assessment of aortic root pathology have all been demonstrated with 3D echocardiography.[58-66]

Aortic Stenosis. Planimetry of aortic valve area by intraoperative 3D TEE (reconstruction technique) has been shown to be accurate compared with invasive (Gorlin equation) and Doppler (continuity equation) methods and more accurate than measures by 2D transesophageal imaging.[60] This improvement results from the variable ability of any single 2D transesophageal imaging plane to image the aortic valve limiting orifice on-axis and the ability to optimally redefine that imaging plane through the limiting orifice with the 3D US data set. Not all 3D approaches may yield similar results, however, as a recent study has suggested that planimetry of the valve area from volume rendered images will underestimate the valve area

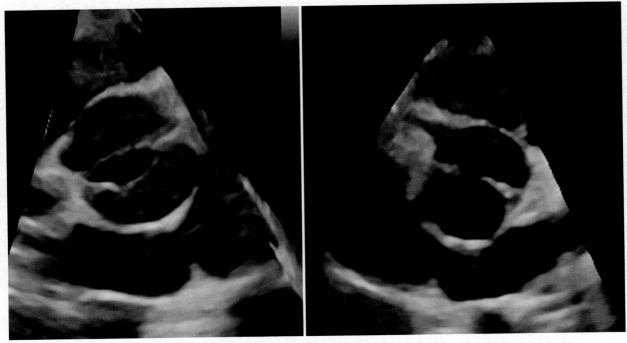

A   B

Figure 4–12. Systolic (A) *and diastolic* (B) *frames from transverse planes through a three-dimensional transthoracic echocardiogram of bicuspid aortic valve and viewed from the left ventricle. (Courtesy of Randolph Martin, MD, Emory Healthcare.)*

compared to transthoracic Doppler, 2D transesophageal, and optimum imaging planes through the valve derived from 3D transesophageal reconstructions.[67] This discrepancy results from several issues related to the representation of the volume rendered image, including the fact that the shading used on the image to convey depth results in a thickening of structures. As the time required for 3D image acquisition, reconstruction, and planimetry of the aortic valve is streamlined, this approach should have a role in the assessment of aortic stenosis in the operating room (OR) in which Doppler methods are more difficult. Because planimetry of the aortic valve from standard 2D TEEs is accurate in many cases, further studies are necessary to determine in which subsets of patients (bicuspid aortic valve, and so on) the 3D approach is of most additive value.

Aortic Insufficiency. The vena contracta and PISA methods described for assessment of MR can be applied to aortic regurgitation and though experience is much more limited, it is assumed that 3D echocardiography would have comparable accuracy in aortic insufficiency as noted for mitral insufficiency.[68] In the absence of other regurgitant valves, aortic insufficiency can also be accurately quantified as the difference in LV and RV stroke volumes calculated by 3D TTE.[69] Aortic valve repair is feasible for certain etiologies of aortic regurgitation.[70,71] Measurements of the ascending aorta,

the sinotubular junction, the perpendicular distance from annulus to coaptation point of the leaflet tips, the distance from annulus to sinotubular junction, and the distance from the sinotubular junction to leaflet coaptation point can provide insights into the mechanisms responsible for aortic insufficiency and incomplete aortic valve closure.[66] These measurements are feasible with 3D TEE and may facilitate the development of new repair techniques and the assessment of the success of aortic valve repair.

LVOT Obstruction

Improved identification of systolic anterior motion of the mitral valve and the location of the predominant septal hypertrophy in hypertrophic cardiomyopathy has been shown with real-time 3D echocardiography.[72] Whereas it is possible that careful 2D scanning might yield similar results, the time for image acquisition with the 3D approach is shorter and its display enhances comprehension of the pathology. 3D echocardiography may also have value in the identification and quantification of LV outflow tract and septal remodeling after surgical myomectomy and percutaneous alcohol septal ablation in patients with hypertrophic cardiomyopathy. Initial applications of this technique in this disease have shown that the enlargement of the outflow tract is greater with the surgical rather than the percutaneous technique.[63]

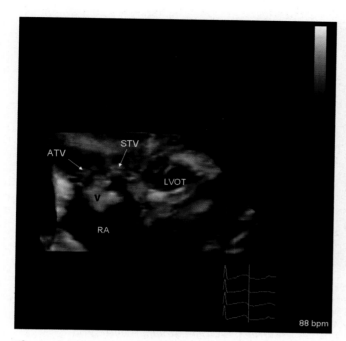

Figure 4–13. Transverse crop from a three-dimensional full-volume transthoracic echocardiogram of a tricuspid valve vegetation. The vegetation is seen to arise from the atrial surface of the septal leaflet. ATV, anterior leaflet of tricuspid valve; LVOT, left ventricular outflow tract; RA, right atrium; STV, septal leaflet of tricuspid valve; v, vegetation.

Endocarditis

Case reports have highlighted the value of 3D echocardiography in infectious endocarditis (Fig. 4–13). These reports suggest that the 3D views of the valves may improve the detection of valve perforations in addition to identifying the number and location of vegetations on both native and prosthetic valves.[73,74] Additional studies suggest that vegetation size measured on real-time 3D TTE is more accurate than 2D TTE.[75] Systematic studies comparing 3D TTE and 3D TEE to the 2D echocardiographic modalities are required to determine if vegetation detection rate is improved and if there is additive value of 3D echocardiography.

Congenital Heart Disease

Some of the greatest potential for 3D echocardiography is in the area of congenital heart disease (CHD) because this noninvasive imaging technique can define and display the complex spatial relationships seen in many of these pathologies. In addition, the shorter time for image acquisition with volumetric 3D echocardiography improves the probability of complete cardiac US imaging assessment of children. A study of 3D echocardiography in 75 patients with suspicion of congenital heart defects reported that the real-time 3D echocardiographic image sets were obtained in all cases in less than 5 minutes and sedation of infants and children was never required.[76] In a more recent report of real-time 3D echo-

cardiography in 70 patients with simple and complex CHD, improved depiction of cardiac and lesion morphology was noted compared to 2D imaging regardless of experience level of the echocardiographer.[77] In this study, in at least 30% of the cases, the 3D echocardiogram added new information compared to the 2D imaging. Other investigators have recently shown that in 28 of 82 patients with CHD (35%), real-time 3D echocardiography provided anatomic information not seen on 2D echocardiography that was helpful in clinical decision making.[78] This additive benefit was most prominent in patients with atrial septal defect, ventricular septal defects, atrioventricular septal defects, and L-transposition of the great vessels. In another 29% of this population, the 3D technique provided additional information compared to 2D echocardiography, but it was deemed not critical to decision making and in 36% of the patients the information was equivalent for the two techniques.

Both reconstruction and volumetric 3D echocardiography have been applied to the detection of atrial septal defects and quantification of defect size[79] (Fig. 4–14). The area or diameters of the defect can be measured from an enface view from either the right atrial or left atrial perspective.[80] When images are of adequate quality, the atrial septal defect size quantified by 3D transthoracic reconstruction was comparable to the same transesophageal technique.[81] Calculation of atrial septal defect shunt volume from 3D transesophageal reconstructions of Doppler color flow through the defect compares favorably to other methods.[82] Visualization of the extent of septal rim and assessment of the proximity of other structures is necessary when considering if a patient with an atrial septal defect is a candidate for percutaneous closure device, and 3D echocardiography may provide value in this assessment. The prospective application of the 3D TEE reconstruction technique in a small number of children with atrioventricular septal defects and left atrioventricular valve failure has demonstrated its superiority compared to standard 2D TEE for identification of valve morphology, function, and cause of leaflet failure.[83] Thus, 3D echocardiography can assist in the planning of repairs of complex congenital lesions.

Another example of one of the many applications of 3D echocardiography in complex CHD is its use in hypoplastic left-sided heart syndrome to understand the mechanisms responsible for tricuspid regurgitation.[84] Quantitative real-time 3D TTE has shown that following Fontan procedures, bidirectional cavopulmonary shunts, and Norwood procedures, significant tricuspid regurgitation can occur resulting from enlarged annular area, reduced systolic annulus area change, systolic annular flattening, and papillary muscle displacement. The observation that the tricuspid regurgitation predominantly results from annular and ventricular abnormalities rather than valve morphologic abnormalities may enable modification of surgical techniques.

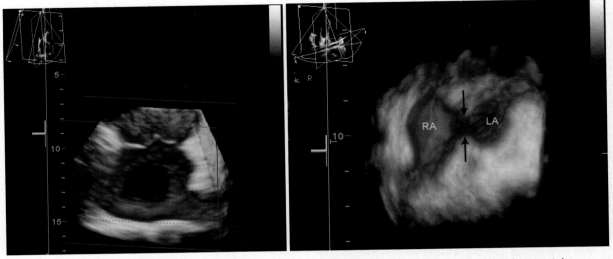

Figure 4–14. Full-volume three-dimensional transthoracic echocardiogram of a secundum atrial septal defect. A, *Sagittal crop through the atrial septum and viewed from the right atrial perspective to visualize the defect "enface."* B, *The volume of ultrasound is cropped obliquely and then viewed from a perspective to visualize a diameter of the atrial septal defect* (between arrows) *and the entrances of the vena cavae into the right atrium. LA, left atrium; RA, right atrium. (Courtesy of Miriam Hospital Echocardiography.)*

Currently in patients with congenital heart lesions, real-time 3D echocardiographic imaging is considered complementary rather than a replacement for 2D echocardiography. Development of higher frequency matrix array transducers with smaller footprints, full Doppler capabilities, and faster frame rates are required before 3D echocardiography can be considered a full substitute.

Other Applications

As would be expected, 3D echocardiography can be applied to almost any current use of 2D echocardiography. Some of these are described in this section. When assessing its additive value, important questions include whether the technology provides additional information that alters diagnosis or outcome and whether the information is obtained in a simpler or faster fashion.

Aortic Dissection

Whereas case reports have demonstrated aortic dissection by 3D echocardiography, one study suggests that the diagnosis of type A aortic dissection by the transthoracic approach can be dramatically enhanced with 3D echocardiography.[85] In this investigation of a small number of patients, the authors suggest that the dissection flaps in transthoracic volumetric 3D echocardiograms could be identified definitively, whereas many of these could not be differentiated from artifact on the 2D echocardiogram.

Stress Echocardiography

The use of single cardiac cycle multiplane image and real-time 3D echocardiography during stress echocardiography offers several advantages over the current practice. First, all ventricular segments are imaged rapidly at each stage, which is particularly important at peak stress, so that all myocardial segments are visualized before reduction in workload and the resolution of transient ischemia-induced wall motion abnormalities (Fig. 4–15). Second, function of all myocardial segments is assessed at the same point in time enabling accurate comparisons. Third, cropping of the images enables display and interpretation of image planes that are on-axis, thus reducing errors that occur with interpretation of oblique cuts of the ventricular walls or rotational motion. Lastly, cropping of the 3D images from each stage allows comparison of reproducible and identical myocardial segments at each stage even if the heart has changed size or shape. The feasibility of the integration of real-time 3D echocardiography with treadmill and dobutamine stress echocardiography (DSE) has been demonstrated.[86,87] Initial applications and comparisons with 2D stress echocardiography have shown a higher rate of noninterpretable segments particularly the anterior and lateral regions resulting in reduced test sensitivity.[88] At present, especially when the left ventricle is enlarged, several image acquisitions from different transducer positions may be necessary to acquire all myocardial segments in the imaging volume. In addition, the large footprint of the matrix array transducer may contribute to the difficulties in visual-

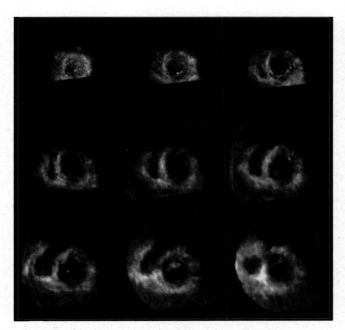

Figure 4-15. Nine simultaneous short-axis views demonstrating the type of display of the three-dimensional volume set that is ideally suited for transthoracic stress echocardiography. The upper left-hand *corner is a short-axis image from the apex, the* lower right-hand *image is from the base of the left ventricle and the image in the middle is from the midventricular level. The distance between each adjacently displayed image is equal.*

izing certain ventricular regions. The limitations of image quality have been reduced with the addition of intravenous (IV) contrast for LV opacification. The fusion of component images from multiple cardiac cycles may lead to image artifacts, particularly during stress and recovery when the heart rate is changing. Before widespread clinical application, increased frame rates will be required to adequately resolve ventricular wall kinetics at the increased heart rates encountered at peak stress.

Myocardial Perfusion

Real-time 3D echocardiographic imaging enables display of myocardial contrast perfusion zones in a single cardiac cycle rather than reliance on a single image plane as is the common practice of 2D myocardial contrast echocardiography (MCE). The extent of perfusion defect and quantification of myocardial perfusion have been demonstrated in both experimental preparations and humans with volumetric 3D echocardiography.[89] The high acoustic power and large number of scan lines that the current matrix array transducers transmit enhance premature microbubble destruction. To enhance microbubble delivery and perfusion detection during real-time 3D echocardiography, modifications to microbubble stability, microbubble infusion techniques, or transducer mechanical index will be required.

Right Ventricular Biopsy

Initial reports of the use of 3D echocardiography have been described for guiding RV biopsy in children.[90] This application highlights the potential role of 3D echocardiography for real-time guidance in a variety of percutaneous cardiac interventions.

Pericardial Effusion

The size of pericardial effusions can be more accurately quantified by 3D echocardiography than 2D techniques. The 3D technique does not rely on the assumption that the fluid is symmetrically distributed. With the 3D echocardiographic method, the pericardial fluid volume is calculated as the difference between the volume of the outer pericardial sac (parietal pericardium) and the heart. Experimental studies using the reconstruction technique have shown excellent accuracies compared to true volume (r = 0.98; SEE 7.7 mL; mean error 1.1 ± 7.8 mL).[91] For accurate quantitation of the fluid, the entire parietal pericardium or outer border of the effusion must be obtained in the image volume.

Intracardiac Masses

Case reports have described the detection of thrombi and other masses within the heart by 3D echocardiography.[92-94] This technique may improve echocardiographic detection of the site of attachment of the mass to cardiac structures and the size of the mass. Studies are required to determine if serial quantification of thrombus volume is an accurate and reproducible method to assess response to therapy.

Left Ventricular Dyssynchrony

The advantages of 3D echocardiography for the assessment of LV dyssynchrony and the response to cardiac resynchronization therapy in heart failure patients are similar to those noted above for stress echocardiography—all segments can be assessed simultaneously. A variety of methods have been proposed for this 3D assessment including quantification of the temporal variability of segmental myocardial Doppler indices, segmental volume change, and the displacement and timing of endocardial contours.[95,96] Potential advantages of the 3D Doppler-echocardiography techniques over 2D techniques for dyssynchrony assessment include reduced time of data acquisition, improved accuracy, and decreased measurement variability; but investigations will be required to confirm these speculations. Improvements in spatial and temporal resolution of the real-time 3D technique are also required to enhance reproducibility of these indices. For example, optimal myocardial Doppler quantitation requires images to be obtained above 100 frames per second.[97] Presently, 3D volumetric image acquisition is not able to achieve this minimal degree of temporal resolution. Thus, if simultaneous myocardial Doppler information is desired, at present, quantitation from up to three simultaneous apical 2D images using the multiplane capabilities of a matrix array transducer maintains the frame rate above the minimal requirement.

Future Considerations

The key to the future of 3D echocardiographic imaging is continued enhancements. Enhancements to transducer technology and computer processing will enable higher frame rate acquisitions with smaller matrix array transducers for real-time 3D echocardiography, and this should lead to improved image quality and color Doppler display. Also such advances will lead to larger volume data acquisitions during a single cardiac cycle with the aim of a real-time full-volume display rather than the current integration of several cardiac cycles. This will remove the artifacts observed with arrhythmias, respirations, and patient motion. Enhancements to the real-time, multiplane approach will include faster automated reconstructions and improvements in automated border detection for automated chamber and function quantification. Technical enhancements and miniaturization are leading to the ability to perform real-time 3D echocardiography with transesophageal transducers. The refinement of real-time 3D TEE will enable the use of echocardiography for monitoring of "beating heart" surgery (without cardiopulmonary bypass [CPB]) for lesions such as atrial septal defects and MVP.[98,99]

As 3D echocardiographic full-volume data acquisition becomes a routine part of the clinical workflow, there is the potential for shortened image acquisition time because a 3D volume of US containing all cardiac structures should be able to be imaged within just a few cardiac cycles from just a few imaging windows. Additional time would then be spent on preparing the image sets for interpretation, mainly by cropping the views into image planes that best display the various cardiac structures. Thus, future efforts will need to focus on development of imaging protocols, standardized image cropping planes, and the training of personnel for this image preparation and quantitation. In addition, enhancements to the 3D image display should lead to development of novel ways to view the images, such as stereoscopic visualization, and the ability to perform "virtual dissections" through the image set both offline and in real time. Because echocardiography has superior temporal resolution compared to other noninvasive cardiac imaging modalities (some of which have superior spatial resolution), there is the potential to enhance noninvasive diagnostic and thera-

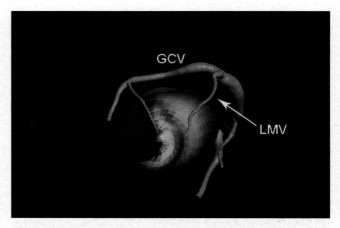

Figure 4–16. *An image integrating three-dimensional transthoracic echocardiography and three-dimensional rotational coronary venous angiography viewed from the lateral apex of the left ventricle. This example displays the left ventricular dyssynchrony map (on a three-dimensional echocardiographic volume of the left ventricle) and the coronary venous anatomy before placement of pacemakers for cardiac resynchronization therapy. The most delayed myocardial segments are coded on the left ventricular volume in orange and the earliest contracting segments are in green. GCV, great cardiac vein; LMV, lateral marginal vein. (Courtesy of Francois Tournoux, MD, Massachusetts General Hospital.)*

peutic cardiac imaging through fusion of modalities, such as cardiac MRI or computed tomographic imaging with 3D echocardiography[100] (Fig. 4–16).

Lastly, as the technique becomes more refined, continued thorough clinical investigations comparing 2D echocardiography and 3D echocardiography will be required to demonstrate the incremental value of 3D echocardiography for detection and quantification of specific cardiac pathologies and for improved cardiac care. This remains a challenge because the 3D US technology will continue to improve at a rapid rate during the duration of these investigations.

Summary

3D echocardiography has many advantages over 2D echocardiography, including improved visualization of complex shapes and spatial relations between cardiac structures; improved quantitation of cardiac volumes, mass, and function; improved visualization of color Doppler flow fields; improved display and assessment of valve dysfunction; and decreased time for image acquisition. Technical improvements including more automation for reconstruction from 2D image planes and enhanced transducer design for better image quality from volumetric data sets are required for its widespread clinical use and for it to replace 2D echocardiography. 3D echocardiography is a technique undergoing rapid evolution.

KEY POINTS

- Understanding the complex shapes and spatial relationships of various cardiac structures is enhanced with 3D echocardiography.

- 3D echocardiography eliminates the need to assume a specific geometric shape of the left ventricle or right ventricle when quantifying volume and ejection fraction.

- 3D echocardiography has the potential to reduce the time required for echocardiographic image acquisition.

- 3D US can be acquired as either a series of 2D images requiring reconstruction into a 3D image or as a 3D volume of US.

- The reconstruction technique requires image acquisition, registration, reconstruction, and rendering before display.

- The volumetric technique requires a rectangular (matrix) array transducer and the images are best displayed after offline cropping of the 3D US data set.

- Multiple 2D image planes can be obtained simultaneously with a matrix array transducer.

- 3D echocardiographic quantitation of LV volume, ejection fraction, mass, and RV volume are more accurate than the 2D approaches, and these measurements derived from 3D echocardiography have reduced measurement variability.

- In CHD, significant benefits of 3D echocardiography compared to 2D echocardiography have been noted in patients with atrial septal defect, ventricular septal defect, atrioventricular septal defects, and L-transposition of the great vessels.

- An important enhancement to the current 3D echocardiographic technique required before broader clinical applications includes higher volume or frame rate acquisitions to improve image quality and resolution.

REFERENCES

1. Dekker DL, Piziali RL, Dong E Jr: A system for ultrasonically imaging the human heart in three dimensions. *Comput Biomed Res* 7(6):544-553, 1974.
2. Moritz WE, Shreve PL: A microprocessor-based spatial locating system for use with diagnostic ultrasound. *Proc IEEE* 64:966-974, 1976.
3. Levine RA, Handschumacher MD, Sanfilippo AJ, et al: Three-dimensional echocardiographic reconstruction of the mitral valve, with implications for the diagnosis of mitral valve prolapse. *Circulation* 80(3):589-598, 1989.
4. King DL, Harrison MR, King DL Jr, et al: Improved reproducibility of left atrial and left ventricular measurements by guided three-dimensional echocardiography. *J Am Coll Cardiol* 20(5)1238-1245, 1992.
5. Siu SC, Rivera JM, Guerrero JL, et al: Three-dimensional echocardiography. In vivo validation for left ventricular volume and function. *Circulation* 88(4 Pt 1):1715-1723, 1993.
6. Gopal AS, Keller AM, Rigling R, et al: Left ventricular volume and endocardial surface area by three-dimensional echocardiography: comparison with two-dimensional echocardiography and nuclear magnetic resonance imaging in normal subjects. *J Am Coll Cardiol* 22(1):258-270, 1993.
7. Sapin PM, Schroeder KD, Smith MD, et al: Three-dimensional echocardiographic measurement of left ventricular volume in vitro: Comparison with two-dimensional echocardiography and cineventriculography. *J Am Coll Cardiol* 22(5):1530-1537, 1993.
8. Jiang L, Vazquez de Prada JA, et al: Three-dimensional echocardiography: in vivo validation for right ventricular free wall mass as an index of hypertrophy. *J Am Coll Cardiol* 23(7):1715-1722, 1994.
9. Handschumacher MD, Lethor JP, Siu SC, et al: A new integrated system for three-dimensional echocardiographic reconstruction: Development and validation for ventricular volume with application in human subjects. *J Am Coll Cardiol* 21(3):743-753, 1993.
10. Siu SC, Rivera JM, Handschumacher MD, et al: Three-dimensional echocardiography: the influence of number of component images on accuracy of left ventricular volume quantitation. *J Am Soc Echocardiogr* 9(2):147-155, 1996.
11. Sugeng L, Spencer KT, Mor-Avi V, et al: Dynamic three-dimensional color flow Doppler: An improved technique for the assessment of mitral regurgitation. *Echocardiography* 20(3):265-273, 2003.
12. Snyder JE, Kisslo J, von Ramm O: Real-time orthogonal mode scanning of the heart. I. System design. *J Am Coll Cardiol* 7(6):1279-1285, 1986.
13. von Ramm OT, Smith SW: Real time volumetric ultrasound imaging system. *J Digit Imaging* 3(4):261-266, 1990.
14. Sheikh K, Smith SW, von Ramm O, Kisslo J: Real-time, three-dimensional echocardiography: feasibility and initial use. *Echocardiography* 8(1):119-125, 1991.
15. Iwakura K, Ito H, Kawano S, et al: Comparison of orifice area by transthoracic three-dimensional Doppler echocardiography versus proximal isovelocity surface area (PISA) method for assessment of mitral regurgitation. *Am J Cardiol* 97(11):1630-1637, 2006.
16. Khanna D, Vengala S, Miller AP, et al: Quantification of mitral regurgitation by live three-dimensional transthoracic echocardiographic measurements of vena contracta area. *Echocardiography* 21(8):737-743, 2004.
17. Siu SC, Levine RA, Rivera JM, et al: Three-dimensional echocardiography improves noninvasive assessment of left ventricular volume and performance. *Am Heart J* 130(4):812-822, 1995.
18. Weyman AE: Cross-sectional scanning: Technical principles and instrumentation (Ch 2). In Weyman AE (ed): *Principles and practice of echocardiography*, 2nd ed. Philadelphia: Lea & Febiger, 1993.
19. Erbel R, Schweizer P, Lambertz H, et al: Echoventriculography—a simultaneous analysis of two-dimensional echocardiography and cineventriculography. *Circulation* 67(1):205-215, 1983.
20. Schnittger I, Fitzgerald PJ, Daughters GT, et al: Limitations of comparing left ventricular volumes by two dimensional echocardiography, myocardial markers and cineangiography. *Am J Cardiol* 50(3):512-519, 1982.
21. Mannaerts HF, Van Der Heide JA, Kamp O, et al: Quantification of left ventricular volumes and ejection fraction using freehand transthoracic three-dimensional echocardiography: Comparison with magnetic resonance imaging. *J Am Soc Echocardiogr* 16(2):101-109, 2003.
22. Fleming SM, Cumberledge B, Kiesewetter C, et al: Usefulness of real-time three-dimensional echocardiography for reliable mea-

surement of cardiac output in patients with ischemic or idiopathic dilated cardiomyopathy. *Am J Cardiol* 95(2):308-310, 2005.

23. Zeidan Z, Erbel R, Barkhausen J, et al: Analysis of global systolic and diastolic left ventricular performance using volume-time curves by real-time three-dimensional echocardiography. *J Am Soc Echocardiogr* 16(1):29-37, 2003.

24. Corsi C, Lang RM, Veronesi F, et al: Volumetric quantification of global and regional left ventricular function from real-time three-dimensional echocardiographic images. *Circulation* 112(8):1161-1170, 2005.

25. Oe H, Hozumi T, Arai K, et al: Comparison of accurate measurement of left ventricular mass in patients with hypertrophied hearts by real-time three-dimensional echocardiography versus magnetic resonance imaging. *Am J Cardiol* 95(10):1263-1267, 2005.

26. Galzerano D, Tammaro P, Cerciello A, et al: Freehand three-dimensional echocardiographic evaluation of the effect of telmisartan compared with hydrochlorothiazide on left ventricular mass in hypertensive patients with mild-to-moderate hypertension: A multicentre study. *J Hum Hypertens* 18(1):53-59, 2004.

27. Prakasa KR, Dalal D, Wang J, et al: Feasibility and variability of three dimensional echocardiography in arrhythmogenic right ventricular dysplasia/cardiomyopathy. *Am J Cardiol* 97(5):703-709, 2006.

28. Sukmawan R, Akasaka T, Watanabe N, et al: Quantitative assessment of right ventricular geometric remodeling in pulmonary hypertension secondary to left-sided heart disease using real-time three-dimensional echocardiography. *Am J Cardiol* 94(8):1096-1099, 2004.

29. Tsang TS, Abhayaratna WP, Barnes ME, et al: Prediction of cardiovascular outcomes with left atrial size: Is volume superior to area or diameter? *J Am Coll Cardiol* 47(5):1018-1023, 2006.

30. Keller AM, Gopal AS, King DL: Left and right atrial volume by freehand three-dimensional echocardiography: In vivo validation using magnetic resonance imaging. *Eur J Echocardiogr* 1(1):55-65, 2000.

31. Poutanen T, Ikonen A, Vainio P, et al: Left atrial volume assessed by transthoracic three dimensional echocardiography and magnetic resonance imaging: Dynamic changes during the heart cycle in children. *Heart* 83(5):537-542, 2000.

32. Jenkins C, Bricknell K, Marwick TH: Use of real-time three-dimensional echocardiography to measure left atrial volume: Comparison with other echocardiographic techniques. *J Am Soc Echocardiogr* 18(9):991-997, 2005.

33. Fabricius AM, Walther T, Falk V, Mohr FW: Three-dimensional echocardiography for planning of mitral valve surgery: current applicability? *Ann Thorac Surg* 78(2):575-578, 2004.

34. Sugeng L, Coon P, Weinert L, et al: Use of real-time 3-dimensional transthoracic echocardiography in the evaluation of mitral valve disease. *J Am Soc Echocardiogr* 19(4):413-421, 2006.

35. Binder TM, Rosenhek R, Porenta G, et al: Improved assessment of mitral valve stenosis by volumetric real-time three-dimensional echocardiography. *J Am Coll Cardiol* 36(4):1355-1361, 2000.

36. Chen Q, Nosir YF, Vletter WB, et al: Accurate assessment of mitral valve area in patients with mitral stenosis by three-dimensional echocardiography. *J Am Soc Echocardiogr* 10(2):133-140, 1997.

37. Zamorano J, Cordeiro P, Sugeng L, et al: Real-time three-dimensional echocardiography for rheumatic mitral valve stenosis evaluation: An accurate and novel approach. *J Am Coll Cardiol* 43(11):2091-2096, 2004.

38. Sebag IA, Morgan JG, Handschumacher MD, et al: Usefulness of three-dimensionally guided assessment of mitral stenosis using matrix-array ultrasound. *Am J Cardiol* 96(8):1151-1156, 2005.

39. Langerveld J, Valocik G, Plokker HW, et al: Additional value of three-dimensional transesophageal echocardiography for patients with mitral valve stenosis undergoing balloon valvuloplasty. *J Am Soc Echocardiogr* 16(8):841-849, 2003.

40. Sitges M, Jones M, Shiota T, et al: Real-time three-dimensional color doppler evaluation of the flow convergence zone for quantification of mitral regurgitation: Validation experimental animal study and initial clinical experience. *J Am Soc Echocardiogr* 16(1):38-45, 2003.

41. Yosefy C, Levine RA, Vaturi M, et al: Real-time 3D echo can enhance assessment of the vena contracta width: Overcoming the problem of oblique measurement in eccentric jets. *Circulation* 110(Suppl III):746, 2004.

42. Yosefy C, Levine RA, Solis-Martin J, et al: Proximal flow convergence region as assessed by real-time 3D echocardiography: Challenging the hemispherical assumption. *J Am Soc Echocardiogr* 20(4):389-396, 2007.

43. Salustri A, Becker AE, van Herwerden L, et al: Three-dimensional echocardiography of normal and pathologic mitral valve: A comparison with two-dimensional transesophageal echocardiography. *J Am Coll Cardiol* 27(6):1502-1510, 1996.

44. Chauvel C, Bogino E, Clerc P, et al: Usefulness of three-dimensional echocardiography for the evaluation of mitral valve prolapse: An intraoperative study. *J Heart Valve Dis* 9(3):341-349, 2000.

45. Ahmed S, Nanda NC, Miller AP, et al: Usefulness of transesophageal three-dimensional echocardiography in the identification of individual segment/scallop prolapse of the mitral valve. *Echocardiography* 20(2):203-209, 2003.

46. Macnab A, Jenkins NP, Ewington I, et al: A method for the morphological analysis of the regurgitant mitral valve using three dimensional echocardiography. *Heart* 90(7):771-776, 2004.

47. Otsuji Y, Handschumacher MD, Schwammenthal E, et al: Insights from three-dimensional echocardiography into the mechanism of functional mitral regurgitation: Direct in vivo demonstration of altered leaflet tethering geometry. *Circulation* 96(6):1999-2008, 1997.

48. Otsuji Y, Handschumacher MD, Liel-Cohen N, et al: Mechanism of ischemic mitral regurgitation with segmental left ventricular dysfunction: Three-dimensional echocardiographic studies in models of acute and chronic progressive regurgitation. *J Am Coll Cardiol* 37(2):641-648, 2001.

49. Hung J, Guerrero JL, Handschumacher MD, et al: Reverse ventricular remodeling reduces ischemic mitral regurgitation: Echo-guided device application in the beating heart. *Circulation* 106(20):2594-2600, 2002.

50. Kwan J, Shiota T, Agler DA, et al: Geometric differences of the mitral apparatus between ischemic and dilated cardiomyopathy with significant mitral regurgitation: Real-time three-dimensional echocardiography study. *Circulation* 107(8):1135-1140, 2003.

51. Ahmad RM, Gillinov AM, McCarthy PM, et al: Annular geometry and motion in human ischemic mitral regurgitation: Novel assessment with three-dimensional echocardiography and computer reconstruction. *Ann Thorac Surg* 78(6):2063-2068; discussion 8, 2004.

52. Watanabe N, Ogasawara Y, Yamaura Y, et al: Geometric deformity of the mitral annulus in patients with ischemic mitral regurgitation: A real-time three-dimensional echocardiographic study. *J Heart Valve Dis* 14(4):447-452, 2005.

53. Daimon M, Shiota T, Gillinov AM, et al: Percutaneous mitral valve repair for chronic ischemic mitral regurgitation: A real-time three-dimensional echocardiographic study in an ovine model. *Circulation* 111(17):2183-2189, 2005.

54. Messas E, Guerrero JL, Handschumacher MD, et al: Chordal cutting: A new therapeutic approach for ischemic mitral regurgitation. *Circulation* 104(16):1958-1963, 2001.

55. Qin JX, Shiota T, McCarthy PM, et al: Importance of mitral valve repair associated with left ventricular reconstruction for patients with ischemic cardiomyopathy: A real-time three-dimensional echocardiographic study. *Circulation* 108(Suppl 1):II241-II246, 2003.

56. Langer F, Rodriguez F, Ortiz S, et al: Subvalvular repair: The key to repairing ischemic mitral regurgitation? *Circulation* 112(9 Suppl):I383-I389, 2005.

57. Acker MA, Bolling S, Shemin R, et al: Mitral valve surgery in heart failure: Insights from the Acorn Clinical Trial. *J Thorac Cardiovasc Surg* 132(3):568-577, 77 e1-e4, 2006.

58. Nanda NC, Roychoudhury D, Chung SM, et al: Quantitative assessment of normal and stenotic aortic valve using transesophageal three-dimensional echocardiography. *Echocardiography* 11(6):617-625, 1994.

59. Menzel T, Mohr-Kahaly S, Kolsch B, et al: Quantitative assessment of aortic stenosis by three-dimensional echocardiography. *J Am Soc Echocardiogr* 10(3):215-223, 1997.

60. Ge S, Warner JG Jr, Abraham TP, et al: Three-dimensional surface area of the aortic valve orifice by three-dimensional echocardiography: Clinical validation of a novel index for assessment of aortic stenosis. *Am Heart J* 136(6):1042-1050, 1998.

61. Fyfe DA, Ludomirsky A, Sandhu S, et al: Left ventricular outflow tract obstruction defined by active three-dimensional echocardiography using rotational transthoracic acquisition. *Echocardiography* 11(6):607-615, 1994.

62. Miyamoto K, Nakatani S, Kanzaki H, et al: Detection of discrete subaortic stenosis by 3-dimensional transesophageal echocardiography. *Echocardiography* 22(9):783-784, 2005.

63. Sitges M, Qin JX, Lever HM, et al: Evaluation of left ventricular outflow tract area after septal reduction in obstructive hypertrophic cardiomyopathy: A real-time 3-dimensional echocardiographic study. *Am Heart J* 150(4):852-858, 2005.

64. Acar P, Jones M, Shiota T, et al: Quantitative assessment of chronic aortic regurgitation with 3-dimensional echocardiographic reconstruction: Comparison with electromagnetic flowmeter measurements. *J Am Soc Echocardiogr* 12(2):138-148, 1999.

65. Shiota T, Jones M, Tsujino H, et al: Quantitative analysis of aortic regurgitation: Real-time 3-dimensional and 2-dimensional color Doppler echocardiographic method—a clinical and a chronic animal study. *J Am Soc Echocardiogr* 15(9):966-971, 2002.

66. Sato Y, Kamata J, Izumoto H, et al: Morphological analysis of aortic root in eccentric aortic regurgitation using anyplane two-dimensional images produced by transesophageal three-dimensional echocardiography. *J Heart Valve Dis* 12(2):186-196, 2003.

67. Handke M, Schafer DM, Heinrichs G, et al: Quantitative assessment of aortic stenosis by three-dimensional anyplane and three-dimensional volume-rendered echocardiography. *Echocardiography* 19(1):45-53, 2002.

68. Fang L, Hsiung MC, Miller AP, et al: Assessment of aortic regurgitation by live three-dimensional transthoracic echocardiographic measurements of vena contracta area: Usefulness and validation. *Echocardiography* 22(9):775-781, 2005.

69. Li X, Jones M, Irvine T, et al: Real-time 3-dimensional echocardiography for quantification of the difference in left ventricular versus right ventricular stroke volume in a chronic animal model study: Improved results using C-scans for quantifying aortic regurgitation. *J Am Soc Echocardiogr* 17(8):870-875, 2004.

70. David TE, Feindel CM, Webb GD, et al: Long-term results of aortic valve-sparing operations for aortic root aneurysm. *J Thorac Cardiovasc Surg* 132(2):347-354, 2006.

71. Alsoufi B, Borger MA, Armstrong S, et al: Results of valve preservation and repair for bicuspid aortic valve insufficiency. *J Heart Valve Dis* 14(6):752-758; discussion 8-9, 2005.

72. Qin JX, Shiota T, Asher CR, et al: Usefulness of real-time three-dimensional echocardiography for evaluation of myectomy in patients with hypertrophic cardiomyopathy. *Am J Cardiol* 94(7):964-966, 2004.

73. Nemes A, Lagrand WK, McGhie JS, ten Cate FJ: Three-dimensional transesophageal echocardiography in the evaluation of aortic valve destruction by endocarditis. *J Am Soc Echocardiogr* 19(3):355 e13-e14, 2006.

74. Kort S: Real-time 3-dimensional echocardiography for prosthetic valve endocarditis: Initial experience. *J Am Soc Echocardiogr* 19(2):130-139, 2006.

75. Asch FM, Bieganski SP, Panza JA, Weissman NJ: Real-time 3-dimensional echocardiography evaluation of intracardiac masses. *Echocardiography* 23(3):218-224, 2006.

76. Balestrini L, Fleishman C, Lanzoni L, et al: Real-time 3-dimensional echocardiography evaluation of congenital heart disease. *J Am Soc Echocardiogr* 13(3):171-176, 2000.

77. Seliem MA, Fedec A, Cohen MS, et al: Real-time 3-dimensional echocardiographic imaging of congenital heart disease using matrix-array technology: Freehand real-time scanning adds instant morphologic details not well delineated by conventional 2-dimensional imaging. *J Am Soc Echocardiogr* 19(2):121-129, 2006.

78. De Castro S, Caselli S, Papetti F, et al: Feasibility and clinical impact of live three-dimensional echocardiography in the management of congenital heart disease. *Echocardiography* 23(7):553-561, 2006.

79. Marx GR, Fulton DR, Pandian NG, et al: Delineation of site, relative size and dynamic geometry of atrial septal defects by real-time three-dimensional echocardiography. *J Am Coll Cardiol* 25(2):482-490, 1995.

80. Mehmood F, Vengala S, Nanda NC, et al: Usefulness of live three-dimensional transthoracic echocardiography in the characterization of atrial septal defects in adults. *Echocardiography* 21(8):707-713, 2004.

81. Acar P, Dulac Y, Roux D, et al: Comparison of transthoracic and transesophageal three-dimensional echocardiography for assessment of atrial septal defect diameter in children. *Am J Cardiol* 91(4):500-502, 2003.

82. Hofmann T, Franzen O, Koschyk DH, et al: Three-dimensional color Doppler echocardiography for assessing shunt volume in atrial septal defects. *J Am Soc Echocardiogr* 17(11):1173-1178, 2004.

83. Barrea C, Levasseur S, Roman K, et al: Three-dimensional echocardiography improves the understanding of left atrioventricular valve morphology and function in atrioventricular septal defects undergoing patch augmentation. *J Thorac Cardiovasc Surg* 129(4):746-753, 2005.

84. Nii M, Guerra V, Roman KS, et al: Three-dimensional tricuspid annular function provides insight into the mechanisms of tricuspid valve regurgitation in classic hypoplastic left heart syndrome. *J Am Soc Echocardiogr* 19(4):391-402, 2006.

85. Htay T, Nanda NC, Agrawal G, et al: Live three-dimensional transthoracic echocardiographic assessment of aortic dissection. *Echocardiography* 20(6):573-577, 2003.

86. Zwas DR, Takuma S, Mullis-Jansson S, et al: Feasibility of real-time 3-dimensional treadmill stress echocardiography. *J Am Soc Echocardiogr* 12(5):285-289, 1999.

87. Pulerwitz T, Hirata K, Abe Y, et al: Feasibility of using a real-time 3-dimensional technique for contrast dobutamine stress echocardiography. *J Am Soc Echocardiogr* 19(5):540-545, 2006.

88. Takeuchi M, Otani S, Weinert L, et al: Comparison of contrast-enhanced real-time live 3-dimensional dobutamine stress echocardiography with contrast 2-dimensional echocardiography for detecting stress-induced wall-motion abnormalities. *J Am Soc Echocardiogr* 19(3):294-299, 2006.

89. Toledo E, Lang RM, Collins KA, et al: Imaging and quantification of myocardial perfusion using real-time three-dimensional echocardiography. *J Am Coll Cardiol* 47(1):146-154, 2006.

90. Scheurer M, Bandisode V, Ruff P, et al: Early experience with real-time three-dimensional echocardiographic guidance of right ventricular biopsy in children. *Echocardiography* 23(1):45-49, 2006.

91. Vazquez de Prada JA, Jiang L, Handschumacher MD, et al: Quantification of pericardial effusions by three-dimensional echocardiography. *J Am Coll Cardiol* 24(1):254-259, 1994.

92. Duncan K, Nanda NC, Foster WA, et al: Incremental value of live/real time three-dimensional transthoracic echocardiography in the assessment of left ventricular thrombi. *Echocardiography* 23(1):68-72, 2006.

93. Lokhandwala J, Liu Z, Jundi M, et al: Three-dimensional echocardiography of intracardiac masses. *Echocardiography* 21(2):159-163, 2004.

94. Chamoun AJ, McCulloch M, Xie T, et al: Real-time three-dimensional echocardiography versus two-dimensional echocardiography in the diagnosis of left ventricular apical thrombi: Preliminary findings. *J Clin Ultrasound* 31(8):412-418, 2003.

95. van der Heide JA, Mannaerts HF, Spruijt HJ, et al: Noninvasive mapping of left ventricular electromechanical asynchrony by three-dimensional echocardiography and semi-automatic contour detection. *Am J Cardiol* 94(11):1449-1453, 2004.

96. Kapetanakis S, Kearney MT, Siva A, et al: Real-time three-dimensional echocardiography: A novel technique to quantify global left ventricular mechanical dyssynchrony. *Circulation* 112(7):992-1000, 2005.

97. Lind B, Nowak J, Dorph J, et al: Analysis of temporal requirements for myocardial tissue velocity imaging. *Eur J Echocardiogr* 3(3):214-219, 2002.

98. Suematsu Y, Takamoto S, Kaneko Y, et al: Beating atrial septal defect closure monitored by epicardial real-time three-dimensional echocardiography without cardiopulmonary bypass. *Circulation* 107(5):785-790, 2003.

99. Suematsu Y, Marx GR, Stoll JA, et al: Three-dimensional echocardiography-guided beating-heart surgery without cardiopulmonary bypass: A feasibility study. *J Thorac Cardiovasc Surg* 128(4):579-587, 2004.

100. Rasche V, Mansour MC, Reddy V, et al: Fusion of three-dimensional x-ray angiography and live three-dimensional echocardiography. *IEEE Transactions on Medical Imaging* 2006; In press.

Chapter 5

Tissue Doppler and Speckle Tracking Echocardiography

OTTO A. SMISETH, MD, PhD • THOR EDVARDSEN, MD, PhD

In daily clinical practice left ventricular (LV) function is commonly evaluated by two-dimensional (2D) and M-mode echocardiography. Despite all obvious advantages, visual evaluation of LV function by 2D echocardiography suffers from being subjective and provides only semi-quantitative data. Furthermore, visual assessment has limited ability to detect more subtle changes in function and changes in timing of myocardial motion throughout systole and diastole. M-mode echocardiography provides quantitative data but does not allow comprehensive evaluation of regional LV function. Tissue Doppler imaging (TDI) and speckle tracking echocardiography (STE) have been introduced as quantitative and more objective methods to quantify regional and global LV systolic and diastolic function. TDI can measure a number of different myocardial functional parameters, that is velocity, acceleration, displacement, strain rate (SR), and strain. STE is an alternative method for measuring myocardial strain and can be used to quantify LV rotation. Both methods can be applied to assess right ventricular (RV) function as well, but validation has been done mostly for the left ventricle.

This chapter will explain the technical principles behind TDI and STE and the physiological meaning of the different parameters. The clinical application of the methodologies will be reviewed. Finally, synchronization of ventricular contraction will be addressed. Application of TDI in stress echocardiography is discussed in Chapter 16.

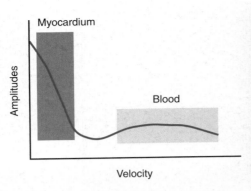

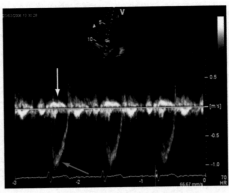

Figure 5–1. *Principle for separation of myocardial velocities from blood flow velocities. The* left panel *illustrates the difference in velocity and amplitude between myocardial and blood velocities. The* right panel *is a recording in the left ventricular outflow tract, which samples both myocardial and blood flow velocities. The* white arrow *points to the high intensity signals from the myocardium and the* red arrow *to the low intensity, but high velocity signals from the blood.*

Physical Principles of Tissue Doppler Echocardiography

Velocity and Displacement Imaging

Velocities by Color Doppler

The Doppler principle has traditionally been used to measure blood flow velocities but may also be used to measure myocardial velocities and other tissue velocities. Separation between velocities in myocardium and blood is possible because of different signal amplitudes and Doppler frequencies. The myocardium is moving at much lower speed than blood, and therefore Doppler frequencies are lower. Furthermore, the amplitude of myocardial signals is much higher than for blood. These differences allow myocardial velocities to be separated from blood flow velocities by using filters, which reject echoes that originate from the blood pool (Fig. 5–1). Velocities can be recorded using color Doppler or pulsed Doppler mode.

Myocardial velocity imaging was first introduced in the early 1990s[1,2] and is now an established clinical method for quantifying LV systolic and diastolic function. Similar to color flow imaging, TDI uses an autocorrelator technique to calculate and display multigated points of color-coded velocities along a series of ultrasound (US) scan lines within a 2D sector. As illustrated in Figure 5–2, myocardial motion can be imaged as color-coded velocities superimposed on a 2D gray scale image in real time. The frame rate for 2D color Doppler is typically from 80 to 200 frames per second, depending on the width of the US sector, and is usually set higher than for the simultaneous gray scale images. Myocardial velocities are automatically decoded into numerical values, which can be stored digitally for later offline analyses.[3] By convention, velocities toward the transducer are color-coded red, and velocities away from the transducer are coded blue. Figure 5–3 shows

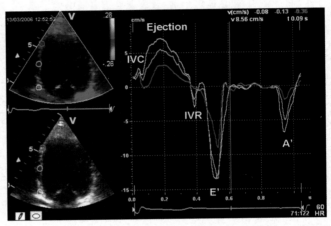

Figure 5–2. *Normal myocardial velocities. Tissue Doppler velocities from the anterior wall of the left ventricle in a healthy individual. A', velocity during atrial-induced filling; E', velocity during early diastolic filling; IVC, isovolumic contraction period; IVR, isovolumic relaxation period.*

2D images from a normal person and from a patient with acute myocardial infarction (AMI).

During normal LV systole the base of the ventricle descends toward the apex and moves back during diastole, whereas the apex is relatively stationary. Therefore, from apical views long-axis motion is dominated by red-encoded velocities in systole and blue-encoded velocities during early filling and atrial-induced filling. Dysfunctional myocardium, however, may show grossly abnormal motion with reversed longitudinal velocities during systole. Assessment of myocardial function by the 2D color display, however, is not useful in practical diagnostics, and velocity analysis should be done as post-processing. In some cases it may be helpful to use the curved M-mode format, which provides a quick view of direction and timing of velocities in different segments (Fig. 5–4). The standard approach, however, is analysis of velocity traces from

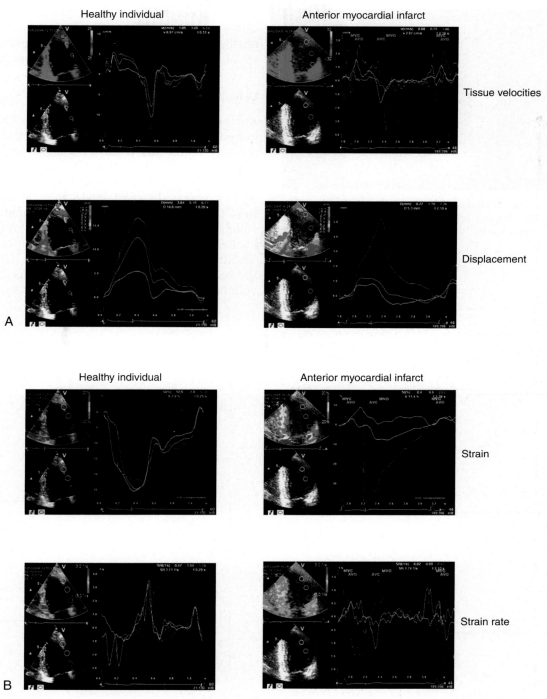

Figure 5–3. Acute myocardial infarction. To the left, recordings from a healthy individual, and to the right, from a patient with anterior myocardial infarction (be aware of different scales). All tissue Doppler modalities are sampled from three identical levels along the anterior left ventricular wall. In ischemic myocardium systolic velocities and displacement are typically reduced (A), and there are reductions in systolic strain and strain rate (B).

multiple regions within a 2D image, as illustrated in Figure 5–2. This analysis allows direct comparison of velocities in different segments on the same image. The most important measures from the velocity traces are peak systolic ejection velocity (S) and peak early diastolic lengthening velocity (E′). One should be aware that velocities obtained with TDI in 2D color mode are mean values of the instantaneous velocity spectrum.[3,4] A schematic presentation of all tissue Doppler modalities (tissue velocities, displacement, SR, and strain) from the apical four-chamber view is demonstrated in Figure 5–5.

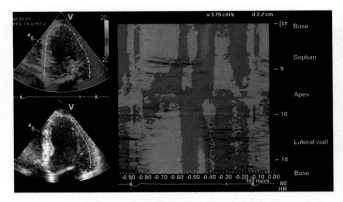

Figure 5-4. Curved M-mode display of myocardial velocities. Tissue Doppler imaging velocities in two-dimensional display in systole from a normal heart (left) *and as curved M-mode* (right).

Assessment of LV function from the parasternal short axis is possible, but only a limited number of segments can be imaged (Fig. 5-6). Therefore, most often apical views are preferred when assessing LV function by TDI.

Velocities by Pulsed Doppler

Another approach is to use spectral tissue Doppler with pulsed-Doppler activated, which is applied mainly to measure mitral and tricuspid annular velocities. It is important to be aware that the pulsed-Doppler mode presents the peaks of the instantaneous velocity spectrum, whereas the color mode provides mean velocities. This implies that velocities measured by the 2D color method described previously are lower than velocities by pulsed Doppler, typically about 25% lower.[5,6] The difference, however, depends on the band width of the velocity spectrum, which is determined by sample volume and by acoustical noise. Figure 5-7 illustrates

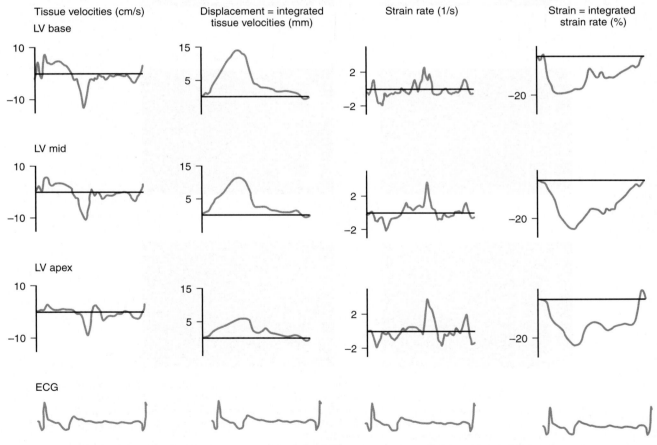

Figure 5-5. Simultaneous presentation of the different tissue Doppler imaging modalities. Recordings are from basal, mid, and apical part of the septum in apical four-chamber view. The first column shows velocity tracings. The second column shows displacement curves obtained by temporal integration of the velocity curves. The third column shows strain rate. The fourth column shows strain, obtained by temporal integration of strain rate. The time axis is the same for all modalities. Velocity and displacement decrease from base to apex, whereas strain and strain rate are relatively similar in magnitude at all levels. ECG, electrocardiogram; LV, left ventricular. (Modified from Skulstad H, Urheim S, Edvardsen T, et al: J Am Coll Cardiol 47:1672-1682, 2006.)

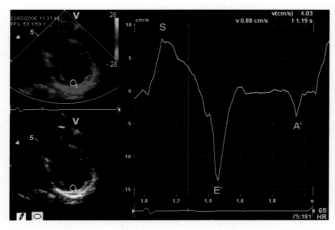

Figure 5-6. *Myocardial velocities from a parasternal short-axis view. A', velocity during atrial-induced velocity; E', velocity during early diastolic filling; S, systolic ejection velocity.*

the difference between velocities by color Doppler and pulsed-Doppler modes. Disadvantages of the pulsed-Doppler method are: (1) it has limited spatial resolution; (2) velocities are obtained from only one region at a time; and (3) it does not allow offline analysis.

Limitations of Velocity Imaging

Angle Dependency. Similar to all other Doppler modalities velocity imaging is angle dependent because only velocity components in the beam direction are recorded. Therefore, it is essential that the US beam is aligned parallel to the LV wall in long-axis imaging and perpendicular to the wall for radial measurements in short-axis imaging. In longitudinal views, velocities should not be measured near the apex because the apical curvature gives large-angle problems. This is a significant limitation when studying patients with coronary artery disease (CAD) because pathology may be limited to the apical segments. Although the velocity amplitude is angle dependent, characteristic features in the temporal velocity pattern are not angle dependent.

Therefore, with the exception of the apical region, velocity imaging is a powerful tool for comparing function between different segments.[7]

Movement of Sample Volume Relative to Myocardium. Tissue Doppler measures velocity within a defined sample volume but not within a defined piece of myocardium. The difference between the two may be significant depending on cardiac motion. This limitation, which applies to all TDI modalities, can in part be compensated for by using tracking algorithms that move the sample volume continuously or in steps during the heart cycle. STE compensates for this limitation.

Reverberations. Reverberations are echoes resulting from multiple reflections within the body and are often caused by relatively motionless tissue layers close to the body surface in transthoracic imaging. In gray scale imaging they are seen as false echoes or reduced contrast. For color TDI, the reverberations may cause a bias in the mean velocity estimate, and often the bias is toward zero velocity. The amount of bias depends on the intensity of the reverberation signal relative to the tissue velocity signal. Still, the sign of the velocity is seldom affected, so it might be difficult to detect reverberations when using the color display.

Tethering Effects and Cardiac Translation. Because myocardium in one region of the ventricle is tethered to neighboring myocardium, velocities in one region are affected by motion in adjacent tissue. In addition, regional velocities may result from motion of the entire heart (translation).[8-10] Therefore, myocardial velocities demonstrate marked regional non-uniformity in the normal ventricle.[11,12] These factors are not limitations of the TDI methodology but reflect a limitation of velocity to serve as a parameter of regional contractility.

Load Dependency. Similar to global ejection fraction (EF), all regional ejection phase indices are load depen-

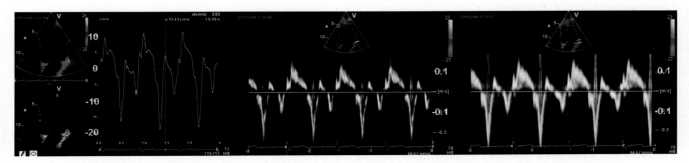

Figure 5-7. *Comparison between velocities by color Doppler and pulsed Doppler modes. All images are recorded from identical position in the same left ventricle. Myocardial color Doppler is shown in the* left panel *and pulsed Doppler in the* middle *and* right panels. *Because the color mode gives mean velocities, amplitudes are smaller than with pulsed-Doppler mode. The recording in the* right panel *is performed with a larger sample volume (12 mm) and higher gain than for the* middle panel *(5 mm). Please note the effect of sample volume and gain on signal amplitudes in systolic and diastolic velocities.*

dent.[9,12] This problem, however, is less important than for EF because the TDI parameters are used primarily to diagnose regional myocardial dysfunction, and regional differences are likely to persist even when there are changes in loading. This is not a limitation of the technology but reflects a fundamental relationship between myocardial fiber shortening and load.

Displacement Imaging

By performing temporal integration of velocities from a particular region one obtains *displacement* curves. This is illustrated in Figure 5–3A. In long-axis views, velocity and displacement increase progressively from apex toward base. Displacement can be displayed in real time as color-coded bands or measured offline from displacement curves. At the present time, this modality has not proven to provide added diagnostic value to velocity imaging.[12] The limitations that are listed for velocity imaging also apply to displacement imaging.

Strain Rate and Strain Imaging

Strain means deformation and is an excellent parameter for quantification of myocardial function. Analogous to LV EF, which quantifies global contractility, myocardial strain quantifies regional contractility. In principle, strain may also be used to quantify diastolic function, but this application has not been well developed.

Using implanted myocardial markers, quantification of myocardial function in terms of strain and SR has been available for a long time in cardiac physiology.[13] The only clinical method to measure myocardial strain has been magnetic resonance imaging (MRI) with tissue tagging, but complexity and cost has limited this methodology to research protocols.[14] More recently SR imaging by TDI has been introduced as a bedside, clinical method.[9,15,16] Strain may also be measured by STE, an emerging technology that is addressed on page 122.

Definitions of Strain and Strain Rate

Strain is a measure of how much an object has been deformed, and several formulas can be used to calculate different types of strain. In cardiac mechanics, the simple approach proposed by Mirsky and colleagues[17,18] is used to calculate strain as percent or fractional change in dimension. This implies that systolic strain is a measure of percentage shortening when measurements are done in the long axis and percent thickening for radial measurements in the short axis. This strain measure is named Lagrangian strain and is given by Equation A. Epsilon (ϵ) is used as symbol of Lagrangian strain: In the formula, L is the current length and L_0 is the original length.

$$L = \frac{L - L_0}{L} = \frac{\Delta L}{L_0} \qquad (A)$$

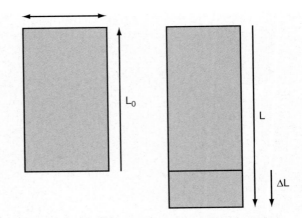

Figure 5–8. *Schematic illustration of myocardial strain. Lagrangian strain equals $\Delta L/L_0$. L, current length; L_0, original length; ΔL, change in length.*

Figure 5–8 illustrates schematically the principles for calculation of Lagrangian strain, and Figure 5–9 shows a typical myocardial strain trace recorded from implanted myocardial markers in an experiment. By convention, lengthening and thickening strains are assigned positive values and shortening and thinning strains negative values. This implies that systolic shortening results in negative strains, and systolic thickening in positive strains.

When strain is measured in one dimension, there will only be shortening and lengthening strains or thickening and thinning strains, respectively. During the heart cycle, however, the LV myocardium goes through a complex three-dimensional (3D) deforma-

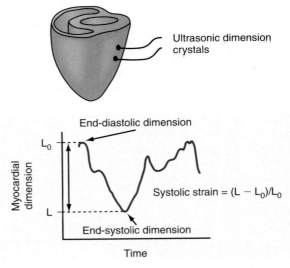

Figure 5–9. *Typical longitudinal myocardial strain trace. The recording shows strain by sonomicrometry in an anesthetized dog. Strain was recorded between two ultrasonic crystals implanted into the myocardium. The figure illustrates calculation of systolic strain. Please note that peak systolic strain equals systolic shortening fraction. L_0, original length; L, current length.*

tion that leads to shear strains, when one border is displaced relative to another. In a clinical context, however, we only assess the one-dimensional myocardial strains.

Calculation of Strain Rate and Strain from Myocardial Velocity Gradient

The theoretical basis for measuring strain by TDI is that myocardial velocity gradient is an estimate of SR, and therefore strain can be calculated as the temporal integral of SR. Using these concepts Heimdal and colleagues[16] introduced real-time SR imaging based on myocardial Doppler velocities. SR can be estimated by TDI as a velocity gradient between two spatial points (x and $x+\Delta x$) as shown in Equation B.

$$SR \approx \frac{v(x) - v(x + \Delta x)}{\Delta x} \qquad (B)$$

Temporal integration of the velocity gradient gives the logarithmic strain estimate denoted *natural strain* (ϵ_N) shown in Equation C. The name refers to the use of the natural logarithm function, ln. Lagrangian strain (ϵ) can be derived from natural strain using the mathematical conversion in Equation D. To accurately determine strain it is necessary to track and follow the motion of the material points (fixed particles) within the myocardium through time. This it is not feasible with TDI, and therefore only estimates of true strain can be obtained by this imaging modality.

$$\epsilon_N = \ln(L/L_0) \qquad (C)$$

$$\epsilon = \exp(\epsilon_N) - 1 \qquad (D)$$

The rationale for using spatial velocity gradient as a marker of myocardial function is that a velocity difference between two adjacent regions implies either compression or lengthening of the tissue in between, and the spatial velocity gradient equals SR. When LV systolic function is studied in the LV long-axis view, SR measures regional shortening rate, and strain measures regional shortening fraction. In the LV short-axis view, SR measures systolic thickening rate. During diastole, SR measures myocardial lengthening and thinning rates, respectively. Because strain is dimensionless, SR has units of 1/s.

SR can be considered a "normalized myocardial velocity," which is not influenced by overall motion of the heart (translation) or by motion caused by contraction in adjacent segments. This is in contrast to *velocity* within a myocardial segment, which is the net result of motion caused by contractions in that segment, motion resulting from tethering to other segments, and cardiac translation.[9,19] The effect of tethering explains why LV longitudinal velocities measured from an apical window increase progressively from the apex toward the

base.[20-22] Strains and SRs, however, are essentially similar between apex and base. Therefore, strain and SR in principle are superior to velocity as markers of regional contractility. However, there are technical issues that make SR imaging more challenging than velocity imaging.

Some authors prefer to express regional myocardial function as spatial velocity gradient rather than SR, in particular for radial strains.[23-25] Because SR by definition equals the spatial velocity gradient, the two measurements are in principle the same parameter.

Limitations of Strain and Strain Rate Imaging

Signal Noise. SR by TDI has significant problems with random noise. This reflects an effect of measuring a difference between velocities because the error is the sum of the errors of the two velocities. The signal-to-noise ratio for SR can be improved by increasing the spatial offset (strain length) for the velocity points, which increases the velocity difference but will reduce the spatial resolution. The problem with random noise can also be reduced by temporal averaging within a heart cycle and by averaging multiple heart cycles. However, these methods for noise reduction represent compromises between optimal signal-to-noise ratio and requirements for high spatial and temporal resolution. The spatial offset for measurement of longitudinal strain and SR is typically between 5 and 12 mm but can be defined by the operator. For transmural strain wall, thickness and translational motion restricts the range for adjustment of strain length. As a rule of thumb the strain length should be set to approximately half the systolic thickness of the wall.[26] SR imaging has limited lateral resolution, which limits the ability to measure separately from subendocardial and subepicardial wall layers. Furthermore, when the sample volume is at the inner or outer LV wall layers, the signal may in part represent velocities in the blood pool and pericardium, respectively. Fortunately, measurement of strain is associated with fewer noise problems than SR because integration tends to eliminate random noise in the SR signal. In the strain signal, however, there may be significant drift within a given heart cycle.

Angle Dependency. Another problem with SR imaging is strong sensitivity to misalignment between the cardiac axis and the US beam. Similar to measurement of blood flow velocity, myocardial velocity is reduced in proportion to the cosine of the angle between the velocity vector and the US beam. Furthermore because myocardium is virtually uncompressible, for example shortening in one axis is always accompanied by thickening in other axis, and this increases measurement problems resulting from misalignment.[9] Therefore, care should be taken to align the US beam parallel to all myocardial segments of interest. It is of special impor-

TABLE 5–1. Myocardial Velocities, Strain Rates, and Strains in Healthy Volunteers*

	Segments							
	Anterior		**Septal**		**Posterior**		**Lateral**	
	Base	*Apex*	*Base*	*Apex*	*Base*	*Apex*	*Base*	*Apex*
Tissue Doppler velocities (cm/s) ($n = 33$)	6.5±1.6	2.8±1.0†	6.7±1.4	2.8±1.1†	6.5±1.4	2.9±1.3†	6.7±1.5	3.2±1.6†
Doppler strain rate (1/s) ($n = 33$)	−1.7±0.4	−1.6±0.4	−1.6±0.4	−1.7±0.3	−1.6±0.3	−1.7±0.3	−1.6±0.3	−1.6±0.3
Doppler strain (%) ($n = 33$)	−19±4	−18±5	−17±3	−19±4	−20±4	−21±2	−18±4	−17±3
MRI strain (%) ($n = 11$)	−17±3	−18±4	−17±3	−19±5	−18±4	−19±3	−18±4	−17±4

*Longitudinal measures from eight segments (two- and four-chamber views).
†$P < 0.05$ compared to the basal segment within the same region.
MRI, magnetic resonance imaging.
Adapted from Edvardsen T, Gerber BL, Garot J, et al: *Circulation* 106:50-56, 2002.

tance to avoid misinterpretation in myocardial areas close to the LV apex resulting from the apical curvature. Angle problems can be reduced by using the smallest possible sector and recording from one wall at a time. Recent studies indicate that the problem with misalignment might be less than anticipated.[12,27]

Reverberations. Reverberations are a major source of error in SR imaging. A small local bias in the velocity will cause large changes in the spatial velocity gradient and therefore in the SR. The only way to avoid reverberation noise is to get better scanning window. When analyzing the SR data, it is important to recognize the reverberation artifacts and to avoid the regions affected. Curved anatomical M-mode can be an effective tool to identify larger reverberation artifacts and for the experienced user can be seen as "unphysiological" color patterns.

Movement of the myocardium relative to the sampling volume and load dependency are limitations as discussed in the section on limitations of velocity imaging.

Preferred TDI Modalities in Clinical Routine

Despite theoretical advantages of SR and strain relative to velocity,[28] there are unresolved technical limitations of these modalities. Therefore, with the present state of the technologies, velocity imaging is preferred as the primary TDI methodology for assessing regional function. Strain and SR imaging may be used as a supplementary method for exploring changes in regional function. Displacement imaging needs more validation before it can be recommended for routine clinical use. Table 5–1 displays LV longitudinal strain and SR values compared to tissue velocities.[15]

Speckle Tracking Echocardiography

STE measures strain by tracking speckles in gray scale echocardiographic images. The speckles are created by interference of US beams in the myocardium and are seen in gray scale B-mode images as a characteristic speckle pattern. The speckles are the result of constructive and destructive interference of US back-scattered from structures smaller than a wavelength of US.[29,30] The speckles function as natural acoustic markers, which can be tracked from frame to frame (Fig. 5–10). By automated measurement of distance between speckles, it is possible to measure angle-independent strain (Figs. 5–11 and 5–12). Measurements can be done simultaneously from multiple regions within an image plane.

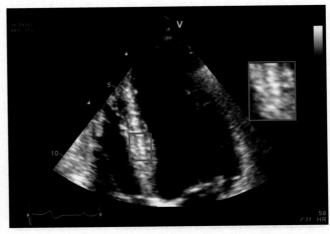

Figure 5–10. *Myocardial speckles. Speckle tracking echocardiography measures strain by tracking speckles in gray scale echocardiographic images. A part of the septum (red box) from a four-chamber view is enlarged.*

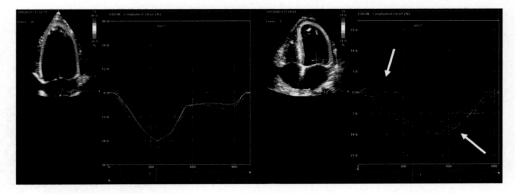

Figure 5–11. Speckle tracking echocardiography showing long-axis strains. The left panel *shows typical strain pattern from a normal left ventricle. The* right panel *shows recordings from a patient with an anterior myocardial infarction. In the apical left ventricular segments* (arrows) *there is lengthening during early systole and there is postsystolic shortening.*

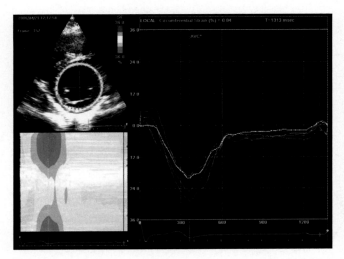

Figure 5–12. Circumferential strain by speckle tracking echocardiography in a normal person.

In contrast to Doppler-based strain, which measures velocities from a fixed point in space with reference to an external probe, STE measures distance between two markers within a defined piece of myocardium. Furthermore, speckle tracking provides a direct measure of strain, whereas TDI calculates strain by integrating SR. The most obvious advantages of STE, however, are independence of insonation angle and of cardiac translation.[31-33] In contrast to Doppler-based strain this enables measurement of circumferential strains from the LV short axis, radial strains in multiple segments, and longitudinal strain from myocardial areas close to the LV apex. Another promising feature is the ability to measure LV rotation and torsion.[32,34] Optimal frame rates are in the order of 80 frames per second, but higher frame rates may be expected with further development of the methodology.[35] Higher frame rates are needed to measure peak velocities and SRs. The clinical value of STE remains to be defined.

Normal Physiology—Left Ventricle

To interpret TDI parameters it is important to understand the physiology of LV function. During normal systole there is longitudinal myocardial shortening, which causes the LV base to descend toward the apex,[35-37] and there is circumferential shortening. Systolic thickening is a result of both longitudinal and circumferential shortening. The systolic descent of the base is approximately 12 to 15 mm in healthy people,[36,37] whereas the apex is relatively stationary, moving only a few millimeters. During diastole there is myocardial lengthening during early diastolic and during atrial-induced filling. In addition, there is a twisting motion (torsion) of the ventricle. When viewed from the LV apex toward base, there is systolic counterclockwise rotation of the apex and clockwise rotation of the base, and there is back-rotation in early diastole. Because apex and base rotate in opposite directions, the ventricle is twisted about its long-axis (Fig. 5–13). This pattern of contraction reflects the spiral orientation of myocardial fibers (Fig. 5–14). In the LV subendocardium the myocardial fibers have an approximately longitudinal orientation with an angle of about 80 degrees with respect to the circumferential direction. The angle decreases toward the midwall, in which the fibers are oriented in the circumferential direction (0 degrees) and decreases further to an oblique fibre orientation of about −60 degrees in the subepicardium (Fig. 5–15). This fiber orientation appears to be essentially similar in humans[38,39] and other mammalian species.[40,41]

LV twist appears to play an important role for normal systolic function, and diastolic untwist may contribute to diastolic suction.[42-45] The magnitude and characteristics of LV twist have been described in different clinical and experimental studies, and it is well established that LV rotation is sensitive to changes in

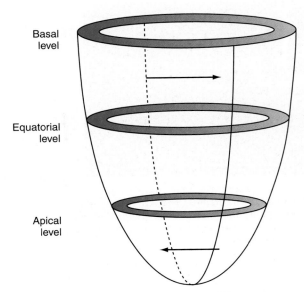

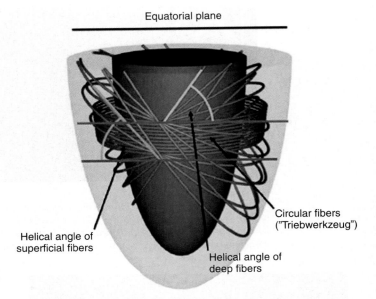

Figure 5–13. *Schematic representation of directions of left ventricular systolic rotation. When viewed from the apex, apical rotation is counterclockwise and basal rotation is clockwise.[33]*

Figure 5–14. *Schematic illustration of the varying fiber orientation through the left ventricular wall. The fibers are obliquely oriented in the subepicardial layers and changes gradually to a circumferential direction in the midwall and further to a longitudinal direction in the subendocardium. (From Anderson RH, Ho SY, Redmann K, et al: Eur J Cardiothorac Surg 28[4]:517-525, 2005.)*

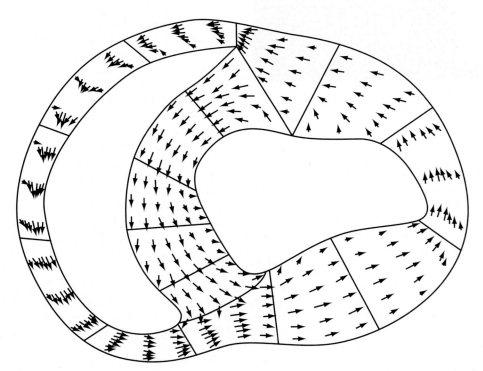

Figure 5–15. *Measured fiber directions in a pig heart. Fiber direction vectors are projected onto a two-dimensional cross-section, viewed from base toward apex. All fibers are drawn as vectors with the same length, so the more longitudinally aligned fibers, particularly in the subendocardium, have a smaller projection onto this plane than the circumferentially aligned midwall fibers. (The apparent inward orientation of some of the subepicardial and subendocardial fibers reflects the taper of the wall, out of the plane of this projection.) (Reprinted from Stevens C, Remme E, LeGrice I, Hunter P: J Biomech 36[5]:737-748, 2003.)*

both regional and global LV function.[46-58] Therefore, assessment of LV rotation represents an interesting approach for quantifying LV function. However, until recently magnetic resonance imaging tagging has been the only clinical method available.[59-67] It has recently been shown that LV rotation and twist can be measured with STE.[32,34] Figure 5–16 shows LV rotation as measured by STE and magnetic resonance imaging tagging. LV twist is calculated as the difference between apical and basal rotations.

In LV short-axis images, TDI shows that the subendocardium moves faster than the subepicardium, which results in a transmural velocity gradient. Figure 5–17 illustrates that this velocity gradient reflects a progressive increase in strain (thickening fraction) when moving the sample volume from the epicardium toward the endocardium. More thickening in subendocardium than subepicardium does not represent a difference in contractility between wall layers but is just a consequence of geometry and tissue incompressibility. As

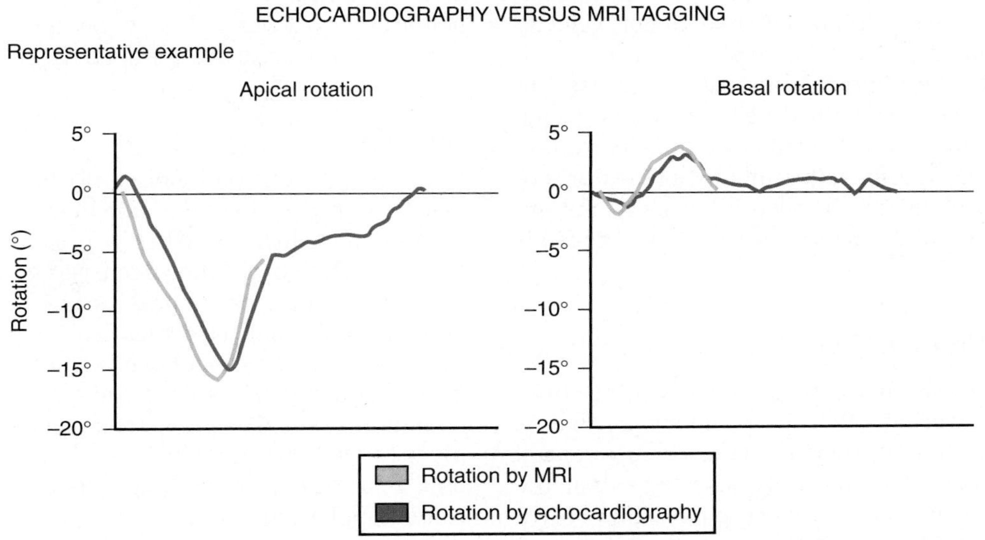

ECHOCARDIOGRAPHY VERSUS MRI TAGGING

Figure 5–16. *Representative traces of left ventricular rotation by speckle tracking echocardiography compared to mechanical resonance imaging (MRI) tagging.[33] Rotation is not feasible for a whole cardiac cycle because of MR tag fading* (yellow line).

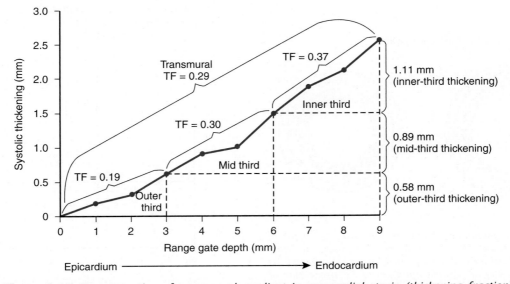

Figure 5–17. *Demonstration of transmural gradient in myocardial strain (thickening fraction) between inner and outer left ventricular wall layers in a dog study. The left ventricular wall was divided into three layers, each 3 mm thick. Systolic thickening was measured by a 10-mHz miniaturized Doppler probe that was sutured to the epicardium. The figure displays systolic thickening fraction layer by layer and demonstrates that the inner layer thickens more than the outer layer. TF, thickening fraction. (Reproduced from Zhu WX, Myers ML, Hartley CJ, et al: Am J Physiol 251[5 Pt 2]:H1045-H1055, 1986.)*

illustrated in Figure 5-18 the transmural gradient in thickening is consistent with the behavior of wall layers in simple spherical and ellipsoidal models.[68,69] In the LV long-axis view, there are also higher velocities and strains in the inner than in the outer wall layers, but the differences are smaller than for radial measurements and are difficult to measure by current TDI technology.[70]

During the cardiac cycle the LV velocity trace has three major velocity spikes[3] (see Fig. 5-2). In the long-axis view, the dominant systolic velocity component is directed toward the LV apex and represents the ejection phase. During diastole there are two major velocity components: an early diastolic velocity and an atrial-induced velocity, both directed toward the LV base. In addition, there are well-defined velocity spikes during isovolumic contraction (IVC) and isovolumic relaxation (IVR).[71] All these velocity spikes are distinct features of the velocity trace and can be seen in virtually any imaging projection, but direction of the velocities depends on projection.

Isovolumic Contraction

As illustrated in Figure 5-2 there is a sharp, but brief velocity spike during IVC. This velocity spike is caused by shortening, which starts before mitral valve closure and is temporarily arrested when the mitral valve reaches its final closing position.[72] Myocardial shortening during IVC can occur because blood is displaced into the bulging mitral leaflets, which causes reduction in LV long and short axis but no real change in LV volume.

In some cases there is a small negative velocity component at the end of IVC (see Fig. 5-2), which reflects normal asynchrony in electromechanical activation.

The high frame rate of TDI enables measurement of myocardial acceleration, and studies of mitral and tricuspid ring motion suggest that IVC acceleration can serve as an index of contractility.[73,74] This is an interesting concept and may be valid for studies of global LV function. However, as recently demonstrated, regional myocardial acceleration does not reflect regional contractility during ischemia.[75] More studies are needed before IVC acceleration can be recommended as a clinical tool to measure contractility.

Ejection

Peak systolic ejection velocity (S) has proven to be a marker of regional systolic function[4,10,76-78] (Fig. 5-19). Myocardial velocity reaches a peak during the early phase of ejection and then decreases gradually. In some cases a second, smaller peak occurs later during ejection. Longitudinal velocities are more reproducible than radial velocities and can be measured in virtually all vascular territories of the left ventricle. Therefore, longitudinal velocities are recommended in the assessment of LV function. Table 5-1 presents normal ejection velocities from LV long axis as assessed by 2D color Doppler mode.

Isovolumic Relaxation

In the LV long-axis there is a negative velocity spike during IVR (see Fig. 5-2). Analogous to the mechanism for the IVC velocity, the IVR velocity is attributed to

SPHERICAL MODEL

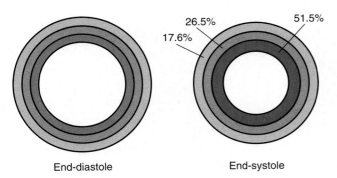

Figure 5-18. Explanation of transmural strain gradient in left ventricular short-axis strain. A spherical model in which the wall is divided into equally spaced layers. The model assumes homogeneity of regional function and conservation of mass. The starting position to the left *simulates end-diastole. To the right, systole is simulated by reducing inner radius by 25%. Note the marked difference between thickening of the inner (51.5%), middle (26.5%), and outer layers (17.6%). The same principle applies to cylindrical models, but the magnitude of the gradient is smaller. (Reproduced from Hexeberg E, Homan DC, Bache RJ: Cardiovasc Res 29[1]:16-21, 1995.)*

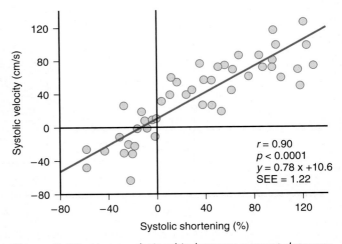

Figure 5-19. Linear relationship between percent decrease in regional segment length shortening (abscissa) and systolic velocities (ordinate). There is a significant correlation between systolic velocities and segment shortening. (From Derumeaux G, Ovize M, Loufoua J, et al: Circulation 97:1970-1977, 1998.)

myocardial lengthening, which starts near end-systole and is temporarily interrupted by aortic valve closure.[72] A the end of IVR there is normally a small positive velocity component that represents slight postsystolic shortening.[79] The etiology of this velocity component is not known, but it may reflect normal intraventricular asynchrony of relaxation.[80] In the diseased ventricle and in particular during myocardial ischemia there may be marked postsystolic shortening, and postsystolic velocity may extend into the diastolic filling phase. Postsystolic velocities and strains in healthy subjects, however, are of low amplitude and occur before mitral valve opening.[79]

Diastole

Assessment of mitral annulus velocities by TDI plays an important role in the evaluation of patients with suspected diastolic dysfunction. Measurements are done from apical views, and velocities may be measured at septal, lateral, anterior, and inferior mitral annular areas. However, most often mitral annulus velocities are measured from an apical four-chamber view and either the septal, the lateral, or an average value of septal and lateral mitral annulus velocities are used. There are two main velocity waves that reflect early diastolic (E′) and atrial-induced (A′) myocardial lengthening (see Fig. 5–2). The E′ wave is often followed by an oppositely directed wave of low amplitude, which reflects changes in geometry associated with redistribution of blood within the LV cavity.[76] Similar to systolic velocities, diastolic velocities progressively decrease from base toward apex.

It is also possible to measure diastolic SR and strains by TDI. As shown in Figure 5–20 there are diastolic strain rates that correspond to the E′ and A′ velocity spikes and strains that reflect early diastolic and atrial-

induced lengthening. In contrast to velocities, SRs and strains are essentially similar at all measurement levels between base and apex. SR and strain by TDI, however, have significant technical limitations and therefore can not be recommended in routine assessment of diastolic function.

Myocardial Ischemia

Myocardial ischemia may be caused by either a reduction in coronary blood flow as in acute coronary syndrome or by an increase in myocardial oxygen demand during stress in patients with coronary artery stenosis. In either case ischemia leads to reduction in regional myocardial function, which ranges from reduced systolic shortening (hypokinesia) to systolic lengthening (dyskinesia). Furthermore, myocardial ischemia leads to postsystolic shortening, that is, segmental shortening after end of LV ejection. Reduced systolic shortening and postsystolic shortening, which are the two hallmarks of ischemic dysfunction, can be quantified by all four TDI modalities.[9,16,78,81-85] In clinical routine, however, velocity imaging is the preferred modality, and strain is used only as a supplementary method. Typical velocity traces in acute myocardial ischemia are shown in Figure 5–3.

The main advantage of strain relative to velocity imaging is that measurements are less influenced by translational motion and tethering, and this makes strain more specific with regard to segmental localization of ischemia.[9,86] Therefore, in patients with acute infarctions, strain better defines the transitional zone between intact and dysfunctional myocardium and is superior to velocity imaging to define anatomical extension of dysfunctional myocardium.[12]

In principle, strain is better than ejection velocity to quantify myocardial function and in particular to differentiate between degrees of ischemic dysfunction.[12] Whereas ejection velocity differentiates well between normal and ischemic myocardium, it has limited ability to differentiate between hypokinetic and dyskinetic myocardium. As demonstrated in Figure 5–21 and Figure 5–22, systolic ejection velocity approaches zero in hypokinetic segments and becomes slightly negative in dyskinetic segments, but the difference is only minor. The strain trace in dyskinetic myocardium, however, is strikingly different from that in hypokinetic myocardium.

By extending velocity analysis to the isovolumic phases, however, velocity imaging may also identify dyskinetic myocardium. In ventricles with preserved systolic function there is a dominantly positive longitudinal velocity during IVC, with only a minor negative velocity component. With severe ischemia, the positive velocity component diminishes and the negative component increases.[71,87] In dyskinetic myocardium, the

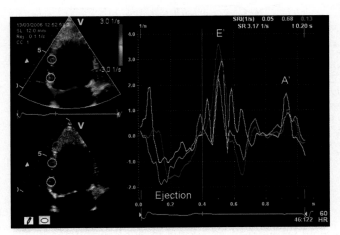

Figure 5–20. *Strain rates from the septum in a healthy individual. The dominant negative trace during systole represents ejection. The two dominant positive spikes are during early diastolic filling (E′) and during atrial-induced filling (A′).*

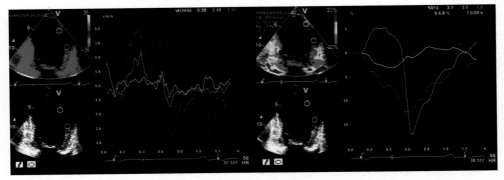

Figure 5–21. *Tissue velocities* (left) *and strains* (right) *from the anterior left ventricular wall in a patient with anterior myocardial infarction. The blue line in both panels is from midpart of the anterior wall. During systole the yellow velocity trace from the apical segment* (left) *approaches zero while the strain trace* (right) *shows systolic lengthening.*

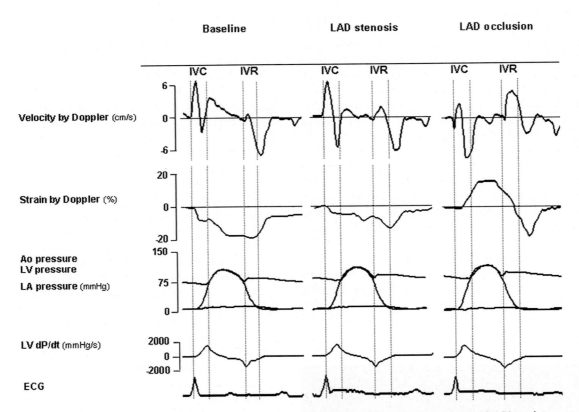

Figure 5–22. *Representative traces during left anterior descending coronary artery (LAD) occlusion in an anesthetized dog showing myocardial Doppler velocities, strain, and pressure traces. Please note that the ejection velocities are relatively similar during LAD stenosis and LAD occlusion, whereas the isovolumic contraction (IVC) and isovolumic relaxation (IVR) velocities are markedly different. During LAD occlusion the large negative velocity spike during IVC corresponds to systolic lengthening as demonstrated in the strain trace. Furthermore, the marked postsystolic velocity during IVR corresponds to late systolic and postsystolic shortening in the strain trace. Ao, aortic; LV, left ventricular; LA, left atrial. (Modified from Skulstad H, Urheim S, Edvardsen T, et al:* J Am Coll Cardiol *47:1672-1682, 2006.)*

positive velocity component is replaced by a large negative IVC velocity (Fig. 5–23). Furthermore, dyskinesia is associated with enhanced postsystolic velocity resulting from postsystolic shortening. Therefore, a typical velocity trace from dyskinetic myocardium has a large negative velocity spike during IVC and a large

positive velocity during IVR with velocities near zero during ejection. One should be aware that myocardial lengthening may not occur in nontransmural infarcts because of shortening of intact subepicardial fibers.

Postsystolic shortening by TDI (see Fig. 5–23) can be used as a marker of acute and stress-induced myocar-

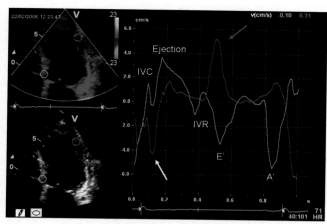

Figure 5-23. *Abnormal myocardial velocities during isovolumic contraction (IVC) and isovolumic relaxation (IVR). Tissue Doppler imaging from a patient with anterior wall infarct involving the apical lateral segment. The red trace is recorded from the infarcted part of the ventricle and demonstrates a negative IVC spike and a large postsystolic shortening velocity. A', atrial-induced filling; E', early diastolic filling.*

TABLE 5-2. Typical Tissue Doppler Imaging Findings in Myocardial Ischemia

Moderate Myocardial Ischemia
By velocity imaging
  Reduced systolic ejection velocity
  Marked postsystolic shortening velocity
By strain imaging
  Reduced systolic shortening
  Postsystolic shortening

Severe Myocardial Ischemia
By velocity imaging
  Systolic ejection velocity near zero
  Marked negative preejection velocity
  Marked postsystolic shortening velocity
By strain imaging
  Systolic lengthening
  Postsystolic shortening

dial ischemia.[3,71,83,88] The mechanism of postsystolic shortening can be either delayed active contraction, passive recoil of dyskinetic myocardium, or a combination of active contraction and passive recoil.[89] When postsystolic shortening occurs in entirely passive or necrotic myocardium, it is analogous to the behavior of a stretched elastic spring that recoils passively when the stretching force is removed. In moderately ischemic myocardium postsystolic shortening results from delayed active contraction.[89] Because postsystolic shortening may occur in actively contracting and in necrotic myocardium, it is non-specific with regard to tissue viability. As suggested by experimental work, postsystolic shortening, which far exceeds systolic lengthening, may be a marker of tissue viability,[90] but the validity of this concept needs to be tested clinically. At the present stage, the clinical value of postsystolic shortening, measured either as a postsystolic velocity or postsystolic strain, is that it serves as a marker of ischemia. One should also remember, however, that postsystolic shortening can be present in a normal LV velocity pattern although the magnitude is less than in an ischemic ventricle.[79,91]

Ischemia is also associated with changes in diastolic myocardial velocities, and measurement of myocardial diastolic velocity patterns could improve the ability of TDI to identify ischemic regions.[78,89,92] The clinical value of assessing diastolic velocities other than IVR velocities remains to be determined.

Displacement imaging and SR imaging can also be used for assessing ischemic dysfunction. In clinical practice, however, they have no proven added value. The most robust TDI methodology is velocity imaging and is recommended as the primary method. Strain assessment may be used as a supplementary method

when there is uncertainty regarding a finding with velocity imaging.

Longitudinal TDI measures have mainly been discussed because apical views give the most extensive imaging of the left ventricle. Similar findings during ischemia can be observed with radial measurements in short-axis images but are restricted to anteroseptal and posterior segments. Some authors present radial measurements as *velocity gradient* instead of SR.[25,93] This is a valid approach but is not used much clinically.

In summary, myocardial ischemia is characterized by reduction in systolic ejection velocity and a postsystolic shortening velocity (Table 5-2). Furthermore, in dyskinetic myocardium there is a marked negative velocity during IVC, which represents systolic lengthening. Strain measurement can be used to verify changes in tissue velocities and is useful to confirm dyskinesia. Furthermore, strain imaging provides a more site-specific measure.

Diastolic Dysfunction

Heart failure with normal LV EF accounts for a large fraction of all heart failure cases, especially in the elderly population.[94] These patients appear to have predominant and occasionally isolated diastolic heart failure. The apparently normal systolic function may reflect a limitation of EF to identify mild systolic dysfunction, as suggested by studies that have shown reduced systolic ejection velocity by TDI. Therefore, some patients with normal EF actually have mild systolic dysfunction.[95-97] In addition, there are patients without heart failure who have impaired diastolic function, such as patients with hypertension or diabetes mellitus.

Assessment of mitral annulus motion by TDI is an essential part of the evaluation of patients with potential diastolic heart failure and diastolic dysfunction. The most important measure is E', which is peak LV lengthening velocity. Peak E' correlates with invasive indices of global LV relaxation (τ) and therefore is a marker of diastolic dysfunction.[98] As described in more detail in Chapter 11, patients with diastolic dysfunction may have three abnormal LV filling patterns, representing different stages of diastolic dysfunction.[99] At an early stage of diastolic dysfunction, there is typically a pattern of "impaired myocardial relaxation," with a decrease in peak transmitral E velocity, a compensatory increase in the atrial-induced (A) velocity and therefore a decrease in the E/A ratio. In patients with advanced cardiac disease, there may be a pattern of "restrictive filling," with elevated peak E velocity, short E deceleration time, and markedly increased E/A ratio. In patients with an intermediate pattern between impaired relaxation and restrictive filling, the E/A ratio and the deceleration time may be normal, so-called "pseudonormalized filling." TDI is a useful tool for differentiating between true normal and pseudonormal filling patterns, as E' is reduced only in the latter case[98] (Figure 5–24). The three filling patterns represent increasing severity of diastolic function, with "impaired relaxation" representing mild dysfunction, restrictive filling representing severe dysfunction, and the pseudonormalized filling is an intermediate form. Therefore, by combining assessment of transmitral flow velocities and E', it is possible to perform staging of diastolic dysfunction during a routine echocardiographic examination. It is important to be aware that the filling pattern is load dependent, and therefore a given patient may change filling pattern because of changes in volume status or blood pressure.

Another application of TDI in heart failure is to serve as a marker of LV filling pressure, which utilizes difference responses of E' and E to elevated LV preload. In the normal ventricle both E and E' are markedly load dependent. In the failing ventricle, however, E' is much less load dependent than transmitral flow velocities.[98,100-102] Thus, when LV filling pressure becomes elevated in a failing ventricle, E increases more than E' and the E/E' ratio becomes elevated. This relative load independence of E' forms the basis for using the E/E' as a marker of elevated LV filling pressure.[101,103-105]

When using E' to assess diastolic function it is important to be aware that most of the validation studies have used the pulsed Doppler mode to assess E', and therefore values are significantly higher than with current color Doppler modes. Pulsed Doppler E' >8 cm/s in older adults and >10 cm/s in younger adults have been regarded as normal values.[5,106]

Restrictive Cardiomyopathy versus Constrictive Pericarditis

Another practical application of TDI in relation to diastolic dysfunction is differentiation between restrictive cardiomyopathy and constrictive pericarditis. With few exceptions, patients with constrictive pericarditis have normal systolic function and normal ventricular relaxation, and therefore E' is normal.[106] In restrictive cardiomyopathy, however, systolic function is impaired. It has been shown that an E' velocity below 8 cm/s is indicative of restrictive cardiomyopathy, whereas substantial overlap was found for transmitral filling velocities between normal; those with constrictive pericarditis and restrictive cardiomyopathy.[107] The lateral part of the mitral annulus in the longitudinal axis has been used for measurements of E'. One should make sure that the sample volume is placed within the myocardium and not affected by the lower pericardial velocities when using these methods.

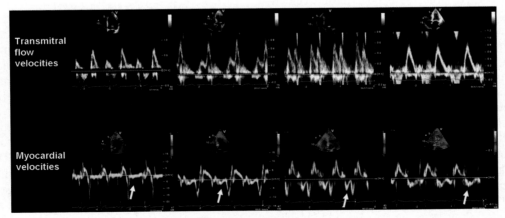

Figure 5–24. Left ventricular filling patterns. Patterns of mitral inflow and mitral annulus velocity from a normal person and patients with patterns of impaired relaxation, pseudonormalized filling, and restrictive filling, respectively. All patients have E' less than −8 cm/s (arrows), whereas the normal person has E' close to −15 cm/s. E', early diastolic filling.

TABLE 5-3. Doppler Echocardiographic Findings in Diastolic Dysfunction

Impaired Relaxation
Reduced transmitral early filling velocity (E) and compensatory increase in atrial-induced (A) velocity, resulting in reduced E/A ratio
Prolonged E wave deceleration time
Reduced early diastolic mitral annulus velocity (E′) by TDI

Pseudonormalized Filling
Normal transmitral E/A ratio and E wave deceleration time
Reduced E′ by TDI

Restrictive Filling
Elevated peak E velocity and increased E/A ratio
Short E deceleration time
Reduced E′ by TDI

TDI, tissue Doppler imaging.

In summary, assessment of E′ in combination with transmitral filling patterns can be used clinically to diagnose diastolic dysfunction (Table 5–3) and to estimate LV filling pressure in patients with heart failure.

Cardiac Synchrony

Normal ventricular activation spreads rapidly through the conduction system, and the result is a synchronized ventricular contraction. The average time delay between onset of QRS signal and the onset of regional ejection motion is 100 to 110 ms in a normal ventricle.[108] In patients with severe heart failure, however, there is often prolonged intraventricular or interventricular conduction, which leads to mechanical dyssynchrony and ineffective cardiac function. Approximately one third of patients with low LV EF and class III to IV heart failure have QRS duration longer than 120 ms. In addition, patients with heart failure may have prolonged atrioventricular (AV) interval.

Effect of Dyssynchrony on Left Ventricular Function

Ventricular dyssynchrony in patients with heart failure most often results from left bundle branch block (LBBB), which impairs both intraventricular and interventricular incoordination of contractile function. Interventricular dyssynchrony is a significant problem during LBBB resulting from associated abnormal septal motion.[109,110] Normally, the septum behaves like a passive membrane during diastole, and septal position is determined by the transseptal pressure gradient. In normal diastole, LV pressure exceeds RV pressure and explains why the septum curves toward the RV at end-diastole. During LBBB, however, the RV starts to contract before the LV,

and therefore end-diastolic RV pressure exceeds LV pressure. This reversal of the transseptal pressure gradient causes a shift of the septum toward the LV. Subsequently, when the LV contracts and causes a rapid rise in LV pressure, the transseptal gradient becomes directed toward the RV, and the septum shifts back toward the RV. Because of this abnormal septal motion, there is loss of septal contribution to LV ejection, which tends to reduce LV stroke volume.

Intraventricular dyssynchrony also tends to reduce LV stroke volume and causes significant waste of myocardial work.[111] In regions in which contraction starts prematurely there is no ejection, and in late activated regions there may be contraction after end of ejection. In addition to a direct negative effect on stroke volume, intraventricular dyssynchrony may cause abnormal myocardial stresses that may lead to local hypertrophy and remodeling. It has been shown that relatively small temporal differences in electrical activation are associated with increased shortening in late activated areas because of abnormal fiber stretch before contraction.[112] Doppler strain analysis suggests that early systolic septal shortening in LBBB causes a pressure rise that stretches the lateral wall and may increase regional shortening via the Frank-Starling mechanism.[113] This in turn leads to increased local work and might be a stimulus to regional hypertrophy.[114]

Cardiac dyssynchrony may also be caused by abnormal AV conduction. The importance of atrioventricular synchrony in congestive heart failure (CHF), however, is not well defined, and there is limited insight into the effects of optimizing atrioventricular synchrony on clinical signs and prognosis.

Selection of Patients for Cardiac Resynchronization Therapy

In patients with ventricular dyssynchrony cardiac function can be improved by electrically activating the right and the left ventricles in a synchronized manner with a biventricular pacing device, a treatment named cardiac resynchronization therapy (CRT). By using two pacing leads, the left ventricle is stimulated at about the same time as the right ventricle. This technology has evolved rapidly over a few years and is now established as effective treatment in selected patients with congestive heart failure, causing improvement of symptoms, reduction of mortality, and reverse LV remodeling.[115,116] Furthermore, CRT tends to reduce mitral regurgitation (MR).[117-119] However, about one third of patients treated with CRT do not show clinical improvement, indicating that we need better methods for identifying those who will benefit from the therapy.[117,120]

Identification of CRT responders can be done by two different principles—by assessing either electrocardiographic or cardiac mechanical signs of dyssynchrony.

At the present time electrocardiographic criteria are used as the main screening tool, and patients are selected for CRT based on morphology and duration of the QRS complex. In clinical trials that have documented clinical benefit of CRT, one of the entry criteria has been QRS duration over 120 ms, and average QRS duration in the large trials has been over 150 ms, most often with LBBB type morphology and sinus rhythm.[121] There is limited documentation of CRT in patients with pure right bundle branch block.

Recent trials, however, have shown that QRS is not a precise marker of LV dyssynchrony because patients with a wide QRS may not have LV dyssynchrony, and patients with a narrow QRS may actually have dyssynchrony.[122-126] This may explain why a substantial fraction of patients with wide QRS are non-responders to CRT therapy in the large trials.[125,127] There is a strong interest in cardiac mechanical markers of dyssynchrony, and different echocardiography modalities have been investigated.

Assessment of Interventricular Dyssynchrony

Interventricular dyssynchrony is measured by Doppler echocardiography as the difference between the left and right ventricular preejection intervals calculated from onset of QRS on electrocardiogram (ECG) to onset of aortic outflow and pulmonary outflow, respectively. A difference in ejection delays >40 ms is considered a sign of interventricular dyssynchrony.[128-130] Interventricular dyssynchrony can also be measured by TDI.[131] One approach is to compare the delay between peak systolic velocity of the RV free wall and the LV lateral wall.[132]

It has been shown that reverse LV remodeling and improved LV function during CRT is associated with reduction of interventricular dyssynchrony.[119,133] The relative importance of interventricular and intraventricular dyssynchrony, however, is not entirely clear and data are somewhat conflicting regarding the clinical importance of measuring interventricular dyssynchrony.[133,134]

Assessment of Intraventricular Dyssynchrony

Intraventricular dyssynchrony can be assessed by M-mode echocardiography from the parasternal short-axis view, and septal-to-posterior wall motion delay has been proposed as a marker of responders to CRT.[130,135] In these studies a majority of patients had nonischemic cardiomyopathy. In patients with ischemic cardiomyopathy, however, there may be previous infarcts and akinesia in the measurement regions, which makes it difficult to define the peaks of septal and posterior wall inward motion. These limitations are significant, and in a study, which included a majority of patients with ischemic cardiomyopathy, septal-to-

posterior wall motion delay did not predict reverse remodeling or clinical improvement with CRT.[136] At the present time septal-to-posterior wall motion cannot be recommended as a routine method for identifying candidates for CRT.

Computerized and contrast enhanced 2D echocardiographic methods may be used to measure septal-to-posterior wall motion delay, but these methods have not proven to be useful in routine diagnostics.[137,138]

TDI is the preferred echocardiographic method to identify mechanical dyssynchrony during a routine examination, and velocity imaging can measure timing of contraction in virtually any myocardial segment. Using apical four-chamber, two-chamber, and long-axis views measurements from multiple segments can be compared. One approach is to assess velocities in the basal parts of six basal and six mid-LV segments and to measure the time from beginning of the QRS signal to *maximum* systolic velocity[129,131] (Fig. 5–25). Regional variability in time to peak systolic velocity expressed as standard deviation for measurements from all 12 segments can predict reverse remodeling with CRT. This dyssynchrony index has demonstrated high sensitivity and specificity to predict LV reverse remodeling.[131,132] Maximal delay in peak velocity between the anterior, inferior, septal, and lateral walls also predicts clinical response to CRT and reverse remodeling.[129,131] Intraventricular dyssynchrony has also been measured as regional differences in the time from onset of QRS to *onset of regional ejection velocity*.[134] Doppler-based strain or SR imaging are currently undergoing testing but have so far not showed any advantages in the assessment of dyssynchrony or to predict responses to CRT.[131]

Tissue tracking and tissue synchronization imaging are modalities that display color-coded maps of myo-

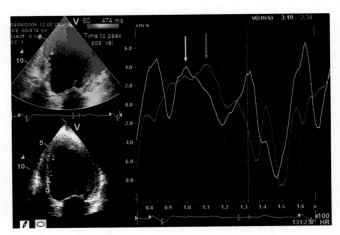

Figure 5–25. Measurement of intraventricular dyssynchrony: Apical four-chamber view of the left ventricle. The tissue Doppler traces from the apical part of the septum (yellow) *show delayed ejection velocity* (yellow arrow) *compared to the corresponding ejection velocity from the apical part of the lateral wall* (white arrow). *The delay is 170 ms. Note the large postsystolic velocity from the septum* (red arrow).

cardial displacement and can also be used to visualize LV dyssynchrony (see Fig. 5–25) and to identify patients likely to benefit from CRT.[139-142] The role of these modalities in clinical routine remains to be defined.

Positioning of the Left Ventricular Pacing Lead

The best hemodynamic responses to biventricular pacing is obtained when the LV pacing lead is positioned at the wall that has most delay in mechanical activation.[143] Most often the LV lead is introduced by a transvenous approach and is positioned in a coronary vein, aiming at the location of latest electromechanical activation. With TDI it is possible to locate the site of latest activation, and most often this is the posterolateral or inferior regions of the left ventricle.[144] Not only TDI,[144] but also STE can be used to optimize lead positioning.[145]

It has been shown that CRT does not reduce LV dyssynchrony in patients with transmural scar tissue in posterolateral segments.[146] This lack of response may be explained by absence of active contraction in scar tissue. Passive scar tissue is stretched during IVC and contracts by a passive recoil mechanism when LV pressure is falling at end-systole. This principle is illustrated in Figure 5–23. Because timing of passive contraction is determined by LV pressure and not by timing of depolarization, it is unlikely that it will be modified by CRT.

In summary, several studies show that TDI can identify responders to CRT. It is important to remember, however, that the size of these studies is small and that larger prospective trials with clinical endpoints are lacking. At the present time TDI may be used as a supplementary method to QRS analysis. Although QRS duration is an imperfect marker of responders to CRT, there is yet no other consensus definition of dyssynchrony that has been sufficiently evaluated. Most likely the TDI indices will prove to have added value, but more documentation is needed.

Right Ventricular Function

The right ventricle has a complex anatomical structure and even in experimental models it has been difficult to quantify RV function. The right ventricle is functionally divided into two parts, the inflow tract and the outflow tract, separated by the crista supraventricularis. Echocardiographic imaging of RV function and measurement of EF have been difficult because of its motion pattern and problems with defining the endocardial surface of the thin RV free wall. In daily cardiology practice RV function is usually evaluated qualitatively by 2D echocardiography.

During systolic contraction there is longitudinal shortening of the RV, with the base descending toward the apex, whereas the apical part is relatively stationary. In addition there is circumferential shortening that squeezes the ventricle. The interventricular septum contributes to RV and to LV function, and the relative contribution can be different in the normal and the diseased heart. The precise role of the septum remains to be determined. Systolic motion of the tricuspid annulus can be measured by M-mode echocardiography, and it has been shown that systolic annulus motion correlates with RV EF measured by radionuclide angiography.[147] This measurement, however, is relatively complicated and is not widely used. Measurement of tricuspid annulus motion by TDI is much easier and faster.

Tissue Doppler echocardiography enables measurement of RV long-axis function as velocity, strain, and SR. Because of the thin wall of the RV, TDI signals from the free wall are often unsatisfactory. Measurements of tricuspid annular motion, however, are usually of good quality and can be performed in most patients. Pulsed-Doppler velocity imaging is a simple and robust method for measuring tricuspid annular velocity. It has been shown that systolic tricuspid annular velocity correlates well with RV EF by radionuclide angiography.[148]

KEY POINTS

- Tissue Doppler echocardiography provides measures of myocardial velocity, displacement, SR and strain.

- Tissue Doppler velocity imaging can be applied clinically to diagnose myocardial ischemia and to evaluate patients with diastolic dysfunction.

- Tissue Doppler velocity imaging is a promising tool in selection of patients for CRT.

- Tissue Doppler strain and SR imaging can be used clinically as supplementary methods to explore findings with velocity imaging, but both modalities have significant technical limitations.

- STE is a promising, angle-independent method for measurement of myocardial strain.

REFERENCES

1. McDicken WN, Sutherland GR, Moran CM, Gordon LN: Colour Doppler velocity imaging of the myocardium. *Ultrasound Med Biol* 18(6-7):651-654, 1992.
2. Sutherland GR, Stewart MJ, Groundstroem KW, et al: Color Doppler myocardial imaging: a new technique for the assessment of myocardial function. *J Am Soc Echocardiogr* 7(5):441-458, 1994.
3. Edvardsen T, Aakhus S, Endresen K, et al: Acute regional myocardial ischemia identified by 2-dimensional multiregion tissue Doppler imaging technique. *J Am Soc Echocardiogr* 13(11):986-994, 2000.
4. Wilkenshoff UM, Hatle L, Sovany A, et al: Age-dependent changes in regional diastolic function evaluated by color Doppler myocardial imaging: a comparison with pulsed Doppler indexes of global function. *J Am Soc Echocardiogr* 14(10):959-969, 2001.

5. Dokainish H: Tissue Doppler imaging in the evaluation of left ventricular diastolic function. *Curr Opin Cardiol* 19(5):437-441, 2004.

6. Stoylen A, Skjaerpe T: Systolic long axis function of the left ventricle. Global and regional information. *Scand Cardiovasc J* 37(5):253-258, 2003.

7. Olstad B, Brodin LA, Berg S: Display of cardiac activation pathways with echocardiography. *Medical Imaging* 3033, 309-315, 1997.

8. Kerber RE, Marcus ML, Wilson R, et al: Effects of acute coronary occlusion on the motion and perfusion of the normal and ischemic interventricular septum. *Circulation* 54(6):928-935, 1976.

9. Urheim S, Edvardsen T, Torp H, et al: Myocardial strain by Doppler echocardiography. Validation of a new method to quantify regional myocardial function. *Circulation* 102(10):1158-1164, 2000.

10. Wilkenshoff UM, Sovany A, Wigstrom L et al: Regional mean systolic myocardial velocity estimation by real-time color Doppler myocardial imaging: a new technique for quantifying regional systolic function. *J Am Soc Echocardiogr* 11(7):683-692, 1998.

11. Galiuto L, Ignone G, DeMaria AN: Contraction and relaxation velocities of the normal left ventricle using pulsed-wave tissue Doppler echocardiography. *Am J Cardiol* 81(5):609-614, 1998.

12. Skulstad H, Urheim S, Edvardsen T, et al: Grading of myocardial dysfunction by tissue Doppler echocardiography a comparison between velocity, displacement, and strain imaging in acute ischemia *J Am Coll Cardiol* 47(8):1672-1682, 2006.

13. Ellis RM, Franklin DL, Rushmer RF: Left ventricular dimensions recorded by sonocardiometry. *Circ Res* 4(6):684-688, 1956.

14. Zerhouni EA, Parish DM, Rogers WJ, et al: Human heart: Tagging with MR imaging—a method for noninvasive assessment of myocardial motion. *Radiology* 169(1):59-63, 1988.

15. Edvardsen T, Gerber BL, Garot J, et al: Quantitative assessment of intrinsic regional myocardial deformation by Doppler strain rate echocardiography in humans: validation against three-dimensional tagged magnetic resonance imaging. *Circulation* 106(1):50-56, 2002.

16. Heimdal A, Stoylen A, Torp H, Skjaerpe T: Real-time strain rate imaging of the left ventricle by ultrasound. *J Am Soc Echocardiogr* 11(11):1013-1019, 1998.

17. Mirsky I, Pasternac A, Ellison RC: General index for the assessment of cardiac function. *Am J Cardiol* 30(5):483-491, 1972.

18. Mirsky I, Parmley WW: Assessment of passive elastic stiffness for isolated heart muscle and the intact heart. *Circ Res* 33(2):233-243, 1973.

19. Uematsu M, Nakatani S, Yamagishi M, et al: Usefulness of myocardial velocity gradient derived from two-dimensional tissue Doppler imaging as an indicator of regional myocardial contraction independent of translational motion assessed in atrial septal defect. *Am J Cardiol* 79(2):237-241, 1997.

20. Bogaert J, Rademakers FE: Regional nonuniformity of normal adult human left ventricle. *Am J Physiol Heart Circ Physiol* 280(2):H610-H620, 2001.

21. Garot J, Bluemke DA, Osman NF, et al: Fast determination of regional myocardial strain fields from tagged cardiac images using harmonic phase MRI. *Circulation* 101(9):981-988, 2000.

22. MacGowan GA, Shapiro EP, Azhari H, et al: Noninvasive measurement of shortening in the fiber and cross-fiber directions in the normal human left ventricle and in idiopathic dilated cardiomyopathy. *Circulation* 96(2):535-541, 1997.

23. Fleming AD, Xia X, McDicken WN, et al: Myocardial velocity gradients detected by Doppler imaging. *Br J Radiol* 67(799):679-688, 1994.

24. Uematsu M, Miyatake K, Tanaka N, et al: Myocardial velocity gradient as a new indicator of regional left ventricular contraction: Detection by a two-dimensional tissue Doppler imaging technique. *J Am Coll Cardiol* 26(1):217-223, 1995.

25. Derumeaux G, Mulder P, Richard V, et al: Tissue Doppler imaging differentiates physiological from pathological pressure-overload left ventricular hypertrophy in rats. *Circulation* 105(13):1602-1608, 2002.

26. Matre K, Fannelop T, Dahle GO, et al: Radial strain gradient across the normal myocardial wall in open-chest pigs measured with Doppler strain rate imaging. *J Am Soc Echocardiogr* 18(10):1066-1073, 2005.

27. Storaa C, Aberg P, Lind B, Brodin LA: Effect of angular error on tissue Doppler velocities and strain. *Echocardiography* 20(7):581-587, 2003.

28. Weidemann F, Jamal F, Kowalski M, et al: Can strain rate and strain quantify changes in regional systolic function during dobutamine infusion, B-blockade, and atrial pacing—implications for quantitative stress echocardiography. *J Am Soc Echocardiogr* 15(5):416-424, 2002.

29. Smith SW, Trahey GE, Hubbard SM, Wagner RF. Properties of acoustical speckle in the presence of phase aberration. Part II: Correlation lengths. *Ultrason Imaging* 10(1):29-51, 1988.

30. Bohs LN, Trahey GE: A novel method for angle independent ultrasonic imaging of blood flow and tissue motion. *IEEE Trans Biomed Eng* 38(3):280-286, 1991.

31. Behar V, Adam D, Lysyansky P, Friedman Z: The combined effect of nonlinear filtration and window size on the accuracy of tissue displacement estimation using detected echo signals. *Ultrasonics* 41(9):743-753, 2004.

32. Notomi Y, Lysyansky P, Setser RM, et al: Measurement of ventricular torsion by two-dimensional ultrasound speckle tracking imaging. *J Am Coll Cardiol* 45(12):2034-2041, 2005.

33. Amundsen BH, Helle-Valle T, Edvardsen T, et al: Noninvasive myocardial strain measurement by speckle tracking echocardiography: validation against sonomicrometry and tagged magnetic resonance imaging. *J Am Coll Cardiol* 47(4):789-793, 2006.

34. Helle-Valle T, Crosby J, Edvardsen T, et al: New noninvasive method for assessment of left ventricular rotation: speckle tracking echocardiography. *Circulation* 112(20):3149-3156, 2005.

35. Leitman M, Lysyansky P, Sidenko S, et al: Two-dimensional strain-a novel software for real-time quantitative echocardiographic assessment of myocardial function. *J Am Soc Echocardiogr* 17(10):1021-1029, 2004.

36. Alam M, Hoglund C, Thorstrand C: Longitudinal systolic shortening of the left ventricle: an echocardiographic study in subjects with and without preserved global function. *Clin Physiol* 12(4):443-452, 1992.

37. Pai RG, Bodenheimer MM, Pai SM, et al: Usefulness of systolic excursion of the mitral anulus as an index of left ventricular systolic function. *Am J Cardiol* 67(2):222-224, 1991.

38. Greenbaum RA, Ho SY, Gibson DG, et al: Left ventricular fibre architecture in man. *Br Heart J* 45(3):248-263, 1981.

39. Sanchez-Quintana D, Garcia-Martinez V, Climent V, Hurle JM: Morphological changes in the normal pattern of ventricular myoarchitecture in the developing human heart. *Ann Anat* 243(4):483-495, 1995.

40. Stevens C, Remme E, LeGrice I, Hunter P: Ventricular mechanics in diastole: material parameter sensitivity. *J Biomech* 36(5):737-748, 2003.

41. Streeter DD Jr, Spotnitz HM, Patel DP, et al: Fiber orientation in the canine left ventricle during diastole and systole. *Circ Res* 24(3):339-347, 1969.

42. McDonald IG. The shape and movements of the human left ventricle during systole: A study by cineangiography and by cineradiography of epicardial markers. *Am J Cardiol* 26(3):221-230, 1970.

43. Rademakers FE, Buchalter MB, Rogers WJ, et al: Dissociation between left ventricular untwisting and filling. Accentuation by catecholamines. *Circulation* 85(4):1572-1581, 1992.

44. Gibbons Kroeker CA, Ter Keurs HE, Knudtson ML, et al: An optical device to measure the dynamics of apex rotation of the left ventricle. *Am J Physiol Heart Circ Physiol* 265(4):H1444-H1449, 1993.

45. Moon MR, Ingels NB Jr, Daughters GT, et al: Alterations in left ventricular twist mechanics with inotropic stimulation and volume loading in human subjects. *Circulation* 89(1):142-150, 1994.

46. Hansen DE, Daughters GT, Alderman EL, et al: Effect of volume loading, pressure loading, and inotropic stimulation on left ventricular torsion in humans. *Circulation* 83(4):1315-1326, 1991.

47. Yun KL, Niczyporuk MA, Daughters GT, et al: Alterations in left ventricular diastolic twist mechanics during acute human cardiac allograft rejection. *Circulation* 83(3):962-973, 1991.

48. Maier SE, Fischer SE, McKinnon GC, et al: Evaluation of left ventricular segmental wall motion in hypertrophic cardiomyopathy with myocardial tagging. *Circulation* 86(6):1919-1928, 1992.

49. Buchalter MB, Rademakers FE, Weiss JL, et al: Rotational deformation of the canine left ventricle measured by magnetic resonance tagging: effects of catecholamines, ischaemia, and pacing. *Cardiovasc Res* 28(5):629-635, 1994.

50. DeAnda A Jr, Komeda M, Nikolic SD, Daughters GT, II, Ingels NB, Miller DC. Left ventricular function, twist, and recoil after mitral valve replacement. *Circulation* 92(9):458-466, 1995.

51. Gibbons Kroeker CA, Tyberg JV, Beyar R: Effects of load manipulations, heart rate, and contractility on left ventricular apical rotation: An experimental study in anesthetized dogs. *Circulation* 92(1):130-141, 1995.

52. Gibbons Kroeker CA, Tyberg JV, Beyar R: Effects of ischemia on left ventricular apex rotation: An experimental study in anesthetized dogs. *Circulation* 92(12):3539-3548, 1995.

53. Knudtson ML, Galbraith PD, Hildebrand KL, et al: Dynamics of left ventricular apex rotation during angioplasty: A sensitive index of ischemic dysfunction. *Circulation* 96(3):801-808, 1997.

54. Stuber M, Scheidegger MB, Fischer SE, et al: Alterations in the local myocardial motion pattern in patients suffering from pressure overload due to aortic stenosis. *Circulation* 100(4):361-368, 1999.

55. Nagel E, Stuber M, Lakatos M, et al: Cardiac rotation and relaxation after anterolateral myocardial infarction. *Coron Artery Dis* 11(3):261-267, 2000.

56. Sandstede JJW, Johnson T, Harre K, et al: Cardiac systolic rotation and contraction before and after valve replacement for aortic stenosis: A myocardial tagging study using MR imaging. *Am J Roentgenol* 178(4):953-958, 2002.

57. Fuchs E, Muller MF, Oswald H, et al: Cardiac rotation and relaxation in patients with chronic heart failure. *Eur J Heart Fail* 6(6):715-722, 2004.

58. Tibayan FA, Rodriguez F, Langer F, et al: Alterations in left ventricular torsion and diastolic recoil after myocardial infarction with and without chronic ischemic mitral regurgitation. *Circulation* 110(11Suppl1):II-109, 2004.

59. Buchalter MB, Weiss JL, Rogers WJ, et al: Noninvasive quantification of left ventricular rotational deformation in normal humans using magnetic resonance imaging myocardial tagging. *Circulation* 81(4):1236-1244, 1990.

60. Maier SE, Fischer SE, McKinnon GC, et al: Evaluation of left ventricular segmental wall motion in hypertrophic cardiomyopathy with myocardial tagging. *Circulation* 86(6):1919-1928, 1992.

61. Stuber M, Scheidegger MB, Fischer SE, et al: Alterations in the local myocardial motion pattern in patients suffering from pressure overload due to aortic stenosis. *Circulation* 100(4):361-368, 1999.

62. Fogel MA, Weinberg PM, Hubbard A, Haselgrove J: Diastolic Biomechanics in Normal Infants Utilizing MRI Tissue Tagging. *Circulation* 102(2):218-224, 2000.

63. Nagel E, Stuber M, Burkhard B, et al: Cardiac rotation and relaxation in patients with aortic valve stenosis. *Eur Heart J* 21(7):582-589, 2000.

64. Nagel E, Stuber M, Lakatos M, et al: Cardiac rotation and relaxation after anterolateral myocardial infarction. *Coron Artery Dis* 11(3):261-267, 2000.

65. Sandstede JJW, Johnson T, Harre K, et al: Cardiac systolic rotation and contraction before and after valve replacement for aortic stenosis: A myocardial tagging study using MR imaging. *Am J Roentgenol* 178(4):953-958, 2002.

66. Setser RM, Kasper JM, Lieber ML, et al: Persistent abnormal left ventricular systolic torsion in dilated cardiomyopathy after partial left ventriculectomy. *J Thorac Cardiovasc Surg* 126(1):48-55, 2003.

67. Fuchs E, Muller MF, Oswald H, et al: Cardiac rotation and relaxation in patients with chronic heart failure. *Eur J Heart Fail* 6(6):715-722, 2004.

68. Hexeberg E, Homans DC, Bache RJ: Interpretation of systolic wall thickening. Can thickening of a discrete layer reflect fibre performance? *Cardiovasc Res* 29(1):16-21, 1995.

69. Arts T, Reneman RS, Veenstra PC. A model of the mechanics of the left ventricle. *Ann Biomed Eng* 7(3-4):299-318, 1979.

70. Hashimoto I, Li X, Hejmadi BA, et al: Myocardial strain rate is a superior method for evaluation of left ventricular subendocardial function compared with tissue Doppler imaging. *J Am Coll Cardiol* 42(9):1574-1583, 2003.

71. Edvardsen T, Urheim S, Skulstad H, et al: Quantification of left ventricular systolic function by tissue Doppler echocardiography: Added value of measuring pre- and postejection velocities in ischemic myocardium. *Circulation* 105(17):2071-2077, 2002.

72. Remme E, Lyseggen E, Nash MP, et al: Mechanism behind the velocity spikes during isovolumic relaxation. *Circulation* 112(17 Suppl):268, 2005.

73. Vogel M, Schmidt MR, Kristiansen SB, et al: Validation of myocardial acceleration during isovolumic contraction as a novel noninvasive index of right ventricular contractility: Comparison with ventricular pressure-volume relations in an animal model. *Circulation* 105(14):1693-1699, 2002.

74. Vogel M, Cheung MM, Li J, et al: Noninvasive assessment of left ventricular force-frequency relationships using tissue Doppler-derived isovolumic acceleration: validation in an animal model. *Circulation* 107(12):1647-1652, 2003.

75. Lyseggen E, Rabben SI, Skulstad H, et al: Myocardial acceleration during isovolumic contraction: relationship to contractility. *Circulation* 111(11):1362-1369, 2005.

76. Isaaz K, Munoz del RL, Lee E, Schiller NB: Quantitation of the motion of the cardiac base in normal subjects by Doppler echocardiography. *J Am Soc Echocardiogr* 6(2):166-176, 1993.

77. Pai RG, Gill KS: Amplitudes, durations, and timings of apically directed left ventricular myocardial velocities: I. Their normal pattern and coupling to ventricular filling and ejection. *J Am Soc Echocardiogr* 11(2):105-111, 1998.

78. Derumeaux G, Ovize M, Loufoua J, et al: Doppler tissue imaging quantitates regional wall motion during myocardial ischemia and reperfusion. *Circulation* 97(19):1970-1977, 1998.

79. Voigt JU, Lindenmeier G, Exner B, et al: Incidence and characteristics of segmental postsystolic longitudinal shortening in normal, acutely ischemic, and scarred myocardium. *J Am Soc Echocardiogr* 16(5):415-423, 2003.

80. Sengupta PP, Khandheria BK, Korinek J, et al: Apex-to-base dispersion in regional timing of left ventricular shortening and lengthening. *J Am Coll Cardiol* 47(1):163-172, 2006.

81. Edvardsen T, Skulstad H, Aakhus S, et al: Regional myocardial systolic function during acute myocardial ischemia assessed by strain Doppler echocardiography. *J Am Coll Cardiol* 37(3):726-730, 2001.

82. Gorcsan J III, Strum DP, Mandarino WA, Pinsky MR: Color-coded tissue Doppler assessment of the effects of acute isch-

emia on regional left ventricular function: comparison with sonomicrometry. *J Am Soc Echocardiogr* 14(5):335-342, 2001.

83. Voigt JU, Exner B, Schmiedehausen K, et al: Strain-rate imaging during dobutamine stress echocardiography provides objective evidence of inducible ischemia. *Circulation* 107(16):2120-2126, 2003.

84. Madler CF, Payne N, Wilkenshoff U, et al: Non-invasive diagnosis of coronary artery disease by quantitative stress echocardiography: Optimal diagnostic models using off-line tissue Doppler in the MYDISE study. *Eur Heart J* 24(17):1584-1594, 2003.

85. Smiseth OA, Stoylen A, Ihlen H: Tissue Doppler imaging for the diagnosis of coronary artery disease. *Curr Opin Cardiol* 19(5):421-429, 2004.

86. Stoylen A, Heimdal A, Bjornstad K, et al: Strain rate imaging by ultrasonography in the diagnosis of coronary artery disease. *J Am Soc Echocardiogr* 13(12):1053-1064, 2000.

87. Pislaru C, Bruce CJ, Belohlavek M, et al: Intracardiac measurement of pre-ejection myocardial velocities estimates the transmural extent of viable myocardium early after reperfusion in acute myocardial infarction. *J Am Coll Cardiol* 38(6):1748-1756, 2001.

88. Kukulski T, Jamal F, Herbots L, et al: Identification of acutely ischemic myocardium using ultrasonic strain measurements. A clinical study in patients undergoing coronary angioplasty. *J Am Coll Cardiol* 41(5):810-819, 2003.

89. Skulstad H, Edvardsen T, Urheim S, et al: Postsystolic shortening in ischemic myocardium: active contraction or passive recoil? *Circulation* 106(6):718-724, 2002.

90. Lyseggen E, Skulstad H, Helle-Valle T, et al: Myocardial strain analysis in acute coronary occlusion: A tool to assess myocardial viability and reperfusion. *Circulation* 112(25):3901-3910, 2005.

91. Pislaru C, Anagnostopoulos PC, Seward JB, et al: Higher myocardial strain rates during isovolumic relaxation phase than during ejection characterize acutely ischemic myocardium. *J Am Coll Cardiol* 40(8):1487-1494, 2002.

92. Gorcsan J III, Strum DP, Mandarino WA, et al: Quantitative assessment of alterations in regional left ventricular contractility with color-coded tissue Doppler echocardiography. Comparison with sonomicrometry and pressure-volume relations. *Circulation* 95(10):2423-2433, 1997.

93. Derumeaux G, Ovize M, Loufoua J, et al: Assessment of nonuniformity of transmural myocardial velocities by color-coded tissue Doppler imaging: characterization of normal, ischemic, and stunned myocardium. *Circulation* 101(12):1390-1395, 2000.

94. How to diagnose diastolic heart failure. European Study Group on Diastolic Heart Failure. *Eur Heart J* 19(7):990-1003, 1998.

95. Garcia EH, Perna ER, Farias EF, et al: Reduced systolic performance by tissue Doppler in patients with preserved and abnormal ejection fraction: new insights in chronic heart failure. *Int J Cardiol* 108(2):181-188, 2006.

96. Wang M, Yip GW, Wang AY, et al: Peak early diastolic mitral annulus velocity by tissue Doppler imaging adds independent and incremental prognostic value. *J Am Coll Cardiol* 41(5):820-826, 2003.

97. Wang M, Yip GW, Wang AY, et al: Tissue Doppler imaging provides incremental prognostic value in patients with systemic hypertension and left ventricular hypertrophy. *J Hypertens* 23(1):183-191, 2005.

98. Sohn DW, Chai IH, Lee DJ, et al: Assessment of mitral annulus velocity by Doppler tissue imaging in the evaluation of left ventricular diastolic function. *J Am Coll Cardiol* 30(2):474-480, 1997.

99. Appleton CP, Hatle LK, Popp RL: Relation of transmitral flow velocity patterns to left ventricular diastolic function: new insights from a combined hemodynamic and Doppler echocardiographic study. *J Am Coll Cardiol* 12(2):426-440, 1998.

100. Hasegawa H, Little WC, Ohno M, et al: Diastolic mitral annular velocity during the development of heart failure. *J Am Coll Cardiol* 41(9):1590-1597, 2003.

101. Nagueh SF, Mikati I, Kopelen HA, et al: Doppler estimation of left ventricular filling pressure in sinus tachycardia. A new application of tissue doppler imaging. *Circulation* 98(16):1644-1650, 1998.

102. Nagueh SF, Sun H, Kopelen HA, et al: Hemodynamic determinants of the mitral annulus diastolic velocities by tissue Doppler. *J Am Coll Cardiol* 37(1):278-285, 2001.

103. Nagueh SF, Middleton KJ, Kopelen HA, et al: Doppler tissue imaging: a noninvasive technique for evaluation of left ventricular relaxation and estimation of filling pressures. *J Am Coll Cardiol* 30(6):1527-1533, 1997.

104. Nagueh SF, Lakkis NM, Middleton KJ, et al: Doppler estimation of left ventricular filling pressures in patients with hypertrophic cardiomyopathy. *Circulation* 99(2):254-261, 1999.

105. Ommen SR, Nishimura RA, Appleton CP, et al: Clinical utility of Doppler echocardiography and tissue Doppler imaging in the estimation of left ventricular filling pressures: A comparative simultaneous Doppler-catheterization study. *Circulation* 102(15):1788-1794, 2000.

106. Garcia MJ, Thomas JD, Klein AL: New Doppler echocardiographic applications for the study of diastolic function. *J Am Coll Cardiol* 32(4):865-875, 1998.

107. Rajagopalan N, Garcia MJ, Rodriguez L, et al: Comparison of new Doppler echocardiographic methods to differentiate constrictive pericardial heart disease and restrictive cardiomyopathy. *Am J Cardiol* 87(1):86-94, 2001.

108. Harris WS, Schoenfeld CD, Weissler AM: Effects of adrenergic receptor activation and blockade on the systolic preejection period, heart rate, and arterial pressure in man. *J Clin Invest* 46(11):1704-1714, 1967.

109. Grines CL, Bashore TM, Boudoulas H, et al: Functional abnormalities in isolated left bundle branch block. The effect of interventricular asynchrony. *Circulation* 79(4):845-853, 1989.

110. Kingma I, Tyberg JV, Smith ER: Effects of diastolic transseptal pressure gradient on ventricular septal position and motion. *Circulation* 68(6):1304-1314, 1983.

111. Nelson GS, Curry CW, Wyman BT, et al: Predictors of systolic augmentation from left ventricular preexcitation in patients with dilated cardiomyopathy and intraventricular conduction delay. *Circulation* 101(23):2703-2709, 2000.

112. Prinzen FW, Hunter WC, Wyman BT, McVeigh ER: Mapping of regional myocardial strain and work during ventricular pacing: experimental study using magnetic resonance imaging tagging. *J Am Coll Cardiol* 33(6):1735-1742, 1999.

113. Breithardt OA, Stellbrink C, Herbots L, et al: Cardiac resynchronization therapy can reverse abnormal myocardial strain distribution in patients with heart failure and left bundle branch block. *J Am Coll Cardiol* 42(3):486-494, 2003.

114. Spragg DD, Leclercq C, Loghmani M, et al: Regional alterations in protein expression in the dyssynchronous failing heart. *Circulation* 108(8):929-932, 2003.

115. Bristow MR, Saxon LA, Boehmer J, et al: Cardiac-resynchronization therapy with or without an implantable defibrillator in advanced chronic heart failure. *N Engl J Med* 350(21):2140-2150, 2004.

116. Cleland JG, Daubert JC, Erdmann E, et al: The effect of cardiac resynchronization on morbidity and mortality in heart failure. *N Engl J Med* 2005 352(15):1539-1549, 2005.

117. Abraham WT, Fisher WG, Smith AL, et al: Cardiac resynchronization in chronic heart failure. *N Engl J Med* 346(24):1845-1853, 2002.

118. Breithardt OA, Sinha AM, Schwammenthal E, et al: Acute effects of cardiac resynchronization therapy on functional mitral regurgitation in advanced systolic heart failure. *J Am Coll Cardiol* 41(5):765-770, 2003.

119. St John Sutton MG, Plappert T, Abraham WT, et al: Effect of cardiac resynchronization therapy on left ventricular size and function in chronic heart failure. *Circulation* 107(15):1985-1990, 2003.

120. Reuter S, Garrigue S, Barold SS, et al: Comparison of characteristics in responders versus nonresponders with biventricular pacing for drug-resistant congestive heart failure. *Am J Cardiol* 89(3):346-350, 2002.

121. Radford MJ, Arnold JM, Bennett SJ, et al: ACC/AHA key data elements and definitions for measuring the clinical management and outcomes of patients with chronic heart failure: a report of the American College of Cardiology/American Heart Association Task Force on Clinical Data Standards (Writing Committee to Develop Heart Failure Clinical Data Standards): developed in collaboration with the American College of Chest Physicians and the International Society for Heart and Lung Transplantation: endorsed by the Heart Failure Society of America. *Circulation* 112(12):1888-1916, 2005.

122. Achilli A, Sassara M, Ficili S, et al: Long-term effectiveness of cardiac resynchronization therapy in patients with refractory heart failure and "narrow" QRS. *J Am Coll Cardiol* 42(12):2117-2124, 2003.

123. Bleeker GB, Schalij MJ, Molhoek SG, et al: Relationship between QRS duration and left ventricular dyssynchrony in patients with end-stage heart failure. *J Cardiovasc Electrophysiol* 15(5):544-549, 2004.

124. Kass DA: Predicting cardiac resynchronization response by QRS duration: the long and short of it. *J Am Coll Cardiol* 42(12):2125-2127, 2003.

125. Leclercq C, Kass DA: Retiming the failing heart: principles and current clinical status of cardiac resynchronization. *J Am Coll Cardiol* 39(2):194-201, 2002.

126. Yu CM, Lin H, Zhang Q, Sanderson JE: High prevalence of left ventricular systolic and diastolic asynchrony in patients with congestive heart failure and normal QRS duration. *Heart* 89(1):54-60, 2003.

127. Bax JJ, Abraham T, Barold SS, et al: Cardiac resynchronization therapy: Part 1—issues before device implantation. *J Am Coll Cardiol* 46(12):2153-2167, 2005.

128. Rouleau F, Merheb M, Geffroy S, et al: Echocardiographic assessment of the interventricular delay of activation and correlation to the QRS width in dilated cardiomyopathy. *Pacing Clin Electrophysiol* 24(10):1500-1506, 2001.

129. Bax JJ, Bleeker GB, Marwick TH, et al: Left ventricular dyssynchrony predicts response and prognosis after cardiac resynchronization therapy. *J Am Coll Cardiol* 44(9):1834-1840, 2004.

130. Pitzalis MV, Iacoviello M, Romito R, et al: Cardiac resynchronization therapy tailored by echocardiographic evaluation of ventricular asynchrony. *J Am Coll Cardiol* 40(9):1615-1622, 2002.

131. Yu CM, Fung JW, Zhang Q, et al: Tissue Doppler imaging is superior to strain rate imaging and postsystolic shortening on the prediction of reverse remodeling in both ischemic and nonischemic heart failure after cardiac resynchronization therapy. *Circulation* 110(1):66-73, 2004.

132. Yu CM, Chau E, Sanderson JE, et al: Tissue Doppler echocardiographic evidence of reverse remodeling and improved synchronicity by simultaneously delaying regional contraction after biventricular pacing therapy in heart failure. *Circulation* 105(4):438-445, 2002.

133. Penicka M, Bartunek J, De BB, et al: Improvement of left ventricular function after cardiac resynchronization therapy is predicted by tissue Doppler imaging echocardiography. *Circulation* 109(8):978-983, 2004.

134. Bader H, Garrigue S, Lafitte S, et al: Intra-left ventricular electromechanical asynchrony. A new independent predictor of severe cardiac events in heart failure patients. *J Am Coll Cardiol* 43(2):248-256, 2004.

135. Pitzalis MV, Iacoviello M, Romito R, et al: Ventricular asynchrony predicts a better outcome in patients with chronic heart failure receiving cardiac resynchronization therapy. *J Am Coll Cardiol* 45(1):65-69, 2005.

136. Marcus GM, Rose E, Viloria EM, et al: Septal to posterior wall motion delay fails to predict reverse remodeling or clinical improvement in patients undergoing cardiac resynchronization therapy. *J Am Coll Cardiol* 46(12):2208-2214, 2005.

137. Breithardt OA, Stellbrink C, Kramer AP, et al: Echocardiographic quantification of left ventricular asynchrony predicts an acute hemodynamic benefit of cardiac resynchronization therapy. *J Am Coll Cardiol* 40(3):536-545, 2002.

138. Kawaguchi M, Murabayashi T, Fetics BJ, et al: Quantitation of basal dyssynchrony and acute resynchronization from left or biventricular pacing by novel echo-contrast variability imaging. *J Am Coll Cardiol* 39(12):2052-2058, 2002.

139. Sogaard P, Hassager C: Tissue Doppler imaging as a guide to resynchronization therapy in patients with congestive heart failure. *Curr Opin Cardiol* 19(5):447-451, 2004.

140. Gorcsan J III, Kanzaki H, Bazaz R, et al: Usefulness of echocardiographic tissue synchronization imaging to predict acute response to cardiac resynchronization therapy. *Am J Cardiol* 93(9):1178-1181, 2004.

141. Yu CM, Zhang Q, Fung JW, et al: A novel tool to assess systolic asynchrony and identify responders of cardiac resynchronization therapy by tissue synchronization imaging. *J Am Coll Cardiol* 45(5):677-684, 2005.

142. Sogaard P, Egeblad H, Kim WY, et al: Tissue Doppler imaging predicts improved systolic performance and reversed left ventricular remodeling during long-term cardiac resynchronization therapy. *J Am Coll Cardiol* 40(4):723-730, 2002.

143. Butter C, Auricchio A, Stellbrink C, et al: Effect of resynchronization therapy stimulation site on the systolic function of heart failure patients. *Circulation* 104(25):3026-3029, 2001.

144. Ansalone G, Giannantoni P, Ricci R, et al: Doppler myocardial imaging to evaluate the effectiveness of pacing sites in patients receiving biventricular pacing. *J Am Coll Cardiol* 39(3):489-499, 2002.

145. Suffoletto MS, Dohi K, Cannesson M, et al: Novel speckle-tracking radial strain from routine black-and-white echocardiographic images to quantify dyssynchrony and predict response to cardiac resynchronization therapy. *Circulation* 113(7):960-968, 2006.

146. Bleeker GB, Kaandorp TA, Lamb HJ, et al: Effect of posterolateral scar tissue on clinical and echocardiographic improvement after cardiac resynchronization therapy. *Circulation* 113(7):969-976, 2006.

147. Kaul S, Tei C, Hopkins JM, Shah PM: Assessment of right ventricular function using two-dimensional echocardiography. *Am Heart J* 107(3):526-531, 1984.

148. Meluzin J, Spinarova L, Bakala J, et al: Pulsed Doppler tissue imaging of the velocity of tricuspid annular systolic motion; A new, rapid, and non-invasive method of evaluating right ventricular systolic function. *Eur Heart J* 22(4):340-348, 2001.

Chapter 6

Intracardiac Echocardiography

THOMAS BARTEL, MD • SILVANA MÜLLER, MD •
THOMAS KONORZA, MD • ACHIM GUTERSOHN, MD •
RAIMUND ERBEL, MD

A variety of noncoronary percutaneous interventional procedures have been developed during the last decade. Many of these require echocardiographic guidance, for example, device closure of interatrial communications, percutaneous transluminal septal myocardial ablation, pulmonary vein ablation, percutaneous left atrial appendage closure, and intraaortic procedures. Conventional fluoroscopy is limited because it cannot distinguish soft tissues and because of its inherent restriction to two-dimensional (2D) cross-sectional imaging. Fluoroscopy does allow visualization of catheters and devices projecting over the cardiac silhouette, but accurate positioning can be difficult with just fluoroscopic guidance. On the other hand, remote posterior areas are difficult to depict with transthoracic echocardiography (TTE), especially when the patient is supine. Although transesophageal echocardiography (TEE) is a well-established diagnostic tool and provides exceptional high-resolution images, TEE's usefulness for interventional procedures is also limited when patients are supine. Nowadays, intracardiac echocardiography (ICE) has become an alternative for safe guidance of a multitude of complex interventional procedures.[1] So far, however, evidence that ICE guidance can improve the safety of these procedures is lacking.

Miniaturized catheter devices that are tipped with ultrasound (US) crystals were primarily introduced for intravascular use. The first attempts to percutaneously introduce intravenous (IV) probes with built in echocardiographic transducers for in vivo intracardiac imaging were reported in the late 1960s. During the following two decades, several intracardiac echocardiographic catheters were developed. Later, intravascular ultrasound (IVUS) was employed to image coronary arteries, the aorta, and peripheral vessels. IVUS-based intracardiac imaging was also used for guiding electrophysiological procedures. Nevertheless, intracardiac IVUS lacks Doppler capabilities and is further limited by inadequate US penetration. For current noncoronary percutaneous interventions in various congenital and acquired cardiac conditions, high-quality, near-field images and Doppler flow analysis are a prerequisite for optimal imaging and also help in avoiding and detecting complications. Thus, technical advances led from IVUS to the development of intraluminal phased-array imaging (IPAI). US imaging using this approach from within large vessels (e.g., vena cava or aorta) is termed IPAI, whereas imaging with the transducer tip in the heart is called ICE. Unfortunately, using these sophisticated techniques solely for diagnostic purposes is considered uneconomic in many countries. But the methods are beneficial; using them as a guiding tool in noncoronary percutaneous interventions is justifiable. Especially the progress in electrophysiological ablation is clearly linked to the advances made with ICE.[2] ICE and IPAI are also exciting research tools. Transfer of the methodology from the realm of research to routine clinical use is ongoing.

Intracardiac Echocardiography: Equipment and Handling Procedures

Current devices are multimodal, phased-array transducer-tipped ICE. The 8 and 10 French (F) AcuNav-catheters—the first intracardiac single plane probe—currently are the tools of choice for ICE. Just like conventional echocardiography, the miniaturized ICE transducer provides a 90-degree-sector image. The ICE probe is connected to standard US units using a connector to the catheter, which then attaches to the US unit like any probe. After covering the connector with a sterile jacket, it can be placed into the sterile field at the catheter table where it is connected to the sterile ICE probe. It is recommended to check the catheter steering mechanism and the function of the transducer in a water bath before insertion. Recently, a further miniaturized version of the catheter has been introduced emphasizing the advantages of ICE and IPAI in comparison with TEE and IVUS (Table 6–1).

Introduction of smaller (8F) US catheters with a longer insertable length facilitates ICE and probably increases safety and patient comfort. The initial clinical experience in pediatric cardiology is promising.[3]

Besides two-dimensional and M-mode imaging, the ICE catheter also permits functional analysis. It possesses complete Doppler capabilities, including pulsed wave, continuous wave, color flow, and tissue Doppler recordings.[4] An access sheath is required for introducing the US catheter into the femoral vessels or the right jugular vein. The disposable ICE catheter can be navigated through the inferior vena cava (IVC; femoral ve-

TABLE 6–1. Technical Characteristics of Different Imaging Techniques

	ICE/IPAI	TEE	IVUS
Frequences	5.0-10.0 MHz	3.5-7.0 MHz	10-20 MHz
Cross-sectional imaging circumferential	90-degree sector	90-degree sector	360 degrees
Maximum penetration depth	12 cm	20 cm	5 cm
M-mode	+	+	−
Doppler capability	Full*	Full*	−
Cardiac imaging	+++	++	+
Imaging of the aorta	+++	+	++

*Full Doppler capability includes color Doppler, spectral Doppler (pulsed wave and continuous wave), and tissue Doppler but does not include power Doppler.

ICE, intracardiac echocardiography; IPAI, intraluminal phased-array imaging; IVUS, intravascular ultrasound; TEE, transesophageal echocardiography.

nous access) or the superior vena cava (SVC; jugular venous access) into the right atrium (RA). This may present a potential risk. Because most patients undergo ICE as part of an interventional procedure, the additional risk remains minimal, however. Special caution is needed when navigating the ICE catheter through the pelvic veins. Although the risk of venous injury or perforation is low, isolated pelvic veins perforation and IVC dissection have been described.[3] Adequate handling of the catheter device includes use of a long access sheath and fluoroscopy: two recommended precautions that enhance patient safety. In that respect, the use of a long sheath reduces fluoroscopy time needed for navigation. Especially the long-access sheath spares the examiner problems associated with pelvic vein navigation, thereby increasing patient safety. In addition, it is recommended to infuse saline solution before ICE. This increases venous pressure and dilates the central veins, facilitating venous puncture and insertion of access sheaths and the ICE catheter. Even intracardiac navigation becomes easier if the heart is well filled. The intracardiac probe does not accommodate a guide wire and is therefore fundamentally different from IVUS catheters. These require guide wires and are therefore relatively safe to manipulate. Obtaining arbitrary views may be difficult, however, especially in the near field. Particularly in the vicinity of the RA, the guide wire can restrict full visualization of lumen and wall and will frequently not allow adequate views of structures of interest, that is, the transition into other chambers, vessel orifices, and so on.

Practical Tips

- Use long-access sheaths to avoid injuring the pelvic veins during navigation.

- Use fluoroscopy as a precaution to safely advance the guide wireless bidirectionally steerable catheter into the heart.

- Infusion of 500 mL saline solution is recommended to dilate the veins and to facilitate catheter passage. Added benefit: Reduced tendency for vagal responses when both the left and the right femoral vein need to be punctured.

To permit adequate imaging of the interatrial septum (IAS) and its neighboring structures, two standardized views are used[1]: a transatrial longitudinal view showing the extent of the IAS from cranial to its distal margins (this view is seen with the catheter retroflexed inside the RA) and[2] a perpendicular transatrial short-axis view for visualizing the anterior part of the IAS and the transition to the aortic valve and the ascending aorta (Fig. 6–1).

The aortic valve is visualized by turning the catheter toward the aorta. One may need to straighten or even slightly anteflect the catheter. The tricuspid valve and

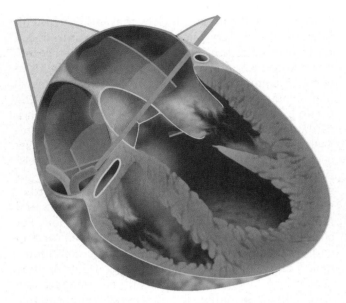

Figure 6–1. Graph showing standard transatrial views for adequate intracardiac imaging.

the right ventricle (RV) are best displayed in a longitudinal view by anteflexing the probe after positioning the tip in the high RA. The left and right pulmonary veins and the left atrial appendage (LAA) are each visualized in a modified transatrial longitudinal view. For depicting the left pulmonary veins and the LAA, the catheter is angulated inferiorly; to visualize the right pulmonary veins, it is turned clockwise and advanced superiorly.

Clockwise rotation of the straightened ICE catheter permits visualization of smallest anatomic details in the near field and to a depth of up to 12 cm. To enter the RV, the tip of the probe is positioned in the mid to upper RA with the piezo-electric crystal facing the free wall of the RA, before the probe is gradually deflected anteriorly. From the RV, the transventricular long-axis view of the left ventricle (LV) is obtained, which shows the interventricular septum proximally, the left ventricular outflow tract (LVOT) and the mitral valve apparatus. By tilting the catheter tip to the right, the transventricular short-axis view of the left ventricle comes into view (Figs. 6–2 and 6–3).

Interpretation of left ventricular wall motion from transventricular views requires care because the catheter is moving inside the RV. By tilting the catheter tip away from the transventricular long-axis view, right ventricular outflow tract (RVOT) and pulmonary valve can be visualized as well (Fig. 6–4).

To avoid ventricular arrhythmias, the catheter has to be carefully navigated inside the right ventricular cavity. The catheter should not be advanced beyond the pulmonary valve. When using the SVC approach, inadvertent catheter passage into the coronary sinus (CS) has to be avoided by all means. A certain expertise in intracardiac catheter manipulation is essential to safely advance the

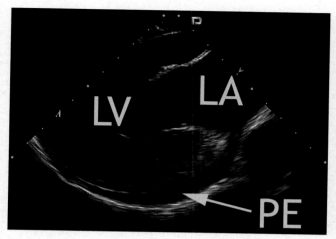

Figure 6–2. *Transventricular long-axis view of the left ventricle and the left atrium in patient with pericardial effusion. LA, left atrium; LV, left ventricle; PE, pericardial effusion.*

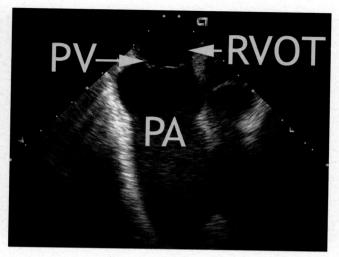

Figure 6–4. *Catheter positioned in the right ventricle provides view of the right ventricular outflow tract and the pulmonary valve. PA, pulmonary artery; PV, pulmonary valve; RVOT, right ventricular outflow tract.*

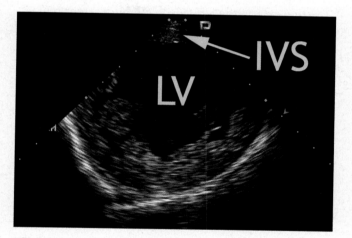

Figure 6–3. *Transventricular short-axis view of the left ventricle. LV, left ventricle; IVS, interventricular septum.*

catheter into the right heart, to orient oneself inside the heart, to obtain standardized views, and to adequately visualize the cardiac anatomy[5] (Table 6–2 and Fig. 6–1).

Although diagnostic potential and limitations of this imaging modality have not been fully evaluated, ICE may find an adequate place in operating rooms (ORs) and catheterization laboratories for online monitoring of complex intracardiac interventions. Nonsurgical cardiac procedures require real-time, high-quality, and near-field views for optimal results. Moreover, continuous progress in the field of percutaneous interventions warrants more effective imaging guidance without a compromise to patient comfort and safety. ICE has been proven an important diagnostic tool for depicting expected or unanticipated aberrant anatomy in patients

TABLE 6–2. Standardized Views

Window	Catheter Position	Standardized Cut Plan
Transatrial	Retroflexed in RA	Longitudinal, cranio-caudal view of IAS, LA, LAA
	Straightened in RA	Short-axis view of the anterior IAS and ascending aorta
	Anteflexed in RA	Longitudinal view of the RV, showing TV, RV
Transventricular	RV	Long-axis view of the LV, IVS, LVOT, LA including LAA
		Short-axis view of the LV
Transvenous	IVC	Aortic view of the abdominal aorta and its side branches
	SVC and RA	Aortic view of the ascending aorta and innominate artery
		Long-axis view of the AV
		Short-axis view of the AV
Intra-aortic	Ascending and descending aorta	Imaging from inside the aorta

AV, aortic valve; IAS, interatrial septum; IVC, inferior vena cava; LA, left atrium; LAA, left atrial appendage; LV, left ventricle; LVOT, left ventricular outflow tract; RA, right atrium; RV, right ventricle; TV, tricuspid valve.

with congenital heart disease (CHD). Tissue motion, intracardiac devices, and their relation to the surrounding structures can be clearly delineated. Additionally, ICE can provide complete Doppler assessment of intracardiac and paracardiac flows, allowing comprehensive hemodynamic evaluation.

Guiding Device Closure of Interatrial Communications

Device closure of interatrial communications is used for preventing paradoxical embolism in patients with a patent foramen ovale (PFO) and for treating severe left-to-right shunts associated with atrial septal defects (ASD). Nevertheless, a certain risk of severe complications remains.[6,7] Some complications are the result of suboptimal device performance, but others may be related to discontinuous echocardiographic monitoring because supine patients do not tolerate continuous monitoring with TEE well unless they are sedated or under general anesthesia. Still, TEE does represent the standard approach to echocardiographic guidance. For device closure, most centers rely to a certain extent on fluoroscopic imaging, although fluoroscopy cannot sufficiently depict the spatial relation between occluder device and cardiac structures in the vicinity of the interatrial communication, neither is it capable of detecting rapid clot formation on the device. More than 10 years of experience make us believe that some specific complications of transcatheter closure can potentially be avoided with improved echocardiographic monitoring. In that respect, ICE can be recommended as an alternative method for guiding percutaneous device closure, especially of ASDs.

Before passing instrumentation through the interatrial communication, the ICE catheter is advanced through the IVC into the RA. The transducer is aimed at the left atrium (LA) to obtain the transatrial longitudinal view. As a first step, guide wire passage through the interatrial communication is observed and adequate position of a long guide wire in the left upper pulmonary vein demonstrated. The entrance of the left upper pulmonary vein into the RA is depicted by angulating the probe from the longitudinal view inferiorly. Although the size of ASDs can be measured by ICE, the validity of this measurement remains to be elucidated. Thus, sizing-balloons must still be used—a mandatory step for estimating the size of the communication before ASD device closure. Balloon sizing does require fluoroscopy. There is an ongoing study evaluating balloon-sizing with ICE in comparison to conventional fluoroscopy based balloon sizing.

Next, the long-access sheath required for occluder device application is inserted over the guide wire. Fluo-

roscopic imaging during that part of the procedure can be reduced to short intermittent checks because placement of the tip of the sheath into the LA can be primarily guided and documented by ICE. Simultaneous echocardiographic and fluoroscopic viewing is recommended during deployment of the closure device:

- ICE displays release of the left-sided counteroccluder opening in the LA.
- The whole system including the long-access sheath with the delivery cable inside and the opened left-sided counteroccluder is slightly pulled back until the open counteroccluder applies some traction on the IAS. ICE depicts the moment when the left-sided counteroccluder matches the IAS closely.
- With the delivery cable still under traction, the long-access sheath is further withdrawn to release the right-sided counteroccluder. ICE demonstrates release of the right-sided counteroccluder inside the RA and the left-sided counteroccluder remaining on the left side of the IAS.
- While monitoring the opening of the right-sided counteroccluder, the delivery cable is carefully pushed forward until the counteroccluder fits also tightly into the IAS but from the right side. Viewing two perpendicular cut plains (transatrial longitudinal and short-axis views) is mandatory to confirm the result and to rule out that one of the counteroccluders is jammed in the interatrial communication (Fig. 6–5).

With the occluder device positioned but still connected to the delivery cable, the "wiggle-maneuver" is monitored. Aiming to ensure that the counteroccluders cannot tilt or slip to the contralateral side, the occluder device is pushed and pulled before release. This will guarantee that the IAS is optimally engaged. Details of this maneuver, which is considered the best technique to avoid unsatisfactory device orientation or embolization, can be nicely shown by ICE. The wiggle-maneuver should be visualized in the transatrial longitudinal view and again in the transatrial short-axis view. In the short-axis view, any compression of the aortic bulb by the occluder device can be ruled out (Fig. 6–6).

It is sensible to also use ICE for monitoring device disconnection from the delivery cable (Fig. 6–7).

Only when released, the device lines up with the IAS, reaching its definitive orientation. The final position of the device should be visualized to ensure the counteroccluders completely enclose the rims of the interatrial communication. After device deployment, color flow imaging can depict any residual shunt. During deployment of the occluder device, it is important to ensure that the device and ICE catheters do not interfere with each other. As a precaution, the ICE catheter should be kept at a distance of at least 1 cm from the occluder device. A closer position would impair

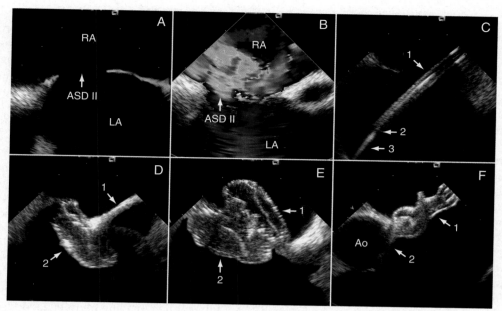

Figure 6–5. *Device closure of an atrial septal defect guided by intracardiac echocardiography.* A, *Atrial septal defect.* B, *Significant left-to-right shunt.* C, *Long-access sheath with indwelling wire:* 1, *long sheath crossing the septum;* 2, *tip of long sheath;* 3, *wire.* D, *Unfolded left-sided countercluder:* 1, *sheath with folded right-sided countercluder inside;* 2, *unfolded left-sided countercluder.* E, *Unfolded countercluders with the device being pulled:* 1, *unfolded right-sided countercluder;* 2, *left-sided countercluder.* F, *Final device position:* 1, *device after release from the delivery cable;* 2, *aorta is shown to be unaffected. Ao, aorta; ASD II, secundum atrial septal defect; LA, left atrium; RA, right atrium. (From Bartel T, Konorza T, Arjumand J, et al:* Circulation *107:795-797, 2003.)*

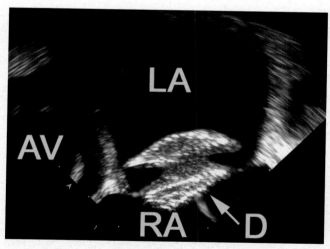

Figure 6–6. *During the "wiggle-maneuver," the occluder device is pushed and pulled by the delivery cable, which is still attached. AV, aortic valve; D, delivery cable, which is being pushed at this moment; LA, left atrium; RA, right atrium.*

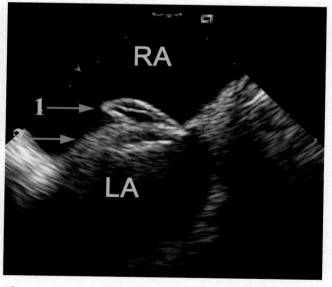

Figure 6–7. *Patent foramen ovale-occluder device before disconnection. LA, left atrium; RA, right atrium; 1, right-sided countercluder; 2, left-sided countercluder.*

optimal imaging of the occluder device. As detailed, continuous intracardiac imaging during each stage of the procedure allows optimal device positioning: this is a prerequisite for safe percutaneous closure of inter-atrial communications. Peri-interventional ICE-based three-dimensional (3D) image reconstruction is also feasible but still has to mature.

Several investigators have demonstrated that ICE can safely guide interventional therapy in interatrial communications and that ICE monitoring is superior to conventional TEE.[8-11] TEE requires general anesthesia with or without endotracheal intubation, whereas ICE permits unlimited echocardiographic viewing in fully conscious and compliant patients. This is of utmost importance because malposition and migration of the device into the systemic or pulmonary circulation or perforation of the cardiac wall and rapid thrombus formation on the device are known to happen on occasion.[6,7,12,13] ICE represents the latest echocardiographic approach. It depicts the fullest detail of both the specific anatomy of the interatrial communication and the instrumentation needed for the procedure. ICE provides better image resolution than TEE and therefore facilitates the procedure, particularly when long continuous or repeated echocardiographic viewing is required or when complications begin to develop. ICE results in much lower procedural stress to the patient, and fluoroscopic and procedural times can be shortened.[8,11] Because many patients with interatrial communications are of reproductive age, reduction of radiation exposure has to be considered a major advantage of ICE. In that respect, patients who undergo ASD closure benefit more from ICE than patients undergoing patent foramen ovale closure because ASD closure is more complex and more time-consuming. It is likely that after completing a comparative assessment of ICE-based balloon-sizing, ICE can also be used to aid sizing in some patients.

Employing ICE in the pediatric population would be desirable. Especially in children, reduction of radiation exposure is of utmost importance to protect all organs, especially the immature reproductive system. In addition, the unresolved issue of potential esophageal injury from TEE probe insertion needs to be taken into account. Several years' experiences show that ICE is a practical and straightforward approach for guiding device closure in children and adolescents.[3,10] Although the potential overall risk related to ICE cannot be conclusively estimated at this time, it appears to be low. Moreover, it is likely that ICE improves the safety of interventional device closure in interatrial communications. From an economic point of view, savings from shorter procedural time and from avoiding general anesthesia need to be weighed against the cost of the ICE catheter. After a brief learning curve, interventional cardiologists who are familiar with echocardiography can fully benefit from the advantages of ICE.

Monitoring of Percutaneous Left Atrial Appendage Closure

ICE guidance for percutaneous left atrial appendage transluminal occlusion (PLAATO) procedures has only been described in a few cases.[14] PLAATO is an option in patients with atrial fibrillation (AFib) in whom oral anticoagulation is contraindicated. Anatomical variation of the LAA, exclusion of thrombi, and the diameter of the ostium are usually assessed by TEE, which is also used for intraprocedural monitoring. As in any

other percutaneous transseptal catheter interventions, one needs to establish access to the atrial appendage by septal puncture prior to PLAATO. This is best done under ICE guidance. The transatrial longitudinal view is used as described for device closure of interatrial communications. Before atrial septal puncture, anatomic anomalies should be ruled out. When tenting of the fossa ovalis identifies contact with the transseptal needle, the pressure on the needle can be slightly increased until the needle perforates the IAS (Fig. 6–8).

Transseptal crossover and advancement of the dilator and sheath are adequately imaged and the ostium of the LAA is easily delineated and measured by ICE. Device positioning, release, potential periprosthetic leaks, and especially the spatial relation of the device to the surrounding structures can be continuously monitored in the transatrial longitudinal view (Fig. 6–9).

In some patients, the transventricular long-axis view can represent an alternative (see Table 6–2).

Intracardiac imaging permits good visualization and confirmation that the device contacts the LAA wall. To prevent device embolization or potential rapid thrombus formation on the device, it is as also mandatory to assure complete device apposition in the LAA. In addition, ICE permits close monitoring for possible procedural complications, such as perforation and pericardial effusion. For guiding PLAATO, superiority of ICE over TEE is not as convincing as for device closure of

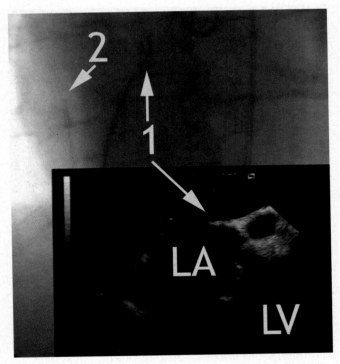

Figure 6–8. Simultaneous fluoroscopic and intracardiac echocardiographic images depict "tenting" of the fossa ovalis while a Brockenbrough needle is advanced from the right atrium. LA, left atrium; LV, left ventricle; 1, Brockenbrough needle; 2, intracardiac echocardiographic catheter placed in the right atrium.

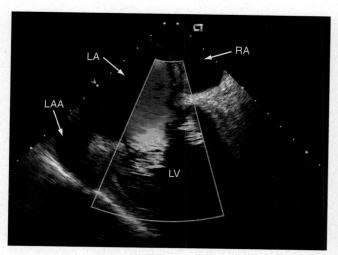

Figure 6–9. *Transatrial longitudinal view: Left atrial appendage and transmitral flow into the left ventricle. LAA, left atrial appendage; LA, left atrium; LV, left ventricle; RA, right atrium.*

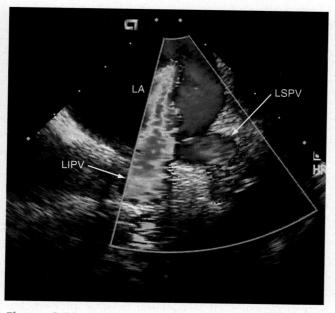

Figure 6–10. *Modified transatrial longitudinal view: Flow from left-sided pulmonary veins into the left atrium. LA, left atrium; LIPV, left inferior pulmonary vein; LSPV, left superior pulmonary vein.*

interatrial communications. The main reason is the relatively large distance between LAA and transducer, which must be placed in the RA. The spatial separation lowers image resolution. In other words, imaging of the LAA cannot be improved by ICE in comparison to TEE. However, as in device closure of interatrial communications, ICE is better tolerated by the patient.

Guiding Radiofrequency Pulmonary Vein Ablation

The rapidly evolving field of interventional electrophysiology creates a demand for guidance by imaging. This is particularly true in view of the fact that currently available techniques, such as fluoroscopy and endocardial electrocardiogram (ECG), may be helpful but have certain limitations. In many cases, angiographic guidance of circular mapping catheters is not sufficiently accurate. After initial puncture of the IAS, high-quality images provided by ICE are capable of guiding transseptal pulmonary vein ablation, a treatment option in atrial fibrillation. Delineation of the endocardium and direct visualization of the pulmonary venous ostium facilitates mapping and radiofrequency ablation by depicting the target area, ensuring electrode/tissue contact, and helping with energy titration (Fig. 6–10).

Angiography-guided placement can result in poor contact between the ablation catheter and the endocardial surface. Inadequate contact reduces heat transfer to the tissue and allows convective heat loss into the circulating blood.

In the transatrial longitudinal view, the left pulmonary veins can be imaged by advancing the probe without tension or steering forces. Clockwise rotation

of the catheter and insertion into the SVC allows the right pulmonary veins to be visualized in a cross-sectional view. Left or right steering permits longitudinal views of the right pulmonary veins. Thus, accurate anatomical positioning of the ablation catheter tip in relation to adjacent endocardial structures is supported[15] (Fig. 6–11).

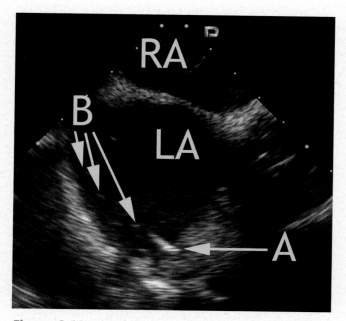

Figure 6–11. *Radiofrequency ablation at the left inferior pulmonary vein. A, tip of the ablation catheter; B, bubbles resulting from radiofrequency delivery; LA, left atrium; RA, right atrium.*

Doppler measurements of pulmonary vein flow velocities before and after ablation are recommended. During the procedure, the ablation zone can be directly visualized, including the evolving tissue injury. Visualization permits assessment of shape, cross-sectional area, wall thickness, and lesion formation[16] and depicts lesion size and continuity.[17] ICE is also useful for monitoring bubble formation during the phase of radiofrequency energy delivery, allowing radiofrequency dose titration to prevent overheating of the catheter tip. After effective ablation, transvenous flow velocities should be interrogated using continuous-wave Doppler to identify the potential presence of a gradient,[18] which can occur as a complication. This illustrates that ICE contributes to the safety of the ablation procedure and to prevention or early detection of potential complications associated with electrophysiological interventions, that is, thrombus formation[19] and development of pulmonary vein stenosis.[18] Peri-interventional monitoring depicts each step of the ablation process, improves efficacy, and also reduces early and late complications.[20] As demonstrated for device closure of interatrial communications, ICE can lower fluoroscopy time and shorten the ablation procedure.

Monitoring of Percutaneous Transluminal Septal Myocardial Ablation

According to the American Society of Echocardiography guidelines, echocardiography plays a definitive role in the preinterventional assessment in hypertrophic obstructive cardiomyopathy and for follow-up after percutaneous transluminal septal myocardial ablation (PTSMA). With intraprocedural myocardial contrast echocardiography (MCE), a more targeted and optimized procedure can be performed.[21] This method permits precise prediction of the extent of myocardial necrosis before alcohol is injected into the selected septal coronary artery side-branch.

ICE represents a new alternative monitoring approach in PTSMA and for demonstrating the effectiveness of the intervention with no need for interrupting the procedure.[14] Transventricular long-axis and short-axis views are most suitable for effective guidance in PTSMA. Systolic anterior motion (SAM) of the anterior mitral valve leaflet is confirmed and the thickness of the ventricular septum is precisely measured by intracardiac M-mode echocardiography. Left ventricular outflow tract and mitral valve are interrogated with Doppler, allowing identification of flow acceleration and mitral regurgitation. Using intracoronary contrast injection, ICE primarily aims to identify and measure the area at risk for alcohol necrosis. Levovist (see Chapter 3) is our preference for depicting the perfusion bed of the target vessel. There-fore, the entire proximal and midseptum and the papillary muscles are visualized to make sure that exclusively those parts of the septum being responsible for the obstruction will be ablated.

ICE images obtained during alcohol injection were shown to reveal progressive appearance of a sharply demarcated triangular septal area with increased echocardiographic density and marked shadowing. In many cases, this echocardiographic-dense area is larger than the area previously delineated by myocardial contrast injection. Alterations of myocardial echocardiographic contrast optical properties during alcohol exposure in addition to the presence of alcohol in the myocardium resulting from capillary leak might explain this highly echogenic and larger than expected area.[14] If the left ventricular outflow tract gradient is adequately lowered after treating the initially targeted septal branch, the result can be considered adequate. Before completion of the procedure, long-axis, 2D, and M-mode images should be obtained for later reference. In summary, one can consider the use of ICE to identify the area at risk for alcohol necrosis, to confirm the septal myocardium responsible for the gradient, and to rule out that the targeted septal branch provides aberrant blood supply to the papillary muscles and/or to the free ventricular wall. Simultaneous echocardiography during the interventional procedure brings major advances to ICE monitoring and also permits more timely therapeutic decision making when needed.

Perioperative and Peri-Interventional Imaging of the Ascending Aorta and Aortic Valve

When a high transesophageal cut plane—also known as "banana view"—is used, TEE depicts the caudal part of the ascending aorta anteriorly to the right pulmonary artery. Unfortunately, ascending aortic flow is not aligned with the Doppler beam in this cut plane. For that reason, perioperative functional assessment of the aortic valve and the ascending aorta by TEE is limited to regurgitant flow detection. Perioperative IPAI and ICE may become alternative approaches for complete morphologic assessment of the ascending aorta and functional evaluation of the aortic valve. The ICE catheter, especially the new 8F version, can be inserted via a jugular venous access and advanced through the SVC into the upper RA. In contrast to transfemoral access, no fluoroscopic guidance is needed because the access sheath guides the catheter sufficiently, making direct catheter navigation superfluous. From the upper RA, aortic bulb and aortic valve can be displayed in the long-axis view and after tilting the tip of the catheter, also in a short-axis view. After the catheter is pulled back into the SVC, a longitudinal cut plane of the

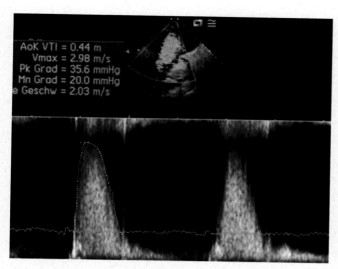

Figure 6–12. Transjugular approach: Intraoperative view from the superior vena cava toward the ascending aorta, depicting aortic valve prosthesis. This approach allows full intraoperative hemodynamic assessment as well.

whole ascending aorta reaching up to the innominate artery can be obtained. In contrast to TEE, systolic flow is mostly aligned with the Doppler beam of the catheter, permitting color flow and pressure gradient recordings of highest image quality. Therefore, ICE/IPAI might be of clinical interest immediately after aortic valve surgery and for guiding antegrade or retrograde percutaneous aortic valve implantation (Fig. 6–12).

Percutaneous aortic valve implantation is an increasingly performed intervention in patients who are not candidates for surgical aortic valve replacement. Typical patients are in markedly reduced general health. Therefore, extensive continuous or repeated TEE monitoring would require general anesthesia. In that respect, ICE monitoring results in much lower procedural stress to patients.

Intraoperative cannulation of the ascending aorta with surgical devices can also be monitored with IPAI views from the SVC. Further development of right heart assist devices could create another potential application. Nevertheless, the clinical experience with the transjugular approach is limited. Only a few case studies were performed, and these lack validation of their qualitative and quantitative data. After the techniques move from the realm of research into the cardiac anesthesiological and surgical practice, more data will become available.

Peri-Interventional Imaging of the Descending Thoracic Aorta

As recently reported, TEE adds incremental information, improving the safety of stent-graft placement in type-B aortic dissection. In addition, IVUS is consid-

ered helpful in patients with complex dissection including abdominal extension.[22] With respect to aortic diseases, the main limitation of IVUS is attributable to its inability to perform Doppler analysis. Flow detection by TEE is also limited if the flow is not aligned with the Doppler beam. In consequence, detecting flow from true to false lumen and vice versa by TEE depends on the alignment of the dissection flap. Therefore, TEE has a low sensitivity for detecting small entries and reentries (Fig. 6–13).

On the other hand, sonographic approaches may help lower the current complication rate of percutaneous stent-graft implantation,[23] thus opening up new opportunities for monitoring interventional therapy in aortic diseases using IPAI. In that respect, IPAI not only combines advantages of TEE and IVUS but also adds capabilities.

The descending thoracic aorta cannot be viewed from any venous access. Peri-interventional sonographic diagnostic methods need to clarify which lumen supplies the side branches, a difficult feat with TEE and even with IVUS images. Thus, the necessity to navigate the aorta with the echocardiographic catheter turns from a disadvantage into an advantage because the Doppler-beam can be aligned with any flow between true and false lumen and with blood flow into small branches. Thus, intraaortic monitoring by IPAI has great potential to become a tool for the effective guidance of aortic stent-graft implantation, that is, in such a manner that all entries are closed. First case reports also suggest that IPAI is capable of safely guiding other diagnostic intra-aortic procedures in aortic diseases.[24]

For intra-aortic employment of the echocardiographic catheter, a very long-access sheath is definitely recommended so that only the tip of the catheter with the

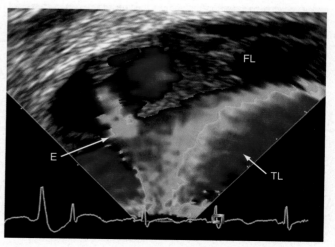

Figure 6–13. Intraluminal phased-array imaging from the true lumen to the false lumen: Thrombus formation in Type B aortic dissection. E, entry; FL, false lumen; TL, true lumen.

transducer sticks out of the sheath. Sheath and indwelling catheter are then jointly pulled back while imaging is performed. The catheter can be rotated intermittently and aimed at the region of interest by tilting its tip.

In type B aortic dissection, the echocardiographic catheter is placed into the true lumen and IPAI performed carefully. IPAI provides scans of the dissection flap when the device is rotated and withdrawn. Detection and precise localization of tears in the dissection membrane must be considered important for therapeutic decision making. In most cases, there are obviously more entries than demonstrable by angiography, IVUS, and TEE. The fact that such data form the basis for optimal stent-graft placement, which aims to close all entries to the false lumen, mandates a detailed analysis of the sensitivity of conventional diagnostic approaches. If overlooked or not properly closed by interventional treatment, even small tears can lead to significant flow into and inside the false lumen, subsequently impairing the desired thrombus formation in the false lumen and thereby impeding healing of the dissection. IPAI depicts more entries than one would expect from conventional diagnostics and demonstrates which abdominal vessels originate from the true and the false lumen. Thrombus formation in the false lumen, a result of effective pressure separation between true and false lumen, can be also displayed.

IPAI can also be used to safely guide percutaneous biopsies of intra-aortic masses suspected to be tumors. In most cases such masses are thrombi. But, if those masses are large and do not respond to anticoagulant therapy an angiosarcoma, which is rare (2 to 3 new cases per 1,000,000 population per year) but on the other hand multicentric and malignant masses must be excluded. To accomplish that, the transducer is aimed at the mass and the radial-jaw-biopsy-forceps (Fig. 6–14).

Under continuous ultrasonographic imaging, targeted biopsies are taken from the depth of the mass. Opening, pushing, and closure of the biopsy forceps can be precisely guided and documented.[24] If handled carefully, interference between echocardiographic catheter and lesion can be avoided. Nevertheless, there is some risk of peripheral embolization during the procedure.

Guiding Intimal Flap Fenestration in the Abdominal Aorta

As demonstrated for intracardiac interventional procedures, high-resolution imaging not only allows delineation of distinct pathology but also optimization of any therapeutic intervention in the abdominal aorta. With the echocardiographic catheter in the IVC, IPAI is an ideal tool to safely guide balloon fenestration of the dissection flap.[25] It provides a longitudinal view of the abdominal aorta neighboring the IVC (Fig. 6–15).

In case of true lumen collapse, IPAI also identifies the position of the smallest true lumen, that is, the location of the highest degree of compression by the false lumen. If there is no reentry in type B dissection or after surgical repair of the ascending aorta in type A dissection, true lumen collapse of the descending aorta can result in renal failure, bowel ischemia, and lower limb ischemia. In these cases, rapid and irreversible tissue destruction leads to rapidly rising lactate and plasma creatinine levels. Acute stent-graft implantation is one option for closing the entry, significantly lower-

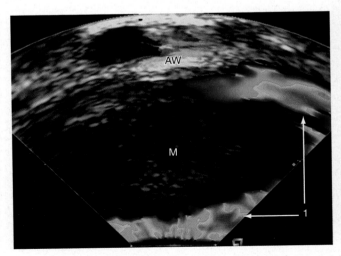

Figure 6–14. Intraluminal phased-array imaging of an intra-aortic mass. AW, aortic wall; M, mass; 1, flow around the mass.

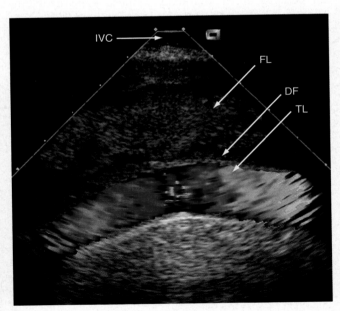

Figure 6–15. Dissection of the abdominal aorta with spontaneous contrast in the false lumen viewed from the inferior vena cava. DF, dissection flap; FL, false lumen; IVC, inferior vena cava; TL, true lumen.

ing the pressure in the false lumen.[26] Aortic stent-graft implantation, however, requires close cooperation with other disciplines. In an acute scenario, the logistics can be prohibitively time consuming. Therefore, fatal necrosis of intestinal tissue cannot be avoided in many cases. Transvenous IPAI could potentially be used to guide stent-graft implantation in the abdominal aorta, but its use for that purposes has never been reported. One alternative option, surgical fenestration, is known to be associated with mortality rates of up to 25%. Mortality figures can even exceed 70% in patients with critical mesenteric or renal ischemia.

Although emergency balloon fenestration, which is another alternative, may be facilitated by IVUS, puncture can result in perforation of the aortic free wall. IVUS is capable of displaying collapse of the true lumen. But it has limited use as a guiding tool for emergency fenestration because it does not provide longitudinal views aligned with the advancing Brockenbrough needle. Additionally one has to consider that puncture of the false lumen may not be possible at the selected location, as the needle may simply slide over the surface of the soft and compliant intimal flap. This can neither be demonstrated by fluoroscopy nor by IVUS. In that case, the needle must be reshaped and advanced with increased pressure. Although less invasive than surgical fenestration, in the past this approach has also been associated with a considerable residual mortality of up to 25%.[27] Therefore, simultaneous fluoroscopic and longitudinal ultrasonographic imaging seems to be the key for directing the needle precisely and with just the proper amount of pressure. After IPAI identification of the optimal position for puncture, the fluoroscopic image of the tip of the echocardiographic catheter serves as a marker for needle orientation. Perforation of the dissection flap is demonstrated by administering an echocardiographic contrast agent into the false lumen via the needle-catheter. The dissection flap is then fenestrated with a conventional balloon-catheter. This step can also be adequately monitored by IPAI.

Peri-Interventional Imaging of the Mitral Valve

Percutaneous transseptal balloon valvuloplasty of the mitral valve can be performed in concentric stenosis when the commissures are fused because of rheumatic heart disease without significant calcification and mitral regurgitation. Suitability of mitral stenosis for balloon valvuloplasty can be assessed using the Wilkins score and a commissural score. As described for PLAATO, atrial septal puncture is guided by the ICE transatrial longitudinal view. In that view, tool positioning in the LA can also be monitored. After introduction of a special guide wire into the LA, the transven-

tricular long-axis view of the left ventricle is obtained. Mitral ring diameter and intercommissural distance are measured, and the fused commissures are visualized. A balloon of appropriate size is selected. The same view is also useful for guiding a balloon through the stenotic mitral valve into the left ventricle. Adhering to the double balloon technique, the distal balloon is inflated. Inflation should be monitored with ICE and fluoroscopy simultaneously. The next steps must be completed quickly to avoid prolonged left ventricular inflow occlusion. Simultaneous echocardiographic and fluoroscopic viewing and documentation are recommended to accomplish this goal. The distal balloon is first inflated and then pulled back toward the stenotic valve. Not before this step is completed, the proximal balloon is inflated and valvuloplasty performed. At this time, ICE demonstrates that the balloon fits tightly into the stenotic valve orifice. The recently introduced single balloon technique[28] may require even closer echocardiographic guidance to precisely position the cylindrical balloon into the stenosis (Fig. 6–16).

After balloon deflation and withdrawal, immediate two-dimensional and Doppler analyses are recommended to show the split commissures and to exclude any injury of the commissures or the mitral valve apparatus. In addition, the degree of mitral regurgitation is reassessed. Intraprocedural ICE viewing may be considered an optional imaging modality, especially if the transthoracic acoustic window is poor. It allows analysis of the valvular anatomy and is ideal when enhanced views are required.[29] ICE is capable of providing excellent imaging and guidance, which results in a low radiation exposure and minimizes the need for contrast angiography.[14]

One would expect the more sophisticated interventional procedures to derive more benefits from ICE. Thus, there is great potential for ICE in percutaneous

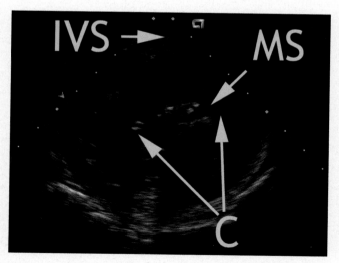

Figure 6–16. *Transventricular short-axis view: Excentric mitral stenosis with calcified commissures. C, commissures; IVS, interventricular septum; MS, mitral stenosis.*

valve implantation techniques and other catheter based "valvular repair" procedures currently under development. Especially transcatheter mitral annuloplasty techniques appear promising, particularly for inoperable patients with congestive heart failure (CHF), a population prone to develop considerable relative mitral regurgitation.

Another future application may arise from increasing importance of minimal invasive and reconstructive mitral valve surgery. Because high image resolution is required to depict filigreed portions of the mitral valvular apparatus, intraoperative ICE monitoring has the potential of facilitating such surgical intervention, probably improving their quality.

Limitations

Adequate handling of the ICE catheter requires a learning curve, even for an interventionalist familiar with left and right heart catheterization and IVUS. If a "noninvasive" cardiologist assists in image acquisition, training and experience in insertion and manipulation of the catheter is needed for safe performance of this procedure. The relatively large probe may limit its use in infants. In addition, the multifrequency probe does not provide harmonic imaging analysis. ICE does, however, eliminate the need for general anesthesia and intubation, thereby lowering costs and increasing patient comfort. On the other hand, ICE raises the cost of the procedure. The high price for one ICE catheter remains an important shortcoming. Today, the catheter is no longer a disposable device. The lumenless catheter can be resterilized with gas. Vanguard AG Medical Services for Europe (Berlin, Germany) is an approved CE-certified company licensed to resterilize ICE catheters. Technical and medical safety and compliance with appropriate legal regulations governing health care products are guaranteed. After more than two years of experience, we can recommend resterilization as a safe procedure, which permits each catheter to be reused approximately three times. Vanguard (Alliance) is cleared by the Food and Drug Administration to reprocess AcuNav as is Sterilmed. Although the image quality may slightly deteriorate from resterilization, each catheter can eventually be used four times, markedly lowering the costs for each use, even when the expenses for resterilization are accounted for.

Finally, the relation between advantages and disadvantages of using ICE and IPAI depends mainly on the expenditure and the risk of the specific interventional procedures. Increasing familiarity of interventionalists with this technique may also impact its use in the clinical practice (Table 6–3).

TABLE 6–3. Usefulness and Effectiveness of Intracardiac and Intravascular Imaging

Procedure	Clinical Benefit
Device closure of ASD	Very high
Device closure of PFO	Moderate
PLAATO	High
Radiofrequency PV ablation	Very high
PTSMA	Moderate
Percutaneous AV implantation	Potentially high
Surgery of the ascending aorta	Undetermined
Interventional therapy of the descending aorta	Potentially high
Balloon mitral valvuloplasty	High
Surgical/interventional mitral valve repair	Undetermined
Pulmonary embolism/detection and fragmentation of thrombi	Undetermined

ASD, atrial septal defect; AV, aortic valve; PFO, patent foramen ovale; PLAATO, percutaneous left atrial appendage transluminal occlusion; PTSMA, percutaneous transluminal septal myocardial ablation; PV, pulmonary vein.

KEY POINTS

As an alternative to TEE and IVUS and in conjunction with fluoroscopy, ICE can guide a variety of noncoronary percutaneous interventional therapeutic interventions.

Interventional procedure	Guidance by ICE
■ Device closure of interatrial communications	View from the RA
■ LAA occlusion (PLAATO)	View from the RA (and RV)
■ Radiofrequency pulmonary vein ablation	View from the RA
■ PTSMA in hypertrophic-obstructive cardiomyopathy	View from the RV
■ Imaging of the ascending aorta	View from the SVC and RA
■ Imaging of the descending thoracic aorta	Intra-aortic view
■ Imaging of the abdominal aorta	View from the IVC
■ Mitral valve angioplasty and repair	View from the RA and RV

REFERENCES

1. Bruce CJ, Packer DL, Seward JB: Intracardiac echocardiography: newest technology. *J Am Soc Echocardiogr* 13:788-795, 2000.
2. Olgin JE, Kalman JM, Chin M, et al: Electrophysiological effects of long, linear atrial lesions placed under intracardiac ultrasound guidance. *Circulation* 96:2715-2721, 1997.
3. Luxenberg DM, Silvestry FE, Herrmann HC, et al: Use of a new 8 French intracardiac echocardiographic catheter to guide device closure of atrial septal defects and patent foramen ovale in small children and adults: initial clinical experience. *J Invasive Cardiol* 17:540-545, 2005.
4. Bruce CJ, Packer DL, Seward JB: Intracardiac Doppler hemodynamics and flow: New vector, phased-array ultrasound-tipped catheter. *Am J Cardiol* 83:1509-1512, 1999.
5. Bartel T, Müller S, Caspari G, Erbel R: Intracardiac and intraluminal echocardiography: Indications and standard approaches. *Ultrasound Med Biol* 28:997-1003, 2002.
6. Du ZD, Hijazi ZM, Kleinman CS, et al: Comparison between transcatheter and surgical closure of secundum atrial septal defect in children and adults. *J Am Coll Cardiol* 39:1836-1844, 2003.
7. Chessa M, Carminati M, Butera G, et al: Early and late complications associated with transcatheter occlusion of secundum atrial septal defect. *J Am Coll Cardiol* 39:1061-1065, 2002.
8. Bartel T, Konorza T, Arjumand J, et al: Intracardiac echocardiography is superior to conventional monitoring for guiding closure of interatrial communications. *Circulation* 107:795-797, 2003.
9. Mullen MJ, Dias BF, Walker F, et al: Intracardiac echocardiography guided device closure of atrial septal defects. *J Am Coll Cardiol* 41:285-292, 2003.
10. Koenig P, Cao QL, Heitschmidt M, et al: Role of intracardiac echocardiographic guidance in transcatheter closure of atrial septal defects and patent foramen ovale using the Amplatzer device. *J Interv Cardiol* 16:51-62, 2003.
11. Bartel T, Konorza T, Neudorf U, et al: Intracardiac echocardiography: An ideal guiding tool for device closure of interatrial communications. *Eur J Echocardiogr* 6:92-96, 2005.
12. Nkomo VT, Theuma P, Maniu VC, et al: Patent foramen ovale transcatheter closure device thrombosis. *Mayo Clin Proc* 76:1057-1061, 2001.
13. Martin F, Sánchez PL, Doherty E, et al: Percutaneous transcatheter closure of patent foramen ovale in patients with paradoxical embolism. *Circulation* 106:1121-1126, 2002.
14. Vaina S, Ligthart J, Vijayakumar M, et al: Intracardiac echocardiography during interventional procedures. *Eurointervention* 1:454-464, 2006.
15. Epstein LM, Mitchell MA, Smith TW, Haines DE: Comparative study of fluoroscopy and intracardiac echocardiographic guidance for the creation of linear atrial lesions. *Circulation* 98:1796-1801, 1998.
16. Tardif JC, Groeneveld PW, Wang PJ, et al: Intracardiac echocardiographic guidance during microwave catheter ablation. *J Am Soc Echocardiogr* 12:41-47, 1999.
17. Roithinger FX, Steiner PR, Goseki Y, et al: Low-power radiofrequency application and intracardiac echocardiography for creation of continuous left atrial linear lesions. *J Cardiovasc Electrophysiol* 10:680-691, 1999.
18. Callans DJ, Ren JF, Schwartzman D, et al: Narrowing of the superior vena cava-right atrium junction during radiofrequency catheter ablation for inappropriate sinus tachycardia: Analysis with intracardiac echocardiography. *J Am Coll Cardiol* 33:1667-1670, 1999.
19. Ren JF, Marchlinski FE, Callans DJ: Left atrial thrombus associated with ablation for atrial fibrillation: Identification with intracardiac echocardiography. *J Am Coll Cardiol* 43:1861-1867, 2004.
20. Marrouche NF, Martin DO, Wazni O, et al: Phased-array intracardiac echocardiography monitoring during pulmonary vein isolation in patients with atrial fibrillation: Impact on outcome and complications. *Circulation* 107:2710-2716, 2003.
21. Faber L, Seggewiss H, Gleichmann U: Percutaneous transluminal septal myocardial ablation in hypertrophic obstructive cardiomyopathy: results with respect to intraprocedural myocardial contrast echocardiography. *Circulation* 98:2415-2421, 1998.
22. Koschyk DH, Nienaber CA, Knap M, et al: How to guide stent-graft implantation in type B aortic dissection? *Circulation* 122(suppl I):I-260-I-264, 2005.
23. Eggebrecht H, Nienaber CA, Neuhäuser M, et al: Endovascular stent-graft placement in aortic dissection: A meta-analysis. *Eur Heart J* 27(4):489-498; Epub Oct. 14, 2005.
24. Bartel T, Eggebrecht H, Erbel R: Safe biopsy of aortic masses guided by intraluminal two-dimensional ultrasonography. *Heart* 90:974, 2004.
25. Bartel T, Eggebrecht H, Ebralidze T, et al: Optimal guidance for intimal flap fenestration in aortic dissection by transvenous two-dimensional and Doppler Ultrasonography. *Circulation* 107:e17-e18, 2003.
26. Eggebrecht H, Herold U, Kuhnt O, et al: Endovascular stent-graft treatment of aortic dissection: Determinants of post-interventional outcome. *Eur Heart J* 26:489-497, 2005.
27. Chavan A, Galanski M, Pichlmaier M: Minimally invasive therapy options in aortic dissections. *Rofo* 172:576-586, 2000.
28. Joseph G, Chandy S, George P, et al: Evaluation of a simplified transseptal mitral valvuloplasty technique using over-the-wire single balloons and complementary femoral and jugular venous approaches in 1,407 consecutive patients. *J Invasive Cardiol* 17(3):132-138, 2005.
29. Salem MI, Makaryus AN, Kort S, et al: Intracardiac echocardiography using the AcuNav ultrasound catheter during percutaneous balloon mitral valvuloplasty. *J Am Soc Echocardiogr* 15:1533-1537, 2002.

Chapter 7

Intravascular Ultrasound: Principles and Clinical Applications

NEIL J. WEISSMAN, MD • GARY S. MINTZ, MD

Technical Background

Intravascular ultrasound (IVUS) is a cardiovascular imaging application that utilizes a miniaturized transducer secured at the end of a flexible catheter that is inserted into arteries for in vivo visualization of vascular anatomy. This technology allows assessment of vascular anatomy literally from the inside out with detailed visualization of all arterial layers. The IVUS catheter can be advanced into various vascular structures, including peripheral arteries to assess peripheral vascular disease, coronary arteries to assess the degree and extent of coronary atherosclerosis and to guide percutaneous intervention, and into the intracardiac chambers (covered in the chapter on intracardiac echocardiography). Intracoronary ultrasound has become the most commonly used form of intravascular imaging and is regularly employed to delineate plaque morphology and distribution, to assess angiographically ambiguous lesions, and to guide transcatheter coronary intervention (Fig. 7–1).

See page 169 for a list of key acronyms for this chapter.

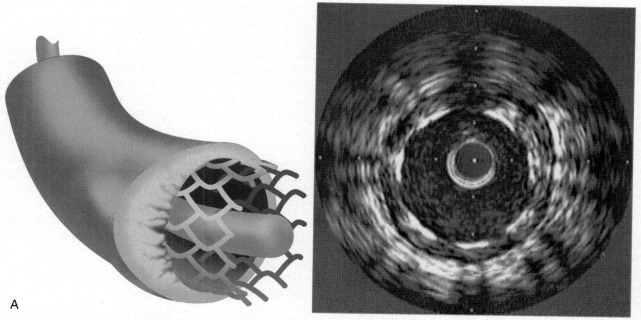

Figure 7–1. A, *Pictorial representation of an intravascular ultrasound catheter inserted into a coronary artery after stent deployment;* B, *actual intravascular ultrasound image of a well deployed coronary stent.*

Types of Intravascular Ultrasound Catheters

IVUS imaging uses a specially adapted ultrasound (US) machine that is dedicated to catheter-based imaging. Historically, most IVUS units in clinical use have been portable, which allows them to be used in various rooms of the catheterization lab as needed. More recent versions, however, are permanently stationed in the catheterization lab and integrated into the laboratory equipment. Regardless of the location of the IVUS machine, all clinical applications require the monitor to be within easy view of the cardiologist and technical staff. The IVUS catheter is attached to the US machine through an interface that ensures sterility of the catheter and allows for motorized pullback. Motorized pullback of the IVUS catheter (or of the transducer within the catheter) at 0.5 mm/sec or 1.0 mm/sec allows calculation of lesion length, ensures adequate time to visualize the lesion, provides a frame of reference for findings with fixed anatomic landmarks (side-branches), and allows comparison between IVUS "runs" done at different times but with similar pullback speeds. It is for these reasons that motorized pullback is recommended for all IVUS examinations.

There are two types of transducers used in IVUS catheters: mechanical and phased array. The mechanical catheter is the most common type of IVUS catheter in clinical use because of its high spatial resolution. It uses a single mechanical transducer that is mounted at the tip of the catheter and rotates quickly (at 1800 rotations per minute [rpm]). Because the IVUS transducer is oriented at a 90-degree angle to the length of the catheter, the images are displayed as cross-sectional views of the artery. The mechanical transducer has the advantage of a simple design and a greater signal-to-noise ratio. These properties account for its high image quality with an overall resolution (with current 40 MHz transducers) of approximately 100 to 120 microns. The primary disadvantage of mechanical transducers is that they require a central drive shaft to rotate the transducer on the tip of the catheter. This drive shaft decreases catheter flexibility. If a mechanical transducer is placed within a tortuous vessel, the drive shaft may be constricted, resulting in nonuniform rotation of the distal transducer, thus creating an artifact of the image termed nonuniform rotational distortion or NURD.

The phased array transducer uses multiple, tiny transducer elements. Each transducer element is permanently affixed along the circumference of the catheter tip and sends and receives US from a small sector. The multiple imaging sectors are then "added together" via the US console to produce a cross-sectional image of the artery, as occurs with the mechanical transducer. Thus, the mechanical and phased-array transducers produce comparable images although the image is formed in a different fashion. Because the phased-array transducer is permanently fixed with no moving parts, it is more flexible and transverses torturous vessels more easily. These transducers do not produce NURD artifact. However, the phased-array transducer does require more complex programming to add the sectors together and thus has a lower temporal resolution (a function of computational speed) and lower spatial resolution. With the advent of higher speed computers, sophisticated software, and additional elements mounted on the catheter tip, the phased-array images have greatly improved within the last few years and now produce images similar to those from mechanical transducers.

Image Formation

An IVUS image is formed when US bounces off of the multiple layers of the artery and returns to the transducer. To understand how an IVUS image is created, the normal arterial structures and the acoustic properties of these structures must first be appreciated.

The coronary artery is a muscular vessel composed of three basic layers: the intima, media, and adventitia. The artery is a conduit for blood flow and is essentially a pipe. The coating of the pipe is the intima, a thin sheet of cell layers which, when young, is just a few cells thick. It is in the intima that atherosclerotic plaque gets deposited causing the intima to greatly enlarge. The intima is directly surrounded by the media, a layer of predominately homogeneous smooth muscle cells that provides the artery with its vascular tone. The final layer is the adventitia. The adventitia surrounds the media and provides additional external support to the artery with several layers of fibrous connective tissue. Because US transmitted from the transducer will "bounce" back whenever it encounters an interface of different acoustic impedance (which is primarily dependent on the density of the tissue), it is fortunate that each of these layers tends to have different acoustic properties, thus allowing each to be visualized. US transmitted from the transducer, while in the lumen and surrounded by blood, will traverse the blood with minimal reflection. When it encounters the intima, there is a large change in acoustic impedance and thus much of the US is bounced back to the transducer and displayed on the screen. The reflected US from the intima is displayed as a single concentric echo. All of the US, however, is not reflected by the intima (unless extremely hard, such as calcified plaque), and some will penetrate through to the media. Because the media is composed of homogeneous smooth muscle cells, US passes through with minimal reflection and appears as a dark zone devoid of echoes. The most outer layer, the adventitia, has numerous layers of collagen fibers, thus creating multiple interfaces from which to reflect sound and is a highly reflective structure. The adventitia will therefore appear bright. As a result of these different acoustic properties of the blood, intima, media, and adventitia, the normal coronary artery has a three-layered appearance, which includes (1) a bright echo from the intima, (2) a dark zone from the media, and (3) bright surrounding echoes from the adventitia.

The typical three-layered appearance of a coronary artery and atherosclerotic deposition is most com-monly seen in clinical practice. It is possible, however, that a truly normal and nondiseased artery will not have this three-layered appearance and will, instead, appear to be mono-layered (blood appears to be touching the adventitia). Because the resolution of IVUS is approximately 100 to 120 microns, the intima has to be at least this thick to be visualized. In Western society, most patients presenting to the cardiac catheterization laboratory have some diffuse thickening of the intima to at least this degree, but if the intima is truly disease free, as in a newborn or an adolescent child, then the intima will be much thinner (one or two cell layers thick or approximately 50 microns) and therefore not be visible with IVUS. Thus, a monolayer is indeed normal, and if the intima is only a single, thin concentric echo within the media, then it is also considered essentially normal.

Image Interpretation

As the atherosclerotic disease accumulates, the intimal zone will thicken on the IVUS image, and the dark anechoic (i.e., lack of echoes) media will outline the size that the artery would be if there were no atherosclerotic disease. Thus, interpretation of an IVUS image involves only a few simple steps: (1) identify the IVUS catheter in the center of the screen and keep in mind that the IVUS catheter is traveling down the lumen within the blood flow, (2) identify the dark stripe of the media that tells the size of the artery in the absence atherosclerotic disease, (3) remember that all of the echoes within the media stripe represent intima or intimal (atherosclerotic) disease and, (4) all of the echoes outside the media are adventitia.

IVUS is uniquely suited to assess atherosclerotic plaque extent, morphology, and distribution. The tomographic cross-sectional view of the artery allows the interpreter to determine concentric from eccentric plaque and to quantitate that distribution. IVUS is far more accurate than angiography for assessing plaque eccentricity, which is critical in selecting some interventional approaches (e.g., directional atherectomy for eccentric lesions). Because US reflects off of tissue to a different extent depending on the acoustic impedance (density) of the tissue, IVUS has the ability to differentiate plaque of different compositions. Hard material (calcium) will reflect more US and appear brighter on the image, whereas soft plaque (fat) will not reflect the US and will appear dark. Calcium is so dense that no US penetrates to the deeper tissues and thus calcium produces acoustic shadows. This shadowing, along with the bright echoes, is the hallmark of calcification. A plaque that is dense enough to produce bright echoes but not so reflective that it causes shadowing is labeled *hard* and is composed primarily of fibrous tissue. A standard approach is to compare the overall brightness of the plaque to the surrounding adventitia; if it is brighter, the plaque is hard and if it is less bright, the plaque is *soft*. Thus, plaque is typically characterized as soft, hard, calcified, or mixed. Obviously, this is a fairly crude classification scheme, but IVUS does not have the differential capability to be an acoustic microscope and this rough classification scheme is appropriate for conventional gray scale IVUS plaque characterization.

Because of its high resolution, IVUS has proven to be a valuable tool to precisely determine arterial lumen, plaque, and vessel (or external elastic membrane [EEM]) size. Angiography permits the measurement of luminal diameters only and typically in only two or three views. IVUS displays the vessel in a tomographic, cross-sectional view (with 180 potential diameters of the lumen and EEM) that lends itself to a more accurate measurement. This, combined with the higher spatial resolution of IVUS, accounts for the superiority of IVUS measurements over angiographic measurements.

The higher resolution of IVUS also allows for better detection of small splits in the plaque that occur spontaneously or after coronary intervention. These small dissections or plaque fissures are part of the mechanism for luminal enlargement with angioplasty and are commonly seen after routine balloon treatment. The small plaque fissures associated with balloon angioplasty differ from large dissections, which extend to the media. These larger dissections extending to the media are often associated with adverse outcomes. IVUS has been shown to be able to detect dissections better than angioplasty because of its high spatial resolution and tomographic imaging.

Intravascular Ultrasound versus Angiography

To fully appreciate and apply IVUS in clinical practice, one needs to have a full understanding of how IVUS and angiography differ. Angiography is often referred to as a "shadow-o-gram" of the lumen because a silhouette of the arterial lumen is obtained by injecting radiopaque dye into the lumen and projecting the shadow from the dye on to cineangiographic film. The shadow-o-gram is then used to extrapolate a luminal narrowing to a plaque accumulation. Furthermore, angiography may result in hazy areas or other types of ambiguous lesions (such as left main stenosis). These hazy or ambiguous lesions may result from irregular plaque, a focal area of calcium, a dissection, or an intraluminal thrombus. IVUS is particularly useful for ambiguous lesions because each of the causes (plaque irregularities, calcium, dissection, or thrombus) appear different on IVUS.

To better understand the differences between IVUS and angiography, one must recognize why IVUS is so good at detecting angiographically silent atherosclerotic disease. It is common to detect atherosclerosis by IVUS in an artery that appears "normal" by angiography. Although it may appear to be a discrepancy at first, it is not, and both the angiography and the IVUS studies are providing complementary and accurate information. The primary difference is that angiography is visualizing just the lumen, whereas IVUS visualizes both the lumen and arterial walls. If the assumption is that all angiographic stenosis are from plaque, then it would make sense to conclude that an angiogram displaying a lumen without any narrowing is free of plaque. However, that may not be true (and usually is not). An angiogram of an artery can be free of any stenosis, but that artery can still have many areas of plaque. This is true because of three phenomena: (1) atherosclerotic plaque is often diffusely distributed, (2) arteries undergo vascular remodeling, and (3) complex atherosclerotic plaques are not appreciated by the two-dimensional silhouette.

If an artery is thought of as a pipe and the pipe is uniformly filled with material, then an angiogram of the pipe would show smooth walls and no focal stenosis. The lack of stenosis or luminal irregularities does not mean there is no material (or plaque) within the artery; it just means the lumen does not have a narrowing. In fact, IVUS has shown that "normal" areas around a stenosis that are often used as a "reference" by angiography may have as much as one third of their cross-sectional area filled with plaque. It has been further verified in autopsy studies and other IVUS studies of healthy donors that most people have diffuse atherosclerotic disease throughout their arteries by mid-life, and this disease often remains angiographically silent because of its diffuse nature.

In addition to diffuse plaque, vascular remodeling is also responsible for the high prevalence of angiographically silent disease. Both pathology and IVUS studies have documented that coronary arteries will enlarge to accommodate focal plaque deposition in an attempt to maintain luminal integrity. Successful compensatory enlargement preserves the luminal dimensions and results in no angiographic (luminal) stenosis. The lack of luminal stenosis occurs even with the deposition of a focal atherosclerotic plaque.

Lastly, complex luminal shapes can result from irregular plaques or the disruption of a plaque (from balloon angioplasty). Although such a lesion may appear hazy, it may not demonstrate a luminal stenosis when viewed from only one or two views and projected as a silhouette. This may be similar to an eccentric lesion, which can fool inexperienced angiographers, unless a large number and variety of views are obtained, each displaying a different severity. However, a lumen with highly irregular borders may not be fully appreciated, even in multiple views. The tomographic images of IVUS are necessary to appreciate the true luminal shape. Therefore, diffuse plaque, vascular remodeling, and irregular plaque can all lead to an inability of angiography to appreciate the plaque that is seen on

IVUS. This is predominately because angiography only visualizes the lumen and does so in limited views using silhouettes of the dye.

Clinical Application

The concepts involved in the use of IVUS to guide coronary interventions are not different from the concepts involved in the use of angiography to guide interventional procedures. From a practical standpoint, the primary uses of IVUS are to assess the severity of a coronary artery stenosis including left main coronary artery (LMCA) disease, to measure lesion length, to measure reference vessel size, to identify complications, to optimize final results, and to assess in-stent restenosis. Unless drug-eluting stents virtually eliminate restenosis, the main clinical indication for IVUS imaging remains in-stent restenosis in order to assess severity and mechanical complications, such as stent underexpansion. Perhaps even more importantly, careful systematic IVUS imaging, including systematic acquisition and volumetric analysis is critical to the understanding of new therapeutic interventions, whether mechanical or pharmacologic, and to ensure adequate stent implantation, whether bare-metal or drug-eluting.

An important reference for the clinical application of IVUS is "Standards for the acquisition, measurement, and reporting of intravascular ultrasound studies: A report of the American College of Cardiology Task Force on Clinical Expert Consensus Documents."[1] This consensus document is the current gold standard for IVUS imaging. These acquisition, measurement, and reporting guidelines should be followed as a general rule and especially in studies in which IVUS is used as an endpoint or as a tool to better understand the mechanisms of treatment effects.

Integration into Practice

Major resistances to the routine use of IVUS include procedural cost, physician education (both how to interpret the images and how to use the information), equipment complexity, and difficulties in integrating IVUS into a busy catheterization laboratory. IVUS will be used routinely only if it is quick to set up, easy to perform, and does not slow down the flow of the clinical cases. Each catheterization laboratory is organized differently. Even tasks performed by the same health care professionals vary from laboratory to laboratory. It is possible to integrate clinical IVUS imaging into a busy laboratory, maintain image acquisition standards, and not add significant time to the overall procedure (i.e., no more than 5 minutes for an average of three runs: pre-intervention, at some time during the procedure, and post-intervention). In general, the integration

of IVUS will be most successful if it is under the administrative structure of the cardiac catheterization laboratory, not the noninvasive imaging laboratory. The temperaments of the two environments are different; interventional procedures cannot be put on hold waiting for equipment and/or personnel, and the individuals involved in IVUS imaging must have an understanding of interventional procedures.

Even in a busy laboratory with constant IVUS use, it is difficult to train all laboratory personnel. Many practical aspects of IVUS imaging (e.g., instrumentation and recording) are foreign to traditional catheterization lab practices. IVUS imaging is facilitated by designating specific IVUS technologists who become responsible for all practical aspects of IVUS imaging: (1) equipment and catheter set-up, (2) image optimization, (3) proper recording of IVUS imaging runs, (4) accurate voice and onscreen alphanumeric documentation, (5) patient and procedure logs, and (6) equipment maintenance, etc. With time, technologists can be trained to interpret images accurately, to provide the iterative feedback necessary for IVUS-based decision making, and to answer questions posed by the primary operators. Measurements should be made offline (from videotape or digital images after the imaging run is complete), not when the catheter is in the vessel; this saves procedure time and minimizes patient ischemia.

The angiographic (i.e., "road-map") monitors can be set up to display IVUS images. Angiographic monitors offer superior resolution, are convenient and readily visible to the operator, and allow the IVUS machine to be placed in a position away from the patient table and out of the way of the nurses providing patient care.

In a busy laboratory with multiple operators, it is important to standardize image acquisition and analysis. The use of a motorized transducer pullback device aids (in fact, enforces) discipline and acquisition standards; there is no question whether the transducer is being advanced or withdrawn. The preferred pullback speed is 0.5 mm/sec; this is the fastest rate at which the trained eye can assimilate the information. However, with focal stenoses, especially ostial stenoses, a slower pullback may be necessary. A motorized transducer pullback does not preclude the addition of careful, manually controlled, interrogation of the lesion. Standardization of image acquisition facilitates offline image analysis and comparison of serial (preintervention versus postintervention or postintervention versus follow-up) studies; it is essential for multicenter studies.

Accurate procedural information is critical. Even when recording verbal commentary, it is helpful if online procedural information is annotated onto the IVUS system's video screen. On-screen labeling should contain three elements: (1) the timing of IVUS imaging (e.g., preintervention, etc.), (2) the procedure being performed, and (3) the target vessel and location. All IVUS instruments have internal clocks, and the time is automatically recorded onto the image. It is helpful to note the time that corresponds to the center of the lesion. In the absence of systematic preintervention imaging, voice annotation or recording the time corresponding to the lesion may be the only way to identify the target lesion on subsequent review. Digital acquisition and storage is preferred, but in the absence of a digital system, good quality videotapes are essential. It is recommended that never-before-used broadcast quality s-VHS tapes be used. There is significant quality difference, and the cost differential is minimal. CDs and videotapes should be stored in a secure place (or digital images should be archived onto the hospital server with regular backup).

Many catheterization laboratories have excessive ambient electrical or radiofrequency noise, which can produce artifacts on the US image. Offenders include monitoring equipment, intra-aortic balloon pumps, and so on. Eliminating these problems requires troubleshooting and working with both the IVUS and non-IVUS equipment vendors. A Doppler FloWire can cause two types of interference. One is electrical, and the other is cross-talk between the two signals. Ultrasonic cross-talk is present whenever two sources of ultrasonic signals are used simultaneously. In addition, in some hospitals the paging system generates a radiofrequency signal that momentarily blanks out the IVUS image. Inexpensive, custom filters will solve this problem.

Standard Intravascular Ultrasound Acquisition Protocol

There are two technical approaches to imaging: motorized or manual interrogation. Regardless of which approach is used, imaging should include careful uninterrupted imaging of (1) at least 10 mm of distal reference, (2) the lesion site(s), and (3) the entire proximal reference back to the aorta. Advantages of motorized pullback are (1) controlled catheter withdrawal so no segment of the vessel is skipped or imaged too quickly by pulling the catheter back too rapidly, (2) the ability to concentrate on the images without having to simultaneously pay attention to catheter manipulation,

(3) ability for length and volumetric measurements, and (4) uniform and reproducible image acquisition for multicenter and serial studies. Disadvantages of motorized pullback are the following: (1) even at slow pullback speeds, it is possible to skip over focal lesions, (2) not enough attention may be paid to important regions of interest, and (3) it is not possible to have the transducer "sit" at one specific site in the vessel. Nonetheless, motorized transducer pullback is especially important in multicenter studies assessing the results of new therapies (both mechanical and pharmacologic).

Manual transducer pullback should be at a slow rate similar to motorized pullback. Advantages are that it is possible to concentrate on specific regions of interest by having the transducer sit at a specific site in the vessel. Disadvantages include the following: (1) it is easy to skip over significant pathology by pulling the transducer back too quickly or unevenly, (2) length and volume measurements cannot be performed, and (3) antegrade and retrograde manual catheter movement can be confusing when the study is reviewed at a later date.

When interrogating aorto-ostial lesions it is important that the guiding catheter be disengaged from the ostium. If not, the true aorto-ostial lumen dimensions may not be identified. In all cases, at least one continuous uninterrupted imaging run should be performed from approximately 10 mm beyond the target lesion to the aorto-ostial junction.

Safety

There have been three large studies evaluating the safety of IVUS. Other than transient spasm, complications appear to be rare (Table 7–1).

Assessment of Stenosis Severity

Coronary angiography underestimates stenosis severity most markedly in vessels with 50% to 75% plaque burden (plaque area divided by arterial area) at necropsy and in patients with multivessel disease.[5-9] Several studies have correlated IVUS with other diagnostic modalities and have demonstrated the diagnostic accuracy of IVUS and can be seen in Table 7–2 and Figure 7–2.

TABLE 7–1. Studies Evaluating the Safety of Intravascular Ultrasound

Study	Number of Patients	Number of Centers	Transient Vessel Spasms	Major Complications
Hausmann and colleagues[2]	2207	28	2.9%	0.4%
Batkoff and colleagues[3]	718	12	0.6%	0.6%
Gorge and colleagues[4]	7085	51	3.0%	0.14%

Data from references 2, 3, and 4.

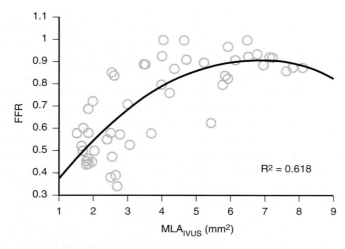

Figure 7–2. *Plots of the relationship between fractional flow reserve (FFR) and the minimal lumen area (MLA) by intravascular ultrasound (IVUS). R, radius. (From Takagi A, Tsurumi Y, Ishii Y, et al: Circulation 100:250-255, 1999.)*

TABLE 7–2. Validation of Intravascular Ultrasound Assessment of Ischemia Producing Stenosis

	Doppler FloWire versus IVUS[10]	
	IVUS MLA ≥ 4.0 mm²	IVUS MLA ≤ 4.0 mm²
CFR < 2.0	2	27
CFR ≥ 2.0	39	4
	SPECT Thallium versus IVUS[11,12]	
	IVUS MLA ≥ 4.0 mm²	IVUS MLA ≤ 4.0 mm²
+ SPECT	4	42
− SPECT	20	1

CFR, coronary flow reserve; IVUS, intravascular ultrasound; MLA, minimum lumen areas; SPECT, single photon emission computed tomography.

For a 5-year period, our laboratory used IVUS to study 756 patients (900 lesions) specifically to quantify the severity of an intermediate stenosis (<70% angiographic diameter stenosis [DS] by visual estimation) in a major epicardial vessel other than the left main artery and not in the setting of a recent myocardial infarction (MI). If the stenosis was deemed significant, intervention was performed; if not, intervention was deferred. We excluded from this analysis: 196 patients (233 lesions) who underwent in-hospital revascularization based on IVUS findings and 260 patients with 310 previously treated lesions. Therefore, in 300 patients (357 de novo intermediate native artery lesions) intervention was deferred based on IVUS findings. In general, based on this data, the criteria for deferred intervention was a minimum lumen area less than 4 mm² or a minimum lumen diameter (MLD) less than 2 mm. Complete follow-up data were available in 99% of the patients; the minimum follow-up in patients who were event free was 12 months. Events occurred in

24 patients. There were two (0.7%) cardiac deaths after 7 and 21 months. Four patients (1.3%) had a MI at a mean follow-up time of 13.5 (range 3 to 15) months. Eighteen (6%) patients had lesion-related revascularization, only three revascularizations (two percutaneous transluminal coronary angioplasty [PTCA] and one coronary artery bypass graft [CABG]) were performed within 6 months after the diagnostic IVUS study. There seemed to be an important difference between lesions with minimum lumen areas above and below 4 mm². In 248 lesions with a minimum lumen cross-sectional area (CSA) greater than 4 mm², the event rate was only 4.4% and the revascularization rate only 2.8%. The predictors for target lesion revascularization (PTCA and CABG) were diabetes mellitus, IVUS lesion lumen area, and IVUS area stenosis (minimum lumen area compared to the mean reference lumen area). These results are shown in Table 7–3.[13]

TABLE 7–3. Predictors of Cardiac Events at Follow-up (PTCA and CABG)

	RR	95% CI	*p* valve
Any Event			
IVUS lumen CSA (mm²)	0.57	0.400-0.842	0.0041
IVUS AS (%)	1.04	1.006-1.082	0.0235
Target Lesion Revascularization			
Diabetes mellitus	2.90	1.003-8.381	0.0493
IVUS lesion lumen CSA (mm²)	0.52	0.331-0.812	0.0042
IVUS AS (%)	1.04	0.999-1.088	0.0553

AS, area stenosis; CABG, coronary artery bypass graft; CI, confidence interval; CSA, cross-sectional area; IVUS, intravascular ultrasound; PTCA, percutaneous transluminal coronary angioplasty; RR, relative risk.
From Abizaid AS, Mintz GS, Mehran R, et al: *Circulation* 100:256-261, 1990.

Thus, based both on comparison to physiologic measures and follow-up data, an IVUS minimum lumen area of 4 mm² is considered to be the threshold for significance. This cutoff only applies to major epicardial vessels excluding the left main artery and excluding saphenous vein grafts. This diagnostic use of IVUS depends on technique. Because of the importance of the minimum lumen CSA, it is necessary to interrogate the lesion carefully to identify the image slice with the smallest lumen, especially in very focal stenoses. Poor technique (too rapid or uneven transducer withdrawal or not interrogating the stenosis carefully) may miss the true minimum lumen CSA. Once the smallest lumen is identified, careful measurement is required. Furthermore, clinical events are determined by lumen size not by the amount of plaque. Therefore, it is important to focus on accurate measurement of lumen dimensions and not to be distracted by the plaque burden. Plaque burden in patients with atherosclerosis tends to be large even in the absence of lumen compromise.

Unusual Lesion Morphology

IVUS is useful in understanding lesions with an unusual angiographic appearance. Three such lesions are filling defects, aneurysms, and spontaneous dissection. Although most filling defects are true thrombi, a small percentage are calcified plaque. Clinical clues that a filling defect represents calcified plaque include (1) no decrease in size with prolonged anticoagulation, thrombolytic agents, or IIb/IIIa inhibitors and (2) severe, diffuse coronary calcification.[14] An example is shown in Figure 7–3.

An IVUS classification of angiographic coronary artery aneurysms has also been created.[15] Of 77 aneurysm-containing lesions, 21 (27%) were classified as true aneurysm; 3 (4%) were classified as pseudoaneurysms (all having previous intervention); 12 (16%) were complex plaques; and the other 41 (53%) were normal arterial segments adjacent to one or more stenoses. Examples are shown in Figures 7–4 through 7–7. Spontaneous dissections are an intramural process that appear as a me-

Moderate calcification

Severe calcification

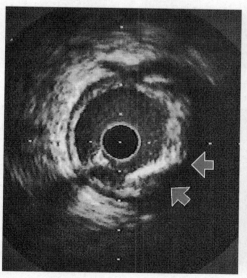
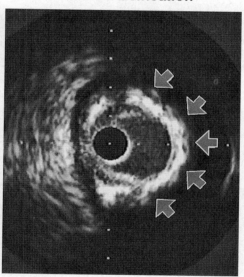

Figure 7–3. *Calcified plaque.*

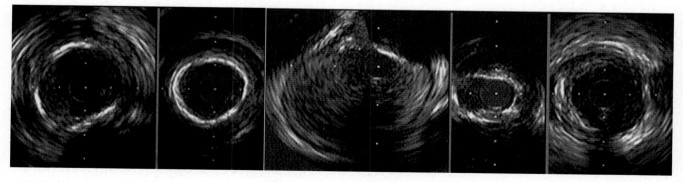

Figure 7–4. *True aneurysm.*

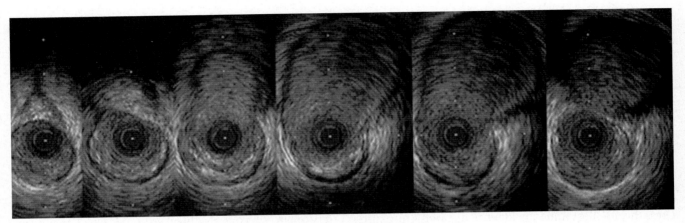

Figure 7–5. Pseudoaneurysm.

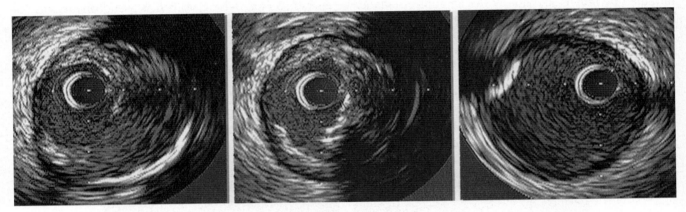

Figure 7–6. Complex plaque.

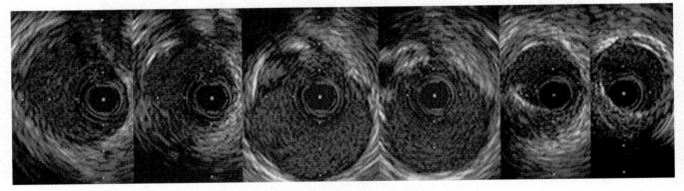

Figure 7–7. Normal arterial segments adjacent to stenoses.

dial dissection with an intramural hematoma occupying the dissected false lumen without intimal tears and without a communication between the true and false lumens.[16] An example is shown in Figure 7–8.

Assessment of Left Main Coronary Artery Disease

Hermiller and colleagues showed that a high percentage (89%) of patients with angiographically normal LMCA had disease by IVUS.[17] These findings were confirmed in studies by Yamagishi, Gerber, and Ge.[18-20]

Hermiller also reported no correlation between IVUS and quantitative coronary angiographic (QCA) lumen dimensions in patients with angiographically detectable LMCA disease.[17] Reasons for the discrepancy between angiography and necropsy or IVUS assessment of LMCA disease include the following (1) diffuse atherosclerotic involvement affects the angiographic DS calculation because of the lack of a normal reference segment; (2) a short LMCA also makes identification of a normal reference segment difficult; (3) unique geometric issues exist in LMCA disease (the correlation between angiography and necropsy

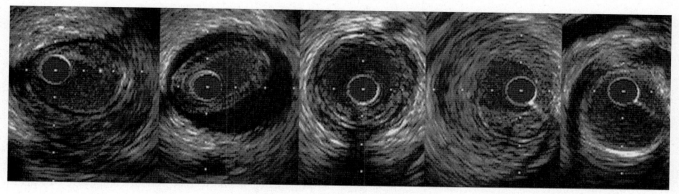

Figure 7–8. Spontaneous dissection.

or IVUS appears to be somewhat better in non-LMCA stenoses); (4) There is significant interobserver and intraobserver variability in the angiographic assessment of LMCA disease.[21-28] In fact, the LMCA is the coronary arterial segment with the greatest variability in angiographic assessment.

We reported 122 patients who underwent angiographic and IVUS assessment of the severity of LMCA disease, who did not have subsequent catheter or surgical intervention and who were followed for 1 year.[29] There was a poor correlation between QCA and IVUS assessment of reference segment and lesion site lumen dimensions. The IVUS minimum lumen diameter was the only independent quantitative predictor of late events. The one-year event (death, MI, or need for revascularization) rate in patients with IVUS-guided deferred treatment of LMCA stenoses was 14% with fewer than 2% having procedure unrelated deaths. (During follow-up, 4 patients died, none had a MI, 3 underwent catheter-based intervention of the LMCA, and 11 underwent bypass surgery.) There were three distinct predictors of these cardiac events: diabetes, a major epicardial vessel, or bypass graft with a QCA DS less than 50% that was left untreated, and LMCA lesion site MLD of less than 5 measured by IVUS. An example is shown in Figure 7–9. In general, we use one of two criteria to defer intervention: either a LMCA minimum lumen area greater than 6 mm^2 or an IVUS DS greater than 50% (compared to the reference lumen dimension). The rationale for these two criteria is as follows. In general, when a parent artery bifurcates into two daughter arteries, the sum of the two daughter arteries is 1.5 times the size of the parent. The LMCA provides flow to the left anterior descending (LAD) and left circumflex coronary artery (LCX), and we previously determined that 4 mm^2 is the minimum lumen area necessary for the LAD and LCX. Similarly, Wolfard and colleagues studied 56 patients with significant stenosis of the LAD or LCX arteries and questionable LMCA morphology.[30] A significant luminal reduction of the LMCA was defined as an IVUS area stenosis greater than 50% or an MLD less than 3 mm. Additionally, 12 patients showed a ruptured plaque within the LMCA. Thirty of these 36 patients were originally thought to be candidates for angioplasty. Based on IVUS findings, 34 of these 36 patients were sent to surgery. No perioperative ischemic complications occurred. This diagnostic use of IVUS also depends on technique. In particular, when assessing ostial LMCA disease (or disease at the aorto-ostial junction of any vessel), it is important to disengage the guiding catheter from the ostium so that the guiding catheter is not mistaken for a calcific lesion with an MLD equal to the inner lumen of the guiding catheter.

No significant LMCA disease

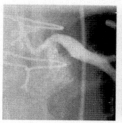
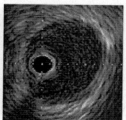

Severe distal LMCA disease

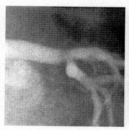
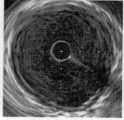
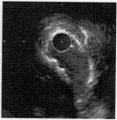

Reference   **Lesion**

Figure 7–9. Normal left main coronary artery (LMCA) compared to LMCA with severe disease.

Assessment of Lesion Length

Assessment of lesion length by IVUS is only possible using motorized transducer pullback. This technique has been validated with IVUS lesion length measurements in vivo.[31] The discrepancy between IVUS and QCA lesion lengths is shown in Figure 7–10. Motorized transducer pullback is also essential for volumetric analysis and for ensuring a consistent relationship between reference segment and target lesion image slices as discussed previously.

Assessment of Reference Lumen Dimensions

Fundamental to the performance of any intervention is the selection of the size of the balloon, stent, etc. In our laboratory, a comparison of IVUS and QCA reference lumen measurements in 3311 nonstial native coronary arteries or saphenous vein graft lesions was done in 164 left main, 959 LAD, 510 left circumflex coronary artery, and 1096 right coronary artery, and 582 saphenous vein graft lesions. The QCA proximal reference lumen diameter was 3.05±0.68 mm; and the IVUS proximal reference lumen diameter was 3.41±0.62 mm (p < 0.0001 versus QCA). The difference between the IVUS and QCA measurements was 0.36±0.64 mm or 15±24%. This difference was greatest in the smallest vessels, decreased asymptotically with increasing vessel size, and was zero at a QCA reference of approximately 4 mm. This analysis suggests that, especially in the smaller-sized arteries (which have higher restenosis rates), (1) the angiographic assessment of reference lumen dimensions is flawed and that (2) an IVUS measurement would indicate that a larger device could be

used. This could result in larger final lumen dimensions without having to resort to midwall or media-to-media device/vessel sizing. Alternatively, some authorities have advocated the use of IVUS "true vessel," "media-to-media," or midwall dimensions for device sizing (see section on percutaneous transluminal coronary angioplasty).

IVUS true vessel, media-to-media, or midwall dimensions, in reality, reflect the amount of angiographically silent disease and therefore, are consistently larger than angiographic reference lumen dimensions. Compensatory dilation of the arterial wall occurs in direct response to the accumulation of atherosclerotic plaque. An absolute reduction in lumen dimensions typically does not occur until the lesion occupies approximately 40% to 50% of the area within the internal elastic membrane (40% to 50% cross-sectional narrowing).[32] As a result, most of the atherosclerotic burden is contained within angiographically normal reference segments.[33]

Percutaneous Transluminal Coronary Angioplasty

The use of stents has increased exponentially and virtually replaced PTCA. Paradoxically, stent availability appears to have improved the efficacy of stand-alone balloon angioplasty. With stents as a safety net, the interventionalist can be more aggressive in his or her attempts to optimize the results of balloon angioplasty. The pilot phase of the Clinical Outcomes Ultrasound Trial (CLOUT) reported that IVUS reference segment midwall dimensions could be used to safely upsize PTCA balloons.[34] (Conversely, attempts to improve on the results of PTCA by routinely using balloons signifi-

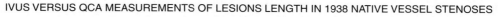

IVUS VERSUS QCA MEASUREMENTS OF LESIONS LENGTH IN 1938 NATIVE VESSEL STENOSES

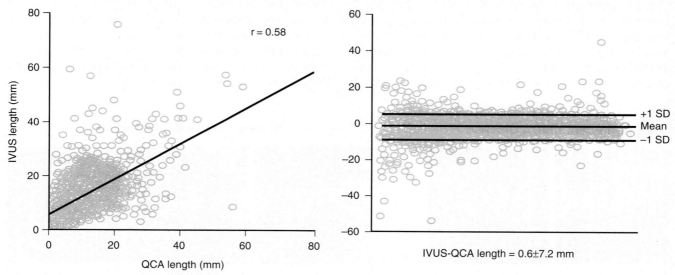

Figure 7–10. Intravascular ultrasound (IVUS) versus quantitative coronary angiographic (QCA) measurements of lesion length in 1938 native vessel stenoses. r, radius; SD, standard deviation.

cantly larger than the angiographic reference segment measurements have resulted in unacceptably high rates of major dissection and ischemic complications.)[35-37] In CLOUT, PTCA was first performed using conventional angiographic balloon sizing; then PTCA was repeated using IVUS balloon sizing. Nominal balloon/artery ratios increased from 1.12 ± 0.15 to 1.30 ± 0.17 ($p < 0.0001$); and QCA measured balloon/artery ratios increased from 1.00 ± 0.12 to 1.12 ± 0.13 ($p < 0.0001$). Acute results were improved (QCA DS decreased from $28\pm15\%$ to $18\pm14\%$, $p < 0.0001$) without an increase in complications. Our laboratory published a study that extended the finding of CLOUT in three important areas: balloon sizing, acute endpoint determination, and long-term follow-up. In CLOUT the proximal and distal reference segment midwall dimensions were measured after angiographic-guided PTCA, and the smaller of the proximal and distal reference segment midwall dimensions was used for balloon sizing.[38] The distal vessel is often small and underperfused preintervention, especially with the IVUS catheter across the lesion. In our report, the preintervention lesion site EEM diameter (often loosely called the media-to-media diameter) was used to select the PTCA balloon size. We enrolled 284 consecutive patients with 438 native coronary artery stenoses in a study of IVUS-guided provisional stenting. The axial center of the target lesion was identified. Maximum and minimum EEM diameters were measured; and the two were averaged to select the balloon size. Any balloon that was approved as semicompliant or noncompliant by the Food and Drug Administration (FDA) was used; the manufacturer-supplied "in-air" nominal inflated balloon diameter had to match the lesion site EEM diameter at the maximum inflated pressure during the PTCA. If necessary, quarter-sized balloons were used for more exact size matching. PTCA balloons were deliberately inflated to greater than 10 atmospheres (atm). If a persistent waist was present, then inflation pressures were increased to a maximum of 18 atm. When the operator felt that the best angiographic result had been achieved, IVUS was repeated. Patients were crossed over to stent implantation if angiography showed fewer than TIMI-3 flow or an NHLBI grade C or greater dissection or if post-PTCA IVUS did not show an optimal result. An optimal IVUS result was defined as (1) a minimum lumen CSA greater than 65% of the average of the proximal and distal reference lumen areas or a minimum lumen CSA greater than 6 mm² and (2) no major dissection. A major dissection was defined as (1) a mobile flap, (2) a dissection involving more than 90% of the vessel circumference, or (3) a dissection causing a suboptimal true lumen CSA (excluding the area subtended by the dissection plane) as previously defined. When necessary, stents were implanted using conventional techniques, followed by high pressure adjunct PTCA. The IVUS criteria for op-timum stent implantation were a minimum stent CSA greater than 80% of the average reference lumen CSA (or an absolute minimum stent CSA > 7.5 mm²) and complete stent-vessel wall apposition. Overall, 206 lesions in 134 patients were treated with PTCA alone. Conversely, 232 lesions in 150 patients crossed over to stent implantation; this included 2 lesions (2 patients) that developed out-of-laboratory abrupt-closure post-PTCA. Reasons for crossover were angiographic or IVUS flow-limiting or lumen compromising dissections in 65 (27.9%) or a suboptimal IVUS minimum lumen CSA (as previously defined) in 167 (72.1%). Long-term follow-up was available in 96% of patients. There were no deaths and one MI. The 1-year target lesion revascularization (TLR) rate was 8.2% for the PTCA group and 15.5% for the stent crossover group ($p = 0.016$).

A similar study was performed at Tubingen, Germany.[39] The authors reported 252 patients who had 271 lesions treated with IVUS-guided balloon angioplasty. IVUS was performed before and after intervention to determine the EEM diameter at the lesion site. The balloon catheter was sized according to the EEM diameter measured by IVUS. The mean balloon diameter was 4.1 ± 0.5 mm, the dilation time 130 ± 60 seconds with a balloon pressure of 7.0 ± 2.0 atm. Clinical acute and 1-year long-term follow-up were obtained for all patients and follow-up angiography in 71% of patients. Acute events occurred post-interventionally in five patients (2%). The cumulative event rate during long-term follow-up was 14%. The angiographic restenosis rate (DS > 50%) after 1 year was 19%.

Stent Implantation

Serial IVUS studies in humans showed (1) that Palmaz-Schatz stents and subsequent tubular-slotted stent designs exhibit almost no chronic recoil, (2) that in-stent restenosis was almost entirely neointimal hyperplasia, (3) that there was no predilection for tissue accumulation within any one segment, and (4) that neointimal thickness was independent of stent size. It is for these reasons that many studies have reported that the absolute final stent dimensions by IVUS—not the relative stent dimensions (i.e., the minimum stent CSA as a percentage of the reference)—are the strongest quantitative predictors of clinical and angiographic in-stent restenosis.[40-43] For example, between June 1996 and September 1997, 2242 consecutive patients with 2853 unselected native coronary artery lesions were treated with either tubular-slotted or multicellular stents at the Washington Hospital Center. Stent implantation was monitored using iterative IVUS with prespecified endpoints; and high-pressure inflations were performed as needed. Prespecified IVUS endpoints were (1) minimum lumen CSA greater than 80% of the mean of the proximal and distal reference lumen CSA or a minimum lumen CSA greater than 7.5 mm², (2) complete stent-vessel wall apposition, and (3) no lumen compromising dissection. Follow-up was available in 94.7% ($n = 2701$ lesions in 2123 patients). The overall incidence of major out-of-hospital events (death, nonfatal MI, TLR) was 13.7%. The overall one-year TLR rate was 11%. Multivariable regression analysis was used to determine the independent predictors of TLR and any adverse cardiac events at one year follow-up. The following variables were entered into the models: diabetes, aorto-ostial lesion location, LAD lesion location, final IVUS lumen CSA, final QCA MLD, and baseline QCA reference lumen diameter. The independent predictors of TLR were history of diabetes (odds ratio [OR] = 2.1; $p = 0.03$), decreasing IVUS final lumen CSA (OR = 0.71; $p = 0.0001$), ostial lesion location (OR = 3.0; $p = 0.005$), and decreasing QCA final MLD (OR = 0.61; $p = 0.04$). Decreasing IVUS final lumen CSA (OR = 0.74; $p = 0.0001$), ostial lesion location (OR = 2.8; $p = 0.05$), and history of diabetes (OR = 1.9; $p = 0.01$) were found to predict any late adverse cardiac events (death/MI/TLR).

Another study, a secondary analysis of the Can Routine Ultrasound Influence Stent Expansion? (CRUISE) trial, suggested that 6.5 mm^2 is the optimum minimum stent CSA in most situations.[43-46] It should be noted that the CRUISE trial enrolled relatively simple lesions in relative larger vessels: 1 or 2 stents/lesion, 1 or 2 lesions/patient, reference artery greater than 3 mm, and a visual residual stenosis less than 10% before enrollment; the actual mean lesion length was 11 mm treated with 1.4 stents/lesion. Thus, whereas a minimum stent CSA of 6.5 mm^2 might be adequate in simple, focal lesions in low-risk patients, a minimum stent CSA of 6.5 mm^2 probably is not adequate in complex lesions in high-risk patients. Conversely, in developing a practical paradigm, it must be recognized that it is impossible to create a 6.5-mm^2 lumen (or larger) in a 2-mm artery.

In-Stent Restenosis

The uses of IVUS in evaluating patients with in-stent restenosis is mostly limited to bare-metal stents and include (1) determining whether in-stent restenosis is severe enough to treat, (2) identifying occult mechanical problems with the stent that (presumably) occurred at the time of implantation, (3) assessing the patterns of in-stent restenosis, and (4) assessing the acute results. Three groups have showed that if a patient with in-stent restenosis can be treated medically, long-term outcome is favorable.[65-67] In fact, Kimura and colleagues showed that lumen dimensions tend to increase in these patient from 1 to 3 years.[65] As in the assessment of intermediate lesions, IVUS can be used to determine if the in-stent restenosis lesion is severe enough to treat. Nishioka and colleagues presented the results of 142 patients with 150 intermediate in-stent restenosis lesions—defined as an angiographic DS of

40% to 75%; 34% of the lesions fit the standard definition of restenosis—angiographic DS of greater than 50%; and 17% of the patients had a positive exercise thallium. Repeat intervention was deferred if the IVUS minimum lumen area measured greater than 3.5 mm^2 regardless of symptoms, noninvasive testing, or angiographic findings. At follow-up, which averaged 32 months, only 10% of patients had events; and the two year event-free survival rate was 96.5%.[67]

There are a number of technical and mechanical complications of stent implantation that can remain unrecognized until the patient presents with in-stent restenosis. Technical and mechanical problems include (1) missing the lesion, (2) stent underexpansion, (3) stent "crush," and (4) having the stent stripped off the balloon during the implantation procedure. Because most stents are radiolucent, some lesions, especially aorto-ostial lesions, can be missed. Incomplete stent expansion during implantation can be missed angiographically because stents are porous and contrast can flow through and around them. Chronic stent recoil is rare.[68,69] If the guide wire is accidentally removed and in recrossing the freshly placed (and presumably not fully implanted) stent, it courses adjacent to the stent and enters the stent through one of the diamonds, subsequent adjunct PTCA can crush part of the stent against the vessel wall. These mechanical problems constitute a minority of in-stent restenosis. However, the treatment of in-stent restenosis must begin by excluding these problems and, if present, by correcting them. Examples are shown in Figures 7–11 through 7–13.

In an analysis of over 1000 consecutive in-stent restenosis lesions, the frequency of these mechanical complications was found to be 4% to 5%. In addition, stent underexpansion was common: 15% had a minimum stent CSA less than 4.5 mm^2 and 25% had a minimum stent CSA between 4.5 and 6 mm.[70] Thus, mechanical problems contributed importantly to a significant percentage of in-stent restenosis lesions; the exact percentage depends on the definition of stent underexpansion. IVUS guidance may help to minimize these mechanical problems and their contribution to restenosis. In addition, it is logical that the treatment of in-stent restenosis lesions should begin with correcting these mechanical problems. The pattern of in-stent restenosis is predictive of recurrence. This was studied systematically in a recent publication by Mehran and colleagues.[71] Four patterns of in-stent restenosis were defined: I focal (10 mm in length), II diffuse (in-stent restenosis > 10 mm within the stent), III proliferative (in-stent restenosis > 10 mm extending outside the stent), and an IV totally occluded in-stent restenosis. TLR increased with a worsening pattern: 19%, 35%, 50%, and 83% in class I to IV, respectively ($p < 0.001$). The TLR rate was 19% for focal in-stent restenosis, 35% for diffuse intrastent restenosis (>10 mm in length and confined to the stent, in 22%), 50% for diffuse proliferative in-stent resteno-

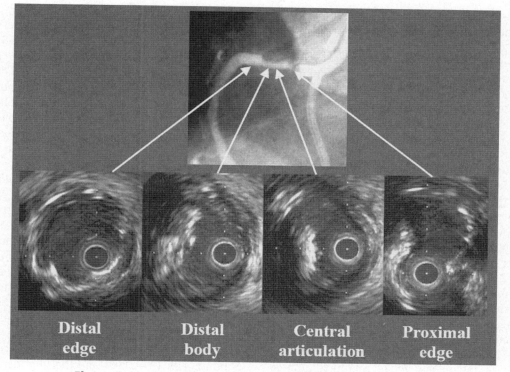

Figure 7-11. *The implanted stent is crushed against the vessel wall.*

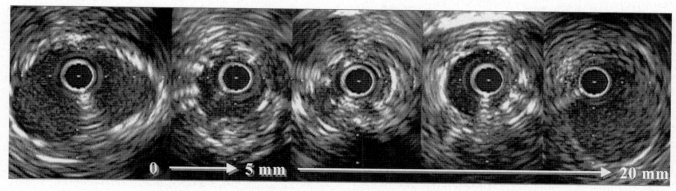

Figure 7-12. *Chronic stent underexpansion in a saphenous vein graft.*

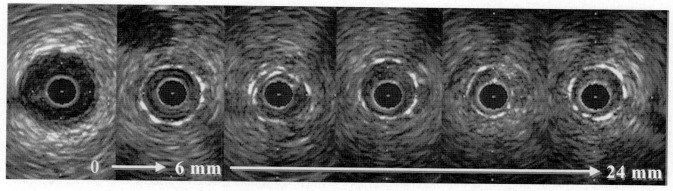

Figure 7-13. *Stent underexpansion in a small left anterior descending coronary artery.*

sis (>10 mm in length and extending into adjacent reference segments, in 30%), and 83% for total occlusions (occurring in 6%). There are a number of considerations in the use of IVUS to treat in-stent restenosis lesions. Before treatment, IVUS is useful in identifying in-stent restenosis lesions associated with mechanical problems (underexpansion or frank mechanical complications). The second observation is that, with the exception of additional stent implantation, conventional catheter-based treatment of in-stent restenosis never recovers the lumen dimension of the original stent implantation procedure.[72-74] The third observation is the phenomenon that has been called "instant" in-stent restenosis. In a study of 32 lesions in which IVUS was repeated, an average of 42 ± 8 minutes after PTCA, excimer laser angioplasty + PTCA, or rotational atherectomy + PTCA, the delayed IVUS minimal lumen CSA decreased by 23%; and in 9 lesions (28%) there was a more than 2 mm^2 decrease in minimum lumen CSA.[75] The mechanism of this early lumen loss appears to be neointimal tissue reintusion back into the stent, rather than stent recoil. In this regard, it is similar to recoil after balloon angioplasty of nonstented lesions. An IVUS substudy of angioplasty versus rotational atherectomy for treatment of diffuse in-stent restenosis trial (ARTIST; randomized comparison of rotational atherectomy versus PTCA in the treatment of in-stent restenosis) involved 41 patients in the atherectomy group and 45 patients in the PTCA group. There was effective debulking of the neointima after rotation; adjunctive low pressure PTCA further enlarged the lumen by decreasing the in-stent neointima without additional stent expansion. In contrast, in the PTCA group, high-pressure dilation resulted in a significant increase in stent area and a larger final lumen area. Neointimal regrowth between intervention and follow-up was not significantly different between the two groups. However, because of the larger stent and lumen areas, the lumen area at follow-up was larger in the PTCA group.[76] Whereas these findings may suggest that re-stenting the in-stent restenosis lesion is an ideal approach, IVUS analysis has shown that any benefit in acute lumen gain is lost at follow-up.[77]

Does Intravascular Ultrasound Reduce Restenosis?

Numerous recent studies have shown that IVUS-guided stent implantation results in a larger final stent size, which is associated with decreased restenosis. CRUISE was a substudy of Stent Antithrombotic Regimen Study (STARS) in which STARS sites elected to perform IVUS-guided stenting, angiography-guided stenting with documentary IVUS, or no IVUS. The nine-month target vessel revascularization rate in the IVUS guided group was 8.5% versus 15.3% in the documentary IVUS group, $p = 0.019$. In a study that randomized patients to IVUS

verus angiographic guided stenting, the IVUS-guided group had a lower clinical restenosis rate: 8.4% versus 12.4% ($p = 0.08$) overall, 4.9% versus 10.8% ($p = 0.02$) in vessels greater than 2.5 mm, and 5.1% versus 20.8% ($p = 0.03$) in saphenous vein grafts.[47] Thrombocyte activity evaluation and effects of Ultrasound guidance in Long Intracoronary stent Placement (TULIP) was a randomized comparison of long lesions. Despite more stents and longer stent length (42 ± 11 mm versus 35 ± 11 mm, $p = 0.001$), the IVUS-guided group had lower angiographic restenosis (23% versus 45%, $p = 0.008$), TLR (10% versus 23%, $p = 0.018$), and major adverse cardiac event (MACE) rates (12% versus 27%, $p = 0.026$).[48] An earlier study (Strategy for Intracoronary Ultrasound-Guided PTCA and Stenting [SIPS]) that randomized patients to angiographic versus IVUS guidance used a provisional stent strategy.[49] Ultimately, half of the patients in each group were treated with PTCA and half with stenting. The 2-year clinically driven TLR was 17% versus 29% ($p = 0.02$) with a 61% probability that IVUS guidance was both less expensive and more effective.[50] In a nonrandomized comparison, Choi[51] showed that IVUS reduced both in-hospital acute closure ($p = 0.04$) and 6-month TLR ($p = 0.08$) and that the increased costs of IVUS guidance were entirely related to the cost of the IVUS catheter. CENIC, the Brazilian Society of Interventional Cardiology Registry, reported the acute results of 3375 patients treated with IVUS-guided stenting and 51,151 patients treated with angiographic-guided stenting. The IVUS-guided group had lower rates of cardiac death (0.4% versus 1.1%, $p < 0.001$), Q wave myocardial infarction (0.06% versus 0.09%, $p = 0.054$), and death/myocardial infarction (0.08% versus 1.7%, $p < 0.001$).[52] Gaster randomized patients to angiography versus IVUS and found a lower frequency of a number of endpoints, such as clinical restenosis and recurrent angina, with no increase in costs.[53] And finally, the Balloon Equivalent to STent (BEST) study took another approach—avoid stenting altogether.[54] 250 patients were randomized to IVUS-guided provisional stenting versus conventional angiographic guidance of deliberate stent implantation. The study was designed to show equivalence between these two strategies and a reduction in the rate of in-stent restenosis in the IVUS-guided provisional stenting group. In the IVUS-guided provisional stenting group, balloon angioplasty was first performed using a balloon sized according to the IVUS lesion site media-to-media dimensions; crossover to stenting was allowed and was necessary in 44%. At follow-up the angiographic restenosis rate was 16.8% in the IVUS-guided provisional stenting group versus 18.1% in the deliberate stenting group; the MACE rate was 16% versus 20%, respectively (both p = nonstented, meeting the primary study endpoint). However, the in-stent restenosis rate was only 5% in the IVUS-guided provisional stenting group, achieving the investigators primary objective of reducing the occurrence of troublesome in-stent restenosis.

To provide a balanced view, it is important to note that there have been two studies (REStenosis after Intravascular ultrasound STenting [RESIST] and randomized comparison of coronary stent implantation under ultrasound or angiographic guidance to reduce stent restenosis [OPTICUS study]) that have shown no benefit from IVUS-guidance in reducing angiographic restenosis.[55,56] It is not clear what has produced these different conclusions especially because a more recent report from RESIST now reports a clinical benefit from IVUS guidance. In this later report the clinical need for revascularization in the IVUS group was 21/79 versus 31/76 in the control group ($p = 0.03$).[57]

Drug-Eluting Stents

The clinical use of IVUS in the era of drug-eluting stents (DESs) remains unknown. Whereas the incremental value of IVUS in a stent that dramatically reduces restenosis is unknown, it is clear that the use of IVUS in drug-eluting stents has greatly advanced our understanding of their mechanism and efficacy.[58-63]

Several randomized trials of sirolimus-eluting stents and of paclitaxel-eluting stents have been completed. They have all shown a marked reduction in intrastent neointimal hyperplasia. RAndomized study with the sirolimus-eluting VElocity balloon-expandable stent in the treatment of patients with de novo native coronary artery Lesions (RAVEL) enrolled 238 patients at 19 centers; a subset of 118 patients at 6 centers underwent IVUS imaging at 6-months follow-up but not at implantation.[78] Patients were randomized (1:1) to either a single bare-metal or sirolimus-eluting Bx Velocity stent. Post-dilation was performed to achieve a residual DS less than 20%. Volumetric IVUS analysis included the stent and 5-mm long proximal and distal adjacent reference segment. Qualitative IVUS showed no persistent dissection at the stent edges, but there was a 21% incidence of malapposition in the sirolimus-eluting group versus 4% in the control group ($p = 0.001$). The 10 patients in the sirolimus-eluting group with malapposition were asymptomatic and event-free at 1 year, whereas 1 of the 2 control patients with malapposition underwent percutaneous revascularization. Because IVUS was not performed at implantation, it was not possible to determine whether the malapposition at follow-up was new or old (i.e., late acquired malapposition).

There are only four possible explanations for malapposition at follow-up: (1) persistent malapposition that was present at implantation; (2) chronic stent recoil without any change in arterial or plaque area; (3) increase in arterial dimension (positive remodeling) that is greater than any increase in persistent plaque mass; and (4) decrease in plaque mass without an equal amount of negative remodeling. Shah and colleagues studied 206 patients with native artery lesions treated with bare-metal tubular-slotted stents who had IVUS performed at index and after 6 ± 3 months of follow-up.[79] There were nine patients (4.4%) with late acquired malapposition. The location of late malapposition was the stent edge in eight of nine patients. Intrastent neointima at follow-up occurred only where the stent was in contact with the vessel wall; areas of malapposed stents were free of intrastent neointima. The authors suggested that late malapposition was the result of positive remodeling without an equal increase in persistent plaque mass.

Sirolimus-Eluting Stent in Coronary Lesions (SIRIUS) was a randomized study comparing sirolimus-eluting stents to bare-metal stents in 1100 patients with a site-specific IVUS substudy in 250 patients. The intrastent intimal hyperplasia volume was reduced from 57 mm^3 to 4 mm^3 and the percentage of neointimal volume was reduced from 34% to 3%. In sirolimus-eluting stents, intimal hyperplasia is greatest at the proximal end (although still markedly less than bare-metal stents), virtually eliminated in the center, and in between in amount at the distal end; 8.7% of the sirolimus-eluting stents had late acquired malappositon, but none of these were associated with any clinical event.

Asian Paclitaxel-Eluting Stent Clinical Trial (ASPECT) was a randomized trial of a paclitaxel-coated stent versus a bare-metal stent. Single de novo lesions in 177 patients were randomized to placebo or one of two doses of paclitaxel (low dose: 1.28 μg/mm^2 and high dose: 3.10 μg/mm^2). Complete poststent implantation and follow-up IVUS was available in 81 patients: 25 control, 28 low dose, and 28 high dose. Intrastent and 5-mm proximal and distal reference segments were analyzed volumetrically.[80] The percentage of IH volume decreased from $30\pm20\%$ in controls to $19\pm17\%$ in low-dose patients to $13\pm13\%$ in high-dose patients. There was one patient with late malapposition in the high-dose group, which was not associated with a clinical event.

Six month volumetric IVUS was the primary endpoint in TAXUS II in both the slow-release and moderate-release formulations of the paclitaxel-eluting stent. Of note, there was almost complete (90%) post-intervention and follow-up IVUS in both groups. The percentage of intimal hyperplasia volume was $7.8\pm9.78\%$ in the moderate-release group (versus $20.5\pm16.7\%$ in the control group) and $7.6\pm9.9\%$ in the slow-release group (versus $23.2\pm18.2\%$ in the control group). The results of TAXUS II were supported by the pivotal TAXUS IV study, which showed a marked reduction in in-stent neointima and virtually no incidences of late acquired malapposition (one to two percent in both the TAXUS group and the bare-metal control group). In the TAXUS studies, there were no adverse edge effects and there was a beneficial distal edge effect with drug-eluting stents causing less luminal loss along the distal edge. Thus, IVUS has been, and will continue to be, instrumental in assessing the efficacy and safety of stents as they are further developed. IVUS will continue to have a role in guiding optimal stent placement, regardless of whether the stent is a bare metal stent or a drug eluting stent.

Assessment of Interventional Complications

It is difficult to describe all of the potential complications of coronary interventions and their IVUS findings. Common examples include dissections, perforations, intramural hematomas, and a stripped stent. There are a number of general statements that can be made about dissections. They tend to occur at the junction of plaque or arterial elements of different compliance: calcific versus noncalcific plaque, fibrotic versus nonfibrotic plaque, and plaque versus normal vessel wall. This also explains the tendency of dissections to occur at the edges of stents. Conversely, there are a number of limitations with IVUS in assessing these complications. In particular, a dissection that is "behind" calcium will not be seen. A dissection that is "propped up" by the IVUS catheter may be more difficult to see, especially if the near-field gain settings are low or if it occurs within the blanking zone of the electronic array catheter. There are no hard and fast rules regarding the treatment of dissections seen by IVUS. In general, dissections that (1) reduce the lumen below the threshold for an optimum result, (2) impinge on the IVUS catheter, and (3) are mobile are treated. Small edge dissections are generally not treated. Some authorities believe that dissections on the endocardial side of the vessel are more benign than dissections on the epicardial side. Intramural hematomas are a variant of a dissection. They tend to occur in normal arcs of the vessel wall proximal or distal to a lesion or opposite the plaque in an extremely eccentric lesion. The EEM expands outward and the internal elastic membrane is pushed inward to cause lumen compromise. Blood accumulates in the space caused by the split in the media. The hematoma can propagate antegrade or retrograde but tends to be stopped by branches or severely diseased parts of the vessel. When contrast accumulates within the split media, a layering of echolucent contrast and echogeneic blood builds up. Careful interrogation can sometimes define an entry point. Intramural hematomas tend to be treated because of the propensity for propagation and lumen compromise.

Practical Recommendations

In practical day-to-day terms, how should IVUS be used during stenting procedures? The following is one suggested algorithm. It begins with preintervention IVUS and concludes with iterative IVUS to optimize the final result. Perform preintervention IVUS to assess stenosis severity, measure reference vessel size, and measure lesion length. From the maximum reference lumen diameter, determine the maximum achievable stent dimension. Select stent length based on distance between proximal and distal references (Fig. 7–14).

After the stent is implanted, repeat IVUS imaging to assess the minimum stent CSA. If the minimum stent CSA is adequate, stop. An adequate stent CSA is one that matches the reference lumen (i.e., no residual luminal stenosis) or one that achieves a minimum stent area (7.5 mm² for a bare-metal stent and at least 5.5 mm² for a drug-eluting stent). If the minimum stent CSA is inadequate, perform additional high-pressure inflations, if necessary using a larger balloon. If additional balloon inflations are performed, recheck the IVUS results.

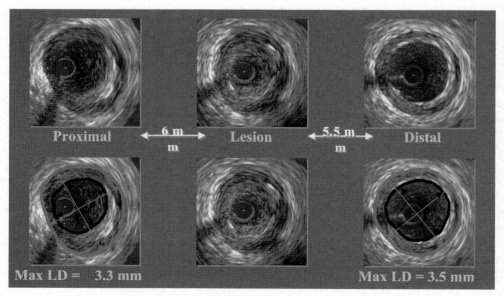

Figure 7–14. The resultant stent size would be 3.5 mm. LD, lumen diameter.

A variation of this strategy has been recommended by Colombo[64] for treating long lesions. He compared full lesion coverage to a strategy of spot-stenting. Long lesions (>15 mm in length) were first treated with balloon angioplasty, and stents were implanted only if the minimum lumen area was less than 5.5 mm^2 or the minimum lumen area was less than 50% of the total arterial (EEM) area at the lesion site. Compared to a matched group treated with full lesion coverage, the restenosis rate was lower after a spot-stenting strategy was used (25% versus 39%, $p < 0.05$).[64] This approach especially makes sense in smaller vessels. The impact of stent length on restenosis is greater in smaller vessels than in larger ones.[45]

Key Acronyms

IVUS	Intravascular ultrasound
PTCA	Percutaneous transluminal coronary angioplasty
DS	Diameter stenosis
EEM	External elastic membrane
QCA	Quantitative coronary angiography
CSA	Cross-sectional area
MLD	Minimum lumen diameter
TLR	Target lesion revascularization

KEY POINTS

■ IVUS provides a unique view of the artery literally from the inside out with high resolution.

■ IVUS images all components of the arterial wall providing information beyond the luminal profile displayed by angiography.

■ This unique in vivo imaging modality has helped health care providers understand the atherosclerotic process, including plaque morphology, vascular remodeling, and plaque rupture.

■ IVUS can guide the use and further understanding of percutaneous intervention to optimize the results.

■ The added information from IVUS is particularly helpful for angiographically ambiguous lesions, unusual lesions, and complex clinical scenarios.

REFERENCES

1. Mintz GS, Nissen SE, Anderson WD, et al: Standards for the acquisition, measurement, and reporting of intravascular ultrasound studies: A report of the American College of Cardiology Task Force on Clinical Expert Consensus Documents. *J Am Coll Cardiol* 37:1478-1492, 2001.

2. Hausmann D, Erbel R, Alibelli-Chemarin M-J, et al: The safety of intracoronary ultrasound: A multicenter survey of 2207 examinations. *Circulation* 91:623-630, 1995.

3. Batkoff BW, Linker DT: The safety of intracoronary ultrasound: Data from a multicenter European registry. *Catheter Cardiovasc Diagn* 38:238-241, 1996.

4. Gorge G, Peters RJG, Pinto F, et al: Intravascular ultrasound: Safety and indications for use in 7085 consecutive patients studied in 32 centers in Europe and Israel. *J Am Coll Cardiol* 27:155A, 1996.

5. Arnett EN, Isner JM, Redwood DR, et al: Coronary artery narrowing in coronary artery disease: Comparison of cineangiographic and necropsy findings. *Ann Intern Med* 91:350-356, 1979.

6. Waller BF: Anatomy, histology, and pathology of the major epicardial coronary arteries relevant to echocardiographic imaging techniques. *J Am Soc Echocardiogr* 2:232-252, 1989.

7. Isner JM, Donaldsen RF: Coronary angiographic and morphologic correlation. In: Waller BF, ed. *Cardiac Morphology*. Philadelphia: Saunders, 1984, pp. 571-592.

8. Marcus ML, Skorton DJ, Johnson MR, et al: Visual estimates of percent diameter coronary stenosis: "A battered gold standard." *J Am Coll Cardiol* 11:882-885, 1988.

9. Hutchins GM, Bulkley BH, Ridolfi RL, et al: Correlation of coronary arteriograms and left ventriculograms with postmortem studies. *Circulation* 56:32-37, 1977.

10. Abizaid A, Mintz GS, Pichard AD, et al: Clinical, intravascular ultrasound, and quantitative angiographic determinants of the coronary flow reserve before and after percutaneous transluminal coronary angioplasty. *Am J Cardiol* 82:423-428, 1998.

11. Nishioka T, Amanullah AM, Luo H, et al: Clinical validation of intravascular ultrasound imaging for assessment of coronary stenosis severity: Comparison with stress myocardial perfusion imaging. *J Am Coll Cardiol* 33:1870-1878, 1999.

12. Takagi A, Tsurumi Y, Ishii Y, et al: Clinical potential of intravascular ultrasound for physiological assessment of coronary stenosis: Relationship between quantitative ultrasound tomography and pressure-derived fractional flow reserve. *Circulation* 20(100):250-255, 1999.

13. Abizaid AS, Mintz GS, Mehran R, et al: Long-term follow-up after percutaneous transluminal angioplasty was not performed based on intravascular ultrasound findings: importance of lumen dimensions. *Circulation* 100:256-261, 1999.

14. Duissaillant GD, Mintz GS, Pichard AD, et al: Intravascular ultrasound identification of calcified intraluminal lesions misdiagnosed as thrombi by coronary angiography. *Am Heart J* 132:687-689, 1996.

15. Maehara A, Mintz GS, Ahmed JM, et al: An intravascular ultrasound classification of angiographic coronary artery aneurysms. *Am J Cardiol* 88:365-370, 2001.

16. Maehara A, Mintz GS, Castagna MT, et al: Intravascular ultrasound assessment of spontaneous coronary artery dissection. *Am J Cardiol* 89:466-468, 2002.

17. Hermiller JB, Buller CE, Tenaglia AN, et al: Unrecognized left main coronary artery disease in patients undergoing interventional procedures. *Am J Cardiol* 71:173-176, 1993.

18. Yamagishi M, Hongo Y, Goto Y, et al: Intravascular ultrasound evidence of angiographically undetected left main coronary artery disease and associated trauma during interventional procedures. *Heart Vessels* 11:262-268, 1996.

19. Gerber TC, Erbel R, Gorge G, et al: Extent of atherosclerosis and remodeling of the left main coronary artery determined by intravascular ultrasound. *Am J Cardiol* 73:666-671, 1994.

20. Ge J, Liu F, Gorge G, et al: Angiographically "silent" plaque in the left main coronary artery detected by intravascular ultrasound. *Coron Artery Dis* 6:805-810, 1956.

21. Fisher LD, Judkins MP, Lesperance J, et al: Reproducibility of coronary arteriographic reading in the Coronary Artery Surgery Study (CASS). *Cathet Cardiovasc Diagn* 8:565-575, 1982.

22. Isner JM, Kishel J, Kent KM, et al: Accuracy of angiographic determination of left main coronary arterial narrowing: Angio-graphic-histologic correlative analysis in 28 patients. *Circulation* 63:1056-1064, 1981.

23. Detre KM, Wright E, Murphy ML, et al: Observer agreement in evaluating coronary angiograms. *Circulation* 52:979-986, 1975.

24. DeRouen TA, Murray JA, Owen W: Variability in the analysis of coronary arteriograms. *Circulation* 55:324-328, 1977.

25. Zir LM, Miller SW, Dinsmore RE, et al: Interobserver variability in coronary angiography. *Circulation* 53:627-632, 1976.

26. Sanmarco ME, Brooks SH, Blankenhorn DH: Reproducibility of a consensus panel in the interpretation of coronary angiograms. *Am Heart J* 96:430-437, 1978.

27. Cameron A, Kemp HG Jr, Fisher LD, et al: Left main coronary artery stenosis: angiographic determination. *Circulation* 68:484-489, 1983.

28. Flemming RM, Kirkeeide RL, Smalling RW, et al: Patterns in visual interpretation of coronary arteriograms as detected by quantitative coronary arteriography. *J Am Coll Cardiol* 18:945-951, 1991.

29. Abizaid AS, Mintz GS, Abizaid A, et al: One year follow-up after intravascular ultrasound assessment of moderate left main coronary artery disease in patients with ambiguous angiograms. *J Am Coll Cardiol* 34:707-715, 1999.

30. Wolfard U, Gorge G, Konorza T, et al: Intravascular ultrasound (IVUS) examination reverses therapeutic decision from percutaneous intervention to a surgical approach in patients with alterations of the left main stem. *Thorac Cardiovasc Surg* 46:281-284, 1998.

31. Fuessl RT, Mintz GS, Pichard AD, et al: In vivo validation of intravascular ultrasound length measurements using a motorized transducer pullback device. *Am J Cardiol* 77:1115-1118, 1996.

32. Glagov S, Weisenberg E, Zarins CK, et al: Compensatory enlargement of human atherosclerotic coronary arteries. *N Engl J Med* 316:1371-1375, 1987.

33. Mintz GS, Painter JA, Pichard AD, et al: Atherosclerosis in angiographically "normal" coronary artery reference segments: An intravascular ultrasound study with clinical correlations. *J Am Coll Cardiol* 25:1479-1485, 1995.

34. Stone GW, Hodgson JM, St. Goar FG, et al: For the CLOUT Investigators. Improved procedural results of coronary angioplasty with intravascular ultrasound guided balloon sizing: The CLOUT Pilot Trial. *Circulation* 95:2044-2052, 1997.

35. Roubin GS, Douglas JS, King SB, et al: Influence of balloon size on initial success, acute complications, and restenosis after percutaneous transluminal coronary angioplasty. *Circulation* 78:557-565, 1988.

36. Nichols AB, Smith R, Berke AD, et al: Importance of balloon size in coronary angioplasty. *J Am Coll Cardiol* 13:1094-1100, 1989.

37. Beatt KV, Serruys PW, Luijten HE, et al: Restenosis after coronary angioplasty: The paradox of increased lumen diameter and restenosis. *J Am Coll Cardiol* 19:258-266, 1992.

38. Abizaid A, Pichard AD, Mintz GS, et al: Acute and long-term results of an IVUS-guided PTCA/provisional stent implantation strategy. *Am J Cardiol* 84:1381-1384, 1999.

39. Schroeder S, Baumbach A, Haase KK, et al: Reduction of restenosis by vessel size adapted percutaneous transluminal coronary angioplasty using intravascular ultrasound. *Am J Cardiol* 83:875-879, 1999.

40. Hoffmann R, Mintz GS, Mehran R, et al: Intravascular ultrasound predictors of angiographic restenosis in lesions treated with Palmaz-Schatz stents. *J Am Coll Cardiol* 31:43-49, 1997.

41. Moussa I, DiMario C, Moses J, et al: The predictive value of different intravascular ultrasound criteria for restenosis after coronary stenting. *J Am Coll Cardiol* 29:60A, 1997.

42. Ziada KM, Kapadia SR, Belli G, et al: Prognostic value of absolute versus relative measures of the procedural result after successful coronary stenting: Importance of vessel size in predicting long-term freedom from target vessel revascularization. *Am Heart J* 141:823-831, 2001.

43. Morino Y, Honda Y, Okura H, et al: An optimal diagnostic threshold for minimal stent area to predict target lesion revascularization following stent implantation in native coronary lesions. *Am J Cardiol* 88:301-303, 2001.

44. Kornowski R, Mintz GS, Kent KM, et al: Increased restenosis in diabetes mellitus after coronary interventions is due to exaggerated intimal hyperplasia: A serial intravascular ultrasound study. *Circulation* 95:1366-1369, 1997.

45. de Feyter PJ, Kay P, Disco C, et al: Reference chart derived from post-stent-implantation intravascular ultrasound predictors of 6-month expected restenosis on quantitative coronary angiography. *Circulation* 100:1777-1783, 1999.

46. Fitzgerald PJ, Oshima A, Hayase M, et al: Final results of the Can Routine Ultrasound Influence Stent Expansion (CRUISE) study. *Circulation* 102:523-530, 2000.

47. Russo RJ, Attubato MJ, Davidson CJ, et al: Angiography versus intravascular ultrasound-directed stent placement: Final results from AVID. *Circulation* 100:I-234, 1990.

48. Oemrawsingh PV, Mintz, GS, Schalij MJ, et al: Intravascular ultrasound guidance improves angiographic and clinical outcome of stent implantation for long coronary artery stenoses. *Circulation* 107:62-67, 2003.

49. Frey AW, Hodgson JM, Muller C, et al: Ultrasound-guided strategy for provisional stenting with focal balloon combination catheter: results from the randomized Strategy for Intracoronary Ultrasound-guided PTCA and Stenting (SIPS) trial. *Circulation* 102:2497-2502, 2000.

50. Mueller C, Hodgson JM, Buettner HJ, et al: Cost-effectiveness of intracoronary ultrasound for percutaneous coronary interventions: Economic analysis of the randomized SIPS Trial. *J Am Coll Cardiol* 39:55A, 2002.

51. Choi JW, Goodreau LM, Davidson CJ: Resource utilization and clinical outcomes of coronary stenting: A comparison of intravascular ultrasound and angiographical guided stent implantation. *Am Heart J* 142:112-118, 2001.

52. Sousa A, Abizaid A, Mintz G, et al: The influence of intravascular ultrasound guidance on the in-hospital outcomes after stent implantation: Results from the Brazilian Society of Interventional Cardiology Registry-CENIC. *J Am Coll Cardiol* 39:54A, 2002.

53. Schiele F, Meneveau N, Gilard M, et al: Final results of the Balloon Equivalent to StenT Study (BEST): Multicenter randomized study comparing intravascular ultrasound guided balloon angioplasty with systematic stent implantation. *Circulation* 106:II-482, 2002.

54. Gaster AL, Slothuus U, Larsen J, et al: Cost-effectiveness analysis of intravascular ultrasound guided percutaneous coronary intervention versus conventional percutaneous coronary intervention. *Scan Cardiovasc J* 35:80-85, 2001.

55. Schiele F, Meneveau N, Vuillemenot A, et al: Impact of intravascular ultrasound guidance in stent deployment on 6-month restenosis rate: a multicenter, randomized study comparing two strategies—with and without intravascular ultrasound guidance. RESIST Study Group. REStenosis after Ivus guided STenting. *J Am Coll Cardiol* 32:320-328, 1998.

56. Mudra H, di Mario C, de Jaegere P, et al: Randomized comparison of coronary stent implantation under ultrasound or angiographic guidance to reduce stent restenosis (OPTICUS Study). *Circulation* 104:1343-1349, 2001.

57. Schiele F, Seronde MF, Meneveau N, et al: Medical costs of intravascular ultrasound optimization of stent deployment: Results of the multicenter randomized "REStenosis after Intravascular ultrasound STenting" (RESIST) study. *Circulation* 102:II-547, 2000.

58. Moussa I, Moses J, DiMario C, et al: Stenting after optimal lesion debulking (SOLD) resigtry. Angiographic and clinical outcome. *Circulation* 98:1604-1609, 1998.

59. Prati F, DiMario C, Moussa I, et al: In-stent neointimal proliferation correlates with the amount of residual plaque burden out-

side the stent: An intravascular ultrasound study. *Circulation* 99:1011-1014, 1999.

60. Matar FA, Mintz GS, Pinnow E, et al: Multivariate predictors of intravascular ultrasound endpoints after directional coronary atherectomy. *J Am Coll Cardiol* 25:318-324, 1995.

61. Mintz GS, Popma JJ, Pichard AD, et al: Patterns of calcification in coronary artery disease: A statistical analysis of intravascular ultrasound and coronary angiography in 1155 lesions. *Circulation* 91:1959-1965, 1995.

62. Mintz GS, Popma JJ, Pichard AD, et al: Limitations of angiography in the assessment of plaque distribution in coronary artery disease. *Circulation* 93:924-931, 1996.

63. Mintz GS, Popma JJ, Pichard AD, et al: Intravascular ultrasound predictors of restenosis following percutaneous transcatheter coronary revascularization. *J Am Coll Cardiol* 27:1678-1687, 1996.

64. Colombo A, De Gregorio J, Moussa I, et al: Intravascular ultrasound-guided percutaneous transluminal angioplasty with provisional spot stenting for treatment of coronary lesions. *J Am Coll Cardiol* 38:1427-1433, 2001.

65. Kimura T, Yokoi H, Nakagawa Y, et al: Three-year follow-up after implantation of metallic coronary-artery stents. *N Engl J Med* 334:561-566, 1996.

66. Lee JH, Lee CW, Park SW, et al: Long-term follow-up after deferring angioplasty in asymptomatic patients with moderate non-critical in-stent restenosis. *Clin Cardiol* 24:551-555, 2001.

67. Nishioka H, Shimada K, Fukuda D, et al: Long term follow-up of intermediate in-stent restenosis lesions following deferral of re-intervention on the basis of intravascular ultrasound findings. *Circulation* 106:II-587, 2002.

68. Hoffmann R, Mintz GS, Dussaillant GR, et al: Patterns and mechanisms of in-stent restenosis: A serial intravascular ultrasound study. *Circulation* 94:1247-1254, 1996.

69. Hong M-K, Park S-W, Lee CW, et al: Intravascular ultrasound comparison of chronic recoil among different stent designs. *Am J Cardiol* 84:1247-1250, 1999.

70. Castagna MT, Mintz GS, Weissman NJ, et al: The contribution of "mechanical" problems to in-stent restenosis. An intravascular ultrasound analysis of 1090 consecutive in-stent restenosis lesions. *Am Heart J* 142:970-974, 2001.

71. Mehran R, Dangas G, Abizaid AS, et al: Angiographic patterns of in-stent restenosis. Classification and implications for long-term outcome. *Circulation* 100:1872-1878, 1999.

72. Mehran R, Mintz GS, Popma JJ, et al: Mechanisms and results of balloon angioplasty for the treatment of in-stent restenosis. *Am J Cardiol* 78:618-622, 1996.

73. Mehran R, Mintz GS, Satler LF, et al: Treatment of in-stent restenosis with excimer laser coronary angioplasty. Mechanisms and results compared to PTCA alone. *Circulation* 96:2183-2189, 1997.

74. Mehran R, Dangas G, Mintz GS, et al: Treatment of in-stent restenosis with excimer laser coronary angioplasty versus rotational atherectomy: Comparative mechanisms and results. *Circulation* 101:2484-2489, 2000.

75. Shiran A, Mintz GS, Waksman R, et al: Early lumen loss after treatment of in-stent restenosis. An intravascular ultrasound study. *Circulation* 98:200-203, 1998.

76. vom Dahl J, Dietz U, Haager PK, et al: Rotational atherectomy does not reduce recurrent in-stent restenosis: Results of the angioplasty versus rotational atherectomy for treatment of diffuse in-stent restenosis trial (ARTIST). *Circulation* 105:583-588, 2002.

77. Morino Y, Limpijankit T, Honda Y, et al: Late vascular response to repeat stenting for in-stent restenosis with and without radiation: an intravascular ultrasound volumetric analysis. *Circulation* 105:2465-2468, 2002.

78. Serruys PW, Degertekin M, Tanabe K, et al: Intravascular ultrasound findings in the multicenter, randomized, double-blind RAVEL (RAndomized study with the sirolimus-eluting VElocity balloon-expandable stent in the treatment of patients with de novo native coronary artery Lesions) trial. *Circulation* 106:798-803, 2002.

79. Shah VM, Mintz GS, Apple S, Weissman NJ: "Background" incidence of late malapposition following bare metal stent implantation. *Circulation* 106:1753-1755, 2002.

80. Hong M-K, Mintz GS, Lee CW, et al: Paclitaxel coating reduces in-stent intimal hyperplasia in human coronary arteries: A serial volumetric intravascular ultrasound analysis from ASPECT. *Circulation* 107:517-520, 2003.

Chapter 8

Hand-Carried Ultrasound

MARTIN E. GOLDMAN, MD • LORI B. CROFT, MD

- Development of Technology
- Applications of Hand-Carried Ultrasound
- "Echo Stethoscope" as Adjunct to Bedside Examination
- Noncardiologists
- Screening Populations
- Screening for Heart Failure
- Economic Implications
- Future Applications of Hand-Carried Ultrasound

The bedside cardiac physical examination uses technology that is almost 200 years old.[1,2] In 1816, embarrassed to examine an obese young woman by putting his head to her chest, René Théophile-Hyacinthe Laënnec rolled a sheet of paper, placed one end over her precordium and the other to his ear. Thus, the stethoscope was born. The binaural (two-ear type) stethoscope was proposed in 1851 by Arthur Leared and developed in 1852 by George Cammann. The sphygmomanometer dates back to 1881, when Samuel Siegfried Karl Ritter von Basch invented the sphygmomanometer. It is with these two ancient tools that the physician approaches a patient at the bedside to this day. In the interim, the explosive growth of medical technology has spawned ultrasound (US) machines that are as small as 3 pounds (1.4 kg) (the iLook-25, SonoSite, Bothell WA), which can be integrated into the point-of-care patient evaluation (Figs. 8–1 and 8–2).

Development of Technology

The American Society of Echocardiography (ASE) defines a hand-carried ultrasound (HCU) device as a small US machine (typically weighing less than 6 pounds), but neither the device nor the context of the examination fulfills the criteria for a state-of-art limited or comprehensive echocardiographic examination.[3] However, since that publication in 2002, advances in US technology have incorporated all the capabilities expected of a full-sized system into a small package. One commercially available 8.4-pound system (3.8 kg) measuring 11.8 × 10.8 × 3.1 inches has the capacity for two-dimensional (2D), M-mode imaging, color flow Doppler, pulsed-wave and continuous-wave Doppler, tissue Doppler imaging (TDI), tissue harmonic imaging, and broadband multifrequency imaging with image processing and digital storage (The MicroMaxx, SonoSite Bothell, WA; see Fig. 8–1).

The first miniaturized handheld US system was proposed in 1978 by Professor J. R. Roelandt.[4] Bulky keyboards, large monitors, and video recorders have now been replaced by touch pads, flat screens, and digital storage devices. Small echocardiographic systems can be separated on the basis of performance capability, size, weight, and cost (Table 8–1). The least sophisticated, small, real-time imaging systems with limited functionality (hand carried or handheld) are light but with basic technology of 2D imaging and some form of color Doppler, primarily for screening echocardiograms. These systems can be applied for screening of left ventricular (LV) function, wall thick-

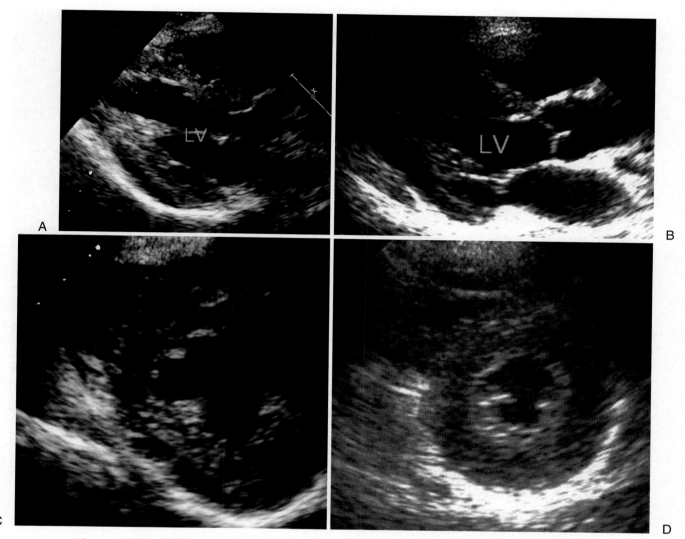

Figure 8–1. *Comparison of images on standard echocardiographic system (Philips IE33) and the MicroMaxx small system. A and C, The long-axis and short-axis views, respectively, from the standard system; B and D, the comparable diagnostic images from the small system. LV, left ventricle.*

TABLE 8–1. Echocardiography System Positioning

	Med Center	Hosp	Cardio	Office	Physical Exam
"Loaded"	+	+	+/−	−	−
Large	+	+	+	−	−
Laptop	+	+	+	+	−
Hand carried	−	−	+	+	+
PDA size	−	−	−	−	+

+, indicated; −, not indicated; Cardio, cardiologist with level 1 to level 2 training; Hosp, primary-care hospital-based system; Med Center, referral medical center; "Loaded," fully capable echo system; PDA, personal digital assistant.

ness, chambers size, hypertrophy, pericardial effusions, and abdominal aortic aneurysms. The other end of the miniature US spectrum is a sophisticated cardiac dedicated system, capable of performing a complete echocardiographic examination including a transesophageal imaging, vascular imaging, and stress echocardiography in a small, laptop-sized box (comparable in capabilities to a full-sized system). Ultimately, the decision of which of two system types to use will vary with the skill and experience of the people performing the imaging and its interpretation (see Tables 8–1 and 8–2). These are the same issues that are paramount to a successful echocardiographic examination regardless of the size of the imaging system. Because the slightly larger, laptop-sized systems are almost comparable to larger standard systems in

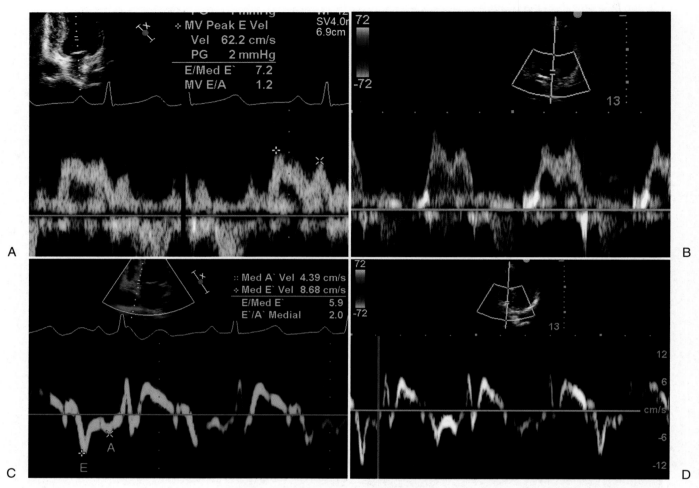

Figure 8–2. *Comparison of diastolic function Doppler interrogation on the standard system and the MicroMaxx small system. A and C, the transmitral E/A (early to atrial velocity ratio) waveforms and the tissue Doppler imaging, respectively from the standard system; B and D, the comparable diagnostic images from the small system.*

TABLE 8–2. Echocardiographic Needs by Training

	3D	TEE	Perf	Strain	DTI	Stress	Color	CW/PW	Quant	2D	M-M
Echocardiologist	+	+	+	+	+	+	+	+	+	+	+
Cardio	−	+	−	−	+	+	+	+	+	+	+
Internist	−	−	−	−	−	−	+	−	−	+	−
ICU	−	−	−	−	−	−	+	−	−	+	−
Anesth	−	+	−	−	−	−	+	+	+	+	−
ER	−	−	−	−	−	−	+	−	−	+	−
Med Stu	−	−	−	−	−	−	+	−	−	+	−
Nurse	−	−	−	−	−	−	+	−	−	+	−
Tech Sch'l	−	−	−	−	−	−	+	+	+	+	−

+, indicated; −, not indicated; 2D, two dimensional; 3D, three dimensional; anesth, anesthesiologist; cardio, cardiologist; color, color flow Doppler; CW/PW, continuous-wave/pulsed-wave Doppler; DTI, Doppler tissue imaging; ER, emergency room; ICU, intensive care unit; med stu, medical student; M-M, m mode; perf, perfusion; quant, quantification; stress, stress echocardiography; TEE, transesophageal echocardiography; tech sch'l, technology training schools.

performance, this chapter will focus on the smaller inexpensive HCU systems with limited capability.

The reliability and accuracy of HCU devices has been validated in studies comparing their performance obtained by skilled technicians or physicians to full-sized systems. Vourvouri demonstrated greater than a 90% concordance between results using a handheld system and a standard full-sized system in the echocardiographic evaluation of LV size and function.[5,6] Additionally, Vourvouri evaluated 300 consecutive patients referred to a cardiologist. Agreement between the hand-carried echocardiographic device and the standard system for the detection of major abnormalities was excellent (98%). The hand-carried devices missed 4% of the major findings.[7] However, because of limitations in penetration and resolution, HCU may underestimate severity of wall motion in difficult-to-image patients. In general, the quality of the study correlated directly with the skill and experience of the personnel acquiring and interpreting the images. Cardiology fellows had 100% agreement between HCU and conventional echocardiography on qualitative assessment of LV systolic function and a 94% concordance for LV end-diastolic dimension and interventricular septal thickness in a 6±2 minute examination.[8]

While the cardiac US technology has become more portable and sophisticated, unfortunately, cardiac auscultatory skills have declined tremendously. A recent study from the Mayo Clinic assessed cardiac auscultation skills before and after an educational 3-day symposium dedicated to improving auscultation. A preconference correct identification score of 26.3%, which improved postconference to only 44.7%, led the authors to conclude that "cardiac auscultatory skills among today's health care professionals are extremely poor regardless of the level and/or type of training of the professional."[9] Thus, there is a growing interest in using hand-carried US equipment not only for supplementing the physical examination, but also for facilitating the rapid triage of emergency department (ED) or patients in the intensive care unit (ICU) and as a screening test for large or underserved populations.

Applications of Hand-Carried Ultrasound

Several general uses for hand-held echocardiographic systems have been explored and include:

1. An "echo stethoscope" to supplement the bedside physical examination or as an adjunct for improving auscultatory skills.
2. For use in mass screening of populations for detection of cardiac disease, as a part of general health screening.

"Echo Stethoscope" as Adjunct to Bedside Examination

Recognizing the limitations of the bedside cardiovascular examination relying on palpation and auscultation, HCU is being used to reenforce auscultation or as a didactic instrument for medical students. However, there is no consensus on the appropriate training protocols and dedicated time required to incorporate didactics for image recognition and hands-on experience. As expected, a meta-analysis found that the accuracy of the hand-carried echocardiogram depended on the training time allocated and level of skill of the personnel performing the echocardiogram ranging from medical students to cardiologists.[10] Diagnoses by medical students trained on a HCU system (OptiGo) for 18 hours were compared with those of a board-certified, experienced cardiologist using a standard physical examination. Medical students correctly identified 75% of abnormal findings compared to 49% by the cardiologists as determined by a standard echocardiogram system.[11]

Croft trained medical students to perform screening echocardiograms in the ER after a 2-week didactic experience, including review of digital images and hands-on supervision. The student's echocardiograms were diagnostic in greater than 90% of the patient's and were interpreted correctly by the students in greater than 80% of patients.[12] Subtle wall motion abnormalities were often missed. For 20 medical house officers participating in a 3-hour training program, the HCU echocardiographic examination substantially improved the assessment of LV function and detection of pericardial effusion over the history and physical examination but was of limited effectiveness for valvular heart disease.[13] However, another study of medical residents using handheld US demonstrated that even a brief training period of only 1 hour significantly improved their diagnosis of LV systolic function and yielded greater than 80% satisfactory quality images.[14]

Medical residents may achieve an acceptable level of performing and interpreting HCU echocardiograms following brief didactic review of anatomy, technology, and supervision while performing 20 to 40 studies.[15] Another successful medical student curriculum incorporated 60 hours of didactics and 40 hours of supervised imaging.[16]

Roelandt suggested that ideally US training should be incorporated in the medical student curriculum to empower them to use US as a part of their physical examination.[17] However, the cost of these devices is still a major limitation. Application of US at the bedside should reinvigorate the lost ardor and skill for the physical examination by providing immediate gratification by identifying the source of a murmur or palpated mass (Figs. 8–3 through 8–5).

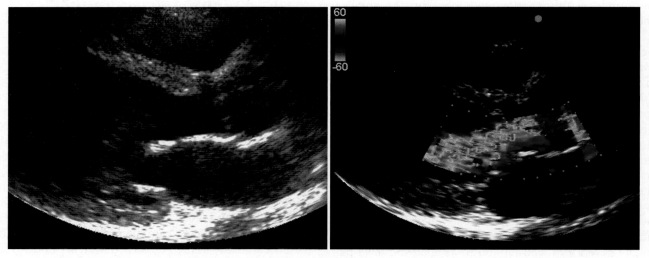

Figure 8–3. Aortic regurgitation. The hand-carried system accurately demonstrated a bicuspid aortic valve and the resulting significant aortic regurgitation, which produced a loud diastolic murmur (A, parasternal long axis with asymmetric closure point of right and noncoronary aortic cusps; B, mosaic aortic regurgitant jet).

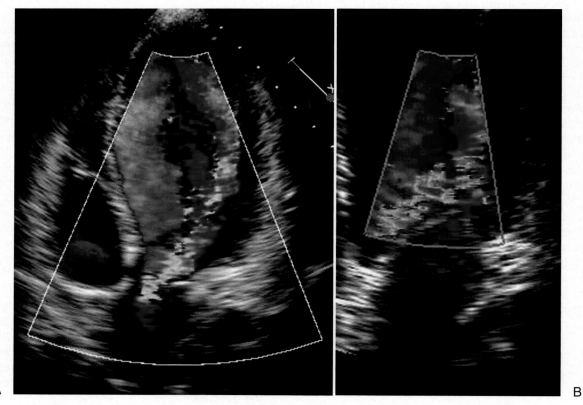

Figure 8–4. Aortic regurgitation. A, A large jet of aortic regurgitation flowing over the anterior mitral valve leaflet from the standard system and B, similar-size jet from the small system.

Noncardiologists

There is a growing practical experience of incorporating HCU into the point of care to supplement the physical examination. The current guidelines for in-dependent competency and the use of handheld US by the ASE recommend at least level 1 training (performing 75 examinations and personally interpreting 150 examinations).[3] However, this time commitment is usually practical only for cardiology training programs. The American College of Emergency Physi-

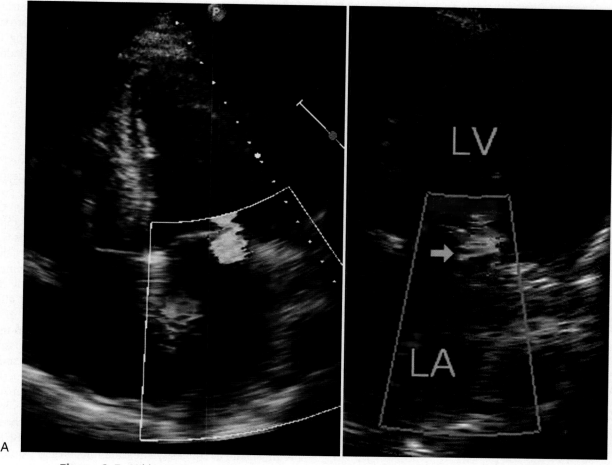

Figure 8–5. *Mild mitral regurgitation.* A, *A small, inaudible jet of mitral regurgitation from the standard system;* B, *similar-sized jet from the small system.* LA, *left atrium;* LV, *left ventricle.*

cians (ACEP) has recognized that echocardiography can provide valuable diagnostic and triage information but that an extended training may not be practical. Furthermore, ACEP encourages point-of-care US for many other organ systems other than the heart (Fig. 8–6). ACEP guidelines published and available online recommend 40 hours of general instruction and performing 25 to 50 cardiac US examinations.[18]

Intensivists who supervise care of a hospital's most complex and unstable patients have also integrated US into their armamentarium. Following 10 1-hour tutorial sessions, intensivists performed limited echocardiograms to assess LV function volume status in 90 patients in the intensive care unit. They successfully performed a diagnostic limited transthoracic echocardiogram (TTE) in 94% of the patients and interpreted them correctly independently in 84% patients, primarily assessing relative volume status and source of hypotension. Importantly, new cardiac information provided a change of management in 37% of patients and additionally useful information was found in 41% of patients.[19]

The general indications for performing an echocardiographic or US examination in the intensive care unit include[20]:

1. Hemodynamic instability
2. Infected endocarditis
3. Aortic dissection rupture
4. Unexplained hypoxemia
5. Source of embolus
6. Central line placement
7. Assessment of pleural effusion and intra-abdominal fluid collections

Obviously, personnel not trained in cardiology may be limited in the performance and interpretation of echocardiograms for many of these clinical situations. Although the HCU device provides important anatomical information in critically ill patients, the lack of color and spectral Doppler or M-mode may be too great a sacrifice for its small size and low cost.[21] However, HCUs may be sophisticated enough to limit the spectrum of a differential diagnosis, thereby expe-

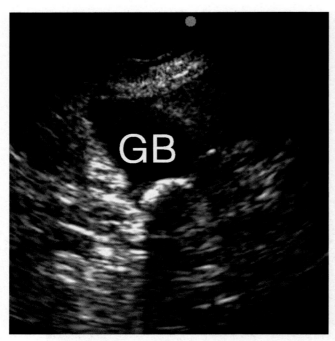

Figure 8–6. Large calcific gallstone detected during emergency department ultrasound investigation with a handheld system of a woman with atypical chest pain. GB, gall-bladder.

diting appropriate treatment and prioritizing other diagnostic tests.

Screening Populations

Screening large populations with low incidence of disease, such as LV hypertrophy in patients with hypertension or in school athletes for asymptomatic disease, is both a time- and cost-effective potential application of HCU.[22,23] HCU has been used to screen for LV hypertrophy with excellent concordance with a standard system.[24] Weidenbener screened 2997 athletes in 21 Indianapolis High Schools and detected 40 cases of mitral valve prolapse (MVP; prevalence 1.4%), 10 with bicuspid aortic valves (0.3%), and 1 with mild hypertrophy of ventricular septum and 1 with a 3-cm mass in the right ventricle.[25] A "limited" echocardiogram with a standard system was able to perform screening echocardiograms in athletes at $15 a test.[26] The cost would be expected to be substantially less with HCU systems.

The HCU could enhance health care delivery in underserved minority populations and developing countries. A general internist evaluated 153 patients at a typical underserved population clinic and found 27 major findings in 19 patients.[27] Such a screening in an indigent community in rural Mexico detected abnormalities in 68% of subjects and obviated the need for further comprehensive echocardiographic evaluation in 90% of patients.[28]

HCU has been used by the military to diagnose and triage in the battlefield (Sonosite 180).[29] The primary care applications of HCU can include noncardiac screening for abdominal aorta aneurysms, gallstones, urinary bladder size, and carotid arterial plaque.

Screening for Heart Failure

B-type natriuretic peptide (BNP) has been advocated as a serum marker, identifying patients with a congestive heart failure (CHF) and LV dysfunction. One study compared the accuracy and cost effectiveness of a predischarge BNP and a comprehensive echocardiography Doppler study for predicting the outcome of patients with congestive heart failure. Only the BNP greater than 250 pg/ml and a mitral E/Ea greater than 15 had incremental value.[30] Echocardiographic Doppler correctly predicted the endpoint in 52 or 54 events with a cost effective ratio of $729.10, in which BNP predicted 47 of 54 events at a cost effective ratio of $49.98.[31] When used to screen dyspneic patients on admission for possible congestive heart failure using a standard echocardiographic system to screen for a LV ejection fraction (EF) greater than 50% had a sensitivity and specificity of 70% and 77% whereas BNP greater than 100 pg/ml was 89% and 73%, respectively[32] (Fig. 8–7). If a standard echocardiographic Doppler examination is not superior to BNP to prognosticate in congestive heart failure, a HCU examination with limited Doppler capability certainly will not be. But a more appropriate application of HCU in the ER has been to supplement the point-of-care physical examination and expedite triage of patients presenting with chest pain or dyspnea (non-asthmatic) not to prognosticate future outcomes. In 100 such patients, the ER physician's diagnosis was changed in 25% of patients and management altered in 15% based on a 5 to 8 minute HCU examination.[33] The HCU was highly concordant ($\kappa = 0.8$) with troponin T test. Also, had 100% sensitivity for the detection of acute coronary syndrome in the patients presenting to the ER with chest pain.[34]

Economic Implications

The limited examination on a relatively inexpensive HCU system can be time efficient and cost effective. In a cardiology clinic, a HCU system (OptiGo, Phillips Medical System) was compared to standard echocardiographic system with a mean examination time of 6.7 ± 1.5 minutes using hand-carried device versus 13.6 ± 2.4 minutes using the standard echocardiographic system.[35] The hand-carried device was considered satisfactory in 85% of patients, and the data was concordant with the stan-

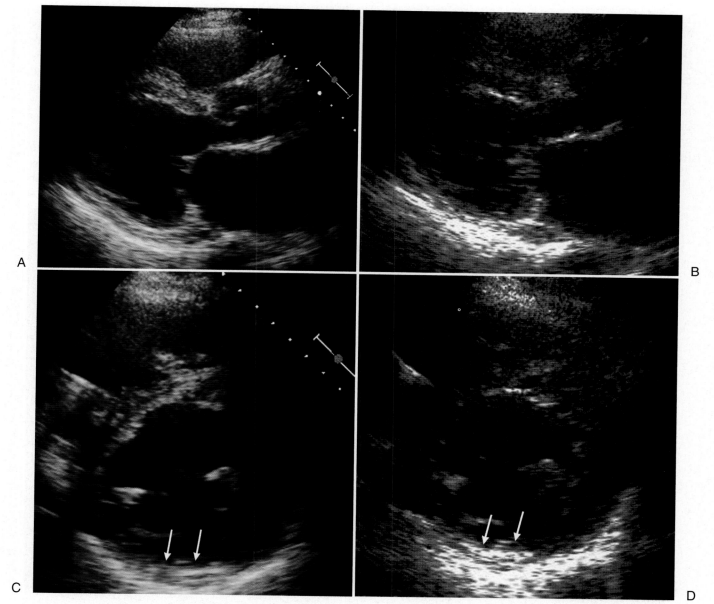

Figure 8–7. *Inferior basal scar. Comparison of images on standard echocardiographic system and the handheld system. A and C, The long-axis and short-axis views, respectively, from the standard system; B and D, the comparable diagnostic images from the small system (arrows pointing to the scar in both short axes).*

dard echocardiographic system in 83.8% of patients. Time for the HCU examination was similar to an estimate of less than 5 minutes by Kimura.[36] Certainly, a cardiologist could incorporate a HCU examination as part of his or her bedside evaluation to great utility and impact on clinical management.[37]

Because of its abilities to save time and eliminate unnecessary examinations, HCU is cost effective. One analysis estimated a 29% reduction in departmental workload at a significant cost saving if all patients with request for LV function assessment underwent HCU initially and only those with abnormal scans under-

went a complete standard echo.[38] The high accuracy of HCU for detection of normal is an efficient tool in eliminating unnecessary examinations.

Future Applications of Hand-Carried Ultrasound

The ASE conservative approach to the use of HCU was largely a result of their concern about the inappropriate use or misapplication of hand-carried devices.[3]

The words *targeted, focused,* and *limited* are often equated with *incomplete, inadequate,* or *inaccurate,* which may reach an appropriate overuse or frank abuse of this and other diagnostic modalities. They felt a limited examination increases the possibility of missing relevant information. ASE believed the appropriate use of HCU is to extend the accuracy of the bedside physical examination.

ASE specifically recommends at least level 1 training to use HCU for cardiovascular diagnosis, which is 75 personally performed examinations and 150 personally interpreted examinations. The ASE strongly recommended that the user should have level 2 training (a total of 150 personally performed examinations and 300 interpreted studies). The ASE reserved the right to revise their report as technology evolves.

ACEP recommended a minimum of 25 with a range of 25 to 50 studies to qualify for emergency cardiac imaging in context of a formal training program.[18] Thus, they promulgated minimal recommendations practical for their training programs and needs.

This approach may be the most practical solution to the dilemma of who uses HCU and what extent of expertise is warranted. The extent of training should be

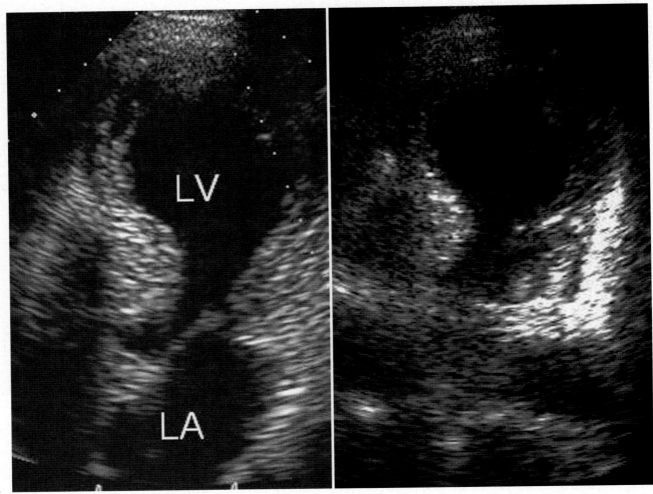

A   B

Figure 8–8. Case study on handheld system. An 82-year-old woman with hypertension presented with half an hour of midback pain, hypotension, and extreme fatigue the day following her granddaughter's wedding. Four months earlier she had a negative maximal stress test for atypical pain. The admission electrocardiogram had new inferior and septal Q waves and poor R wave progression across the precordium. Before cardiac enzymes were known, the emergent handheld echo-Doppler exam demonstrated a hyperdynamic base and ballooning of the rest of the left ventricle. Transmitral Doppler flow was abnormal as was the tissue Doppler imaging. Cardiac angiography was performed without waiting for the enzymes results, which showed normal coronary arteries. Medical therapy was instituted. Cardiac enzymes subsequently were positive and high. This woman probably had cathecholamine-induced takatsubo cardiomyopathy, which is described following an extreme emotional reaction probably generating diffuse microcirculatory vasospasm. The images from a standard system (left) show apical ballooning on a four-chamber view (A), abnormal transmitral flow (C), and tissue Doppler imaging (E) compared to the small MicroMaxx on the right (B, D, and F). LA, left atrium; LV, left ventricle.

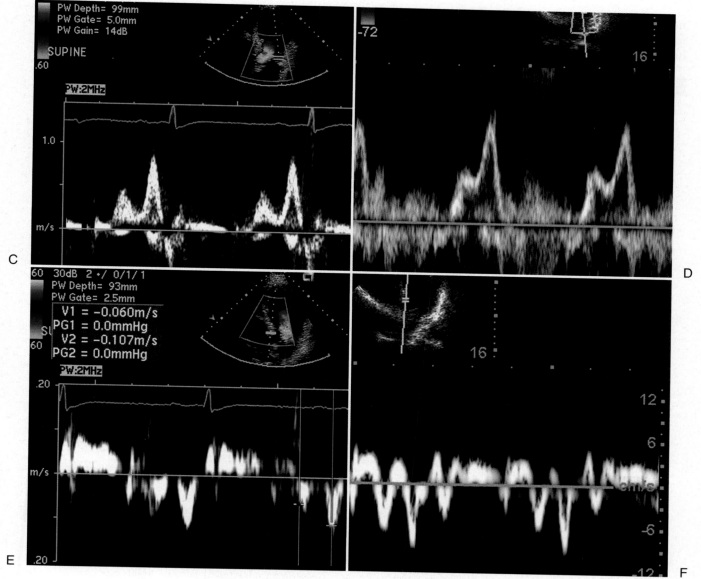

Figure 8–8, cont'd. For legend see opposite page.

commensurate with expected application (see Table 8–2). Cardiologists sophisticated in echocardiography (echocardiologists) who may want to use a sophisticated, smaller system will require level 1 to level 2 skills to obtain images, gradients, and diagnose severity of valvular disease; all that is expected of a full standard systems examination. However, in the ER, when a patient in a coma who is hypotensive presents acutely, rapid detection of cardiac activity or tamponade may dramatically alter care (Fig. 8–8). The necessary training for recognizing cardiac movement or effusions may be similar to those recommended by the emergency physicians. For augmenting and supplementing a physical examination, a brief course with didactic and 20 to 40 supervised patient or simulated examinations could be incorporated into the medical school or residency curriculum.

Unfortunately, the cost of current systems is still prohibitive for routine incorporation to a medical student's basic medical equipment bag. However, one prototype device design is already as low as $3000, incorporating a mechanical scanning transducer to a USB 2.0 port of a personal computer.[39] The future may deliver a small infrared transducer beaming wirelessly to a personal digital assistant (PDA)–sized device priced under $1000.

With the increasing number of older patients, there will be an increased incidence of valvular heart disease and murmurs on physical examination.[40] Integration of HCU into the medical school physical examination curriculum could empower future clinicians with the basic skills for image acquisition and interpretation. Inexpensive HCU cardiac examinations may effectively triage those patients requiring full echocardiographic examinations, thereby expediting care, assuring appropriate utilization of expensive technologies, and reducing health care costs.

KEY POINTS

- HCU refers to small, light weight systems, with basic 2D imaging capability.

- HCU is best suited as an adjunct to supplement the bedside physical examination.

- HCU is ideal for inexpensive screening large populations with low prevalence of disease.

- Training guidelines for image acquisition and interpretation vary by specialty and need.

- Small but technologically complete laptop-sized systems are currently available.

REFERENCES

1. The telltale heart: diagnosing cardiovascular illness. History of stethoscopes and sphygmomanometers. Available at http://www.hhmi.org/biointeractive/museum/exhibit98/content/b6_17info.html.
2. History of the stethoscope. Doctor secrets! Medical Information Clear Simple Quick. Available at http://www.doctorsecrets.com/amazing-medical-facts/sthethoscope-history/history-of-the-stethoscope.html.
3. Seward RB, Douglas PS, Erbel R, et al: Hand-carried cardiac ultrasound (HCU) device: recommendations regarding new technology. A report from the echocardiography task force on new technology of the nomenclature and standards committee of the American Society of Echocardiography. J Am Soc Echocardiogr 15:369-373, 2002.
4. Roelandt J, ten Cate FJ, Hugenholtz PG, et al: The ultrasonic stethoscope: a miniature hand held device for real time cardiac imaging. Circulation 58:II-75, 1978.
5. Vourvouri EC, Poldermans D, DeSutter J, et al: Experience with an ultrasound stethoscope. J Am Soc Echocardiogr 15:80-85, 2002.
6. Vourvouri EC, Schinkel AFL, Roelandt JRTC, et al: Screening for left ventricular dysfunction using a hand-carried cardiac ultrasound device. Eur J Heart Fail 5:767-774, 2003.
7. Vourvouri EC, Poldermans D, Deckers JW, et al: Evaluation of a hand carried cardiac ultrasound device in an outpatient cardiology clinic. Heart 91:171-176, 2005.
8. Lemola K, Yamada E, Jagasia D, Kerber RE: A hand-carried personal ultrasound device for rapid evaluation of left ventricular function: Use after limited echo training. Echocardiography 20(4):309-312, 2003.
9. March SK, Bedynek JL Jr, Chizner MA: Teaching cardiac auscultation: effectiveness of a patient-centered teaching conference on improving cardiac auscultatory skills. Mayo Clin Proc 80(11):443-448, 2005.
10. Kobal SL, Trento L, Baharami S, et al: Comparison of effectiveness of hand-carried ultrasound to bedside cardiovascular physical examination. Am J Cardiol 96:1002-1006, 2005.
11. Kobal SL, Atar S, Siegel RJ: Hand-carried ultrasound improves the bedside cardiovascular examination. Chest 126:693-701, 2004.
12. Croft LB, Cohen BL, Dorants TM, et al: The echo stethoscope: Is it ready for prime time by medical students? J Am Coll Cardiol 39:448A, 2002.
13. Alexander JH, Peterson ED, Chen AY, et al: Feasibility of point-of-care echocardiography by internal medicine housestaff. Am Heart J 147:476-481, 2004.
14. Kimura BJ, Amundson SA, Willis CL, et al: Usefulness of a hand-held ultrasound device for bedside examination of left ventricular function. Am J Cardiol 90:1038-1039, 2002.
15. Hellmann DB, Whiting-O'Keefe Q, Shapiro EP, et al: The rate at which residents learn to use hand-held echocardiography at the bedside. Am J Med 118:1010-1018, 2005.
16. DeCara JM, Kirkpatrick JN, Spencer KT, et al: Use of hand-carried ultrasound devices to augment the accuracy of medical student beside cardiac diagnoses. J Am Soc Echocardiogr 18:257-263, 2005.
17. Roelandt JRTC. Ultrasound stethoscopy: A renaissance of the physical examination? Heart 89:971-974, 2003.
18. American College of Emergency Physicians. Use of ultrasound imaging by emergency physicians. 2001. Available at http://www.acep.org/webportal/PracticeResources/PolicyStatements/.
19. Manasia AR, Nagaraj HM, Kodali RB, et al: Feasibility and potential clinical utility of goal-directed transthoracic echocardiography performed by noncardiologist intensivists using a small hand-carried device (SonoHeart) in critically ill patients. J Cardiothorac Vasc Anesth 19(2):155-159, 2005.
20. Beaulieu Y, Marik PE: Bedside ultrasonography in the ICU. Chest 128:881-895, 2005.
21. Goodkin GM, Spevack DM, Tunick PA, Kronzon I: How useful is hand-carried bedside echocardiography in critically ill patients. J Am Coll Cardiol 37:2019-2022, 2001.
22. Sheps SG, Frohlich ED: Limited echocardiography for hypertensive left ventricular hypertrophy. Hypertension 29:560-563, 1997.
23. Kimura BJ, DeMaria AN: Indications for limited echocardiographic imaging: a mathematical model. J Am Soc Echocardiogr 13:855-861, 2000.
24. Vourvouri EC, Poldermans D, Schinkel AF: Left ventricular hypertrophy screening using a hand-held ultrasound device. Eur Heart J 19:1516-1521, 2002.
25. Weidenbener CJ, Krauss MD, Waller BF, et al: Incorporation of screening echocardiography in the preparticipation exam. Clin J Sports Med 5:86-89, 1995.
26. Murry PM, Cantwell JD, Heath DL, Shoop J: The role of limited echocardiography in screening athletes. Am J Cardiol 76:849-850, 1995.
27. Kirkpatrick JN, Davis A, DeCara JM, et al: Hand-carried cardiac ultrasound as a tool to screen for important cardiovascular disease in an underserved minority health care clinic. J Am Soc Echocardiography 17:399-403, 2004.
28. Kobal SL, Lee SS, Willner R, et al: Hand-carried cardiac ultrasound enhances healthcare delivery in developing countries. Am J Cardiol 94:539-541, 2004.
29. Parker PJ, Adams SA, Williams D, Shepherd A. Forward surgery on operation Telic-Iraq 2003. JR Army Med Corps 151:186-191, 2005.
30. Dokainish H, Zoghbi A, Lakkis NM, et al: Incremental predictive power of B-type natriuretic peptide and tissue Doppler echocardiography in the prognosis of patients with congestive heart failure. J Am Coll Cardiol 45:1223-1226, 2005.
31. Dokainish H, Zoghbi WA, Ambriz E, et al: Comparative cost-effectiveness of B-type natriuretic peptide and echocardiography for predicting outcome in patients with congestive heart failure. Am J Cardiol 97:400-403, 2005.
32. Steg PG, Joubin L, McCord J, et al: B-Type Natriuretic Peptide and Echocardiographic determination of ejection fraction in the diagnosis of congestive heart failure in patients with acute dyspnea. Chest 128:21-29, 2005.
33. Duvall WL, Croft LB, Goldman ME: Can hand-carried ultrasound devices be extended for use by the noncardiology medical community? Echocardiography 20(5):471-476, 2003.

34. Atar S, Feldman A, Darawshe A, et al: Utility and diagnostic accuracy of hand-carried ultrasound for emergency room evaluation of chest pain. *Am J Cardiol* 94:408-409, 2004.

35. Giannotti G, Mondillo S, Galderisi M, et al: Hand-held echocardiography: added value in clinical cardiological assessment. *Cardiovasc Ultrasound* 24(3):7, 2005.

36. Kimura BJ, DeMaria AN: Technology insight: hand-carried ultrasound cardiac assessment—evolution, not revolution. *Nat Clin Pract Cardiovasc Med* 2(4):217-223, 2005.

37. DeGroot-de Laat LE, ten Cate FJ, Vourvouri EC, et al: Impact of hand-carried cardiac ultrasound on diagnosis and management during cardiac consultation rounds. *Eur J Echocardiogr* 6:196-201, 2005.

38. Greaves K, Jeetley P, Hickman M, et al: The use of hand-carried ultrasound in the hospital setting—a cost-effective analysis. *J Am Soc Echocardiogr* 18:620-625, 2005.

39. Saijo Y, Nitta S, Kobayashi K, et al: Development of an ultraportable echo device connected to USB port. *Ultrasonics* 42:699-703, 2004.

40. Croft LB, Donnio R, Shapiro R, et al: Age-related prevalence of cardiac valvular abnormalities warranting infectious endocarditis prophylaxis. *Am J Cardiol* 94:386-389, 2004.

Part Two

The Left Ventricle

Quantitative Evaluation of Left Ventricular Structure, Wall Stress, and Systolic Function

GERARD P. AURIGEMMA, MD • WILLIAM H. GAASCH, MD

■ Definitions and Theoretical Considerations

■ Assessment of Left Ventricular Mass, Volume, and Geometry
   M-Mode Echocardiography
   Two-Dimensional Echocardiography
   Alternative Methods for Quantitation of Left Ventricular Structure and Function

■ Assessment of Left Ventricular Systolic Function
   Ejection Fraction
   Fractional Shortening and Related Indices
   Stress-Shortening Relations
   Pressure-Volume Analysis

■ Potential Limitations

The quantitation of left ventricular (LV) systolic function, size, and geometry is critical to the proper evaluation and management of patients with all types of heart disease.[1] For example, the assessment of LV function in patients with coronary artery disease (CAD) provides better prognostic information than does knowledge of the number of diseased vessels (Fig. 9–1). Even when only one or two vessels are diseased, a low ejection fraction (EF) is associated with a higher mortality than that seen in patients with three-vessel disease and a normal EF.[2] Large LV systolic and diastolic volumes are also associated with a poor prognosis; thus, a patient with a reduced EF after a myocardial infarction (MI) can be categorized according to subsequent risk based on the absolute end-systolic volume (ESV; Fig. 9–2).[3] Furthermore, information concerning LV size and geometry has important therapeutic implications, in view of the salutary effects of therapy with angiotensin converting enzyme (ACE) inhibitors on postinfarction remodeling and prognosis in patients with a reduced EF.[4,5]

Similarly, in cardiomyopathy of any cause, mortality remains high in patients with an EF less than 35%, even with medical therapy. A depressed EF is uniformly present in patients with idiopathic dilated cardiomyopathy and results from a combination of afterload excess and depressed contractility. In this setting, indices of LV geometry, such as the relative wall thickness (RWT) or the mass/volume (M/V) ratio (Fig. 9–3),

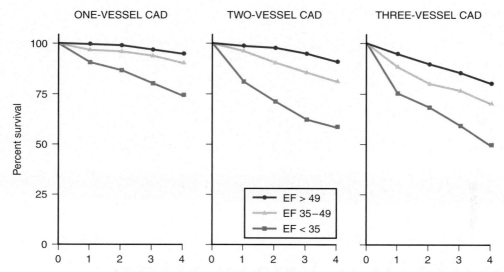

Figure 9–1. The relation between left ventricular ejection fraction (EF) and survival in patients with single-, double-, and triple-vessel coronary artery disease. The negative impact of a low EF is seen in all three groups. Survival is better in patients with three-vessel CAD and a normal EF than in those with one- or two-vessel disease and a low EF. (Adapted from Mock MB, Rindqvist I, Fisher LD, et al: Circulation 66:562-567, 1982. In Aurigemma GP, Gaasch WH, Villegas B, Meyer TE: Curr Probl Cardiol 20:368, 1995.)

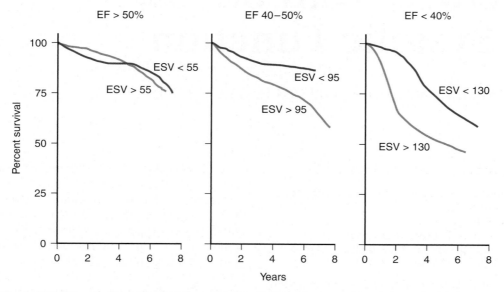

Figure 9–2. The relation between left ventricular end-systolic volume (ESV) and survival in patients with normal, near-normal, and abnormal ejection fraction (EF). Data were obtained from patients with a history of myocardial infarction. End-systolic volume (ESV) is a major predictor of survival when the EF is less than 50%. (Adapted from White HD, Norris RM, Brown MA, et al: Circulation 76:44-51, 1987. In Aurigemma GP, Gaasch WH, Villegas B, Meyer TE: Curr Probl Cardiol 20:369, 1995.)

provide prognostic information that is independent of the EF. Conversely, it is important to identify the significant percentage of patients with congestive heart failure (CHF) symptoms who have a normal EF.[6-8]

Measurement of LV volume, mass, and function can provide data that are necessary to define the optimal time for surgery in patients with volume overload hypertrophy owing to chronic, severe mitral re-

gurgitation (MR) or aortic regurgitation (AR). In this regard, the prognostic usefulness of ventricular end-diastolic volume (EDV) and ESV, the EF, the ratio of EDV to mass, systolic stress-shortening relations, and end-systolic pressure-volume (P-V) relations has been tested in a variety of clinical studies. The ESV and EF appear to provide the most useful clues to prognosis.[9-15] Certainly, a most important determinant of

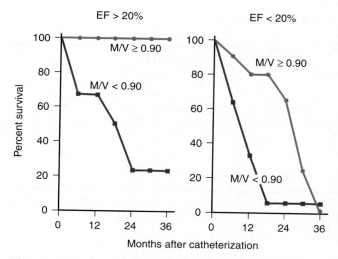

Figure 9–3. *The relation between left ventricular mass/ volume (M/V) ratio and survival in patients with an ejection fraction (EF) higher than and less than 20%. Data were obtained from patients with dilated cardiomyopathy. Patients with a normal M/V ratio exhibit better survival than those with a low ratio; this trend is seen in EF categories. (Adapted from Feild BJ, Baxley WA, Russell RO Jr, et al: Circulation 47:1022-1031, 1973. In Aurigemma GP, Gaasch WH, Villegas B, Meyer TE: Curr Probl Cardiol 20:370, 1995.)*

postoperative survival is the level of LV systolic function (Fig. 9–4).

In pressure overload hypertrophy owing to aortic stenosis (AS), an assessment of systolic function is perhaps less important than in the regurgitant lesions. Although severe depression of the EF may indicate an increased surgical risk, patients with an EF as low as 20% to 25% can show substantial clinical improve-

ment after aortic valve replacement.[16-18] In such patients, excessive systolic loads are usually responsible for the low EF; this situation is termed *inadequate hypertrophy* or *afterload excess*. Alternatively, *excessive* or *inappropriate hypertrophy*, indicated by a high RWT, appears to identify a group of patients having a high perioperative risk[19,20]; in this situation, a normal or high EF does not seem to be beneficial. In AS, therefore, indices of LV geometry[20] (RWT) appear to provide prognostic clues that are not reflected in the EF.

It is well established that increased LV mass is a strong predictor of cardiovascular morbidity and cardiovascular and all-cause mortality, even when age, blood pressure, and other risk factors are considered[21-27] (see Chapter 32). Some investigators have suggested that LV geometry provides prognostic information that is incremental to the extent of LV hypertrophy.[24-26] For example, an increased ratio of LV wall thickness to cavity dimension[27] identifies patients at higher risk for cardiovascular morbidity and mortality (Table 9–1); whether this incremental risk is truly independent of LV mass has been called into question by other data.[28]

Thus, a substantial body of clinical research has demonstrated the prognostic value of indices of LV volume, mass, geometry, and function. Most if not all of these indices are routinely available to the clinician from standard M-mode and two-dimensional (2D) and Doppler echocardiography. In this chapter the echocardiographic techniques for evaluating LV geometry, stress, and systolic function are reviewed. Principles and methods are discussed, and clinical applications to patients with pressure and volume overload hypertrophy are emphasized.

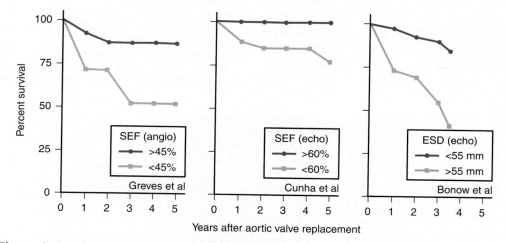

Figure 9–4. *Relation of preoperative ventricular function to postoperative survival. These and other published data (see text) indicated that preoperative ventricular function is an important determinant of postoperative survival. ESD (echo), end-systolic dimension by echocardiography; SEF (angio), systolic ejection fraction by angiography; SEF (echo), systolic ejection fraction by echocardiography. (Adapted from Hoshino PK, Gaasch WH: Arch Intern Med 146:349-352, 1986. Copyright © 1986 American Medical Association. In Aurigemma GP, Gaasch WH, Villegas B, Meyer TE: Curr Probl Cardiol 20:371, 1995.)*

TABLE 9–1. Relation between Morbid Events and the Pattern of Left Ventricular Geometry

| | Normal Left Ventricular Mass | | | Left Ventricular Hypertrophy | |
	RWT < 0.45 (N = 150)	RWT ≥ 0.45 (N = 34)	RWT < 0.45 (N = 40)	RWT ≥ 0.45 (N = 29)	P
CV deaths (%)	0	3	10	21	<0.001
CV events (%)	11	15	23	31	0.03
All deaths (%)	1	6	10	24	<0.01

The prognostic value of LVH for morbid events in men (at an average of 10.2 years of follow-up) is striking. For all end points, the RWT provides incremental value for assessing risk. *P*-value obtained by analysis of variance.
CV, cardiovascular; LVH, left ventricular hypertrophy; RWT, relative wall thickness.
From Koren M, Devereux R, Casale PN, et al: *Ann Intern Med* 114:345–352, 1991.

Definitions and Theoretical Considerations

The systolic pumping of the left ventricle is a complex process that involves a coordinated contraction of subendocardial, midwall, and subepicardial muscle fibers. These fibers are arranged in a complex, helical fashion. At the equator of the ventricle, midwall fibers are oriented circumferentially; contraction of these fibers mainly contributes to a decrease in the minor axis (or dimension) of the ventricle and is responsible for generation of much of the stroke volume (SV; Fig. 9–5). Longitudinally oriented fibers in the subendocardium and subepicardium contribute to shortening of the long axis of the ventricle, also contributing to SV. In addition to circumferential and long-axis shortening, the apex of the left ventricle rotates counterclockwise during systolic contraction, and the base rotates clockwise (as viewed from the apex).[29,30] Such "twist," like fiber shortening, appears to be influenced by the contractile state of the myocardium. In concert with these shortening and twisting motions, wall thickening contributes to volume displacement and generation of the SV.[31]

Preload, afterload, contractility, and geometry influence shortening and thickening.

The pumping activity of the left ventricle provides oxygenated blood to the tissues of the body; therefore, the SV can be used as a parameter of the pump performance of the ventricle (Table 9–2). Because LV systolic pressure and SV are inversely related, using stroke work as an index of ventricular performance can be

TABLE 9–2. Aspects of Ventricular Function

Pump Performance
The pumping activity of the left ventricle that results in the delivery of oxygenated blood to the tissues. Stroke volume and stroke work are parameters of pump performance.

Ventricular Function
Left ventricular performance assessed relative to end-diastolic fiber length (or related parameter).

Myocardial Contractility
A basic property of the myocardium that reflects its active state, rather than loading conditions.

Contractile Function
A descriptor of ventricular performance or function that is affected by inotropic state, fiber length, or load.

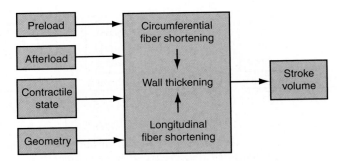

Figure 9–5. Circumferential and longitudinal fibers contribute to wall thickening and volume displacement. These functions are influenced by left ventricular preload, afterload, contractile state, and geometry. (From Aurigemma GP, Gaasch WH, Villegas B, Meyer TE: Curr Probl Cardiol 20:374, 1995.)

more appropriate; a stroke work parameter credits the ventricle for the development of pressure and for shortening. When performance is assessed relative to end-diastolic fiber length or a related parameter, ventricular function can be described. Thus, a ventricular function curve can be generated by plotting stroke work against end-diastolic pressure, diameter, volume, or wall stress. Volume loading therefore produces an increment in stroke work (i.e., performance) through use of the Frank-Starling mechanism. By contrast, increased myocardial contractility also can produce an increment in stroke work, but in this case performance is augmented through a change in inotropic state rather than by a change in end-diastolic fiber length. In other words, contractility refers to a basic property of the myocardium that reflects the intensity of its active state. The use of the term *contractility* should be restricted to situations in which a change in performance or EF cannot be ascribed to a change in preload or afterload. *Contractile function* is a more general term used to describe changes in performance or function that could be affected by changes in inotropic state, fiber length, or loads. Thus, a change in the EF might best be classified as a change in contractile function; this term is often used interchangeably with systolic function. To fully describe the ventricle, it is necessary to define several additional terms that refer to its mechanical properties.

Stress is defined as the force per unit cross-sectional area (CSA) of a material. It is an engineering term used to compare loads borne by different-sized elements of a material; the total load is less important than the load per unit of material. If the same load is borne by a smaller amount of material, the stress on that material is higher. In a spherical model of the left ventricle, wall stress (σ) is directly proportional to the transmural pressure (P) and inversely proportional to the product of chamber radius (R) and wall thickness (Th):

$$\sigma = PR/2Th$$

In the left ventricle, geometry is much more complex, and several components of stress exist within the wall (Fig. 9–6). Of these, meridional and circumferential stresses have most commonly been used in the analysis of LV mechanics. The meridional stress vector is oriented in the longitudinal or apex-to-base direction and represents the component of the load resisting long-axis shortening; circumferential stress is oriented along the equator, perpendicular to the long axis (see Fig. 9–6) and represents the component of the load resisting minor-axis shortening. Meridional stress (σ_m) can be calculated as

$$\sigma_m = P \cdot LVID / [4 \cdot Th(1 + LVID/Th)]$$

in which P is pressure (mm Hg), Th is wall thickness, and $LVID$ is cavity dimension.[32] This stress parameter does not require measurement of the long axis of the LV cavity. Circumferential stress (σ_c) can be calculated as

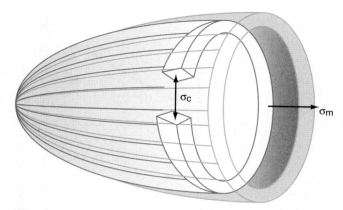

Figure 9–6. Schematic of the left ventricle (LV) (represented as a truncated ellipsoid) illustrating the major stress vectors. Meridional stress (σ_m) is the force acting along the long axis of the LV; meridional stress opposes long-axis shortening. Circumferential stress (σ_c) is the force acting in the equatorial direction; circumferential stress opposes circumferential fiber shortening, and circumferentially oriented fibers are located in the midwall of the left ventricle. The inner shell represents the left ventricle in systole, and the outer, the ventricle in diastole. (From Aurigemma GP, Gaasch WH, Villegas B, Meyer TE: Curr Probl Cardiol *20:375, 1995.)*

$$\sigma_c = P \cdot a^2[1 + (b^2/r^2)]/(b^2 - a^2)$$

in which P is end-systolic pressure (mm Hg), a is the internal (endocardial) radius, b is the external (epicardial) radius, and r is the midwall radius.[33] Other approaches to the calculation of circumferential stress, using minor- and major-axis dimensions, have been evaluated.[34] Formulas for calculation of meridional and circumferential stress using 2D echocardiographic data are as follows[35]:

$$\sigma_m = 1.33P \, A_m/A_c \cdot 10^3 \text{ kdyn/cm}^2$$

$$\sigma_c = \frac{1.33P\sqrt{A_c}}{\sqrt{A_m + A_c} - \sqrt{A_c}}\left[\frac{\dfrac{4(A_c)^{3/2}}{\pi L^2}}{\sqrt{A_m + A_c} - \sqrt{A_c}}\right]$$

in which A_t is the short-axis area subtended by the LV epicardium and right side of the septum, A_c is the cavity (endocardial) area, and $A_m = A_t - A_c$ or myocardial area, and L is the LV cavity length, obtained from the apical four-chamber view. 2D and M-mode methods yield somewhat different results, with M-mode-derived σ_m being higher than 2D-derived values, even in normal subjects. In spherical ventricles, σ_m by any method tends to overestimate afterload.[36]

The determination of wall stress requires assessment of LV pressure. Invasively determined values may be combined with echocardiographic dimensions, but they are often not available or simultaneously obtained. Three methods have been proposed for using noninvasive recordings to ascertain LV systolic pressures; LV diastolic pressures (and therefore diastolic stress) cannot be reliably determined noninvasively. Although

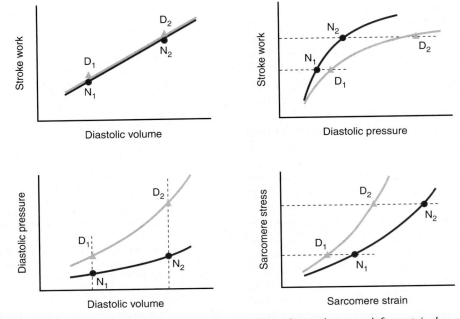

Figure 9–7. The effect of diastolic dysfunction on the relation between left ventricular systolic performance and preload. Classic ventricular function curves relating stroke work to end-diastolic volume are shown in the top left panel; stroke work is related to end-diastolic pressure in the top right panel; diastolic pressure-volume curves are shown below. When the left ventricular end-diastolic pressure is used as an index of preload, ventricular systolic function in diastolic heart failure (D1, D2) appears to be less than normal (N1, N2). These results are extrapolated to sarcomere stress-shortening relations. For a given level of sarcomere stress (point 1 to point 2), there is much less sarcomere strain in patients with diastolic failure (D1, D2) than in normal (N1, N2). (From Aurigemma GP, Zile MR, Gaasch WH: Circulation 113:296-304, 2006.)

these methods assume that there is no LV outflow gradient, the first and easiest method assumes that end-systolic LV pressure can be approximated by peak arterial pressure.[32] Thus, cuff systolic blood pressure is substituted for LV end-systolic pressure. The second method involves calibration of an externally recorded pulse recording using cuff systolic and diastolic pressures, with calculation of arterial pressures at the dicrotic notch.[37] The third involves the substitution of mean arterial pressure, derived from cuff recording, for end-systolic pressure, given the close correlation between these two values, as shown by Rozich.[38]

Because wall stress parameters incorporate appropriate size normalization, they allow comparison among the mechanical properties of different hearts. End-systolic wall stresses, calculated using end-systolic pressures (or the surrogates discussed earlier) and dimensions, are taken as indices of LV afterload, whereas end-diastolic wall stress, calculated using end-diastolic pressure and dimension, is a measure of LV preload.

Preload is the force (i.e., load) acting to stretch the resting myofibril. Preload is commonly estimated as the LV end-diastolic pressure, diameter, or volume, but to be more precise, this force should be normalized for each unit CSA of muscle and expressed as end-diastolic wall stress. In this manner, LV preload is analogous to the preload on a strip of isolated cardiac muscle in a myograph. This force, which acts to stretch the myocar-

dium, is resisted by the stiffness of the muscle. Thus, the extent to which the myocardial fiber is stretched depends on an interaction between preload and muscle stiffness.[39] Because preload influences initial fiber length, it affects LV systolic performance. This phenomenon, which operates on a beat-to-beat basis, is generally referred to as Starling's law of the heart or the Frank-Starling mechanism.

The preload reserve of the ventricle depends on the baseline hemodynamic conditions and the stiffness of the myocardium. Thus, in the upright posture, normal human subjects exhibit a substantial preload reserve, whereas in the recumbent posture they may exhibit a minimal preload reserve. The difference in preload reserve is related to difference in the baseline EDV, which is lower in the upright posture than it is when the subject is recumbent, owing to the differences in venous return. This fact should be kept in mind when interpreting exercise studies; the EDV of the normal left ventricle generally increases during upright exercise, but it may not during recumbent exercise. Moreover, the ability to recruit the Frank-Starling mechanism may also be limited in hypertrophied ventricles that have abnormal ventricular compliance characteristics (Fig. 9–7). Thus, in patients with AS or hypertensive heart disease, there may be little or no increment in LV EDV during exercise, and consequently the EF may not increase normally.[40-42] Such limited preload reserve occurs as a result of a steep diastolic PV relation in which large changes in filling pressure cause only small changes in volume.[43,44] This mechanism may even underlie marginal LV function in the basal state.[39]

Despite a low EF, many dilated hearts (particularly those with compensated MR or AR) generate a normal or high SV. In this instance, although the Frank-Starling mechanism may be a contributing factor, the large SV is primarily a function of the large EDV. In other words, the presence of a large LV chamber does not necessarily indicate use of preload reserve at the fiber level. Many such hearts retain the ability to use preload reserve to augment SV. By contrast, in end-stage heart failure, preload reserve may be exhausted.

Afterload can be thought of as the force (i.e., stress) developed by the myocardium after the onset of contraction. As described by the Laplace relation, afterload (systolic wall stress) is directly related to LV systolic pressure and radius and inversely related to wall thickness. Afterload varies with time, and thus it can be calculated at the instant of aortic valve opening, at the end of ejection, or at any instant throughout systole. Whereas LV systolic pressure and systemic vascular resistance (SVR) can affect afterload, neither of these should be considered the equivalent of afterload.[45-47] Likewise, aortic input impedance influences systolic pressure and stress, but impedance is not the equivalent of afterload.[48]

In AS, the LV systolic pressure may exceed 250 mm Hg, but if there is an appropriate increase in LV wall thickness, the force borne by each unit of heart muscle might remain near normal (i.e., afterload is normal).[46-47,49] On the other hand, an acute increase in systolic pressure or chamber size can result in an increased afterload.[50] By virtue of the inverse relation between load and shortening, an acute increase in afterload generally causes a decrease in shortening, and vice versa.

Contractility can be defined as the quality of cardiac muscle that determines performance independent of loading conditions. Contractility is easiest to study and define in isolated heart muscles when loading conditions are held constant. For example, if resting length is held constant, the addition of digitalis or norepinephrine to an isolated muscle preparation results in an increase in the extent and velocity of force development and shortening; such increased performance under constant loading conditions reflects an augmented inotropic state (i.e., increased contractility). In many cardiac diseases, abnormal LV pump function may be caused by disordered loading conditions, depression of contractility, or both. For this reason, it may be difficult to determine the exact cause of decreased fiber shortening. Accordingly, there has been considerable interest in the development of a sensitive index of contractility that is not affected by changes in loading conditions.[51-52] Unfortunately, there is no completely load-independent index of basal contractile state. Thus,

directional changes in contractility (during acute hemodynamic interventions) are relatively easy to demonstrate, but it is not possible to define a basal level of contractility in patients with chronic heart disease.

Assessment of Left Ventricular Mass, Volume, and Geometry

Remodeling of the left ventricle in valvular heart disease, heart failure, and hypertensive heart disease is characterized by changes in LV mass and geometry. Descriptors of LV geometry include the RWT, short axis/long axis ratio, and mass/volume ratio. These descriptors are easily obtained by M-mode and 2D echocardiography. As suggested earlier, alterations in LV geometry have been used to assist risk stratification in a variety of diseases and to describe more completely remodeling changes effected by valve replacement. In patients with idiopathic dilated cardiomyopathy, for example, a poorer survival is associated with larger short-axis dimension and a greater ratio of short/long axes (i.e., a more spherical LV geometry).[53] The RWT, when used to estimate the "adequacy" of LV hypertrophy in patients with idiopathic dilated cardiomyopathy, also predicts the increase in contractility in response to dobutamine infusion[54]; cardiomyopathy patients with a diminution in RWT appear to have an attenuated contractile response to dobutamine infusion. In the following section, the methods used to calculate LV mass and describe LV geometry are reviewed.

M-Mode Echocardiography

Mass

Whereas newer and more costly tomographic methods, such as ultrafast computed tomography (CT) and magnetic resonance imaging (MRI), permit more precise quantitation, echocardiography remains the most commonly used technique for estimating LV mass and geometry. This subject has recently been reviewed by the Chamber Quantification Writing Group of the American Society of Echocardiography (ASE).[55] M-mode echocardiography is universally available and relatively low cost, and there is a considerable body of evidence supporting its accuracy in LV mass quantitation.[56-57] Quantitation of mass (see also Chapter 32) is based on the geometric assumption that the ventricle is a prolate ellipsoid with a 2:1 long axis/short axis ratio.[58] In practical terms, LV mass estimates are most accurate in ventricles with normal shape,[58] specifically, a long axis/short axis ratio that approximates 2:1. It is assumed, of course, that minor-axis dimensions are measured in a region free of wall motion abnormalities. This assumption is invalidated in ischemic heart disease with focal wall motion abnormality or in right ventricular (RV) overload. Estimates of myocardial mass and volume are derived from LV minor-axis dimensions obtained with the transducer in the parasternal position (Fig. 9–8). Under 2D echocardiographic guidance, the ultrasound (US) beam is aligned so that it is perpendicular to the interventricular septum and posterior wall at a level slightly below the mitral leaflet tips; the chamber dimension is obtained from the parasternal long-axis view.[55] This approach maximizes the LV cavity dimension and ensures that proper beam orientation with respect to the papillary muscles is obtained. LV mass is estimated from measurements of septal and posterior wall thickness and LV cavity di-

mensions at end-diastole using the anatomically validated cube formula[55]:

$$LV\ mass = 0.8[1.04(ST_d + LVID_d + PWT_d)^3$$

$$- LVIDd^3] + 0.6\ g$$

in which ST_d is the diastolic septal thickness, $LVID_d$ is the diastolic LV cavity dimension, PWT_d is the diastolic posterior wall thickness, and 1.04 is the specific gravity of myocardium. The measurements are made using the leading-edge American Society of Echocardiography standard technique.[56] As shown by Devereux and colleagues[57] LV mass estimates made with American Society of Echocardiography measurements overestimate true anatomic LV weights by 20%, necessitating a correction factor of 0.8. The chamber quantification recommendations note that direct measurements by 2D echocardiography may be substituted for 2D-derived M-mode measurements.[55] It is important to note, however, that direct 2D measurements will yield lower values than 2D-directed M-mode measurements.[55] The accuracy of three-dimensional (3D) methods for calculating LV mass has been demonstrated (see Chapter 4).

Volume

A simple estimate of LV volume may be obtained from the minor-axis dimension, derived by M-mode echocardiography as

$$V = LVID^3$$

The geometric assumptions are similar to those used for LV mass calculation. However, in the dilated, spherical left ventricle encountered in long-standing valvular regurgitation or dilated cardiomyopathy, the ratio of length to minor-axis dimension decreases, leading to significant overestimation of LV volumes by this simple method. Teichholz and colleagues[59] derived a formula that attempts to correct for this problem:

$$V_d = [7/(2.4 + LVID_d)] \cdot LVID_d^3$$

LV volumes derived with this formula correlate well with single-plane angiographic estimates.[58] The Teichholz method produces the most accurate volume estimates of any of the M-mode formulas.[60] Because M-mode echocardiography provides minor-axis dimensions of the left ventricle in systole and diastole, the Teichholz method may be used to compute LV volumes at end-systole and end-diastole and thus to derive SV and cardiac output (CO). A compelling advantage of this method is that LV volume can be determined rapidly from easily obtained M-mode measurements.

Relative Wall Thickness

M-mode estimates of myocardial mass and volume are derived from LV minor-axis dimensions obtained with the transducer in the parasternal position (see Fig. 9–8).

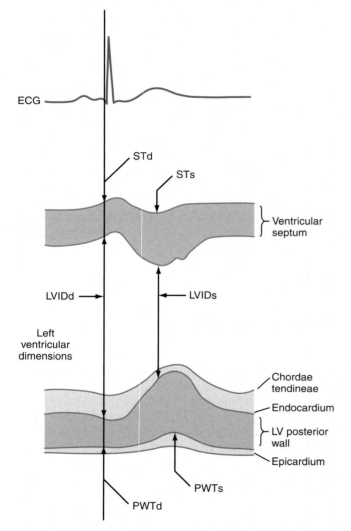

Figure 9–8. Schematic of an M-mode echocardiogram obtained using two-dimensional echocardiographic guidance. Measurements are made coincident with the Q wave of the simultaneous electrocardiogram. ECG, echocardiogram; LV, left ventricular; LVIDd, left ventricular internal dimensions in diastole; LVIDs, left ventricular internal dimensions in systole; PWTd, posterior wall thickness in diastole; PWTs, posterior wall thickness in systole; STd, ventricular septal thickness in diastole; STs, ventricular septal thickness in systole. (From Aurigemma GP, Gaasch WH, Villegas B, Meyer TE: Curr Probl Cardiol 20:381, 1995.)

These same measurements are used to describe LV geometry. Although the amount of LV mass is an important predictor of subsequent cardiac events in hypertensive disease, the geometry and pattern of LV hypertrophy also provide insight into the pathophysiology of hypertensive hypertrophy[55] and may confer prognostic information (see Chapter 34).[24-26] The most commonly used index of the pattern of hypertrophy is the RWT,[27] which is calculated as

$$RWT = 2 \cdot PWT/LVID$$

in which *PWT* is the posterior wall thickness and *LVID* is the LV internal dimension, respectively; RWT may be measured in diastole or systole. RWT also has been expressed as *h/R*, in which *h* is wall thickness and *R* is cavity radius.

Ford[61] and others[47-48] have shown that in the normal or compensated ventricle, the RWT increases in direct proportion to elevations in systolic pressure (Fig. 9-9). Assuming that there is not a substantial shape change as the ventricle enlarges (i.e., during normal growth), the relation is independent of absolute chamber size.[47] It is also assumed that the magnitude and transmural distribution of stresses are the same in normal ventricles of different size. Systolic dysfunction with dilation is usually associated with a lower RWT; in contrast, chronic pressure overload produces an increment in wall thickness with little change in the chamber radius (a high relative wall thickness).[62]

In untreated hypertensive patients, LV mass and relative wall thickness determinations may be used to subdivide the population into four general categories (Fig. 9-10):

1. Concentric hypertrophy (elevations in both LV mass and RWT),
2. Eccentric hypertrophy (elevation in LV mass with normal RWT),
3. Concentric remodeling (normal mass but abnormally high RWT), and
4. Normal LV mass and RWT.

In a population of untreated hypertensive patients, the majority had normal LV mass and normal RWT; concentric hypertrophy was the least common abnormal pattern observed.[27]

What is the clinical relevance of the mass and geometry subcategories? Patients with concentric hypertrophy have a relatively high incidence of adverse cardiovascular and noncardiovascular events compared with patients with eccentric hypertrophy.[25-27] In addition, concentric geometry, even without hypertrophy, appears to be associated with adverse consequences during follow-up (see Table 9-1). Thus, in hypertensive disease, as noted earlier, incremental information regarding risk for both cardiovascular and noncardiovascular events is provided by assessing geometry and LV mass. The RWT may provide insight into the appropriateness of hypertrophy. There is occasionally more muscle mass than would be required for the observed pressure; thus, a high RWT, such as is encountered in hypertrophic cardiomyopathies, "hypertensive hypertrophic cardiomyopathy of the elderly,"[63-66] uncommonly in hypertension, and not infrequently in AS,[62] indicates excessive or inappropriate LV hypertrophy. In our experience, RWT values greater than 0.8 are uncommon in AS, but when present, they appear to represent inappropriate hypertrophy. Indeed, values exceeding 0.8 predict a systolic pressure in excess of 300 mm Hg, a pressure rarely seen, even in adults with AS[62] (see Fig. 9-9). Extreme concentric hypertrophy, with exceedingly high values for RWT, has been described in elderly patients undergoing aortic valve replacement for AS.[20]

The interaction among shape, load, and function is complex and important because each one may influence the others. A decompensated heart clearly demonstrates abnormalities of all three-low RWT, high afterload, and reduced function—yet it is not possible to state which abnormality is primary. Does the ventricle dilate, thereby raising afterload and reducing pump performance or is shortening impaired first, leading to dilation, which then raises afterload? Human studies shed little light because of the lengthy time course of disease and other confounding factors; animal studies suggest that all three events may occur in concert.[67]

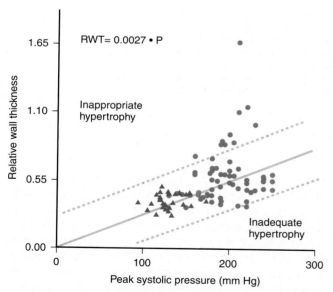

Figure 9-9. *Relationship between relative wall thickness (RWT; equivalent to the ratio of thickness to radius) and level of systolic pressure in patients with aortic stenosis (red circles). In normal hearts (blue triangles), RWT increases in direct proportion to the level of systolic pressure. Individuals with a higher thickness-to-radius ratio than predicted by the level of pressure are considered to have inappropriate (or excessive) hypertrophy; by contrast, individuals whose thickness-to-radius ratio is less than that predicted by the level of pressure have inadequate hypertrophy. In normal hearts, the relationship between peak pressure (P) and RWT, as defined by Ford,[69] is RWT = 0.0027P.*

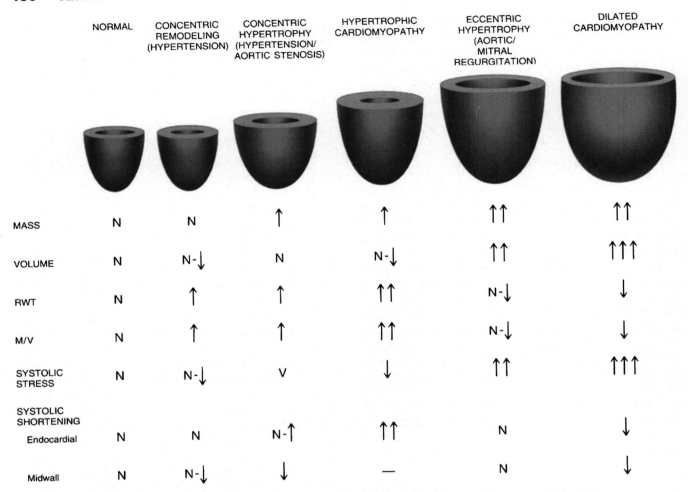

	NORMAL	CONCENTRIC REMODELING (HYPERTENSION)	CONCENTRIC HYPERTROPHY (HYPERTENSION/ AORTIC STENOSIS)	HYPERTROPHIC CARDIOMYOPATHY	ECCENTRIC HYPERTROPHY (AORTIC/ MITRAL REGURGITATION)	DILATED CARDIOMYOPATHY
MASS	N	N	↑	↑	↑↑	↑↑
VOLUME	N	N-↓	N	N-↓	↑↑	↑↑↑
RWT	N	↑	↑	↑↑	N-↓	↓
M/V	N	↑	↑	↑↑	N-↓	↓
SYSTOLIC STRESS	N	N-↓	V	↓	↑↑	↑↑↑
SYSTOLIC SHORTENING						
Endocardial	N	N	N-↑	↑↑	N	↓
Midwall	N	N-↓	↓	—	N	↓

Figure 9-10. *Left ventricular (LV) volume, mass, and geometry, stress, and systolic shortening in various cardiac disorders. Different cardiac disorders are classified with respect to LV mass, volume, relative wall thickness (RWT), and mass/volume (M/V) ratio, and stress and shortening as normal (N), increased (up arrows), or decreased (down arrows). N, normal. (Redrawn from Aurigemma GP, Gaasch WH, Villegas B, Meyer TE:* Curr Probl Cardiol *20:385, 1995.)*

Two-Dimensional Echocardiography

2D echocardiography permits acquisition of data with excellent spatial orientation because the left ventricle can be sampled in real time at multiple levels. In many laboratories, therefore, 2D echocardiography is the principal noninvasive means for quantitation of LV volume and for the assessment of global and regional systolic function. LV mass and volume quantitation by 2D echocardiography requires high-quality images and true long- and short-axis images of the left ventricle. A variety of geometric models is used to approximate the shape of the left ventricle and to compute LV volumes, including the prolate ellipse model, the hemiellipse model, and others that represent a combination of geometric shapes. Detailed review of the geometric principles underlying these volumes for formulas may be found elsewhere.[55,58,68] This chapter emphasizes the applications most suited for clinical use.

Mass

Theoretically, 2D echocardiographic assessment of LV mass can improve on the limitations of M-mode methods; mean wall thickness can be back-calculated from planimetered short-axis myocardial area, which helps avoid reliance on single-dimensional determinations. One of the most practical 2D methods for mass calculation, the area-length method, approximates the left ventricle as a cylinder-hemiellipsoid; volume is calculated for both the inner and outer "shells" (the LV cavity and total myocardial area, respectively), as shown schematically in Figure 9-11:

$$V = 5/6 \, A \times L$$

in which *A* is planimetered short-axis area obtained at the high papillary muscle level, and *L* is the LV length obtained from the apical four-chamber view; area and length measurements are made at end-diastole. In this

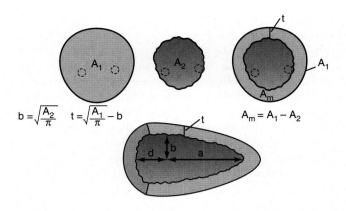

$$b = \sqrt{\frac{A_2}{\pi}} \quad t = \sqrt{\frac{A_1}{\pi}} - b \qquad A_m = A_1 - A_2$$

LV mass (AL) = 1.05 { [$\frac{5}{6}$ A$_1$ (a + d + t)] − [$\frac{5}{6}$ A$_2$ (a + d)] }

Figure 9–11. Schematic illustrating the technique used to calculate left ventricular (LV) mass with the area-length (AL) method. Endocardial and epicardial borders are traced (and papillary muscles excluded). Myocardial area (A_m) and mean wall thickness (t) are back-calculated from the LV cavity area (A_2) and total area (A_1), and minor axis radius (b). The sum a + d is equivalent to the diastolic LV cavity length, which is measured from the apical four-chamber view. (Adapted from Schiller N, Shah P, Crawford M, et al: J Am Soc Echocardiogr 2:358-367, 1989. In Aurigemma GP, Gaasch WH, Villegas B, Meyer TE: Curr Probl Cardiol 20:389, 1995.)

way, total LV and internal (LV cavity) volume are determined; myocardial volume is the difference between the inner and outer shells.[69-70] Myocardial volume is then multiplied by the specific gravity of myocardium (1.04 g/mL) to compute myocardial mass. The model has been validated by comparing echocardiographic and anatomic LV mass in 21 patients who underwent 2D echocardiographic studies shortly before death[70]; there was an excellent correlation between anatomic and echocardiographic mass (r = 0.93 and standard error = 31 g). It is important to note that phantom-generated regression equations were used to correct clinical mass measurements for each 2D echocardiographic machine. Although more complicated 2D and 3D echocardiographic methods, as previously mentioned, have been associated with greater accuracy for LV mass determination, the cylinder-hemiellipsoid area-length method represents a relatively simple and practical approach that yields acceptable results.[58]

Volume

As noted earlier, a variety of geometric approaches is described for the quantitation of LV volume from 2D echocardiography. There are theoretical advantages for use of the Simpson's rule algorithm, and this approach is preferable when ventricular shape is distorted, such as with an apical aneurysm. The Simpson's rule approach, also known as the *method of discs,* is predicated on the fact that the volume of the whole left ventricle (or of any object) may be computed as the

sum of individual "slice" volumes. In general, the accuracy of the measurement varies directly with the number of slices:

$$V = \sum_{i=1}^{n} A_i T$$

V is total volume (cavity or myocardial), *A* is planimetered area, and *T* is slice thickness. Myocardial volume is then multiplied by the specific gravity of myocardium to estimate myocardial mass. It is best to compute LV volume from two orthogonal apical views with the LV length divided equally along that length[55,68,70]; apical four- and two-chamber views at end-diastole should be recorded to maximize ventricular length. The use of the cylinder-hemiellipsoid (area-length) method for calculating the volume component represents a reasonable alternative to the method of discs.

In general, LV volumes derived from 2D echocardiographic measurements are smaller than those obtained by contrast angiography.[58,59] There are several explanations for these findings, including foreshortening of the maximal length of the left ventricle on 2D echocardiography; differences in measurement of the LV long axis; and the fact that angiographic contrast material fills intermyocardial interstices, contributing to overall LV cavity volume, whereas echocardiography does not account for this volume.[58]

Geometry

Compared with M-mode echocardiography, 2D echocardiography offers improved spatial orientation because the left ventricle can be sampled in real time at multiple levels. Accordingly, 2D echocardiography may be used to quantify the LV mass and chamber volumes of abnormally shaped ventricles, and because measurements of LV length are possible, this technique provides more extensive description of LV geometry. Estimates of both the short axis/long axis ratio and the volume/mass ratio[71-74] are possible with 2D echocardiography. In patients with normal LV mass and function, the short axis/long axis ratio ranges from 0.45 to 0.62.[72-74] In untreated hypertensive patients with normal LV systolic function, the short axis/long axis ratios range from 0.52 ± 0.04 in patients with concentric remodeling to 0.63 ± 0.03 in patients with eccentric hypertrophy. The short axis/long axis ratio also provides information regarding ventricular compensation in valvular heart disease. As in patients with dilated cardiomyopathy, in whom the ventricle becomes more spherical, patients with poorly compensated AS and AR (those with low EFs) tend to have higher short axis/long axis ratios.[74] A high ratio in turn alters the relationship of meridional to circumferential stresses, a change in the distribution of afterload that may affect overall pump performance[74] (see Fig. 9–10).

The end-diastolic volume/mass ratio in normal men and women, as defined by 2D echocardiography, is approximately 0.8.[73] It has been traditionally assumed that the ratio of LV volume to mass is relatively constant from the most basal to the most apical slices of the left ventricle. A study using the technique of ultrafast computed tomography, which can provide approximately eight tomographic slices through the left ventricle, showed that in normal subjects, the volume/mass ratio decreased from approximately 0.8 at the most basal slice, a finding consistent with results of 2D echocardiography, to approximately 0.25 at the most apical slice. LV mass exceeds LV volume at each slice location.[75]

It is important to emphasize that 2D echocardiographic methods have limitations that militate against their routine use for quantitation in the clinical setting[55] (Table 9–3). M-mode echocardiography samples at approximately 1000 frames per second, whereas the frame rate for 2D echocardiography is orders of magnitude less: 30 to 60 frames per second under optimal conditions. There is considerable image degradation when stop frames are used, making precise endocardial definition problematic. Near-field artifact and poor lateral resolution make it difficult to reliably identify endocardium around the entire ventricular perimeter. Apical views often do not yield images of sufficient quality for manual tracing and computations tend to be tedious. The use of intravenous (IV) contrast has improved the accuracy of LV volume determinations.

In view of the limitations discussed earlier, there is considerable interest in the development of online, beat-to-beat volumetric quantitation. One potential solution is the technique of automated boundary detection, which uses integrated backscatter to define a border between echocardiographic picture elements (pixels) assigned to myocardium or LV cavity.[76-79] Thus, the area of the LV cavity can be displayed for each frame, plotted with respect to time, and the fractional area change computed; the technique may be applied to images obtained from either parasternal or apical windows. Several validation studies have been performed with this technique[77-79] and have shown an excellent correlation between online LV cavity areas and offline manual planimetry of the corresponding 2D echocardiographic images (Fig. 9–12). Further software development permits online estimation of beat-to-beat LV volumes (using the area-length or Simpson's rule methods), the rate of rise in ventricular volume (dV/dt), time to peak positive dV/dt, and time to peak negative dV/dt.

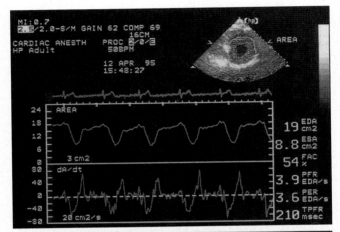

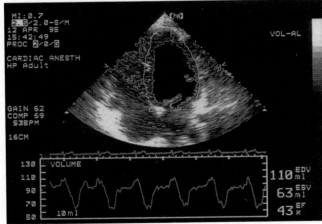

Figure 9–12. Technique of automated boundary detection and its application to the study of cardiac volumes and ejection fraction (EF) in clinical practice. Top, A parasternal short-axis image with corresponding end-diastolic and end-systolic areas (EDA and ESA, respectively); the fractional area change for each beat is also displayed below the two-dimensional image. Bottom, In an apical four-chamber view, the corresponding beat-to-beat volume display is shown. From these measurements, the EF can be computed beat to beat. End-diastolic and end-systolic volumes (EDV and ESV, respectively) are given in milliliters.

TABLE 9–3. Limitations of Ultrasound Methods for Mass and Volume Quantitation

General
All methods require high-quality images with good endocardial definition.
Most methods require geometric assumptions about left ventricular shape and are applicable only to normally shaped hearts.

M-Mode Echocardiography
Small errors in measurement may lead to large errors in mass/volume determinations.
May be insensitive to small changes in mass (20 to 40 g) observed in response to antihypertensive treatment.

Two-Dimensional Echocardiography
Limited frame rate, making timing of cardiac events difficult.
Considerable degradation when images are stop-framed.
Apical images may foreshorten true left ventricular length.
Tedious, labor-intensive computations.

As mentioned previously 3D echocardiography (see Chapter 4) has been shown to provide the most accurate US determination of LV volume, mass, and EF, largely because the need for geometric assumptions and on-axis views will be eliminated.[55,80-84]

Alternative Methods for Quantitation of Left Ventricular Structure and Function

In addition to cardiac US, the clinician may use other noninvasive and invasive techniques to measure LV size and function. A brief review of some of the more commonly used techniques is therefore appropriate.

Doppler Echocardiography

Routine Doppler measurements of flow velocity may be combined with echocardiographic dimensional data to determine SV and CO.[85,86] This technique is known as the time velocity integral (TVI) method. The appeal of this method is that, unlike M-mode and 2D echocardiographic measurements, TVI measurements do not require geometric assumptions about cardiac shape.

To compute SV using the TVI method, an integral of the systolic pulsed wave flow envelope in the aortic outflow tract is computed (Fig. 9–13). To obtain this velocity spectrum, the transducer is placed in the apical position with the sample volume positioned at the level of the aortic valve annulus. Although the TVI may be obtained in other locations, such as the pulmonary artery (PA) or LV inflow, accuracy seems to be best

with measurements made in the proximal ascending aorta. The cross-sectional linear dimension of the proximal ascending aorta is obtained in the same approximate location that the pulsed or continuous wave Doppler velocity spectrum is recorded, using the parasternal long-axis window (see Fig. 9–13). SV is then the product of the TVI and CSA of the aortic annulus, which is assumed to be circular:

$$CSA = \pi(D/2^2)$$

$$SV = CSA \cdot TVI$$

in which *CSA* is the cross-sectional area of the aortic annulus, *D* is the linear dimension of the annulus, and *TVI* is the time velocity integral. SV and CO obtained by the TVI method correlate well with results of concurrent thermodilution CO determinations in patients who were without left-sided valvular regurgitation.[85,86] The Doppler TVI method is highly dependent on accurate measurements of aortic annular diameter because the CSA formula involves squaring the annular dimension; it is also assumed that the Doppler beam is oriented parallel to flow. This method can be particularly useful for following changes in a single patient-beat to beat, or over weeks to months.

Doppler echocardiographic assessments of LV function do not depend on measurements of ventricular size (and thus avoid the attendant geometric assumptions and sources of error); they rely on information derived from flow velocities.[86] This information includes measurement of LV SV, CO, and peak flow veloc-

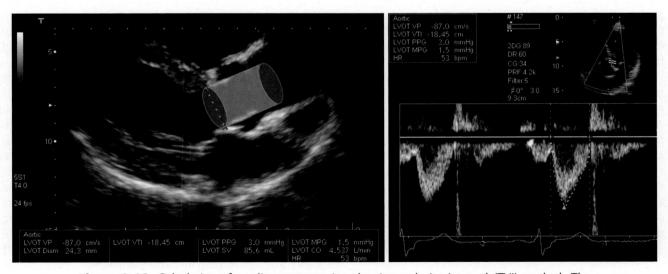

Figure 9–13. Calculation of cardiac output using the time velocity integral (TVI) method. The pulsed wave Doppler-derived TVI (also called velocity time integral [VTI]) is displayed. The left ventricular outflow tract (LVOT) dimension is approximately 24 mm, and radius 12 mm. p times the square of the annular radius yields the LVOT cross-sectional area, and the TVI is 18.5 cm by planimetry. The stroke volume is 84 mL per beat (LVOT cross-sectional area multiplied by the TVI), and yields a cardiac output of 4.5 L/min at the patient's heart rate of 53 bpm.

ity of aortic ejection, all of which, being ejection phase indices, are dependent on afterload. One approach to the noninvasive assessment of the rate of rise of ventricular pressure (dP/dt) has used the continuous wave profile of the mitral regurgitant flow.[87-89]

As we have seen, SV, and thereby CO, may be calculated by measuring the area under the flow velocity contour and multiplying it by the CSA of the annulus.[85] Accuracy is dependent on recording velocity parallel to flow and, most importantly, on the aortic diameter measurement used to calculate the CSA. This method also requires that there be no significant aortic or mitral valve disease.

Magnetic Resonance Imaging

In many respects, MRI is the ideal method to quantitate LV mass and volume. It combines the attributes of ultrafast computed tomography (noninvasive and permitting true tomographic imaging throughout the entire cardiac volume) with several unique advantages. MRI does not require contrast administration or ionizing radiation, and there is no limitation to image plane selection; thus, the heart may be imaged not only in the familiar contrast ventriculography views but also in the long- and short-axis planes used in standard transthoracic echocardiography (TTE). MRI usually provides images with excellent contrast between myocardium and the blood pool so that manual or even semiautomated computerized mass and volume quantitation is possible.[84,90] For these reasons, MRI has provided the most accurate noninvasive estimates of LV mass and volume to date,[84,91] even in ventricles distorted by myocardial infarction.[92] Gradient echocardiographic techniques display the heart in cine loop fashion at up to 64 frames per cardiac cycle; this technique can be used to quantitate EF and regional function and to estimate the severity of valvular regurgitation.[93-97]

Although MRI can be used to estimate mass, volume, and EF,[95,97] US and radionuclide techniques are currently much more commonly used for this purpose. At present, however, the use of MRI in adult clinical practice is usually confined to answering questions regarding anatomic abnormalities, such as disorders involving the aorta, the pericardium, congenital heart disease, cardiac masses, and right ventricular dysplasia.[96,98] This will likely change with further reduction in scan times and the refinement of software packages, which facilitate mass and volume quantitation.

Assessment of Left Ventricular Systolic Function

As shown in Figure 9-5, the major factors affecting LV systolic performance and function are preload, afterload, myocardial contractile (or inotropic) state, and heart rate. Nonuniform contraction can also be important; thus, regional variations in mechanical function, as occur in coronary heart disease or even with electronic ventricular pacing, can affect SV. Only if synchronous contraction is present, heart rate is stable, and loading conditions are constant does a change in performance indicate a change in contractility. These traditional concepts relating preload, afterload, and contractility are generally considered in the assessment of an acute response to altered hemodynamic conditions. Thus, an isolated increase in preload is said to produce an increment in performance through the Frank-Starling mechanism, whereas an isolated increase in afterload is said to produce a decrease in the SV (or EF) by virtue of the inverse force-shortening relation. Unfortunately, in the intact heart, especially in patients with chronic heart disease, it is virtually impossible to produce an *isolated* change in preload or afterload. For example, nitrates are classified as vasodilators and agents that primarily affect preload, but the associated decrease in LV volume and arterial pressure leads to a reduction in afterload. Likewise, a pure arterial vasodilator also reduces heart size (and preload) by augmenting the SV. It is apparent, therefore, that preload and afterload are intimately related, and that it is an oversimplification to assume that isolated changes in preload or afterload occur in patients with chronic heart disease.

Most interventions that produce an acute change in preload or afterload also result in a length-dependent change in intrinsic myocardial contractility,[99] which further complicates the assessment of global systolic function. Therefore, acute changes in preload produce changes in performance through the Frank-Starling mechanism *and* through this length-dependent activation. The importance of this phenomenon in the chronically enlarged or diseased heart is unknown.

It is usually not difficult to detect an acute change in LV performance or contractile function, but it is harder to determine the major mechanism or mechanisms responsible for the change. Chronic changes in LV volume, mass, and geometry are even more difficult to interpret because such changes tend to limit our use of the traditional interrelationships of preload, afterload, and contractility. Indeed, there is no acceptable index of basal contractility that can be used in patients with chronic heart disease, nor can LV end-diastolic pressure or even absolute EDV be used as a surrogate for fiber stretch in chronically diseased hearts. For these and other reasons, the evaluation of contractile function and the distinction between a compensated and a decompensated ventricle often rest on empiric observations coupled with analyses based on physiologic principles. In the following section the use and limitations of several clinically useful approaches to the evaluation of contractile function are discussed (Table 9-4).

TABLE 9–4. Clinical Methods Used to Evaluate Systolic Function

Ejection fraction
Fractional shortening at endocardium and midwall
Stress-shortening relations
Pressure-volume analysis

Ejection Fraction

The EF is the most widely used measure of LV systolic function. This parameter is defined as the change in LV volume (i.e., SV) divided by the initial volume (i.e., EDV):

$$EF = (EDV - ESV)/EDV$$

in which *EDV* is end-diastolic volume and *ESV* is end-systolic volume; these may be obtained by either M-mode or 2D echocardiography.[55] The EF, representing volume strain, is appropriately normalized; it can be used as an index of systolic function that is independent of the size of the patient or the ventricle.

The normal ventricle ejects more than half of its EDV; the average EF, as determined by 2D echocardiography, varies from 63% to 69%.[55,71] In patients with coronary disease or idiopathic cardiomyopathy, it is generally conceded that values in the range of 40% to 50% are abnormal but of little clinical significance.[1] However, in patients with MR, an EF in this range may denote significant depression in contractile function.[100]

Hemodynamic Determinants of the Ejection Fraction

Acute changes in LV loading conditions are known to exert a major influence on the EF. Thus, an acute increase in preload and/or a decrease in afterload results in a higher EF. By contrast, an acute decrease in preload and/or an increase in afterload reduces the EF. Under such circumstances, it can be difficult to decide whether a change in contractility has occurred. If, however, alterations in load are associated with a change in the EF that is opposite to the expected result, it is possible to conclude that a simultaneous change in contractility (i.e., inotropic state) also occurred. For example, an increased EF in the presence of increased afterload likely represents increased contractility because an increase in afterload would normally be expected to cause a lower EF. Despite its load sensitivity, the EF can therefore provide useful information, even during acute hemodynamic interventions. In this regard, the concept of preload reserve is important.

In patients with chronic heart disease, the EF can be an important index of contractile function, in part because of its sensitivity to increased afterload. As LV

dysfunction develops and dilation occurs, afterload tends to increase, as dictated by the Laplace relationship, and the EF falls. Such a decline in the EF can be useful in identifying LV dysfunction early in the course of a disease; it does not, however, identify the underlying mechanism or mechanisms. Therefore, in patients with chronic heart disease, the EF must be interpreted with consideration of the magnitude and time course of changes in loading conditions that evolve during progression of the disease. For example, early in the course of AR, LV preload and afterload tend to be increased; these changes affect the EF in opposite directions, and it remains within the normal range. As the ventricle remodels and eccentric hypertrophy develops, the loads normalize despite LV enlargement; if myocardial contractility is preserved, the EF remains normal. As the hemodynamic burden increases (or contractile dysfunction develops), the afterload increases and the EF decreases. Thus, even a modest decline in the EF can be an important early marker of LV dysfunction.

In decompensated AS, LV systolic pressures increase in parallel with an increase in wall stress, as predicted by the Laplace relationship. As wall stress progressively rises, EF decreases. Carabello and colleagues[16] have shown that patients with critical AS, congestive heart failure, and decreased EF owing to high levels of wall stress ("afterload mismatch") may anticipate improvement in systolic function following afterload reduction associated with valve replacement[16,100,101] (Fig. 9–14). By contrast, those patients whose reduction in EF is out of proportion to the high levels of wall stress are thought to have developed cardiomyopathic changes in addition to excess afterload; such patients generally do not experience functional improvement after valve replacement.[16,101] This subgroup of patients may be identifiable by a low transvalvular gradient (usually less than 30 mm Hg) in association with severe stenosis of the aortic valve.[16] In the clinical setting, making the proper diagnosis can be challenging. Because the Gorlin equation is flow dependent, patients with primary LV dysfunction and coexistent (mild) calcific AS can be difficult to distinguish from those with LV dysfunction caused by unrelieved severe aortic AS. Dobutamine echocardiography is increasingly used to help make this distinction and to assess prognosis.[102]

Fractional Shortening and Related Indices

The fractional change (percentage) in minor-axis dimension is a widely used index of systolic performance; fractional shortening is usually derived from M-mode echocardiographic tracings (see Fig. 9–8). This measurement is particularly useful because LV circumferential fiber shortening is responsible for most of the SV. In this regard, fractional shortening is similar to the EF; in the absence of focal wall motion abnormalities, the two indices correlate closely, although the absolute

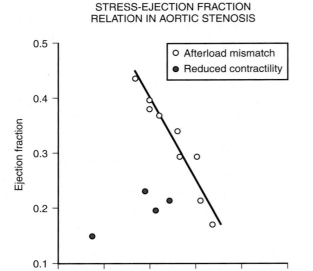

STRESS-EJECTION FRACTION
RELATION IN AORTIC STENOSIS

○ Afterload mismatch
● Reduced contractility

Figure 9–14. Relationship between ejection fraction (EF) and end-systolic stress in patients undergoing cardiac catheterization for critical aortic stenosis and severe congestive heart failure. All patients were free of significant coronary artery disease. Patients falling close to the regression line relating EF to stress (open circles) are thought to have left ventricular (LV) dysfunction owing to excessive wall stress (afterload). These patients experienced a gratifying functional recovery after aortic valve replacement. In contrast, the four subjects who fell below the regression line (blue circles) have depressed EF beyond that predicted by the level of afterload and are considered to have depressed contractility as well. These patients did not experience functional recovery after valve replacement. (Adapted from Carabello BA, Green LH, Grossman W, et al: Circulation 62:42, 1980. In Aurigemma GP, Gaasch WH, Villegas B, Meyer TE: Curr Probl Cardiol 20:416, 1995.)

values for fractional shortening are obviously less than that for EF. Fractional shortening, measured at the endocardium (FS_{endo} [%]), is calculated as

$$FS_{endo} = 100 \times (LVID_d - LVID_s)/(LVID_d)$$

Normal values for FS_{endo} exceed 25%.[55] As is the case with EF, FS_{endo} is influenced by factors in addition to contractile state and should be interpreted in the light of loading conditions; increases in preload and decreases in afterload increase fractional shortening.

A refinement of fractional shortening, the velocity of circumferential shortening (V_{cf}) reflects the mean velocity of ventricular shortening at the level of the LV minor axis, and it is also calculated from M-mode echocardiographic dimensions:

$$V_{cf} = FS_{endo}/ET$$

in which *ET* is the ejection time derived either from the duration of aortic valve opening, from the period

of aortic forward flow (pulsed-wave or continuous-wave Doppler), or from a carotid pulse tracing. The V_{cf} is expressed in circumferences per second (the lower limit of normal is 1.1 c/sec); because V_{cf} measures the velocity rather than the extent of shortening, it is theoretically a more sensitive index of contractility than FS_{endo} and may be an earlier marker of abnormality in chronic disease states. As with the EF and fractional shortening, this parameter is normalized for LV chamber size and may be used to make comparisons between patients. V_{cf} has been shown to be relatively insensitive to acute changes in preload.[103,104] However, it is also possible that this preload insensitivity may be a result of acute elevations in preload increasing heart size (and pressure) and thus increasing afterload. Thus, augmentation in afterload may offset the increased shortening caused by the increased preload. A further refinement in V_{cf}, the rate-corrected V_{cf},[102] may be obtained by dividing V_{cf} by the square root of the preceding RR interval. This index is designed to allow comparison between patients with differing heart rates. The incremental value of velocity of shortening methods (e.g., V_{cf}, rate-corrected V_{cf}), compared with extent of shortening (e.g., fractional shortening) may be marginal.[105]

Standard M-mode measurements also may be used to estimate circumferential fractional shortening at the midwall (FS_{mw} [%]), using the same standard M-mode echocardiographic measurements. FS_{mw} is calculated using a modified two-shell cylindrical model.[106] This method assumes constant LV mass throughout the cardiac cycle and does not require the assumption that inner and outer wall thickening fractions are equal.[107,108] Most important, in contrast to FS_{endo}, FS_{mw} is not influenced by LV geometry (RWT) and therefore has particular use in the evaluation of the hypertrophied heart with increased RWT (see Fig. 9–16).

Normal systolic function includes the excursion of the mitral annulus toward the relatively immobile apex; thus, the long axis of the left ventricle shortens during systole.[43] An assessment of the longitudinal (or long-axis) shortening of the left ventricle can be made using M-mode measurements under 2D echocardiographic guidance.[43,108] Using the apical window, the transducer is oriented to maximize apical endocardial to mitral annular distance. M-mode tracings are made with the cursor directed through the lateral aspects of the mitral annulus; recordings of multiple cardiac cycles are made on strip chart paper,[109] and mitral annular excursion is normalized for initial diastolic length.

Several investigators have used mitral annular excursion and long-axis shortening as a descriptor of ventricular systolic function. Keren and LeJemtel[110] showed that the principal systolic mitral annular excursion toward the apex coincides with the systolic component of pulmonary venous flow; this systolic phase of mitral annular motion is markedly attenuated in patients with dilated cardiomyopathy. Jones and Gibson[109] showed that in the normal left ventricle mitral annular excursion toward the apex precedes circumferential shortening, which leads to a more spherical LV shape early in systole.[109] These investigators also showed that mitral annular descent was reduced in patients with mitral disease who had undergone valve replacement.[109] In patients with "compensated" hypertensive heart disease, that is, LV hypertrophy and normal EF, long-axis shortening is depressed compared with normal controls.[108] Similar findings have been reported using the technique of MRI tagging, as will be described later.[111]

Other US techniques have been employed in recent years to investigate LV systolic and diastolic function. Doppler tissue imaging applies a modification of pulsed Doppler methods to the assessment of myocardial systolic motion.[112,113] In this way, the velocity of myocardial tissue or of the mitral annulus, and not just the total excursion, may be measured. The velocity of the diastolic mitral annular motion has been applied to the study of LV diastolic function (Chapters 5 and 11).[112-113] This technique is now being employed to evaluate the extent of systolic dyssynchrony and to evaluate the appropriateness of biventricular pacemaker implantation[114,115] and patients with acute ischemia.[116]

Stress-Shortening Relations

On the basis of extensive experimental and clinical experience, the myocardial force-velocity relation provides a framework for evaluating the contractile state and function of the left ventricle. A most important advantage of assessing function with a stress-shortening analysis is that it avoids afterload dependency, the major limitation of the EF alone. Unfortunately, end-diastolic fiber length (or the degree to which the resting fiber is stretched) is difficult if not impossible to measure; LV end-diastolic pressure, EDV, or even wall stress fails to provide an absolute measure of fiber length. For this reason, length is generally omitted and the simpler force-velocity or stress-shortening relation is used as a substitute for the force-length-velocity relation.

Both systolic stress (the force per unit CSA of myocardium) and shortening (fractional change in length or volume) are appropriately normalized and allow accurate comparisons among hearts of different sizes.[117] Therefore, contractile function in pressure overload hypertrophy, volume overload hypertrophy, and dilated and hypertrophic cardiomyopathies may be assessed within the framework of the stress-shortening relation.

A major limitation of the simple stress-shortening analysis is the assumption that differences in resting length do not substantially influence the stress-shortening relation. In this regard, a distinction must be made between acute interventions and chronic steady-state conditions. Changes in fiber length and appropriate use of preload reserve certainly occur during acute or short-term hemodynamic interventions. However, under chronic conditions (e.g., chronic compensated volume overload), this may not be the case.[118] After the acute or subacute phase, when the compensatory remodeling process is complete and chronic changes in LV volume and mass are established, end-diastolic fiber length may not be substantially different from normal.[119] In pressure overload or concentric hypertrophy, end-diastolic sarcomere lengths may even be less than normal.[120,121] In such hearts, high chamber stiffness apparently limits use of the preload reserve. It appears, therefore, that assumptions about chronic changes in fiber length are unwarranted.

Midwall Stress-Shortening Analysis

The analysis of midwall stress-shortening relations may be superior to that of endocardial stress-shortening relations, especially for comparison of contractile state between hearts differing in LV geometry (Figs. 9–15 and 9–16). The first advantage of midwall measurements is that the (circumferential) stress vector and the shortening transient are oriented in the same direction because circumferential fibers predominate in the midwall of the LV.[122-123]

Second, the values for midwall (but not endocardial) shortening are consonant with experimental data indicating that myocardial fibers shorten by approximately 15% to 20%. Circumferential midwall strain ranges from 9% ± 2% in the anesthetized, open-chest dog (implanted markers)[124] to 30% ± 7% in conscious humans (MRI tagging).[125] We believe that the experimental results represent an underestimate of strain, but MRI techniques likely overestimate true myocardial shortening. All methods indicate that circumferential shortening at the endocardium exceeds that seen at the midwall. We believe that studies designed to assess myocardial contractile function should ideally be based on midwall stress-shortening data and not on endocardial shortening parameters, which may be contaminated by altered ventricular geometry.

An example of the usefulness of a midwall stress-shortening analysis is shown in Figure 9–17. The endocardial stress-shortening relation is normal in patients with pressure overload hypertrophy owing to AS; thus, LV function is normal. By contrast, the midwall stress-shortening relation is abnormal in approximately one

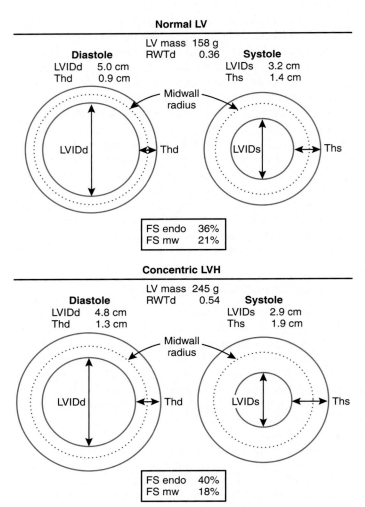

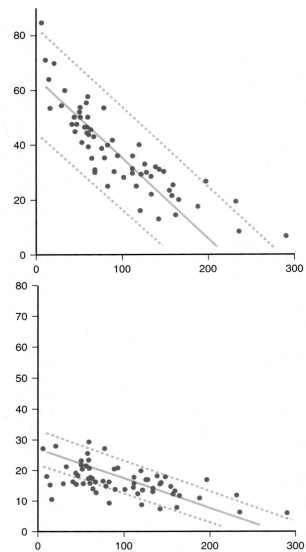

Figure 9–15. *Left ventricular (LV) shortening in normal LV (top) and in concentric left ventricular hypertrophy (LVH) (bottom), illustrating the added insight into systolic function provided by midwall shortening. LV endocardial dimension (LVID), wall thickness (Th), relative wall thickness (RWT), and LV mass are measured in diastole (d). The systolic dimensions (s) are shown at right. The midwall circumference is indicated by the dotted line. Systolic shortening refers to the percent reduction in the circumference that occurs from diastole to systole. FS endo, the percent reduction of the endocardial circumference (dark inner circle), and FS mw, the percent reduction of the midwall circumference (dotted line), are in the normal range. However, concentric LVH (elevated relative wall thickness dimension (RWTd) and LV mass) is associated with an increased value for FS endo, but a diminution in FS mw, compared with normal LV, owing to the nonuniformity of systolic thickening. Myocardial fibers in the inner (subendocardial) layers contribute more to systolic thickening than those in the outer (epicardial) layers; this effect is exaggerated when concentric geometry is present.*

Figure 9–16. *Endocardial and midwall stress-shortening relations in pressure overload hypertrophy. The top panel shows fractional shortening at the endocardium versus circumferential stress in a consecutive series of patients with severe, symptomatic aortic stenosis who were free of segmental wall motion abnormalities. All patients fall within the 95% confidence intervals of the stress-shortening relationship, suggesting normal contractile function. In contrast, the bottom panel shows midwall shortening versus circumferential stress in the same population. A substantial portion (approximately one third) of these patients demonstrates a diminution in contractility by the midwall analysis.*

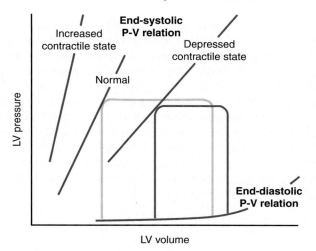

Figure 9–17. Left ventricular (LV) pressure-volume (P-V) loops. The yellow loop indicates a normal ventricle. An acute decrease in contractile state is shown in purple; the loop is displaced to the right, and the end-systolic P-V line shifts downward and to the right. The effect of an acute increase in contractile state is illustrated by the line on the left; the slope of the end-systolic P-V line is increased (the corresponding loop is not shown). (From Aurigemma GP, Gaasch WH, Villegas B, Meyer TE: Curr Probl Cardiol 20:418, 1995.)

third of the patients, indicating a subtle depression of myocardial function in these individuals.[43]

Pressure-Volume Analysis

By plotting LV pressure against volume throughout the entire cardiac cycle, a P-V loop can be generated (Fig. 9–18). The height of the loop is determined by systolic pressure, and its width is determined by SV; thus, the area within the loop is a measure of stroke work. By definition, such loops incorporate EDV and ESV; thus, the SV and the EF are displayed. The bottom limb of the loop (i.e., the diastolic P-V curve) describes ventricular diastolic compliance. Therefore, the P-V loop can provide a simple yet comprehensive description of ventricular pump function.[126] Such loops can be generated from a variety of techniques that provide ventricular volume data in conjunction with LV pressure.[127-129] Online, beat-to-beat determinations of LV volumes with automated edge detection can be combined with LV pressure measurements to yield real-time pressure-volume loops, useful in both clinical and research settings[129-131] (Fig. 9–19).

By manipulating LV volume and/or arterial pressure, multiple coordinates of the maximal ratio of pressure to volume or dimension (which occurs near end-ejection) can be obtained; these coordinates exhibit a nearly linear direct relation. The slope of this relation (E_{max}) is relatively insensitive to acute changes in loading conditions. The relation shifts upward and to the left during positive inotropic interventions, and it shifts downward to the right when the ventricle is depressed; the slope of the relation generally increases with the former and decreases with the latter (see Figs. 9–18 and 9–19).

This end-systolic index of contractility is sensitive to acute changes in contractility, but its reliability is diminished in chronically diseased hearts, especially dilated hearts. In large ventricles the end-systolic P-V curve can be displaced down and to the right (depressed E_{max}), in the absence of a depressed contractility. For this reason, E_{max} should be normalized for heart

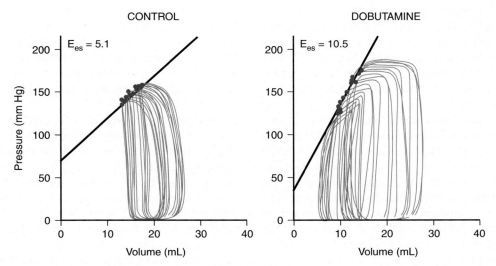

Figure 9–18. Pressure-volume loops with inferior vena caval occlusion at baseline and with 3 μg/kg/min of dobutamine infusion in an intact canine model. Volume was assessed online with transesophageal echocardiographic border detection using a Simpson's rule algorithm. End-systolic elastance (E_{es}) or the slope of the end-systolic pressure-volume (P-V) relation, increased with positive inotropic modulation, which is consistent with increased contractility. (Courtesy Dr. John Gorcsan III.)

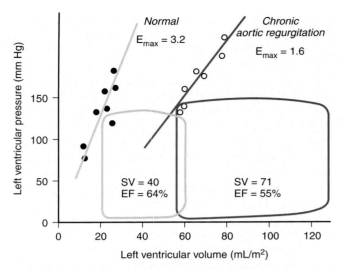

Figure 9–19. Left ventricular pressure-volume loops and end-systolic pressure-volume lines illustrate the effects of chronic aortic regurgitation on ventricular size and function. Moderate ventricular enlargement is present, ejection fraction (EF) is normal, and stroke volume (SV) is high. Such data are consistent with compensated aortic regurgitation. However, the slope of the end-systolic pressue-volume relation (E_{max}) is reduced. This apparent inconsistency may be resolved by considering the effect of chamber size on E_{max}. If the slope is normalized for chamber size (end-diastolic volume), the result indicates that E_{max} is similar in the two ventricles. (Adapted from Shen WF, Roubin G, Choong CYP, et al: Circulation 71:31-38, 1985. In Aurigemma GP, Gaasch WH, Villegas B, Meyer TE: Curr Probl Cardiol 20:420, 1995.)

size,[132-134] as illustrated in Figure 9–19. In this example of chronic AR, there is modest LV enlargement, the ESV is less than 60 mL/m² the EF is normal, and the total SV is high. Such data indicate that the ventricle is compensated, albeit larger than normal. However, the depressed slope of the end-systolic P-V relation inappropriately suggests depressed contractility. These disparate conclusions can be reconciled if the effect of chamber dilation on E_{max} is considered.[132-134] Thus, if the slope is normalized for chamber size, it approximates that seen in the normal heart.

Recognizing this limitation, end-systolic stress-volume or stress-dimension relations should not be a major criterion for the diagnosis of chronic contractile dysfunction. Certainly, it is not useful as a measure of basal contractility, and it has limited applicability in comparisons among normal and diseased hearts. The raw P-V or stress-dimension data provide important diagnostic information and, with few exceptions, the simple measurement of the ESV or dimension identifies a depressed ventricle.

An example of the usefulness of echocardiography pressure-dimension loops is shown in Figure 9–20. This example illustrates the effect of mitral valve re-

placement on LV size and function in compensated and decompensated chronic MR. In compensated MR the chamber is enlarged but the end-systolic dimension is only 42 mm, systolic stress is minimally increased, and the fractional shortening is normal (35%). After valve replacement the stress-dimension loop returns to near normal. In decompensated MR the EDV and ESV are markedly increased and fractional shortening is low (26%). After mitral valve replacement there is persistent LV enlargement and a further decline in shortening. A similar analysis has been used in patients with AR.[135] (See also Chapter 19.)

Potential Limitations

It is worthwhile to briefly reiterate some of the practical limitations of echocardiographic evaluation of LV structure and function. It is axiomatic that quantitation of mass and volumes requires high-quality echocardiographic images, with good endocardial definition for a variety of reasons, such high-quality images may not be available in many patients encountered in clinical practice. As noted previously, M-mode (and most 2D) quantitative methods require that the ventricle not have major shape distortion. Meticulous attention to beam orientation is also imperative for M-mode quantitation of the LV; every millimeter of inaccuracy in LV chamber dimension results in an 8-g difference in LV mass[80]; a 1-mm inaccuracy in LV wall thickness measurement results in a 15-g difference in LV mass. Moreover, experience with the technique of 3D echocardiography[81,82] raises significant questions about whether US beam orientation is truly orthogonal to the long axis of the LV in routine clinical practice. These findings may help to explain why, for the individual patient, serial M-mode echocardiographic studies may be insensitive to the 20- to 40-g changes in LV mass that are observed, on average, in response to antihypertensive treatment.[136,137]

As noted previously, 2D echocardiographic methods also have limitations, including limited frame rate (which renders precise timing of cardiac events difficult), near-field artifacts, and poor lateral resolution. Apical views often do not yield images of sufficient quality for manual tracing, and foreshortening of the long axis of the left ventricle leads, in part, to volume estimates lower than those obtained by contrast ventriculography. Despite these important limitations, however, quantitative US techniques find widespread clinical and research applications because of their portability and low cost, and because results are immediately obtainable.

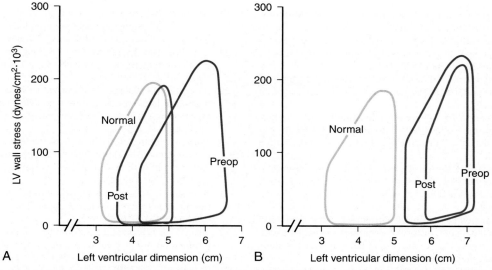

Figure 9–20. *Left ventricular (LV) stress-dimension loops in two cases of mitral regurgitation, before (Preop) and after (Post) mitral valve replacement. A, The preoperative loop indicates compensated ventricular function; the end-diastolic dimension is 6.5 cm, the end-systolic dimension is 4.2 cm, systolic stress is minimally elevated, and fractional shortening is normal (35%). After valve replacement the end-diastolic dimension and end-systolic wall stress return to normal but fractional shortening decreases (29%). B, The preoperative loop indicates a decompensated ventricle; the end-diastolic and end-systolic dimensions are markedly increased (7.3 cm and 5.4 cm, respectively) and fractional shortening is low (26%). After valve replacement there is persistent LV enlargement and a further decline in fractional shortening. These examples illustrate the LV response to mitral valve replacement in compensated and decompensated mitral regurgitation. (From Aurigemma GP, Gaasch WH, Villegas B, Meyer TE:* Curr Probl Cardiol *20:421, 1995.)*

KEY POINTS

■ Assessment of LV mass, volume, and geometry is critical for the management of patients and the assessment of prognosis.

■ Current noninvasive methods, M-mode echocardiography, 2D echocardiography, and 3D echocardiography are utilized for assessment of mass, volume, and shape. Each has strengths and limitations.

■ Assessment of LV systolic function generally involves computation of the EF, but other aspects of systolic function, such as SV and CO, can be calculated as well.

■ A major limitation of EF is its dependence on load; this limitation is particularly important in the assessment of systolic function in valvular heart disease.

■ There are compelling advantages to use of mid-wall shortening as an index of systolic function when the left ventricle has undergone hypertrophic remodeling in response to hypertension.

REFERENCES

1. Gaasch WH: Diagnosis and treatment of heart failure based on LV systolic or diastolic dysfunction. *JAMA* 271:1276-1280, 1994.
2. Mock MB, Rindqvist I, Fisher LD, et al: Survival of medically treated patients in the coronary artery surgery (CASS) registry. *Circulation* 66:562-567, 1982.
3. White HD, Norris RM, Brown MA, et al: Left ventricular end systolic volume as the major determinant of survival after recovery from myocardial infarction. *Circulation* 76:44-51, 1987.
4. Pfeffer MA, Braunwald E, Moye LA, et al: Effect of captopril on mortality and morbidity in patients with left ventricular dysfunction after myocardial infarction: Results of the survival and ventricular enlargement trial. *N Engl J Med* 327:669-677, 1992.
5. The SOLVD Investigators: Effect of enalapril on survival in patients with reduced left ventricular ejection fractions and congestive heart failure. *N Engl J Med* 325:293-302, 1991.
6. Gottdiener JS, Arnold AM, Aurigemma GP, et al: Predictors of congestive heart failure in the elderly: The Cardiovascular Health Study. *J Am Coll Cardiol* 35:1628-1637, 2000.
7. Aurigemma GP, Gottdiener JS, Shemanski L, et al: Predictive value of systolic and diastolic function for incident congestive heart failure in the elderly: The Cardiovascular Health Study. *J Am Coll Cardiol* 37:1042-1048, 2001.
8. Gottdiener JS, McClelland RL, Marshall R, et al: Outcome of congestive heart failure in elderly persons: influence of left

ventricular systolic function. The Cardiovascular Health Study. *Ann Intern Med* 137(8):31-39, 2002.

9. Bonow RO, Carabello B, DeLeon A, et al: ACC/AHA guidelines for the management of patients with valvular heart disease. *J Am Coll Cardiol* 32(5):1486-1588, 1998.

10. Schuler G, Peterson KL, Johnson A, et al: Temporal response of left ventricular performance to mitral valve surgery. *Circulation* 59:1218-1231, 1979.

11. Gaasch WH, Carroll JD, Levine HJ, et al: Chronic aortic regurgitation: Prognostic value of left ventricular end-systolic dimension and end-diastolic radius/thickness ratio. *J Am Coll Cardiol* 1:775-782, 1983.

12. Zile MR, Gaasch WH, Carroll JD, et al: Chronic mitral regurgitation: Predictive value of preoperative echocardiographic indexes of left ventricular function and wall stress. *J Am Coll Cardiol* 3:235-242, 1984.

13. Bonow RO, Lakatos E, Maron BJ, Epstein SE. Serial long-term assessment of the natural history of asymptomatic patients with chronic aortic regurgitation and normal left ventricular systolic function. *Circulation* 84(4):625-635, 1991.

14. Carabello BA, Usher BW, Hendrix GH, et al: Predictors of outcome for aortic valve replacement in patients with aortic regurgitation and left ventricular dysfunction: A change in the measuring stick. *J Am Coll Cardiol* 10:991-997, 1987.

15. Crawford MH, Souchek J, Oprian CA, et al: Determinants of survival and left ventricular performance after mitral valve replacement. *Circulation* 81:1173-1181, 1990.

16. Carabello BA, Green LH, Grossman W, et al: Hemodynamic determination of prognosis of aortic valve replacement in critical aortic stenosis and advanced congestive heart failure. *Circulation* 62:42, 1980.

17. Connolly HM, Oh JK, Schaff HV, et al: Severe aortic stenosis with low transvalvular gradient and severe left ventricular dysfunction: Result of aortic valve replacement in 52 patients. *Circulation* 101:1940-1946, 2000.

18. Collinson J, Henein M, Flather M, et al: Valve replacement for aortic stenosis in patients with poor left ventricular function: Comparison of early changes with stented and stentless valves. *Circulation* 100(19 suppl):II1-5, 1999.

19. Orsinelli DA, Aurigemma GP, Battista S, et al: Left ventricular hypertrophy and mortality after aortic valve replacement for aortic stenosis: A high risk subgroup identified by preoperative relative wall thickness. *J Am Coll Cardiol* 22:1679-1683, 1993.

20. Aurigemma G, Battista S, Orsinelli D, et al: Abnormal left ventricular intracavitary flow acceleration in patients undergoing aortic valve replacement for aortic stenosis: A marker for high postoperative morbidity and mortality. *Circulation* 86:926-936, 1992.

21. Casale PN, Devereux RB, Milner M, et al: Value of echocardiographic measurement of left ventricular mass in predicting cardiovascular morbid events in hypertensive men. *Ann Intern Med* 105:173-178, 1986.

22. Levy D, Garrison RJ, Savage D, et al: Prognostic implications of echocardiographically determined left ventricular mass in the Framingham Heart Study. *N Engl J Med* 322:1561-1566, 1990.

23. Levy D, Garrison RJ, Savage D, et al: Left ventricular mass and incidence of coronary heart disease in an elderly cohort. *Ann Intern Med* 110:101-107, 1990.

24. Koren M, Devereux R, Casale PN, et al: Relation of LV mass and geometry to morbidity and mortality in uncomplicated essential hypertension. *Ann Intern Med* 114:345-352, 1991.

25. Verdecchia P, Schillaci G, Borgioni C, et al: Adverse prognostic significance of concentric remodeling of the left ventricle in hypertensive patients with normal left ventricular mass. *J Am Coll Cardiol* 25:871-878, 1995.

26. Devereux R: Left ventricular geometry, pathophysiology and prognosis. *J Am Coll Cardiol* 25:885-887, 1995.

27. Ganau A, Devereux RB, Roman MJ, et al: Patterns of left ventricular hypertrophy and geometric remodeling in essential hypertension. *J Am Coll Cardiol* 19(7):550-558, 1992.

28. Krumholz HM, Larson M, Levy D: Prognosis of left ventricular geometric patterns in the Framingham Heart Study. *J Am Coll Cardiol* 25:879, 1995.

29. Buchalter MB, Weiss JL, Rogers WJ, et al: Noninvasive quantification of left ventricular rotational deformation in normal humans using magnetic resonance imaging myocardial tagging. *Circulation* 81:1236-1244, 1990.

30. Notomi Y, Setser RM, Shiota T, et al: Assessment of left ventricular torsional deformation by Doppler tissue imaging: validation study with tagged magnetic resonance imaging. *Circulation* 111(9):141-147, 2005.

31. Dumesnil J: A mathematical model of the dynamic geometry of the intact left ventricle and its application to clinical data. *Circulation* 59:1024-1034, 1979.

32. Reichek N, Wilson J, St. John Sutton M, et al. Noninvasive determination of left ventricular end-systolic stress: Validation of the method and initial application. *Circulation* 65:99-108, 1982.

33. Gaasch WH, Zile MR, Hoshino PK, et al: Stress-shortening relations and myocardial blood flow in compensated and failing canine hearts with pressure overload hypertrophy. *Circulation* 79:872-883, 1989.

34. St. John Sutton M, Plappert T, Hirshfeld JW, et al: Assessment of left ventricular mechanics in patients with asymptomatic aortic regurgitation: A two-dimensional echocardiographic study. *Circulation* 69:259-270, 1984.

35. Mirsky I: Review of the various theories for evaluation of left ventricular wall stress. In Mirsky I, Chiston DN, Sandler H, (eds): *Cardiac Mechanics: Physiological, Chemical, and Mathematical Considerations.* New York, John Wiley, 1974.

36. Douglas PS, Reichek N, Plappert T, et al: Comparison of echocardiographic methods for assessment of left ventricular shortening and wall stress. *J Am Coll Cardiol* 9:945-951, 1987.

37. Colan SD, Borow KM, Neumann A: Use of the calibrated carotid pulse tracing for calculation of left ventricular pressure and wall stress throughout ejection. *Am Heart J* 109:1306-1310, 1985.

38. Rozich JD, Carabello BA, Usher BW, et al: Mitral valve replacement with and without chordal preservation in patients with chronic mitral regurgitation. *Circulation* 86:1718-1726, 1992.

39. Gaasch WH, Battle WE, Oboler AD, et al: Left ventricular stress and compliance in man: With special reference to normalized ventricular function curves. *Circulation* 45:746-762, 1972.

40. Clyne CA, Arrighi JA, Maron BJ, et al: Systemic and LV responses to exercise stress in asymptomatic patients with valvular aortic stenosis. *Am J Cardiol* 68:1469-1476, 1991.

41. Cuocolo A, Sax F, Brush J, et al: Left ventricular hypertrophy and impaired diastolic filling in essential hypertension. *Circulation* 81:978-986, 1990.

42. Kitzman D, Higginbotham M, Cobb F, et al: Exercise intolerance in patients with heart failure and preserved LV systolic function. *J Am Coll Cardiol* 7:1065-1072, 1991.

43. Aurigemma GP, Zile MR, Gaasch WH: Contractile behavior of the left ventricle in diastolic heart failure: with emphasis on regional systolic function. *Circulation* 113:296-304, 2006.

44. Bonow RO, Udelson JE: LV diastolic dysfunction as a cause of congestive heart failure. *Ann Intern Med* 117:502-510, 1992.

45. Schwinger RH, Bohm M, Koch A, et al: The failing heart is unable to use the Frank-Starling mechanism. *Circ Res* 74:959-969, 1994.

46. Ross J Jr: Afterload mismatch and preload reserve: A conceptual framework for the analysis of ventricular function. *Prog Cardiovasc Dis* 18:255-264, 1976.

47. Grossman W, Jones D, McLaurin LP: Wall stress and patterns of hypertrophy in the human left ventricle. *J Clin Invest* 56:56-64, 1975.

48. Pouleur H, Covell JW, Ross J Jr: Effects of alterations in aortic input impedance on the force-velocity-length relationship in the intact canine heart. *Circ Res* 45:126-135, 1979.

49. Gaasch WH: LV radius to wall thickness ratio. *Am J Cardiol* 43:1189-1194, 1979.

50. Goldfine H, Aurigemma GP, Zile MR, Gaasch WH: Left ventricular length-force-shortening relations before and after surgical correction of chronic mitral regurgitation. *J Am Coll Cardiol* 31:180-185, 1998.

51. Carabello BA, Spann JF: The uses and limitations of end-systolic indices of left ventricular function. *Circulation* 69:1058-1064, 1984.

52. Sagawa K: The end-systolic pressure-volume relationship of the ventricle: Definitions, modifications, and clinical use. *Circulation* 61:1223-1227, 1981.

53. Douglas PS, Morrow R, Ioli A, et al: Left ventricular shape, afterload and survival in idiopathic dilated cardiomyopathy. *J Am Coll Cardiol* 13:311-315, 1989.

54. Borow KM, Lang RM, Neumann A, et al: Physiologic mechanisms governing hemodynamic responses to positive inotropic therapy in patients with dilated cardiomyopathy. *Circulation* 77:625-637, 1988.

55. Lang RM, Bierig M, Devereux RB, et al: Recommendations for chamber quantification: A report from the American Society of Echocardiography's Guidelines and Standards Committee and the Chamber Quantification Writing Group, developed in conjunction with the European Association of Echocardiography, a branch of the European Society of Cardiology. *J Am Soc Echocardiogr* 18(2):1440-1463, 2005.

56. Devereux R, Reichek N: Echocardiographic determination of left ventricular mass in man. Anatomic validation of the method. *Circulation* 55:613-618, 1977.

57. Devereux RB, Alonso D, Lutas E, et al: Echocardiographic assessment of left ventricular hypertrophy: Comparison to necropsy findings. *Am J Cardiol* 57:450-458, 1986.

58. Vuille C, Weyman AE: Left ventricle I: General considerations, assessment of chamber size and function. In Weyman AE (ed): *Principles and Practice of Echocardiography,* 2nd ed. Philadelphia, Lea & Febiger, 1994, pp. 575-624.

59. Teichholz LE, Kreulen T, Herman MV, et al: Problems in echocardiographic volume determinations: Echocardiographic-angiographic correlations in the presence or absence of asynergy. *Am J Cardiol* 37:7-12, 1976.

60. Kronik G, Slany J, Mosslacher H: Comparative value of eight M-mode echocardiographic formulas for determining left ventricular stroke volume. *Circulation* 60:1308-1316, 1979.

61. Ford LE: Heart size. *Circ Res* 39:297, 1976.

62. Aurigemma G, Silver K, McLaughlin M, et al: Impact of chamber geometry and gender on LV systolic function in patients over 60 years of age with aortic stenosis. *Am J Cardiol* 74:794-798, 1994.

63. Topol E, Traill T, Fortuin N: Hypertensive hypertrophic cardiomyopathy of the elderly. *N Engl J Med* 312:277-283, 1985.

64. Pearson AC, Gudipati CV, Labovitz A: Systolic and diastolic flow abnormalities in elderly patients with hypertensive hypertrophic cardiomyopathy. *J Am Coll Cardiol* 12:989-995, 1988.

65. Lewis JF, Maron BJ: Elderly patients with hypertrophic cardiomyopathy: A subset with distinctive LV morphology and progressive clinical course late in life. *J Am Coll Cardiol* 13:36-45, 1989.

66. Fay WP, Taliercio CP, Ilstrup DM, et al: Natural history of hypertrophic cardiomyopathy in the elderly. *J Am Coll Cardiol* 16:821-826, 1990.

67. Litwin SE, Katz SE, Weinberg EO, et al: Serial echocardiographic Doppler assessment of left ventricular geometry and function in rats with pressure-overload hypertrophy: Chronic angiotensin converting enzyme inhibition attenuates the transition to heart failure. *Circulation* 91:2642-2649, 1995.

68. Schiller N, Shah P, Crawford M, et al: Recommendations for quantitation of the left ventricle by two-dimensional echocardiography. *J Am Soc Echocardio*gr 2:358-367, 1989.

69. Schiller NB: Considerations in the standardization of measurement of LV myocardial mass by two-dimensional echocardiography. *Hypertension* 9(suppl II):II33-II35, 1987.

70. Reichek NR, Helak J, Plappert T, et al: Anatomic validation of left ventricular mass from clinical two-dimensional echocardiography: Initial results. *Circulation* 67:348-352, 1983.

71. Wahr DW, Schiller NB: Left ventricular volumes determined by two-dimensional echocardiography in a normal adult population. *J Am Coll Cardiol* 1:863-868, 1983.

72. St. John Sutton MG, Plappert T, Crosby L, et al: Effects of reduced left ventricular mass on chamber architecture, load, and function: A study of anorexia nervosa. *Circulation* 72:991-1000, 1985.

73. Byrd BF, Wahr D, Wang YS, et al: Left ventricular mass and volume/mass ratio determined by two-dimensional echocardiography in normal adults. *J Am Coll Cardiol* 6:1021-1025, 1985.

74. Douglas PS, Reichek N, Hackney K, et al: Contribution of afterload, hypertrophy, and geometry to left ventricular ejection fraction in aortic valve stenosis, pure aortic regurgitation and idiopathic dilated cardiomyopathy. *Am J Cardiol* 59:1398-1404, 1987.

75. Feiring A, Rumberger J, Reiter S, et al: Determination of left ventricular mass in dogs with rapid-acquisition cardiac computed tomographic scanning. *Circulation* 72:1355-1364, 1985.

76. Perez JE, Waggoner AD, Barzilai B, et al: On-line assessment of ventricular function by automatic boundary detection and ultrasonic backscatter imaging. *J Am Coll Cardiol* 19:313-320, 1992.

77. Perez JE, Klein SC, Prater DM, et al: Automated on-line quantitation of left ventricular dimensions and function by echocardiography with backscatter imaging and lateral gain compensation. *Am J Cardiol* 70:1200-1205, 1992.

78. Vandenburg BF, Rath LS, Stuhlmiller P, et al: Estimation of left ventricular cavity area with an on-line semiautomated echocardiographic edge detection system. *Circulation* 86:159-166, 1992.

79. Mor-Avi VV, Spencer KT, Lang RM: Acoustic quantification today and its future horizons. *Echocardiography* 16:85-94, 1999.

80. King DL: Three-dimensional echocardiography: Use of additional spatial data for measuring left ventricular mass. *Mayo Clin Proc* 69:293-295, 1994.

81. King DL, Gopal AS, Keller AM, et al: Three-dimensional echocardiography advances for measurement of ventricular volume and mass. *Hypertension* 23:172, 1994.

82. King DL, Harrison MR, King DL Jr, et al: Ultrasound beam orientation during standard two-dimensional imaging: Assessment by three dimensional echocardiography. *J Am Soc Echocardiogr* 5:567-576, 1992.

83. Schmidt MA, Ohazama CJ, Agyeman KO, et al: Real-time three-dimensional echocardiography for measurement of left ventricular volumes. *Am J Cardiol* 84:1434-1439, 1999.

84. Mor-Avi V, Sugeng L, Weinert L, et al: Fast measurement of left ventricular mass with real-time three-dimensional echocardiography: Comparison with magnetic resonance imaging. *Circulation* 110:1814-1818, 2004.

85. Gardin JM, Tomasso CL, Talano JV: Evaluation of dilated cardiomyopathy by pulsed Doppler echocardiography. *Am Heart J* 106:1057-1065, 1983.

86. Lewis JF, Kuo LC, Nelson JG, et al: Pulsed Doppler echocardiographic determination of stroke volume and cardiac output: Clinical validation of two new methods using the apical window. *Circulation* 70:425-431, 1984.

87. Bargiggia GS, Bertucci C, Recusani F, et al: A new method for estimating left ventricular dP/dt by continuous wave Doppler-

echocardiography: Validation studies at cardiac catheterization. *Circulation* 80:1287-1292, 1989.

88. Pai RG, Bansal RC, Shah P: Doppler-derived rate of left ventricular pressure rise. *Circulation* 82:514-520, 1990.

89. Chen C, Rodriguez L, Guererro JL, et al: Noninvasive measurement of the instantaneous first derivative of left ventricular pressure using continuous wave Doppler echocardiography. *Circulation* 83:2101-2110, 1991.

90. Aurigemma GP, Reichek N, Venugopal R, et al: Automated left ventricular mass, volume, and shape from 3D MRI: In vitro validation. *Am J Card Imaging* 5:257-263, 1991.

91. Maddahi J, Crues J, Berman DS, et al: Noninvasive quantification of left ventricular myocardial mass by gated proton nuclear magnetic resonance imaging. *J Am Coll Cardiol* 10:682-692, 1987.

92. Shapiro EP, Rogers WJ, Beyar R, et al: Determination of left ventricular mass by magnetic resonance imaging in hearts deformed by acute infarction. *Circulation* 79:706-711, 1989.

93. Utz JA, Herfkens RJ, Heinsimer JA: Cine MR determination of left ventricular ejection fraction. *Am J Roentgenol* 148:839-849, 1987.

94. Aurigemma G, Reichek N, Schiebler M, Axel L: Evaluation of mitral regurgitation by cine magnetic resonance imaging. *Am J Cardiol* 66:621-625, 1990.

95. Aurigemma G, Reichek N, Schiebler M, Axel L: Evaluation of aortic regurgitation by cardiac cine magnetic resonance imaging: Planar analysis and comparison to Doppler echocardiography. *Cardiology* 78(4):340-347, 1991.

96. Lima JAC, Desai MY. Cardiovascular magnetic resonance imaging: Current and emerging applications. *J Am Coll Cardiol* 44:1164-1171, 2004.

97. Chuang ML, Hibberd MG, Beaudin RA, et al: Importance of imaging method over imaging modality in noninvasive determination of left ventricular volumes and ejection fraction. *J Am Coll Cardiol* 35:477-484, 2000.

98. Carlson MD, White RD, Trohman RG, et al: Right ventricular outflow tract ventricular tachycardia: Detection of previously unrecognized anatomic abnormalities using cine magnetic resonance imaging. *J Am Coll Cardiol* 24:720-727, 1994.

99. Allen DG, Kentish JC: The cellular basis of the length tension relation in cardiac muscle. *J Mol Cell Cardiol* 17:821-828, 1985.

100. Ross J Jr: Afterload mismatch in aortic and mitral valve disease: Implications for surgical therapy. *J Am Coll Cardiol* 5:811-826, 1985.

101. St. John Sutton M, Plappert T, Spiegel A, et al: Early postoperative changes in LV chamber size, architecture, and function in aortic stenosis and aortic regurgitation and their relation to intraoperative changes in afterload: A prospective two-dimensional echocardiographic study. *Circulation* 76:77-89, 1987.

102. DeFilippi CR, Willett DL, Brickner ME, et al: Usefulness of dobutamine echocardiography in distinguishing severe from nonsevere valvular aortic stenosis in patients with depressed left ventricular function and low transvalvular gradients. *Am J Cardiol* 75:191-194, 1995.

103. Colan SD, Borow KM, Neuman AS: The left ventricular endsystolic wall stress-velocity of fiber shortening relation: A load independent index of myocardial contractility. *J Am Coll Cardiol* 4:715-724, 1984.

104. Quinones MA, Gaasch WH, Alexander JK: Influences of acute changes in preload, afterload, contractile state, and heart rate on ejection and isovolumic indices of myocardial contractility in man. *Circulation* 53:293-300, 1976.

105. Aurigemma GP, Meyer TE, Sharma M, et al: Evaluation of extent of shortening versus velocity of shortening at the endocardium and midwall in hypertensive heart disease. *Am J Cardiol* 83:792-794, 1999.

106. Shimizu G, Zile M, Blaustein AS, Gaasch WH: Left ventricular chamber filling and midwall fiber lengthening in patients with

left ventricular hypertrophy: Overestimation of fiber velocities by conventional midwall measurements. *Circulation* 71:266-272, 1985.

107. deSimone G, Devereux RB, Roman MJ, et al: Assessment of left ventricular function by the midwall fractional shortening/end systolic stress relation in human hypertension. *J Am Coll Cardiol* 23:1444-1451, 1994.

108. Aurigemma GP, Silver KH, Fox MA, et al: Depressed midwall and long axis shortening in hypertensive left ventricular hypertrophy with normal ejection fraction. *J Am Coll Cardiol* 26:195-202, 1995.

109. Jones CR, Gibson D: Functional importance of the long axis dynamics of the human left ventricle. *Br Heart J* 65:215-220, 1990.

110. Keren G, LeJemtel T: Mitral annulus motion: Relation to pulmonary venous and transmitral flows in normal subjects and in patients with dilated cardiomyopathy. *Circulation* 78:621-629, 1988.

111. Palmon L, Reichek N, Yeon S, et al: Intramural myocardial shortening in hypertensive left ventricular hypertrophy with normal pump function. *Circulation* 89:122-131, 1994.

112. Sutherland GR, Stewart MJ, Groundstroem KWE, et al: Color Doppler myocardial imaging: A new technique for the assessment of myocardial function. *J Am Soc Echocardiogr* 7:441-458, 1994.

113. Abraham TP, Nishimura RA: Myocardial strain: can we finally measure contractility? *J Am Coll Cardiol* 37:731-734, 2001.

114. Sogaard P, Egeblad H, Kim WY, et al: Tissue doppler imaging predicts improved systolic performance and reversed left ventricular remodeling during long-term cardiac resynchronization therapy. *J Am Coll Cardiol* 40:723-730, 2002.

115. Bax JJ, Ansalone G, Breithardt OA, et al: Echocardiographic evaluation of cardiac resynchronization therapy: ready for routine clinical use? *J Am Coll Cardiol* 44:1-9, 2004.

116. Edvardsen T, Gerber BL, Bluemke GJ, et al: Quantitative assessment of intrinsic regional myocardial deformation by Doppler strain rate echocardiography in humans: validation against three-dimensional tagged magnetic resonance imaging. *Circulation* 106:10-16, 2002.

117. Mirsky I, Pasternac A, Ellison RC: General index for the assessment of cardiac function. *Am J Cardiol* 30:483-491, 1972.

118. Ross J Jr: Adaptations of the left ventricle to chronic valvular overload. *Circ Res* 35:64-70, 1974.

119. Ross J Jr, Sonnenblick EH, Taylor RR, et al: Diastolic geometry and sarcomere lengths in the chronically dilated canine left ventricle. *Circ Res* 28:49-56, 1971.

120. Sonnenblick EH: Correlation of myocardial ultrastructure and function. *Circulation* 38:29-44, 1968.

121. Laks MM, Morady F, Swan HJC: Canine right and left ventricular cell and sarcomere lengths after banding the pulmonary artery. *Circ Res* 24:705-710, 1969.

122. Greenbaum R, Ho S, Gibson D: Left ventricular fibre architecture in man. *Br Heart J* 45:248-263, 1981.

123. Streeter D, Spotnitz H, Patel D: Fiber orientation in the canine left ventricle during diastole and systole. *Circ Res* 24:339-346, 1969.

124. Villareall FJ, Lew WYW, Waldman LK et al: Transmural myocardial deformation in the ischemic canine left ventricle. *Circ Res* 68:368-381, 1991.

125. Clark NR, Reichek N, Bergey P, et al: Circumferential myocardial shortening in the normal human left ventricle. Assessment by magnetic resonance imaging using spatial modulation of magnetization. *Circulation* 84:67-74, 1991.

126. Sagawa K, Maughan L, Suga H, Sunagawa K: *Cardiac Contractility and the Pressure-Volume Relationship.* New York, Oxford University Press, 1988.

127. Magorien DJ, Shaffer P, Bush CA, et al: Assessment of left ventricular pressure-volume relations using gated radionuclide an-

giography, echocardiography and micromanometer pressure recordings. *Circulation* 67:844-852, 1983.

128. McKay RG, Aroesty JM, Heller GV, et al: Left ventricular pressure-volume diagrams and end-systolic pressure-volume relations in human beings. *J Am Coll Cardiol* 3:301-312, 1984.

129. Gorcsan J III, Gasior TA, Mandarino WA: Assessment of the immediate effects of cardiopulmonary bypass on left ventricular performance by on-line pressure-area relations. *Circulation* 89:180-190, 1994.

130. Gorcsan J III, Denault A, Gasior TA, et al: Rapid estimation of LV contractility from end systolic relations by echocardiographic automated border detection and femoral artery pressure. *Anesthesiology* 81:553-562, 1994.

131. Katz WE, Gasior TA, Reddy SC, Gorcsan J III: Utility and limitations of biplane transesophageal echocardiography for estimation of LV stroke volume. *Am Heart J* 128:389-396, 1994.

132. Sagawa K: The ventricular pressure-volume diagram revisited. *Circ Res* 43:677-680, 1978.

133. Bogen DK, Ariel Y, McMahon TA, Gaasch WH: Measurement of peak systolic elastance in intact canine circulation with servo pump. *Am J Physiol* 1249:H585-H593, 1985.

134. Berko B, Gaasch WH, Tanigawa N, et al: Disparity between ejection and end systolic indexes of left ventricular contractility in mitral regurgitation. *Circulation* 75:1310-1319, 1987.

135. Gaasch WH, Carroll JD, Levine HJ, et al: Chronic aortic regurgitation: Prognostic value of left ventricular end-systolic dimension and end-diastolic radius/thickness ratio. *J Am Coll Cardiol* 1:775-782, 1983.

136. Gottdiener JS, Livengood SV, Meyer PS, et al: Should echocardiography be performed to assess the effects of antihypertensive therapy? Test-retest reliability of echocardiography for measurement of left ventricular mass and function. *J Am Coll Cardiol* 25:424-430, 1995.

137. Dahloff B, Pennert K, Hanson L: Reversal of left ventricular hypertrophy in hypertensive patients: A meta-analysis of 109 treatment studies. *Am J Hypertens* 5:95-110, 1992.

Chapter 10

Ventricular Shape and Function

FLORENCE H. SHEEHAN, MD

Ventricular Structure

The role of the heart is to propel blood forward at a rate appropriate for organ perfusion and bodily function. Study of the structure-function relationship of the left ventricle (LV) and the right ventricle (RV) is like peeling an onion. The development of new methods enables exploration of additional layers of complexity and formulation of more comprehensive models incorporating myocardial fiber and sheet organization,[1] global chamber geometry, regional stresses and strains, and the effects of electrical activation. Science has

advanced far from the early muscle dissections, and current research is performed using finite element analysis on supercomputers. Nevertheless, the input data for such analyses includes the basic knowledge of muscle anatomy gained decades ago from painstaking dissections.

Nearly all of our knowledge of ventricular fiber anatomy is for the LV, which can easily be modeled as an ellipsoid or cylinder. Streeter and colleagues described the divergence of fiber angle between the epicardium and endocardium, between the base and apex, and between diastole and systole, comparing the interweaving helical fiber pattern to a wicker basket.[2] Delineating the helical layers of fibers was key to understanding ejection. Myocardial fibers shorten 15%, inadequate for the more circular fibers to achieve a normal ejection fraction (EF) by narrowing the ventricle. Contraction of the helical fiber layers contributes to LV stroke volume (SV) by shortening the ventricle.[3] Because of the lack of a middle layer, circular fibers are sparser in the RV, which consequently relies more heavily on longitudinal shortening[4-5] (Fig. 10–1). More recently studies in the normal live human heart using magnetic resonance imaging (MRI) tagging have confirmed that the myocardial strain pattern of wall thickening, circumferential shortening, and longitudinal shortening is related to the fiber orientation and shape of the LV.[6]

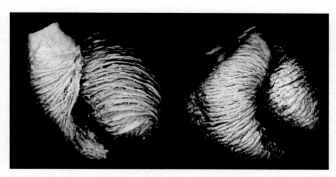

Figure 10-1. *Stenocostal view of the middle layer in a normal* (left) *and malformed* (right) *heart. Note the lack of a middle layer in the normal right ventricle and the presence of a well-defined middle layer of fibers in the right ventricle of the malformed heart. (From Sanchez-Quintana D, Garcia-Martinez V, Hurle JM:* Acta Anat (Basel) *138(4):352-358, 1990. With permission from S. Karger AG, Basel, Switzerland).*

Fibers in the subendocardium of the LV follow a right-handed helix, whereas fibers in the subepicardium spiral left-handed.[2] The contraction of these fibers causes counterclockwise twisting of the LV apex relative to the base about its long axis (as viewed from the apex).[7] This torsional deformation is the "wringing" motion of the heart described centuries ago. During systole, the magnitude of torsion is linearly related to the ejection of blood.[8] However, the LV undergoes much of its untwisting during isovolumic relaxation.[8,9] This recoil is a restoring force important for diastolic function and may be the mechanism of diastolic suction.[9,10] In the interventricular septum, generally considered part of the LV, there are longitudinal fibers belonging to the RV (Fig. 10-2). The RV chamber is considered to have two parts, the sinus and the conus.

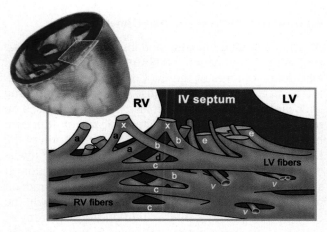

Figure 10-2. *Bifurcation of myocardial fibers at anterior interventricular sulcus region* (inset). *Details of typical fiber branchings: a, Right ventricular (RV) fiber groups branching into RV trabeculae, x; c, superficial fiber paths of the RV and left ventricular (LV) walls; d, fiber groups from RV wall branching into septum; e, fiber groups from LV wall branching into septum; v, vessels. IV, interventricular. (From Fox CC, Hutchins GM:* Johns Hopkins Med J *130:289-299, 1972.)*

Fibers in the sinus are mostly oriented obliquely with an average major radius of curvature of nearly 4 cm, whereas fibers in the outflow track are circumconal with a small radius of curvature of 0.8 cm.[11] Contraction of the RV proceeds with a peristaltic pattern from sinus to infundibulum.[12] Torsion also occurs for the RV, as would be expected from the tight interlacing of its fibers.

Models of LV mechanics have been developed to quantify the relationship between fiber structure and function. The models vary in complexity, but even one that simplifies the shape of the LV to a cylinder was able to relate observed fiber orientations and torsion angles to fractional shortening values.[13] *Ventricular remodeling* is the term applied to the compensatory hypertrophy and dilatation that maintain cardiac output (CO) in overload states and encompasses changes in chamber dimensions, wall thickness, and shape caused by microscopic changes in myocytes and the extracellular matrix. In the LV, the shape changes have been attributed to redistribution of stress.[14]

The distribution of stress in the heart is determined by the three-dimensional (3D) structure of the ventricular walls, the material properties of the myofibers and the collagen matrix, and the boundary conditions imposed by cavity pressure and intracardiac and extracardiac structures. It is of fundamental importance to measure the distribution of wall stress in the myocardium because it affects ventricular function, myocardial oxygen demand, coronary blood flow, vulnerability to injury, remodeling, and action potential shape.[15,16] To date, no method has been developed for directly measuring regional stresses in the intact myocardium because of the tissue injury that implanted transducers would cause. Instead the analysis of regional ventricular stress is currently performed using mathematical modeling of the determinants.

Finite element analysis has been used as a parametric framework to characterize the heart's regional function as a 3D continuum. It is a powerful engineering tool that may be applied to estimate stress and deformation in structures, such as the heart with complex geometry, material properties, and loading conditions because it overcomes limitations of closed-form stress equations that must assume that the heart has a regular, symmetrical geometry.[17] These assumptions would preclude study of the RV were it not for finite element analysis. Models have been developed for 3D finite element analysis of the canine LV and RV geometry utilizing nonuniform fiber distribution[18] and to study ventricular wall motion and regional strain in normal subjects and patients.[19-23] Models have also been developed to incorporate descriptions of macroscopic and microscopic anatomy, such as muscle fiber orientation and myocardial sheet organization,[1] and enable deformation stress analyses of the mechanics and electrical dynamics of the beating heart.[24,25] The heart is a mechanical organ, and as such its functionality relies on its form.

Regional Systolic Function in Two and Three Dimensions

The Left Ventricle

Echocardiography is well suited to the assessment of regional LV systolic function for both clinical and research applications. Every region of the ventricle can be examined at high spatial and temporal resolution, allowing a more comprehensive visualization than with other imaging modalities. Furthermore, echocardiography is portable, safe, and relatively inexpensive so that serial studies can be obtained without risk to the patient to follow disease progression or response to therapy. Quantitative methods have been developed for measurement of systolic function both for diagnosis and for evaluation of treatment efficacy and prognosis in patients with ischemic heart disease. These methods also allow analysis of the structure-function relationship of the LV and mitral valve, of asynchrony in the timing of contraction, and of the heart's compensatory response to disease processes. Thus, echocardiographic examination offers high informational content for both clinical and research applications.

Semi-Quantitative Assessment in Two Dimensions

In clinical practice, visual assessment of two-dimensional (2D) echocardiograms provides a rapid evaluation of regional systolic function. In each imaging plane the LV contour is divided into several segments. Each segment is assigned a numerical value indicating its degree of asynergy. The American Heart Association recently recommended a model for dividing the LV into 17 segments.[26] The locations of the segments follow the perfusion territory of the three major epicardial arteries to facilitate the diagnosis of ischemic dysfunction.

The severity of dysfunction is scored visually in each segment as 1 for normal contraction or hyperkinesis, 2 for hypokinesis, 3 for akinesis, 4 for dyskinesis, and 5 for aneurysmal segments.[27] Some investigators use the system developed for angiography which assigns 1 for normal motion, 2 for mild or moderate hypokinesis, 3 for severe hypokinesis or akinesis, 4 for dyskinesis, and 5 for aneurysmal segments.[28] Gibson and colleagues recommended evaluating wall thickening and motion in scoring segmental function because of reports that wall motion varies widely in normal subjects.[29] Hyperkinesis can be distinguished from normal motion and may be assigned a negative value (e.g., −1) to indicate that its contribution to global function is opposite to that of segments with depressed func-

tion.[30] A global wall motion score is then calculated by summing or averaging the readings in all of the segments. The region of infarction can be evaluated separately from the noninfarct region by averaging the scores in the appropriate subset of segments.[31]

In clinical validation studies, the echocardiographic score agreed exactly with the score obtained from contrast ventriculograms in 44% of segments; agreement within one functional class was seen in 68% to 88%.[32-37] That is, agreement is higher for distinguishing normal from abnormal contraction than in identifying grades of abnormality. Comparable results were obtained in comparisons of radionuclide ventriculography versus 2D echocardiography.[34,38] In a significant minority of patients, however, the discordance is two or three classes. In one study, the global wall motion score by 2D echocardiography and by angiography correlated with r = .70.[36]

Factors affecting the accuracy of qualitative assessment of wall motion include image quality and correct positioning of the image plane relative to the LV and the comparison imaging modality. Unlike contrast and radionuclide ventriculography, 2D echocardiography is tomographic, producing images of discrete slices of the heart. Therefore, the different modalities do not obtain exactly comparable views of each segment. The training and experience of the observer are also important. Exact agreement within and between observers ranges from 81% to 95% percent.[39-42] However, allowance of a one-grade error—for example, combining normal with hypokinesis or dyskinesis with aneurysm—improves intraobserver and interobserver agreement to 98% to 99%. To minimize observer variability, most studies report readings made by consensus between two or more observers.

Quantitative Analysis in Two Dimensions

As a tomographic imaging modality, 2D echocardiography allows delineation of both the endocardial and epicardial contours of the LV. Consequently it is possible to calculate not only those parameters reflecting endocardial displacement but also parameters based on measuring wall thickness. The analysis of function, both regional and global, measures the alteration of the LV between end-diastole and end-systole. Some investigators have also studied the extent of contraction at specific phases, such as during isovolumic contraction or relaxation.[43] Frame-by-frame analysis through the cardiac cycle provides information on the synchrony of regional function. This can be taken to the "fourth dimension" (4D) by performing 3D analyses of the LV at multiple time points through the cardiac cycle.

The ultimate goal is to measure shortening in the direction of myocardial fibers—for example, using strain analysis—to obtain more accurate assessment of performance and tissue viability independent of translational motion.[44,45] Until recently these measurements could only be performed using MRI tagging.[21] Echocardiographic strain analysis by tracking tissue patterns now provides longitudinal and radial strain, although not circumferential strain.[46]

Wall Motion Analysis. Displacement of the LV endocardium between end-diastole and end-systole is measured and normalized for patient-to-patient differences in heart size by dividing by the LV dimension at end-diastole to produce a unitless shortening fraction. Unlike the EF, wall motion may have negative values that indicate paradoxical outward motion during systole.

Because it was not possible to track specific points on the LV by ultrasound (US) over time until the recent development of speckle tracking,[46] a plethora of methods were invented that model rather than measure wall motion. Most wall motion analysis methods for echocardiography employ a radial coordinate system. Motion is assumed to proceed from all points on the endocardial contour toward a single point, the center of area. There is little evidence supporting this assumption, but the radial approach seems inherently suited to analysis of short-axis images. The radial method has also been applied to contours from apical views.[47]

In methods based on a rectangular coordinate system, motion is measured along hemiaxes constructed at intervals along and perpendicular to the long axis of the ventricle. Rectangular coordinate system methods are applied only to apical views.[48-50] Justification for the rectangular coordinate system approach derives from an angiographic study that tracked landmarks felt to represent trabeculae and found that endocardial displacement at the apex results from apical obliteration because the lateral walls contract toward the long axis.[51]

Two methods have been developed for modeling wall motion without using a coordinate system. Gibson and colleagues divided the end-diastolic contour into a number of evenly spaced points and measure the distance from each to the nearest point on the end-systolic contour.[52] In the centerline method, a center line is drawn midway between the end-diastolic and end-systolic contours. Motion is measured along 100 chords evenly spaced along and perpendicular to the center line and normalized by the end-diastolic perimeter length[53-56] (Fig. 10–3). Because they make no assumptions concerning the geometry of the LV contour, both of these methods can be applied to chambers of diverse shapes. For example, the centerline method has been used to measure wall motion in the RV and from different views of the LV, unaffected by distortions of ventricular shape resulting from disease processes.

Motion can be measured in one dimension as the linear distance between the end-diastolic and end-systolic contours and normalize to yield a shortening fraction. Alternatively, function can be measured in

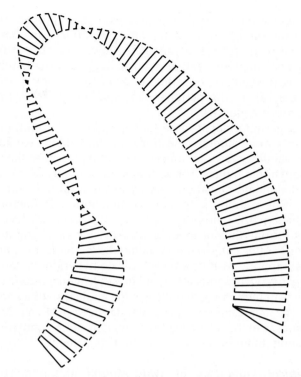

Figure 10–3. *Centerline method for regional wall motion analysis. End-diastolic and end-systolic endocardial contours of the left ventricle from the apical four-chamber echocardiographic view. One hundred equidistant chords are constructed perpendicular to the centerline (not shown). The motion at each chord is normalized by the end-diastolic perimeter to yield a dimensionless chord fractional shortening.*

regions of the LV: the change in the area of a region between end-diastole and end-systole normalized by the end-diastolic area yields a regional EF. Studies have shown that such an area parameter is less subject to variability in delineating the EF contour, probably because the variability at individual contour points is "averaged out" over the region.[50,57,58]

Definition of Coronary Artery Territories. The principal challenge to regional assessment lies in the definition of the regions. Although the perfusion territories of the major epicardial coronary arteries have been mapped,[59] studies have shown that dysfunction in patients with ischemic heart disease may extend beyond the defined territory of the stenosed artery.[30,60-64] This may result from multivessel disease, border zone dysfunction, and/or variable coronary anatomy.

The impact of variable coronary anatomy on the measurement of regional LV function is significant because dysfunction may be underestimated if the central ischemic region straddles two adjacent segments, each of which also contains some normally contracting myocardium.[53] One solution to this problem is to measure wall motion at many discrete points around the ventricular contour and then average the motion of points lying within the region of interest. This approach is flexible enough to adjust for variable coronary anatomy while retaining the advantage of lower variability for regional analyses and has been applied successfully using the centerline method to analyze function in the center of, on the periphery of, and remote from the ischemic region.[53,65]

It is important to note that the motion of multiple points from different locations on the contour cannot be validly averaged unless the motion values have comparable ranges. For wall motion, the normal mean and standard deviation vary by location on the ventricle. One solution is to convert the shortening fraction values to a Z score, that is, to units of standard deviations from the mean of a normal reference population.[58] After conversion, a value of zero indicates normal motion, positive values indicate hyperkinesis, and negative values indicate hypokinesis. The magnitude of the wall motion value indicates the clinical significance of the abnormality. These standardized wall motion values can be averaged over regions and compared among different regions and different patients.

Clinical Validation of Wall Motion Methods. The various methods for wall motion analysis have been validated clinically using empirical criteria. The principal criteria are high sensitivity and specificity in distinguishing patients with diseased hearts from normal subjects. The results of such testing depend on the patient populations used for testing. For example, the diagnostic accuracy of a new method will appear to be much higher if the diseased patients have myocardial infarction (MI) than if they merely suffer from chronic stable angina, simply because the latter have near-normal function. Consequently the relative merits of the various methods of wall motion analysis are best assessed from comparative studies of two or more methods. Angiographic studies have shown that the radial and centerline methods have higher diagnostic accuracy than methods based on a rectangular coordinate system. One study of 2D echocardiograms in the subcostal view reported that the centerline method is less likely to diagnose abnormality in normal subjects than the radial method.[47] In contrast, another echocardiographic study found that a rectangular coordinate system approach yielded higher diagnostic accuracy than either the radial or centerline methods.[49]

The homogeneity of the normal group is the second empirical criterion. A narrow normal range, reflected by a small standard deviation (SD), enhances sensitivity in diagnosing abnormality. For example, in calculating sample size for a clinical trial, the number of patients per group is proportional to the square of the SD. To evaluate the sensitivity with which a method can detect abnormal function, divide the normal mean by the normal SD. If the quotient is greater than 2, then akinesis is unlikely to lie within the normal range (de-

fined as the mean ±2 SD). If, on the other hand, akinesis differs from the normal mean by less than 2 SD, then a patient's motion must be dyskinetic or aneurysmal to be considered definitely abnormal. Such a method will be relatively insensitive to lesser degrees of dysfunction.

Translational Motion. During systole the LV rotates about its long axis and translates anteriorly.[66,67] Whether to "correct" for translation by realigning the end-systolic contour relative to the end-diastolic contour is controversial. Using a fixed reference system may cause artifactual hypokinesis in a normal heart,[68-70] but using a floating reference (i.e., realigning) may present a dysfunctional segment as normal.[68] One study reported that fixed and floating reference systems yielded equal accuracy in detecting the presence of wall motion abnormalities, but the fixed reference system was superior for localizing the abnormality.[71] Another study found that a floating reference provides superior sensitivity and specificity in the apical four-chamber view, whereas optimal results were obtained with a fixed reference in the short-axis view.[72] Yet another dilemma is choosing the method of realignment.[73] Hence many investigators prefer thickening for analyzing regional systolic function.[74]

Wall Thickening. This parameter is computed as the change in wall thickness from end-diastole to end-systole normalized by the end-diastolic dimension. Normal myocardium thickens during systole. Dysfunctional myocardium exhibits decreased thickening or even thinning. Wall thickening is independent of artifact as a result of cardiac translation as long as each thickness measurement is made wholly at one time point.[66] Wall thickness must be measured orthogonal to the myocardial wall because analysis at oblique angles will overestimate wall thickness. Some investigators advocate 3D analysis to ensure orthogonality.[75] Only two methods are used for wall thickening analysis. The radial method measures wall thickness along radii extending from an origin usually located at the center of area or at the midpoint of an anatomically defined diameter.[50,66,68] This method is most suitable for analyzing short-axis views with their near-circular contours.[76] In the centerline method, a center line is drawn midway between the endocardial and epicardial contours. Wall thickness is measured along chords constructed perpendicular to and evenly spaced along the center line (i.e., in the direction of the local radial vector)[55,77,78] (Fig. 10-4).

The accuracy of measuring wall thickness from echocardiograms was established initially using M-mode imaging of postmortem specimens.[79] The accuracy of wall thickening measurements from 2D echocardiogram has been validated for the calculation of ventricular mass.[80,81] However, 3D analysis of LV strain

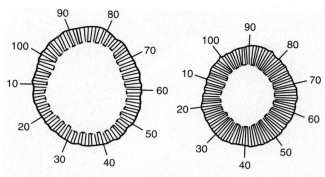

Figure 10-4. *Centerline method for regional wall thickening analysis in a short-axis view. Left ventricular endocardial and epicardial contours at end-diastole (left) and end-systole (right) traced from a short-axis echocardiographic view. Wall thickness is measured at each of one hundred equidistant chords constructed perpendicular to the centerline (not shown). Wall thickening is computed as the systolic change in thickness and normalized by the end diastolic thickness.[78]*

in man using MRI tagging has now shown that wall thickening primarily reflects radial strain and does not fully characterize regional contractile function.[6]

Comparison of Wall Motion versus Wall Thickening. The advantages of wall thickening are that it is independent of the degree of hypertrophy, unlike wall motion, and therefore can be applied in patients with hypertrophied LVs[82] and that it is independent of translational artifact. The disadvantages of wall thickening are that it does not reflect the contribution of epicardial motion to stroke volume,[73] and it requires delineation of the epicardial contours and the endocardial contours, which doubles the workload and introduces error and variability.

The performance of wall motion and wall thickening have been compared in several studies.[50,63,71,77,83-85] Although both akinesis and the absence of wall thickening are rare in normal subjects, wall thickening is more heterogeneous (i.e., has a higher coefficient of variation). The normal range, defined as mean ±2 SD, is more likely to encompass 0% thickening than 0% motion. The higher wall thickening variability results in large part from point-to-point differences in end-diastolic wall thickness and can be reduced by using the end-diastolic perimeter length to normalize the observed change in wall thickness.[77] Nevertheless wall thickening has proved to be more sensitive in diagnosing MI in man.[84,86]

Midwall Motion. When the LV is modeled as a thick-walled cylinder contracting radially and longitudinally, it can be shown mathematically that wall thickening, midwall shortening, and longitudinal axis shortening are related, but internal radius shortening (i.e., wall motion) is significantly influenced by the degree of LV hypertrophy.[82] In ventricles with normal wall thick-

ness, wall motion and wall thickening correlate closely.[87] However, the relative contribution of wall thickening but not of wall motion to ventricular power during ejection increases with increasing hypertrophy.[88] Consequently function is overestimated by analysis of wall motion from endocardial contours in patients with LV hypertrophy and is more appropriately measured from analysis of midwall shortening or wall thickening.[89,90] Midwall shortening is calculated from M-mode or from 3D reconstructions by assuming the conservation of mass throughout the cardiac cycle[89,91]: This construct allows for migration of the midwall toward the epicardium because of the greater shortening of subendocardial fibers compared with subepicardial fibers.[92] Midwall shortening lends itself to stress-shortening analysis—for example, to compare the function of groups of patients with pressure overload hypertrophy because such analysis requires that both stress and shortening be measured in the same direction, which is true at the midwall as a result of the predominance of circumferential fibers.[44,93]

Strain Analysis. Strain analysis offers assessment of regional myocardial function independent of cardiac translation. Strain values are uniform in different regions of the heart, an aid to differentiating normal from abnormal contraction.[94] The strain measurement by tissue Doppler imaging (TDI) is angle dependent as a result of use of the Doppler effect.[95] However, speckle tracking is based on B-mode imaging and has been validated recently against sonomicrometry in experimental animals and by comparison with MRI tagging in patients for measurement of regional function in long- and short-axis views.[96] Clinical experience with this new technique has focused on analysis of regional dyssynchrony, using the variation in regional time-to-peak-strain to predict response to cardiac resynchronization therapy in patients with heart failure.[97] The technique can also be applied to assess LV rotation.[98] However, accuracy is limited at the base because the LV moves longitudinally in and out of the image plane. This may present a problem if torsion is calculated as the difference in rotation between the base and apex.

Three-Dimensional Analysis of Regional Left Ventricular Function

2D echocardiography provides visualization of many structures in the beating heart; however, interpretive skills are needed for the observer to mentally formulate the heart's complex anatomy. In 3D echocardiography the spatial location and orientation of each image plane is recorded with the image so that information from multiple images can be analyzed jointly. This permits multiplanar image data to be assembled into 3D displays that facilitate the assessment and communication of anatomic relations. The 3D format also enables the quantification of the size, shape, and function of cardiac structures with minimal geometric assumptions, a particular advantage when dealing with disease-distorted anatomy or complex shapes, such as the RV. Although 3D echocardiography was conceptualized in 1961, most of the advances were made during the past decade after fast and inexpensive computers became more readily available; Belohlavek and colleagues have reviewed the earlier work.[99]

3D echocardiography is often equated with volumetric imaging to obtain spatial visualization of cardiac anatomy.[100,101] In this mode, dense image data sets are acquired and processed to permit the shape of the structures to be appreciated visually using 3D display formats, such as surface rendering in which shading indicates topography. The image data set can be opened at any cut plane to provide a surgeon's eye view of the heart's interior. The third dimension can also be appreciated using stereoscopy or holography.[102,103] Volumetric imaging is primarily used to search visually for structural abnormalities, such as congenital defects or deformed valves, although volumetric data sets can also be analyzed to measure volume or a defect's size. Automated detection of the LV endocardium is now commercially available, which enables segmental function to be measured in terms of the volume contained in a pyramid defined by the area of the segment on the surface and the center of gravity (Fig. 10–5); segmental volume time curves are generated throughout the cardiac cycle for assessment of asynchrony.[104]

In the surface-modeling mode of 3D echocardiogram, the surface of the targeted structure is reconstructed based on tracings of its border from multiple image planes. All chambers, valves, and intracardiac structures, such as the papillary muscles and chordae tendineae, can be reconstructed for quantitative analysis of size, shape, function, and spatial relationships between structures. Surface modeling provides superior accuracy in measuring ventricular volume and mass and for accurate, reproducible measurement of a variety of cardiac descriptors. However, quantification currently requires manual image analysis. Then the traced borders are used to reconstruct the LV as a 3D surface using one of the numerous methods that have been developed.[105-107] Analysis of regional function from surface models requires reconstructions that faithfully represent the 3D shape—not just the volume—of the LV. 3D wall thickening analysis also requires accurate epicardium reconstruction.

The same questions apply in 3D as in 2D. One must still decide on whether to measure wall motion or wall thickening and what model to apply, whether to correct for translational motion, and how to define "regional." Indeed with a 3D surface there are more ways to correct for translation[108] and more data points to deal with. In seven publications on regional LV function

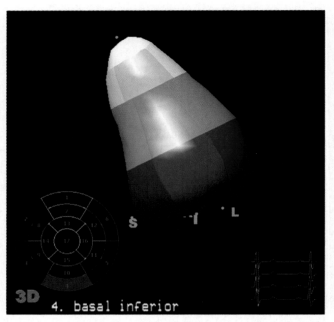

Figure 10–5 A mathematical model of the left ventricular (LV) endocardial surface obtained using semiautomated border tracking from a volumetric three-dimensional echocardiographic data set. Following identification of a few anatomical landmarks the model is segmented into the standard 16 or 17 segments. The volume of each segment (relative to the LV center of gravity) can be calculated for each frame in the cardiac cycle and presented as regional volume-time curves. (From Monaghan MJ: Heart 92:131-136, 2006. Reprinted with permission from the BMJ Publishing Group.)

measured from a 3D reconstruction, the number of regions ranged from 5 to 36, and none followed the recommended 17-segment model. Another issue that must be addressed in 3D analysis is the need to measure wall thickness orthogonal to the ventricular wall. Thickness is overestimated in oblique image planes, such as short-axis slices near the apex. One approach that was developed and validated for MRI but theoretically applicable to ultrasound, is to divide the myocardial space into elements whose volumes are divided by the mean of the endocardial and epicardial areas of the element.[109] The centersurface method is the 3D version of the centerline method; thickness is measured along chords drawn orthogonal to a medial surface constructed midway between the endocardial and epicardial reconstructions[110] (Fig. 10–6). Color-coding the 3D reconstruction enables rapid visual appreciation of the location and severity of regional dysfunction and its extent in terms of the area of involvement.

The Right Ventricle

A major impetus driving interest in quantifying regional LV function came in the early and mid-1980s, when thrombolytic therapy for treatment of acute myocardial infarction (AMI) was under intense interna-

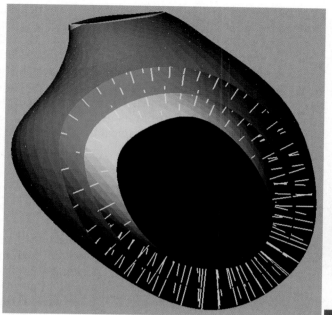
A

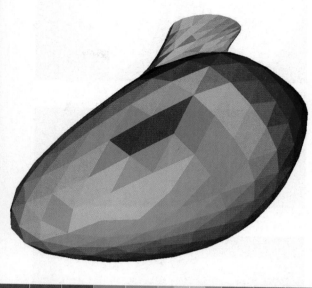
B

Figure 10–6. *The center surface method permits measurement of wall thickness in three-dimensional orthogonal to the local myocardial wall.*[176] *A, The close and distant thirds of the left ventricle have been "cut away" to provide a tomographic view. A medial surface (green) is constructed midway between the endocardium (yellow) and the epicardium (blue). Chords are drawn perpendicular to the center surface and extended to the endocardial and epicardial surfaces. The length of each chord is the local wall thickness. B, Example of the visual presentation of regional left ventricular function in three dimensions. The wall thickening at each vertex has been converted into units of standard deviations from the mean of a normal reference population. Cool colors represent levels of hypokinesis; warm colors, hyperkinesis (color scale developed by S Maza). Visualization as an overlay on the patient's three-dimensional surface facilitates appreciation of the location, extent, and severity of dysfunction.*

tional study to prove coronary reperfusion reduces mortality by reducing infarct size and salvaging ischemic myocardium. Interest in the RV seemed to diminish with recognition of this chamber's resilience to even prolonged coronary occlusion, even though RV function has a significant impact on prognosis independent of the LV.[111,112]

For semi-quantitative assessment of regional function the free wall in the short-axis view is commonly divided into anterior, lateral, and inferior segments; global RV EF correlated well with the wall motion score index computed by averaging all of the segmental scores.[113] In the registry of arrhythmogenic RV dysplasia, wall motion was assessed in the same seven anatomically defined regions in echocardiography as in angiography.[114]

For quantitative wall motion analysis, few of the geometric models developed for the LV have been applied to the RV. Radial coordinate systems do not fit long-axis views of either ventricle well, and they also do not fit short-axis views of the RV as a result of the sharp angles at the junction of the septal and free walls. Rectangular coordinates do not fit crescentic contours well either. In contrast, the centerline method—which does not rely on geometric assumptions about RV

shape—has been successfully applied to angiographic, echocardiographic, and MRI studies.[78,115-117]

The heterogeneity of normal RV wall motion is well documented from MRI tagging studies.[19] These studies have confirmed greater long-axis than short-axis shortening,[118,119] torsion,[120] and an overall motion of the RV free wall toward the interventricular septum[19] (Fig. 10–7). However, a problem facing those interested in regional RV function is not the measurement itself but the lack of any consensus on how the contour should be segmented. The standardized segmentation developed for the LV was designed to enhance recognition of ischemic dysfunction by relating segment location to the three coronary artery perfusion territories.[26] Because ischemia in the RV produces regional dysfunction out of proportion to the size of infarction, it is difficult to develop a segmentation plan based on ischemic dysfunction patterns for the RV comparable to that for the LV.[111]

Consequently investigators have developed methods as needed for the question being addressed. The diversity of methodology is most prevalent in studies involving 3D analysis or conditions other than ischemic heart disease. In four studies of normal subjects, arrhythmogenic RV dysplasia, or congenital heart disease (CHD),

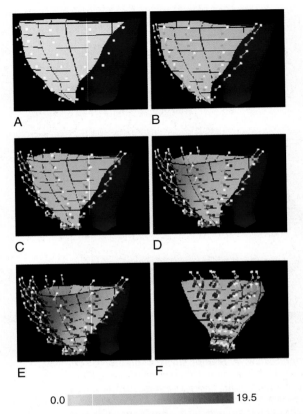

A   B

C   D

E   F

0.0 ▭▭▭▭▭▭▭ 19.5

Figure 10–7. Normal displacement of the right ventricular (RV) free wall. A-E, The free wall is shown through four phases of systole. The left ventricular (LV) wall is drawn shaded for reference. F, Septal wall at end-systole from the vantage point of the LV. The line segments show that displacement is nonuniformly distributed, with the greatest amount at the base of the RV. (From Haber I, Metaxas DN, Axel L: Med Image Anal 4(4):335-355, 2000. With permission from Elsevier.)

the RV was divided into 4 circumferential regions, 3 vertical regions, or 9 to 12 regions created by subdividing short-axis slices.[117,121-123] One study carefully justified its segmentation plan: McConnell and colleagues observed a pattern of regional RV dysfunction in patients with acute pulmonary embolism (PE) by centerline analysis of RV wall motion (Fig. 10–8). They also proposed diagnostic criteria for visual assessment of function in four regions of the RV free wall and then demonstrated the accuracy of these criteria.[124] It may be appropriate to use different segmentation plans for different disease entities. However, all investigators studying a given disease should employ the same plan so that results will be comparable.

Given the lack of a segmentation plan, concern about the anatomic location of standard views, and the inaccuracy of geometric models for calculating RV volume from 2D echocardiograms,[125] a number of investigators have developed surrogate parameters of global RV function based on a single view. The analysis is usually performed on the apical four-chamber view, appropriate given the predominantly longitudinal con-

tractile pattern of the RV.[118,119] The most common parameters are fractional area change and tricuspid annular descent.[126] Fractional area change from a short-axis view has also been shown to correlate with outcome.[127] However, the single-view approach to the RV may incur error when nonvisualized regions fail to contract similarly as assumed. For example, tricuspid annular descent deviated from its usually tight correlation with EF in a patient with apical dyskinesis.[128]

Ventricular Shape

The Left Ventricle

It has long been established that the LV becomes more spherical when it dilates to compensate for volume loading.[14,129] This compensatory mechanism allows more even distribution of regional stress and improves ventricular efficiency. More recently it has been recognized that similar changes occur on a regional level in patients with recent MI. Measurement of the magnitude of these changes provides information on the mechanism, magnitude, and time course of remodeling and its effect on prognosis.

The analysis of global LV shape from 2D endocardial contours is performed using general mathematical models. One approach is to determine the degree of roundness of the LV contour by computing its eccentricity.[130,131] Sphericity is assessed by determining the ratio of the long-axis length to the short-axis diameter.[132] To avoid variability in measuring the axis lengths, sphericity is also computed as the ratio of the end-diastolic volume to the volume of a sphere with equivalent long-axis length or the ratio of the end-diastolic volume to the volume of the sphere with equivalent surface area. In an experimental heart failure model, shape measurements based on axis length and area-to-perimeter ratios were less sensitive to incipient ventricular decompensation than the volume-to-surface area ratio.[133] Analysis of sphericity index from a 3D echocardiographic data set benefits from more accurate measurement of long-axis length and was found to identify patients destined to undergo remodeling after MI.[134] Other popular methods of shape analysis relate volume or a surrogate of volume, such as cavity area, to an idealized LV shape.[130,133] The disadvantages of these approaches to shape analysis are (1) these methods measure only global shape and thus provide little additional mechanistic information, (2) an unlimited number of shapes can present with the same ratio because it lacks any regional information about the LV; and (3) disease processes, particularly pertaining to regional ischemia, may vary LV shape from elliptical.

Curvature analysis is free of geometric assumptions, provides some regional shape information, and can compare shape to a population-derived normal value.[135]

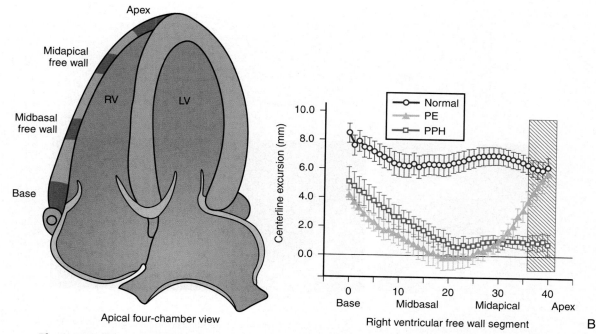

Figure 10–8. *A, Schematic diagram of the apical four-chamber view from a transthoracic two-dimensional echocardiogram. Qualitative wall motion scores were assigned at four locations of the right ventricular free wall (shaded areas). B, Segmental right ventricular free wall excursion (mean ± 1 SEM) by centerline analysis as a function of right ventricular free wall segment. Centerline excursion in patients with acute pulmonary embolism (PE) was near normal (p = NS versus normal), p greater than 0.03 versus primary pulmonary hypertension (PPH) at the apex (hatched area), but abnormal at the midfree wall and base (p < 0.02 versus normal). Centerline excursion in patients with primary pulmonary hypertension was reduced compared with that in normal subjects in all segments (p < 0.03). LV, left ventricle; NS, not significant; RV, right ventricle; SEM, standard error of the mean. (From McConnell MV, Solomon SD, Rayan ME, et al: Am J Cardiol 78(4):469-473, 1996. With permission from Excerpta Medical Inc.)*

However, curvature is sensitive to noise in border tracing unless averaged over a longer portion of the contour, in which case this parameter becomes relatively insensitive to local shape.[136] Because regional shape abnormalities affect curvature not in the region itself but at its limits, interpretation of this parameter is less than intuitive. Furthermore the method assumes an anatomical correspondence between each point on the patient's ventricle and the same numbered point in the normal reference ventricles. Curvature analysis applied to a long-axis contour can identify shape differences between patients with ischemic heart disease affecting different coronary beds and the values provide information on regional ventricular function.[137,138] The curvature of the short-axis contour can identify patients prone to infarct expansion, worsening dysfunction and death.[139] Perhaps its most useful application, however, has been identification of patients with pulmonary hypertension from changes in the curvature of the interventricular septum from short-axis images[140,141] (Fig. 10–9).

Another approach to LV shape analysis is to represent the endocardial contour as the weighted sum of shape terms using Fourier analysis.[142] Although this method was able to identify shape differences between aortic versus mitral regurgitation (MR), the technique is inefficient, requiring a fairly large number of terms to describe a LV in terms of geometric shapes, such as a dumbbell. One comparative analysis showed that the formula, Eccentricity $= \sqrt{L^2 + D^2}/L$, in which L is the long-axis length measured from the apex to mid-aortic valve and D is the short-axis length, is more sensitive to shape changes than indices of sphericity, curvature, or Fourier terms.[131]

Eigenshape or principal component analysis promises greater efficiency than Fourier analysis by deriving the shape terms from analysis of a population of LVs; therefore each term has a ventricular shape. For example, the "first" eigenshape is the average LV, and subsequent eigenshapes represent dimensions of variability around the average. On testing, however, the eigenshape method was unable to distinguish between normal subjects and patients with recent anterior, inferior, or lateral MI or with dilated cardiomyopathy unless the EF was considered.[143] Furthermore, neither Fourier nor eigenshape analysis provide an easy format for measuring the depth of an aneurysm because these methods express abnormality by the magnitudes of coefficients for multiple global terms whose shapes are increasingly complex.

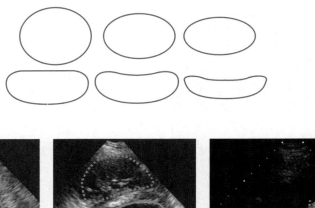

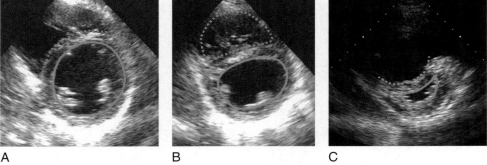

Figure 10–9. Top, *Discrete shapes used to describe the shape sequence model. Shape factor is the pointer into this sequence and varies from a value of one for a perfect circle to seven for an indented ellipse.* Bottom, *Short-axis echocardiographic views of a normal subject (A), a patient with tetralogy of Fallot with pulmonary regurgitation (B), and patient with pulmonary hypertension (C) illustrating the variation in the shape of the left ventricle (solid green contour) and of the right ventricle (dotted green contour) according to the level of hemodynamic load. (A from Azancot A, Caudell TP, Allen HD, et al:* Am J Cardiol *56:520-526, 1985.)*

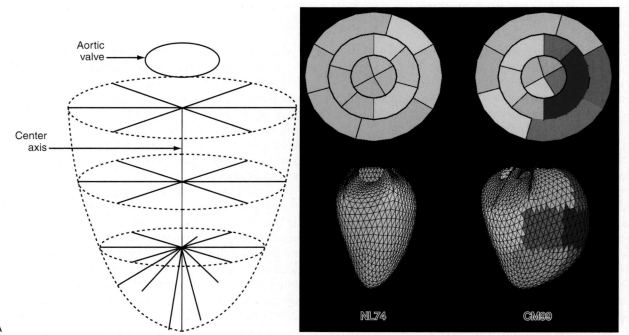

Figure 10–10. A, *The center axis method measures regional shape in terms of radial distance from a center axis to the endocardial surface. To normalize for heart size, the distance from the center axis to the reconstructed surface is divided by center axis length. The left ventricle is divided into 16 segments whose shape is calculated as the mean radial distance of the points lying within that segment to the center axis. B, The severity of shape abnormality is displayed using a color scale allowing visual appreciation of the difference between a normal subject (NL74) and anterior and anterolateral dilatation in a patient with idiopathic dilated cardiomyopathy (CM99).*

The center-axis method measures the distance between the 3D LV surface and its long axis, providing an easy-to-understand metric and graphic display[144] (Fig. 10–10). Despite the assumption that the longest distance from the centroid of the mitral annulus is the LV apex, center-axis shape measurements established a significant relationship between regional LV shape and the severity of functional MR (see Clinical Applications).[145]

The methods described above all share one major simplification. They compute shape from the patient's LV alone instead of comparing the patient's heart with a composite normal or with itself in serial studies. However, this visual comparison is what observers instinctively perform to evaluate shape abnormalities and measure their magnitude and location. From a computational point of view the comparison is performed by aligning the index and reference contours (if 2D) or surfaces (if 3D) according to concordant shape and/or anatomic landmarks. Alignment is usually done using the method of least squares, which minimizes the sum of the squared distances between corresponding points on the two surfaces being compared. Because the squared penalty term tends to force an alignment that spreads a regional shape abnormality over the rest of the surface, least squares is useful for defining the average *normal* heart but not for measuring the severity of a local deformation. An alternative alignment method has been developed and validated for analyzing 3D shape changes in serial studies of the same patient (Fig. 10–11); however, it cannot be applied for diagnosing shape abnormality by comparing a patient with a normal reference group because there are not enough anatomic landmarks on the LV to guide the alignment.[146]

The Right Ventricle

Study of the RV has been impeded by its complex shape, which has resisted simple geometric modeling. Most of the studies of RV shape have been performed to develop a method of measuring volume by angiography or 2D echocardiogram, modalities whose limited perspective necessitated comparing the RV to various geometric figures.[147-149] Whereas LV volume can be accurately measured from 2D imaging by assuming an ellipsoid shape, none of the 2D models proposed for estimating RV volume from echocardiographic images has gained clinically acceptable levels of accuracy. Another problem is that RV shape can change substantially in congenital heart disease, so that a given model may better fit normal subjects than diseased hearts or vice versa,[150] resulting in variable accuracy.

In 3D imaging, the borders traced to compute RV volume using Simpson's approach define an RV surface whose base is truncated to exclude its two valve orifices. This truncated RV model can also be applied for

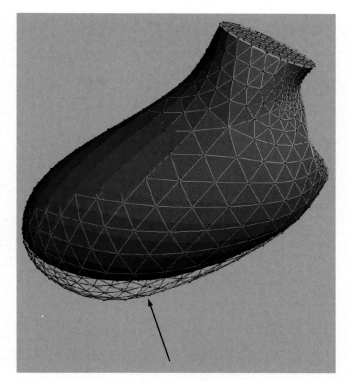

Figure 10–11. *The alignment method measures regional shape in terms of distance between the patient's heart and a reference such as normal average heart.[177] Here a normal end-diastolic left ventricular endocardial surface (mesh) has been deformed at the inferoapical wall (arrow) and aligned with its original, undeformed self (red surface) along regions of similar shape. The magnitude of shape abnormality can be quantified using the center surface algorithm.*

3D shape analysis. In one study of remodeling in pulmonary hypertension, regional geometry was measured in terms of segmental volumes at five levels from apex to base.[151] Nielson and colleagues used this approach in their elegant biventricular finite element model to investigate the relationship of RV shape to fiber orientation.[18] Young and colleagues extended this method to describe the 3D geometry of the LV and RV in experimental MR in terms of distances, arc lengths, surface areas, and surface curvatures among regions defined by the nodes of the finite-element model[152] (Fig. 10–12). Marcus and colleagues characterized RV shape from the curvature of borders in three orthogonal cross sections (coronal, sagittal, and transverse) and found that the contraction pattern was more predictive of RV hypertension in neonates than RV shape.[153] However, the RV surface that this method reconstructed was only validated for volume measurement not for shape.

Because of the difficulty in modeling the RV, research to analyze change in RV geometry in response to disease processes has been limited in scope. Studies of the impact of RV overload in congenital heart disease, pulmonary hypertension, and other conditions have concentrated on the shape of the LV and interven-

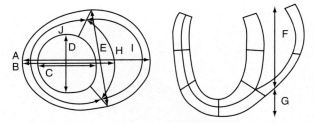

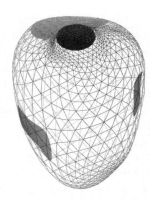

Figure 10–12. *Method of measuring left ventricular (LV) and right ventricular (RV) shape change from finite-element model. A, LV lateral epicardium to RV free-wall epicardium; B, LV lateral epicardium to RV septum endocardium; C, lateral-to-septal LV endocardium; D, anterior-to-posterior LV endocardium; E, anterior-to-posterior RV-LV insertions; F, RV apex to RV base (longitudinal); G, RV apex to LV apex (longitudinal); H, RV endocardial septum (arc length); I, RV free-wall endocardium (arc length); J, LV free-wall midwall (arc length). (From Young AA, Orr R, Smaill BH, Dell-Italia LJ: Am J Physiol 271: H2689-H2700, 1996. Reproduced with permission from American Physiological Society.)*

Figure 10–13. *In the piecewise smooth subdivision method, borders of anatomic landmarks can be carried through to the final surface reconstruction. Left, Wire mesh display of borders traced of the left ventricular endocardium (black), mitral annulus (blue-filled circles), aortic valve (green-filled circles), and papillary muscles (red). Right, On the fitted surface, the location of the papillary muscle insertions are displayed in red.*

tricular septum and its flattening or reverse curvature rather than on the RV[140] (see Fig. 10–9). At one time it was felt that regional RV wall stress analysis was impractical as a result of the RV's "convoluted shape."[154]

Instead of reconstructing the entire chamber, several investigators studying RV shape have focused on just one wall of the RV. Sacks and colleagues reconstructed the entire free wall of a normal canine RV in 3D from MRI data and characterized not only its regional curvature but also the change in curvature through the cardiac cycle.[155] Moses and Axel reconstructed the septum and developed an analytical tool for quantifying the curvature of its RV surface throughout the cardiac cycle from MRI data.[156] Although the interventricular septum is considered to be part of the LV, a complete description of the RV as a chamber should include examination of this surface and the free wall. Indeed virtually all ventricular shape studies in diseases involving the RV have focused on septal shape and its impact on LV rather than on RV function. For example, the degree of septal bulge into the LV cavity reflects the ratio of RV:LV pressure[140] and depresses LV function in RV volume overload.[157]

Because an infinite number of shapes can hold the same volume, 3D shape should be analyzed from anatomically accurate reconstructions of the targeted chamber. The piecewise smooth subdivision surface (PSSS) method is the only method validated for accuracy in reproducing 3D endocardial LV and RV shape and in measuring volume.[107,158] An additional advantage of this method is that anatomic landmarks identified on the images are conveyed to the final surface and can be used in computing parameters of geometry and shape (Fig. 10–13). When the PSSS method was applied to reconstruct the RVs of patients with pulmonary regurgitation following repair for tetralogy of Fallot

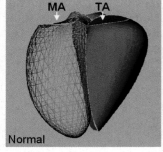

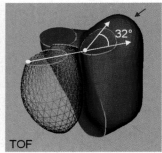

Figure 10–14. *Reconstructions of the left ventricular (green mesh) and right ventricular (red surface) endocardium of a normal subject (left) and a patient with repaired tetralogy of Fallot (TOF) (right). The patient with tetralogy of Fallot has severe right ventricular dilatation resulting from pulmonary regurgitation, and the left ventricle looks diminished in comparison. The shape of the right ventricle is characterized by widening at the apex (green arrow) and basal bulging (blue arrow) associated with tilting of the tricuspid annulus (TA) relative to the mitral annulus (MA) (white arrows).*

(TOF), two shape changes were seen: (1) bulging at the base lateral to the tricuspid annulus and (2) tilting of the tricuspid annulus[159,160] (Fig. 10–14). Similar shape changes were seen in pulmonary hypertension. These shape changes would have been difficult to recognize from short-axis images alone, such as are prepared from volumetric 3D echocardiographic data sets and probably would be excluded from analysis using RV models that truncate the base. Thus, assessment of RV shape in volume or pressure overload conditions should be performed on systems that permit analysis of long-axis and short-axis images (Fig. 10–15).

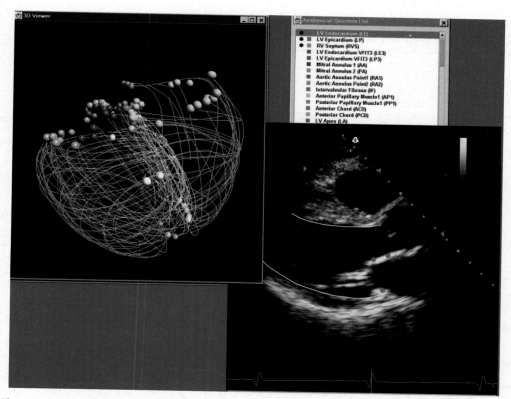

Figure 10–15. System for image analysis. The two-dimensional images are reviewed (right), and the borders of the target organ and associated anatomic landmarks are traced. Using position and orientation information from the tracking system, the x,y coordinates of each border are transformed into x, y, z coordinates for display in a three-dimensional window (left) in which short axis and long axis and oblique image borders can be reviewed together. Here the red and green borders are traced from the left ventricular endocardium and epicardium, the blue and violet from the right ventricle, and the spheres from valve orifices, ventricular apices, and other anatomic landmarks.

Clinical Applications

Regional Systolic Function

Analysis of regional ventricular function as a diagnostic aid is most useful when entertaining the diagnosis of a disease that causes a localized, regional abnormality rather than diffuse, global dysfunction. Thus, although regional abnormalities of LV function have been described in valvular disease,[161] wall motion analysis is most commonly applied in ischemic heart disease.

Diagnosis of Myocardial Infarction

Soon after the development of 2D echocardiography, its potential utility for diagnosing acute myocardial infarction was recognized,[162,163] as discussed in Chapters 13 and 14. Its sensitivity has been quite high in most studies, whether function was assessed qualitatively or quantitatively (Table 10–1). In general, wall thickening discriminates normal from infarcted myocardium better than does wall motion,[61,164] and transmural infarctions are better detected than subendocardial infarctions involving less than 20% of the wall thickness.[61] Histopathology studies have shown that myocardial segments with greater than 14% fibrosis are akinetic.[165] Thus, measurements of regional function are sensitive to the presence of infarction.

2D echocardiographic examination is quite accurate in localizing the infarction as well. In infarct patients the location of the dyssynergic segment agrees with the electrocardiographic infarct site in most patients (see Table 10–1). Discrepancies are a result of the presence of multivessel disease, history of previous infarction, or overlap between the perfusion territories of the right and circumflex coronary arteries. Thus, MI can be diagnosed and localized with excellent accuracy from visual inspection of wall motion. Indeed the relationship between infarction and dysfunction is so close that the lack of a wall motion or wall thickening defect rules out clinically significant infarction.[166]

TABLE 10–1. Accuracy of Regional Systolic Function Analysis in Diagnosing Myocardial Infarction

Study Group	Method	Threshold	Diagnosis Sens (%)	Diagnosis Spec (%)	Location Accuracy %	Reference
Human: 37 AMI	Semi-quantitative	Abnormal	100	—	97	Heger and colleagues[178]
Human: 26 TMMI, 6 SEMI	Semi-quantitative	Hypo, ak, dys	—	—	90	Nixon and colleagues[179]
Human: 66 AMI	Semi-quantitative	Hypo, ak, dys	—	—	94	Visser and colleagues[180]
Human: 20 MI, 18 normal	Area change	<2 SD	95	89	—	Parisi and colleagues[71]
Human: 20 MI, 18 normal	Hemiaxis shortening	<2 SD	85	78	—	Parisi and colleagues[71]
Human: 20 MI, 18 normal	Perimeter shortening	<2 SD	90	72	—	Parisi and colleagues[71]
Human: 15 MI	Semi-quantitative	Hypo, ak, dys	90	54	—	Weiss and colleagues[181]
Human: 48 AMI	Semi-quantitative	Hypo, ak, dys	—	—	96	Visser and colleagues[182]
Human: 18 angina, 12 SEMI	Semi-quantitative	Akinesis	50	100	—	Loh and colleagues[40]
Human: 18 angina, 12 SEMI	Semi-quantitative	Severe hypo	83	100	—	Loh and colleagues[40]
Human: 32 angina, 33 AMI	Semi-quantitative	Abnormal	94	84	—	Horowitz and colleagues[166]
Dog: 27	Area change	<2 SD	77	83	79	O'Boyle and colleagues[164]
Dog: 27	Wall thickening	<2 SD	81	100	88	O'Boyle and colleagues[164]
Human: 9 TMMI 6 SEMI	Wall motion Wall motion	<2 SD <2 SD	100 33	— —	— —	Henschke and colleagues[86]
Human: 9 TMMI 6 SEMI	Wall thickening Wall thickening	<2 SD <2 SD	89 83	— —	— —	Henschke and colleagues[86]
Human: 6 SEMI	Epicardial motion	<2 SD	0	—	—	Henschke and colleagues[86]
Human: 95 AMI	Semi-quantitative	Hypo, ak, dys	94	—	95	Van Reet and colleagues[183]
Human: 31 TMMI 9 SEMI	Semi-quantitative Semi-quantitative	Hypo, ak, dys Hypo, ak, dys	100 56	— —	— —	Widimsky and colleagues[184]
Dog: 24 MI, 5 nl	Wall thickening	≤0	71	100	—	Pandian and colleagues[185]
Dog: 24 MI, 5 nl	Wall motion	≤0	63	80	—	Pandian and colleagues[185]
Human: 32 AMI	Semi-quantitative	Hypo, ak, dys	100	—	93	Aebischer and colleagues[186]
Human: 73 TMMI	Semi-quantitative	Hypo, ak, dys	—	—	88	Widimsky and colleagues[187]
Human: 92 AMI	Semi-quantitative	Hypo, ak, dys	93	—	74	Otto and colleagues[42]

ak, akinesis; AMI, acute myocardial infarction; dys, dyskinesis; hypo, hypokinesis; MI, myocardial infarction; SD, standard deviation; SEMI, subendocardial MI; sens, sensitivity; spec, specificity; TMMI, transmural MI.
Data from references 40, 42, 71, 86, 164, 166, 178-187.

Assessment of Infarct Size

The hypothesis underlying infarct size assessment is that the pattern of dysfunction reflects the extent of infarction. However, many investigators have found that the circumferential extent of dysfunction exceeds the extent of infarction in patients.[60-64,167] One reason is that about 30% of infarct patients have multivessel disease, and 15% have had a previous infarction.[168] Even in single-vessel occlusion the region of dysfunction extends outside the perfusion territory of the occluded artery and into the normally perfused border zone.[60,64] The width of the border zone is small, less than 1 cm.[68,169] Function does not drop precipitously at each side of the infarction but rather declines gradually.[55,169] Because there is no clear separation between dysfunction in the viable, perfused border zone and dysfunction within the infarcted region, infarct size is estimated by applying an empirical threshold to the regional function measurements.

Reports on the accuracy of infarct size estimation have a wide range of results (see Table 10-2). In general, wall motion analysis tends to overestimate infarct size compared to wall thickening, but both parameters yield similarly close estimates of infarct size.[55,164] The results are similar for qualitative and for quantitative assessment of function. Most studies report a high correlation between infarct size and the extent of regional dysfunction, but rarely has the regression line approached the line of identity.

Assessment of Myocardial Viability

Echocardiography has been useful for evaluation of myocardial viability (see Chapter 16) and to document the magnitude of recovery and its time course after revascularization. In evaluating the response to revascularization, serial studies offer a diagnostic advantage because the influence of baseline variability between patients is minimized by having each patient as his or her own control. In practice, however, care must be taken to reproduce imaging conditions, such as patient position, sonographer, and imaging plane, to prevent study-to-study variability from obscuring the change in function.

Ventricular Shape

Many studies have been published reporting global and/or regional shape abnormalities in various cardiac diagnoses. However, the strongest application of ventricular shape analysis has been to improve our understanding of disease processes or to elucidate response to a therapeutic intervention.

Functional Valvular Regurgitation

3D echocardiography has unparalleled potential for elucidating the mechanism of disease processes as a result of its high spatial and temporal resolution. For example, 4D analysis of the annulus has permitted characterization of how the normal mitral valve achieves area reduction during systole through a combination of perimeter shortening and shape modulation.[170] Such techniques permit measurement of the extent to which annular dynamics or static dimensions may be altered by disease processes, such as ischemic heart disease or cardiomyopathy. 3D shape analysis of the components of the mitral apparatus has demonstrated the dependence of valve function on geometry by relating the severity of functional MR to regional antero-lateral LV dilatation, with resultant papillary muscle displacement and chordal angle widening, in patients with idiopathic dilated cardiomyopathy[145] (Fig. 10-16). In patients with ischemic heart disease the development of functional MR is associated primarily with inferior MI and outward displacement of the posterior papillary muscle causing leaflet tethering[171] (Fig. 10-17). In a similar manner to the LV, RV remodeling may negatively impact prognosis by affecting tricuspid valve function. Approximately one third of patients with repaired tetralogy of Fallot have moderate to severe tricuspid regurgitation,[172] which may be attributable to progressive RV and tricuspid annulus dilatation and other shape changes.

Outcome of Surgical Procedures

Analysis of LV or RV shape is of particular interest following surgical reconstructions of congenital anomalies because these patients are now surviving long enough for late complications to appear. In late survivors of tetralogy of Fallot repair, impaired clinical status has been associated with moderate or severe LV or RV dysfunction, and one mechanism of RV dysfunction is outflow track aneurysm or akinesis related to the use of a transannular patch during repair.[173,174] A second area of interest is LV reconstruction in patients with anterior postinfarction aneurysm: regional wall motion and curvature analysis demonstrated that aneurysmectomy and LV patch plasty reconstruction resulted in normalized outward convexity of the LV wall.[175]

TABLE 10–2. Evaluation of Myocardial Infarction by Two-Dimensional Echocardiography

Study Group	N	Timing	Echocardio-graphic View	Method	Threshold	Infarct Size Parameter	Corr Coeff	SEE	Reference
colspan Estimation of Infarct Size
Dog	25	5.5 hrs	1 LAX + 3 SAX	Semi-quantitative	Hypo, ak, dys	Tc99	0.90	—	Meltzer and colleagues[188]
Man	20	2-4 days	4 SAX	Semi-quantitative	Hypo, ak, dys	Thallium-201	0.87	—	Nixon and colleagues[179]
Man	29	2-4 days	4 SAX	Semi-quantitative	Hypo, ak, dys	Tc99	0.74	—	Nixon and colleagues[179]
Man	60	<12 hrs	3 LAX +5 SAX	Semi-quantitative	Hypo, ak, dys	Peak CK-MB	0.87	—	Visser and colleagues[180]
Man	15	varied	3 SAX	Semi-quantitative	Ak, dys	Postmortem	0.90	—	Weiss and colleagues[181]
Man	48	<12 hrs	3 apical	Semi-quantitative	Hypo, ak, dys	Peak CK-MB	0.81	—	Visser and colleagues[182]
Dog	20	2 hrs	1 LAX +3 SAX	Wall thickening	<0	Histopathology	0.50	5.9 %	Nieminen and colleagues[167]
Dog	20	48 hrs	1 LAX +3 SAX	Wall thickening	<0	Histopathology	0.73	4.9 %	Nieminen and colleagues[167]
Dog	24	20 min	2 SAX	Wall thickening	<0	Histopathology	0.92	—	Pandian and colleagues[63]
Dog	24	2 days	2 SAX	Wall thickening	<0	Histopathology	0.94	—	Pandian and colleagues[63]
Dog	27	Varied	3 SAX	Area change	<2 SD	Histopathology	0.76	16 %	O'Boyle and colleagues[164]
Dog	27	Varied	3 SAX	Wall thickening	<2 SD	Histopathology	0.77	16 %	O'Boyle and colleagues[164]
Dog	10	6 hrs	4 SAX	Semi-quantitative	Abnormal	Histopathology	0.75	13.5%	Kemper and colleagues[189]
Man	61	<12 hrs	4 LAX +3 SAX	Semi-quantitative	Hypo, ak, dys	Peak CK	0.39	—	Nishimura and colleagues[190]
Dog	11	6 hrs	3 SAX +3 apical	Semi-quantitative; endocardial surface map	Abnormal	Histopathology	0.91	—	Guyer and colleagues[191]
Man	20	<1 yr	3 SAX +2 apical	Semi-quantitative; endocardial surface map	Abnormal	Postmortem	0.94	25 cm^2	Wilkins and colleagues[192]
Dog	10	72 hrs	5 SAX	Radial shortening at ES	<15%	Histopathology	0.77	—	Mann and colleagues[193]
Dog	10	72 hrs	5 SAX	Radial shortening over cardiac cycle	<15%	Histopathology	0.81	—	Mann and colleagues[193]

2D, two dimensional; ak, akinesis; CI, confidence interval; CK, creatine kinase; CK-MB, creatine kinase, MB fraction; COM, center of mass (method of realignment for translation); Corr Coef, correlation coefficient; dys, dyskinesis; ES, end systole; hypo, hypokinesis; LAX, long axis; SAX, short-axis view; SD, standard deviations; SEE, standard error of estimate; Tc99, [99]technetium pyrophosphate scintigraphy.
Data from references 55, 63, 68, 164, 167, 169, 179-182, 188-194.

TABLE 10–2. **Evaluation of Myocardial Infarction by Two-Dimensional Echocardiography—cont'd**

Correlation with the Size of the Risk Region

Study Group	N	Timing	Echocardio-graphic View	Method	Threshold	Infarct Size Parameter	Corr Coeff	SEE	Reference
Dog	24	20 min	2 SAX	Wall thickening	<0	Angiography	0.83	—	Pandian and colleagues[63]
Dog	24	2 days	2 SAX	Wall thickening	<0	Angiography	0.85	—	Pandian and colleagues[63]
Dog	10	6 hrs	4 SAX	Semi-quantitative	Abnormal	Echocardio-graphic contrast	0.73	14.6%	Kemper and colleagues[189]
Dog	11	3 hrs		Wall motion	<10%	Echocardio-graphic contrast	0.92	1.7 %	Kaul and colleagues[194]
Dog	11	3 hrs	4 SAX	Wall motion	<20%	Echocardio-graphic contrast	0.79	3.3 %	Kaul and colleagues[194]
Dog	11	3 hrs	4 SAX	Circumference	Ak, dys	Echocardio-graphic contrast	0.66	2.5 %	Kaul and colleagues[194]
Dog	11	3 hrs	4 SAX	Wall motion over cardiac cycle	<95% CI	Echocardio-graphic contrast	0.92	1.7 %	Kaul and colleagues[194]
Dog	12	2 hrs	1 SAX	Wall thickening: referenced to contrast defect	<95% CI	Echocardio-graphic contrast	0.84	3.8 %	Force and colleagues[68]
Dog	12	2 hrs	1 SAX	Wall thickening: COM method	<95% CI	Echocardio-graphic contrast	0.68	5.4 %	Force and colleagues[68]

Study Group	N	Timing	Echocardio-graphic View	Method	Threshold	Infarct Size Parameter	Risk Region Size		
							Estimated	True	Reference
Dog	18	60 mins	1 SAX	Wall thickening	<95% CI	Microsphere	174*	135*	Buda and colleagues[169]
Dog	16	60 mins	1 SAX	Wall motion	<2 SD	Microsphere	45.9	37.5	McGillem and colleagues[55]
Dog	16	60 mins	1 SAX	Wall motion	<95% CI	Microsphere	25.6	37.5	McGillem and colleagues[55]
Dog	16	60 mins	1 SAX	Wall motion	Dys	Microsphere	13.1	37.5	McGillem and colleagues[55]
Dog	16	60 mins	1 SAX	Wall thickening	<2 SD	Microsphere	37.3	37.5	McGillem and colleagues[55]
Dog	16	60 mins	1 SAX	Wall thickening	<95% CI	Microsphere	19.1	37.5	McGillem and colleagues[55]
Dog	16	60 mins	1 SAX	Wall thickening	Dys	Microsphere	20.6	37.5	McGillem and colleagues[55]

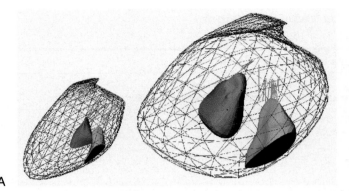

A

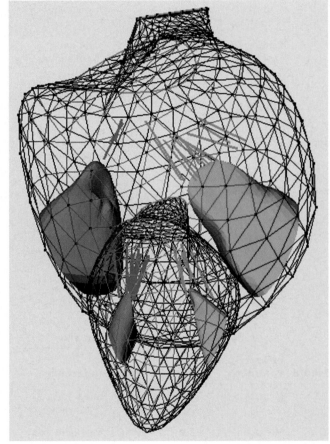

B

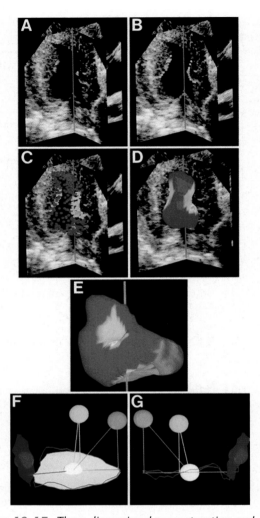

Figure 10–16. A, *Reconstructions of the left ventricular en-docardium and the papillary muscles at end-diastole of a normal subject (left) and a patient with idiopathic dilated car-diomyopathy. The principal chordae tendineae proceeding from each papillary muscle head are displayed as pink or green line segments. The reconstructions enable visualization of the enlargement of the left ventricle and the outward dis-placement of the papillary muscle insertions. B, Alignment of the normal (front) and cardiomyopathic (back) ventricles to demonstrate the divergence of the angle of the chordae ten-dineae to the mitral annulus (horizontal in this view). Chordae are normally nearly vertical, but with left ventricular dilata-tion the angle between anterior and posterior chordae is wid-ened.[145]*

Figure 10–17. Three-dimensional reconstruction and analy-sis of the mitral apparatus. A, Reconstruction of two intersect-ing echocardiographic images of a live dog heart in three di-mensions with a texture mapping algorithm. Images intersect the left ventricle from two different angles: one through the anterior papillary muscle and another through the posterior muscle. B, Points on images in A are traced with different colors to identify different features: red, endocardium; yellow, papillary muscle indentation; blue, region of papillary muscle tips; and green, mitral leaflets. C, Reconstruction of points from full data set. D, Surface of the left ventricular chamber with color mapping from adjacent structures. E, Entire left ventricular endocardial surface with papillary indentations (yellow), closed mitral leaflet surface (green with blue annular ring), and outflow tract (purple with pink annular ring). F, Dia-gram of the mitral apparatus as reconstructed in mid systole. This view shows the mitral annulus as a thin blue line. Projec-tion of the annulus onto the surface of the least-squares fitted x-y plane (light gray). The centroid of the mitral annulus is white, and the centroid of aortic annulus is red. The diagram is oriented so that the two papillary muscles (yellow and green) lie above the plane of the mitral annulus. The altitude above plane (axial distance) and angular relationships to cen-troid and to each other are illustrated by connecting lines. G, View of the same mitral reconstruction looking directly into the x-y plane of the mitral annulus (visible only as a horizontal green line). The altitude of the papillary tips above the plane is appreciated. (Reprinted from Otsuji Y, Handschumacher MD, Schammenthal E, et al: Circulation 96:1999-2008, 1997. With permission from Lippincott Williams & Wilkins.)*

KEY POINTS

- Because the heart is a mechanical organ, its function is closely related to its structure, from fiber orientation to the spatial geometry of components of the mitral apparatus.

- Visual assessment of regional left ventricular function is performed at 16 segments corresponding to coronary artery perfusion territories.

- For quantitative analysis regional left ventricular function can be measured in terms of endocardial wall motion, wall thickening, or midwall motion in patients with hypertrophy. Recently regional strain analysis became available using the technique of speckle tracking.

- 3D echocardiography has two modes. Volumetric imaging provides realistic visualization of cardiac structures. Surface modeling provides superior accuracy for quantifying volumes, function, and the opportunity to evaluate ventricular shape and the spatial relationships between cardiac structures.

- 2D methods for ventricular shape analysis fall into two types. The simpler methods (e.g., for computing sphericity) assume a regular ellipsoid shape to the LV. The more complex methods (e.g., for Fourier, eigenshape, or curvature analysis) express shape in terms that may be perplexing.

- 3D shape analysis of LV shape is in its infancy. Most reports on RV shape examined interventricular septal curvature in the short-axis view as a gauge of pulmonary hypertension severity.

- Early applications of function and shape analysis were methods of gauging parameters, such as infarct size, that can now be quantified directly using other imaging techniques. 3D analysis provides quantification of the relationship between function and shape and is providing insight into the mechanism of disease processes and the effect of surgical interventions.

REFERENCES

1. Hunter PJ, Mcculloch AD, ter Keurs HE: Modeling the mechanical properties of cardiac muscle. *Prog Biophys Mol Biol* 69:289-331, 1998.
2. Streeter DD, Jr: Gross morphology and fiber geometry of the heart. In: Berne RM, Sperelakis N, Geiger S, (eds): *Handbook of Physiology*. Section 2, vol. 1. The cardiovascular system (American Physiology Society). Baltimore: Williams & Wilkins, 1979, pp. 61-112.
3. Sallin EA: Fiber orientation and ejection fraction in the human left ventricle. *Biophysical J* 9:954-964, 1969.
4. Sanchez-Quintana D, Garcia-Martinez V, Hurle JM: Myocardial fiber architecture in the human heart. *Acta Anat* 138:352-358, 1990.
5. Rushmer RF, Crystal DK, Wagner C: The functional anatomy of ventricular contraction. *Circ Res* 1:162-170, 1953.
6. Bogaert J, Rademakers FE: Regional nonuniformity of normal adult human left ventricle. *Am J Physiol* 280:H610-H620, 2001.
7. Hansen DE, Daughters GT, Alderman EL, et al: Torsional deformation of the left ventricular midwall in human hearts with intramyocardial markers: Regional heterogeneity and sensitivity to the inotropic effects of abrupt rate changes. *Circ Res* 62:941-952, 1988.
8. Beyar R, Yin F, Hausknecht M, et al: Dependence of left ventricular twist-radial shortening relations on cardiac cycle phase. *Am J Physiol* 257:H1119-H1126, 1989.
9. Yun KL, Miller DC: Torsional deformation of the left ventricle. *J Heart Valve Dis* 4 (Suppl. II):S214-S222, 1995.
10. Shapiro EP, Rademakers FE: Importance of oblique fiber orientation for left ventricular wall deformation. *Technol Health Care* 5:21-28, 1997.
11. Armour JA, Randall WC: Structural basis for cardiac function. *Am J Physiol* 218:1517-1523, 1970.
12. Geva T, Powell AJ, Crawford EC, et al: Evaluation of regional differences in right ventricular systolic function by acoustic quantification echocardiography and cine magnetic resonance imaging. *Circulation* 98:339-345, 1998.
13. Arts T, Reneman RS: The importance of the geometry of the heart to the pump. In: ter Keurs HE, Noble M, (eds): *Starling's Law of the Heart Revisited*. Dordrecht: Kluwer Acad Publishers, 1988, pp. 94-111.
14. Dodge HT, Frimer M, Stewart DK: Functional evaluation of the hypertrophied heart in man. *Circ Res* 34-35 (Suppl II):II-122-II-127, 1974.
15. McCulloch AD: Cardiac biomechanics. In: Bronzino JD (ed): *Biomedical Engineering Handbook*. Boca Raton: CRC Press: IEEE Press, 1995, pp. 418-439.
16. McCulloch AD, Omens JH: Factors affecting the regional mechanics of the diastolic heart. In: Glass L, Hunter R, Mcculloch AD, (eds): *Theory of Heart: Biomechanics, Biophysics, and Nonlinear Dynamics of Cardiac Function*. New York: Springer-Verlag, 1991, pp. 87-119.
17. Hunter PJ, Nielsen PMF, Smaill BH, LeGrice IJ: An anatomical heart model with applications to myocardial activation and ventricular mechanics. *Crit Rev Biomed Eng* 20:403-426, 1992.
18. Nielsen PMF, Le Grice IJ, Smaill BH, Hunter PJ: Mathematical model of geometry and fibrous structure of the heart. *Am J Physiol Heart Circ Physiol* 260(29):H1365-H1378, 1991.
19. Haber I, Metaxas DN, Axel L: Three-dimensional motion reconstruction and analysis of the right ventricle using tagged MRI. *Med Image Anal* 4:335-355, 2000.
20. Young AA, Dokos S, Powerll KA, et al: Regional heterogeneity of function in nonischemic dilated cardiomyopathy. *Cardiovasc Res* 49:308-318, 2001.
21. Young AA, Kramer CM, Ferrari VA, et al: Three-dimensional left ventricular deformation in hypertrophic cardiomyopathy. *Circulation* 90:854-867, 1994.
22. Walker JC, Ratcliffe MB, Zhang P, et al. MRI-based finite-element analysis of left ventricular aneurysm. *Am J Physiol Heart Circ Physiol* 289:692-700, 2005.
23. Cupps BP, Moustakidis P, Pomerantz BJ, et al: Severe aortic insufficiency and normal systolic function: Determining regional left ventricular wall stress by finite-element analysis. *Ann Thorac Surg* 76:668-675, 2003.
24. McCulloch AD, Waldman L, Rogers J: Large-scale finite element analysis of the beating heart. *Crit Rev Biomed Eng* 20:427-449, 1992.
25. Vetter FJ, Mcculloch AD: Three-dimensional analysis of regional cardiac function: A model of rabbit ventricular anatomy. *Prog Biophys Mol Biol* 69:157-183, 1998.
26. Cerqueira MD, Weissman NJ, Dilsizian V, et al: Standardized myocardial segmentation and nomenclature for tomographic imaging of the heart. *Circulation* 105:539-542, 2002.
27. Schiller NB, Shah PM, Crawford M, et al: Recommendations for quantitation of the left ventricle by two-dimensional echocardiography. *J Am Soc Echocardiogr* 2:358-367, 1989.

28. Herman MV, Gorlin R. Implications of left ventricular asynergy. *Am J Cardiol* 23:538-547, 1969.

29. Gibson RS, Bishop HL, Stamm RB, et al: Value of early two dimensional echocardiography in patients with acute myocardial infarction. *Am J Cardiol* 49:1110-1119, 1982.

30. Stamm RB, Gibson RS, Bishop HL, et al: Echocardiographic detection of infarct-localized asynergy and remote asynergy during acute myocardial infarction: Correlation with the extent of angiographic coronary disease. *Circulation* 67:233-244, 1983.

31. Bourdillon PDV, Broderick TM, Sawada SG, et al: Regional wall motion index for infarct and noninfarct regions after reperfusion in acute myocardial infarction: Comparison with global wall motion index. *J Am Soc Echocardiogr* 2:398-407, 1989.

32. Kisslo J, Robertson D, Gilbert B, et al: A comparison of real-time, two-dimensional echocardiography and cineangiography in detecting left ventricular asynergy. *Circulation* 55:134-141, 1977.

33. Ohuchi Y, Kuwako K, Umeda T, Machii K. Real-time, phased-array, cross-sectional echocardiographic evaluation of left ventricular asynergy and quantitation of left ventricular function: A comparison with left ventricular cineangiography. *Jpn Heart J* 21:1-15, 1980.

34. Hecht HS, Taylor R, Wong M, Shah PM: Comparative evaluation of segmental asynergy in remote myocardial infarction by radionuclide angiography, two-dimensional echocardiography, and contrast ventriculography. *Am Heart J* 101:740-749, 1981.

35. Freeman AP, Giles RW, Walsh WF, et al: Regional left ventricular wall motion assessment: Comparison of two-dimensional echocardiography and radionuclide angiography with contrast angiography in healed myocardial infarction. *Am J Cardiol* 56:8-12, 1985.

36. Shiina A, Tajik AJ, Smith HC, et al: Prognostic significance of regional wall motion abnormality in patients with prior myocardial infarction: a prospective correlative study of two-dimensional echocardiography and angiography. *Mayo Clin Proc* 61:254-162, 1986.

37. Lundgren C, Bourdillon PDV, Dillon JC, Feigenbaum H: Comparison of contrast angiography and two-dimensional echocardiography for the evaluation of left ventricular regional wall motion abnormalities after acute myocardial infarction. *Am J Cardiol* 65:1071-1077, 1990.

38. Ginzton L, Conant R, Brizendine M, et al: Exercise subcostal two-dimensional echocardiography: a new method of segmental wall motion analysis. *Am J Cardiol* 53:805-811, 1984.

39. Bhatnagar SK, Al-Yusuf AR: Significance of early two-dimensional echocardiography after acute myocardial infarction. *Int J Cardiol* 5:575-584, 1984.

40. Loh IK, Yzhar C, Beeder C, et al: Early diagnosis of nontransmural myocardial infarction by two-dimensional echocardiography. *Am Heart J* 104:963-968, 1982.

41. Deutsch HJ, Curtius JM, Leischik R, et al: Reproducibility of assessment of left ventricular function using intraoperative transesophageal echocardiography. *Thoracic Cardiovasc Surg* 41:54-58, 1993.

42. Otto C, Stratton JR, Maynard C, et al: Echocardiographic evaluation of segmental wall motion early and late after thrombolytic therapy in acute myocardial infarction: The Western Washington Tissue Plasminogen Activator Emergency Room Trial. *Am J Cardiol* 65(3):132-138, 1990.

43. Gibson DG, Prewitt TA, Brown DJ: Analysis of left ventricular wall movement during isovolumic relaxation and its relation to coronary artery disease. *Br Heart J* 38:1010-1019, 1976.

44. de Simone G, Devereux RB: Rationale of echocardiographic assessment of left ventricular wall stress and midwall mechanics in hypertensive heart disease. *Eur J Echocardiogr* 3:192-198, 2002.

45. Hexeberg E, Homans DC, Bache RJ: Interpretation of systolic wall thickening: Can thickening of a discrete layer reflect fibre performance? *Cardiovasc Res* 29:16-21, 1995.

46. Langeland S, D'hooge J, Wouters PF, et al: Experimental validation of a new ultrasound method for the simultaneous assessment of radial and longitudinal myocardial deformation independent of insonation angle. *Circulation* 112:2157-2162, 2005.

47. Ginzton LE, Berntzen R, Lobodzinski S, et al: Computerized quantitative segmental wall motion analysis during exercise: Radial vs. centerline left ventricular segmentation. In: *Computers in Cardiology.* Long Beach: IEEE Computer Society, 1985, pp. 157-160.

48. Rein A, Sapoznikov D, Lewis N, et al: Regional left ventricular ejection fraction from real-time two-dimensional echocardiography. *Inter J Cardiol* 2:61-70, 1982.

49. Assmann PE, Slager CJ, van der Border SG, et al: Comparison of models for quantitative left ventricular wall motion analysis from two-dimensional echocardiograms during acute myocardial infarction. *Am J Cardiol* 71:1262-1269, 1993.

50. Moynihan PF, Parisi AF, Feldman EL: Quantitative detection of regional left ventricular contraction abnormalities by two-dimensional echocardiography: I. Analysis of methods. *Circulation* 63:752-760, 1981.

51. Slager CJ, Hooghoudt TEH, Serruys PW, et al: Quantitative assessment of regional left ventricular motion using endocardial landmarks. *J Am Coll Cardiol* 7:317-327, 1986.

52. Gibson DG, Sanderson JE, Traill TA, et al: Regional left ventricular wall movement in hypertrophic cardiomyopathy. *Br Heart J* 40:1327-1333, 1978.

53. Sheehan FH, Bolson EL, Dodge HT, et al: Advantages and applications of the centerline method for characterizing regional ventricular function. *Circulation* 74:293-305, 1986.

54. Wohlgelernter D, Cleman M, Highman A, et al: Regional myocardial dysfunction during coronary angioplasty: Evaluation by two-dimensional echocardiography and 12 lead electrocardiography. *J Am Coll Cardiol* 7:1245-1254, 1986.

55. McGillem MJ, Mancini GBJ, DeBoe SF, Buda AJ: Modification of the centerline method for assessment of echocardiographic wall thickening and motion: A comparison with areas of risk. *J Am Coll Cardiol* 11:861-866, 1988.

56. Ginzton LE: Stress echocardiography and myocardial contrast echocardiography. *Cardiol Clin* 7:493-509, 1989.

57. Sheehan FH, Stewart DK, Dodge HT, et al: Variability in the measurement of regional ventricular wall motion from contrast angiograms. *Circulation* 68:550-559, 1983.

58. Gelberg HJ, Brundage BH, Glantz S, Parmley WW: Quantitative left ventricular wall motion analysis: A comparison of area, chord and radial methods. *Circulation* 59:991-1000, 1979.

59. Jugdutt BI, Hutchins GM, Bulkley BH, Becker LC: Myocardial infarction in the conscious dog: Three-dimensional mapping of infarct, collateral flow and region at risk. *Circulation* 60:1141-1150, 1979.

60. Kerber RE, Marcus ML, Ehrhardt J, et al: Correlation between echocardiographically demonstrated segmental dyskinesis and regional myocardial perfusion. *Circulation* 52:1097-1104, 1975.

61. Lieberman AN, Weiss JL, Jugdutt BI, et al: Two-dimensional echocardiography and infarct size: Relationship of regional wall motion and thickening to the extent of myocardial infarction in the dog. *Circulation* 63:739-746, 1981.

62. Wyatt HL, Meerbaum S, Heng MK: Experimental evaluation of the extent of myocardial dyssynergy and infarct size by two-dimensional echocardiography. *Circulation* 63:607-614, 1981.

63. Pandian NG, Koyanagi S, Skorton DJ, et al: Relations between 2-dimensional echocardiographic wall thickening abnormalities, myocardial infarct size and coronary risk area in normal and hypertrophied myocardium in dogs. *Am J Cardiol* 52:1318-1325, 1983.

64. Hutchins GM, Bulkley BH, Ridolfi RL, et al: Correlation of coronary arteriograms and left ventriculograms with postmortem studies. *Circulation* 56:32-37, 1977.

65. Sheehan FH, Doerr R, Schmidt WG, et al: Early recovery of left ventricular function after thrombolytic therapy for acute myo-

cardial infarction: An important determinant of survival. *J Am Coll Cardiol* 12:289-300, 1988.

66. Pandian NG, Skorton DJ, Collins SM, et al: Heterogeneity of left ventricular segmental wall thickening and excursion in 2-dimensional echocardiograms of normal human subjects. *Am J Cardiol* 51:1667-1673, 1983.

67. Assmann PE, Slager CJ, Dreysse ST, et al: Two-dimensional echocardiographic analysis of the dynamic geometry of the left ventricle: The basis for an improved model of wall motion. *J Am Soc Echocardiogr* 1:393-405, 1988.

68. Force T, Kemper A, Perkins L, et al: Overestimation of infarct size by quantitative two-dimensional echocardiography: The role of tethering and of analytic procedures. *Circulation* 73:1360-1368, 1986.

69. Feneley M, Farnsworth A, Shanahan M, Cheng V: Mechanisms of the development and resolution of paradoxical interventricular septal motion after uncomplicated cardiac surgery. *Am Heart J* 114:106-114, 1987.

70. Feneley M, Gavaghan T: Paradoxical and pseudoparadoxical interventricular septal motion in patients with right ventricular volume overload. *Circulation* 74:230-238, 1986.

71. Parisi A, Moynihan P, Folland E, Feldman C: Quantitative detection of regional left ventricular contraction abnormalities by two-dimensional echocardiography. II. Accuracy in coronary artery disease. *Circulation* 63(4):761-767, 1981.

72. Schnittger I, Fitzgerald P, Gordon E, et al: Computerized quantitative analysis of left ventricular wall motion by two-dimensional echocardiography. *Circulation* 70(2):242-254, 1984.

73. Zoghbi WA, Charlat ML, Bolli R, et al: Quantitative assessment of left ventricular wall motion by two-dimensional echocardiography: Validation during reversible ischemia in the conscious dog. *J Am Coll Cardiol* 11:851-860, 1988.

74. Kittleson MD, Knowlen GG, Johnson LE: Early and late global and regional left ventricular function after experimental transmural myocardial infarction: Relationships of regional wall motion, wall thickening, and global performance. *Am Heart J* 114:70-78, 1987.

75. Beyar R, Shapiro EP, Graves WL, et al: Quantification and validation of left ventricular wall thickening by a three-dimensional volume element magnetic resonance imaging approach. *Circulation* 81:297-307, 1990.

76. Erbel R, Schweizer P, Meyer J, et al: Sensitivity of cross-sectional echocardiography in detection of impaired global and regional left ventricular function: Prospective study. *Int J Cardiol* 7:375-389, 1985.

77. Sheehan FH, Feneley MP, DeBruijn NP, et al: Quantitative regional wall thickening analysis by transesophageal echocardiography. *J Thorac Cardiovasc Surg* 103:347-354, 1992.

78. Yang P, Otto C, Sheehan F: The effect of normalization in reducing variability in regional wall thickening. *J Am Soc Echocardiogr* 10:197-204, 1997.

79. Heikkila J, Nieminen MS: Echoventriculography in acute myocardial infarction. IV:Infarct size and reliability by pathologic anatomic correlations. *Clin Cardiol* 3:26-35, 1980.

80. Feneley M, Hickie J: Validity of echocardiographic determination of left ventricular systolic wall thickening. *Circulation* 70(2):226-232, 1984.

81. Weiss RJ, Buda AJ, Pasyk S, et al: Noninvasive quantification of jeopardized myocardial mass in dogs using 2-dimensional echocardiography and thallium-201 tomography. *Am J Cardiol* 52:1340-1344, 1983.

82. Dumesnil J, Shoucri R, Laurenceau J, Turcot J: A mathematical model of the dynamic geometry of the intact left ventricle and its application to clinical data. *Circulation* 59:1024-1034, 1979.

83. Sandor T, Henschke C, Risser TA, et al: Quantitative analysis of left ventricular wall motion and thickness using two-dimensional echocardiography. *Int J Biomed Comput* 14: 431-439, 1983.

84. Ren JF, Kotler MN, Hakki AH, et al: Quantitation of regional left ventricular function by two-dimensional echocardiography in normals and patients with coronary artery disease. *Am Heart J* 110(3):552-560, 1985.

85. Haendchen RV, Wyatt HL, Maurer G, et al: Quantitation of regional cardiac function by two-dimensional echocardiography. I. Patterns of contraction in the normal left ventricle. *Circulation* 67:1234-1245, 1983.

86. Henschke CI, Risser TA, Sandor T, et al: Quantitative computer-assisted analysis of left ventricular wall thickening and motion by 2-dimensional echocardiography in acute myocardial infarction. *Am J Cardiol* 52:960-964, 1983.

87. Sasayama S, Franklin D, Ross J Jr, et al: Dynamic changes in left ventricular wall thickness and their use in analyzing cardiac function in the conscious dog: A study based on a modified ultrasonic technique. *Am J Cardiol* 38:870-879, 1976.

88. Azancot I, Masquet C, Bourthoumieux A, et al: Myocardial hypertrophy, rate of change of free wall thickness and directional components of ventricular power in man. *J Physiol (Paris)* 77:695-703, 1981.

89. Shimizu G, Zile MR, Blaustein AS, Gaasch WH: Left ventricular chamber filling and midwall fiber lengthening in patients with left ventricular hypertrophy: overestimation of fiber velocities by conventional midwall measurement. *Circulation* 71:266-272, 1985.

90. Aurigemma GP, Silver KH, McLaughlin M, et al: Impact of chamber geometry and gender on left ventricular systolic function in patients >60 years of age with aortic stenosis. *Am J Cardiol* 74:794-798, 1994.

91. Jung HO, Sheehan FH, Bolson EL, et al: Evaluation of midwall systolic function in left ventricular hypertrophy: A comparison of 3D versus 2D echo indices. *J Am Soc Echocardiogr* 19:802-810, 2006.

92. Gallagher KP, Osakada G, Hess OM, et al: Subepicardial segmental function during coronary stenosis and the role of myocardial fiber orientation. *Circ Res* 50:352-359, 1982.

93. Aurigemma GP, Silver KH, McLaughlin M, et al: Gender influences the pattern of left ventricular hypertrophy in elderly patients with aortic stenosis (abstr.). *Circulation* (Suppl 1):I-538, 1992.

94. Edvardsen T, Gerber BL, Garot J, et al: Quantitative assessment of intrinsic regional myocardial deformation by Doppler strain rate echocardiography in humans: Validation against three-dimensional tagged magnetic resonance imaging. *Circulation* 106:50-56, 2002.

95. Urheim S, Edvardsen T, Torp H, et al: Myocardial strain by Doppler echocardiography: Validation of a new method to quantify regional myocardial function. *Circulation* 102:1158-1164, 2000.

96. Amundsen BH, Helle-Valle T, Edvardsen T, et al: Noninvasive myocardial strain measurement by speckle tracking echocardiography. *J Am Coll Cardiol* 47:789-793, 2006.

97. Suffoletto MS, Dohi K, Cannesson M, et al: Novel speckle-tracking radial strain from routine black-and-white echocardiographic images to quantify dyssynchrony and predict response to cardiac resynchronization therapy. *Circulation* 113:960-968, 2006.

98. Helle-Valle T, Crosby J, Edvardsen T, et al: New noninvasive method for assessment of left ventricular rotation: Speckle tracking echocardiography. *Circulation* 112:3149-3156, 2005.

99. Belohlavek M, Foley DA, Gerber TC, et al: Three- and four-dimensional cardiovascular ultrasound imaging: A new era for echocardiography. *Mayo Clin Proc* 68:221-240, 1993.

100. Matsumoto M, Inoue M, Tamura S, et al: Three-dimensional echocardiography for spatial visualization and volume calculation of cardiac structures. *J Clin Ultrasound* 9:157-165, 1981.

101. Roelandt J, ten Cate FJ, Vletter WB, et al: Ultrasonic dynamic three-dimensional visualization of the heart with a multiplane transesophageal imaging transducer. *J Am Soc Echocardiogr* 7:217-229, 1994.

102. Matsumoto M, Matsuo H, Kitabatake A, et al: Three-dimensional echocardiograms and two-dimensional echocardiographic images at desired planes by a computerized system. *Ultrasound Med Biol* 3:163-178, 1977.

103. Vannan MA, Cao QL, Pandian NG, et al: Volumetric multiplexed transmission holography of the heart with echocardiographic data. *J Am Soc Echocardiogr* 8:567-575, 1995.

104. Corsi C, Lang RM, Veronesi F, et al: Volumetric quantification of global and regional left ventricular function from real-time three-dimensional echocardiographic images. *Circulation* 112:1161-1170, 2005.

105. Gopal A, Keller A, Rigling R, et al: Left ventricular volume and endocardial surface area by three-dimensional echocardiography: Comparison with two-dimensional echocardiography and nuclear magnetic resonance imaging in normal subjects. *J Am Coll Cardiol* 22:258-270, 1993.

106. Handschumacher MD, Lethor JP, Siu SC, et al: A new integrated system for three-dimensional echocardiographic reconstruction: Development and validation for ventricular volume with application in human subjects. *J Am Coll Cardiol* 21:743-753, 1993.

107. Legget ME, Leotta DF, Bolson EL, et al: System for quantitative three dimensional echocardiography of the left ventricle based on a magnetic field position and orientation sensing system. *IEEE Trans Biomed Eng* 45:494-504, 1998.

108. Potel MJ, MacKay SA, Rubin JM, et al: Three-dimensional left ventricular wall motion in man. Coordinate systems for representing wall movement direction. *Invest Radiol* 19:499-509, 1984.

109. Lima JA, Jeremy R, Guier W, et al: Accurate systolic wall thickening by nuclear magnetic resonance imaging with tissue tagging: Correlation with sonomicrometers in normal and ischemic myocardium. *J Am Coll Cardiol* 21:1741-1751, 1993.

110. Hubka M, Lipiecki J, Bolson EL, et al: Three-dimensional echocardiographic measurement of left ventricular wall thickness: In vitro and in vivo validation. *J Am Soc Echocardiogr* 15:129-135, 2002.

111. Laster SB, Ohnishi Y, Saffitz JE, Goldstein JA: Effects of reperfusion on ischemic right ventricular dysfunction. *Circulation* 90:1398-1409, 1994.

112. Zornoff LAM, Skali H, Pfeffer MA, et al: Right ventricular dysfunction and risk of heart failure and mortality after myocardial infarction. *J Am Coll Cardiol* 39:1450-1455, 2002.

113. Lebeau R, Di Lorenzo M, Sauve C, et al: Two-dimensional echocardiography estimation of right ventricular ejection fraction by wall motion score index. *Can J Cardiol* 20:169-176, 2004.

114. Yoerger DM, Marcus F, Sherrill D, et al: Echocardiographic findings in patients meeting Task Force criteria for arrhythmogenic right ventricular dysplasia. *J Am Coll Cardiol* 45:860-865, 2005.

115. Sheehan FH, Mathey DG, Wygant J, et al: Measurement of regional right ventricular wall motion from biplane contrast angiograms using the centerline method. In: *Computers in Cardiology*. Long Beach, CA: IEEE Computer Society, 1985, pp. 149-152.

116. Nakasato M, Akiba T, Sato S, et al: Right and left ventricular function assessed by regional wall motion analysis in patients with tetralogy of Fallot. *Int J Cardiol* 58:127-134, 1997.

117. Tulevski II, Zijta FM, Smeijers AS, et al: Regional and global right ventricular dysfunction in asymptomatic or minimally symptomatic patients with congenitally corrected transposition. *Cardiol Young* 14:168-174, 2004.

118. Fayad ZA, Ferrari VA, Kraitchman DL, et al: Right ventricular regional function using MR tagging: Normals versus chronic pulmonary hypertension. *Magn Reson Med* 39:116-123, 1998.

119. Naito H, Arisawa J, Harada K, et al: Assessment of right ventricular regional contraction and comparison with the left ventricle in normal humans: A cine magnetic resonance study with presaturation myocardial tagging. *Br Heart J* 74:186-191, 1995.

120. Young AA, Fayad ZA, Axel L: Right ventricular midwall surface motion and deformation using magnetic resonance tagging. *Am J Physiol* 271:H2677-H2688, 1996.

121. Menteer J, Weiinberg PM, Fogel MA: Quantifying regional right ventricular function in tetralogy of Fallot. *J Cardiovasc Mag Res* 7:753-761, 2005.

122. Klein SS, Graham TPJ, Lorenz CH: Noninvasive delineation of normal right ventricular contractile motion with magnetic resonance imaging myocardial tagging. *Ann Biomed Eng* 26:756-763, 1998.

123. Bomma C, Dal D, Tandri H, et al: Regional differences in systolic and diastolic function in arrhythmogenic right ventricular dysplasia/cardiomyopathy using magnetic resonance imaging. *Am J Cardiol* 95:1507-1511, 2005.

124. McConnell MV, Solomon SD, Rayan ME, et al: Regional right ventricular dysfunction detected by echocardiography in acute pulmonary embolism. *Am J Cardiol* 78:469-473, 1996.

125. Helbing WA, Bosch HG, Maliepaard C, et al: Comparison of echocardiographic methods with magnetic resonance imaging for assessment of right ventricular function in children. *Am J Cardiol* 76:589-594, 1995.

126. Kaul S, Tei C, Hopkins J, Shah P: Assessment of right ventricular function using two-dimensional echocardiography. *Am Heart J* 107:526-531, 1984.

127. Ghio S, Recusani F, Klersy C, et al: Prognostic usefulness of the tricuspid annular plane systolic excursion in patients with congestive heart failure secondary to idiopathic or ischemic dilated cardiomyopathy. *Am J Cardiol* 85:837-842, 2000.

128. Smith JL, Bolson EL, Wong SP, et al: Three-dimensional assessment of two-dimensional technique for evaluation of right ventricular function by tricuspid annulus motion. *Int J Cardiovasc Imaging* 19:189-197, 2003.

129. Burton AC: The importance of the shape and size of the heart. *Am Heart J* 54:801-810, 1957.

130. Gibson DG, Brown DJ: Continuous assessment of left ventricular shape in man. *Br Heart J* 37:904-910, 1975.

131. Rehman AU, D'Cruz IA: Quantitative echocardiographic assessment of left ventricular shape. *Echocardiography* 14:171-180, 1997.

132. D'Cruz IA, Aboulatta H, Killam H, et al: Quantitative two-dimensional echocardiographic assessment of left ventricular shape in ischemic heart disease. *J Clin Ultrasound* 17:569-572, 1989.

133. Tomlinson CW: Left ventricular geometry and function in experimental heart failure. *Can J Cardiol* 3:305-310, 1987.

134. Mannaerts HFJ, van der Heide JA, Kamp O, et al: Early identification of left ventricular remodelling after myocardial infarction, assessed by transthoracic 3D echocardiography. *Eur Heart J* 25:680-687, 2004.

135. Mancini GBJ, McGillem MJ: Quantitative regional curvature analysis: Validation in animals of a method for assessing regional ventricular remodeling in ischemic heart disease. *Int J Cardiovasc Imaging* 7:73-78, 1991.

136. Van Eyll C, Pouleur H, Raigoso J, et al: Curvature analysis of ventriculograms: How useful is it to assess progression of left ventricular remodeling and dysfunction? *Comput Cardiol*. Chicago, IEEE Computer Society Press, 1991, pp. 577-580.

137. Mancini GBJ, DeBoe SF, Anselmo E, et al: Quantitative regional curvature analysis: an application of shape determination for the assessment of segmental left ventricular function in man. *Am Heart J* 113:326-334, 1987.

138. Fantini F, Barletta G, di Donato M, et al: Alterations in left ventricular shape in patients with angina and single-vessel coronary disease. *Coron Artery Dis* 5:901-908, 1994.

139. Jugdutt BI: Identification of patients prone to infarct expansion by the degree of regional shape distortion on an early two-dimensional echocardiogram after myocardial infarction. *Clin Cardiol* 13:28-40, 1990.

140. Azancot A, Caudell TP, Allen HD, et al: Echocardiographic ventricular shape analysis in congenital heart disease with right ventricular volume or pressure overload. *Am J Cardiol* 56:520-526, 1985.

141. King ME, Braun H, Goldblatt A, et al: Interventricular septal configuration as a predictor of right ventricular systolic hypertension in children: a cross-sectional echocardiographic study. *Circulation* 68:68-75, 1983.

142. Kass DA, Traill TA, Keating M, et al: Abnormalities of dynamic ventricular shape change in patients with aortic and mitral valvular regurgitation: Assessment by Fourier shape analysis and global geometric indexes. *Circ Res* 62:127-138, 1988.

143. Sampson PD, Bookstein FL, Sheehan FH, Bolson EL: Eigenshape analysis of left ventricular outlines from contrast ventriculograms. *Advances in Morphometrics.* New York: Plenum Press, 1996, pp. 211-233.

144. Munt BI, Leotta DF, Martin RW, et al: Left ventricular shape analysis from three dimensional echocardiograms. *J Am Soc Echocardiogr* 11:761-769, 1998.

145. Aikawa K, Sheehan FH, Otto CM, et al: The severity of functional mitral regurgitation depends on the shape of the mitral apparatus: A three dimensional echo analysis. *J Heart Valve Dis* 11:627-636, 2002.

146. Hubka M, McDonald JA, Wong S, et al: Monitoring change in the three-dimensional shape of the human left ventricle. *J Am Soc Echocardiogr* 17:404-410, 2004.

147. Czegledy FP, Katz J: A new geometric description of the right ventricle. *J Biomed Eng* 15:387-391, 1993.

148. Yim PJ, Ha B, Ferreiro JI, et al: Diastolic shape of the right ventricle of the heart. *Anat Rec* 250:316-324, 1998.

149. Matsumori M, Ito T, Toyono M, et al: Influence of right ventricular volume and pressure overloads on assessment of left ventricular volume using two-dimensional echocardiography in infants and children with congenital heart diseases. *Am J Cardiol* 80:965-968, 1997.

150. Helbing WA, Rebergen SA, Maliepaard C, et al: Quantification of right ventricular function with magnetic resonance imaging in children with normal hearts and congenital heart disease. *Am Heart J* 130:828-837, 1995.

151. Sukmawan R, Akasaka T, Watanabe N, et al: Quantitative assessment of right ventricular geometric remodeling in pulmonary hypertension secondary to left-sided heart disease using real-time three-dimensional echocardiography. *Am J Cardiol* 94:1096-1099, 2004.

152. Young AA, Orr R, Smaill BH, Dell'Italia LJ: Three-dimensional changes in left and right ventricular geometry in chronic mitral regurgitation. *Am J Physiol* 271:H2689-H2700, 1996.

153. Marcus EN, Munoz RA, Margossian R, et al: Echocardiographic assessment of the right ventricular response to hypertension in neonates on the basis of average-shaped contraction models. *J Am Soc Echocardiogr* 15:1145-1153, 2002.

154. Leman RB, Spinale FG, Dorn GWI, et al: Supernormal ejection performance is isolated to the ipsilateral congenitally pressure-overloaded ventricle. *J Am Coll Cardiol* 13:1314-1319, 1989.

155. Sacks MS, Chuong CJ, Templeton GH, Peshock R: In vivo 3-D reconstruction and geometric characterization of the right ventricular free wall. *Ann Biomed Eng* 21:263-275, 1993.

156. Moses DA, Axel L: Quantification of the curvature and shape of the interventricular septum. *Magn Reson Med* 52:154-163, 2004.

157. Louie EK, Lin SS, Reynertson SI, et al: Pressure and volume loading of the right ventricle have opposite effects on left ventricular ejection fraction. *Circulation* 92:819-824, 1995.

158. Hubka M, Bolson EL, McDonald JA, et al: Three-dimensional echocardiographic measurement of left and right ventricular mass and volume: In vitro validation. *Int J Cardiovasc Imaging* 18:111-118, 2002.

159. Urnes K, Sheehan FH: Three-dimensional remodeling of the right ventricle varies under different loading conditions (abstr.). *J Am Soc Echocardiogr* 18:564, 2005.

160. Sheehan FH, Ge S, Vick GW III: The right ventricle in tetralogy of Fallot remodels to a different 3D shape from dilated cardiomyopathy (abstr.). *J Am Soc Echocardiogr* 18:515, 2005.

161. Osbakken MD, Bove AA, Spann JF: Left ventricular regional wall motion and velocity of shortening in chronic mitral and aortic regurgitation. *Am J Cardiol* 47:1005-1009, 1981.

162. Sabia P, Abbott RD, Afrookteh A, et al: Importance of two-dimensional echocardiographic assessment of left ventricular systolic function in patients presenting to the emergency room with cardiac-related symptoms. *Circulation* 84:1615-1624, 1991.

163. Peels CH, Visser CA, Kupper AJ, et al: Usefulness of two-dimensional echocardiography for immediate detection of myocardial ischemia in the emergency room. *Am J Cardiol* 65:687-691, 1990.

164. O'Boyle JE, Parisi AF, Nieminen M, et al: Quantitative detection of regional left ventricular contraction abnormalities by 2-dimensional echocardiography: Comparison of myocardial thickening and thinning and endocardial motion in a canine heart. *Am J Cardiol* 51:1732-1738, 1983.

165. Ideker RE, Behar VS, Wagner GS, et al: Evaluation of asynergy as an indicator of myocardial fibrosis. *Circulation* 57:715-725, 1978.

166. Horowitz RS, Morganroth J, Parrotto C, et al: Immediate diagnosis of acute myocardial infarction by two-dimensional echocardiography. *Circulation* 65(2):223-329, 1982.

167. Nieminen M, Parisi AF, O'Boyle JE, et al: Serial evaluation of myocardial thickening and thinning in acute experimental infarction: identification and quantification using two-dimensional echocardiography. *Circulation* 66:174-180, 1982.

168. TIMI Research Group: Immediate vs delayed catheterization and angioplasty following thrombolytic therapy for acute myocardial infarction. *J Am Med Assoc* 260:2849-2858, 1988.

169. Buda AJ, Zotz RJ, Gallagher KP: Characterization of the functional border zone around regionally ischemic myocardium using circumferential flow-function maps. *J Am Coll Cardiol* 8:150-158, 1986.

170. Kaplan SR, Bashein B, Sheehan FH, et al: Three-dimensional echocardiographic assessment of annular shape changes in the normal and regurgitant mitral valve. *Am Heart J* 139:378-387, 2000.

171. Otsuji Y, Handschumacher MD, Schammenthal E, et al: Insights from three-dimensional echocardiography into the mechanism of functional mitral regurgitation: Direct in vivo demonstration of altered leaflet tethering geometry. *Circulation* 96:1999-2008, 1997.

172. Mahle WT, Parks WJ, Fyfe DA, Sallee D: Tricuspid regurgitation in patients with repaired tetralogy of Fallot and its relation to right ventricular dilatation. *Am J Cardiol* 92:643-645, 2003.

173. Davlouros PA, Kilner PJ, Hornung TS, et al: Right ventricular function in adults with repaired tetralogy of Fallot assessed with cardiovascular magnetic resonance imaging: Detrimental role of right ventricular outflow aneurysms or akinesia and adverse right-to-left ventricular interaction. *J Am Coll Cardiol* 40:2044-2052, 2002.

174. Geva T, Sandweiss BM, Gauvreau K, et al: Factors associated with impaired clinical status in long-term survival of tetralogy of Fallot repair evaluated by magnetic resonance imaging. *J Am Coll Cardiol* 43:1068-1074, 2004.

175. Dor V, Montiglio F, Sabatier M, et al: Left ventricular shape changes induced by aneurysmectomy with endoventricular circular patch plasty reconstruction. *Eur Heart J* 15:1063-1069, 1994.

176. Bolson EL, Sheehan FH, Legget ME, et al: Applying the Center-Surface model to 3-D reconstructions of the left ventricle for regional function analysis. *Comput Cardiol*, Los Alamitos, CA, IEEE Computer Society Press, 1995, pp. 63-66.

177. Hubka M, Wong SP, McDonald JA, et al: Shape analysis of left ventricular remodeling following myocardial infarction using three-dimensional echocardiography. *Computers in Cardiology* 27:127-130, 2000.

178. Heger JJ, Weyman AE, Wann LS, et al: Cross-sectional echocardiography in acute myocardial infarction: Detection and localization of regional left ventricular asynergy. *Circulation* 60:531-538, 1979.

179. Nixon JV, Narahara KA, Smitherman TC: Estimation of myocardial involvement in patients with acute myocardial infarction by two-dimensional echocardiography. *Circulation* 62:1248-1255, 1980.

180. Visser CA, Lie KI, Kan G, et al: Detection and quantification of acute, isolated myocardial infarction by two dimensional echocardiography. *Am J Cardiol* 47:1020-1025, 1981.

181. Weiss JL, Bulkley BH, Hutchins GM, Mason SJ: Two-dimensional echocardiographic recognition of myocardial injury in man: Comparison with postmortem studies. *Circulation* 63:401-408, 1981.

182. Visser CA, Kan G, Lie KI, et al: Apex two dimensional echocardiography: Alternative approach to quantification of acute myocardial infarction. *Br Heart J* 47:461-467, 1982.

183. Van Reet RE, Quinones MA, Poliner LR, et al: Comparison of two-dimensional echocardiography with gated radionuclide ventriculography in the evaluation of global and regional left ventricular function in acute myocardial infarction. *J Am Coll Cardiol* 3(2):243-252, 1984.

184. Widimsky P, Gregor P, Cervenka V, Visek V: Two-dimensional echocardiography in acute transmural and non-transmural myocardial infarction. *Cor Vasa* 26(1):12-19, 1984.

185. Pandian NG, Skorton DJ, Collins SM, et al: Myocardial infarct size threshold for two-dimensional echocardiographic detection: Sensitivity of systolic wall thickening and endocardial motion abnormalities in small versus large infarcts. *Am J Cardiol* 55:551-555, 1985.

186. Aebischer N, Bise AC, Gabathuler J, Lerch R: Valeur pronostique de l'echocardiographie bidimensionnelle au stade aigu de l'infarctus du myocarde. *Schweiz Med Wochenschr* 115:1641-1646, 1985.

187. Widimsky P, Kopsa P, Cervenka V, et al: The possibility of non-invasive identification of occluded coronary artery in acute myocardial infarction. *Cor Vasa* 28:428-437, 1986.

188. Meltzer RS, Woythaler JN, Buda AJ, et al: Two dimensional echocardiographic quantification of infarct size alteration by pharmacologic agents. *Am J Cardiol* 44:257-262, 1979.

189. Kemper AJ, O'Boyle JE, Sharma S, et al: Hydrogen peroxide contrast-enhanced two-dimensional echocardiography: Real-time in vivo delineation of regional myocardial perfusion. *Circulation* 68:603-611, 1983.

190. Nishimura RA, Tajik AJ, Shub C, et al: Role of two-dimensional echocardiography in the prediction of in-hospital complications after acute myocardial infarction. *J Am Coll Cardiol* 4:1080-1087, 1984.

191. Guyer DE, Foale RA, Gillam LD, et al: An echocardiographic technique for quantifying and displaying the extent of regional left ventricular dyssynergy. *J Am Coll Cardiol* 8:830-835, 1986.

192. Wilkins GT, Southern JF, Choong CY, et al: Correlation between echocardiographic endocardial surface mapping of abnormal wall motion and pathologic infarct size in autopsied hearts. *Circulation* 77:978-987, 1988.

193. Mann DL, Foale RA, Gillam LD, et al: Early natural history of regional left ventricular dysfunction after experimental myocardial infarction. *Am Heart J* 115:538-546, 1988.

194. Kaul S, Pandian NG, Gillam LD, et al: Contrast echocardiography in acute myocardial ischemia. III. An in vivo comparison of the extent of abnormal wall motion with the area at risk for necrosis. *J Am Coll Cardiol* 7:383-392, 1986.

Chapter 11

Assessment of Diastolic Function by Echocardiography

MILIND Y. DESAI, MD • ALLAN L. KLEIN MD

Introduction

Heart failure (HF) is a major public health problem in the Western world, adding a significant burden to patients, health care providers, and society. Over the years, our concept of the natural history of HF has evolved to recognize that cardiovascular disease can result in systolic and diastolic dysfunction of the ventricles.[1,2] To date, echocardiography remains the most robust and widely studied technique to accurately assess diastolic function.[3] This chapter discusses the state-of-the-art echocardiographic techniques in optimal assessment of diastolic function. The role of echocardiography in specific cardiac diseases, which may cause diastolic dysfunction, is highlighted.

Physiology of Diastole

The cardiac cycle is broadly divided into two phases: systole and diastole. Diastole is the time period that extends from closure of the aortic valve to the termination of the mitral inflow and is itself divided into the following periods: an isovolumic relaxation, early rapid filling, diastasis (slow filling), and atrial systole.[4] These phases are shown relating left ventricular (LV) and left atrial (LA) pressure tracings and mitral inflow, tricuspid inflow, pulmonary vein and hepatic venous Doppler echocardiography profiles[4a] (Fig. 11–1).

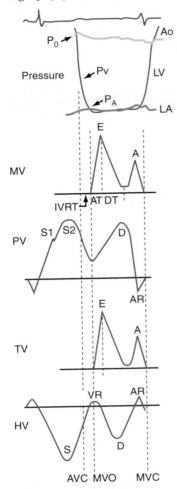

Figure 11–1. Diastole using Doppler echocardiography: combined schematic displaying left atrial (LA), left ventricular (LV), and aortic (Ao) pressures during diastole. Instantaneous LV pressure (P_v) falls exponentially through the isovolumic relaxation period (IVRT) from the P_0 (LV pressure at aortic valve closure [AVC]) to P_A (LV pressure at mitral valve opening [MVO]). Transmitral (MV) Doppler demonstrates an early rapid-filling wave (E) broken into an acceleration time (AT) and a deceleration time (DT), a diastasis period with little inflow, and an atrial contraction wave (A) associated with an elevation of LA pressure above LV pressure until mitral valve closure (MVC) is induced by the onset of ventricular systole. Pulmonary vein (PV) demonstrates a systolic wave (S1) related to atrial relaxation and mitral annular descent (S2), a diastolic wave (D) associated with atrial emptying through an open mitral valve, and an atrial reversal wave (AR) associated with atrial systole causing regurgitation of flow back up the pulmonary veins. Transtricuspid (TV) inflow has a similar pattern velocity to transmitral. Hepatic vein (HV) flow is similar to pulmonary vein flow, with a more prominent reversal of flow between the S and D waves associated with ventricular systole (VR). (From Klein AL, Asher CR: Diseases of the pericardium, restrictive cardiomyopathy, and diastolic dysfunction. In Topol EJ, Califf RM, Prystowsky EN, et al (eds): Textbook of Cardiovascular Medicine, 3rd ed. Philadelphia, Lippincott, Williams & Wilkins, 2007, pp 420-459.)

Isovolumic Relaxation

By definition, this period extends from the time of aortic valve closure to mitral valve opening and occurs without a change in LV volume.[5] It is an energy-dependent process, which occurs until mid-diastole. Ventricular pressure (P_v) decay during the isovolumic period follows an approximately exponential curve that can be characterized by its starting pressure (P_0) and its time constant (τ).[6] This curve can be fitted with the assumption of a either a zero asymptote $Pv = (P_0 e^{-t/\tau})$ or nonzero asymptote $Pv = (P_0 e^{-t/\tau} + P_b)$ (to account for subatmospheric pressure and the effects of pericardial pressure), where P_b is the left ventricular pressure at the time of aortic closure or peak negative dp/dt, t is the time after the onset of relaxation and a τ is the time constant of relaxation.

A low τ value is suggestive of fast relaxation, whereas a high value represents slow relaxation. Isovolumic relaxation ends when the LV pressure falls below the LA pressure, resulting in mitral valve opening and the start of the rapid filling phase.[7]

Rapid Filling

The rapid filling phase occurs from mitral valve opening until mitral valve closure, when the LV pressure falls below LA pressure.[7] Continued relaxation and elastic recoil lead to a continuous fall in LV pressure, resulting in development of a left-atrial-to-left-ventricular pressure gradient and resultant blood acceleration.[7] This gradient is influenced by the level of LA pressure at mitral valve opening and the rate of decline of LV pressure.[8] Blood rapidly enters the left ventricle from the left atrium during the early filling period with approximately 70% of the stroke volume (SV) received by the left ventricle during the first third of diastole.[9] Active ventricular suction (pulling of blood) may play an important role in the rapid filling phase.[10] Ventricular suction may occur because of the recoil of the compressed elastic elements during contraction.[11] Rapid filling ends as atrial and ventricular pressures equilibrate.[7]

Diastasis (Slow Filling)

Diastasis, or the slow filling period, occurs between the rapid filling phase and atrial contraction and accounts for less than 5% of filling. After rapid filling, LA and LV pressures are almost equal, yielding no immediate forward driving gradient.[7]

Atrial Systole

The atrial filling phase of diastole occurs when the LA pressure rises above ventricular pressure, forcing or pushing blood across the mitral valve and a small amount of regurgitation into the pulmonary veins. This late diastolic transmitral flow increases ventricular end-diastolic volume by 25% in normals with only a small rise in mean pulmonary venous pressure. Diastole ends with onset of ventricular systole when the rapid increase in ventricular pressure closes the mitral valve.[7]

Determinants of Diastolic Function

The following are the major parameters of diastolic function: (1) active myocardial relaxation; (2) LV compliance; (3) left atrial (including atrial function), pulmonary vein, and mitral valve characteristics; and (4) heart rate.[7] Along with that, the pericardium also plays an important role in determining the diastolic function of the heart.[4a]

Myocardial relaxation, which occurs during isovolumic relaxation and early diastolic filling, is an active process involving the use of intracellular adenosine triphosphate (ATP) and calcium by the myocardium.[12] Many factors affect isovolumic relaxation, including internal loading forces (cardiac fiber), external loading states (wall stress, arterial impedence), and reduced or inhibited myocardial contractility (metabolic, neurohormonal, or pharmacologic).

Ventricular compliance is the ratio of change in volume to change in pressure (dV/dP), and stiffness is the reverse of compliance (dP/dV). From a conceptual standpoint, we can divide compliance into two components: intrinsic myocardial and chamber. Compliance is the net result of a variety of factors: viscoelastic nature of the myocardium; chamber size, shape, and wall thickness; right ventricular (RV) and LV pressure-volume interaction; pleural pressure and pericardial characteristics; and any active incomplete myocardial relaxation.[13] Intrinsic myocardial stiffness relates to the amount of collagen within the myocardium. Collagen plays an essential role in converting the contractile force of the myocytes into intraventricular pressure and determining overall ventricular size and shape.[14,15] Pressure-induced hypertrophy is associated with increased collagen content and secondarily increased overall stiffness. Evaluation of ventricular compliance has been studied and quantified extensively using pressure volume loops that demonstrate the degree to which pressure and volume change vis-à-vis each other over a wide range of physiologic pressures and volumes[16-18] (Fig. 11–2). The volume of blood that enters the left ventricle is in large part determined by pulmonary vein or left atrial and mitral valve characteristics.[7] The pressure gradient between the pulmonary veins or left atrium and the left ventricle and the rate of myocardial relaxation and ventricular suction are responsible for early rapid filling.[10,19] Hence, diseases of the mitral valve, such as mitral stenosis (MS), delay LV filling and prevent early rapid filling.[7]

The left atrium predominantly acts as a passive reservoir of blood during early LV filling and as an active pump at end-diastole.[20] Atrial systolic function (active phase) may be essential to maintain cardiac output (CO) in disease states.[21,22] In young and healthy normal individuals, the atrial contribution is less than 20% of the total volume, whereas in older normal subjects, the atrial "kick" accounts for a greater proportion of the total LV filling.[23] Atrial contractile function has delayed recovery (stunning) following electrical cardioversion.[24] Decreased atrial systolic function as a result of infiltration plays a role in the reduction in forward transmitral atrial contraction wave by Doppler echocardiography as seen in advanced cardiac amyloidosis.[25]

Heart rate (HR) has a direct impact on cardiac output in cases of diastolic dysfunction.[26,27] As HR increases, the diastolic filling period preferentially decreases with respect to the systolic ejection period. As ventricular filling is functionally delayed, adequacy of inflow deteriorates and cardiac output paradoxically falls. Catecholamines may enhance relaxation and increase HR, thus decreasing the diastolic period.[28]

Other factors that affect diastolic function include neurohormonal activation, conduction abnormalities, and the stiffness of the pericardium. LV relaxation may be impaired by conduction abnormalities that cause segmental asynchrony.[29] This may contribute to decreased exercise tolerance in patients with left bundle branch block or right ventricular paced rhythms. The pericardium considerably affects diastolic function as commonly seen in constrictive pericarditis.[30]

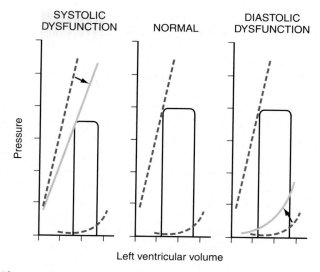

Figure 11–2. Schematic representation of ventricular pressure-volume loops. The center panel demonstrates the normal situation. Note the exponential nature of the curve through late diastole. In systolic dysfunction (left), the end-systolic pressure line is displayed downward and is manifested by a decreased ability of the left ventricle to generate high pressures for a given volume. Diastolic dysfunction involves an upward and leftward shift of the exponential curve, a result of elevated filling pressures for a given volume. (From Katz AM: Am Coll Cardiol 11:438-445, 1988.)

Definition of Diastolic Dysfunction

Heart failure (HF) is most often secondary to impairment of LV systolic function. However, a significant percentage of cases of HF result from abnormalities of diastolic function or diastolic HF. Lack of symptoms in the presence of a normal ejection fraction is known as diastolic dysfunction. There may be different structural and functional aspects of systolic and diastolic HF. The main difference between these conditions is that in systolic heart failure, there is LV cavity enlargement, eccentric hypertrophy, and abnormal systolic and diastolic function; whereas in diastolic heart failure, there is normal cavity size, concentric hypertrophy, and abnormal diastolic function.[31] A recent study from the Mayo Clinic has actually shown that diastolic HF has increased over a 15-year period, while the death rate has remained unchanged.[31a]

Patients with HF secondary to diastolic dysfunction generally have a better prognosis than patients with systolic dysfunction[32]; however, they may have recurrent HF, hospitalizations, and recurrent chest pain even despite coronary revascularization.[1,33,34] The prognosis of diastolic HF varies, depending on the population studied with an annual mortality rate varying approximately 10% per year, which is lower than patients with systolic dysfunction at 19%.[35] The lower mortality rate with diastolic function has been shown in a large number of population-based studies including the Veterans Administration Cooperative Study (V-HeFT) and Coronary Artery Surgery Study (CASS).[35,36] The addition of coronary artery disease (CAD) in patients with HF adds considerable risk to diastolic dysfunction, however, it does not approach the risk of patients with low ejection fractions (EFs).[32] A study by Senni and colleagues showed similar mortality in older patients with diastolic and systolic dysfunction.[37] Thus, although diastolic HF is often not clinically well recognized, it is associated with increases in morbidity and all-cause mortality.[37a] Because diastolic dysfunction is common as an isolated disease in the elderly and also increases the burden of HF among patients with systolic dysfunction, these observations have major implications for the future, particularly given the increasing age of the population. These recent studies further emphasize the importance of recognizing diastolic dysfunction. However, it is to be noted that systolic and diastolic dysfunction are frequently observed concurrently in the same patient.[2]

Differentiation between systolic and diastolic HF cannot be made on the basis of history, physical examination, electrocardiogram (ECG), or chest radiograph alone because these clinical markers have same frequency of occurrence in these two forms of HF.[38,39] The following criteria (Table 11–1) for primary diastolic HF were proposed by the Working Group for the European Society of Cardiology (1) presence of signs or symptoms of HF; (2) presence of normal or only mildly abnormal LV systolic function; (3) evidence of abnormal LV relaxation, filling, or diastolic stiffness.[6] These diagnostic criteria have three major flaws. First, the requirement that there be signs or symptoms of HF. It

TABLE 11–1. Definition of Diastolic Dysfunction

1. Definition by Working Group for the European Society of Cardiology
   a. Presence of signs or symptoms of HF
   b. Presence of normal (LVEF > 45%) or only mildly abnormal left ventricular systolic function
   c. Evidence of abnormal LV relaxation, filling, or diastolic stiffness.

2. Definition by Vasan and colleagues
   a. Definite diastolic heart failure requires definitive evidence of HF; objective evidence of normal systolic function, with an EF greater than 50% within 72 hours of the HF event; and objective evidence of diastolic dysfunction on cardiac catheterization.
   b. If objective evidence of diastolic dysfunction is lacking but the first two criteria are present, this fulfills the criteria for probable diastolic heart failure. If the first criterion is present and EF is greater than 50% but not assessed within 72 hours of the HF event, this fulfills the criteria for possible diastolic heart failure.
   c. Possible diastolic heart failure can be upgraded to probable diastolic heart failure if one of a number of additional criteria is present.

HF, heart failure; EF, ejection fraction; LV, left ventricular; LVEF, left ventricular ejection fraction.

is well recognized that the mere presence of breathlessness and fatigue is not specific for the presence of HF. It would be more prudent to include the term signs *and* symptoms of HF or to use specific diagnostic criteria, such as the Framingham criteria. Second, the term *systolic function* is not specific. The working group defined systolic function as being normal when LV EF is greater than 45%. Because EF is not a measure of contractility or a load-independent measurement of systolic function, the second requirement would be more precise if stated simply as a normal EF. Third, the requirement that a measurable abnormality in diastolic function be present. Similar to measurements of systolic function, measurements of ventricular relaxation, filling, and compliance are load dependent. Therefore, their poor specificity, sensitivity, and predictive accuracy, limit the application of this requirement in the clinical setting. Vasan and colleagues refined these criteria and divided them into definite, probable, and possible diastolic HF.[40] Definite diastolic HF requires definitive evidence of HF; objective evidence of normal systolic function, with an EF greater than 50% within 72 hours of the HF event; and objective evidence of diastolic dysfunction on cardiac catheterization. If objective evidence of diastolic dysfunction is lacking, but the first two criteria are present, this fulfills the criteria for probable diastolic HF. If the first criterion is present and EF is greater than 50% but not assessed within 72 hours of the HF event, this fulfills the criteria for possible diastolic HF. Possible diastolic HF can be upgraded to probable diastolic HF if one of a number of additional criteria is present. The clinical application of these guidelines is limited, because they are both complex and empiric. Controversy exists whether measurements of LV relaxation or compliance by cardiac catheterization or Doppler echocardiography are actually needed when LV hypertrophy or concentric remodeling is present.[41] Recently further definitions of diastolic HF or HF with preserved EF have been proposed.[34,41a,41b]

Echocardiographic Evaluation of Diastolic Function

Echocardiography has been the mainstay for understanding the physiology of diastolic function and identifying the pathophysiology of diastolic dysfunction. In current practice, the clinician has a number of techniques in the evaluation of diastolic function, including the traditional Doppler techniques, which includes mitral inflow and pulmonary vein flow and the newer modalities, such as tissue Doppler imaging and color M-mode Doppler. Table 11–2 provides the common diastolic filling variables that can be measured in clinical practice. Table 11–3 provides the clinical utility and technical limitations of various echocardiographic techniques in assessment of diastolic function. A framework of the different imaging modalities is shown in Figure 11–3 in normals and patients with different stages of diastolic dysfunction.

Doppler Techniques in Assessment of Diastolic Filling Patterns

There is a large body of scientific evidence validating the typical patterns of diastolic filling in normal subjects and those with diastolic dysfunction. These filling patterns generally are not characteristic of a particular disease process, but represent the end product of a complex set of pathophysiologic events. Furthermore, these patterns can also be affected by operator-related issues (e.g., precise placement of the sample volume) and physiologic factors (e.g., HR and fluid status) and are not a reflection of true diastolic function.[42]

Transmitral Flow Assessment

The most traditional technique of assessment of LV filling patterns involves using pulsed-wave Doppler mitral flow velocity recordings.[43] The following are the variables derived from mitral flow interrogation: peak early diastolic transmitral flow velocity (E), peak late diastolic transmitral flow velocity (A), early filling deceleration time (DT), and A-wave duration (Adur). Normal mitral flow velocity curves vary with loading conditions, age, and HR.

Normal individuals demonstrate a rapidly accelerating E wave, relatively rapid deceleration, and an A

TABLE 11–2. Diagnostic Criteria for Diastolic Function

Normal Filling	Impaired (or Abnormal) Relaxation or Stage 1	Pseudonormal Pattern or Stage 2	Restrictive Filling or Stages 3 and 4
DT 160-240 msec (but can be lower, especially in young people)	DT > 240 msec	DT 160-240 msec	DT < 160 msec
IVRT 70-90 msec; E/A: 1-2	IVRT > 90 msec; E/A < 1	IVRT < 90 msec; E/A: 1-1.5 Reversal of E/A ratio (to <1) with preload reduction (e.g., Valsalva maneuver)	IVRT < 70 ms; E/A > 1.5 Decreased E/A ratio with preload reduction (e.g., Valsalva)
Mitral A duration ≥ PVa duration	Mitral A duration ≥ or < PVa duration (depending on LVEDP)	Mitral A duration < PVa duration; PVa velocity ↑ (>35 cm/s)	Mitral A duration < PVa duration; PVa velocity ↑ (≥35 cm/s, usually but not always)
PVs2 ≥ PVd (PVs2 can be smaller than PVd in young people)	PVs2 > > PVd	PVs2 < PVd	PVs2 < < PVd
No anatomic abnormalities	—	2D echocardiographic evidence of structural heart disease (↓ EF, ↑ LA, LVH)	2D echocardiographic evidence of structural heart disease

2D, two dimensional; A, filling wave due to atrial contraction; DT, deceleration time; E, early rapid filling wave; EF, ejection fraction, IVRT, isovolumic relaxation time; LA, left atrial; LVEDP, left ventricular end-diastolic pressure; LVH, left ventricular hypertrophy; PVa, atrial flow reversal velocity; PVd, diastolic velocity; PVs2, systolic velocity. Note: Restrictive filling can also be considered when DT is less than 150 msec.
Adapted from Oh JK: *The Echo Manual,* 3rd ed. Philadelphia, Lippincott, Williams & Wilkins, 2007, pp. 120-142.

TABLE 11–3. Utility of Different Echocardiographic Techniques in Assessment of Diastolic Function

	Clinical Utility	Technical Points	Limitations
Mitral inflow	Can assess LV compliance, relaxation, filling pressures. Short DT associated with poor prognosis. Best used with combined systolic and diastolic heart failure.	Sample volume between 1 and 2 mm, velocity filter at 200 Hz, sweep speed between 50 and –100 mm/s. Can measure E and A waves, DT, IVRT. A duration can be measured at mitral annulus.	Preload dependent. E/A ratio can be pseudonormalized.
Pulmonary vein flow	Can assess LV compliance, relaxation, filling pressures. Blunted systolic/diastolic velocities associated with poor prognosis. Best used with combined systolic and diastolic heart failure. AR used to assess pseudonormalization.	Sample volume box between 3 and 4 mm, velocity placed 1-2 cm into the PV, filter at 200 Hz, sweep speed between 50 and 100 mm/s. Can measure S, D, and AR waves.	Relatively preload independent Technically difficult to obtain in all patients. Blunted S/D from other conditions including atrial fibrillation and mitral regurgitation.
Tissue Doppler imaging	Can assess LV compliance, relaxation, filling pressures. E/Ea > 15 associated with elevated filling pressures. Best used with primary diastolic heart failure.	Sample volume box between 4 and 5 mm at all four mitral annuli, filter at 200 Hz, sweep speed between 50 and 100 mm/s. Can measure S, Ea, and Aa waves.	Relatively preload independent. Angle and translation dependent. Different velocities at annuli (lateral > medial).
Color M-mode	Can assess LV compliance, relaxation, filling pressures. E/Vp > 1.5 associated with elevated filling pressures. Best used with primary diastolic heart failure.	Slope of flow propagation (first aliasing velocity) for 4 cm into LV. The 2D depth is reduced to 16 cm. The color velocity scale is set for color aliasing by moving the baseline up so that it is in the 40 cm/s range. The M-mode sweep should be recorded at a speed of 100 mm/s. Can measure Vp slope.	Relatively preload independent. Technically difficult to obtain in all patients. Influenced by LV geometry.

2D, two-dimensional; A, filling wave due to atrial contraction; AR, atrial reversal; D, diastolic flow; DT, deceleration time; IVRT, isovolumic relaxation time; LV, left ventricular; PV, pulmonary vein; S, systolic flow; Vp, velocity of propagation.

wave significantly smaller than the E wave. The E/A ratio is greater than one, the mitral DT (reflecting LV compliance) is typically between 160 and 240 ms, and the isovolumic relaxation time (IVRT) is between 70 and 90 ms. With normal aging, there is slowing of LV relaxation and, hence, the gradual decrease of E wave and increase of A wave. In most individuals, E and A waves become approximately equal in the sixth decade of life[44] (Fig. 11–4).

The evolution of traditional diastolic parameters with progressively worsening diastolic function, occurs in the following manner: For patients with diastolic dysfunction, three abnormal filling patterns are

initially recognized[26,45] (see Fig. 11–3). In stage 1 diastolic dysfunction (abnormal relaxation), there is a low E wave and a high A wave, resulting in an E/A ratio less than 1. DT is prolonged and is usually greater than 240 msec and IVRT is greater than 90 ms. Stage 2 diastolic dysfunction or pseudonormal pattern, results is associated with a normal appearance of the transmitral inflow with an E/A ratio between 1 and 1.5, a DT between 160 and 240 msec and a IVRT between 60 and 100 msec. With disease progression (Stage 3 diastolic dysfunction or restrictive filling), there is a very high E wave, a low A wave, and a significantly decreased DT. The E/A ratio is usually

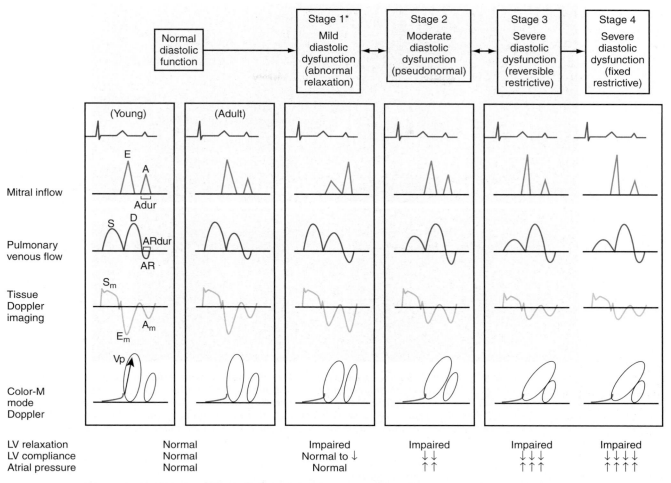

Figure 11–3. *Stages of diastolic function. Schematic representation of the typical patterns seen with mitral inflow, pulmonary venous flow, tissue Doppler echocardiography, and color M-mode propagation velocity (Vp) for normal (young and adult), impaired relaxation, pseudonormal, and restrictive diastolic function. The stages of diastolic dysfunction can be determined using an integrated approach with these four different modalities for assessment of diastolic flow pattern. *Stage 1 can be divided into Stage 1A and Stage 1B depending on an elevated LV end-diastolic pressure. A, late mitral filling; A_M, diastolic filling during atrial contraction; D, diastolic filling; E, early mitral filling; E_M, early diastolic; S, systolic filling; S_M, systolic; Vp, propagation velocity. (Adapted from Garcia MJ, Thomas JD, Klein AL: J Am Coll Cardiol 32:865-875, 1998.)*

greater than two with a DT less than 160 ms, and IVRT less than 70 ms.

Further observations have subcategorized this last pattern to either reversible or fixed restrictive pattern (Stage 4) depending on the response to the Valsalva maneuver or other preload reducing maneuvers.[46] The major challenge in the interpretation of Doppler mitral inflow patterns is in distinguishing the normal from pseudonormal pattern. To accurately assess and stratify the degree of diastolic abnormality, further measurements are generally necessary. There are several traditional methods that are useful in distinguishing normal from pseudonormal patterns, including pulmonary venous (PV) flow measurements and the Valsalva maneuver.

Pulmonary Venous Flow

PV flow velocity variables provide an integrated approach with mitral inflow in the evaluation of diastolic dysfunction. The four useful variables from the PV flow interrogation are peak systolic PV flow velocity (S), peak diastolic PV flow velocity (D), peak PV atrial reversal flow velocity (AR), and AR duration (ARdur). Figure 11–3 shows a schematic representation of the PV variables in normal diastolic function and in various stages of diastolic dysfunction.[47]

The flow from the PV to the LA occurs in three phases: systolic phase (peak early and late systolic PV flow velocity); early diastolic phase (peak diastolic PV flow velocity); and retrograde flow during the late diastole with

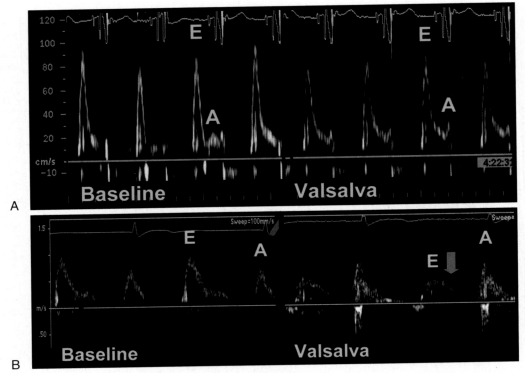

Figure 11–4. Effect of Valsalva maneuver on mitral inflow in a patient with different stages of diastolic dysfunction. A, A patient with Stage 3 diastolic dysfunction. Notice after Valsalva maneuver, the E wave remains the same, consistent with irreversible diastolic dysfunction (Stage 4). B, The patient has Stage 2 diastolic dysfunction, and with Valsalva, there is blunting of the E wave and appearance of Stage 1 diastolic dysfunction. A, atrial component of diastolic filling; E, early diastolic filling.

atrial contraction (AR). With a normal LA pressure, the majority of the flow into LA occurs in systole. However, when the mean LA pressure increases, the majority of the antegrade flow occurs in diastole with a concomitant reduction in systolic flow. A decreased systolic fraction of less than 40% is associated with an elevated mean LA pressure greater than 15 mmHg.[47a] Similar to mitral inflow, the pulmonary vein flow demonstrates a U-shaped curve, suggesting preload dependence. Pulmonary vein AR and ARdur provides incremental value in assessing diastolic function. An AR velocity greater than 35 cm/s and an ARdur at least 30 msec longer than the mitral inflow A-wave duration is predictive of a left ventricular end-diastolic pressure (LVEDP) greater than 15 mm Hg.[48] However, it may be difficult to optimally assess PV flow because of multiple reasons. A frequent reason is inadequate PV flow profiles, commonly because of body habitus and operator dependence. Blunting of PV systolic waves may be present in young healthy individuals as a result of rapid diastolic "suction" and AR may be absent in advanced diastolic dysfunction as a result of the loss of atrial function.[49,50] Therefore, newer modalities, including color M-mode Doppler and tissue Doppler imaging (TDI), have evolved to provide additional information for the assessment of diastolic function and evaluation of LV filling pressures[44] (see Fig. 11–3).

Mitral Inflow at Peak Valsalva Maneuver

Because preload affects interpretation of diastolic dysfunction, the Valsalva maneuver is another supplement to the measurement of mitral inflow parameters (see Fig. 11–4). The strain phase of the Valsalva maneuver is a simple approach used to decrease LA pressure. During this phase, E wave velocity normally decreases by 20% with a smaller decrease in A velocity.[51] In patients with pseudonormal mitral inflow patterns, Valsalva strain lowers LA pressure and unmasks the underlying impaired LV relaxation, resulting in a measured E/A less than one.[52] Patients with restrictive filling patterns or individuals who are preload-sensitive will revert to a pseudonormal or even impaired relaxation pattern. Patients with restrictive filling patterns without any change with Valsalva have severe irreversible or fixed diastolic dysfunction. Much like PV Doppler variables, the primary limitation in the use of Valsalva to assess diastology is obtaining adequate signals for measurement. Ommen and colleagues[52] were able to obtain satisfactory Doppler data in only 61% of patients during a Valsalva maneuver. In addition, the inherent limitations in performance of an adequate Valsalva maneuver limit its utility in routine practice.

Evaluation of the Right Heart by Doppler

Diastolic function of the right-sided heart can be evaluated by the interrogation of the tricuspid inflow, hepatic vein (see Fig. 11–1), and superior vena cava (SVC) flow.[53] The Doppler flow patterns in the hepatic veins and superior vena cava are somewhat similar to the PV flow patterns.[54,55] In addition to the systole (S), diastole (D), and AR waves, a second reversed flow is often seen between the S and the D wave at the end of ventricular contraction (VR).[56] Right-sided flow velocities normally increase during inspiration and decrease with Valsalva.[56,57] As with the PV flow, the S wave is related to right atrial (RA) relaxation and tricuspid annular descent, and the D is related to early RV filling velocity (E). The magnitude of AR and VR varies according to RV stiffness, RA contractility, and central venous pressure.[58] The effect of respiration of the right-sided flows is useful in differentiating constriction from restriction and estimating right-sided filling pressures.[54,55]

Other Echocardiographic Techniques

Tissue Doppler Imaging for Evaluation of Diastolic Function

The Doppler principle states that the velocity of a moving object will alter the frequency of a reflected sound wave. Ultrasonic Doppler technique is a direct application of this effect and is based on the analysis of the amount of frequency alteration of ultrasound (US) waves reflected by a moving body. This US principle has been applied in cardiovascular medicine for many years, predominantly for blood flow velocity measurement within the heart and great vessels.[59] In conventional Doppler color imaging, wall filters are employed to eliminate high-amplitude, low-frequency signals reflected from myocardium in favor of the low-amplitude, high-frequency signals reflected from moving red blood cells. Because these low Doppler shift frequencies are produced by the contracting myocardium, they are expected to contain potential information for the assessment of myocardial properties. TDI is an echocardiographic technique that directly measures myocardial velocities. In TDI, wall filters are bypassed to specifically measure the velocities of the myocardium, which typically range from 0 to 20 cm/s. Doppler gain settings also must be increased to adequately visualize TDI waveforms.

TDI was first described in 1989 by Isaaz who demonstrated that low myocardial velocities at the posterior mitral annulus correlated with abnormal posterior wall motion on LV angiography.[60] In the evaluation of diastolic function, Sohn and colleagues[61] demonstrated that E_a correlated with invasive indices of myocardial relaxation (τ), while Nagueh and colleagues[62] showed that the pulsed Doppler peak early mitral inflow velocity (E) divided by TDI early diastolic mitral annular velocity (E_a or E_m) resulted in a ratio (E/E_a) that correlated with pulmonary capillary wedge pressure (PCWP). Ommen and colleagues[52] corroborated this work, demonstrating that the E/E_a is useful in estimating mean LV filling pressures. The E/E_a ratio has since been demonstrated to be useful in estimating LV filling pressures in patients with hypertrophic cardiomyopathy (HCM),[63] sinus tachycardia,[64] atrial fibrillation,[65] and postcardiac transplantation.[66]

Techniques of Tissue Doppler Imaging. Pulsed and color TDI have been used for the assessment of myocardial function; however, both techniques show advantages and disadvantages. Using pulsed Doppler techniques we can (1) obtain high quality Doppler signals; (2) measure, mean and instantaneous local acceleration; and (3) obtain quantitative wall motion information (i.e., velocity, acceleration, and displacement). However, the pulsed Doppler technique has many shortcomings including (1) the need for manual mapping; (2) a limited spatial resolution making it difficult to distinguish subendocardial from subepicardial myocardial velocities; (3) difficulty in simultaneous recording of different ventricular wall segments; and (4) recognition that important qualitative differences exist between the various echocardiographic machines in terms of obtained signals. On the other hand, using color TDI of the myocardium, we can superimpose wall motion velocity on the two-dimensional (2D) echocardiographic imaging by velocity color coding. 2D color Doppler imaging of the myocardium (1) enables rapid visual qualitative assessment of wall dynamics, (2) provides a good spatial resolution to differentiate between velocity profiles of subendocardial and subepicardial layers, and (3) allows simultaneous analysis of various myocardial regions. However, it is limited by poor temporal resolution. In contrast, M-mode color-coded tissue imaging is characterized by a high spatial and temporal resolution, but sampling is only performed along a single line.

In the assessment of diastolic function, velocities typically are measured at the annuli or myocardium in the longitudinal axis to minimize the effect of cardiac translation.[61,67] From either the apical four-chamber or two-chamber acoustic windows, the region of interest is placed at the level of the mitral annulus on the septal, lateral, anterior, or posterior aspect. Recordings are obtained during apnea to minimize translation-induced motion artifacts. In clinical TDI applications, three waveforms are visualized per cardiac cycle: the peak systolic wave (Sm), early diastolic wave (Em), and end-diastolic wave produced by atrial contraction (Am) (see Fig. 11–3).

In evaluation of velocities in healthy subjects. the annular early diastolic wave velocities recorded in the short-axis view were higher at the level of posterior wall than at the anteroseptal wall.[68] Garcia and colleagues[68] found an average value of 6.3±1.7 cm/s for Em at the anteroseptal wall versus 9.3±3 cm/s at the posterior wall. In the apical view, myocardial diastolic velocities recorded by TDI are higher at the base than at the mid-left ventricle or at the apex, which is almost stationary.[69,70] Although TDI velocities decrease with age, a healthy 50-year-old adult has spectral TD values of 10 cm/s or greater, and color TD values of generally 6 cm/s or greater for Sm, Em, and Am.

Tissue Doppler Imaging and Diastolic Function in Ischemic Heart Disease.

Many patients with ischemic heart disease demonstrate abnormal diastolic function recorded by pulsed Doppler TDI despite having normal systolic function.[60] Recent studies have also shown a reduced Em and Em/Am ratio in ischemic or infarcted segments.[71,72] One study also showed that the number of segments with abnormal E_a/A_a ratio was higher in ischemic patients with a decreased transmitral Doppler E/A ratio compared with those with a normal transmitral E/A ratio. Recording diastolic TDI has also been shown to be a sensitive method for detecting transient myocardial ischemia—for example, during inflation of an angioplasty balloon.[73,74]

Relationship of E_a to Active Relaxation. E_a is a relatively preload independent measure of myocardial relaxation in patients with cardiac disease, as compared to early transmitral velocity.[61,62] It has been shown that in patients with abnormal relaxation, saline loading led to a pseudonormal transmitral pattern whereas TDI E_a and E_a/A_a remained unchanged. Also, the authors showed that the time constant of relaxation (τ) was better linearly related to E_a and E_a/A_a than to transmitral velocity variables.[61] A value of E_a less than 8.5 cm/s with a ratio E_a/A_a less than 1 identified a pseudonormalized transmitral velocity pattern with a 88% sensitivity and 67% specificity (Fig. 11–5). Another study[62] included three groups of patients: 34 normal subjects, 40 asymptomatic patients with normal EF and transmitral E/A less than 1 (abnormal relaxation), and 51 patients with HF and E/A ratio greater than 1 (pseudonormal). It was shown that E_a was lower with a decreased E_a/A_a in both impaired relaxation and pseudonormal compared with normals; the ratio E/E_a was similar between normals and pa-

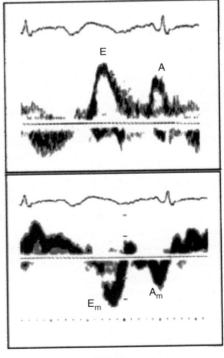

Normal

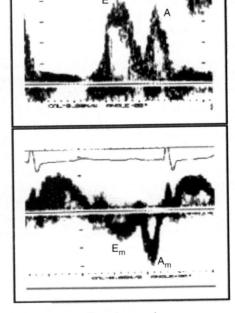

Pseudonormal

Figure 11–5. Standard pulsed Doppler transmitral inflow (upper panels) *showing the early (E) and atrial (A) filling velocities, and myocardial axial velocities* (lower panels) *recorded at the basal lateral wall in a healthy volunteer and in a patient with severe aortic stenosis, left ventricular hypertrophy, and elevated filling pressures (pseudonormal). Early diastolic myocardial velocity (E_m) is significantly reduced, as well as the early-to-atrial velocity ratio (E_m/A_m) in the pseudonormal patient. A_m, atrial velocity. (From Garcia MJ, Thomas JD, Klein AL: J Am Coll Cardiol 32[4]:865-875, 1998.)*

tients with impaired relaxation but was significantly higher in the patients with pseudonormal transmitral pattern. Also, in 60 patients in whom mean PCWP was measured (Fig. 11–6), the authors found a good correlation between the ratio E/E_a and mean PCWP (correlation coefficient $r = 0.87$). An E/E_a ratio greater than 10 indicated a PCWP greater than 12 mm Hg with a 91% sensitivity and a 81% specificity.[62] In another study of 50 patients who had a heart transplant, a significant correlation between the mitral annular E_a/A_a ratio and the PCWP ($r = 0.80$) and between the tricuspid annular E_a/A_a ratio and right atrial pressure ($r = 0.79$) was demonstrated. A mitral annular E_a/A_a ratio equal to 8 identified patients with PCWP equal to 15 mm Hg with a 87% sensitivity and a 81% specificity.[66] Another study also reported[75] a linear correlation between pulsed DTI-derived E/A at any site on the LV posterior wall and the time constant τ measured invasively by catheterization (correlation coefficients ranging from 0.69 to 0.81, $P < 0.0001$), whereas no significant correlation was found between τ and the transmitral early diastolic velocity. Given that in patients with elevated LV filling pressures, the cardiac myocytes are under strain, B-type natriuretic peptide (BNP) levels can be useful in determining the presence of elevated filling pressures. A recent study demonstrated that BNP had a significant correlation ($r = 0.51$) with mitral E/E_a. Other investigators have shown that BNP and mitral E/E_a are similarly accurate in diagnosing clinical HF in patients hospitalized for dyspnea; but a comprehensive Doppler assessment using 2D, conventional Doppler, and TDI variables appeared more specific than BNP.[76] In patients with indwelling pulmonary artery (PA) catheters, E/E_a and BNP were highly and equally sensitive for PCWP greater than 15 mm Hg, but E/E_a was more specific. Hence, E_a appears to be better and more directly related to active myocardial relaxation as compared to standard transmitral flow variables.[44,77]

Restrictive versus Constrictive Physiology. E_a can also be used to distinguish between restrictive and constrictive physiology[78] (Fig. 11–7). It has been demonstrated that E_a measured by pulsed Doppler at the level of the lateral part of the mitral annulus was significantly lower in 7 patients with restrictive cardiomyopathy than in 15 normal subjects and 8 patients with constrictive pericarditis. In another study, abnormal pulsed TDI velocity pattern was reported in 12 patients with constrictive pericarditis versus a group of 20 normal subjects.[79] A cutoff of $Ea \geq 8$ cm/s was useful in separating constrictive pericarditis from restriction in another study.[67]

Diastolic Function in Left Ventricular Hypertrophy Assessed by Tissue Doppler Imaging. TDI has been demonstrated as a better discriminator between normal controls and patients with primary or secondary LV hypertrophy with a decrease in E_a and in ratio E_a/A_a and with a prolonged time from the electrocardiogram Q wave to the onset of E_a in pathologic groups.[69,80] Differences in the onset of diastolic myocardial velocity waves between the different myocardial components of the cardiac base has been reported both in primary and secondary LV hypertrophy.[69,80] The etiology of LV volume overload leading to LV hypertrophy may result in different TDI velocity patterns.[80] Abe and colleagues[81] have reported lower E_a and prolonged time to E_a onset in patients with chronic aortic regurgitation when compared with those with mitral regurgitation. Myocardial early diastolic velocities have been demonstrated to decrease with age.[80,82] However, it has been shown that the difference between normal controls and patients with LV hypertrophy remained significant even after accounting for age.[82]

Tissue Doppler Assessment of Diastolic Function and Prognosis. Recently, there has been tremendous interest in the prognostic implications of TD diastolic variables. One study demonstrated that after first acute myocardial infarction, E_a and E/E_a were univariate predictors of death or hospital readmission. Another population-based study[83] showed that patients with increasing degrees of diastolic dysfunction (using a comprehensive Doppler-echocardiography assessment including TD variables) have increasingly worse outcome. E/E_a has been demonstrated to be a strong multivariate predictor of patient outcome when assessed a mean of 1.6 days after acute myocardial infarction (AMI).[84] Recent work from the ADEPT study in 225

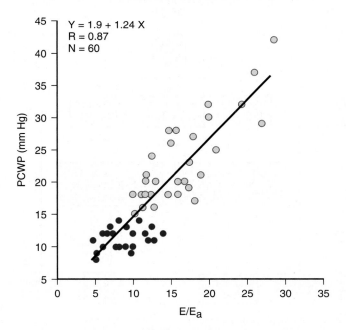

Figure 11–6. Relation of early transmitral velocity to tissue Doppler mitral annular early diastolic velocity (E/E_a) to pulmonary capillary wedge pressure (PCWP) in 60 patients. The solid dots *indicate patients with impaired relaxation. The open dots* indicate patients with a pseudonormalized pattern *of diastolic filling. (From Nagueh S, Middleton JK, Kopelen HA, et al:* J Am Coll Cardiol *30[6]:1527-1533, 1997.)*

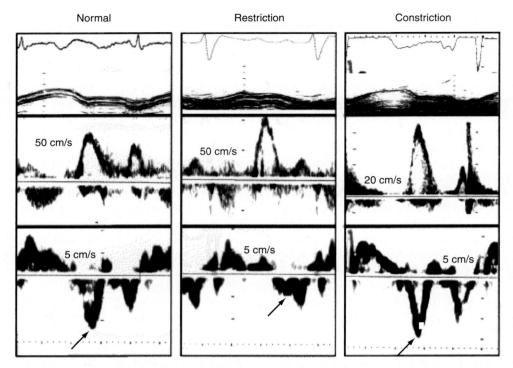

Figure 11-7. *Representative samples of mitral annular M-mode tracings, tissue Doppler imaging velocities in the longitudinal axis and transmitral Doppler flow velocities in a normal volunteer, a patient with restrictive cardiomyopathy and a patient with constrictive pericarditis. A marked difference in early diastolic longitudinal axis velocities, despite similar early transmitral flow velocities, is appreciated. (From Garcia MJ, Thomas JD, Klein AL:* J Am Coll Cardiol *32[4]:865-875, 1998.)*

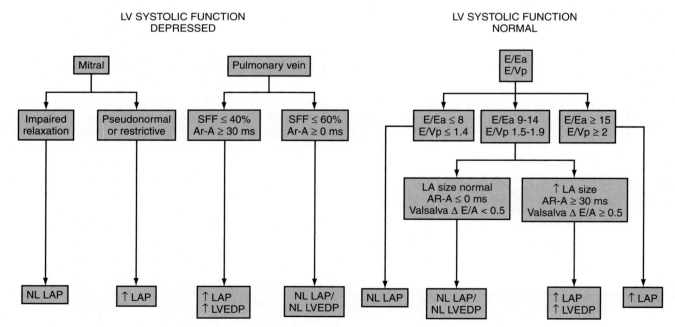

Figure 11-8. *Schemata for assessment of left atrial (LA) pressure and left ventricular end-diastolic pressures (LVEDP) in patients with normal and depressed LV systolic function. Ar-A, difference in duration of the atrial reversal wave of mitral inflow; E/A, ratio of early to atrial diastolic filling velocities; E/Ea, ratio of transmitral Doppler to annular tissue Doppler early diastolic velocities; E/Vp, ratio of early diastolic filling to velocity of propagation from color M-mode. LV, left ventricular; NL LAP, normal left atrial pressure; SFF, systolic filling fraction. (Adapted from Nagueh SF, Zoghbi WA:* ACC Current J Rev *10[4]:45-49, 2001).*

patients who had symtomatic HF demonstrated that E/Ea predicted mortality, transplantation, and hospitalization for HF and was incremental to deceleration time and EF.[84a] An overall schemata utilizing the different imaging modalities in estimating filling pressures is displayed in Figure 11–8.

Strain Rate Imaging in Evaluation of Diastolic Function

Strain and strain rate (SR) are measures of myocardial mechanical properties. Myocardial strain is a dimensionless index of change in myocardial length in response to an applied force and is expressed as fractional or percentage change (Fig. 11–9). SR is the time derivative of strain with unit of per second (s^{-1}). By convention, myocardial lengthening or thinning gives a positive strain value and shortening or thickening gives a negative value.[85] Strain parameters can be derived noninvasively from either magnetic resonance imaging

(MRI) tagging techniques[86,87] or echocardiography, using M-mode[85] or Doppler tissue velocity data.[88,89] Measurement of myocardial SR by TDI originally was described as the (radial) myocardial velocity gradient. SR values are calculated from the tissue velocities at two points at a fixed distance in the direction of one US beam. The distance between the points (the "offset") is usually approximately 8 mm, taking into account the trade-off between less noise with larger offsets and more spatial resolution with smaller offsets. In a further step, SR can be integrated numerically over time to yield strain itself. Hence, local strain can be directly extracted from tissue Doppler data. This has been well validated by sonomicrometry.[90] By echocardiography, SR and strain (see Fig. 11–9) can be obtained only in the direction of the US beam in the longitudinal, radial, and circumferential imaging planes. In the longitudinal plane this is obtained by imaging along the long axis of the left ventricle (e.g., the septum in an apical four-chamber view), in which systolic shortening yields

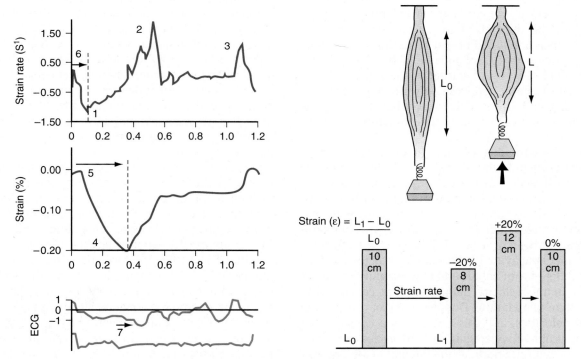

Figure 11–9. *Schematic representation of potential quantitative parameters obtained from echocardiography derived strain rate (SR) tracing (left). Both amplitude and timing of mechanical events can be used to assess regional function by SR imaging. SR tracing (upper): 1, peak systolic SR; 2, peak early diastolic SR; 3, peak late diastolic SR; 6, time to peak systolic SR. Strain tracing (middle) is obtained by integrating the SR signal. This procedure is automatic in most custom or commercially available analysis packages: 4, peak systolic strain; 5, time to peak. SR signal showing low systolic SR but presence of postsystolic SR (lower) (7). Schematic illustrating concept of strain and SR (right). Strain (ε) is change in length normalized to initial length of muscle (upper right corner). Thus, decrease in length (such as occurring in muscle contraction) would result in negative strain, increase in length (muscle relaxation) would result in positive strain, and rate at which length changes occur would be SR. ECG, electrocardiogram; L_0, initial length of muscle; L_1, final length. (From Yip G, Abraham T, Belohlavek M, Khandheria BK: J Am Soc Echocardiogr 16[12]:1334-1342, 2003.)*

negative SR and strain values. In the radial plane, this is done by imaging across the thickness of myocardial walls (e.g., the posterior wall from a parasternal window), in which systolic thickening yields positive SR and strain values. In the circumferential plane, this is performed by imaging in the short-axis view. However, only septal and lateral segments will be aligned to display circumferential deformation. Thus, circumferential strain is rarely used for clinical purposes.

Acquisition of Images for Strain and Strain Rate Analysis. Doppler tissue velocity images of three to four cardiac cycles are acquired at end-expiration.[91] To optimize the tissue velocity signals, a clear differentiation between the myocardium and the blood pool is obtained using the gain controls in the 2D image. Pulse repetition frequency setting is also adjusted to avoid any aliasing within the myocardial wall (usually 1 to 2 kHz). The frame rate is maximized using the machine frame rate controls and reducing sector size if possible. High frame rates provide superior quality TDI and strain rate imaging (SRI) signals. Every attempt should be made to acquire images at or above 150 frames/s. The upper velocity range for the myocardial velocities should also be maximized to a level just below the highest velocity recorded at rest or during stress echocardiography so as to enhance sensitivity of velocity measurement. The usual setting of the upper limit of the velocity scale is approximately 14 to 20 cm/s for both resting and stress TDI. Myocardial velocity data can then be analyzed in real time or offline to yield various strain variables.[91]

There are a number of limitations of strain imaging.[92] These include the following: (1) Only deformation in the direction of the US beam is measured, although myocardial deformation in reality occurs in all directions. The assumption that measurement in one direction is representative for the other strain components has not been proven.[93] (2) Angle errors affect SR measurements heavily. (3) SR data are calculated from a small difference of values and thus magnify the noise inherent in the velocity data. They are considerably noisier than blood flow Doppler data or raw tissue Doppler velocities, and this constitutes a considerable practical problem. Averaging several cycles (in sinus rhythm) is helpful. Strain, as the integral of SR, appears much less noisy. Observer variability has been reported to range 10% to 15% for peak SR and systolic strain measured by two observers.[86] (4) Although strain and SR distinguish local deformation from transmitted motion ("tethering" or translation), they do not distinguish active or passive local deformation.

Normal Values of Myocardial Strain and Strain Rate. Isolated myocardial fibers shorten by approximately 15% after excitation. This value is much less than the normal value of LV EF. Typical values for normal systolic *longitudinal* strain and peak systolic strain rate in humans are $-19\pm6\%$ and -1.27 ± 0.39 s^{-1}, respectively.[86] Typical values for normal systolic *radial* strain and SR in humans are $41\pm4.4\%$ and 2.3 ± 0.3 s^{-1}, respectively. In a comparative study of pharmacological and bicycle exercise stress, SR increases linearly with HR and dp/dt of the left ventricle by approximately 80% to 100%. Strain increased slightly at low stress levels (by about 15% to 20%) and returned close to baseline values at peak stress.[92]

Assessment of Diastolic Function by Strain Echocardiography. Assessment of transmitral and pulmonary vein blood flow is utilized to detect global changes in LV filling. On the other hand, myocardial velocity profiles measure local wall motion and have the potential of identifying local changes induced by filling. E-wave changes in myocardial diastolic parameters will usually mirror the changes in global filling detected in the transmitral and pulmonary vein flow. However, when there are regional abnormalities in diastolic function, changes in the E′ peak velocity will better reflect regional impairment in relaxation whereas changes in compliance are better reflected by early diastolic changes in the regional strain curve. Regional abnormalities in myocardial diastolic motion may be detectable despite mitral and pulmonary vein velocities being normal. Garcia-Fernandez and colleagues[72] demonstrated in an experimental model of acute ischemia that up to 40% of segments may have measurable regional diastolic motion abnormalities whereas blood pool indices remain normal.

One advantage of the new US deformation strain indices for the study of diastolic events is that they offer high real-time temporal resolution of deformation (sampling rates of ≈200 frames/s) compared with other noninvasive imaging modalities (Fig. 11–10). This is important when studying diastole, as high-amplitude, short-lived deformations occur during this time period.[94,95] SR imaging has shown the normal sequence of regional changes in deformation during diastole to be complex.[94] Regional lengthening begins in the mid-inferior septal segment and might happen before aortic valve closure and may have propagated to the apex by the time of mitral valve opening. The basal segments are the last to start to lengthen in early diastole. Their lengthening is associated with the onset of flow into the left ventricle. On the other hand, in the free walls, changes in deformation are more variable. After the cessation of early lengthening as a result of early filling, there is a reverse lengthening wave caused by passive recoil, which starts at the apex and spreads toward the base. During diastasis there are usually no measurable changes in deformation. Diastasis is followed by a base-apex wave of lengthening that is

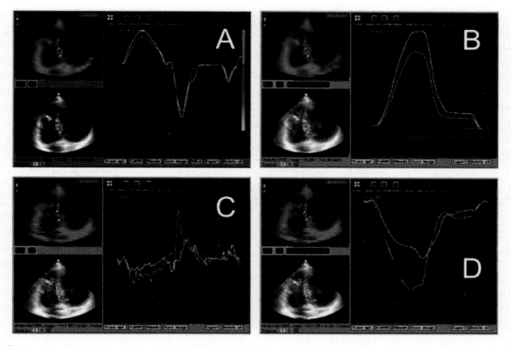

Figure 11-10. A, *Normal patterns of Doppler tissue echocardiography velocity;* B, *displacement;* C, *strain rate;* D, *strain;* blue, green, *and* red curves *represent basal, mid, and apical segments, respectively. (From Sun JP, Popovic ZB, Greenberg NL, et al:* J Am Soc Echocardiogr *17[2]:132-138, 2004.)*

caused by atrial filling of the ventricle. This normal pattern may be markedly altered in disease. However, in describing regional deformation changes during filling, not only regional radial and longitudinal deformation must be examined, but also an attempt should be made to resolve regional twisting/untwisting occurring during IVRT. To do this, circumferential shear strain must be measured. Circumferential radial shear strain can be shown to be abnormal in diseased segments. Recently, strain imaging has been shown to differentiate between control subjects and patients with hypertension and among patients with hypertension, to differentiate between those with and without diastolic dysfunction.[96,97] Regional abnormalities in the amount of deformation during early filling are also a frequent finding in cardiomyopathies. A complex pattern of alterations in SR profiles has been demonstrated to occur for patients with restrictive filling when compared with both patients with constriction and control subjects.[98] SR imaging indices have been shown to be better than regional velocity profile data in detecting regional abnormalities in patients with asymmetric septal hypertrophy and in discriminating HCM from physiologic hypertrophy. SR imaging has also been shown to be better than either gray-scale M-mode or velocity data in detecting changes in regional function either after septal ablation[99] or in detecting the regression of hypertrophy after antioxidant treatment for HCM.

Color M-Mode Doppler

As discussed in the previous portions of this chapter, the LV pressure drops without LV filling during isovolumic relaxation. The time constant of LV pressure decline (τ) is an index of LV relaxation that is relatively independent of HR and preload. After mitral valve opening, LV filling occurs with variable LV pressures (auxotonic relaxation). Measurements made during auxotonic relaxation are determined both by active relaxation and passive chamber stiffness, with the latter becoming increasingly important toward the end of ventricular filling.[100] The active processes during early diastole lead to a rapid LV pressure drop during isovolumic relaxation and fast active filling at low pressures during early auxotonic relaxation. As early as the 1930s, the normal ventricular relaxation was thought to result in "active suction" of the blood into the left ventricle. However, only in the early 1980s, the presence of diastolic intraventricular pressure gradients (IVPGs) were confirmed.[101,102] The gradients between the ventricular base (mitral valve) and apex were suggested to exert a suction effect ("recoil"). It was later demonstrated that these gradients were diminished by ischemia and related to systolic function.[103] With the demonstration of IVPGs during early diastole in filling and in nonfilling heart beats, their potential role as an index for isovolumic and early auxotonic ventricular relaxation was established.[104] Because pressure gradients in fluids imply fluid acceleration and fluid currents, a noninvasive index of fluid acceleration would, in theory, reflect these IVPGs. The color M-mode velocity propagation index (Vp) can potentially fulfill this promise.

Acquisition of Color M-Mode Images. Color M-mode Doppler is a pulsed Doppler technique in which mean velocities are color encoded and displayed in time (on the horizontal axis) and depth along the entire scan line (on the vertical axis). Acquisition is made in the four-chamber view. To visualize the direction of the inflowing blood, a large color box is placed from the mitral valve to the apex. The scan line should ideally go through the center of the mitral valve and along the central part of the blood column.[105,106] Switching to M-mode and with the chart recorder set at a sweep rate of 100 mm/s, an M-mode spatial-temporal velocity map with the shape of a flame is displayed (see Fig. 11–3). By digital processing, for each pixel of the displayed color M-mode map, time, depth, and numerical velocity can be determined. The Euler equation enables the calculation of instantaneous pressure gradients along the inflow tract in a noninvasive way, however, it is too cumbersome for routine practice.[106] Therefore, for clinical practice, the spatial-temporal velocity information is expressed as distance to time ratios (cm/s) and is known as the flow propagation velocity (FPV) because it has the dimensions of velocity and it has been interpreted as the distance the flow-wave (E-wave) propagates into the left ventricle as a function of time. The following techniques have been proposed for determining FPV: (1) Stugaard and colleagues measured the time delay between onset of maximal flow velocity at the mitral valve tips and at 3.7 cm toward the apex.[107] This technique requires offline postprocessing using dedicated software to decode the color of each pixel into numerical values. It depends on two individual pixels, and the reliance on accurate measurement of apical flow constitutes its primary limitation.[108] (2) Brun and colleagues measured slopes of the isovelocity lines formed by transition of no color to color (black to red).[109] The technique was later modified by Garcia and colleagues who traced the slope of the first "aliasing" velocity (red to blue) from the mitral valve plane to 4 cm distal in the LV (Vp in cm/s). The latter technique only requires online adaptation of the Nyquist range limit or baseline to obtain aliasing.[110] Both techniques rely on a large number of pixels and the measurements can be performed online. (3) The Takatsuji method of FPV calculation depends on offline, progressive scaling down of the Nyquist range by specific software. The slope between the site of the highest velocity at the mitral valve, connected with the point in which aliasing becomes apparent when the Nyquist range is further scaled down by 30% (regardless of the depth of this point) is defined as Vp.[111]

Flow Propagation Velocity and Hemodynamics. It has been demonstrated that despite worsening relaxation, E wave increases as a result of increasing filling pressures (pseudonormalization), but Vp does not rise.[111] This indirectly suggests preload independence. In invasive canine studies, significant preload alteration[107,112] did not induce significant change in propagation velocity. Recently, preload independence has also been demonstrated in human patients with and without LV systolic dysfunction.[112,113] There is an inverse relationship between Vp and the isovolumetric time constant of relaxation (τ). In dogs, Stugaard and colleagues showed a significant reduction of Vp in parallel with an increase in τ during induction of diastolic failure with regional[107] or global ischemia and with high dose propranolol.[114] Similar highly significant correlations between Vp and changes in τ during esmolol and dobutamine infusion were obtained by Garcia and colleagues in dogs.[112] Invasive studies in humans also show a consistent high inverse correlation between tau and the propagation rate Vp. Takatsuji and colleagues[111] found a strong inverse relation in 40 patients undergoing cardiac catheterization ($r = -0.82$; $P < 0.001$), similar to values reported by Garcia and colleagues ($r = -0.86$; $P < 0.001$),[112] and Brun and colleagues ($r = -0.73$; $P < 0.0001$).[109]

Clinical Use of Color M-Mode Doppler. In normal adults, little loss in blood velocities occurs between the basal ventricle and the apical region. The color M-mode flame appears at the apical region before early flow at the mitral valve level has stopped. The slope of the displayed filling wave is relatively steep. With impaired relaxation, the slope of the first filling wave is less steep; velocity loss makes the maximal velocities reside at the level of the mitral tips and mostly do not reach the apical region. With further reduction in diastolic relaxation and elevation of filling pressures as a result of reduced compliance, the slope of the early filling wave will stay reduced; the wave usually gets blurry as a result of low flow velocities in the apical region, which can continue after early mitral inflow has stopped or even after mitral valve closure. Brun and colleagues have been the first to show that velocity propagation is related to wall relaxation.[109] The progressive decrease of Vp runs in parallel with the increase of the isovolumic relaxation constant τ, irrespective of rising filling pressures.[111] Nishihara and colleagues have confirmed that the strong correlation between τ and Vp is also valid in HCM.[115] Using his acquisition method, Garcia and colleagues have proposed a cut-off value of 55 cm/s and 45 cm/s to define impaired relaxation in the young, respectively, midaged adults.[44]

Estimation of Filling Pressures and Prognosis. Combined indices of 1/Vp, as a preload independent surrogate for τ, with preload and relaxation-dependent mitral inflow parameters, provide close prediction of mean PCWP pressure.[110,113,116,117] In a direct comparison, the

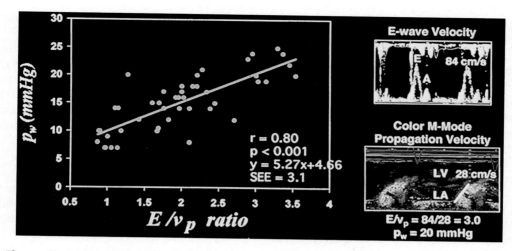

Figure 11–11. Linear regression between the dimensionless index: peak early transmitral flow velocity/flow propagation velocity (E/Vp) and capillary wedge pressure (Pw). SEE, standard error of the estimate. (From Garcia MJ, Ares MA, Asher CR, et al: J Am Coll Cardiol 29[2]:448-454, 1997.)

combination of IVRT and Vp turned out to be more accurate.[117] With an r-value of 0.89 ($P < 0.0001$), the reported accuracy of this combination is reasonable: $PCWP = 4.5 \times (10^3/[\{2 \times IVRT\} + Vp]) - 9$ (in mmHg, 1 SEE = 3.3).[116] Reported positive and negative predictive values for $(10^3/[\{2 \times IVRT\} + Vp]) > 5.5$ to predict $PCWP > 15$ are 100% and 94%, respectively.[116] However, E/Vp is the most widely used index. In a heterogeneous group comprising normal, ischemic, hypertrophic, and dilated hearts, PCWP was calculated as follows: $PCWP = [5.27 \times E/Vp] + 4.6$ (in mmHg, 1 SEE = 3.1) ($r = 0.80$, $P < 0.001$)[110] (Fig. 11–11). Reported positive and negative predictive values for E/Vp greater than 1.5 to predict PCWP greater than 12 mm Hg are 93% and 70%, respectively.[113] Correlation between E/Vp and PCWP outperforms correlations with maximal E ($r = 0.62$) and E/A ($r = 0.52$), independent of EF. Nagueh and colleagues have confirmed that the same formula is valid in HCM.[63,118] The E/Vp ratio has also been applied to assess filling pressures in atrial fibrillation with reasonable accuracy, averaged over three heart beats E/Vp yields a 100% specificity and 72% sensitivity in predicting a PCWP greater than 15 mm Hg.[119] It favorably corresponds to NYHA-class and elevated values of brain natriuretic peptide in this group.[120]

Limitations of Vp as a Preload Independent Index for Relaxation. Reliability and reproducibility of the three different acquisition and reading methods constitute a major limitation for the application of Vp. In a direct comparison of the three methods, large differences in obtained numerical values and in interobserver and intraobserver reproducibility of Vp were generated.[108] The method described by Garcia and colleages[110] is advocated because of the acceptable and superior reproducibility compared to the other methods.[108] Reported intraobserver and interobserver variability varies from less than 10%; in the lower (pathological)

ranges of Vp and up to 20% in the "higher" (normal) range of Vp and for TEE acquisitions.[110,112,116,119] Moreover, it does not require dedicated software, and therefore is the most feasible technique for rapid, online measurements.

All conditions associated with altered intraventricular flow patterns, giving rise to significant turbulence or significant local pressure gradient formation, constitute a limitation to the application of the technique: significant aortic regurgitation, mitral stenosis, artificial mitral valves, and intracavity obstructions. Merging of early and late inflow as a result of tachycardia or atrioventricular conduction delay could lead to erroneous measurements. Marked variations on both transmitral inflow and Vp recordings can be seen during atrial fibrillation and in some patients during respiration. In these patients, it should be recommended to average more than three cardiac cycles.

Clinical Utility of Diastolic Function Assessment

The clinical utility of echocardiographic assessment of diastolic function in specific diseases is discussed in this section.

Myocardial Diseases

Dilated cardiomyopathy manifests with a multitude of diastolic filling patterns and differences in diastolic function may explain differences in clinical symptoms between patients with similar degree of systolic dysfunction. When systolic dysfunction is present, the elevated end-systolic volume results in a shift along the pressure-volume curve to a steeper segment. This means that for a given diastolic pressure-volume relationship, compliance is reduced at higher LV volumes. Thus, the expected pattern of diastolic filling in advanced dilated cardiomyopathy is that of reduced compliance: a high E velocity, rapid deceleration slope, low A velocity, and an E/A ratio greater than 1 (Stage 3).

Cardiac amyloidosis is associated with abnormal LV and RV diastolic function. As the disease process worsens following impaired relaxation, there is worsening of compliance, resulting in pseudonormal and restrictive patterns associated with a progressive decrease in compliance with progressive deposition of amyloid fibrils in the myocardium.[121] There are associated abnormalities of RV diastolic function.[53] In patients with RV free wall thickness of less than 7 mm, there is abnormal relaxation, and when the right ventricular wall is greater than 7 mm in thickness, restrictive physiology is present. Patients with a mean wall thickness of 15 mm had a median survival of 0.4 years compared to a median survival of 2.4 years for those with a mean wall thickness of 12 mm.[122] Patients with a DT of the mitral early filling wave at baseline study of 150 msec or less had a significantly reduced survival compared to those whose DT was greater than 150 msec[123] (Fig. 11–12). A new Doppler index combining systolic and diastolic performance (Tei index) has shown significant prognostic importance in cardiac amyloidosis.[124] RV enlargement has also been identified as an independent predictor of poor outcomes among patients with primary amyloidosis.[125] Newer diagnostic tools, including strain and SR imaging, have been used to characterize patients with cardiac amyloidosis before the onset of congestive

symptoms and with preserved LV function and tissue Doppler velocities.[126]

Patients with HCM often have a pattern of LV diastolic filling consistent with impaired relaxation. Some studies have suggested that Doppler evaluation of LV diastolic filling can be used to assess the effects of medical therapy (e.g., beta-blockers or calcium channel blockers) on diastolic function in this disease.

Left Ventricular Hypertrophy

In left ventricular hypertrophy (LVH), the predominant abnormality is impaired relaxation, resulting in a pattern of reduced early diastolic filling and an enhanced atrial contribution to filling (see Chapter 34). The Doppler velocity curve typically shows a prolonged IVRT, reduced acceleration to a reduced E velocity, prolonged early diastolic deceleration slope, an increased A velocity, and an E/A ratio less than 1. When LV systolic dysfunction supervenes, the elevated LVEDP and elevated LA pressure may result in pseudonormalization of this pattern with an enhanced E velocity (related to a higher mitral valve opening gradient) and reduced A velocity (resulting from the elevated LVEDP).

Ischemic Cardiac Disease

In patients with coronary artery disease and no prior myocardial infarction (MI), induction of ischemia results in diastolic dysfunction before systolic dysfunction. Diastolic filling curves with ischemia induced by balloon inflation during percutaneous transluminal angioplasty show rapid onset of a reduced E velocity, with resolution of these changes as ischemia is relieved. In acute myocardial infarction, a pattern of delayed relaxation is seen acutely. At follow-up, one of several patterns of LV filling may be observed. With successful reperfusion and little myocardial damage, LV diastolic filling returns to normal. With an infarction but preserved LV systolic function, the pattern of impaired relaxation often persists. With a large infarction and significant LV systolic dysfunction, the pseudonormalized pattern of high E velocity and low A velocity as a result of a combination of reduced compliance, a high LVEDP, and a shift along the diastolic pressure volume curve (increased end-systolic volume) can be seen.

Pericardial Disease

With both pericardial tamponade and pericardial constriction, cardiac filling is impaired by pericardial extrinsic constraint, and there is marked reciprocal respiratory variation of LV and RV filling. In the case of tamponade physiology, filling is impaired in both early and late diastole. With constrictive pericarditis, early diastolic filling tends to be normal, with marked impairment of filling late in diastole when the heart has expanded to the maximum allowed by the fibrotic peri-

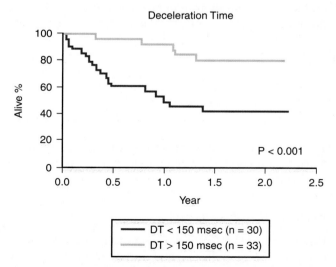

SURVIVAL CURVES IN CARDIAC AMYLOIDOSIS
CARDIAC DEATHS

Deceleration Time

— DT < 150 msec (n = 30)
— DT > 150 msec (n = 33)

Figure 11–12. Survival in 63 patients with cardiac amyloidosis subdivided on the basis of the deceleration time (DT) of 150 msec. Patients with a shortened deceleration time of less than 150 msec (blue line) had significantly reduced survival compared with patients with a deceleration time of greater than 150 msec. (From Klein AL, Hatle LK, Taliercio CP, et al: Circulation 83:808-816, 1991.)

cardial encasement. Utility of TDI in separating restrictive from constrictive physiology is described previously in the chapter (see p. 247).

Emerging Techniques in Assessment of Diastolic Function

Torsion Echocardiography: Emergence of Speckle Tracking

LV torsion (or twist) plays an important role with respect to LV ejection and filling.[127-129] During the cardiac cycle, there is a systolic twist and an early diastolic untwist of the LV about its long axis due to oppositely directed apical and basal rotations. As viewed from the LV apex, systolic apical rotation is counterclockwise and basal rotation, clockwise. LV rotation is sensitive to changes in both regional and global LV function.[128,130-132] Therefore, assessment of LV rotation represents an interesting approach for quantifying LV function. However, MRI tagging has been the only clinically available method thus far,[131,133-137] and implementation has therefore been limited by complexity and cost.

A newly developed speckle tracking imaging (STI) technique (Fig. 11-13) has presented us the possibility of enhancing the accuracy of displacement estimation by filtering out random speckles and then performing autocorrelation to estimate motion of stable structures[138-140] (see Chapter 5). This non-Doppler assessment of cardiac

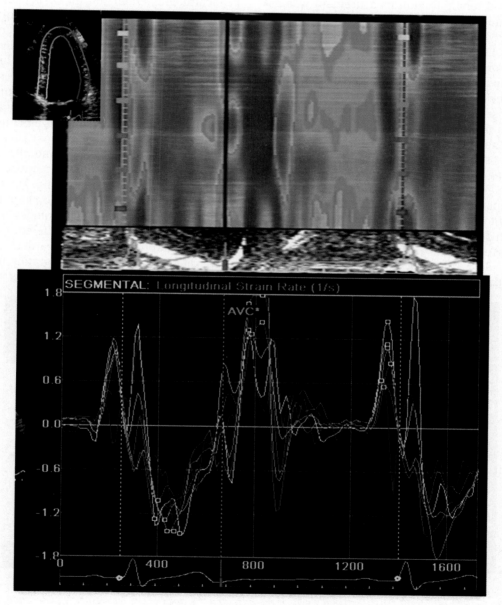

Figure 11–13. *Speckle tracking imaging to derive regional longitudinal strain rate: color coding of six left ventricular segments in a four-chamber view (inset); color M-mode map of longitudinal strain rate (top); strain rate tracing averaged over individual left ventricular segments (bottom). AVC, aortic valve closure (end-systole).*

mechanics could rival MRI or TDI in measuring LV torsion and may prove more versatile in assessing patients in clinical and research settings. Motion analysis by speckle tracking has been attempted using block matching and autocorrelation search algorithms.[141,142] Speckle motion has been closely linked to underlying tissue motion when small displacements are involved. On the basis of this displacement estimation technique, LV rotation (angle-displacement about the central axis of LV in the short-axis view) for assessment of LV torsion can be measured[41a] (Fig. 11-14).

Validation of Speckle Tracking

The accuracy and consistency of speckle tracking imaging method for LV torsion measurement was assessed in comparison with tagged MRI and TDI in 15 patients.[143,144] LV torsion was defined as the net difference of LV rotation at the basal and apical planes. Data on 13 of 15 patients were usable for speckle tracking analysis, and LV torsion profile estimated by speckle tracking imaging strongly correlated with those by tagged MRI. The speckle tracking imaging torsional velocity profile also correlated well with that by the TDI method (Fig. 11-15).

In another study, apical and basal rotation by speckle tracking was measured from short-axis images by automatic frame-to-frame tracking of gray-scale speckle patterns in mongrel dogs and healthy humans and compared to sonomicrometry (dogs) and MRI (humans).[145,146] In dogs, the mean peak apical rotation was −3.7±1.2 degrees and −4.1±1.2 degrees, and basal rotation was 1.9±1.5 degrees and 2.0±1.2 degrees by sonomicrometry and speckle tracking, respectively.

Apical rotation by both methods decreased during left anterior descending coronary artery occlusion ($P < 0.007$), whereas basal rotation was unchanged. In healthy humans, apical rotation was −11.6±3.8 degrees and −10.9±3.3 degrees, and basal rotation was 4.8±1.7 degrees and 4.6±1.3 degrees by MRI tagging and speckle tracking echocardiography (STE), respectively. Torsion measurement by STE showed good correlation and agreement with sonomicrometry ($r = 0.94$; $P < 0.001$) and MRI ($r = 0.85$; $P < 0.001$).

Summary

Echocardiography remains the cornerstone of the study of diastology. Additional lessons regarding the fundamentals of diastolic dysfunction have occurred with the use of newer US-based technologies, including strain, SR, tissue tracking, and torsion imaging. These technologies have allowed for earlier recognition of diastolic dysfunction and aided in distinguishing primary forms of pathological hypertrophy and restrictive cardiomyopathies and predicting preclinical deterioration to HF in select patient groups. These applications appear to have finally overcome the limitations of standard Doppler techniques separating the effects of preload and relaxation in LV filling. Further studies are needed to standardize and develop automated measuring methods and to establish ranges of values from larger patient populations. While it is expected that echocardiographic techniques, cardiac magnetic resonance imaging, computed tomography (CT), and BNP levels will continue to provide insights into the patho-

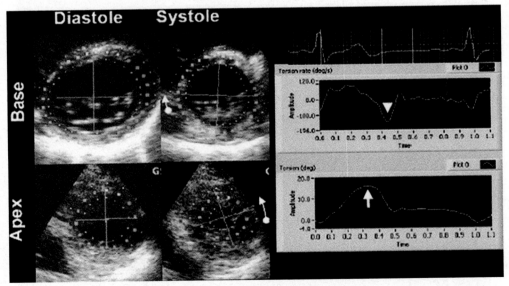

Figure 11–14. *Quantitation of torsion and torsion velocity (rate) by speckle tracking imaging. Images to the left represent cross-sectional views of the base and the apex of the left ventricle superimposed with speckle tracking imaging-generated markers of left ventricular torsion. Images to the right represent torsion rate and torsion signal. Arrowhead and arrow mark peak negative torsion velocity and peak systolic torsion, respectively. (From Thomas JD, Popovic ZB: J Am Coll Cardiol 48[10]:2012-2025, 2006.)*

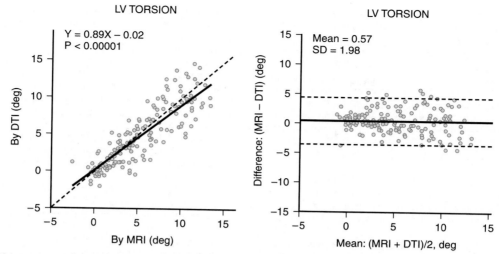

Figure 11–15. Regression analysis by repeated-measures regression models and limits of agreement analysis for LV torsion. Correlation and identity lines depicted as solid and dashed lines, respectively, in left panel. In right panel, solid line indicates mean, and dotted lines indicate 2-SD limits. (From Notomi Y, Setser RM, Shiota T, et al: Circulation 111[9]:1141-1147, 2005.)

physiology of diastology and related diseases and improve diagnosis and management strategies, we anticipate that the next frontier in diastology will occur in the development of better treatment options.

KEY POINTS

■ Diastolic HF is as common as systolic heart failure (HF) and has significant morbidity and mortality.

■ There is a controversy whether the best term is diastolic HF or HF with preserved EF.

■ Diastole is divided into the following periods: isovolumic relaxation, early rapid filling, diastasis, and atrial systole

■ The major parameters of diastolic function include: active myocardial relaxation, LV compliance, left atrial function, pulmonary vein flow, mitral valve characteristics, and HR.

■ The definition of diastolic HF includes signs or symptoms of HF, normal or only mildly abnormal LV systolic function, and evidence of abnormal LV relaxation, filling, or diastolic stiffness.

■ Echocardiographic techniques for evaluation of diastolic function include mitral inflow, pulmonary venous flow, tissue Doppler imaging, and color M-Mode Doppler.

■ For patients with diastolic dysfunction, four abnormal filling patterns are recognized: Stage 1 (mild) or abnormal relaxation, Stage 2 (moderate) or pseudonormal, Stage 3 (severe) or restrictive, or Stage 4 (severe) or irreversible restrictive.

■ Tissue Doppler imaging and color M-mode Doppler evaluation of LV diastolic filling are less preload dependent than mitral inflow or PV flow.

■ Peak early mitral inflow velocity (E) divided by TDI early diastolic mitral annular velocity (E_a) resulted in a ratio (E/E_a) that correlates with PCWP. Similarly, peak early mitral inflow velocity (E) divided by color M-mode flow propagation resulted in a ratio (E/Vp) that correlates with PCWP.

■ An E/E_a ratio greater than 15 or E/Vp greater than 1.5 suggests elevated LV filling pressures.

■ Mitral inflow and PV flow can adequately assess LV filling pressures in patients with systolic HF. Tissue Doppler imaging and color M-mode are needed when there is primary diastolic HF (normal EF).

■ A short mitral inflow DT is generally associated with a poor prognosis in most diseases, except for hypetrophic cardiomyopathy.

■ Strain and strain rate (SR) are measures of myocardial mechanical properties. Myocardial strain is a dimensionless index of change in myocardial length in response to an applied force and is expressed as fractional or percentage of change. SR is the time derivative of strain with unit of per second (s^{-1}).

■ Echocardiographic assessment of diastolic function in useful in hypertension, ischemic heart disease, cardiomyopathies, and pericardial diseases.

■ 2D strain or speckle tracking are emerging techniques in the study of muscle mechanics.

■ LV torsion (or twist) plays an important role with respect to LV ejection and filling.

REFERENCES

1. Brogan WC 3rd, Hillis LD, Flores ED, et al: The natural history of isolated left ventricular diastolic dysfunction. *Am J Med* 92(6):627-630, 1992.

2. Gaasch WH: Diagnosis and treatment of heart failure based on left ventricular systolic or diastolic dysfunction. *JAMA* 271(16):1276-1280, 1994.

3. How to diagnose diastolic heart failure. European Study Group on Diastolic Heart Failure. *Eur Heart J* 19(7):990-1003, 1998.

4. Zile MR: Diastolic dysfunction: detection, consequences and treatment. Part 1: Definition and determinants of diastolic function. *Mod Concepts Cardiovasc Dis* 58(12):67-72, 1989.

4a. Klein AL, Asher CR: Diseases of the pericardium, restrictive cardiomyopathy, and diastolic dysfunction. In Topol EJ, Califf RM, Prystowsky EN, et al (eds): *Textbook of Cardiovascular Medicine*, 3rd ed. Philadelphia, Lippincott, Williams & Wilkins, 2007, pp. 420-459.

5. Thomas JD, Flachskampf FA, Chen C, et al: Isovolumic relaxation time varies predictably with its time constant and aortic and left atrial pressures: Implications for the noninvasive evaluation of ventricular relaxation. *Am Heart J* 124:1305-1313, 1992.

6. Weiss JL, Frederikson JW, Weisfeldt JL: Hemodynamic determinants of the time-course of fall in canine left ventricular pressure. *J Clin Invest* 8:751-776, 1976.

7. Little WC, Downes TR: Clinical evaluation of left ventricular diastolic performance. *Prog Cardiovasc Dis* 32(4):273-290, 1990.

8. Choong CY, Abascal VA, Thomas JD, et al: Combined influence of ventricular loading and relaxation in the transmitral flow velocity profile in dogs measured by Doppler echocardiography. *Circulation* 78:672-683, 1988.

9. Thomas JD, Weyman AE: Echo-Doppler evaluation of ventricular diastolic function: Physics and physiology. *Circulation* 77:977-990, 1991.

10. Robinson T, Factor S, Sonnenblick E: The heart as a suction pump. *Sci Am* 254:84, 1986.

11. Nikolic S, Yellin EL, Tamura K, et al. Passive properties of the canine left ventricle: Diastolic stiffness and restoring forces. *Circ Res* 62:1210-1222, 1988.

12. Pouleur H: Diastolic dysfunction and myocardial energetics. *Eur Heart J* 1990;11(Suppl C):30-34, 1990.

13. Gaasch WH, Quinones MA, Waisser E, et al: Diastolic compliance of the left ventricle in man. *Am J Cardiol* 36(2):193-201, 1975.

14. Janicki J, Matsubara B: Myocardial collagen and left ventricular diastolic function. In: Gaasch W, LeWinter M, (eds): *Left Ventricular Diastolic Dysfunction and Heart Failure*, Philadelphia, Lea & Febiger, 1994, pp. 125-140.

15. Matsubara B, Hennigar J, Janicki J: Structural and functional role of myocardial collagen. *Circulation* 84:II-212, 1991.

16. Gilbert JC, Glantz SA: Determinants of left ventricular filling and the diastolic pressure-volume relation. *Circ Res* 64:827-852, 1989.

17. Cheng CP, Igarashi Y, Little WC: Mechanism of augmented rate of left ventricular filling during exercise. *Circ Res* 70(1):9-19, 1992.

18. Tyberg JV, Misbach GA, Glantz SA, et al: A mechanism for shifts in the diastolic, left ventricular, pressure-volume curve: the role of the pericardium. *Eur J Cardiol* 7(Suppl):163-175, 1978.

19. Suga H, Goto Y, Igarashi Y, et al: Ventricular suction under zero source pressure for filling. *Am J Physiol* 251(1 Pt 2):H47-H55, 1986.

20. Toutouzas P, Stefanadis C, Boudoulas H: 1st international symposium on left atrial function: introduction. *Eur Heart J Suppl* 2 (supplement K):K1-K3, 2000.

21. Ito T, Suwa M, Hirota Y, et al: Influence of left atrial function on Doppler transmitral and pulmonary venous flow patterns in dilated and hypertrophic cardiomyopathy: Evaluation of left atrial appendage function by transesophageal echocardiography. *Am Heart J* 131(1):122-130, 1996.

22. Pollick C, Taylor D: Assessment of left atrial appendage function by transesophageal echocardiography. Implications for the development of thrombus. *Circulation* 84(1):223-231, 1991.

23. Klein AL, Burstow DJ, Tajik AJ, et al: Effects of age on left ventricular dimensions and filling dynamics in 117 normal persons. *Mayo Clin Proc* 69(3):212-224, 1994.

24. Grimm RA, Leung DY, Black IW, et al: Left atrial appendage "stunning" after spontaneous conversion of atrial fibrillation demonstrated by transesophageal Doppler echocardiography. *Am Heart J* 130(1):174-176, 1995.

25. Plehn JF, Friedman BJ: Diastolic dysfunction in amyloid heart disease: restrictive cardiomyopathy or not? *J Am Coll Cardiol* 13(1):54-56, 1989.

26. Appleton CP, Carucci MJ, Henry CP, et al: Influence of incremental changes in heart rate on mitral flow velocity: Assessment in lightly sedated, conscious dogs. *J Am Coll Cardiol* 17:227-236, 1991.

27. Harrison MR, Clifton GD, Pennell AT, et al: Effect of heart rate on left ventricular diastolic transmitral flow velocity patterns assessed by Doppler echocardiography in normal subjects. *Am J Cardiol* 67(7):622-627, 1991.

28. Walsh RA: Sympathetic control of diastolic function in congestive heart failure. *Circulation* 82(2 Suppl):I52-I58, 1990.

29. Tanabe A, Mohri T, Ohga M, et al: The effects of pacing-induced left bundle branch block on left ventricular systolic and diastolic performances. *Jpn Heart J* 31(3):309-317, 1990.

30. Hatle LK, Appleton CP, Popp RL: Differentiation of constrictive pericarditis and restrictive cardiomyopathy by Doppler echocardiography. *Circulation* 79(2)3:57-370, 1989.

31. Zile MR, Baicu CF, Bonnema DD: Diastolic heart failure: definitions and terminology. *Prog Cardiovasc Dis* 47(5):307-313, 2005.

31a. Owan TE, Hodge DO, Herges RM, et al: Trends in prevalence and outcome of heart failure with preserved ejection fraction. *N Engl J Med* 355(3):251-259, 2006.

32. Vasan RS, Benjamin EJ, Levy D: Prevalence, clinical features and prognosis of diastolic heart failure: an epidemiologic perspective. *J Am Coll Cardiol* 26(7):1565-1574, 1995.

33. Kramer K, Kirkman P, Kitzman D, et al: Flash pulmonary edema: association with hypertension and reoccurrence despite coronary revascularization. *Am Heart J* 140(3):451-455, 2000.

34. Smith GL, Masoudi FA, Vaccarino V, et al: Outcomes in heart failure patients with preserved ejection fraction: mortality, readmission, and functional decline. *J Am Coll Cardiol* 41(9):1510-1518, 2003.

35. Cohn JN, Johnson G. Heart failure with normal ejection fraction: The V-HeFT study. *Circulation* 81(Suppl II):III48-III53, 1990.

36. Judge KW, Pawitan Y, Caldwell J, et al: Congestive heart failure symptoms in patients with preserved left ventricular systolic function: analysis of the CASS registry. *J Am Coll Cardiol* 18(2):377-382, 1991.

37. Senni M, Tribouilloy CM, Rodeheffer RJ, et al: Congestive heart failure in the community: a study of all incident cases in Olmsted County, Minnesota, in 1991. *Circulation* 98(21):2282-2289, 1998.

37a. Aurigemma GP: Diastolic heart failure—A common and lethal condition by any name. *N Engl J Med* 355(3):308-310, 2006.

38. McDermott MM, Feinglass J, Sy J, et al: Hospitalized congestive heart failure patients with preserved versus abnormal left ventricular systolic function: clinical characteristics and drug therapy. *Am J Med* 99(6):629-635, 1995.

39. Echeverria HH, Bilsker MS, Myerburg RJ, et al: Congestive heart failure: echocardiographic insights. *Am J Med* 75(5):750-755, 1983.

40. Vasan RS, Levy D: Defining diastolic heart failure: A call for standardized diagnostic criteria. *Circulation* 101(17):2118-2121, 2000.

41. Zile MR, Gaasch WH, Carroll JD, et al: Heart failure with a normal ejection fraction: is measurement of diastolic function necessary to make the diagnosis of diastolic heart failure? *Circulation* 104(7):779-782, 2001.

41a. Hunt SA, Abraham WT, Chin MH, et al: ACC/AHA 2005 Guideline Update for the Diagnosis and Management of Chronic Heart Failure in the Adult: a report of the American College of Cardiology/American Heart Association Task Force on Practice Guidelines (Writing Committee to Update the 2001 Guidelines for the Evaluation and Management of Heart Failure): developed in collaboration with the American College of Chest Physicians and the International Society for Heart and Lung Transplantation: endorsed by the Heart Rhythm Society. *Circulation* 112(12): e154-235, 2005.

41b. Heart Failure Society of America: Evaluation and management of patients with heart failure and preserved left ventricular ejection fraction. *J Card Fail* 12(1):e80-e85, 2006.

42. Appleton CP, Jensen JL, Hatle LK, et al: Doppler evaluation of left and right ventricular diastolic function: A technical guide for obtaining optimal flow velocity recordings. *J Am Soc Echocardiogr* 10:271-292, 1997.

43. Kitabatake A, Inoue M, Asao M, et al: Transmitral blood flow reflecting diastolic behavior of the left ventricle in health and disease—a study by pulsed Doppler technique. *Jpn Circ J* 46(1):92-102, 1982.

44. Garcia MJ, Thomas JD, Klein AL: New Doppler echocardiographic applications for the study of diastolic function. *J Am Coll Cardiol* 32(4):865-875, 1998.

45. Nishimura RA, Abel MD, Hatle LK, et al: Assessment of diastolic function of the heart: background and current applications of Doppler echocardiography. Part II. Clinical studies. *Mayo Clin Proc* 64(2):181-204, 1989.

46. Nishimura RA, Abel MD, Hatle LK, et al: Assessment of diastolic function of the heart: background and current applications of Doppler echocardiography. Part II. Clinical studies. *Mayo Clin Proc* 64(2):181-204, 1989.

47. Appleton CP, Gonzalez MS, Basnight MA: Relationship of left atrial pressure and pulmonary venous flow velocities: importance of baseline mitral and pulmonary venous flow velocity patterns studied in lightly sedated dogs. *J Am Soc Echocardiogr* 7(3 Pt 1):264-275, 1994.

47a. Kuecherer HF, Muhiudeen IA, Kusumoto FM, et al: Estimation of mean left atrial pressure from transesophageal pulsed Doppler echocardiography of pulmonary venous flow. *Circulation* 82(4):1127-1139, 1990.

48. Rossvoll O, Hatle LK: Pulmonary venous flow velocities recorded by transthoracic Doppler ultrasound: Relation to left ventricular diastolic pressures. *J Am Coll Cardiol* 21(7):1687-1696, 1993.

49. Appleton CA, Hatle LK, Popp RL: Relation of transmitral flow velocity patterns to left ventricular diastolic function: New insights from a combined hemodynamic and Doppler echocardiographic study. *J Am Coll Cardiol* 12:426-440, 1988.

50. Plehn JF, Southworth J, Cornwell GGd: Brief report: atrial systolic failure in primary amyloidosis. *N Engl J Med* 327(22):1570-1573, 1992.

51. Appleton CP, Firstenberg MS, Garcia MJ, et al: The echo-Doppler evaluation of left ventricular diastolic function. A current perspective. *Cardiol Clin* 18(3):513-546, ix, 2000.

52. Ommen SR, Nishimura RA, Appleton CP, et al: Clinical utility of Doppler echocardiography and tissue doppler imaging in the estimation of left ventricular filling pressures: A comparative simultaneous doppler-catheterization study. *Circulation* 102(15):1788-1794, 2000.

53. Klein AL, Hatle LK, Burstow DJ, et al: Comprehensive Doppler assessment of right ventricular diastolic function in cardiac amyloidosis. *J Am Coll Cardiol* 15(1):99-108, 1990.

54. Klein AL, Cohen GI: Doppler echocardiographic assessment of constrictive pericarditis, cardiac amyloidosis, and cardiac tamponade. *Cleve Clin J Med* 59(3):278-290, 1992.

55. Cohen GI, Pietrolungo JF, Thomas JD, et al: A practical guide to assessment of ventricular diastolic function using Doppler echocardiography. *J Am Coll Cardiol* 27(7):1753-1760, 1996.

56. Klein AL, Leung DY, Murray RD, et al: Effects of age and physiologic variables on right ventricular filling dynamics in normal subjects. *Am J Cardiol* 84(4):440-448, 1999.

57. Appleton CP, Hatle LK, Popp RL: Superior vena cava and hepatic vein Doppler echocardiography in healthy adults. *J Am Coll Cardiol* 10:1032-1039, 1987.

58. Zoghbi WA, Habib GB, Quinones MA: Doppler assessment of right ventricular filling in a normal population. Comparison with left ventricular filling dynamics. *Circulation* 82(4):1316-1324, 1990.

59. Hatle L, Angelsen B: *Doppler Ultrasound in Cardiology*, Philadelphia, Lea & Febiger, 1985.

60. Isaaz K, Thompson A, Ethevenot G, et al: Doppler echocardiographic measurement of low velocity motion of the left ventricular posterior wall. *Am J Cardiol* 64(1):66-75, 1989.

61. Sohn DW, Chai IH, Lee DJ, et al: Assessment of mitral annulus velocity by Doppler tissue imaging in the evaluation of left ventricular diastolic function. *J Am Coll Cardiol* 30(2):474-480, 1997.

62. Nagueh SF, Middleton KJ, Kopelen HA, et al: Doppler tissue imaging: a noninvasive technique for evaluation of left ventricular relaxation and estimation of filling pressures. *J Am Coll Cardiol* 30(6):1527-1533, 1997.

63. Nagueh SF, Lakkis NM, Middleton KJ, et al: Doppler estimation of left ventricular filling pressures in patients with hypertrophic cardiomyopathy. *Circulation* 99(2):254-261, 1999.

64. Nagueh SF, Mikati I, Kopelen HA, et al: Doppler estimation of left ventricular filling pressure in sinus tachycardia. A new application of tissue Doppler imaging. *Circulation* 98(16):1644-1650, 1998.

65. Sohn DW, Song JM, Zo JH, et al: Mitral annulus velocity in the evaluation of left ventricular diastolic function in atrial fibrillation. *J Am Soc Echocardiogr* 12(11):927-931, 1999.

66. Sundereswaran L, Nagueh SF, Vardan S, et al: Estimation of left and right ventricular filling pressures after heart transplantation by tissue Doppler imaging. *Am J Cardiol* 82(3):352-357, 1988.

67. Rajagopalan N, Garcia MJ, Rodriguez L, et al: Comparison of new Doppler echocardiographic methods to differentiate constrictive pericardial heart disease and restrictive cardiomyopathy. *Am J Cardiol* 87(1):86-94, 2001.

68. Garcia MJ, Rodriguez L, Ares M, et al: Myocardial wall velocity assessment by pulsed Doppler tissue imaging: Characteristic findings in normal subjects. *Am Heart J* 132:648-656, 1996.

69. Pai RG, Gill KS. Amplitudes, durations, and timings of apically directed left ventricular myocardial velocities: I. Their normal pattern and coupling to ventricular filling and ejection. *J Am Soc Echocardiogr* 11(2):105-111, 1998.

70. Galiuto L, Ignone G, DeMaria AN: Contraction and relaxation velocities of the normal left ventricle using pulsed-wave tissue Doppler echocardiography. *Am J Cardiol* 81(5):609-614, 1998.

71. Alam M, Wardell J, Andersson E, et al: Effects of first myocardial infarction on left ventricular systolic and diastolic function with the use of mitral annular velocity determined by pulsed wave doppler tissue imaging. *J Am Soc Echocardiogr* 13(5):343-352, 2000.

72. Garcia-Fernandez MA, Azevedo J, Moreno M, et al: Regional diastolic function in ischaemic heart disease using pulsed wave Doppler tissue imaging. *Eur Heart J* 20(7):496-505, 1999.

73. Bach DS, Armstrong WF, Donovan CL, et al: Quantitative Doppler tissue imaging for assessment of regional myocardial velocities during transient ischemia and reperfusion. *Am Heart J* 132(4):721-725, 1996.

74. Derumeaux G, Loufoua J, Pontier G, et al. Tissue Doppler imaging differentiates transmural from nontransmural acute myocardial infarction after reperfusion therapy. *Circulation* 103:589-596, 2001.

75. Oki T, Tabata T, Yamada H, et al: Clinical application of pulsed Doppler tissue imaging for assessing abnormal left ventricular relaxation. *Am J Cardiol* 79(7):921-928, 1997.

76. Dokainish H, Zoghbi WA, Lakkis NM, et al: Comparative accuracy of B-type natriuretic peptide and tissue Doppler echocar-

diography in the diagnosis of congestive heart failure. *Am J Cardiol* 93(9):1130-1135, 2004.

77. Farias CA, Rodriguez L, Garcia MJ, et al: Assessment of diastolic function by tissue Doppler echocardiography: comparison with standard transmitral and pulmonary venous flow. *J Am Soc Echocardiogr* 12(8):609-617, 1999.

78. Garcia MJ, Rodriguez L, Ares M, et al: Differentiation of constrictive pericarditis from restrictive cardiomyopathy: Assessment of left ventricular diastolic velocities in longitudinal axis by Doppler tissue imaging. *J Am Coll Cardiol* 27(1):108-114, 1996.

79. Oki T, Tabata T, Yamada H, et al: Right and left ventricular wall motion velocities as diagnostic indicators of constrictive pericarditis. *Am J Cardiol* 81(4):465-470, 1998.

80. Naqvi TZ, Neyman G, Broyde A, et al: Comparison of myocardial tissue Doppler with transmitral flow Doppler in left ventricular hypertrophy. *J Am Soc Echocardiogr* 14(12):1153-1160, 2001.

81. Abe M, Oki T, Tabata T, et al: Difference in the diastolic left ventricular wall motion velocities between aortic and mitral regurgitation by pulsed tissue Doppler imaging. *J Am Soc Echocardiogr* 12(1):15-21, 1999.

82. Rodriguez L, Garcia M, Ares M, et al: Assessment of mitral annular dynamics during diastole by Doppler tissue imaging: comparison with mitral Doppler inflow in subjects without heart disease and in patients with left ventricular hypertrophy. *Am Heart J* 131(5):982-987, 1996.

83. Redfield MM, Jacobsen SJ, Burnett JC Jr, et al: Burden of systolic and diastolic ventricular dysfunction in the community: appreciating the scope of the heart failure epidemic. *JAMA* 289(2):194-202, 2003.

84. Hillis GS, Moller JE, Pellikka PA, et al: Noninvasive estimation of left ventricular filling pressure by E/e′ is a powerful predictor of survival after acute myocardial infarction. *J Am Coll Cardiol* 43(3):360-367, 2004.

84a. Thomas JD, Popovic ZB: Assessment of left ventricular function by cardiac ultrasound. *J Am Coll Cardiol* 48(10):2012-2025, 2006.

85. Weidemann F, Jamal F, Sutherland GR, et al: Myocardial function defined by strain rate and strain during alterations in inotropic states and heart rate. *Am J Physiol Heart Circ Physiol* 283(2):792-799, 2002.

86. Voigt JU, Arnold MF, Karlsson M, et al: Assessment of regional longitudinal myocardial strain rate derived from Doppler myocardial imaging indexes in normal and infarcted myocardium. *J Am Soc Echocardiogr* 13(6):588-598, 2000.

87. Jamal F, Kukulski T, Strotmann J, et al: Quantification of the spectrum of changes in regional myocardial function during acute ischemia in closed chest pigs: An ultrasonic strain rate and strain study. *J Am Soc Echocardiogr* 14(9):874-884, 2001.

88. Derumeaux G, Ovize M, Loufoua J, et al: Assessment of non-uniformity of transmural myocardial velocities by color-coded tissue Doppler imaging: characterization of normal, ischemic, and stunned myocardium. *Circulation* 101(12):1390-1395, 2000.

89. Firstenberg MS, Greenberg NL, Smedira NG, et al: The effects of acute coronary occlusion on noninvasive echocardiographically derived systolic and diastolic myocardial strain rates. *Curr Surg* 57(5):466-472, 2000.

90. Urheim S, Edvardsen T, Torp H, et al: Myocardial strain by Doppler echocardiography. Validation of a new method to quantify regional myocardial function. *Circulation* 102(10):1158-1164, 2000.

91. Yip G, Abraham T, Belohlavek M, et al: Clinical applications of strain rate imaging. *J Am Soc Echocardiogr* 16(12):1334-1342, 2003.

92. Voigt JU, Flachskampf FA: Strain and strain rate. New and clinically relevant echo parameters of regional myocardial function. *Z Kardiol* 93(4):249-258, 2004.

93. Waldman LK, Fung YC, Covell JW: Transmural myocardial deformation in the canine left ventricle. Normal in vivo three-dimensional finite strains. *Circ Res* 57(1):152-163, 1985.

94. Stoylen A, Slordahl S, Skjelvan GK, et al: Strain rate imaging in normal and reduced diastolic function: comparison with pulsed Doppler tissue imaging of the mitral annulus. *J Am Soc Echocardiogr* 14(4):264-274, 2001.

95. Voigt JU, Lindenmeier G, Werner D, et al: Strain rate imaging for the assessment of preload-dependent changes in regional left ventricular diastolic longitudinal function. *J Am Soc Echocardiogr* 15(1):13-19, 2002.

96. Yuda S, Short L, Leano R, et al: Myocardial abnormalities in hypertensive patients with normal and abnormal left ventricular filling: A study of ultrasound tissue characterization and strain. *Clin Sci (Lond)* 103(3):283-293, 2002.

97. Marwick TH: Measurement of strain and strain rate by echocardiography: ready for prime time? *J Am Coll Cardiol* 47(7):1313-1327, 2006.

98. Palka P, Lange A, Donnelly JE, et al: Differentiation between restrictive cardiomyopathy and constrictive pericarditis by early diastolic doppler myocardial velocity gradient at the posterior wall. *Circulation* 102(6):655-662, 2000.

99. Abraham TP, Nishimura RA, Holmes DR Jr, et al: Strain rate imaging for assessment of regional myocardial function: results from a clinical model of septal ablation. *Circulation* 105(12):1403-1406, 2002.

100. Zile MR, Brutsaert DL: New concepts in diastolic dysfunction and diastolic heart failure: Part I: diagnosis, prognosis, and measurements of diastolic function. *Circulation* 105(11):1387-1393, 2002.

101. Ling D, Rankin JS, Edwards CD, et al: Regional diastolic mechanics of the left ventricle in the conscious dog. *Am J Physiol* 236(2):H323-H330, 1979.

102. Courtois M, Kovacs SJ Jr, Ludbrook PA: Transmitral pressure-flow velocity relation: Importance of regional pressure gradients in the left ventricle during diastole. *Circulation* 78:661-671, 1988.

103. Courtois M, Sandor KJ, Ludbrook PA: Physiological early diastolic intraventricular pressure gradient is lost during acute myocardial ischemia. *Circulation* 81:1688-1696, 1990.

104. Nikolic SD, Feneley MP, Pajaro OE, et al. Origin of regional pressure gradients in the left ventricle during early diastole. *Am J Physiol* 268(2 Pt 2):H550-H557, 1995.

105. Greenberg NL, Castro PL, Drinko J, et al: Effect of scanline orientation on ventricular flow propagation: assessment using high frame-rate color Doppler echocardiography. *Biomed Sci Instrum* 36:203-208, 2000.

106. Greenberg NL, Vandervoort PM, Firstenberg MS, et al. Estimation of diastolic intraventricular pressure gradients by Doppler M-mode echocardiography. *Am J Physiol Heart Circ Physiol* 280(6):2507-2515, 2001.

107. Stugaard M, Smiseth OA, Risoe C, et al: Intraventricular early diastolic filling during acute myocardial ischemia, assessment by multigated color m-mode Doppler echocardiography. *Circulation* 88(6):2705-2713, 1993.

108. Sessoms MW, Lisauskas J, Kovacs SJ: The left ventricular color M-mode Doppler flow propagation velocity V(p): in vivo comparison of alternative methods including physiologic implications. *J Am Soc Echocardiogr* 15(4):339-348, 2002.

109. Brun P, Tribouilloy C, Duval AM, et al: Left ventricular flow propagation during early filling is related to wall relaxation: A color M-mode Doppler analysis. *J Am Coll Cardiol* 20:420-432, 1992.

110. Garcia MJ, Ares MA, Asher C, et al: An index of early left ventricular filling that combined with pulsed Doppler peak E velocity may estimate capillary wedge pressure. *J Am Coll Cardiol* 29:448-454, 1997.

111. Takatsuji H, Mikami T, Urasawa K, et al: A new approach for evaluation of left ventricular diastolic function: Spatial and

temporal analysis of left ventricular filling flow propagation by color M-mode Doppler echocardiography. *J Am Coll Cardiol* 27(2):365-371, 1996.

112. Garcia MJ, Smedira NG, Greenberg NL, et al: Color M-mode Doppler flow propagation velocity is a preload insensitive index of left ventricular relaxation: animal and human validation. *J Am Coll Cardiol* 35(1):201-208, 2000.

113. Firstenberg MS, Levine BD, Garcia MJ, et al: Relationship of echocardiographic indices to pulmonary capillary wedge pressures in healthy volunteers. *J Am Coll Cardiol* 36(5):1664-1669, 2000.

114. Stugaard M, Risoe C, Ihlen H, et al: Intracavitary filling pattern in the failing left ventricle assessed by color M-mode echocardiography. *J Am Coll Cardiol* 24:663-670, 1994.

115. Nishihara K, Mikami T, Takatsuji H, et al: Usefulness of early diastolic flow propagation velocity measured by color M-mode Doppler technique for the assessment of left ventricular diastolic function in patients with hypertrophic cardiomyopathy. *J Am Soc Echocardiogr* 13(9):801-808, 2000.

116. Gonzalez-Vilchez F, Ares M, Ayuela J, et al. Combined use of pulsed and color M-mode Doppler echocardiography for the estimation of pulmonary capillary wedge pressure: An empirical approach based on an analytical relation. *J Am Coll Cardiol* 34(2):515-523, 1999.

117. Gonzalez-Vilchez F, Ayuela J, Ares M, et al: Comparison of Doppler echocardiography, color M-mode Doppler, and Doppler tissue imaging for the estimation of pulmonary capillary wedge pressure. *J Am Soc Echocardiogr* 15(10 Pt 2):1245-1250, 2002.

118. Nagueh SF, Lakkis NM, Middleton KJ, et al: Changes in left ventricular diastolic function 6 months after nonsurgical septal reduction therapy for hypertrophic obstructive cardiomyopathy. *Circulation* 99(3):344-347, 1999.

119. Nagueh SF, Kopelen HA, Quinones MA: Assessment of left ventricular filling pressures by Doppler in the presence of atrial fibrillation. *Circulation* 94:2138-2154, 1996.

120. Oyama R, Murata K, Tanaka N, et al: Is the ratio of transmitral peak E-wave velocity to color flow propagation velocity useful for evaluating the severity of heart failure in atrial fibrillation? *Circ J* 68(12):1132-1138, 2004.

121. St. John Sutton MG, Reichek N, Kastor JA, et al: Computerized M-mode echocardiographic analysis of left ventricular dysfunction in cardiac amyloid. *Circulation* 66(4):790-799, 1982.

122. Cueto-Garcia L, Reeder GS, Kyle RA, et al: Echocardiographic findings in systemic amyloidosis: spectrum of cardiac involvement and relation to survival. *J Am Coll Cardiol* 6:737-743, 1985.

123. Klein AL, Hatle LK, Taliercio CP, et al: Prognostic significance of Doppler measures of diastolic function in cardiac amyloidosis. A Doppler echocardiography study. *Circulation* 83(3):808-816, 1991.

124. Tei C, Dujardin KS, Hodge DO, et al: Doppler Index combining systolic and diastolic myocardial performance: Clinical value in cardiac amyloidosis. *J Am Coll Cardiol* 28:658-664, 1996.

125. Patel AR, Dubrey SW, Mendes LA, et al: Right ventricular dilation in primary amyloidosis: an independent predictor of survival. *Am J Cardiol* 80(4):486-492, 1997.

126. Koyama J, Ray-Sequin PA, Falk RH: Longitudinal myocardial function assessed by tissue velocity, strain, and strain rate tissue Doppler echocardiography in patients with AL (primary) cardiac amyloidosis. *Circulation* 107(19):2446-2452, 2003.

127. Rademakers FE, Buchalter MB, Rogers WJ, et al: Dissociation between left ventricular untwisting and filling. Accentuation by catecholamines. *Circulation* 85(4):1572-1581, 1992.

128. Gibbons Kroeker CA, Tyberg JV, Beyar R: Effects of load manipulations, heart rate, and contractility on left ventricular apical rotation. An experimental study in anesthetized dogs. *Circulation* 92(1):130-141, 1995.

129. Moon MR, Ingels NB Jr, Daughters GT 2nd, et al: Alterations in left ventricular twist mechanics with inotropic stimulation and volume loading in human subjects. *Circulation* 89(1):142-150, 1994.

130. Hansen DE, Daughters GT 2nd, Alderman EL, et al: Effect of volume loading, pressure loading, and inotropic stimulation on left ventricular torsion in humans. *Circulation* 83(4):1315-1326, 1991.

131. Maier SE, Fischer SE, McKinnon GC, et al: Evaluation of left ventricular segmental wall motion in hypertrophic cardiomyopathy with myocardial tagging. *Circulation* 86(6):1919-1928, 1992.

132. Buchalter MB, Rademakers FE, Weiss JL, et al: Rotational deformation of the canine left ventricle measured by magnetic resonance tagging: Effects of catecholamines, ischaemia, and pacing. *Cardiovasc Res* 28(5):629-635, 1994.

133. Stuber M, Scheidegger MB, Fischer SE, et al: Alterations in the local myocardial motion pattern in patients suffering from pressure overload due to aortic stenosis. *Circulation* 100(4):361-368, 1999.

134. Nagel E, Stuber M, Burkhard B, et al: Cardiac rotation and relaxation in patients with aortic valve stenosis. *Eur Heart J* 21(7):582-589, 2000.

135. Nagel E, Stuber M, Lakatos M, et al: Cardiac rotation and relaxation after anterolateral myocardial infarction. *Coron Artery Dis* 11(3):261-267, 2000.

136. Buchalter MB, Weiss JL, Rogers WJ, et al: Noninvasive quantification of left ventricular rotational deformation in normal humans using magnetic resonance imaging myocardial tagging. *Circulation* 81(4):1236-1244, 1990.

137. Setser RM, Kasper JM, Lieber ML, et al: Persistent abnormal left ventricular systolic torsion in dilated cardiomyopathy after partial left ventriculectomy. *J Thorac Cardiovasc Surg* 126(1):48-55, 2003.

138. Behar V, Adam D, Lysyansky P, et al: The combined effect of nonlinear filtration and window size on the accuracy of tissue displacement estimation using detected echo signals. *Ultrasonics* 41(9):743-753, 2004.

139. Reisner SA, Lysyansky P, Agmon Y, et al: Global longitudinal strain: a novel index of left ventricular systolic function. *J Am Soc Echocardiogr* 17(6):630-633, 2004.

140. Leitman M, Lysyansky P, Sidenko S, et al: Two-dimensional strain-a novel software for real-time quantitative echocardiographic assessment of myocardial function. *J Am Soc Echocardiogr* 17(10):1021-1029, 2004.

141. Bohs LN, Trahey GE: A novel method for angle independent ultrasonic imaging of blood flow and tissue motion. *IEEE Trans Biomed Eng* 38(3):280-286, 1991.

142. Bohs LN, Geiman BJ, Anderson ME, et al: Speckle tracking for multi-dimensional flow estimation. *Ultrasonics* 38(1-8):369-375, 2000.

143. Notomi Y, Lysyansky P, Setser RM, et al: Measurement of ventricular torsion by two-dimensional ultrasound speckle tracking imaging. *J Am Coll Cardiol* 45(12):2034-2041, 2005.

144. Notomi Y, Setser RM, Shiota T, et al: Assessment of left ventricular torsional deformation by Doppler tissue imaging: validation study with tagged magnetic resonance imaging. *Circulation* 111(9):1141-1147, 2005.

145. Amundsen BH, Helle-Valle T, Edvardsen T, et al: Noninvasive myocardial strain measurement by speckle tracking echocardiography: Validation against sonomicrometry and tagged magnetic resonance imaging. *J Am Coll Cardiol* 47(4):789-793, 2006.

146. Helle-Valle T, Crosby J, Edvardsen T, et al: New noninvasive method for assessment of left ventricular rotation: speckle tracking echocardiography. *Circulation* 112(2):3149-3156, 2005.

Chapter 12

Echocardiographic Digital Image Processing and Approaches to Automated Border Detection

JOHAN G. BOSCH, PhD

Digital image processing techniques nowadays can be found in any ultrasonography machine or offline analysis system. Moreover, ultrasonography machines have evolved from mainly analog, video-type technology into fully digital, computerized systems. Digital image storage and digital processing of echocardiographic images, both for image enhancement and for analysis, are widely practiced. Several forms of automated image analysis and automated border detection (ABD) techniques (also known as edge detection, border delineation, or edge finding) are commercially available for two-dimensional (2D) and three-dimensional (3D) echocardiographic data. However, ABD is still in full development.

ABD can potentially supply the echocardiologist with quantitative, more objective tools for research and clinical practice. However, ultrasonography is a difficult imaging modality for interpretation, for both humans and computers. This chapter provides the clinician with an overview of available tools, some insights into the background of different techniques with their possibilities and limitations, and supplies some practical guidelines for the choice and use of techniques.

Digital Image Processing and Automated Border Detection: Definition and Motivation

Digital image processing concerns all manipulation of images by a computer. More specifically, it refers to enhancement or analysis of images. Image enhancement aims at improvement of images for visual interpretation or for further automated analysis. This can range from a simple contrast adjustment to sophisticated filtering.

Image analysis generally involves the derivation of some quantitative measures or parameters from images. In a narrower sense, this often refers to automatic localization and outlining (border detection) of certain structures or to tracking the motion of such structures. In echocardiography, the left ventricular (LV) myocardium is of prime interest. Outlining of the LV endocardial border allows quantitative measurements of LV cavity area and calculation of volume, local wall displacement and velocity, and so on. Combination with the epicardial border allows calculation of wall thickening and LV mass. Tracking the motion of tissue or borders over the cycle allows the calculation of displacement, relative shortening (strain), and so on.

Besides quantitative measurements, visual estimation of parameters (such as ejection fraction [EF]) or semi-quantitative classification (e.g., wall motion scoring for stress echocardiography) still plays a dominant role in clinical practice. Eyeballing can be done fast, without much ado, and some experts reach an admirable accuracy. In general, however, it is inaccurate, irreproducible, subjective, and hard to learn.[1] Visual estimation of quantifiable measures should be discouraged for any purpose beyond a rough classification, whenever a quantitative alternative is present. Quantitative analysis is advisable when repetitive interpretations are done, when more subtle differences are sought, when interpretation experience is limited, and whenever scientific research is the goal.

The classic method of outlining the borders is manual drawing. Any ultrasonography machine or offline analysis system has facilities for this, using a mouse, trackball, or similar device. Manual drawing, however, is known to have high interobserver and intraobserver variability; it is strenuous and time consuming for the operator and requires expertise and dexterity. Concerning consistency and workload, manual drawing is especially hard to perform practically when large sets of images are involved—for example, analyzing one or more complete cardiac cycles, for several cross sections and over multiple stages (as in stress echocardiography) or analyzing the hundreds of 2D frames in a full-cycle 3D data set. In principle, ABD can provide solutions to these problems. Potentially, any measurement that requires manual drawing of borders or indication of landmark points may benefit from automated detection techniques. Moreover, if ABD could be performed online and in real time, it would open possibilities for real-time monitoring of parameters, such as LV area and volume.

Procedures, such as stress echocardiography, that currently rely on visual scoring of wall motion and comparison between different stages could benefit enormously from automated analysis; the lack of quantification and the large interobserver and intraobserver and interinstitution variabilities[2] are perceived as important limitations. The potential of real-time 3D echocardiography for volume estimation and regional wall motion quantification also depends largely on automated analysis. Some promising developments for these fields are described.

Digital Image Storage, Communication, and Compression

The basis of digital image processing and analysis is the availability of images in digital form. Digital image storage and related subjects are discussed in more detail in the chapters on the digital echocardiography laboratory; in this chapter, an overview of properties of importance for image processing is given. The generation of ultrasonographic images (ultrasound [US] physics, radiofrequency signal processing, and instrumentation) is beyond the scope of this chapter. Excellent descriptions on these subjects can be found in many handbooks.[3-6]

Digital Images

Digital images are bitmaps, large rectangular matrices of dots or pixels (picture elements) in which the brightness or color at each position is represented by a numeric (digital) value. Brightness level is also referred to as intensity or gray value. A cineloop or movie is a sequence of such images, typically at a frame rate of 20 to 200 images per second. A digital representation makes it possible to store and process images in a computer, hence, digital image processing. Inside the ultrasonography system, echocardiographic images are always created as digital images. For display on a video monitor and recording on VCR, these digital images are converted into an analog video signal. Nowadays, most ultrasonography machines are totally digitized and support the storage and communication of digital images and cineloops. Digital images do not degrade when copied, transmitted, or stored for longer periods. Digital images can be stored on digital media such as MOD, CD-R, or DVD, transported over networks, stored in large databases, and linked with any other patient information. The main drawback is still the large amount of data storage that is involved—a 2-hour VCR tape carries the equivalent of about 200 gigabytes of uncompressed color images. With image compression and selection, we can limit the storage requirements considerably.

Analog video, as is used in TVs and VCRs, consists of a continuously varying electrical signal (the video signal) that represents the brightness along horizontal lines in the image. Such a signal is subject to noise and degradation when it is transmitted or stored on a VCR tape. Frame rate and resolution are generally lower than for the original digital images.

For image processing and analysis, digital images are a prerequisite. If only analog video output or VCR tape is available, it is possible to redigitize the analog signal with the help of computer devices named frame grabbers or video digitizers. Note that this introduces unwanted image deterioration in the form of noise and jitter, loss of spatial and temporal detail, loss of separation between image, graphics, and color overlays and loss of additional information, such as calibration and patient information. Therefore, the use of analog video should be strongly discouraged for analysis purposes.

Storage Formats and Image Communication

Digital Imaging and Communications in Medicine

The current method of choice for digital image storage and exchange is Digital Imaging and Communications in Medicine (DICOM)[7]. DICOM is a generally accepted international standard for medical images. Originally developed for radiography, DICOM now encompasses extensions for most medical image modalities, including all types of US imaging. The DICOM standard (current version: 2006) is still being extended and improved to better support new developments in medical imaging. As its name implies, DICOM is a communication standard rather than a file format; it defines the way in which medical imaging devices, such as ultrasonography ma-

chines, picture archiving and communications systems (PACS) servers, and printers, communicate to transport, store, retrieve, find, or print images and associated patient information. All major manufacturers have committed themselves to support DICOM; eventually, this should allow easy networking in multivendor environments, workable PACS systems and easy and transparent offline viewing and analysis. Ultimately, this will lead to the digital integrated patient record, which contains the full patient file, including patient history, laboratory reports, images of all modalities, and other information. DICOM covers every detail of medical image handling for a multitude of imaging modalities and uses—all captured in substandards that are defined by subcommittees and working groups. Therefore, DICOM is a complicated standard: The full description covers several thousands of pages.[8] A readable explanation of DICOM for echocardiographers is given by Thomas.[9]

Note that the statement that devices are DICOM compliant is rather meaningless in itself; DICOM defines a multitude of services and imaging modalities. For each piece of equipment, a DICOM conformance statement defines precisely which services are supplied and supported for what modalities and to what extent. To verify interoperability between devices, the conformance statements should be compared—not a simple job for a novice in DICOM.[10]

Proprietary Formats

Several manufacturers also use their own proprietary formats for storage of digital image runs with associated patient and image information. Such formats include DSR[11] (Philips/Agilent/HP) and CLP (GE Vingmed). These digital formats may have certain advantages in a single-vendor environment, but they complicate exchange with other departments or hospitals, use of PACS, offline analysis systems, and so on.

General Purpose Formats

Other widely used general purpose image formats, such as BMP, TIF, GIF, and JPEG, are often used for export of screen shots or single images for use in reports, presentations, and papers. For movies, AVI, MPEG, and QuickTime are popular formats. These general purpose formats generally lack the possibility for storage of additional patient information and can lead to significant image quality degradation because of lossy compression. Therefore, they should not be used for primary image storage or archiving.

Image Compression

For reducing the data storage requirements, image compression can be employed. A distinction should be made between lossless and lossy image compression. For lossless compression techniques (such as run length encoding [RLE], lossless JPEG, or general purpose file compression, such as LZW [used in the ubiquitous ZIP or TAR file compression utilities]), reversing the compression will produce a perfect copy of the original image. Unfortunately, lossless compression generally only reduces file sizes by a factor of 2 to 5.

Lossy compression can reach much higher compression ratios (up to 20 to 100) at the cost of a certain amount of image degradation, generally by eliminating information for which the eye is least sensitive. This degradation may be acceptable visually (JPEG factor 20 has been found to produce only diagnostically nonsignificant degradation[12]), especially when compared with the degradation associated with VCR storage. However, the compression artifacts may certainly influence digital image processing and analysis. Severely lossy compression is not advisable for archiving or when digital image postprocessing is foreseen. Lossy compression techniques include Lossy JPEG, fractal and wavelet compression, and MPEG.

DICOM currently[8] supports RLE, JPEG (lossless and lossy), JPEG2000, and MPEG2 compression schemes.

Digital Image Processing

Digital image processing[13,14] is a science by itself and cannot be discussed here in great detail. Medical image processing is a thriving subdiscipline with many applications and innovations that have become valuable tools in the hands of the clinician. Several good handbooks on medical image processing, with special attention to ultrasonography, are available.[15,16]

Image Enhancement: Level Manipulations and Filtering

Image enhancement deals with the improvement of images, either for visual interpretation or as a preprocessing for analysis. Most of the techniques described here are available in any general purpose program for manipulating digital images (such as photo editors) and on most ultrasonography machines and offline analysis programs. Nowadays, the simpler manipulations are mostly applied in processing of 3D images.

The simplest class of operations is level manipulations: operations that change the brightness level (or color or transparency) of each pixel without considering any neighboring pixels. These operations are also known as lookup-table (LUT) operations because the original brightness of the pixel is simply used to look up the new value in a conversion table. Operations of this class include brightness level manipulations and pseudocoloring. In 3D visualization, such look-up table operations are the main tools to control the appearance of the volume rendering, in terms of brightness, transparency, and surface extraction.

Brightness Level Manipulations

This class includes all one-to-one conversions of image brightness levels (input) to display brightness levels (output), either linear or nonlinear. Examples are digital contrast and brightness adjustments, image inversion, gamma correction, and so on. Some examples are given in Figure 12–1. Note that many level manipulations may result in clipping (see Fig. 12–1C, D, and E) and in reduction of the effectively used number of brightness levels. The extreme example is thresholding (see Fig. 12–1E), in which all brightness levels above a threshold are set to white and all below to black.

Pseudocolors

Pseudocoloring involves a direct conversion of brightness levels to a color scale, generally labeled with fancy names such as Rainbow, Ocean, or Harvest. As the eye is more sensitive to color differences than to intensities, this may reveal subtle contrast differences. It can be visually pleasing, but it is highly suggestive because it clusters similar gray values into color groups. Because brightness levels in ultrasonography by themselves do not represent any physical property and are highly dependent on signal attenuation and local gain settings, the borders that are suggested visually by these colors have no practical significance.[17] This technique is also applied sometimes to highlight brightness values above some threshold with a color—for example, to visualize the arrival of contrast agents in perfusion imaging. Similar objections apply—this may be highly suggestive.

Filtering

Filtering is the generic name for image operations that consider pixels within their neighborhood and deal with the spatial or temporal aspects of the image. Filtering operations include smoothing (noise reduction), and sharpening (edge enhancement). Smoothing or low-pass filtering (e.g., uniform, Gaussian) is used in many ABD methods to reduce the speckle noise and get more or less homogeneous regions; high-pass edge enhancing or detection filters (e.g., Sobel, Laplacian) are often used to find (candidate) border points. Note that most smoothing methods slightly change the positions of edges and differentiate poorly between noise and weak signals. High-pass filters tend to be sensitive to noise. In general, filtering does not improve the appearance of ultrasonographic images without simultaneously removing valuable information. Smoothing

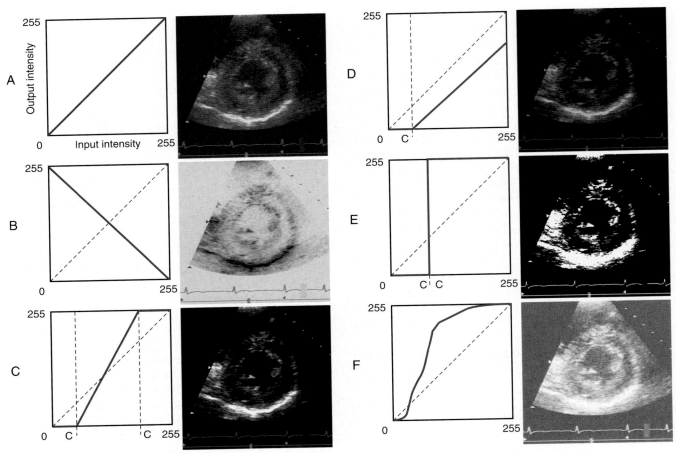

Figure 12–1. *Image brightness conversions and their results.* A, *Identity: no change;* B, *inversion;* C, *increased contrast (note clipping);* D, *decreased brightness;* E, *thresholding;* F, *histogram equalization.*

and sharpening filters may be available on your (3D) ultrasonography machine for real-time use: Keep the aforementioned caveats in mind when using this option.

Image Interpretation: The Interpretation Pyramid

The interpretation of highly complex information, like medical images, is an extremely complicated task. We humans tend to underestimate it considerably: For us, vision is a natural process that we perform instantly and automatically. From the study of human perception, we know that vision is anything but a simple, straightforward process. Think of the many well-known optical illusions: there is a lot of hidden interpretation going on. In the interpretation of images, a certain number of information abstraction levels can be distinguished. This is generally known as the image interpretation pyramid (Fig. 12–2). The levels of this pyramid give us more insight into the mechanisms of different automated techniques and their limitations. A good analogy is found in the interpretation of handwriting or spoken language. This analogy is described in Table 12–1. For interpretation of a written text, one has to know about the alphabet, spelling, vocabulary, syntax, semantics, the subject of the text, the intentions of the source, and adornments, such as humor, sarcasm, and metaphors. These last aspects concern real-world knowledge that has nothing to do with language—it refers to the domain that the text is discussing. In practice, this is not just a simple bottom-up process of combining letters into words into sentences into significance. Text can be fragmented; there are imperfections, such as misspellings and ambiguities, unknown words, and missing domain knowledge, that necessitate interactions and feedback between all levels, and even guessing, to come to a consistent interpretation.

Cardiac Image Interpretation

In image interpretation, we have a similar hierarchy. At the base, we find the raw image information (pixels). Going up, we encounter image features, such as local texture and gradients; structures, such as regions (groups of adjacent pixels with similar properties) and edges (lines of sudden change, between regions); objects, such as a square or a person; and a scene, such

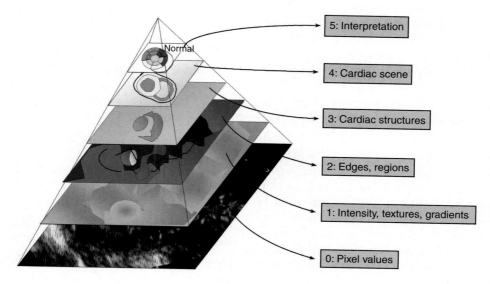

Figure 12-2. The image interpretation pyramid.

TABLE 12-1. **Abstraction Level Hierarchy**

Level	General	Speech	Image	Cardiac	Associated Operations
0	Raw data	Samples	Pixels	Pixels	Image generation
1	Features	Amplitude, frequency	Intensity, texture, gradients	Intensity, texture, gradients	Preprocessing, filtering, feature extraction
2	Structures	Phonemes	Edges, regions	Edges, regions	Linking, merging, matching, clustering
3	Objects	Words	World entities, borders, objects	Cardiac structures (lumen, endocardium valve)	Model relaxation, border finding, classification
4	Object sets	Sentences	Scene	Cardiac scene	Scene modeling, interobject relationships
5	Interpretation	Significance	Scene interpretation	Interpretation and diagnosis	High-level interpretation, expert systems, rules

as a football match. At the top we have significance, such as finding out who's winning; this requires specific knowledge on behavior of the players and audience, rules of the play, and so on.

Interpretation of medical images, especially of a complex, dynamic organ like the heart, is still more difficult because it requires expert knowledge about the 3D anatomic structures in the heart, their dynamic behavior, pathology and anatomic variability between patients, and the intricacies of the imaging modality involved. This last point specifically is not to be underestimated for ultrasonography.

Again, interpretation is not a simple bottom-up process. Missing or ambiguous information, disturbances, such as noise and artifacts, and higher-level knowledge of anatomy, physiology, and pathology, are involved and necessitate feedback and interactions between levels.

Clearly, different sorts of knowledge are applied at each level to come to a valid interpretation, and only the lower levels have to do with image properties; higher levels concern sizes and shapes of cardiac parts, anatomic models of the heart, physiology, congenital or pathologic conditions, and so on. ABD systems generally have limited knowledge at the higher interpretation levels and resolve this in one of three ways:

1. They use coarse, simplifying assumptions regarding the objects. For example, the left ventricle is a dark, round object in the middle of the image; the endocardial contour is convex; the endocardium is the strongest edge in the image; the cardiac wall will not move more than x pixels per frame. Most of such assumptions will hold only to some extent or are overly general.

2. They limit themselves to a subset of the problem domain, for aspects like cross sections (e.g., only short axis at mid-papillary level), image quality (no dropouts, low noise), anatomy (e.g., no congenital defects), or imaging equipment or settings (scale, gain, or frequency).

3. They require the user to handle the high-level aspects by initializing, guiding, or correcting the system.

One should make a distinction between ABD and automated tracking of borders and other structures. In detection, a structure is found in an image based on certain characteristics. In tracking, a structure that is indicated somehow in an image is followed over a series of images by finding the positions that best resemble the original. Such approaches can supply valuable temporal analyses and are often more reliable than pure detection approaches.

Rules for a Well-Behaved Automated Border-Detection Method

No practical system can do without the intervention of the user. Ideally, there is only one desired and necessary interaction: When multiple interpretations could be correct, the user should have the final decision. In practice, a computer system can never have all the high-level knowledge that the physician has, and it requires the physician's intervention to handle such blind spots. Systems with little high-level knowledge and models, however, rely heavily on the user to handle their shortcomings and mistakes. This improper use of the qualities of the expert user is mostly experienced as irritating.

With these limitations in mind, we can formulate a few criteria for a good and well-behaved ABD method.

1. The method should generate "correct" contours. Because this judgment may be subjective (in the light of multiple possible interpretations), a system should preferably be able to adapt to the expert user's general ideas about correct contours.

2. The contours should be reproducible; this seems obvious for an automatic system, but almost all systems require some type of user interaction (parameter choices, indicating a start point or region, corrections), which will lead to some variability in results. This interobserver and intraobserver difference should possibly be smaller than the interobserver and intraobserver variabilities associated with similar manual work.

3. The method should be user friendly; it should only address the user for high-level expert decisions, not for handling "stupid" mistakes or do repetitive corrections. Some implications are:

   - It should not generate physically or anatomically impossible solutions; unlikely solutions

should be marked as such. It should supply alternative solutions when relevant.

   - It should not override user-drawn contours (apart from clean-up of minor imperfections).

   - It should allow for easy, intelligent, minimized control and correction (e.g., by applying the intent of the correction throughout the whole image set).

Automated Border Detection in Echocardiography

Problems and Pitfalls of Border Detection in Ultrasonography

Ultrasonography is a particularly difficult imaging modality for interpretation. Inexperienced users mostly find it hard to interpret, at least harder than other tomographic modalities, such as computed tomography (CT) and magnetic resonance imaging (MRI). Ultrasonography exhibits several specific properties that impede automated analysis.

1. Pixel intensity does not directly reflect any physical property of the tissue visualized, in contrast to the Lambert-Beer law for radiography or the Hounsfield units for computed tomography. In ultrasonography, images are formed by sound reflection and scattering, resulting in a combination of interference patterns (US speckle patterns) and reflections at tissue transitions or inhomogeneities. Different tissues are often distinguishable only by subtle differences in texture (speckle patterns) or coherent behavior of texture over time rather than by different intensity values.

2. Ultrasonographic image information is anisotropic and position dependent. Reflection intensity, lateral and radial point spread functions, and signal-to-noise (S/N) ratio are dependent on both the depth and the angle of incidence of the US beam, and on the user-controlled time gain compensation (depth gain) settings.

3. Image disturbances (artifacts) are caused by side lobes, reverberations, clutter, and so on. Many of these problems are associated with high gain settings, which are often necessary in obese or older patients.

4. Parts of the anatomy are not imaged because of dropouts (for structures parallel to the US beam), shadowing (behind acoustically dense structures), scan sector limitations, and limited echocardiographic windows. Still-frame images generally miss some information; the human eye compensates for this when viewing a sequence

of images. It resolves ambiguities and interpolates the missing parts by exploiting the temporal coherence of structures and speckle, which allows discrimination between noise, artifacts, and anatomy.

5. The limited temporal resolution and the scanning process may introduce artifacts. The sequential scanning of lines combines information from different time moments into one image. For quickly moving structures, this may lead to spatial distortion. Sharp transitions between "older" and "newer" image parts may appear. This is particularly prominent in real-time 3D US, in which information from different heartbeats is stitched together to include a complete object (such as the left ventricle).

6. In two-dimensional ultrasonography, the exact spatial localization of the cross-sectional plane is generally not known. This in contrast to 3D techniques (3D US, magnetic resonance imaging or computed tomography), in which the 3D context is known and this information is often employed in model positioning for the detection. In 2D cardiac ultrasonography, the choice of the imaged cross section depends both on the skill and precision of the sonographer and on the available echocardiographic window, which is limited by ribs etc. Apart from volume measurement errors, this may also result in detection problems if the ABD method relies on assumptions of shape and the presence or absence of other structures, such as valves or papillary muscles.

Practical Considerations for Automated Border Detection

Practical considerations for appropriate border detection (either automatic or manual) are listed in Table 12–2, subdivided into three categories.

Acquisition and Image Quality

The primary requirement for automated analysis is optimal image quality. For ABD this is even more crucial than for manual tracing or visual analysis. If the border cannot be seen, an intelligent guess or interpolation is the only option (for computer *and* human). Therefore, one should take every precaution to optimize image quality, standardize system settings, and reduce variability in settings and cross sections.

Select a depth such that the object of interest is in focus, fits well inside the scan sector, and fills most of it. Try to adjust acoustic power, overall gain, and time gain control such that the endocardium is best and most homogeneously visualized. Remember that stop-

TABLE 12–2. Practical Considerations for Automated Border Detection

Acquisition and Image Quality
Optimize border visualization
Limit variation in system settings (gain, power, time gain control, lateral gain control)
Limit variation in cross sections (use landmarks)
Proper region of interest and depth
High frame rate
Digital storage (preferably lossless); no filtering
No spatial or temporal subsampling or small regions of interest for storage

Border Definitions and Consistency
Inventory of desired calculations
Standardize border drawing definitions:
   Inclusion or exclusion of papillary muscles, trabecular structures, valves, etc.
   Position of edges: leading, peak, trailing
Exclusion criteria and special cases
   Image quality: foreshortening, dropouts, artifacts, noise
   Pathologies: hypertrophy, dilation, cardiac masses, etc.
   Congenital deformations, etc.
Assess interobserver and intraobserver variabilities
   To test standardization
   To check errors against study goal, estimate patient population size for significance
   Include acquisition protocol?

Choice of Detection Technique
Check specifics of technique against problem:
   Views or cross sections
   Cardiac objects (left ventricle, right ventricle, endocardium, epicardium)
   Border definitions
   Single frame, ED/ES, full-cycle, multicycle
   Real time online or offline with corrections
   Dependence on image quality, artifacts, settings
   Amount and types of user interaction
Is manual analysis a practical alternative?

frame images are much harder to interpret than moving sequences; individual frames may be much less pleasing than the cineloop suggests.

A high frame-rate (at least 25 frames per second) is advisable, both for full-cycle analysis and for proper selection of end-diastolic (ED) and end-systolic (ES) frames in case of ED/ES analysis. For most tissue tracking or speckle tracking techniques, a higher frame rate (above 50) is advised because such techniques rely on local correlations between consecutive frames, which quickly become less reliable for lower frame rates.

For image storage, use digital images whenever possible—do not redigitize from videotape. Avoid lossy compression with high compression rates, image subsampling (resolution reduction), and temporal subsampling (frame rate reduction). When selecting a region of interest for storage, make sure that it will contain the object completely over the full time range.

Contour Definitions and Consistency

Before attempting manual or automated detection, make sure that proper criteria are defined for the desired contours. This may depend on the desired calculations to be performed from the contour. Trabecular structures, papillary muscles, or valves can either be included or excluded for certain calculations (LV volume, regional wall motion, LV mass). Many topics need to be standardized: whether leading, maximum, or trailing edges are drawn; what to do in case of foreshortening, dropout, and so on.[17,18] When possible, perform interobserver and intraobserver comparisons and try to reach consensus between observers before starting a large study. In some cases, this should include the image acquisition protocol, to assess interoperator and intraoperator variability in the choice of cross section, ultrasonographic system settings, and other factors.

Choice of Detection Technique

When considering an automated technique for border detection, it is wise to check the following against the specifications of the automated method: the imaging modes involved (M-mode, B-mode, 3D, harmonics, contrast etc); the views or cross sections involved, the object to be detected (e.g., left ventricle, right ventricle, atrium); the type of contour to be found (blood-tissue border or other, such as epicardium); single-frame, ED/ES, full-cycle or multicycle analysis; the brand and type of echocardiographic machine used, and online or offline availability of the detection; possibilities for user correction of the boundaries; dependency on system gain, image quality, and common artifacts, such as dropouts or noise; and amount of user interaction needed. In case no suitable automated technique is found for a certain analysis, manual measurements might provide the only practical alternative.

Overview of Automated Border-Detection Methods

Ever since the invention of echocardiography, methods have been devised for the automated analysis of these images. Literally hundreds of methods have been reported,[19,20] most of which have only academic value.[21] An excellent overview was recently published by Noble and Boukerroui.[19] I do not try to present a complete categorization here and limit the discussion to the main directions of research, based on the levels of the interpretation described previously. I will refrain from any comparisons on reported success scores, as there are no standard test data sets for this purpose or standard test criteria. Detected contours are generally compared with contours manually drawn by one or more experts or derived values, such as area or volume, are com-

pared with some alternative measurement. Most of these values are hard to compare between studies. One should note that good results on one or two cases can never be proof of a method's merit: No matter how naive the method, one can always find some images on which it will work. Robustness of a method can only be assessed by applying it on large sets of clinical-quality images. In general, one should distrust the practical value of methods that have been tested only on a few patients.

A listing of representative techniques is given in Table 12–3. For each level, the most basic technique is given first. This one is often applied by methods that focus on other levels. Not surprisingly, older techniques generally operate on a lower level. Of level five, few true examples currently exist. The terms *knowledge-based, intelligent,* and *model-driven* are widely misused, even for the most basic techniques at any level.

Feature-Based Method: Integrated Backscatter

A method for ABD that has gained much clinical attention in the past is acoustic quantification (AQ),[22] which is available on several Philips (formerly Hewlett-Packard, Agilent) ultrasonography machine models (Fig. 12–3). AQ is not an ABD system in the strict sense as described previously because it merely does a blood/border/tissue pixel classification by thresholding the integrated backscatter energy of the radiofrequency US signal. Therefore, it fits into the lower hierarchical levels of the image interpretation pyramid. A real-time plot of lumen area and its derivative over time can be generated and a real-time frame-to-frame monoplane volume calculation. Its use of the radiofrequency data, the online real-time applicability, and widespread availability make it a valuable tool. When used with care in images of good quality, it can

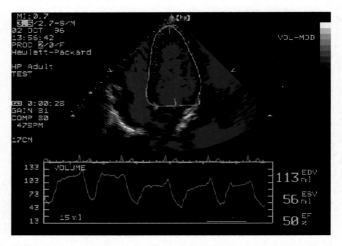

Figure 12–3. Acoustic quantification on Philips (Hewlett-Packard) equipment. (Courtesy Philips Medical Systems Ultrasound, Andover, Mass.)

TABLE 12–3. Overview of Automated Border-Detection Methods at Different Abstraction Levels

Level Name	Basic Technique(s)	Advanced Techniques
1. Preprocessing	Heavy smoothing for noise or speckle reduction[68] Contrast stretching Histogram equalization	Spatiotemporal smoothing[69] Morphologic filters[70] Texture filters: inverse difference moment,[71] wavelet transforms,[72] Fourier-based filters[73] Radiofrequency data processing: integrated backscatter (AQ)[22]
2. Edge or region detection	Global or local thresholding[69] Simple edge detectors such as difference-of-boxes[75, 76]	Advanced edge detectors: Marr-Hildreth,[77] Canny,[78–80] rank-based operator[81] Pattern or profile matching[56] Matched filters,[82] arc filters[74] Tracking: optical flow,[34-36] block similarity[37-39] Region detection: region growing,[73] fuzzy clustering, resolution pyramids, neural nets, Markov random fields[83]
3. Geometric objects or models	Implicit models: e.g., radial search for candidate points,[68] interpolation/linking, smoothing/shape filtering	Classification of edge points by fuzzy reasoning[77] Dynamic programming optimization[40,79,84,85] Simulated annealing,[80] self-organizing maps (SOM, Kohonen)[81] Snakes/balloons/active contours/deformable contours, etc.[53,75,78,79,86] Active shape models (ASM)[56,57]
4. Anatomic structure or scene models	None or implicit: Hard-coded Manually positioned User-drawn	Single geometrical shape models—2D, 2D+T, 3D, 3D+T Model positioning/landmark finding techniques: row/column sums,[76,77] arc filters,[74] template matching; Hough transform[80]; fuzzy logic[72] Shape parameters (2D+T)[20] 3D shape neural nets[87] Composite models (several objects and their relation, for example, ventricles and septum)—2D, 2D+T, 3D, 3D+T Point distribution models[57] Multiple active contours[78] Fuzzy neural nets (2D)[88]
5. Interpretation, high-level knowledge	None User intervention: correction of contours, etc.	Adaptation of models to image and user[20,61] Use of patient group derived models: neural nets,[70] SOM,[81] appearance eigenvariations (AAM)[54-62] Learning behavior over all cases analyzed Rule-based analysis Pathology awareness Multiple hypothesis generation

2D, two-dimensional; 3D, three-dimensional; AAM, active appearance models; AQ, acoustic quantification; ASM, active shape models; PDM, point distribution models; SOM, self organizing maps; T, time.

give useful results. However, AQ also suffers from some serious drawbacks,[23,24] which are typical for a low-level method, and can be summarized:

1. The AQ borders are sensitive to image quality (noise, dropouts) and gain settings (time gain control, lateral gain control) and often difficult to control for the user. Cardiac cycle-dependent intensity changes can influence area change calculations.[23]

2. It is mostly impossible to eliminate tissue parts within the ventricle (valve, papillary muscle, and trabecular structures) or to exclude dropout regions from the ventricle, and noise and artifacts may cause serious problems, especially in difficult patients. Reported success scores in larger patient populations vary widely.

3. The contours are irregular, which can be expected for a thresholding-type technique; this implies that they are not directly suitable for regional wall motion calculations. Postprocessing of the contours can supply such information,[25] but this disregards the image information and is generally inferior to techniques that fit a model directly to the image data.

Most of these problems are exemplary for a low-level method that does not use any geometric models or knowledge about cardiac anatomy. The use of harmonic imaging has been shown to improve AQ border delineation[26,27] but does not eliminate most of these problems.

A spin-off of AQ is known as color kinesis (CK)[28,29] (Fig. 12–4). This technique is in essence a method of

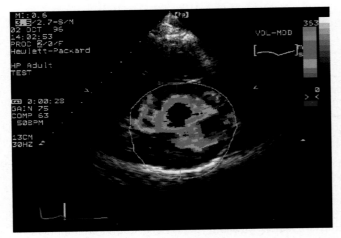

Figure 12–4. Color kinesis image on Philips (Hewlett-Packard) equipment. (Courtesy Philips Medical Systems Ultrasound, Andover, Mass.)

presenting the time sequence of AQ contours in a single image, by color-coding the consecutive displacements of the border. This method renders a rainbow-like band around the contour in which each color represents some time-offset from ED or ES. Provided there is little global heart translation, this can give a good impression of wall motion patterns in systole or diastole, especially when these motions are analyzed per region.[29,30] Of course, all limitations of AQ apply here as well, plus the concern of overall heart translation, making this technique also challenging to apply accurately.

AQ has been applied in clinical studies for many purposes, especially for looking at LV function (lumen area, volume, and fractional area change). Studies on right ventricular (RV) function have been reported as well.[31] CK has been used for studying wall motion patterns in several patient groups, systolic and diastolic function, regional wall motion in stress echocardiography, and other parameters.[29,32,33]

Structure-Based Method: Tissue Tracking

A good example of a structure-based method can be found among the different 2D tissue tracking methods. Such approaches track the motion of certain structures by finding correspondence between regions in consecutive images. Tracking is not a border detection approach as such because it tracks motion of tissue instead of finding a blood-tissue border, but it can be used for quite similar purposes. Most approaches rely on straightforward region similarity measures like normalized cross correlation or sum of absolute differences. An alternative approach, optical flow, was already proposed in an early stage for 2D tissue tracking[34] and recently has gained new interest.[35,36] In general, such tissue tracking techniques can provide motion information in the form of displacement of some set of points (generally along a user-drawn line) or calculate a complete 2D displacement vector field. By calculating time integrals, total relative deformation (strain) can be calculated as well in all directions. As a 2D approach, it can overcome the principal limitation of tissue Doppler imaging (TDI). TDI supplies a direct physical (Doppler) velocity measurement that can be performed with extreme temporal resolution, but it can only give a one-dimensional motion estimate (in the direction of the US beam). 2D speckle tracking may therefore supplement or be an alternative to TDI.[37]

As an example of a structure-based tracking method, the approach of Lysyansky, Friedman and colleagues[38,39] for 2D tissue tracking is described. This method forms the basis of the 2D speckle tracking software in the EchoPAC analysis system (GE-Vingmed Medical Systems, Horten, Norway) (Fig. 12–5).

The user loosely traces an approximate endocardial contour in one frame of a cycle. A band outside this contour is used as the region of interest. Within this region (Fig. 12–5A), the speckle structure is analyzed and speckles of high intensities are identified as natural targets (Fig. 12–5A and B). These targets are tracked

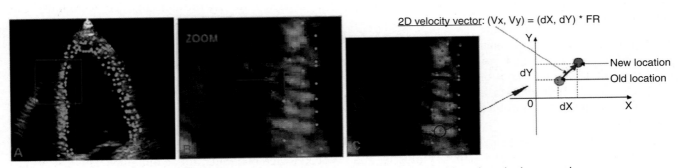

Figure 12–5. Two-dimensional strain imaging. A, In a region defined by a loosely drawn endocardial contour (red dots), natural acoustic markers are identified in the myocardium (green dots). B, Zoomed display of found acoustic markers (green dots: center of each marker). C, These markers are tracked from frame to frame and their displacements define two-dimensional velocity vectors. FR, frame rate. (From Leitman M, Lysyansky P, Sidenko S, et al: J Am Soc Echocardiogr 17:1021-1029, 2004.)

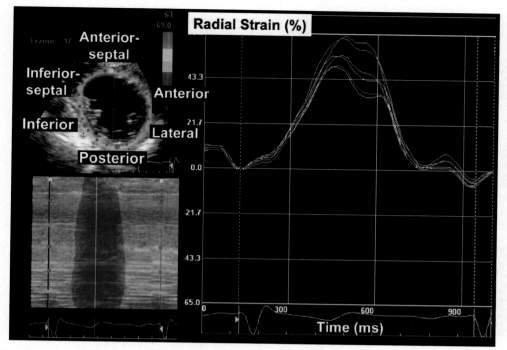

Figure 12-6. An example of radial time-strain curves in a normal control subject from the mid-ventricular short-axis view. Radial strain was calculated by speckle tracking from multiple circumferential points over a cardiac cycle. These data were averaged to six time-strain plots to represent standard segments. Note that time to peak strain in a normal subject occurs synchronously over a narrow time range. (From Suffoletto MS, Dohi K, Cannesson M, et al: Circulation 113:960-968, 2006.)

over consecutive frames (Fig. 12-5C) by block matching with a sum of absolute differences similarity criterion.[37,39] From the resulting velocity field, local displacement and strain are calculated (Fig. 12-6).

Similar speckle tracking approaches from other vendors are available. A prerequisite for successful application is a sufficiently high frame rate and good image quality.

Object-Based Method: Echo-CMS

Many techniques for model-based or object-based detection of borders exist; these are generally based on some deformable model (snake, balloon) in combination with an edge detector, a motion model, and an optimization strategy.

As an example of a clear-cut object-based (pattern and geometric model–based) ABD method, we describe the Echo-CMS system (developed by the Division of Image Processing, Radiology, Leiden University Medical Center). The system has been designed for practical use, with the main intent of quantifying endocardial frame-to-frame wall motion and lumen volume. For short-axis views, a straightforward edge-based dynamic programming border detection with a circular shape model is used; detected contours are propagated as models into following frames.[40] In the different long-axis views (apical four-chamber, two-chamber, and

parasternal long axis), a more sophisticated semiautomatic pattern-based approach is used.[20] For the analysis of one or more complete beats (Fig. 12-7A), one ED and ES contour must be manually drawn (see Fig. 12-7B). Next, three landmark points characterizing the position of the LV (apex and mitral valve attachment points, which are the end points of the contour) are extracted from the contours and interpolated or extrapolated linearly over the cycles. The user is required to inspect these markers over the cycles and may then redefine, if necessary, intermediate positions in which the true position deviates from the estimated position. Now, the automated contour detection is started. From the manually drawn ED and ES contours, models are extracted describing the geometrical shape of the ventricle over the cycle and the intensity profiles in a neighborhood of the drawn contours. All models (phase, pose, geometry, and edge profiles) are interpolated over the cycle and extrapolated over other cycles (see Fig. 12-7C, D, and E). The resulting geometry models are positioned over the images (Fig. 12-8A and B), which are resampled along straight lines perpendicular to the models. For each point of all scan lines (see Fig. 12-8C, left), a cost value is calculated representing the likelihood of this point as a contour point: Unlikely points will have high costs. The cost is calculated from a combination of edge detectors, match differences with the edge profile models, and local edge

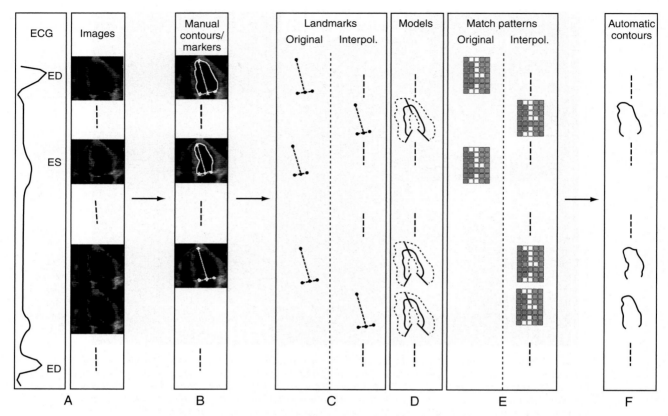

Figure 12–7. *Echo-CMS semiautomatic border detection procedure.* A, *Electrocardiogram (ECG) and original images;* B, *manual drawing of two contours and inspection of markers;* C, *generation of pose models (landmarks);* D, *generation of shape models;* E, *generation of profile models (match patterns);* F, *automatically detected contours. ED, end-diastole; ES, end-systole.*

reliability measures. Through this rectangular array of cost values (see Fig. 12–8C, *center*), an optimal connective path is determined using a dynamic programming approach. Cumulative costs for all connective paths are calculated, applying position-dependent penalties for deviation from a straight path. In this way, local stiffness of parts of the border is modeled. The path with overall lowest cost is selected as optimal (see Fig. 12–8C, *right*) and by inversion of the resampling process converted into a new contour (see Fig. 12–8D).

After detection of all contours (see Fig. 12–7F), the user may apply any corrections by overdrawing part of a contour. Consecutively, all models are updated with the extra user-defined information, which is interpolated and extrapolated over the sequence, followed by a redetection of all nonmanual contours.

In short, this method uses full-cycle models for the 2D pose, shape, and local stiffness properties of the wall and for the intensity profiles of the edges. Case-specific and user-specific information is incorporated by collecting information from all user-defined contours. Drawbacks are the need for two manually defined borders and the marker manipulations. This method has been applied in studies on wall motion patterns for cardiac resynchronization therapy by bi-

ventricular pacing[41,42] and regional wall motion quantification for myocardial viability,[43] stress echocardiography,[44] and for LV remodeling.[45] The system has some strong features, including tracking of structures other than blood-tissue borders (user-defined positions); temporal and spatial coherence; and basic knowledge of LV anatomy and appearance. For research purposes, it has been shown to be a valuable tool, but it is mainly focused on frame-to-frame or multibeat analyses of wall motion patterns. For ED/ES analyses, it offers no extra benefits because the ED/ES contours need to be defined manually.

Similar techniques are now available, such as the Axius Velocity Vector Imaging[46,47] approach commercialized by Siemens Medical Solutions (Malvern, Penn.). This technique, which appears to be based on the work of Pedrizzetti and Tonti[48] requires a user-drawn initial border and tracks the points of this border over one or more heart cycles. It applies a template matching by cross-correlation along lines perpendicular to the initial border and applies a one-dimensional path finding in the temporal direction for each point, by searching a maximum likelihood over its neighborhood in the following frames. Consecutively, it tracks the motion of all points along the direction of the bor-

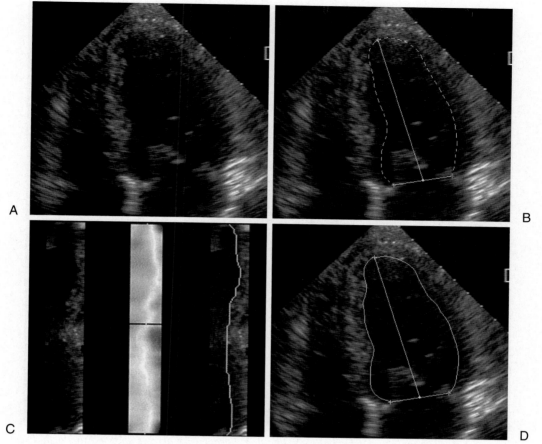

Figure 12–8. *Echo-CMS dynamic programming border detection. A, Original image; B, image with landmarks and shape model; C, scan value matrix (left), cost value matrix (middle), and detected path (right); D, image with detected contour.*

der (tangential) as well. Combining these perpendicular and tangential displacements supplies a 2D velocity vector in each point (Fig. 12–9, *left*). From the resulting borders, volumes are calculated, but also TDI-like velocity, strain, and strain rate (SR) plots are generated (see Fig. 12–9, *right*). Because this method makes only limited use of object models (mainly spatiotemporal continuity and temporal cyclic behavior), it could be placed between the structure-based and object-based method levels. The technique does not rely on speckle tracking or radiofrequency information and can be applied online or offline on B-mode images of most transducers and systems. Initial clinical validation shows promising results especially for cardiac resynchronization therapy.[46,47]

Three-Dimensional Models: Three-Dimensional Active Surface Detection

Recently, some practical methods for segmentation of four-dimensional (4D) (3D+ time) US images have emerged as well. The semiautomatic analysis tools, such as 4D-LV-Analysis (commercialized by TomTec Imaging Systems GmbH, Unterschleissheim, Germany),

are probably most widely used and have shown good results in comparison to MRI.[49-51] In our lab, a four-dimensional semiautomatic approach[52] was developed based on similar principles as the Echo-CMS described previously, which can derive a 4D segmentation with limited user interaction.

As an example, we will describe in this section the semiautomatic 4D detection as implemented in the Philips QLAB analysis package. This method is based on the active surface detection technique described by Gérard and colleagues.[53] A deformable surface is described as a two-simplex mesh; for each mesh vertex, the internal energy is determined by the local surface smoothness, and external energy by nearby image gradients combined with image intensity. The 3D mesh is initialized in the ED and ES 3D images by manually indicating five markers for mitral valve and apex in the two-chamber and four-chamber cross sections. A standard LV 3D shape is fit affinely to the manual points to define an initial mesh and the active surface optimization is started from there in a coarse-to-fine manner. First, rigid-body and affine transforms are applied, then local mesh deformations and mesh refinement.

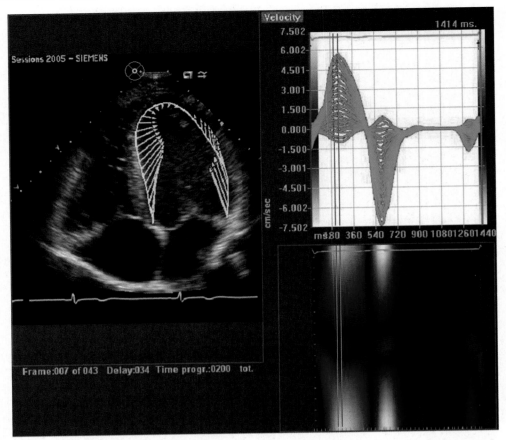

Figure 12–9. *Siemens Axius Velocity Vector Imaging. Border with arrows showing the local direction of border motion* (left). *Velocity for all points on border as function of time, and displayed as a tissue Doppler imaging–style color map* (right). *(Courtesy Siemens Medical Solutions, Malvern, Penn.)*

After ED and ES surfaces have been found, the detection can be extended over the full cycle. For all remaining phases, an initial mesh is generated by propagating the ED and ES shapes using a 4D statistical heart motion model. The active surface optimization is then applied in each 3D image separately (Fig. 12–10). The found shapes can be manually edited conveniently by 3D mesh dragging. A wide range of analytical parameters is derived from the 3D shapes, concerning global and regional volumes and wall motion indexes. It has been validated successfully against several other modalities.[51,53]

The method is fast and reasonably robust and supplies a practical tool for analysis of the 3D endocardial volume. One should note that as a result of the nature of the detection approach and its spatiotemporal smoothness constraints, the found surfaces and graphs are always relatively rounded and smooth. Furthermore, it may be hard to apply manual corrections because this disturbs the nice temporal continuity of shapes and graphs: Such corrections are not propagated over the temporal sequence.

Population Model–Based Method: Active Appearance Models

A relatively new class of techniques called active appearance models (AAMs) holds great promise. These techniques were originally developed by Cootes and colleagues[54,55] for facial recognition and medical image analysis, as an extension of the active shape model (ASM) approach.[56,57] AAMs have been applied to 2D and 3D magnetic resonance imaging[58,59] and echocardiography[59,60] with promising results. These techniques derive the typical shape and appearance of an echocardiogram from a large set of example images with expert-drawn contours. Principal component analysis (PCA) on a point-distribution model extracts the average organ shape and the principal variations (so-called *eigenvariations*) of shape. By warping all examples to the average shape, an average image (Fig. 12–11) and principal image variations (Fig. 12–12) can be found. By applying another PCA, simultaneous shape and intensity eigenvariations are modeled in an appearance model. Such an appearance model can synthetically generate "prob-

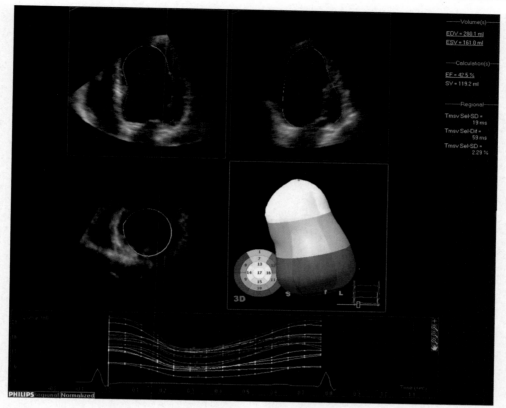

Figure 12-10. *Semiautomatic three-dimensional active surface border detection (Philips QLAB 3DQ advanced). (Courtesy Philips Medical Systems Ultrasound, Andover, Mass.)*

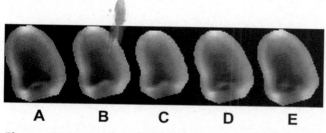

Figure 12-11. *Active appearance model: average four-chamber images of left ventricle from 65 patients, at different moments in the cardiac phase. A, End-diastole; B, mid-systole; C, end-systole; D, end of rapid filling; E, start of atrial filling.*

able" echocardiographic images similar to the variations shown in Figure 12-12. By deforming the model along the characteristic model eigenvariations, using a gradient descent minimization of the difference between the synthetic and the real image, the desired structure can be found (Fig. 12-13). This can be done fast and fully automatically with good results.

This technique has some significant advantages: It models both average organ shape and all variations over a population of examples; it models the complete organ appearance, including typical artifacts; it captures the expert's definition of proper border definition; it can model complex shapes (e.g., LV endocardium plus LV epicardium, right ventricle, valves); it is not limited to blood-tissue borders; and it is easily custom-izable for different types of images. Limitations of this technique are its dependence on the training data, the selected population of examples, and the quality of the expert contours.

A recent commercial application that employs a similar approach is the Axius Auto Ejection Fraction software (Auto EF) by Siemens Medical Solutions (Malvern, Penn.). Auto EF is based on the work of Comaniciu and others[61,62] It comprises a fully automated endocardial contour detection approach for the apical four-chamber and two-chamber cross sections, which employs a population-based statistical model of endocardial shape and appearance in end-diastole and end-systole. After a rough determination of the position of the ventricle, the appearance model matches to the image and finds the endocardial contour for the estimated ED and ES frames. Using a special robust information fusion approach, the contour is tracked over the complete sequence from both frames, merging the motion estimated from the images (by an optical flow approach) with a dynamics model. The PCA-based shape model is strongly adapted to the current patient, and the motion estimates and their varying confidence (Fig. 12-14) are combined with expected shape dynamics using a Kalman filter-based tracking. From the found contours, ED and ES volumes and ejection fraction are calculated, and a full-cycle volume curve. Initial clinical evaluations show promising results.[63]

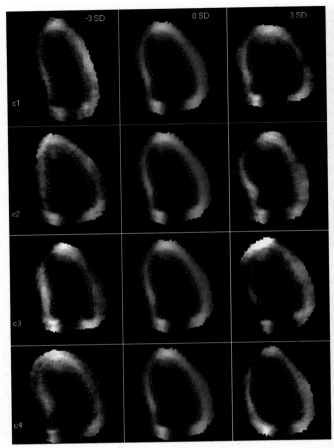

Figure 12–12. Active appearance model eigenvariations. Eigenvariations one to four (c1-c4) of four-chamber left ventricle at end-diastole (top to bottom). Average minus three standard deviations (−3SD), average (0 SD), average plus three standard deviations (3SD) (left to right). Note the simultaneous shape and intensity variations.

Future Promise

In recent years, several instrumental developments have had important beneficial effects on the feasibility of ABD, and the ABD methods themselves have improved considerably. Recently, several useful tools for ABD have become available commercially[39,46,49,53,62] and in the near future, further improvements in the applicability of ABD can be expected.

In the instrumental field, the complete digitization of the image formation and storage has improved image quality considerably. Front-end improvements, resulting in harmonic imaging, higher frame rates, and so on have also contributed considerably. The advent of real-time 3D imaging turned ultrasonography into a truly 3D modality and also has greatly boosted developments toward automated analysis. The continuous increase in computing power and the advent of novel algorithms have enabled such developments. In general, any further improvement in image quality is likely to enhance ABD as well.

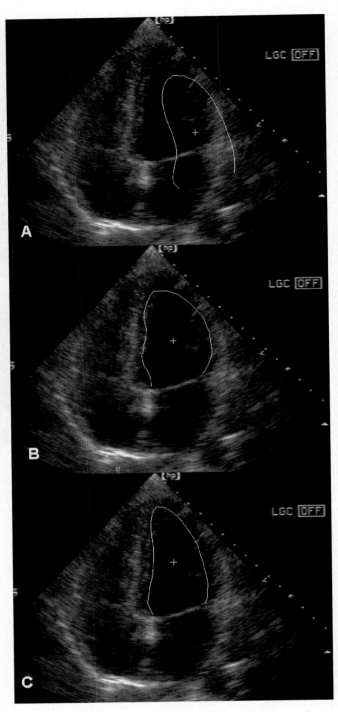

Figure 12–13. Active appearance model matching results on end-systolic left ventricular four-chamber image. A, Image with initial model; B, intermediate iteration; C, final matching result.

Contrast

One development that has not yet fulfilled its promises is the use of contrast. Ultrasonographic contrast agents can be used for luminal opacification to improve visualization of the endocardial border or for myocardial opacification. Contrary to what is often suggested,[64] contrast has not yet shown to directly enhance ABD.

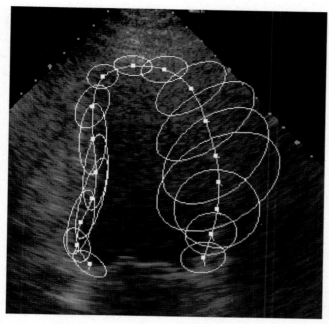

Figure 12–14. *Siemens Axius AutoEF detection process. Border point candidates with 95% confidence ellipses corresponding to the local measurement uncertainty. (From Comaniciu D, Zhou XS, Krishnan S: IEEE Trans Med Imaging 23[7]:849-860, 2004.)*

Although lumen opacification may boost the visual interpretation, application of contrast still has many pitfalls. The transient nature of the opacification, incomplete or inhomogeneous filling of the cavity, shadowing, and local destruction of microbubbles (causing swirling patterns of "white" and "black" blood), especially make it hard to model the lumen appearance for any detection method. Next-generation contrast agents or special-purpose border detection techniques may provide solutions.

Developments in Image Processing

Population Model–Based Techniques

As seen in the section on AAMs, this type of technique that holds considerable promise is currently entering the arena of commercial ABD applications.[62] These techniques can model the complete appearance of a cardiac echocardiographic scene, including patient variabilities. Because both shape variations over a large patient set and image appearance variations can be modeled, these techniques may handle typical artifacts, locally differing edge patterns, and other problems although restricting themselves to probable shapes. Furthermore, these models can be separated into patient-specific, view-specific, and pathology-specific parts,[65] allowing more precise and flexible models and opening views to automated classification.[66]

Intelligent Systems

At the interpretation level, the domain of artificial intelligence is entered. Work in this field, especially in conjunction with image interpretation, is still in its infancy.[67] Many high-level interpretation problems will need solutions from the field of artificial intelligence: formal reasoning from rule-based expert knowledge; generating multiple hypotheses with measures of confidence; reasoning with pathologic or congenital conditions during detection; checking overall consistency of an interpretation and taking action to resolve conflicts; opportunistically choosing an optimal detection strategy for the image data presented; and learning from operator corrections and actions. Ultimately, such developments should lead to an intelligent "automated image interpretation assistant" for echocardiographers.

KEY POINTS

- ABD is starting to play an important role in 2D and 3D clinical echocardiography and will allow more quantitative results.

- Optimal image quality and rigorous standardization of image acquisition and analysis is absolutely essential for reliable ABD.

- Digital image storage with lossless or no compression is highly recommended.

- Application of ABD in clinical research should be applied with care. The user should be aware of the possibilities and limitations of the technique, should be able to distinguish imaging and detection artifacts from pathology, and should remain critical about the outcome.

- Modeling of anatomical and pathological variability over patient groups plays an increasingly important role in ABD techniques.

- 2D tissue tracking approaches are gaining importance and will complement TDI applications and wall motion analysis by border detection.

- Instrumental hardware improvements, more elaborate 3D and 4D modeling and analysis techniques and artificial intelligence approaches have boosted, and will further improve, clinical feasibility of ABD.

REFERENCES

1. Foster E, Cahalan MK: The search for intelligent quantitation in echocardiography: "Eyeball," "trackball" and beyond. *J Am Coll Cardiol* 22:848-850, 1993.
2. Hoffman R, Lethen H, Marwick TH, et al: Analysis of interinstitutional observer agreement in interpretation of dobutamine stress echocardiograms. *J Am Coll Cardiol* 27:330-336, 1996.
3. Feigenbaum H, Armstrong WF, Ryan T: Physics and instrumentation. In: *Feigenbaum's echocardiography*, 6th ed. Philadelphia, Lippincott, 2005, pp. 11-45.

4. Geiser EA: Echocardiography: Physics and instrumentation. In Skorton DJ, Schelbert HR, Wolf GL, Brundage BH (eds): *Marcus Cardiac Imaging: A Companion to Braunwald's Heart Disease.* Philadelphia, WB Saunders, 1996, pp. 273-291.

5. Weyman AE: Physical principles of ultrasound. In Weyman AE (ed): *Principles and Practice of Echocardiography.* Philadelphia, Lea & Febiger, 1994, pp. 3-28.

6. Weyman AE: Cross-sectional scanning: Technical principles and instrumentation. In Weyman AE (ed): *Principles and Practice of Echocardiography.* Philadelphia, Lea & Febiger, 1994, pp. 29-55.

7. Kennedy TE, Nissen SE, Simon R, et al: Digital Cardiac Imaging in the 21st Century: A Primer. Bethesda, Md, American College of Cardiology, Cardiac and Vascular Information Working Group, 1997.

8. DICOM Standards Committee: Digital Imaging and Communications in Medicine (DICOM), 2006 ed. Rosslyn, VA, National Electrical Manufacturers Association, 2006.

9. Thomas JD: The DICOM image formatting standard: What it means for echocardiographers. *J Am Soc Echocardiogr* 8:319-327, 1995.

10. Waitz AS: An echocardiographer's guide to determining whether DICOM disk interchange can be achieved between two systems. In Kennedy TE, Nissen SE, Simon R, et al (eds): *Digital Cardiac Imaging in the 21st Century: A Primer.* Bethesda, Md, American College of Cardiology, Cardiac and Vascular Information Working Group, 1997, pp. 138-145.

11. Anonymous: Digital Storage and Retrieval (DSR) File Format Specification V 0.18 (Report Nr. 77450-99000). Andover, Mass, Agilent Technologies, Healthcare Solutions Group, Imaging Systems Division (ISY), 2000.

12. Karson TH, Chandra S, Morehead AJ, et al: JPEG compression of digital echocardiographic images: Impact on image quality. *J Am Soc Echocardiogr* 8:306-318, 1995.

13. Gonzalez RC, Woods RE: *Digital image processing*, 2nd ed. Englewood Cliffs, NJ, Prentice-Hall, 2002.

14. Sonka M, Hlavac V, Boyle R: *Image Processing, Analysis and Machine Vision*, 2nd ed. Pacific Grove, Calif, International Thomson-Brooks/Cole, 1999.

15. Skorton DJ, Schelbert HR, Wolf GL, Brundage BH: *Marcus Cardiac Imaging: A Companion to Braunwald's Heart Disease*, 2nd ed. Philadelphia, WB Saunders, 1996.

16. Sonka M, Fitzpatrick JM: *Handbook of Medical Imaging*, vol 2. *Medical Image Processing and Analysis*. Bellingham, Wash, SPIE-The International Society for Optical Engineering, 2000.

17. Vuille C, Weyman AE: Left ventricle I: General considerations, assessment of chamber size and function. In Weyman AE (ed): *Principles and Practice of Echocardiography.* Philadelphia, Lea & Febiger, 1994, pp. 575-624.

18. Nidorf SM, Weyman AE: Left ventricle II: Quantification of segmental dysfunction. In Weyman AE (ed): *Principles and Practice of Echocardiography.* Philadelphia, Lea & Febiger, 1994, pp. 625-655.

19. Noble JA, Boukerroui D: Ultrasound image segmentation: A survey. *IEEE Trans Med Imaging* 25:987-1010, 2006.

20. Bosch JG, van Burken G, Nijland F, Reiber JHC: Overview of automated quantitation techniques in 2D echocardiography. In Reiber JHC, van der Wall EE (eds): *What's New in Cardiovascular Imaging.* Dordrecht, The Netherlands, Kluwer, 1998, pp. 363-376.

21. Sheehan F, Wilson DC, Shavelle D, Geiser EA: Echocardiography. In Sonka M, Fitzpatrick JM (eds): *Handbook of Medical Imaging*, vol 2. *Medical Image Processing and Analysis*. Bellingham, WA, SPIE-The International Society for Optical Engineering, 2000, pp. 609-674.

22. Perez JE, Waggoner AD, Barzilai B, et al: On-line assessment of ventricular function by automatic boundary detection and ultrasonic backscatter imaging. *J Am Coll Cardiol* 19:313-320, 1992.

23. Marcus R, Bednarz J, Coulden R, et al: Ultrasonic backscatter system for automated on-line endocardial boundary detection: Evaluation by ultrafast computed tomography. *J Am Coll Cardiol* 22:839-847, 1993.

24. Bosch JG, Reiber JH, van Burken G, et al: Automated contour detection and acoustic quantification. *Eur Heart J* 16 (Suppl J):35-41, 1995.

25. Chandra S, Garcia MJ, Morehead AJ, et al: Spatiotemporal Fourier filtration of acoustic quantification endocardial border using carthesian vs. polar coordinate system. In Murray A (ed): *Proceedings, Computers in Cardiology*, Los Alamitos, Calif, IEEE Computer Society Press, 1994, pp. 17-20.

26. Spencer KT, Bednarz J, Rafter PG, et al: Use of harmonic imaging without echocardiographic contrast to improve two-dimensional image quality. *Am J Cardiol* 82:794-799, 1998.

27. Tsujita-Kuroda Y, Zhang G, Sumita Y, et al: Validity and reproducibility of echocardiographic measurement of left ventricular ejection fraction by Acoustic Quantification with Tissue Harmonic Imaging technique. *J Am Soc Echocardiogr* 13:300-305, 2000.

28. Lang RM, Vignon P, Weinert L, et al: Echocardiographic quantification of regional left ventricular wall motion with color kinesis. *Circulation* 93:1877-1885, 1996.

29. Koch R, Lang RM, Garcia MJ, et al: Objective evaluation of regional left ventricular wall motion during dobutamine stress echocardiographic studies using segmental analysis of color kinesis images. *J Am Coll Cardiol* 34:409-419, 1999.

30. Vignon P, MorAvi V, Weinert L, et al: Quantitative evaluation of global and regional left ventricular diastolic function with color kinesis. *Circulation* 97:1053-1061, 1998.

31. Helbing WA, Bosch HG, Maliepaard C, et al: On-line automated border detection for echocardiographic quantification of right ventricular size and function in children. *Pediatr Cardiol* 18:261, 1997.

32. Carey CF, Mor-Avi V, Koch R, et al: Effects of inotropic stimulation on segmental left ventricular relaxation quantified by color kinesis. *Am J Cardiol* 85:1476-1480, 2000.

33. Mor-Avi V, Spencer KT, Lang RM: Acoustic quantification today and its future horizons. *Echocardiography* 16:85-94, 1999.

34. Mailloux GE, Langlois F, Simard PY, Bertrand M: Restoration of the Velocity Field of the Heart from Two-Dimensional Echocardiograms. *IEEE Trans Med Imaging* 8:143-153, 1989.

35. Meunier J: Tissue motion assessment from 3D echographic speckle tracking. *Phys Med Biol* 43:1241-1254, 1998.

36. Sühling M, Arigovindan M, Jansen C, et al: Myocardial Motion Analysis from B-mode Echocardiograms. *IEEE Trans Im Processing* 14(4):525-536, 2005.

37. Suffoletto MS, Dohi K, Cannesson M, et al: Novel speckle-tracking radial strain from routine black-and-white echocardiographic images to quantify dyssynchrony and predict response to cardiac resynchronization therapy. *Circulation* 113:960-968, 2006.

38. Behar V, Adam D, Lysyansky P, Friedman Z: The combined effect of nonlinear filtration and window size on the accuracy of tissue displacement estimation using detected echo signals. *Ultrasonics* 41:743-753, 2004.

39. Leitman M, Lysyansky P, Sidenko S, et al: Two-dimensional strain: A novel software for real-time quantitative echocardiographic assessment of myocardial function. *J Am Soc Echocardiogr* 17:1021-1029, 2004.

40. Bosch JG, Savalle LH, van Burken G, Reiber JHC: Evaluation of a semiautomatic contour detection approach in sequences of short-axis two-dimensional echocardiographic images. *J Am Soc Echocardiogr* 8:810-821, 1995.

41. Auricchio A, Ghanem A, Groethus F, et al: Echocardiographic analysis of left ventricular contraction patterns in left bundle branch block and congestive heart failure (abstract). *J Card Fail* 5(Suppl 1):3, 1999.

42. Breithardt OA, Stellbrink C, Kramer AP, et al: Echocardiographic quantification of left ventricular asynchrony predicts an acute hemodynamic benefit of cardiac resynchronization therapy. *J Am Coll Cardiol* 40(3):536-545, 2002.

43. Nijland F, Kamp O, Verhorst PMJ, et al: Myocardial viability: impact on left ventricular dilatation after acute myocardial infarction. *Heart* 87(1):17-22, 2002.

44. Cain P, Short L, Baglin T, et al: Development of a fully quantitative approach to the interpretation of stress echocardiography using radial and longitudinal myocardial velocities. *J Am Soc Echocardiogr* 15(8):759-767, 2002.

45. Warda HM, Bax JJ, Bosch JG, et al: Effect of intracoronary aqueous oxygen on left ventricular remodeling after anterior wall ST-elevation acute myocardial infarction. *Am J Cardiol* 96(1):22-24, 2005.

46. Vannan MA, Pedrizzetti G, Li P, et al: Effect of cardiac resynchronization therapy on longitudinal and circumferential left ventricular mechanics by velocity vector imaging: description and initial clinical application of a novel method using high-frame rate b-mode echocardiographic images. *Echocardiography* 22(10):826-830, 2005.

47. Cannesson M, Tanabe M, Suffoletto MS, et al: Velocity vector imaging to quantify ventricular dyssynchrony and predict response to cardiac resynchronization therapy. *Am J Cardiol* 98(7):949-953, 2006.

48. Pedrizzetti G, Tonti G: Method of tracking position and velocity of objects' borders in two or three dimensional digital images, particularly in echographic images. US Patent 2005/0074153, April 2005.

49. Kühl HP, Schreckenberg M, Rulands D, et al: High-resolution transthoracic real-time three-dimensional echocardiography. Quantitation of cardiac volumes and function using semi-automatic border detection and comparison with cardiac magnetic resonance imaging. *J Am Coll Cardiol* 43:2083-2090, 2004.

50. Nikitin NP, Constantin C, Loh PH, et al: New generation 3-dimensional echocardiography for left ventricular volumetric and functional measurements: Comparison with cardiac magnetic resonance. *Eur J Echocardiogr* 7:365-372, 2006.

51. Jenkins C, Chan J, Hanekom L, Marwick TH: Accuracy and feasibility of online 3-dimensional echocardiography for measurement of left ventricular parameters. *J Am Soc Echocardiogr* 19:1119-1128, 2006.

52. van Stralen M, Bosch JG, Voormolen MM, et al: Left ventricular volume estimation in cardiac 3D ultrasound: a semi-automatic border detection approach. *Acad Radiol* 12:1241-1249, 2005.

53. Gérard O, Billon AC, Rouet JM, et al: Efficient model-based quantification of left ventricular function in 3-D echocardiography. *IEEE Trans Med Imaging* 21(9):1059-1068, 2002.

54. Cootes TF, Edwards GJ, Taylor CJ: Active Appearance Models. In *Proceedings, European Conference Computer Vision*. Berlin, Springer, 1998, pp. 484-498.

55. Cootes TF, Taylor CJ: Statistical models of appearance for medical image analysis and computer vision. *Proc. SPIE Medical Imaging 2001, Image Processing*, Vol 4322. Bellingham WA, SPIE, 2001, pp. 236-248.

56. Cootes TF, Hill A, Taylor CJ, Haslam J: Use of active shape models for locating structures in medical images. *Image Vision Computing* 12:355-366, 1994.

57. Parker AD, Hill A, Taylor CJ, et al: Application of point distribution models to the automated analysis of echocardiograms. In Murrary A (ed): *Proceedings, Computers in Cardiology*. Los Alamitos, Calif, IEEE Computer Society Press, 1994, pp. 25-28.

58. Mitchell SC, Lelieveldt BPF, van der Geest RJ, et al: Multistage hybrid active appearance model matching: Segmentation of left and right ventricles in cardiac MR images. *IEEE Trans Med Imaging* 20(5):415-423, 2001.

59. Mitchell SC, Bosch JG, Lelieveldt BPF, et al: 3-D active appearance models: segmentation of cardiac MR and ultrasound images. *IEEE Trans Med Imaging* 21(9):1167-1178, 2002.

60. Bosch JG, Mitchell SC, Lelieveldt BPF, et al: Automatic segmentation of echocardiographic sequences by active appearance motion models. *IEEE Trans Med Imaging* 21(11):1374-1383, 2002.

61. Comaniciu D, Zhou XS, Krishnan S: Robust real-time tracking of myocardial border: an information fusion approach. *IEEE Trans Med Imaging* 23(7):849-860, 2004.

62. Georgescu B, Zhou XS, Comaniciu D, Rao B: Real-time multi-model tracking of myocardium in echocardiography using robust information fusion. In Barillot C, Haynor DR, Hellier P (eds): *Medical Image Computing and Computer-Assisted Intervention—MICCAI 2004, Lecture Notes in Computer Science 3216*, Berlin, Springer, 2004, pp. 777-785.

63. Cannesson M, Suffoletto MS, Tanabe M, et al: A novel two-dimensional echocardiographic image analysis system using artificial intelligence shape and pattern recognition for rapid automated ejection fraction (abstract) *J Am Coll Cardiol* 47:251A, 2006.

64. Kamp O, Sieswerda GT, Visser CA: State-of-the-art: Stress echocardiography entering the next millennium. In Reiber JHC, van der Wall EE (eds): *What's New in Cardiovascular Imaging*. Dordrecht, The Netherlands, Kluwer, 1998, pp. 351-362.

65. Costen N, Cootes TF, Edwards GJ, Taylor CJ: Simultaneous extraction of functional face subspaces. In *Proceedings, IEEE Computer Vision & Pattern Recognition*. Los Alamitos, Calif, IEEE Computer Society Press, 1999, pp. 492-497.

66. Bosch JG, Nijland F, Mitchell SC, et al: Computer-aided diagnosis via model-based shape analysis: Automated classification of wall motion abnormalities in echocardiograms. *Acad Radiol* 12(3):358-367, 2005.

67. Bovenkamp EGP, Dijkstra J, Bosch JG, Reiber JHC: Multi-agent segmentation of IVUS images. *Pattern Recognition* 37(4):647-663, 2004.

68. Grube E, Mathers F, Backs B, Luederitz B: Automatische und halbautomatische Konturfindung des linken Ventrikels im zwei-dimensionalen Echokardiogramm: In-vitro Untersuchungen an formalinfixierten Schweineherzen. *Z Kardiol* 74:15-22, 1985.

69. Ezekiel A, Garcia EV, Areeda JS, Corday SR: Automatic and intelligent left ventricular contour detection from two-dimensional echocardiograms. In Ripley K (ed): *Proceedings, Computers in Cardiology*. Los Alamitos, Calif, IEEE Computer Society Press, 1985, pp. 261-264.

70. Klingler JW, Vaughan CL, Fraker TD, Andrews LT: Segmentation of echocardiographic images using mathematical morphology. *IEEE Trans Biomed Eng* 35:925-934, 1988.

71. Montilla G, Barrios V, Roux C, et al: Border detection in echocardiography images using texture analysis. In Murray A (ed): *Proceedings, Computers in Cardiology*. Los Alamitos, Calif, IEEE Computer Society Press, 1992, pp. 643-646.

72. Setarehdan SK, Soraghan JJ: Automatic left ventricular feature extraction and visualisation from echocardiographic images. In Murray A (ed): *Proceedings, Computers in Cardiology*. Los Alamitos, Calif, IEEE Computer Society Press, 1996, pp. 9-12.

73. Verlande M, Flachskampf FA, Schneider W, et al: 3D reconstruction of the beating left ventricle and mitral valve based on multiplanar TEE. In Murray A (ed): *Proceedings, Computers in Cardiology*. Los Alamitos, Calif, IEEE Computer Society Press, 1991, pp. 285-288.

74. Geiser EA, Wilson DC, Wang DX, et al: Autonomous epicardial and endocardial boundary detection in echocardiographic short-axis images. *J Am Soc Echocardiogr* 11:338-348, 1998.

75. Hozumi T, Yoshida K, Yoshioka H, et al: Echocardiographic estimation of left ventricular cavity area with a newly developed automated contour tracking method. *J Am Soc Echocardiogr* 10:822-829, 1997.

76. Monteiro AP, Marques de Sa JP, Abreu-Lima C: Automatic detection of echocardiographic LV-contours: A new image enhancement and sequential tracking method. In Ripley K (ed): *Proceedings, Computers in Cardiology*. Los Alamitos, Calif, IEEE Computer Society Press, 1988, pp. 453-456.

77. Feng J, Lin W-C, Chen C-T: Epicardial boundary detection using fuzzy reasoning. *IEEE Trans Med Imaging* 10:187-199, 1991.

78. Chalana V, Linker DT, Haynor DR, Kim Y: A multiple active contour model for cardiac boundary detection on echocardiographic sequences. *IEEE Trans Med Imaging* 15:290-298, 1996.

79. Dong L, Pelle G, Brun P, Unser M: Model-based boundary detection in echocardiography using dynamic programming technique. In *Proceedings, SPIE Medical Imaging V.* Bellingham, Wash, SPIE-The International Society for Optical Engineering, 1991, pp. 178-187.

80. Friedland N, Adam D: Echocardiographic myocardial edge detection using an optimization protocol. In Ripley K (ed): *Proceedings, Computers in Cardiology.* Los Alamitos, Calif, IEEE Computer Society Press, 1989, pp. 379-382.

81. Belohlavek M, Manduca A, Behrenbeck T, et al: Image analysis using modified self-organizing maps: Automated delineation of the left ventricular cavity in serial echocardiograms. In Hoehne KH, Kikinis R (eds): *Proceedings of the 4th International Conference on Visualisation in Biomedical Computing.* VBC '96, Berlin, Springer, 1996, p. 247-252.

82. Detmer PR, Bashein G, Martin RW: Matched filter identification of left-ventricular endocardial borders in transesophageal echocardiograms. *IEEE Trans Med Imaging* 9:396-404, 1990.

83. Herlin IL, Nguyen C, Graffigne C: Stochastic segmentation of ultrasound images. In *Proceedings of the 11th IAPR International Conference on Pattern Recognition A: Computer Vision and Applications.* Los Alamitos, Calif, IEEE Computer Society Press, 1992, pp. 289-292.

84. Dias JMB, Leitao JMN: Wall position and thickness estimation from sequences of echocardiographic images. *IEEE Trans Med Imaging* 15:25-38, 1996.

85. Gustavsson T, Molander S, Pascher R, et al: A model-based procedure for fully automated boundary detection and 3D reconstruction from 2D echocardiograms. In Murray A (ed): *Proceedings, Computers in Cardiology.* Los Alamitos, Calif, IEEE Computer Society Press, 1994, pp. 209-212.

86. Cohen LD: Note on active contour models and balloons. *CVGIP Image Understanding* 53:211-218, 1991.

87. Coppini G, Poli R, Valli G: Recovery of the 3-D shape of the left ventricle from echocardiographic images. *IEEE Trans Med Imaging* 14:301-317, 1995.

88. Brotherton T, Pollard T, Simpson P, DeMaria A: Echocardiogram structure and tissue classification using hierarchical fuzzy neural networks. In *Proceedings, IEEE Conference on Acoustics, Speech, and Signal Processing.* New York, Computer Society Press, 1994, pp. 573-576.

Part Three

Ischemic Heart Disease

The Role of Echocardiographic Evaluation in Patients Presenting with Acute Chest Pain in the Emergency Room

SARAH WEEKS, MD • KIRSTEN E. FLEISCHMANN, MD, MPH

Background and Principles

Coronary artery disease (CAD) accounted for 1.1 million hospital discharges in 2000,[1] and in the United States alone, several million patients present each year to the emergency department (ED) with a chief complaint of chest pain. The challenge for the clinician is to identify those patients with a serious cause of chest pain requiring intervention, particularly when acute coronary syndromes (ACSs) present with atypical symptoms, or diagnostic changes in the electrocardio-

TABLE 13-1. Goals of Echocardiography in Evaluation of Patients with Acute Chest Pain

Diagnosis of Acute Coronary Syndrome
Determination of coronary vascular territory involved
Assessment of the area of myocardium at risk
Evaluation of global ventricular function

Exclusion of Other Causes of Chest Pain
Aortic dissection
Pericarditis (with effusion)
Aortic stenosis
Hypertrophic cardiomyopathy

gram (ECG) or cardiac enzyme markers are lacking. Time is also of the essence when it comes to a patient with chest pain. Early treatment of myocardial injury and other serious diagnoses improves morbidity and mortality. Efficient diagnosis not only aids the patient but also reduces hospitalization time and costs.

The diagnosis of myocardial infarction (MI) is generally based on patient history, electrocardiographic findings, and cardiac enzyme levels.[2] Use of serum cardiac markers (Troponin, CKMB) has become central to the evaluation of chest pain and or dyspnea in the ED. Unfortunately, these markers often take hours from symptom onset to exceed the normal range and are not elevated in ACSs that are not associated with frank myocardial necrosis. Depending on the particular cardiac marker, enzyme levels can also be elevated in the absence of ACS, depending on renal function and underlying disease process. Electrocardiographic changes are frequently nonspecific.

Given these limitations, echocardiography can be a useful adjunct in assessing the patient with chest pain. The evaluation of left ventricular (LV) systolic function, diastolic function, and more recently, myocardial perfusion may aid in the diagnosis and triage of patients with chest pain. Echocardiography may also be useful in the diagnosis of other etiologies of chest pain, including: aortic dissection, aortic stenosis (AS), hypertrophic cardiomyopathy (HCM), and pericardial effusion (Table 13-1). This chapter will focus on the current application of echocardiography for early diagnosis of ACS.

Echocardiography and the Physiology of Acute Ischemia

Acute ischemia is associated with a number of biochemical and physiologic changes in myocardial tissue.[3] The ischemic cascade begins with biochemical changes causing subsequent abnormalities in diastolic dysfunction and then systolic dysfunction. These abnormalities may precede the development of symptoms, electrocardiographic changes or the increase in cardiac marker

levels.[4] The ability to detect myocardial ischemia earlier in the cascade of events has lead to an interest in the use of echocardiography in patients presenting with chest pain without a clear diagnosis of ACS.

Technical Aspects of Echocardiography in the Emergency Department

Image Acquisition

EDs are often loud and busy places, making the echocardiogram a more challenging examination than in the controlled environment of the echocardiographic lab. Transthoracic echocardiographic (TTE) examination of patients with chest pain should focus on the evaluation of biventricular function and the presence of regional wall motion abnormalities. The study should also serve to screen for nonischemic causes of cardiac chest pain, such as aortic stenosis, hypertrophic cardiomyopathy, pericardial effusion, and aortic dissection (although sensitivity for the latter diagnosis is limited and a negative TTE is not sufficient to rule out the diagnosis). The more recently developed use of myocardial contrast agents to identify areas with abnormal myocardial perfusion should also be considered.

The standard two-dimensional (2D) TTE views necessary for assessment of regional wall motion are the parasternal long-axis and short-axis views and the apical four-chamber, two-chamber, and three-chamber views (Fig. 13-1). If adequate image quality cannot be achieved from the parasternal or apical views, subcostal views can be extremely helpful. Off-axis or foreshortened views make the interpretation of regional wall motion abnormalities difficult and increase the likelihood of error.

The use of echocardiographic contrast agents can be invaluable in defining endocardial borders for wall motion analysis. Commercially available intravenous (IV) echocardiographic contrast agents contain gas-filled microbubbles, which are small enough to pass through the pulmonary circulation, resulting in opacification of the right and left ventricles. This results in enhancement of endocardial borders (Fig. 13-2).

A well-trained, experienced sonographer or echocardiographer is essential in the emergency setting. The sonographer should acquire necessary images in an efficient manner with attention to proper patient positioning, transducer selection, and technical settings. The technical settings may vary dependent on the patient characteristics, such as the use of lower-frequency settings in obese patients. Second harmonic imaging increases the signal-to-noise ratio resulting in clearer imaging. The use of echocardiographic contrast requires changes in technical settings for endocardial definition versus myocardial perfusion, particularly in mechanical index.

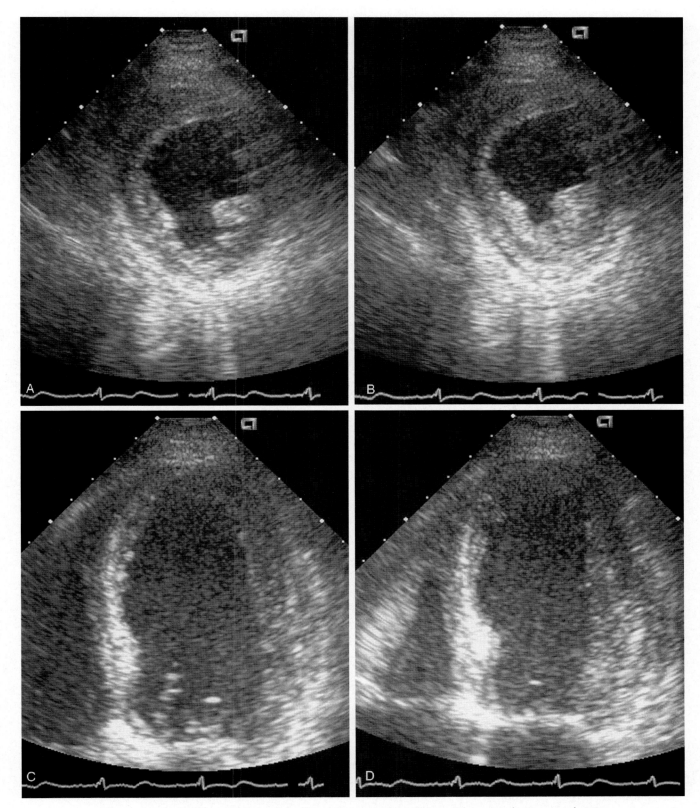

Figure 13–1. Still frames from the echocardiogram of a patient with acute chest pain, showing severe hypokinesis of the anterior, septal, and apical walls, in the parasternal short axis (A, diastole; B, systole) and the apical four chamber (C, diastole; D, systole).

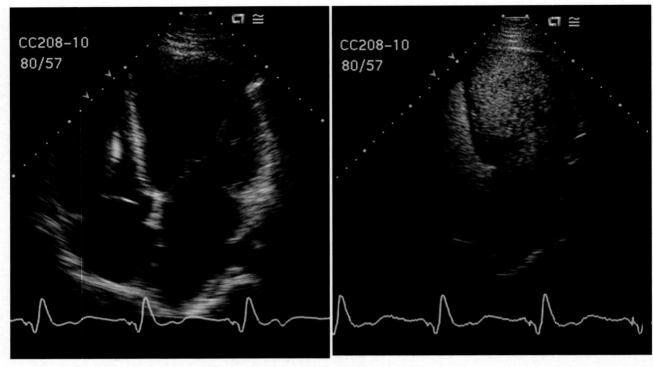

Figure 13-2. Improvement in left ventricular endocardial border delineation, particularly at the apex, with the use of intravenous echocardiographic contrast and second harmonic imaging (A, without contrast; B, with contrast).

The advancement of echocardiographic technology has substantially reduced the number of patients with inadequate echocardiographic images. In an early study by Horowitz and colleagues on the use of echocardiography in patients with acute chest pain, adequate images were obtained in 81% of patients.[5] A Danish multicenter study of 7001 patients after acute myocardial infarction (AMI) from the early 1990s reported assessable images in 93%. The use of intravenous echocardiographic contrast agents significantly increases endocardial border definition.[6] Hundley and colleagues compared volumetric assessment with contrast echocardiography with cardiac magnetic resonance imaging (MRI). The correlation for volumes and ejection fraction (EF) was greater than 92%.[7]

Stress Echocardiography

Echocardiographic imaging in conjunction with exercise or pharmacologic stress to assess for ischemia is safe and effective in patients presenting without myocardial infarction (MI) or unstable angina. Exercise stress can be performed using a standard treadmill protocol (i.e., Bruce) or a supine bicycle protocol. The advantage of bicycle protocols is the ability to image wall motion throughout exercise, as the patient exercises on an echocardiographic table that can be tilted into a left lateral position. The supine bicycle protocol increases the energy expenditure, typically in 30 Watt

increments every 3 minutes. This allows for image comparison at low, medium, and high workload. Additional Doppler information including pulmonary artery (PA) systolic pressure estimate, outflow tract, and valvular gradients can be obtained.

For a treadmill study patients are imaged at baseline and just after peak exercise only. For maximum sensitivity, it is essential that the echocardiographic imaging begin immediately after exercise terminates, before heart rate (HR) decreases significantly. This stress modality is primarily for assessment of global and regional systolic function.

For patients unable to exercise adequately, pharmacologic stress testing can be performed. Dobutamine is the agent most studied and therefore, most commonly utilized in North America. Baseline images are obtained, followed by the infusion of dobutamine at incremental levels (usually 5, 10, 20, 30, and 40 μg/kg/min) of 3 minutes duration. The test is terminated when the patient's HR reaches 85% of maximum predicted HR or develops evidence of myocardial ischemia, hypotension, significant arrhythmia, significant LV outflow tract obstruction, or drug-related side effects. Patients who do not reach target HR despite 40 μg/kg/min of dobutamine can perform handgrip maneuvers or be given intravenous atropine in doses of 0.1 to 0.25 mg up to a total of 1 mg, unless contraindications exist.

Endocardial definition is essential for reliable wall motion assessment. Images during stress decrease in quality due to cardiac movement and hyperventilation. The use of second harmonic imaging has increased the sensitivity for the diagnosis of CAD in patients with poor image quality from 64% to 92%. Specificity is unchanged with second harmonic imaging.[8] The use of echocardiographic contrast agents has also increased the sensitivity of stress echocardiography for the diagnosis of CAD. Rainbird and colleagues[9] analyzed 300 consecutive patients undergoing dobutamine stress echocardiogram (DSE). The percentage of wall segments visualized increased from 94.4% to 99.8% with the use of LV opacification during peak exercise ($p < 0.01$). There was no decrease in segment visualization from rest to peak exercise as was the case if an echocardiographic contrast agent was not used.

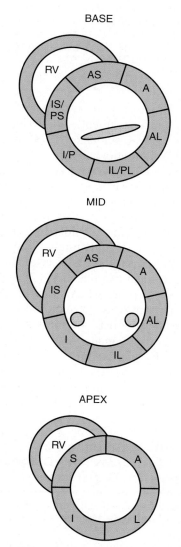

BASE

MID

APEX

Figure 13–3. A 16-segment model for evaluation of regional wall motion as recommended by the American Society of Echocardiography. A, anterior; AL, anterolateral; AS, anteroseptal; I, inferior; IL inferolateral; IS, inferoseptal; PL, posterolateral; PS, posteroseptal. (Adapted from Schiller NB, Shah PM, Crawford M, et al: J Am Soc Echocardiogr 2:358-367, 1989.)

Image Interpretation

Accurate interpretation of regional wall motion also requires an experienced echocardiographer. Wall thickening and systolic endocardial motion are evaluated for each LV segment, leading to its classification as hyperkinetic, normal, hypokinetic, akinetic, or dyskinetic.

The American Society of Echocardiography recommends a 16-segment model of regional wall motion evaluation[10] (Fig. 13–3). This model is consistent with the models used in nuclear and magnetic resonance imaging. Each segment is assigned a score based on visual assessment of contractility: normal, 1; hypokinesis, 2; akinesis, 3; dyskinesis, 4; and aneurysmal, 5. The wall motion score index (WMSI), a semi-quantitative measure of regional wall motion abnormality, is calculated by averaging wall motion scores for visualized segments. For example, a left ventricle with normal systolic function has a WMSI of 1, while a dysfunctional ventricle will have an increasing WMSI proportional to the severity. This score correlates with myocardial infarct size on clinicopathologic studies[11] and to perfusion defect size on single photon emission computed tomographic (SPECT) imaging.[12] A similar 14-segment wall motion index predicts long-term survival in patients with chest pain.[13]

Evaluation of stress-induced regional wall motion abnormalities is based on detailed comparison of rest and stress images; which is facilitated by simultaneous, synchronized display of images. The accuracy of digital images compared to videotape recorded images for the diagnosis of CAD is comparable, but interobserver and intraobserver agreement are improved with digital imaging.[14] Mohler and colleagues[15] prospectively compared digital images with videotape images in 117 patients presenting with chest pain. Overall agreement in regional wall motion assessment was 94%.

Recent refinements in tissue Doppler imaging (TDI) and the measurement of myocardial velocity allow for quantitative analysis of regional function.[16] Although not routine at present, as technology evolves, quantitative analysis will likely become part of the assessment of stress echocardiography.

Myocardial Contrast Echocardiography

Over the last decade, the concept of myocardial contrast echocardiography (MCE) has developed. This technique allows for the assessment of myocardial perfusion with the use of intravenous echocardiographic contrast agents and regional wall motion with endocardial border definition as described previously (see Chapter 3). Myocardial perfusion is assessed by the injection of microbubbles at the bedside, in real time, with rapid image acquisition. These microbubbles are delivered to small myocardial vessels with normal perfusion. Areas that are hypoperfused lack the echocardiographic enhancement generated by the contrast

APICAL FOUR CHAMBER

Rest   Stress   Stress

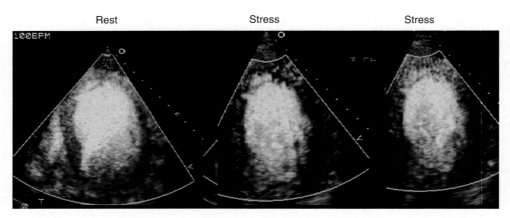

Figure 13–4. An example of a positive stress echocardiogram using intravenous echocardiographic contrast material for assessment of myocardial perfusion. At the far left, there is abnormal perfusion of the basal septum and basal lateral wall at rest (myocardium appears darker in this area). In the middle panel, there is an inducible perfusion defect of the mid to distal septum, and apex at stress (myocardium appears dark when compared to rest images). The far right panel shows partial reperfusion of the defect. (From Wei et al: Am J Cardiol 91:1293-1298, 2003.)

agent. The difference in areas with and without adequate perfusion is achieved by destruction of the bubbles at timely intervals, allowing for image acquisition as the areas of normal perfusion increase in signal intensity compared to areas with hypoperfusion. The destruction of bubbles occurs with the use of high-intensity pulses (mechanical index 1) synchronized to end-systole, while imaging occurs at a mechanical index of approximately 0.5 (Fig. 13–4).

The ability to analyze perfusion has added a new potential dimension to the echocardiographic assessment. Recent studies have demonstrated that MCE is comparable to SPECT for the detection of CAD in a high-risk population.[17] Patients scheduled for coronary angiography underwent intermediate triggered MCE and SPECT imaging at rest and after dipyridamole infusion. Seventy-eight percent of patients studied had confirmed stenosis of greater than 50%. There was no difference in the sensitivity of MCE compared with SPECT (91% versus 88%). Economic analysis has suggested a cost saving for the use of MCE over SPECT.[18]

Clinical Applications

Triage of Patients with Chest Pain

Several studies have assessed 2D TTE in evaluating patients with chest pain.[19-26] In the 1980s, Horowitz and colleagues[27] studied 80 patients with acute chest pain in the absence of prior MI, valvular heart disease, cardiomyopathy, or significant pericardial effusion. Echocardiograms were performed within 8 hours of admission and used a five-segment model for wall mo-

tion analysis. Nineteen percent of patients had inadequate images for assessment. Ninety-four percent of patients with clinical evidence of MI were found to have regional wall motion abnormalities. In comparison, the initial ECG was diagnostic of AMI in only 45%, and CKMB was elevated in 52%. This study was completed before the routine use of troponin as a cardiac marker. The specificity was 84%, as 27 out of 32 patients without clinical evidence of infarction had normal wall motion. Of note, none of the patients with normal wall motion on the initial echocardiogram had an in-hospital clinical complication (Table 13–2).

Subsequently, a prospective study of 180 consecutive patients presenting with symptoms suggestive of myocardial ischemia was performed.[28] Echocardiograms were technically inadequate in 6% of patients. A 12-segment model was used for assessment of regional systolic function. Of the 30 patients with confirmed MI, 27 had regional wall motion abnormalities (sensitivity 90%). In comparison, the initial ECG had a sensitivity

TABLE 13–2. Alternate Imaging Techniques for Chest Pain Diagnosis in the Emergency Department

Dissection: Transesophageal echocardiography, computed tomography angiography, magnetic resonance angiography, aortogram
Coronary artery disease: computed tomography angiography, nuclear perfusion imaging, left-sided heart catheterization
Pericarditis/Myocarditis: cardiac magentic resonance imaging
Pulmonary embolus: ventilation-perfusion scan, computed tomography angiography, pulmonary angiography

of 30%. All patients that suffered from in-hospital complications had regional wall motion abnormalities on the initial echocardiogram, as compared with only 31% having ST elevation on initial ECG.

Patients with a clear current of injury pattern on ECG generally benefit from prompt reperfusion therapy. However, in patients with chest pain, but without clear cut ECG or cardiac marker abnormalities on presentation, additional triage is often helpful. Sabia and colleagues[28] proposed in the early 1990s that these patients undergo 2D echocardiography. Those patients with technically adequate examinations and without regional wall motion abnormalities could be safely discharged. Applying this strategy to a group of study patients would have reduced hospital admissions by 32%, hospital stay by 23%, and cost by 24%. Using this approach, two patients with small MIs, without complications, would have been sent home. Using conventional strategies, two patients with large MIs were sent home, one of whom suffered a serious complication. The authors concluded that 2D echocardiography was superior to conventional criteria at that time in the diagnosis and risk assessment of patients presenting with suspected MI. Importantly, however, this strategy has not been validated in an external cohort of patients.

Myocardial Contrast Echocardiography

A recent prospective study by Kang and colleagues[29] enrolled 114 consecutive patients presenting to the ED with chest pain on exertion or at rest. Patients with ST elevation or Q waves on ECG were excluded. Echocardiography and MCE were performed to evaluate regional wall motion and myocardial perfusion. The sensitivity and specificity of a myocardial perfusion defect for the diagnosis of AMI were 93% and 63%, respectively. For the diagnosis of unstable angina the sensitivity was 59% with a specificity of 96%. The authors concluded that the use of MCE to predict clinically confirmed ACS was more sensitive than the use of ECG, cardiac troponins, or echocardiographic assessment of regional wall motion abnormalities alone.

MCE has been compared to the use of the Thrombolysis In Myocardial Infarction (TIMI) risk score for risk stratification of patients presenting with chest pain.[30] Over 900 patients with suspected cardiac chest pain and a nondiagnostic ECG underwent MCE for perfusion and regional wall motion. A modified TIMI risk score (without cardiac markers) was calculated immediately on arrival. This score was unable to differentiate between patients at intermediate and those at high risk. However, only 2 out of 523 patients with normal regional function had a primary event. In patients with abnormal regional function, myocardial perfusion was able to differentiate patients between intermediate and high-risk groups (see Fig. 13–4).

Use of Echocardiography in Chest Pain Units and Clinical Algorithms

Chest pain centers specializing in evaluation of patients presenting with acute chest pain have become increasingly popular.[31] Use of clinical algorithms has been evaluated by clinical outcomes. For example, Gibler and colleagues developed a "Heart ER Program"; a diagnostic and treatment program for patients with chest pain in an urban tertiary care ED.[32] Over 1000 patients with symptoms suggestive of ACS were enrolled over 32 months. Patients with known CAD, acute ST segment shift, hemodynamic instability, or clinical presentation consistent with unstable angina were admitted directly. Remaining patients underwent a 9-hour observation period during which cardiac markers (CKMB) were evaluated on arrival and every 3 hours thereafter for a total of three measurements. Patients had continuous ST segment monitoring. 2D echocardiography and graded exercise testing were performed on all patients at the end of the 9-hour observation period. The results determined the disposition of the patient. The vast majority of patients were discharged from the ED (82.1%), whereas only 15% were admitted for further evaluation. Of patients admitted, 34% were found to have a cardiac etiology for their symptoms (Tables 13–3 and 13–4).

DSE has also been studied in a clinical algorithm for chest pain assessment in the ED.[33] Patients with normal ECG and cardiac markers underwent rest 2D echocardiograms. If the rest images were normal, a dobutamine stress protocol was used with a trained nurse and sonographer. The test was completed in an average time of 5.4 hours from presentation. Using clinical follow-up and cardiac catheterization data for comparison, the protocol was found to have a sensitivity of 89.5%, a specificity of 88.9%, and a negative predictive value of 98.5%.

More recently, a group in Italy evaluated 6723 patients in the ED presenting with chest pain and a nondiagnostic ECG.[34] Patients were triaged using a clinical chest pain score, and those at low risk were discharged home. Patients with intermediate scores were admitted to an observational unit. If ECG and cardiac markers remained nondiagnostic over 6 hours, patients underwent further evaluation with either scintigraphy, exer-

TABLE 13–3. Essential Features of a Successful Chest Pain Unit

Telemetry capabilities
Timely serial cardiac marker measurements and electrocardiogram testing
Access to timely investigations such as treadmill testing, echocardiography, computed tomography, nuclear imaging, and angiography
Bed availability to hold majority of patients 6–12 hours

TABLE 13–4. A Sampling of Clinical Studies for Use of Echocardiography in the Assessment of Chest Pain

Year	Authors	Sample Size	Population	Result
1984	Nishimura and colleagues[19]	61	Patients within 12 hours of an AMI	Increased wall motion score index was predictive of in-hospital complications
1990	Peels and colleagues[20]	43	Acute chest pain with nondiagnostic ECG and no history of CAD	88% sensitive 78% specific for diagnosis of ischemia when compared to angiography
1991	Sabia and colleagues[21]	171	Patients presenting with cardiac symptoms	LV systolic dysfunction predicts both short-term and long-term cardiac events
1994	Fleischmann and colleagues[24]	513	Patients presenting with chest pain	Moderate LV systolic dysfunction and significant valvular regurgitation independently predict survival
1997	Trippi and colleagues[22]	163	Patients presenting with chest pain, normal markers and nondiagnostic ECG	Dobutamine stress echo has a NPV of 98.5% for coronary artery ischemia
2005	Kang[29]	114	Patients presenting with chest pain at rest	Myocardial perfusion defect on contrast echocardiography was associated with an odds ratio of 21 for the diagnosis of AMI
2005	Tong[30]	957	Patients with chest pain and nondiagnostic ECG	Contrast echocardiography provides short-term and long-term prognostic information prior to results of cardiac markers

AMI, acute myocardial infarction; CAD, coronary artery disease; ECG, electrocardiogram; LV, left ventricular; NPV, negative predictive value.

cise treadmill testing, or dobutamine echocardiography. In general, older patients or those with multiple risk factors or nondiagnostic ECGs had SPECT imaging, younger patients and those with more than two risk factors and normal ECGs underwent exercise treadmill testing (ETT) and those unable to exercise or with uncertain or nondiagnostic ETT or SPECT results had DSEs. Although the multiple types of testing performed make interpretation of their results more difficult, this protocol enabled them to make the early diagnosis of CAD in 22% of their chest pain unit patients, with early discharge in 78%.

A subsequent manuscript reported on approximately 500 patients with recent chest pain, but without ischemic ECG changes or definite evidence of CAD after a 6-hour work-up including troponin levels. Patients unable to exercise, or with left bundle-branch block or poor echocardiographic windows were excluded. Patients had exercise echocardiography and exercise methoxyisobutyl isonitrile (MIBI) radionuclide imaging within 24 hours and patients with abnormal troponin levels at any time or positive stress tests were recommended for angiography. Endpoints for the study were a greater than 50% stenosis on catheterization or cardiovascular events at 6 months. The exercise echocardiogram was positive in 20% of the cohort, the exercise MIBI in 24%. Fourteen patients with negative exercise echocardiograms were ultimately diagnosed with CAD versus 13 patients with negative exercise MIBI. The sensitivity of exercise echo and exercise MIBI for the ultimate diagnosis of CAD in this study was similar (85% versus 86%), while the specificity of exercise echocardiogram was slightly higher (95% versus 90%), leading to a higher likelihood ratio for a positive exercise echocardiogram test.[35]

Cost-Effectiveness

Cost-effectiveness data for echocardiography in patients presenting to the ED with acute chest pain are scarce. More general cost-effectiveness analyses of diagnostic strategies for patients with chest pain have found the preferred initial strategy to be noninvasive testing for patients with low to intermediate pretest probability of CAD, and coronary angiography for those with high pretest probability. For example, in one study,[36] the incremental cost of exercise echocardiography compared with exercise electrocardiography in 55-year old men with atypical angina was $41,900 per quality-adjusted life-year (QALY), a range generally considered cost-effective in comparison to other accepted interventions. In comparison, exercise SPECT cost $54,800 per QALY as compared with exercise electrocardiography for these patients. However, in higher risk patients, such as 55-year-old men with typical angina, the incremental cost-effectiveness ratio of routine coronary angiography compared with exercise echocardiography was only $36,400 per QALY saved, making angiography an attractive strategy from a cost-effectiveness standpoint. The incremental cost-effectiveness ratio of exercise electrocardiography compared with no testing was $57,700 per QALY saved for 55-year-old men with nonspecific chest pain. The authors concluded that exercise electrocardiography or exercise echocardiography resulted in reasonable cost-effectiveness ratios for patients at mild to moderate risk for CAD.

Assessment of the Need for Urgent Coronary Angiography

Coronary angiography is still generally regarded as the gold standard test for diagnosing obstructive epicardial CAD. Patients with a nondiagnostic ECG and a high pretest probability of CAD often proceed directly to angiography and possible percutaneous coronary intervention (PCI). This technique leads to prompt diagnosis, however in most cases, does not yield information about the functional significance of stenoses found. Functionality of lesions can be assessed in the catheterization suite with the use of pressure or flow wires, but this is often time consuming and costly. Echocardiographic findings may assist in the decision regarding the need for urgent coronary angiography. Normal global and regional function could lead to a more conservative approach, with later stress imaging to rule out significant coronary stenosis. Conversely, the finding of a new wall motion abnormality may prompt more urgent coronary angiography.

MCE for perfusion assessment may also be beneficial in the decision for need and timing of coronary angiography. Angiographic flow does not necessitate the presence of tissue perfusion. Recently, several studies have evaluated the use of contrast echocardiography to assess microvascular reperfusion after AMI. A study by Greaves and colleagues[37] performed contrast echocardiography in 15 patients postprimary PCI for AMI. Analysis showed that a perfused hypokinetic or akinetic segment was 50 times more likely to recover function than a nonperfused segment. MCE predicted segmental myocardial recovery with a sensitivity of 88%, a specificity of 74%, and positive and negative predictive values of 83% and 81%, respectively. MCE outperformed other known modalities, such as TIMI frame rate, myocardial blush grade and percentage of ST segment resolution.

Color and pulsed Doppler TTE was performed to evaluate distal left anterior descending coronary artery (LAD) reperfusion in 56 consecutive patients with a first anterior AMI before coronary intervention.[38] Patients with a peak velocity of less than 21 cm/s had a sensitivity, specificity, and accuracy of 82%, 93%, and 91%, respectively. If confirmed in larger series, this would potentially enable noninvasive evaluation of distal LAD reperfusion in the acute phase of anterior myocardial infarction before mechanical intervention.

Risk Stratification and Analysis of Long-Term Clinical Outcome

A number of studies have demonstrated incremental utility of echocardiography, beyond clinical assessment and electrocardiography in predicting clinical outcomes of patients with acute chest pain.[39-40] In a prospective study of patients visiting a large urban ED, Fleischmann and colleagues[39] identified echocardiographic predictors of serious predischarge complications (significant recurrent myocardial ischemia, heart failure, and arrhythmia) in patients with chest pain. Doppler echocardiograms, an average of 21 hours after presentation, assessed biventricular, regional and valvular function. In univariate analysis, LV function (OR 2.9), right ventricular function (OR 2.7), LV end diastolic dimension (OR 1.6), LV end systolic dimension (OR 1.4), and wall motion index (OR 3.0) predicted complications. Wall motion index was an independent predictor of complications beyond clinical and electrocardiographic variables.

The long-term survival of 448 patients in this study was examined.[13] Over a follow-up period of 35.0 + 12.1 months, independent predictors of survival were: moderate or severe LV dysfunction and more than mild valvular regurgitation. These echocardiographic findings offered incremental prognostic value over clinical and ECG findings in patients presenting with acute chest pain. Kaplan-Meier survival curves stratified by LV function and the grade of mitral regurgitation (MR) in this study are shown in Figure 13–5 and Figure 13–6, respectively.

DSE has been shown to predict subsequent cardiac events in patients with known or suspected CAD.[41] A cohort of 860 patients was assessed using the 16-segment model for wall motion and followed for 52 months. The independent predictors of cardiac events were: history of congestive heart failure (HR 2.51), percentage of abnormal segments at peak

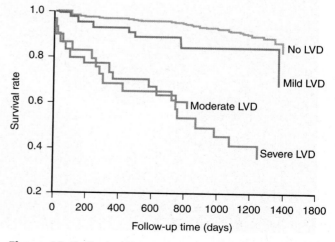

Figure 13–5. Kaplan-Meier survival curves for patients presenting with chest pain stratified by left ventricular dysfunction (LVD). (From Fleischmann KE, Lee RT, Come PC, et al: Am J Cardiol 80:1266-1272, 1997. From Excerpta Medica Inc.)

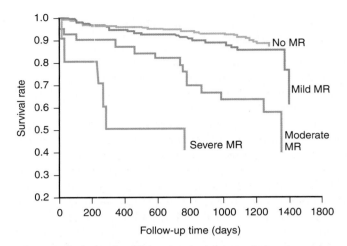

Figure 13–6. *Kaplan-Meier survival curves for patients presenting with chest pain stratified by grade of mitral regurgitation (MR) (on a 4+ scale). (From Fleischmann KE, Lee RT, Come PC, et al: Am J Cardiol 80:1266-1272, 1997. From Excerpta Medica Inc.)*

stress (HR 1.23), and abnormal LV end-systolic volume response to stress (HR 1.98).

Evaluation of Other Causes of Chest Pain

Although the assessment of global and regional ventricular function is the core of the echocardiogram for the patient presenting with chest pain, it is essential to provide also a rapid screen for other nonischemic causes of chest pain.

Aortic dissection is a life-threatening diagnosis that may be detected on TTE, although sensitivity is limited. An intimal flap may be identified in the aortic root, proximal ascending aorta, and arch or descending abdominal aorta (Fig. 13–7). It is important to note that the sensitivity of transthoracic imaging for aortic dissection is only 79%; compared to 99% for transesophageal echocardiograms (TEE).[42] Therefore, a negative TTE is not sufficient to exclude the diagnosis if clinical suspicion exists. Other potential clues to aortic dissection would include aortic regurgitation, a dilated proximal aorta, and the presence of a pericardial effusion.

Effusive pericarditis can be diagnosed on TTEs. The subcostal window is especially useful in patients with limited apical and parasternal image quality. The potential hemodynamic consequences of a pericardial effusion may be evaluated by scanning for signs of right atrial collapse, right ventricular collapse, exaggerated respiratory variation in tricuspid and/or mitral valve inflow velocities, and inferior vena cava size and respiratory variation. The use of echocardiographic guidance for pericardiocentesis has been shown to enhance the safety of the procedure.[43]

Screening for aortic stenosis involves 2D imaging for calcification and restricted movement and Doppler measurement of transvalvular gradients. Similarly, signs of hypertrophic obstructive cardiomyopathy include hypertrophy (asymmetric), the presence of systolic anterior motion of the anterior mitral valve leaflet, and Doppler evidence of a dynamic gradient in the LV outflow tract.

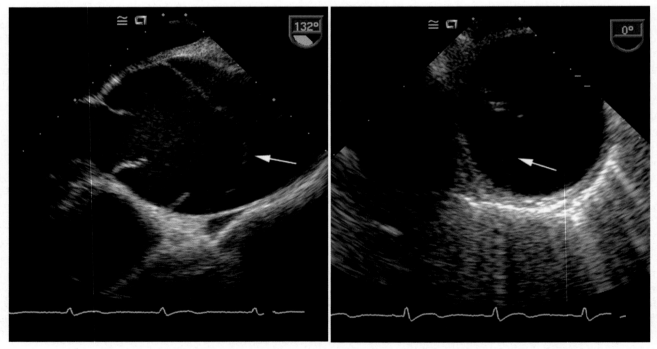

Figure 13–7. *Transesophageal images of a Type A aortic dissection involving the aortic arch. A, Three-chamber close-up view of the aortic valve and proximal ascending aorta revealing a dissection flap. B, A short-axis view of the aortic arch with the presence of the dissection flap.*

Limitations

Ischemia Evaluation

Echocardiographic evaluation of patients with suspected ACS has several limitations. Between episodes of cardiac ischemia, the patient's wall motion may be completely normal, so, normal LV systolic function in a pain free patient cannot rule out cardiac ischemia as the cause of the patient's symptoms. In addition, small areas of ischemic myocardium, particularly in the subendocardium, may not result in a discernible wall motion abnormality, leading to false negatives. Stress testing should be considered after infarction is ruled out. Emerging strategies using MCE to evaluate perfusion may help stratify these patients.

The presence of preexisting LV dysfunction makes the evaluation of new regional wall motion abnormalities more difficult and may lower specificity of this technique.

Image Quality

Detection of regional wall motion abnormalities requires adequate visualization of endocardial borders, which may be difficult in patients with morbid obesity, chest wall deformity, chest trauma, or recent thoracic surgery. The use of second harmonic imaging with echocardiographic contrast administration may improve endocardial border delineation in such patients and make echocardiographic evaluation in the ED more feasible.

Personnel Availability

Ready availability of skilled sonographers and echocardiographers is essential to expanding the use of echocardiography in the evaluation of patients with chest pain in the ED. Both are generally available during usual working hours in most hospitals. However, it may not be economically practical to have personnel on site 24 hours a day for most community hospitals or even tertiary medical centers. Contacting "on-call" sonographers and echocardiographers outside the hospital is inevitably associated with delays in the management of such patients. The national shortage of sonographers complicates the situation further.[44]

One approach to this problem is to train ED personnel to perform echocardiograms, but successful implementation of this approach has been hampered by difficulty in gaining and maintaining sufficient experience in performing echocardiographic studies in the context of the rotating shift system in most EDs.

Digital tele-echocardiography systems, which allow transmission of digital images over a high-speed network to an experienced echocardiographer outside the hospital for immediate evaluation, may aid in ensuring adequate image interpretation. In future, greater real-time interaction between the off-site interpreting physician and the on-site sonographer may be possible, helping to ensure complete acquisition of all required images.

Future Developments

Tele-Echocardiography

Electronic transmission of images has been used successfully in a variety of telemedicine projects. Successful use in nonemergent settings has been reported in the difficult diagnostic cases, such as patients with congenital heart disease requiring special expertise.[45-47] Trippi and colleagues[22] used DSE in the ED to determine which patients presenting with chest pain could be safely discharged. In this study, echocardiograms were digitized into a quad-screen systolic eight-frame cineloop format (resolution 320 by 240 pixels), transmitted to the interpreting physician over the standard telephone line using a proprietary "lossless" format predating current digital imaging and communications in medicine (DICOM) standards.[48,49]

Technologic developments since that time, including higher memory capacity and faster microprocessors and network connections via the Internet or dedicated lines, may result in more widespread use. Of course, transmission of patient-specific data also will require proper encryption and adequate safeguards to ensure patient privacy.

Tissue Doppler Imaging

Tissue Doppler imaging (TDI),[50-52] color kinesis (CK),[53,54] and vector analysis are areas of promise (Fig. 13–8). Currently used for research purposes, these techniques have potential to aid in evaluation of regional wall motion.

Summary

TTE can provide useful information in the diagnosis and triage of patients presenting with acute chest pain. Depending on the situation, stress echocardiography or transesophageal echocardiography may provide additional information. The echocardiogram elicits information about global function, regional function, valvular function, and pericardial effusion. This not only helps to triage patients with suspected ACS but also can provide information on both short- and long-term outcomes. Newer techniques utilizing echocardiographic contrast agents for left ventricular opacification and myocardial perfusion have further enhanced the bedside echocardiographic assessment of patients with chest pain.

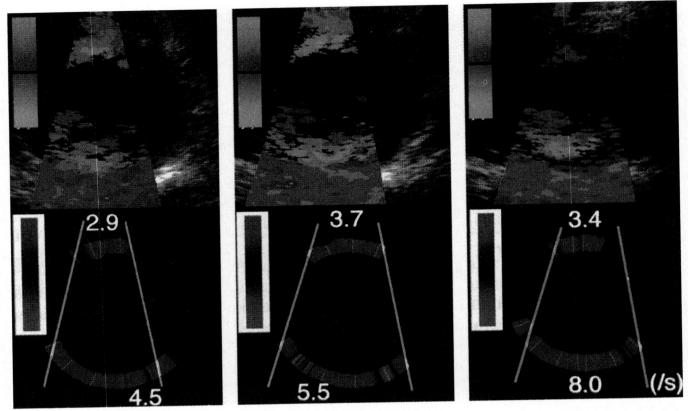

Figure 13–8. Tissue Doppler imaging (TDI) (top) and myocardial velocity gradient (MVG) (bottom) *images of the left ventricle in the parasternal short-axis view from a patient with left anterior descending coronary artery obstruction; at baseline (left), with low dose (10 µg/kg/min) dobutamine (middle), and high dose (30 µg/kg/min) dobutamine (right). In the tissue Doppler imaging (TDI) images, the anteroseptal wall is color-coded blue because it is moving away from the transducer during systole. Similarly, the posterior wall is color-coded red because it is moving toward the transducer. The MVG is derived from TDI, and it is defined as the slope of the regression line of the intramyocardial velocity profile across the myocardium. It reflects regional wall thickening and has been shown to be independent of the translational motion of the heart. In the MVG images, thickening of the myocardium is color-coded red, and thinning of the myocardium is color-coded blue. Calculated segmental MVGs are shown beside the corresponding segments. In this patient, MVG undergoes a dose-responsive increase in the posterior segment and no significant change in the anteroseptal segment supplied by the diseased coronary artery. (From Tsutsui H, Uemastu M, Shimizu H, et al: J Am Coll Cardiol 31:89-93, 1998. From American College of Cardiology.)*

KEY POINTS

■ Acute chest pain results in millions of ED visits annually. Early diagnosis improves patient outcomes and reduces hospital costs.

■ Echocardiography can help screen for the presence of myocardial ischemia with the assessment of wall motion. Wall motion abnormalities occur prior to the onset of symptoms or ECG changes in the ischemic cascade.

■ The presence of aortic valve disease, LV or right ventricular dysfunction, elevated pulmonary pressures, or pericardial effusion could all be valuable in diagnosis of the patient with chest pain.

■ Myocardial contrast agents are now commonly used not only for LV opacification and better endocardial definition but also for perfusion assessment. MCE has a sensitivity of greater than 90% for the presence of AMI.

■ Stress echocardiography is a safe and cost-effective way to assess for the presence of significant CAD.

■ Treadmill stress echocardiograms require rapid acquisition of images after peak exercise to maintain sensitivity.

■ Bicycle echocardiography can assess for evidence of inducible ischemia, as well as the effect of exercise on valvular disease, shunt, or pulmonary artery pressure.

■ DSEs have been utilized for the assessment of chest pain in patients with normal cardiac markers and normal ECG. The negative predictive valve has been shown to be greater than 98%.

■ For patients at intermediate risk of CAD, stress echocardiography has been shown to be cost-effective over routine treadmill testing or SPECT imaging.

■ Echocardiograms performed early in the evaluation of patients with chest pain are prognostic for in-hospital complications as well as long-term prognosis.

REFERENCES

1. Hall MJ, Owens MF: 2000 National Hospital Discharge Survey, *Advanced Data* 329:1-18, 2002.
2. Alpert JS, Thygesen KA, Antman E, Bassand JP: Myocardial infarction redefined—a consensus document of The Joint European Society of Cardiology/American College of Cardiology Committee for the redefinition of myocardial infarction. *J Am Coll Cardiol* 36:959-969, 2000.
3. Tennant R, Wiggers CJ: The effect of coronary artery occlusion on myocardial contraction. *Am J Physiol* 112:351-361, 1935.
4. Hauser AM, Gangadharan V, Ramos RG, et al: Sequence of mechanical, electrocardiographic and clinical effects of repeated coronary artery occlusion in human beings: Echocardiographic observations during coronary angioplasty. *J Am Coll Cardiol* 5:193-197, 1985.
5. Horowitz RS, Morganroth J, Parrotto C, et al: Immediate diagnosis of acute myocardial infarction by two-dimensional echocardiography. *Circulation* 65:323-329, 1982.
6. Senior R, Andersson O, Caidahl K, et al: Enhanced left ventricular endocardial border delineation with an intravenous injection of Sonovue, a new echocardiographic contrast agent: A European multicenter study. *Echocardiography* 17:705-711, 2000.
7. Hundley WG, Kizibash AM, Afridi I, et al: Administration of an intravenous perfluorocarbon contrast agent improves echocardiographic determination of left ventricular volumes and ejection fraction: Comparison with cine magnetic resonance imaging. *J Am Coll Cardiol* 32:1426-1432, 1998.
8. Franke A, Hoffman R, Keuhl HP, et al: Non-contrast second harmonic imaging improves interobserver agreement and accuracy of dobutamine stress echocardiography in patients with impaired image quality. *Heart* 83:133-140, 2000.
9. Rainbird AJ, Mulvagh SL, Oh JK, et al: Contrast dobutamine stress echocardiography: clinical practice assessment in 300 consecutive patients. *J Am Soc Echocardiogr* 14:378-385, 2001.
10. Schiller NB, Shah PM, Crawford M, et al: Recommendations for the quantification of the left ventricle by two-dimensional echocardiography. American Society of Echocardiography Committee on Standards, Subcommittee on Quantification of Two-Dimensional Echocardiograms. *J Am Soc Echocardiogr* 2:358-367, 1989.
11. Shen WK, Khandheria BK, Edwards WD, et al: Value and limitations of two-dimensional echocardiography in predicting myocardial infarct size. *Am J Cardiol* 68:1143-1149, 1991.
12. Oh JK, Gibbons RJ, Christian TF, et al: Correlation of regional wall motion abnormalities detected by two-dimensional echocardiography with perfusion defect determined by technetium 99 m sestamibi imaging in patients treated with reperfusion therapy during acute myocardial infarction. *Am Heart J* 131:32-37, 1996.
13. Fleischmann KE, Lee RT, Come PC, et al: Impact of valvular regurgitation and ventricular dysfunction on long term survival in patients with chest pain. *Am J Cardiol* 80:1266-1272, 1997.
14. Takeuchi M, Sonoda S, Miura Y, et al: Reproducibility of dobutamine digital stress echocardiography. *J Am Soc Echocardiogr* 10:344-351, 1997.
15. Mohler ER, Ryan T, Segar DS, et al: Comparison of digital with videotape echocardiography in patients with chest pain in the emergency department. *J Am Soc Echocardiogr* 9:501-507, 1996.
16. Malder CF, Payne N, Wilkenshoff U, et al: Non-invasive diagnosis of coronary artery disease by quantitative stress echocardiography. *Eur Heart J* 24:1584-1594, 2003.
17. Jeetley P, Hickman M, Kamp O, et al: Myocardial contrast echocardiography for the detection of coronary artery stenosis. *J Am Coll Cardiol* 47:141-145, 2006.
18. Tardif JC, Dore A, Chan KL, et al: Economic impact of contrast stress echocardiography on the diagnosis and initial treatment of patients with suspected coronary artery disease. *J Am Soc Echocardiogr* 15:1335-1345, 2002.
19. Nishimura RA, Tajik AJ, Shub C, et al: Role of two-dimensional echocardiography in the prediction of in-hospital complications after acute myocardial infarction. *J Am Coll Cardiol* 4:1080-1087, 1984.
20. Peels CH, Visser CA, Kupper AJ, et al: Usefulness of two-dimensional echocardiography for immediate detection of myocardial ischemia in the emergency room. *Am J Cardiol* 65:687-691, 1990.
21. Sabia P, Abbott RD, Afrookteh A, et al: Importance of two-dimensional echocardiographic assessment of left ventricular systolic function in patients presenting to the emergency room with cardiac-related symptoms. *Circulation* 84:1615-1624, 1991.
22. Trippi JA, Lee KS, Kopp G, et al: Dobutamine stress tele-echocardiography for evaluation of emergency department patients with chest pain. *J Am Coll Cardiol* 30:627-632, 1997.
23. Colon PJ 3rd, Guarisco JS, Murgo J, et al: Utility of stress echocardiography in the triage of patients with atypical chest pain from the emergency department. *Am J Cardiol* 82:1282-1284, A10, 1998.
24. Fleischmann KE, Goldman L, Robiolio PA, et al: Echocardiographic correlates of survival in patients with chest pain. *J Am Coll Cardiol* 23:1390-1396, 1994.
25. Fleischmann KE, Lee RT, Come PC, et al: Clinical and echocardiographic correlates of health status in patients with acute chest pain. *J Gen Intern Med* 12:751-756, 1997.
26. Saeian K, Rhyne TL, Sagar KB: Ultrasonic tissue characterization for diagnosis of acute myocardial infarction in the coronary care unit. *Am J Cardiol* 74:1211-1215, 1994.
27. Horowitz RS, Morganroth J, Parrotto C, et al: Immediate diagnosis of acute myocardial infarction by two-dimensional echocardiography. *Circulation* 65:323-329, 1982.
28. Sabia P, Afrookteh A, Touchstone DA, et al: Value of regional wall motion abnormality in the emergency room diagnosis of acute myocardial infarction: A prospective study using two-dimensional echocardiography. *Circulation* 84:I85-I92, 1991.
29. Kang D, Kang S, Song J, et al: Efficacy of myocardial contrast echocardiography in the diagnosis and risk stratification of acute coronary syndrome. *Am J Cardiol* 96:1498-1502, 2005.
30. Tong KL, Kaul S, Wang XQ, et al: Myocardial contrast echocardiography versus Thrombolysis In Myocardial Infarction score in patients presenting to the emergency department with chest pain and a nondiagnostic electrocardiogram. *J Am Coll Cardiol* 46:920-927, 2005.
31. Storrow AB, Gibler WB: Chest pain centers: Diagnosis of acute coronary syndromes. *Ann Emerg Med* 35:449-461, 2000.
32. Gibler WB, Runyon JP, Levy RC, et al: A rapid diagnostic and treatment center for patients with chest pain in the emergency department. *Ann Emerg Med* 25:1-8, 1995.
33. Savonitto S, Ardissino D, Granger CB, et al: Prognostic value of the admission electrocardiogram in acute coronary syndromes. *JAMA* 281:707-713, 1999.
34. Conti A, Paladini B, Magazzini S, et al: Chest pain unit management of patients at low and not low-risk for coronary artery disease in the emergency department. A 5-year experience in the Florence area. *Eur J Emerg Med* 9:31-36, 2002.
35. Conti A, Sammicheli L, Gallini C, et al: Assessment of patients with low-risk chest pain in the emergency department: Head-to-head comparison of exercise stress echocardiography and exercise myocardial SPECT. *Am Heart J* 149:894-901, 2005.
36. Kuntz KM, Fleischmann KE, Hunink MG, et al: Cost-effectiveness of diagnostic strategies for patients with chest pain. *Ann Intern Med* 130:709-718, 1999.
37. Greaves K, Dixon SR, Fejka M, et al: Myocardial contrast echocardiography is superior to other known modalities for assessing myocardial reperfusion after acute myocardial infarction. *Heart* 89:139-144, 2003.
38. Lee S, Otsuji Y, Minagoes S, et al: Correlation between distal left anterior descending artery flow velocity by transthoracic Doppler

echocardiography and corrected TIMI frame count before mechanical reperfusion in patients with anterior acute myocardial infarction. *Circ J* 69:1022-1028, 2005.

39. Fleischmann KE, Lee TH, Come PC, et al: Echocardiographic prediction of complications in patients with chest pain. *Am J Cardiol* 79:292-298, 1997.

40. Kontos MC, Arrowood JA, Paulsen WH, et al: Early echocardiography can predict cardiac events in emergency department patients with chest pain. *Ann Emerg Med* 31:550-557, 1998.

41. Chuah SC, Pellikka PA, Roger VL, et al: Role of dobutamine stress echocardiography in predicting outcome in 860 patients with known or suspected coronary artery disease. *Circulation* 97:1474-1480, 1998.

42. Erbel R, Daniel W, Visser C, et al: Echocardiocardiography in the diagnosis of aortic dissection. *Lancet* 333:457-461, 1989.

43. Callahan JA, Seward JB, Nishimura R, et al: Two-dimensional echocardiographically guided pericardiocentesis: experience in 117 consecutive patients. *Am J Cardiol* 55:476-479, 1985.

44. Lockhart ME, Robbin ML, Berland LL, et al: The sonographer practitioner: one piece to the radiologist shortage puzzle. *J Ultrasound Med* 22:861-864, 2003.

45. Fisher JB, Alboliras ET, Berdusis K, et al: Rapid identification of congenital heart disease by transmission of echocardiograms. *Am Heart J* 131:1225-1227, 1996.

46. Caldwell MA, Miles R, Barrington W: Long distance transmission of diagnostic cardiovascular information. *Biomed Sci Instrumen* 32:1-6, 1996.

47. Scholz TD, Kienzle MG: Optimizing utilization of pediatric echocardiography and implications for telemedicine. *Am J Cardiol* 83:1645-1648, 1999.

48. Trippi JA, Kopp G, Lee KS, et al: The feasibility of dobutamine stress echocardiography in the emergency department with telemedicine interpretation. *J Am Soc Echocardiogr* 9:113-118, 1996.

49. Trippi JA, Lee KS, Kopp G, et al: Emergency echocardiography telemedicine: An efficient method to provide 24-hour consultative echocardiography. *J Am Coll Cardiol* 27:1748-1752, 1996.

50. Uematsu M, Miyatake K, Tanaka N, et al: Myocardial velocity gradient as a new indicator of regional left ventricular contraction: Detection by a two-dimensional tissue Doppler imaging technique. *J Am Coll Cardiol* 26:217-223, 1995.

51. McDicken WN, Sutherland GR, Moran CM, et al: Colour Doppler velocity imaging of the myocardium. *Ultrasound Med Biol* 18:651-654, 1992.

52. Miyatake K, Yamagishi M, Tanaka N, et al: New method for evaluating left ventricular wall motion by color-coded tissue Doppler imaging: In vitro and in vivo studies. *J Am Coll Cardiol* 25:717-724, 1995.

53. Tsutsui H, Uematsu M, Shimizu H, et al: Comparative usefulness of myocardial velocity gradient in detecting ischemic myocardium by a dobutamine challenge. *J Am Coll Cardiol* 31:89-93, 1998.

54. Lang RM, Vignon P, Weinert L, et al: Echocardiographic quantification of regional left ventricular wall motion with color kinesis. *Circulation* 93:1877-1885, 1996.

Echocardiography in the Coronary Care Unit: Management of Acute Myocardial Infarction, Detection of Complications, and Prognostic Implications

IVOR L. GERBER, MD, MBChB • ELYSE FOSTER, MD

299

Applicable Modes of Echocardiography in the Coronary Care Unit

Transthoracic echocardiography (TTE) provides a rapid bedside assessment of wall motion and global left ventricular (LV) function, and it excludes the presence of major complications. In the patient presenting with chest pain who has a nondiagnostic electrocardiogram (ECG), identification of a segmental wall motion abnormality assists in the determination of definitive therapy. In the patient with an established myocardial infarction (MI), early evaluation of LV ejection fraction (EF), regional wall motion, diastolic function, and mitral regurgitation (MR) greatly assist with management. When recurrent pain complicates reperfusion therapy, electrocardiographic changes may be nonspecific. In this situation, echocardiography helps differentiate between recurrent ischemia and pericarditis. The cause of hemodynamic instability in patients with MI, including pump failure and mechanical complications, often can be established by bedside TTE without invasive monitoring.

One of the most common uses of echocardiography in the coronary care unit (CCU) is for the evaluation of regional wall motion abnormalities, which carries diagnostic, therapeutic, and prognostic implications.[1,2] Despite advances in echocardiographic imaging, assessment of regional wall motion remains a challenge with interobserver variability. The use of left-sided contrast improves interobserver agreement,[3] and although it has an additional cost, it is considerably cheaper than other imaging modalities, such as magnetic resonance imaging (MRI). Other newer methods under investigation to improve the sensitivity for the detection of regional wall motion abnormalities include color kinesis (CK),[4] tissue Doppler imaging (TDI),[5] and Doppler-derived strain and strain rate (SR) analysis.[6-8] These modalities are discussed further in Chapter 5.

Handheld echocardiographic instruments are of great clinical utility in the emergency department (ED), CCU, and cardiology outpatient clinics for the triage of acutely unwell patients. These instruments play a role in particular for targeted evaluation of global and regional LV and right ventricular (RV) systolic function and for the detection of pericardial effusion. Several studies have shown the utility of these systems,[9-11] but they are not yet comparable to full-service systems, and care should be exercised to ensure that clinicians using and reporting studies with these instruments are appropriately trained (see Chapter 8).

In patients with severe hemodynamic compromise, TTE may be limited by mechanical ventilation, recent cardiac surgery, and an inability to adequately position the patient. Whereas the use of left-sided contrast agents have greatly limited the need for further imaging modalities in this situation, transesophageal echocardiography (TEE) has proven to be efficacious, especially in ruling out complications related to cardiac rupture and for the assessment of global and regional ventricular function.[12-14] With careful sedation and close monitoring, TEE can be performed safely early after acute myocardial infarction (AMI).[15,16]

Stress echocardiography has assumed an increasingly important role in the postinfarction period for the assessment of myocardial viability and inducible myocardial ischemia. Dobutamine stress echocardiography (DSE), using low doses that do not significantly alter hemodynamics, has been shown to improve function in viable myocardial segments. Higher doses of dobutamine and exercise echocardiography can be used to detect residual ischemia. DSE should be used with caution early after MI as a result of reports of free wall rupture in association with high-dose dobutamine stress testing within the first week following MI.[17-19]

Myocardial contrast echocardiography (MCE) is a major advance in the assessment of global and regional LV function and in the assessment of myocardial perfusion and viabiltiy.[20] This technique has recently been shown to be superior to routine evaluation for the detection of acute coronary syndromes (ACSs).[21] Because perfusion abnormalities precede wall motion abnormalities in the ischemic cascade, MCE has a higher sensitivity for the detection of coronary artery disease (CAD).[20] With continued refinement, it is likely this technique will gain widespread acceptance (see Chapter 3).

Saline contrast may be indicated for enhancement of tricuspid regurgitant jets to estimate pulmonary artery (PA) pressures and to exclude a patent foramen ovale (PFO) in patients with cerebral embolization or hypoxemia especially in the setting of RV infarction.[22]

Three-dimensional (3D) echocardiography has proved to be an important research tool, and it is gaining more widespread clinical use. Recent reports have demonstrated the clinical feasibility of volumetric analysis of real-time 3D echocardiographic data that allows fast, semiautomated, dynamic measurement of LV volume and automated detection of regional wall motion abnormalities[23] and real-time 3D echocardiographic perfusion imaging.[24] It is likely that real-time 3D echocardiography will continue to play a greater role in the assessment of patients with coronary artery disease.

Pathophysiology and Echocardiographic Correlations

Timing and Evolution of Infarction

The effects of acute coronary ligation of experimental MI have been well described, and the sequence of events in myocardial ischemia are known as the ischemic cascade.[25] The first effects associated with heterogeneity of flow to the left ventricle are biochemical changes followed by a perfusion defect. This is followed by regional ventricular dysfunction, characterized by abnormal diastolic relaxation, impaired systolic wall thickening, and reduced endocardial motion. The subsequent development of ischemic ST segment depression on the ECG and the clinical development of angina are relatively late manifestations and do not occur consistently. Echocardiography, especially MCE, is therefore ideally suited for the evaluation of myocardial ischemia. Echocardiography is more sensitive than electrocardiography and evaluates the location and extent of ischemia and the functional consequences.

Approximately 30 minutes following an acute coronary occlusion, a wavefront of myocardial necrosis begins to proceed from endocardium to epicardium, resulting in a transmural MI over a period of 4 to 6 hours.[26] This final expression of prolonged myocardial ischemia is irreversible myocardial injury with significant short- and long-term implications. Initially, the regional myocardium affected becomes akinetic with maintained normal wall thickness. During the subsequent 4 to 6 weeks, when greater than 50% of the wall thickness is affected (transmural or Q-wave MI), the affected myocardial segments become thinned and echogenic as a result of scar formation. When less than 50% of the wall thickness is affected (nontransmural, or non–Q-wave MI), there may be an area of hypokinesis rather than akinesis, and wall thinning is less prominent. After transmural MI, alterations in LV structure and function occur, commonly referred to as LV remodeling, described in detail later in this chapter.

Reperfusion Therapy, Myocardial Stunning, and Infarct Size

The demonstration by DeWood and colleagues[27] that an acute coronary thrombosis was responsible for most AMIs, led to one of the major therapeutic advances in cardiology: the use of thrombolytic therapy for AMI. The theoretical basis for the use of early reperfusion is grounded in the work of early investigators in this field who showed that timely restoration of coronary flow (i.e., coronary reperfusion) salvages myocardium. However, improvement in flow had variable immediate effects on wall motion abnormalities, with most showing improvement but others showing no improvement or even worsening.[28] After reperfusion there is no significant correlation between infarct size and extent of regional dyskinesis or area of systolic wall thinning by two-dimensional (2D) echocardiography performed up to 10 days after reperfusion.[29,30] Thus, echocardiographic wall motion abnormalities as a predictor of infarct extent appeared to be more accurate following permanent occlusion than after occlusion with reperfusion.

There are several plausible explanations for the lack of correlation between infarct size and regional wall motion abnormalities in reperfused myocardium. Most often echocardiographic assessment results in an overestimation of infarct size. After restoration of flow, there may be persistent postischemic dysfunction in viable myocardial segments, known as myocardial stunning, in which the wall motion abnormality persists even though irreversible damage has not occurred. The pathophysiologic basis for this phenomenon is covered in several excellent reviews.[31,32] Wall motion abnormalities 2 weeks after reperfusion correlate better with infarct size,[30] which suggests that return of function of stunned myocardium may be delayed. The rate at which reperfusion occurs also affects function, and it may be relevant in terms of the type of therapy chosen in the acute postinfarction period. In a canine model of infarction, sudden complete reperfusion resulted in increased wall thickness and slow return of function over a 7-day period, which is consistent with cell swelling and reperfusion injury (albeit reversible). In contrast, staged partial reperfusion (followed by complete reperfusion) did not lead to an immediate increase in wall thickness, with functional recovery being seen as early as 30 minutes.[33] Thus, echocardiography early after a reperfused MI (i.e., within 2 weeks) may overestimate the eventual area of necrosis because of stunning, reperfusion injury, or both. Infarct size also may be overestimated if the abnormal motion of infarcted myocardium impairs endocardial motion of adjacent normal myocardium owing to a "tethering" effect.[34]

Alternately, the area of necrosis may be underestimated in the presence of a nontransmural infarction that subtends less than 25% of the wall thickness, with the salvaged normal subepicardial region resulting in overall normal segmental function.[35] In patients with old infarctions (>6 months), echocardiographic infarct size tends to underestimate the volume of necrosis when measured at autopsy.[36] In some cases, the ventricular remodeling process may be responsible for the change in the tendency from early (<2 weeks) overestimation to late (>6 months) underestimation of infarct size.[37]

To identify postischemic ventricular dysfunction or "stunned myocardium," investigators examined the effect of inotropic stimulation on the function of reperfused, viable myocardium and compared it with the effect on infarcted tissue. Serial 2D echocardiography during dopamine infusion demonstrated an increase in the contractility of the viable myocardium, with improvements in systolic wall thickening and endocardial motion. This improvement in regional function was shown to be associated with an improvement in regional myocardial blood flow.[38] This study and others provided the experimental basis for the clinical use of dobutamine in detecting myocardial viability, described in further detail elsewhere. More recent echocardiographic methods for determining myocardial viability are ultrasonic tissue characterization[39] and MCE.[40] With ultrasonic tissue characterization, viable myocardium shows cyclic variation of integrated backscatter confirmed by the integrity of the microvasculature identified by MCE, whereas in nonviable myocardium this variation is diminished or lost. MCE using sonicated iodinated contrast media identifies segments with persistent flow deficits despite reperfusion of the epicardial vessel. The areas of no reflow are believed to be a result of microvascular damage and correspond to nonviable segments.

Echocardiography in the Diagnosis and Localization of Acute Myocardial Infarction

Diagnostic Role of Echocardiography

The accuracy of an echocardiographic diagnosis of a MI is dependent on its ability to detect wall motion abnormalities in the involved segment. The severity of the wall motion abnormality depends on the transmural extent of the infarction, and the circumferential limits depend on the arterial distribution and collateral blood supply. Images of the left ventricle adequate for segmental analysis of wall motion can be obtained in greater than 90% of patients by skilled sonographers, and the use of left-sided contrast agents have increased the percentage of patients in whom technically adequate images can be obtained.[41-43] Pulse inversion harmonic imaging is a new modality that increases detection of myocardial contrast by canceling linearly transmitted signals. This modality has recently been shown to provide improved endocardial definition relative to tissue harmonic imaging for specific regions of the endocardium, in particular the base and the anterior wall.[44]

The most widely used scoring system for grading the severity of a wall motion abnormality is that recommended by the American Society of Echocardiography,[45] as shown in Table 14-1. Several studies have examined the specificity of echocardiographic wall motion abnormalities for diagnosis of acute coronary syndromes showing a higher specificity for infarction than ischemia.[46,47] 2D echocardiographic evidence of a wall motion abnormality is present in 90% to 100% of patients with a Q-wave infarction compared with 75% to 85% in patients with a non–Q-wave infarction.[46,48,49] Other causes of segmental dysfunction must be recognized, and a false-positive diagnosis can often be avoided if wall thickening is examined in addition to endocardial motion. The inward motion of the endocardial surface may be delayed or paradoxical owing to abnormal conduction in the presence of Wolff-Parkinson-White syndrome,[50] a left bundle branch block (LBBB),[51] or RV pacing.[52] Paradoxical septal motion also is present in RV volume overload and follow-

TABLE 14–1. Scoring System for Grading Wall Motion[45]

Score	Wall Motion	Endocardial Motion*	Wall Thickening*
1	Normal	Normal	Normal (>30%)
2	Hypokinesis	Reduced	Reduced (<30%)
3	Akinesis	Absent	Absent
4	Dyskinesis	Outward	Thinning
5	Aneurysmal	Diastolic deformity	Absent or thinning

*In systole.

ing open-heart surgery.[53] In these conditions, the systolic thickening of the septum or other involved segment (e.g., posterolateral wall in Wolff-Parkinson-White syndrome) should be preserved.[54] Nonischemic causes of segmental dysfunction that result in reduced systolic thickening and endocardial motion include focal myocarditis,[55] idiopathic cardiomyopathy, and the apical ballooning syndrome (Takotsubo cardiomyopathy).[56] Newer techniques for the evaluation of regional wall motion include tissue Doppler imaging, myocardial strain rate imaging, and tissue characterization. These techniques are discussed in more detail in Chapter 5.

MCE, using new perfluorocarbon- or nitrogen-based agents, evaluate the integrity of capillary flow in the myocardium. Tong and colleagues[57] reported on the diagnostic and prognostic value of MCE in 957 patients presenting to the emergency department with suspected cardiac chest pain and a nondiagnostic ECG. Only 2 of 523 patients with normal regional function had an early primary event, and regional function provided incremental prognostic value over the modified Thrombolysis In Myocardial Infarction (TIMI) score for predicting intermediate and late events. In patients with abnormal regional function, myocardial perfusion further classified patients into intermediate and high-risk groups. The authors suggested that patients with both abnormal regional function and abnormal myocardial perfusion are at high risk for early cardiac events and could be triaged even before cardiac serum markers become available. Although this is a promising technology, expertise in the acquisition and interpretation of the images may not be widely available, and the cost effectiveness requires further study.

Localization of Infarction

The classification of AMI according to electrocardiographic patterns has been based largely on comparing autopsy findings with the distribution of pathological Q waves during the chronic phase of infarction. However, the hypothesis that ST segment elevation during acute infarction has a similar significance for localization of AMI to that of the distribution of the Q waves during chronic phase of infarction has never been verified.[58] Clinical studies have documented the accuracy of echocardiography in identifying the site of coronary occlusion. Echocardiographic localization has significant advantages over electrocardiographic localization, particularly for apical and lateral wall infarction. Otto and colleagues[59] suggested that echocardiographic imaging may be more precise than electrocardiography for localization of infarction, with an 81% concordance between echocardiography and angiography compared with 76% for electrocardiography. The presence of preexisting wall motion abnormalities and surgical grafts or collateral circulation altering the distribution of flow must be taken into account.

In 1989, the American Society of Echocardiography recommended a 16-segment model for LV segmentation.[45] Recently, in an attempt to establish segmentation standards applicable to all types of imaging, including echocardiography, nuclear perfusion imaging, cardiovascular magnetic resonance, and cardiac computed tomography (CT), a 17-segment model has been proposed.[60] This new model includes the apical cap, which is the segment beyond the end of the LV cavity, and is generally only seen with some contrast and myocardial perfusion studies. With routine echocardiographic studies, the 16-segment model can be used, without the apical cap. The LV segments and the approximate and most common coronary arterial distri-

bution in relation to these segments are depicted in Figures 14–1 and 14–2, respectively. The anterior, anterolateral, anteroseptal, and apical (anterior and septal) segments correspond to the left anterior descending artery (LAD) distribution. Isolated disease in a diagonal branch of the LAD artery results in a discrete wall motion abnormality in the portion of the anterolateral wall supplied by that vessel. The lateral wall and lateral apex are in the distribution of the left circumflex artery. The inferolateral wall is supplied by the posterior descending artery. In 80% of the population, the posterior descending artery arises from the right coronary artery (RCA) and supplies the inferolateral wall and the inferior free wall and inferior septum (right dominant). In the other 20% of patients, the posterior descending artery arises from the circumflex artery (left dominant system). The right ventricle is supplied by the RCA via its acute marginal branches. In general, infarctions in the LAD distribution tend to be more apically situated, whereas those in the RCA and the circumflex distribution are more basal in their location. The extent of apical involvement and its distribution depends, to a degree, on the relative supply from the left anterior and posterior descending arteries. It should be noted that the extent of the segmental wall motion is related to the exact coronary anatomy in an individual patient, which may be variable. In addition, the presence of collaterals and previous bypass surgery alters the distribution of ischemia and infarction relative to the involved arterial supply.

Direct visualization of the ostia of the left main coronary artery (LMCA) and RCA, the proximal LAD

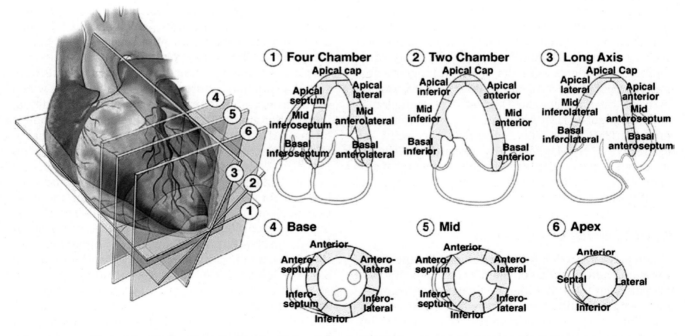

Figure 14–1. Segmental analysis of left ventricular walls, based on schematic views, in parasternal and apical views. (From Lang RM, Bierig M, Devereux RB, et al: J Am Soc Echocardiogr 18[12]:1440-1463, 2005.)

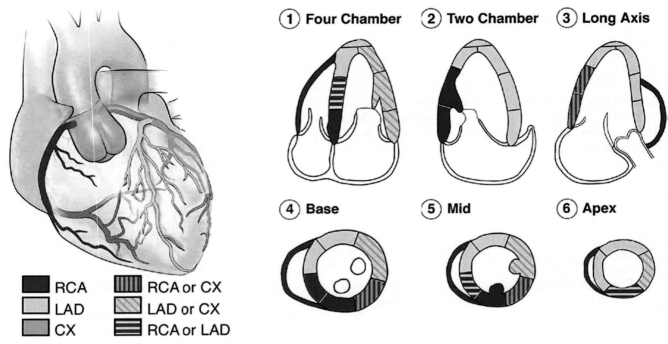

Figure 14–2. Typical coronary artery distribution of blood flow shown in the apical and parasternal short-axis views. CX, circumflex; LAD, left anterior descending; RCA, right coronary artery. (From Lang RM, Bierig M, Devereux RB, et al: J Am Soc Echocardiogr 18[12]:1440-1463, 2005.)

artery can be achieved in most adults with TTE and TEE, and this may be useful to exclude anomalous coronary artery origins. Transthoracic Doppler echocardiography may also be useful to determine coronary artery flow. Otsuka and colleagues[61] recently showed that the detection of reverse flow in the distal RCA and the inferior septal branches using transthoracic Doppler echocardiography detected an occluded RCA with a sensitivity and specificity of 100% and 98%, respectively. Lee and colleagues[62] showed in a study of 46 consecutive patients with first acute anterior MI that diastolic peak distal LAD artery flow velocity equal to 25 cm/s by transthoracic Doppler echocardiography could distinguish TIMI 3 flow in the LAD coronary artery from TIMI 2 flow with a sensitivity, specificity, and accuracy of 77%, 94%, and 89%, respectively. The use of contrast agents may expand the feasibility of this technology to localize a coronary artery stenosis and quantify coronary flow.[62]

Right Ventricular Infarction

Although RV infarction was first described in the 1930s, it was only after the hemodynamic consequences were recognized in the 1970s that RV infarction was considered a clinical entity.[63]

RV infarction occurs in up to 50% of inferior MI, but hemodynamic compromise develops in fewer than one-half of such cases.[64] The right ventricle is predomi-

nantly supplied by acute marginal branches of the RCA, and occlusion of the RCA proximal to the origin of these branches results in ischemic dysfunction of the right ventricle. When the occlusion is distal to the right atrial (RA) branches, augmented RA contractility enhances RV function and cardiac output (CO). Conversely, more proximal occlusions result in ischemic depression of RA contractility, which impairs RV filling and function, resulting in more severe hemodynamic compromise. Much less commonly, RV infarction occurs in association with acute anteroseptal MI as a result of a variation of coronary artery anatomy in which RV branches arise from the LAD artery.[65] In addition, the anterior apex of the right ventricle may be supplied by the LAD "wrapping" around the apex of the heart. Isolated RV infarction has been reported to occur in less than 3% of autopsy studies of AMI.[66-68]

The diagnosis of RV infarction should be suspected in a patient with jugular venous distention and clear lung fields in the setting of an inferior MI. The clinical importance of RV infarction is emphasized by the much higher incidence of hemodynamic compromise, arrhythmias, and in-hospital mortality than MI involving only the left ventricle.[69] The electrocardiographic sign of 1-mm ST segment elevation in V_{4R} is sensitive and specific for the diagnosis, but these changes may resolve within 12 hours and do not provide information as to the extent of involvement or its hemodynamic impact.[70]

Echocardiography plays a vital role in the evaluation of patients with suspected RV infarction[71] (Table 14–2). In an early report, Sharpe and colleagues[72] described the M-mode echocardiographic findings of RV infarction including RV enlargement and paradoxical septal motion. The 2D echocardiographic signs of RV infarction include RV dilation, decreased RV function, segmental wall motion abnormalities, and paradoxical septal motion.[73] In many cases, the inferior wall motion abnormality may be relatively small with preserved overall LV function. Tissue Doppler echocardiography may provide complementary evidence for RV infarction. In a recent study of 60 patients with a first acute inferior MI, a tricuspid valve annulus peak systolic velocity less than 12 cm/s had a sensitivity, specificity, and negative predictive value of 81%, 82%, and 92%, respectively, for RV infarction.[74] Reduced RV compliance may be detected by an increased A wave velocity on the hepatic vein flow signal and by a short pressure half-time of the pulmonary regurgitant jet (<150 msec); the latter has been shown to be a predictor of in-hospital events in patients with RV infarction.[75] Characteristic echocardiographic features of RV failure with high RA pressures include bowing of the interatrial septum into the left atrium (LA) and dilation of the inferior vena cava with lack of inspiratory collapse. These echocardiographic indicators of RV function correlate with clinical status and prognosis.[76]

Echocardiography also plays a crucial role in detecting complications of RV infarction, including ventricular septal rupture, severe tricuspid regurgitation (as a result of papillary muscle ischemic dysfunction or rupture and functional regurgitation resulting from tricuspid valve annular dilatation). In addition, severe hypoxemia resulting from right-to-left shunting across a patent foramen ovale may occur with large RV infarction associated with elevated RA pressures.[64]

In most cases of RV infarction, RV function improves and returns to near normal within 3 to 12 months regardless of the patency of the infarct-related artery,[77,78] although the improvement may not be complete when compared to a control group.[79] Experimental evidence suggest this unique feature of RV functional recovery is a result of the beneficial effects of collaterals and the more favorable oxygen supply-demand characteristics compared to the left ventricle.[77] Because the acutely ischemic dysfunctional right ventricle represents predominantly viable myocardium, which may spontaneously recover or respond favorably to successful reperfusion even late after the onset of occlusion, it has been suggested that the term *RV infarction* is largely a misnomer, and the term *RV ischemic dysfunction* be used.[80] However, it is important to recognize that RV infarction is associated with high in-hospital mortality, and early pharmacological[81] or mechanical[82] reperfusion enhances recovery of RV function with an improved clinical course and survival.

Detecting Complications of Acute Myocardial Infarction

The prognosis of MI is directly related to the extent of necrosis. A large infarction encompassing greater than 40% of the heart is likely to result in severe pump failure. In the hemodynamically unstable patient, it is critical to exclude rupture, a situation that is potentially amenable to surgery, before concluding that cardiogenic shock is on the basis of pump failure (Table 14–3). In most cases, TTE (supplemented when necessary by TEE) is sufficient to exclude papillary muscle, free wall, and ventricular septal ruptures, but it should be recognized that in some cases multiple mechanical complications of MI may occur in the same patient.[83]

TABLE 14–2. Echocardiographic Signs of Right Ventricular Infarction

Primary
Right ventricular dilation
Segmental wall motion abnormality of the right ventricular free wall
Decreased descent of the right ventricular base
Tricuspid vave annulus peak systolic velocity <12 cm/s

Secondary
Paradoxical septal motion
Tricuspid regurgitation
Tricuspid papillary muscle rupture
Pulmonary regurgitant jet pressure half-time ≤150 msec
Dilated inferior vena cava
Right-to-left interatrial septal bowing
Right-to-left shunting across patent foramen ovale

TABLE 14–3. Echocardiography in Complications of Myocardial Infarction

Hemodynamic States
Hypovolemia
Right ventricular infarction
Globally reduced left ventricular contractility

Mechanical Complications
Papillary muscle rupture and severe mitral regurgitation
Ventricular septal rupture
Free wall rupture and tamponade

Other
Left ventricular aneurysm
Mural thrombus
Pericardial effusion

Hemodynamic Classification of Myocardial Infarction Using Doppler Echocardiography

In 1967, Killip and Kimball[84] classified patients with AMI into four groups depending on the clinical manifestations of cardiac failure on admission. In 1976, Forrester and colleagues[85,86] classified patients with AMI using right-sided heart catheterization into four groups based on cardiac index and pulmonary capillary wedge pressure (PCWP). Both classifications predicted in-hospital mortality independently of the patient's age, gender, precipitating factors, and location of the MI. Although invasive measurement of PCWP and CO remains common in patients with AMI complicated by cardiac failure or cardiogenic shock, recent data suggests the use of invasive catheters may be associated with increased mortality when used in critically ill patients.[87,88]

A carefully performed Doppler echocardiographic study can provide sufficient information to determine a patient's hemodynamic category after infarction. A hemodynamic classification on the basis of these well-studied parameters is given in Table 14-4. The noninvasive measurement of CO and PCWP in patients with AMI and cardiac failure is useful to guide therapy and for prognosis.

A simple echocardiographic method of estimating CO is to measure the velocity time integral of aortic flow by pulsed wave or continuous wave Doppler. Recently, automated CO measurements, based on the digital velocities from color flow mapping, have become available and can be performed with TTE[89] and TEE.[90]

In patients with AMI, various measures of LV diastolic function have been shown to accurately estimate PCWP when compared to invasive measurements. Earlier studies demonstrated the value of transmitral Doppler to estimate PCWP. In a study of postinfarction patients with LV EF less than 35%, a mitral deceleration time of less than 120 msec was highly predictive of a PCWP greater than 20 mm Hg.[91]

Subsequent studies showed the value of pulmonary venous flow Doppler to estimate PCWP. In subjects older than 40 years of age with normal filling pressures, pulmonary venous peak velocities and velocity time integrals (VTIs) are higher during systole than during diastole, and the duration of the pulmonary venous A wave is less than that of the mitral A wave. With high filling pressures, diastolic filling predominates and the A wave duration exceeds that of the mitral A wave.[92] In patients with AMI, a systolic fraction of pulmonary venous flow less than 45% was highly associated with a PCWP greater than 18 mm Hg.[89] In a study comparing pulmonary venous flow Doppler to transmitral Doppler to estimate PCWP in patients with AMI, the deceleration time of the diastolic component of pulmonary venous flow had a better correlation with PCWP than the mitral deceleration time. The sensitivity and specificity of a diastolic component pulmonary venous deceleration time less than 160 msec in predicting a

TABLE 14-4. Hemodynamic Classification of Myocardial Infarction* by Doppler Echocardiography

Hemodynamic Category	LVEF	RVEF	LVOT VTI	Mitral E/A Dominance	Pulmonary Venous Flow	PASP (TR velocity)	IVC
Normal	Nl	Nl	≈20 cm	A wave†	S > D†	Nl	Nl
Hyperdynamic	Nl to ↑	Nl	>20 cm	A wave†	S > D†	Nl to slight ↑	Nl
Hypovolemia	Variable	Nl	<20 cm	A wave†	S > D†	Nl to ↓	Small, spontaneous collapse
Mild LV failure	Mild ↓	Nl to ↓	Mild ↓	E wave	S < D	Mild ↑	Nl to plethoric
Severe LV failure	Mod ↓	Nl to ↓	Mod ↓	E wave	S << D	Mod ↑	Nl to plethoric
Cardiogenic shock	Severe ↓	Nl to ↓	Sev ↓	E wave	S << D	Mod ↑	Nl to plethoric
RV infarction	Variable‡	↓	↓	A wave†	S > D†	↓	Sev plethora w/o collapse
MR	Nl to ↑	Nl to ↓	↓	E wave	SFR	↑	Nl to plethoric
VSD	Nl to ↑	Nl to ↓	↓	Variable	S < D	↑	Nl to plethoric

*As described by Pasternak, Braunwald, and Sobol.[102]
†In the infarction age group.
‡Dependent on extent of LV infarction.
↓, decreased; ↑, increased; D, diastolic; E/A, ratio of early to late (atrial) left ventricular diastolic inflow velocity; IVC, inferior vena cava; LVEF, left ventricular ejection fraction; LVOT, left ventricular outflow tract; mod, moderate; MR, mitral regurgitation; Nl, normal; PASP, pulmonary artery systolic pressure; RV, right ventricular; RVEF, right ventricular ejection fraction; S, systolic; SFR, systolic flow reversal; TR, tricuspid regurgitation; VSD, ventricular septal defect; VTI, velocity time integral; w/o, without.

TABLE 14–5. Incidence of Pericardial Effusion after Infarction

First Author (Year)	Number of Patients	Number with Effusion (%)	Comments
Pierard (1986)[108]	66	17 (26)	Anterior > inferior
Galve (1986)[107]	138	39 (28)	Anterior > inferior; peaked on third day
Charlap (1989)[106]	172	30 (17)	Echocardiogram at 72 hours
Sugiura (1994)[105]	185	44 (24)	Inferior MIs only; higher incidence with RV infarct
Widimsky (1995)[109]	192	82 (43)	Peaked fifth day; CHF or death more common; no increase with thrombolysis or heparin
Mazzoni (2000)[110]	545	51 (9)	Hyperechoic effusions often associated with adverse events
Sugiura (1998)[111]	214	45 (21)	Pericardial effusion still relatively common after primary percutaneous coronary angioplasty

CHF, congestive heart failure; MI, myocardial infarction; RV, right ventricular.

PCWP greater than or equal to 18 mm Hg were 97% and 96%, respectively, compared with 86% and 59%, respectively, for a mitral deceleration time of less than 130 msec.[93]

Several newer parameters of LV diastolic function have been studied in postinfarction patients. Tissue Doppler imaging measuring mitral annular velocities is a well validated method for estimating PCWP.[94,95] The measurement of peak mitral early diastolic filling velocity/flow propagation velocity (E/FPV) by color M-mode Doppler in patients with AMI has been shown to be strongly correlated with PCWP. A recent study showed an E/FPV greater than or equal to 2 predicted a PCWP of greater than or equal to 18 mm Hg with a sensitivity and specificity of 95% and 98%, respectively.[96]

The Tei index, defined as the sum of isovolumic contraction and relaxation times divided by ejection time, expresses global LV function. In patients with AMI, the Tei index has been shown to correlate significantly with the PCWP and the cardiac index. A Tei index greater than or equal to 0.60 diagnosed impaired hemodynamics (PCWP greater than or equal to 18 mm Hg and/or cardiac index $\leq$2.2 L/min/m^2) with a sensitivity, specificity, and accuracy of 86%, 82%, and 83%, respectively.[97] In addition, a Tei index greater than or equal to 0.55 can distinguish pseudonormal/restrictive mitral flow from normal mitral flow with a sensitivity, specificity, and accuracy of 84%, 100%, and 88%, respectively.[98]

Elevated pulmonary artery systolic pressure is associated with increased mortality in AMI.[99] Doppler echocardiographic measurement of pulmonary artery systolic pressure using tricuspid regurgitant jets has been well validated in the literature,[100] and the size and respiratory dynamics of the inferior vena cava can be used to estimate RA pressure.[101]

Combining these parameters with measurements (quantitative or qualitative) of LV and RV function,

color flow Doppler interrogation for MR, and assessment of mechanical complications, results in a comprehensive evaluation of the hemodynamic state after infarction.[102] When the data are incomplete from a transthoracic examination, one should not hesitate to employ TEE given its established safety even in the critically ill patient. Of course, the hemodynamic information available from an echocardiographic examination is available only at a single point in time, and continued invasive monitoring may be necessary in patients with ongoing instability.

Postinfarction Pericarditis and Pericardial Effusion

Postinfarction pericarditis most often occurs between 3 and 10 days following a Q wave MI with a mean incidence of 25% and is less common when thrombolytic therapy has been used.[103] Onset after 10 days is usually considered Dressler's syndrome, which has an incidence of 5% or less.[104] Chest pain caused by pericarditis typically is pleuritic and may be accompanied by the auscultatory finding of a pericardial friction rub, although the presence of a pericardial friction rub is not necessary for the diagnosis.[103]

A pericardial effusion is common after infarction and although it is thought to result from epicardial inflammation, it is not pathognomonic of pericarditis. Several investigators have reported on the incidence of pericardial effusion following infarction,[105-111] as summarized in Table 14–5. In these studies, pericardial effusion was associated with larger infarctions as measured by wall motion scores[105,108] or degree of creatine kinase elevation.[106,108] The incidence of congestive heart failure (CHF) and mortality is higher in those patients with effusions apparent on echocardiography.[109] In a study of 214 consecutive patients with a first Q wave AMI treated with primary percutaneous coronary angioplasty, pericardial effusion was a relatively common finding (21%),[111] which is a similar incidence to studies of thrombolytic therapy. In almost all cases the effusions are small, hypoanechoic, and hemodynamically insignificant. Thus, the effusion did not cause the increase in morbidity and mortality but serves as yet another marker of a large infarction. Larger effusions or echocardiographic dense effusions representing hemorrhage should always prompt urgent consideration of free wall rupture.[110]

Acute Mitral Regurgitation

Acute mitral valve incompetence in the setting of MI is usually a result of necrosis and rupture of papillary muscle tissue (Fig. 14–3). Incomplete coaptation of the mitral valve leaflets secondary to LV remodeling and distortion of ventricular architecture may also cause MR, and this is discussed in more detail later in the chapter.

The clinical recognition of MR in the setting of MI may be confounded by several variables. Up to 50% of patients with hemodynamically significant MR do not have an audible murmur owing to rapid equalization of LV and left atrial pressures (especially in a low output state) or because the murmur is obscured by lung sounds in a patient with pulmonary edema or mechanical ventilation.[112] In those patients with a new systolic murmur and evidence of cardiac failure, the main differential diagnosis is papillary muscle rupture and acute ventricular septal rupture. In this situation, TTE is highly accurate in establishing the cause,[113] but TEE may be necessary to determine the precise anatomic defect.

Detection and grading of MR is accomplished with 2D, M-mode, color, and spectral Doppler techniques. 2D imaging may detect abnormalities in the mitral valve apparatus, including flail leaflets and/or ruptured papillary muscle. Even if not clearly visualized, papillary muscle rupture should be suspected when there is an eccentric jet of MR with a relatively normal-sized left atrium. Although color flow parameters are those most often used, accurate grading of MR severity should encompass other echocardiographic Doppler signs as well.[114] In the patient with pulmonary edema, the unexpected findings of a small infarction, a hyperdynamic left ventricle, or increased early mitral inflow velocity[115] should prompt a careful search for MR even when color flow Doppler is initially unrevealing.

Papillary muscle necrosis with rupture and acute severe MR is a life-threatening complication of MI that requires surgical intervention. In a review of papillary muscle rupture, 15 of 17 cases occurred in patients with inferior infarction and rupture of the posteromedial papillary muscle.[116] The more frequent involvement of the posteromedial papillary muscle is a result of its blood supply from a single coronary artery (posterior descending artery) compared to the dual coronary artery supply of the anterolateral papillary muscle (LAD and circumflex arteries) (Fig. 14–4). Chordae to both leaflets arise from each of the papillary muscles so that in cases of "complete" rupture of the entire trunk of a papillary muscle, both leaflets are affected. In less severe cases, the rupture is "incomplete," and only a single head is torn. The 2D echocardiographic findings include prolapse of one or both leaflets, a flail leaflet, and liberation of a portion of the papillary muscle.[117] In some patients, the ruptured muscle may remain tethered to the chordae and chaotic motion is present. Spectral and color flow Doppler imaging of the jet is usually easily accomplished with surface imaging, but an eccentric path of flow may complicate its identification, and TEE is superior in this regard.[13]

When only a single head of the papillary muscle is affected (incomplete rupture), medical stabilization often is possible. When rupture is complete, involving

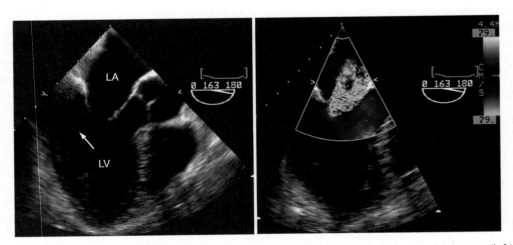

Figure 14–3. Transesophageal echocardiogram of a patient with papillary muscle rupture (left) and associated severe mitral regurgitation shown on the right. The ruptured papillary muscle (arrow) can be seen within the body of the left ventricle. LA, left atrium; LV, left ventricle.

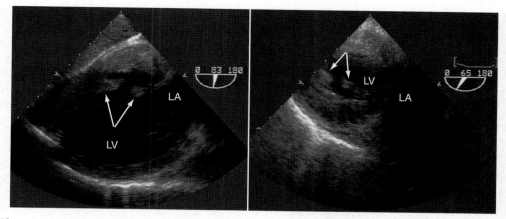

Figure 14–4. Transesophageal echocardiograms (transgastric views) of posteromedial papillary muscle rupture (left), which is more common as a result of its single blood supply, and anterolateral papillary muscle rupture (right), which is less common as a result of a dual blood supply. LA, left atrium; LV, left ventricle.

the main trunk of the papillary muscle, the complication is uniformly fatal without immediate recognition and prompt surgical repair.[117,118]

Ventricular Septal Rupture

Ventricular septal defect owing to myocardial rupture has a reported incidence during the prethrombolytic era of 1% to 2% of all AMIs and up to 5% of all fatal infarctions.[119] In the Global Utilization of Streptokinase and Tissue Plasminogen Activator for Occluded Coronary Arteries (GUSTO-1) trial, the incidence of ventricular septal rupture was only 0.2% (84 of 41,021 enrolled patients), suggesting that thrombolytic therapy has reduced the incidence of rupture.[120] Primary percutaneous coronary intervention has also recently been reported to reduce the incidence of ventricular septal rupture.[121] Ruptures occur only in the presence of transmural infarction and result from hemorrhage within the necrotic zone. Independent risk factors for the development of a ventricular septal defect are similar to those for papillary muscle rupture and include first infarction, advanced age (>65), hypertension, and female gender.[122,123] In addition, there is a higher incidence in patients without a history of prior angina and with infarcts in the distribution of a single vessel.[122,123] Thus, septal rupture is more likely following abrupt occlusion of a single artery that vascularizes a territory for which there is little collateral flow. Unlike papillary muscle rupture, ventricular septal rupture occurs with equal frequency among patients with anterior (LAD) and inferior (RCA) infarctions but less frequently in those with lateral (left circumflex artery) infarctions.[124]

In the prethrombolytic era, ventricular septal rupture usually presented 3 to 6 days after AMI, whereas most ventricular septal ruptures associated with early thrombolytic therapy occur at a peak incidence time within 24 hours after treatment.[120] Thus, although timely thrombolytic therapy reduces the rate of rupture, it tends to occur earlier after thrombolysis. Thrombolytic therapy that is delayed more than 12 hours following the onset of chest pain may increase the incidence of ventricular septal rupture.[125]

Patients with ventricular septal rupture usually present with recurrent chest pain, dyspnea, and sudden hypotension or shock. A new harsh pansystolic murmur is present in approximately 50% of patients but may be difficult to distinguish clinically from acute severe MR and may be relatively soft with LV failure or pulmonary hypertension. Particular ECG changes may be associated with an increased likelihood of septal rupture. It has recently been shown that in patients with anterior myocardial infarction with ST segment elevation in all inferior ECG leads in addition to anterior leads, ventricular septal rupture occurred in 9 of 21 patients (43%), but those ECG changes were present in only 10 of 275 patients (3.6%) of those who did not have septal rupture.[126]

Bedside echocardiography is highly sensitive and specific in the diagnosis of ventricular septal rupture.[117] Infarct expansion is readily diagnosed by echocardiography and typically occurs before rupture. Ventricular septal rupture resulting from occlusion of the RCA usually occurs in the basal inferior septum, (Fig. 14–5), and ventricular septal rupture after acute anterior MI most often occurs in the distal one third of the septum (Fig. 14–6). Ventricular septal ruptures may be multiple and often have a serpiginous course through the myocardium. When ventricular septal rupture is clinically suspected, it is often necessary to use nonconventional imaging planes, first with color Doppler to locate the defect and then with 2D imaging. The width of the jet by color flow Doppler correlates with the size of the defect as measured at surgery.[127] Although the peak gradient across the ventricular septal defect measured with continuous wave Doppler allows an estimate of RV systolic pressure, the measurement should be used with caution in patients with complex defects resulting

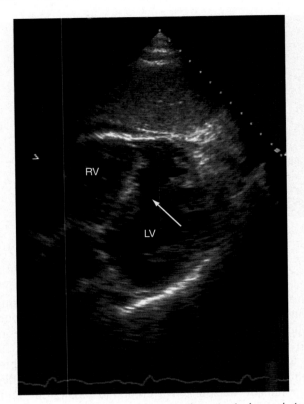

Figure 14–5. Transthoracic echocardiogram (subcostal view) showing a large ventricular septal defect resulting from a rupture in a patient with a large inferior myocardial infarction. The area of discontinuity can be visualized as a large, irregularly shaped area of myocardial dropout (arrow). Note the dilated right ventricle consistent with right ventricular infarction or right ventricular volume/pressure overload. LV, left ventricle; RV, right ventricle.

in indirect tracts through the myocardium.[127] Associated echocardiographic findings of elevated RV pressure include RV dilation, decreased RV systolic function, and paradoxical septal motion. Signs of increased RA pressure include RA dilation, bowing of the interatrial septum toward the left throughout the cardiac cycle, and plethora of the inferior vena cava. When TTE is suboptimal, TEE is highly accurate with improved delineation of the site of defect, the morphology, and presence of multiple defects.[128]

Although ventricular septal rupture carries a high mortality rate, with and without urgent surgery, echocardiography may help risk stratify patients. Complex septal ruptures and RV involvement are significant determinants of adverse clinical outcome.[128] Rupture of the posterior septum after inferior MI is associated with a higher mortality rate, related to the degree of associated RV dysfunction.[124,129] Moreover, posterior septal ruptures tend to be more complex and associated with remote myocardial involvement. In contrast, anterior septal defects more often have a direct course and involve a discrete myocardial region. The strongest indicator of poor prognosis is the development of cardiogenic shock associated with as much as a 90% mortality rate.[129] Early surgery appears to improve survival when cardiogenic shock is present, with the SHOCK trial investigators reporting a survival rate of 19% in the surgically treated group compared to 5% in the medically treated group.[124] When the patient can be stabilized medically, operative mortality may be improved when surgical repair is delayed until 6 weeks following the event.[123] In select patients, a conservative

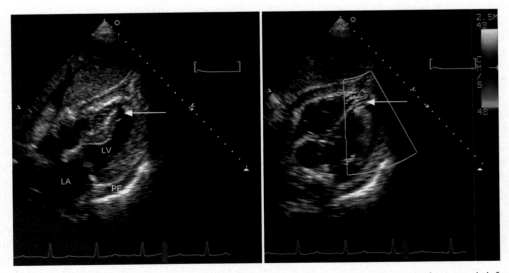

Figure 14–6. Transthoracic echocardiogram (subcostal view) showing a ventricular septal defect resulting from rupture involving the apical septum (left). Color flow Doppler demonstrates left-to-right shunting across the septal defect (right). Also note the small circumferential pericardial effusion. LA, left atrium; LV, left ventricle; PE, pericardial effusion.

approach may be appropriate and associated with a good midterm outcome. A recent report described 7 patients out of 27 with post-MI ventricular septal rupture who did not undergo surgery and were followed up for a mean of approximately 3 years. All seven patients had single vessel disease, small defect size (on average 9.8 mm), minimal left-to-right shunt, and preserved RV function.[130] In certain clinical situations, percutaneous device closure should be considered, with case reports of successful short-term outcome.[131]

Rupture of the Ventricular Free Wall and Pseudoaneurysm

Rupture of the free wall of the left ventricle is the second most common mechanical cause of death in acute ST segment elevation MI after cardiogenic shock as a result of pump failure and is usually a fatal event.[132]

Risk factors for free wall rupture are similar to those for papillary muscle and ventricular septal rupture; however, this complication is more likely to occur in patients with a transmural MI involving the inferolateral wall associated with a left circumflex occlusion[133] or with a LAD occlusion.[134] Early successful reperfusion appears to decrease the risk of rupture. In a study of 1300 patients, the overall incidence of cardiac rupture was lower in those receiving thrombolytic therapy (1.7%) than in those in the conventional therapy group (2.7%). Among patients who received thrombolytic therapy, patients older than 70 years of age and women had higher rates of rupture.[135,136] Moreover, patients in whom reperfusion was unsuccessful have a significantly higher rate of rupture than those who were successfully reperfused (5.9% versus 0.5%).[137] Conversely, late reperfusion appears to increase the risk of myocardial rupture though decreasing overall mortality.[138,139] The intensity of post-thrombolytic anticoagulation with heparin or hirudin does not appear to affect the rate of rupture.[136] A recent study comparing primary percutaneous angioplasty with fibrinolytic therapy showed a significantly lower risk of free wall rupture in patients treated with primary percutaneous coronary angioplasty.[140]

Ventricular free wall rupture usually presents clinically as an acute catastrophic event rapidly leading to death. However, recent pathologic and clinical studies have suggested that some cases may take a subacute or chronic course.[141] Intramural hematoma or hemorrhage at the junction of the necrotic and the normal myocardium results in a small endocardial rent. The tear usually takes a circuitous pathway through the myocardium, ending in a small epicardial opening. A prodrome of persistent or recurrent chest pain (in the absence of an elevation in creatinine kinase), repetitive large volume emesis, unexplained agitation, hypotension, or syncope may be associated with the initial small tear.[142,133] A small amount of hemorrhage into the pericardial space may precede the final catastrophic event. Patients diagnosed during this subacute phase and taken promptly to surgery have a greater chance of survival. In a prospective study of 608 consecutive patients with AMI, subacute free wall rupture (death occurring 30 minutes to a few days after the first clinical indication of the event) was identified in 2.5%, whereas acute free wall rupture (death within 30 minutes) occurred in 4.1% cases. The long-term outcome of survivors who underwent urgent surgery was good.[141]

Echocardiography has a high sensitivity for diagnosing rupture.[142] An echocardiographic feature of risk for rupture is infarct expansion with significant wall thinning at the infarct site. A small pericardial effusion is a common finding after an uncomplicated transmural MI, but increasing size of a pericardial effusion and the presence of thrombus in the pericardial space significantly increases the specificity for rupture (>98%), as shown in Figure 14–7.[139,142,143] The absence of pericar-

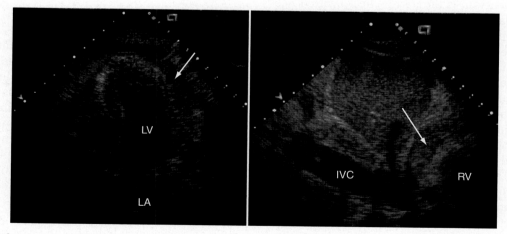

Figure 14–7. Transthoracic echocardiogram showing a hemorrhagic pericardial effusion with thrombus within the pericardial space (arrow) in an apical four-chamber view on the left and a subcostal view on the right. Note the dilated and plethoric inferior vena cava. IVC, inferior vena cava; LA, left atrium; LV, left ventricle; RV, right ventricle.

dial effusion virtually excludes rupture. An intrapericardial thrombus appears as an echo-dense mass; it may be mobile, undulating within the pericardial space or immobile, impinging on the cardiac chambers.[144] Direct visualization of the myocardial tear with TTE is relatively uncommon, reported in up to 40% of patients.[134] When the diagnosis is uncertain, the use of left heart contrast may clearly delineate the tear.[145]

The mortality rate of free wall rupture in the absence of surgical intervention has been reported to be high,[146] although recent series report as much as a 50% survival rate in patients who underwent pericardiocentesis and conservative medical management.[134,147] The in-hospital mortality rate for those who undergo surgical repair is in the range of 40%.[134,139] Those who survive until hospital discharge appear to have a good long-term prognosis.[141] Thus, early echocardiographic diagnosis with prompt surgical or percutaneous drainage is mandatory in patients who develop postinfarction myocardial rupture.

A pseudoaneurysm is a contained rupture of the LV free wall. It usually represents a complication of an AMI, but it may also occur after cardiac surgery, chest trauma, and endocarditis.[117] The majority of pseudoaneurysms are located in the inferoposterior or inferolateral regions (associated with right coronary or left circumflex coronary occlusions), and rarely occur within the ventricular septum.[148]

It is important to distinguish a pseudoaneurysm, which has a high likelihood of spontaneous rupture, from a true aneurysm, which seldom ruptures. The walls of the pseudoaneurysm are composed of organizing thrombus from hemorrhage into the pericardial space after cardiac rupture and varying amounts of the epicardium and parietal pericardium. In contrast, the wall of a true aneurysm consists of dense fibrous tissue with excellent tensile strength (Fig. 14–8). An often described distinguishing echocardiographic feature of a pseudoaneurysm is the narrow neck, with a neck diameter-to-maximum aneurysm diameter ratio less than 0.5, compared with the broader "entrance" to the body of a true aneurysm. However, this sign may not always be reliable and has been reported to be only 60% sensitive in distinguishing a pseudoaneurysm from a true aneurysm.[148] This is particularly the case with aneurysms at the base of the heart most commonly after inferior MI. Spectral and color Doppler imaging demonstrate characteristic flow in and out of the pericardial cavity at the site of the tear (Fig. 14–9) and abnormal flow within the pseudoaneurysm.

Surgical repair is the preferred treatment, although conservative medical treatment in certain high-risk patients may not be associated with an increased risk of cardiac rupture.[148,149] Percutaneous closure of a pseudoaneurysm is a potential approach in carefully selected patients (Fig. 14–10).

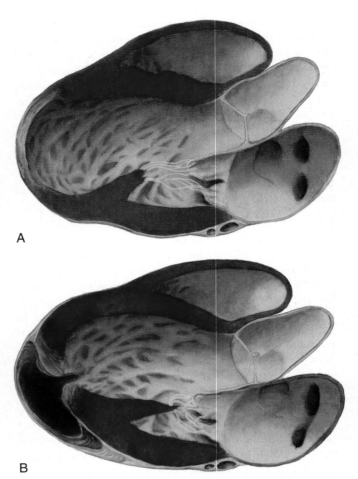

Figure 14–8. *The difference between a true aneurysm* (A) *and a false aneurysm* (B). *Note that in the true aneurysm there is continuity of myocardium in the region of dilation* (arrows), *in contrast to the loss of this continuity in the pseudoaneurysm with an abrupt area of rupture* (arrow). *(Modified from MacKenzie JW, Lemole GM:* Tex Heart Inst J *21:296-301, 1994.)*

Infarct Expansion and True Aneurysm Formation

Infarct expansion represents acute remodeling with an increase in the circumferential extent of the area of infarction, which results from stretching and thinning of the infarcted zone. This process typically occurs 24 to 72 hours after acute transmural MI.[150] Early clinical studies demonstrated that infarct expansion with a consequent increase in LV volume and wall stress was associated with an in-hospital mortality rate up to 40%.[150] Although any region of the left ventricle may be affected, it is more common after anteroapical MI.

Echocardiographic features of infarct expansion include an aneurysmal bulge of the myocardium with reduced local wall thickness. An area of thin necrotic wall, with low tensile strength, typically precedes me-

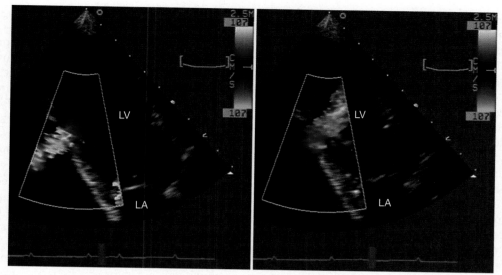

Figure 14–9. *Transthoracic echocardiogram in the apical three-chamber view demonstrating rupture of the midinferolateral wall with flow from the left ventricular cavity into the pseudoaneurysm in systole* (left) *and from the pseudoaneurysm into the left ventricular cavity in diastole* (right). *The wall of the pseudoaneurysm is not shown. LA, left atrium; LV, left ventricle.*

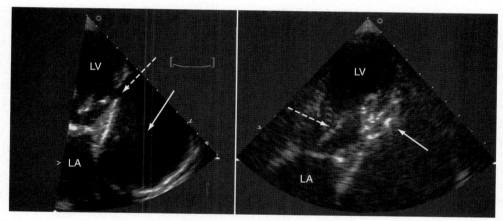

Figure 14–10. *Transthoracic echocardiogram in the apical four-chamber view demonstrating a large pseudoaneurysm of the midinferolateral wall, shown on the* left. *Solid arrow,* pseudoaneurysm; *dotted arrow,* site of free wall rupture. *The appearance after transcatheter closure is shown on the* right. *Solid arrow,* amplatzer device; *dotted arrow,* catheter. *LA, left atrium; LV, left ventricle.*

chanical complications including ventricular septal rupture, free-wall rupture, and papillary muscle rupture.

In the absence of rupture, the final expression of infarct expansion is aneurysm formation that occurs only with transmural infarction and a full-thickness scar. A true aneurysm is defined as a deformity of the thinned infarct segment that is apparent during diastole, as well as during systole, and demonstrates a diastolic contour abnormality. In contrast, a dyskinetic myocardial segment deforms during systole, extending beyond the normal contour of the myocardium. The involved myocardial segment is scarred with thin walls (<7 mm) and increased echogenicity owing to the increased collagen content.[151] The wall of the aneurysm may eventually calcify.

The reported incidence of aneurysm formation after AMI ranges considerably, from 5% to 40%.[152-157] Most aneurysms occur in the LV apex and anterior wall, and less commonly in the inferior wall. Aneurysms of the lateral wall are uncommon. Although the use of thrombolytic therapy, per se, has not been convincingly shown to reduce the frequency of aneurysm formation, a study of 205 patients presenting with AMI reported a significantly reduced incidence of aneurysm formation in those patients receiving thrombolytic therapy and exhibiting a patent infarct-related artery compared to those who received thrombolytic therapy but without a patent infarct-related artery.[154]

Serial 2D echocardiographic studies show that aneurysmal dilation is present as early as 5 days after MI, and new aneurysms after 3 months are unlikely.[156] Spontaneous rupture of an acute aneurysm is rare, and late rupture virtually never occurs. Aneurysms may vary in size, and small aneurysms may be difficult to visualize by echocardiography. Technically, the detection of an apical aneurysm is highly dependent on the skill of the operator. Routine employment of high-frequency transducers with a shallow focal point enhances near-field resolution and aids examination of the LV apex. Left-sided contrast agents also may enable detection of small apical aneurysms. Using these methods, the sensitivity of TTE for detection of apical aneurysms should approach 100%. It should be noted that TEE may not provide adequate visualization of the LV apex and, therefore, in our experience, is less sensitive than surface imaging.

Echocardiographic recognition of a LV aneurysm is clinically relevant for the following reasons: First, the early formation of an aneurysm adversely affects early (in-hospital) and late (1 year) mortality and is associated with an increased incidence of cardiac failure. Second, thrombi are frequently found within aneurysms and are associated with systemic embolization, and third, aneurysms may cause life-threatening ventricular arrhythmias.[156] In patients with heart failure or ventricular arrhythmias, aneurysmectomy may be recommended, and echocardiography plays an important role in patient selection. When considering aneurysmectomy, it is important to ensure the basal portions of the left ventricle have normal function. A basal (residual) shortening fraction or EF greater than 18% or 40%, respectively, is more likely to be associated with a satisfactory result.[158,159] Newer surgical approaches to managing ventricular aneurysms include reduction myoplasty and Dor myoplasty.[160] Echocardiography also plays an important role in assessing the feasibility of these techniques.

Left Ventricular Thrombus

A prerequisite for LV thrombus formation is the presence of a segmental wall motion abnormality, most commonly the LV apex resulting from occlusion of the LAD coronary artery. Studies in the prethrombolytic era reported incidence rates of thrombus formation after anterior MI, especially those involving the apex, of up to 56%, but thrombi were rarely reported in inferior infarction.[161] In general, thrombolytic therapy has decreased the rate of mural thrombus development, although thrombus formation may still occur after lytic therapy and concurrent antithrombin and antiplatelet agents[162-167] (Table 14–6). In the Gruppo Italiano per lo Studio della Streptochinasi nell'Infarta Miecardico (GISSI-2) trial there was no significant difference between the four treatment groups (recombinant tissue plasminogen activator ± heparin, streptokinase ± heparin), with respect to thrombus formation with an overall incidence of 28%.[168] The tendency for reperfusion therapy to decrease infarct size is likely to lower the risk of thrombus formation. The incidence of LV thrombus may also be reduced by mechanical reperfusion. In a recent study of 92 consecutive patients with acute ST elevation MI treated with primary percutaneous coronary intervention and glycoprotein IIb/IIIa inhibitors and who underwent echocardiography within 3 days of presentation, LV thrombus was seen in only 4%, and all cases occurred in anterior MI (4/37, 11%).[169] Almost identical results were shown by Kalra and Jang[170] in a study of 71 consecutive patients.

The peak timing of thrombus formation after AMI is 3 days, but thrombus may occur as early as within a few hours in large areas of apical akinesis and may occur a few weeks after a MI. The echocardiographic appearance of a mural thrombus is that of a mass distinct from the endocardium and protruding to a vari-

TABLE 14–6. Effect of Thrombolytic Therapy on Incidence of Left Ventricular Thrombus in Anterior Wall Myocardial Infarction

First Author (Year)	Number of Patients	Agent	Mean Time to Rx (hr)	Treated (%)	Untreated (%)	P
Eigler (1984)[164]	22	SK	<3	1/12 (8)	7/10 (70)	<0.005
Stratton (1985)[157]	83	SK*	4.7	7/45 (16)	6/38 (16)	NS
Natarajan (1988)[166]	45	SK	<6	0/27 (0)	8/18 (44)	<0.05
Lupi (1989)[165]	63	SK	≤3	4/19 (22)	30/44 (54)	<0.05
Bhatnagar (1991)[167]	118	r-TPA	<4	3/54 (5.5)	8/44 (18)†	<0.05
Mooe (1996)[162]	99	SK	NA	34/74 (46)	10/25 (40)	NS
Domenicucci (1999)[163]	222	SK, alteplase	NA	26/97 (27)	71/125 (57)	<0.005

*Intracoronary.
†Received heparin.
NA, not available; NS, not significant; r-TPA, recombinant tissue plasminogen activator; Rx, treatment; SK, streptokinase.

able extent into the LV cavity. Under ideal conditions, the surface of the thrombus can be distinguished clearly from the underlying endocardium, and the mass can be visualized in two different imaging planes. The tissue characteristics of an acute thrombus are usually similar to that of the myocardium. A chronic thrombus may have increased reflectivity, demonstrate a layered appearance corresponding to the lines of Zahn, and contain areas of calcification. The base of attachment to the wall may be broad in the case of a sessile thrombus and narrow in a pedunculated thrombus. Occasionally, thrombus may have a cystic appearance with a relative echocardiographic lucency to the center of the thrombus (Fig. 14-11). False-positive echocardiographic diagnoses are usually a result of pseudotendons (i.e., false chordae) spanning the LV apex, coarse trabeculations associated with LV hypertrophy, or near-field artifacts (commonly present with low-frequency transducers). High-frequency transducers with a short focus point can sometimes differentiate true thrombus from these other phenomena. Left-sided contrast agents may outline the contours of the thrombus, creating a filling defect[171] with improved detection of thrombus.

The greatest concern with a mural thrombus is the potential for systemic embolization. The likelihood of an embolic event is highest in the first 2 weeks after an AMI and reduces over the following 6 weeks. After this time, there is endothelialization of the thrombus associated with reduced embolic potential. When multiple characteristics of the thrombus are analyzed, mobility of the thrombus is most closely associated (positive predictive value, 85%) with embolic events, and when both mobility and protrusion of the thrombus into the LV cavity occur, embolic rates of up to 40% have been reported.[172-174] Anticoagulant therapy appears to decrease the risk of embolic events and enhances the resolution of thrombus, although spontaneous resolution also may occur.[175,176] In any given patient, the morphology may spontaneously change while on anticoagulation from sessile to pedunculated and vice versa; mobility may resolve spontaneously.[177,178] This emphasizes the need to follow patients with LV thrombus with serial echocardiography as thrombectomy should be considered in selected patients in whom a high-risk thrombus morphology is detected.

Postmyocardial Infarction Risk Stratification

Despite advances in the management of AMI, patients who survive are at increased risk of cardiac morbidity and mortality. Echocardiography has a pivotal role in the evaluation of patients with AMI. Routine echocardiographic measures after AMI include assessment of LV volume, systolic and diastolic function, regional wall motion abnormalities, and the presence and de-

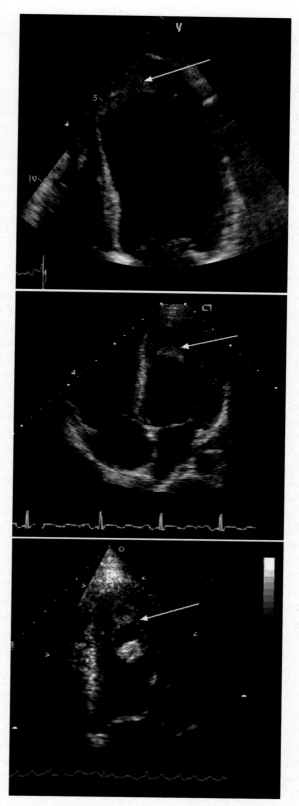

Figure 14-11. Top, *Acute thrombus* (arrow) *in the left ventricular apex. Note that the thrombus is homogeneous in texture, without evidence of calcification.* Middle, *Protruding thrombus, a feature that is associated with increased embolic risk.* Bottom, *Uncommonly, thrombus may be cystic in appearance.*

gree of MR. In addition, evaluation of myocardial viability and residual ischemia guides revascularization strategies.

Left Ventricular Systolic Function

Echocardiographic measures of global LV systolic function including LV EF and LV end-systolic volume are well established predictors of prognosis after AMI[179] and can be accurately measured by echocardiography in the vast majority of patients. Although LV EF is a powerful predictor of outcome, the EF may be normal as a result of regional hyperkinesis in the noninfarcted segments despite extensive myocardial damage, such as in inferior MI.

Regional Wall Motion Score

Semiquantitative assessment of regional systolic function using wall motion score index is an alternative to EF for the assessment of LV systolic function. An echocardiographic wall motion score has been the most widely used measure of functional infarct size in clinical practice. The total score is derived by assigning a grade of 1 through 5 (see Table 14–1) to each myocardial segment that is adequately visualized. For a segment to be scored, the majority of the endocardium within that segment must be apparent, and wall thickening and endocardial motion should be examined. The scores for each segment are added and then divided by the number of segments graded for a total wall motion score. Several studies have demonstrated that a higher wall motion score index (12 to 24 hours after admission) is associated with a higher rate of in-hospital complications, including malignant arrhythmias, pump failure, and death.[125,180] A higher wall motion score index also predicts a higher rate of complications, including free wall rupture, ventricular septal rupture, papillary muscle rupture, and death from cardiogenic shock.[180] A higher wall motion score, signifying a more extensive infarction, also is predictive of late mortality.[180,181] In a study of 767 patients with AMI, echocardiography was performed at a median of 1 day after admission, and patients were followed for a median of 19 months. Whereas both LV EF and wall motion score index were powerful predictors of all-cause mortality by univariate analysis, wall motion score index was an independent predictor of death, primarily in patients with non–ST segment elevation MI. In addition, mortality was high in patients with extensive regional wall motion abnormalities but relatively preserved EF, most likely as a result compensatory regional hyperkinesis.[1] Diastolic wall motion abnormality assessed early after MI by color kinesis has been shown to be associated with neurohormonal activation and angiographic severity of coronary artery disease and also provides independent prognostic information.[182]

Wall motion abnormalities remote from the infarction site may be present early in the course of the infarction or may develop in the presence of postinfarction angina, suggesting de novo ischemia. The echocardiographic finding of remote asynergy at or soon after clinical presentation is strong evidence of multivessel disease. Abnormal wall motion in a second (or even third) coronary distribution is possibly a result of (1) previous infarction, (2) increased myocardial oxygen demands placed on the noninfarcted segment as a result of increased wall stress outstripping its oxygen supply, (3) a cessation in its collateral blood supply that originated from the newly occluded vessel, or (4) simultaneous infarctions in multiple coronary beds, the least likely cause.[183]

Left Ventricular Diastolic Function

Doppler echocardiography for the assessment of LV diastolic function has been shown to provide accurate prognostic information in the early phase after AMI (Table 14–7). The ratio of early (E wave) to late (A wave) transmitral peak velocities and a shortened deceleration time of early transmitral flow were one of the earliest measures of LV diastolic function shown to be powerful predictors of outcome.[184-186] In a study of 125 consecutive patients with AMI, Moller and colleagues[187] demonstrated that pseudonormal and restrictive filling patterns were related to progressive LV dilatation and predicted cardiac mortality. Specifically, 1-year survival was 100% in patients with normal filling, 89% in those with impaired relaxation, 50% in those with a pseudonormal pattern, and 35% in those with a restrictive pattern. Color M-mode flow propagation velocity and pulsed-wave tissue Doppler have also been shown to be powerful predictors of cardiac mortality and readmission to hospital because of heart failure.[188] In a tissue Doppler study of 250 patients with AMI, an E/e′ ratio greater than 15 predicted all-cause mortality incremental to LV EF, age, and a restrictive filling transmitral filling pattern.[189] In addition, this study showed that measurement of E/e′ allowed risk stratification among patients with normal and reduced LV systolic function. The value of serial echocardiography after MI is emphasized by the finding that patients with a persistently abnormal or a deterioration of LV filling pattern as opposed to improved or normal filling are at increased risk of cardiac death and readmission as a result of heart failure after AMI.[190]

In contrast to Doppler indices of LV diastolic function, left atrial volume is a more stable parameter integrating the effects of elevated left filling pressures from preexisting cardiovascular conditions and acute disease. Beinart and colleagues[191] demonstrated that left atrial volume measured within 48 hours of an AMI is an independent predictor of 5-year mortality and was a more powerful predictor than LV volumes and the pres-

Chapter 14: Echocardiography in the Coronary Care Unit **317**

TABLE 14-7. The Role of Diastolic Functional Parameters in Prognosis after Myocardial Infarction

First Author (Year)	n	Comment
Pozzoli (1995)[184]	107	Patients with cardiac events had significantly higher mitral E/A ratios and shorter mitral deceleration time
Sakata (1997)[185]	206	Decreased mitral A wave was associated with high in-hospital mortality and congestive heart failure
Nijland (1997)[186]	95	1-yr survival rate: restrictive filling, 50%; nonrestrictive filling, 100%.
Moller (2000)[190]	110	Patients with a persistently abnormal or a deterioration of left ventricular filling pattern as opposed to improved or normal filling are at increased risk of cardiac death and readmission as a result of heart failure
Moller (2000)[187]	125	Restrictive filling and pseudonormal filling independently predicted death
Hillis (2004)[189]	250	Ratio of mitral E wave to early mitral annulus diastolic velocity (E/e′) >15 was the most powerful independent predictor of survival
Moller (2001)[188]	67	Ratio of mitral E wave velocity to color M-mode flow propagation velocity ≥1.5 was a significant predictor of the composite of cardiac death and readmission for heart failure

ence of MR. Similarly, Moller and colleagues[192] showed left atrial volume index was a powerful predictor of mortality and remained an independent predictor after adjustment for clinical factors, LV systolic function, and Doppler-derived parameters of diastolic function.

Left Ventricular Remodeling

After transmural MI, alterations in LV structure and function occur, commonly referred to as LV remodeling.[193] The early phase of LV remodeling is confined to the infarct zone and consists primarily of infarct expansion, whereas the late phase involves changes in the entire myocardium and may continue for months. The major factors that determine the magnitude and duration of the remodeling process include the size and location of the initial infarct (usually a complication of a larger anterior infarction), the patency and time to restoration of flow in the infarct-related artery, neurohormonal activation, and the ability of the extracellular matrix to form a stable, mature collagen scar.[194] The major clinical significance of remodeling is the resultant ventricular dilatation with reduced contractility, associated with an increased incidence of cardiac failure, arrhythmias, and death. In addition, remodeling may also cause MR as a result of apical and lateral displacement of the papillary muscles, a process that is associated with increased mortality and risk of cardiac failure. The use of beta-blockers and angiotensin-converting enzyme (ACE) inhibitors after AMI have been shown to prevent or retard remodeling.[195,196]

Echocardiography plays a major role in predicting ventricular remodeling and functional recovery. Although thrombolysis and percutaneous coronary artery interventions frequently restore patency of the infarct related artery, myocardial perfusion may be absent,

which is associated with adverse outcomes. MCE is an accurate measure of reperfusion at a microvascular level, has been shown to predict LV function after myocardial infarction,[197,198] and may predict functional recovery after AMI.[199-202] Echocardiography during low-dose dobutamine infusion is used to detect myocardial viability in segments that have persistent dysfunction following reperfusion.[203] Low dose DSE can detect contractile reserve of dysfunctional myocardium and predict LV dilatation[204,205] and functional recovery.[206,207] In a study directly comparing MCE and low dose DSE in 21 patients 2 to 4 weeks after an anterior MI who underwent successful primary angioplasty, myocardial perfusion was predictive of regional and global LV remodeling rather than of functional recovery, whereas contractile reserve assessed by DES was predictive of functional recovery rather than LV remodeling.[208]

Stress Echocardiography

Echocardiography during higher dose dobutamine infusion or with dynamic stress can be used to detect residual ischemia and provides superior prognostic value to exercise electrocardiography in the postinfarction period.[209] A normal stress echo provides favorable prognostic information in patients with preserved EF after MI, with a reported 5-year survival of 94%. In addition, a 95% 1-year survival after AMI was reported in patients with a negative stress echocardiogram compared with 85% and 75% in those with high- and low-dose ischemia, respectively.[210] Caution should be exercised in the first week after a transmural infarction because cases of myocardial rupture during high-dose dobutamine infusion have been reported.[18,19] Stress echocardiography is discussed in further detail in Chapters 15 and 16.

Mitral Regurgitation

MR is common among patients presenting with AMI, and the prevalence increases twofold in patients with heart failure.[211] Earlier studies reported a prevalence of MR in AMI by angiography of 2% to 19%,[212] whereas echocardiographic studies report a widely varying prevalence of 8% to 74%.[213-215] The different reported prevalences of MR may be a result of different sensitivities of the two imaging modalities and the timing of imaging.[212] In addition, some recent studies included patients with troponin positive acute coronary syndromes, which previously may not have been considered an AMI.

MR diagnosed in AMI may be a result of preexisting MR, for example as a result of structural leaflet disease (such as mitral valve prolapse), which need to be differentiated from ischemic causes directly related to the MI, such as papillary muscle rupture (discussed in detail previously). Ischemic MR can be defined as valvular incompetence associated with myocardial ischemia or infarction in the absence of primary leaflet or chordal pathology and may vary from trivial to severe (Fig. 14–12). Papillary muscle dysfunction represents malfunction of the scarred papillary muscle and of the underlying ventricular wall. This results in retraction of the anterior or posterior leaflet and malcoaptation. The LV remodeling process that occurs after a transmural MI may also result in apical and posterior displacement of the LV wall supporting the papillary muscle and the papillary muscle itself, with abnormal mitral leaflet coaptation and MR. In addition, dilatation of the mitral annulus to varying degrees usually also contributes to the MR. It is important to realize that depending on the site of the infarction and the degree of remodeling, one mitral leaflet may be more involved than the other (the posterior leaflet is more commonly involved) and the jet of MR may therefore be eccentric, which is a common cause for underestimating the severity of MR.

The presence of ischemic MR in AMI is associated with an adverse prognosis and increases mortality even when mild, with a graded relationship between severity and reduced survival.[216] In a recent study of 417 patients with AMI, mild MR (present in 29%) and moderate or severe MR (present in 6%) diagnosed by echocardiography were independently associated with increased 1-year mortality.[217]

In patients requiring surgical myocardial revascularization, it is generally accepted that mitral valve surgery is necessary for severe ischemic MR and not for mild MR, but it is controversial how to treat moderate ischemic MR.[218] A recent study demonstrated that coronary artery bypass graft (CABG) surgery alone may be sufficient to correct moderate MR when regurgitant severity decreases during DSE.[219]

Summary

Early experimental models employing echocardiography for the detection and quantitation of ischemia and infarction helped investigators elucidate the pathophysiology. This work was directly transferable into the CCU and provided the basis for the clinical, diagnostic, and prognostic role of echocardiography. Advances in echocardiography, especially color flow Doppler imaging, increased the capabilities of echocardiography in detecting the occurrence of complications, such as ventricular septal defect and papillary muscle rupture. Newer modalities, including MCE and 3D echocardiography, continue to show promise in the comprehensive evaluation of patients admitted to the CCU, including accurate assessment of myocardial perfusion, regional wall motion abnormalities, and LV function.

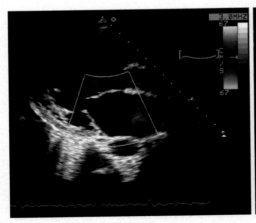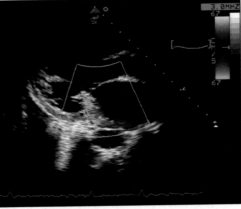

Figure 14–12. Ischemic mitral regurgitation in a patient with an inferolateral myocardial infarction. Note the normal thickening in systole of the anterior interventricular septum compared to the lack of thickening of the akinetic inferolateral wall (systolic frame on the right compared with the end-diastolic frame on the left), with a resultant posteriorly directed jet of mitral regurgitation.

Based on a wealth of accumulated data on the diagnostic and prognostic value of echocardiography in the CCU, the portability and noninvasive nature, and continuing advances in technology, will ensure echocardiography remains the noninvasive imaging modality of choice in the CCU.

KEY POINTS

- The principle advantages of TTE in the CCU include its portability, noninvasive nature, and the wealth of anatomic and hemodynamic information provided.

- The use of left-sided contrast agents have increased the percentage of patients in whom technically adequate images can be obtained.

- TTE provides key prognostic information after MI.

- All mechanical complications of MI can be detected by echocardiography.

- Echocardiography is the gold-standard imaging modality for the evaluation of ischemic MR.

- TEE is safe in the early postinfarction period and provides complementary information to TTE when needed.

- Pharmacologic stress echocardiography with dobutamine allows the identification of viable myocardium and residual ischemia after MI, which helps determine optimal revascularization strategies.

- Handheld echocardiographic instruments provide a rapid bedside assessment of wall motion, global ventricular function, and pericardial effusion.

- MCE allows a comprehensive assessment of global and regional LV function, myocardial perfusion, and myocardial viability, and can predict functional recovery after MI.

- Ongoing advances in echocardiographic imaging, including 3D echocardiography, will see real-time 3D echocardiography play an increasing role in the assessment of patients with coronary artery disease.

REFERENCES

1. Moller JE, Hillis GS, Oh JK, et al: Wall motion score index and ejection fraction for risk stratification after acute myocardial infarction. *Am Heart J* 151(2):19-25, 2006.
2. Marwick TH, Mehta R, Arheart K, et al: Use of exercise echocardiography for prognostic evaluation of patients with known or suspected coronary artery disease. *J Am Coll Cardiol* 30(1):83-90, 1997.
3. Hoffmann R, von Bardeleben S, Kasprzak JD, et al: Analysis of regional left ventricular function by cineventriculography, cardiac magnetic resonance imaging, and unenhanced and contrast-enhanced echocardiography: a multicenter comparison of methods. *J Am Coll Cardiol* 47(1):21-28, 2006.
4. Mor-Avi V, Jacobs LD, Weiss RJ, et al: Color encoding of endocardial motion improves the interpretation of contrast-enhanced echocardiographic stress tests by less-experienced readers. *J Am Soc Echocardiogr* 19(1):48-54, 2006.
5. Borges AC, Kivelitz D, Walde T, et al: Apical tissue tracking echocardiography for characterization of regional left ventricular function: comparison with magnetic resonance imaging in patients after myocardial infarction. *J Am Soc Echocardiogr* 16(3):54-62, 2003.
6. Pellerin D, Sharma R, Elliott P, et al: Tissue Doppler, strain, and strain rate echocardiography for the assessment of left and right systolic ventricular function. *Heart* 89(Suppl 3):iii9-iii17, 2003.
7. Greenberg NL, Firstenberg MS, Castro PL, et al: Doppler-derived myocardial systolic strain rate is a strong index of left ventricular contractility. *Circulation* 105(1):99-105, 2002.
8. Urheim S, Edvardsen T, Torp H, et al: Myocardial strain by Doppler echocardiography. Validation of a new method to quantify regional myocardial function. *Circulation* 102(10):158-164, 2000.
9. Mondillo S, Giannotti G, Innelli P, et al: Hand-held echocardiography: Which usefulness? Who user? *Int J Cardiol* 111(1):1-5, 2005.
10. Hellmann DB, Whiting-O'Keefe Q, Shapiro EP, et al: The rate at which residents learn to use hand-held echocardiography at the bedside. *Am J Med* 118(9):1010-1018, 2005.
11. Giannotti G, Mondillo S, Galderisi M, et al: Hand-held echocardiography: added value in clinical cardiological assessment. *Cardiovasc Ultrasound* 3(1):7, 2005.
12. Esakof DD, Vannan MA, Pandian NG, et al: Visualization of left ventricular pseudoaneurysm with panoramic transesophageal echocardiography. *J Am Soc Echocardiogr* 7:174-178, 1994.
13. Zotz RJ, Dohmen G, Genth S, et al: Diagnosis of papillary muscle rupture after acute myocardial infarction by transthoracic and transesophageal echocardiography. *Clin Cardiol* 16:665-670, 1993.
14. Chirillo F, Totis O, Cavarzerani A, et al: Transesophageal echocardiographic findings in partial and complete papillary muscle rupture complicating acute myocardial infarction. *Cardiology* 81:54-58, 1992.
15. Foster E, Schiller NB: Transesophageal echocardiography in the critical care patient. *Cardiol Clin* 11:489-503, 1993.
16. Foster E, Schiller NB: The role of transesophageal echocardiography in critical care: UCSF experience. *J Am Soc Echocardiogr* 5:368-374, 1992.
17. Smart SC, Knickelbine T, Stoiber TR, et al: Safety and accuracy of dobutamine-atropine stress echocardiography for the detection of residual stenosis of the infarct-related artery and multivessel disease during the first week after acute myocardial infarction. *Circulation* 95:1394-1401, 1997.
18. Daniels CJ, Orsinelli DA: Cardiac rupture with dobutamine stress echocardiography. *J Am Soc Echocardiogr* 10:979-981, 1997.
19. Orlandini AD, Tuero EI, Diaz R, et al: Acute cardiac rupture during dobutamine-atropine echocardiography stress test. *J Am Soc Echocardiogr* 13:152-153, 2000.
20. Lepper W, Belcik T, Wei K, et al: Myocardial contrast echocardiography. *Circulation* 109(25):132-135, 2004.
21. Kaul S, Senior R, Firschke C, et al: Incremental value of cardiac imaging in patients presenting to the emergency department with chest pain and without ST-segment elevation: a multicenter study. *Am Heart J* 148(1):29-36, 2004.
22. Cox D, Taylor J, Nanda NC: Refractory hypoxemia in right ventricular infarction from right-to-left shunting via a patent foramen ovale: Efficacy of contrast transesophageal echocardiography. *Am J Med* 91:653-655, 1991.
23. Corsi C, Lang RM, Veronesi F, et al: Volumetric quantification of global and regional left ventricular function from real-time three-dimensional echocardiographic images. *Circulation* 112(8):161-170, 2005.
24. Toledo E, Lang RM, Collins KA, et al: Imaging and quantification of myocardial perfusion using real-time three-dimensional echocardiography. *J Am Coll Cardiol* 47(1):46-54, 2006.

25. Otto CM: *Textbook of Clinical Echocardiography*, 3rd ed. Philadelphia, Elsevier Saunders, 2004.

26. Reimer KA, Jennings RB: Myocardial ischemia, hypoxia and infarction. In Fozzard HA (ed): *The Heart and Cardiovascular System*. New York, Raven Press, 1986, pp. 1122-1202.

27. DeWood MA, Apores J, Notske R, et al: Prevalence of total coronary occlusion during the early hours of transmural myocardial infarction. *N Engl J Med* 303:897-902, 1980.

28. Kerber RE, Marcus ML, Abboud FM: Echocardiography in experimentally-induced myocardial ischemia. *Am J Med* 63:21-28, 1977.

29. Kerber RE, Pandian N, Taylor A: Late effects of coronary reperfusion on regional left ventricular function. Can infarct size be estimated noninvasively? *Adv Cardiol* 34:77-84, 1986.

30. Isobe M, Nagai R, Takaku F, et al: Infarct sizing after reperfusion by two-dimensional echocardiography and serum cardiac myosin light chain II in conscious dogs: Dissociation between early left ventricular wall motion and ultimate infarct size. *Jpn Circ J* 53:1100-1107, 1989.

31. Bolli R: Mechanism of myocardial "stunning." *Circulation* 82:723-738, 1990.

32. Bolli R: Myocardial "stunning" in man. *Circulation* 86:1671-1691, 1992.

33. Yamazaki S, Fujibayashi Y, Rajagopalan RE, et al: Effects of staged versus sudden reperfusion after acute coronary occlusion in the dog. *J Am Coll Cardiol* 7:564-572, 1986.

34. Force T, Kemper A, Perkins L, et al: Overestimation of infarct size by quantitative two-dimensional echocardiography: The role of tethering and of analytic procedures. *Circulation* 73:1360-1368, 1986.

35. Mann DL, Gillam LD, Mich R, et al: Functional relation between infarct thickness and regional systolic function in the acutely and subacutely infarcted canine left ventricle. *J Am Coll Cardiol* 14:481-488, 1989.

36. Wilkins GT, Southern JF, Choong CY, et al: Correlation between echocardiographic endocardial surface mapping of abnormal wall motion and pathologic infarct size in autopsied hearts. *Circulation* 77:978-987, 1988.

37. Feigenbaum H: *Echocardiography*, 6th ed. Philadelphia, Lea & Febiger, 2005.

38. Arnold JM, Braunwald E, Sandor T, et al: Inotropic stimulation of reperfused myocardium with dopamine: Effects on infarct size and myocardial function. *J Am Coll Cardiol* 6:1026-1034, 1985.

39. Yamada S, Komuro K: Integrated backscatter for the assessment of myocardial viability. *Curr Opin Cardiol* 21(5):33-37, 2006.

40. Hayat SA, Senior R: Contrast echocardiography for the assessment of myocardial viability. *Curr Opin Cardiol* 21(5):73-78, 2006.

41. Yong Y, Wu D, Fernandes V, et al: Diagnostic accuracy and cost-effectiveness of contrast echocardiography on evaluation of cardiac function in technically very difficult patients in the intensive care unit. *Am J Cardiol* 89(6):11-18, 2002.

42. Reilly JP, Tunick PA, Timmermans RJ, et al: Contrast echocardiography clarifies uninterpretable wall motion in intensive care unit patients. *J Am Coll Cardiol* 35:485-490, 2000.

43. Yu EH, Sloggett CE, Iwanochko RM, et al: Feasibility and accuracy of left ventricular volumes and ejection fraction determination by fundamental, tissue harmonic, and intravenous contrast imaging in difficult-to-image patients. *J Am Soc Echocardiogr* 13:216-224, 2000.

44. Vancon AC, Fox ER, Chow CM, et al: Pulse inversion harmonic imaging improves endocardial border visualization in two-dimensional images: comparison with harmonic imaging. *J Am Soc Echocardiogr* 15(4):302-308, 2002.

45. Schiller NB, Shah PM, Crawford M, et al: Recommendations for quantitation of the left ventricle by two-dimensional echocardiography. American Society of Echocardiography Committee on Standards, Subcommittee on Quantitation of Two-Dimensional Echocardiograms. *J Am Soc Echocardiogr* 2:358-367, 1989.

46. Horowitz RS, Morganroth J, Parrotto C, et al: Immediate diagnosis of acute myocardial infarction by two-dimensional echocardiography. *Circulation* 65:323-329, 1982.

47. Peels CH, Visser CA, Kupper AJ, et al: Usefulness of two-dimensional echocardiography for immediate detection of myocardial ischemia in the emergency room. *Am J Cardiol* 65:687-691, 1990.

48. Nixon JV, Narahara KA, Smitherman TC: Estimation of myocardial involvement in patients with acute myocardial infarction by two-dimensional echocardiography. *Circulation* 62:1248-1255, 1980.

49. Weiss JL, Bulkley BH, Hutchins GM, et al: Two-dimensional echocardiographic recognition of myocardial injury in man: Comparison with postmortem studies. *Circulation* 63:401-408, 1981.

50. Kuecherer HF, Abbott JA, Botvinick EH, et al: Two-dimensional echocardiographic phase analysis. Its potential for noninvasive localization of accessory pathways in patients with Wolff-Parkinson-White syndrome [see comments]. *Circulation* 85:130-142, 1982.

51. Shah KD, Daxini BV: Noninvasive and invasive evaluation of left bundle branch block (LBBB). *Acta Cardiol* 45:125-131, 1990.

52. Xiao HB, Brecker SJ, Gibson DG: Differing effects of right ventricular pacing and left bundle branch block on left ventricular function. *Br Heart J* 69:166-173, 1993.

53. Force T, Bloomfield P, O'Boyle JE, et al: Quantitative two-dimensional echocardiographic analysis of motion and thickening of the interventricular septum after cardiac surgery. *Circulation* 68:1013-1020, 1983.

54. Corya BC, Rasmussen S, Feigenbaum H, et al: Systolic thickening and thinning of the septum and posterior wall in patients with coronary artery disease, congestive cardiomyopathy, and atrial septal defect. *Circulation* 55:109-114, 1977.

55. Ramamurthy S, Talwar KK, Goswami KC, et al: Clinical profile of biopsy proven idiopathic myocarditis. *Int J Cardiol* 41:225-232, 1993.

56. Akashi YJ, Musha H, Kida K, et al: Reversible ventricular dysfunction takotsubo cardiomyopathy. *Eur J Heart Fail* 7(7):171-176, 2005.

57. Tong KL, Kaul S, Wang XQ, et al: Myocardial contrast echocardiography versus Thrombolysis In Myocardial Infarction score in patients presenting to the emergency department with chest pain and a nondiagnostic electrocardiogram. *J Am Coll Cardiol* 46(5):20-27, 2005.

58. Porter A, Strasberg B, Vaturi M, et al: Correlation between electrocardiographic subtypes of anterior myocardial infarction and regional abnormalities of wall motion. *Coron Artery Dis* 11(6):89-93, 2000.

59. Otto CM, Stratton JR, Maynard C, et al: Echocardiographic evaluation of segmental wall motion early and late after thrombolytic therapy in acute myocardial infarction: The Western Washington Tissue Plasminogen Activator Emergency Room Trial. *Am J Cardiol* 65:132-138, 1990.

60. Lang RM, Bierig M, Devereux RB, et al: Chamber Quantification Writing Group; American Society of Echocardiography's Guidelines and Standards Committee; European Association of Echocardiography. Recommendations for chamber quantification: a report from the American Society of Echocardiography's Guidelines and Standards Committee and the Chamber Quantification Writing Group, developed in conjunction with the European Association of Echocardiography, a branch of the European Society of Cardiology. *J Am Soc Echocardiogr* 18(12):440-463, 2005.

61. Otsuka R, Watanabe H, Hirata K, et al: A novel technique to detect total occlusion in the right coronary artery using retrograde flow by transthoracic Doppler echocardiography. *J Am Soc Echocardiogr* 18(7):704-709, 2005.

62. Lee S, Otsuji Y, Minagoe S, et al: Noninvasive evaluation of coronary reperfusion by transthoracic Doppler echocardiography in patients with anterior acute myocardial infarction before coronary intervention. *Circulation* 108(22):763-768, 2003.

63. Cohn JN, Guiha NH, Broder MI, et al: Right ventricular infarction. Clinical and hemodynamic features. *Am J Cardiol* 33:209-214, 1974.

64. Goldstein JA: Pathophysiology and management of right heart ischemia. *J Am Coll Cardiol* 40(5):41-53, 2002.

65. Tahirkheli NK, Edwards WD, Nishimura RA, et al: Right ventricular infarction associated with anteroseptal myocardial infarction: a clinicopathologic study of nine cases. *Cardiovasc Pathol* 9(3):75-79, 2000.

66. Setaro JF, Cabin HS: Right ventricular infarction. *Cardiol Clin* 10(1):69-90, 1992.

67. Kinch JW, Ryan TJ: Right ventricular infarction. *N Engl J Med* 330(17):211-217, 1994.

68. Goldstein JA: Right heart ischemia: Pathophysiology, natural history, and clinical management. *Prog Cardiovasc Dis* 40(4):25-41, 1998.

69. Zehender M, Kasper W, Kauder E, et al: Right ventricular infarction as an independent predictor of prognosis after acute inferior myocardial infarction. *N Engl J Med* 328(14):81-88, 1993.

70. Fijewski TR, Pollack ML, Chan TC, et al: Electrocardiographic manifestations: right ventricular infarction. *J Emerg Med* 22(2):89-94, 2002.

71. Kozakova M, Palombo C, Distante A: Right ventricular infarction: the role of echocardiography. *Echocardiography* 18(8):701-707, 2001.

72. Sharpe DN, Botvinick EH, Shames DM, et al: The noninvasive diagnosis of right ventricular infarction. *Circulation* 57:483-490, 1987.

73. Cecchi F, Zuppiroli A, Favilli S, et al: Echocardiographic features of right ventricular infarction. *Clin Cardiol* 7:405-412, 1984.

74. Ozdemir K, Altunkeser BB, Icli A, et al: New parameters in identification of right ventricular myocardial infarction and proximal right coronary artery lesion. *Chest* 124(1):19-26, 2003.

75. Cohen A, Logeart D, Costagliola D, et al: Usefulness of pulmonary regurgitation Doppler tracings in predicting in-hospital and long-term outcome in patients with inferior wall acute myocardial infarction. *Am J Cardiol* 81:276-281, 1998.

76. Goldberger JJ, Himelman RB, Wolfe CL, et al: Right ventricular infarction: Recognition and assessment of its hemodynamic significance by two-dimensional echocardiography. *J Am Soc Echocardiogr* 4:140-146, 1991.

77. Laster SB, Shelton TJ, Barzilai B, et al: Determinants of the recovery of right ventricular performance following experimental chronic right coronary artery occlusion. *Circulation* 88(2):696-708, 1993.

78. Dell'Italia LJ, Lembo NJ, Starling MR, et al: Hemodynamically important right ventricular infarction: follow-up evaluation of right ventricular systolic function at rest and during exercise with radionuclide ventriculography and respiratory gas exchange. *Circulation* 75(5):996-1003, 1987.

79. Ketikoglou DG, Karvounis HI, Papadopoulos CE, et al: Echocardiographic evaluation of spontaneous recovery of right ventricular systolic and diastolic function in patients with acute right ventricular infarction associated with posterior wall left ventricular infarction. *Am J Cardiol* 93(7):911-913, 2004.

80. Goldstein JA: Right versus left ventricular shock: a tale of two ventricles. *J Am Coll Cardiol* 41(8):280-282, 2003.

81. Mattioli AV, Fini M, Mattioli G: Right ventricular dysfunction after thrombolysis in patients with right ventricular infarction. *J Am Soc Echocardiogr* 13:655-660, 2000.

82. Bowers TR, O'Neill WW, Grines C, et al: Effect of reperfusion on biventricular function and survival after right ventricular infarction. *N Engl J Med* 338(14):33-40, 1998.

83. Walts PA, Gillinov AM: Survival after simultaneous left ventricular free wall, papillary muscle, and ventricular septal rupture. *Ann Thorac Surg* 78(5): e77-e78, 2004.

84. Killip T 3rd, Kimball JT: Treatment of myocardial infarction in a coronary care unit. A two year experience with 250 patients. *Am J Cardiol* 20(4):457-464, 1967.

85. Forrester JS, Diamond G, Chatterjee K, et al: Medical therapy of acute myocardial infarction by application of hemodynamic subsets (first of two parts). *N Engl J Med* 295(24):356-362, 1976.

86. Forrester JS, Diamond GA, Swan HJ: Correlative classification of clinical and hemodynamic function after acute myocardial infarction. *Am J Cardiol* 39(2):137-145, 1977.

87. Connors AF Jr, Speroff T, Dawson NV, et al: The effectiveness of right heart catheterization in the initial care of critically ill patients. SUPPORT Investigators. *JAMA* 276(11):889-897, 1996.

88. Dalen JE, Bone RC: Is it time to pull the pulmonary artery catheter? *JAMA* 276(11):916-918, 1996.

89. Hozumi T, Yoshida K, Mori I, et al: Noninvasive assessment of hemodynamic subsets in patients with acute myocardial infarction using digital color Doppler velocity profile integration and pulmonary venous flow analysis. *Am J Cardiol* 83:1027-1032, 1999.

90. Akamatsu S, Oda A, Terazawa E, et al: Automated cardiac output measurement by transesophageal color Doppler echocardiography. *Anesth Analg* 98(5):232-238, 2004.

91. Giannuzzi P, Imparato A, Temporelli PL, et al: Doppler-derived mitral deceleration time of early filling as a strong predictor of pulmonary capillary wedge pressure in postinfarction patients with left ventricular systolic dysfunction. *J Am Coll Cardiol* 23:1630-1637, 1994.

92. Rossvoll O, Hatle LK: Pulmonary venous flow velocities recorded by transthoracic Doppler ultrasound: Relation to left ventricular diastolic pressures. *J Am Coll Cardiol* 21:1687-1696, 1993.

93. Yamamuro A, Yoshida K, Hozumi T, et al: Noninvasive evaluation of pulmonary capillary wedge pressure in patients with acute myocardial infarction by deceleration time of pulmonary venous flow velocity in diastole. *J Am Coll Cardiol* 34:90-94, 1999.

94. Ommen SR, Nishimura RA, Appleton CP, et al: Clinical utility of Doppler echocardiography and tissue Doppler imaging in the estimation of left ventricular filling pressures: A comparative simultaneous Doppler-catheterization study. *Circulation* 102(15):788-794, 2000.

95. Nagueh SF, Middleton KJ, Kopelen HA et al: Doppler tissue imaging: a noninvasive technique for evaluation of left ventricular relaxation and estimation of filling pressures. *J Am Coll Cardiol* 30(6):527-533, 1997.

96. Ueno Y, Nakamura Y, Kinoshita M, et al: Noninvasive estimation of pulmonary capillary wedge pressure by color M-mode Doppler echocardiography in patients with acute myocardial infarction. *Echocardiography* 19(2):95-102, 2002.

97. Takasaki K, Otsuji Y, Yoshifuku S, et al: Noninvasive estimation of impaired hemodynamics for patients with acute myocardial infarction by Tei index. *J Am Soc Echocardiogr* 17(6):615-621, 2004.

98. Abd-El-Rahim AR, Otsuji Y, Yuasa T, et al: Noninvasive differentiation of pseudonormal/restrictive from normal mitral flow by Tei index: A simultaneous echocardiography-catheterization study in patients with acute anteroseptal myocardial infarction. *J Am Soc Echocardiogr* 16(12):231-236, 2003.

99. Moller JE, Hillis GS, Oh JK, et al: Prognostic importance of secondary pulmonary hypertension after acute myocardial infarction. *Am J Cardiol* 96(2):199-203, 2005.

100. Himelman RB, Stulbarg M, Kircher B, et al: Noninvasive evaluation of pulmonary artery pressure during exercise by saline-enhanced Doppler echocardiography in chronic pulmonary disease. *Circulation* 79:863-871, 1989.

101. Kircher BJ, Himelman RB, Schiller NB: Noninvasive estimation of right atrial pressure from the inspiratory collapse of the inferior vena cava. *Am J Cardiol* 66:493-496, 1990.

102. Pasternak RC, Braunwald E, Sobol BE: Acute myocardial infarction. In Braunwald E (ed): *Heart Disease: A Textbook of Cardiovascular Medicine*, 4th ed. Philadelphia, WB Saunders, 1992, p. 1250.

103. Oliva PB, Hammill SC, Talano JV: Effect of definition on incidence of postinfarction pericarditis. It is time to redefine postinfarction pericarditis? *Circulation* 90(3):537-541, 1994.

104. Welin L, Vedin A, Wilhelmsson C: Characteristics, prevalence, and prognosis of postmyocardial infarction syndrome. *Br Heart J* 50(2):40-45, 1983.

105. Sugiura T, Iwasaka T, Tarumi N, et al: Clinical significance of pericardial effusion in Q-wave inferior wall acute myocardial infarction. *Am J Cardiol* 73:862-864, 1994.

106. Charlap S, Greenberg S, Greengart A, et al: Pericardial effusion early in acute myocardial infarction. *Clin Cardiol* 12:252-254, 1989.

107. Galve E, Garcia-Del-Castillo H, Evangelista A, et al: Pericardial effusion in the course of myocardial infarction: Incidence, natural history, and clinical relevance. *Circulation* 73:294-299, 1986.

108. Pierard LA, Albert A, Henrard L, et al: Incidence and significance of pericardial effusion in acute myocardial infarction as determined by two-dimensional echocardiography. *J Am Coll Cardiol* 8:517-520, 1986.

109. Widimsky P, Gregor P: Pericardial involvement during the course of myocardial infarction. A long-term clinical and echocardiographic study. *Chest* 1081:89-93, 1995.

110. Mazzoni V, Taiti A, Bartoletti A, et al: The spectrum of pericardial effusion in acute myocardial infarction: an echocardiographic study. *Ital Heart J* 1(1):45-49, 2000.

111. Sugiura T, Takehana K, Hatada K, et al: Pericardial effusion after primary percutaneous transluminal coronary angioplasty in first Q-wave acute myocardial infarction. *Am J Cardiol* 81(9):1090-1093, 1998.

112. Tcheng JE, Jackman J Jr, Nelson CL, et al: Outcome of patients sustaining acute ischemic mitral regurgitation during myocardial infarction. *Ann Intern Med* 117:18-24, 1992.

113. Smyllie JH, Sutherland GR, Geuskens R, et al: Doppler color flow mapping in the diagnosis of ventricular septal rupture and acute mitral regurgitation after myocardial infarction. *J Am Coll Cardiol* 15:1449-1455, 1990.

114. Zoghbi WA, Enriquez-Sarano M, Foster E, et al: Recommendations for evaluation of the severity of native valvular regurgitation with two-dimensional and Doppler echocardiography. *J Am Soc Echocardiogr* 16(7):777-802, 2003.

115. Thomas L, Foster E, Hoffman JI, et al: The Mitral Regurgitation Index: An echocardiographic guide to severity. *J Am Coll Cardiol* 33:2016-2022, 1999.

116. Nishimura RA, Schaff HV, Shub C, et al: Papillary muscle rupture complicating acute myocardial infarction: analysis of 17 patients. *Am J Cardiol* 51(3):373-377, 1983.

117. Buda AJ: The role of echocardiography in the evaluation of mechanical complications of acute myocardial infarction. *Circulation* 84(3 Suppl):I109-I121, 1991.

118. Nishimura RA, Schaff HV, Gersh BJ, et al: Early repair of mechanical complications after acute myocardial infarction. *JAMA* 256:47-50, 1986.

119. Heitmiller R, Jacobs ML, Daggett WM: Surgical management of postinfarction ventricular septal rupture. *Ann Thorac Surg* 41(6):683-691, 1986.

120. Crenshaw BS, Granger CB, Birnbaum Y, et al: Risk factors, angiographic patterns, and outcomes in patients with ventricular septal defect complicating acute myocardial infarction. GUSTO-I (Global Utilization of Streptokinase and TPA for Occluded Coronary Arteries) Trial Investigators. *Circulation* 101:27-32, 2000.

121. Yip HK, Fang CY, Tsai KT, et al: The potential impact of primary percutaneous coronary intervention on ventricular septal rupture complicating acute myocardial infarction. *Chest* 125(5):1622-1628, 2004.

122. Leavey S, Galvin J, McCann H, et al: Post-myocardial infarction ventricular septal defect: An angiographic study. *Ir J Med Sci* 163:182-183, 1994.

123. Lemery R, Smith HC, Giuliani ER, et al: Prognosis in rupture of the ventricular septum after acute myocardial infarction and role of early surgical intervention. *Am J Cardiol* 70:147-151, 1992.

124. Menon V, Webb JG, Hillis LD, et al: Outcome and profile of ventricular septal rupture with cardiogenic shock after myocardial infarction: A report from the SHOCK Trial Registry. Should we emergently revascularize Occluded Coronaries in cardiogenic shock? *J Am Coll Cardiol* 36(3 suppl A):1110-1116, 2000.

125. Nishimura RA, Tajik AJ, Shub C, et al: Role of two-dimensional echocardiography in the prediction of in-hospital complications after acute myocardial infarction. *J Am Coll Cardiol* 4:1080-1087, 1984.

126. Hayashi T, Hirano Y, Takai H, et al: Usefulness of ST-segment elevation in the inferior leads in predicting ventricular septal rupture in patients with anterior wall acute myocardial infarction. *Am J Cardiol* 96(8):1037-1041, 2005.

127. Helmcke F, Mahan Ed, Nanda NC, et al: Two-dimensional echocardiography and Doppler color flow mapping in the diagnosis and prognosis of ventricular septal rupture. *Circulation* 81:1775-1783, 1990.

128. Vargas-Barron J, Molina-Carrion M, Romero-Cardenas A, et al: Risk factors, echocardiographic patterns, and outcomes in patients with acute ventricular septal rupture during myocardial infarction. *Am J Cardiol* 95(10):1153-1158, 2005.

129. Moore CA, Nygaard TW, Kaiser DL, et al: Postinfarction ventricular septal rupture: The importance of location of infarction and right ventricular function in determining survival. *Circulation* 74:45-55, 1986.

130. Sivadasan Pillai H, Tharakan J, Titus T, et al: Ventricular septal rupture following myocardial infarction. Long-term survival of patients who did not undergo surgery. Single-centre experience. *Acta Cardiol* 60(4):403-407, 2005.

131. Burrell CJ, Zacharkiw LA, DeGiovanni JV: Percutaneous device closure of post-infarction ventricular septal defect with aneurysm. *Heart* 90(7):731, 2004.

132. Keeley EC, de Lemos JA: Free wall rupture in the elderly: Deleterious effect of fibrinolytic therapy on the ageing heart. *Eur Heart J* 26(17):1693-1694, 2005.

133. Oliva PB, Hammill SC, Edwards WD: Cardiac rupture, a clinically predictable complication of acute myocardial infarction: Report of 70 cases with clinicopathologic correlations [see comments]. *J Am Coll Cardiol* 22:720-726, 1993.

134. Slater J, Brown RJ, Antonelli TA, et al: Cardiogenic shock due to cardiac free-wall rupture or tamponade after acute myocardial infarction: A report from the SHOCK Trial Registry. Should we emergently revascularize occluded coronaries for cardiogenic shock? *J Am Coll Cardiol* 36(3 suppl A):1117-1122, 2000.

135. Bueno H, Martinez-Selles M, Perez-David E, et al: Effect of thrombolytic therapy on the risk of cardiac rupture and mortality in older patients with first acute myocardial infarction. *Eur Heart J* 26(17):1705-1711, 2005.

136. Becker RC, Hochman JS, Cannon CP, et al: Fatal cardiac rupture among patients treated with thrombolytic agents and adjunctive thrombin antagonists: Observations from the Thrombolysis and Thrombin Inhibition in Myocardial Infarction 9 Study. *J Am Coll Cardiol* 33:479-487, 1999.

137. Nakamura F, Minamino T, Higashino Y, et al: Cardiac free wall rupture in acute myocardial infarction: Ameliorative effect of coronary reperfusion. *Clin Cardiol* 15:244-250, 1992.

138. Honan MB, Harrell F Jr, Reimer KA, et al: Cardiac rupture, mortality and the timing of thrombolytic therapy: A meta-analysis [see comments]. *J Am Coll Cardiol* 16:359-367, 1990.

139. Raitt MH, Kraft CD, Gardner CJ, et al: Subacute ventricular free wall rupture complicating myocardial infarction. *Am Heart J* 126:946-955, 1993.

140. Moreno R, Lopez-Sendon J, Garcia E, et al: Primary angioplasty reduces the risk of left ventricular free wall rupture compared with thrombolysis in patients with acute myocardial infarction. *J Am Coll Cardiol* 39(4):598-603, 2002.

141. Purcaro A, Costantini C, Ciampani N, et al: Diagnostic criteria and management of subacute ventricular free wall rupture complicating acute myocardial infarction. *Am J Cardiol* 80(4):397-405, 1997.

142. Lopez-Sendon J, Gonzalez A, Lopez de Sa E, et al: Diagnosis of subacute ventricular wall rupture after acute myocardial infarction: Sensitivity and specificity of clinical, hemodynamic and echocardiographic criteria. *J Am Coll Cardiol* 19:1145-1153, 1992.

143. Brack M, Asinger RW, Sharkey SW, et al: Two-dimensional echocardiographic characteristics of pericardial hematoma secondary to left ventricular free wall rupture complicating acute myocardial infarction. *Am J Cardiol* 68:961-964, 1991.

144. Purcaro A, Costantini C, Ciampani N, et al: Diagnostic criteria and management of subacute ventricular free wall rupture complicating acute myocardial infarction. *Am J Cardiol* 80:397-405, 1997.

145. Wilkenshoff UM, Ale Abaei A, Kuersten B, et al: Contrast echocardiography for detection of incomplete rupture of the left ventricle after acute myocardial infarction. *Z Kardiol* 93(8):624-629, 2004.

146. Pappas PJ, Cernaianu AC, Baldino WA, et al: Ventricular free-wall rupture after myocardial infarction. Treatment and outcome. *Chest* 99:892-895, 1991.

147. Figueras J, Cortadellas J, Evangelista A, et al: Medical management of selected patients with left ventricular free wall rupture during acute myocardial infarction. *J Am Coll Cardiol* 29:512-518, 1997.

148. Yeo TC, Malouf JF, Oh JK, et al: Clinical profile and outcome in 52 patients with cardiac pseudoaneurysm. *Ann Intern Med* 128:299-305, 1998.

149. Frances C, Romero A, Grady D: Left ventricular pseudoaneurysm. *J Am Coll Cardiol* 32:557-561, 1998.

150. Eaton LW, Weiss JL, Bulkley BH, et al: Regional cardiac dilatation after acute myocardial infarction: Recognition by two-dimensional echocardiography. *N Engl J Med* 300:57-62, 1979.

151. Siu SCB WA: Left Ventricle III: Coronary artery disease-clinical manifestations and complications. In Weyman AE (ed): *Principles and Practice of Echocardiography*, 2nd ed. Philadelphia, Lea & Febiger, 1994, pp. 656-686.

152. Ba'albaki HA, Clements SD Jr: Left ventricular aneurysm: A review. *Clin Cardiol* 12(1):5-13, 1989.

153. Faxon DP, Ryan TJ, Davis KB, et al: Prognostic significance of angiographically documented left ventricular aneurysm from the Coronary Artery Surgery Study (CASS). *Am J Cardiol* 50(1):157-164, 1982.

154. Tikiz H, Balbay Y, Atak R, et al: The effect of thrombolytic therapy on left ventricular aneurysm formation in acute myocardial infarction: relationship to successful reperfusion and vessel patency. *Clin Cardiol* 24(10):656-662, 2001.

155. Tikiz H, Ramazan A, Balbay Y, et al: Left ventricular aneurysm formation after anterior myocardial infarction: clinical and angiographic determinants in 809 patients. *Int J Cardiol* 82(1):7-14; discussion 14-16, 2002.

156. Visser CA, Kan G, Meltzer RS, et al: Incidence, timing and prognostic value of left ventricular aneurysm formation after myocardial infarction: A prospective, serial echocardiographic study of 158 patients. *Am J Cardiol* 57:729-732, 1986.

157. Stratton JR, Speck SM, Caldwell JH, et al: Late effects of intracoronary streptokinase on regional wall motion, ventricular aneurysm and left ventricular thrombus in myocardial infarction: Results from the Western Washington Randomized Trial. *J Am Coll Cardiol* 5:1023-1028, 1985.

158. Visser CA, Kan G, Meltzer RS, et al: Assessment of left ventricular aneurysm resectability by two-dimensional echocardiography. *Am J Cardiol* 56:857-860, 1985.

159. Ryan T, Petrovic O, Armstrong WF, et al: Quantitative two-dimensional echocardiographic assessment of patients undergoing left ventricular aneurysmectomy. *Am Heart J* 111:714-720, 1986.

160. Sartipy U, Albage A, LIndblom A: The Dor procedure for left ventricular reconstruction. Ten-year clinical experience. *Eur J Cardiothorac Surg* 27(6):1005-1010, 2005.

161. Greaves SC, Zhi G, Lee RT, et al: Incidence and natural history of left ventricular thrombus following anterior wall acute myocardial infarction. *Am J Cardiol* 80(4):442-448, 1997.

162. Mooe T, Teien D, Karp K, et al: Long term follow up of patients with anterior myocardial infarction complicated by left ventricular thrombus in the thrombolytic era. *Heart* 75:252-256, 1996.

163. Domenicucci, S, Chiarella, F, Bellotti, P, et al: Long-term prospective assessment of left ventricular thrombus in anterior wall acute myocardial infarction and implications for a rational approach to embolic risk. *Am J Cardiol* 839:519-524, 1999.

164. Eigler N, Maurer G, Shah PK: Effect of early systemic thrombolytic therapy on left ventricular mural thrombus formation in acute anterior myocardial infarction. *Am J Cardiol* 54:261-263, 1984.

165. Lupi G, Domenicucci S, Chiarella F, et al: Influence of thrombolytic treatment followed by full dose anticoagulation on the frequency of left ventricular thrombi in acute myocardial infarction. *Am J Cardiol* 64:588-590, 1989.

166. Natarajan D, Hotchandani RK, Nigam PD: Reduced incidence of left ventricular thrombi with intravenous streptokinase in acute anterior myocardial infarction: Prospective evaluation by cross-sectional echocardiography. *Int J Cardiol* 20:201-207, 1988.

167. Bhatnagar SK, al-Yusuf AR: Effects of intravenous recombinant tissue-type plasminogen activator therapy on the incidence and associations of left ventricular thrombus in patients with a first acute Q wave anterior myocardial infarction. *Am Heart J* 122:1251-1256, 1991.

168. Turpie AG, Robinson JG, Doyle DJ, et al: Comparison of high-dose with low-dose subcutaneous heparin to prevent left ventricular mural thrombosis in patients with acute transmural anterior myocardial infarction. *N Engl J Med* 320:352-357, 1989.

169. Rehan A, Kanwar M, Rosman H, et al: Incidence of post myocardial infarction left ventricular thrombus formation in the era of primary percutaneous intervention and glycoprotein IIb/IIIa inhibitors. A prospective observational study. *Cardiovasc Ultrasound* 4:20, 200.

170. Kalra J, Jang IK: Prevalence of early left ventricular thrombus after primary coronary intervention for acute myocardial infarction. *J Thromb Thrombolysis* 10(2):133-136, 2000.

171. Thanigaraj S, Schechtman KB, Perez JE: Improved echocardiographic delineation of left ventricular thrombus with the use of intravenous second-generation contrast image enhancement. *J Am Soc Echocardiogr* 12:1022-1026, 1999.

172. Chesebro JH, Ezekowitz M, Badimon L, et al: Intracardiac thrombi and systemic thromboembolism: Detection, incidence, and treatment. *Annu Rev Med* 36:579-605, 1985.

173. Visser CA, Kan G, Meltzer RS, et al: Embolic potential of left ventricular thrombus after myocardial infarction: A two-dimensional echocardiographic study of 119 patients. *J Am Coll Cardiol* 5:1276-1280, 1985.

174. Domenicucci S, Bellotti P, Chiarella F, et al: Spontaneous morphologic changes in left ventricular thrombi: A prospective two-dimensional echocardiographic study. *Circulation* 75:737-743, 1987.

175. Keating EC, Gross SA, Schlamowitz RA, et al: Mural thrombi in myocardial infarctions. Prospective evaluation by two-dimensional echocardiography. *Am J Med* 74:989-995, 1983.

176. Kouvaras G, Chronopoulos G, Soufras G, et al: The effects of long-term antithrombotic treatment on left ventricular thrombi in patients after an acute myocardial infarction. *Am Heart J* 119:73-78, 1990.

177. Domenicucci S, Chiarella F, Bellotti P, et al: Long-term prospective assessment of left ventricular thrombus in anterior wall acute myocardial infarction and implications for a rational approach to embolic risk. *Am J Cardiol* 839:519-524, 1999.

178. Glikson M, Agranat O, Ziskind Z, et al: From swirling to a mobile, pedunculated mass—the evolution of left ventricular thrombus despite full anticoagulation. Echocardiographic demonstration. *Chest* 103(1):281-283, 1993.

179. White HD, Norris RM, Brown MA, et al: Left ventricular end-systolic volume as the major determinant of survival after recovery from myocardial infarction. *Circulation* 76(1):44-51, 1987.

180. Kan G, Visser CA, Koolen JJ, et al: Short and long term predictive value of admission wall motion score in acute myocardial infarction. A cross sectional echocardiographic study of 345 patients. *Br Heart J* 56:422-427, 1986.

181. Shiina A, Tajik AJ, Smith HC, et al: Prognostic significance of regional wall motion abnormality in patients with prior myocardial infarction: A prospective correlative study of two-dimensional echocardiography and angiography. *Mayo Clin Proc* 61:254-262, 1986.

182. Husic M, Norager B, Egstrup K, et al: Diastolic wall motion abnormality after myocardial infarction: relation to neurohormonal activation and prognostic implications. *Am Heart J* 150(4):767-774, 2005.

183. Stamm RB, Gibson RS, Bishop HL, et al: Echocardiographic detection of infarct-localized asynergy and remote asynergy during acute myocardial infarction: correlation with the extent of angiographic coronary disease. *Circulation* 67:233-244, 1983.

184. Pozzoli M, Capomolla S, Sanarico M, et al: Doppler evaluations of left ventricular diastolic filling and pulmonary wedge pressure provide similar prognostic information in patients with systolic dysfunction after myocardial infarction. *Am Heart J* 129:716-725, 1995.

185. Sakata K, Kashiro S, Hirata S, et al: Prognostic value of Doppler transmitral flow velocity patterns in acute myocardial infarction. *Am J Cardiol* 79:1165-1169, 1997.

186. Nijland F, Kamp O, Karreman AJ, et al: Prognostic implications of restrictive left ventricular filling in acute myocardial infarction: a serial Doppler echocardiographic study. *J Am Coll Cardiol* 30:1618-1624, 1997.

187. Moller JE, Sondergaard E, Poulsen SH: Pseudonormal and restrictive filling patterns predict left ventricular dilation and cardiac death after a first myocardial infarct: a serial color M-mode Doppler echocardiographic study. *J Am Coll Cardiol* 36(6):1841-1846, 2000.

188. Moller JE, Sondergaard E, Poulsen SH, et al: Color M-mode and pulsed wave tissue Doppler echocardiography: powerful predictors of cardiac events after first myocardial infarction. *J Am Soc Echocardiogr* 14(8):757-763, 2001.

189. Hillis GS, Moller JE, Pellikka PA, et al: Noninvasive estimation of left ventricular filling pressure by E/e′ is a powerful predictor of survival after acute myocardial infarction. *J Am Coll Cardiol* 43(4):360-367, 2004.

190. Moller JE, Poulsen SH, Sondergaard E, et al: Impact of early changes in left ventricular filling pattern on long-term outcome after acute myocardial infarction. *Int J Cardiol* 89(2-3):207-215, 2003.

191. Beinart R, Bovko V, Schwamm E, et al: Long-term prognostic significance of left atrial volume in acute myocardial infarction. *J Am Coll Cardiol* 44(2):327-334, 2004.

192. Moller JE, Hillis GS, Oh JK, et al: Left atrial volume: a powerful predictor of survival after acute myocardial infarction. *Circulation* 107(17):2207-2212, 2003.

193. de Kam PJ, Nicolosi GL, Voors AA, et al: Prediction of 6 months left ventricular dilatation after myocardial infarction in relation to cardiac morbidity and mortality. Application of a new dilatation model to GISSI-3 data. *Eur Heart J* 23(7):536-542, 2002.

194. St John Sutton M, Scott CH: A prediction rule for left ventricular dilatation post-MI? *Eur Heart J* 23(7):509-511, 2002.

195. Jugdutt BI, Khan MI, Jugdutt SJ, et al: Combined captopril and isosorbide dinitrate during healing after myocardial infarction. Effect on ventricular remodeling, function, mass and collagen. *J Am Coll Cardiol* 25:1089-1096, 1995.

196. Senior R, Basu S, Kinsey C, et al: Carvedilol prevents remodeling in patients with left ventricular dysfunction after acute myocardial infarction. *Am Heart J* 137(4 Pt 1):646-652, 1999.

197. Greaves K, Dixon SR, Fejka M, et al: Myocardial contrast echocardiography is superior to other known modalities for assessing myocardial reperfusion after acute myocardial infarction. *Heart* 89(2):139-144, 2003.

198. Balcells E, Powers ER, Lepper W, et al: Detection of myocardial viability by contrast echocardiography in acute infarction predicts recovery of resting function and contractile reserve. *J Am Coll Cardiol* 41(5):827-833, 2003.

199. Hillis GS, Mulvagh SL, Pellikka PA, et al: Comparison of intravenous myocardial contrast echocardiography and low-dose dobutamine echocardiography for predicting left ventricular functional recovery following acute myocardial infarction. *Am J Cardiol* 92(5):504-508, 2003.

200. Main ML, Magalski A, Morris BA, et al: Combined assessment of microvascular integrity and contractile reserve improves differentiation of stunning and necrosis after acute anterior wall myocardial infarction. *J Am Coll Cardiol* 40(6):1079-1084, 2002.

201. Mengozzi G, Rossini R, Palagi C, et al: Usefulness of intravenous myocardial contrast echoardiography in the early left ventricular remodeling in acute myocardial infarction. *Am J Cardiol* 90(7):713-719, 2002.

202. Jeetley P, Swinburn J, Hickman M, et al: Myocardial contrast echocardiography predicts left ventricular remodelling after acute myocardial infarction. *J Am Soc Echocardiogr* 17(10):1030-1036, 2004.

203. Pierard LA: Comparison of approaches in the assessment of myocardial viability and follow-up of PTCA/CABG. The role of echocardiography. *Int J Card Imaging* 1:11-17, 1993.

204. Coletta C, Sestili A, Seccareccia F, et al: Influence of contractile reserve and inducible ischaemia on left ventricular remodelling after acute myocardial infarction. *Heart* 89(10):1138-1143, 2003.

205. Nijland F, Kamp O, Verhorst PM, et al: Myocardial viability: impact on left ventricular dilatation after acute myocardial infarction. *Heart* 87(1):17-22, 2002.

206. Bolognese L, Buonamici P, Cerisano G, et al: Early dobutamine echocardiography predicts improvement in regional and global left ventricular function after reperfused acute myocardial infarction without residual stenosis of the infarct-related artery. *Am Heart J* 139(1 Pt 1):153-163, 2000.

207. Smart SC, Sawada S, Ryan T, et al: Low-dose dobutamine echocardiography detects reversible dysfunction after thrombolytic therapy of acute myocardial infarction. *Circulation* 88(2):405-415, 1993.

208. Abe Y, Muro T, Sakanoue Y, et al: Intravenous myocardial contrast echocardiography predicts regional and global left ventricular remodelling after acute myocardial infarction: comparison with low dose dobutamine stress echocardiography. *Heart* 91(12):1578-1583, 2005.

209. Greco CA, Salustri A, Seccareccia F, et al: Prognostic value of dobutamine echocardiography early after uncomplicated acute myocardial infarction: a comparison with exercise electrocardiography. *J Am Coll Cardiol* 29(2):261-267, 1997.

210. Sicari R, Landi P, Picano E, et al: Exercise-electrocardiography and/or pharmacological stress echocardiography for non-invasive risk stratification early after uncomplicated myocardial infarction. A prospective international large scale multicentre study. *Eur Heart J* 23(13):1030-1037, 2002.

211. Trichon BH, Felker GM, Shaw LK, et al: Relation of frequency and severity of mitral regurgitation to survival among patients with left ventricular systolic dysfunction and heart failure. *Am J Cardiol* 91(5):538-543, 2003.

212. Bursi F, Enriquez-Sarano M, Jacobsen SJ, et al: Mitral regurgitation after myocardial infarction: a review. *Am J Med* 119(2):103-112, 2006.

213. Bursi F, Enriquez-Sarano M, Nkomo VT, et al: Heart failure and death after myocardial infarction in the community: the emerging role of mitral regurgitation. *Circulation* 111(3):295-301, 2005.

214. Bhatnagar SK, al Yusuf AR: Significance of a mitral regurgitation systolic murmur complicating a first acute myocardial infarction in the coronary care unit—assessment by colour Doppler flow imaging. *Eur Heart J* 12(12):1311-1315, 1991.

215. Barzilai B, Gessler C Jr, Perez JE, et al: Significance of Doppler-detected mitral regurgitation in acute myocardial infarction. *Am J Cardiol* 61(4):220-223, 1988.

216. Levine RA, Schwammenthal E: Ischemic mitral regurgitation on the threshold of a solution: from paradoxes to unifying concepts. *Circulation* 112(5):745-758, 2005.

217. Feinberg MS, Schwammenthal E, Shlizerman L, et al: Prognostic significance of mild mitral regurgitation by color Doppler echocardiography in acute myocardial infarction. *Am J Cardiol* 86(9):903-907, 2000.

218. Gorman RC, Gorman JH 3rd: Why should we repair ischemic mitral regurgitation? *Ann Thorac Surg* 81(2):785; author reply 785-786, 2006.

219. Roshanali F, Mandegar MH, Yousefnia MA, et al: Low-dose dobutamine stress echocardiography to predict reversibility of mitral regurgitation with CABG. *Echocardiography* 23(1):31-37, 2006.

Chapter 15

Exercise Echocardiography

ROSARIO V. FREEMAN, MD, MS

The author acknowledges Pamela Marcovitz, MD, the previous author of this chapter in *The Practice of Clinical Echocardiography*, 2nd edition.

Stress echocardiography integrates echocardiographic imaging with exercise electrocardiogram (ECG) testing to aid in the evaluation of ischemic, valvular, and cardiopulmonary heart disease. By providing direct, real-time visualization of myocardial function, the accuracy for stress echocardiography to detect the extent and location of myocardial ischemia is excellent, particularly when baseline ECG abnormalities render standard exercise ECG testing nondiagnostic.[1,2] In addition to the initial diagnosis of coronary artery disease (CAD), stress echocardiography can monitor disease progression and assess the clinical response to medical therapy in those with known disease.[3] Stress echocardiography also provides information on myocardial viability, risk stratification, and prognostication.[3] Nonischemia applications include management of cardiopulmonary, congenital, and valvular heart disease. Future advances utilize three-dimensional (3D) imaging, tissue Doppler interrogation with stress and strain imaging for additional measures of myocardial function, and the potential to integrate coronary flow reserve data with myocardial perfusion imaging.

The premise of stress echocardiography is provocation of myocardial ischemia by one of various cardiac stressors.[4] Nonexercise cardiac stressors include pharmacologic and pacing protocols (see Chapter 16). Exercise stressors include various treadmill and bicycle ergometry protocols. Images are acquired either during peak exercise or, because of imaging difficulty resulting from patient motion, immediately following exercise cessation.

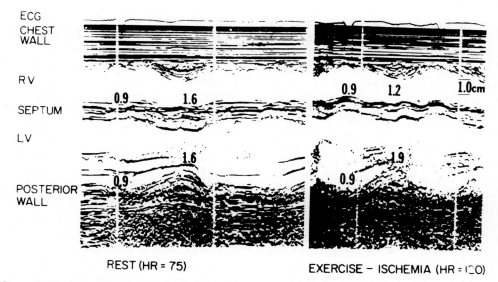

Figure 15–1. Stress test with M-mode. ECG, electrocardiogram; HR, heart rate; LV, left ventricle; RV, right ventricle. (From Mason SJ, Weiss JL, Weisfeldt ML, et al: Circulation 59[1]:50-59, 1979.)

Imaging data is then integrated with ECG data, exercise tolerance, and patient symptoms for final interpretation.

The capability of echocardiography to detect myocardial ischemia was shown over three decades ago in animal models demonstrating concordance between regional wall motion abnormalities and the severity and duration of perfusion impairment.[5-7] Early corroborating human studies identified lesions in the left anterior descending (LAD) artery distribution, demonstrating reduced septal motion via M-mode imaging.[8] In one of the earliest human descriptions of inducible ischemia using echocardiography in concert with bicycle exercise, septal wall motion abnormalities seen with M-mode imaging were correlated with LAD lesions[9] (Fig. 15–1). However, the inability to image more than a discrete portion of the myocardium with M-mode was limiting. The advent of two-dimensional (2D) echocardiography in the 1980s allowing for tomographic cardiac imaging increased utility for ischemia assessment. Advances in transducer performance, harmonic imaging, and digital loop grabbers have dramatically improved image quality and simplified interpretation. Increased availability and the relative ease of establishing a laboratory have made stress echocardiography an easily accessible, first line diagnostic tool.[10,11] Within the United States last year alone, over three million stress echocardiographic studies were performed.

Physiologic Principles of Exercise Echocardiography

In the absence of ischemia, exercise provokes an increase in regional wall thickening and systolic function. In the presence of a hemodynamically significant coro-

nary stenosis, increases in myocardial oxygen demand result in a relative disparity in oxygen supply. Transient hypoperfusion leads to mechanical dysfunction of the affected myocardium. Stress echocardiography is well suited for assessing the response to ischemia by directly visualizing myocardial function, assessing the physiologic significance of a coronary narrowing. Localization of the stenosis based on the myocardial segments affected is reasonable as coronary artery anatomy and myocardial distribution are relatively maintained among humans[12] (see Fig. 14–2).

Myocardial ischemia progresses in a well-defined sequence of events, termed the *ischemic cascade,* initiated by regional hypoperfusion of a distal coronary bed.[13] Metabolic changes occur within the affected myocardium. Following this, there are alterations in diastolic function with subsequent systolic dysfunction of affected segments. Only in the later stages of ischemia are characteristic ECG changes (ST segment depression) and angina manifest[14-17] (Fig. 15–2). Standard

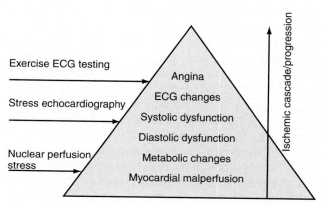

Figure 15–2. Ischemic cascade. ECG, electrocardiogram.

exercise ECG testing detects ischemia in the later stages of the ischemic cascade, contributing to the acknowledged limitations in diagnostic accuracy (decreased sensitivity). In contrast, imaging modalities identify ischemia earlier, at onset of systolic dysfunction. With cessation of the stressor and restoration of adequate coronary flow, induced abnormalities typically recover rapidly but may be persistent if ischemia is severe or prolonged. Echocardiographic imaging during angioplasty in humans demonstrates onset of regional systolic dysfunction as early as 19 seconds following balloon inflation with ischemic ECG changes and angina occurring 30 to 40 seconds after inflation. Resolution of these abnormalities typically occurs within 10 to 20 seconds after balloon deflation.[14,17,18] Angioplasty balloon inflation models demonstrate ischemia during dynamic obstruction. Imaging during provoked ischemia with a fixed coronary obstruction has shown similar temporal progression with onset of mechanical dysfunction preceding ECG changes and angina.[15,19]

In the absence of a physiologically significant coronary narrowing, the myocardial response to stress is augmentation of systolic function with increased inward motion, termed *hyperdynamic* function. However, myocardium perfused by coronary beds distal to an occlusion will demonstrate regional contractile abnormalities if an increase in myocardial oxygen demand produces a transient oxygen deficit.

Myocardial responses to ischemia include:

1. *Hypokinesis:* myocardial thickening with inward motion less than 5 mm or relatively less than the rest of the myocardium
2. *Akinesis:* absence of thickening or inward motion
3. *Dyskinesis:* thinned myocardium with paradoxical outward systolic motion

The myocardial response to exercise is representative of coronary disease status. In the absence of disease, baseline systolic function is generally normal and myocardial response is hyperdynamic (Fig. 15–3). In ischemic but noninfarcted myocardium, the stress response is concordant with ischemia severity. In more severe cases, hypokinesis progresses to akinesis. Following an infarction, the appearance of the myocardium is altered. Acutely infarcted myocardium appears hypokinetic or akinetic with normal wall thickness as postinfarct remodeling has not yet occurred. When blood flow is restored to acutely infarcted myocardium, return of function is variable both temporally and spatially. Regions of transmural infarct subject to prolonged ischemia are likely to remain hypocontractile. Chronically infarcted regions with transmural injury appear thinned and akinetic with persistent akinesis or dyskinesis. Myocardium subjected to only a short duration of coronary flow limitation, may return to a normal contractile state. However, recovery may be delayed for days up to months, termed *myocardial*

stunning. Prediction of recovery of stunned segments is feasible with low dose dobutamine stress echocardiography (DSE) (see Chapter 16).

Studies of coronary disease severity demonstrate that the effect on ventricular wall motion and thickening are proportional to the severity of impaired coronary blood flow.[19-21] The greater the occlusion severity or area affected, the greater the likelihood of provoking a perceptible abnormality. For intermediate range lesions or isolated single-vessel disease in which only a few myocardial segments are affected, abnormalities during ischemia may be subtle or transient. Assuming an adequate stressor is used, the coronary narrowing in which systolic dysfunction is generally perceptible is in the range of 50% to 60%; akinesis is seen when a greater than 80% reduction in coronary flow is present.[20,22,23] However, this range is not absolute, as a visual estimate of stenosis severity may not necessarily correlate with the physiologic significance of an occlusion, particularly in the case of intermediate range lesions.

Exercise Stressors Used for Stress Echocardiography

Exercise stress is preferred over nonexercise stressors in individuals able to exercise maximally, as it allows for a contextual understanding of results relative to patient symptoms and functional capacity. Exercise stressors should be used unless the patient is unlikely to achieve at least 5 metabolic equivalent units (METS) or is unable to use the exercise equipment. The types of exercise protocols most widely utilized are treadmill and bicycle ergometry (upright or supine). The type of stress employed varies according to equipment availability and the patient's familiarity with the form of exercise. In the United States, treadmill protocols remain the predominant form; whereas in Europe, bicycling is a more familiar activity and more commonly used for diagnostic purposes.

Regardless of the type of exercise stress, an adequate workload is necessary to provide a diagnostic study. The most common hemodynamic target is a peak heart rate (HR) based on patient age and gender, calculated as 85% of the maximal predicted HR: (220 − patient's age − [an additional 10 if female]). If necessary, workload can be augmented to reach target with other measures, such as hyperventilation or handgrip exercise.[24] Although handgrip exercise alone can produce an increase in afterload adequate to induce ischemia, in practice it is difficult to implement as patients often are unable to sustain handgrip exercise for more than 2 to 4 minutes. It is institution and physician dependent whether exercise is discontinued once hemodynamic targets are achieved or whether the patient is asked to continue to maximum exercise capacity.

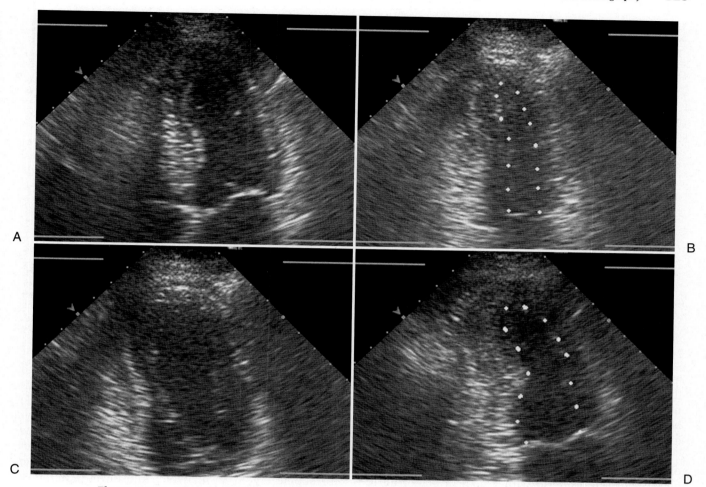

Figure 15–3. *Normal exercise echocardiogram study. Following exercise stress, there is hyperdynamic function of all segments with a decrease in chamber size (endocardial border traced in dotted line). A, Apical four-chamber view at rest; B, apical four-chamber view at stress; C, apical two-chamber view at rest; D, apical two-chamber view at stress.*

With treadmill exercise protocols, baseline echocardiographic images are obtained in a left lateral decubitus position to facilitate acoustic access (Table 15–1). The patient then proceeds with exercise according to standardized protocols.[25,26] Less voluntary effort is needed with treadmill versus bicycle protocols as the treadmill proceeds at prespecified speeds, and the patient paces with the treadmill belt. Most patients who are reasonably active perform the Bruce protocol. However, in patients with mobility restrictions or limited exercise tolerance, the Cornell or Naughton protocols are other options to allow for at least 6 to 12 minutes of continuous exercise. The treadmill portion is halted if significant symptoms develop (severe angina, ataxia, dizziness, pallor), there are concerning ECG changes, arrhythmias, or hemodynamic targets are achieved.[27]

Because patient motion limits imaging during active treadmill use, stress imaging is typically performed immediately following exercise cessation without a cooldown period. The duration of ischemia induced abnormalities is variable and dependent on the severity of coronary occlusion, number of vessels affected, existence of collateral blood flow, and workload achieved.[28,29] Although induced abnormalities can persist for some time after exercise cessation, most reverse within minutes of relative oxygen deficit restoration. Therefore, expeditious imaging is critical to maximize the likelihood of identifying transient ischemia. Reasonable agility is required as patients need to transition to the imaging table, reassume a left lateral decubitus position, and allow time for imaging within 60 to 90 seconds after exercise completion. Immediate postimaging imaging is "all-or-nothing." If prolonged delays in patient transfer occur or acoustic windows are suboptimal, transient ischemia may not be identified. This is particularly true in the case of intermediate range occlusions or single-vessel disease

TABLE 15-1. Exercise Stress Protocols for Echocardiography

Treadmill	Upright Bicycle	Supine Bicycle
1. Patient on imaging bed Image parasternal LAX Image parasternal SAX Image apical four-chamber view Image apical two-chamber view	1. Patient on imaging bed Image parasternal LAX Image parasternal SAX	1. Patient on integrated imaging bed Image parasternal LAX Image parasternal SAX Image apical four-chamber view Image apical two-chamber view
2. Patient moves to treadmill	2. Patient moves to bicycle	2. Patient remains on integrated bed
3. Exercise commences	3. Image apical rest views	3. Exercise commences
4. Exercise cessation	4. Exercise commences	4. Imaging at each stage end
5. Patient moves to imaging bed Postexercise imaging	5. Imaging at each stage end	5. Exercise cessation
	6. Exercise cessation	6. Postexercise imaging
	7. Patient moves to imaging bed Postexercise imaging	

LAX, long-axis view; SAX, short-axis view.

in which induced abnormalities may be fleeting. Although feasibility of peak stress imaging on the treadmill has been demonstrated, the minimal incremental benefit coupled with difficulties in obtaining reproducible results limit widespread use.[30]

For upright bicycle ergometry, baseline images are obtained in a left lateral decubitus position. Patients perform bicycle exercise with a goal of achieving increases in wattage, lasting 2 to 3 minutes per stage. Because the workload is effort driven, achievement of maximal workload is more patient dependent than treadmill protocols. Bicycle protocols allow for maintenance of a relatively stationary position for simultaneous image acquisition during active exercise.[29,32] Imaging concurrent with peak stress is an advantage over immediate posttreadmill imaging, increasing the sensitivity for detecting transient abnormalities.[29,33-35] If apical windows are not easily accessible during exercise, use of subcostal views is an alternative.[31] Although a more lordotic position is needed to avoid apical foreshortening, most myocardial segments can be visualized. After exercise completion, the patient reassumes a left lateral decubitus position for further imaging. An alternative to upright bicycle is supine bicycle ergometry with use of integrated imaging stretchers that allow for patient rotation and positioning such that transition to a separate imaging bed is obviated, resulting in time savings.

In the United States, treadmill stress is favored over bicycle ergometry because of the widespread availability of treadmills in hospital settings, and the familiarity of walking as a form of exercise. Treadmill ECG testing, as an established diagnostic modality, is also well validated, providing a wealth of prognostic information

referenced to exercise duration and ECG response to exercise. Patients performing treadmill exercise are generally able to achieve a higher workload than bicycle exercise, increasing the likelihood of attaining hemodynamic targets. During bicycle protocols, if quadriceps fatigue precedes maximal workload, patients may prematurely discontinue exercise. This is particularly true for supine ergometry in which the lower extremities must be supported against gravity, with development of angina at a lower workload.

In Europe, where bicycling as a more common form of exercise, upright bicycle protocols are more favored. Guided by a real-time evaluation of wall motion, bicycle protocols allow for ischemia detection at its onset, allowing for identification of the ischemic threshold and the theoretical advantage of increased safety over treadmill protocols, which use ECG changes or symptom onset to identify the time point to discontinue exercise. Real-time identification of ischemia may allow for increased detection of subtle or transient ischemia in those with single-vessel disease or intermediate range lesions. Bicycle protocols also offer the ability to obtain and optimize imaging without the all-or nothing constraints of a narrow immediate poststress imaging window. The choice of which stressor to employ should be individualized to the ability of the patient to perform the exercise, the experience level of the personnel administering the study, and the availability of equipment. In published reports comparing the accuracy of the different exercise protocols, the incremental difference is minimal.[33,35,36] Regardless of the stressor employed, as long as an adequate workload is achieved, the overall accuracy is likely comparable.[37]

Methodology

Equipment

The current standard for laboratories performing exercise echocardiography includes high-quality instruments with a digital frame grabber, harmonic imaging capability for image enhancement, and an offline analysis system. Dependent on the type of stress employed, appropriate equipment (treadmill or bicycle ergometer) should be available, as should imaging beds with lateral cutouts to facilitate apical imaging. A cardiac arrest cart and defibrillator should be easily accessible.

Digital frame grabbers and split screen displays allow side-by-side comparison of rest and stress images to facilitate identification of regional wall motion abnormalities. Digital frame capture rates range from 20 to 100 msec intervals, which can be looped and replayed continuously for analysis.[38,39] These intervals allow for variable capture within the cardiac cycle ranging from systole alone to the entire cardiac cycle length. Most systems acquire eight frame digital loops per view with 50 msec allowed for each frame. This duration is generally adequate; however, if the HR exceeds 150 beats per minute, image quality may be enhanced by reducing the capture interval to 30 to 40 msec. An approximately 10 to 20 second digital clip per view is needed for adequate wall motion analysis. These clips can then be displayed in a continuous loop format for review and comparison. Image gating to the ECG allows for analysis of endocardial motion at the same point in the cardiac cycle between the baseline and stress images to identify interval changes in regional function. A videotaped backup recording of the study is helpful to ensure that the digital loops accurately reflect myocardial motion.[40]

Procedure

A brief history is taken to document symptoms and atherosclerosis risk factors. The medication list is confirmed and basic laboratory findings are reviewed. Patients should refrain from oral intake for 4 hours before the procedure. Medications, which may impact workload achieved (i.e., atrioventricular nodal blocking agents), should be temporarily held for 1 to 2 doses, but if the purpose of the study is to diagnose ischemia while on active therapy or if the risk of an adverse event off of the medication is deemed too high, then the study may ensue on the medication. Telemetry leads are placed at standard limb and precordial sites, slightly displacing leads that interfere with acoustic windows. One ECG lead is concurrently displayed on the echocardiography monitor to correlate wall motion changes with ECG abnormalities. Information on HR, rhythm, exercise capacity, and blood pressure are recorded (Table 15–2). If significant ischemia develops,

TABLE 15–2. Standard Exercise Electrocardiogram Testing: Measurement Parameters

Hemodynamic and Symptomatic Parameters
1. Blood pressure and heart rate response
2. Exercise duration
3. Heart rate recovery following exercise cessation
4. Time to onset and resolution of angina
5. Other cardiopulmonary symptoms (presyncope, dyspnea)

ECG Parameters
1. ST segment elevation/depression and slope
2. Arrhythmias
3. Number of leads involved
4. Time to onset and resolution of ST abnormalities

ECG, electrocardiogram.
Adapted from Gibbons RJ, Balady GJ, Bricker JT, et al: *J Am Coll Cardiol* 40(8):1531-1540, 2002.

the study may be discontinued at the discretion of the supervising medical professional, depending on patient symptoms and severity of the abnormality. The most common ECG criterion for myocardial ischemia is greater than 1-mm horizontal or downsloping ST depression at least 60 ms after the end of the QRS complex.[27]

Optimal acoustic windows are located and baseline echocardiographic images obtained. If anatomic abnormalities are seen, a brief study should be performed to detect any undiagnosed conditions that may affect the study. Examples include unknown ventricular dysfunction, significant valvular abnormalities, or pericardial effusion. The baseline screening examination also allows for assessment of image quality and optimal acoustic windows. If image quality is suboptimal, as can be seen in up to 20% of cases, an intravenous (IV) line can be placed and transpulmonary contrast can be used to enhance endocardial border definition (Fig. 15–4). Contrast use can be particularly helpful in the assessment of anterior and lateral wall motion, regions that may be more difficult to see in larger patients or those with pulmonary disease. Because peak contrast effects with transpulmonary agents last only 1 to 2 minutes after injection, separate injections are needed for baseline and stress images. For treadmill studies, contrast is usually injected during peak exercise so it is in place during poststress imaging.

Imaging

Myocardial segments are imaged in multiple views to fully evaluate the heart and avoid misdiagnosis resulting from an oblique image plane. The four basic views used for stress echocardiography are concordant with standard transthoracic tomographic planes and include the parasternal short- and long-axis views and the apical four- and two-chamber views. Subcostal views are not commonly used but may be substituted

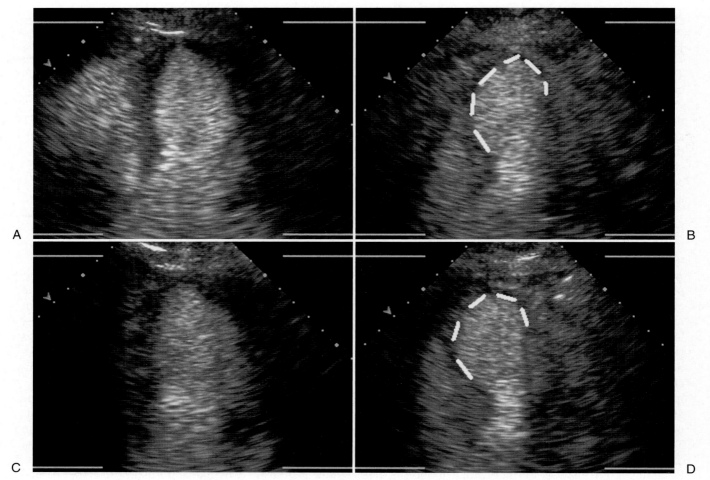

A

B

C

D

Figure 15–4. *Example of abnormal treadmill stress echocardiogram with contrast (A-D). A 56-year-old without prior history of coronary artery disease went 8 minutes on a standard Bruce protocol. Definity transpulmonary contrast was used to enhance the endocardial border. Following exercise, aneurysmal dilation, and hypokinesis was seen in the distal inferior wall, apex and distal anterior wall (highlighted with dashes). A, Apical four-chamber view at rest; B, apical four-chamber view at stress; C, apical two-chamber view at rest; D, apical two-chamber view at stress.*

in the rare instance when they provide better images, such with intervening lung tissue as a result of chronic pulmonary disease.[31] Because induced abnormalities may normalize quickly, the imaging sequence for the immediate posttreadmill images usually starts with apical windows for more complete ventricular evaluation, then moving to the parasternal windows. However, views and sequencing can and should be tailored as needed. Once baseline images are obtained, acoustic windows are identified and marked to minimize need for transducer repositioning during poststress imaging. Several digital loops are acquired in each view in rapid sequence to optimize subsequent image loop selection for comparison. Vigorous cardiac contraction and exaggerated respiration increases translational and rotational movement of the heart through the scanning sector. Patients with excessive cardiac motion resulting from exaggerated respiratory effort

should briefly halt respiration at end- or mid-expiration to aid in maintaining a relatively constant imaging plane. This maneuver also aids in imaging those in whom variably interpositioned lung tissue interferes.

Doppler

Doppler echocardiography is not routinely performed during ischemia evaluation. Rapid HR and additional time requirements for imaging beyond immediate poststress imaging do not allow for reliable data acquisition. However, research-based Doppler applications during peak stress imaging have provided additive information on left ventricular (LV) function. These Doppler-derived indicators of myocardial response to stress include LV ejection velocities, aortic systolic ejection rates, and transmitral filling velocities.[41,42] Increased research applications of tissue Doppler to measure myocardial velocities have shown utility as well and may play a role in supplementing standard wall motion analysis. However, in its current state, the additional time demands of Doppler interrogation coupled with the relatively small incremental gain in information has limited widespread use.

Tailored Doppler interrogation integrated with exercise echocardiography can provide valuable clinical information for the evaluation of valvular heart disease with the capability to provide estimates of transvalvular pressure gradients and pulmonary pressures. In patients with significant valvular lesions who have equivocal symptoms or are asymptomatic, exercise echocardiography provides objective data on exercise tolerance, symptom provocation, hemodynamic effects of exercise, and the pulmonary pressure response to exercise.[43] This data can then be used in assessing candidacy and timing for intervention. Although direct color Doppler interrogation of regurgitant valve lesions at high HRs is possible, it is often of limited value resulting from signal aliasing.

Room Layout

The layout of the room is critical to the success of the procedure. The narrow time window between exercise cessation and recording of the poststress images neces-

sitates spatial optimization to maximize time savings and facilitate image acquisition. A typical floor plan minimizes the number of steps and impediments to transfer for completing portions of the study[44] (Fig. 15–5). Blood pressure cuffs and ECG lines should be long enough to enable easy transfer to and from the imaging table. There should be adequate space around the imaging bed for the ECG and echocardiography instruments, sonographer, and medical professional supervising the study. Patients should receive clear instructions on the maneuvers required after termination of exercise to avoid introducing unnecessary delay. Often, it helps to have a practice session so that the patient knows what is expected after stress completion. Emergency medical equipment and supplies should be easily available but on the periphery so as not to be obstructive.

Personnel

Staffing for exercise echocardiography requires at least two people, a sonographer to obtain the images and a medical professional to monitor the patient and evaluate for symptom onset.[45] The exercise portion of the study should be supervised either directly by a physician or by a properly trained nurse, exercise physiologist, or physician assistant. If not directly supervising the study, a physician should be in the immediate vicinity and avail-

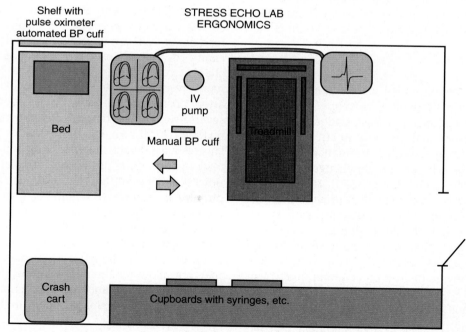

Figure 15–5. Room layout. Stress echocardiography laboratory equipment set-up. Beginning at the bottom of the figure and moving clockwise: storage cupboards with intravenous (IV) equipment, crash cart, imaging bed with shelf above for pulse oximeter and automated blood pressure (BP) cuff, echocardiography machine with frame grabber, IV pump for pharmacologic stress echocardiography, manual BP cuff, treadmill, electrocardiography (EKG) machine. The patient moves between the imaging bed and the treadmill, requiring no more than two steps in each direction (yellow arrows). (Modified from Marcovitz PA: Exercise Echocardiography, in the Practice of Clinical Echocardiography. Philadelphia, WB Saunders, 2002.)

able for emergencies.[27] In many laboratories, physician supervision is a requirement, either physically present or more remotely, observing from a monitor. Regardless of the personnel used, considerable skill on the part of the supervisor, sonographer, and/or technician is needed to facilitate an adequate study.

There is a significant learning curve for both physicians and sonographers associated with the technical challenges of image acquisition, study implementation, and interpretation. Sonographers should have completed training in standard transthoracic imaging with an additional 3 months of training in exercise echocardiography and should possess basic knowledge of coronary anatomy and myocardial distribution to aid in optimizing imaging.[46] It is recommended that sonographers complete at least 50 stress studies to claim proficiency and perform more than 10 studies per month to maintain appropriate skill level. Physicians responsible for the supervision and interpretation of studies should be at least Level II trained in echocardiography. The committee on physician training from the American Society of Echocardiography recommends physicians undergo supervised overreading of at least 100 studies to attain a minimum competence level for independent interpretation, with interpretation of more than 15 studies per month to maintain skills.[46-49] Although these volumes are reasonable for interpretation of routine studies, more specialized applications, such as the evaluation of valvular heart disease or myocardial viability, warrant more clinical expertise and volume.[48]

Interpretation

A normal study is one in which there is normal resting wall motion and a hyperdynamic response to exercise (see Fig. 15–3). Following stress, endocardial wall thickening and myocardial response to stress are compared to baseline images. With abnormal studies, location, extent, and severity of interval changes are noted and recorded (Table 15–3 and Fig. 15–6). During interpretation, comment should be made if provoked abnormalities are concordant with a probable coronary artery distribution. Regional wall motion is assessed and reported following standardized nomenclature for the myocardial segments as described in American Society of Echocardiography guidelines on chamber quantification (see Fig. 14-1).[12] Several factors can affect myocardial appearance and response to stress. These include:

1. Compensatory hyperdynamic function of nonischemic regions
2. Tethering of nonischemic regions
3. Balanced ischemia
4. Lack of hyperdynamic response to stress

With prolonged ischemia, compensatory hyperdynamic function in regions remote to ischemic zones may

TABLE 15–3. Interpretation of Myocardial Response to Stress

Resting Myocardial Appearance	Myocardium Response to Exercise	Interpretation
Normal	Hyperdynamic	Nonischemic
Normal	Hypokinetic or akinetic	Ischemic
Normal	Unchanged (lack of hyperdynamic response)	Microvascular ischemia or balanced ischemia
Hypokinetic	Akinetic	Infarcted myocardium
Akinetic	Dyskinetic	Transmural infarct

manifest as a result of a physiologic response to maintain overall cardiac output (CO).[50] If pronounced, this may mask stress-induced abnormalities in ischemic segments. Not only ischemic segments demonstrate abnormal function following a stressor. Nonischemic segments adjacent to ischemic myocardium may also exhibit decreased motion despite the presence of adequate blood flow. Termed *tethering*, this may lead to overestimation of ischemic burden.[51] Stress-induced global hypokinesis, or a lack of hyperdynamic response to exercise, can be seen in patients with disease in all major epicardial coronary arteries, or balanced ischemia. However, other markers of CAD are usually identifiable, such as significantly decreased exercise tolerance, ischemic ECG changes, or angina. Occasionally, a lack of hyperdynamic response occurs in the absence of major coronary artery obstruction: those with LV hypertrophy, diabetes, severe arterial hypertension, and hypertrophic cardiomyopathy (HCM). Angiographic studies in these patient subsets have demonstrated a reduction in coronary flow reserve despite the presence of normal epicardial blood flow. It is believed that microvascular disease is a more prominent feature, with smaller, patches of ischemia failing to manifest in frank mechanical dysfunction. Because heterogeneity in wall motion is absent in these individuals, the diagnostic accuracy to identify ischemia is lowered.[52,53] Although current diagnostic techniques may not allow for the definitive diagnosis of microvascular ischemia, advances in myocardial contrast perfusion imaging may increase understanding of this disease process in the future.

To date, interpretation of stress echocardiography examinations remains largely qualitative with visualized wall motion abnormalities the core marker of ischemia. This approach, although generally adequate for patient management, is subject to interpreter bias and experience level. In studies on the concordance of interpretation between experts, reliability and reproducibility of results is largely dependent on interpreter

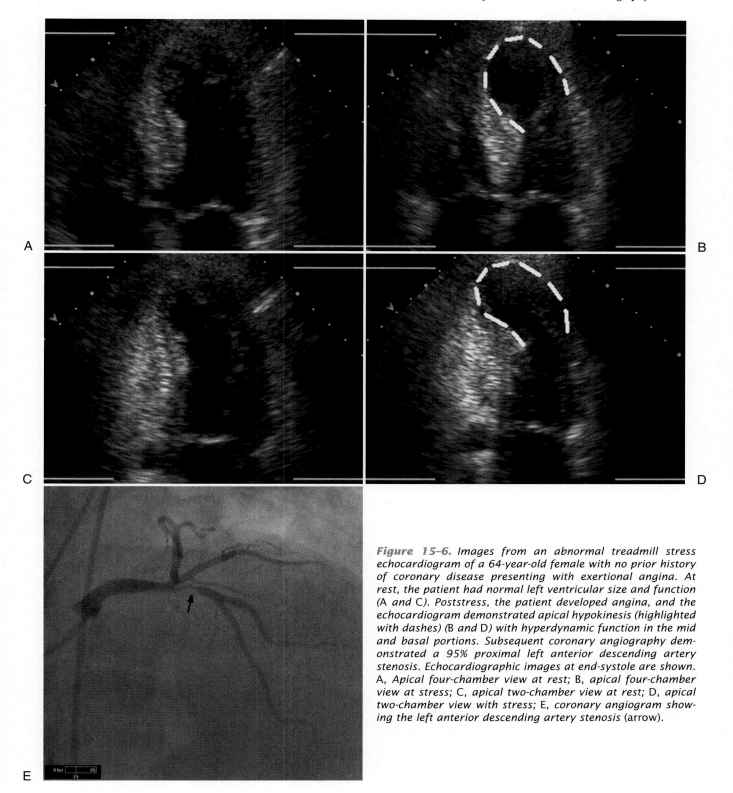

Figure 15–6. *Images from an abnormal treadmill stress echocardiogram of a 64-year-old female with no prior history of coronary disease presenting with exertional angina. At rest, the patient had normal left ventricular size and function (A and C). Poststress, the patient developed angina, and the echocardiogram demonstrated apical hypokinesis (highlighted with dashes) (B and D) with hyperdynamic function in the mid and basal portions. Subsequent coronary angiography demonstrated a 95% proximal left anterior descending artery stenosis. Echocardiographic images at end-systole are shown. A, Apical four-chamber view at rest; B, apical four-chamber view at stress; C, apical two-chamber view at rest; D, apical two-chamber view with stress; E, coronary angiogram showing the left anterior descending artery stenosis (arrow).*

experience.[49] Adequate physician and sonographer training and conservative interpretation criteria improve diagnostic sensitivity, consistency, reliability, and validity.[47,54] A logical approach to interpretation is essential. Echocardiographers should be cognizant of the patient's clinical history when assessing wall motion. For example, in patients with prior coronary bypass surgery or a history suggesting collateralized vessels, the pattern of wall motion should take into account this history. Similarly, in individuals with prior infarcts, the potential effects of tethering on adjacent nonischemic regions should be evaluated.

Interpreters should be vigilant for findings commonly diagnosed as abnormal but which do not actually signify ischemia. Such false-positive findings include abnormal septal motion relative to other segments due to ventricular pacing, an intrinsic conduction abnormality, or postoperative changes. Another common false septal abnormality is stress-induced early relaxation of the anteroseptal region relative to other segments.[55] This early relaxation can usually be timed in the cardiac cycle to just before mitral valve opening and is not indicative of ischemia. Other commonly overdiagnosed regions include the basal inferior wall. Without prior bypass revascularization, an isolated basal wall motion abnormality should be scrutinized closely.[49] A logical approach suggests the unlikelihood of an isolated proximal wall abnormality with normal or hyperdynamic mid and distal segments.

False-negative studies are most commonly encountered as a consequence of procedural difficulties, such as when workload is inadequate and the ischemic threshold is not met, inexperienced interpreters, or with poor endocardial border definition and inferior image quality. Specific regions more subject to false-negatives, or missed ischemia, include lateral wall segments, particularly in obese patients, and those with significant interposed lung tissue in which imaging is hindered.

In the setting of a significant residual occlusion with chronic ischemia, stress echocardiography can be used to evaluate for the presence of viable myocardium, which appears hypokinetic. Minimally adequate blood flow may meet basal metabolic needs but is insufficient to support normal function. The distinction between viable or frankly infarcted myocardium is important for patient management as revascularization of viable tissue improves long-term survival with improvement in systolic function and reduction in the ischemic burden.[56] Following a low level of stress, there is mild augmentation in wall motion but with higher levels of the stress, affected segments become ischemic with hypokinesis or akinesis. This "biphasic" response is the hallmark of viable myocardium. Because of the subtlety in interval wall motion changes (see Fig. 14–1) identified in viability testing, exercise stressors have not proven reliable, and available protocols uniformly utilize pharmacologic stressors (see Chapter 16).

A more quantitative approach to exercise echocardiography would, in theory, provide more standardized interpretation but is labor intensive to implement. The most commonly utilized semi-quantitative application is the *Wall Motion Score Index*. The left ventricle is divided up into segments and regional wall motion in each segment is visually assessed.[12,57] Wall motion is graded between 1 and 4 depending on the severity of abnormality. A score of 1 is normal motion, 2 is hypokinetic, 3 is akinetic, and 4 is dyskinetic, with a score of 0 for hyperkinetic segments. The total sum is divided by the number of segments evaluated to obtain a global wall motion score index. Alternatively, individual coronary artery distributions can be assigned a regional wall motion score index, and the location and severity of coronary occlusions assessed. Similar to qualitative interpretation, overscoring of nonischemic segments tethered to ischemic myocardium may lead to overestimation of ischemic burden. In the presence of other factors, which affect normal coronary flow, such as collateral blood flow from chronic coronary disease or bypass grafting surgery, diagnostic accuracy can also be adversely affected.

Computer driven algorithms offer the potential for decreasing the time demands of quantitative analysis (see Chapter 10). The *centroid* and *centerline* algorithms gauge wall motion referenced to a baseline within the left ventricle. With the centroid method, multiple radii extending from a geometric center of mass to the endocardial and epicardial surfaces of the left ventricle are generated, and the relative difference in wall motion between the rest and stress images are compared. With the centerline method, distance measurements of the endocardium and epicardium perpendicular to the midpoint of the myocardium are compared. Relative wall thickening and motion are then assessed. Although these methods are more automated, subjective decision making on the part of the interpreter is still needed in marking the endocardial and epicardial borders. Availability of automated endocardial border recognition algorithms is increasing; however, superior image quality for accurate border delineation is needed (see Chapter 12). This requisite need is paradoxical as excellent qualitative interpretation is usually possible when image quality is superior without the time demands of quantitative measurement. Although a quantitative tool is an attractive concept to increase ease and reliability for interpretation, no currently available tools are adequate candidates to supplant standard qualitative analysis in the clinical setting.[58]

Diagnostic Accuracy of Exercise Echocardiography

The diagnostic accuracy of cardiac stress testing is generally reported as the sensitivity and specificity to detect angiographically identified lesions. When reporting diagnostic accuracy, consideration of the stenosis severity cutoff with which to denote disease presence should be evaluated. Stenoses threshold criteria create artificial distinctions in a process that in fact represents a spectrum. If the cutoff is set higher (i.e., >70% versus >50% for disease presence), patients with true ischemia but less severe occlusion would be erroneously labeled false-positive A higher setpoint increases sensitivity by increasing the likelihood of a true positive and reducing false-negatives.[20,21,59-63] Inherent in this approach are the acknowledged limitations of angiographic evaluation as a measure of hemodynamic significance.[64,65] However, limited data using quantitative angiography demonstrate excellent correlation of results, with the relative discrepancy compared to visual estimates not likely significant.[19,22,23]

Diagnostic accuracy is also affected by factors that introduce bias. Early reports on exercise echocardiography suffered from reporting bias, in which the newer modality is favored over the old. In initial studies, accuracy of standard ECG testing was compared with and without echocardiographic imaging. Because the exercise ECG portion was the same, imaging was only additive so that "worse" performance was impossible. Reporting bias was also reflected in the test populations used. Most early validation studies were performed at higher volume centers with increased clinical expertise. Such studies often recruited selected patients with prior myocardial infarction (MI), known multivessel disease, or LV dysfunction: with the high pretest probability of disease, sensitivity was increased. With acceptance of the validity of a test modality, posttest referral bias also occurs where only positive tests are referred for confirmatory testing (in this case, angiography), and negative tests are accepted as correct without verification. This source of bias most greatly affects test specificity.[66] With accepted use of a modality and its more general application, there is a drift in sensitivity and specificity as the pretest probability of disease drops. This has been seen with nuclear perfusion stress testing, a more established modality, for which larger cohort data are now available.[67]

Diagnostic accuracy also depends on the disease prevalence in the tested population, the definition of significant disease, and the criteria used to define a positive test. In interpretation, inclusion of borderline or equivocal findings (identifying a lack of a hyperdynamic response as ischemia) increases the likelihood of identifying disease and therefore raises sensitivity but at the expense of specificity by concurrently increasing false-positives. Interpreter experience is a crucial factor in accuracy of reading. If image quality is suboptimal or if there is excessive delay in transfer to the imaging bed, diagnostic accuracy suffers and sensitivity is decreased[29,34,35,37,63] (Table 15–4).

Several patient-dependent factors are relevant to diagnostic accuracy. Testing patients with a higher pre-

TABLE 15–4. Factors Affecting Exercise Echocardiography Interpretation and Accuracy

Lowered Specificity (False Positive Errors)	Lowered Sensitivity (False Negative Errors)
Hypertensive response to stress	Poor image quality
Basal inferior wall abnormalities	Excessive postexercise delay to imaging
Tethered segments	Single vessel disease
Lack of hyperdynamic response	Testing points with lower pretest disease probability
Early septal relaxation	Lateral wall abnormalities
Interventricular conduction delay or paced rhythms	Inadequate workload (suboptimal effort or meds)
Valvular heart disease with loss of contractile reserve	Multivessel disease with balanced ischemia
Cardiomyopathies	Mild or intermediate severity stenoses
Inexperienced personnel	Inexperienced personnel

test probability of CAD increases sensitivity by increasing the likelihood a positive result is correct. If a patient has single-vessel disease, the ischemic zone is relatively smaller and ischemia more difficult to detect, increasing the likelihood of a false-negative study and lowering sensitivity. Compared to the overall sensitivity of exercise echocardiography for detecting coronary artery disease (~84%), individuals with single-vessel disease and normal LV function have a lower test sensitivity for ischemia identification (~75%)[21,63,68,69] (Table 15–5). Patients who are unable to achieve a high workload are less likely to provoke an oxygen mismatch and unmask a critical coronary lesion to obtain an accurate diagnostic result.[28,29] This often occurs in those taking medications which lower the HR response to exercise (i.e., atrioventricular nodal blocking agents).

Understanding these issues, initial reports on the diagnostic accuracy of exercise echocardiography focused on the feasibility of the modality to produce an accurate and reproducible result. With advances in imaging techniques and the advent of digital capture, contemporary reports of exercise echocardiography document that feasibility approaches 95% to 99%, when performed in experienced laboratories using current instrumentation.[59-61,70-76] Overall, exercise echocardiography is both sensitive and specific for ischemia identification, with an accuracy of 85% to 90%, comparable to nuclear im-

TABLE 15–5. Selected Studies on Diagnostic Accuracy of Exercise Echocardiography

First Author (Year)	Mode	Number of Patients	Sensitivity	Sensitivity*	Specificity	Accuracy
Limacher (1983)[70]	TME	73	91%	64%	88%	90%
Armstrong (1986)[1]	TME	95	88%	—	87%	87%
Armstrong (1987)[21]	TME	123	88%	81%	86%	88%
Ryan (1988)[60]	TME	64	78%	76%	100%	86%
Pozzoli (1991)[62]	UBE	75	71%	61%	96%	80%
Marwick (1992)[63]	TME	150	84%	79%	86%	85%
Quinones (1992)[74]	TME	112	74%	59%	88%	78%
Hecht (1993)[34]	SBE	180	93%	84%	86%	91%
Ryan (1993)[32]	UBE	309	91%	86%	78%	87%
Mertes (1993)[106]	SBE	79	84%	87%	85%	85%
Marwick (1994)[208]	BE	86	88%	82%	80%	85%
Beleslin (1994)[76]	TME	136	88%	88%	82%	88%
Williams (1994)[77]	UBE	70	88%	89%	84%	86%
Roger (1995)[68]	TME	127	88%	—	72%	—
Marwick (1995)[147]	TME/UBE	161	80%	75%	81%	81%
Luotolahti (1996)[78]	UBE	118	94%	94%	70%	92%
Roger (1997)[66]	TME	340	78%	—	41%	69%
Hoffmann (1993)[79]	SBE	66	80%	79%	88%	82%
Marangelli (1994)[59]	TME	80	89%	76%	91%	90%
Dagianti (1995)[33]	SBE	60	76%	70%	94%	87%

*Sensitivity for detection of one vessel coronary disease.
TME, treadmill echocardiography; UBE, upright bicycle ergometry; SBE, supine bicycle ergometry; V, vessel.

aging techniques[77-79] (see Table 15–5). A meta-analysis of over 2600 patients drawing from 24 studies reported overall sensitivity of 85% and specificity of 77%.[80] In this meta-analysis, comparative summary receiver operating characteristic (ROC) curves demonstrated superiority of exercise echocardiography to exercise ECG testing and comparable sensitivity to exercise single photon emission computed tomography (SPECT) imaging studies, with a slight edge to echocardiography in specificity. In a re-review of this meta-analysis, ROC curves demonstrate superior diagnostic accuracy of echocardiography at higher specificity level. However, when specificity is reduced (higher sensitivity is valued) nuclear modalities perform better, resulting in overall comparable discriminatory ability[81] (Fig. 15–7).

Comparison with Other Stress Modalities

Exercise ECG testing is the most established modality of stress testing, widely available and well validated for initial CAD diagnosis, cardiac risk assessment, and prognostication. However, if baseline ECG abnormalities are present, exercise ECG testing may be nondiagnostic.[52,82] Furthermore, ST segment changes during exercise can be effected by factors other than ischemia, such as endogenous estrogen, which can have a digoxin-like effect on the ECG, and hyperventilation, which can cause diffuse ST segment abnormalities.[83] Diagnostic accuracy for exercise ECG testing is reasonable when applied to appropriate patient populations. In a recent review of 58 exercise ECG studies involving nearly 12,000 patients

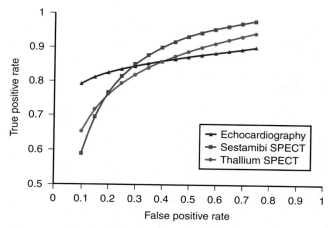

Figure 15–7. *Receiver operator characteristic curves for exercise echocardiography compared to nuclear single photo emission computed tomography (SPECT) stress testing.*[81] *The true positive rate (sensitivity) is plotted on the y-axis and the false positive rate (1-specificity) is plotted on the x-axis. When specificity is reduced (higher sensitivity is valued) nuclear modalities perform better. In contrast, when test specificity is valued, echocardiography tends to outperform nuclear modalities. (From Kymes SM, Bruns DE, Shaw LJ, et al: J Nucl Cardiol 7[6]:604, 2000.)*

undergoing both coronary angiography and exercise testing, the mean sensitivity was 67% with a mean specificity of 72%.[27] Factors that affect these reports include the decrease in sensitivity when equivocal findings were deemed a normal study and the previously discussed biases. The greatest diagnostic value for exercise ECG testing is seen in its relatively higher specificity, with an excellent negative predictive value.

With the addition of direct imaging of the heart during stress, either with echocardiography or nuclear SPECT, overall diagnostic accuracy for ischemia is improved. However, imaging requires additional equipment, space, and personnel with specialized expertise. With the added time demands and costs, it is logistically impossible and cost ineffective to replace all exercise ECG tests with imaging studies. Exercise ECG tests

should therefore be targeted for those individuals with a higher likelihood of a nondiagnostic ECG portion.

Stress echocardiography and nuclear studies provide reasonably comparable information with regards to ischemia diagnosis, identification of myocardial viability, and prognostic information.[80,84] For both modalities, diagnostic accuracy is dependent on disease prevalence in the population tested, and the criteria to define significant disease and a positive test. Accuracy for both modalities is improved in the setting of multivessel disease, increased disease severity, a higher ischemic workload achieved, and more experienced readers. However, substantive differences do exist. Because echocardiographic imaging is performed in real time, stress echocardiography can provide concurrent data on valvular function and pulmonary pressures during testing and offers the theoretical advantage of increased safety by identifying preexisting conditions, which may impact testing, such as valvular heart disease. The time requirements are disparate. For exercise echocardiography, unless transpulmonary contrast is needed, intravenous access is not needed and a study can be performed within 1 to 2 hours, whereas, nuclear studies require at a minimum, several hours to complete imaging (Table 15–6).

For a variety of reasons, contemporary comparisons between echocardiography and nuclear modalities are lacking. Because comparative studies tend to occur in centers where expertise in a particular modality is favored, results of single-center direct comparisons are of questionable validity. Stress echocardiography is a relatively newer modality, and availability of patient databases for longitudinal comparisons are lacking. The earliest comparative studies used thallium scintography, which does not reflect contemporary practice in which sestamibi or thallium SPECT, which reduce imaging artifacts, are more commonly used. More recent studies document comparable performance.[62,74,85,86] A meta-analysis of 44 studies showed a pooled sensitivity of 85% for echocardiography and 87% for nuclear stress testing.[80] In 112 patients who underwent both

TABLE 15–6. Comparison: Different Exercise Test Modalities

Exercise ECG	Exercise SPECT	Exercise Echocardiography
Largest historical database	Larger historical database	Relatively newer test modality
Portable	Additional time requirement (≈4 hours)	Additional time requirement (≈30 minutes)
Versatile	Increased personnel training	Increased personnel training
Limited with baseline ECG abnormalities	Increased expertise	Increased expertise
	Equipment requirements	Equipment requirements
	Patient transfer during the test	Patient transfer during the test
	Most sensitive modality	Most specific modality
	Significant increase in cost (≈5 times higher than ECG)	Significant increase in cost (≈2.5 times higher than ECG)
		Ability to directly visualize wall motion

ECG, electrocardiogram; SPECT, single photon emission computed tomography.

stress modalities with angiographic correlation using highly experienced readers, concordance between the two modalities was excellent (82%), with comparable sensitivity and a slight edge in specificity for echocardiography.[74] Sensitivity for single-vessel disease was lower than multivessel disease for both modalities (61% nuclear versus 58% for echocardiography).[74] Similar concordance has been reported elsewhere (84%), especially in those with a history of a prior infarction in which the concordance rate approached 91%.[62]

For ischemia evaluation, stress echocardiography differs from nuclear perfusion studies by assessing the functional consequences of ischemia rather than an alteration in regional myocardial perfusion. As such, when resting wall motion abnormalities are present, identification of subtle ischemia may be relatively more difficult to interpret with stress echocardiography rather than detecting changes in regional perfusion, resulting in a slight advantage in sensitivity for nuclear studies. Generally, advantages of nuclear stress studies include slightly higher sensitivity, particularly in single-vessel disease, higher technical success rate, less interobserver variability, and better accuracy for detecting new areas of myocardial ischemia when resting wall motion abnormalities are present. Factors favoring stress echocardiography included shorter test times, greater patient convenience, higher specificity, versatility, the absence of radiation exposure, and lower cost. Ultimately, the choice is dependent on the expertise of local personnel, facilities, and cost-effectiveness consideration.

Cost-Effectiveness

Care providers should be aware of and incorporate into their clinical practice, the relative costs of ordered procedures to provide an informed decision on the most appropriate test to obtain. Cost considerations for the different cardiac stress modalities include the patient's incurred costs, Medicare and insurer reimbursement charges, and the additional costs of further diagnostic testing prompted by the study. Prior comparative cost analyses highlight the importance of assessing the pretest probability of disease when selecting which diagnostic modality to use. For example, if pretest probability is high, then the most cost-effective course may be to proceed to direct angiography. For those with a normal baseline ECG and low pretest probability but where stress testing is warranted (and a negative study is valued), an exercise ECG study may be cost effective.

Several papers comment on the cost-effectiveness of different forms of cardiac stress testing.[87-89] Medicare fees provide comparative and relative costs for professional and technical fees for the different modalities.[27] Not surprisingly, the "test-only" cost for exercise ECG

testing is the least, approximately 3.3 relative value units (RVUs), with imaging additive, approximately 2.3 times higher for echocardiography and 5.3 times higher for nuclear testing.[27] However, these test-only costs do not account for the increased accuracy and the consequential reduced need for confirmatory downstream testing that imaging confers. When these issues are accounted for, cost-based analyses favor stress imaging studies, particularly when the likelihood of a nondiagnostic stress ECG study was high.[87-90] Because the Medicare reimbursement costs for stress echocardiography studies are roughly half those of nuclear testing with comparable diagnostic accuracy, exercise echocardiography may reasonably be considered a rational initial test of choice when considering an imaging stress modality, especially when considering the comparable diagnostic accuracy and prognostic information from both modalities.[88-91]

The diagnostic value of any testing modality is greatest when it significantly increases (based on a positive result) or lowers (based on a negative result) suspicion for CAD. As such, the greatest value for testing is seen in those patients with an intermediate range pretest probability of disease (in the range of 20% to 80%). In patients with a low pretest probability, such as those with atypical symptoms or few cardiovascular risk factors, a positive test is more likely to be a false-positive. Similarly, in individuals with a high pretest probability, a negative result may be looked on with skepticism, such that direct coronary angiography could be considered. Stress testing in these patients does have utility in cases in which multiple lesions are suspected or moderate lesions are present, and a functional study is needed to assess whether a blockage correlates with ischemia after a stressor is introduced.

Providers should be aware of the direct and downstream costs of the different diagnostic options and the relative expertise in the different modalities at their institutions. Current diagnostic schemes and pathways have not yet incorporated newer technologies of cardiac magnetic resonance imaging (MRI) or multislice computed tomography (CT) angiography with the clinical impact of these technologies yet to be realized.

Safety

Other than those known to be associated with physical exercise and the potential risk incurred from provoked ischemia, there are no adverse effects associated with exercise echocardiography. Major complications are rare, with myocardial infarction reported in 1/2500 studies and death in 1/10,000.[27,92] Contraindications to exercise echocardiography include those normally associated with exercise ECG testing (Table 15–7). Relative contraindications include active use of beta-blockers or other atrioventricular nodal blocking agents, which may lead to a submaximal HR response to exercise.

TABLE 15-7. Contraindications for Exercise Echocardiography

Absolute Contraindications	Relative Contraindications
Acute myocardial infarction (within 48 hours)	Left main coronary stenosis
High-risk unstable angina	Severe arterial hypertension (SBP > 200 mm Hg, DBP > 110 mm Hg)
Uncontrolled cardiac arrhythmias with symptoms or hemodynamic compromise	Poor acoustic windows/image quality (not aided by transpulmonary contrast)
Symptomatic severe aortic stenosis	Mental or physical impairment leading to inability to adequately exercise
Symptomatic heart failure	Tachyarrhythmias or bradyarrhythmias
Acute pulmonary embolus	Atrioventricular nodal blocking agents
Acute aortic dissection	Hypertrophic cardiomyopathy
Acute myocarditis or pericarditis	

DBP, diastolic blood pressure; SBP, systolic blood pressure.

Applications

Coronary Artery Disease

Diagnosis

The primary application of exercise echocardiography is in the diagnosis and management of CAD. In patients with symptoms consistent with unstable angina, stress testing should be performed within 3 to 7 days of symptom onset as long as heart failure is absent, and the ECG remains normal. Symptomatic patients with a higher pretest probability of disease, those with ischemic ECG changes or positive cardiac serum biomarkers, should be considered for direct coronary angiography. Exercise echocardiography is valuable for distinguishing between ischemic and nonischemic cardiopulmonary disease, such as pulmonary hypertension, valvular heart disease, and structural abnormalities. Dyspnea is a common presentation of atypical angina. In an exercise echocardiographic study of 443 patients with unexplained dyspnea, ischemia was demonstrated in 42% of dyspneic patients and in 58% of those with both angina and dyspnea, with a higher subsequent incidence of cardiac death and infarction.[93] Accurate diagnosis in these patients is important to establish an appropriate treatment course.

Historically, in patients presenting to the hospital with chest discomfort, the site of initial evaluation is in the emergency department (ED) with subsequent hospital admission to rule out an acute myocardial infarction (AMI) before risk stratification. In the last decade, intermediate- and lower-risk patients are increasingly managed with triage to a chest pain unit, usually within the ED.[94] Different models exist, but the basic premise is to provide efficient triage and risk stratification with expedited exercise stress testing in those patients in whom an acute coronary syndrome (ACS) is ruled out. This approach has been effective in identifying higher-risk individuals while concurrently reducing need for inpatient

stays.[95] Although the choice of which modality to use is institution dependent, reports demonstrate improved accuracy with exercise echocardiography compared to exercise ECG testing.[96] Nuclear SPECT testing is a reasonable option as it may provide a small advantage in sensitivity. A recent study comparing exercise echocardiography and nuclear SPECT testing in 503 ED patients demonstrated higher accuracy (93% versus 89%), specificity (95% versus 90%), and positive predictive value (81% versus 67%) for echocardiography, with a small advantage for nuclear SPECT in sensitivity.[97] Given the superior performance over exercise ECG testing and the comparable diagnostic accuracy with nuclear SPECT, exercise echocardiography is an attractive option for an initial diagnostic study, especially when considering timeliness, cost savings, and versatility.

The use of exercise testing for CAD diagnosis in asymptomatic individuals is controversial. Cardiovascular prognosis in low-risk or intermediate-risk patients is excellent and false-positive findings may instigate a diagnostic pathway with unnecessary additional testing. Moreover, the adverse psychological impact of a positive cardiac stress test should be considered along with potential data misuse affecting employment and insurance coverage. Therefore, pretest risk stratification is warranted. Judicious testing of asymptomatic individuals in high-risk subsets, such as those with diabetes or vascular disease may be considered, particularly in those who are contemplating higher-risk activities such as a new exercise regimen.

Known Coronary Artery Disease

Cardiac stress testing in those with a recent myocardial infarct allows for assessment of injury extent, residual ischemia, and identification of other critical coronary lesions. This is crucial for guidance on future therapy and acquisition of prognostic information. In patients with recent infarcts who did not undergo angiography, a submaximal predischarge stress test 3 to 7 days following the event is recommended for risk assessment.[27,94] Submaximal protocols have lower hemodynamic endpoints, such as achievement of 5 METS or 70% of the predicted maximum HR.[98] As early as 2 to 3 weeks following hospital discharge after an infarct, symptom-limited stress tests can be performed reasonably safely, with the reported incidence of nonfatal infarct less than 1% and fatal infarct approximately 0.03%.[27,99] Historically, standard exercise ECG testing was obtained; however, with the ECG abnormalities that are frequently present following an acute infarct, the sensitivity of exercise ECG testing for detecting new ischemia is poor, in the range of only 50% to 70%.[74] Sensitivity for exercise echocardiography is also somewhat limited by tethering effects from the infarcted myocardium; however, overall diagnostic accuracy is significantly improved over exercise ECG testing, with visual localization of the ischemic territory, comparable to that seen with nuclear stress studies.

In individuals under consideration for revascularization (either percutaneously or surgically), preprocedure ischemia evaluation and documentation of myocardial viability of hypocontractile segments is recommended, allowing for targeting of vascular territories for intervention.[100,101] Revascularizing frankly infarcted tissue exposes the patient to procedural risk with little clinical benefit as myocardial recovery is unlikely. Viability protocols are well established for pharmacologic stressors (predominantly dobutamine) (see Chapter 16).[102] Data for treadmill exercise viability testing are nearly absent, but limited data using low-level bicycle ergometry demonstrate feasibility.[103-105] Tethering effects from resting wall motion abnormalities increase difficulty in interpretation, and the all or nothing posttreadmill imaging approach limits utility when trying to identify subtle interval changes in function. A stationary patient position and ability to image during active exercise with bicycle ergometry increases feasibility of exercise testing for viability, but accuracy is not as high as seen with pharmacologic applications. In 52 postinfarct patients who underwent low-level supine bicycle exercise and low dose dobutamine echocardiography, sensitivity for predicting functional recovery with exercise was 81% with specificity of 92%, compared to 91% and 86% for dobutamine, respectively.[104] More investigation is needed to validate this method as a reliable assessment of myocardial viability.

Following percutaneous revascularization, stress testing can evaluate the effects of intervention by documenting improvement in exercise tolerance and regional function.[106-108] In 36 patients evaluated before and after angioplasty, exercise duration and workload improved after the procedure. Although 17 patients had persistent regional wall motion abnormalities, most demonstrated improved function compared to baseline.[108] Asymptomatic restenosis typically represents intermediate range, single-vessel lesions and is therefore often difficult to diagnose. As such, ECG testing is an insensitive predictor of restenosis, with sensitivities ranging 40% to 55%.[27] Echocardiographic imaging improves diagnostic accuracy.[106,108-110] In 86 patients evaluated 6 months after revascularization, the overall sensitivity for exercise echocardiography to detect restenosis was 83% compared to only 42% for exercise ECG.[106] Studies comparing nuclear perfusion imaging stress to exercise echocardiography following percutaneous intervention are lacking, but limited data available show comparable performance, with 89% concordance.[111] However, in contemplating revascularization in an asymptomatic individual, cardiac stress testing for restenosis surveillance is controversial when considering clinical relevance and long-term benefit.

The utility of exercise echocardiography following coronary artery bypass revascularization includes both assessment of graft patency and evaluation of residual coronary disease.[112-114] The presence of inducible ischemia has been correlated with stenotic vessels, obstructed grafts, and diseased native vessels with excellent diagnostic accuracy.[114] In a series of 125 patients, sensitivity for exercise echocardiography was 98% compared to 41% for exercise ECG testing and was more closely correlated with the regional distribution of compromised vascular supply.[113] Following surgery, the clinical yield of exercise testing in asymptomatic patients with successful surgical revascularization is low in the first few years after intervention but is more useful when disease likelihood is high, at least 5 years after surgery and/or in the setting of risk factors such as diabetes mellitus, recurrent angina, and chronic dialysis.

Prognosis

Determinants of prognosis in ischemic heart disease are ejection fraction, location of disease, and disease severity.[115,116] Independent prognostic factors from the exercise ECG include exercise duration, achieved workload, induced ST segment abnormalities, and hemodynamic response to exercise, including HR recovery.[27,117-119] With visual assessment of ventricular function and ischemia, exercise echocardiography is well situated to provide additional data incremental to exercise ECG testing.[120-126] Poorer outcome is generally seen in those with resting wall motion abnormalities, larger ischemic regions, shorter exercise duration, and shorter ischemia onset time.[127-135] The results of cardiac stress testing should be put into the context of risk factors and symptoms, i.e., a positive test result with higher pretest probability, such as in diabetics, carries more prognostic information. In those without known coronary disease, the negative predictive value of a normal exercise echocardiogram is excellent, with likelihood of a major cardiac event less than 1% over the next 1 to 4 years.[136,137]

Ideally, prognostic data should be used to identify higher-risk individuals to direct diagnostic resources. However, prospective studies of the natural history following an acute infarct with an abnormal stress study response are not currently feasible as most care providers, when faced with a positive study, will refer for angiography and revascularization. Understanding this, in patients with known disease, exercise echocardiography has been used as a prognostic tool for both hard events (recurrent myocardial infarction, death) and soft events (need for revascularization). Important prognostic determinants following an infarct include ejection fraction, new remote induced ischemia (evidence of multivessel disease), lower functional capacity, and hypotensive exercise response. Exercise echocardiography identifies those at higher risk with a positive predictive value in the range of 63% to 80% and negative predictive value 78% to 95%. Accuracy is generally improved over exercise ECG testing because resting ECG abnormalities are generally present.[36,69,115,138,139]

Women

Diagnostic testing for coronary disease in women in general is not optimal. Women tend to have less obstructive coronary lesions and more often have only single-vessel involvement. Women are on average a decade older on presentation with more comorbidities and functional debilitation. Moreover, there has been a relative paucity of female representation in cardiovascular trials. In a meta-analysis of studies published between 1966 and 1995, only 27 studies included at least 50 women who underwent exercise testing and angiography, of which only 3 used exercise echocardiography.[140] Poor study representation and inadequate test validation has adversely affected reported accuracies.

The choice of which modality to obtain should take into account the relative limitations of each approach. Exercise ECG testing in women produces a high incidence of false-positive findings, often resulting from resting ST-T wave abnormalities, hypertension-induced abnormalities, and estrogen effects on the ECG.[27,141] Studies have documented a 40% rate of false-positive

ST segment depressions in women compared to 10% in men.[142-144] Because of isotope scatter and attenuation, nuclear imaging tests also have limitations. The accuracy of thallium-201 perfusion imaging is reduced with obscuration of the inferior wall in obese patients and the anterior wall in large-breasted women. However, artifacts have been lessened with increased used of technecium-99m, a higher-energy radioisotope with better tissue penetration.[145] Exercise echocardiography is less subject to false-positives abnormalities (more specific). However, measures to ensure adequate workload should be employed to increase the likelihood of a diagnostic study. A low clinical threshold to use transpulmonary contrast for endocardial border enhancement is needed, particularly when the anterior or lateral walls are poorly seen.

Limitations in the different modalities are reflected in published reports of diagnostic accuracy. In a meta-analysis of 19 standard exercise ECG studies that included at least 50 women, the weighted mean sensitivity was only 61% with specificity of 70%.[140] Imaging increased diagnostic accuracy with a weighted mean sensitivity of 86% and specificity of 79% for echocardiography and respective percentages of 78% and 64% for nuclear imaging.[140] Overall accuracy of exercise echocardiography in women (sensitivity range 79% to 86%) is presented in Table 15–8. Because the likelihood of a nondiagnostic exercise ECG study is higher in women, recent publications have advocated using imaging stress studies as the initial study.[146,147] A cost analysis balancing cost with the lowest number of false-negatives and fewest inappropriate angiography referrals found exercise echocardiography had the best overall accuracy at the lowest cost.[147] However, uniform referral would be logistically difficult, and the negative predictive value of a normal exercise ECG study remains high.

Concordant with the general population, stress echocardiography in women provides valuable prognostic information.[140,148-151] In 4234 women, LV function and the extent of wall motion abnormalities was predictive of cardiac death.[149] These findings were reiterated in a community based study of 1188 women in which those with resting wall motion abnormalities or exercise-

TABLE 15–8. Diagnostic Accuracy of Exercise Echocardiography in Women

First Author (Year)	Mode	Number of Points	Sensitivity	Specificity	Accuracy
Sawada (1989)[73]	TME or UBE	57	86%	86%	86%
Williams (1994)[77]	UBE	70	88%	84%	86%
Marwick (1995)[147]	TME or UBE	161	80%	81%	81%
Roger (1997)[66]	TME or UBE	96	79%	37%	63%

TME, treadmill echocardiography; UBE, upright bicycle ergometry.

induced ischemia predicted a higher rate of myocardial infarction and death.[152] Prospective, female-specific investigations for coronary disease diagnosis are lacking. The ongoing Women Ischemia Syndrome Evaluation (WISE) study, by the National Heart, Lung, and Blood Institute (NHLBI), is the largest prospective female-specific study to date, studying different modalities of cardiac diagnostic testing, and evaluating the influence of menopausal status and hormones on diagnostic test results in nearly 1000 women.[141] Future results from this study should shed light on the gender-specific issues that affect variances on diagnostic accuracy for all cardiac stress testing modalities.

Risk Stratification before Noncardiac Surgery

Given the hemodynamic burden associated with surgery, preoperative risk stratification in intermediate-risk to high-risk asymptomatic individuals (e.g., those with vascular disease, renal insufficiency, diabetes, prior ischemic heart disease, or congestive heart failure aids in decision making, particularly when surgery is elective and in evaluating need for presurgical revascularization.[153] Patients with peripheral vascular disease generally carry a significant cardiovascular risk factor profile. Because cardiac events are the main source of perioperative morbidity and mortality in patients undergoing vascular surgery, with death or myocardial infarct occurring in approximately 10%, this population has the greatest published experience in preoperative risk stratification. Preoperative evaluation for vascular surgery also provides opportunity for preemptive revascularization to limit potential long-term sequelae of coronary disease. Exercise stress is usually obviated because of concurrent lower extremity vascular disease. Therefore, pharmacologic stress testing is usually utilized, with a positive test associated with a 10% to 20% risk of a perioperative event or spontaneous event in subsequent years.

Hypertrophic Cardiomyopathy

Applications of exercise echocardiography in patients with HCM primarily include assessment of left ventricular outflow tract (LVOT) obstruction severity (see Chapter 28). Timing of intervention in patients with nonobstructive HCM is often equivocal. Demonstration of a significant increase in LVOT gradient with exercise can be seen in as many as 20% of patients after exercise and 48% with both exercise and inhalation of amyl nitrate. Making this diagnosis is important as those with inducible gradients have both higher morbidity (necessitating intervention) and mortality.[154] Exercise echocardiography also aids in the identification of occult systolic dysfunction, described in up to 44% of HCM patients.[155] In athletic

individuals with the appearance of HCM, exercise echocardiography aids in differentiating HCM from athlete's heart by demonstrating an absence of an exercise-induced LVOT gradient and an appropriate hyperdynamic response to exercise.[154]

During testing, standard exercise protocols are used, with cessation of exercise if symptoms develop or if a significant gradient in excess of 50 mm Hg is provoked. Rest and stress velocities of the LVOT are measured using continuous-wave Doppler from the apical views.[154] Exercise induced regional wall motion abnormalities that develop in the absence of coronary disease are thought to be associated with microvascular ischemia and are a predictor of developing worsening resting systolic dysfunction, suggesting potential need for earlier intervention. Following intervention, stress echocardiography has been used to document a reduction in the LVOT gradient and monitor efficacy of treatment.

Dilated Cardiomyopathy

Both pharmacologic and exercise stress echocardiography have been safely used in the study of patients with dilated cardiomyopathy, but there is a predominance for pharmacologic testing. Applications include identification of viable myocardium following an infarct, as described previously, and earlier identification of patients at risk for developing systolic dysfunction, such as myocarditis patients and cancer survivors exposed to potentially cardiotoxic agents.[154] Recently, exercise echocardiography also has been proposed as an approach to better identify candidates for resynchronization therapy, with adverse changes in ventricular dyssynchrony during exercise correlating with a decline in cardiac output and worsening of mitral regurgitation.[156,157] However, standard protocols are not yet available, and the reproducibility of these measures have yet to be established.

Following cardiac transplantation, transplant vasculopathy is a major source of morbidity and mortality. Surveillance testing includes noninvasive pharmacologic stress testing and intravascular ultrasound during coronary angiography. Limited data with exercise echocardiography demonstrate reasonable specificity, in the range of 86% to 95% but poor sensitivity[158,159] (Table 15-9). Diagnostic accuracy of dobutamine echocardiography is improved over exercise testing, and also provides prognostic information on subsequent cardiac events (see Chapter 31).[160]

Valvular Heart Disease

Stress echocardiography is a valuable adjunct in the management of patients with valvular heart disease by assessing the dynamic response of valvular function to changes in physiologic demand.[161-163] Inter-

TABLE 15–9. Diagnostic Accuracy of Exercise Echocardiography for Transplant Vasculopathy

First Author (Year)	Mode	Number of Points	Sensitivity	Specificity	Accuracy
Collings (1994)[159]	TME	51	25	86	69
Cohn (1996)[158]	UBE	51	26	95	73

TME, treadmill echocardiography; UBE, upright bicycle ergometry.

vention, including pharmacologic, percutaneous, or surgical, should be considered with onset of cardiopulmonary symptoms during testing, such as exertional dyspnea, heart failure, arrhythmias, angina, or syncope.[43] In asymptomatic patients or those with equivocal symptoms, stress echocardiography allows for assessment of:

1. Exercise tolerance and contextual evaluation of a patient's clinical status
2. Symptom provocation
3. Induced pulmonary hypertension
4. Evaluation of ventricular function
5. Direct evaluation of stenosis or regurgitant severity
6. Evaluation for exercise induced arrhythmias

For patients with significant, symptomatic aortic stenosis (AS), current guidelines advocate aortic valve replacement without need for provocative exercise testing.[43] Exercise testing is contraindicated for symptomatic patients, due to the risk of hemodynamic compromise. However, in asymptomatic patients or those with equivocal symptoms, exercise testing can be performed relatively safely when supervised by an experienced physician.[95,164-171] The exercise test should be ended promptly if there is only a minimal increase in blood pressure or the patient experiences symptoms. Standard exercise ECG testing alone has limited accuracy for ischemia evaluation given the commonly present baseline ECG abnormalities. Instead of ischemia evaluation, stress echocardiography provides valuable information on hemodynamic significance and symptom provocation.[164,166,170,171]

In mitral stenosis (MS) patients with equivocal symptoms and only a moderate transmitral gradient, a significant increase in pulmonary pressure during exercise indicates greater hemodynamic severity. Intervention should be considered when the systolic pulmonary pressure exceeds 50 mm Hg at rest or 60 mm Hg during exercise.[43] During stress, direct measurements of Doppler-derived transmitral pressure gradients and mitral valve area estimation are of limited utility. Because of alterations in atrial-ventricular filling, there is a decrease in the transmitral pressure half-time resulting in a rapid deceleration of LV filling velocity rather than a true increase in the estimated the mitral valve area. In this situation, mitral valve area should be calculated from the continuity equation.[162,172-175]

Disease progression of chronic aortic and mitral regurgitation can be insidious. Timing of surgical intervention in asymptomatic patients is predicated on evidence of adverse hemodynamic effects on the left ventricle with impaired systolic function or enlargement.[43] In patients with normal indices at rest, hemodynamic significance may manifest as abnormalities in exercise tolerance or an increase in pulmonary pressures.[43,162,176] Additionally, in patients with normal resting systolic function and chronic regurgitant lesions, an exercise-induced loss of contractile reserve has been shown to be a marker of impending dysfunction and should prompt consideration of surgical intervention.[177]

Other Applications

Exercise protocols in the pediatric population are adjusted to account for decreased stature with similar indices of exercise tolerance, ECG changes and identification of regional wall motion abnormalities.[178,179] Ischemic heart disease is less prevalent in children, and therefore exercise echocardiography is primarily targeted at arrhythmia evaluation and assessment of the hemodynamic significance of valvular and congenital abnormalities.

In adults with chronic pulmonary disease, exercise-induced pulmonary hypertension and serial evaluation of pulmonary pressures is a valuable adjunct to patient management. In patients with chronic autoimmune disease who may have underlying pulmonary arterial disease, although resting pulmonary pressures may be normal, exercise induced pulmonary hypertension may allow identification of patients who may benefit from earlier instigation of disease modifying therapy.[180,181]

Future Directions

Several research applications seek to address the relative limitations of stress echocardiography. Quantitative approaches to interpretation should increase reproducibility and accuracy, particularly for relatively less experienced readers. Currently, with advances in automated border recognition, acoustic quantification, and color kinesis, which allow for online analysis without manual endocardial boundary tracing, the time demands of interpretation may be shortened with potential improvement of endocardial motion analysis.[182,183]

Conceptually, diagnosis of induced diastolic dysfunction may increase test sensitivity as it allows for ischemic identification at an earlier time point on the ischemic cascade.[184] Diastolic interrogation is feasible with bicycle ergometry or pharmacologic stressor applications. Given the individual heterogeneity in mitral inflow patterns, load dependency of the parameters, and the time constraints of immediate poststress imaging in treadmill exercise applications, the utility of diastolic function assessment is only supplemental to systolic evaluation.[184-186] As with any Doppler application, limitations include underestimation of velocities with nonparallel intercept angles and inaccurate velocity measurement resulting from increased translational cardiac motion.

Tissue Doppler interrogation evaluates myocardial tissue velocity referenced to the transducer, allowing for differentiation of normal and hypokinetic motion (see Chapter 5).[42,187-191] Speckle tracking allows for simultaneous tracking of two or more adjacent points, or "speckles," and evaluating relative velocity between the points rather than referenced to the transducer, which allows for an evaluation of interval change in velocities.

Strain and strain rate (SR) imaging are measures derived from tissue Doppler velocities.[192] Conceptually, strain rate refers to the speed of myocardial deformation and strain represents relative deformation. Alterations in these measures suggest an interval change in function. Available systems allow for offline analysis of prerecorded samples for time savings during active scanning. Because of background imaging noise and respiratory artifact, strain and strain rate imaging have been difficult to implement during exercise stress, with one study documenting noninterpretable data in as many as 36% of subjects.[193] In its current state, the time demand for strain rate imaging data analysis remains lengthy, but automated analysis is in progress.[42,191,194]

Newly introduced myocardial contrast agents allow for the assessment of coronary flow reserve integrated with concurrent wall motion analysis.[195-203] In a prospective study comparing myocardial contrast pharmacologic echocardiography with nuclear SPECT, there was no significant difference in sensitivity for coronary disease detection.[201] Primarily a research tool, published reports with exercise stressors are lacking. A potentially valuable application of myocardial contrast imaging may be in the identification of viable myocardium (see Chapter 3).

The potential advantage of real-time three-dimensional (3D) imaging is the ability for tomographic imaging of the heart within a few cardiac cycles with subsequent image reconstruction of the heart. Because sensitivity of exercise echocardiography decreases the longer the interval from exercise cessation to image acquisition, a single-image acquisition time point allows for evaluation at a higher workload. 3D reconstruction allows for evaluation of any myocardial segment and when coupled with the time savings, should improve sensitivity for ischemia detection. This is pertinent as even the most experienced sonographers require approximately 30 seconds for image acquisition with current protocols. Early feasibility of 3D imaging has been demonstrated with pharmacologic stress echocardiography.[204-206] 3D imaging with exercise is relatively limited by translational motion of the heart and exaggerated respiratory cardiac motion, but advances may allow for future application[207] (see Chapter 4).

KEY POINTS

■ Exercise echocardiography integrates real-time echocardiographic imaging with exercise (ECG) testing to aid in the evaluation of ischemic, valvular, and cardiopulmonary heart disease.

■ Images are acquired either during peak exercise for bicycle ergometry protocols or immediately following exercise for treadmill protocols. Imaging data is integrated with ECG data, exercise tolerance, and patient symptoms for final interpretation.

■ When image quality is poor, transpulmonary contrast can aid endocardial border definition dramatically.

■ Stress echocardiography and stress nuclear studies provide comparable information on ischemia diagnosis, myocardial viability, and prognostication. General factors favoring echocardiography include shorter test times, greater patient convenience, versatility, absence of radiation exposure, and lower cost.

■ Future advances may include 3D imaging, tissue Doppler stress and strain imaging, and the potential to evaluate coronary flow reserve utilizing myocardial perfusion imaging.

REFERENCES

1. Armstrong WF, O'Donnell J, Dillon JC, et al: Complementary value of two-dimensional exercise echocardiography to routine treadmill exercise testing. *Ann Intern Med* 105:829-835, 1986.
2. Hlatky MA, Pryor DB, Harrel FE Jr, et al: Factors affecting sensitivity and specificity of exercise echocardiography. *Am J Med* 77:64, 1984.
3. Marwick TH, Shaw L, Case C, et al: Clinical and economic impact of exercise electrocardiography and exercise echocardiography in clinical practice. *Eur Heart J* 24(12):1153-1163, 2003.

4. Ross J Jr: Assessment of ischemic regional myocardial dysfunction and its reversibility. *Circulation* 74:1186-1190, 1986.

5. Kerber RE, Marcus ML, Abboud FM: Echocardiography in experimentally-induced myocardial ischemia. *Am J Med* 63(1):21-28, 1977.

6. Kerber RE, Marcus ML, Ehrhardt J, et al: Correlation between echocardiographically demonstrated segmental dyskinesis and regional myocardial perfusion. *Circulation* 52(6):1097-1104, 1975.

7. Kerber RE, Marcus ML, Ehrhardt J, Abboud FM: Effect of intra-aortic balloon counterpulsation on the motion and perfusion of acutely ischemic myocardium. An experimental echocardiographic study. *Circulation* 53(5):853-859, 1976.

8. Gordon MJ, Kerber RE: Interventricular septal motion in patients with proximal and distal left anterior descending coronary artery lesions. *Circulation* 55(2):38-41, 1977.

9. Mason SJ, Weiss JL, Weisfeldt ML, et al: Exercise echocardiography: Detection of wall motion abnormalities during ischemia. *Circulation* 59(1):50-59, 1979.

10. Lauer MS: The "exercise" part of exercise echocardiography. *J Am Coll Cardiol* 39(8):1353-1355, 2002.

11. Picano E: Stress echocardiography: A historical perspective. *Am J Med* 114(2):126-130, 2003.

12. Lang RM, BM, Devereux RB, et al: Recommendations for chamber quantification: a report from the American Society of Echocardiography's Guidelines and Standards Committee and the Chamber Quantification Writing Group, developed in conjunction with the European Association of Echocardiography, a branch of the European Society of Cardiology. *J Am Soc Echocardiogr* 18(12):1440-1463, 2005.

13. Battler A, Froelicher VF, Gallagher KP, et al: Dissociation between regional myocardial dysfunction and ECG changes during ischemia in the conscious dog. *Circulation* 62:735-744, 1980.

14. Wohlgelernter D, Cleman M, Highman HA, et al: Regional myocardial dysfunction during coronary angioplasty: evaluation by two-dimensional echocardiography and 12 lead electrocardiography. *J Am Coll Cardiol* 7(8):1245-1254, 1986.

15. Sugishita Y, Kosseki S, Matsuda M, et al: Dissociation between regional myocardial dysfunction and ECG changes during myocardial ischemia induced by exercise in patients with angina pectoris. *Am Heart J* 106(1 Pt 1):1-8, 1983.

16. Nesto RW, Kowalchuck GJ: The ischemic cascade: Temporal sequence of hemodynamic, electrocardiographic, and symptomatic expressions of ischemia. *Am J Cardiol* 59(7):23C-30C, 1987.

17. Hauser AM, Gangadharan V, Ramos RG, et al: Sequence of mechanical, electrocardiographic and clinical effects of repeated coronary artery occlusion in human beings: echocardiographic observations during coronary angioplasty. *J Am Coll Cardiol* 5(2pt1):193-197, 1985.

18. Visser CA, David GK, Kan G, et al: Two-dimensional echocardiography during percutaneous transluminal coronary angioplasty. *Am J Cardiol* 111:1035-1041, 1986.

19. Sheikh KH, Bengston JR, Helmy S, et al: Relation of quantitative coronary lesion measurements to the development of exercise-induced ischemia assessed by exercise echocardiography. *J Am Coll Cardiol* 15(5):1043-1051, 1990.

20. Beleslin BD, Ostojic M, Djordjevic-Dikic A, et al: Integrated evaluation of relation between coronary lesion features and stress echocardiography results: the importance of coronary lesion morphology. *J Am Coll Cardiol* 33(3):717-726, 1999.

21. Armstrong WF, O'Donnell J, Ryan T, Feigenbaum H: Effect of prior myocardial infarction and extent and location of coronary disease on accuracy of exercise echocardiography. *J Am Coll Cardiol* 10(3):31-38, 1987.

22. Salustri A, Amese M, Boersma E, et al: Correlation of coronary stenosis by quantitative coronary arteriography with exercise echocardiography. *Am J Cardiol* 75(4):87-90, 1995.

23. Agati L, Arata L, Luongo R, et al: Assessment of severity of coronary narrowings by quantitative exercise echocardiography and comparison with quantitative arteriography. *Am J Cardiol* 67(15):1201-1207, 1991.

24. Strizik B, Chiu S, Ilercil A, et al: Usefulness of isometric handgrip during treadmill exercise stress echocardiography. *Am J Cardiol* 90(4):420-422, 2002.

25. Fletcher GF, Balady G, Froelicher VF, et al: Exercise standards: A statement for healthcare professionals from the American Heart Association Writing Group. *Circulation* 91:580-615, 1995.

26. Pina IL, Balady GJ, Hanson P, et al: Guidelines for clinical exercise testing laboratories: a statement for healthcare professionals from the Committee on Exercise and Cardiac Rehabilitation, American Heart Association. *Circulation* 91:912-921, 1995.

27. Gibbons RJ, Balady GJ, Bricker, JT, et al: ACC/AHA Guideline update for exercise testing: a report of the American College of Cardiology/American Heart Association Task Force on Practice Guidelines. *J Am Coll Cardiol* 40(8):1531-1540, 2002.

28. Kloner RA, Allen J, Cox TA, et al: Stunned left ventricular myocardium after exercise treadmill testing in coronary artery disease. *Am J Cardiol* 68(4):329-334, 1991.

29. Presti CF, Armstong W, Feigenbaum H: Comparison of echocardiography at peak exercise and after bicycle exercise in evaluation of patients with known or suspected coronary artery disease. *J Am Soc Echocardiogr* 1(2):119-126, 1988.

30. Peteiro J, Garrido I, Monserrat L, et al: Comparison of peak and post-exercise treadmill echocardiography with the use of harmonic imaging acquisition. *J Am Soc Echocardiogr* 17:1044-1049, 2004.

31. Ginzton LE, Conant R, Brizendine M, et al: Exercise subcostal two-dimensional echocardiography: A new method of segmental wall motion analysis. *Am J Cardiol* 53:805-811, 1984.

32. Ryan T, Segar DS, Sawada DG, et al: Detection of coronary artery disease with upright bicycle exercise echocardiography. *J Am Soc Echocardiogr* 6:186-197, 1993.

33. Dagianti A, Penco M, Agati L, et al: Stress echocardiography: comparison of exercise, dipyridamole and dobutamine in detecting and predicting the extent of coronary artery disease. *J Am Coll Cardiol* 26:18-25, 1995.

34. Hecht HS, DeBord L, Sotomayor N, et al: Supine bicycle stress echocardiography: Peak exercise imaging is superior to postexercise imaging. *J Am Soc Echocardiogr* 6(3 pt 1):265-271, 1993.

35. Badruddin SM, Ahmad A, Mickelson J, et al: Supine bicycle versus post-treadmill exercise echocardiography in the detection of myocardial ischemia: A randomized single-blind crossover trial. *J Am Coll Cardiol* 33(6):1485-1490, 1999.

36. Applegate RJ, Dell'Italia LJ, Crawford MH: Usefulness of two-dimensional echocardiography during low-level exercise testing early after uncomplicated acute myocardial infarction. *Am J Cardiol* 60(1):10-14, 1987.

37. Modesto K, Rainbird A, Klarich, et al: Comparison of supine bicycle exercise and treadmill exercise Doppler echocardiography in evaluation of patients with coronary artery disease. *Am J Cardiol* 91:1245-1248, 2003.

38. Armstrong WF, West SR, Dillon JC, Feigenbaum H: Assessment of location and size of myocardial infarction with contrast-enhanced echocardiography. II. Application of digital imaging techniques. *J Am Coll Cardiol* 4(1):141-148, 1984.

39. Hecht HS, DeBord L, Shaw R, et al: Digital supine bicycle stress echocardiography: A new technique for evaluating coronary artery disease. *J Am Coll Cardiol* 21(4):50-56, 1993.

40. Attenhofer CH, Pellikka PA, Oh JK, et al: Is review of videotape necessary after review of digitized cine-loop images in stress echocardiography? A prospective study in 306 patients. *J Am Soc Echocardiogr* 10(2):179-184, 1997.

41. Hunziker PR, Picard MH, Jander N, et al: Regional wall motion assessment in stress echocardiography by tissue Doppler bull's eyes. *J Am Soc Echocardiogr* 12:196-202, 1999.

42. Pasquet A, Armstrong G, Beachler L, et al: Use of segmental tissue Doppler velocity to quantitate exercise echocardiography. *J Am Soc Echocardiogr* 12(11):901-912, 1999.

43. Bonow RO, Carabello BA, Chatterjee K, et al: ACC/AHA 2006 guidelines for the management of patients with valvular heart disease—executive summary: a report of the American College of Cardiology/American Heart Association Task Force on Practice Guidelines (Writing Committee to Develop Guidelines for the Management of Patients With Valvular Heart Disease). *J Am Coll Cardiol* 48:598-675, 2006.

44. Marcovitz PA: Exercise Echocardiography. In *The Practice of Clinical Echocardiography*. Pennsylvania, WB Saunders Company, 2002, pp. 275-300.

45. Ketteler T, Krahwinkel W, Godke J, et al: Stress echocardiography: personnel and technical equipment. *Eur Heart J* D:D43-D48, 1997.

46. Armstrong WF, Pellikka PA, Ryan T, et al: Stress echocardiography: recommendations for performance and interpretation of stress echocardiography. Stress Echocardiography Task Force of the Nomenclature and Standards Committee of the American Society of Echocardiography. *J Am Soc Echocardiogr* 11(1):97-104, 1998.

47. Varga A, Picano E, Dodi C, et al: Madness and method in stress echo reading. *Eur Heart J* 20:1271-1275, 1999.

48. Imran MB, Palinkas A, Pasanisi EM, et al: Optimal reading criteria in stress echocardiography. *Am J Cardiol* 90(4):44-45, 2002.

49. Hoffmann R, Lethen H, Marwick T, et al: Analysis of interinstitutional observer agreement in interpretation of dobutamine stress echocardiograms. *J Am Coll Cardiol* 27:330-336, 1996.

50. Buda AJ, Lefkowitz CA, Gallagher KP: Augmentation of regional function in nonischemic myocardium during coronary occlusion measured with two-dimensional echocardiography. *J Am Coll Cardiol* 16:175-180, 1990.

51. Guth BD, White FC, Gallagher KP, Bloor CM: Decreased systolic wall thickening in myocardium adjacent to ischemic zones in conscious swine during brief coronary artery occlusion. *Am Heart J* 107:458, 1984.

52. Cortigiani L, Bigi R, Rigo F, et al: Diagnostic value of exercise electrocardiography and dipyridamole stress echocardiography in hypertensive and normotensive chest pain patients with right bundle branch block. *J Hypertens* 21(11):2189-2194, 2003.

53. Picano E, Palinkas A, Amyot R: Diagnosis of myocardial ischemia in hypertensive patients. *J Hypertens* 19:1177-1183, 2001.

54. Picano E, Lattanzi F, Orlandini A, et al: Stress echocardiography and the human factor: the importance of being expert. *J Am Coll Cardiol* 17(3):666-669, 1991.

55. Obeidat O, Arida M, Al-Mallah M, et al: Segmental early relaxation phenomenon: Incidence, clinical characteristics, and significance in stress echocardiography. *Chest* 125(4):1218-1223, 2004.

56. Marwick TH: Stress echocardiography. *Heart* 89(1):113-118, 2003.

57. Schiller NB, Shah PM, Crawford M, et al: Recommendations for quantitation of the left ventricle by two-dimensional echocardiography. American Society of Echocardiography Committee on standards, subcommittee on quantitation of two-dimensional echocardiograms. *J Am Soc Echocardiogr* 2:358-367, 1989.

58. Pellikka PA: Stress echocardiography for the diagnosis of coronary artery disease: Progress towards quantification. *Curr Opin Cardiol* 20(5):395-398, 2005.

59. Marangelli V, Iliceto S, Piccinni G, et al: Detection of coronary artery disease by digital stress echocardiography: Comparison of exercise, transesophageal atrial pacing and dipyridamole echocardiography. *J Am Coll Cardiol* 24:117-124, 1994.

60. Ryan T, Vasey CG, Presti CF, et al: Exercise echocardiography: detection of coronary artery disease in patients with normal left ventricular wall motion at rest. *J Am Coll Cardiol* 11(5):993-999, 1988.

61. Crouse LJ, Harbrecht JJ, Vacek JL, et al: Exercise echocardiography as a screening test for coronary artery disease and correlation with coronary arteriography. *Am J Cardiol* 67(15):213-218, 1991.

62. Pozzoli MM, Fioretti P, Salustri A, et al: Exercise echocardiography and technecium-99m MIBI single photon emission computed tomography in the detection of coronary artery disease. *Am J Cardiol* 67:350-355, 1991.

63. Marwick TH, Nemec JJ, Pashkow FJ, et al: Accuracy and limitations of exercise echocardiography in a routine clinical setting. *J Am Coll Cardiol* 19(1):74-81, 1992.

64. White CW, Wright CB, Doty DB, et al: Does visual interpretation of the coronary arteriogram predict the physiological importance of a coronary stenosis? *N Engl J Med* 310:819-824, 1984.

65. Topol EJ, Nissen SE: Our preoccupation with coronary luminology: The dissociation between clinical and angiographic findings in ischemic heart disease. *Circulation* 92:2333, 1995.

66. Roger VL, Pellikka PA, Bell MR, et al: Sex and verification bias. Impact on the diagnostic value of exercise echocardiography. *Circulation* 95:405-410, 1997.

67. Detrano R, Jenosi A, Lyons KP, et al: Factors affecting sensitivity and specificity of a diagnostic test: the exercise thallium scintigram. *Am J Med* 84:699-710, 1988.

68. Roger VL, Pellikka PA, Oh JK, et al: Stress echocardiography. Part I. Exercise echocardiography: techniques, implementation, clinical applications, and correlations. *Mayo Clin Proc* 70(1):5-15, 1995.

69. Ryan T, Armstrong WF, O'Donnell JA, Feigenbaum H: Risk stratification after acute myocardial infarction by means of exercise two-dimensional echocardiography. *Am Heart J* 1144(6):305-316, 1987.

70. Limacher MC, Quinones MA, Poliner LR, et al: Detection of coronary artery disease with exercise two-dimensional echocardiography. Description of a clinically applicable method and comparison with radionuclide ventriculography. *Circulation* 67:1211-1218, 1983.

71. Oberman A, Fan PH, Nanda NC, et al: Reproducibility of two-dimensional exercise echocardiography. *J Am Coll Cardiol* 14(4):923-928, 1989.

72. Robertson WS, Feigenbaum H, Armstrong WF, et al: Exercise echocardiography: A clinically practical addition in the evaluation of coronary artery disease. *J Am Coll Cardiol* 2(6):1085-1091, 1983.

73. Sawada SG, Ryan T, Fineberg NS, et al: Exercise echocardiographic detection of coronary artery disease in women. *J Am Coll Cardiol* 14(6):440-447, 1989.

74. Quinones MA, Verani MS, Haichin RM, et al: Exercise echocardiography versus 201Tl single-photon emission computed tomography in evaluation of coronary artery disease. Analysis of 292 patients. *Circulation* 85:1026-1031, 1992.

75. Roger VL, Pellikka PA, Oh JK, et al: Identification of multivessel coronary artery disease by exercise echocardiography. *J Am Coll Cardiol* 24(1):109-114, 1994.

76. Beleslin BD, Ostojic M, Stepanovic J, et al: Stress echocardiography in the detection of myocardial ischemia. Head to head comparison of exercise, dobutamine and dipyridamole tests. *Circulation* 90:1168-1176, 1994.

77. Williams MJ, Marwick TH, O'Gorman D, Foale RA: Comparison of exercise echocardiography with an exercise score to diagnose coronary artery disease in women. *Am J Cardiol* 74(5):35-38, 1994.

78. Luotolahti M, Saraste M, Hartiala J: Exercise echocardiography in the diagnosis of coronary artery disease. *Ann Med* 28:73-77, 1996.

79. Hoffmann R, Lethen H, Kleinhans E, et al: Comparative evaluation of bicycle and dobutamine stress echocardiography with perfusion scintigraphy and bicycle electrocardiogram for identification of coronary artery disease. *Am J Cardiol* 72:555-559, 1993.

80. Fleischmann KE, Hunink MG, Kuntz KM, Douglas PS: Exercise echocardiography or exercise SPECT imaging? A meta-analysis of diagnostic test performance. *JAMA* 280(10):913-920, 1998.

81. Kymes SM, Bruns DE, Shaw LJ, et al: Anatomy of a meta-analysis: A critical review of "Exercise echocardiography or exercise SPECT imaging? A meta-analysis of diagnostic test performance." *J Nucl Cardiol* 7:599-615, 2000.

82. Cortigiani L, Bigi R, Gigli G, et al: Prognostic implications of intraventricular conduction defects in patients undergoing stress echocardiography for suspected coronary artery disease. *Am J Med* 115:12-18, 2003.

83. Detrano R, Gianrossi R, Froelicher V: The diagnostic accuracy of the exercise electrocardiogram: a meta-analysis of 22 years of research. *Prog Cardiovasc Dis* 32:173-206, 1989.

84. Lee TH, Boucher CA: Clinical practice. Noninvasive tests in patients with stable coronary artery disease. *N Engl J Med* 244:1840-1845, 2001.

85. Geleijnse ML, Elhendy A: Can stress echocardiography compete with perfusion scintigraphy in the detection of coronary artery disease and cardiac risk assessment? *Eur J Echocardiogr* 1(1):12-21, 2000.

86. O'Keefe JH Jr, Barnhart CS, Bateman TM: Comparison of stress echocardiography and stress myocardial perfusion scintigraphy for diagnosing coronary artery disease and assessing its severity. *Am J Cardiol* 175(11):25d-34d, 1995.

87. Shaw LJ, Heller GV, Travin MI, et al: Cost analysis of diagnostic testing for coronary artery disease in women with stable chest pain. *J Nucl Cardiol* 6:559-569, 1999.

88. Garber AM, Solomon NA: Cost-effectivness of alternative test strategies for the diagnosis of coronary artery disease. *Ann Intern Med* 130:719-728, 1999.

89. Kuntz KM, Fleischmann KE, Hunink MG, et al: Cost effectiveness of diagnostic strategies for patients with chest pain. *Ann Intern Med* 130:709-718, 1999.

90. Marwick TH: Cost-effectiveness of stress echocardiography for assessment of coronary artery disease: What we know and what we need to know. *Eur J Echocardiogr* 1:22-31, 2000.

91. Kim C, Kwok YS, Saha S, et al: Diagnosis of suspected coronary artery disease in women: A cost-effectiveness analysis. *Am Heart J* 137:1019-1027, 1999.

92. Gibbons L, Blair SN, Kohl HW, Cooper K: The safety of maximal exercise testing. *Circulation* 80:846-852, 1989.

93. Bergeron S, Ommen SR, Bailey KR, et al: Exercise echocardiographic findings and outcome of patients referred for evaluation of dyspnea. *J Am Coll Cardiol* 43(12):2242-2246, 2004.

94. Braunwald E, Antman EA, Beasley JW, et al: ACC/AHA 2002 guideline update for the management of patients with unstable angina and non-ST-segment elevation myocardial infarction: a report of the American College of Cardiology/American Heart Association Task Force on Practice Guidelines (Committee on the Management of Patients with Unstable Angina). *J Am Coll Cardiol* 40:1366-1374, 2002.

95. Ramakrishna G, Milavetz JJ, Zinsmeister AR, et al: Effect of exercise treadmill testing and stress imaging on the triage of patients with chest pain: CHEER substudy. *Mayo Clin Proc* 80(3):322-329, 2005.

96. Jeetley P, Burden L, Senior R: Stress echocardiography is superior to exercise ECG in the risk stratification of patients presenting with acute chest pain with negative Troponin. *Eur J Echocardiogr* 7(2):155-164, 2006.

97. Conti A, Sammicheli L, Gallini C, et al: Assessment of patients with low-risk chest pain in the emergency department: Head-to-head comparison of exercise stress echocardiography and exercise myocardial SPECT. *Am Heart J* 149(5):894-901, 2005.

98. Hamm LF, Crow RS, Stull GA, Hannan P: Safety and characteristics of exercise testing early after acute myocardial infarction. *Am J Cardiol* 63(17):1193-1197, 1989.

99. Jain A, Myers GH, Sapin PM, O'Rourke RA: Comparison of symptom limited and low level exercise tolerance tests early after myocardial infarction. *J Am Coll Cardiol* 22(7):1816-1820, 1993.

100. Eagle KA, Guyton RA, Davidoff R, et al: ACC/AHA Guidelines on coronary artery bypass surgery: executive summary: a report of the American College of Cardiology. American Heart Association Task Force on Practice Guidelines. *J Am Coll Cardiol* 34(4):1262-1347, 1999.

101. Smith SC Jr, Dove JT, Jacobs AK, et al: ACC/AHA Guidelines on percutaneous coronary interventions: executive summary: A report of the American College of Cardiology. American Heart Association Task Force on Practice Guidelines. *J Am Coll Cardiol* 37(8):2215-2239, 2001.

102. Armstrong WF, Zoghbi WA: Stress echocardiography: Current methodology and clinical applications. *J Am Coll Cardiol* 45(11):739-747, 2005.

103. Haghani K, Shapiro S, Ginzton LE: Low-level exercise echocardiography identifies contractile reserve in patients with a recent myocardial infarction: Comparison with dobutamine stress echocardiography. *J Am Soc Echocardiogr* 15(7):671-677, 2002.

104. Hoffer EP, Dewe W, Celentano C, Pierard LA: Low-level exercise echocardiography detects contractile reserve and predicts reversible dysfunction after acute myocardial infarction: comparison with low-dose dobutamine echocardiography. *J Am Coll Cardiol* 34(4):989-997, 1999.

105. Lancellotti P, Hoffer EP, Pierard LA: Detection and clinical usefulness of a biphasic response during exercise echocardiography early after myocardial infarction. *J Am Coll Cardiol* 41(7):1142-1147, 2003.

106. Mertes H, Erbel R, Nixdorff U, et al: Exercise echocardiography for the evaluation of patients after nonsurgical coronary artery revascularization. *J Am Coll Cardiol* 21:1087-1093, 1993.

107. Labovitz AJ, Lewen M, Kern MJ, et al: The effects of successful PTCA on left ventricular function: assessment by exercise echocardiography. *Am Heart J* 117(5):1003-1008, 1989.

108. Broderick T, Sawada S, Armstrong WF, et al: Improvement in rest and exercise-induced wall motion abnormalities after coronary angioplasty: an exercise echocardiographic study. *J Am Coll Cardiol* 15(3):591-599, 1990.

109. Hecht HS, DeBord L, Shaw R, et al: Usefulness of supine bicycle stress echocardiography got detection of restenosis after percutaneous transluminal coronary angioplasty. *Am J Cardiol* 71:293-296, 1993.

110. Crouse LJ, Vacek JL, Beauchamp GD, Kramer PH: Use of exercise echocardiography to evaluate patients after coronary angioplasty. *Am J Cardiol* 78(10):1163-1166, 1996.

111. Fioretti PM, Pozzoli MM, Ilmer B, et al: Exercise echocardiography versus thallium-201 SPECT for assessing patients before and after PTCA. *Eur J Cardiol* 13:213, 1992.

112. Sawada SG, Judson WE, Ryan T, et al: Upright bicycle exercise echocardiography after coronary artery bypass grafting. *Am J Cardiol* 64(18):1123-1129, 1989.

113. Crouse LJ, Vacek JL, Beauchamp GD, et al: Exercise echocardiography after coronary artery bypass grafting. *Am J Cardiol* 70(6):572-576, 1992.

114. Kafka H, Leach AJ, Fitzgibbon GM: Exercise echocardiography after coronary artery bypass surgery: Correlation with coronary angiography. *J Am Coll Cardiol* 25:1019-1023, 1995.

115. Jaarsma W, Visser CA, Kupper AJ, et al: Usefulness of two-dimensional exercise echocardiography shortly after myocardial infarction. *Am J Cardiol* 57:86-90, 1986.

116. Ryan T, Armstrong WF, O'Donnell JA, Feigenbaum H: Risk stratification after acute myocardial infarction by means of exercise two-dimensional echocardiography. *Am Heart J* 114(6):1305-1316, 1987.

117. Chen MS, Blackstone EH, Pothier CE, Lauer MS: Heart rate recovery and impact of myocardial revascularization on long-term mortality. *Circulation* 110(18):851-857, 2004.

118. Vivekananthan DP, Blackstone EH, Pothier CE, Lauer MS: Heart rate recovery after exercise is a predictor of mortality, independent of the angiographic severity of coronary disease. *J Am Coll Cardiol* 42(5):831-838, 2003.

119. Watanabe J, Thamilarasan M, Blackstone EH, et al: Heart rate recovery immediately after treadmill exercise and left ventricular systolic dysfunction as predictors of mortality: The case of stress echocardiography. *Circulation* 104:1911-1916, 2001.

120. Peteiro J, Monserrrat L, Pineiro M, et al: Comparison of exercise echocardiography and the Duke treadmill score for risk stratification in patients with known or suspected coronary artery disease and normal resting electrocardiogram. *Am Heart J* 151(6):324e1-10, 2006.

121. Krivokapich J, Child JS, Gerber RS, et al: Prognostic usefulness of positive or negative exercise stress echocardiography for predicting coronary events in ensuing twelve months. *Am J Cardiol* 71(8):646-651, 1993.

122. Elhendy A, Arruda AM, Mahoney DW, Pellikka PA: Prognostic stratification of diabetic patients by exercise echocardiography. *J Am Coll Cardiol* 37(6):1551-1557, 2001.

123. Peteiro JC, Monserrat L, Bouzas A, et al: Risk stratification by treadmill exercise echocardiography. *J Am Soc Echocardiogr* 19(7):894-901, 2006.

124. Marwick TH, Case C, Vasey C, et al: Prediction of mortality by exercise echocardiography: a strategy for combination with the duke treadmill score. *Circulation* 103(21):566-571, 2001.

125. Mazur W, Rivera JM, Khoury AF, et al: Prognostic value of exercise echocardiography: validation of a new risk index combining echocardiographic, treadmill, and exercise electrocardiographic parameters. *J Am Soc Echocardiogr* 16(4):318-325, 2003.

126. Elhendy A, Mahoney DW, McCully RB, et al: Use of a scoring model combining clinical, exercise test, and echocardiographic data to predict mortality in patients with known or suspected coronary artery disease. *Am J Cardiol* 93(10):223-228, 2004.

127. Sicari R, Pasanisi E, Venneri L, et al: Stress echo results predict mortality: a large-scale multicenter prospective international study. *J Am Coll Cardiol* 41(4):589-595, 2003.

128. Arruda AM, Das MK, Roger VL, et al: Prognostic value of exercise echocardiography in 2,632 patients > or = 65 years of age. *J Am Coll Cardiol* 37(4):1036-1041, 2001.

129. Elhendy A, Mahoney DW, Burger KN, et al: Prognostic value of exercise echocardiography in patients with classic angina pectoris. *Am J Cardiol* 94(5):559-563, 2004.

130. McCully RB, Roger VL, Mahoney DW, et al: Outcome after abnormal exercise echocardiography for patients with good exercise capacity: Prognostic importance of the extent and severity of exercise-related left ventricular dysfunction. *J Am Coll Cardiol* 39(8):1345-1352, 2002.

131. Olmos LI, Dakik H, Gordon R, et al: Long-term prognostic value of exercise echocardiography compared with exercise 201Tl, ECG, and clinical variables in patients evaluated for coronary artery disease. *Circulation* 98(24):2679-2686, 1998.

132. Yao SS, Qureshi E, Sherrid MV, Chaudhry FA: Practical applications in stress echocardiography: risk stratification and prognosis in patients with known or suspected ischemic heart disease. *J Am Coll Cardiol* 42(6):1084-1090, 2003.

133. McCully RB, Roger VL, Ommen SR, et al: Outcomes of patients with reduced exercise capacity at time of exercise echocardiography. *Mayo Clin Proc* 79(6):750-757, 2004.

134. D'Andrea A, Severino S, Caso P, et al: Risk stratification and prognosis of patients with known or suspected coronary artery disease by use of supine bicycle exercise stress echocardiography. *Ital Heart J* 6(7):565-572, 2005.

135. Elhendy A, Mahoney DW, Khandheria BK, et al: Prognostic significance of the location of wall motion abnormalities during exercise echocardiography. *J Am Coll Cardiol* 40(9):1623-1629, 2002.

136. McCully RB, Roger VL, Mahoney DW, et al: Outcome after normal exercise echocardiography and predictors of subsequent cardiac events: Follow-up of 1,325 patients. *J Am Coll Cardiol* 31(1):44-49, 1998.

137. Sawada SG, Ryan T, Conley MJ, et al: Prognostic value of a normal exercise echocardiogram. *Am Heart J* 120(1):49-55, 1990.

138. Quintana M, Lindvall K, Ryden L, Brolund E: Prognostic value of predischarge exercise stress echocardiography after acute myocardial infarction. *Am J Cardiol* 76:1115-1121, 1995.

139. Chetlin MD, Armstrong WF, Aurigemma GP, et al: ACC/AHA/ASE 2003 Guideline update for the clinical application of echocardiography: a report of the American College of Cardiology/American Heart Association Task Force on Practice Guidelines. *J Am Coll Cardiol* 42(5):954-970, 2003.

140. Kwok Y, Kim C, Grady D, et al: Meta-analysis of exercise testing to detect coronary artery disease in women. *Am J Cardiol* 83(5):660-666, 1999.

141. Shaw LJ, Bairey Merz CN, Pepine CJ, et al: Insights from the NHLBI-Sponsored Women's Ischemia Syndrome Evaluation (WISE) Study: Part I: gender differences in traditional and novel risk factors, symptom evaluation, and gender-optimized diagnostic strategies. *J Am Coll Cardiol* 47(3 suppl):S4-S20, 2006.

142. Sketch MD, Mohuiddin SM, Lynch JD, et al: Significant sex differences in the correlation of electrocardiographic exercise testing and coronary arteriograms. *Am J Cardiol* 36(2):169-173, 1975.

143. Cox JL, Teskey RJ, Lalonde LD, Iles SE: Noninvasive testing in women presenting with chest pain: Evidence for diagnostic uncertainty. *Can J Cardiol* 11:885-890, 1995.

144. Curzen N, Patel D, Clarke D, et al: Women with chest pain: Is exercise testing worthwhile? *Heart* 76:156-160, 1996.

145. Shaw LJ, Miller DD, Romeis JC, et al: Gender differences in the noninvasive evaluation of patients with suspected coronary artery disease. *Ann Intern Med* 120:559-566, 1994.

146. Mieres JH, Shaw LJ, Arai A, et al: Role of noninvasive testing in the clinical evaluation of women with suspected coronary artery disease: Consensus statement from the Cardiac Imaging Committee, Council on Clinical Cardiology, and the Cardiovascular Imaging and Intervention Committee, Council on Cardiovascular Radiology and Intervention, American Heart Association. *Circulation* 111(5):682-696, 2005.

147. Marwick TH, Anderson T, Williams MJ, et al: Exercise echocardiography is an accurate and cost-efficient technique for detection of coronary artery disease in women. *J Am Coll Cardiol* 26(2):35-41, 1995.

148. Arruda-Olson AM, Juracan EM, Mahoney DW, et al: Prognostic value of exercise echocardiography in 5,798 patients: is there a gender difference? *J Am Coll Cardiol* 39(4):625-631, 2002.

149. Shaw LJ, Vasey C, Sawada S, et al: Impact of gender on risk stratification by exercise and dobutamine stress echocardiography long-term mortality in 4,234 women and 6,898 men. *Eur Heart J* 26:447-456, 2005.

150. Sanfilippo J, Abdollah H, Knott TC, et al: Stress echocardiography in the evaluation of women presenting with chest pain syndrome: A randomized, prospective comparison with electrocardiographic stress testing. *Can J Cardiol* 21(5):405-412, 20205.

151. Heupler S, Mehta R, Lobo A, et al: Prognostic implications of exercise echocardiography in women with known or suspected coronary artery disease. *J Am Coll Cardiol* 30(2):414-420, 1997.

152. Vasey CG, Usedom JE, Allen SM, Koch GG: Prognostic value of exercise echocardiography in women in the community setting. *Am J Cardiol* 85(2):58-60, 2000.

153. Eagle KA, Brundage BH, Chaitman BR et al: Guidelines for perioperative cardiovascular evaluation for noncardiac surgery: a report of the American College of Cardiology/American Heart Association task force on practice guidelines. *J Am Coll Cardiol* 27:910-948, 1996.

154. Wu WC, Bhavsar J, Aziz GF, Sadaniantz A: An overview of stress echocardiography in the study of patients with dilated or hypertrophic cardiomyopathy. *Echocardiography* 21(5):467-475, 2004.

155. Okeie K, Shimizu M, Yoshio H, et al: Left ventricular systolic dysfunction during exercise and dobutamine stress in patients with hypertrophic cardiomyopathy. *J Am Coll Cardiol* 36:856-863, 2000.

156. Bordachar P, Lafitte S, Reuter S, et al: Echocardiographic assessment during exercise of heart failure patients with cardiac resynchronization therapy. *Am J Cardiol* 97(11):1622-1625, 2006.

157. Lafitte S, Bordachar P, Lafitte M, et al: Dynamic ventricular dyssynchrony: An exercise-echocardiography study. *J Am Coll Cardiol* 47(11):2253-2259, 2006.

158. Cohn JM, Wilensky RL, O'Donnell JA, et al: Exercise echocardiography, angiography and intracoronary ultrasound after cardiac transplantation. *Am J Cardiol* 77:1216-1219, 1996.

159. Collings CA, Pinto FJ, Valantine HA, et al: Exercise echocardiography in heart transplant recipients: A comparison with angiography and intracoronary ultrasonography. *J Heart Lung Transplant* 13:604-613, 1994.

160. Aranda JM Jr, Hill J: Cardiac transplant vasculopathy. *Chest* 118(6):792-800, 2000.

161. Wang A, Jaggers J, Ungerleider RM, et al: Exercise echocardiographic comparison of pulmonary autograft and aortic homograft replacements for aortic valve disease in adults. *J Heart Valve Dis* 12(2):202-208, 2003.

162. Wu WC, Aziz G, Sadaniantz A: The use of stress echocardiography in the assessment of mitral valvular disease. *Echocardiography* 21(5):51-58, 2004.

163. Bach DS: Stress echocardiography for evaluation of hemodynamics: Valvular heart disease, prosthetic valve function, and pulmonary hypertension. *Prog Cardiovasc Dis* 39:543-554, 1997.

164. Clyne CA, Arrighi JA, Maron BJ, et al: Systemic and left ventricular responses to exercise stress of asymptomatic patients with valvular aortic stenosis. *Am J Cardiol* 68:1469-1476, 1991.

165. Atwood JE, Kawanishi S, Myers J, Froelicher VF: Exercise testing in patients with aortic stenosis. *Chest* 93(5):1083-1087, 1988.

166. Otto CM, Pearlman AS, Kraft CD, et al: Physiologic changes with maximal exercise in asymptomatic valvular aortic stenosis assessed by Doppler echocardiography. *J Am Coll Cardiol* 20(5):160-167, 1992.

167. Chambers J: Exercise testing to guide surgery in aortic stenosis. *Heart* 82:7-8, 1999.

168. Otto CM, Burwash I, Legget ME, et al: Prospective study of asymptomatic valvular aortic stenosis: Clinical, echocardiographic, and exercise predictors of outcome. *Circulaton* 95:2262-2270, 1997.

169. Linderholm H, Osterman G, Teien D: Detection of coronary artery disease by means of exercise ECG in patients with aortic stenosis. *Acta Med Scand* 218:181-188, 1985.

170. Alborino D, Hoffman JL, Fournet PC, Bloch A: Value of exercise testing to evaluate the indication for surgery in asymptomatic patients with valvular aortic stenosis. *J Heart Valve Dis* 11(2):204-209, 2002.

171. Lancellotti P, Lebois F, Simon M, et al: Prognostic importance of quantitative exercise Doppler echocardiography in asymptomatic valvular aortic stenosis. *Circulation* 112(9 Suppl):I377-I382, 2005.

172. Sagar KB, Wann LS, Paulson WJ, Lewis S: Role of exercise Doppler echocardiography in isolated mitral stenosis. *Chest* 92(1):7-30, 1987.

173. Braverman AC, Thomas JD, Lee RT: Doppler echocardiographic estimation of mitral valve area during changing hemodynamic conditions. *Am J Cardiol* 68:1485-1490, 1991.

174. Leavitt JL, Coats MH, Falk RH: Effects of exercise on transmitral gradient and pulmonary artery pressure in patients with mitral stenosis or a prosthetic mitral valve: A Doppler echocardiographic study. *J Am Coll Cardiol* 17(7):520-526, 1991.

175. Tunnick PA, Freedberg RS, Gargiulo A, Kronzon I: Exercise Doppler echocardiography as an aid to clinical decision making in mitral valve disease. *J Am Soc Echocardiogr* 5:225-230, 1992.

176. Tribouilloy C, Shen WF, Leborgne L, et al: Comparative value of Doppler echocardiography and cardiac catheterization for management decision-making in patients with left-sided valvular regurgitation. *Eur Heart J* 17(2):272-280, 1996.

177. Leung DY, Griffin BP, Stewart WJ, et al: Left ventricular function after valve repair for chronic mitral regurgitation: Predictive value of preoperative assessment of contractile reserve by exercise echocardiography. *J Am Coll Cardiol* 28:1198-1205, 1996.

178. Pahl E, Duffy CE, Chaudhry FA: The role of stress echocardiography in children. *Echocardiography* 17(5):507-512, 2000.

179. Pahl E, Seghal R, Chrystof D, et al: Feasibility of exercise stress echocardiography for the follow-up of children with coronary involvement secondary to Kawasaki disease. *Circulation* 91(1):122-128, 1995.

180. Alkotob ML, Soltani P, Sheatt MA, et al: Reduced exercise capacity and stress-induced pulmonary hypertension in patients with scleroderma. *Chest* 130(1):176-181, 2006.

181. Collins N, Bastian B, Jones C, et al: Abnormal pulmonary vascular responses in patients registered with a systemic autoimmunity database: Pulmonary Hypertension Assessment and Screening Evaluation using stress echocardiography (PHASE-I). *Eur J Echocardiogr* 7(6):439-446, 2006. Epub 2006 Jan 20.

182. Mor-Avi V, Jacobs LD, Weiss RJ, et al: Color encoding of endocardial motion improves the interpretation of contrast-enhanced echocardiographic stress tests by less-experienced readers. *J Am Soc Echocardiogr* 19(1):48-54, 2006.

183. Vitarelli A, Sciomer S, Penco M, et al: Assessment of left ventricular dyssynergy by color kinesis. *Am J Cardiol* 81(12A):86G-90G, 1998.

184. Ha JW, Oh JK, Pellikka PA, et al: Diastolic stress echocardiography: A novel noninvasive diagnostic test for diastolic dysfunction using supine bicycle exercise Doppler echocardiography. *J Am Soc Echocardiogr* 18(1):63-68, 2005.

185. Burgess MI, Jenkins C, Sharman JE, Marwick TH: Diastolic stress echocardiography: hemodynamic validation and clinical significance of estimation of ventricular filling pressure with exercise. *J Am Coll Cardiol* 47(9):1891-1900, 2006.

186. von Bibra H TA, Klein A, et al: Regional diastolic function by pulsed Doppler myocardial mapping for the detection of left ventricular ischemia during pharmacologic stress testing. *J Am Coll Cardiol* 36(2):444-452, 2000.

187. Goebel B, Arnold R, Koletzki E, et al: Exercise tissue Doppler echocardiography with strain rate imaging in healthy young individuals: Feasibility, normal values and reproducibility. *Int J Cardiovasc Imaging* 23(2):149-155, 2007.

188. Reuss CS, Moreno CA, Appleton CP, Lester SJ: Doppler tissue imaging during supine and upright exercise in healthy adults. *J Am Soc Echocardiogr* 18(12):1343-1348, 2005.

189. Madler CF, Payne N, Wilkenshoff U, et al: Non-invasive diagnosis of coronary artery disease by quantitative stress echocardiography: optimal diagnostic models using off-line tissue Doppler in the MYDISE study. *Eur Heart J* 24(17):1584-1594, 2003.

190. Galiuto L, Ignone G, DeMaria A: Contraction and relaxation velocities of the normal left ventricle using pulsed wave tissue Doppler echocardiography. *Am J Cardiol* 81:609-614, 1998.

191. Smiseth O, Stoylen A, Halfdan I: Tissue Doppler imaging for the diagnosis of coronary artery disease. *Curr Opin Cardiol* 19:421-429, 2004.

192. Sutherland GR, Di Salvo G, Claus P, et al: Strain and strain rate-imaging: A new clinical approach to quantifying regional myocardial function. *J Am Soc Echocardiogr* 17:788-802, 2004.

193. Davidavicius G, Kowalski M, Williams I, et al: Can strain and strain rate measurement be performed during both dobutamine

and exercise echocardiography, and do regional deformation responses differ with different forms of stress testing? *J Am Soc Echocardiogr* 16:299-308, 2003.

194. Abraham T, Belohlavek M, Thomson H, et al: Time to onset of regional relaxation: Feasibility, variability, and utility of a novel index of regional myocardial function by strain rate imaging. *J Am Coll Cardiol* 39:1531-1537, 2002.

195. Shimoni S, Zoghbi W, Xie F, et al: Real-time assessment of myocardial perfusion and wall motion during bicycle and treadmill exercise echocardiography: comparison with single photon emission computed tomography. *J Am Coll Cardiol* 37(3):741-747, 2001.

196. Laskar R, Grayburn PA: Assessment of myocardial perfusion with contrast echocardiography at rest and with stress: An emerging technology. *Prog Cardiovasc Dis* 43:245-258, 2000.

197. Moir S, Haluska B, Jenkins C, et al: Comparison of specificity of quantitative myocardial contrast echocardiography for diagnosis of coronary artery disease in patients with versus without diabetes mellitus. *Am J Cardiol* 96(2):187-192, 2005.

198. Moir S, Haluska B, Jenkins C, et al: Incremental benefit of myocardial contrast to combined dipyridamole-exercise stress echocardiography for the assessment of coronary artery disease. *Circulation* 110(9):1108-1113, 2004.

199. Moir S, Marwick TH: Combination of contrast with stress echocardiography: A practical guide to methods and interpretation. *Cardiovasc Ultrasound* 2:15, 2004.

200. Mulvagh SL, DeMaria AN, Feinstein SB, et al: Contrast echocardiography: Current and future applications. *J Am Soc Echocardiogr* 13(4):331-342, 2000.

201. Jeetley P HM, Kamp O, et al: Myocardial contrast echocardiography for the detection of coronary artery stenosis: A prospective multicenter study in comparison with single-photon emission computed tomography. *J Am Coll Cardiol* 47(1):141-145, 2006. Epub 2005 Dec 15.

202. Jeetley P, Swinburn J, Hickman M, et al: Myocardial contrast echocardiography predicts left ventricular remodelling after acute myocardial infarction. *J Am Soc Echocardiogr* 17(10):1030-1036, 2006.

203. Hickman M, Jeetley P, Senior R: Usefulness of myocardial contrast echocardiography derived coronary flow reserve to accurately determine severity of left anterior descending coronary artery stenosis. *Am J Cardiol* 93(9):1159-1162, 2004.

204. Takuma S, Cardinal C, Homma S: Real-time three-dimensional stress echocardiography: A review of current applications. *Echocardiography* 17(8):791-794, 2000.

205. Ahmad M, Xie T, McColloch M, et al: Real-time three-dimensional dobutamine stress echocardiography in assessment of ischemia: Comparison with two-dimensional dobutamine stress echocardiography. *J Am Coll Cardiol* 37:1303-1309, 2001.

206. Pulerwitz T, Hirata K, Abe Y, et al: Feasibility of using a real-time 3-dimensional technique for contrast dobutamine stress echocardiography. *J Am Soc Echocardiogr* 19(5):540-545, 2006.

207. Zwas DR, Takuma S, Mullis-Jansson S, et al: Feasibility of real-time 3-dimensional treadmill stress echocardiography. *J Am Soc Echocardiogr* 12:285-289, 1999.

208. Marwick TH, D'Hondt A, Mairesse GH, et al: Comparative ability of dobutamine and exercise stress in inducing myocardial ischaemia in active patients. *Br Heart J* 72:31-38, 1994.

Chapter 16

Stress Echocardiography with Nonexercise Techniques: Principles, Protocols, Interpretation, and Clinical Applications

THOMAS H. MARWICK, MBBS, PhD

TABLE 16–1. Indications for Nonexercise Stressors

Unable to Exercise	Able to Exercise
Inability to exercise maximally	Specific indications
Diagnosis of coronary artery disease, decision making	Coronary spasm
Risk stratification	Myocardial viability
Situations preventing exercise	Developing indications
Angiography laboratory, operating room	Onset of ischemia
	New technologies
	(TDI, CK, contrast)

CK, color kinesis; TDI, tissue Doppler imaging.

Background

Indications for Nonexercise Stress Testing

The performance of a maximal level of exercise is a critical determinant of the sensitivity of all stress modalities for the detection of coronary artery disease (CAD). Unfortunately, many patients—fully 30% to 40% at some tertiary centers—either cannot exercise at all or cannot exercise maximally,[1] but these patients may still need to undergo stress testing for diagnostic, decision-making, or prognostic purposes. The most common causes of limited exercise capacity are vascular disease and orthopedic problems. Other situations warranting nonexercise stress testing include severe cardiopulmonary disease (CPD) and general debility, especially among the elderly, in whom pharmacologic testing has been shown to be well tolerated and reliable.[2-5]

Although the inability of a patient to exercise maximally constitutes the main indication for the use of nonexercise stressors, such stressors are also indicated in other situations (Table 16–1). The most important of these situations include circumstances in which pharmacologic stress may offer diagnostic data, which are not available from exercise stress, for example, the diagnosis of coronary spasm using ergonovine testing.[6,7] A similar scenario involves patients early or late after myocardial infarction (MI), after which left ventricular (LV) dysfunction may not be permanent. The diagnostic challenge in this situation is that while stunned myocardium improves sponta-

neously, the revascularization of hibernating myocardium has implications for functional capacity and prognosis. Echocardiography can be used with dobutamine[8] or dipyridamole[9,10] stress, or both[11] for the identification of viable myocardium.

Pharmacologic stress is more appropriate than exercise in some environments, such as the cardiac catheterization laboratory or operating room (OR). Finally, nonexercise methods have been used in preference to exercise echocardiography even in patients who are able to exercise because of their relative technical ease. The incremental nature of these stressors means that the time course of ischemia can be identified; these data are not available using posttreadmill stress and are more difficult to obtain with bicycle exercise testing. Although the decision to use a nonexercise stress may not be justifiable with routine echocardiographic imaging at present, the facilitation of adjunctive techniques (which may be less feasible during exercise than nonexercise stress)—such as tissue Doppler, color kinesis (CK), and contrast echocardiography—could in the future justify the use of nonexercise techniques in patients who are able to exercise.

Choice and Mechanism of Action of Nonexercise Stressors

The two general groups of nonexercise stress agents induce ischemia by increasing myocardial work and oxygen consumption (exercise-simulating agents) or by influencing coronary perfusion and therefore myocardial oxygen supply (vasoactive agents). The latter include the coronary vasodilators dipyridamole and adenosine, which cause ischemia by provoking coronary steal, and ergonovine, which can be used to provoke coronary spasm. In addition, nonpharmacologic approaches, including hand-grip and the cold pressor test, have been used.[12,13] Hand-grip testing is often combined with dobutamine-atropine testing,[14] but the cold pressor test has not been widely adopted clinically because of limited efficacy and discomfort.

Exercise-Simulating Agents

The exercise simulators include dobutamine and other sympathomimetic agents, pacing, and atropine (usually used as an adjunct to the other approaches), all of which increase cardiac work and myocardial oxygen requirement. The induction of ischemia and regional dysfunction reflects the inability of the diseased coronary circulation to respond to this increased oxygen demand, a process that parallels the response to exercise. Because increased cardiac workload and oxygen demand is the usual mechanism underlying ischemia in most ambulatory situations, the exercise-simulating agents are often considered to be a more physiologic means of stressing the heart. However, additional mechanisms include effects on cardiac metabolism producing an "oxygen-wasting" effect[15-17] and concurrent "supply" ischemia resulting from reduction of subendocardial perfusion and maldistribution of coronary flow.[18]

Vasoactive Agents

The use of dipyridamole in combination with myocardial perfusion imaging is based on the induction of maximal coronary vasodilation in all territories. Flow heterogeneities (and therefore apparent perfusion defects) develop if a coronary stenosis limits the regional hyperemic response.[19] This process does not involve the provocation of ischemia in a functional or metabolic sense. In contrast, the development of regional wall motion abnormalities at stress echocardiography necessitates the induction of ischemia.

The chief mechanism of vasodilator-induced ischemia is coronary steal.[19] Horizontal steal involves blood flowing to nonstenosed from stenosed territory, resulting from reduced collateral flow into the stenosed territory because of depressurization of vessels supplying the collaterals, which result from increased runoff. Vertical steal occurs because vasodilator-induced depressurization of the microcirculation causes subendocardial vessels to collapse under the greater extravascular pressure in this region and "stealing" flow to the subepicardium from the subendocardium. Other mechanisms of vasodilator-induced ischemia, unrelated to coronary steal, include reduced coronary supply because of coronary spasm, systemic hypotension, or collapse of the stenosis. Under conditions of maximal coronary hyperemia, driving pressure is the main determinant of myocardial perfusion because vasodilator reserve is exhausted. Hence, systemic hypotension may accentuate hypoperfusion resulting from coronary steal. Stenosis "collapse" may be provoked if profound microcirculatory vasodilation causes a reduction of lateral pressure induced by increased flow. Finally, myocardial oxygen demand may be increased in response to increased cardiac workload because of increased sympathetic activity secondary to angina.

Agents Used to Identify Myocardial Viability

In the presence of dysfunctional but viable myocardium, regional function is enhanced by the inotropic effect of low-dose dobutamine; this appears to require both recruitable perfusion and an increment in metabolism.[20] Viable myocardium supplied by a patent infarct-related vessel (generally corresponding to stunned myocardium) demonstrates a sustained improvement during the infusion, which then reverses after the test. Viable tissue supplied by a stenosed infarct-related artery (which may involve stunned or chronically malperfused tissue) is characterized by an initial improvement, occurring at low doses (<20 μg/kg/min), low heart rates (HRs), or both, followed by deterioration of regional function as the chronotropic effect becomes more prominent and myocardial work increases.[8] If the region is supplied by a critically stenosed artery, however, it may be possible for the territory to become ischemic before there is a noticeable enhancement of contractility. Moreover, the ability of the myocardium to thicken is determined by the amount of infarcted tissue within the segment.[21]

Myocardial viability may also be inferred from the contractile response to dipyridamole. The mechanism of this is also putative but probably relates to myocardial congestion with interstitial fluid as a result of vasodilation. A so-called mini-Starling effect may be caused by this congestive process, producing additional tension on the myofibrils.[22]

Principles of Nonexercise Stress Techniques

Pharmacology and Physiopathology of Nonexercise Stress Techniques

Exercise-Simulating Agents

The exercise simulating agents include dobutamine, dopamine, epinephrine, and isoproterenol. Of these, dobutamine has become the most commonly administered exercise simulating agent, and the majority of published data on pharmacologic stress echocardiography have involved this agent. Dopamine stimulates alpha receptors and, if it extravasates, may cause localized limb ischemia resulting from vasoconstriction. Dopamine may also be a less effective precipitant of myocardial ischemia than is dobutamine.[23] Although other sympathomimetic agents have been used for stress testing, epinephrine and isoproterenol are probably the more arrhythmogenic. This side effect is dose dependent, but its avoidance by conservative dosing may compromise the sensitivity of the test by limiting the amount of stress on the heart.

Dobutamine is predominantly a beta-1 agonist, and normal areas become hyperkinetic in response to its inotropic effect. Segments supplied by a stenosed coronary artery may become akinetic or dyskinetic, but more subtly, are unable to augment their thickening and excursion. Vasodilation and chronotropy appear at higher doses,[23] usually at the 20 μg/kg/min level of the routine dobutamine stress protocols, reflecting the stimulation of other receptors to a lesser degree. This chronotropic response appears to be the most important factor in terms of precipitating ischemia; most dobutamine stress protocols cause a mean HR increment of 40 to 50 beats per minute and mean peak HRs of 110 to 120 beats per minute.[24-30] However, reflex bradycardia may occur in response to hypertension. Blood pressure (BP) normally rises in response to the inotropic effect of the drug, but high doses cause vasodilation and therefore cause BP to fall at peak doses. Increases in myocardial oxygen demand resulting from increased cardiac work and a weak vasodilator effect lead to the development of coronary hyperemia in territories supplied by normal coronary arteries. Although this response is probably less than that induced by coronary vasodilators, the coronary hyperemic response to dobutamine stress permits its combination with perfusion scintigraphy.[30-33] The detection of myocardial perfusion defects in the presence of coronary disease may be augmented by partial volume effects as a result of thinning of the ischemic wall.

Vasoactive Agents

The principal coronary vasodilators are dipyridamole and adenosine, which differ with respect to the onset and duration of their effects. Dipyridamole increases endogenous adenosine levels by reducing cellular reuptake and metabolism and thereby acts indirectly.[19] This indirect mechanism causes some delay between the administration of this agent and the timing of peak vasodilation, and this indirect action may account for interindividual variations in the magnitude of its effects. Adenosine acts directly on the vasculature, its vasodilator efficacy being equivalent to that of papaverine.[34] The potency and speed of onset of adenosine cause its side effects to be more intense but also more short-lived than those of dipyridamole.

Ergonovine stress echocardiography is not widely practiced, although its use as a test for coronary spasm is well validated. This agent has a direct effect on the vessel; responsiveness to acetylcholine may be related to loss of nitric oxide production at the site of disease.

Exercise Simulation Using Pacing Stress

Several nonpharmacologic stressors have been used, including "physiologic" stresses, such as the cold pressor test, which are poorly tolerated. Pacing is an alternative means of increasing cardiac work; pacing-induced tachycardia increases myocardial oxygen consumption and causes myocardial ischemia in the setting of significant coronary stenoses.[35,36] The reduction of subendocardial perfusion with pacing[36] may also contribute to the development of ischemia.

Ventricular pacing is not favored because it causes both abnormal regional contractility and abnormal perfusion, so that pacing stress techniques generally involve atrial stimulation, either transvenously or via the esophagus. Of the transesophageal pacing approaches, the "pill" electrode has formerly been studied; although this technique is effective, it may cause significant discomfort. Attachment of pacing electrodes to transesophageal echocardiography (TEE) probes has been reported in trials[37,38] but has not moved into commercial production. A small esophageal pacing catheter offers enhanced contact between the electrodes and the esophagus. The technique causes less discomfort than other pacing techniques because of the presence of smaller pacing thresholds,[39] but it is not widely used.

Pacing stress may be useful in patients in whom the pharmacologic approaches are contraindicated or associated with side effects. Additional attractions that might justify its use in preference to pharmacologic testing include the capacity to achieve a target HR in virtually all patients, the potential to immediately terminate the tachycardia if the patient develops complications (in contrast to pharmacologic methods, which require a period of time for the effects to dissipate), and the ability to perform measurements in the ischemic ventricle at a low heart rate (after cessation of pacing). Using atrial pacing stress, ischemic myocardium has been shown to have reduced ventricular compliance.[40] Sudden termination of stress during ischemia may also be of value in the combination of stress testing with color-flow Doppler, as the use of low frame rates may pose a problem at high HRs. Despite the benefits of transesophageal atrial pacing, its availability for many years,[41] and recent data showing correlation with dobutamine echocardiography, despite a shorter test duration and better patient tolerance,[39] this technique has not become widely used because it remains somewhat invasive.

Combined Approaches

Atropine reduces the depressant effect of vagal stimulation on HR and may be particularly useful when reflex reduction of the HR occurs in response to BP elevation. Atropine is combined with dobutamine in patients who fail to develop an adequate degree of tachycardia in response to dobutamine, the most common situation involving patients taking beta-receptor antagonists.[42-44] Tachycardia (and therefore ischemia resulting from increased oxygen demand) may be obtained by combining atropine with dipyridamole.[45-47] In both circumstances, the addition of atropine to other stressors has been associated with an increment in sensitivity. Indeed, there is a trend toward earlier use of atropine during the dobutamine protocol,[48,49] especially in beta-blocked patients. Early administration of atropine should not be allowed to interfere with the assessment of the low-dose response, so this agent is not administered before the end of the 20 μg/kg/min dose. A simple guide is that patients who fail to attain a HR of 70 beats per minute or fail to increase HR by 5 beats per minute at this dose rarely achieve target HR and might as well have the atropine early so as to avoid a prolonged test.[48] Of course, while nondiagnostic results resulting from a submaximal HR response can be avoided by the use of atropine, this adjunct does not help the results of submaximal tests that reflect premature termination of pharmacologic stress as a result of side effects.

The rationale for combining dobutamine and dipyridamole reflects their different mechanisms. The sequence of drug administration can be used to produce a stepwise stress on the heart. The initial administration of dipyridamole permits detection of the most severe coronary stenoses resulting from the development of coronary steal. The subsequent incremental administration of dobutamine progressively increases oxygen demand, permitting the identification of progressively more moderate stenoses.[50] The combination has also been used to enhance the accuracy of detection of myocardial viability.[11] While the combination of these techniques has afforded higher levels of sensitivity than the individual tests can provide, this is obtained at the cost of an unacceptably long stress protocol.[50]

Echocardiographic Approach to Nonexercise Stress Techniques

Image Acquisition

The technical challenges of pharmacologic and pacing stress, although less extreme than those posed by exercise echocardiography, mandate the use of the best available equipment. The development of harmonic imaging has made a major impact on endocardial visualization[51-53] and therefore the feasibility of stress echocardiography.[54] Although few patients (<2%) have completely uninterpretable images, failure to detect the endocardium in every myocardial segment is common, and contrast is indicated if two segments are obscured (Fig. 16-1).

Typically, transthoracic images are obtained in the standard views (parasternal long- and short-axis and apical four- and two-chamber), to which the apical long-axis is routinely added, which may overcome technical problems with parasternal imaging. An apical short axis is often worthwhile but may be difficult to maintain in the same plane during the stress. Of the complementary imaging techniques, including contrast, strain and three-dimensional (3D) imaging, the evaluation of coronary flow reserve in the left anterior descending (LAD) artery, is the simplest addition, although this seems to be most feasible in combination with adenosine.[55]

TEE has been employed in combination with both pharmacologic[56-58] and pacing stress[37,38,59] usually for patients with inadequate transthoracic images. During transesophageal imaging with pharmacologic stress, the standard imaging planes are approximated as closely as possible by recording transverse and longitudinal esophageal and transgastric short- and long-axis views. During pacing with electrodes attached to the TEE probe, the need to stimulate the esophagus inhibits the ability to move the transducer, so that imaging is performed in the transgastric planes only.

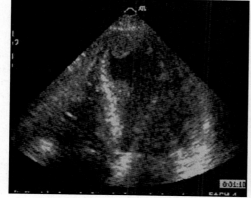
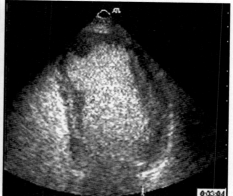

Figure 16-1. Use of myocardial contrast for left ventricular opacification during stress echocardiography. Compared with harmonic imaging (A), the postcontrast end-diastolic apical four-chamber image (B) shows significant improvement of lateral wall resolution.

Although the constraints of a busy stress echocardiography schedule may preclude the performance of a detailed examination in every patient, a "screening" M-mode, pulsed wave (especially for LV inflow), and color Doppler echocardiographic examination should be performed at the beginning of every study. Tissue Doppler images at baseline are obtained for the assessment of filling pressure[60] and dyssynchrony.[61] Time should also be taken to optimize two-dimensional (2D) echocardiographic images, gain settings (for endocardial detection), and image size (to obtain the best spatial resolution and frame rate). During the stress, the patient is imaged continuously, and the images are stored digitally and on videotape. When the study is performed for the diagnosis of coronary disease, the default quad-screen display is set up with a resting image, a low-dose image (10 μg/kg/min dobutamine, 0.56 mg/kg dipyridamole, or a small HR increment with pacing), and two high-dose images (40 μg/kg/min dobutamine or 0.84 mg/kg dipyridamole with or without atropine), or a peak and early poststress image. However, the ability to save images at multiple stages enables easy alteration of this display. For example, when the clinical question pertains to the possibility of viable myocardium, two low-dose images should be displayed (5 and 10 μg/kg/min dobutamine) and one high-dose image.

Image Processing

Both videotape and digital techniques are used for interpretation and archiving of stress echocardiograms. Digital image processing facilitates image display and interpretation by allowing a side-by-side display of resting, low-dose, and high-dose images and the ability to review individual frames (which is useful to evaluate the temporal sequence of contraction). However, all studies should be recorded on videotape as well as in digital format, to provide a backup in case technical problems with the digital capture (especially triggering) or corruption of the archived data threaten loss of the study. Indeed, routine review of videotape has a significant impact on diagnosis, probably by permitting review of off-axis images and regions that are not adequately represented by saving a single cardiac cycle.[62]

Qualitative Interpretation

The interpretation of stress echocardiograms for clinical purposes is based on a qualitative evaluation of regional function at rest and stress.[63] Some standardization is obtained by scoring regional wall motion and thickening in a number of segments. The American Heart Association has proposed a unified 17-segment model, which includes the apical cap, to facilitate comparison between imaging modalities.[64] Unfortunately, this template ignores the small but important detail that the true apex is often not identified at echocardiography, so the most widely used template remains the 16-segment model (anterior, septal, lateral, and inferior at the apex, with these segments and anteroseptal and posterior segments at the base and midpapillary muscle level).[65] Despite this standardization, however, the expertise of the physician interpreting the test is critical, and even accomplished echocardiographers require a significant learning period. In a study of echocardiographers learning dipyridamole stress echocardiography, Picano and colleagues[66] reported that 100 supervised studies were required to bring the accuracy of novices to the level of experts. Despite many technical advances in stress echocardiography in the last two decades, this learning curve remains important.

The standard qualitative algorithm for interpretation of pharmacologic stress echocardiography is summarized in Table 16–2. With the exception of the low-dose responses, which denote myocardial viability, it may also be applied to pacing or other stressors.

TABLE 16–2. Interpretation of Myocardial Viability and Ischemia Using Dobutamine Echocardiography

Diagnosis	Resting Function	Low Dose	Peak/Poststress Function
Normal	Normal	Normal	Hyperkinetic
Ischemic	Normal	Normal (unless severe CAD)	Reduction versus rest Reduction versus other segments Delayed contraction
Viable, patent IRA	Hypo/akinetic	Improvement	Sustained improvement
Viable, stenosed IRA	Hypo/akinetic	Improvement	Reduction (compared with low dose)
Infarction	A/dyskinetic	No change	No change

CAD, coronary artery disease; IRA, infarct-related artery.

Regional wall motion at rest may be classified as normal, hypokinetic, akinetic, or dyskinetic. Severe hypokinesia may be difficult to distinguish from akinesia; a useful guide is based on endocardial excursion, with less than 2 mm identifying akinesia and

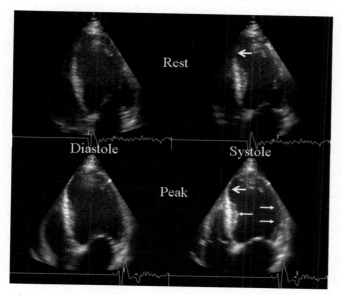

Figure 16–2. *End-diastolic and end-systolic freeze-frame images illustrating left ventricular enlargement at dobutamine echocardiography in a patient with left ventricular dysfunction and multivessel coronary artery disease. There is a resting wall motion abnormality in the apex (large arrow), which is unchanged with stress. At peak stress, there is left ventricular enlargement with reduction of systolic motion and thickening of the lateral (and to a lesser degree the septal) wall.*

less than 5 mm indicating hypokinesia. Regions that fail to thicken or that move only in late systole (after movement of the adjacent myocardium) may be moving passively and should be considered akinetic, irrespective of endocardial excursion. Segments with resting akinesis or dyskinesis are most likely composed of infarcted myocardium, if the wall is thinned and dense,[67] but in the absence of thinning, they are likely to consist of viable tissue. Indeed, hypokinetic segments are not identified as being infarcted on the basis that residual contraction implies the presence of residual viability. Because the process of thinning and fibrosis takes some time after infarction, myocardium of normal thickness is commonly seen after recent or nontransmural infarction. Improvement of abnormal function in response to low doses of dobutamine (5 or 10 μg/kg/min) or dipyridamole (0.28 or 0.56 mg/kg) suggests the presence of viable myocardium (Fig. 16–2). This finding is more reliable if the segment subsequently deteriorates, which indicates ischemia.

The global LV responses to dobutamine stress include an increase in cardiac output (CO) and reduction of LV cavity size. LV dilation implies multivessel or left main coronary artery (LMCA) disease (see Fig. 16–2), but this is less commonly seen with pharmacologic than exercise stress,[68] probably because of reduction of LV loading. Together with an extreme inotropic response, this afterload reduction may produce cavity obliteration (Fig. 16–3), and although this response is favorable prognostically (presumably reflecting a low

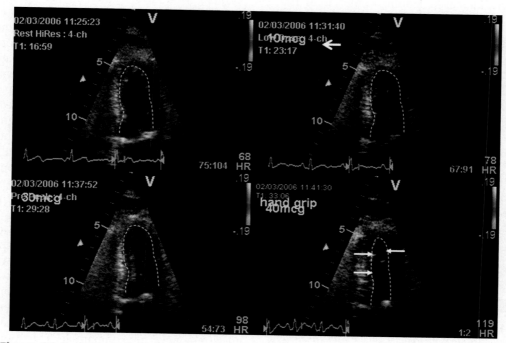

Figure 16–3. *End-systolic freeze-frame images of apical four-chamber views illustrating marked reduction in left ventricular volume at peak stress, with close to cavity obliteration. The resulting low transmural wall stress may prevent the induction of ischemia despite the presence of coronary artery disease.*

probability of multivessel disease),[69] it may impair sensitivity both because of reducing transmural wall stress and because endocardial excursion is reduced and small areas of wall motion are unrecognized.[70] Use of intravenous (IV) beta-blockade allows the HR to slow rapidly after stress, filling the LV cavity and revealing wall motion abnormalities, which were unidentified at peak stress[71]; a similar outcome can be obtained by poststress imaging.

The normal response to inotropic stress is to increase endocardial excursion, speed of contraction, and degree of myocardial thickening. A deterioration of function from rest, or after an initial enhancement of function, indicates ischemia (Fig. 16–4). Variants of overt deterioration include delayed contraction ("tardokinesis") and reduced myocardial thickening. Caution should be applied in the assessment of peri-infarct zones, which may fail to improve function with stress or even appear dyskinetic if the infarct bulges as result of tethering by the infarcted zone. Examination of wall thickening may assist in distinguishing peri-infarct ischemia and tethering.

The evaluation of segments with abnormal resting function is more difficult. Akinetic or even dyskinesic segments may still be viable if they augment in response to either low-dose dipyridamole or dobutamine. Care must be taken to avoid misinterpretation based on differences in image planes, especially if the wall motion abnormality is localized. Deterioration of augmenting myocardium identifies ischemia, but in the absence of augmentation, a deterioration of function probably reflects increased loading rather than ischemia.[72] Segments with resting hypokinesia often reflect nontransmural infarction, although some normal segments may be mildly hypokinetic, and it is important to be wary of overinterpretation, especially in the posterior wall. Analysis of myocardial deformation using two-dimensional strain techniques have suggested that the pattern of impaired longitudinal function with preserved radial or rotational motion may be used to identify nontransmural infarction, as measured by gadolinium enhanced magnetic resonance imaging (MRI). Hypokinetic segments are also the most challenging for the identification of ischemia; those demonstrating a stress-induced improvement are classified as normal, and those showing a deterioration (compared with either rest or low-dose) are identified as ischemic. However, differentiation between degrees of hypokinesia may be difficult, even with side-by-side cine-loop analysis. Some caution needs to be applied in the interpretation of regional variations in the degree of hyperkinesis because these may occur in normal patients.[73] The diagnosis in hypokinetic regions that fail to improve function in response to stress is debated; if adjacent segments mount a hyperkinetic response, these are characterized as ischemic.

The greatest limitations of the current application of stress echocardiography are concerns related to subjectivity and reproducibility. Although single-center studies have suggested that the interobserver variation in interpretation is small,[74] interinstitution variability (while similar to that of other imaging techniques) is significant.[75] Interinstitution variability is particularly a problem in studies of poor image quality and in patients with mild ischemia. This discordance has been progressively reduced by definition of standard reading criteria[76] and more recently by the adoption of harmonic imaging.[77] The following reading guidelines are useful for controlling variation: minor degrees of hypokinesia are not identified as ischemia (especially if only apparent at peak and not at poststress readings); focal abnormalities that do not follow angiographic territories are ignored; abnormalities are corroborated whenever possible with another view; basal inferior and septal segments are not identified as abnormal in the absence of a neighboring abnormal segment; studies are read by multiple observers whenever possible; and reading is blinded to all other data.

Finally, a standard sequence is found to be valuable in the interpretation of stress echocardiograms. First, review the resting data or previous transthoracic echocardiogram for nonwall motion data that may color interpretation, including M-mode and Doppler components. On the digital images, check that images are triggered correctly and the prestress, peak stress, and poststress views are comparable. Then briefly review all of the side-by-side displays to see if there are new wall motion abnormalities or obvious changes in cavity size (suggesting multivessel disease) or cavity shape. Seg-

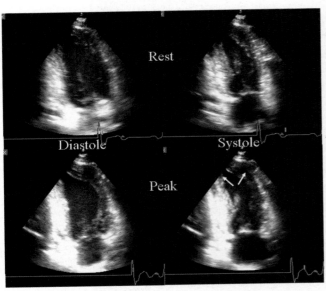

Figure 16–4. Apical two-chamber views illustrating the development of myocardial ischemia (reduced wall thickening, arrows) of the apex during dobutamine stress echocardiography. End-diastolic images are given on the left and systolic images on the right, with resting images above and peak dose below.

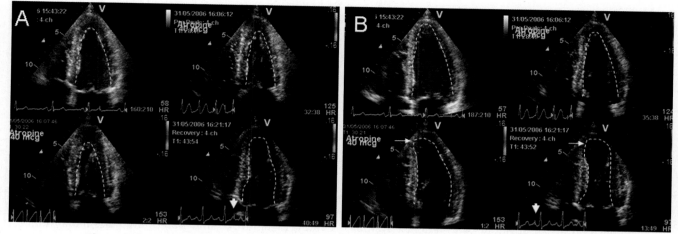

Figure 16–5. *Apical four-chamber views illustrating the phenomenon of early relaxation. A, Homogeneous contraction with reduction of apical cavity volume. B, An apical shape change after the end of systole (see broad arrow on electrocardiogram).*

mental analysis is carried out by careful comparison of regional function in each of the 16 segments, comparing the same site at rest and at stress. Both wall motion and thickening are compared, using both cine-loop and frame-by-frame review of the digital images. Freezing the images and stepping through one frame at a time is invaluable—delayed contraction is a hallmark of ischemic tissue, which is not apparent to the unaided eye,[78] but is often recognizable when images are reviewed frame-by-frame. The reader should think twice about identifying resting- or stress-induced wall motion abnormalities in segments that move rapidly and smoothly immediately after the QRS. Focusing on the first part of systole may minimize the contribution of rotational or translational movement, and assessing the timing of contraction may also avoid false-positive interpretations provoked by early relaxation (Fig. 16–5). The ability to save multiple cycles in each view has reduced the need to review videotaped stress images, but these remain of value for nonstandard views and to check on uncertainties arising from the digitized images. The site, extent (number of abnormal segments), severity (segmental wall motion score), time of onset and offset of ischemia, and the effect of ischemia on global LV function should be recorded.

Technical Aspects of Nonexercise Stress Techniques

General Considerations

Patients are instructed to fast, partly because nausea is a side effect with some agents (especially dipyridamole and adenosine), and in case complications ensue with attending aspiration risks. For dipyridamole stress testing, coffee, tea, and cola drinks should be avoided for 12 hours before the examination because xanthines antagonize the effects of dipyridamole on adenosine metabolism and by direct competitive inhibition of adenosine.

For diagnostic testing, patients should be instructed to stop anti-ischemic drugs on the day of the procedure, but medications may be continued if testing is being performed to assess the adequacy of therapy. Intravenous access is secured, and monitoring electrodes may be moved away from the echocardiographic windows. Two personnel (sonographer and physician) are mandatory for performance of these protocols, and many centers involve a nurse as well. Clinical and electrocardiographic monitoring during the tests parallels the monitoring undertaken during exercise stress testing. In addition to the usual resuscitation equipment, intravenous beta-blocking agents and nitrates should be available to treat severe ischemia. For dipyridamole stress, aminophylline should be available for the treatment of severe ischemia.

Exercise-Simulating Agents

Protocols for Administration of Sympathomimetic Agents

Dobutamine has been administered using various empiric regimens, but none is clearly superior to the others. The most widely used is an incremental administration from 5 to 40 μg/kg/min in 2-minute or 3-minute stages.[24-30] Variants include maximal doses of up to 50 μg/kg/min and down to 20 μg/kg/min; lower-dose rates administered over longer periods are able to attain similar hemodynamic effects to the high-dose protocols.[29] New accelerated dobutamine protocols are currently being used to reduce the duration of the test, but whichever regimen is applied, a reasonable (i.e.,

2-minute to 3-minute) period at peak HR is desirable because ischemic wall motion abnormalities may take a short time to become apparent. If atropine is added to induce an increase in HR, the usual dose is 1 to 2 mg total in 0.25-mg increments.

Hemodynamic Responses to Sympathomimetics

Low doses of dobutamine enhance LV contractility, usually without the development of tachycardia. At doses greater than 20 µg/kg/min, systolic BP increases, and HR augments to more than 100 beats per minute. HR can be expected to increase to about 120 beats per minute in most patients, reflecting a increment of 40 to 50 beats per minute. In normotensive patients, systolic BP usually increases to about 170 mm Hg (i.e., by 30 to 40 mm Hg) without a significant change of diastolic pressure. The systolic pressure response may be marked in hypertensive patients and blunted in patients with LV dysfunction or multivessel coronary disease. The peak rate-pressure product reaches 16,500 to 20,000. Although the development of ischemia at lower dobutamine doses and cardiac workloads indicates the presence of more extensive coronary disease, there is too much overlap for the hemodynamic response to be a reliable predictor of one-vessel, two-vessel, or three-vessel disease.

The hemodynamic response to dobutamine shows significant variability between patients. Beta-blockade may attenuate the physiologic response through competitive antagonism at the receptor. Patients taking beta-blockers have a significantly lower HR response (usually about 100 beats per minute), and a lower double product (to levels of around 14,000), although this may be avoided by use of atropine. Peak systolic pressure is less during dobutamine than exercise,[25] so the cardiac stress imposed at maximal dobutamine dosage is less than that obtainable with maximal exercise testing. In comparisons between dobutamine and exercise stress in the same patients, systolic BP levels were comparable, but peak HR and double product were significantly greater during exercise.[29,79-84] These disparities have important implications for the relative sensitivity of dobutamine and exercise echocardiography.

Side Effects of Stress Testing with Sympathomimetic Agents

Other than the development of myocardial ischemia, dose-limiting side effects generally reflect intense adrenergic stimulation. Consequently, dobutamine stress is contraindicated in patients with severe hypertension and serious arrhythmias. Serious side effects are rare during dobutamine stress testing. In more than 1000 dobutamine studies reported by Mertes and colleagues,[85] no patients died or suffered

MI or sustained tachyarrhythmias. Similarly, in 650 studies with dobutamine and atropine reported by Poldermans and colleagues,[86] no patients died or suffered MI, and cardiac arrhythmias were most likely in patients with LV dysfunction or preexisting ventricular arrhythmias. In a multicenter study reported by Picano and colleagues,[46] nine major cardiac events occurred in nearly 3000 studies (three from MI or severe ischemia, five from ventricular tachyarrhythmias, and one with hypotension). In my experience, serious side effects of dobutamine stress occurred in 3 per 1000 patients,[87] a similar result to that of a large German study.[88] Nonetheless, case reports of fatalities have been reported from ventricular fibrillation and cardiac rupture,[89] and safety in patients at highest risk—those with severe LV dysfunction—has been described only in small populations.[90] Nonetheless, considering that the sickest patients (those unable to exercise and with questions of myocardial viability) undergo the test, this safety profile is reasonable. This may reflect the detection of ischemia by online imaging, permitting termination before serious problems arise.

The most frequent serious but nonfatal complications are MI and arrhythmias (atrial fibrillation and ventricular tachycardia). Other problems include palpitations (atrial and ventricular extra systoles), hypertension, anxiety (sometimes manifested as dyspnea or vagal reactions), tremor, and urinary urgency. Hypotension may arise from the vasodilator effect of high-dose dobutamine, the development of outflow tract obstruction, or the development of severe ischemia.[91-94] Unlike hypotension during exercise testing, it does not denote the presence of serious coronary disease or LV dysfunction,[95] and in particular, the finding of a left ventricular outflow tract (LVOT) gradient does not appear to be prognostically meaningful. The frequency of these side effects has varied from 5%, if only serious, dose-limiting side effects are considered,[24] to 82% if all side effects are included.[29] Variability also relates to the type of stress protocol, the incidence being lower if the test is terminated for attainment of a target HR or at detection of ischemia[24] or if submaximal test responses are excluded.[25]

Vasodilator Stress Protocols

Stress Protocols

Dipyridamole is administered into a large proximal arm vein to minimize local discomfort from this strongly alkaline compound. Various dipyridamole administration regimens have been used. For myocardial perfusion imaging, the most commonly administered dose is 0.56 mg/kg intravenously,[96] but the sensitivity of dipyridamole echocardiography is optimal if an additional 2 minutes of infusion are added if the initial response is negative, and no major side effects have appeared.[97,98] Because the time of onset of ischemia correlates with the severity of coronary disease and prognosis, images are recorded every 2 minutes from the conclusion of the first dose until 18 minutes from the start. Digital images are saved at rest, before the start of the second dose (8 minutes), after the second dose (12 minutes, which is the most common time for the onset of ischemia), and at 16 minutes. Aminophylline (in aliquots of 50 to 75 mg intravenously) is used to reverse the effects of dipyridamole if severe ischemia or side effects arise; the threshold for using this agent is influenced by the overall LV function and the clinical state of the patient.

Because exogenous adenosine is able to act directly, it rapidly achieves steady state, and its biologic effects are of rapid onset.[34] A fixed dose schedule of 0.14 or 0.17 mg/kg/min or incremental protocols (3-minute stages starting at 0.10 mg/kg/min, increasing to 0.14 and 0.18 mg/kg/min) have been used for echocardiographic studies.[99-102] The use of aminophylline is rarely required for side effects because these resolve within a minute of stopping the infusion.

Hemodynamic Responses to Vasodilators

The mechanism of action of vasodilator agents is chiefly through the phenomenon of coronary steal. There is a small contribution of increasing oxygen demand from tachycardia,[22] which may be a response to angina and side effects rather than arising from the agents themselves. Similarly, BP is usually little changed by these stressors, which may cause hypotension. The addition of atropine leads to an augmentation of HR and cardiac work,[45,47] effectively combining reduced coronary supply with increased oxygen demand.

Side Effects of Dipyridamole and Adenosine

Side effects during dipyridamole stress usually follow completion of the infusion, rarely preclude completion of the study, and usually resolve spontaneously. Minor side effects, including flushing and headache occur in about two thirds of patients studied with high-dose dipyridamole.[103] Severe or prolonged myocardial ischemia is infrequent but can be treated with nitrates or aminophylline. Serious side effects are very rare—probably less frequent than with dobutamine,[46,104] but severe myocardial ischemia and MI, bronchospasm, complete heart block, and even death have been reported. Dipyridamole stress is contraindicated with atrioventricular (AV) block and bronchospasm, although patients with chronic obstructive airway disease with no or minimal airway reactivity may undergo the test.

The side effect profile of adenosine is similar to dipyridamole, and although the intensity and frequency of side effects with adenosine is greater, they are of shorter duration. Some form of side effects occur in most patients undergoing adenosine stress.[105] In a high-dose protocol,[102] side effects prevented about one third of patients from achieving peak dose, a comparable frequency to that found with dobutamine. As the effect of adenosine is transient, cessation of the infusion is usually the only treatment required for side effects.

Vasoconstrictor Protocols

Ergonovine stress may be useful for the diagnosis of coronary spasm, the frequency of which seems to show geographic variation. In the West, spasm is recorded in 4% of patients in whom it is suspected clinically, although smokers and patients with some coronary disease are at higher risk.[106] Ergonovine testing has been most widely used in the angiography laboratory,[106] because spasm can be visualized directly, and intracoronary nitrates infused to treat severe spasm. However, ergonovine stress appears to be safe when applied noninvasively in patients without significant stenoses,[107-109] and the test has been applied to some patient groups without previous angiography.[6,7] The standard protocol involves repeated bolus doses of ergonovine maleate at 5-minute intervals up to a total cumulative dose of 0.35 mg, unless ischemia is detected.

Pacing Stress

Stress Protocols

The use of an implanted pacemaker to alter the HR during testing is often necessary to achieve target HR in the presence of atrioventricular block. Ventricular stimulation produces dyssynchronous contraction, but interpretable images are obtainable if image quality is sufficient to evaluate thickening, and atrial pacing poses no problems for interpretation.[110] The test endpoints are the same as those for other nonexercise stressors; in the absence of these endpoints, pacing at peak HR is continued for 3 minutes. No protocol has been uniformly accepted. Pacing is used in combination with dobutamine to obtain the inotropic response to stress, and therefore maintain a 3-minute incremental protocol when pacing is added, usually starting at 100 beats per minute.

Transesophageal pacing requires topical pharyngeal anesthesia and mild sedation and is rarely used. Use of a short protocol minimizes the risk of electrode movement and loss of capture. Atropine is often required to overcome atrioventricular block.

Hemodynamic Responses

The hemodynamic response to pacing is more controllable than with pharmacologic agents. HRs of 160 beats per minute are attainable, but systolic BP is stable, giving a rate-pressure product of 15,000 to 20,000. Use of transesophageal pacing in an awake patient may itself provoke hemodynamic changes and hence ischemia, so that "resting" TEE images may not be truly acquired at rest.

Side Effects

Fewer side effects occur during transesophageal pacing than with pharmacologic stress. Esophageal discomfort, gagging, or nausea are uncommon with modern pacing electrodes. Angina may be provoked by stress but is usually self-limiting after cessation of pacing. Atrial flutter or fibrillation may also be precipitated. Esophageal injury is theoretically possible in response to high levels of stimulation over a prolonged period, but this has not been reported clinically.

Accuracy of Nonexercise Stress Echocardiography for Diagnosis of Coronary Artery Disease

Dobutamine Stress Echocardiography

Table 16–3* summarizes studies of more than 100 patients that examine the sensitivity and specificity of dobutamine echocardiography for the detection of CAD. Atropine appears to enhance the sensitivity of the test, as does transesophageal imaging. No single feature accounts for false-positive results, although the most frequent site of false-positive results is the basal inferior wall.[120]

The use of a 50% or 70% stenosis cutoff is arbitrary and does not take into account stenosis location or vessel size, both of which clearly influence the likelihood of an abnormal response. This concern has been addressed in several studies that have compared the results of dobutamine echocardiography with stenosis diameter at quantitative coronary angiography.[121-123] The angiographic cutoff value with the best predictive value for a positive dobutamine test was a luminal diameter of 1.07 mm, percent diameter stenosis of 52%, and percent area stenosis of 75%, of which minimal lumen diameter was found to have the best predictive value for a positive dobutamine stress test (odds ratio, 51; sensitivity, 94%; specificity, 75%).[121] Stenoses smaller than 1 mm in diameter can be identified with a sensitivity of 86%.[122,123]

The use of myocardial fractional flow reserve (the ratio of mean hyperemic distal coronary to aortic pressure) as a functional index of coronary stenosis severity takes into account collateral flow and overcomes the limitations of comparing stress echocardiography with the anatomic severity of stenosis. The degree of

dobutamine-induced dyssynergy correlates significantly better with myocardial fractional flow reserve than percent stenosis or minimal lumen diameter, and the sensitivity of dobutamine echocardiography is significantly lower for lesions in vessels smaller than 2.6 mm than for larger vessels.[122]

The existence of a regional wall motion abnormality identifies the presence of coronary disease, so dobutamine echocardiography demonstrates higher sensitivities in patients with MI. In patients with single-vessel disease, the sensitivity of dobutamine echocardiography (40% to 70%) is lower than in multivessel disease. As dobutamine produces a less potent stress on the heart than exercise, dobutamine echocardiography is probably more susceptible to external influences than exercise echocardiography or myocardial perfusion scintigraphy. This may be pertinent to the extrapolation of results from clinical trials (in which patients were carefully supervised and tested under optimal conditions, off therapy), to routine clinical practice, in which patients are often tested on therapy and are more likely to have a "suboptimal" test result because of inability to complete the protocol or interference by beta-blocker therapy.[30]

Dipyridamole Stress Echocardiography

The reported accuracy of vasodilator stress echocardiography in studies of more than 100 patients is summarized in Table 16–4.* The low-dose (0.56 mg/kg) protocol is associated with lower sensitivity than the high-dose regimen. Atropine appears to enhance sensitivity,[45,126] although this is only about 50% in patients with single-vessel disease. Transesophageal imaging enhances the accuracy of this test.[127] The greater variation in the sensitivity of stress echocardiography with vasodilators than dobutamine and exercise stress seems to relate to patient selection[128] and the definition of "significant" disease; many of the more favorable results pertain to populations with a high percentage of patients with more severe coronary disease. The specificity is excellent.

Investigators have sought to address the accuracy of dipyridamole stress with physiologic rather than anatomic criteria of significant stenosis.[129] In 30 patients with isolated stenoses of the left anterior descending coronary artery, predictors of an abnormal dipyridamole echocardiogram were a stenotic flow reserve of less than 2.8, stenosis diameter greater than 59%, lumen diameter less than 1.35 mm, and coronary flow reserve less than 2, of which stenotic flow reserve was the only independent predictor of ischemia. This study was interesting on two grounds: First, it implies that dipyridamole identifies fewer mild stenoses than dobutamine

---

*See references 24, 28, 30, 47, 50, 82, 111-119.

*See references 45, 47, 50, 82, 113, 114, 119, 124, 125.

TABLE 16-3. Sensitivity and Specificity of Echocardiography with Dobutamine Stress (Studies of >100 Patients)

Study	Patients, N	Dobutamine Protocol, μg/kg/min	Significant Stenosis Diameter, %	Multivessel Disease, n (% all CAD)	Myocardial Infarction, n (% all CAD)	Sensitivity: Overall, % (n)	Sensitivity: SVD, % (n)	Specificity, % (n)
Sawada and colleagues[24]	103	30	>50	14 (40)	35 (43)	95 (81)	89 (38)	77 (22)
Marcovitz and Armstrong[28]	141	30	>50	47 (43)	—	96 (109)	95 (62)	66 (32)
Marwick and colleagues[30]	217	40	>50	74 (52)	0 (0)	72 (142)	66 (68)	83 (75)
Takeuchi and colleagues[111]	120	30	>50	37 (50)	62 (84)	85 (74)	73 (37)	93 (46)
Beleslin and colleagues[82]	136	40	>50	11 (9)	41 (34)	82 (119)	82 (108)	77 (27)
Ostojic and colleagues[50]	150	40	>50	16 (12)	38 (29)	75 (131)	—	79 (19)
Pingitore and colleagues[47]	110	40 + atropine	>50	42 (46)	25 (27)	84 (92)	—	89 (18)
Ling and colleagues[112]	183	40 + atropine	>70	109 (74)	105 (71)	95 (148)	—	51 (35)
San Roman and colleagues[113]	102	40 + atropine	>50	34 (54)	0 (0)	77 (63)	68 (29)	95 (39)
Anthopoulos and colleagues[114]	120	40 + atropine	>50	48 (40)	38 (30)	87 (89)	74 (19)	84 (31)
Dionisopoulos and colleagues[115]	288	40 + atropine	>50	122 (58)	—	87 (209)	80 (70)	89 (79)
Elhendy and colleagues[116]	96 females	40 + atropine	>50	142 (61)	214 (70)	76 (62)	64	94 (34)
	210 males					73 (171)	56	77 (39)
Hennessy and colleagues[117]	219	40 + atropine	>50	113 (66)	55 (24)	82 (170)	74 (57)	65 (49)
Nagel and colleagues[118]	208	40 + atropine	>50	70 (64)	0 (0)	74 (107)	67 (39)	70 (101)
Beleslin and colleagues[119]	168	40	>50	0 (0)	40 (24)	61 (153)	61 (153)	88 (25)

SVD, single vessel disease; TEE, transesophageal echocardiography.
Data from references 24, 28, 30, 47, 50, 82, 111-119.

TABLE 16–4. Accuracy of Vasodilator (Dipyridamole and Exercise) Echocardiography (Studies of >100 Patients)

Study	Patients, N	Agent Dose	Definition of CAD, %	Multivessel Disease, n (% all CAD)	Myocardial Infarction, n (% all CAD)	Sensitivity, % (n)	Specificity, % (n)
Picano and colleagues[124]	445	Dipyridamole, 0.84 mg/kg*	>50	119 (46)	0 (0)	96 (256)	96
Severi and colleagues[125]	429	Dipyridamole, 0.84 mg/kg*	>75	114 (46)	0	75 (246)	90
Picano and colleagues[45]	130	Dipyridamole, 0.84 mg/kg + atropine	>50	—	—	87 (94)	94
Ostojic and colleagues[50]	150	Dipyridamole, 0.84 mg/kg*	>50	16 (12)	38 (29)	71 (131)	89
Beleslin and colleagues[82]	136	Dipyridamole, 0.84 mg/kg*	>50	11 (9)	41 (34)	74 (119)	94 (17)
San Roman and colleagues[113]	102	Dipyridamole, 0.84 mg/kg*	>50	34 (54)	0 (0)	77 (63)	97
Pingitore and colleagues[47]	110	Dipyridamole, 0.84 mg/kg + atropine	>50	—	—	82 (92)	94
Anthopoulos and colleagues[114]	120	Adenosine, 0.14 μg/kg/min*	>50	48 (40)	38 (30)	66 (89)	90 (31)
Beleslin and colleagues[119]	168	Dipyridamole, 0.84 mg/kg*	>50	0 (0)	40 (24)	61 (153)	88 (25)

*Low-dose positivity permits conclusion of study before stated "peak" dose.
Data from references 47, 50, 82, 113, 114, 119, 124, 125.

echocardiography, and second, it identified angiographic variables of stenosis severity to relate to dipyridamole echocardiographic results better than intracoronary Doppler variables. Other studies have confirmed that the optimal angiographic cutoff point for dipyridamole stress echocardiography is 60%, as compared with 58% for dobutamine and 54% for exercise echocardiography.[119]

Vasodilator Stress with Adenosine Echocardiography

The reported accuracy of adenosine stress echocardiography is variable. Favorable results are more likely with multivessel disease or prior infarction; the sensitivity is 60% or less in patients with a normal electrocardiogram[100] or without prior infarction.[102] The intense coronary vasodilation induced by adenosine[130,131] or dipyridamole[132] permits the comparison of rest and hyperemic images using contrast echocardiography. Similarly, coronary flow reserve may be measured at adenosine stress transthoracic echocardiography (TTE) or TEE.[133] The longer time course and less predictable peak flow with dipyridamole make this a less attractive agent, and if this is selected, high dose is certainly required.[55]

Pacing Stress Echocardiography

Studies that have combined atrial pacing with echocardiography (Table 16–5) show favorable results, although the number of studies and patients within studies is limited.[37,38,41,134-136] The accuracy of both transesophageal imaging and pacing probably reflects the benefits of high-quality images as much as the role of pacing stress

because similar favorable findings have been obtained using TEE with dobutamine and dipyridamole. The discrepancy between the reported accuracy, feasibility, and patient acceptance of pacing stress[43] contrasts with the limited application of the test. The following are important issues that influence the continued use of pharmacologic stress. First, the evidence base for diagnostic, management, and prognostic information using pharmacologic agents is greater than with pacing stress. Second, the pacing test is unlikely to be useful for the detection of viable myocardium, and even when this is not needed from a clinical standpoint, the biphasic response has been shown to facilitate the distinction of ischemia in the setting of resting wall motion abnormalities. Third, most patients and some clinicians look at the test as being excessively invasive. This test has several niche applications: patients with hypertension or rhythm contraindications to dobutamine, potentially unstable patients (because the stress can be stopped suddenly), or patients with chronotropic incompetence of various causes.

Comparison between Nonexercise Stressors for the Diagnosis of Coronary Artery Disease

Selection of the Optimal Pharmacologic Stress

Both dobutamine and vasodilator stress echocardiography are effective for the diagnosis of CAD, and meta-analyses by Picano and colleagues[137] have proposed that the accuracy of the tests is comparable. However, variations in the study groups make it difficult to compare the relative efficacy of the stressors by merely comparing the

TABLE 16–5. Sensitivity and Specificity of Atrial Pacing Stress Echocardiography (Studies >50 Patients)

Study	Patients, N	Method	Feasibility, %	Definition of CAD, %	Sensitivity: Overall, % (n)	Sensitivity: SVD, % (n)	Specificity, % (n)
Iliceto and colleagues[41]	85	TTE	95	>75	91 (56)	80 (20)	88 (25)
Lambertz and colleagues[38]	50	TEE	100	>50	93 (41)	85 (20)	100 (9)
Kamp and colleagues[37]	71	TEE	99	>50	83 (52)	69 (13)	94 (18)
Marangelli and colleagues[134]	80	TTE	77	>75	83 (35)	75 (16)	76 (25)
Michael and colleagues[135]	65	TTE	—	>50	87	—	88
Schroder and colleagues[136]	69	TTE	52	>50	82 (69)	82 (69)	—

TEE, transesophageal echocardiography; TTE, transthoracic echocardiography.
Data from references 37, 38, 41, 134, 160.

results of individual studies, and the limitations of meta-analyses for assessment of therapies likely applies to their application to diagnostic testing.[138]

Figure 16–6 summarizes the accuracy of stress echocardiography with a variety of stressors, and Table 16–6 summarizes large head-to-head comparisons of the tests in the same patients, under the same conditions.[50,82,113,114,139] The feasibility of dobutamine and vasodilator stress are similar. The sensitivity of dobutamine stress echocardiography (DSE) exceeds that of vasodilator stress; the main source of discrepancy appears to be patients with single-vessel coronary disease, among whom dobutamine appears to be superior. This difference parallels a significantly greater cardiac workload with dobutamine compared with vasodilator stress.

The contraindications to inotropes and vasodilators vary, so their selection may be individualized; patients with hypertension or arrhythmias should undergo a vasodilator stress, and patients with bronchospasm or conduction disorders should be submitted to inotropic stress. However, in the majority of patients who do not have these contraindications, dobutamine appears to be the most sensitive agent for pharmacologic stress echocardiography.

Selection of Pacing Rather than Other Nonexercise Stress

There are few comparative data between pacing and pharmacologic stress. Pacing is reportedly less feasible (77% versus 96%, $P < 0.0001$) but more sensitive (83% versus 43%, $P = 0.0005$) than dipyridamole echocardiography. Atrial pacing showed more favorable safety, duration, and patient acceptance than dobutamine echocardiography.[39]

Assessment of Disease Significance Using Nonexercise Echocardiography

The use of stress echocardiography for identification of the "culprit" coronary lesion is often constrained by the assumptions inherent in allocating territories of the heart to individual coronary vessels. The most ambiguous areas in this respect are the apex (usually supplied by the left anterior descending coronary artery) and the posterior wall (usually supplied by the left circumflex artery). Because of the equivocal involvement of the right coronary or left circumflex vessels in the posterior territory, investigators have examined the ability to discern the presence of coronary disease in the anterior and posterior circulations. Although in the preharmonic imaging era, the lateral wall was a source of false-negative results, the accuracy of dobutamine echocardiography in this area has improved (Fig. 16–7).

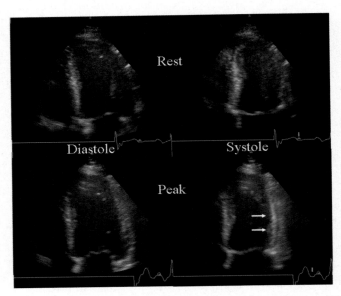

Figure 16–6. Lateral wall ischemia. Freeze-frame images in the apical four-chamber view demonstrate normal thickening at rest (top), with reduced thickening at peak stress (arrows).

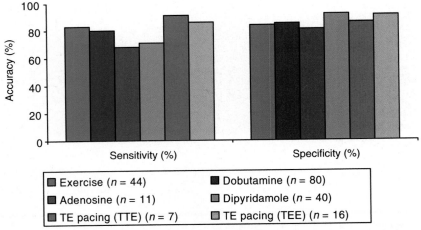

Figure 16–7. Meta-analysis of sensitivity and specificity of stress echocardiography performed with various stress modalities.

TABLE 16-6. Studies Comparing Sensitivity and Specificity of Dobutamine and Vasodilator Stress Echocardiography (>100 Patients)

Study	Patients, N	CAD, n (%)	Multivessel Disease, n (% all CAD)	Myocardial Infarction, n (% all CAD)	Sensitivity: Dobutamine, %	Sensitivity: Dipyridamole, %	Specificity: Dobutamine, %	Specificity: Dipyridamole, %
Beleslin and colleagues[82]	136	119 (88)	11 (9)	41 (34)	82	74	77	94
Ostojic and colleagues[50]	150	131 (87)	16 (12)	38 (29)	75	71	79	89
Anthopoulos and colleagues[114*]	120	89 (74)	48 (40)	38 (30)	87	66	84	90
San Roman and colleagues[113]	102	63 (62)	34 (54)	0 (0)	77	77	95	97
Fragasso and colleagues[139]	101	56 (56)	37 (65)	0 (0)	88	61	80	91

*Adenosine used instead of dipyridamole.
CAD, coronary artery disease.
Data from references 50, 82, 113, 114, 139.

The recognition of multivessel disease at stress echocardiography may be important in planning revascularization rather than medical therapy. The ability of stress echocardiography to predict multivessel disease is greatest in patients with a history of previous MI, under which circumstances its sensitivity for the correct identification of disease is 80% to 85%, and its specificity is 88%.[24,140] In contrast, the sensitivity for multivessel disease in patients without previous infarction is approximately 70%,[24] exceeding the levels reported in this situation using exercise echocardiography. A close correlation has been demonstrated between the extent of ischemia defined by dobutamine echocardiography and perfusion scintigraphy, although both underestimate the angiographic extent of disease,[30] a reflection of the difficulties of assessing the functional implications of disease extent on anatomic grounds.

In addition to the "space coordinate" (extent of abnormal segments),[19] another indication of the extent of coronary disease is the "time coordinate" (ischemic threshold). Multivessel disease may be predicted if ischemia has an early onset (similar to the "ischemia-free" time at exercise testing), corresponding to its occurrence at a low dose or provocation at a low HR and rate-pressure product.[25,103,141] This corresponds to a lower ischemic threshold at exercise testing[125] and a worse prognosis.

Prognostic Evaluation Using Nonexercise Echocardiography

Prediction of Cardiac Events in Patients Undergoing Major Noncardiac Surgery

CAD is highly prevalent in patients with vascular disease,[142] and cardiac events are the leading cause of perioperative complications at vascular surgery.[143] However, whereas postoperative unstable angina and heart failure are frequent in patients with vascular disease, "hard" endpoints (death, MI) occur in less than 10% of patients in the perioperative period.[144] Severe coronary disease is also the major contributor to late deaths after vascular surgery, so the screening of vascular patients for significant coronary disease is important for both perioperative and late risk stratification.

The American Heart Association and American College of Cardiology guidelines emphasize that the first step in preoperative risk stratification is clinical evaluation.[145] Patients with unstable coronary syndromes within the last 6 months constitute a high-risk group and warrant careful functional testing or possibly angiography and preoperative intervention. The nature of the planned surgery is important; extensive risk evaluation is best directed toward vascular, major orthopedic, and major abdominal operations, which engender

significant cardiac risk. Those with previous bypass surgery (within 5 years) or negative coronary investigations within 2 years are at low risk and do not require reinvestigation in the absence of recurrent symptoms. Finally, the patient history has an important influence on risk; a simple score derived from the patient's age, presence of diabetes, angina, prior infarction, and congestive heart failure (CHF) has been shown to identify low-risk patients.[146] In more than 4300 patients[147] undergoing high-risk surgery, history of ischemic heart disease, congestive heart failure or cerebrovascular disease, insulin treatment, and preoperative serum creatinine level greater than 2 mg/dL were markers of risk; patients with none, one, two, or three or more of these factors had major cardiac complication rates of approximately 0.5%, approximately 1%, approximately 5%, and approximately 10%, respectively. Inactive patients are usually asymptomatic even in the presence of significant coronary disease, so nonexercise stress imaging techniques are required if screening is to be undertaken.

Table 16–7 summarizes the results of large studies of dipyridamole and dobutamine echocardiography for preoperative risk stratification.[141,148-153] The predictive value of a negative test is high, but that of a positive test is intermediate (from 20% to 70%)—reflecting the role of not only coronary stenoses but also medical treatment and anesthetic intervention in the genesis of events at surgery. Positive tests may be further stratified by paying attention to the ischemic threshold and the clinical risk factor status (Fig. 16–8).

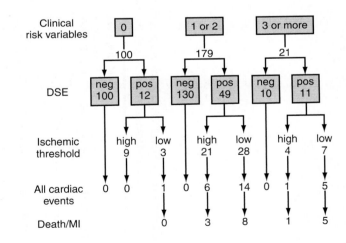

300 Preop patients

Figure 16–8. Evaluation of risk in patients undergoing vascular surgery. Patients without clinical predictors of risk rarely have a positive dobutamine study (DSE), are unlikely to suffer events, and usually do not require testing. The presence of ischemia is predictive of events, especially if the patient has multiple clinical risk factors or a low ischemic threshold. MI, myocardial infarction; neg, negative; pos, positive; preop, preoperative. (From Poldermans D, Arnese M, Fioretti PM, et al: J Am Coll Cardiol 26:648-653, 1995.)

TABLE 16-7. Use of Stress Echocardiography to Predict Events in Patients Undergoing Vascular Surgery (>100 Patients)

Study	Stress	Patients, *N*	Events, *n*	Predictive Value, %		Events
				Positive Test	Negative Test	
Tischler and colleagues[148]	Dipyridamole	109	8	78	99	MI, UAP, CHF
Sicari and colleagues[149]	Dipyridamole	121	9	25	98	Death, MI, UAP
Rossi and colleagues[150]	Dipyridamole	110	10		100	Death, MI, UAP
Pasquet and colleagues[151]	Dipyridamole	129	9	30	97	Death, MI, UAP
Poldermans and colleagues[152]	Dobutamine + atropine	131	15	43	100	Death, MI, UAP, CHF
Poldermans and colleagues[153]	Dobutamine + atropine	181	18	32	100	Death, MI, UAP, CHF
Poldermans and colleagues[141]	Dobutamine + atropine	300	27	38	100	MI, AP, LVF

AP, angina pectoris; CHF, congestive heart failure; LVF, left ventricular failure; MI, myocardial infarction; UAP, unstable angina pectoris. Data from references 141, 148-153.

Prognostic Evaluation of Patients with Stable Coronary Disease

Major cardiac events are infrequent in stable chronic coronary disease (less than 1% per year), but some patients have a more favorable prognosis with intervention. The detection of left main or multivessel disease at coronary angiography is often used to identify subgroups likely to benefit from revascularization, but this procedure is too costly and invasive to be used in all patients. As in the case of preoperative risk stratification, clinical data (including the severity of angina, prior infarction, heart failure, and diabetes) may identify high- and low-risk subgroups,[154,155] and additional investigations are of most value in those at intermediate or greater risk. Exercise capacity and ST segment depression at exercise testing offer important prognostic information in patients who are able to exercise,[156,157] and exercise single photon emission computed tomography (SPECT)[158] or exercise echocardiography have been shown to provide incremental data in some patients.[159]

The prognostic implications[160] of pharmacologic stress echocardiography are summarized in Table 16–8.[160-167] Ischemia is an independent predictor of adverse outcomes, incremental to clinical and resting echocardiographic data. Ischemic threshold adds significantly to simple assessment of test positivity, for example cardiac events occurred in 41% of patients with wall motion abnormalities occurring at low-dose dipyridamole, and

26% of those with high-dose responses. Ischemia is a better predictor of cardiac events than coronary anatomy.[167] The prognostic value of pharmacologic stress appears to be preserved within various subgroups, including hypertensive patients.[168]

Dobutamine and dipyridamole offer comparable risk stratification in patients at low to moderate risk of cardiac events,[169] and similar to that of SPECT.[169] The prognostic components of both tests include the presence, severity, and extent of induced ischemia. Perhaps the most important aspect of the prognostic literature is that a negative test portends extremely low risk, evidenced by an event rate of 1% or less per year. However, there are some exceptions—patients with diabetes are a high-risk group, among whom even patients with a negative test retain some risk, especially in the subset who are unable to exercise.[170] Likewise, the protection from ischemia provided by antianginal drug therapy does not necessarily translate to protection against subsequent cardiac events, so the predictive value of a negative test on treatment is less than in patients off treatment.[171]

Prognostic Evaluation of Patients after Myocardial Infarction

Although the current era of early intervention has led to a reduction in the use of stress echocardiography following MI, there is little to choose between the efficacy of invasive and noninvasive strategies. If the latter

TABLE 16-8. Use of Stress Echocardiography to Predict Events in Patients with Chronic Stable Coronary Disease

Study	Stress	Patients, N	Mean Follow-up, mo	Predictive Value, %		Comments
				Positive Test	Negative Test	
Poldermans and colleagues[161]	Dobutamine	430	17	26	87	—
Kamaran and colleagues[162]	Dobutamine	210	16	43	92	—
Marcovitz colleagues[163]	Dobutamine	291	15	10-17	99	—
Schroder and colleagues[160]	Dobutamine	134	19	31	94	—
Steinberg and colleagues[281]	Dobutamine —	120 —	60 —	67 13	67 95	All events Hard events
Senior and colleagues[164]	Dobutamine	121	15	45	88	—
Chuah and colleagues[165]	Dobutamine	860	52	14	96	—
Poldermans and colleagues[166]	Dobutamine	1659	36	8-20	96	Hard events
Picano and colleagues[167]	Dipyridamole (high dose)	539	36	26	94	—
	Dipyridamole (low dose)	539	36	41	94	—
Schroder and colleagues[160]	Dipyridamole	134	19	27	92	—

Data from references 160-167, 281.

is chosen, clinical features, such as age and the presence of heart failure, should be used in the initial risk assessment. The extent of infarcted and ischemic myocardium are major determinants of outcome.[172] Stress echocardiography permits the assessment of ischemia as homozonal dyssynergy (peri-infarct ischemia) or heterozonal dyssynergy (multivessel disease), and infarction may also be estimated.

Table 16–9 summarizes the prognostic implications of positive and negative nonexercise stress echocardiography after infarction.[173-178] The presence of ischemia and its time of onset are important predictors of cardiac events;[175] in elderly patients, ischemia was an independent predictor of mortality.[179] All tests have proven to be effective for the detection of multivessel disease[140,173,180] and predictive for the subsequent development of cardiac events.

Evaluation of Therapy Using Nonexercise Echocardiography

Medical Therapy

The identification of ischemia with stress echocardiography is dependent on the development of ischemia. This is a disadvantage to the extent that antianginal therapy reduces the sensitivity of stress echocardiography, particularly when dipyridamole stress is used.[128] Patients on beta-blockers account for most patients who fail to attain a HR greater than 85% of age-predicted maximum. With dobutamine echocardiography, the interaction between dobutamine and beta-blockers involves competitive inhibition, and if enough dobutamine is administered, this effect may be overcome, leading several studies to suggest that concurrent drug therapy has no effect.[181] Atropine can be used to enhance the sensitivity of dobutamine stress testing, without reducing specificity or inducing serious side effects.

The interaction between medical therapy and the development of ischemia may be of use in evaluating the adequacy of therapy.[182-184] Testing on medical therapy may compromise the reliability of a negative test. Sequential testing is limited by the subjectivity of wall motion scoring, and this application requires a reliable quantitative approach.

Follow-Up after Coronary Interventions

After angioplasty and bypass surgery, chest wall pains may be difficult to distinguish from recurrent symptoms resulting from restenosis or graft closure. The American Heart Association and American College of Cardiology guidelines recommend the use of a stress imaging test after revascularization.[185] Stress echocardiography performed before and after angioplasty has

TABLE 16-9. Application of Nonexercise Stressors to Postinfarction Risk Evaluation (>100 Patients)

Study	Year	Patients, N	Timing	Stress	Follow-up, months	Outcomes	Predictive Value, % Positive	Predictive Value, % Negative	Relative Risk	P
Bolognese and colleagues[173]	92	217		Dipyridamole	24	Cardiac death	30	99	2.78	NS
						Cardiac death, reinfarction	80	98	3.47	NS
						Cardiac death, reinfarction, angina	33	90	3.24	0.0001
Sclavo and colleagues[174]	92	103	5-8 days	Dipyridamole	14.5	Cardiac death	0	97	—	NS
						Cardiac death, reinfarction	0	96	—	NS
						Cardiac death, reinfarction, angina	22	89	1.94	NS
Picano and colleagues[175]	93	925	10 days	Dipyridamole	14	Cardiac death	6	98	3.05	<0.002
Chiarella and colleagues[176]	94	251	70 hours	Dipyridamole	13 days	Cardiac death	2	99	2.05	NS
						Cardiac death, reinfarction	8	98	4.11	<0.04
						Cardiac death, reinfarction, angina	40	97	13.46	<0.0001
Picano and colleagues[177]	95	1080	10 days	Dipyridamole	14	Reinfarction	6	97	1.91	<0.02
						Cardiac death, reinfarction	11	98	5.15	<0.02
						Cardiac death, reinfarction, angina	24	88	2.08	<0.03
						Cardiac death, reinfarction	11	100	—	<0.02
						Cardiac death, reinfarction, angina	54	79	2.55	<0.0001
Picano and colleagues[178]	98	314	12 days	Dobutamine	9	Cardiac death	5	98	2.24	NS
						Cardiac death, reinfarction	7	96	1.76	NS
						Cardiac death, reinfarction, angina	15	90	1.45	NS

Data from references 173-178.

been shown to confirm resolution of ischemia using dipyridamole[186,187] and dobutamine stress,[188,189] and stress echocardiography can be used effectively for the diagnosis of restenosis.[190,191] Stress echocardiography has been shown to be accurate after bypass surgery, and if the patient cannot exercise, pacing or pharmacologic stresses can reasonably be used.[192,193] Echocardiography may be used to confirm the improvement of dysfunctional but viable myocardium.[194]

Assessment of Myocardial Viability Using Nonexercise Echocardiography

Clinical Significance

LV dysfunction after MI results not only from scarring but also from stunned and hibernating myocardium. Stunning shows spontaneous resolution of dysfunction,[195] but hibernating tissue requires myocardial revascularization to resume normal function.[196,197] Myocardial revascularization in patients with viable myocardium may improve cardiac function or overall functional capacity and avoid subsequent cardiac events from this inherently unstable tissue. Clinical decisions about whether to revascularize, which vessel to revascularize, and how to do it may be influenced by the detection of viable myocardium.

The recovery of function is an imperfect gold standard for defining viability (and thereby the performance of noninvasive testing) because it is influenced by the adequacy of revascularization, bypass graft closure, and restenosis, but it has the attraction of having direct clinical relevance. Conventional techniques used for the detection of myocardial scar and viability (Q waves on the electrocardiogram [ECG], regional LV dysfunction at ventriculography, and "fixed" perfusion defects at conventional scintigraphic procedures) do not reliably exclude the presence of residual viable myocardium. More accurate alternatives include positron emission tomography (PET) and thallium scintigraphy using rest-redistribution or stress-redistribution-reinjection protocols, both of which have a high negative predictive value.[198] A positive test result is less predictive of functional recovery, probably manifesting the sensitivity of these tests for small regions of viable myocardium that may not be able to contribute to regional function when revascularized.

Use of Dobutamine Echocardiography for the Diagnosis of Viable Myocardium

Administration of sympathomimetic agents has been shown to reverse postischemic LV dysfunction.[199-202] The typical response of viable myocardium is to increase thickening in response to low doses of dobutamine; in the presence of a stenosed infarct-related ar-

tery, function subsequently deteriorates as the tissue becomes ischemic. Indeed, there is a balance between the recovery of function and the development of ischemia—the latter may compromise the functional recovery of areas that are marginally perfused at rest. The high-dose response (>20 μg/kg/min) has been shown to be a less reliable predictor of recovery.[8] Although some investigators start at lower doses or use only a low-dose protocol for the assessment of viability and others use 5-minute rather than 3-minute increments,[203] there does not appear to be a clear benefit in favor of any of these alternatives.

Dipyridamole enhances both segmental shortening and load-independent indices of ventricular function in stunned myocardium.[204] The mechanism of this phenomenon is unclear, but a local Frank-Starling response (whereby augmentation of myocardial blood volume leads to increased sarcomere separation) appears to be the most likely explanation. Additionally, an indirect sympathomimetic response to dipyridamole-induced ischemia may contribute to improvement of regional function, as may resolution of ischemia secondary to improvement of coronary perfusion. Dipyridamole is used for this purpose in low-dose and "infra-low-dose" protocols;[10] the choice of agent is dependent on local expertise and preference.

Viable segments are characterized by reduced resting function, which augments in response to low-dose dobutamine (usually 7.5 to 10 μg/kg/min, although this is extended to 20 μg/kg/min if long-acting beta-blockers such as carvedilol are being used). There is continued augmentation if there is a patent infarct-related artery or the tissue is well collateralized. In the presence of a stenosed infarct-related artery, an increasing proportion of segments become ischemic as the HR increases.[205] This initial improvement followed by deterioration in function constitutes the "biphasic response," which is strongly predictive of eventual functional recovery of the tissue.[205] A uniphasic response or a classic ischemic response is less predictive of the recovery of resting function. Because the biphasic response is the most reliable finding (Fig. 16–9), the preference is to induce ischemia whenever possible by proceeding to maximal stress (i.e., 40 μg/kg/min dobutamine with or without atropine), rather than using a discreet "viability" or low-dose protocol. In patients with severe LV dysfunction, this approach warrants caution, and early termination may be needed if ischemia is progressive or if other responses might induce instability. Finally, viability studies are the most difficult to interpret; usually multiple low doses are compared, using videotape if there is uncertainty.

The response of regional function to dobutamine is influenced by the extent of viable tissue, the degree of residual stenosis, the extent and magnitude of collaterals, the size of the risk area (which influences tethering), and the presence of drug therapy.[206] The uniphasic response is ambiguous—it may be caused by part of

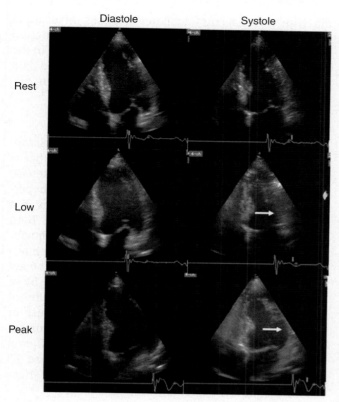

Figure 16-9. *Apical four-chamber diastolic* (right) *and systolic* (left) *views at rest* (top), *with low-dose dobutamine* (middle), *and with peak-dose dobutamine* (bottom), *illustrating a "biphasic" response to dobutamine stress (reduced systolic thickening at rest, increment with low dose, and deterioration at peak dose) in the lateral wall.*

the wall augmenting (i.e., admixture of scar and normal tissue) or all of the wall mounting a partial response (i.e., viable myocardium). The ability to discriminate the extent of subendocardial damage, with its implications for the likelihood of subsequent functional recovery, is poor. The augmentation of function

is dependent on delivery of more substrate; thus, tissue supplied by more severe stenosis may become ischemic before it augments function, which may compromise the recognition of viability.

The accuracy of dobutamine for prediction of regional functional recovery has been studied in a number of small trials.* The overall sensitivity of dobutamine (≈80%) appears greater than that of dipyridamole stress (≈60%), although the specificity of the former is less (78% versus 87%). Nuclear approaches are more sensitive but less specific than these techniques (Fig. 16-10).

Prediction of Recovery of Global Function and Outcome

Improvements in ejection fraction (EF), exercise capacity, and outcome are goals of revascularization, whereas most studies have focused on improvement of LV function within individual segments. However, stress echocardiography can be used to predict improved global LV function after revascularization. Identification of 4 of 16 viable (biphasic) segments at dobutamine echocardiography gives an 89% sensitivity and 81% specificity for prediction of a significant (5%) improvement in ejection fraction.[207] The global ventricular response to low-dose dobutamine is a strong predictor of global functional recovery.[208] A large number of thinned and akinetic segments or large ventricular volumes imply a low likelihood of recovery.[209] The revascularization of patients with adequate amounts of viable myocardium (usually >25% of LV mass) is associated with improved functional class. Viable myocardium may influence outcome in two ways. First, revascularized viable tissue may lead to improved function and thereby improved outcome.[210] Second, nonrevascularized viable

---

*See references 8, 10, 30, 67, 70, 87, 110, 202, 275, 276, 279, 282, 283, 285.

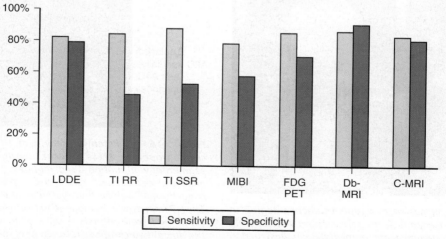

Figure 16-10. *Meta-analysis of sensitivity and specificity of different techniques for assessing viability. C-MRI, contrast magnetic resonance imaging; Db-MRI, dobutamine stress magnetic resonance imaging; FDG PET, fluorodeoxyglucose positron emission tomography; LDDE, low dose dobutamine echocardiography; MIBI, [(99m)Tc]methoxyisobutylisonitrile SPECT; Tl RR, thallium rest-redistribution; Tl SSR, thallium stress-rest-redistribution.*

tissue may be unstable and act as a substrate for recurrent events,[211] including mortality.[210]

New Technologies That May Solve Limitations of Stress Echocardiography

Image Quality

Contrast Echocardiography for Left Ventricular Opacification

Although perfect image quality is certainly not essential for a stress echocardiographic study to be interpretable, it certainly favors concordance between observers[75] and facilitates an accurate diagnosis of disease extent and distinction of ischemia and scar. The use of contrast echocardiography may facilitate delineation of the endocardial border, even when harmonic imaging has been used.[54] The implications of this finding are addressed in another chapter.

Contrast Echocardiography for Assessment of Myocardial Perfusion

The comparison of myocardial perfusion at rest and during hyperemia is now possible with either high or low mechanical index imaging.[212] The low mechanical index approach allows real-time imaging, which is probably easier during stress than intermittent imaging, and bubble destruction with a high energy flash allows appreciation of refill, which depends on perfusion (Fig. 16–11). All stressors produce coronary hyperemia to some degree, although the vasodilator stressors have the most marked effect, and the lack of tachycar-

dia with these agents facilitates imaging. Myocardial contrast data increase the sensitivity of wall motion assessment[213-221] (Table 16–10) and is comparable to the accuracy of SPECT.[222] In addition, there are limited data to show an improvement of prognostic assessment.[223]

Three-Dimensional Echocardiography

Comparison of images in the same plane is a basic requirement of stress echocardiography, and one that is easier to satisfy during pharmacologic than exercise stress because the patient is immobile and not hyperventilating. Moreover, foreshortening of the apex is a significant problem with two-dimensional echo. Both limitations may be addressed with 3D echocardiography, and in addition, subsegmental areas may be interrogated by 3D echocardiography (Fig. 16–12). The accuracy of 3D echocardiography is supported by a limited evidence base.[224,225] Although the feasibility of this technique is likely to be enhanced by the use of contrast for LV opacification (LVO),[226,227] the current version of this technology has limitations in temporal and spatial resolution. A prudent strategy is to use 3D echocardiography as an adjunct to standard stress echocardiography.

Quantitative Approaches to Interpretation

The current qualitative algorithm for interpretation of stress echocardiograms requires a significant level of expertise on the part of the observer. A less subjective

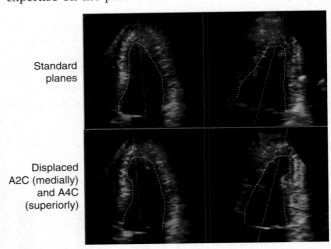

Standard planes

Displaced A2C (medially) and A4C (superiorly)

Figure 16–12. Potential benefit of three-dimensional echocardiography to stress echocardiography by identifying subsegmental wall motion abnormalities. The upper panels demonstrate peak-stress end-systolic freeze-frame images in conventional apical four-chamber and two-chamber views. They demonstrate homogeneous contraction. The lower panels demonstrate off-axis images, with septal displacement of the apical two-chamber (see red axis marker on four-chamber view) and slight superior displacement of the apical four-chamber (see green axis marker on two-chamber view). This demonstrates an apical shape-change consistent with left anterior descending territory ischemia. A2C, apical two-chamber view; A4C, apical four-chamber view.

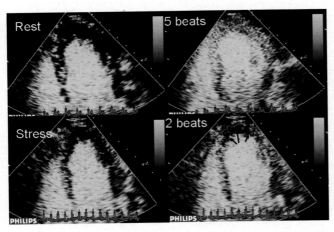

Rest   5 beats

Stress   2 beats

PHILIPS   PHILIPS

Figure 16–11. Use of destruction-replenishment imaging to identify evidence of ischemia from perfusion as well as wall-motion. Left frames demonstrate immediate postdestruction image (note lack of myocardial contrast) at rest (above) and at peak stress (below). Right frames demonstrate return of contrast after sufficient time to allow for refill of myocardium. Note the apical subendocardial perfusion defect (arrows) in this patient who did not demonstrate abnormal wall motion.

TABLE 16-10. Sensitivity and Specificity of Myocardial Contrast Echocardiography for the Detection of Significant Coronary Stenoses

	Myocardial Contrast		Wall Motion			
	Sensitivity (CAD)	Specificity (no CAD)	Sensitivity (CAD)	Specificity (no CAD)	Stress	Angio
Cwajg and colleagues[213]	87% (32)	—(13)	—	—	Db/Ex	All 45
Shimoni and colleagues[214]	75% (28)	100% (16)	75%	—	Ex	44/101
Heinle and colleagues[215]	75% (12)	67% (3)	—	—	Adeno	15/123
Wei and colleagues[216]	100% (15)	—	—	—	Adeno	15/54
Rocchi and colleagues[217]	89% (12)	88% (N segts)	68%	100%	Dipy	12/25
Olszowska and colleagues[218]	97% (44)	93% (N segts)	89%	94%	Db	All 44
Moir and colleagues[219]	91% (43)	70% (27)	74%	81%	Dipy-Ex	70/85
Elhendy and colleagues[220]	91% (127)	51% (43)	70%	74%	Db	All 170
Peltier and colleagues[221]	86% (22)	69% (13)	—	—	Dipy	All 35

Adeno, adenosine; Angio, angiogram; CAD, coronary artery disease; Db, dobutamine; Dipy, Dipyridamole; Ex, exercise; segts, segments. Data from references 213-221.

means of interpretation could improve feasibility and reproducibility. Either semiquantitative or fully quantitative strategies of examining wall motion can be used to evaluate global and regional LV function. Global indices (ejection fraction or end-systolic volume) are insensitive to mild degrees of ischemia and are not an answer to the shortcomings of qualitative interpretation. Wall motion scoring offers a semi-quantitative regional approach, which may improve the reproducibility of observers, but this does not constitute a major deviation from the regional approach used by most experienced readers and does not measure function independent of the observer.

Quantitation of regional function may be based on following either longitudinal or radial myocardial motion. The simplest approach involves tracing of endocardial (and/or epicardial) interfaces and their superimposition using a fixed or floating reference system and measurement of endocardial excursion or myocardial thickening. The limitations of this approach may be solved by some technical advances. Although excellent border definition of both endocardium and epicardium (especially in the apical views) is not always obtainable, even with harmonic imaging, contrast echocardiography may be of value. Failure to compensate for rotational or translational cardiac movement may be associated with false-positive results; correction for cardiac movement is possible,[228] but may compromise sensitivity. Third, the tedious and time-consuming process of tracing multiple systolic and diastolic frames may be automated by recent developments in edge tracking, including with acoustic quantification.[229] The feasibility and accuracy of

this approach has now been documented in several studies.[230,231]

Myocardial tissue Doppler may provide another means of quantifying regional function. This approach is that it can be used to quantify motion in the longitudinal (base-apex) direction, which corresponds to the contribution of longitudinal subendocardial muscle fibers.[232] Pulsed-wave Doppler, although useful for resting imaging,[233] is less feasible during stress because of the need to acquire all values online within a limited time at peak stress. Tissue velocity profiles within each segment of a color myocardial Doppler image may be obtained by postprocessing, but this requires a high frame rate (at least 80 to 100 frames per second) to ensure that true peak systolic velocity is captured. The development of ischemia causes a reduction of peak velocity and transmyocardial velocity gradient and a delay in the development of peak velocity. Peak velocity has been shown to correlate with wall motion interpretation,[234,235] and ischemia at dual isotope SPECT.[236] More recently, normal ranges at peak stress have been described, and these ranges have been applied to the identification of angiographically defined coronary disease,[237] providing comparable accuracy to an expert reader. This technique appears to be more amenable to dobutamine than exercise stress, but much greater problems pertain to its angle dependency and susceptibility to tethering and translational movement.

The development of strain rate (SR) and strain rate imaging have addressed the problems of tethering and translation. The measurement of myocardial shortening by this site-specific technique has been extensively validated,[238,239] and it appears that strain is an analog of regional ejection fraction, while strain rate corresponds to dP/dt.[240] Strain rate imaging has been successfully applied to the assessment of augmentation at low-dose dobutamine echocardiogram[241,242] (Fig. 16–13), but signal noise is a particular problem to its application with peak-dose dobutamine, and only one small study has suggested it to be superior to wall motion assessment.[243] Deformation indices

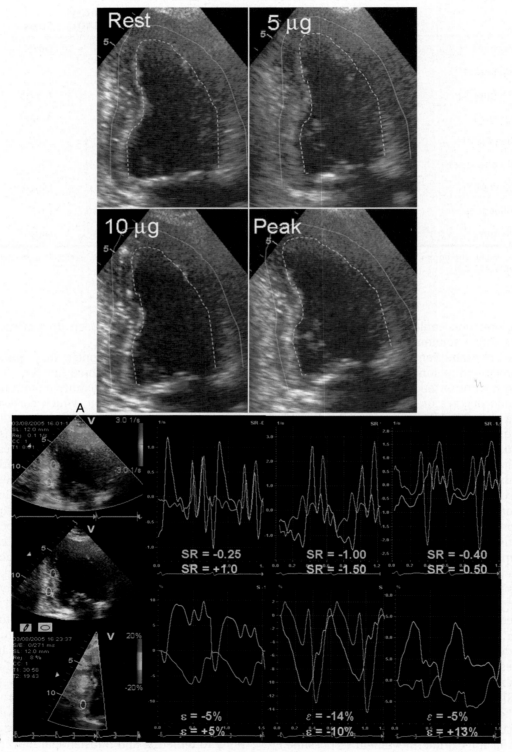

Figure 16–13. *Application of myocardial deformation imaging to stress echocardiography. End-systolic freeze-frame images in the apical two-chamber view (A) show less thickening in the inferior wall at rest, which improves with low-dose and deteriorates again at peak. However, these changes are subtle and the response is more readily identified from deformation imaging (B). The basal inferior segment (yellow) shows positive strain and strain rate (lengthening) at rest, shortening at low dose, and lengthening again at peak. ε, strain; SR, strain rate.*

may now be measured from speckle-tracking (two-dimensional strain).[244] This offers smoother curves and avoids angle dependency. However, its role in the diagnosis of ischemia remains undefined.

Stress Doppler Echocardiography

The use of Doppler to directly evaluate coronary flow adds incremental information to stress echocardiography but seems most feasible with vasodilator stress. Doppler responses to stress can examine systolic or diastolic blood flow alterations caused by ischemia. Unfortunately, this information is of limited value—changes in stroke volume occur mainly in the presence of extensive ischemia,[245] and stress-induced alterations in global cardiac function are not specific for coronary disease. Similarly, ischemia-induced mitral regurgitation (MR)[29] is uncommon.[246] However, the use of Doppler to assess low output aortic stenosis (AS) is potentially useful in discriminating the relative contribution of impaired LV function and a stenosed valve; generally, the presence of LV contractile reserve is the most reassuring funding.[247] A stenotic valve usually demonstrates an increment of aortic valve gradient with a stable valve area (Fig. 16–14).

LV relaxation may be altered by the development of myocardial ischemia.[248] Reductions in passive LV filling (i.e., impaired relaxation secondary to ischemia) may be identified during dobutamine stress echocardiography,[249] but are more feasible with stressors that provoke ischemia without tachycardia, such as dipyridamole and pacing.[250] Tissue Doppler assessment may be of value in examining regional diastolic function with less influence from left atrial pressure (LA).[251] Changes of diastolic function in response to stress are not specific for ischemia and may be a result of LV hypertrophy. An increment of filling pressure with exercise may be a means of identifying the contribution of increased filling pressure to dyspnea,[252] but the value of assessing this during pharmacologic stress is undefined.

Alternatives to Nonexercise Stress Echocardiography

Exercise Stress Testing

In patients who are unable to exercise maximally, a nonexercise stressor is mandatory, as the sensitivity of exercise echocardiography is low. In patients who *are* able to exercise, exercise echocardiography is increasingly used instead of the stress electrocardiogram. Although this is contrary to the American Heart Association and American College of Cardiology guidelines,[185] this strategy may be cost-effective.[253] The advantages of pharmacologic approaches are feasibility, better image quality, and ability to image the heart during stepwise increments of stress and at peak stress. Pharmacologic stressors probably give similar accuracy to exercise stress* (Table 16–11). The reported greater feasibility of nonexercise techniques may be colored by greater expertise in pharmacologic than in exercise echocardiography at some centers. The greater extent of ischemia with exercise than with dobutamine may reflect the greater cardiac workload imposed by exercise—this more extensive ischemia may lead the observer to be more confident in the results of exercise, despite the image quality being better with dobutamine. Electrocardiographic data are useful with exercise stress and less so with pharmacologic stressors, and data about exercise are readily extrapolated to everyday life. Exercise capacity data are prognostically important. As exercise echocardiography offers more data than the nonexercise approaches, the use of exercise-simulating techniques is limited to patients who are unable to perform maximal exercise. However, the new techniques that are adjunctive to stress echocardiography (for example, contrast, tissue Doppler, and acoustic quantification echocardiography) are more easily performed in the stationary patient and may lead to an increase in the number of nonexercise studies in the future. The sensitivity and specificity of the tests in meta-analyses are compared in Figure 16–15.

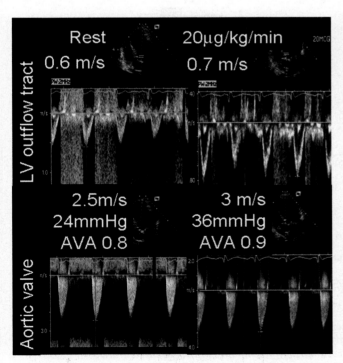

Figure 16–14. Use of Doppler imaging with low-dose dobutamine stress to evaluate low output aortic stenosis in a patient with contractile reserve. Note the stable outflow tract velocity with an increment of valvular velocity. AVA, aortic valve area; LV, left ventricular.

---

*See references 79, 80, 82, 84, 134, 254-256.

TABLE 16–11. Sensitivity and Specificity of Echocardiography with Exercise and Nonexercise Methodologies

Study	Patients, N	CAD, n	CAD Diameter, %	Multivessel, n (% all CAD)	Myocardial Infarction, n (% all CAD)
Picano and colleagues[254]	55	34	>70	18 (53)	6 (18)
Hoffmann and colleagues[84]	66	50	>70	21 (42)	0 (0)
Cohen and colleagues[79]	52	37	>70	21 (57)	11 (30)
Beleslin and colleagues[82]	136	119	>50	11 (9)	41 (34)
Marangelli and colleagues[134]	60	35	>75	19 (54)	—
Marwick and colleagues[80]	86	56	>50	34 (61)	0 (0)
Dagianti and colleagues[255]	60	25	>70	15 (60)	0 (0)
Rallidis and colleages[256]	85	85	>70	40 (47)	42 (49)

CAD, coronary artery disease.
Data from references 79, 80, 82, 84, 134, 254-256.

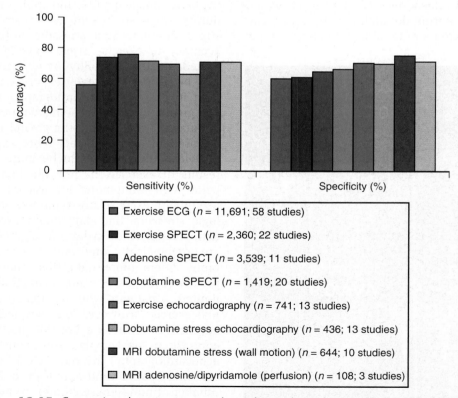

Exercise ECG (*n* = 11,691; 58 studies)

Exercise SPECT (*n* = 2,360; 22 studies)

Adenosine SPECT (*n* = 3,539; 11 studies)

Dobutamine SPECT (*n* = 1,419; 20 studies)

Exercise echocardiography (*n* = 741; 13 studies)

Dobutamine stress echocardiography (*n* = 436; 13 studies)

MRI dobutamine stress (wall motion) (*n* = 644; 10 studies)

MRI adenosine/dipyridamole (perfusion) (*n* = 108; 3 studies)

Figure 16–15. Comparison between stress echocardiography techniques with nuclear and magnetic resonance imaging in meta-analyses of each technique. ECG, electrocardiogram; MRI, magnetic resonance imaging; SPECT, single-photon emission computed tomography. (Data obtained from O'Rourke RA, Fuster V, Alexander RW, Roberts R [eds]: Hurst's the Heart: Manual of Cardiology, 11th ed. New York, McGraw Hill, 2005.)

TABLE 16–11. Sensitivity and Specificity of Echocardiography with Exercise and Nonexercise Methodologies—cont'd

Sensitivity, %				Specificity, %				
Exercise	Dobu-tamine	Dipyri-damole	Atrial Pacing	Exercise	Dobu-tamine	Dipyri-damole	Atrial Pacing	Comments
76	—	72	—	81	—	100	—	Exercise and dipyridamole comparable
80	79	—	—	87	81	—	—	Exercise and dobutamine comparable
78	86	—	—	87	87	—	—	Exercise and dobutamine comparable
80	82	74	—	82	77	94	—	Exercise, dobutamine and dipyridamole comparable
89	—	43	83	91	—	92	76	Exercise has best balance of sensitivity and specificity
88	54	—	—	80	83	—	—	Exercise superior with submaximal dobutamine
76	72	52	—	94	97	97	—	Myocardial infarction excluded
77	67	—	—	—	—	—	—	Only known CAD

Pharmacologic Stress Echocardiography versus Perfusion Scintigraphy

Nuclear perfusion imaging is the most widely used technique for the noninvasive diagnosis of CAD and is technically easier to perform and interpret than stress echocardiography. However, nuclear imaging has disadvantages pertaining to specificity, cost, and patient convenience. As there is a substantial variation in the reported accuracy of both stress echocardiography and nuclear imaging, based on variations in the population studied, their relative accuracy in those who are unable to exercise can best be addressed by direct comparison.

Diagnosis of Coronary Artery Disease

Scintigraphy and echocardiography have a concordance rate of 80% to 90% for the presence or absence of disease in most studies. Studies comparing stress echocardiography and scintigraphy using dipyridamole, adenosine, dobutamine, or atrial pacing stress are summarized in Table 16–12.[30,102,257-261] Using dobutamine or pacing stress, the sensitivities are comparable, with most studies showing slightly greater sensitivity with scintigraphy. This difference is most evident in patients with single-vessel disease,[262] a finding that might be expected from the identification of flow heterogeneity with perfusion imaging, which is an earlier event in the ischemic cascade than regional dysfunction, identified by echocardiography. Similarly, antianginal therapy may compromise the results of echocardiography because it prevents the development of ischemia[128] with less effect on perfusion scintigraphy.[263] Vasodilator stress echocardiography is significantly less sensitive than perfusion scintigraphy.[264] This difference is most marked in patients with single-vessel coronary disease and reflects failure to develop coronary steal in the absence of extensive coronary disease. This difference is less prominent in patients with multivessel disease.

The specificities of stress echocardiography and perfusion scintigraphy are comparable, with most series showing a small benefit for echocardiography. Two important sources of false-positive results are patients with left bundle branch block (LBBB) and patients with LV hypertrophy. Stress echocardiography appears to show greater specificity in patients with left bundle branch block.[265] Patients with hypertensive hypertrophy are prone to false-positive results with SPECT but not stress echocardiography.[139]

Good scintigraphy is always better than poor stress echocardiography, and good stress echocardiography is always better than poor scintigraphy.

Prognostic Assessment

Although a substantial amount of literature regarding the individual predictive abilities of echocardiography and perfusion imaging is available, comparative data are sparse. In patients undergoing surgery for vascular disease, dipyridamole stress thallium imaging has been shown to have a negative predictive value of more than 90% in most studies.[145] The occurrence of unexpected cardiac events in some patients probably results from intracoronary thrombus formation on nonsignificant stenoses (which do not cause abnormal perfusion results). The predictive value of ischemia at scintigraphy ranges from 30% to 50%, this result being attributable to positive perfusion studies in the context of mild (prognostically benign) coronary disease and false-

TABLE 16-12. Comparison of Pharmacologic Stress Echocardiography and Single Photon Emission Computed Tomography for Diagnosis of Coronary Artery Disease (>50 Patients)

Study	Patients, N	Stress	Dose	Sensitivity, %		Single-Vessel Disease		Specificity	
				Echo-cardiography	Nuclear Imaging	Echo-cardiography	Nuclear Imaging	Echo-cardiography	Nuclear Imaging
Marwick and colleagues[102]	97	Adenosine	0.18 mg/kg/min	58	86	52	81	87	71
Marwick and colleagues[30]	217	Dobutamine	40 μg	72	76	66	74	83	67
Senior and colleagues[257]	61	Dobutamine	40 μg	93	95	86	86	94	71
Ho and colleagues[258]	54	Dobutamine	40 μg	93	98	—	—	73	73
Huang and colleagues[259]	93	Dobutamine	40 μg	93	90	—	—	77	81
Santoro and colleagues[260]	60	Dobutamine	40 μg	61	91	—	—	96	81
San Roman and colleagues[261]	102	Dobutamine	40 μg + atropine	78	87	—	—	88	70
Santoro and colleagues[260]	60	Dipyridamole	0.84 mg/kg	55	97	—	—	96	89
San Roman and colleagues[261]	102	Dipyridamole	0.84 mg/kg	81	87	—	—	94	70

Data from references 30, 102, 257-261.

positive results. Overall, these results are comparable to those of pharmacologic stress echocardiography (see Table 16–7). Direct comparisons of stress echocardiography and SPECT for the prediction of perioperative cardiac events have shown their prognostic value to be similar.[151,266] A meta-analysis of published work concluded that dobutamine echocardiography and SPECT (mainly with dipyridamole stress), had comparable levels of accuracy, with cost-effectiveness in favor of echocardiography.[267]

In patients with chronic stable coronary disease and after MI, the relative prognostic roles of stress echocardiography and myocardial perfusion scintigraphy appear comparable. Ischemia may be difficult to identify within segments having abnormal resting function, and this is a source of discrepancy from the findings of perfusion scintigraphy. Preliminary data comparing dipyridamole stress echocardiography and [(99m)Tc]methoxyisobutylisonitrile-SPECT (MIBI-SPECT) in patients after recent MI have shown the finding of ischemia at echocardiography (and not at scintigraphy) to be predictive of subsequent hard events.[268]

Diagnosis of Viable Myocardium

The comparison of positron emission tomography, thallium reinjection techniques, and dobutamine echocardiography from meta-analyses is summarized in Figure 16–10; Table 16–13 summarizes matched data.[269-280] Most comparative studies show SPECT techniques to be more sensitive but of lower specificity for the prediction of functional recovery.

TABLE 16–13. Comparison of Nuclear and Stress Echocardiographic Techniques for Prediction of Viability (Evidenced by Improvement of Regional Left Ventricular Function)*

Study	Thallium Technique	Dobutamine Protocol, μg/kg/min	Sensitivity, %		Specificity	
			Thallium SPECT	Dobutamine Echocardiography	Thallium SPECT	Dobutamine Echocardiography
Marzullo and colleagues[269]	Rest-redistribution	Low dose, 10	86	82	92	92
Charney and colleagues[270]	Rest-redistribution	Low dose, 10	95	71	85	93
Kostopoulos and colleagues[271]	Rest-redistribution	Low dose, 10	90	87	69	94
Qureshi and colleagues[272]	Rest-redistribution	High dose, 40	90	74	56	89
Nagueh and colleagues[273]	Rest-redistribution	High dose, 40	91	68	43	83
Senior and collagues[274]	Stress (dobutamine)-rest/NTG	Low dose, 10	92	87	78	82
Arnese and colleagues[275]	Stress (dobutamine) reinjection	Low dose, 10	89	74	48	95
Perrone-Filardi and colleagues[276]	Stress (dobutamine) reinjection	Low dose, 10	100	79	22	83
Bax and colleagues[277]	Stress (dobutamine) reinjection	Low dose, 10	93	85	43	63
Haque and colleagues[278]	Stress (exercise) reinjection	Low dose, 20	100	94	40	80
Vanoverschelde and colleagues[279]	Stress (exercise) reinjection	High dose, 40	72	88	73	77
Elsasser and colleages[280]	Stress (dobutamine) reinjection	High dose, 40	87	95	98	80

*Average ejection fraction 38%.
NTG, nitroglycerin; SPECT, single photon emission computed tomography.
Data from references 269-280.

KEY POINTS

- Nonexercise stress with dobutamine, vasodilators, and pacing are all feasible, although interest in the latter has not been sustained, and all demonstrate satisfactory levels of accuracy.

- Despite greater ease in gathering images, pharmacologic stress is less potent than exercise stress. The resulting lesser extent of ischemia may paradoxically make the interpretation of these studies more difficult than exercise.

- The adoption of new technologies such as myocardial contrast, 3D and myocardial deformation techniques is easier with pharmacologic than exercise stress.

- Subjective interpretation remains the Achilles' heel of stress echocardiography—perhaps even more so with pharmacologic stress echocardiogram because of the subtleties of interpreting augmentation of function in viability studies. Measurement of myocardial velocity and deformation offer potential support to interpretation but remain in evolution.

REFERENCES

1. Marwick TH: Current status of non-invasive techniques for the diagnosis of myocardial ischemia. *Acta Clin Belg* 47:1-5, 1992.
2. Poldermans D, Fioretti PM, Boersma E, et al: Dobutamine-atropine stress echocardiography in elderly patients unable to perform an exercise test. Hemodynamic characteristics, safety, and prognostic value. *Arch Intern Med* 154:2681-2686, 1994.
3. Anthopoulos LP, Bonou MS, Kardaras FG, et al: Stress echocardiography in elderly patients with coronary artery disease: Applicability, safety and prognostic value of dobutamine and adenosine echocardiography in elderly patients. *J Am Coll Cardiol* 28:52-59, 1996.
4. Hashimoto A, Palmar EL, Scott JA, et al: Complications of exercise and pharmacologic stress tests: differences in younger and elderly patients. *J Nucl Cardiol* 6:612-619, 1999.
5. Ferrara N, Leosco D, Abete P, et al: Dipyridamole echocardiography as a useful and safe test in the assessment of coronary artery disease in the elderly. *J Am Geriatr Soc* 39:993-999, 1991.
6. Song JK, Lee SJ, Kang DH, et al: Ergonovine echocardiography as a screening test for diagnosis of vasospastic angina before coronary angiography. *J Am Coll Cardiol* 27:1156-1161, 1996.
7. Morales MA, Lombardi M, Distante A, et al: Ergonovine-echo test to assess the significance of chest pain at rest without ECG changes [see comments]. *Eur Heart J* 16:1361-1366, 1995.
8. Smart SC, Sawada S, Ryan T, et al: Low-dose dobutamine echocardiography detects reversible dysfunction after thrombolytic therapy of acute myocardial infarction. *Circulation* 88:405-415, 1993.
9. Picano E, Marzullo P, Gigli G, et al: Identification of viable myocardium by dipyridamole-induced improvement in regional left ventricular function assessed by echocardiography in myocardial infarction and comparison with thallium scintigraphy at rest. *Am J Cardiol* 70:703-710, 1992.
10. Varga A, Ostojic M, Djordjevic-Dikic A, et al: Infra-low dose dipyridamole test. A novel dose regimen for selective assessment of myocardial viability by vasodilator stress echocardiography. *Eur Heart J* 17:629-634, 1996.
11. Picano E, Ostojic M, Varga A, et al: Combined low dose dipyridamole-dobutamine stress echocardiography to identify myocardial viability. *J Am Coll Cardiol* 27:1422-1428, 1996.
12. Mitamura H, Ogawa S, Hori S, et al: Two dimensional echocardiographic analysis of wall motion abnormalities during handgrip exercise in patients with coronary artery disease. *Am J Cardiol* 48:711-719, 1981.
13. Fujita T, Ajisaka R, Yukisada K, et al: Quantitative analysis of left ventricular function by cold pressor two-dimensional echocardiography in patients with coronary artery disease. *Jpn Heart J* 27:813-824, 1986.
14. Afridi I, Main ML, Parrish DL, et al: Usefulness of isometric hand grip exercise in detecting coronary artery disease during dobutamine atropine stress echocardiography in patients with either stable angina pectoris or another type of positive stress test. *Am J Cardiol* 82:564-568, 1998.
15. Vasu MA, O'Keefe DD, Kapellakis GZ, et al: Myocardial oxygen consumption: effects of epinephrine, isoproterenol, dopamine, norepinephrine, and dobutamine. *Am J Physiol* 235:H237-H241, 1978.
16. Vanoverschelde JL, Wijns W, Essamri B, et al: Hemodynamic and mechanical determinants of myocardial O2 consumption in normal human heart: effects of dobutamine. *Am J Physiol* 265:H1884-H1892, 1993.
17. Mairesse GH, Vanoverschelde JL, Robert A, et al: Pathophysiologic mechanisms underlying dobutamine-induced myocardial ischemia. *Am Heart J* 136:63-70, 1998.
18. Warltier DC, Zyvoloski M, Gross GJ, et al: Redistribution of myocardial blood flow distal to a dynamic coronary arterial stenosis by sympathomimetic amines: Comparison of dopamine, dobutamine and isoproterenol. *Am J Cardiol* 48:269-279, 1981.
19. Picano E, Lattanzi F: Dipyridamole echocardiography. A new diagnostic window on coronary artery disease. [Review]. *Circulation* 83:III19-III26, 1991.
20. Sun KT, Czernin J, Krivokapich J, et al: Effects of dobutamine stimulation on myocardial blood flow, glucose metabolism, and wall motion in normal and dysfunctional myocardium. *Circulation* 94:3146-3154, 1996.
21. Sklenar J, Ismail S, Villanueva FS, et al: Dobutamine echocardiography for determining the extent of myocardial salvage after reperfusion. An experimental evaluation. *Circulation* 90:1502-1512, 1994.
22. Picano E: Stress echocardiography. From pathophysiological toy to diagnostic tool. [Review]. *Circulation* 85:1604-1612, 1992.
23. McGillem MJ, DeBoe SF, Friedman HZ, Mancini GBJ: The effects of dopamine and dobutamine on regional function in the presence of rigid coronary stenoses and subcritical impairments of reactive hyperemia. *Am Heart J* 115:970-977, 1988.
24. Sawada SG, Segar DS, Ryan T, et al: Echocardiographic detection of coronary artery disease during dobutamine infusion. *Circulation* 83:1605-1614, 1991.
25. Cohen JL, Greene TO, Ottenweller J, et al: Dobutamine digital echocardiography for detecting coronary artery disease. *Am J Cardiol* 67:1311-1318, 1991.
26. Previtali M, Lanzarini L, Ferrario M, et al: Dobutamine versus dipyridamole echocardiography in coronary artery disease. *Circulation* 83:III27-III31, 1991.
27. Salustri A, Fioretti PM, Pozzoli MM, et al: Dobutamine stress echocardiography: Its role in the diagnosis of coronary artery disease. *Eur Heart J* 13:70-77, 1992.
28. Marcovitz PA, Armstrong WF: Accuracy of dobutamine stress echocardiography in detecting coronary artery disease. *Am J Cardiol* 69:1269-1273, 1992.
29. Mazeika PK, Nadazdin A, Oakley CM: Dobutamine stress echocardiography for detection and assessment of coronary artery disease. *J Am Coll Cardiol* 19:1203-1211, 1992.
30. Marwick T, D'Hondt AM, Baudhuin T, et al: Optimal use of dobutamine stress for the detection and evaluation of coronary

artery disease: Combination with echocardiography or scintigraphy, or both? *J Am Coll Cardiol* 22:159-167, 1993.

31. Mason JR, Palac RT, Freeman ML, et al: Thallium scintigraphy during dobutamine infusion: nonexercise—dependent screening test for coronary disease. *Am Heart J* 107:481-485, 1984.

32. Hays JT, Mahmarian JJ, Cochran AJ, Verani MS: Dobutamine thallium-201 tomography for evaluating patients with suspected coronary artery disease unable to undergo exercise or vasodilator pharmacologic stress testing. *J Am Coll Cardiol* 21:1583-1590, 1993.

33. Pennell DJ, Underwood SR, Swanton RH, et al: Dobutamine thallium myocardial perfusion tomography. *J Am Coll Cardiol* 18:1471-1479, 1991.

34. Wilson RF, Wyche K, Christensen BV, et al: Effects of adenosine on human coronary arterial circulation. *Circulation* 82:1595-1606, 1990.

35. Pasternac A, Gorlin R, Sonnenblick EH, et al: Abnormalities of ventricular motion induced by atrial pacing in coronary artery disease. *Circulation* 45:1195-1205, 1972.

36. Becker L: Effect of tachycardia on left ventricular blood flow distribution during coronary occlusion. *Am J Physiol* 230:1072-1077, 1976.

37. Kamp O, De Cock CC, Kupper AJ, et al: Simultaneous transesophageal two-dimensional echocardiography and atrial pacing for detecting coronary artery disease. *Am J Cardiol* 69:1412-1416, 1992.

38. Lambertz H, Kreis A, Trumper H, Hanrath P: Simultaneous transesophageal atrial pacing and transesophageal two-dimensional echocardiography: a new method of stress echocardiography [see comments]. *J Am Coll Cardiol* 16:1143-1153, 1990.

39. Lee CY, Pellikka PA, McCully RB, et al: Nonexercise stress transthoracic echocardiography: transesophageal atrial pacing versus dobutamine stress. *J Am Coll Cardiol* 33:506-511, 1999.

40. Iliceto S, Amico A, Marangelli V, et al: Doppler echocardiographic evaluation of the effect of atrial pacing—induced ischemia on left ventricular filling in patients with coronary artery disease. *J Am Coll Cardiol* 11:953-961, 1988.

41. Iliceto S, Sorino M, D'Ambrosio G, et al: Detection of coronary artery disease by two-dimensional echocardiography and transesophageal atrial pacing. *J Am Coll Cardiol* 5:1188-1197, 1987.

42. McNeill AJ, Fioretti PM, el-Said SM, et al: Enhanced sensitivity for detection of coronary artery disease by addition of atropine to dobutamine stress echocardiography. *Am J Cardiol* 70:41-46, 1992.

43. Fioretti PM, Poldermans D, Salustri A, et al: Atropine increases the accuracy of dobutamine stress echocardiography in patients taking beta-blockers. *Eur Heart J* 15:355-360, 1994.

44. Chen L, Ma L, de Prada VA, et al: Effects of beta-blockade and atropine on ischemic responses in left ventricular regions subtending coronary stenosis during dobutamine stress echocardiography. *J Am Coll Cardiol* 28:1866-1876, 1996.

45. Picano E, Pingitore A, Conti U, et al: Enhanced sensitivity for detection of coronary artery disease by addition of atropine to dipyridamole echocardiography. *Eur Heart J* 14:1216-1222, 1993.

46. Picano E, Mathias W Jr, Pingitore A, et al: Safety and tolerability of dobutamine-atropine stress echocardiography: A prospective, multicentre study. Echo Dobutamine International Cooperative Study Group [see comments]. *Lancet* 344:1190-1192, 1994.

47. Pingitore A, Picano E, Colosso MQ, et al: The atropine factor in pharmacologic stress echocardiography. Echo Persantine (EPIC) and Echo Dobutamine International Cooperative (EDIC) Study Groups. *J Am Coll Cardiol* 27:1164-1170, 1996.

48. Hepner AM, Bach DS, Armstrong WF: Early chronotropic incompetence predicts the need for atropine during dobutamine stress echocardiography. *Am J Cardiol* 79:365-366, 1997.

49. Lewandowski TJ, Armstrong WF, Bach DS: Reduced test time by early identification of patients requiring atropine during dobu-

50. Ostojic M, Picano E, Beleslin B, et al: Dipyridamole-dobutamine echocardiography: A novel test for the detection of milder forms of coronary artery disease. *J Am Coll Cardiol* 23:1115-1122, 1994.

51. Belohlavek M, Tanabe K, Mulvagh SL, et al: Image enhancement by noncontrast harmonic echocardiography. Part II. Quantitative assessment with use of contrast-to-speckle ratio. *Mayo Clin Proc* 73:1066-1070, 1998.

52. Mulvagh SL, Foley DA, Belohlavek M, Seward JB: Image enhancement by noncontrast harmonic echocardiography. Part I. Qualitative assessment of endocardial visualization. *Mayo Clin Proc* 73:1062-1065, 1998.

53. Caidahl K, Kazzam E, Lidberg J, et al: New concept in echocardiography: harmonic imaging of tissue without use of contrast agent [see comments]. *Lancet* 352:1264-1270, 1998.

54. Franke A, Hoffmann R, Kuhl HP, et al: Non-contrast second harmonic imaging improves interobserver agreement and accuracy of dobutamine stress echocardiography in patients with impaired image quality. *Heart* 83:133-140, 2000.

55. Lim HE, Shim WJ, Rhee H, et al: Assessment of coronary flow reserve with transthoracic Doppler echocardiography: Comparison among adenosine, standard-dose dipyridamole, and high-dose dipyridamole. *J Am Soc Echocardiogr* 13:264-270, 2000.

56. Panza JA, Laurienzo JM, Curiel RV, et al: Transesophageal dobutamine stress echocardiography for evaluation of patients with coronary artery disease. *J Am Coll Cardiol* 24:1260-1267, 1994.

57. Baer FM, Voth E, Deutsch HJ, et al: Predictive value of low dose dobutamine transesophageal echocardiography and 18-FDG postiron emission tomography for recovery of regional left ventricular function after successful revascularization. *J Am Coll Cardiol* 28:60-69, 1996.

58. Baer FM, Voth E, LaRosee K, et al: Comparison of dobutamine transesophageal echocardiography and dobutamine magnetic resonance imaging for detection of residual myocardial viability. *Am J Cardiol* 78:415-419, 1996.

59. Stempfle HU, Kruger TM, Brandl BC, et al: Simultaneous transesophageal echocardiography and atrial pacing: assessment of the functional significance of coronary artery disease before surgical treatment of an abdominal aneurysm. *Clin Investig* 72:206-208, 1994.

60. Ommen SR, Nishimura RA, Appleton CP, et al: Clinical utility of Doppler echocardiography and tissue Doppler imaging in the estimation of left ventricular filling pressures: A comparative simultaneous Doppler-catheterization study. *Circulation* 102:1788-1794, 2000.

61. Bleeker GB, Bax JJ, Schalij MJ, van der Wall EE: Tissue Doppler imaging to assess left ventricular dyssynchrony and resynchronization therapy. *Eur J Echocardiogr* 6:382-384, 2005.

62. Attenhofer CH, Pellikka PA, Oh JK, et al: Is review of videotape necessary after review of digitized cine-loop images in stress echocardiography? A prospective study in 306 patients. *J Am Soc Echocardiogr* 10:179-184, 1997.

63. Armstrong WF, Pellikka PA, Ryan T, et al: Stress echocardiography: recommendations for performance and interpretation of stress echocardiography. Stress Echocardiography Task Force of the Nomenclature and Standards Committee of the American Society of Echocardiography. *J Am Soc Echocardiogr* 11:97-104, 1998.

64. Cerqueira MD, Weissman NJ, Dilsizian V, et al: Standardized myocardial segmentation and nomenclature for tomographic imaging of the heart: a statement for healthcare professionals from the Cardiac Imaging Committee of the Council on Clinical Cardiology of the American Heart Association. *Circulation* 105:539-542, 2002.

65. Schiller NB, Shah PM, Crawford M, et al: Recommendations for quantitation of the left ventricle by two-dimensional echocardiog-

raphy. American Society of Echocardiography Committee on Standards, Subcommittee on Quantitation of Two-Dimensional Echocardiograms. [Review]. *J Am Soc Echocardiogr* 2:358-367, 1989.

66. Picano E, Lattanzi F, Orlandini A, et al: Stress echocardiography and the human factor: the importance of being expert. *J Am Coll Cardiol* 17:666-669, 1991.

67. Furukawa T, Haque T, Takahashi M, Kinoshita M: An assessment of dobutamine echocardiography and end-diastolic wall thickness for predicting post-revascularization functional recovery in patients with chronic coronary artery disease. *Eur Heart J* 18:798-806, 1997.

68. Attenhoffer CH, Pellikka PA, Oh JK, et al: Comparison of ischemic response during exercise and dobutamine echocardiography in patients with left main coronary artery disease. *J Am Coll Cardiol* 27:1171-1177, 1996.

69. Secknus MA, Niedermaier ON, Lauer MS, Marwick TH: Diagnostic and prognostic implications of left ventricular cavity obliteration response to dobutamine echocardiography. *Am J Cardiol* 81:1318-1322, 1998.

70. Yuda S, Khoury V, Marwick TH: Influence of wall stress and left ventricular geometry on the accuracy of dobutamine stress echocardiography. *J Am Coll Cardiol* 40:1311-1319, 2002.

71. Mathias W Jr, Tsutsui JM, Andrade JL, et al: Value of rapid beta-blocker injection at peak dobutamine-atropine stress echocardiography for detection of coronary artery disease. *J Am Coll Cardiol* 41:1583-1589, 2003.

72. Arnese M, Fioretti PM, Cornel JH, et al: Akinesis becoming dyskinesis during high-dose dobutamine stress echocardiography: a marker of myocardial ischemia or a mechanical phenomenon? *Am J Cardiol* 73:896-899, 1994.

73. Carstensen S, Ali SM, Stensgaard-Hansen FV, et al: Dobutamine-atropine stress echocardiography in asymptomatic healthy individuals. The relativity of stress-induced hyperkinesis. *Circulation* 92:3453-3463, 1995.

74. Oberman A, Fan PH, Nanda NC, et al: Reproducibility of two-dimensional exercise echocardiography. *J Am Coll Cardiol* 14:923-928, 1989.

75. Hoffmann R, Lethen H, Marwick T, et al: Analysis of interinstitutional observer agreement in interpretation of dobutamine stress echocardiograms. *J Am Coll Cardiol* 27:330-336, 1996.

76. Hoffmann R, Lethen H, Marwick T, et al: Standardized guidelines for the interpretation of dobutamine echocardiography reduce interinstitutional variance in interpretation. *Am J Cardiol* 82:1520-1524, 1998.

77. Hoffmann R, Marwick TH, Poldermans D, et al: Refinements in stress echocardiographic techniques improve inter-institutional agreement in interpretation of dobutamine stress echocardiograms. *Eur Heart J* 23:821-829, 2002.

78. Strotmann JM, Escobar Kvitting JP, et al: Anatomic M-mode echocardiography: A new approach to assess regional myocardial function—A comparative in vivo and in vitro study of both fundamental and second harmonic imaging modes. *J Am Soc Echocardiogr* 12:300-307, 1999.

79. Cohen JL, Ottenweller JE, George AK, Duvvuri S: Comparison of dobutamine and exercise echocardiography for detecting coronary artery disease. *Am J Cardiol* 72:1226-1231, 1993.

80. Marwick TH, D'Hondt AM, Mairesse GH, et al: Comparative ability of dobutamine and exercise stress in inducing myocardial ischaemia in active patients. *Br Heart J* 72:31-38, 1994.

81. Previtali M, Lanzarini L, Fetiveau R, et al: Comparison of dobutamine stress echocardiography, dipyridamole stress echocardiography and exercise stress testing for diagnosis of coronary artery disease. *Am J Cardiol* 72:865-870, 1993.

82. Beleslin BD, Ostojic M, Stepanovic J, et al: Stress echocardiography in the detection of myocardial ischemia. Head-to-head comparison of exercise, dobutamine, and dipyridamole tests. *Circulation* 90:1168-1176, 1994.

83. Rallidis L, Cokkinos P, Tousoulis D, Nihoyannopoulos P: Comparison of dobutamine and treadmill exercise echocardiography in inducing ischemia in patients with coronary artery disease. *J Am Coll Cardiol* 30:1660-1668, 1997.

84. Hoffmann R, Lethen H, Kleinhans E, et al: Comparative evaluation of bicycle and dobutamine stress echocardiography with perfusion scintigraphy and bicycle electrocardiogram for identification of coronary artery disease. *Am J Cardiol* 72:555-559, 1993.

85. Mertes H, Sawada SG, Ryan T, et al: Symptoms, adverse effects, and complications associated with dobutamine stress echocardiography. Experience in 1118 patients. *Circulation* 88:15-19, 1993.

86. Poldermans D, Fioretti PM, Boersma E, et al: Safety of dobutamine-atropine stress echocardiography in patients with suspected or proven coronary artery disease. *Am J Cardiol* 73:456-459, 1994.

87. Secknus MA, Marwick TH: Evolution of dobutamine echocardiography protocols and indications: safety and side effects in 3,011 studies over 5 years. *J Am Coll Cardiol* 29:1234-1240, 1997.

88. Zahn R, Lotter R, Nohl H, et al: [Feasibility and safety of dobutamine stress echocardiography: experiences with 1,000 studies]. *Zeitschrift fur Kardiologie* 85:28-34, 1996.

89. Orlandini AD, Tuero EI, Diaz R, et al: Acute cardiac rupture during dobutamine-atropine echocardiography stress test. *J Am Soc Echocardiogr* 13:152-153, 2000.

90. Cornel JH, Balk AH, Boersma E, et al: Safety and feasibility of dobutamine-atropine stress echocardiography in patients with ischemic left ventricular dysfunction. *J Am Soc Echocardiogr* 9:27-32, 1996.

91. Rosamond TL, Vacek JL, Hurwitz A, et al: Hypotension during dobutamine stress echocardiography: initial description and clinical relevance. *Am Heart J* 123:403-407, 1992.

92. Marcovitz PA, Bach DS, Mathias W, et al: Paradoxic hypotension during dobutamine stress echocardiography: clinical and diagnostic implications. *J Am Coll Cardiol* 21:1080-1086, 1993.

93. Heinle SK, Tice FD, Kisslo J: Hypotension during dobutamine stress echocardiography: is it related to dynamic intraventricular obstruction? *Am Heart J* 130:314-317, 1995.

94. Tanimoto M, Pai RG, Jintapakorn W, Shah PM: Mechanisms of hypotension during dobutamine stress echocardiography in patients with coronary artery disease. *Am J Cardiol* 76:26-30, 1995.

95. Lieberman EB, Heinle SK, Wildermann N, et al: Does hypotension during dobutamine stress echocardiography correlate with anatomic or functional cardiac impairment? *Am Heart J* 129:1121-1126, 1995.

96. Albro PC, Gould KL, Westcott RJ, et al: Non-invasive assessment of coronary stenoses by myocardial imaging during pharmacologic coronary vasodilation. III Clinical trial. *Am J Cardiol* 42:751-760, 1978.

97. Picano E, Distante A, Masini M, et al: Dipyridamole-echocardiography test in effort angina pectoris. *Am J Cardiol* 56:452-456, 1985.

98. Picano E, Lattanzi F, Masini M, et al: Usefulness of the dipyridamole-exercise echocardiography test for diagnosis of coronary artery disease. *Am J Cardiol* 62:67-70, 1988.

99. Zoghbi WA: Use of adenosine echocardiography for diagnosis of coronary artery disease. *Am Heart J* 122:285-292; discussion 302, 1991.

100. Zoghbi WA, Cheirif J, Kleiman NS, et al: Diagnosis of ischemic heart disease with adenosine echocardiography. *J Am Coll Cardiol* 18:1271-1279, 1991.

101. Tawa CB, Baker WB, Kleiman NS, et al: Comparison of adenosine echocardiography, with and without isometric handgrip, to exercise echocardiography in the detection of ischemia in patients with coronary artery disease. *J Am Soc Echocardiogr* 9:33-43, 1996.

102. Marwick T, Willemart B, D'Hondt AM, et al: Selection of the optimal nonexercise stress for the evaluation of ischemic regional myocardial dysfunction and malperfusion. Comparison of dobutamine and adenosine using echocardiography and 99mTc-MIBI single photon emission computed tomography [see comments]. *Circulation* 87:345-354, 1993.

103. Picano E, Lattanzi F, Masini M, et al: High dose dipyridamole echocardiography test in effort angina pectoris. *J Am Coll Cardiol* 8:848-854, 1986.

104. Picano E, Marini C, Pirelli S, et al: Safety of intravenous high-dose dipyridamole echocardiography. The Echo-Persantine International Cooperative Study Group. *Am J Cardiol* 70:252-258, 1992.

105. Cerqueira MD, Verani MS, Schwaiger M, et al: Safety profile of adenosine stress perfusion imaging: Results from the Adenoscan Multicenter Trial Registry [see comments]. *J Am Coll Cardiol* 23:384-389, 1994.

106. Harding MB, Leithe ME, Mark DB, et al: Ergonovine maleate testing during cardiac catheterization: a 10-year perspective in 3,447 patients without significant coronary artery disease or Prinzmetal's variant angina. *J Am Coll Cardiol* 20:107-111, 1992; published erratum appears in *J Am Coll Cardiol* 21(3):848, 1993.

107. Song JK, Park SW, Kang DH, et al: Diagnosis of coronary vasospasm in patients with clinical presentation of unstable angina pectoris using ergonovine echocardiography [see comments]. *Am J Cardiol* 82:1475-1478, 1998.

108. Song JK, Park SW, Kim JJ, et al: Values of intravenous ergonovine test with two-dimensional echocardiography for diagnosis of coronary artery spasm. *J Am Soc Echocardiogr* 7:607-615, 1994.

109. Previtali M, Ardissino D, Barberis P, et al: Hyperventilation and ergonovine tests in Prinzmetal's variant angina pectoris in man. *Am J Cardiol* 63:17-20, 1989.

110. Picano E, Alaimo A, Chubuchny V, et al: Noninvasive pacemaker stress echocardiography for diagnosis of coronary artery disease: a multicenter study. *J Am Coll Cardiol* 40:1305-1310, 2002.

111. Takeuchi M, Araki M, Nakashima Y, Kuroiwa A: Comparison of dobutamine stress echocardiography and stress thallium-201 single-photon emission computed tomography for detecting coronary artery disease. *J Am Soc Echocardiogr* 6:593-602, 1993.

112. Ling LH, Pellikka PA, Mahoney DW, et al: Atropine augmentation in dobutamine stress echocardiography: Role and incremental value in a clinical practice setting. *J Am Coll Cardiol* 28:551-557, 1996.

113. San Roman JA, Vilacosta I, Castillo JA, et al: Dipyridamole and dobutamine-atropine stress echocardiography in the diagnosis of coronary artery disease. Comparison with exercise stress test, analysis of agreement, and impact of antianginal treatment. *Chest* 110:1248-1254, 1996.

114. Anthopoulos LP, Bonou MS, Kardaras FG, et al: Stress echocardiography in elderly patients with coronary artery disease: Applicability, safety and prognostic value of dobutamine and adenosine echocardiography in elderly patients. *J Am Coll Cardiol* 28:52-59, 1996.

115. Dionisopoulos PN, Collins JD, Smart SC, et al: The value of dobutamine stress echocardiography for the detection of coronary artery disease in women. *J Am Soc Echocardiogr* 10:811-817, 1997.

116. Elhendy A, Geleijnse ML, van Domburg RT, et al: Gender differences in the accuracy of dobutamine stress echocardiography for the diagnosis of coronary artery disease. *Am J Cardiol* 80:1414-1418, 1997.

117. Hennessy T, Diamond P, Holligan B, et al: Correlation of myocardial histologic changes in hibernating myocardium with dobutamine stress echocardiographic findings. *Am Heart J* 135:952-959, 1998.

118. Nagel E, Lehmkuhl HB, Bocksch W, et al: Noninvasive diagnosis of ischemia-induced wall motion abnormalities with the use of high-dose dobutamine stress MRI: Comparison with dobutamine stress echocardiography. *Circulation* 99:763-770, 1999.

119. Beleslin BD, Ostojic M, Djordjevic-Dikic A, et al: Integrated evaluation of relation between coronary lesion features and stress echocardiography results: the importance of coronary lesion morphology. *J Am Coll Cardiol* 33:717-726, 1999.

120. Bach DS, Muller DW, Gros BJ, Armstrong WF: False positive dobutamine stress echocardiograms: characterization of clinical, echocardiographic and angiographic findings. *J Am Coll Cardiol* 24:928-933, 1994.

121. Baptista J, Arnese M, Roelandt JR, et al: Quantitative coronary angiography in the estimation of the functional significance of coronary stenosis: correlations with dobutamine-atropine stress test. *J Am Coll Cardiol* 23:1434-1439, 1994.

122. Bartunek J, Marwick TH, Rodrigues AC, et al: Dobutamine-induced wall motion abnormalities: correlations with myocardial fractional flow reserve and quantitative coronary angiography. *J Am Coll Cardiol* 27:1429-1436, 1996.

123. Segar DS, Brown SE, Sawada SG, et al: Dobutamine stress echocardiography: correlation with coronary lesion severity as determined by quantitative angiography. *J Am Coll Cardiol* 19:1197-1202, 1992.

124. Picano E, Severi S, Lattanzi F: The diagnostic and prognostic value of echo-dipyridamole in patients with suspected coronary disease. *Giornale Italiano di Cardiologia* 21:621-632, 1991.

125. Severi S, Picano E, Michelassi C, et al: Diagnostic and prognostic value of dipyridamole echocardiography in patients with suspected coronary artery disease. Comparison with exercise electrocardiography. *Circulation* 89:1160-1173, 1994.

126. Lanzarini L, Fetiveau R, Poli A, et al: Results of dipyridamole plus atropine echo stress test for the diagnosis of coronary artery disease. *Int J Card Imaging* 11:233-240, 1995.

127. Agati L, Renzi M, Sciomer S, et al: Transesophageal dipyridamole echocardiography for diagnosis of coronary artery disease. *J Am Coll Cardiol* 19:765-770, 1992.

128. Lattanzi F, Picano E, Bolognese L, et al: Inhibition of dipyridamole-induced ischemia by antianginal therapy in humans. Correlation with exercise electrocardiography. *Circulation* 83:1256-1262, 1991.

129. Danzi GB, Pirelli S, Mauri L, et al: Which variable of stenosis severity best describes the significance of an isolated left anterior descending coronary artery lesion? Correlation between quantitative coronary angiography, intracoronary Doppler measurements and high dose dipyridamole echocardiography. *J Am Coll Cardiol* 31:526-533, 1998.

130. Porter TR, Xie F, Kilzer K, Deligonul U: Detection of myocardial perfusion abnormalities during dobutamine and adenosine stress echocardiography with transient myocardial contrast imaging after minute quantities of intravenous perfluorocarbon-exposed sonicated dextrose albumin. *J Am Soc Echocardiogr* 9:779-786, 1996.

131. Porter TR, Kricsfeld A, Deligonul U, Xie F: Detection of regional perfusion abnormalities during adenosine stress echocardiography with intravenous perfluorocarbon-exposed sonicated dextrose albumin. *Am Heart J* 132:41-47, 1996.

132. Kaul S, Senior R, Dittrich H, et al: Detection of coronary artery disease with myocardial contrast echocardiography: Comparison with 99mTc-sestamibi single-photon emission computed tomography. *Circulation* 96:785-792, 1997.

133. Hamouda MS, Kassem HK, Salama M, et al: Evaluation of coronary flow reserve in hypertensive patients by dipyridamole transesophageal doppler echocardiography. *Am J Cardiol* 86:305-308, 2000.

134. Marangelli V, Iliceto S, Piccinni G, et al: Detection of coronary artery disease by digital stress echocardiography: Comparison

of exercise, transesophageal atrial pacing and dipyridamole echocardiography. *J Am Coll Cardiol* 24:117-124, 1994.

135. Michael TA, Antonescu A, Bhambi B, Balasingam S: Accuracy and usefulness of atrial pacing in conjunction with transthoracic echocardiography in the detection of cardiac ischemia. *Am. J Cardiol* 77:187-190, 1996.

136. Schroder K, Voller H, Dingerkus H, et al: Comparison of the diagnostic potential of four echocardiographic stress tests shortly after acute myocardial infarction: submaximal exercise, transesophageal atrial pacing, dipyridamole, and dobutamine-atropine. *Am J Cardiol* 77(11):909-914, 1996.

137. Picano E, Bedetti G, Varga A, Cseh E: The comparable diagnostic accuracies of dobutamine-stress and dipyridamole-stress echocardiographies: a meta-analysis. *Coron Artery Dis* 11:151-159, 2000.

138. Lelorier J, Gregoire G, Benhaddad A, et al: Discrepancies between meta-analyses and subsequent large randomized, controlled trials. *N Engl J Med* 337:536-542, 1997.

139. Fragasso G, Lu C, Dabrowski P, et al: Comparison of stress/rest myocardial perfusion tomography, dipyridamole and dobutamine stress echocardiography for the detection of coronary disease in hypertensive patients with chest pain and positive exercise test. *J Am Coll Cardiol* 34:441-447, 1999.

140. Berthe C, Pierard LA, Hiernaux M, et al: Predicting the extent and location of coronary artery disease in acute myocardial infarction by echocardiography during dobutamine infusion. *Am J Cardiol* 58:1167-1172, 1986.

141. Poldermans D, Arnese M, Fioretti PM, et al: Improved cardiac risk stratification in major vascular surgery with dobutamine-atropine stress echocardiography. *J Am Coll Cardiol* 26:648-653, 1995.

142. Hertzer NR, Beven EG, Young JR, et al: Coronary artery disease in peripheral vascular patients. A classification of 1000 coronary angiograms and results of surgical management. *Ann Surg* 199:223-233, 1984.

143. Mangano DT: Perioperative cardiac morbidity. *Anesthesiology* 72:153-184, 1990.

144. Mangano DT, London MJ, Tubau JF, et al: Dipyridamole thallium-201 scintigraphy as a preoperative screening test: A reexamination of its predictive capacity. *Circulation* 84:493-502, 1991.

145. Eagle KA, Brundage BH, Chaitman BR, et al: Guidelines for perioperative cardiovascular evaluation for noncardiac surgery. Report of the American College of Cardiology/American Heart Association Task Force on Practice Guidelines. Committee on Perioperative Cardiovascular Evaluation for Noncardiac Surgery. *Circulation* 93:1278-1317, 1996.

146. Eagle KA, Singer DE, Brewster DC: Dipyridamole thallium scanning in patients undergoing vascular surgery. Optimizing preoperative evaluation of cardiac risk. *JAMA* 257:2185-2189, 1987.

147. Lee TH, Marcantonio ER, Mangione CM, et al: Derivation and Prospective Validation of a Simple Index for Prediction of Cardiac Risk of Major Noncardiac Surgery. *Circulation* 100:1043-1049, 1999.

148. Tischler MD, Lee TH, Hirsch AT: Prediction of major cardiac events after peripheral vascular surgery using dipyridamole echocardiography. *Am J Cardiol* 68:593-599, 1991.

149. Sicari R, Picano E, Lusa AM, et al: The value of dipyridamole echocardiography in risk stratification before vascular surgery: A multicenter study. *Eur Heart J* 16:842-847, 1995.

150. Rossi E, Citterio F, Vescio MF, et al: Risk stratification of patients undergoing peripheral vascular revascularization by combined resting and dipyridamole echocardiography. *Am J Cardiol* 82:306-310, 1998.

151. Pasquet A, D'Hondt AM, Verhelst R, et al: Comparison of dipyridamole stress echocardiography and perfusion scintigraphy for cardiac risk stratification in vascular surgery patients. *Am J Cardiol* 82:1468-1474, 1998.

152. Poldermans D, Fioretti PM, Forster T, et al: Dobutamine stress echocardiography for assessment of perioperative cardiac risk in patients undergoing major vascular surgery. *Circulation* 87:1506-1512, 1993.

153. Poldermans D, Fioretti PM, Forster T, et al: Dobutamine-atropine stress echocardiography for assessment of perioperative and late cardiac risk in patients undergoing major vascular surgery. *Eur J Vasc Surg* 8:286-293, 1994.

154. Pryor DB, Shaw L, McCants CB, et al: Value of the history and physical in identifying patients at increased risk for coronary artery disease. *Ann Intern Med* 118:81-90, 1993.

155. Weiner DA, Ryan TJ, McCabe CH, et al: Prognostic importance of a clinical profile and exercise test in medically-treated patients with coronary artery disease. *J Am Coll Cardiol* 3:772-779, 1984.

156. Mark DB, Hlatky MA, Harrell FE, et al: Exercise treadmill score for predicting prognosis in coronary artery disease. *Ann Intern Med* 106:793-800, 1987.

157. Shaw LJ, Peterson ED, Shaw LK, et al: Use of a prognostic treadmill score in identifying diagnostic coronary disease subgroups. *Circulation* 98:1622-1630, 1998.

158. Berman DS, Hachamovitch R, Kiat H, et al: Incremental value of prognostic testing in patients with known or suspected ischemic heart disease: A basis for optimal utilization of exercise technetium-99m sestamibi myocardial perfusion single-photon emission computed tomography. *J Am Coll Cardiol* 26:639-647, 1990.

159. Marwick TH, Mehta R, Arheart K, Lauer MS: Use of exercise echocardiography for prognostic evaluation of patients with known or suspected coronary artery disease. *J Am Coll Cardiol* 30:83-90, 1997.

160. Schroder K, Wieckhorst A, Voller H: Comparison of the prognostic value of dipyridamole and dobutamine stress echocardiography in patients with known or suspected coronary artery disease. *Am J Cardiol* 79:1516-1518, 1997.

161. Poldermans D, Fioretti PM, Boersma E, et al: Dobutamine-atropine stress echocardiography and clinical data for predicting late cardiac events in patients with suspected coronary artery disease. *Am J Med* 97:119-125, 1994.

162. Kamaran M, Teague SM, Finkelhor RS, et al: Prognostic value of dobutamine stress echocardiography in patients referred because of suspected coronary artery disease. *Am J Cardiol* 76:887-891, 1995.

163. Marcovitz PA, Shayna V, Horn RA, et al: Value of dobutamine stress echocardiography in determining the prognosis of patients with known or suspected coronary artery disease. *Am J Cardiol* 78:404-408, 1996.

164. Senior R, Soman P, Khattar RS, Lahiri A: Prognostic value of dobutamine stress echocardiography in patients undergoing diagnostic coronary arteriography. *Am J Cardiol* 79:1610-1614, 1997.

165. Chuah SC, Pellikka PA, Roger VL, et al: Role of dobutamine stress echocardiography in predicting outcome in 860 patients with known or suspected coronary artery disease. *Circulation* 97:1474-1480, 1998.

166. Poldermans D, Fioretti PM, Boersma E, et al: Long-term prognostic value of dobutamine-atropine stress echocardiography in 1737 patients with known or suspected coronary artery disease: A single-center experience. *Circulation* 99:757-762, 1999.

167. Picano E, Severi S, Michelassi C, et al: Prognostic importance of dipyridamole-echocardiography test in coronary artery disease. *Circulation* 80:450-457, 1989.

168. Cortigiani L, Paolini EA, Nannini E: Dipyridamole stress echocardiography for risk stratification in hypertensive patients with chest pain. *Circulation* 98:2855-2859, 1998.

169. Pingitore A, Picano E, Varga A, et al: Prognostic value of pharmacological stress echocardiography in patients with known or suspected coronary artery disease: A prospective, large-scale, multicenter, head-to-head comparison between dipyridamole and dobutamine test. Echo-Persantine International Cooperative

(EPIC) and Echo-Dobutamine International Cooperative (EDIC) Study Groups. *J Am Coll Cardiol* 34:1769-1777, 1999.

170. Marwick TH, Case C, Sawada S, et al: Use of stress echocardiography to predict mortality in patients with diabetes and known or suspected coronary artery disease. *Diabetes Care* 25:1042-1048, 2002.

171. Sicari R, Cortigiani L, Bigi R, et al: Prognostic value of pharmacological stress echocardiography is affected by concomitant antiischemic therapy at the time of testing. *Circulation* 109:2428-2431, 2004.

172. Candell-Riera J, Permanyer-Miralda G, Castell J, et al: Uncomplicated first myocardial infarction: strategy for comprehensive prognostic studies. *J Am Coll Cardiol* 18:1207-1219, 1991.

173. Bolognese L, Sarasso G, Aralda D, et al: High dose echocardiography test early after uncomplicated acute myocardial infarction: Correlation with exercise testing and coronary angiography. *J Am Coll Cardiol* 14:357-363, 1989.

174. Sclavo MG, Noussan P, Pallisco O, Presbitero P: Usefulness of dipyridamole-echocardiographic test to identify jeopardized myocardium after thrombolysis. Limited clinical predictivity of dipyridamole-echocardiographic test in convalescing acute myocardial infarction: correlation with coronary angiography. *Eur Heart J* 13:1348-1355, 1992.

175. Picano E, Landi P, Bolognese L, et al: Prognostic value of dipyridamole echocardiography early after uncomplicated myocardial infarction: a large-scale, multicenter trial. The EPIC Study Group. *Am J Med* 95:608-618, 1993.

176. Chiarella F, Domenicucci S, Bellotti P, et al: Dipyridamole echocardiographic test performed 3 days after an acute myocardial infarction: Feasibility, tolerability, safety and in-hospital prognostic value. *Eur Heart J* 15:842-850, 1994.

177. Picano E, Pingitore A, Sicari R, et al: Stress echocardiographic results predict risk of reinfarction early after uncomplicated acute myocardial infarction: Large-scale multicenter study. Echo Persantine International Cooperative (EPIC) Study Group. *J Am Coll Cardiol* 26:908-913, 1995.

178. Picano E, Sicari R, Landi P, et al: Prognostic value of myocardial viability in medically-treated patients with global left ventricular dysfunction early after acute uncomplicated myocardial infarction: A dobutamine stress echocardiographic study. *Circulation* 98:1078-1084, 1998.

179. Camerieri A, Picano E, Landi P, et al: Prognostic value of dipyridamole echocardiography early after myocardial infarction in elderly patients. Echo Persantine Italian Cooperative (EPIC) Study Group. *J Am Coll Cardiol* 22:1809-1815, 1993.

180. Iliceto S, Caiati C, Ricci A, et al: Prediction of cardiac events after uncomplicated myocardial infarction by cross-sectional echocardiography during transesophageal pacing. *Int J Cardiol* 28:95-104, 1990.

181. Salustri A, Fioretti PM, McNeill AJ, et al: Pharmacological stress echocardiography in the diagnosis of coronary artery disease and myocardial ischaemia: a comparison between dobutamine and dipyridamole. *Eur Heart J* 13:1356-1362, 1992.

182. Lombardi M, Morales MA, Michelassi C, et al: Efficacy of isosorbide-5-mononitrate versus nifedipine in preventing spontaneous and ergonovine-induced myocardial ischaemia. A double-blind, placebo-controlled study. *Eur Heart J* 14:845-851, 1993.

183. Dodi C, Pingitore A, Sicari R, et al: Effects of antianginal therapy with a calcium antagonist and nitrates on dobutamine-atropine stress echocardiography. Comparison with exercise electrocardiography. *Eur Heart J* 18:242-247, 1997.

184. Varga A, Preda I: Pharmacological stress echocardiography for exercise independent assessment of anti-ischaemic therapy [editorial; comment]. *Eur Heart J* 18:180-181, 1997.

185. Gibbons RJ, Abrams J, Chatterjee K, et al: ACC/AHA 2002 guideline update for the management of patients with chronic stable angina—summary article: a report of the American College of Cardiology/American Heart Association Task Force on Practice Guidelines (Committee on the Management of Patients With Chronic Stable Angina). *Circulation* 107:149-158, 2003.

186. Massa D, Pirelli S, Gara E, et al: Exercise testing and dipyridamole echocardiography test before and 48 h after successful coronary angioplasty: prognostic implications. *Eur Heart J* 10(Suppl G):13-7, 1989.

187. Picano E, Pirelli S, Marzilli M, et al: Usefulness of high-dose dipyridamole echocardiography test in coronary angioplasty. *Circulation* 80:807-815, 1989.

188. McNeill AJ, Fioretti PM, el-Said SM, et al: Dobutamine stress echocardiography before and after coronary angioplasty. *Am J Cardiol* 69:740-745, 1992.

189. Akosah KO, Porter TR, Simon R, et al: Ischemia-induced regional wall motion abnormality is improved after coronary angioplasty: demonstration by dobutamine stress echocardiography. *J Am Coll Cardiol* 21:584-589, 1993.

190. Pirelli S, Danzi GB, Alberti A, et al: Comparison of usefulness of high-dose dipyridamole echocardiography and exercise electrocardiography for detection of asymptomatic restenosis after coronary angioplasty. *Am J Cardiol* 67:1335-1338, 1991.

191. Heinle SK, Lieberman EB, Ancukiewicz M, et al: Usefulness of dobutamine echocardiography for detecting restenosis after percutaneous transluminal coronary angioplasty. *Am J Cardiol* 72:1220-1225, 1993.

192. Bjoernstad K, Aakhus S, Lundbom J, et al: Digital dipyridamole stress echocardiography in silent ischemia after coronary artery bypass grafting and/or after healing of acute myocardial infarction. *Am J Cardiol* 72:640-646, 1993.

193. Elhendly A, Geleijnse ML, Roelandt JR, et al: Assessment of patients after coronary artery bypass grafting by dobutamine stress echocardiography. *Am J Cardiol* 77:1234-1236, 1996.

194. Ghods M, Pancholy S, Cave V, et al: Serial changes in left ventricular function after coronary artery bypass: implications in viability assessment. *Am Heart J* 129:20-23, 1995.

195. Kloner RA, Bolli R, Marban E, et al: Medical and cellular implications of stunning, hibernation and preconditioning: An NHLBI workshop. *Circulation* 97:1848-1867, 1998.

196. Rahimtoola SH: The hibernating myocardium. *Am Heart J* 117:2113-2115, 1989.

197. Ross J Jr: Myocardial perfusion-contraction matching. Implications for coronary heart disease and hibernation. *Circulation* 83:1076-1083, 1991.

198. Bonow RO: Identification of viable myocardium. *Circulation* 94:2674-2680, 1996.

199. Mercier JC, Lando U, Kanmatsuse K, et al: Divergent effects of inotropic stimulation on the ischemic and severely depressed reperfused myocardium. *Circulation* 66:397-403, 1982.

200. Buda AJ, Zotz RJ, Gallagher KP: The effect of inotropic stimulation on normal and ischemic myocardium after coronary occlusion. *Circulation* 76:163-172, 1987.

201. Ellis SG, Wynne J, Braunwald E, et al: Response of reperfusion-salvaged, stunned myocardium to inotropic stimulation. *Am Heart J* 107:13-19, 1984.

202. Bolli R, Zhu WX, Myers ML, et al: Beta-adrenergic stimulation reverses post-ischemic myocardial dysfunction without producing subsequent functional deterioration. *Am J Cardiol* 56:946-951, 1985.

203. Weissman NJ, Rose GA, Foster GP, Picard MH: Effects of prolonging peak dobutamine dose during stress echocardiography. *J Am Coll Cardiol* 29:526-530, 1997.

204. Stahl LD, Aversano TR, Becker LC: Selective enhancement of function of stunned myocardium by increased flow. *Circulation* 74:843-851, 1986.

205. Afridi I, Kleiman NS, Raizner AE, Zoghbi WA: Dobutamine echocardiography in myocardial hibernation. Optimal dose and accuracy in predicting recovery of ventricular function after coronary angioplasty. *Circulation* 91:663-670, 1995.

206. Kaul S. Response of dysfunctional myocardium to dobutamine. "The eyes see what the mind knows." *J Am Coll Cardiol* 27:1608-1611, 1996.

207. Cornel JH, Bax JJ, Elhendy A, et al: Biphasic response to dobutamine predicts improvement of global left ventricular function after surgical revascularization in patients with stable coronary artery disease: Implications of time course of recovery on diagnostic accuracy. *J Am Coll Cardiol* 31:1002-1010, 1998.

208. Pasquet A, Lauer MS, Williams MJ, et al: Prediction of global left ventricular function after bypass surgery in patients with severe left ventricular dysfunction. Impact of pre-operative myocardial function, perfusion, and metabolism. *Eur Heart J* 21:125-136, 2000.

209. Marwick TH, Zuchowski C, Lauer MS, et al: Functional status and quality of life in patients with heart failure undergoing coronary bypass surgery after assessment of myocardial viability. *J Am Coll Cardiol* 33:750-758, 1999.

210. Afridi I, Grayburn PA, Panza JA, et al: Myocardial viability during dobutamine echocardiography predicts survival in patients with coronary artery disease and severe left ventricular systolic dysfunction. *J Am Coll Cardiol* 32:921-926, 1998.

211. Williams MJ, Odabashian J, Lauer MS, et al: Prognostic value of dobutamine echocardiography in patients with left ventricular dysfunction. *J Am Coll Cardiol* 27:132-139, 1996.

212. Moir S, Marwick TH: Combination of contrast with stress echocardiography: A practical guide to methods and interpretation. *Cardiovasc Ultrasound* 2:15, 2004.

213. Cwajg J, Xie F, O'Leary E, et al: Detection of angiographically significant coronary artery disease with accelerated intermittent imaging after intravenous administration of ultrasound contrast material. *Am Heart J* 139:675-683, 2000.

214. Shimoni S, Zoghbi WA, Xie F, et al: Real-Time assessment of myocardial perfusion and wall motion during bicycle and treadmill exercise echocardiography: comparison with single photon emission computed tomography. *J Am Coll Cardiol* 37:741-747, 2001.

215. Heinle SK, Noblin J, Goree-Best P, et al: Assessment of myocardial perfusion by harmonic power Doppler imaging at rest and during adenosine stress: comparison with (99m)Tc-sestamibi SPECT imaging. *Circulation* 102:55-60, 2000.

216. Wei K, Crouse L, Weiss J, et al: Comparison of usefulness of dipyridamole stress myocardial contrast echocardiography to technetium-99m sestamibi single-photon emission computed tomography for detection of coronary artery disease (PB127 Multicenter Phase 2 Trial results). *Am J Cardiol* 91:1293-1298, 2003.

217. Rocchi G, Fallani F, Bracchetti G, et al: Non-invasive detection of coronary artery stenosis: a comparison among power-Doppler contrast echo, 99Tc-Sestamibi SPECT and echo wall-motion analysis. *Coron Artery Dis* 14:239-245, 2003.

218. Olszowska M, Kostkiewicz M, Tracz W, Przewlocki T: Assessment of myocardial perfusion in patients with coronary artery disease. Comparison of myocardial contrast echocardiography and 99mTc MIBI single photon emission computed tomography. *Int J Cardiol* 90:49-55, 2003.

219. Moir S, Haluska BA, Jenkins C, et al: Incremental benefit of myocardial contrast to combined dipyridamole-exercise stress echocardiography for the assessment of coronary artery disease. *Circulation* 110:1108-1113, 2004.

220. Elhendy A, O'Leary EL, Xie F, et al: Comparative accuracy of real-time myocardial contrast perfusion imaging and wall motion analysis during dobutamine stress echocardiography for the diagnosis of coronary artery disease. *J Am Coll Cardiol* 44:2185-2191, 2004.

221. Peltier M, Vancraeynest D, Pasquet A, et al: Assessment of the physiologic significance of coronary disease with dipyridamole real-time myocardial contrast echocardiography. Comparison with technetium-99m sestamibi single-photon emission computed tomography and quantitative coronary angiography. *J Am Coll Cardiol* 43:257-264, 2004.

222. Jeetley P, Hickman M, Kamp O, et al: Myocardial contrast echocardiography for the detection of coronary artery stenosis: A prospective multicenter study in comparison with single-photon emission computed tomography. *J Am Coll Cardiol* 47:141-145, 2006.

223. Tsutsui JM, Elhendly A, Anderson JR, et al: Prognostic value of dobutamine stress myocardial contrast perfusion echocardiography. *Circulation* 112:1444-1450, 2005.

224. Matsumura Y, Hozumi T, Arai K, et al: Non-invasive assessment of myocardial ischaemia using new real-time three-dimensional dobutamine stress echocardiography: Comparison with conventional two-dimensional methods. *Eur Heart J* 26:1625-1632, 2005.

225. Ahmad M, Xie T, McCulloch M, et al: Real-time three-dimensional dobutamine stress echocardiography in assessment stress echocardiography in assessment of ischemia: comparison with two-dimensional dobutamine stress echocardiography. *J Am Coll Cardiol* 37:1303-1309, 2001.

226. Pulerwitz T, Hirata K, Abe Y, Otsuka R, Herz S, Okajima K et al: Feasibility of using a real-time 3-dimensional technique for contrast dobutamine stress echocardiography. *J Am Soc Echocardiogr* 19:540-545, 2006.

227. Takeuchi M, Otani S, Weinert L, et al: Comparison of contrast-enhanced real-time live 3-dimensional dobutamine stress echocardiography with contrast 2-dimensional echocardiography for detecting stress-induced wall-motion abnormalities. *J Am Soc Echocardiogr* 19:294-299, 2006.

228. Bates JR, Ryan T, Rimmerman CR, et al: Color coding of digitized echocardiograms: Description of a new technique and application in detecting and correcting for cardiac translation. *J Am Soc Echocardiogr* 7:363-369, 1994.

229. Perez JE, Miller JG, Holland MR, et al: Ultrasonic tissue characterization: integrated backscatter imaging for detecting myocardial structural properties and on-line quantitation of cardiac function. *Am J Card Imaging* 8:106-112, 1994.

230. Lang RM, Vignon P, Weinert L, et al: Echocardiographic quantitation of regional left ventricular wall motion with color kinesis. *Circulation* 93:1877-1885, 1996.

231. Koch R, Lang RM, Garcia MJ, et al: Objective evaluation of regional left ventricular wall motion during dobutamine stress echocardiographic studies using segmental analysis of color kinesis images. *J Am Coll Cardiol* 34:409-419, 1999.

232. Greenbaum RA, Ho SY, Gibson DG, et al: Left ventricular fibre architecture in man. *Br Heart J* 45:248-263, 1981.

233. Nagueh SF, Mikati I, Kopelen HA, et al: Doppler estimation of left ventricular filling pressure in sinus tachycardia. A new application of tissue Doppler imaging. *Circulation* 98:1644-1650, 1998.

234. Pasquet A, Armstrong G, Beachler L, et al: Analysis of segmental myocardial Doppler velocity as a quantitative adjunct to exercise echocardiography. *J Am Soc Echocardiogr* 12:901-912, 1999.

235. Wilkenshoff UM, Sovany A, Wigstrom L, et al: Regional mean systolic myocardial velocity estimation by real-time color Doppler myocardial imaging: a new technique for quantifying regional systolic function. *J Am Soc Echocardiogr* 11:682-692, 1998.

236. Pasquet A, Armstrong G, Rimmerman CM, Marwick TH: Correlation of myocardial Doppler velocity response to exercise with independent evidence of myocardial ischemia by dual isotope single photon emission computed tomography. *Am J Cardiol* 85:536-542, 2000.

237. Cain P, Baglin T, Case C, et al: Application of tissue Doppler to interpretation of dobutamine echocardiography: comparison with quantitative coronary angiography. *Am J Cardiol* 87:525-531, 2001.

238. Urheim S, Edvardsen T, Torp H, et al: Myocardial strain by Doppler echocardiography. Validation of a new method to quantify regional myocardial function. *Circulation* 102:1158-1164, 2000.

239. Edvardsen T, Gerber BL, Garot J, et al: Quantitative assessment of intrinsic regional myocardial deformation by Doppler strain rate echocardiography in humans: validation against three-dimensional tagged magnetic resonance imaging. *Circulation* 106:50-56, 2002.

240. Greenberg NL, Firstenberg MS, Castro PL, et al: Doppler-derived myocardial systolic strain rate is a strong index of left ventricular contractility. *Circulation* 105:99-105, 2002.

241. Hoffmann R, Altiok E, Nowak B, et al: Strain rate measurement by Doppler echocardiography allows improved assessment of myocardial viability inpatients with depressed left ventricular function. *J Am Coll Cardiol* 39:443-449, 2002.

242. Hanekom L, Jenkins C, Jeffries L, et al: Incremental value of strain rate analysis as an adjunct to wall-motion scoring for assessment of myocardial viability by dobutamine echocardiography: A follow-up study after revascularization. *Circulation* 112:3892-3900, 2005.

243. Voigt JU, Exner B, Schmiedehausen K, et al: Strain-rate imaging during dobutamine stress echocardiography provides objective evidence of inducible ischemia. *Circulation* 107:2120-2126, 2003.

244. Leitman M, Lysyansky P, Sidenko S, et al: Two-dimensional strain-a novel software for real-time quantitative echocardiographic assessment of myocardial function. *J Am Soc Echocardiogr* 17:1021-1029, 2004.

245. Sabbah HN, Khaja F, Brymer JF, et al: Non-invasive evaluation of left ventricular performance based on peak aortic blood flow acceleration measured by a continuous-wave Doppler velocity meter. *Circulation* 74:323-329, 1986.

246. Heinle SK, Tice FD, Kisslo J: Effect of dobutamine stress echocardiography on mitral regurgitation. *J Am Coll Cardiol* 25:122-127, 1994.

247. Monin JL, Quere JP, Monchi M, et al: Low-gradient aortic stenosis: operative risk stratification and predictors for long-term outcome: a multicenter study using dobutamine stress hemodynamics. *Circulation* 108:319-324, 2003.

248. Nishimura RA, Abel MD, Hatle LK, Tajik AJ: Assessment of diastolic function of the heart: Background and current applications of Doppler echocardiography. Part II Clinical studies. *Mayo Clin Proc* 64:181-204, 1989.

249. el-Said ES, Roelandt JR, Fioretti PM, et al: Abnormal left ventricular early diastolic filling during dobutamine stress Doppler echocardiography is a sensitive indicator of significant coronary artery disease. *J Am Coll Cardiol* 24:1618-1624, 1994.

250. Lattanzi F, Picano E, Masini M, et al: Transmitral flow changes during dipyridamole-induced ischemia. A Doppler-echocardiographic study. *Chest* 95:1037-1042, 1989.

251. von Bibra H, Tuchnitz A, Klein A, et al: Regional diastolic function by pulsed Doppler myocardial mapping for the detection of left ventricular ischemia during pharmacologic stress testing: A comparison with stress echocardiography and perfusion scintigraphy. *J Am Coll Cardiol* 36:444-452, 2000.

252. Sheikh KH, Bengtson JR, Helmy S, et al: Relation of quantitative coronary lesion measurements to the development of exercise-induced ischemia assessed by exercise echocardiography [see comments]. *J Am Coll Cardiol* 15:1043-1051, 1990.

253. Marwick TH, Shaw L, Case C, et al: Clinical and economic impact of exercise electrocardiography and exercise echocardiography in clinical practice. *Eur Heart J* 24:1153-1163, 2003.

254. Picano E, Lattanzi F, Masini M, et al: Comparison of the high-dose dipyridamole-echocardiography test and exercise two-dimensional echocardiography for diagnosis of coronary artery disease. *Am J Cardiol* 59:539-542, 1987.

255. Dagianti A, Penco M, Agati L, et al: Stress echocardiography: comparison of exercise, dipyridamole and dobutamine in detecting and predicting the extent of coronary artery disease [see comments]. *J Am Coll Cardiol* 26:18-25, 1995; published erratum appears in *J Am Coll Cardiol* 26(4):1114, 1995.

256. Rallidis L, Cokkinos P, Tousoulis D, Nihoyannopoulos P: Comparison of dobutamine and treadmill exercise echocardiography in inducing ischemia in patients with coronary artery disease. *J Am Coll Cardiol* 30:1660-1668, 1997.

257. Senior R, Sridhara BS, Anagnostou E, et al: Synergistic value of simultaneous stress dobutamine sestamibi single-photon-emission computerized tomography and echocardiography in the detection of coronary artery disease. *Am Heart J* 128:713-718, 1994.

258. Ho FM, Huang PJ, Liau CS, et al: Dobutamine stress echocardiography compared with dipyridamole thallium-201 single-photon emission computed tomography in detecting coronary artery disease. *Eur Heart J* 16:570-575, 1995.

259. Huang PJ, Ho YL, Wu CC, et al: Simultaneous dobutamine stress echocardiography and thallium-201 perfusion imaging for the detection of coronary artery disease. *Cardiology* 88:556-562, 1997.

260. Santoro GM, Sciagra R, Buonamici P, et al: Head-to-head comparison of exercise stress testing, pharmacologic stress echocardiography, and perfusion tomography as first-line examination for chest pain in patients without history of coronary artery disease [see comments]. *J Nucl Cardiol* 5:19-27, 1998.

261. San Roman JA, Rollan MJ, Vilacosta I, et al: [Echocardiography and MIBI-SPECT scintigraphy during dobutamine infusion in the diagnosis of coronary disease]. *Rev Esp Cardiol* 48:606-614, 1995.

262. Pozzoli MM, Fioretti PM, Salustri A, et al: Exercise echocardiography and technetium 99m MIBI single photon emission computed tomography in the detection of coronary artery disease. *Am J Cardiol* 67:350-355, 1991.

263. Leppo J, Boucher CA, Okada RD, et al: Serial thallium-201 myocardial imaging after dipyridamole infusion: Diagnostic utility in detection of coronary stenoses and relation to regional wall motion. *Circulation* 66:649-657, 1982.

264. Armstrong WF: Stress echocardiography for detection of coronary artery disease. *Circulation* 84:I43-I49, 1991.

265. Mairesse GH, Marwick TH, Arnese M, et al: Improved identification of coronary artery disease in patients with left bundle branch block by use of dobutamine stress echocardiography and comparison with myocardial perfusion tomography. *Am J Cardiol* 76:321-325, 1995.

266. Van Damme H, Pierard L, Gillain D, et al: Cardiac risk assessment before vascular surgery: a prospective study comparing clinical evaluation, dobutamine stress echocardiography, and dobutamine Tc-99m sestamibi tomoscintigraphy. *Cardiovasc Surg* 5:54-64, 1997.

267. Shaw LJ, Eagle KA, Gersh BJ, Miller DD: Meta-analysis of intravenous dipyridamole-thallium-201 imaging (1985 to 1994) and dobutamine echocardiography (1991 to 1994) for risk stratification before vascular surgery [see comments]. *J Am Coll Cardiol* 27:787-798, 1996.

268. van Daele ME, McNeill AJ, Fioretti PM, et al: Prognostic value of dipyridamole sestamibi single-photon emission computed tomography and dipyridamole stress echocardiography for new cardiac events after an uncomplicated myocardial infarction. *J Am Soc Echocardiogr* 7:370-380, 1994.

269. Marzullo P, Parodi O, Reisenhofer B, et al: Value of rest thallium-201/technetium-99m sestamibi scans and dobutamine echocardiography for detecting myocardial viability. *Am J Cardiol* 71:166-172, 1993.

270. Charney R, Schwinger ME, Chun J, et al: Dobutamine echocardiography and resting-redistribution thallium-201 scintigraphy predicts recovery of hibernating myocardium after coronary revascularization. *Am Heart J* 128:864-869, 1994.

271. Kostopoulos KG, Kranidis AI, Bouki KP, et al: Detection of myocardial viability in the prediction of improvement in left ven-

tricular function after successful coronary revascularization by using the dobutamine stress echocardiography and quantitative SPECT rest-redistribution-reinjection 201TI imaging after dipyridamole infusion. *Angiology* 47:1039-1046, 1996.

272. Qureshi U, Nagueh SF, Afridi I, et al: Dobutamine echocardiography and quantitative rest-redistribution 201Tl tomography in myocardial hibernation. Relation of contractile reserve to 201Tl uptake and comparative prediction of recovery of function. *Circulation* 95:626-635, 1997.

273. Nagueh SF, Vaduganathan P, Ali N, et al: Identification of hibernating myocardium: comparative accuracy of myocardial contrast echocardiography, rest-redistribution thallium-201 tomography and dobutamine echocardiography. *J Am Coll Cardiol* 29:985-993, 1997.

274. Senior R, Glenville B, Basu S, et al: Dobutamine echocardiography and thallium-201 imaging predict functional improvement after revascularisation in severe ischaemic left ventricular dysfunction. *Br Heart J* 74:358-364, 1995.

275. Arnese M, Cornel JH, Salustri A, et al: Prediction of improvement of regional left ventricular function after surgical revascularization. A comparison of low-dose dobutamine echocardiography with 201Tl single-photon emission computed tomography. *Circulation* 91:2748-2752, 1995.

276. Perrone-Filardi P, Pace L, Prastaro M, et al: Assessment of myocardial viability in patients with chronic coronary artery disease. Rest-4-hour-24-hour 201Tl tomography versus dobutamine echocardiography [see comments]. *Circulation* 94:2712-2719, 1996.

277. Bax JJ, Cornel JH, Visser FC, et al: Prediction of recovery of myocardial dysfunction after revascularization. Comparison of fluorine-18 fluorodeoxyglucose/thallium-201 SPECT, thallium-201 stress-reinjection SPECT and dobutamine echocardiography. *J Am Coll Cardiol* 28:558-564, 1996.

278. Haque T, Furukawa T, Takahashi M, Kinoshita M: Identification of hibernating myocardium by dobutamine stress echocardiography: comparison with thallium-201 reinjection imaging. *Am Heart J* 130:553-563, 1995.

279. Vanoverschelde JL, D'Hondt AM, Marwick T, et al: Head-to-head comparison of exercise-redistribution-reinjection thallium single-photon emission computed tomography and low dose dobutamine echocardiography for prediction of reversibility of chronic left ventricular ischemic dysfunction. *J Am Coll Cardiol* 28:432-442, 1996.

280. Elsasser A, Muller KD, Vogt A, et al: Assessment of myocardial viability: Dobutamine echocardiography and thallium-201 single-photon emission computed tomographic imaging predict the postoperative improvement of left ventricular function after bypass surgery. *Am Heart J* 135:463-475, 1998.

281. Steinberg EH, Madmon L, Patel CP, et al: Long-term prognostic significance of dobutamine echocardiography in patients with suspected coronary artery disease: Results of a 5-year follow-up study. *J Am Coll Cardiol* 29:969-973, 1997.

Chapter 17

Echocardiographic Evaluation of Coronary Blood Flow: Approaches and Clinical Applications

NOZOMI WATANABE, MD

Coronary flow velocity and coronary flow velocity reserve measurements provide useful clinical and physiological information. Previously, coronary flow velocity has been assessed invasively by Doppler flow wire technique in the cardiac catheterization lab. Recent technological advances in Doppler echocardiography provide noninvasive coronary flow detection by Doppler transthoracic echocardiography (TTE).[1,2] Accuracy of this new noninvasive transthoracic coronary flow and coronary flow reserve measurements has been validated compared to Doppler flow wire.[3-7] Doppler TTE is widely available in the clinical setting, and this technique can be performed in an outpatient setting. The majority of the clinical data regarding this technique has been reported by European and Japanese groups, but Takeuchi and colleagues did a unique investigation testing the feasibility of transthoracic coronary flow detection in relatively obese U.S. population[8] and found a similar success rate for recording coronary flow and coronary flow reserve. Intravenous (IV) contrast injection helps in detection of the coronary signal.[9-12] This new noninvasive imaging technique of the coronary arteries promises to expand the field of diagnostic echocardiography and bring new insight into the pathophysiology of ischemic heart disease.

Coronary Anatomy

It is important to understand the coronary arterial anatomy for assessment of coronary flow by Doppler TTE (Fig. 17–1). The coronary arteries provide oxygenated blood to the myocardium. The left and right coronaries originate from the left and right coronary sinuses of the aortic root. The left main coronary artery (LMCA) bifurcates into the left anterior descending (LAD) artery, which runs over the anterior interventricular sulcus, and the left circumflex (LCx) artery in the left atrioventricular (AV) sulcus. The LAD artery often extends beyond the apex. In this situation, the LAD artery extends up the posterior interventricular sulcus. The septal branches arise at an acute angle from the LAD artery, coursing close to the endocardium on the right side of the interventricular septum. The LCx artery is the other principal vessel originating from the left main coronary artery. It is covered by the left atrial (LA) appendage in its proximal portion, and then courses along the left atrioventricular sulcus. The right coronary artery (RCA) has its origin at the right coronary aortic sinus and follows the right atrioventricular sulcus. The posterior descending artery lies in the posterior interventricular sulcus.

Doppler Evaluation of Coronary Flow

Technical Aspects

There are some important technical issues for detecting coronary flow signals. First, a good high-resolution and high-sensitivity ultrasound (US) system, with a high-frequency transducer is required (7 to 12 MHz for mid to distal LAD artery, 2 to 5 MHz for proximal LAD artery, RCA, and LCx artery). Second, in color Doppler imaging, the Doppler velocity range should be set in the range of 10 to 30 cm/s to detect the coronary flow signal because the blood flow velocity is relatively slow. In cases in which it is difficult to detect a coronary flow signal, intravenous injection of contrast agent enhances the Doppler signal intensity.[5,9] The contrast enhancer used in the most studies was Levovist (Shering). Levovist, at a concentration of 300 mg/mL, was administrated intravenously by using an infusion pump. The infusion rate is adjusted from 0.5 to 2 mL/min, according to the quality and intensity of the Doppler signal enhancement achieved. By positioning the Doppler sample volume in the coronary flow stream under the guidance of color Doppler flow imaging, the characteristic coronary flow spectrum, with biphasic predominantly diastolic flow velocities, can be recorded. In

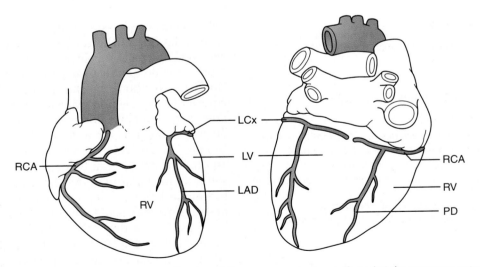

Figure 17–1. Anatomical position of epicardial coronary arteries. Left and right coronary arteries originate from the left and right coronary sinuses respectively. Left anterior descending artery (LAD) runs over the anterior interventricular sulcus toward apex. Left circumflex artery (LCx) runs along the left atrioventricular sulcus. Right coronary artery (RCA) runs along the right atrioventricular sulcus, and the posterior descending artery (PD) runs in the posterior interventricular sulcus. Thus, landmarks for searching coronary flow by transthoracic echocardiography are interventricular sulcus and atrioventricular sulcus. LV, left ventricle; RV, right ventricle.

pulsed-Doppler technique, angle correction is required depending on the direction of coronary flow.

Detection

Left Main and Proximal Coronary Arteries

Patients should be examined in the left lateral decubitus position. To visualize the left main trunk and proximal left anterior descending artery, start with the image plane at the level of the aortic root, in a short axis view (Fig. 17–2A). This part of the exam can be performed using a relatively low-frequency transducer (2 to 4 MHz). The left main trunk is identified as a tubular structure that originates from the left coronary sinus. By adjusting the orientation of the ultrasound beam toward the distal side of the left main trunk, the proximal LAD artery, which runs from the bifurcation toward the anterior wall of the heart, can be visualized using color Doppler flow mapping. At the level of the left main bifurcation, the proximal circumflex artery is detected by rotating the transducer clockwise.

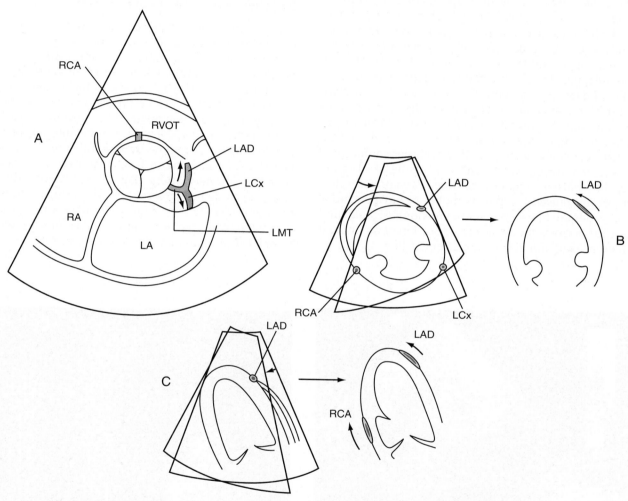

Figure 17–2. *Schematic illustrations of coronary flow detection by transthoracic Doppler echocardiography. A, Proximal portion of left and right coronary arteries in short-axis view at the level of coronary sinus. The left main trunk (LMT) originates from the left coronary sinus, and the right coronary artery (RCA) originates from the right coronary sinus. B, Position of three coronary arteries in left ventricular short-axis view. Cross-sectional coronary arteries can be observed by color Doppler. Left anterior descending artery (LAD) is positioned at anterior interventricular sulcus. LAD signal can be seen longer by counterclockwise rotation. RCA (posterior descending artery) is seen at the position of posterior interventricular sulcus. Left circumflex artery (LCx) is seen in a varied position but generally can be found at lateral wall of the left ventricle (LV) (3-o'clock to 5-o'clock position). C, Detection of distal portion of left anterior descending artery by apical view. Posterior descending artery is visualized in posterior interventricular sulcus. In apical long-axis view, cross-sectional LAD flow can be found. The flow signal becomes longer by adjusting the transducer to look at the interventricular sulcus (clockwise rotation). LA, left atrium; RA, right atrium; RVOT, right ventricular outflow tract.*

The proximal RCA, which originates from right coronary sinus, can be identified at the aortic root, in short-axis or long-axis views.

Left Anterior Descending Coronary Artery

In the short-axis images of the left ventricle, mid portion of the LAD artery can be identified as a cross section of the tubular structure containing the color Doppler flow signal, located in the anterior interventricular sulcus (Fig. 17–2B,C). The color Doppler signal in the LAD artery, which typically appears as a red color, is mainly seen in diastole. After confirming its position, rotate the transducer counterclockwise to image the left ventricle in a long-axis view aligned with the intraventricular sulcus under the guidance of color Doppler flow imaging. To visualize the distal portion of the LAD artery, image the left ventricle in a long-axis view starting from the apex and searching for the coronary flow signal around the intraventricular sulcus. In this view, pericardial fluid may appear similar to a coronary flow signal near the epicardium. However, pericardial fluid is seen mainly in systole and can easily be discriminated by pulsed-Doppler recording. The coronary flow pattern by pulsed Doppler is biphasic, but pericardial fluid generally has a systolic, bidirectional signal. Once the LAD artery is found as a cross section of the tubular structure containing the color Doppler flow signal, ro-

tate the transducer clockwise (toward two-chamber view position) to detect the flow signal in the long-axis view (Fig. 17–3). Coronary flow detection in the distal portion of the LAD artery is important, as coronary flow reserve should be measured distal to any stenosis. Coronary blood flow velocity profiles are recorded by positioning a pulsed sample volume on the color flow signal. The incident angle between the Doppler beam and direction of blood flow should be used to correct the velocity scale.

Posterior Descending Coronary Artery

The posterior descending coronary artery usually is the distal extension of the RCA and runs along the posterior interventricular sulcus toward the apex. After obtaining an apical two-chamber image of the left ventricle, angle the ultrasound beam superiorly to image the posterior interventricular sulcus. In this situation a lower frequency probe is recommended because this area is far from the transducer, compared to the anterior interventricular sulcus. Carefully examine this area using color Doppler flow imaging to locate the right posterior descending coronary artery (Fig. 17–4). Though the success rate in detecting coronary flow velocity profile in the right posterior descending coronary artery is lower compared with the LAD artery, a contrast-enhanced Doppler technique improves the success rate.[13]

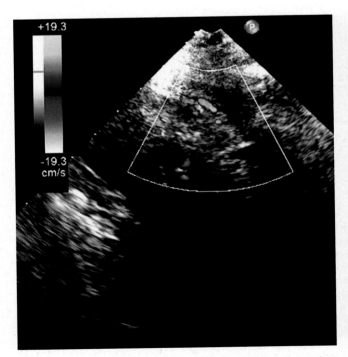

Figure 17–3. *Distal portion of the left anterior descending artery by color Doppler echocardiography. In modified apical long-axis view, left anterior descending artery flow signal appears as red color signal in diastole.*

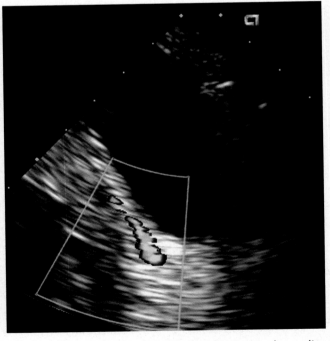

Figure 17–4. *Right coronary artery (posterior descending artery) by color Doppler echocardiography. In modified two-chamber view, posterior descending artery appears as red color signal in diastole.*

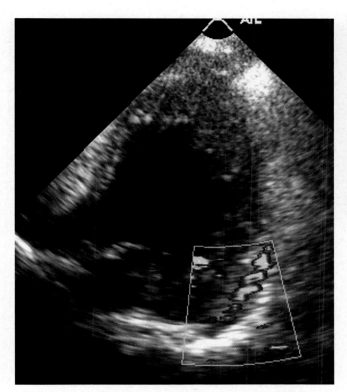

Figure 17–5. Left circumflex artery by color Doppler echocardiography. Left circumflex artery flow signal is seen at the epicardial side in the lateral wall in modified four-chamber view.

Left Circumflex Coronary Artery

The LCx artery can be found in the modified four-chamber view. It is normally distinguished as a color flow signal running along the basal lateral wall[14] (Fig. 17–5). However, visualization of circumflex arteries is relatively difficult because of their anatomical variations, and furthermore, these vessels are distant from the transducer, as well as the RCA.

Assessment of Coronary Flow Profile

Doppler spectral tracings of coronary flow velocity can be recorded by pulsed-Doppler technique by positioning a sample volume (1.5 to 2.5 mm wide) on the color Doppler signal. Angle correction is needed in each examination. Coronary flow velocity provides some useful clinical information, such as coronary flow direction, coronary flow velocity, and coronary flow pattern. Normal coronary flow is characterized by a biphasic flow profile, which consists of a small systolic and a large diastolic flow signal (Fig. 17–6). It should be noted that pulsed-Doppler recording provides coronary flow velocity and not the absolute volume of coronary blood flow. Coronary flow reserve by Doppler TTE is

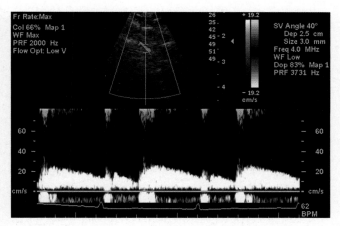

Figure 17–6. Coronary flow velocity profile in normal subject. Coronary flow velocity profile is characterized by biphasic flow pattern with small systolic and large diastolic components.

derived from changes in the velocity of coronary blood flow, which has been shown to correlate with absolute coronary flow reserve.

Clinical Applications

Phasic Flow Characteristics and Coronary Stenosis

Resting coronary flow pattern is characterized by a diastolic dominant biphasic flow. In severe coronary stenosis, diastolic flow decreases and hence, diastolic to systolic flow velocity ratio (DSVR) decreases at rest.[15] Cutoff points of 1.6 for peak DSVR and 1.5 for mean DSVR have high sensitivities and specificities in the detection of severe coronary stenosis (>85%)[16] and of myocardial ischemia compared to thallium[201] single photon emission computed tomography (SPECT).[17]

Coronary Flow Velocity Reserve Measurement

Coronary flow reserve is expressed as a ratio of maximum flow to resting flow (Fig. 17–7). With a normal coronary artery, a vasodilatory stimulus results in an approximately fourfold increase in flow rate compared to baseline. With progressive coronary stenosis, baseline flow remains normal until the coronary artery is narrowed by 80% to 85% diameter stenosis. However, coronary flow reserve begins to decrease at 40% to 50% diameter stenosis.[18] Coronary flow reserve decreases to two times baseline at approximately 75% diameter stenosis, which indicates myocardial ischemia.

Coronary flow velocity reserve can be alternatively assessed as the ratio of hyperemic to basal coronary flow velocity after drug-induced coronary vasodilatation. Measurements of coronary flow velocity reserve

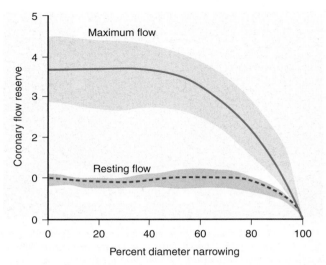

Figure 17–7. Coronary flow reserve and percent diameter stenosis. With progressive coronary stenosis, baseline flow remains normal until the coronary artery is narrowed by 80% to 85% diameter stenosis. However, coronary flow reserve begins to decrease at 40% to 50% diameter stenosis for a vasodilatory stimulus, increasing flow normally to four times baseline. Coronary flow reserve decreases to two times baseline at approximately 75% diameter stenosis. (From Gould KL, Lipscomb K: Am J Cardiol 34:48-55, 1974.)

by Doppler TTE have already been established as feasible and accurate.[3,5,6]

After recording baseline spectral Doppler signals in the distal portion of the LAD artery, administrate the vasodilator, either adenosine 140 μg/kg/min as an intravenous infusion for about 1 minute or dipyridamole 0.56 mg/kg intravenously for about 4 minutes, to achieve maximum flow. Then spectral Doppler signals are recorded during hyperemic conditions (Fig. 17–8) with measurement of the mean diastolic velocity and peak diastolic velocity of each flow spectrum. Coronary flow velocity reserve by transthoracic-Doppler technique is measured from only diastolic mean velocities and not mean velocities throughout the entire cardiac cycle because, in some cases, it is difficult to obtain a complete Doppler spectral envelope throughout the cardiac cycle because of cardiac motion. However, previous studies have reported that the ratio of hyperemic to basal mean

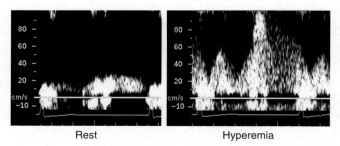

Figure 17–8. Coronary flow velocity reserve measurement by pulsed-Doppler echocardiography in patient with a normal coronary artery. Both systolic and diastolic flow velocity increase during hyperemia.

diastolic velocity and peak diastolic velocity was useful in the evaluation of functional coronary stenosis. Coronary flow velocity reserve is defined as the ratio of hyperemic to basal peak diastolic coronary flow velocity or the ratio of hyperemic to basal mean diastolic coronary flow velocity. Adenosine starts to act generally in 30 seconds, and the coronary flow velocity comes to maximum in 1 minute. Dipyridamole starts to act in 4 to 6 minutes and has a prolonged duration of action (about 30 minutes after administration). The short-acting effect is an advantage of adenosine. Although both vasodilators can cause flushing, headache, hypotension, or bradycardia, the adverse effects of adenosine alleviate immediately after finishing the infusion.

In the clinical setting, some factors that are related to coronary risk factors have been known to affect coronary flow reserve. Passive smoking has been reported to reduce coronary flow reserve in healthy nonsmokers, not in active smokers.[19] Another study demonstrated that coronary flow reserve was significantly higher in nonsmokers than in smokers, and interestingly, oral antioxidant vitamin C increased coronary flow reserve in nonsmokers but not in smokers.[20] Patients with hypertension showed lower coronary flow reserve than normotensive controls,[21] coronary flow reserve is reduced in diabetic patients, especially in patients with retinopathy,[22,23] and coronary flow reserve decreased after a single high-fat meal in young healthy men.[24] Another study showed that in premenopausal women, coronary flow reserve varies during the menstrual cycle, and in postmenopausal women, coronary flow reserve increases after acute estrogen replacement.[25]

Noninvasive Diagnosis of Coronary Stenosis

Coronary Flow Velocity Reserve Measurement Approach

Coronary flow velocity reserve defined as a mean diastolic velocity increase with hyperemia less than 2 had a sensitivity of 91% to 92% and a specificity of 75% to 86% for the presence of significant LAD artery stenosis.[26,27] Comparing with thallium[201] SPECT, a mean coronary flow reserve greater than or equal to 2 predicted reversible perfusion defects, with a sensitivity and specificity of 92% and 90%, respectively.[28] Coronary flow reserve improves after coronary stenting[29] and a coronary flow reserve less than 2 had high sensitivity (91%) and specificity (95%) in the diagnosis of in-stent restenosis after coronary intervention.[30] Furthermore, Voci and colleagues reported that a coronary flow reserve less than 1, which may reflect coronary steal phenomenon, could discriminate high-risk patients with severe stenosis from patients with nonsevere stenosis.[31] For coronary stenosis in the right coronary territory, coronary flow velocity reserve measured in the posterior descending coronary artery is useful.

Detection of the posterior descending artery is more difficult than LAD artery, but the use of an intravenous contrast injection improves Doppler signal recording.[13] Using the cutoff value of 2 for coronary flow velocity reserve in the RCA, the sensitivity and specificity for detection of significant stenosis were 84% to 91% and 83% to 91%, respectively.[6,13,27] Coronary flow velocity reserve less than 2 in the LCx artery has been reported to have a sensitivity of 92% and specificity of 96% for reversible perfusion defect detected by SPECT.[14] Although each coronary risk factor influences the result of coronary flow velocity reserve, a cutoff value less than 2 was still adequate in terms of the diagnosis of significant coronary stenosis. A cutoff value less than 2 for coronary flow reserve had a sensitivity of 90%, a specificity of 93%, a positive predictive value of 77%, and a negative predictive value of 97% for the presence of significant coronary stenosis in a population that included patients with various coronary risk factors.[32]

Prestenotic to Stenotic Flow Velocity Ratio

The location of the coronary artery stenosis can be identified based on "aliasing" of color Doppler. In the diagnosis of significant restenosis (>50%) after coronary intervention in the LAD artery, a prestenotic to stenotic mean diastolic flow velocity ratio less than 0.45 had a sensitivity of 86% and a specificity of 93%.[33] Flow velocity measurements were possible for in-stent stenosis with high sensitivity and specificity as well.[34] Another study has investigated three major coronary vessels by color Doppler and pulsed-Doppler echocardiography. Overall sensitivity and specificity was 82% and 92%, respectively, for the detection of >50% stenosis. The sensitivity and specificity were 73% and 92%, respectively, for LAD artery, 63% and 96% for the RCA, and 38% and 99% for LCx artery.[35]

Detection of Total Occlusion by Retrograde Coronary Flow

Following occlusion of a major epicardial coronary artery, blood flow to the previously supplied myocardium must arrive via coronary collateral vessels. The retrograde blood flow velocity distal to a totally occluded coronary vessel represents collateral flow to the occluded region. Retrograde LAD flow by Doppler TTE had a sensitivity of 93% and a specificity of 100% for the detection of total LAD occlusion[36] (Fig. 17–9). Retrograde flow in LAD or septal artery had a sensitivity of 96% and a specificity of 100% for the detection of total LAD occlusion.[37] Retrograde coronary flow detection is also useful in the RCA. Detection of reverse flow in the distal RCA and the inferior septal branches had a sensitivity of 100% and a specificity of 97.8% for identification of occluded RCA.[38] Coronary flow veloc-

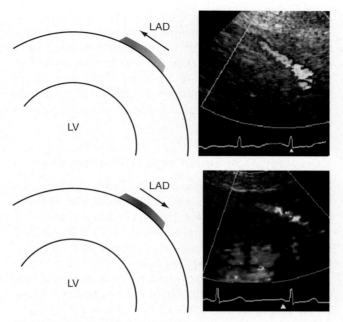

Figure 17–9. Antegrade and retrograde flow signals. Normal left anterior descending artery (LAD) flow (upper panel); retrograde left anterior descending artery flow in patient with total LAD occlusion (lower panel). In total LAD occlusion, retrograde coronary flow signal, which reflects the collateral flow, is observed as blue color. LV, left ventricle. (From Watanabe N, Akasaka T, Yamaura Y, et al: J Am Coll Cardiol 38:1328-1332, 2001.

ity reserve measurements are expected to contribute to the noninvasive diagnosis of coronary heart disease in combination with conventional dobutamine stress echocardiography (DSE). Coronary flow velocity reserve measurements are feasible during dobutamine stress[39] or before dobutamine stress[40] and provide useful additional information in the clinical diagnosis of coronary stenosis.

Coronary Flow Measurements in Acute Coronary Syndrome

Suboptimal coronary reperfusion with thrombolysis in myocardial infarction (TIMI) grade 2 coronary blood flow in acute myocardial infarction (AMI) adversely affects patient prognosis and requires additional procedures, such as thrombolysis or percutaneous coronary intervention (PCI). Doppler TTE enables a rapid noninvasive differentiation of TIMI 3 from TIMI 2 coronary reperfusion in patients with AMI in the acute phase before emergent coronary intervention. The diagnosis of TIMI 3 based on a diastolic peak distal LAD flow velocity of at least 25 cm/s by Doppler TTE had a sensitivity, specificity, and accuracy of 77%, 94%, and 89%, respectively.[41] Voci and colleagues have proposed the "open perforator hypothesis," that presence of the perforator signals in the anterior-apical wall by color Doppler TTE reflects adequate myocardial reperfusion, and hence, perforators are early noninvasive markers of myocardial viability.[42] In the coronary care unit (CCU), noninvasive transthoracic detection of coronary flow patterns are useful in the direct monitoring of coronary flow augmentation during intra-aortic balloon pumping.[43] Evaluation of coronary flow by Doppler TTE gives important physiological information in addition to the conventional diagnostic examination in acute coronary syndrome (ACS).

Coronary Flow in No-Reflow Phenomenon

In no-reflow after coronary revascularization for acute myocardial infarction, coronary flow velocity shows a characteristic to-and-fro pattern, which consists of systolic reversal and rapid diastolic deceleration (Fig. 17–10). This low systolic flow velocity and rapid deceleration time of diastolic coronary blood flow spectrum immediately after primary coronary intervention reflects a greater degree of microvascular damage in the risk area, and evaluation of coronary flow profile after revascularization is useful in predicting recovery of regional left ventricular (LV) function. Optimal cutoff values to predict viable myocardium were 6.5 cm/s for average systolic velocity and 600 ms for diastolic deceleration time (sensitivity, 79%; specificity, 89% and sensitivity, 86%; specificity, 89%, respectively).[44,45] Doppler TTE allows us to record the temporal sequence of coronary flow pattern after coronary intervention. Persistence of abnormal coronary flow pattern can predict left ventricular remodeling after myocardial infarction.[46,47]

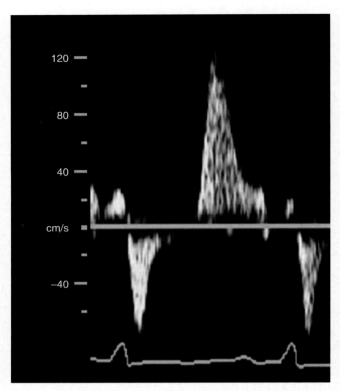

Figure 17–10. *To-and-fro pattern of coronary flow profile in no-reflow phenomenon. Coronary flow velocity pattern in no-reflow is characterized by a systolic reversal flow followed by a diastolic flow with rapid deceleration. Short deceleration time is a predictor of long-term prognosis.*

Impaired Coronary Circulation in Hypertrophic Cardiomyopathy

Coronary flow reserve is reduced in hypertrophic cardiomyopathy (HCM).[48] Several reports have shown the unique coronary flow pattern in hypertrophic cardiomyopathy, which is characteristic with systolic flow reversal and high velocity diastolic flow. Coronary flow abnormalities in hypertrophic cardiomyopathy are related to myocardial thickness rather than the degree of outflow obstruction.[48-51] This characteristic is seen in intramyocardial small coronary arteries as well as in epicardial coronary arteries.[52] This unique pattern is speculated to be related to the myo-

TABLE 17–1. **Alternate Approaches for Evaluation of the Coronary Arteries**

	Advantage	Disadvantage
X-ray angiography	Full coverage of the coronary arteries; high resolution	Invasive; needs nephrotoxic contrast agents
Transthoracic Doppler echocardiography	Noninvasive; portable; cost-effective; physiologic assessment of coronary stenosis (coronary flow reserve measurement)	Limited sites of coronary detection; low success rate in RCA and LCx (need contrast agent)
Multislice CT	Noninvasive; relatively high resolution; plaque characterization	Radiation exposure, motion artifacts; not available at calcified lesion; need a beta-blocker before examination, expensive; nephrotoxic contrast agents
MRI	Noninvasive; soft-tissue characterizing; coronary flow reserve measurement	Expensive; motion artifacts; interpretable segments are limited by the size of the artery

CT, computed tomography; LCx, left circumflex artery; MRI, magnetic resonance imaging; RCA, right coronary artery.

cardial ischemia and chest pain in hypertrophic cardiomyopathy. Noninvasive Doppler examination of coronary circulation would contribute to further evaluation.

Alternate Approaches

There are advantages and disadvantages for each imaging modalities in the assessment of coronary flow. The greatest advantage of Doppler TTE coronary imaging is that this examination is totally noninvasive and can be easily performed at the bedside, repetitively. The pulsed-Doppler technique is a simple and reliable method for detection of coronary flow profiles. Advantages and disadvantages of each coronary imaging examination are summarized in Table 17–1.

KEY POINTS

- For evaluation of coronary blood flow by Doppler echocardiogram, it is important to choose a transducer with adequate frequency and set the velocity range of color Doppler around ±20 cm/s.
- The coronary flow signal is mainly observed during diastole.
- The normal coronary flow pattern is characterized by diastolic dominant biphasic flow.
- Coronary flow reserve can be measured by adenosine intravenous infusion.
- Coronary flow reserve decreases (ratio of hyperemia to rest <2) when significant coronary stenosis is present.
- In acute myocardial infarction, a coronary flow peak velocity less than 25 cm/s predicts poor reperfusion with TIMI flow 2.

REFERENCES

1. Voci P, Testa G, Plaustro G: Imaging of the distal left anterior descending coronary artery by transthoracic color-Doppler echocardiography. *Am J Cardiol* 81:74G-78G, 1998.
2. Tries HP, Lambertz H, Lethen H: Transthoracic echocardiographic visualization of coronary artery blood flow and assessment of coronary flow reserve in the right coronary artery: A first report of 3 patients. *J Am Soc Echocardiogr* 15:739-742, 2002.
3. Hozumi T, Yoshida K, Akasaka T, et al: Noninvasive assessment of coronary flow velocity and coronary flow velocity reserve in the left anterior descending coronary artery by Doppler echocardiography: Comparison with invasive technique. *J Am Coll Cardiol* 32:1251-1259, 1998.
4. Voudris V, Athanassopoulos G, Vassilikos V, et al: Usefulness of flow reserve in the left internal mammary artery to determine graft patency to the left anterior descending coronary artery. *Am J Cardiol* 83:1157-1163, 1999.
5. Caiati C, Montaldo C, Zedda N, et al: Validation of a new noninvasive method (contrast-enhanced transthoracic second harmonic echo Doppler) for the evaluation of coronary flow reserve:

6. comparison with intracoronary Doppler flow wire. *J Am Coll Cardiol* 34:1193-1200, 1999.
7. Ueno Y, Nakamura Y, Takashima H, et al: Noninvasive assessment of coronary flow velocity and coronary flow velocity reserve in the right coronary artery by transthoracic Doppler echocardiography: Comparison with intracoronary Doppler guidewire. *J Am Soc Echocardiogr* 15:1074-1079, 2002.
8. Lethen H, Flachskampf FA, Schneider R, et al: Frequency of deep vein thrombosis in patients with patent foramen ovale and ischemic stroke or transient ischemic attack. *Am J Cardiol* 80:1066-1069, 1997.
9. Takeuchi M, Lodato JA, Furlong KT, et al: Feasibility of measuring coronary flow velocity and reserve in the left anterior descending coronary artery by transthoracic Doppler echocardiography in a relatively obese American population. *Echocardiography* 22:225-232, 2005.
10. Caiati C, Montaldo C, Zedda N, et al: New noninvasive method for coronary flow reserve assessment: Contrast-enhanced transthoracic second harmonic echo Doppler [see comments]. *Circulation* 99:771-778, 1999.
11. Lambertz H, Tries HP, Stein T, Lethen H: Noninvasive assessment of coronary flow reserve with transthoracic signal-enhanced Doppler echocardiography. *J Am Soc Echocardiogr* 12:186-195, 1999.
12. Bartel T, Muller S, Baumgart D, et al: Improved high-frequency transthoracic flow velocity measurement in the left anterior descending coronary artery after intravenous peripheral injection of levovist. *J Am Soc Echocardiogr* 12:252-256, 1999.
13. Caiati C, Zedda N, Montaldo C, et al: Contrast-enhanced transthoracic second harmonic echo Doppler with adenosine: A noninvasive, rapid and effective method for coronary flow reserve assessment [see comments]. *J Am Coll Cardiol* 34:122-130, 1999.
14. Watanabe H, Hozumi T, Hirata K, et al: Noninvasive coronary flow velocity reserve measurement in the posterior descending coronary artery for detecting coronary stenosis in the right coronary artery using contrast-enhanced transthoracic Doppler echocardiography. *Echocardiography* 21:225-233, 2004.
15. Fujimoto K, Watanabe H, Hozumi T, et al: New noninvasive diagnosis of myocardial ischemia of the left circumflex coronary artery using coronary flow reserve measurement by transthoracic Doppler echocardiography: comparison with thallium-201 single photon emission computed tomography. *J Cardiol* 43:109-116, 2004.
16. Crowley JJ, Shapiro LM: Noninvasive analysis of coronary artery poststenotic flow characteristics by using transthoracic echocardiography. *J Am Soc Echocardiogr* 11:1-9, 1998.
17. Higashiue S, Watanabe H, Yokoi Y, et al: Simple detection of severe coronary stenosis using transthoracic Doppler echocardiography at rest. *Am J Cardiol* 87:1064-1068, 2001.
18. Daimon M, Watanabe H, Yamagishi H, et al: Physiologic assessment of coronary artery stenosis without stress tests: noninvasive analysis of phasic flow characteristics by transthoracic Doppler echocardiography. *J Am Soc Echocardiogr* 18:949-955, 2005.
19. Gould KL, Lipscomb K: Effects of coronary stenoses on coronary flow reserve and resistance. *Am J Cardiol* 34:48-55, 1974.
20. Otsuka R, Watanabe H, Hirata K, et al: Acute effects of passive smoking on the coronary circulation in healthy young adults. *JAMA* 286:436-441, 2001.
21. Teramoto K, Daimon M, Hasegawa R, et al: Acute effect of oral vitamin C on coronary circulation in young healthy smokers. *Am Heart J* 148:300-305, 2004.
22. Bartel T, Yang Y, Muller S, et al: Noninvasive assessment of microvascular function in arterial hypertension by transthoracic Doppler harmonic echocardiography. *J Am Coll Cardiol* 39:2012-2018, 2002.
23. Nahser PJ Jr, Brown RE, Oskarsson H, et al: Maximal coronary flow reserve and metabolic coronary vasodilation in patients with diabetes mellitus. *Circulation* 91:635-640, 1995.

23. Akasaka T, Yoshida K, Hozumi T, et al: Retinopathy identifies marked restriction of coronary flow reserve in patients with diabetes mellitus. *J Am Coll Cardiol* 30:935-941, 1997.

24. Hozumi T, Eisenberg M, Sugioka K, et al: Change in coronary flow reserve on transthoracic Doppler echocardiography after a single high-fat meal in young healthy men. *Ann Intern Med* 136:523-528, 2002.

25. Hirata K, Shimada K, Watanabe H, et al: Modulation of coronary flow velocity reserve by gender, menstrual cycle and hormone replacement therapy. *J Am Coll Cardiol* 38:1879-1884, 2001.

26. Hozumi T, Yoshida K, Ogata Y, et al: Noninvasive assessment of significant left anterior descending coronary artery stenosis by coronary flow velocity reserve with transthoracic color Doppler echocardiography. *Circulation* 97:1557-1562, 1998.

27. Takeuchi M, Ogawa K, Wake R, et al: Measurement of coronary flow velocity reserve in the posterior descending coronary artery by contrast-enhanced transthoracic Doppler echocardiography. *J Am Soc Echocardiogr* 17:21-27, 2004.

28. Daimon M, Watanabe H, Yamagishi H, et al: Physiologic assessment of coronary artery stenosis by coronary flow reserve measurements with transthoracic Doppler echocardiography: Comparison with exercise thallium-201 single piston emission computed tomography. *J Am Coll Cardiol* 37:1310-1315, 2001.

29. Pizzuto F, Voci P, Mariano E, et al: Assessment of flow velocity reserve by transthoracic Doppler echocardiography and venous adenosine infusion before and after left anterior descending coronary artery stenting. *J Am Coll Cardiol* 38:155-162, 2001.

30. Pizzuto F, Voci P, Mariano E, et al: Noninvasive coronary flow reserve assessed by transthoracic coronary Doppler ultrasound in patients with left anterior descending coronary artery stents. *Am J Cardiol* 91:522-526, 2003.

31. Voci P, Pizzuto F, Mariano E, et al: Usefulness of coronary flow reserve measured by transthoracic coronary Doppler ultrasound to detect severe left anterior descending coronary artery stenosis. *Am J Cardiol* 92:1320-1324, 2003.

32. Matsumura Y, Hozumi T, Watanabe H, et al: Cut-off value of coronary flow velocity reserve by transthoracic Doppler echocardiography for diagnosis of significant left anterior descending artery stenosis in patients with coronary risk factors. *Am J Cardiol* 92:1389-1393, 2003.

33. Hozumi T, Yoshida K, Akasaka T, et al: Value of acceleration flow and the prestenotic to stenotic coronary flow velocity ratio by transthoracic color Doppler echocardiography in noninvasive diagnosis of restenosis after percutaneous transluminal coronary angioplasty. *J Am Coll Cardiol* 35:164-168, 2000.

34. Watanabe N, Akasaka T, Yamaura Y, et al: Transthoracic Doppler echocardiography can detect coronary flow signals through the coronary stents: Noninvasive direct visualization of in-stent coronary restenosis. *J Echocardiogr* 2:61-67, 2004.

35. Saraste M, Vesalainen RK, Ylitalo A, et al: Transthoracic Doppler echocardiography as a noninvasive tool to assess coronary artery stenoses—a comparison with quantitative coronary angiography. *J Am Soc Echocardiogr* 18:679-685, 2005.

36. Watanabe N, Akasaka T, Yamaura Y, et al: Noninvasive detection of total occlusion of the left anterior descending coronary artery with transthoracic Doppler echocardiography. *J Am Coll Cardiol* 38:1328-1332, 2001.

37. Hirata K, Watanabe H, Hozumi T, et al: Simple detection of occluded coronary artery using retrograde flow in septal branch and left anterior descending coronary artery by transthoracic Doppler echocardiography at rest. *J Am Soc Echocardiogr* 17:108-113, 2004.

38. Otsuka R, Watanabe H, Hirata K, et al: A novel technique to detect total occlusion in the right coronary artery using retrograde flow by transthoracic Doppler echocardiography. *J Am Soc Echocardiogr* 18:704-709, 2005.

39. Takeuchi M, Miyazaki C, Yoshitani H, et al: Assessment of coronary flow velocity with transthoracic Doppler echocardiography during dobutamine stress echocardiography. *J Am Coll Cardiol* 38:117-123, 2001.

40. Florenciano-Sanchez R, de la Morena-Valenzuela G, Villegas-Garcia M, et al: Noninvasive assessment of coronary flow velocity reserve in left anterior descending artery adds diagnostic value to both clinical variables and dobutamine echocardiography: A study based on clinical practice. *Eur J Echocardiogr* 6:251-259, 2005.

41. Lee S, Otsuji Y, Minagoe S, et al: Noninvasive evaluation of coronary reperfusion by transthoracic Doppler echocardiography in patients with anterior acute myocardial infarction before coronary intervention. *Circulation* 108:2763-2768, 2003.

42. Voci P, Mariano E, Pizzuto F, et al: Coronary recanalization in anterior myocardial infarction: The open perforator hypothesis. *J Am Coll Cardiol* 40:1205-1213, 2002.

43. Takeuchi M, Nohtomi Y, Yoshitani H, et al: Enhanced coronary flow velocity during intra-aortic balloon pumping assessed by transthoracic Doppler echocardiography. *J Am Coll Cardiol* 43:368-376, 2004.

44. Kawamoto T, Yoshida K, Akasaka T, et al: Can coronary blood flow velocity pattern after primary percutaneous transluminal coronary angioplasty [correction of angiography] predict recovery of regional left ventricular function in patients with acute myocardial infarction? *Circulation* 100:339-345, 1999.

45. Yamamuro A, Akasaka T, Tamita K, et al: Coronary flow velocity pattern immediately after percutaneous coronary intervention as a predictor of complications and in-hospital survival after acute myocardial infarction. *Circulation* 106:3051-3056, 2002.

46. Hozumi T, Kanzaki Y, Ueda Y, et al: Coronary flow velocity analysis during short term follow up after coronary reperfusion: Use of transthoracic Doppler echocardiography to predict regional wall motion recovery in patients with acute myocardial infarction. *Heart* 89:1163-1168, 2003.

47. Shintani Y, Ito H, Iwakura K, et al: Usefulness of impairment of coronary microcirculation in predicting left ventricular dilation after acute myocardial infarction. *Am J Cardiol* 93:974-978, 2004.

48. Yoshida K, Hozumi T, Takemoto Y, et al: Impaired coronary circulation in patients with apical hypertrophic cardiomyopathy: noninvasive analysis by transthoracic Doppler echocardiography. *Echocardiography* 22:723-729, 2005.

49. Akasaka T, Yoshikawa J, Yoshida K, et al: Phasic coronary flow characteristics in patients with hypertrophic cardiomyopathy: A study by coronary Doppler catheter. *J Am Soc Echocardiogr* 7:9-19, 1994.

50. Celik S, Dagdeviren B, Yildirim A, et al: Determinants of coronary flow abnormalities in obstructive type hypertrophic cardiomyopathy: noninvasive assessment by transthoracic Doppler echocardiography. *J Am Soc Echocardiogr* 17:744-749, 2004.

51. Celik S, Dagdeviren B, Yildirim A, et al: Comparison of coronary flow velocities between patients with obstructive and nonobstructive type hypertrophic cardiomyopathy: Noninvasive assessment by transthoracic Doppler echocardiography. *Echocardiography* 22:1-7, 2005.

52. Watanabe N, Akasaka T, Yamaura Y, et al: Intramyocardial coronary flow characteristics in patients with hypertrophic cardiomyopathy: Non-invasive assessment by transthoracic Doppler echocardiography. *Heart* 89:657-658, 2003.

Part Four

Valvular Heart Disease

Chapter 18

Quantification of Valvular Regurgitation

JUDY HUNG, MD

Quantification of valvular regurgitation plays an important role in clinical practice. The introduction of Doppler techniques to echocardiography in the early 1980s transformed the diagnosis and management of valvular heart disease, allowing for accurate quantification of valvular regurgitation performed noninvasively. Velocity of blood flow across cardiac valves could be measured, providing assessment of regurgitant flows and pressure across cardiac chambers. The addition of color flow mapping to the Doppler examination allowed for color-coded spatial mapping of blood flow, significantly improving quantitation of valvular regurgitation and making it a key component of an echocardiogram. This chapter reviews the current methods in clinical practice for valvular quantification.

Color Doppler techniques are the most commonly applied method for quantification of valvular regurgitation in clinical practice. The regurgitant color Doppler flow pattern has three components: the proximal flow convergence or proximal isovelocity surface area (PISA), the vena contracta, and the distal jet[1] (Fig. 18–1A). Principles of fluid dynamics can be applied to these components of regurgitant flow in which flow can be considered to approach a finite orifice with flow distal to the orifice entering a constrained receiving chamber. The proximal flow convergence region occurs proximal to the regurgitant orifice (proximal to the leaflets). The vena contracta represents the narrowest point at or just downstream from the leaflets. The vena contracta represents the effective orifice area and not the anatomic orifice area. The latter is defined as an orifice at the level of the leaflets, whereas the effective orifice area is defined by the narrowest point of the flow steam, which typically occurs just downstream from the leaflets as flow continues to converge for a short distance beyond the anatomic orifice[1,2] (Fig. 18–1B). The final component is the distal regurgitant jet, which represents the regurgitant flow once it has passed the leaflets and into the receiving chamber. This distal jet is most readily detected and measured but

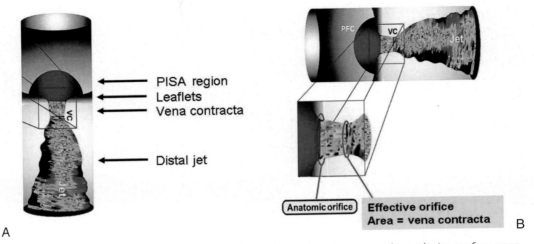

A

B

Figure 18–1. A, *The three components of a regurgitant jet: the proximal isovelocity surface area region also referred to as proximal flow convergence region, vena contracta (VC), and distal jet. B, The effective regurgitant orifice area is the orifice area defined by the narrowest regurgitant flow stream and typically occurs distal to the anatomic orifice defined by the valve leaflets. PISA, proximal isovelocity surface area. (Adapted from Roberts BJ, Grayburn P: J Am Soc Echocardiogr 16:1002-1006, 2003).*

also most subject to external influences present in the receiving chamber.

Quantification of Mitral Regurgitation

Color Doppler Methods

Distal Jet Area Method

A standard method for assessing mitral regurgitation (MR) is measurement of the distal MR jet area as it enters the left atrium (LA).[3,4,4a,4b] The MR jet is defined as the turbulent mosaic color flow within the LA during systole emanating from the mitral leaflets (Fig. 18–2). Care should be taken to avoid including the low-velocity (nonturbulent) blood flows in the LA surrounding the turbulent jet as this will falsely increase the MR jet area. The maximal jet area is traced in multiple views and an average of the areas is calculated.

The distal jet area method is a relatively simple and commonly applied technique for the qualitative assessment of MR. However, there are a number of technical and physiological factors that should be taken into account. Assessing the severity of MR by distal MR jet is based on the assumption that the color Doppler display of MR flow velocities can be a surrogate for MR regurgitant volume. On an empiric basis, this has been validated against angiographic standards. It is important to keep in mind limitations using the color display of the MR flow velocities as a substitute for mitral regurgitant volume. First of all, measurement of the regurgitant jet is taken at the maximal instantaneous point in time, whereas regurgitant volume includes the duration of regurgitant flow. In addition, as MR flow occurs in a pulsatile manner, the

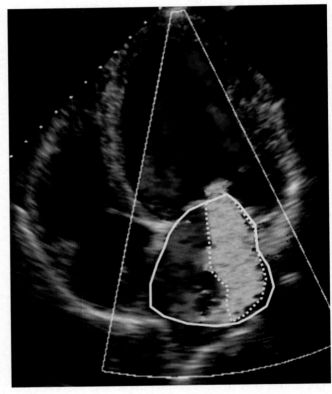

Figure 18–2. *Mitral regurgitation assessed by distal jet area method. Mitral regurgitation jet area is traced (dashed line) and divided by left atrial area (solid line).*

flow rate is not constant, and hence the relationship between jet velocity and flow rate will vary. Because the MR flow is entering a constrained chamber (LA), the behavior of the MR jet is influenced by a number of factors including physical containment from the left atrial wall, entrainment of blood pool in the LA into the MR flow, and flow influences from the pulmonary veins.

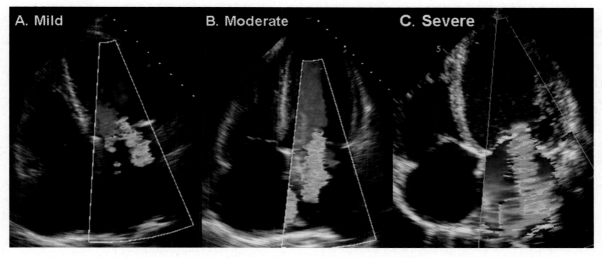

Figure 18–3. *Increasing degrees of mitral regurgitation from mild* (A), *moderate* (B), *and severe* (C) *as assessed by jet area method.*

Eccentric MR jets are subject to impingement from the left atrial wall, which can result in a decrease in the size of the mitral regurgitant jet. In addition, wall jets are subject to the Coandă effect, which is the tendency of flow to track along a wall, particularly a curved convex surface like the wall of the left atrium. This effect influences the direction and ultimately the display of the MR jet.[5,6] Eccentric jets in which the MR jet courses out of the plane of the ultrasound (US) beam will also be missed or underestimated. Because of the limitations with eccentric jets, the jet area method is probably best applied to centrally directed jets.[7] Machine settings can also influence the distal MR jet. A gain setting that is too high, in which there is random color noise present, can overestimate the size of the jet. In contrast, too low gain settings will underestimate the jet size. Low Nyquist settings can also overestimate the true MR jet because lower velocity blood flows present in the LA will be merged into the true MR jet. In general, Nyquist limits should be at least 50 cm/s for color flow mapping of MR regurgitant jets.

Importantly, distal jet area is influenced by hemodynamic conditions.[8-12] Studies have demonstrated the size of the regurgitant jet depends to some extent on the driving pressure across the mitral valve, which is dictated by the left ventricular (LV) systolic pressure to left atrial pressure gradient.[8,12] As this gradient is maximal at midsystole, the MR jet tends to be maximal at this time point in the cardiac cycle. Hemodynamic conditions, which alter systemic arterial pressure or left atrial pressure, can influence the overall jet size.[9,11]

Typically, the distal MR jet area is normalized relative to the left atrial area. Comparison studies suggest that normalization for LA size correlates better than absolute jet area compared to angiographic standards.[5,13] The MR jet area and left atrial area are measured in the same systolic frame to obtain a ratio of jet area to left atrial area (JA/LAA)[13,14] (see Fig. 18–2). Figure 18–3 shows examples of jet areas corresponding to mild to severe MR. The

maximal MR jet area is traced, and then this area divided by the left atrial area measured from the same frame. MR JA/LAA ratios of less than 20% correspond to mild MR, whereas ratios of greater than 40% correspond to severe MR[7] (Table 18–1). One factor that impacts the accuracy of the JA/LAA method is the assumption that there is a relatively linear relationship between JA size and LAA. However, this is not always the case, and there are situations where the actual MR volume is greater than suggested by the JA/LAA, such as in cases of chronic MR in which there has been extensive LA remodeling. Table 18–2 summarizes validation studies for distal jet area methods against comparable standards.

Vena Contracta Method

The vena contracta (VC) is the narrowest portion of the mitral regurgitant jet and provides a simple linear measurement of the proximal MR jet[1,15-21a] (Fig. 18–4). The

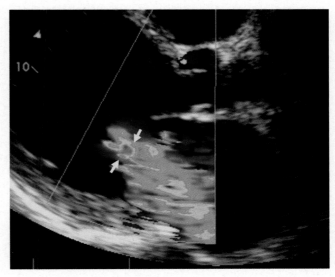

Figure 18–4. *The vena contracta* (arrows) *of the mitral regurgitant jet.*

TABLE 18–1. Qualitative and Quantitative Parameters Useful in Grading Mitral Regurgitation Severity

	Mild	Moderate	Severe
Structural Parameters			
LA size	Normal*	Normal or dilated	Usually dilated†
LV size	Normal*	Normal or dilated	Usually dilated†
Mitral leaflets or support apparatus	Normal or abnormal	Normal or abnormal	Abnormal/flail leaflet/ruptured papillary muscle
Doppler Parameters			
Color flow jet area‡	Small, central jet (usually <4 cm² or <20% of LA area)	Variable	Large central jet (usually >10 cm² or >40% of LA area) or variable size wall—Impinging jet swirling in LA
Mitral inflow—PW	A wave dominant¶	Variable	E wave dominant¶ (E usually 1.2 m/s)
Jet density—CW	Incomplete or faint	Dense	Dense
Jet contour—CW	Parabolic	Usually parabolic	Early peaking–triangular
Pulmonary vein flow	Systolic dominance**	Systolic blunting**	Systolic flow reversal§
Quantitative Parameters††			
VC width (cm)	<0.3	0.3-0.69	≥0.7
R Vol (mL/beat)	<30	30-44, 45-59	≥60
RF (%)	<30	30-39, 40-49	≥50
EROA (cm²)	<0.20	0.20-0.29, 0.30-0.39	≥0.40

*Unless there are other reasons for left atrium or left ventricle dilation. Normal two-dimensional measurements: left ventricle minor axis ≤2.8 cm/m²; left ventricle end-diastolic volume ≤82 mL/m²; maximal left atrium antero-posterior diameter ≤2 cm/m²; maximal left atrium volume ≤36 mL/m².

†Exception: acute mitral regurgitation.

‡At a Nyquist limit of 50-60 cm/s.

§Pulmonary venous systolic flow reversal is specific but not sensitive for severe mitral regurgitation.

¶Usually older than 50 years of age or in conditions of impaired relaxation, in the absence of mitral stenosis or other causes of elevated left atrium pressure.

**Unless other reasons for systolic blunting (e.g., atrial fibrillation, elevated left atrial pressure).

††Quantitative parameters can help sub-classify the moderate regurgitation group into mild to moderate and moderate to severe.

CW, continuous wave; EROA, effective regurgitant orifice area; LA, left atrium; LV, left ventricle; PW, pulsed wave; RF, regurgitant fraction; R Vol, regurgitant volume; 2D, two-dimensional; VC, vena contracta.

Data from Zoghbi WA, Enriquez-Sarano M, Foster E, et al: *J Am Soc Echocardiogr* 16:777-802, 2003.

TABLE 18–2. Summary of Methods for Doppler Evaluation of Mitral Valve Regurgitation

			Mitral Regurgitation			
Author	**Method**	**Comparison Standard**	**Results**	**N**	**Date**	**Journal**
Omoto and colleagues[4]	Jet area	Angiography	—	72 Both AR and MR	1984	*Jpn Heart J*
Miyatake and colleagues[3]	Jet area	Angiography	r = 0.87	109	1986	*J Am Coll Cardiol*
Helmcke and colleagues[13]	Jet area/ LAA	Angiography	r = 0.78	147	1987	*Circulation*
Spain and colleagues[14]	Jet area	Angiography	r = 0.76	47	1989	*J Am Coll Cardiol*
Fehske and colleagues[15]	VC	Angiography	r = 0.94 r = 0.83 (RV)	78	1994	*Am J Cardiol*
Heinle and colleagues[21]	VC-TEE	Pulsed Doppler	r = 0.81 (RV)	35	1998	*Am J Cardiol*
Castello and colleagues[4b]	JA TEE	Angiography	r = 0.90	80	1992	*J Am Coll Cardiol*
Hall and colleagues[20]	VC	Pulsed Doppler	r = 0.85 (RV)	80	1997	*Circulation*
Mele and colleagues[21a]	VC/proximal jet	Angiography Pulsed Doppler	r = 0.85 to 0.91 r = 0.86	33 47	1995	*Circulation*
Omoto and colleagues[4a]	Jet area-TEE	Angiography	—	37	1992	*Circulation*
Grayburn and colleagues[19]	VC-TEE	Angiography	Single plane TEE Sens 100% Spec 95% Multiplane TEE Sens 98%	80	1998	*Am J Cardiol*
Recusani and colleagues[23]	PISA in-vitro model	Electromagnetic flow meter	r = 0.94-0.99 (flow rate) r = 0.795-0.96 (EROA)	—	1991	*Circulation*
Bargiggia and colleagues[24]	PISA	Angiography	r = 0.91 (flow rate) r = 0.93 (RV)	52	1991	*Circulation*
Utsunomiya and colleagues[25]	PISA In vitro	Flow meter	—	226	1991	*J Am Coll Cardiol*
Dujardins and colleagues[40]	Pulsed Doppler	Angiography	r = 0.79 (EROA) r = 0.80 (RV) r = 0.78 (RF)	180	1997	*Circulation*

MRI, magnetic resonance imaging; sens, sensitivity.
Data from references 3-4b, 13-15, 19-21a, 23-25, 37-39, 40-41a.

Continued

TABLE 18–2. Summary of Methods for Doppler Evaluation of Mitral Valve Regurgitation—cont'd

			Mitral Regurgitation			
Kizilbash and colleagues[41a]	Pulsed Doppler	MRI	r = 0.82 (RF)	22	1998	*Am J Cardiol*
Tribouilloy and colleagues[39]	Pulsed Doppler	Angiography	RF by echo 45.8 mL ± 19.2% RF by angio 41.3 ± 17.8%	27	1991	*Br Heart J*
Rokey and colleagues[37]	Pulsed Doppler	Angiography	r = 0.91	25	1986	*J Am Coll Cardiol*
Blumlein and colleagues[38]	Pulsed Doppler	Angiography Scintigraphy	r = 0.82 r = 0.89	27	1986	*Circulation*
Ascah and colleagues[41]	Pulsed Doppler	Electromagnetic flow meter	r = 0.84 (RV) r = 0.83 (RF)	7 (exp. model)	1985	*Circulation*

angio, angiogram; echo, echocardiogram; EROA, effective regurgitant orifice area; exp. model, experimental canine model; MRI, magnetic resonance imaging; r, correlation coefficient; RF, regurgitant fraction; sens, sensitivity; spec, specificity; TEE, transesophageal echocardiogram; VC-TEE, vena contracta from transesophageal echocardiogram.
Data from references 3-4b, 13-15, 19-21a, 23-25, 37-41, 41b.

VC can be considered to be a surrogate measure of the effective regurgitant orifice area because it essentially represents the anterior-posterior dimension of the effective regurgitant orifice area. When measuring the VC, it is important to perform it in views orthogonal to the coaptation line of the mitral leaflets, such as the parasternal long-axis or apical long-axis views because this will provide the optimal color resolution of the VC as imaged in the anterior-posterior plane (Fig. 18–5). Views that display the MR jet along the coaptation line, such as the two-chamber view (medial-lateral dimension), will falsely increase the width of the VC.

Because the VC measurement inherently is within a narrow range, small differences in measurement can make a large impact on MR degree. Care must be taken to optimize the VC region for measurement by magnifying and adjusting depth and sector settings for optimal color Doppler resolution. In addition, it can be difficult to define the narrowest portion of the MR jet as in some cases, the neck of the proximal MR jet is not easily seen or is obscured by the leaflets. Measuring the width of the proximal jet either at the level of the leaflets or just distal to the coaptation line can sometimes circumvent this. The VC is felt to be less influenced by physiologic loading conditions and hence may be more reproducible than jet area methods.[15] Figure 18–6 shows the tighter ranges demonstrated by VC measurement compared with MR jet area against angiography. In vitro studies have demonstrated that VC is less dependent on hemodynamic factors than distal jet area.[16] Another potential advantage of VC measurement over jet area may be in eccentric jets in which the proximal jet will be less affected by wall

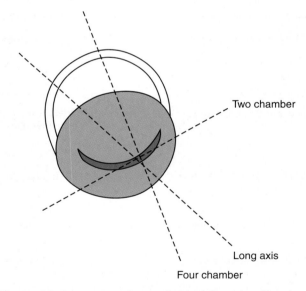

Two chamber

Long axis

Four chamber

Figure 18–5. Imaging planes of apical four-chamber, apical two-chamber, and long-axis views as related to mitral valve orifice.

impingement. Table 18–2 summarizes validation studies of the VC method against comparable standards.

Table 18–1 shows values for VC corresponding to MR degree. VC measurements of less than 3 mm correspond to mild MR; 0.3 to 0.69 moderate MR; and greater than 0.7 severe MR. There is a broad range for VC considered to be in the moderate range, which limits the VC as a quantitative measure. Despite this, VC remains a clinically useful semi-quantitative measure of MR, which is simple in concept and measurement.

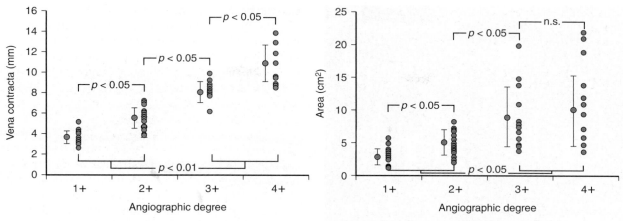

Figure 18–6. Decreased variability in measurements for vena contracta compared with jet area measurements. (From Fehske W et al: Am J Cardiol 73[4]:268-274, 1994.)

Proximal Isovelocity Surface Area Method

The PISA method is based on the fluid dynamic principle that as flow approaches a circular finite orifice, it forms concentric hemispherical shells with gradually decreasing surface area and increasing velocity[22] (Fig. 18–7). This principle can be applied to mitral regurgitant flow in which the PISA region is the hemispheric shell that forms proximal to the mitral leaflets on the LV side, and the finite orifice is the mitral regurgitant orifice at the level of the leaflets[2,11,23-26] By the conservation of mass principle, the flow rate of each of the isovelocity shells equals the flow rate at the regurgitant orifice. Assuming a hemispheric shape for the isovelocity shells, then flow rate is equal to the surface area of a hemisphere, which is equal to $2\pi r^2$ multiplied by the aliasing velocity (where r is the radius of the hemispherical shell). The flow rate of the hemispheric shell equals the MR flow rate at the orifice by the conservation of mass principle. Once flow rate is calculated, the MR regurgitant orifice area and regurgitant volume can be derived using the following formulas: regurgitant orifice area (ROA) is equal to the MR flow rate divided by the peak MR velocity by continuous wave (CW) Doppler.

$$ROA = \frac{PISA \ flow \ rate}{MR \ velocity}$$

Because ROA is calculated from an instantaneous peak flow rate, ROA obtained using the PISA method represents a maximal instantaneous ROA. To calculate regurgitant volume, the ROA is multiplied by the velocity time integral (VTI) of the mitral regurgitant jet:

$$RV = ROA \times VTI \ [MR \ jet]$$

The regurgitant fraction is calculated as regurgitant volume divided by the stroke volume (SV).

$$RF = \frac{RV}{SV}$$

SV can be calculated from 2D calculations of ventricular volumes as the end-diastolic volume minus the end-systolic volume.

To optimize measurement of the radius, r, baseline shifting of the Nyquist limit is recommended (Fig. 18–8). The baseline is shifted toward the direction of the regurgitant flow. The Nyquist limit should be relatively low compared to the regurgitant velocity or the hemispherical assumption can be invalid.[27] Hence, it is important to measure the radius of the PISA region at Nyquist limits much lower than flow rates. In general, 20 to 40 cm/s are Nyquist limit ranges in which there is an optimal balance of maximal radius resolution and integrity of the PISA shape. Low Nyquist limits overestimate the size of the PISA region in which case, there will be elongation in the axial dimension. Conversely, high Nyquist limits will minimize the PISA region making accurate measurements difficult.[25,28-32]

Mitral regurgitant flow rate and ROA can be dynamic throughout systole depending on the etiology of mitral

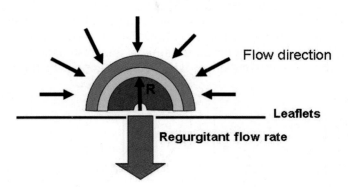

Figure 18–7. Proximal isovelocity surface area (PISA): Fluid dynamic theory predicts that as flow approaches a circular, finite orifice, it forms a series of concentric hemispheric shells with gradually decreasing area and increasing velocity. Arrows refer to direction of flow as it approaches the PISA region. r is the radius of a hemispherical shell. By principle of conservation of mass: Flow through the regurgitant orifice is equal to flow through the isovelocity surface, which equals $2\pi r^2$ multiplied by the aliasing velocity.

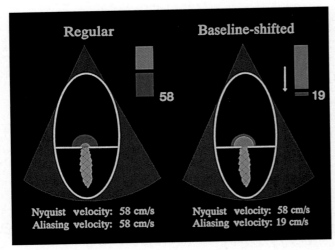

Figure 18–8. *Baseline shifting of the Nyquist limit toward the direction of the regurgitant flow results in a larger proximal isovelocity surface area (PISA) zone for optimal measurement of the PISA region radius (right panel). (Courtesy Robert A. Levine, MD.)*

regurgitation,[33,34] which can be an important consideration when deciding at what time point during systole to measure the PISA radius. For example, with functional MR, there is typically a bimodal pattern with peak MR flow rates in early and late systole, whereas MR flow rate is the least during midsystole. In patients with mitral valve prolapse, peak MR flow occurs midsystole to late systole. For rheumatic disease, the MR flow rate is constant during systole. PISA radius measurement should be avoided early or late in systole because these are times when the mitral leaflets are just closing or about to open, and the flow rate may not be at equilibrium. As a general rule, the PISA radius measurement should occur at the same time as the peak MR velocity (as measured by continuous wave Doppler). This usually occurs at midsystole or at the T wave in the electrocardiogram (ECG) pattern. In practice, in can be difficult to precisely align in time the peak MR velocity with a PISA region, which would be suitable for accurate measurement. In these situations, it is best to aim for accurate PISA region radius measurement at a time point that is close to the peak MR velocity.

Accuracy and reproducibility of the PISA method is highly dependent on careful attention to technique of acquisition and measurements. The PISA region should be magnified with sector and depth optimized for color Doppler resolution, with the PISA region and mitral leaflets encompassing most of the sector. Measurement of the PISA should be aligned parallel to flow rate direction because this optimizes Doppler resolution. An MR regurgitant orifice area of 0.40 cm² or greater is consistent with severe MR, whereas a regurgitant orifice area less than 0.20 cm² is consistent with mild MR. Table 18–2 summarizes validation studies of the PISA method against comparable standards.

Geometric Factors Influencing PISA Method. In theory, the PISA method provides an accurate quantitative measure of MR. However, there are technical and practical aspects to the PISA method that should be considered. The PISA region is influenced by the surrounding geometry of the orifice.[22] This principle is important when examining eccentrically directed PISA regions, such as occurs with a flail mitral leaflet. This typically will result in an overestimation of the PISA radius resulting from distortion of the PISA region as a result of constraint from the left atrial wall, which results in a falsely increased radius.[27] To overcome this, an angle correction factor can be applied to the surface area calculation.[22] Angle correction is performed by multiplying the surface area calculation by α divided by 180, in which α is the angle between the mitral leaflet and end of the PISA region confined by the left atrial wall.[35] However, angle correction for eccentric PISA regions adds additional complexity to the MR flow rate calculation, creating additional opportunities for measurement error. Furthermore, it is not always possible to accurately measure the α-angle because of LV wall confinement.

Technical Factors. One should measure the radius of the PISA region at Nyquist velocities, which are reliably displayed by color Doppler flow mapping. One of the major limitations of the PISA method has been that the calculated results vary widely when the radius is measured at different distances from the orifice because of varying three-dimensional (3D) shapes of the isovelocity surface. The contour of the PISA region changes depending on location of flow rate relative to the regurgitant orifice.[22,31,32] The contour flattens out close to the orifice, whereas the contour assumes an elongated or more oval shape furthest from the orifice. These variations in PISA contour results in systematic overestimation at flow rates farthest from the orifice and underestimation closest to the orifice (Fig. 18–9). In addition, measurement of the radius should be avoided along the sides of the PISA region as flow here is perpendicular to the ultrasound beam, resulting in underestimation of the velocity component with a frank dropout of flow

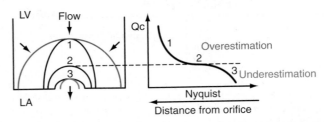

Figure 18–9. *Effect of proximal isovelocity surface area (PISA) radius on PISA shape and flow calculation. LA, left atrium; LV, left ventricle; Qc, flow calculation. (Adapted from Schwammenthal E, Chen C, Geisler C, et al: J Am Coll Cardiol 27:161-172, 1996.)*

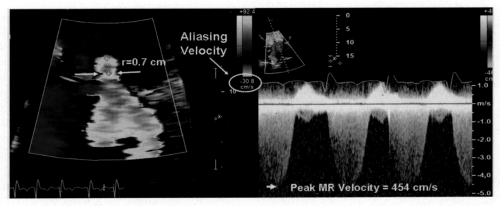

Figure 18–10. *On the left the proximal isovelocity surface area (PISA) region is displayed after baseline shifting and magnification. The arrows point to the drop out in Doppler flow along the sides of the PISA region where the flow is perpendicular to the ultrasound beam. The radius of the PISA zone measures 0.7 cm. The aliasing velocity is 30.8 cm/s as displayed by the Nyquist limit. The peak regurgitant flow rate is equal to $2 \times \pi \times (0.7\ cm)^2 \times 30.8\ cm/s$, which is equal to 95 mL/s. The regurgitant orifice area is equal to $132\ cm^3/s \div 454\ cm/s$, which is equal to $0.21\ cm^2$. MR, mitral regurgitation.*

signals at angles perpendicular to flow.[22] This dropout of color display where flow is perpendicular gives the PISA region a rounded appearance at its base (Fig. 18–10A). Figure 18–11 shows an ideal zone for PISA radius measurement to occur.

In vitro studies have demonstrated that regurgitant orifice shape can impact the shape of the PISA region.[25] This is an important factor to consider when applying the use of a hemispherical formula to the PISA contour, which assumes a circular regurgitant

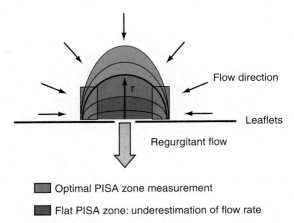

Optimal PISA zone measurement

Flat PISA zone: underestimation of flow rate

Oval PISA zone: overestimation of flow rate

Flow direction nonparallel

Figure 18–11. *The proximal isovelocity surface area (PISA) region is optimally measured where the region is hemispherical. Flows farthest away from the orifice assume an elongated or oval contour, overestimating flows whereas flows closest to the orifice assume a flat contour, underestimating flows. Measurement of the radius should be avoided along the sides of the PISA region because flow here is perpendicular to the ultrasound beam, resulting in underestimation of the velocity component with frank drop out of flow display at angles perpendicular to flow.*

orifice. However, the regurgitant orifice may not be circular, particularly in view of the elliptical coaptation zone of the mitral leaflets; this may be especially important in functional MR, in which there is symmetric tethering of the mitral leaflets. Because of the hemispherical assumption, the PISA method may underestimate regurgitant flow rate, especially with rectangular regurgitant orifices.[25] Application of a hemielliptical formula to the PISA region has shown improved accuracy of MR quantification.[26,36] However, the hemielliptical surface area formula is complex, requiring measurement of a radius in three orthogonal planes, which are then integrated for surface area calculation. This adds considerable complexity to the PISA method and has limited clinical application.

The PISA region appears less influenced by changes in machine settings, such as gain, wall filter, frame rate, or packet size, compared to color jet area distal methods.[28]

Volumetric Methods Using Pulsed Doppler

Volumetric methods utilize pulse wave Doppler techniques to calculate flow rates and SVs. The SV across a valve annulus can be calculated as the velocity time integral (VTI) across the valve annulus multiplied by the cross-sectional area (CSA) of the annulus. Thus, the MR regurgitant volume can be calculated from the flow across the regurgitant valve compared to a normal cardiac valve.[37-41a] Although many combinations can be employed, a common way to derive MR volume is:

$$\text{MR volume} = \text{mitral inflow} - \text{aortic outflow}$$

Mitral inflow volume is calculated as VTI of mitral inflow multiplied by the CSA of the mitral annulus (Fig. 18–12). The VTI of mitral inflow should be measured at the level of the mitral annular plane because this is

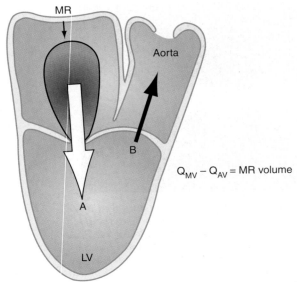

Figure 18-12. Schematic demonstrating volumetric method for calculating mitral regurgitant volume. Mitral inflow (Q_{MV}) minus the aortic outflow (Q_{AV}) equals the mitral regurgitant (MR) volume, provided there is no significant aortic regurgitation. LV, left ventricle.

$$Q_{MV} - Q_{AV} = MR \text{ volume}$$

where CSA is measured (Fig. 18-13). The CSA of the mitral annulus is assumed to be circular and calculated as πr^2, in which r is the diameter measured in the apical four-chamber view divided by 2. Anatomically, the mitral annulus is D-shaped and more shaped like an ellipse rather than a circle. However, using a circular assumption for the annulus is reasonable in patients who have developed at least moderate MR given the annular dilation that occurs with development of moderate or greater MR. Alternatively, the mitral annulus can also be calculated as an ellipse in which the area is πab, with a and b being the diameters measured in the apical two- and four-chamber views divided by 2 to obtain the ra-

dius. Aortic outflow is calculated as VTI of aortic outflow multiplied by the CSA of left ventricular outflow tract (LVOT). This method assumes that there is no aortic regurgitation (AR); otherwise pulmonary artery outflow can be used, assuming no significant pulmonary regurgitation. The MR regurgitant volume can also be obtained by calculating LV SV and subtracting aortic outflow volume, assuming no aortic insufficiency is present. Table 18-2 summarizes validation of volumetric methods using pulsed Doppler against comparable standards.

Although, straightforward in concept, volumetric methods are subject to increased variability related to the number of measurements necessary to calculate cardiac flows from pulsed Doppler and annular areas. For reproducible results, these methods generally require significant training. In addition, as the radius is squared for calculation of area, small errors in measurement are amplified,[37] and accurate resolution of the annulus is important in minimizing measurement errors.

Supportive Evidence in the Assessment of Mitral Regurgitation

Pulmonary Venous Inflow Pattern

The pulmonary venous inflow pattern provides confirmatory data in assessing MR severity. Normal pulmonary venous inflow has forward flow during both systole and diastole with a brief reversal of flow during atrial contraction (Fig. 18-14). Systolic flow (S wave) has two components, S_1 and S_2. The S wave is slightly larger than the diastolic (D) wave. Pulmonary veins are sampled in the apical four-chamber view with the sample volume placed approximately 1 cm from the orifice. Studies have demonstrated feasibility of imaging the pulmonary venous inflow pattern by transthoracic imaging.[42-44] Transthoracic imaging has a reported success rate of 95% for pulmonary venous systolic and diastolic flow velocity and 90% for the atrial reversal wave. Systolic flow reversal as detected by transthoracic imaging had a sensitivity of 61% and specificity of 92% for severe MR as measured by PISA method.[45] Limitations with transthoracic echocardiographic (TTE) imaging of the pulmonary venous inflow pattern occur in which increased depth settings have resulted in inadequate pulse-wave Doppler sampling.

Changes in the systolic pulmonary venous pattern can estimate the degree of MR severity. As MR increases, the systolic wave becomes blunted decreasing to less than the diastolic wave. As the MR volume increases, there is eventual reversal of first the S_2 wave (see Fig. 18-14) and then the entire systolic wave.[46] Changes in pulmonary venous pattern with increasing MR volume relates to initial blunting of the systolic wave from the propagation wave formed by the MR volume into the LA, with overt reversal of pulmonary

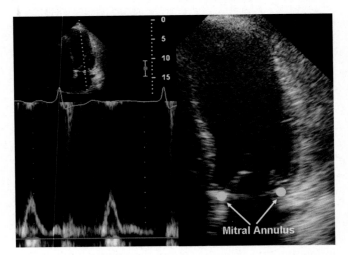

Figure 18-13. Mitral inflow measured at the level of the mitral annulus (left). Diameter of the mitral annulus (yellow dots) measured in mid-diastole (right).

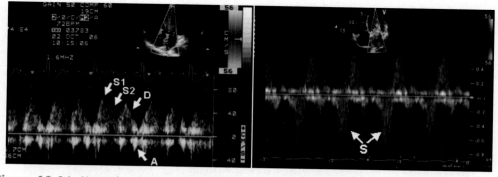

Figure 18–14. Normal pulmonary venous pattern (left). *Pulmonary venous inflow into the left atrium occurs both in systole (S1 and S2) and diastole (D) with brief reversal of flow during atrial contraction (A). Reversal of S2 component* (arrows) *with severe mitral regurgitation* (right).

systolic flow with increasing MR volume. Others have suggested that pulmonary venous inflow is best imaged with transesophageal echocardiographic (TEE) techniques. Studies using transesophageal echocardiography have demonstrated sensitivities of 82% to 90% and specificity of 100% for systolic flow reversal as indicative of severe MR.[47,48]

Systolic blunting of pulmonary veins without reversal of flow also provides confirmatory evidence of significant MR. However, the presence of systolic blunting is nonspecific because it can occur in a number of clinical situations in which there is elevated LA pressures, such as in LV dysfunction or atrial fibrillation.[49,50] Consequently the presence of systolic blunting is not a specific sign of MR severity and should be interpreted with this in mind. On the other hand, systolic flow reversal is a fairly specific sign of severe MR.[45-48] Flow reversal can be difficult to demonstrate with transthoracic imaging. In addition, the MR jet itself can flow directly into the pulmonary vein, contaminating the pulmonary venous Doppler signal. In eccentric MR jets, the right and left pulmonary veins can be differentially affected, depending on the direction of the jet. It is best to pulse Doppler both right and left pulmonary veins to obtain a complete sampling.[46,51]

Continuous Wave Doppler Pattern

CW Doppler of the MR jet provides an indirect assessment of MR severity. The more intense the CW signal of the MR, the greater number of red blood cell reflectors and hence MR volume. In addition, the more complete the MR CW signal, the greater likelihood the MR is significant. Studies have demonstrated that the signal intensity of the MR CW tracing correlates with MR severity comparing against an angiographic standard.[52,53] Rapid equilibration of the LV-LA gradient occurring with severe MR can result in a V-shaped pattern to the normal parabolic CW MR jet. CW intensity and pattern should be used as supportive evidence for MR severity because signal intensity and shape can vary greatly with machine settings as well as alignment of the CW beam along the regurgitant jet.

Other Supportive Factors

Valve morphology can provide important clues in the assessment of MR. Apical tenting of the mitral leaflets is associated with functional MR, which develops in the setting of LV cardiomyopathy.[54-57] The presence of valvular vegetations, flail portion, and frank papillary muscle rupture are associated with severe MR. Increased left atrial and LV size are associated with significant MR, presumably as a result of a volume effect in increasing chamber size. However, left-sided chamber enlargement results from a number of clinical situations, such as arrhythmias and cardiomyopathy, and hence is not specific for MR severity. An elevated right ventricular (RV) systolic pressure also suggests clinically important MR as a result of the regurgitant volume effect on the pulmonary vasculature. An increased E wave velocity is also supportive of significant MR.

Quantification of Aortic Regurgitation

Assessment of AR is based on Doppler techniques using color Doppler and spectral Doppler methods. As with MR, it is important to have an integrative approach toward assessment of AR severity.

Color Doppler Methods

Proximal Jet Methods

Color Doppler assessment of AR should primarily be assessed using the proximal AR jet. The proximal jet is measured just distal to the level of the leaflets in the LVOT and is a more robust measure of assessing AR severity than distal AR jet length or area methods. The proximal jet can be measured as either a jet width or jet area. The proximal jet width is best measured in the parasternal long-axis view (Fig. 18–15). Apical views should be avoided in measuring jet width as the proxi-

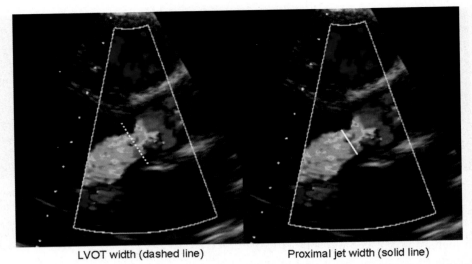

LVOT width (dashed line)   Proximal jet width (solid line)

Figure 18–15. Left ventricular outflow tract width (dashed line) (left). Proximal jet width (solid line) (right).

mal jet can be obscured by the aortic leaflets. Furthermore, the resolution of the proximal jet in the parasternal windows is generally better than in the apical windows. The proximal jet width can be obscured in heavily calcified aortic leaflets. Proximal jet width has been shown to correlate fairly well with angiography. However, the correlation improved when normalized for LVOT diameter.[58,59] In clinical practice, using the ratio of proximal jet width to LVOT diameter is recommended (see Fig. 18–15). Ratios of less than 10% cor-

respond to trace AR; 10% to 25% to mild AR; 25% to 60% to moderate MR; and greater than 60% to severe AR[7] (Fig. 18–16 and Table 18–3).

In addition to proximal jet width, proximal jet area is also a useful measure of AR severity. The proximal jet area is measured in the short-axis view with depth and sector optimized for color Doppler resolution. As with proximal jet width, correlations with angiography improves with normalization for aortic area measured in the same frame as the proximal jet area[58] (Fig. 18–17).

A limitation with proximal jet area involves acoustic shadowing of the AR jet if the aortic leaflets are calcified, a frequent associated finding. In addition, it can be difficult to align the imaging plane in the short-axis view at the level of the LVOT just distal to the leaflets.

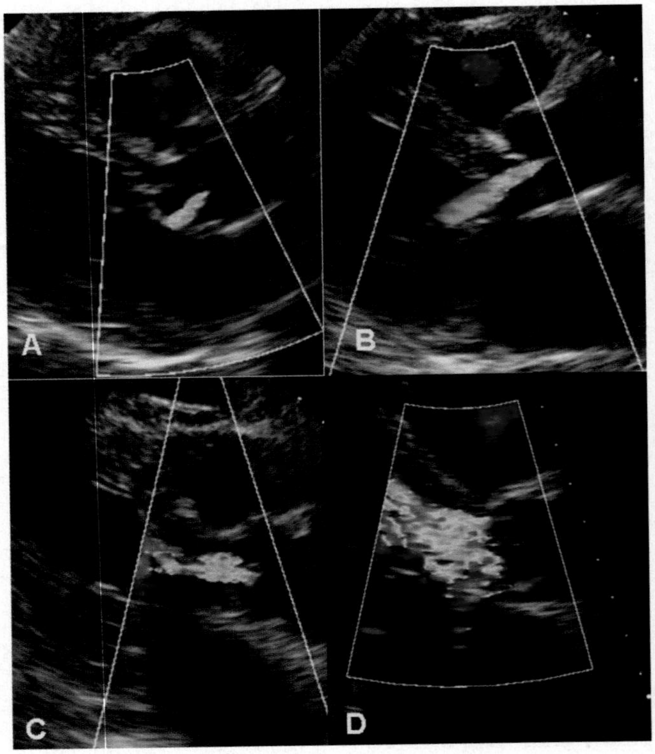

Figure 18–16. Jet widths representing trace (A), mild (B), moderate (C), and severe (D) aortic regurgitation.

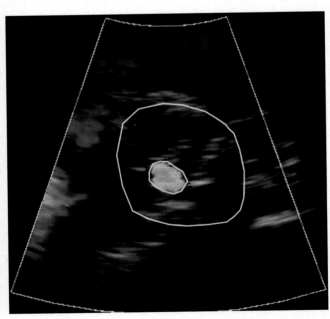

Figure 18–17. Proximal jet area normalized to left ventricular outflow tract area.

TABLE 18-3. Qualitative and Quantitative Parameters Useful in Grading Aortic Regurgitation Severity

	Mild	Moderate	Severe
Structural Parameters			
LA size	Normal*	Normal or dilated	Usually dilated†
Aortic leaflets	Normal or abnormal	Normal or abnormal	Abnormal/flail or wide coaptation defect
Doppler Parameters			
Jet width in LVOT—color flow	Small in central jets	Intermediate	Large in central jets; variable in eccentric jets
Jet density—CW	Incomplete or faint	Dense	Dense
Jet deceleration rate—CW (PHT)§	Slow, >500	Medium 500-200	Steep, <200
Diastolic flow reversal in descending aorta—PW	Brief, early diastolic reversal	Intermediate	Prominent holodiastolic reversal
Quantitative Parameters¶			
VC width, cm‡	<0.3	0.3-0.60	>0.6
Jet width/LVOT width, %‡	<25	25-45, 46-64	≥65
Jet CSA/LVOT CSA, %	<5	5-20, 21-59	≥60
R Vol, mL/beat	<30	30-44, 45-59	≥60
RF, %	<30	30-39, 40-49	≥50
EROA, cm²	<0.10	0.10-0.19, 0.20-0.29	≥0.30

*Unless there are other reasons for left ventricle dilation. Normal two-dimensional measurements: left ventricle minor axis ≤2.8 cm/m²; left ventricle end-diastolic volume ≤82 ml/m².
†Exception: would be acute aortic regurgitation, in which chambers have not had time to dilate.
‡At Nyquist limit of 50-60 cm/s.
§Pressure half-time is shortened with increasing left ventricle diastolic pressure and vasodilator therapy, and may be lengthened in chronic adaptation to severe aortic regurgitation.
¶Quantitative parameters can subclassify the moderate regurgitation group into mild-to-moderate and moderate-to-severe regurgitation as shown.
CSA, cross-sectional area; CW, continuous wave Doppler; EROA, effective regurgitant orifice area; LA, left atrium; LVOT, left ventricular outflow tract; PHT, pressure half-time; PW, pulsed wave Doppler; R Vol, regurgitant volume; RF, regurgitant fraction; VC, vena contracta.
Data from Zoghbi WA, Enriquez-Sarano M, Foster E, et al: *J Am Soc Echocardiogr* 16:777-802, 2003.

Comparison of proximal jet area to proximal jet width have demonstrated reduced reproducibility with proximal jet area methods, likely related to this.[60]

Distal Jet Length and Area

The distal extent of the AR jet into the LV (jet length) was one of the earliest applications of Doppler techniques to assess AR severity. Initial studies examining distal jet length and area demonstrated excellent correlations compared with angiography.[4] However, subsequent studies have shown jet length to be influenced significantly by the driving pressure from the aorta to left ventricle.[58,61,62] In addition, entrainment of the jet from surrounding blood pool in the LVOT can also influence the extent of the jet, making the distal AR jet appear falsely large. Figure 18–18 shows the relatively poor correlation of AR jet length to angiographic assessment of AR compared to AR proximal jet width.[58] Eccentric AR jets can also be truncated by the LV wall

or mitral valve leaflets.[63] As with MR, the Coandă effect can also influence the direction and size of eccentric AR wall jets. Machine and technical factors, such as gain settings and alignment of the ultrasound beam to the jet, have also been shown to impact on distal jet length and area.[64,65] Relying solely on the distal jet length or area should be avoided when assessing AR.

Vena Contracta

The VC of the AR jet can also be measured as a semiquantitative measure of AR. The VC occurs at the level of the leaflets and is the narrowest portion of the AR jet, just before the proximal jet (Fig. 18–19). Because it is often obscured by the leaflets, it can be difficult to measure accurately. It can also be difficult to distinguish separately from the proximal jet width if a "neck" is not apparent. VCs of less than 0.3 cm correspond to mild AR, 0.3 to 0.60 correspond to moderate AR and greater than 0.6 to severe AR (see Table 18–3).[7]

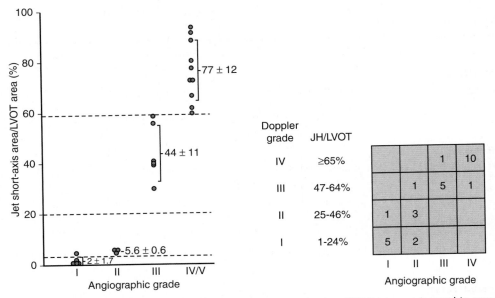

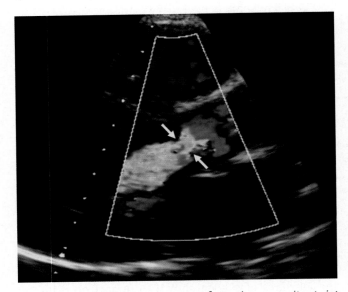

Figure 18–18. *Poor correlation of length of aortic regurgitation (AR) jet to angiographic assessment of AR compared to AR proximal jet width (left). Comparison of Doppler and angiographic grades based on jet height (JH) to left ventricular outflow tract (LVOT) diameter (right). (Adapted from Perry GJ, Helmcke F, Nanda NC, et al:* J Am Coll Cardiol 9:952-999, 1987.)

Figure 18–19. *Vena contracta of aortic regurgitant jet (arrows).*

Proximal Flow Convergence or PISA Method

Studies have demonstrated feasibility and accuracy applying the PISA method to quantitating AR.[66-68] The PISA region is imaged ideally in apical or right parasternal views. The Nyquist limit should be shifted in the direction of the AR jet to optimize measurement of the PISA radius. The peak flow rate is calculated as $2\pi r^2$ multiplied by the aliasing velocity.

The EROA is obtained by dividing the peak AR flow rate by the peak instantaneous AR velocity obtained by CW Doppler. The regurgitant volume is calculated from the EROA by multiplying by, the VTI of the AR jet.

Application of the PISA method to AR has been less used than in MR because of the smaller PISA region and difficulty in parallel alignment of the Doppler beam in parasternal windows. In addition, the PISA region can be obscured by the aortic leaflets, especially if the leaflets are calcified. An AR regurgitant volume of less than 30 mL/beat or EROA of less than 0.10 cm² is consistent with mild AR. An AR regurgitant volume of greater than 60 mL or EROA of greater than 0.30 cm² are consistent with severe AR[7] (see Table 18–3).

Volumetric Methods Using Pulsed Doppler

The aortic regurgitant volume can be estimated using two-dimensional (2D) and pulsed Doppler methods. The aortic regurgitant volume is calculated as mitral inflow minus aortic outflow. Mitral inflow is calculated as VTI of mitral inflow multiplied by the mitral annular area, assuming there is no more than mild MR; otherwise flow across the pulmonary valve can be used. Mitral annular area is calculated as $\pi(d/2)^2$, in which d is the diameter of the mitral annulus measured in the apical four-chamber view in mid-diastole. The mitral annular area can also be assumed to be elliptical in which case, the area is calculated as

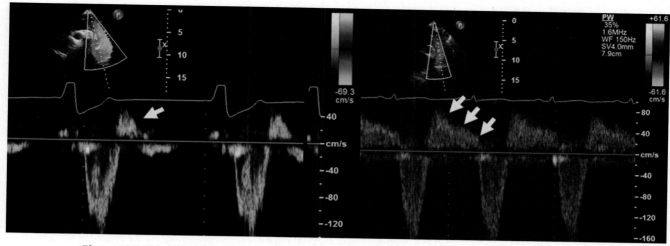

Figure 18–20. Brief diastolic flow in normal patient (arrow) (left). Pandiastolic flow reversal in descending thoracic aorta with severe aortic regurgitation (arrows) (right).

πab, in which *a* is half of the diameter in the apical four-chamber view, and *b* is half of the diameter in the apical two-chamber view. Aortic inflow is calculated as VTI of LVOT inflow multiplied by the LVOT area. The LVOT area is calculated as $\pi(LVOT\ diameter/2)^2$.

Supportive Evidence in the Assessment of Aortic Regurgitation

Flow Reversal in Aorta

The presence of diastolic flow reversal in the aorta provides physiologic evidence of significant AR. As the AR volume increases, there is retrograde flow into the left ventricle across the aortic valve resulting in diastolic flow in the aorta. The presence of pandiastolic flow reversal in the aorta is an indication of moderate or greater AR. It is important that the diastolic flow reversal occurs throughout most of diastole because there can be brief early diastolic flow in the ascending and descending aorta resulting from elastic recoil in a normal aortic Doppler pattern, especially in young children and adults (Fig. 18–20). Pandiastolic flow reversal appears to be most specific for significant AR in the descending aorta either in the abdominal aortic (Fig. 18–21) or descending thoracic aorta.[69-72] In a small series, the presence of diastolic flow reversal with an end-diastolic velocity of at least 32 cm/s correlated well with the presence of severe AR compared to cardiac magnetic resonance imaging (MRI).[69] In addition, calculation of regurgitant fraction based on the ratio of reversed to forward velocity time integrals in the proximal descending aorta has been proposed for measurement of AR severity.[69,73,74]

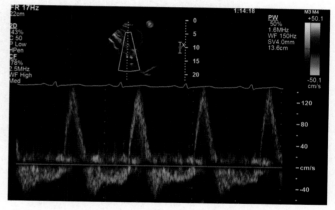

Figure 18–21. Pandiastolic flow reversal in the abdominal aorta consistent with severe aortic regurgitation.

Aortic Deceleration Time (Pressure Half-Time)

The rate of deceleration of the AR jet in diastole provides supportive evidence in assessing AR degree.[75-79] Patients with severe AR will have a shorter rate of decay of pressure resulting from the rapid rise in left ventricular end-diastolic pressure (LVEDP) and decrease in aortic diastolic flow compared to patients with lesser degrees of AR. The rate of pressure decay is measured by determining the pressure half time (PHT) and is obtained by determining the time it takes for the aortic diastolic pressure to decrease by one-half (Fig. 18–22). PHT less than 200 m/s are consistent with severe AR, whereas PHT of greater than 500 m/s are generally associated with mild AR. The PHT has been demonstrated to correlate reasonably well with correlation coefficients ranging from 0.85 to 0.91 with angiographic grading or experimental models of AR.[75,78,79] PHT assessment is less reliable in the setting of chronic AR in which the

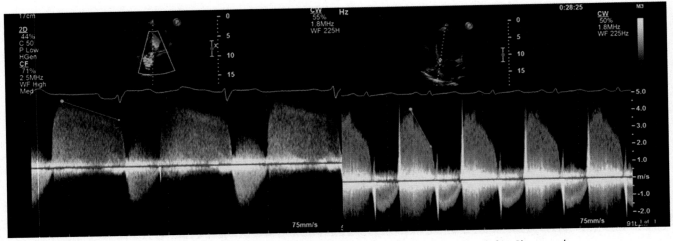

Figure 18–22. *Pressure half time in patient with mild aortic regurgitation* (left). *Shortened pressure half time in severe aortic regurgitation* (right).

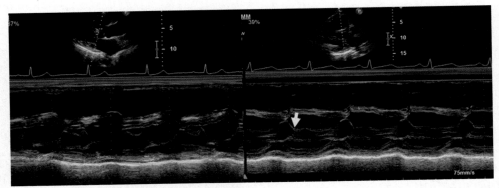

Figure 18–23. *M-mode recording showing normal closure of mitral valve* (left). *Premature closure of mitral valve before the end of diastole* (arrow) *with severe aortic regurgitation* (right).

left ventricle has been able to adapt to the chronic volume load.[76,80,81] Conditions, which influence LV chamber compliance, will affect PHT, lessening the usefulness of PHT as a specific and reliable indicator of AR severity.[80] In addition, PHT can underestimate AR in which LVEDP is elevated as a result of concurrent conditions, such as LV systolic dysfunction. The use of PHT may be best in acute AR, before changes in LV compliance occur with chronic volume load.

Other Supportive Factors

Abnormal valve morphology, such as the presence of vegetations or prolapse, is often associated with significant AR. The presence of a dilated aortic root with incomplete closure of the aortic cusps are signs of functional AR.[82] LV chamber enlargement and LV hypertrophy provide confirmatory evidence of significant AR but are not specific because they are also present in a number of other cardiac conditions. Premature mitral valve closure in which the mitral leaflets close during diastole, before ventricular systole, is a result of the rapid rise in LV diastolic pressures from the aortic regurgitant volume. This rapid rise in LV diastolic pressures results in closure of the mitral leaflets and is indicative of acute severe AR. Premature

mitral valve closure is best demonstrated by M-mode because the greater temporal resolution with M-mode compared to two-dimensional imaging allows delineation of the early closure of the valve[83,84] (Fig. 18–23). When the AR jet is directed eccentrically toward the anterior mitral leaflet, superior bowing deformity of the anterior leaflet can occur and often is a sign of moderate or greater AR.[85,86]

Tricuspid Regurgitation

As with left-sided regurgitant lesions, tricuspid regurgitation (TR) is assessed primarily with color Doppler techniques. Quantification of TR has been less well characterized than left-sided regurgitation resulting from the lack of a gold standard.

Color Doppler Methods

Jet Area Methods

The most common method of quantifying TR is to measure the distal TR jet area[87-89] (Fig. 18–24). The TR jet area must be taken to include only the turbulent por-

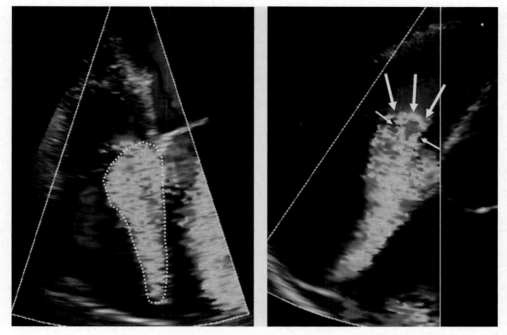

Figure 18–24. *Tricuspid regurgitation assessed by distal jet area* (dashed line) (left). *Proximal isovelocity surface area* (large arrows) *and vena contracta* (small arrows) *of proximal tricuspid regurgitant jet* (right).

tions of the jet or right atrial blood pool will be included and overestimate the overall degree of TR. In rare circumstances in which there is little gradient between the RV and RA, the TR flow may actually appear laminar.

The distal jet area ratio is influenced by physiologic conditions and machine settings. As with other valvular regurgitation, eccentric jets may underestimate the full extent of the distal TR jet resulting from wall confinement and the Coandă effect. Distal TR jet area should be ideally assessed with central jets. The

TR jet area for assessment of severity has been validated against angiographic criteria and clinical criteria with reasonable correlations.[88,90-92] TR jet length has also been proposed as a measurement of regurgitant severity with reasonable correlation with angiography.[93] Although normalization for right atrial size has not been demonstrated to improve reproducibility or accuracy in assessing TR degree,[92] a TR area less than 5 cm^2 is consistent with mild TR. A TR area greater than 10 cm^2 is consistent with severe TR (Fig. 18–25 and Table 18–4).[7]

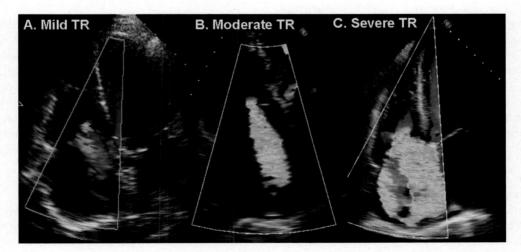

Figure 18–25. *Increasing degrees of tricuspid regurgitation from mild* (A), *moderate* (B), *and severe* (C) *as assessed by jet area method. TR, tricuspid regurgitation.*

TABLE 18–4. Echocardiographic and Doppler Parameters Used in Grading Tricuspid Regurgitation Severity

Parameter	Mild	Moderate	Severe
Tricuspid valve	Usually normal	Normal or abnormal	Abnormal/flail leaflet/poor coaptation
RV/RA/IVC size	Normal*	Normal or dilated	Usually dilated†
Jet area—central jets (cm²)‡	<5	5-10	>10
VC width (cm)§	Not defined	Not defined, but <0.7	>0.7
PISA radius (cm)¶	≤0.5	0.6-0.9	>0.9
Jet density and contour—CW	Soft and parabolic	Dense, variable contour	Dense, triangular with early peaking
Hepatic vein flow**	Systolic dominance	Systolic blunting	Systolic reversal

*Unless there are other reasons for RA or RV dilation, Normal two-dimensional measurements from the apical four-chamber view: right ventricle medio-lateral end-diastolic dimension ≤4.3 cm; right ventricle end-diastolic area ≤35.5 cm², maximal right atrium medio-lateral and supero-inferior dimensions ≤4.6 cm and 4.9 cm, respectively; maximal right atrium volume ≤33 mL/m².
†Exception: acute tricuspid regurgitation.
‡At a Nyquist limit of 50-60 cm/s. Not valid in eccentric jets. Jet area is not recommended as the sole parameter of tricuspid regurgitation severity as a result of its dependence on hemodynamic and technical factors.
§At a Nyquist limit of 50-60 cm/s.
¶Baseline shift with Nyquist limit of 28 cm/s.
**Other conditions may cause systolic blunting (e.g., atrial fibrillation, elevated right atrium pressure).
CW, continuous wave Doppler; IVC, inferior vena cava; PISA, proximal isovelocity surface area; RA, right atrium; RV, right ventricle; VC, vena contracta width.
Data from Zoghbi WA, Enriquez-Sarano M, Foster E, et al: *J Am Soc Echocardiogr* 16:777-802, 2003.

Proximal Jet Geometry

The VC of the proximal jet is a simple measurement that can be performed to assess TR degree (see Fig. 18-24). The VC is measured in the apical windows with depth and sector optimized for color Doppler resolution. A VC greater than 6.5 mm identified severe TR with specificity of 93% and sensitivity of 89%. There is a large degree of overlap of VCs corresponding to mild to moderate TR, which limits its clinical utility in these ranges.[92,94]

The PISA method has been applied to TR with studies demonstrating comparable efficacy to other Doppler methods, such as jet area and VC.[88,90,95] Practically, PISA is not widely applied to TR as the experience and validation has been less than with left-sided valve regurgitation. Table 18-5 summarizes validation studies of TR distal jet area, VC, and PISA methods.

Supportive Evidence in the Assessment of Tricuspid Regurgitation

Hepatic Vein Systolic Flow Reversal

In patients in sinus rhythm, hepatic vein systolic flow reversal provides physiological evidence of severe TR,[96-98] because the tricuspid regurgitant volume is large enough to result in systolic flow reversal into the inferior cava and hepatic veins (Fig. 18-26). Hepatic vein flow is recorded from the subcostal window using pulsed Doppler with the sample volume positioned in the central hepatic vein. Care is needed to ensure a stable sampling position with respiration. Some studies have also proposed a ratio of forward to reverse hepatic vein flow to quantitate TR severity.[96,98] The presence of flow reversal shows an 80% sensitivity of severe TR. Another study has shown a positive predictive value of 91% and a negative predictive value of 78%.[91] In settings where the compliance of the right atrium is abnormal or in patients who are not in sinus rhythm, hepatic vein systolic flow reversal can occur without significant tricuspid regurgitation.

Right-Sided Chamber Enlargement

Right-sided chamber enlargement provides supportive evidence of significant TR, although it is not a specific sign. Abnormalities in valve morphology, such as vegetations or flail portions, can also provide clues to the severity of TR. In addition, the presence of incomplete closure of the tricuspid valve in which the coaptation line occurs above the annular plane by 1 cm or greater suggests the presence of significant TR.[99,100] Inferior vena cava or hepatic vein dilation are also associated with severe TR.

Continuous Wave Doppler

With severe TR in which there is rapid equilibration of pressures across the tricuspid valve, the CW Doppler profile loses its normal parabolic shape becoming more V shaped as the TR Doppler signal falls more rapidly in the latter half of systole[101] (Fig. 18-27).

TABLE 18–5. Summary of Methods for Doppler Evaluation of Tricuspid Valve Regurgitation

			Tricuspid Regurgitation			
Author	**Method**	**Comparison Standard**	**Result**	**N**	**Date**	**Journal**
Tunon and colleagues[89]	Jet area Right atrial area	Angiography	r = 0.924 (combined)	35	1994	*Eur Heart Journal*
Mugge and colleagues[87]	Jet length Jet area Regurgitant Index	Thermodilution	<5 cm² JA (78% sens) (700% spec) mild TR >10% (92% sens) (91% spec) moderate TR 5-10 (89 sens) severe TR No change with RAD	40	1990	*Am J Cardiol*
Gonzalez-Vilchez and colleagues[92]	Jet area	Angiography	r = 0.80 Severe TR (jet area > 10 cm²) Sens 92%, Spec 91% Mild TR (jet area < 5 cm²) Sens 78%, Spec 100%	54	1994	*Int J of Cardiology*
Tribouilloy and colleagues[66]	VC	PISA Hep flow reversal	VC > 6.5 (89% sens) (94% spec) severe TR	71	1998	*J Am Coll Cardiology*
Rivera and colleagues[94]	VC	Pulsed Doppler	r = 0.75 (Q) r = 0.74 (ROA)	40	1994	*Am Heart Journal*
Rivera and colleagues[95]	PISA	Pulsed-Doppler volumetric method	r = 0.95 (RV) r = 0.96 (Q)	45	1996	*Am Heart Journal*

Hep, hepatic; PISA, proximal isovelocity surface area; Q, volume flow rate; r, correlation coefficient; ROA, regurgitant orifice area; RV, regurgitant volume; sens, sensitivity; spec, specificity; TR, tricuspid regurgitation; VC, vena contracta.
Data from references 66, 87, 89, 92, 94, 95.

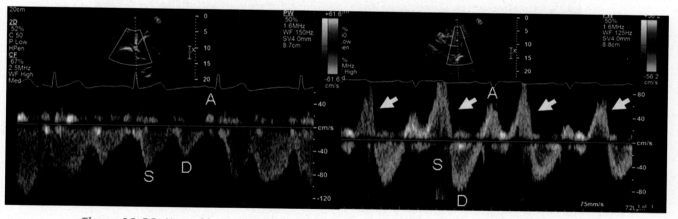

Figure 18–26. *Normal hepatic Doppler pattern* (left). *Systolic flow reversal in the hepatic vein (arrows) with severe tricuspid regurgitation* (right). *A, atrial contraction; D, diastolic wave; S, systolic wave.*

Pulmonary Regurgitation

There is less data available on quantification of pulmonary valve regurgitation compared to the other cardiac valves. This most likely reflects the lesser clinical impact of pulmonary regurgitation (PR) in adults. However, pulmonary regurgitation is increasingly becoming more important, especially in repaired congenital heart disease. Pulmonary regurgitation is primarily assessed in a qualitative manner using color Doppler techniques. The pulmonary regurgitant jet is typically low velocity flow, without aliasing, as the gradient across the pulmonic valve in diastole is low. In clinical practice, pulmonary regurgitation is assessed in a qualitative manner using color Doppler.

The pulmonary regurgitant jet length is commonly used as a measure of PR with a length of 10 mm or less

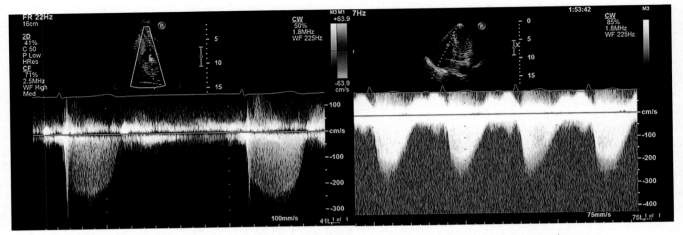

Figure 18–27. Typical parabolic continuous wave pattern of tricuspid regurgitant jet. With severe tricuspid regurgitation in which there is rapid equilibration of pressures across the valve, the tricuspid regurgitant pattern appears more V shaped.

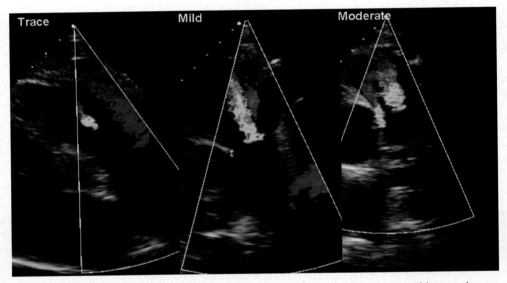

Figure 18–28. Increasing degrees of pulmonary regurgitation from trace to mild to moderate.

beyond the pulmonary annulus considered to be trace. The proximal jet width is probably a more reliable method for determining PR degree.[102] Figure 18–28 displays color Doppler patterns for trace to moderate degrees of pulmonary regurgitation. Severe PR is often best demonstrated by pulsed-wave Doppler in which there is rapid deceleration of the slope of the pulmonary regurgitation Doppler profile and often laminar flow is present because of nonobstructed pulmonary regurgitant flow (Fig. 18–29). In lesser degrees of PR, the spectral Doppler pattern is turbulent, reflecting disorganized velocities across the valve. Table 18–6[7] summarizes echocardiographic criteria corresponding to the degrees of pulmonary regurgitation.

Supportive evidence, such as an enlarged right ventricular outflow tract and morphology of the pulmonary leaflets, should also be included in the overall assessment of pulmonary regurgitation. Qualita-tive Doppler assessment of PR has been directly compared with pulmonary regurgitant function calculated by cardiac MRI. Doppler-derived pulmonary regurgitation index and color Doppler width of the pulmonary regurgitant jet had correlations with pulmonary regurgitant fractions from cardiac MRI of 0.82 and 0.72, respectively.[103] PHT of the pulmonary regurgitant gradient by CW Doppler has been proposed as a measure of PR severity with a cutoff value of less than 100 msec corresponding to a regurgitant fraction of at least 20% as measured by cardiac MRI.[104] In addition, the pulmonary regurgitant fraction can be measured by subtracting the forward flow across the pulmonary artery from the total net flow (forward and reverse).[105] Although validated with hemodynamic data, regurgitant fraction calculated by Doppler showed significant overlap between groups based on regurgitant severity.

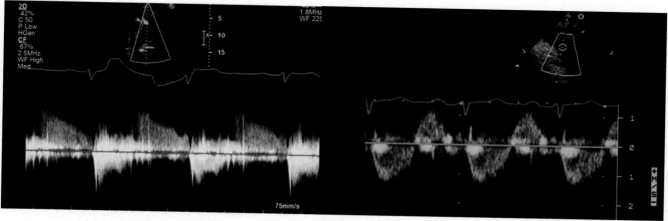

Figure 18–29. Turbulent flow pattern present in moderate or less PR (left). Rapid deceleration and laminar diastolic flow consistent with severe PR (right).

TABLE 18–6. Echocardiographic and Doppler Parameters Used in Grading Pulmonary Regurgitation Severity

Parameter	Mild	Moderate	Severe
Pulmonic valve	Normal	Normal or abnormal	Abnormal
RV size	Normal*	Normal or dilated	Dilated
Jet size by color Doppler‡	Thin (usually <10 mm in length) with a narrow origin	Intermediate	Usually large, with a wide origin; may be brief in duration
Jet density and deceleration rate—CW¶	Soft; slow deceleration	Dense; variable deceleration	Dense; steep deceleration; early termination of diastolic flow
Pulmonic systolic flow compared to systemic flow—PW§	Slightly increased	Intermediate	Greatly increased

*Unless there are other reasons for right ventricle enlargement. Normal two-dimensional measurements from the apical four-chamber view: right ventricle medio-lateral end-diastolic dimension ≤4.3 cm; right ventricle end-diastolic area ≤35.5 cm².
†Exception: acute PR.
‡At a Nyquist limit of 50-60 cm/s.
§Cutoff values for regurgitant volume and fraction are not well validated.
¶Steep deceleration is not specific for severe pulmonic regurgitation.
CW, continuous-wave Doppler; PR, pulmonic regurgitation; PW, pulse wave Doppler; RF, regurgitant fraction; RV, right ventricle.
Data from Zoghbi WA, Enriquez-Sarano M, Foster E, et al: *J Am Soc Echocardiogr* 16:777-802, 2003.

KEY POINTS

■ The assessment of MR is performed in an integrative manner, taking into account Doppler methods and supportive evidence.

■ Distal jet area and VC methods provide semi-quantitative methods for assessing MR.

■ With eccentric MR, jet area methods may underestimate MR degree resulting from wall impingement.

■ MR severity is measured by calculating ROA, RV, and RF using PISA or volumetric methods, when technically possible in moderate or greater degrees of MR.

■ Pulmonary venous systolic flow reversal Doppler pattern provides additional evidence of MR severity.

■ Supportive evidence, including left atrial and LV chamber enlargement, elevated pulmonary pressures, and peak mitral E wave velocity, are included in the overall assessment of MR.

■ AR is assessed in an integrative manner, taking into account Doppler methods and supportive evidence.

■ Color Doppler assessment of AR is based primarily on the proximal jet, measured in the LVOT adjacent to the plane of the aortic leaflets and normalized to LVOT width.

■ Use of aortic regurgitant jet length or area should be avoided.

■ Pandiastolic flow reversal in the descending aorta provides confirmatory evidence of moderate to severe AR.

■ PHT is most specific in acute AR. In chronic AR, with left ventricular remodeling and a change in compliance, the PHT is not as specific a measure of AR severity.

■ Supportive evidence, such as LV chamber enlargement and premature mitral leaflet closure, should be included in the overall assessment of AR.

■ In clinical practice, distal jet area and VC methods are most commonly used to assess TR degree.

■ In addition to color Doppler methods, it is important to include valve morphology, hepatic vein flow profile, CW Doppler profile, and right-sided chamber enlargement in the overall TR assessment.

■ PR is primarily assessed qualitatively using the width of the proximal pulmonary regurgitant jet and the spectral Doppler flow signal.

■ Severe PR has a rapid deceleration slope and laminar Doppler profile.

REFERENCES

1. Roberts BJ, Grayburn PA: Color flow imaging of the vena contracta in mitral regurgitation: technical considerations. *J Am Soc Echocardiogr* 16:1002-1006, 2003.
2. Yoganathan AP, Cape EG, Sung HW, et al: Review of hydrodynamic principles for the cardiologist: Applications to the study of blood flow and jets by imaging techniques. *J Am Coll Cardiol* 12:1344-1353, 1988.
3. Miyatake K, Izumi S, Okamoto M, et al: Semiquantitative grading of severity of mitral regurgitation by real-time two-dimensional Doppler flow imaging technique. *J Am Coll Cardiol* 7:82-88, 1986.
4. Omoto R, Yokote Y, Takamoto S, et al: The development of real-time two-dimensional Doppler echocardiography and its clinical significance in acquired valvular diseases. With special reference to the evaluation of valvular regurgitation. *Jpn Heart J* 25:325-340, 1984.
4a. Omoto R, Kyo S, Matsumura M, et al: Evaluation of biplane color Doppler transesophageal echocardiography in 200 consecutive patients. *Circulation* (85)4:1237-1247, 1992.
4b. Castello RP, Lenzen P, Aguirre F, Labovitz AJ: Quantitation of mitral regurgitation by transesophageal echocardiography with Doppler color flow mapping: correlation with cardiac catheterization. *J Am Coll Cardiol* 19(7):1516-1521, 1992.
5. Chen CG, Thomas JD, Anconina J, et al: Impact of impinging wall jet on color Doppler quantification of mitral regurgitation. *Circulation* 84:712-720, 1991.
6. Enriquez-Sarano M, Tajik AJ, Bailey KR, Seward JB: Color flow imaging compared with quantitative Doppler assessment of severity of mitral regurgitation: influence of eccentricity of jet and mechanism of regurgitation. *J Am Coll Cardiol* 21:1211-1219, 1993.
7. Zoghbi WA, Enriquez-Sarano M, Foster E, et al: Recommendations for evaluation of the severity of native valvular regurgitation with two-dimensional and Doppler echocardiography. *J Am Soc Echocardiogr* 16:777-802, 2003.
8. Hoit BD, Jones M, Eidbo EE, et al: Sources of variability for Doppler color flow mapping of regurgitant jets in an animal model of mitral regurgitation. *J Am Coll Cardiol* 13:1631-1636, 1989.
9. Maciel BC, Moises VA, Shandas R, et al: Effects of pressure and volume of the receiving chamber on the spatial distribution of regurgitant jets as imaged by color Doppler flow mapping. An in vitro study. *Circulation* 83:605-613, 1991.
10. Yellin EL, Yoran C, Sonnenblick EH, et al: Dynamic changes in the canine mitral regurgitant orifice area during ventricular ejection. *Circ Res* 45:677-683, 1979.
11. Rivera JM, Mele D, Vandervoort PM, et al: Physical factors determining mitral regurgitation jet area. *Am J Cardiol* 74:515-516, 1994.
12. Simpson IA, Valdes-Cruz LM, Sahn DJ, et al: Doppler color flow mapping of simulated in vitro regurgitant jets: evaluation of the effects of orifice size and hemodynamic variables. *J Am Coll Cardiol* 13:1195-1207, 1989.
13. Helmcke F, Nanda NC, Hsiung MC, et al: Color Doppler assessment of mitral regurgitation with orthogonal planes. *Circulation* 75:175-183, 1987.
14. Spain MG, Smith MD, Grayburn PA, et al: Quantitative assessment of mitral regurgitation by Doppler color flow imaging: Angiographic and hemodynamic correlations. *J Am Coll Cardiol* 13:585-590, 1989.
15. Fehske W, Omran H, Manz M, et al: Color-coded Doppler imaging of the vena contracta as a basis for quantification of pure mitral regurgitation. *Am J Cardiol* 73:268-274, 1994.
16. Baumgartner H, Schima H, Kuhn P: Value and limitations of proximal jet dimensions for the quantitation of valvular regurgitation: An in vitro study using Doppler flow imaging. *J Am Soc Echocardiogr* 4:57-66, 1991.
17. Lesniak-Sobelga A, Olszowska M, Pienazek P, et al: Vena contracta width as a simple method of assessing mitral valve regurgitation. Comparison with Doppler quantitative methods. *J Heart Valve Dis* 13:608-614, 2004.
18. Zhou X, Jones M, Shiota T, et al: Vena contracta imaged by Doppler color flow mapping predicts the severity of eccentric mitral regurgitation better than color jet area: A chronic animal study. *J Am Coll Cardiol* 30:1393-1398, 1997.
19. Grayburn PA, Fehske W, Omran H, et al: Multiplane transesophageal echocardiographic assessment of mitral regurgitation by Doppler color flow mapping of the vena contracta. *Am J Cardiol* 74:912-917, 1994.
20. Hall SA, Brickner ME, Willett DL, et al: Assessment of mitral regurgitation severity by Doppler color flow mapping of the vena contracta. *Circulation* 95:636-642, 1997.
21. Heinle SK, Hall SA, Brickner ME, et al: Comparison of vena contracta width by multiplane transesophageal echocardiography with quantitative Doppler assessment of mitral regurgitation. *Am J Cardiol* 81:175-179, 1998.
21a. Mele D, Vandervoort P, Palacios I, et al: Proximal jet size by Doppler color flow mapping predicts severity of mitral regurgitation. Clinical studies. *Circulation* 91(3):746-754, 1995.
22. Vandervoort PM, Thoreau DH, Rivera JM, et al: Automated flow rate calculations based on digital analysis of flow convergence proximal to regurgitant orifices. *J Am Coll Cardiol* 22:535-541, 1993.
23. Recusani F, Bargiggia GS, Yoganathan AP, et al: A new method for quantification of regurgitant flow rate using color Doppler flow imaging of the flow convergence region proximal to a discrete orifice. An in vitro study. *Circulation* 83:594-604, 1991.
24. Bargiggia GS, Tronconi L, Sahn DJ, et al: A new method for quantitation of mitral regurgitation based on color flow Doppler imaging of flow convergence proximal to regurgitant orifice. *Circulation* 84:1481-1489, 1991.
25. Utsunomiya T, Ogawa T, Doshi R, et al: Doppler color flow "proximal isovelocity surface area" method for estimating volume flow rate: Effects of orifice shape and machine factors. *J Am Coll Cardiol* 17:1103-1111, 1991.
26. Rivera JM, Vandervoort PM, Thoreau DH, et al: Quantification of mitral regurgitation with the proximal flow convergence method: A clinical study. *Am Heart J* 124:1289-1296, 1992.
27. Rodriguez L, Anconina J, Flachskampf FA, et al: Impact of finite orifice size on proximal flow convergence. Implications for Dop-

pler quantification of valvular regurgitation. *Circ Res* 70:923-930, 1992.

28. Utsunomiya T, Ogawa T, Tang HA, et al: Doppler color flow mapping of the proximal isovelocity surface area: A new method for measuring volume flow rate across a narrowed orifice. *J Am Soc Echocardiogr* 4:338-348, 1991.

29. Utsunomiya T, Doshi R, Patel D, et al: Calculation of volume flow rate by the proximal isovelocity surface area method: simplified approach using color Doppler zero baseline shift. *J Am Coll Cardiol* 22:277-282, 1993.

30. Enriquez-Sarano M, Miller FA Jr, Hayes SN, et al: Effective mitral regurgitant orifice area: Clinical use and pitfalls of the proximal isovelocity surface area method. *J Am Coll Cardiol* 25:703-709, 1995.

31. Schwammenthal E, Chen C, Giesler M, et al: New method for accurate calculation of regurgitant flow rate based on analysis of Doppler color flow maps of the proximal flow field. Validation in a canine model of mitral regurgitation with initial application in patients. *J Am Coll Cardiol* 27:161-172, 1996.

32. Moises VA, Maciel BC, Hornberger LK, et al: A new method for noninvasive estimation of ventricular septal defect shunt flow by Doppler color flow mapping: imaging of the laminar flow convergence region on the left septal surface. *J Am Coll Cardiol* 18:824-832, 1991.

33. Schwammenthal E, Chen C, Benning F, et al: Dynamics of mitral regurgitant flow and orifice area. Physiologic application of the proximal flow convergence method: Clinical data and experimental testing. *Circulation* 90:307-322, 1994.

34. Enriquez-Sarano M, Sinak LJ, Tajik AJ, et al: Changes in effective regurgitant orifice throughout systole in patients with mitral valve prolapse. A clinical study using the proximal isovelocity surface area method. *Circulation* 92:2951-2958, 1995.

35. Pu M, Vandervoort PM, Griffin BP, et al: Quantification of mitral regurgitation by the proximal convergence method using transesophageal echocardiography. Clinical validation of a geometric correction for proximal flow constraint. *Circulation* 92:2169-2177, 1995.

36. Hopmeyer J, He S, Thorvig KM, et al: Estimation of mitral regurgitation with a hemielliptic curve-fitting algorithm: In vitro experiments with native mitral valves. *J Am Soc Echocardiogr* 11:322-331, 1998.

37. Rokey R, Sterling LL, Zoghbi WA, et al: Determination of regurgitant fraction in isolated mitral or aortic regurgitation by pulsed Doppler two-dimensional echocardiography. *J Am Coll Cardiol* 7:1273-1278, 1986.

38. Blumlein S, Bouchard A, Schiller NB, et al: Quantitation of mitral regurgitation by Doppler echocardiography. *Circulation* 74:306-314, 1986.

39. Tribouilloy C, Shen WF, Slama MA, et al: Non-invasive measurement of the regurgitant fraction by pulsed Doppler echocardiography in isolated pure mitral regurgitation. *Br Heart J* 66:290-294, 1991.

40. Dujardin KS, Enriquez-Sarano M, Bailey KR, et al: Grading of mitral regurgitation by quantitative Doppler echocardiography: calibration by left ventricular angiography in routine clinical practice. *Circulation* 96:3409-3415, 1997.

41. Ascah KJ, Stewart WJ, Jiang L, et al: A Doppler-two-dimensional echocardiographic method for quantitation of mitral regurgitation. *Circulation* 72:377-383, 1985.

41a. Kizilbash AM, Hundley WG, Willett DL, et al: Comparison of quantitative Doppler with magnetic resonance imaging for assessment of the severity of mitral regurgitation. *Am J Cardiol* 81(6):792-795, 1998.

42. Masuyama T, Nagano R, Nariyama K, et al: Transthoracic Doppler echocardiographic measurements of pulmonary venous flow velocity patterns: Comparison with transesophageal measurements. *J Am Soc Echocardiogr* 8:61-69, 1995.

43. Jensen JL, Williams FE, Beilby BJ, et al: Feasibility of obtaining pulmonary venous flow velocity in cardiac patients using transthoracic pulsed wave Doppler technique. *J Am Soc Echocardiogr* 10:60-66, 1997.

44. Keren G, Bier A, Sherez J, et al: Atrial contraction is an important determinant of pulmonary venous flow. *J Am Coll Cardiol* 7:693-695, 1986.

45. Enriquez-Sarano M, Dujardin KS, Tribouilloy CM, et al: Determinants of pulmonary venous flow reversal in mitral regurgitation and its usefulness in determining the severity of regurgitation. *Am J Cardiol* 83:535-541, 1999.

46. Klein AL, Obarski TP, Stewart WJ, et al: Transesophageal Doppler echocardiography of pulmonary venous flow: A new marker of mitral regurgitation severity. *J Am Coll Cardiol* 18:518-526, 1991.

47. Castello R, Pearson AC, Lenzen P, Labovitz AJ: Effect of mitral regurgitation on pulmonary venous velocities derived from transesophageal echocardiography color-guided pulsed Doppler imaging. *J Am Coll Cardiol* 17:1499-1506, 1991.

48. Kamp O, Huitink H, van Eenige MJ, et al: Value of pulmonary venous flow characteristics in the assessment of severity of native mitral valve regurgitation: An angiographic correlated study. *J Am Soc Echocardiogr* 5:239-246, 1992.

49. Appleton CP, Galloway JM, Gonzalez MS, et al: Estimation of left ventricular filling pressures using two-dimensional and Doppler echocardiography in adult patients with cardiac disease. Additional value of analyzing left atrial size, left atrial ejection fraction and the difference in duration of pulmonary venous and mitral flow velocity at atrial contraction. *J Am Coll Cardiol* 22:1972-1982, 1993.

50. Bartzokis T, Lee R, Yeoh TK, et al: Transesophageal echo-Doppler echocardiographic assessment of pulmonary venous flow patterns. *J Am Soc Echocardiogr* 4:457-464, 1991.

51. Pieper EP, Hellemans IM, Hamer HP, et al: Value of systolic pulmonary venous flow reversal and color Doppler jet measurements assessed with transesophageal echocardiography in recognizing severe pure mitral regurgitation. *Am J Cardiol* 78:444-450, 1996.

52. Utsunomiya T, Patel D, Doshi R, et al: Can signal intensity of the continuous wave Doppler regurgitant jet estimate severity of mitral regurgitation? *Am Heart J* 123:166-171, 1992.

53. Jenni R, Ritter M, Eberli F, et al: Quantification of mitral regurgitation with amplitude-weighted mean velocity from continuous wave Doppler spectra. *Circulation* 79:1294-1299, 1989.

54. Godley RW, Wann LS, Rogers EW, et al: Incomplete mitral leaflet closure in patients with papillary muscle dysfunction. *Circulation* 63:565-571, 1981.

55. Otsuji Y, Gilon D, Jiang L, et al: Restricted diastolic opening of the mitral leaflets in patients with left ventricular dysfunction: Evidence for increased valve tethering. *J Am Coll Cardiol* 32:398-404, 1998.

56. Yiu SF, Enriquez-Sarano M, Tribouilloy C, et al: Determinants of the degree of functional mitral regurgitation in patients with systolic left ventricular dysfunction: A quantitative clinical study. *Circulation* 102:1400-1406, 2000.

57. Nesta F, Otsuji Y, Handschumacher MD, et al: Leaflet concavity: a rapid visual clue to the presence and mechanism of functional mitral regurgitation. *J Am Soc Echocardiogr* 16:1301-1308, 2003.

58. Perry GJ, Helmcke F, Nanda NC, et al: Evaluation of aortic insufficiency by Doppler color flow mapping. *J Am Coll Cardiol* 9:952-959, 1987.

59. Dolan MS, Castello R, St Vrain JA, et al: Quantitation of aortic regurgitation by Doppler echocardiography: a practical approach. *Am Heart J* 129:1014-1020, 1995.

60. Willems TP, Steyerberg EW, van Herwerden LA, et al: Reproducibility of color Doppler flow quantification of aortic regurgitation. *J Am Soc Echocardiogr* 10:899-903, 1997.

61. Reimold SC, Thomas JD, Lee RT: Relation between Doppler color flow variables and invasively determined jet variables in patients with aortic regurgitation. *J Am Coll Cardiol* 20:1143-1148, 1992.

62. Smith MD, Grayburn PA, Spain MG, DeMaria AN: Observer variability in the quantitation of Doppler color flow jet areas for mitral and aortic regurgitation. *J Am Coll Cardiol* 11:579-584, 1988.

63. Masuyama T, Kitabatake A, Kodama K, et al: Semiquantitative evaluation of aortic regurgitation by Doppler echocardiography: Effects of associated mitral stenosis. *Am Heart J* 117:133-139, 1989.

64. Thomas JD, Liu CM, Flachskampf FA, et al: Quantification of jet flow by momentum analysis. An in vitro color Doppler flow study. *Circulation* 81:247-259, 1990.

65. Krabill KA, Sung HW, Tamura T, et al: Factors influencing the structure and shape of stenotic and regurgitant jets: An in vitro investigation using Doppler color flow mapping and optical flow visualization. *J Am Coll Cardiol* 13:1672-1681, 1989.

66. Tribouilloy CM, Enriquez-Sarano M, Fett SL, et al: Application of the proximal flow convergence method to calculate the effective regurgitant orifice area in aortic regurgitation. *J Am Coll Cardiol* 32:1032-1039, 1998.

67. Sato Y, Kawazoe K, Kamata J, et al: Clinical usefulness of the effective regurgitant orifice area determined by transesophageal echocardiography in patients with eccentric aortic regurgitation. *J Heart Valve Dis* 6:580-586, 1997.

68. Sato Y, Kawazoe K, Nasu M, Hiramori K: Clinical usefulness of the proximal isovelocity surface area method using echocardiography in patients with eccentric aortic regurgitation. *J Heart Valve Dis* 8:104-111, 1999.

69. Reimold SC, Maier SE, Aggarwal K, et al: Aortic flow velocity patterns in chronic aortic regurgitation: Implications for Doppler echocardiography. *J Am Soc Echocardiogr* 9:675-683, 1996.

70. Diebold B, Peronneau P, Blanchard D, et al: Non-invasive quantification of aortic regurgitation by Doppler echocardiography. *Br Heart J* 49:167-173, 1983.

71. Takenaka K, Dabestani A, Gardin JM, et al: A simple Doppler echocardiographic method for estimating severity of aortic regurgitation. *Am J Cardiol* 57:1340-1343, 1986.

72. Sutton DC, Kluger R, Ahmed SU, et al: Flow reversal in the descending aorta: A guide to intraoperative assessment of aortic regurgitation with transesophageal echocardiography. *J Thorac Cardiovasc Surg* 108:576-582, 1994.

73. Touche T, Prasquier R, Nitenberg A, et al: Assessment and follow-up of patients with aortic regurgitation by an updated Doppler echocardiographic measurement of the regurgitant fraction in the aortic arch. *Circulation* 72:819-824, 1985.

74. Tribouilloy C, Avinee P, Shen WF, et al: End diastolic flow velocity just beneath the aortic isthmus assessed by pulsed Doppler echocardiography: A new predictor of the aortic regurgitant fraction. *Br Heart J* 65:37-40, 1991.

75. Teague SM, Heinsimer JA, Anderson JL, et al: Quantification of aortic regurgitation utilizing continuous wave Doppler ultrasound. *J Am Coll Cardiol* 8:592-599, 1986.

76. Padial LR, Oliver A, Vivaldi M, et al: Doppler echocardiographic assessment of progression of aortic regurgitation. *Am J Cardiol* 80:306-314, 1997.

77. Griffin BP, Flachskampf FA, Siu S, et al: The effects of regurgitant orifice size, chamber compliance, and systemic vascular resistance on aortic regurgitant velocity slope and pressure half-time. *Am Heart J* 122:1049-1056, 1991.

78. Labovitz AJ, Ferrara RP, Kern MJ, et al: Quantitative evaluation of aortic insufficiency by continuous wave Doppler echocardiography. *J Am Coll Cardiol* 8:1341-1347, 1986.

79. Beyer RW, Ramirez M, Josephson MA, Shah PM: Correlation of continuous-wave Doppler assessment of chronic aortic regurgitation with hemodynamics and angiography. *Am J Cardiol* 60:852-856, 1987.

80. Griffin BP, Flachskampf FA, Reimold SC, et al: Relationship of aortic regurgitant velocity slope and pressure half-time to severity of aortic regurgitation under changing haemodynamic conditions. *Eur Heart J* 15:681-685, 1994.

81. Ishii M, Jones M, Shiota T, et al: What is the validity of continuous wave Doppler grading of aortic regurgitation severity? A chronic animal model study. *J Am Soc Echocardiogr* 11:332-337, 1998.

82. Movsowitz HD, Levine RA, Hilgenberg AD, Isselbacher EM: Transesophageal echocardiographic description of the mechanisms of aortic regurgitation in acute type A aortic dissection: Implications for aortic valve repair. *J Am Coll Cardiol* 36:884-890, 2000.

83. Ambrose JA, Meller J, Teichholz LE, Herman MV: Premature closure of the mitral valve. Echocardiographic clue for the diagnosis of aortic dissection. *Chest* 73:121-123, 1978.

84. Pridie RB, Benham R, Oakley CM: Echocardiography of the mitral valve in aortic valve disease. *Br Heart J* 33:296-304, 1971.

85. Trappe HJ, Daniel WG, Frank G, Lichtlen PR: Comparisons between diastolic fluttering and reverse doming of anterior mitral leaflet in aortic regurgitation. *Am Heart J* 114:1399-1406, 1987.

86. Robertson WS, Stewart J, Armstrong WF, et al: Reverse doming of the anterior mitral leaflet with severe aortic regurgitation. *J Am Coll Cardiol* 3:431-436, 1984.

87. Mugge A, Daniel WG, Herrmann G, et al: Quantification of tricuspid regurgitation by Doppler color flow mapping after cardiac transplantation. *Am J Cardiol* 66:884-887, 1990.

88. Grossmann G, Stein M, Kochs M, et al: Comparison of the proximal flow convergence method and the jet area method for the assessment of the severity of tricuspid regurgitation. *Eur Heart J* 19:652-659, 1998.

89. Tunon J, Cordoba M, Rey M, et al: Assessment of chronic tricuspid regurgitation by colour Doppler echocardiography: A comparison with angiography in the catheterization room. *Eur Heart J* 15:1074-1084, 1994.

90. Tribouilloy CM, Enriquez-Sarano M, Bailey KR, et al: Quantification of tricuspid regurgitation by measuring the width of the vena contracta with Doppler color flow imaging: A clinical study. *J Am Coll Cardiol* 36:472-478, 2000.

91. Shapira Y, Porter A, Wurzel M, et al: Evaluation of tricuspid regurgitation severity: Echocardiographic and clinical correlation. *J Am Soc Echocardiogr* 11:652-659, 1998.

92. Gonzalez-Vilchez F, Zarauza J, Vazquez de Prada JA, et al: Assessment of tricuspid regurgitation by Doppler color flow imaging: angiographic correlation. *Int J Cardiol* 44:275-283, 1994.

93. Miyatake K, Okamoto M, Kinoshita N, et al: Evaluation of tricuspid regurgitation by pulsed Doppler and two-dimensional echocardiography. *Circulation* 66:777-784, 1982.

94. Rivera JM, Mele D, Vandervoort PM, et al: Effective regurgitant orifice area in tricuspid regurgitation: Clinical implementation and follow-up study. *Am Heart J* 128:927-933, 1994.

95. Rivera JM, Vandervoort P, Mele D, et al: Value of proximal regurgitant jet size in tricuspid regurgitation. *Am Heart J* 131:742-747, 1996.

96. Diebold B, Touati R, Blanchard D, et al: Quantitative assessment of tricuspid regurgitation using pulsed Doppler echocardiography. *Br Heart J* 50:443-449, 1998.

97. Zema MJ, Caccavano M: Two dimensional echocardiographic assessment of aortic valve morphology: feasibility of bicuspid valve detection. Prospective study of 100 adult patients. *Br Heart J* 48:428-433, 1982.

98. Sakai K, Nakamura K, Satomi G, et al: Hepatic vein blood flow pattern measured by Doppler echocardiography as an evalua-

tion of tricuspid valve insufficiency. *J Cardiogr* 13:33-43, 1983.

99. Gibson TC, Foale RA, Guyer DE, Weyman AE: Clinical significance of incomplete tricuspid valve closure seen on two-dimensional echocardiography. *J Am Coll Cardiol* 4:1052-1057, 1984.

100. Sagie A, Schwammenthal E, Padial LR, et al: Determinants of functional tricuspid regurgitation in incomplete tricuspid valve closure: Doppler color flow study of 109 patients. *J Am Coll Cardiol* 24:446-453, 1994.

101. Gupta M, Sasson Z: The Mechanisms and Importance of Tricuspid Regurgitation and Hepatic Pulsations in Dilated Cardiomyopathy: A Review. *Echocardiography* 8:195-206, 1991.

102. Zoghbi WA, Farmer KL, Soto JG, et al: Accurate noninvasive quantification of stenotic aortic valve area by Doppler echocardiography. *Circulation* 73:452-459, 1986.

103. Li W, Davlouros PA, Kilner PJ, et al: Doppler-echocardiographic assessment of pulmonary regurgitation in adults with repaired tetralogy of Fallot: Comparison with cardiovascular magnetic resonance imaging. *Am Heart J* 147:165-172, 2004.

104. Silversides CK, Veldtman GR, Crossin J, et al: Pressure half-time predicts hemodynamically significant pulmonary regurgitation in adult patients with repaired tetralogy of fallot. *J Am Soc Echocardiogr* 16:1057-1062, 2003.

105. Goldberg SJ, Allen HD: Quantitative assessment by Doppler echocardiography of pulmonary or aortic regurgitation. *Am J Cardiol* 56:131-135, 1985.

Chapter 19

Timing of Intervention for Chronic Valve Regurgitation: The Role of Echocardiography

CATHERINE M. OTTO, MD

The timing of intervention to correct valve dysfunction remains controversial in patients with chronic aortic regurgitation (AR) or mitral regurgitation (MR). In patients with symptoms resulting from severe regurgitation and a low anticipated surgical risk, all agree that intervention is appropriate.[1] However, there is less agreement about management of asymptomatic patients with severe regurgitation, symptomatic patients with comorbid conditions or only moderate regurgitation, and patients with a higher expected surgical risk.[2-4]

Key Factors in Clinical Decision Making

Decision making in patients with chronic valve regurgitation is based on integration of several types of clinical data. In the decision-making process, the risks and benefits of intervention are balanced against the risks and benefits of watchful waiting. The balance is shifted toward intervention when disease is more severe, the risk of intervention is low, and long-term outcome data show a benefit of intervention compared to medical therapy. Conversely, the balance is shifted toward watchful waiting when the disease is well tolerated in terms of symptoms and physiology; intervention requires use of a prosthetic valve; or when outcomes are equally good with or without intervention.

The key factors in decision making can be divided into four groups: valve factors, patient factors, intervention choices, and long-term outcomes with and without intervention (Table 19–1). This chapter will focus on echocardiographic evaluation of the valve factors including the morphology of the valve and supporting structures, regurgitant severity, and the left ventricular (LV) response to chronic volume overload.

In clinical practice, echocardiographic evaluation is only one component of patient evaluation. The first step in decision making in patients with valvular heart disease is assessment of symptom status. Symptoms resulting from valve regurgitation are an accepted indication for intervention. In fact, symptoms are the primary indication for intervention in over 75% of patients with chronic AR and the majority of patients with MR. Patient comorbidities also are an important consideration because surgical risk depends more on comorbid conditions, such as pulmonary, renal or hepatic dysfunction, than on age or gender per se.[5] Surgery might be appropriate earlier in the disease course in an otherwise healthy patient with a low operative risk, whereas surgery might be deferred until there are definite symptoms or signs of ventricular dysfunction

in a patient at high surgical risk. Patient preference also contributes to the decision-making process. When patients are educated and informed about the risks and benefits of intervention, some prefer to accept the risks of surgery and undergo intervention early in the disease course, whereas others prefer to defer surgery until absolutely necessary.

The options for intervention clearly impact decision making. When the only choice for relief of valve regurgitation is surgical implantation of a prosthetic valve, the threshold for intervention is high. In addition to operative risk, the balance is shifted toward watchful waiting because of the risks of a prosthetic valve: long-term anticoagulation with a mechanical valve and tissue degeneration with a bioprosthesis. The threshold for intervention for chronic MR has been lowered by the availability of mitral valve repair, which has a lower operative mortality and better short- and long-term outcomes compared to mitral valve replacement. The threshold may be lowered even more if percutaneous approaches to MR are successful.[6-10] However, this shift has not occurred for AR because most patients still require a prosthetic valve.

The foundation for an evidence-based approach to management of patients with chronic valve regurgitation is an accurate understanding of the clinical outcomes with and without intervention in equivalent patient groups. Unfortunately, our knowledge base currently has large gaps. There are only a few prospective studies on the natural history of chronic AR and MR, with the endpoint being surgical intervention or cardiovascular death. Instead, published data primarily consist of surgical studies that compare symptom severity and ventricular function before and after surgical intervention or compare long-term survival after different surgical procedures, albeit rarely in a randomized study design. Most of the data focuses on survival, complications and LV function with little data on functional status or quality of life. However, even in the absence of ideal data, the available outcome data have been analyzed, in conjunction with expert opinion, to develop recommendations for management of patients with chronic valvular regurgitation.[1,11]

TABLE 19–1. Factors Important in Making Decisions about the Timing of Surgical Intervention for Chronic Left-Sided Valve Regurgitation

Valve Factors
Cause of regurgitation
Severity of regurgitation
Left ventricular dilation and systolic dysfunction
Pulmonary hypertension
Atrial fibrillation

Patient Factors
Symptoms
Comorbidities
Patient preferences

Interventions Available
Medical therapy
Percutaneous intervention
Surgical repair
Bioprosthetic valve
Mechanical prosthesis

Outcomes
Operative mortality and morbidity
Long-term survival
Quality of life
Functional status and exercise tolerance
Complications of the disease process or intervention

Pathophysiology of Chronic Valve Regurgitation

Valve Hemodynamics

Valve regurgitation may result from disruption or a defect in the valve tissue or from inadequate valve closure. Examples of primary valve tissue defects include leaflet perforation resulting from endocarditis or chordal rupture resulting from myxomatous valve disease. Valve closure can be impaired with normal valve anatomy, if the supporting structures are enlarged or dis-

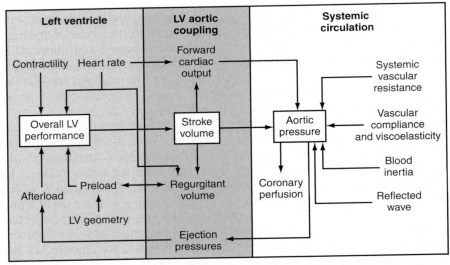

Figure 19–1. *Physiologic framework for understanding the pathophysiology of chronic aortic regurgitation. LV, left ventricular. (Modified from Borow KM, Marcus RH: J Am Coll Cardiol 17:898-900, 1991.)*

torted so the leaflets no longer meet when closed. Examples of abnormal valve closure include AR resulting from dilation of the aortic sinuses or MR resulting from LV dysfunction.

The amount of backflow across a regurgitant valve depends on a complex interaction between the size of the regurgitant orifice and the pressures in the chambers on both sides of the valve.[12] With AR, regurgitant severity depends on characteristics of the systemic circulation and left ventricle and valve anatomy (Fig. 19–1). With MR, LV function and left atrial impedance affect regurgitation severity. In addition, the extent of inadequate leaflet closure often is dynamic, changing both during a single cardiac cycle—for example with late systolic MR resulting from leaflet prolapse—and with varying physiologic conditions—for example an increase in MR resulting from a higher LV systolic pressure.

The severity of valve regurgitation can be described in several ways. The amount of blood flow retrograde across the valve is called regurgitant volume, and the ratio of this volume to total LV stroke volume (SV) is called regurgitant fraction. The anatomic size of the regurgitant flow stream (regurgitant orifice area [ROA]) also is clinically useful, with the recognition that "orifice area" may be a concept, rather than an anatomic feature of the valve, particularly when anatomy is complex, as with MR in which backflow may occur at multiple sites along the valve closure plane.

Compensated Ventricular Hypertrophy

It is intuitive that chronic valve regurgitation imposes a volume load on the ventricle.

Valve regurgitation results in LV volume overload because the total SV ejected during systole includes both the forward flow, delivered to the systemic vascu-

lature, and the regurgitant flow back into the left ventricle (for AR) or left atrium (for MR). This increase in total SV is achieved by progressive ventricular enlargement or "compensatory" LV dilation when AR is present. With MR, the initial compensatory response is an increase in ejection fraction (EF), with dilation occurring only late in the disease course.[13,14] In addition to volume overload, chronic AR imposes a pressure load on the ventricle with an increase in afterload resulting from ejection of the increased SV into the high resistance aorta[12,15] (Fig. 19–2).

LV mass increases in response to volume and/or pressure overload with an increase in both myocyte mass and the extracellular matrix. Ventricular hypertro-

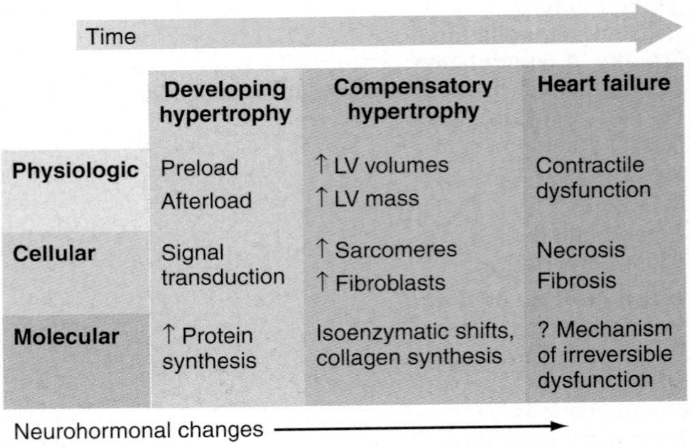

	Developing hypertrophy	Compensatory hypertrophy	Heart failure
Physiologic	Preload Afterload	↑ LV volumes ↑ LV mass	Contractile dysfunction
Cellular	Signal transduction	↑ Sarcomeres ↑ Fibroblasts	Necrosis Fibrosis
Molecular	↑ Protein synthesis	Isoenzymatic shifts, collagen synthesis	? Mechanism of irreversible dysfunction

Time →

Neurohormonal changes →

Figure 19–2. *Stages of the ventricular response to chronic pressure or volume overload resulting from valve regurgitation. There are changes at the physiologic, cellular, and molecular levels during the transition from developing to compensatory hypertrophy and eventual heart failure. Systemic neurohormonal changes parallel these changes in the ventricle. LV, left ventricle.*

phy, defined as an increased LV mass, is associated with differing ventricular geometry, depending on the specific valve lesion. Volume overload tends to result in a dilated chamber with normal wall thickness, termed eccentric hypertrophy: pressure overload typically results in a thick-walled, nondilated chamber, termed concentric hypertrophy. The normal shape of the left ventricle is initially maintained with chronic MR, whereas with AR the apex dilates more than the base, resulting in increased sphericity of the ventricular chamber, even early in the disease course. The typical pressure and volume changes in chronic valve regurgitation are shown in Figure 19–3.

At the cellular level, the volume of individual myocytes increases because mature cardiac myocytes rarely undergo cell division. This increase in cell size occurs with sarcomeres added in series in response to volume overload, resulting in increased length of the myocytes. In contrast, sarcomeres tend to be added in parallel in response to pressure overload, resulting in increased diameter of the myocytes.[16] Changes in the extracellular matrix contribute to the anatomic and physiologic changes seen with chronic ventricular overload.[17] The

interstitial fibers of the myocardium are important in distributing and modulating the force generated by the myocytes. In addition, they limit the maximum passive length of the myocytes.[18,19]

The molecular mechanisms involved in the tissue response to mechanical stretch and ventricular pressure are poorly understood. Potential pathways for signal transduction include the focal adhesion complex that connects the internal cytoskeleton to the extracellular matrix, disruption of the normal cell-cell or cell-extracellular matrix contact, and extracellular matrix kinases.[16] Involvement of more than one or different signalling pathways might explain the different responses to specific valve lesions. The myocyte response then includes changes in production or degradation of myosin heavy chain and re-expression of fetal gene products, including beta-myosin heavy chain and skeletal alpha-actin. The extracellular matrix responds to mechanical stretch with increased fibroblast proliferation and enhanced production of matrix proteins, such as collagen and fibronectin, and alterations in matrix metalloproteinases and their inhibitors.[18-24]

With compensated ventricular hypertrophy in response to chronic valve regurgitation, LV wall stress is maintained in the normal range as the increased myocardial mass "compensates" for the increased ventricular size and pressure (see Chapter 9). With compensated hypertrophy, ventricular contractility and systolic performance are normal, with a normal EF. After surgical intervention, ventricular mass and volume typically return toward normal and ventricular function remains normal.

Transition to Contractile Dysfunction

At some point in the disease course, these compensatory mechanisms fail and contractility decreases. Ventricular decompensation is easily recognized if it coincides with symptom onset or is associated with a fall in EF. However, in a subset of patients, impaired ventricular contractility occurs in the absence of clinical symptoms and with a relatively normal EF. Contractile dysfunction resulting from chronic regurgitation primarily occurs with severe regurgitation, usually in association with significant LV dilation. The mechanisms of the transition to contractile dysfunction are an area of active research.[25] In experimental models and in human studies of aortic stenosis (AS), myocardial microtubule density is increased suggesting contractile dysfunction may be related to excess viscous load on the sarcomeres.[26-29] Aberrant myocardial branching, abnormal beta$_1$-integrin deposition, and loss of the normal attachment between the myocyte and extracellular matrix have also been noted.[30] Clinically, the challenge is to identify the patient at risk of contractile dysfunction so that intervention can be performed before LV dysfunction becomes irreversible.

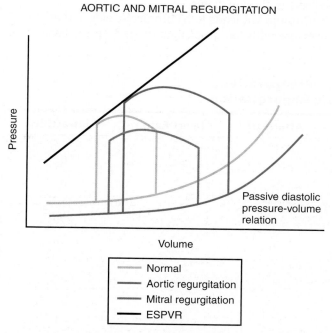

AORTIC AND MITRAL REGURGITATION

Passive diastolic pressure-volume relation

Pressure / Volume

Normal
Aortic regurgitation
Mitral regurgitation
ESPVR

Figure 19–3. *Schematic diagram of pressure volume loops in left ventricular volume overload, compared to normal. With chronic volume overload, the passive diastolic pressure volume relationship is shifted downward and to the right. Ventricular volumes are increased and ejection fraction is normal or increased. The slope of the end-systolic pressure volume relationship (ESPVR) remains normal until a decline in contractility occurs. Note that aortic regurgitation differs from mitral regurgitation in that ventricular volumes are larger and systolic pressures are higher, resulting in combined pressure and volume overload. (From Otto CM:* Valvular Heart Disease, *2nd ed. Philadelphia, Saunders, 2004.)*

Measures of Ventricular Systolic Function

Measurement of ventricular contractility is problematic in the clinical setting because ventricular systolic performance depends on preload, afterload, heart rate (HR), and contractility (see Chapter 9). Although there is no ideal clinical measure of ventricular contractility, end-systolic indices are less load dependent than diastolic or ejection phase measurements[31] (Table 19–2). The LV parameters that currently are used clinically for decision making in patients with chronic valve regurgitation include:

- End-systolic minor-axis dimension or end-systolic volume.
- End-diastolic minor-axis dimension or end-diastolic volume.
- EF.

The rate of rise in ventricular pressure in early systole (dP/dt) also may be helpful in some settings. More sophisticated measures of ventricular function, such as end-systolic circumferential wall stress, the relationship between wall stress and the velocity of circumferential fiber shortening, or elastance (the slope of the end-systolic pressure-volume relationship with altered loading conditions), all have been used in clinical research studies but are not widely used in clinical practice. Doppler or cardiac magnetic resonance myocardial strain rate (SR) analysis is a promising approach that is currently under evaluation.[32]

Because EF is load dependent, some investigators suggest that EF be indexed for end-systolic wall stress, a measure of afterload. The change in indexed EF from rest to exercise may help identify early systolic dysfunction.[33]

Other Consequences of Chronic Regurgitation

In addition to LV dilation and eventual contractile dysfunction, chronic valve regurgitation results in other major physiologic consequences. As in patients with heart failure due to other causes, neurohormonal changes parallel the anatomic and physiologic changes in ventricular performance. Elevated levels of brain natriuretic peptide (BNP) have been demonstrated in patients with symptoms resulting from chronic valve regurgitation and may be an early marker of ventricular decompensations.[34-37] However, interpretation of changes in BNP levels in an individual patient with chronic valve dysfunction is confounded by changes in BNP resulting from other causes of systolic or diastolic dysfunction, such as hypertension and coronary disease, that often coexist in these patients.

Chronic MR leads to a chronically elevated left atrial pressure with left atrial dilation and an increased risk

TABLE 19–2. Physiologic Framework for Assessing Preoperative Predictors of Surgical Outcome in Chronic Aortic Regurgitation

	Preload	Afterload	Heart Rate	Contractility
Severity of Aortic Regurgitation Regurgitant volume	+	+	+	0
Regurgitant fraction	+	+	+	0
End-Diastolic Indexes Volume (dimension)	+	+	+	+/0
Pressure	+	+	+	+/0
Ejection Phase Indexes Rest data	+	+	+	+
Exercise response	+	+	+	+
End-Systolic Indexes Volume (dimension)	0	+	+/0	+
Pressure-volume slope	0	0	+/0	+
Wall stress/volume ratio	0	+	0	+
Wall stress—ejection fraction relationship	+	0	+	+
Wall stress—Vcf$_c$ relationship	0	0	0	+

Vcf$_c$, rate-corrected velocity of fiber shortening; +, dependent; 0, independent.
From Borow KM: *J Am Coll Cardiol* 10:1165-1170, 1987.

of atrial fibrillation (AFib) and systemic embolic events. Left atrial enlargement also may be seen with AR, although this typically is a late finding related to decompensation with elevated diastolic ventricular pressures. AFib is associated with considerable morbidity, so that intervention optimally is timed to prevent progression to permanent AFib.

Pulmonary hypertension results from the passive increase in pulmonary diastolic pressure as left atrial pressure rises, with superimposed reactive changes in the pulmonary vasculature (see Chapter 35). Pulmonary hypertension in patients with MR often resolves after successful valve surgery. Irreversible changes in the pulmonary vasculature can occur with long-standing pulmonary hypertension, with no improvement after surgical intervention. Thus, pulmonary pressures are an important consideration in the timing of valve surgery for chronic regurgitation.

In patients with ventricular hypertrophy, there typically is a corresponding increase in coronary blood flow. With AR, coronary blood flow also is affected by the decreased diastolic perfusion pressure resulting from the lower diastolic pressure in the aorta. Although coronary artery dimensions increase in proportion to the degree of hypertrophy, resulting in an increase in resting myocardial blood flow, the maximal blood flow achieved with coronary vasodilation is not increased so that coronary flow reserve is diminished. Thus, an imbalance in myocardial oxygen demand and supply may result in clinical signs and symptoms of coronary ischemia.[38-40]

The role of the peripheral vasculature in the pathophysiology of chronic regurgitation is unclear. In patients with chronic regurgitation, ventricular afterload includes the impedance of the systemic circuit and end-systolic wall stress. However, there are few studies on the ventricular-vascular interaction in chronic valve regurgitation.

Aortic Regurgitation

Causes

AR may result from primary disease of the valve leaflets or from enlargement of the aortic root. In patients undergoing surgery for chronic AR, the cause of it is about equally divided between primary leaflet disease and aortic root enlargement. The most common causes overall are a bicuspid aortic valve (22%), endocarditis (17%), aortic dissection (10%), and Marfan syndrome (6%). Other less common leaflet abnormalities include congenital valve defects other than bicuspid valve, rheumatic aortic valve disease (typically with concurrent mitral valve involvement), and aortitis.[41] Aortic root involvement resulting in AR may result

from Marfan syndrome or related connective tissue disorders. Aortic enlargement also may be seen in patients with systemic inflammatory diseases, such as ankylosing spondylitis and reactive arthritis or with syphilitic aortitis. However, the cause of AR remains undetermined in 34% of patients with AR severe enough to require valve surgery. Many of these patients have long-standing hypertension, suggesting abnormal aortic root geometry and/or elasticity may be a contributing factor.

The cause of AR is an important factor in timing of surgical intervention because surgery may be indicated for aortic root dilation, independent of regurgitant severity. Conversely, concurrent aortic root replacement is appropriate in patients undergoing replacement of a bicuspid aortic valve if the maximum dimension of the ascending aorta is greater than 45 mm.[1,42,43] In patients with acute severe AR resulting from endocarditis or aortic dissection, emergent surgery typically is needed, and the criteria used for decision making with chronic regurgitation are not applicable.

Natural History

Prospective studies on long-term clinical outcome in adults with chronic severe AR show a rate of onset of symptoms of only about 6% per year[33,44] (Fig. 19–4). Although endocarditis on a bicuspid valve accounts for 17% to 30% of endocarditis cases and about 1200 deaths per year in the United States, the risk of endocarditis with a bicuspid valve is only intermediate (about 0.4 per 1000 patient-years) and endocarditis prophylaxis is no longer recommended. In most patients with

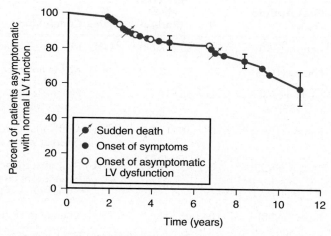

Figure 19–4. Natural history of chronic severe aortic regurgitation. This life table analysis shows the clinical course of 104 initially asymptomatic patients with severe aortic regurgitation. At 11 years, 58+9% of the patients were alive and asymptomatic with normal left ventricular (LV) systolic function. Brackets indicate SEE. (From Bonow RO, Lakatos E, Maron BJ, Epstein SE: Circulation 84:1625-1635, 1991.)

chronic asymptomatic AR of any cause, watchful waiting with patient education, periodic echocardiography, and cardiac risk factor modification is appropriate.

A small subset of patients (<5% per year) develops asymptomatic LV dysfunction, with irreversible changes in ventricular contractility. Thus, the major goal of echocardiographic monitoring is to identify patients with impending, but not yet irreversible, LV contractile dysfunction. The second goal of periodic monitoring is prevention of sudden death, which occurs in less than 1% per year, predominantly in association with excessive LV dilation.

Predictors of Outcome after Aortic Valve Replacement

The parameters used for recommending surgery in asymptomatic adults with AR have been derived from surgical series comparing ventricular function before and after valve replacement and from multivariate analysis of the preoperative predictors of operative mortality and long-term survival Table 19–3.[45]

Clinical predictors of outcome include age, gender, symptom severity, and exercise tolerance.[46-49] As with other types of chronic valve disease, symptoms are a strong predictor of clinical outcome and intervention is recommended for even mild symptoms, when regurgitation is severe.[50] In asymptomatic patients, the best predictors of outcome are LV size and systolic function[33,44,46,49-67] (Fig. 19–5). Chronic LV pressure and volume overload result in significant LV dilation with a normal EF. EF falls only late in the disease course, and it is clear that patients with a higher EF have better surgical outcomes than those with lower EFs. Even a modest fall in EF signifies contractile dysfunction so that current guidelines recommend surgical intervention when the EF falls below 50%.

Similarly, there is a curvilinear relationship (Fig. 19–6) between the preoperative degree of LV dilation and the postoperative EF.[48] End-systolic ventricular size (measured as a minor-axis dimension or as a volume) is less load dependent and thus a more robust predictor of outcome compared end-diastolic measurements. Although there is no clear breakpoint in the data, the clinical consensus is that valve replacement is appropriate when the end-systolic dimension reaches 55 mm. Most women develop symptoms at a LV dimension smaller than the recommendations for surgical intervention.[68] Thus, particular attention to symptom onset is important in women with chronic regurgitation. Some experts recommend using a somewhat lower value (typically 50 mm) as the indicator for intervention in women given their smaller body size.

TABLE 19–3. Timing of Valve Replacement in Chronic Severe Aortic Regurgitation*

				A. Prospective Studies in Patients Who Were Initially Asymptomatic
First Author (Year)	**N**	**Age (yrs) Mean (Range)**	**% Male**	**Conclusions**
Henry (1980)[52]	37	35 (17-64)	54%	ESD and FS predicted which patients became symptomatic and required AVR.
Bonow (1983)[54]	77	37 (16-67)	—	AVR is not needed until symptoms or LV dysfunction occurs.
Siemienczuk (1989)[61]	50	48±16	—	Patients can be risk stratified for "early progression to AVR" based on measurement of LV size and function.
Bonow (1991)[44]	104	36 (17-67)	86%	Multivariate predictors of outcome (death, ventricular dysfunction or symptoms) were: age, initial ESD, rate of change in ESD, rest EF.
Tornos (1995)[47]	101	41±14	80%	Risk of surgery was 12% at 5 years and 24% at 10 years. Predictors of symptom onset or LV dysfunction were: ESD > 50 mm; radionuclide ejection fraction < 60%.
Borer (1998)[33]	104	46±15	79%	Change in EF from rest to exercise normalized to end-systolic wall stress.
Tarasoutchi (2003)[66]	75	28±9	76%	Probability of developing symptoms within 10 years was 58% with an LV EDD ≥ 70 mm and 76% with an LV ESD ≥ 50 mm.

*All studies included only patients with severe aortic regurgitation and excluded patients with coexisting cardiac conditions (e.g., aortic stenosis, other valvular disease, coronary artery disease).

AVR, aortic valve replacement; AR, aortic regurgitation; CHF, congestive heart failure; EDD, left ventricular end diastolic dimension; EF, angiographic ejection fraction; ES, end systolic; ESS, end systolic stress; ESD, left ventricular end-systolic dimension by echocardiography; ESV, end-systolic volume; FS, percent fractional shortening by echocardiography; LV, left ventricular; RR, relative risk.

Data from references 33, 44, 47-50, 52-62, 64-66.

TABLE 19-3. Timing of Valve Replacement in Chronic Severe Aortic Regurgitation—cont'd

B. Surgical Series Comparing Preoperative Variables to Postoperative Ejection Fraction and Outcome

First Author (Year)	N	Age (yrs) Mean (Range)	% Male	Conclusions
Henry (1980)[53]	49	46 (19-68)	82%	Preoperative ESD > 55 mm and FS < 25% were associated with poor outcome post-AVR.
Fioretti (1983)[55]	47	47 (22-75)	62%	Preoperative ESD ≥ 55 does not preclude AVR.
Bonow (1984)[56]	37	41 (20-46)	89%	Duration of preoperative LV dysfunction is an important predictor of reversibility of LV function.
Daniel (1985)[57]	84	46 (18-71)	77%	Preoperative ESD > 55 or FS < 25% does not reliably predict outcome after AVR.
Taniguchi (1987)[58]	62	43 (18-64)	77%	Preoperative LV-ES volume index was most important predictor of subsequent cardiac death.
Carabello (1987)[59]	14	49±6	—	Preoperative ESD correlated best with postoperative EF.
Bonow (1988)[60]	61	43 (19-72)	84%	Long-term improvement in LV function is related to early reduction in EDD postoperatively.
Taniguchi (1990)[62]	35	43 (15-60)	86%	The postoperative increase in EF correlated with the decrease in ESS. Contractile dysfunction persisted.
Pirwitz (1994)[64]	27	(18-72)	78%	The peak systolic pressure to ESV ratio was the strongest predictor of postoperative functional class.
Klodas (1997)[50]	289	50±16 (Group A) 61±14 (Group B)	79%	Operative mortality was higher (7.8% versus 1.2%) and 10-year survival lower (45±5% versus 78±4%) in the 128 patients (Group B) with NYHA Class III/IV symptoms compared to the 161 patients (Group A) with Class I/II symptoms.
Tornos (1998)[48]	87	51±13	82%	Risk of CHF at 10 yrs was 24%. Predictors of CHF were: age > 50 years (RR 10.4), preoperative EF < 40% (RR 10.6), end-systolic diameter > 50 mm (RR 74).
Turina (1998)[49]	192	44	—	Multivariate predictors of survival at a mean follow up of 14 years were age ($P = 0.0004$), ↑ LV end-systolic volume ($P = 0.0004$), higher NYHA class ($P = 0.01$), previous endocarditis ($P = 0.006$).
Tornos (2006)[65]	170	50±14	79%	In patients operated in accordance with current guidelines, compared to those operated late, 10-year survival was higher (85±5% versus 64±5%).

AVR, aortic valve replacement; AR, aortic regurgitation; CHF, congestive heart failure; EDD, left ventricular end diastolic dimension; EF, angiographic ejection fraction; ES, end systolic; ESD, left ventricular end-systolic dimension by echocardiography; ESV, end-systolic volume; FS, percent fractional shortening by echocardiography; LV, left ventricular; RR, relative risk.
Data from references 33, 44, 47-50, 52-62, 64-66.

LV size returns toward normal and systolic function typically improves after aortic valve replacement (AVR). The reduction in afterload and increase in EF associated with valve replacement is similar to that seen with aortic stenosis. Even when extreme LV dilation is present (end-diastolic dimension ≥ 80 mm), surgical intervention improves long-term outcome, although EF may not fully normalize, and there is a higher late mortality compared to patients with earlier intervention.[46]

Echocardiographic Approach

Aortic Valve and Root

The first step in echocardiographic evaluation of the patient with AR is imaging of the valve and aortic root. Typically two-dimensional (2D) transthoracic imaging is adequate, although transesophageal imaging is appropriate when image quality is suboptimal. In patients with a new diagnosis of AR, evaluation includes a diligent search for valvular vegetations

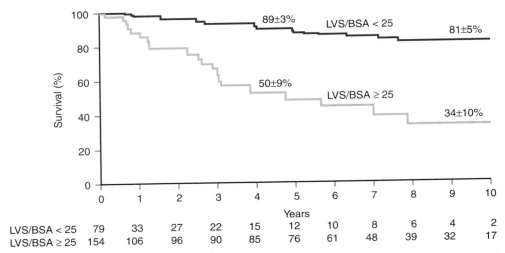

Figure 19–5. *Survival with conservative treatment in patients with severe aortic regurgitation stratified according to left ventricular systolic dimension indexed to body surface area (LVS/BSA). Survival of patients with baseline values ≥25 mm/m² was lower than expected (P < 0.001) and different from that of patients with values less than 25 mm/m² (P < 0.001), whose survival was not different from expected (P = 0.52). (From Dujardin KS, Enriquez-Sarano M, Schaff HV, et al: Circulation 99:1851-1857, 1999.)*

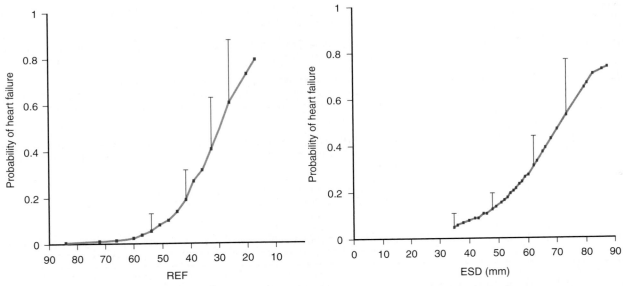

Figure 19–6. *Probability of heart failure during follow-up (y-axis) plotted against (left) preoperative radionuclide ejection fraction (REF) and (right) preoperative end-systolic diameter (ESD) in 87 consecutive patients undergoing aortic valve replacement for severe aortic regurgitation and normal coronary arteries. (From Tomos MP, Olona M, Permanyer-Miralda G, et al: Am Heart J 136[4]:681-687, 1998.)*

and clinical consideration of the diagnosis of endocarditis or an aortic dissection. The pattern of AR also provides clues about the cause of disease. Regurgitation often is eccentric with a bicuspid valve. A central jet suggests stretched leaflets resulting from aortic root disease. A regurgitant jet at a site with no visible anatomic abnormality may be due to a leaflet fenestration.

With chronic regurgitation, care is taken to identify the number of leaflets in systole in a short-axis view, as a bicuspid valve may appear to have three leaflets

when closed if there is a raphe in one leaflet.[43,69,70] With a bicuspid valve, leaflet morphology is described as anterior-posterior, when there is fusion of the right and left coronary cusps, so both coronary arteries arise from the larger anterior sinus, or right-left when there is fusion of the right and noncoronary cusps, with the coronary arteries each coming off a separate sinus.

A rheumatic valve is characterized by fusion at the commissures with a triangular central opening in systole. If rheumatic disease is suspected, careful evaluation of the mitral valve is helpful as rheumatic valve disease typically involves the mitral valve first, then the aortic valve. AR resulting from a systemic inflammatory disease often shows aortic dilation with thickening of the aortic wall, extending to the base of the anterior mitral leaflet—the subaortic bump (see Chapter 36).

The aortic root is measured in all patients with significant AR at the annulus level, the sinuses of Valsalva, the sinotubular junction, and in the mid-ascending aorta. The left ventricular outflow tract (LVOT) diameter (or annulus) dimension also is useful for surgical planning of valve type and size and may prompt consideration of an annular enlargement procedure if the expected valve size would result in patient prosthesis mismatch.[71] The presence and pattern of root dilation helps distinguish Marfan syndrome (effacement of the sinotubular junction) from other diseases of the aorta (see Chapter 38). In patients with Marfan syndrome, the maximum aortic diameter is used for decisions about timing of surgical intervention. Because of the importance of aortic dimension in decision making, other approaches (cardiac computed tomography [CT] or magnetic resonance imaging [MRI]) often are needed to fully delineate aortic anatomy and confirm the degree of dilation when the ascending aorta is not well seen by echocardiography. Additional imaging approaches are particularly important in patients with Marfan syndrome or a bicuspid aortic valve.

Regurgitant Severity

Evaluation of AR based on the American Society of Echocardiography (ASE) guidelines begins with color Doppler visualization and measurement of the vena contracta (VC).[72,73] If more than mild regurgitation is present, with a VC greater than 2 mm, the continuous wave (CW) Doppler AR signal and the flow pattern in the descending aorta are examined. In most cases, these simple approaches are adequate for clinical decision making. For example, in a patient with a bicuspid

valve, a wide VC, holodiastolic flow reversal in the proximal abdominal aorta and a dense CW Doppler signal, regurgitation clearly is severe and further quantitation is not necessary. Conversely, in a patient with a narrow VC, faint CW Doppler signal and normal diastolic flow in the descending aorta, only mild regurgitation is present. When these simple measures suggest moderate regurgitation, further quantitation may be helpful, although decisions about surgical intervention are primarily based on LV size and systolic function (Fig. 19–7).

Calculation of regurgitant volume, regurgitant fraction, and regurgitant orifice area are most helpful in patients with AR when it is unclear if regurgitation is the cause of LV dilation and dysfunction or to concurrent primary myocardial or coronary artery disease (see Chapter 18).

Left Ventricular Size and Systolic Function

The most critical aspect of echocardiographic evaluation of the patient with chronic AR is accurate measurement of LV size and systolic function. Transthoracic imaging is optimal because it is more difficult to obtain standard image planes from the transthoracic approach. In the future, quantitative three-dimensional (3D) imaging may be helpful (see Chapter 4) but the current standard is two-dimensional and M-mode imaging.

LV minor-axis internal dimensions are measured from the parasternal long-axis view, taking care to ensure the measurement is centered and perpendicular to the long-axis of the ventricular chamber. Two-dimensional or 3D imaging is used to optimize alignment; but the most accurate measurements are still made using guided M-mode recordings because the rapid sampling rate allows clear identification of the endocardial borders.

LV volumes and EF are measured using the apical biplane approach based on endocardial border tracing at end-diastole and end-systole in apical four-chamber

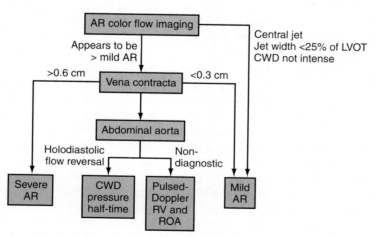

Figure 19-7. Flow chart illustrating the clinical approach to evaluation of aortic regurgitant severity by echocardiography. AR, aortic regurgitation; CWD, continuous-wave Doppler; LVOT, left ventricular outflow tract; ROA, regurgitant orifice area; RV, regurgitant volume. (From Otto CM: Textbook of Clinical Echocardiography, 3rd ed. Philadelphia, Elsevier, 2004.)

and two-chamber view. An echocardiographic stretcher with an apical cutoff with positioning of the patient is a steep left lateral decubitus position allows image acquisition from the true LV apex, avoiding foreshortening with underestimation of ventricular volumes. If image quality is suboptimal, left-sided contrast can be fused to enhance endocardial definition.

On serial studies, review of previous images minimizes measurement variability resulting from changes in the echocardiographic image plane, measurement site or foreshortening of the apical views. Measurements also may vary as a result of physiologic changes in preload, afterload, and heart rate, so that blood pressure and heart rate at the time of imaging study should be recorded. Small changes in measurements may not be clinically significant. Decision making is based on consistent directional changes on serial studies. If measurements are approaching a value that would indicate surgical intervention, a repeat evaluation at a shorter time interval or confirmation by an alternate imaging technique is appropriate.

Other Findings

Echocardiographic evaluation also includes assessment of the anatomy and function of the mitral valve and calculation of pulmonary pressures. Mitral valve prolapse (MVP) is associated with bicuspid aortic valve disease in a subset of patients and some patients being followed for chronic AR develop acute severe MR resulting from chordal rupture. Pulmonary hypertension resulting from AR solely is rare so that the finding of elevated pulmonary pressures should prompt consideration of other causes, such as primary pulmonary disease.

Exercise Echocardiography.

Typically the information needed for clinical decision making in patients with chronic AR is derived from the clinical history and resting echocardiogram; exercise testing is not routinely needed. However, exercise testing is appropriate when it is unclear whether the patient has symptoms or to establish baseline exercise tolerance. The hemodynamic response to exercise also may be helpful for evaluation of functional capacity before participation in athletic activities.[1]

Exercise echocardiographic evaluation of regurgitant severity is unlikely to be useful because aortic regurgitant severity rarely changes with exercise. Any increase in instantaneous retrograde flow resulting from higher aortic pressures is offset by a lower systemic vascular resistance and by the shorter diastolic interval, so that regurgitant volume per beat may go down, whereas regurgitant volume per minute remains unchanged.

Some centers advocate exercise evaluation of EF, by echocardiography or radionuclide angiography, to detect early systolic dysfunction. A smaller rest-exercise change in EF, indexed to end-systolic stress, is a predictor of symptoms onset and cardiac events[33] (Fig. 19–8).

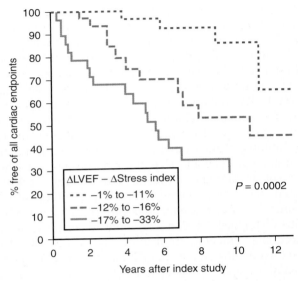

Figure 19–8. *In 104 initially asymptomatic adults with severe aortic regurgitation, this life table analysis shows freedom from cardiac events at follow-up (cardiac death, operable symptoms, and/or subnormal left ventricle performance at rest). The LVEF-ESS index includes a performance descriptor (left ventricular ejection fraction) and a loading descriptor (end-systolic wall stress). The rest to exercise change (Δ) in ejection fraction was normalized for the change in ESS. This LVEF-ESS index was the strongest predictor of clinical outcome using a multivariate Cox model analysis. Outcomes for patients stratified into tertiles of this index are shown. LVEF-ESS, left ventricular ejection fraction-end-systolic wall stress. (From Borer JS, Hochreiter C, Herrold EM, et al: Circulation 97(6):525-534, 1998.)*

However, this approach is not practical, is prone to measurement error, and is not included in current practice guidelines.

Alternate Approaches

Evaluation of aortic regurgitant severity at cardiac catheterization is based on measurement of total SV by angiography and forward SV by the thermodilution or Fick method. This approach is rarely used given the accuracy of echocardiography.

Instead, the current recommendation is to consider cardiac MRI for evaluation of aortic regurgitant severity when echocardiography is nondiagnostic. Regurgitant volume and fraction can be determined by cardiac MRI based on either of two methods. Regurgitant volume can be calculated as the difference between LV and right ventricular SVs measured from endocardial borders at end-diastole and end-systole from image slices that include the entire ventricle chamber. More commonly, regurgitant volume and fraction also are calculated from the volume flow rate (Q-flow) antegrade and retrograde in the ascending aorta.[74-76] Although similar to echocardiographic detection of holodiastolic flow reversal in the descending thoracic aorta, the Q-flow approach is quantitative and more accurate. Cardiac MRI also provides accurate ventricular volumes and EF and a 3D assessment of aortic root anatomy and dimensions (Fig. 19–9).

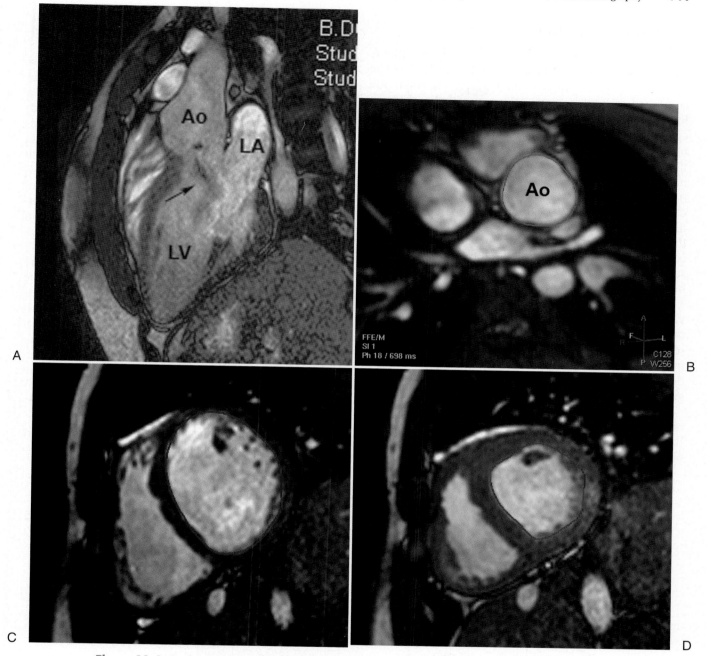

Figure 19–9. In this 19-year-old man with a great vessel switch operation in infancy for transposition of the great arteries, cardiac magnetic resonance imaging was requested because echocardiography showed left ventricular dilation (EDD 6.9 cm, ESD 5.0 cm) greater than expected for the severity of aortic regurgitation (regurgitant volume 48 mL, regurgitant fraction 31%, orifice area 0.15 cm²). In the long-axis image (A) the dilated neo-aorta and the dark jet of aortic regurgitation can be seen. An area of interest was selected over the proximal ascending aorta (B) for calculation of antegrade and retrograde flow rates. Using this approach, the regurgitant volume was 55 mL. However, there is substantial left ventricular dilation so that regurgitant fraction is only 30%. Endocardial borders were traced at end-diastole (C) and end-systole (D) in a series of short-axis left ventricular images from apex to base to calculate a left ventricular ejection fraction of 49%. Total left ventricular stroke volume by Q-flow in the aorta (182 mL) and by LV volumes (195 mL) were similar. Ao, aorta; LA, left atrium; LV, left ventricle.

Clinical Decision Making

The approach to clinical decision making in patients with chronic severe AR is shown in Figure 19–10. The optimal timing of surgical intervention is when the combined risk of surgery and a prosthetic valve is lower than the risk of continued watchful waiting. Because the primary option for treatment of AR is valve replacement with a tissue or mechanical prosthesis, the threshold for intervention is high. Tissue valves have limited longevity, with a shorter durability in younger patients. Mechanical valves are durable but require chronic warfarin anticoagulation, which is inconvenient and is associated with risks of bleeding and thrombosis. In asymptomatic patients, surgery is indicated only if data convincingly show that the risk of sudden death or irreversible LV systolic dysfunction is higher than the risk of watchful waiting.

In patients with chronic severe AR, surgical intervention is appropriate when symptoms are present, regardless of LV size or systolic function. Aortic valve replacement for asymptomatic severe AR is appropriate in patients undergoing other cardiac surgical procedures, such as aortic root surgery or coronary bypass grafting (CABG).[1]

In patients with a bicuspid aortic valve, aortic root replacement is indicated for a dimension over 5 cm or if the rate of increase is 0.5 cm per year or greater, even if other criteria for valve surgery are not present. In bicuspid valve patients undergoing valve replacement for aortic stenosis or AR, aortic root replacement is appropriate when the dimension is over 4.5 cm.[1]

In asymptomatic patients with severe AR, the most robust clinical marker of early LV systolic dysfunction is an EF of 50% or less. Severe LV dilation is also a marker of early LV dysfunction, defined as an end-systolic dimension greater than 55 mm or an end-diastolic dimension greater than 75 mm.[1] In patients with a normal EF, the findings of a progressive increase in ventricular size resulting in end-systolic and end-diastolic dimensions greater than 50 and 70 mm, respectively, are of concern and may warrant surgical intervention. Adherence to these guidelines for intervention in asymptomatic patients with evidence of LV dysfunction has been shown to improve long-term outcomes[65] (Fig. 19–11). When ventricular dimensions or EF are used to recommend surgery, the variability in these measurements must be considered. Data are most convincing when serial studies, with side-by-side comparison of measurements, show a consistent directional change. Because natural history studies show that recovery of ventricular function occurs as long as intervention is performed within 6 to 12 months of the onset of contractile dysfunction, my practice is to repeat borderline measurements after 2 to 3 months before making a final decision about surgical intervention.[56]

When symptom status is unclear based on the clinical history, other findings that justify valve surgery include:

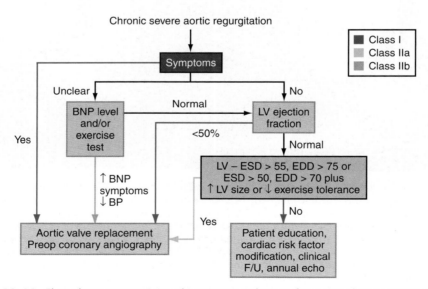

Figure 19–10. Flow chart summarizing the recommendations for surgical intervention in adults with severe valvular aortic regurgitation. Additional factors may be important in clinical decision making in patients with aortic root dilation, patients undergoing other cardiac procedures, and in adolescents and young adults. The class of each recommendation (shown by the colors of the arrows) is based on the 2006 American College of Cardiology and American Heart Association Guidelines for Valve Disease in which Class I means that aortic valve replacement should be performed; Class IIa means that it is reasonable to perform aortic valve replacement; and Class IIb means that aortic valve replacement may be considered. BNP, brain natriuretic peptide; BP, blood pressure; echo, echocardiogram; EDD, left ventricular end-diastolic dimension; ESD, left ventricular end-systolic dimension; F/U, follow-up; LV, left ventricle; Preop, preoperative.

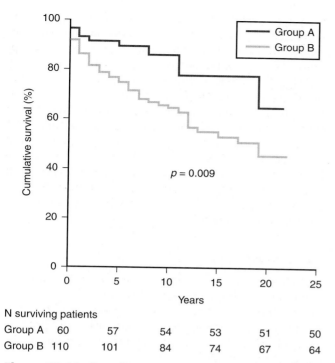

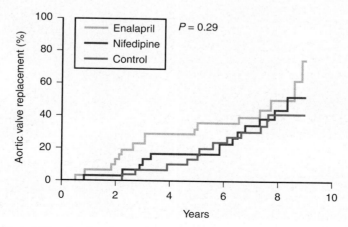

N surviving patients					
Group A	60	57	54	53	51	50
Group B	110	101	84	74	67	64

Figure 19–11. Overall survival in 60 patients with chronic severe aortic regurgitation who underwent early aortic valve replacement for left ventricular dysfunction before symptom onset (Group A) compared to 110 patients who were operated on late with regard to guideline recommendations (Group B). (From Tomos P, Sambola A, Permanyer-Miralda G, et al: J Am Coll Cardio 47(5):1012-1017, 2006.)

(1) a decrease in exercise tolerance compared to expected norms for age or the patient's previous baseline or (2) an abnormal hemodynamic response to exercise. Recent studies suggest that an elevation in serum BNP level is another marker of ventricular decompensation.[77]

In patients with chronic severe AR, who do not meet criteria for intervention, watchful waiting with periodic echocardiographic monitoring is appropriate. The fre-

quency of echocardiography is adjusted based on regurgitant severity and the degree of LV dilation. With only mild AR, periodic monitoring if needed only if the aortic valve is abnormal (e.g., bicuspid) or aortic root enlargement is present. With moderate AR, reevaluation in 2 to 3 years is reasonable. With severe AR and normal LV size and EF, annual echocardiography is recommended. If there is an interval increase in ventricular dimensions or EF or if these parameters are approaching the limits established for surgical intervention, more frequent monitoring, at 3-month to 6-month intervals is warranted. With any degree of AR, reevaluation also is appropriate for any change in symptoms or physical examination findings or for any major change in clinical status, such as pregnancy or need for major noncardiac surgery.

Medical therapy for chronic AR is controversial. Several small studies using echocardiographic measures and one randomized outcomes trial suggest that afterload reduction therapy may reduce regurgitant severity, slow the progression of LV dilation, and delay the need for surgical intervention.[78,79] However, a more recent randomized trial showed no benefit of therapy with an angiotensin converting enzyme (ACE) inhibitor or nifedipine compared to placebo[67] (Fig. 19–12). It is possible that differences in dosage, hemodynamic effects, or timing in the disease course account for the different results in these studies, but clear benefit has not been firmly established.

Mitral Regurgitation

Causes and Mechanisms

Normal function of the mitral valve depends on normal anatomy and dynamics of the left atrium, mitral annulus, mitral leaflets, chordae, papillary muscles, and

Figure 19–12. Probability of aortic valve replacement in 95 patients with asymptomatic chronic severe aortic regurgitation and normal left ventricular function randomized to nifedipine (20 mg every 12 hours), enalapril (20 mg every day), or no treatment, according to the Kaplan-Meier Method. (From Evangelista A, Tornos P, Sambola A, et al: New Engl J Med 953(13):1342-1349, 2005.)

left ventricle and on a normal spatial relationship between these components of the valve apparatus.[80-82] Thus, a wide range of disease processes can result in regurgitation of the mitral valve. The most common primary diseases of the valve leaflets and chords are myxomatous mitral valve disease (MVP), rheumatic disease, and endocarditis. Congenital abnormalities, such as a cleft anterior mitral leaflet or parachute mitral valve, often are seen in association with other congenital lesions. The mitral leaflets may be affected by systemic diseases, such as systemic lupus erythematosus (SLE), hypereosinophilic syndrome, amyloidosis, or rheumatoid arthritis. Radiation therapy or methylsergide therapy also may result in leaflet fibrosis.

With primary diseases of the mitral leaflets, regurgitation may result from excessive leaflet motion, for example with MVP or a flail leaflet segment (Fig. 19–13). Alternatively, regurgitation may result from restricted leaflet motion, for examples with chordal shortening and fusion resulting from rheumatic disease. Regurgitation also may result from defects in the leaflet tissue, for example perforation resulting from endocarditis or shortening in leaflet length, for example with rheumatic disease or an infiltrative process.

Secondary, or "functional," MR occurs when the leaflets and chords are relatively normal, but systolic coaptation (coverage of the orifice by the two leaflets) and apposition (degree of overlap between the leaflets when closed) are reduced.[83,84] For example, with ischemic disease and inadequate contraction of the posterior-lateral wall, motion of the posterior leaflet in systole is restricted, or tethered, resulting from the increased distance from the posterior-lateral papillary muscle to the annulus. The resulting inadequate coaptation and apposition is associated with a posteriorly directed jet of MR as the anterior leaflet "slides" behind the posterior leaflet[78,85-87] (Fig. 19–14). In patients with dilated cardiomyopathy, the angle between the papillary muscles and annular plane becomes less acute, resulting in inadequate central coaptation and a central jet of MR[88-90] (Fig. 19–15). Dilation of the mitral annulus also may contribute to MR with both ischemic regurgitation and dilated cardiomyopathy.[91] Mitral annular calcification is commonly associated with mild to moderate MR.

Natural History

The clinical course of patients with secondary MR depends primarily on the natural history of the primary disease process, such as coronary artery disease (CAD) or dilated cardiomyopathy. In patients with primary MR, the clinical course also varies depending on the cause of regurgitation.

Most of the studies on disease progression with chronic primary MR have focused on patients with myxomatous mitral valve disease[92-102] (Table 19–4). The rate of hemodynamic progression has not been well defined as many patients are first diagnosed only when regurgitation is severe. It is likely that a gradual increase in regurgitant severity occurs in most patients, resulting from a gradual increase in the degree of leaflet

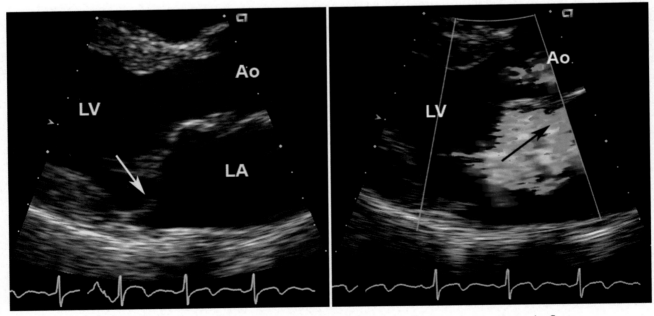

Figure 19–13. *The mechanism of regurgitation with mitral valve prolapse is excessive leaflet motion as illustrated in this parasternal long-axis view showing* (A) *prolapse of the posterior mitral leaflet* (arrow) *with* (B) *and anteriorly directed jet of mitral regurgitation* (arrow) *showing jet direction. Ao, aorta; LA, left atrium; LV, left ventricle.*

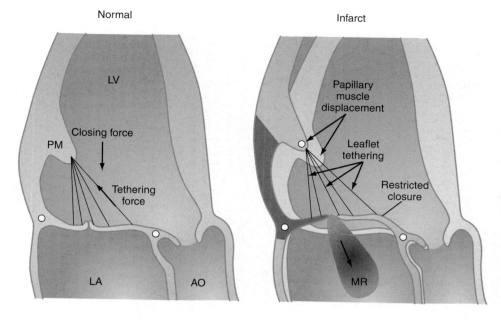

Normal

Infarct

Figure 19–14. This diagram illustrates the mechanism of ischemic mitral regurgitation. Balance of forces acting on mitral leaflets in systole (left). Effect of PM displacement (right). Dark shading indicates inferobasal myocardial infarction; light shading, normal baseline. AO, aorta; LA, left atrium; LV, left ventricle; MR, mitral regurgitation; PM, papillary muscle. (Modified from Liel-Cohen N, Guerrero JL, Otsuji Y, et al: Circulation 101:2756-2763, 2000.)

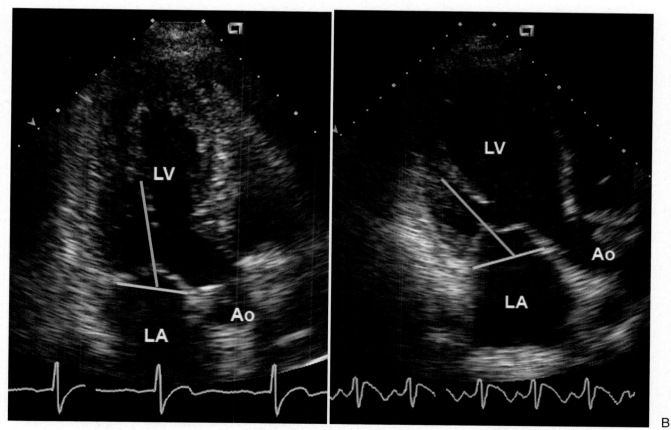

Figure 19–15. Illustration of the mechanism of functional mitral regurgitation with dilated cardiomyopathy (see also Figures 10–16 and 27–8). Echocardiographic images in an apical long-axis view at end-systole in a normal patient (A) and in a patient with dilated cardiomyopathy and severe mitral regurgitation (B). The mitral annulus plane is indicated by the yellow line. Notice that the leaflets are "tented" at end-systole in the patient with dilated cardiomyopathy, with a greater area between the annulus plane and leaflet closure line. The blue line shows the angle from the papillary muscle, through the coaptation point of the anterior and posterior mitral leaflets, to the mitral annulus. Notice that the alignment of the papillary muscle is abnormal in the dilated cardiomyopathy case. Ao, aorta; LA, left atrium; LV, left ventricle.

TABLE 19-4. Natural History of Severe Mitral Regurgitation

First Author (Year)	n	Etiology of MR	% Male	Age (yrs)	Symptoms at Entry	LV-EF (%)	ESD	Long-Term Outcome	Predictors of Outcome
Ling (1996)[100]	229	Flail leaflet	70%	66±13	53% Severe MR in 87%	65±9	19±4 mm/m²	Surgery or death: 90±3% at 10 yrs; CHF: 63±8% 10 years; AF: 30±12% 10 year; Annual mortality rate = 6.3%	Age, NYHA Class, EF, left atrium size
Rosen (1994)[92]	31	MVP	61%	51±13	Asymptomatic severe MR in all	57±6	40±5 mm	Surgery 28% at 5 years (for symptom onset)	Ex Δ RV-EF
Delahaye (1991)[93]	54	Ischemic 13%, MVP 44%, rheumatic 15%, endocarditis 9%	70%	59±19	Severe MR in 91%	56±17	42±9 mm	Actuarial survival: 52±7% at 5 years, 33±9% at 8 years	Ischemic MR, LV-EF
Grigioni (2001)[94]	109	Ischemic post Q-wave MI	70%	71±11	NYHA Class III-IV in 47%, chest pain in 31%	33±14	28±6 mm/m²	Actuarial survival at 5 years 38±5% compared to 61±6% in acute MI patients without MR	Age, EF, NYHA Class, diabetes, atrial fibrillation, creatinine, and MR severity
Enriquez-Sarano (2005)[96]	456	MVP 80%	63%	63±14	Asymptomatic	70±8	34±6 mm	Freedom from CV death, CHF, Afib—33±3% at 5 years	Age, diabetes, regurgitant orifice area
Rosenhek (2006)[95]	132	MVP	51%	55±15	Asymptomatic	66±5	34±5 mm	Survival without MV-surgery: 92±2% at 2 years, 78±4% at 4 years, 65±5% at 6 years, 55±6% at 8 years	Surgery performed based on current guidelines for LV size and function

Afib, atrial fibrillation; AR, aortic regurgitation; CHF, congestive heart failure; CV, cardiovascular; EF, ejection fraction; ESD, end-systolic dimension; LA, left atrial; LV, left ventricle; MI, myocardial infarction; MR, mitral regurgitation; MV, mitral valve; MVP, mitral valve prolapse; NYHA, New York Heart Association.

Data from references 92-96, 100.
Adapted from Otto CM: *Valvular Heart Disease*, 2nd ed. Philadelphia, Saunders, 2004.

prolapse as the patient ages.[103] A more sudden stepwise increase also can occur related to chordal rupture with an abrupt increase in regurgitation, the degree of which depends on whether a primary or secondary chord ruptures.[100,104] Acute severe regurgitation typically requires urgent intervention.

In patients with ischemic MR, more severe MR is associated with poorer outcomes than milder or absent regurgitation.[105] In addition, the severity of MR predicted clinical outcome in a prospective study of 456 patients with chronic severe MR, predominantly resulting from MVP, who were initially asymptomatic and had normal LV function. Those who had a regurgitant orifice area of 0.4 cm² or greater had an increased risk of cardiac death (risk ratio 5.21, 95% confidence interval 1.98 to 14.40)[96] (Fig. 19–16).

In addition to heart failure and valve replacement, other adverse clinical outcomes with chronic MR include AFib with an increased risk of systemic embolic events, pulmonary hypertension with eventual right-sided heart failure, and an increased risk of sudden death. AFib and pulmonary hypertension are prevented by early intervention to relieve regurgitation. There is an increased risk of sudden death in patients with MVP, with an estimated risk of 1% to 2.5% over 6 years of follow up or a risk 10 to 100 times normal. The risk of sudden death is highest in patients with moderate to severe MR, LV dysfunction, AFib, redundant or flail leaflets, and more functional limitation.[102,106,107]

Predictors of Outcome after Mitral Valve Surgery

Clinical Factors

The cause of regurgitation is one of the strongest predictors of outcome after surgical intervention for MR[108-120] (Table 19–5). Long-term outcome is more favorable after surgery in patients with myxomatous mitral valve disease compared to other causes of regurgitation. With rheumatic disease, the success rate for valve repair is lower than with myxomatous disease. With ischemic MR and with regurgitation resulting from dilated cardiomyopathy, long-term outcomes depend more on the underlying disease process than on MR per se. Other baseline factors associated with long-term outcome after mitral valve surgery include older age, female sex, the presence of coronary disease, and involvement of other valves Table 19–6.

Left Ventricular Function. LV systolic function is a strong predictor of postoperative long-term survival, functional status and EF. Evaluation of ventricular contractility is problematic given the altered loading conditions resulting from. Thus, as with AR, clinical recommendations are based on studies comparing postoperative EF to preoperative measure of ventricular volume and EF[121-126] (Fig. 19–17). The current recommended breakpoints for considering surgical intervention in patients with chronic MR are an end-systolic dimension of 40 mm or less and an EF of 60% or less.[1]

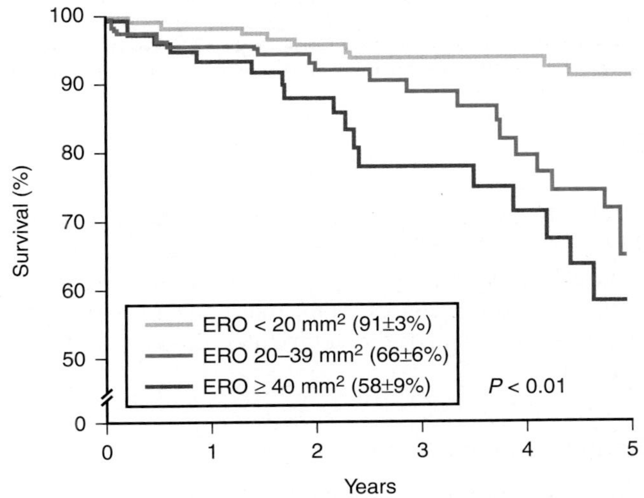

Figure 19–16. Kaplan-Meier estimates of the mean (±SE) rates of overall survival among 456 patients with asymptomatic mitral regurgitation under medical management, according to the effective regurgitant orifice (ERO). Values in parentheses are survival rates at 5 years. (From Enriquez-Sarano M, Avierinos JF, Messika-Zeitoun D, et al: New Engl J Med 352[9]:875-883, 2005.)

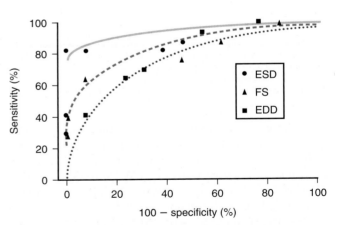

Figure 19–17. Left ventricle (LV) contractility was determined in a series of patients with chronic severe mitral regurgitation by measurement of elastance (Emax). The clinical value of echocardiographic left ventricular end-diastolic dimension (EDD), end-systolic dimension (ESD), and fractional shortening (FS) for identification of impaired contractility is shown using receiver operator curves. An LV-ESD of 40 mm had the best sensitivity (82%) and specificity (100%) for prediction of impaired contractility, defined by reduced elastance. (From Flemming MA, Oral H, Rothman ED, et al: Am Heart J 140, 476-482, 2000.)

TABLE 19–5. Hospital Mortality and Long-Term Outcome after Mitral Valve Repair

First Author (Year)	Etiology of MR	n	Mean Age (years)	Hospital Mortality		Long-Term Survival
Michel (1991)[108]	Myxomatous	156	51	1.3%		84% at 11 years
Jebara (1992)[109]	Myxomatous	79	>70	3.8%		81% at 5 years
David (1993)[110]	Myxomatous	184	57	<1%		94% at 8 years
Gramaglia (1994)[111]	Myxomatous	125	55±16	1.6%	MV repair MVR	95.2% at 5 years 93.7% at 5 years
Mohty (2001)[112]	Myxomatous	917	65±13	—	MVR AL-MVP PL-MVP	31±6% at 15 years 42±5% 41±6%
Fernandez (1993)[113]	Rheumatic	340	?	6.8%		44±3.7% at 14 years
Bernal (1993)[114]	Rheumatic	327	45±13	3.4%		78% at 16 years
Chauvaud (2001)[115]	Rheumatic	951	26	2%		89±19% at 10 years 8±18% at 20 years
Choudhary (2001)[116]	Rheumatic (88%)	818	23±11	4%		93±1% at 11 years
Kay (1986)[117]	Ischemic	101	62±8	≈10%	EF > 40% EF 21%-40% EF < 20%	58±12% at 10 years 33±10% at 10 years 16±14% at 10 years
Hendren (1991)[118]	Ischemic	65	66±10	9.1%		Restrictive motion: 48% at 3 years Prolapse: 96% at 3 years
Lee (1996)[119]	Mixed	226	63±10	1.8%		71±6% at 7 years
Moss (2003)[120]	Myxomatous (60%)	322	61±12	2.8%		Based comparison to a propensity matched group undergoing MV replacement, MV repair patients had significantly improved survival (RR 0.46; 95% CI; 0.28 to 0.75)

AL, anterior leaflet; CI, confidence interval; EF, ejection fraction; MV, mitral valve; MVR, mitral valve replacement; MR, mitral regurgitation; PL, posterior leaflet; RR, relative risk.
Data from references 108-120.
Adapted from Otto CM: *Valvular Heart Disease*, 2nd ed. Philadelphia, Saunders, 2004.

In patients with more severe LV dilation or systolic dysfunction, the degree of improvement after intervention is attenuated, and severe LV dilation or dysfunction and ventricular function may deteriorate further after valve surgery. This decline or lack of improvement in EF after intervention likely is multifactorial related to irreversible contractile dysfunction, which may have been partially masked by altered loading conditions, the abrupt increase in afterload resulting from loss of the low resistance mitral backflow, suboptimal intraoperative myocardial protection, and loss of annular papillary muscle continuity when valve replacement is necessary. Outcomes are poor when LV end-systolic dimension is over 55 mm or EF is less than 30% before intervention, so that medical therapy is the preferred approach in this subgroup.

Other adverse physiologic consequences of chronic MR also are associated with a worse prognosis after surgical interventions. These include increasing left atrial size, the onset of AFib, more severe pulmonary hypertension, and right ventricular dilation and dysfunction.

Surgical Approach

Outcomes with mitral valve repair are superior to those with valve replacement.[120,127-130] Operative mortality is lower and long-term event-free survival is better when mitral valve repair is performed. Although this data is derived largely from observation studies comparing patients who underwent repair to those who underwent replacement, these findings are reproducible be-

TABLE 19–6. Predictors of Outcome after Surgery for Mitral Regurgitation

Clinical Factors
Age
Gender
Functional Status
Symptoms
Etiology of mitral regurgitation

Comorbid Disease
Coronary artery disease
Other valve involvement

Left Ventricular Systolic Function
End-systolic volume or dimension
Ejection fraction
Wall stress
Left ventricular sphericity
Left ventricular maximum dP/dt

Surgical Procedure
Mitral valve replacement with or without chordal preservation
Mitral valve repair

Other
Left atrial size
Left ventricular end-diastolic pressure
Pulmonary artery pressure
Right ventricular ejection fraction

Adapted from Otto CM: *Valvular Heart Disease*, 2nd ed. Philadelphia, Saunders, 2004.

tween centers and have been confirmed based on nonrandomized groups matched by propensity score[120] (Fig. 19–18).

The mechanism of improved outcomes with mitral valve repair is thought to be preservation of the continuity between the mitral annulus and papillary muscles. The normal relationship between the mitral apparatus and left ventricle helps maintain normal ventricular geometry and long-axis systolic shortening (see Chapter 20)[123,126,131-141] (Table 19–7).

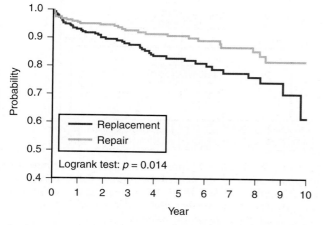

Figure 19–18. Kaplan-Meier survival curves for 322 mitral valve repair patients operated between 1991 and 2000 in British Columbia, Canada, matched by propensity score to an equal number of mitral valve replacement patients. (From Moss RR, Humphries KH, Gao M, et al: Circulation 108 [Suppl 1]:II90-II97, 2003.)

Echocardiographic Approach

Mitral Valve Anatomy

The first step in echocardiographic evaluation of the patient with MR is evaluation of valve anatomy to determine the cause of valve dysfunction. The thickness, redundancy, and motion of both anterior and posterior leaflets are described, with specific attention to the location and severity of any prolapsing or flail segments. Measurement of annulus size in long-axis and four-chamber views may be helpful.

Transthoracic imaging typically is adequate for initial evaluation and serial studies, although transesophageal imaging may be needed when surgical intervention is planned to determine the likelihood of a successful valve repair.[142,143] The long-axis view shows the central segment of both the anterior and posterior leaflets. Medial and lateral angulation shows additional leaflet segments. The short-axis view allows assessment of leaflet thickness, redundancy, and localization of any areas of calcification. In the four-chamber view, the saddle shape of the annulus may result in a leaflet closure line that appears on the left atrial side of the valve. However, given this knowledge of the 3D anatomy of the mitral annulus, the four-chamber view still is useful for evaluation of prolapse and flail segments. The two-chamber view is particularly helpful as it shows the central segment of the anterior leaflet and the lateral and medial scallops of the posterior leaflet. Real-time 3D imaging of the valve provides an understandable view of valve anatomy, but the utility of this approach is limited by image resolution, artifact, and difficulty of image acquisition. Research 3D applications, based on reconstruction of valve anatomy from traced borders, have enhanced the understanding of the mechanisms of MR but are rarely needed for clinical decision making.

Myxomatous mitral disease is diagnosed based on the characteristic findings of diffuse leaflet thickening and redundancy with systolic prolapse of one or more leaflet segments. A flail leaflet segment is differentiated from prolapse based on the direction of the leaflet tip at end-systole either toward the apex (prolapse) or toward the left atrial posterior wall (flail). Rheumatic disease is characterized by thickening at the edges of the leaflets, often with slight diastolic doming even when the degree of stenosis is not significant and by thickening and shortening of the mitral chords. Regurgitation as a result of ischemic disease is diagnosed on echocardiography based on LV regional wall motion abnormalities with restricted motion of the posterior leaflet. However, the etiology of MR should be considered to be ischemic in all patients with known coronary disease unless definitive findings for primary leaflet disease are present. The cause of regurgitation in patients with hypertrophic or dilated cardiomyopathy is evident from the other findings in these conditions.

TABLE 19-7. **Left Ventricular Function after Surgery for Mitral Regurgitation (Selected Studies)**

First Author (Year)	Type of Surgery	*n*	Preoperative EF (%)	Postoperative EF (%)	*P*-value
Kennedy (1979)[131]	MVR	7	55±12	43±15	<0.05
David (1984)[132]	MVR	15	55±9	48±14	<0.01
	MVR + chordal pres	12	53±14	52±16	NS
Goldman (1987)[133]	MVR	8	64±11	40±9	<0.0001
	Valve repair	10	44±20	49±16	NS
Miki (1988)[134]	MVR	20	54±7	52±8	NS
	MVR + chordal pres	12	54±8	59±8	NS
Crawford (1990)[123]	MVR	48	56±15	45±13	<0.001
Rozich (1992)[135]	MVR	7	60±2	36±2	<0.05
	MVR + chordal pres	8	63±1	61±2	NS
Enriquez-Sarano (1995)[137]	MVR	214	60±12	49±15	0.0001
	MVR repair	195	63±9	54±11	0.0001
Corin (1995)[138]	MVR	6	60±10	48±10	0.01
	MVR repair	8	64±5	61±16	NS
Starling (1995)[139]	MV repair	15	58±12	53±16	NS
Leung (1996)[140]	MV repair	74	64±9	55±10	<0.001
Matsumura (2003)[141]	MV repair	171	66±10	63±11	<0.0001

MV, mitral valve; MVR, mitral valve replacement; NS, not significant; pres, preservation.
Data from references 123, 131-135, 137-141.
Adapted from Otto CM: *Valvular Heart Disease,* 2nd ed. Philadelphia, Saunders, 2004.

Regurgitant Severity

Mitral regurgitant severity is initially evaluation by color and CW Doppler.[72,73] A small color jet with a narrow VC (<3 mm) from both parasternal and apical views and a weak CW signal are consistent with mild regurgitation and further evaluation is not needed. A wide color jet (VC of 7 mm or greater) and a dense CW Doppler signal indicate severe regurgitation (Fig. 19–19).

With an intermediate VC width (or when decision making requires a quantitative measure of regurgitant severity), regurgitation volume, regurgitant fraction, and regurgitation orifice area are calculated. The proximal isovelocity surface area (PISA) approach is most useful for central, holosystolic jets. When regurgitation is only late-systolic or with an asymmetric PISA, approaches that integrate flow throughout systole are more appropriate. Forward SV is calculated with Doppler in the left ventricular outflow tract. Total SV is calculated from transmitral Doppler SV or from apical biplane LV diastolic and systolic volumes. Ideally, results are congruent using either Doppler or LV volume derived total SV. Severe MR is defined as a regurgitant volume equal to 60 mL, a regurgitant fraction equal to 50%, and a regurgitant orifice area equal to 0.4 cm² (see Chapter 18).

Color Doppler visualization of jet geometry also may be helpful in determining the etiology of regurgitation.

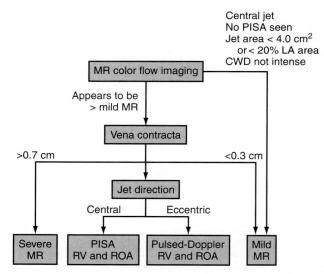

Figure 19–19. Clinical approach to evaluation of mitral regurgitant severity by echocardiography. CWD, continuous-wave Doppler; LA, left atrial; MR, mitral regurgitation; PISA, proximal isovelocity surface area approach; ROA, regurgitant orifice area; RV, regurgitant volume.

Both the PISA and VC identify the site of regurgitation, which may be multiple in some cases. The direction of the jet within the left atrium typically is opposite the affected leaflet—an anteriorly directed jet implies posterior leaflet disease and vice versa. Ischemic regurgitation typically is posteriorly directed. Central regurgitation is seen with dilated cardiomyopathy.

Left Ventricular Size and Systolic Function

As with AR, the most important measurements for serial evaluation of the patient with chronic severe MR are ventricular size and systolic function. Care is needed in measuring minor-axis dimensions perpendicular to the LV long axis at the mitral chordal level, using M-mode to enhance recognition of the endocardial border. EF is calculated using the apical biplane approach, using contrast enhancement, if endocardial definition is suboptimal. Changes in ventricular dimensions or EF are most convincing when studies are compared side by side and when serial studies show a consistent directional change in the measurements.

With MR, it is especially important to ensure accuracy in LV measurements because the values used for timing of surgical intervention would be considered normal in patients without severe MR. Because a "normal" LV end-systolic dimension and EF are cause for concern only when MR is severe, accurate quantitation of regurgitant severity also is critical in these patients.

Other Findings

Progressive left atrial enlargement resulting from chronic MR provides additive information when considering surgical intervention. In addition, to a single anterior-posterior dimension at end-systole, measurement of left atrial volume from tracing the atrium in an apical four-chamber view is useful. Atrial thrombi are less common with AFib resulting from MR than with mitral stenosis but can still occur and are not reliably detected by transthoracic imaging. Transesophageal imaging is required to exclude atrial thrombus before cardioversion.

Pulmonary hypertension is one of the primary adverse effects of chronic MR and significant elevation at rest or with exercise is an indication for intervention. Pulmonary systolic pressure is measured using the standard echocardiographic approach based on the tricuspid regurgitant jet velocity and the respiratory variation in diameter of the inferior vena cava. The velocity of the pulmonic regurgitant jet is a measure of pulmonary diastolic pressure.

The aortic valve may be involved depending on the etiology of MR. The aortic valve is affected in about one third of rheumatic mitral valve cases and in five percent of MVP cases. With systemic diseases that cause infiltration or inflammation, multivalve disease is common.

Exercise Echocardiography

Exercise echocardiography is helpful in selected patients when symptoms seem to be more severe than expected for the degree of MR at rest. Particularly with

MVP, the degree of regurgitation may increase with exercise, resulting in symptoms of exertional dyspnea and decreased exercise tolerance even with only moderate regurgitation is present at rest.[144] Quantitative measurement of regurgitant volume in the first few seconds after exercise is challenging. Instead, the tricuspid regurgitant jet is recorded for measurement of pulmonary pressures. An increase in pulmonary pressure greater than expected for age and the level of exertion indicates exercise induced severe MR. An exercise pulmonary systolic pressure greater than 60 mm Hg is an indication for surgical intervention. A normal increase in LV EF with exercise predicts preservation of EF after valve surgery.[145]

Alternate Approaches

Cardiac catheterization rarely is used to quantitate mitral regurgitant severity. LV angiography with visualization of left atrial opacification is qualitative and shows considerable interobserver variability. Calculation of regurgitant volume based on the difference between angiographic total LV SV and thermodilution or Fick forward SV has wide measurement variability resulting from the clinical variability in both these SV determinations.

Cardiac MRI offers the potential for quantitation of MR based on the difference between LV (total) and RV (forward) SV or based on the difference between LV (total) SV and the antegrade volume flow rate in the aorta.[146] Regurgitant severity also can be measured based on flow rates through the mitral annulus.[147] When echocardiographic measures of LV size or function are suboptimal, cardiac MRI offers an alternate accurate approach to measurement of LV volumes and EF.[148]

Radionuclide angiography for measurement of LV EF at rest and with exercise has been used in some clinical studies, but this approach is not recommended in current guidelines.

Clinical Decision Making

The ideal timing of intervention in adults with chronic MR is when the risk of intervention is lower than the risk of watchful waiting[95] (Fig. 19–20). As with AR, the primary consideration is the LV response to chronic volume overload with the goal of intervening just before the onset of contractile dysfunction. However, because mitral valve repair is possible in many patients, intervention often is appropriate earlier in the disease course because the risk of surgery is low, long-term outcomes are excellent, and a prosthetic valve is not needed (Fig. 19–21).

In the asymptomatic patient with severe MR, surgical intervention is recommended when the LV end-systolic dimension is 40 mm or greater or when EF is 60% or less. Note that these values for ventricular size and EF are both within the normal range. Thus, quantitative evaluation of regurgitant severity is especially

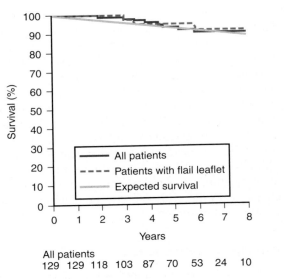

All patients
129 129 118 103 87 70 53 24 10

Patients with flail leaflet
56 55 53 43 37 32 28 10 4

A

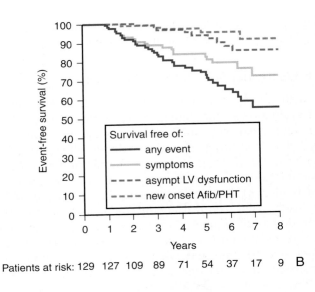

Patients at risk: 129 127 109 89 71 54 37 17 9 B

Figure 19–20. A, *Kaplan-Meier overall survival of 129 patients with asymptomatic severe degenerative mitral regurgitation managed according to a watchful waiting strategy* (solid blue line *indicates total patient population; dotted red line* indicates patients with flail leaflet). *Survival functions did not differ significantly from expected cumulative survival* (solid yellow line). *This analysis includes perioperative and postoperative deaths for those patients who required valve replacement during follow-up.* B, *Kaplan-Meier event-free survival.* Solid blue line *shows survival free of any event to indicate surgery.* Yellow line *shows survival free of symptoms.* Dashed red line *shows survival free of asymptomatic left ventricular (asympt LV) dysfunction.* Dotted green line *shows survival free of asymptomatic development of atrial fibrillation (Afib) and/or pulmonary hypertension (PHT) to indicate surgery. (From Rosenhek R, Rader F, Klar U, et al:* Circulation *113(18):2238-2244, 2006.)*

important because watchful waiting is appropriate if regurgitation is only moderate or mild in severity. Intervention also is reasonable in many patients with severe MR and new onset AFib or pulmonary hypertension (pulmonary systolic pressure >50 mm Hg at rest or >60 mm Hg with exercise), even when ventricular size and function are normal. Some centers with a high level of expertise in mitral valve repair surgery also advocate surgical intervention when severe regurgitation is present if the likelihood of valve repair is greater than 90% regardless of LV size and function, pulmonary pressures, or cardiac rhythm. Again, caution is needed to confirm that regurgitation is truly severe and that valve anatomy and surgical expertise will ensure a successful valve repair.

Intervention is recommended for symptomatic severe MR as long as the EF is 30% or higher and end-systolic dimension is 55 mm or less. However, it may be "too late" for intervention once EF falls below 30% or when severe LV dilation is present. In patients with chronic MR (unlike AR), EF typically is unchanged or falls after intervention. When ventricular function is severely reduced before intervention, surgical risk is high, and there is less benefit of eliminating MR.[149] In some cases, intervention may be harmful with a further reduction in ventricular performance resulting from an abrupt increase in afterload as the low resistance flow into the left atrium is eliminated. Because LV function is better maintained with mitral valve repair, than with valve replacement, in patients with symptomatic severe MR and a low EF, intervention is still reasonable if the likelihood of valve repair is high. When valve repair is not likely, it remains controversial whether intervention will be beneficial.

Management of patients with ischemic MR and with MR secondary to dilated cardiomyopathy remains controversial. Some studies suggest that bypass grafting alone provides better outcomes than combined valve repair, when there is ischemic disease, but other studies suggest concurrent valve repair is beneficial.[150-155] In patients with dilated cardiomyopathy, some centers advocate mitral repair for functional MR, but most centers focus on optimal medical management and cardiac resynchronization therapy in this patient group.[156-159]

Although it seems physiologically plausible that afterload reduction therapy might reduce mitral regurgitant severity and delay the need for valve surgery, published data do not provide convincing support for this approach in patients with primary valve disease.[160-164] Hypertension should be treated but additional medical therapy in this group of patients is not

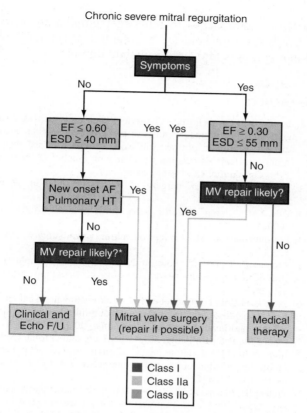

Figure 19–21. *Flowchart summarizing the recommendations for surgical intervention in adults with severe valvular mitral regurgitation. Mitral valve repair likely is defined as greater than 90% likelihood of repair without residual mitral regurgitation at an experienced surgical center. The class of each recommendation is based on the 2006 American College of Cardiology and American Heart Association Guidelines for Valve Disease in which Class I means that mitral valve surgery should be performed; Class IIa means that it is reasonable to perform mitral valve surgery; and Class II means that mitral valve surgery may be considered. AF, atrial fibrillation; echo, echocardiogram; EF, ejection fraction; ESD, left ventricular end-systolic dimension; F/U, follow-up; LV, left ventricle; MV, mitral valve; pulmonary HT, pulmonary hypertension (defined as a systolic pressure >50 mm Hg at rest or >60 mm Hg with exercise).*

recommended. When MR is secondary to LV dilation and systolic dysfunction, mitral regurgitant severity often improves as medical therapy for heart failure is optimized. The presumed mechanism of this improvement is ventricular remodeling with a more normal alignment of the papillary muscles and mitral annulus. Any reduction in the LV to left atrial systolic pressure gradient appears to play only a minor role.[165-167] Biventricular pacing for heart failure also is associated with a reduction in mitral regurgitant severity.[168,169] The relative roles of ventricular resynchronization versus remodeling in the mechanism of this benefit have not been elucidated.

Pulmonic Regurgitation

Pulmonic regurgitation (PR) severe enough to warrant surgical intervention is primarily due to congenital heart disease (CHD). Currently, the most common cause of severe PR in adults is a previous tetralogy of Fallot repair.[170-172] The criteria for surgical intervention are analogous to those for AR, with the primary indications being symptoms resulting from severe regurgitation and evidence of progressive right ventricular dilation and systolic dysfunction. The rationale for early intervention in AR likely applies to PR. Similarly, improvement in ventricular function after relief of regurgitation is plausible because, like AR, PR imposes a pressure and volume load on the ventricle. However, clinical data confirming these physiologic suppositions is lacking.

In addition, many patients have residual right ventricular volume overload after the initial surgical repair, which can be difficult to distinguish from progressive chamber enlargement that occurred subsequently, as a result of PR. Because echocardiography provides only qualitative estimates of right ventricular volumes and EF, cardiac MRI often is used in conjunction with echocardiographic monitoring to determine the optimal timing of intervention. Preliminary studies suggest that pulmonic valve replacement be considered when the right ventricular end-diastolic volume index reaches 150 mL/M^2 or there is a significant fall in EF; however, further validation of this approach is needed.[173] Current guidelines for adults with severe PR recommend pulmonary valve replacement for significant symptoms.[1]

Tricuspid Regurgitation

Tricuspid regurgitation (TR) in adults most often is secondary to pulmonary hypertension and left-sided heart disease or is the consequent of endocarditis. Ebstein's anomaly also is seen and is discussed in Chapter 43.[174]

Although some patients tolerate severe tricuspid regurgitation, others develop symptoms of right heart-sided failure with peripheral edema and ascites, in conjunction with a low forward cardiac output (CO). The indications for surgical intervention are not well defined, in large part because of the suboptimal results of tricuspid valve replacement. Mechanical valves in the tricuspid position have a high rate of valve thrombosis, whereas tissue valves are prone to accelerated degeneration. Thus, tricuspid valve repair or annuloplasty is preferred, whenever possible.[1]

In adolescents and young adults, tricuspid valve surgery is recommended for a significant decrease in exercise tolerance. With severe regurgitation and only mild symptoms, surgery is reasonable when valve repair is likely or when there is new onset AFib. When an atrial septal defect is associated with Ebstein's anomaly, closure is appropriate when cyanosis or clinical symptoms are present.

In adults, tricuspid regurgitation most often is secondary to pulmonary hypertension resulting from either primary pulmonary disease (e.g., cor pulmonale) or from mitral valve dysfunction. In patients undergoing mitral valve surgery, tricuspid valve repair is recommended when severe regurgitation is present. Even when tricuspid regurgitation is only moderate, tricuspid annuloplasty should be considered at the time of mitral valve surgery, especially in patients with rheumatic valve disease, pulmonary hypertension, or annular dilation.[175-177] In adults with primary tricuspid valve disease that is not amenable to repair, tricuspid valve replacement is reserved for severe symptomatic regurgitation refractory to medical therapy.[1]

KEY POINTS

■ Evaluation of the etiology of regurgitation and quantitation of severity is essential for decision making in patients with chronic valve regurgitation.

■ Symptoms are the indication for surgical intervention in most patients with chronic regurgitation, but some patients have impaired ventricular contractility in the absence of symptoms.

■ The most useful clinical parameters for detection of early systolic dysfunction are echocardiographic measurement of LV end-systolic dimension and EF.

■ AR results in significant LV dilation due to chronic volume and pressure overload. Valve replacement is recommended in asymptomatic patients with severe regurgitation when end-systolic dimension reaches 55 mm, or EF is lower than 50%.

■ Earlier intervention is appropriate with MR, when valve repair is highly likely. Intervention is recommended for asymptomatic severe MR, when end-systolic dimension reaches 40 mm or when EF is 60% or less.

■ Exercise echocardiography may be helpful to assess functional capacity, elicit subtle symptoms, and assess the change in pulmonary pressures with exercise, particularly in patients with MR.

■ The role of serum markers, such as BNP levels, in chronic regurgitation is not yet established.

■ Criteria for intervention for chronic tricuspid or pulmonic regurgitation include symptoms and evidence of progressive right ventricular enlargement.

■ Cardiac MRI may provide quantitative measures of regurgitant severity and LV function, when echocardiography is nondiagnostic.

■ Newer approaches to relief of regurgitation may change the threshold for intervention if the risk of intervention is low and results are durable.

REFERENCES

1. Bonow RO, Carabello BA, Chatterjee K, et al: ACC/AHA 2006 guidelines for the management of patients with valvular heart disease: A report of the American College of Cardiology/American Heart Association Task Force on Practice Guidelines. *J Am Coll Cardiol* 48:e1-e148, 2006.
2. Otto CM: Timing of surgery in mitral regurgitation. *Heart* 89:100-105, 2003.
3. Otto CM: Timing of aortic valve surgery. *Heart* 84:211-218, 2000.
4. Enriquez-Sarano M: Timing of mitral valve surgery. *Heart* 87:79-85, 2002.
5. Ambler G, Omar RZ, Royston P, et al: Generic, simple risk stratification model for heart valve surgery. *Circulation* 112:224-231, 2005.
6. Fann JI, St Goar FG, Komtebedde J, et al: Beating heart catheter-based edge-to-edge mitral valve procedure in a porcine model: Efficacy and healing response. *Circulation* 110:988-993, 2004.
7. Maniu CV, Patel JB, Reuter DG, et al: Acute and chronic reduction of functional mitral regurgitation in experimental heart failure by percutaneous mitral annuloplasty. *J Am Coll Cardiol* 44:1652-1661, 2004.
8. Rogers JH, Macoviak JA, Rahdert DA, et al: Percutaneous septal sinus shortening: a novel procedure for the treatment of functional mitral regurgitation. *Circulation* 113:2329-2334, 2006.
9. Webb JG, Harnek J, Munt BI, et al: Percutaneous transvenous mitral annuloplasty: Initial human experience with device implantation in the coronary sinus. *Circulation* 113:851-855, 2006.
10. Munt B, Webb J: Percutaneous valve repair and replacement techniques. *Heart* 92:1369-1372, 2006.
11. Iung B, Gohlke-Barwolf C, Tornos P, et al: Recommendations on the management of the asymptomatic patient with valvular heart disease. *Eur Heart J* 23:1252-1266, 2002.
12. Borow KM, Marcus RH: Aortic regurgitation: The need for an integrated physiologic approach [editorial; comment]. *J Am Coll Cardiol* 17:898-900, 1991.
13. Carabello BA, Zile MR, Tanaka R, et al: Left ventricular hypertrophy due to volume overload versus pressure overload. *Am J Physiol* 263:H1137-H1144, 1992.
14. Carabello BA: The pathophysiology of mitral regurgitation. *J Heart Valve Dis* 9:600-608, 2000.
15. Carabello BA: Aortic regurgitation. A lesion with similarities to both aortic stenosis and mitral regurgitation [comment]. *Circulation* 82:1051-1053, 1990.
16. Lorell BH, Carabello BA: Left ventricular hypertrophy: pathogenesis, detection, and prognosis. *Circulation* 102:470-479, 2000.
17. Sigusch HH, Campbell SE, Weber KT: Angiotensin II-induced myocardial fibrosis in rats: Role of nitric oxide, prostaglandins and bradykinin. *Cardiovasc Res* 31:546-554, 1996.
18. Carver W, Nagpal ML, Nachtigal M, et al: Collagen expression in mechanically stimulated cardiac fibroblasts. *Circ Res* 69:116-122, 1991.
19. Borer JS, Truter S, Herrold EM, et al: Myocardial fibrosis in chronic aortic regurgitation: molecular and cellular responses to volume overload. *Circulation* 105:1837-1842, 2002.
20. Wang X, Li F, Campbell SE, et al: Chronic pressure overload cardiac hypertrophy and failure in guinea pigs: II. Cytoskeletal remodeling. *J Mol Cell Cardiol* 31:319-331, 1999.
21. Schunkert H, Jahn L, Izumo S, et al: Localization and regulation of c-fos and c-jun protooncogene induction by systolic wall

stress in normal and hypertrophied rat hearts. *Proc Natl Acad Sci U S A* 88:11480-11484, 1991.

22. Feldman AM, Weinberg EO, Ray PE, et al: Selective changes in cardiac gene expression during compensated hypertrophy and the transition to cardiac decompensation in rats with chronic aortic banding. *Circ Res* 73:184-192, 1993.

23. Matsuo T, Carabello BA, Nagatomo Y, et al: Mechanisms of cardiac hypertrophy in canine volume overload. *Am J Physiol* 275:H65-H74, 1998.

24. Imamura T, McDermott PJ, Kent RL, et al: Acute changes in myosin heavy chain synthesis rate in pressure versus volume overload. *Circ Res* 75:418-425, 1994.

25. Borer JS, Truter SL, Gupta A, et al: Heart failure in aortic regurgitation: The role of primary fibrosis and its cellular and molecular pathophysiology. *Adv Cardiol* 41:16-24, 2004.

26. Tagawa H, Koide M, Sato H, et al: Cytoskeletal role in the transition from compensated to decompensated hypertrophy during adult canine left ventricular pressure overloading. *Circ Res* 82:751-761, 1998.

27. Zile MR, Koide M, Sato H, et al: Role of microtubules in the contractile dysfunction of hypertrophied myocardium. *J Am Coll Cardiol* 33:250-260, 1999.

28. Koide M, Hamawaki M, Narishige T, et al: Microtubule depolymerization normalizes in vivo myocardial contractile function in dogs with pressure-overload left ventricular hypertrophy. *Circulation* 102:1045-1052, 2000.

29. Zile MR, Green GR, Schuyler GT, et al: Cardiocyte cytoskeleton in patients with left ventricular pressure overload hypertrophy. *J Am Coll Cardiol* 37:1080-1084, 2001.

30. Ding B, Price RL, Goldsmith EC, et al: Left ventricular hypertrophy in ascending aortic stenosis mice: Anoikis and the progression to early failure. *Circulation* 101:2854-2862, 2000.

31. Borow KM: Surgical outcome in chronic aortic regurgitation: A physiologic framework for assessing preoperative predictors. *J Am Coll Cardiol* 10:1165-1170, 1987.

32. Greenberg NL, Firstenberg MS, Castro PL, et al: Doppler-derived myocardial systolic strain rate is a strong index of left ventricular contractility. *Circulation* 105:99-105, 2002.

33. Borer JS, Hochreiter C, Herrold EM, et al: Prediction of indications for valve replacement among asymptomatic or minimally symptomatic patients with chronic aortic regurgitation and normal left ventricular performance. *Circulation* 97:525-534, 1998.

34. Yusoff R, Clayton N, Keevil B, et al: Utility of plasma N-terminal brain natriuretic peptide as a marker of functional capacity in patients with chronic severe mitral regurgitation. *Am J Cardiol* 97:1498-1501, 2006.

35. Detaint D, Messika-Zeitoun D, Avierinos JF, et al: B-type natriuretic peptide in organic mitral regurgitation: Determinants and impact on outcome. *Circulation* 111:2391-2397, 2005.

36. Detaint D, Messika-Zeitoun D, Chen HH, et al: Association of B-type natriuretic peptide activation to left ventricular end-systolic remodeling in organic and functional mitral regurgitation. *Am J Cardiol* 97:1029-1034, 2006.

37. Sutton TM, Stewart RA, Gerber IL, et al: Plasma natriuretic peptide levels increase with symptoms and severity of mitral regurgitation. *J Am Coll Cardiol* 41:2280-2287, 2003.

38. Kaufmann P, Vassalli G, Lupi-Wagner S, et al: Coronary artery dimensions in primary and secondary left ventricular hypertrophy. *J Am Coll Cardiol* 28:745-750, 1996.

39. Nitenberg A, Foult JM, Antony I, et al: Coronary flow and resistance reserve in patients with chronic aortic regurgitation, angina pectoris and normal coronary arteries. *J Am Coll Cardiol* 11:478-486, 1988.

40. Eberli FR, Ritter M, Schwitter J, et al: Coronary reserve in patients with aortic valve disease before and after successful aortic valve replacement. *Eur Heart J* 12:127-138, 1991.

41. Roberts WC, Ko JM, Moore TR, et al: Causes of pure aortic regurgitation in patients having isolated aortic valve replacement

at a single US tertiary hospital (1993 to 2005). *Circulation* 114:422-429, 2006.

42. Fedak PW, Verma S, David TE, et al: Clinical and pathophysiological implications of a bicuspid aortic valve. *Circulation* 106:900-904, 2002.

43. Lewin MB, Otto CM: The bicuspid aortic valve: Adverse outcomes from infancy to old age. *Circulation* 111:832-834, 2005.

44. Bonow RO, Lakatos E, Maron BJ, et al: Serial long-term assessment of the natural history of asymptomatic patients with chronic aortic regurgitation and normal left ventricular systolic function. *Circulation* 84:1625-1635, 1991.

45. Maurer G: Aortic regurgitation. *Heart* 92:994-1000, 2006.

46. Klodas E, Enriquez Sarano M, Tajik AJ, et al: Aortic regurgitation complicated by extreme left ventricular dilation: Long-term outcome after surgical correction. *J Am Coll Cardiol* 27:670-677, 1996.

47. Tornos MP, Olona M, Permanyer Miralda G, et al: Clinical outcome of severe asymptomatic chronic aortic regurgitation: A long-term prospective follow-up study. *Am Heart J* 130:333-339, 1995.

48. Tornos MP, Olona M, Permanyer-Miralda G, et al: Heart failure after aortic valve replacement for aortic regurgitation: prospective 20-year study. *Am Heart J* 136:681-687, 1998.

49. Turina J, Milincic J, Seifert B, et al: Valve replacement in chronic aortic regurgitation. True predictors of survival after extended follow-up. *Circulation* 98:II100-II106, 1998.

50. Klodas E, Enriquez SM, Tajik AJ, et al: Optimizing timing of surgical correction in patients with severe aortic regurgitation: role of symptoms. *J Am Coll Cardiol* 30:746-752, 1997.

51. Dujardin KS, Enriquez-Sarano M, Schaff HV, et al: Mortality and morbidity of aortic regurgitation in clinical practice. A long-term follow-up study. *Circulation* 99:1851-1857, 1999.

52. Henry WL, Bonow RO, Rosing DR, et al: Observations on the optimum time for operative intervention for aortic regurgitation. II. Serial echocardiographic evaluation of asymptomatic patients. *Circulation* 61:484-492, 1980.

53. Henry WL, Bonow RO, Borer JS, et al: Observations on the optimum time for operative intervention for aortic regurgitation. I. Evaluation of the results of aortic valve replacement in symptomatic patients. *Circulation* 61:471-483, 1980.

54. Bonow RO, Rosing DR, McIntosh CL, et al: The natural history of asymptomatic patients with aortic regurgitation and normal left ventricular function. *Circulation* 68:509-517, 1983.

55. Fioretti P, Roelandt J, Bos RJ, et al: Echocardiography in chronic aortic insufficiency. Is valve replacement too late when left ventricular end-systolic dimension reaches 55 mm? *Circulation* 67:216-221, 1983.

56. Bonow RO, Rosing DR, Maron BJ, et al: Reversal of left ventricular dysfunction after aortic valve replacement for chronic aortic regurgitation: influence of duration of preoperative left ventricular dysfunction. *Circulation* 70:570-579, 1984.

57. Daniel WG, Hood WP Jr, Siart A, et al: Chronic aortic regurgitation: Reassessment of the prognostic value of preoperative left ventricular end-systolic dimension and fractional shortening. *Circulation* 71:669-680, 1985.

58. Taniguchi K, Nakano S, Hirose H, et al: Preoperative left ventricular function: minimal requirement for successful late results of valve replacement for aortic regurgitation. *J Am Coll Cardiol* 10:510-518, 1987.

59. Carabello BA, Usher BW, Hendrix GH, et al: Predictors of outcome for aortic valve replacement in patients with aortic regurgitation and left ventricular dysfunction: A change in the measuring stick. *J Am Coll Cardiol* 10:991-997, 1987.

60. Bonow RO, Dodd JT, Maron BJ, et al: Long-term serial changes in left ventricular function and reversal of ventricular dilatation after valve replacement for chronic aortic regurgitation. *Circulation* 78(5 Pt1):1108-1120, 1988.

61. Siemienczuk D, Greenberg B, Morris C, et al: Chronic aortic insufficiency: Factors associated with progression to aortic valve replacement. *Ann Intern Med* 110:587-592, 1989.

62. Taniguchi K, Nakano S, Kawashima Y, et al: Left ventricular ejection performance, wall stress, and contractile state in aortic regurgitation before and after aortic valve replacement. *Circulation* 82:798-807, 1990.

63. Taniguchi K, Nakano S, Matsuda H, et al: Timing of operation for aortic regurgitation: Relation to postoperative contractile state. *Ann Thorac Surg* 50:779-785, 1990.

64. Pirwitz MJ, Lange RA, Willard JE, et al: Use of the left ventricular peak systolic pressure/end-systolic volume ratio to predict symptomatic improvement with valve replacement in patients with aortic regurgitation and enlarged end-systolic volume. *J Am Coll Cardiol* 24:1672-1677, 1994.

65. Tornos P, Sambola A, Permanyer-Miralda G, et al: Long-term outcome of surgically treated aortic regurgitation: influence of guideline adherence toward early surgery. *J Am Coll Cardiol* 47:1012-1017, 2006.

66. Tarasoutchi F, Grinberg M, Spina GS, et al: Ten-year clinical laboratory follow-up after application of a symptom-based therapeutic strategy to patients with severe chronic aortic regurgitation of predominant rheumatic etiology. *J Am Coll Cardiol* 41:1316-1324, 2003.

67. Evangelista A, Tornos P, Sambola A, et al: Long-term vasodilator therapy in patients with severe aortic regurgitation. *N Engl J Med* 353:1342-1349, 2005.

68. Klodas E, Enriquez Sarano M, Tajik AJ, et al: Surgery for aortic regurgitation in women: Contrasting indications and outcomes compared with men. *Circulation* 94:2472-2478, 1996.

69. Roberts WC, Ko JM: Frequency by decades of unicuspid, bicuspid, and tricuspid aortic valves in adults having isolated aortic valve replacement for aortic stenosis, with or without associated aortic regurgitation. *Circulation* 111:920-925, 2005.

70. Schaefer BM, Lewin MB, Stout KK, Otto CM: Usefulness of bicuspid aortic valve phenotype to predict elastic properties of the ascending aorta. *Am J Cardiol* 99:686-690, 2007.

71. Pibarot P, Dumesnil JG: Prosthesis-patient mismatch: Definition, clinical impact, and prevention. *Heart* 92:1022-1029, 2006.

72. Otto CM: *Textbook of Clinical Echocardiography*, 3rd ed. Philadelphia: Elsevier Saunders, 2004.

73. Zoghbi WA, Enriquez-Sarano M, Foster E, et al: Recommendations for evaluation of the severity of native valvular regurgitation with two-dimensional and Doppler echocardiography. *J Am Soc Echocardiogr* 16:777-802, 2003.

74. Gelfand EV, Hughes S, Hauser TH, et al: Severity of mitral and aortic regurgitation as assessed by cardiovascular magnetic resonance: Optimizing correlation with Doppler echocardiography. *J Cardiovasc Magn Reson* 8:503-507, 2006.

75. Wagner S, Auffermann W, Buser P, et al: Diagnostic accuracy and estimation of the severity of valvular regurgitation from the signal void on cine magnetic resonance images. *Am Heart J* 118:760-767, 1989.

76. Dulce MC, Mostbeck GH, O'Sullivan M, et al: Severity of aortic regurgitation: Interstudy reproducibility of measurements with velocity-encoded cine MR imaging. *Ann Thorac Surg* 185:235-240, 1992.

77. Eimer MJ, Ekery DL, Rigolin VH, et al: Elevated B-type natriuretic peptide in asymptomatic men with chronic aortic regurgitation and preserved left ventricular systolic function. *Am J Cardiol* 94:676-678, 2004.

78. Levine HJ, Gaasch WH: Vasoactive drugs in chronic regurgitant lesions of the mitral and aortic valves. *J Am Coll Cardiol* 28:1083-1091, 1996.

79. Scognamiglio R, Rahimtoola SH, Fasoli G, et al: Nifedipine in asymptomatic patients with severe aortic regurgitation and normal left ventricular function [see comments]. *N Engl J Med* 331:689-694, 1994.

80. Perloff JK, Roberts WC: The mitral apparatus: Functional anatomy of mitral regurgitation. *Circulation* 46:227-239, 1972.

81. Roberts WC: Morphologic features of the normal and abnormal mitral valve. *Am J Cardiol* 51:1005-1028, 1983.

82. He S, Fontaine AA, Schwammenthal E, et al: Integrated mechanism for functional mitral regurgitation—leaflet restriction versus coapting force: In vitro studies. *Circulation* 96:1826-1834, 1997.

83. Otsuji Y, Handschumacher MD, Schwammenthal E, et al: Insights from three-dimensional echocardiography into the mechanism of functional mitral regurgitation: Direct in vivo demonstration of altered leaflet tethering geometry. *Circulation* 96:1999-2008, 1997.

84. Kwan J, Shiota T, Agler DA, et al: Geometric differences of the mitral apparatus between ischemic and dilated cardiomyopathy with significant mitral regurgitation: Real-time three-dimensional echocardiography study. *Circulation* 107:1135-1140, 2003.

85. Otsuji Y, Handschumacher MD, Liel-Cohen N, et al: Mechanism of ischemic mitral regurgitation with segmental left ventricular dysfunction: Three-dimensional echocardiographic studies in models of acute and chronic progressive regurgitation. *J Am Coll Cardiol* 37:641-648, 2001.

86. Gorman JH III, Jackson BM, Gorman RC, et al: Papillary muscle discoordination rather than increased annular area facilitates mitral regurgitation after acute posterior myocardial infarction. *Circulation* 96(Suppl):II-124-II-127, 1997.

87. Levine RA, Schwammenthal E: Ischemic mitral regurgitation on the threshold of a solution: From paradoxes to unifying concepts. *Circulation* 112:745-758, 2005.

88. Aikawa K, Sheehan FH, Otto CM, et al: The severity of functional mitral regurgitation depends on the shape of the mitral apparatus: A three-dimensional echo analysis. *J Heart Valve Dis* 11:627-636, 2002.

89. Yiu SF, Enriquez-Sarano M, Tribouilloy C, et al: Determinants of the degree of functional mitral regurgitation in patients with systolic left ventricular dysfunction: A quantitative clinical study. *Circulation* 102:1400-1406, 2000.

90. Nielsen SL, Nygaard H, Fontaine AA, et al: Papillary muscle misalignment causes multiple mitral regurgitant jets: An ambiguous mechanism for functional mitral regurgitation. *J Heart Valve Dis* 8:551-564, 1999.

91. Keren G, Sonnenblick EH, LeJemtel TH: Mitral anulus motion. Relation to pulmonary venous and transmitral flows in normal subjects and in patients with dilated cardiomyopathy. *Circulation* 78:621-629, 1988.

92. Rosen SE, Borer JS, Hochreiter C, et al: Natural history of the asymptomatic/minimally symptomatic patient with severe mitral regurgitation secondary to mitral valve prolapse and normal right and left ventricular performance. *Am J Cardiol* 74:374-380, 1994.

93. Delahaye JP, Gare JP, Viguier E, et al: Natural history of severe mitral regurgitation. *Eur Heart J* 12(Suppl B):5-9, 1991.

94. Grigioni F, Enriquez-Sarano M, Zehr KJ, et al: Ischemic mitral regurgitation: Long-term outcome and prognostic implications with quantitative Doppler assessment. *Circulation* 103:1759-1764, 2001.

95. Rosenhek R, Rader F, Klaar U, et al: Outcome of watchful waiting in asymptomatic severe mitral regurgitation. *Circulation* 113:2238-2244, 2006.

96. Enriquez-Sarano M, Avierinos JF, Messika-Zeitoun D, et al: Quantitative determinants of the outcome of asymptomatic mitral regurgitation. *N Engl J Med* 352:875-883, 2005.

97. Duren DR, Becker AE, Dunning AJ: Long-term follow-up of idiopathic mitral valve prolapse in 300 patients: a prospective study. *J Am Coll Cardiol* 11:42-47, 1988.

98. Marks AR, Choong CY, Sanfilippo AJ, et al: Identification of high-risk and low-risk subgroups of patients with mitral-valve prolapse. *N Engl J Med* 320:1031-1036, 1989.

99. Zuppiroli A, Rinaldi M, Kramer Fox R, et al: Natural history of mitral valve prolapse. *Am J Cardiol* 75:1028-1032, 1995.

100. Ling LH, Enriquez-Sarano M, Seward JB, et al: Clinical outcome of mitral regurgitation due to flail leaflet. *N Engl J Med* 335:1417-1423, 1996.

101. Nishimura RA, McGoon MD, Shub C, et al: Echocardiographically documented mitral-valve prolapse. Long-term follow-up of 237 patients. *N Engl J Med* 313:1305-1309, 1985.

102. Grigioni F, Enriquez-Sarano M, Ling LH, et al: Sudden death in mitral regurgitation due to flail leaflet. *J Am Coll Cardiol* 34:2078-2085, 1999.

103. Kolibash AJ: Progression of mitral regurgitation in patients with mitral valve prolapse. *Herz* 13:309-317, 1988.

104. Grigioni F, Enriquez-Sarano M, Ling LH, et al: Sudden death in mitral regurgitation due to flail leaflet. *J Am Coll Cardiol* 34:2078-2085, 1999.

105. Grigioni F, Detaint D, Avierinos JF, et al: Contribution of ischemic mitral regurgitation to congestive heart failure after myocardial infarction. *J Am Coll Cardiol* 45:260-267, 2005.

106. Kligfield P, Ameisen O, Okin PM, et al: Relationship of the electrocardiographic response to exercise to geometric and functional findings in aortic regurgitation. *Am Heart J* 113:1097-1102, 1987.

107. Zuppiroli A, Mori F, Favilli S, et al: Arrhythmias in mitral valve prolapse: Relation to anterior mitral leaflet thickening, clinical variables, and color Doppler echocardiographic parameters. *Am Heart J* 128:919-927, 1994.

108. Michel PL, Iung B, Blanchard B, et al: Long-term results of mitral valve repair for non-ischaemic mitral regurgitation. *Eur Heart J* 12(Suppl B):39-43, 1991.

109. Jebara VA, Dervanian P, Acar C, et al: Mitral valve repair using Carpentier techniques in patients more than 70 years old. Early and late results. *Circulation* 86:II53-II59, 1992.

110. David TE, Armstrong S, Sun Z, et al: Late results of mitral valve repair for mitral regurgitation due to degenerative disease. *Ann Thorac Surg* 56:7-12, 1993.

111. Gramaglia B, Imazio M, Checco L, et al: Mitral valve prolapse. Comparison between valvular repair and replacement in severe mitral regurgitation. *J Cardiovasc Surg (Torino)* 40:93-99, 1999.

112. Mohty D, Orszulak TA, Schaff HV, et al: Very long-term survival and durability of mitral valve repair for mitral valve prolapse. *Circulation* 104:I1-I7, 2001.

113. Fernandez J, Joyce DH, Hirschfeld KJ, et al: Valve-related events and valve-related mortality in 340 mitral valve repairs. A late phase follow-up study. *Eur J Cardiothorac Surg* 7:263-270, 1993.

114. Bernal JM, Rabasa JM, Vilchez FG, et al: Mitral valve repair in rheumatic disease. The flexible solution. *Circulation* 88(4 Pt1) 1746-1753, 1993.

115. Chauvaud S, Fuzellier JF, Berrebi A, et al: Long-term (29 years) results of reconstructive surgery in rheumatic mitral valve insufficiency. *Circulation* 104:I12-I15, 2001.

116. Choudhary SK, Talwar S, Dubey B, et al: Mitral valve repair in a predominantly rheumatic population. Long-term results. *Tex Heart Inst J* 28:8-15, 2001.

117. Kay GL, Kay JH, Zubiate P, et al: Mitral valve repair for mitral regurgitation secondary to coronary artery disease. *Circulation* 74:88-98, 1986.

118. Hendren WG, Nemec JJ, Lytle BW, et al: Mitral valve repair for ischemic mitral insufficiency [see comments]. *Ann Thorac Surg* 52:1246-1251, 1991.

119. Lee EM, Shapiro LM, Wells FC: Importance of subvalvular preservation and early operation in mitral valve surgery. *Circulation* 94:2117-2123, 1996.

120. Moss RR, Humphries KH, Gao M, et al: Outcome of mitral valve repair or replacement: A comparison by propensity score analysis. *Circulation* 108(Suppl 1):II90-II97.

121. Phillips HR, Levine FH, Carter JE, et al: Mitral valve replacement for isolated mitral regurgitation: Analysis of clinical course and late postoperative left ventricular ejection fraction. *Am J Cardiol* 48:647-654, 1981.

122. Zile MR, Gaasch WH, Carroll JD, et al: Chronic mitral regurgitation: Predictive value of preoperative echocardiographic indexes of left ventricular function and wall stress. *J Am Coll Cardiol* 3(2 Pt 1):235-242, 1984.

123. Crawford MH, Souchek J, Oprian CA, et al: Determinants of survival and left ventricular performance after mitral valve replacement. Department of Veterans Affairs Cooperative Study on Valvular Heart Disease. *Circulation* 81:1173-1181, 1990.

124. Enriquez-Sarano M, Tajik AJ, Schaff HV, et al: Echocardiographic prediction of left ventricular function after correction of mitral regurgitation: Results and clinical implications [see comments]. *J Am Coll Cardiol* 24:1536-1543, 1994.

125. Enriquez-Sarano M, Tajik AJ, Schaff HV, et al: Echocardiographic prediction of survival after surgical correction of organic mitral regurgitation. *Circulation* 90:830-837, 1994.

126. Flemming MA, Oral H, Rothman ED, et al: Echocardiographic markers for mitral valve surgery to preserve left ventricular performance in mitral regurgitation. *Am Heart J* 140:476-482, 2000.

127. David TE, Omran A, Armstrong S, et al: Long-term results of mitral valve repair for myxomatous disease with and without chordal replacement with expanded polytetrafluoroethylene sutures. *J Thorac Cardiovasc Surg* 115:1279-1285, 1998.

128. Carpentier AF, Lessana A, Relland JY, et al: The "physio-ring": An advanced concept in mitral valve annuloplasty. *Ann Thorac Surg* 60:1177-1185, 1995.

129. Cosgrove DM III, Arcidi JM, Rodriguez L, et al: Initial experience with the Cosgrove-Edwards Annuloplasty System. *Ann Thorac Surg* 60:499-503, 1995.

130. Gillinov AM, Cosgrove DM, Blackstone EH, et al: Durability of mitral valve repair for degenerative disease. *J Thorac Cardiovasc Surg* 116:734-743, 1998.

131. Kennedy JW, Doces JG, Stewart DK: Left ventricular function before and following surgical treatment of mitral valve disease. *Am Heart J* 97:592-598, 1979.

132. David TE, Burns RJ, Bacchus CM, et al: Mitral valve replacement for mitral regurgitation with and without preservation of chordae tendineae. *J Thorac Cardiovasc Surg* 88(5 Pt 1):718-725, 1984.

133. Goldman ME, Mora F, Guarino T, et al: Mitral valvuloplasty is superior to valve replacement for preservation of left ventricular function: An intraoperative two-dimensional echocardiographic study. *J Am Coll Cardiol* 10:568-575, 1987.

134. Miki S, Kusuhara K, Ueda Y, et al: Mitral valve replacement with preservation of chordae tendineae and papillary muscles. *Ann Thorac Surg* 45:28-34, 1988.

135. Rozich JD, Carabello BA, Usher BW, et al: Mitral valve replacement with and without chordal preservation in patients with chronic mitral regurgitation. Mechanisms for differences in postoperative ejection performance. *Circulation* 86:1718-1726, 1992.

136. Enriquez-Sarano M, Schaff HV, Orszulak TA, et al: Congestive heart failure after surgical correction of mitral regurgitation. A long-term study. *Circulation* 92:2496-2503, 1995.

137. Enriquez-Sarano M, Schaff HV, Orszulak TA, et al: Valve repair improves the outcome of surgery for mitral regurgitation. A multivariate analysis. *Circulation* 91:1022-1028, 1995.

138. Corin WJ, Sutsch G, Murakami T, et al: Left ventricular function in chronic mitral regurgitation: Preoperative and postoperative comparison. *J Am Coll Cardiol* 25:113-121, 1995.

139. Starling MR: Effects of valve surgery on left ventricular contractile function in patients with long-term mitral regurgitation. *Circulation* 92:811-818, 1995.

140. Leung DY, Griffin BP, Stewart WJ, et al: Left ventricular function after valve repair for chronic mitral regurgitation: Predictive

value of preoperative assessment of contractile reserve by exercise echocardiography. *J Am Coll Cardiol* 28:1198-1205, 1996.

141. Matsumura T, Ohtaki E, Tanaka K, et al: Echocardiographic prediction of left ventricular dysfunction after mitral valve repair for mitral regurgitation as an indicator to decide the optimal timing of repair. *J Am Coll Cardiol* 42:458-463, 2003.

142. Kongsaerepong V, Shiota M, Gillinov AM, et al: Echocardiographic predictors of successful versus unsuccessful mitral valve repair in ischemic mitral regurgitation. *Am J Cardiol* 98:504-508, 2006.

143. Omran AS, Woo A, David TE, et al: Intraoperative transesophageal echocardiography accurately predicts mitral valve anatomy and suitability for repair. *J Am Soc Echocardiogr* 15:950-957, 2002.

144. Messika-Zeitoun D, Johnson BD, Nkomo V, et al: Cardiopulmonary exercise testing determination of functional capacity in mitral regurgitation: physiologic and outcome implications. *J Am Coll Cardiol* 47:2521-2527, 2006.

145. Lee R, Haluska B, Leung DY, et al: Functional and prognostic implications of left ventricular contractile reserve in patients with asymptomatic severe mitral regurgitation. *Heart* 91:1407-1412, 2005.

146. Kon MW, Myerson SG, Moat NE, et al: Quantification of regurgitant fraction in mitral regurgitation by cardiovascular magnetic resonance: Comparison of techniques. *J Heart Valve Dis* 13:600-607, 2004.

147. Westenberg JJ, Doornbos J, Versteegh MI, et al: Accurate quantitation of regurgitant volume with MRI in patients selected for mitral valve repair. *Eur J Cardiothorac Surg* 27:462-466, 2005.

148. Westenberg JJ, van der Geest RJ, Lamb HJ, et al: MRI to evaluate left atrial and ventricular reverse remodeling after restrictive mitral annuloplasty in dilated cardiomyopathy. *Circulation* 112:I437-I442, 2005.

149. Acker MA, Bolling S, Shemin R, et al: Mitral valve surgery in heart failure: Insights from the Acorn Clinical Trial. *J Thorac Cardiovasc Surg* 132:568-577, 2006.

150. Kang DH, Kim MJ, Kang SJ, et al: Mitral valve repair versus revascularization alone in the treatment of ischemic mitral regurgitation. *Circulation* 114:I499-I503, 2006.

151. Guy TS, Moainie SL, Gorman JH III, et al: Prevention of ischemic mitral regurgitation does not influence the outcome of remodeling after posterolateral myocardial infarction. *J Am Coll Cardiol* 43:377-383, 2004.

152. Enomoto Y, Gorman JH III, Moainie SL, et al: Surgical treatment of ischemic mitral regurgitation might not influence ventricular remodeling. *J Thorac Cardiovasc Surg* 129:504-511, 2005.

153. Diodato MD, Moon MR, Pasque MK, et al: Repair of ischemic mitral regurgitation does not increase mortality or improve long-term survival in patients undergoing coronary artery revascularization: A propensity analysis. *Ann Thorac Surg* 78:794-799, 2004.

154. Gillinov AM, Wierup PN, Blackstone EH, et al: Is repair preferable to replacement for ischemic mitral regurgitation? *J Thorac Cardiovasc Surg* 122:1125-1141, 2001.

155. Grossi EA, Bizekis CS, LaPietra A, et al: Late results of isolated mitral annuloplasty for "functional" ischemic mitral insufficiency. *J Card Surg* 16:328-332, 2001.

156. Chen FY, Adams DH, Aranki SF, et al: Mitral valve repair in cardiomyopathy. *Circulation* 98:II124-II127, 1998.

157. Bolling SF, Pagani FD, Deeb GM, et al: Intermediate-term outcome of mitral reconstruction in cardiomyopathy. *J Thorac Cardiovasc Surg* 115:381-386, 1998.

158. Wu AH, Aaronson KD, Bolling SF, et al: Impact of mitral valve annuloplasty on mortality risk in patients with mitral regurgitation and left ventricular systolic dysfunction. *J Am Coll Cardiol* 45:381-387, 2005.

159. Spoor MT, Geltz A, Bolling SF: Flexible versus nonflexible mitral valve rings for congestive heart failure: Differential durability of repair. *Circulation* 114:I67-I71, 2006.

160. Host U, Kelbaek H, Hildebrandt P, et al: Effect of ramipril on mitral regurgitation secondary to mitral valve prolapse. *Am J Cardiol* 80:655-658, 1997.

161. Tischler MD, Rowan M, LeWinter MM: Effect of enalapril therapy on left ventricular mass and volumes in asymptomatic chronic, severe mitral regurgitation secondary to mitral valve prolapse. *Am J Cardiol* 82:242-245, 1998.

162. Dujardin KS, Enriquez-Sarano M, Bailey KR, et al: Effect of losartan on degree of mitral regurgitation quantified by echocardiography. *Am J Cardiol* 87:570-576, 2001.

163. Gupta DK, Kapoor A, Garg N, et al: Beneficial effects of nicorandil versus enalapril in chronic rheumatic severe mitral regurgitation: Six months follow up echocardiographic. *J Heart Valve Dis* 10:158-165, 2001.

164. Levine RA: Dynamic mitral regurgitation—more than meets the eye. *N Engl J Med* 351:1681-1684, 2004.

165. Hamilton MA, Stevenson LW, Child JS, et al: Sustained reduction in valvular regurgitation and atrial volumes with tailored vasodilator therapy in advanced congestive heart failure secondary to dilated (ischemic or idiopathic) cardiomyopathy. *Am J Cardiol* 67:259-263, 1991.

166. Lowes BD, Gill EA, Abraham WT, et al: Effects of carvedilol on left ventricular mass, chamber geometry, and mitral regurgitation in chronic heart failure. *Am J Cardiol* 83:1201-1205, 1999.

167. Rosario LB, Stevenson LW, Solomon SD, et al: The mechanism of decrease in dynamic mitral regurgitation during heart failure treatment: Importance of reduction in the regurgitant orifice size. *J Am Coll Cardiol* 32:1819-1824, 1998.

168. Sutton MG, Plappert T, Hilpisch KE, et al: Sustained reverse left ventricular structural remodeling with cardiac resynchronization at one year is a function of etiology: quantitative Doppler echocardiographic evidence from the Multicenter InSync Randomized Clinical Evaluation (MIRACLE). *Circulation* 113:266-272, 2006.

169. Porciani MC, Macioce R, Demarchi G, et al: Effects of cardiac resynchronization therapy on the mechanisms underlying functional mitral regurgitation in congestive heart failure. *Eur J Echocardiogr* 7:31-39, 2006.

170. Murphy JG, Gersh BJ, Mair DD, et al: Long-term outcome in patients undergoing surgical repair of tetralogy of Fallot. *N Eng J Med* 329:593-599, 1993.

171. Hazekamp MG, Kurvers MM, Schoof PH, et al: Pulmonary valve insertion late after repair of Fallot's tetralogy. *Eur J Cardiothorac Surg* 19:667-670, 2001.

172. Geva T: Indications and timing of pulmonary valve replacement after tetralogy of Fallot repair. *Semin Thorac Cardiovasc Surg Pediatr Card Surg Annu* 11-22, 2006.

173. Dave HH, Buechel ER, Dodge-Khatami A, et al: Early insertion of a pulmonary valve for chronic regurgitation helps restoration of ventricular dimensions. *Ann Thorac Surg* 80:1615-1620, 2005.

174. Celermajer DS, Bull C, Till JA, et al: Ebstein's anomaly: Presentation and outcome from fetus to adult. *J Am Coll Cardiol* 23:170-176, 1994.

175. McCarthy PM, Bhudia SK, Rajeswaran J, et al: Tricuspid valve repair: Durability and risk factors for failure. *J Thorac Cardiovasc Surg* 127:674-685, 2004.

176. Dreyfus GD, Corbi PJ, Chan KM, et al: Secondary tricuspid regurgitation or dilatation: Which should be the criteria for surgical repair? *Ann Thorac Surg* 79:127-132, 2005.

177. Duran CM: Tricuspid valve surgery revisited. *J Card Surg* 9:242-247, 1994.

Chapter 20

Intraoperative Echocardiography in Mitral Valve Repair

WILLIAM J. STEWART, MD • BRIAN P. GRIFFIN, MD

The advent of transesophageal echocardiography (TEE) and innovations in ultrasound (US) technology have led to progressive improvement in the outcomes of valve surgery, especially mitral valve repair. Echocardiography has been used extensively in the operating room (OR) since the early 1980s. It is an essential element of every valve reconstruction operation.

Indications for Intraoperative Echocardiography

Intraoperative echocardiography (IOE) has both diagnostic and monitoring functions that are useful in valve surgery, especially valve-sparing operations. The diagnostic functions of IOE are used before cardiopulmonary bypass (CPB; prepump) to determine the mechanism and severity of the mitral valvular dysfunction, identify lesions of other valves, and refine the surgical mission. After CPB (postpump), the diagnostic strengths of IOE are used again to determine the success of the surgical mission. IOE is essential in performing mitral valve repair and many other types of innovative heart surgery.[1] In addition to its use in valve surgery, the diagnostic function of IOE also is used in the surgical management of congenital heart disease,[2,3] hypertrophic cardiomyopathy (HCM),[4,5] reconstruction of the ascending aorta,[6,7] and many other surgeries[8] (Table 20-1).

The monitoring function of IOE is used to determine the hemodynamic status of the patient before and after cardiac surgery, and during noncardiac surgery, for assessing intravascular volume and ventricular contractility. Perioperative monitoring of left ventricular (LV) function is important in patients with impaired contractility who are undergoing any kind of cardiac surgery, including myocardial revascularization[9,10] and in those with significant cardiac disease undergoing high-risk noncardiac surgery, such as reconstructive surgery of the descending thoracic and abdominal aorta (see Chapter 2).[11-13] IOE also is used to help position intravascular and intracardiac catheters,[14,15] including intraaortic balloon pumps and retrograde cardioplegia implanted via the coronary sinus. It is also used in patient selection and monitoring during alternative surgical approaches, such as limited access (minimally invasive) surgery done through smaller incisions, endoscopic or port access surgery, robotic surgery, and off-pump coronary artery bypass grafting without CPB.[16,17] When postpump echocardiography detects intracardiac air,[18,19] further venting of the cardiac chambers can be done to prevent embolization to the coronary blood vessels[20] or the brain.[21] When there is difficulty weaning a patient from CPB or hypotension in the early postoperative period, echocardiography is a useful diagnostic and monitoring tool.[22,23]

Postpump Intraoperative Echocardiography

The most frequent indication for IOE is the postpump assessment of valve reconstruction surgery to determine whether the desired surgical result has been obtained. The availability of online feedback concerning the adequacy of the surgical result has allowed surgeons to become more innovative in repair techniques.

TABLE 20-1. Indications for Intraoperative Echocardiography

Mitral Disease
Assess feasibility and success of mitral repair for mitral regurgitation.
Assess feasibility and success of commissurotomy for mitral stenosis.
Determine need for mitral surgery in patients undergoing revascularization or aortic surgery.
Assess presence of disease of other valves or other cardiac structures.

Aortic Disease
Assess feasibility and success of aortic valve repair.
Assess size of prosthesis.
Assess feasibility and success of homograft implantation or Ross procedure.

Tricuspid Disease
Assess need for and feasibility and success of tricuspid repair.

Prosthetic Function
Determine presence and site of paravalvular leak.
Assess perivalvular tissue for abscesses or infection.
Assess site and presence of pannus or thrombus.

Revascularization
Assess regional wall motion and global left ventricular function before and after revascularization.
Determine sequence of graft placement.
Detect and assess complications of infarction (ventricular septal defect, mitral regurgitation).

Surgery on Aorta
Assess size and extent of aneurysm.
Determine the mechanism and severity of associated aortic regurgitation.
Determine presence and complications of aortic dissection.
Determine presence and extent of aortic atheroma.

Transplantation/Devices
Assess left ventricular function and suture lines postoperatively.
Assess appropriate sizing, function, and hemodynamic changes with ventricular assist devices.

Congenital Heart Surgery
Determine connections (ventriculoarterial, atrioventricular).
Assess systemic and nonsystemic ventricular size and function.
Assess anatomy of shunts and valvular anatomy.

Monitoring
Assess ventricular volume and function.
Monitor drug effects on ventricular function.
Diagnose presence and location of ischemia.

Immediately after valve repair and before the chest is closed, the echocardiographer can determine whether the repair is adequate or if there is residual regurgitation or other complications present, requiring further repair or prosthetic implantation. Making this determination before the chest is closed allows the surgeon to perform further surgical procedures during a second run of CPB (a "second pump run") to optimize the surgical outcome. This second pump run eliminates the need for another surgical procedure at a later time, which would require another thoracotomy and create an increased mortality risk for the patient. In various studies, 6% to 11% of patients undergoing valve surgery had inadequate results based on postpump echocardiographic imaging and required further surgery.[1,24]

Prepump Intraoperative Echocardiography

It is axiomatic that all elective patients undergoing cardiac surgery have a full diagnostic workup and a definite surgical plan before arriving in the OR. Despite this, there are findings on the prepump echocardiogram that alter management by refining the preoperative diagnosis and the surgical mission. In a series of 436 consecutive patients with various valve problems, the surgical procedure was changed in 40 cases (9.2%) on the basis of prepump echocardiograms. In another series of 154 consecutive patients undergoing valvular surgery, 29 patients (19%) had significant new findings by prepump IOE, and these findings changed the operative plan in 14 patients (9%). The changes were more common in mitral than aortic operations, and most frequently involved an increase in the severity of the valvular regurgitation compared with preoperative studies.[24] In a large series reported by Click and colleagues, there was a 14% incidence of changes in the operation based on the prepump IOE, a frequency which does not appear to be decreasing over the years studied.[25]

Even in patients in whom no major change in plan occurs, the prepump echocardiogram provides an updated understanding of the specific valvular anatomy and the mechanism of dysfunction, which helped to refine the surgical technique. These changes result from the improvement in resolution of TEE over preoperative transthoracic echocardiography (TTE) or cardiac catheterization and from changes in hemodynamic conditions or ischemia between the time of preoperative testing and the time of surgery. Another study of 1918 consecutive cases showed a low prevalence (2.5%) of findings that were discordant between IOE and operative findings. In only 0.3% of patients were the discrepancies sufficiently severe to warrant a change in the operative procedure.[26]

Technique of Intraoperative Echocardiography

IOE may be performed from either the transesophageal or epicardial imaging windows (Table 20–2).

Transesophageal Echocardiography

TEE is the most widely used technique for IOE. Figure 20–1 illustrates the experience with IOE at the Cleveland Clinic Foundation from 1984 through 1999. TEE became available in 1987 and progressively supplanted the epicardial route for most studies. Compared with epicardial echocardiography, TEE has the advantage of allowing image acquisition without interfering with the surgical field or procedure. Immediately after induction of anesthesia and endotracheal intubation, the TEE probe is inserted and left in place throughout the operation.

Although the technique of intraoperative TEE is similar to its use in the echocardiography laboratory, there are additional potential pitfalls. First, it is occasionally difficult to pass the probe, particularly if the patient has been draped and the ether screen has been positioned. Usually, this problem can be overcome using a laryngoscope and direct vision.

TABLE 20–2. Relative Advantages of Epicardial and Transesophageal Approaches to Intraoperative Echocardiography

	Epicardial	Transesophageal
Indications	LVOT gradients; HOCM; congenital, aortic atheroma; when TEE is impossible or nondiagnostic	All others
Transducer	3.5-7.5 MHz transthoracic (standard TTE) sector scan; use higher frequencies for epiaortic scanning and congenital cases	3.5-7.5 MHz transesophageal
Advantages	Excellent images, especially of LVOT and septum; rapid imaging in emergency	Does not interfere with sterile field; continuous imaging possible
Disadvantages	Requires plastic covers for sterile preparation of probe; interferes with operative field and procedure; imaging of posterior structures difficult with prosthetic shadowing; may interfere with hemodynamics; requires >1 person	May be difficult to intubate esophagus once patient is draped; occasionally impossible to obtain images (e.g., result of hiatal hernia, air); imaging of anterior structures difficult; contraindicated with esophageal abnormalities

HOCM, hypertrophic obstructive cardiomyopathy; LVOT, left ventricular outflow tract; TEE, transesophageal echocardiography; TTE, transthoracic echocardiography.

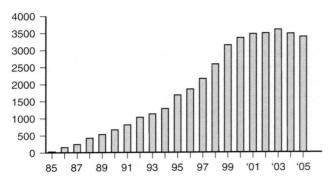

Figure 20–1. Cleveland Clinic Foundation experience with intraoperative echocardiography from 1984 to 2005. The total number of intraoperative echocardiograms per year is shown (bars). The number of intraoperative echocardiography (IOE) per year increased from 45 studies during 1985 to 3398 studies during the year 2005.

Inadequate imaging occurs with the transesophageal approach for a number of reasons. Anatomic causes include a hiatal hernia or the presence of an echodense structure, such as a mechanical valve prosthesis, that can cause shadowing of other cardiac structures. With all TEE studies, there is a blind spot, approximately 2 to 4 cm in size in the middle portion of the ascending aorta caused by interposition of the trachea between the esophagus and the ascending aorta. Interference from electrical apparatus, such as electrocautery, leads to distortion of two-dimensional (2D) imaging and renders spectral and color Doppler signals impossible to interpret. Fortunately, imaging may be resumed once the electrocautery is discontinued. Also, while the patient is on CPB, the absence of cardiac motion causes suboptimal images until the heart is filled with blood again and starts to eject during rewarming.

Epicardial Echocardiography

In epicardial imaging, images of the heart are acquired by placing a standard transthoracic transducer directly on the epicardium. Sterility is maintained using a double plastic sleeve. Intervening air is eliminated by using sterile acoustic gel inside the layers of plastic and by moistening the epicardial surface. An acoustic standoff, such as a sterile bag or glove filled with saline, is sometimes used if the structures of interest are superficial in the first centimeter of depth below the probe.

Epicardial echocardiography often provides better image quality than TEE of anterior structures, such as the ascending aorta, aortic arch, and the right ventricular outflow tract (RVOT) and left ventricular outflow tract (LVOT), and it is especially accurate in measuring the outflow tract velocities. An epicardial approach when IOE is needed clinically is used, but images obtained by TEE are inadequate during an open-chest procedure. In addition, epicardial imaging is needed in

infants who are too small for the available TEE probes. Progressively fewer procedures are performed using an epicardial imaging window. The major current indication for an epicardial approach is in the evaluation of the ascending aorta of patients with suspected ascending atheroma, on the basis of clinical suspicion, calcification on chest x-ray (CXR) study, or palpation by the surgeon. Identification of the severity and location of atheroma helps the surgical team optimize the location and methods of cannulation, including the use of an alternative cannulation sites, such as the subclavian or femoral artery.

In 1987, we described the following four standard transducer positions (Fig. 20–2) useful for epicardial imaging[27]:

1. *Parasternal equivalent.* The transducer is placed on the most anterior portion of the heart, the right ventricular outflow tract. Image planes are similar to those for transthoracic imaging from the left parasternal imaging window. Long-axis and short-axis views of the left ventricles are obtained. The heart is scanned in the short axis from base to apex. By imaging more medially, the tricuspid valve and right ventricle also may be imaged.

2. *Aorta-pulmonary sulcus.* The transducer is placed in the sulcus between the pulmonary artery and ascending aorta, with the long side of the trans-

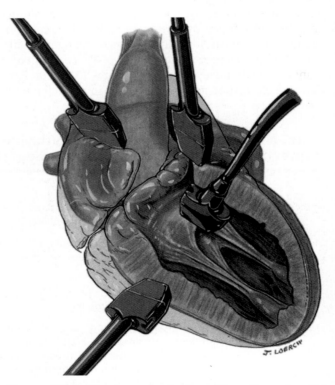

Figure 20–2. The four standard positions for epicardial transducer placement. (From Cosgrove DM, Stewart WJ: Curr Probl Cardiol 14:359-415, 1989.)

ducer against the left side of the ascending aorta. This view looks similar to a parasternal long axis equivalent but is angled more from left anterior to right and posterior. It provides excellent images of the LVOT, aorta, aortic valve, mitral valve, and left atrium.

3. *Subcostal equivalent.* The transducer is placed at the most inferior portion of the thoracotomy incision, with its face against the most inferior portion of the right ventricular free wall, pointing superiorly and slightly to the left. The four-chamber view is used to evaluate all four chambers, mitral and tricuspid valves, pulmonary artery, and the systemic veins. Angling medially allows imaging of the venae cavae, atria, and atrial septum. Angling superiorly and leftward visualizes the right ventricular outflow tract. Angling laterally to the left brings in the LV apex. Rotating the transducer by about 45 degrees allow subcostal equivalent views of the left heart structures in short axis.

4. *Aorta-superior vena cava position.* The long side of the transducer is placed against the right side of the ascending aorta, pointing inferiorly and to the left, to image the LVOT, left atrium, and the aortic and mitral valves. This view is the best way to determine LV outflow gradients by orienting the continuous wave (CW) Doppler beam parallel to flow.

The epicardial window allows excellent imaging of intracardiac structures, such as the cardiac valves and myocardium. High-velocity jets may be measured by CW Doppler either with an imaging transducer or a stand-alone, nonimaging transducer.

The epicardial window also has the disadvantages of interrupting the operation itself and requiring an individual to be scrubbed for surgery who is adept at image acquisition.

Equipment

Ideally, an US machine devoted solely to IOE should be available. In addition to interfacing with transesophageal and transthoracic transducers, the machine should be capable of recording M-mode and two-dimensional imaging and all Doppler modalities. A facility should be available near the OR for cleaning and disinfecting the probes. Transthoracic probes from 3.0 to 7.5 MHz may be useful for different purposes, depending on the objectives of the study, using the lower frequency for general cardiac imaging and the higher frequency for infant congenital cases and aortic atheroma investigation. A stand-alone CW Doppler probe should also be available, especially for recording outflow tract velocities. Sterile sleeves and acoustic gel should be available for epicardial imaging. The ultrasonic machine should

have a capability for cine-loop display and retrieval to compare prepump with postpump images. Cables should be available to input the electrocardiographic signal from the OR monitoring system into the US machine. Many institutions have the capability of transmitting images from the OR to a remote site, such as the echocardiography laboratory, to allow oversight or second opinions to be obtained in selected cases. Digital storage of images allows rapid retrieval to demonstrate findings to the surgical personnel and to facilitate comparison of the preoperative and postoperative images.[28]

Personnel

IOE is a highly demanding technical field requiring specialized personnel skilled in transesophageal and epicardial imaging. This field requires familiarity with the phases of cardiac surgery and their effects on hemodynamics as manifested by echocardiographic and Doppler studies. The American Society of Echocardiography (ASE) suggests that those learning TEE be in the phase of developing level 3 experience, which is equivalent to experience in performing at least 300 echocardiographic studies. In busy ORs, in which a large volume of intraoperative studies are being undertaken, an echocardiographic technologist or other ancillary support person, working under the aegis of the echocardiographer, can facilitate and improve the efficiency of acquiring multiple studies, some of which may be needed simultaneously.

Intraoperative Echocardiography Examination

IOE examinations should be performed in a standard comprehensive manner so that the acquisition of critical information is not omitted. It is important to do a complete TEE study, using imaging planes that allow good views of each intracardiac valve and chamber and the great vessels.[29] The entire prepump examination should be recorded to provide a durable record of the examination, especially as a reference for postpump studies and for medical-legal purposes. In cases in which comparison with postpump findings is likely, storing key images in a cine-loop facilitates rapid comparison at the end of the operation. In diagnostic (as opposed to monitoring) studies, the structure of interest to the primary surgical mission should first be examined thoroughly in multiple planes, using imaging and Doppler modalities. If the echocardiographic study must thereafter be abbreviated because of pressing demands of the surgical agenda or the need to limit anesthetic and cross-clamp time, the primary concern, the raison d'être of the echocardiographic study, has at least been addressed. Other structures of interest should then be examined, including long- and short-axis views of all four chambers, all four valves, and the great vessels. The entire aorta should be examined in all cases. We also advocate a routine intravenous (IV) contrast injection to look for intracardiac shunting. The number of times the probe is passed through the gastroesophageal junction should be minimized, as should all unnecessary manipulation of the probe, to reduce the risk of mucosal trauma, esophageal tears, and pharyngeal trauma that are reported in a small percentage of cases.[30]

Once the prepump study is completed, a written report of the examination detailing significant findings should be made. Although US has not been demonstrated to cause any significant damage to cardiac structures during prolonged examinations,[30] it is advisable to put the machine on freeze so that no US energy is transmitted when imaging is not required. After cessation of CPB, a second comprehensive examination should be carried out and a second or updated report generated.

The intraoperative examination has several aspects that are different from a TEE or TTE study in the outpatient echocardiography laboratory:

1. The echocardiogram is performed simultaneously with the operation; therefore, the room conditions, including the lighting and the space for the machine, may be suboptimal. For example, radiofrequency interference from other machines may mar the quality of images for long periods.

2. The hemodynamic milieu may change quickly, and the echocardiographic appearance may differ from images acquired outside the OR. Changes in hemodynamics, such as intravascular volume, preload, and afterload, substantially affect the severity of valvular lesions and ventricular performance. If necessary, the hemodynamic situation should be manipulated to match "street conditions," to determine the true or potential severity of a valvular lesion.

3. The surgeon who requests the intraoperative study may request online interpretation. Care must be maintained to make only diagnoses and conclusions that have been verified by examination from multiple imaging planes under appropriate imaging and hemodynamic conditions.

Prepump Intraoperative Echocardiography in Patients Undergoing Valve Repair for Mitral Regurgitation

The prepump echocardiogram assessment of mitral regurgitation (MR) (Table 20–3) usually confirms findings made previously by preoperative echocardiography or cardiac catheterization. However, because of its

TABLE 20–3. Intraoperative Assessment of Repair and Reconstructive Valve Operations

Prepump
Assess severity of stenosis/regurgitation.
Assess mechanism of regurgitation and potential reparability of valve.
Measure dimensions of annulus, chambers, and valves.
Assess whether lesions other than the primary lesion require surgery.
Determine biventricular function.

Postpump
Assess severity and mechanism of residual regurgitation/stenosis.
Detect systolic anterior motion of the mitral valve and left ventricular outflow obstruction.
Determine change in severity of other valve lesions.
Assess biventricular function.
Detect iatrogenic complications.

improved resolution over TTE, TEE often improves on the accuracy and resolution of preoperative TTE of the component structures, the mitral valve, and the regurgitant jet. There are four main goals of IOE in mitral valve disease:

1. To assess the severity of MR and determine the need for mitral valve surgery.

2. To assess the mechanism of MR and determine if a repair rather than prosthetic replacement is feasible and to determine the technique of repair.

3. To determine the presence of other significant disease that may require surgical attention, such as tricuspid or aortic valve disease or intraluminal thrombi.

4. To assess left and right ventricular function to compare with the postpump study.

Severity of Mitral Regurgitation

The severity of MR is assessed by IOE in the same manner as the use of echocardiography for other applications in other parts of the hospital (see Chapter 1).[31-35] The intraoperative assessment of MR agrees with the preoperative assessment by contrast ventriculography or TTE,[36,37] however, it may reflect change, depending on different loading conditions. In patients with ischemic MR, agreement between preoperative studies and the intraoperative assessment is less, possibly because of more hemodynamic dependence or differing degrees of ischemia. One study of patients with ischemic MR showed that in 11% of patients the preoperative and intraoperative assessments of MR severity differed by more than one grade, with discordance occurring in both directions.[38] Discordance was more common in patients with clinical instability or those who received thrombolysis. MR is a dynamic lesion, affected greatly by loading conditions. Reduction of afterload or intravascular volume at the time of the operation may reduce the true severity of the regurgitation. When less than expected MR is found, the intravascular blood volume should be expanded and systemic vascular resistance increased transiently using repeated boluses of IV phenylephrine, usually 100 μg every 30 to 60 seconds. The velocity of MR, and therefore display of its jet by color Doppler, depends on the pressure difference between the left atrium and left ventricle, which is higher with hypertension. The size of the jet in the left atrium is also sensitive to changes in color gain (directly proportional) and pulse repetition frequency (inversely proportional; see Chapter 18), so spatial mapping should be performed at a Nyquist setting of 50 to 60 cm/s.

The transesophageal imaging window has advantages over epicardial imaging in the assessment of MR. A mitral prosthesis or severe mitral calcification causes acoustic shadowing of the regurgitant jet when the transducer is placed anteriorly, as in epicardial imaging or TTE. Excellent agreement, however, has been reported between the epicardial and transesophageal approaches in assessing MR.[39]

Semiquantitation of MR on a scale from 0 to 4+[31,32] is determined based on a weighted average of several criteria:

1. The size of the left atrial flow disturbance, based on the depth of penetration and area of the regurgitant jet in the left atrial cavity assessed in multiple imaging planes; a multiplane probe facilitates this process, especially in eccentric jets.

2. The geometry of the jet; eccentric jets tends to have a higher regurgitant volume than free jets of the same area.[33]

3. The size of the proximal convergence zone, by use of the proximal isovelocity surface area (PISA) technique. More severe regurgitation is associated with a larger radius of the proximal flow convergence.[34] Flow convergence can be used to calculate regurgitant flow, orifice area, and volume.

4. The width of the proximal portion of the regurgitant jet (vena contracta [VC]) on the left atrial side of the orifice is also useful and may be less load sensitive than mapping of the regurgitant jet in the atrium.[40]

5. The pulmonary venous pulsed Doppler tracing. Severe MR often leads to systolic reversal of flow in the pulmonary veins,[35] which is 69% sensitive and 98% specific in predicting a regurgitant orifice area (ROA) of greater than 0.3 cm².[41] Blunting of pulmonary vein flow is somewhat reliable in predicting severe MR for patients in normal rhythm with normal LV function but is unreliable in patients with severe LV dysfunction or atrial fibrillation (AFib). A normal pulmonary vein flow pattern is useful in excluding severe MR and predicting a ROA of less than 0.3 cm². Importantly, in patients in whom the right and left pulmonary vein flow pattern is discordant (23% of patients), the more abnormal pattern is most predictive of MR severity.

6. Quantification of mitral regurgitant volume (RV) from the difference between Doppler echocardiography measurements of antegrade flow through the mitral and the aortic valves. Regurgitant fraction (RF) is the proportion of total mitral flow (MF) that is regurgitant:

$$RF\ (\%) = RV/MF$$

LVOT flow and mitral valve flow can be assessed by the product of annular cross-sectional area (CSA) derived from echocardiogram and velocity derived from pulsed-Doppler measurements at the same site. Mitral cross-sectional area is derived from two orthogonal diameters of the annulus, which is elliptic in shape.[42] This method has not been used routinely because of the time-consuming nature of the measurements required and the ease and general reliability of semiquantitative techniques (see Chapter 18).

Other methods of assessing the severity of MR in the OR include surgical palpation of the left atrium for the thrill of a mitral regurgitant jet, evaluation of the size of v waves on the left atrial pressure tracing, fluid filling of the arrested left ventricle, and contrast echocardiography. These methods lack sensitivity and are not as reliable or as convenient as color flow Doppler techniques.[37,43,44]

The size of the ROA can be derived from Doppler echocardiography techniques in the OR,[45] using either the antegrade flow difference method or the flow convergence method. The maximum ROA is calculated by dividing regurgitant flow rate by the maximum mitral regurgitant flow velocity (V_{max}) obtained from CW Doppler. The ROA is greater than 0.4 cm² in severe MR and greater than 0.30 cm² in moderately severe MR.

The flow convergence, or PISA, technique analyzes flow proximal (on the LV side) to the regurgitant orifice, assuming a hemispheric shape.[45,46] In this area, blood accelerates predictably as it moves toward the regurgitant orifice and forms a series of concentric shells of decreasing area and increasing velocity that are depicted clearly and easily measured on the color image because of the color aliasing of the accelerating flow. Because the surface area of a hemiellipse can be calculated from $2\pi r^2$ for blood flow moving at velocity (*v*) and at a radius (*r*) from the regurgitant orifice (Fig. 20–3), flow rate (*Q*) can be calculated as follows:

$$Q = 2\pi r^2 v$$

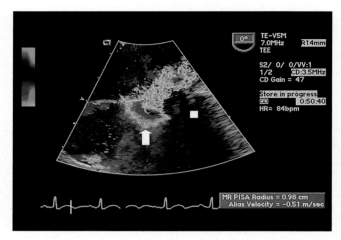

Figure 20–3. *Proximal convergence zone of a patient with severe mitral regurgitation (MR). The hemisphere produced by flow at an aliasing velocity (v) of 51 cm/s is shown (arrow). The radius (R) of the hemisphere is approximately 1 cm. The mitral regurgitation maximum velocity (not shown) was 540 cm/s. The calculated regurgitant orifice area is 0.59 cm², indicating severe MR.*

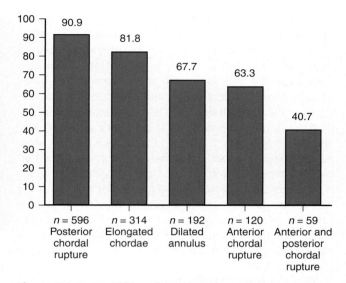

Figure 20–5. *Feasibility of mitral valve repair by mechanism of regurgitation in myxomatous mitral valve disease. (From Stewart WJ:* ACC Heart House Learning Center Highlights *10:2-7, 1995.)*

The PISA method provides excellent estimation of regurgitant flow when the flow convergence is centrally located, well away from the walls; however, this method overestimates regurgitant flow when the proximal flow is constrained by the LV wall. Use of appropriate correction factors can compensate for this problem.[47]

Mechanism of Mitral Regurgitation

Assessment of the cause (Fig. 20–4) and mechanism (Fig. 20–5) of MR[48] is of great importance in determining the suitability of the mitral valve for repair. Mitral valve repair is most likely in patients with MR resulting from myxomatous degeneration and is least likely in patients with regurgitation resulting from endocarditis or rheumatic valvular fibrosis. Repair is now successful

in greater than 90% of all patients with myxomatous disease. The probability of repair, however, is affected by the mechanism of regurgitation, especially whether the posterior leaflet, the anterior leaflet, or both leaflets are involved. Repair is most likely with posterior prolapse or flail, whereas isolated anterior leaflet prolapse and extensive chordal or leaflet disruption substantially reduce the likelihood of successful repair.[49] The presence of mitral annular calcification also reduced the feasibility and likelihood of successful repair.[50]

An Organized Approach to Imaging the Mitral Valve

To adequately assess the pathophysiologic mechanism responsible for MR, it is essential to perform a thorough examination of the mitral valve and mitral apparatus and to determine the origin and geometry of the regurgitant jet. The long-axis imaging planes are best for determining which mitral leaflet is involved. Long-axis views of the mitral valve are obtained by imaging from midesophageal TEE planes. Figure 20–6 shows the "multiplane protractor" with all of the multiplane angles superimposed on the mitral valve.[51] Most basilar long-axis views around the entire multiplane sweep allow portions of both leaflets to be examined individually. The midesophageal intercommissural view[29] at approximately 50 to 60 degrees in most patients, an imaging plane parallel to a line between the commissures, is useful for determining which portion of the anterior or posterior leaflet is involved. Long-axis imaging at a multiplane angle of about 135 degrees cuts perpendicular to this intercommissural line.

The short-axis views also are useful for determining which portion of the anterior or posterior leaflet is in-

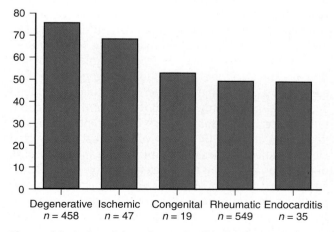

Figure 20–4. *Feasibility of mitral repair by etiology of valve disease at the Cleveland Clinic Foundation. (From Stewart WJ:* ACC Heart House Learning Center Highlights *10:2-7, 1995.)*

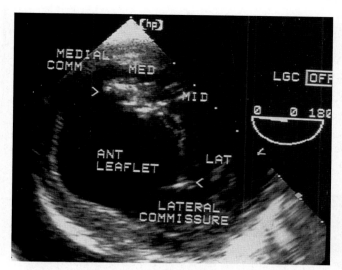

Figure 20–6. *The anatomy of the mitral valve in systole from a transverse transgastric short-axis view of the mitral valve. The medial and lateral commissures (COMM) and the positions of the medial (MED), middle (MID), and lateral (LAT) scallops of the posterior leaflet are shown. ANT, anterior. (From Stewart WJ, Griffin B, Thomas JD: Am J Cardiol Imaging 9:121-128, 1995.)*

cle.[52] In assessing the mitral valve and in providing the results to the surgeon, giving an accurate localization of the abnormality is important. A prospective study of 50 patients used a segmental approach to the mitral valve, breaking each leaflet into three segments, and found that TEE was 96% accurate for localization compared with surgical findings.[53] Other researchers have shown that localization of the defect to the posterior leaflet by TEE is 78% sensitive and 92% specific in myxomatous disease, with accuracy being least when the medial rather than the lateral or middle scallop is involved.[54] Assessment of the mechanism of MR is performed by analyzing the motion of the valve leaflets with two-dimensional echocardiography (Fig. 20–7) and the direction of the regurgitant jet with color flow imaging[55] (Table 20–4). Three types of leaflet motion (Fig. 20–8) may be associated with MR: (1) *excessive motion,* as seen with prolapse or flail valve caused by

volved. These views may be obtained from either the transgastric short-axis view or the epicardial parasternal short-axis equivalent view.[51] The posterior leaflet has three divisions or scallops: the lateral, middle, and medial, respectively numbers P1, P2, and P3. The anterior leaflet is not scalloped but has a central portion known as the *bare area* between the insertions of the chordae from the anterolateral and posteromedial papillary muscles. In a similar way, the posterior leaflet is also supported, about half each by chordae from the anterolateral and posteromedial papillary muscles. The papillary muscles lie below each mitral commissure. The papillary muscles and chordae usually are well visualized from the transgastric long-axis views of the left ventri-

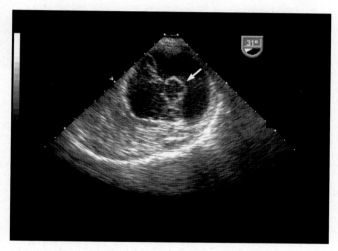

Figure 20–7. *Transgastric short-axis view of the mitral valve in a patient with severe prolapse of the middle scallop of the posterior leaflet (arrow).*

TABLE 20–4. **Determination of the Mechanism of Mitral Regurgitation from Analysis of Jet Direction and Leaflet Mobility**

	Leaflet Motion		
Jet Direction	**Excessive**	**Restrictive**	**Normal**
Anterior	Prolapse/flail of posterior leaflet	—	Perforation in posterior leaflet
Posterior	Prolapse/flail of anterior leaflet	Restriction of posterior > anterior leaflet	Apical tethering from LV dilation
Central	Prolapse/flail of both leaflets	Equal restriction of both leaflets	Apical tethering from LV dilation, annular dilation
Commissural	Rupture of commissural chordae or papillary muscle	—	—
Eccentric origin	—	—	Leaflet perforation or cleft

LV, left ventricular.

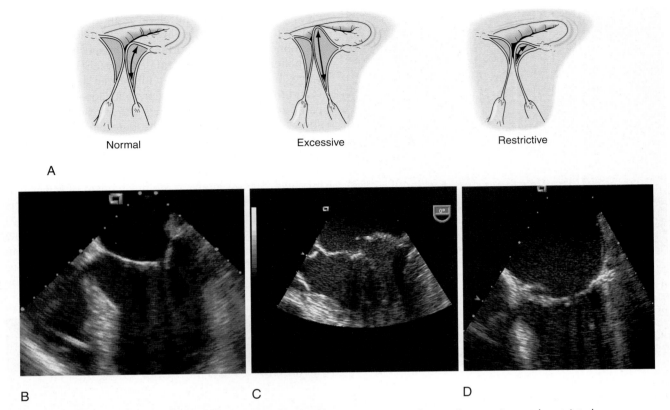

Figure 20–8. Morphology and echocardiographic appearance of normal, excessive, and restricted motion of the mitral valve, each of which can cause mitral regurgitation. Lower panels transesophageal echocardiography show transverse views of patients with mitral regurgitation resulting from (B) apical tethering of normal leaflets as a result of ischemic or functional mitral regurgitation, (C) posterior leaflet flail resulting from ruptured chordae, and (D) restricted leaflet motion as a result of previous chest radiation.

chordal rupture or elongation, (2) *restricted motion,* as seen in rheumatic disease and papillary muscle infarction, and (3) *normal motion,* as seen with leaflet perforation and ventricular-annular dilation.

IOE has been shown to be highly sensitive and specific in determining the mechanism of MR in patients undergoing mitral valve surgery. In a study of 286 patients undergoing mitral valve surgery in whom the echocardiography mechanism was correlated with the surgical findings, echocardiography was highly accurate (86%) in determining the mechanism of MR.[55] Echocardiography was least accurate in ascertaining the mechanism of MR in patients with leaflet perforation, bileaflet prolapse, or ventricular-annular dilation.

Excessive Leaflet Motion

Excessive leaflet motion occurs with elongation or disruption of any portion of the mitral valve or of the mitral apparatus, including the papillary muscles and chordae. Myxomatous disease, endocarditis, and papillary muscle infarction all can lead to this abnormality.

With excessive leaflet motion, the regurgitant jet is directed *away* from the affected leaflet. Thus, prolapse or flail of the posterior leaflet leads to an anteriorly directed jet (Fig. 20–9). In bileaflet prolapse, the excessive motion is often asymmetric, and the jet direction is away from the more severely affected leaflet. When the amount of prolapse or flail is completely balanced between both leaflets, a central jet direction occurs. If the chordae to the commissures are ruptured, then a jet originating at the commissures is seen in the transgastric short-axis view. Jets originating at the commissure also are seen in infarction of a papillary muscle, most commonly the posteromedial one.[56] Excess motion with severe MR results when the head of a papillary muscle ruptures in an acute myocardial infarction (AMI). This type of rupture may be differentiated from acute chordal rupture by detecting a mass attached to the flail leaflet that is a portion of the muscle and by the appropriate clinical setting (Fig. 20–10).

Precise delineation of which portion of the valve has excess motion is important in planning the surgical repair. Rupture of the posterior chordae is the most

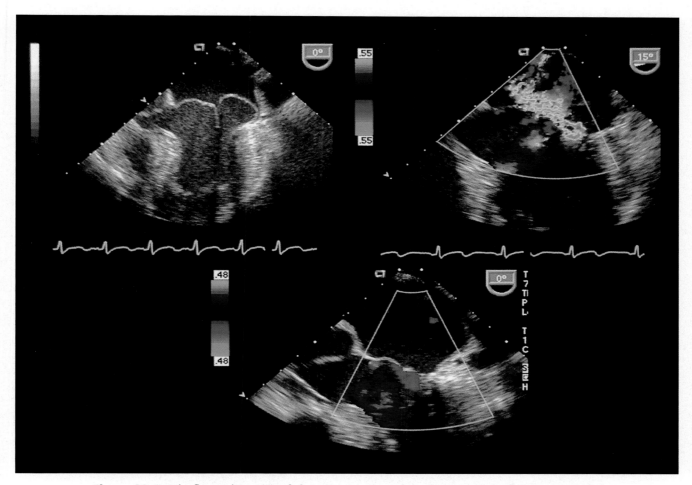

Figure 20–9. *Bileaflet prolapse* (A) *of the posterior more than the anterior leaflet causing severe mitral regurgitation* (B) *before mitral valve repair and no mitral regurgitation after successful mitral valve repair* (C). *The jet is deflected opposite the leaflet that has the most excessive leaflet motion.*

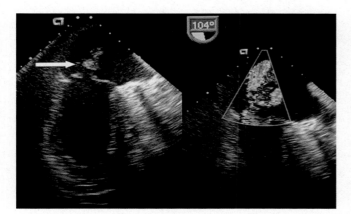

Figure 20–10. *Papillary muscle rupture with resulting severe mitral regurgitation. The ruptured portion of muscle is seen prolapsing into the left atrium* (arrow) *on the* left *panel, and the mitral regurgitation jet is seen on the* right *panel.*

common abnormality and is repaired by quadrilateral resection of the posterior leaflet (Fig. 20–11). Elongation of the chordae is repaired by chordal transfer or by implantation of artificial chordae. Papillary muscle

elongation or disruption may be repaired by reimplantation, supporting, or shortening the affected muscle.[49] Postoperative prognosis is best in those with excessive leaflet motion.

Restricted Leaflet Motion

This pattern, involving leaflet thickening, is seen most commonly in rheumatic disease, but it also can result from ischemic heart disease, the chronic phase of lupus, radiation-induced valvular disease, or acquired disease caused by ergot derivatives or the fen-phen combination (fenfluramine and phentermine). If both leaflets are equally affected by the pathologic process, the jet direction is central. More commonly in rheumatic disease, the posterior leaflet is more severely affected than the anterior leaflet, and the relatively normal anterior leaflet overrides the restricted posterior leaflet. The direction of the regurgitant jet in this situation is posterior, *toward* the affected leaflet. The surgical approach to this condition includes débridement of the valve tissue and chordae, commissurotomy, and

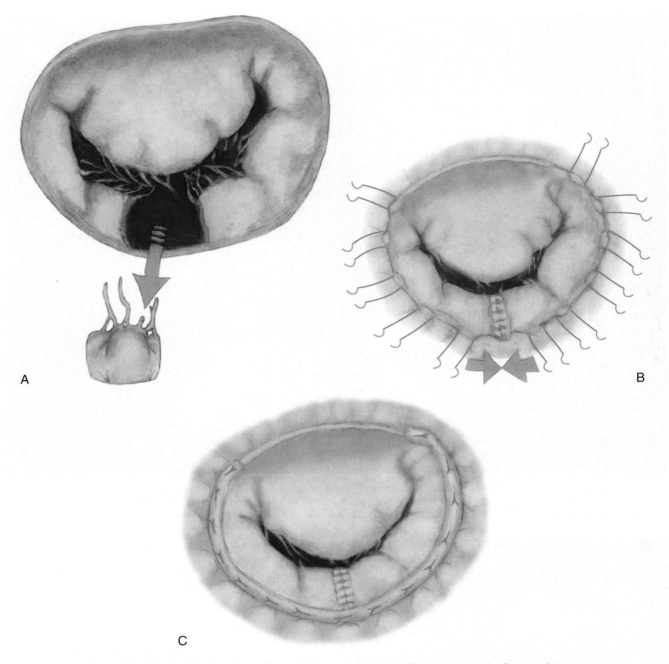

Figure 20–11. *Artist's drawings of a quadrilateral resection of the posterior leaflet (A) of the posterior mitral valve leaflet, after placement of annular sutures (B) and as the annular ring is implanted (C).*

annuloplasty. This type of repair is more technically demanding and is less often successful.

Normal Leaflet Motion

In ischemic heart disease, the leaflets are usually structurally normal, but they are *tethered,* and their motion is relatively restricted, owing to apical displacement of the posteromedial papillary muscle. The leaflets themselves are not thickened but fail to coapt adequately

(Fig. 20–12). The surgical approach to this problem usually involves placement of an annuloplasty ring to reduce the size of the mitral annulus. Surgical treatment of ischemic regurgitation with apical tethering is less successful in that residual regurgitation is often more significant than after myxomatous valve repair.

Normal leaflet motion is commonly seen in patients with MR secondary to LV dilation of any cause, such as disease of other valves, dilated cardiomyopathy, or severe ischemic cardiomyopathy. We have previously

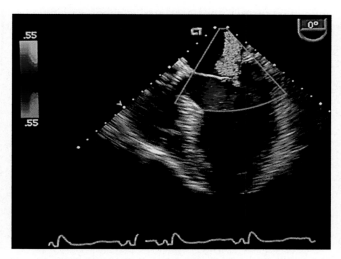

Figure 20–12. Ischemic mitral regurgitation with relative restriction of normal mitral leaflets and a central to posteriorly directed jet of mitral regurgitation. This is the same patient as shown in the left lower panel of Figure 20–8.

termed this category *ventricular-annular dilation.* Ventricular enlargement causes displacement of the mitral coaptation point toward the apex with resultant impaired coaptation. Annular dilation is seen in these patients, but it occurs in proportion to LV dilation, in contrast to myxomatous or rheumatic MR patients whose annulus size is often abnormally large. Annuloplasty with ring insertion is commonly used in the surgical management of these patients. An Alfieri stitch to support the valve also has been used instead of or in addition to the annuloplasty. There has been an upsurge in interest in the surgical management of severe MR in patients with dilated cardiomyopathy. Excellent functional improvement with a relatively low operative mortality has been reported even in selected patients with severe MR and severe LV dysfunction.

Another type of MR with normal leaflet motion results from perforation of a valve leaflet, which occurs most commonly because of endocarditis or because of a congenital cleft in the valve. Occasionally, after attempted repair, it is iatrogenic. The jet origin is eccentric, arising from the midportion of the leaflets rather than from the coaptation line. The prejet flow acceleration also may be seen away from the coaptation line, along the affected leaflet. Leaflet perforation may be repaired in some instances by suture closure or with pericardial patch.[57]

One study of 248 patients undergoing mitral valve surgery showed that TEE was greater than 90% accurate for definition of the mechanism of regurgitation, localizing the origin of regurgitation, and in detecting a flail segment. TEE was 88% accurate in detecting ruptured chordae. The TEE findings of valve function were highly predictive not only of valve reparability but also of long-term survival, which were independent of age, gender, ejection fraction (EF), and coronary artery disease (CAD).[58]

Other Valve Disease and Biventricular Function during Mitral Repair

The severity of aortic and tricuspid valvular disease is assessed by intraoperative TEE using color flow mapping to determine the severity of the dysfunction and the necessity of valve surgery. These decisions should be made preoperatively, but diagnostic information should be refined intraoperatively, as previously mentioned. Intraoperative diagnosis is particularly important in patients with active endocarditis because of the greater potential for interval change. Significant tricuspid regurgitation (TR) or aortic regurgitation (AR) usually requires operative intervention; however, IOE tends to underestimate the degree of TR because of optimization of the hemodynamics that usually results in a reduction of right-sided pressures and volume. Because the preoperative echocardiogram is generally performed under ambulatory conditions, it is a better guide to decision making with regard to tricuspid valve repair, as opposed to the intraoperative findings alone.

Regional and global LV function is best assessed using TEE from long- and short-axis transgastric views and various midesophageal long-axis views. The long- and short-axis views from any epicardial imaging window also show the left and right ventricle well. Right ventricular function is assessed by TEE in the midesophageal 45-degree view at the level of the short axis of the aortic valve, from the midesophageal transverse four-chamber view, or from a longitudinal transgastric view rotated clockwise to obtain a long-axis image of the right ventricle.

Determining the Need for Mitral Valve Surgery in Patients Undergoing Cardiac Surgery for Other Reasons

IOE is increasingly used to determine the need for a mitral valve operation in patients undergoing aortic valve surgery or revascularization procedures; this is especially true in the assessment of patients in whom the severity of the MR preoperatively is significantly different by cardiac catheterization and echocardiography, when the severity of MR over time is variable (such as in ischemic heart disease), and when the MR is of moderate severity.

The following questions must be considered when determining the need for mitral valve surgery in addition to the primary surgery:

1. How severe is the MR?
2. Is there a primary abnormality of the mitral valve (such as a torn chord or prolapse)?

3. Will the MR change as a consequence of the primary operation?

4. Is the valve repairable or is prosthetic replacement necessary?

5. What is the additional risk imposed by the additional mitral valve procedure?

The final decision on what surgery is indicated is made by the surgeon; however, when the surgical plans are changed in the OR, telephone consultation with the referring clinical doctor is advisable.

In many patients, especially those in whom the regurgitation is secondary to apical tethering from ischemic heart disease with LV dilation, the severity of the regurgitation may be variable. Sometimes, the severity of regurgitation detected at the time of operation is different from that recorded preoperatively. Frequently the difference in severity results from a true physiologic change. Compared with ambulatory conditions, the loading conditions during surgery often entail a lower intravascular volume and less peripheral vasoconstriction, both of which may reduce the severity of valvular regurgitation and reduce stenotic valve gradients. On other occasions this discrepancy reflects the superior ability of esophageal and epicardial echocardiography to visualize MR compared to TTE.

When approaching patients whose regurgitation is less than is expected or borderline in severity for the decision to do mitral surgery, it is often useful to increase afterload with multiple boluses of phenylephrine (100 μg every 30 to 120 seconds), to recheck the severity of regurgitation at a mean arterial pressure that is transiently as high as 120 mm Hg. Patients with 3+ or more MR at rest or during this afterload stress test are generally considered candidates for a mitral valve operation. The threshold for surgery on the mitral valve also is affected by other factors, including whether there is a primary structural abnormality of the valve. If the valve appears to be repairable, the threshold for surgery is lower, given the relatively low morbidity and mortality associated with repair as compared with valve replacement, whereas the threshold for surgery is higher in patients with valves that are not reparable. In patients undergoing surgery for aortic stenosis, improvement in the severity of the MR can be expected postoperatively; therefore, the threshold for concomitant mitral surgery is higher.[59,60] On any patient with valvular disease, a postpump assessment is made regardless of whether a surgical intervention on the mitral valve has been performed.

Postpump Intraoperative Echocardiography in Mitral Repair

The most significant indication for IOE in mitral valve repair (see Table 20–3) is to determine the competency of the repair immediately after CPB. If the repair is inadequate, further repair or replacement can be performed immediately during the same thoracotomy.

Timing

To make a relevant assessment of valvular performance, postpump IOE assessment of valvular function should be done after loading conditions and ventricular function has reached its postoperative plateau, when the patient has returned to relatively normal loading conditions. The most appropriate time to image after repair is when the patient is off CPB, the intravascular volume is replete, and the loading conditions are similar to those in the ambulatory state. Imaging can be initiated earlier than that, after the aortic cross-clamp is off and the left ventricle is at least partially filled, but abnormal findings at this time may result from abnormal LV geometry. In particular, the surgeon should not act on these findings unless they are subsequently confirmed by further imaging after the cessation of CPB.

Intraoperative Findings

In most cases, with an experienced surgeon, mitral valve repair leads to a competent mitral valve with mild or no residual MR; however, there are potential complications of mitral valve repair that are readily recognized by postpump IOE. Many of these complications may not be apparent clinically or may take longer to accurately diagnose without echocardiography. If left untreated, these complications may interfere with the long-term success of the procedure and require early reoperation. Complications seen after mitral valve repair by intraoperative echocardiography are shown in Table 20–5. In early experience with over 6000 patients,[1] the frequency of needing a second run of CPB in mitral repair was 7%, which was higher than the frequency in aortic repair (14.7%) and myectomy (17.9%) but lower than the frequency in tricuspid repair (5.1%), congenital heart disease (4.9%), and aortic aneurysm surgery (3.6%).

Incomplete Mitral Repair

Significant residual MR is the most common postpump problem detected by IOE. Moderate (2+) or more MR, either at rest or following afterload challenge with phenylephrine as previously described, is generally considered excessive after mitral repair and is an indication for a further surgical procedure. The incidence of this complication varies with the cause of the valvular regurgitation, the complexity of the repair, the experience of the surgeon, and the threshold of the operative team to accept a suboptimal result. When residual MR is found, further repair of the valve may lead to an improved result with reduction or elimination of MR, particularly when the echocardiographer can define the mechanism of the residual regurgitation. In some patients, further

TABLE 20–5. Management of Abnormal Findings on Doppler Echocardiography after Mitral Valve Repair

Complication	Management
Residual mitral regurgitation	Define mechanism. If ≤1+, accept. If 2+, give phenylephrine to recheck MR with increased afterload; if >2+, further surgery is required.
Systolic anterior motion with LVOT obstruction	Assess LVOT gradient and MR. Increase ventricular volume, stop positive inotropes. If these measures are not successful, further surgery is needed to revise repair.
Dehisced ring or leaflet perforation	Another pump run is needed to redo annuloplasty.
Residual mitral stenosis	Quantify severity. If mean gradient >5 mm Hg or area <1.5 cm², consider further surgery.
Significant tricuspid regurgitation	If 3+ or more, consider further repair.
Regional left ventricular dysfunction	Assess intracardiac air; if not resolved after further time on pump, consider coronary bypass.
Global (right or left) ventricular dysfunction	Assess volume status, afterload, and response to medications. Assessment for coronary air emboli.

LVOT, left ventricular outflow tract; MR, mitral regurgitation.

repair is impossible or fails, and the patient requires a third pump run to implant a prosthesis.

If the regurgitation is mild (1+) or less on the postpump IOE, then the result is usually accepted, though individual surgeons vary in their willingness to accept even mild amounts of regurgitation. The severity of MR detected by immediate postpump IOE correlates well with angiographic or TTE and TEE estimates of severity obtained later.[61,62] Rarely, changes in the early postoperative period, such as progressive chordal rupture, suture dehiscence, or early postoperative endocarditis, may cause acute worsening of the MR. Thus, IOE is a reliable measure of the severity of MR and the need for further intervention.

Other considerations in deciding whether residual MR should be accepted or subjected to another surgical procedure include the mechanism of the MR, the overall condition of the patient, and LV function. Postpump determination of the mechanism of the residual MR helps the surgeon to determine whether a further reparative procedure could lessen the regurgitation and yet conserve the valve. More MR than is usually desirable might be accepted when other surgical procedures, such as aortic valve replacement or coronary artery bypass grafting, have also been accomplished, particularly in elderly patients or those with significant LV dysfunction. For example, in patients with extensive mitral annular calcification, mitral prosthetic insertion may be technically more difficult and more hazardous for the patient than accepting a moderate amount of residual MR.[63]

In various studies of patients undergoing mitral valve repair, 4% to 11% have needed a second pump run. In about half of these (e.g., 3% of the total, less than half

of the 8% in one study) had persistent MR that was greater than 2+.[36] In most of the patients in whom immediate failure of mitral repair is treated with a further run of CPB, further repair can be accomplished successfully, whereas a smaller percentage (10% to 15%) of the patients having a second pump run underwent mitral prosthetic implantation. In one study, inadequate repair was associated with a degenerative cause of the MR and with the absence of an annuloplasty ring implantation at the time of initial repair.[64] In another study, the need for reoperation because of inadequate repair or systolic anterior motion (SAM) of the mitral valve was more common in patients with anterior mitral leaflet or bileaflet prolapse, as opposed to those with posterior prolapse.[65] In still another study with an 11% incidence of second pump runs, interscallop malcoaptation of the posterior leaflet was the most common cause of the initially persistent MR.[66] In the previously cited large retrospective study by Click and colleagues, the incidence of changes based on the postpump IOE was 6%, although only one third of those returned to CPBB for further surgery.[25]

Impact on Clinical Outcome

IOE has a positive impact on prognosis and the incidence of reoperation after mitral repair in large centers and in smaller community hospitals. Reoperations are lower when IOE is used[67] and the percentage of valves which are repaired is improved[68] by the use of IOE.

The severity of residual MR after mitral valve repair, as assessed by IOE, is important for prognosis, as shown by several studies. In one of these studies, moderate or greater MR was associated with a higher incidence of congestive heart failure (CHF), repeat valve surgery, or postoperative death.[38] In a study of ischemic MR, residual regurgitation by postpump IOE was a strong predictor of survival after mitral valve repair.[24] Postoperative recurrence of MR in ischemic heart disease, however, correlates more with the degree of apical tethering, annular dilation, and contractile impairment, rather than the technical success of the repair procedure.[69] In another study, patients with 3+ MR as determined by postpump IOE who did not undergo a further pump run at the time of initial operation required reoperation within 5 days because of hemodynamic instability and the frequent inability to wean off mechanical ventilation.[36]

Patients who undergo a second pump run for an initially inadequate repair have an in-hospital complication rate that is similar to that of patients who require a single pump run.[70,71] In one study, residual MR of 1+ or 2+ did not increase hospital complications when compared with trivial or no regurgitation postoperatively. There was a trend for patients with 1+ or 2+ MR, however, to need more reoperations in late follow-up than those with trivial or no MR.[72]

Other Complications of Mitral Valve Repair

Systolic Anterior Motion of the Mitral Valve

Significant LV outflow obstruction caused by SAM of the mitral valve has been recognized as a complication of surgery since the early days of mitral valve repair.[73,74] This abnormality simulates the physiology seen in hypertrophic obstructive cardiomyopathy, even though septal hypertrophy is absent. The SAM of the mitral valve after mitral repair in these patients is dynamic and exacerbated by reducing the size of the ventricular chamber or augmenting contractility. SAM may cause pressure gradients of 100 mm Hg or more, severe hypotension, severe MR, and inability to wean the patient from CPB but in many cases is mild and not the cause of congestive preload or decreased forward flow. Fortunately, this series of complications is readily recognized and quantified by an experienced echocardiographer on the postpump echocardiogram study (Fig. 20–13). If it is not recognized, in some, but not all, patients it will cause postoperative problems and require reoperation. SAM was initially reported in 2% to 9% of patients undergoing mitral valve repair,[36,65,75] but it is now less common because of the ability to prevent it with better design of the initial repair procedure.

Several mechanisms have been proposed to explain SAM following mitral valve repair. These mechanisms include anterior displacement of the posterior ventricular wall, anterior displacement of the posterior mitral leaflet, and narrowing of the angle between the mitral and aortic valves.[76] It is clear that SAM occurs primarily in patients with degenerative mitral valve disease, those with large mitral leaflets, and in the presence of a hyperdynamic, small ventricle.[65] SAM is usually seen only after annuloplasty ring insertion, but it has been reported after a suture annuloplasty.[65] It is seen more commonly with stiff than flexible annuloplasty rings.[65,75] One quantitative study has shown that SAM is associated with anterior displacement of the mitral coaptation line. The anterior displacement is reduced or disappears after successful revision of the repair and elimination of SAM.[76] The ratio of the length of the anterior and posterior leaflets during coaptation and the distance from the coaptation line to the septum on preoperative TEE were shown to be predictors of SAM. The smaller the ratio between anterior and posterior leaflet and the narrower the distance between the coaptation point and the septum, the greater the likelihood of SAM.[77]

When severe, SAM is easily recognized and may involve both leaflets. The LV outflow gradient and the severity of MR are important indicators of the hemodynamic severity. The best TEE view for measurement of the LV outflow gradient is the deep transgastric imaging window, which puts the heart in an orientation similar to a transthoracic apical five-chamber image and allows alignment of the CW Doppler cursor with the LVOT jet. When this examination cannot be reliably performed with the transesophageal approach, the gradient can be measured with epicardial echocardiography. In many circumstances, the appearance on midesophageal images of marked SAM and significant persistent MR mandates a second pump run, without having to quantitate the gradient itself.

The initial management of patients with SAM and LV outflow obstruction after mitral repair should be to increase intracardiac volume by fluid repletion and to stop any positive inotropic agents that are being administered.[65] Systemic afterload can be supported by a pure alpha agonist (phenylephrine), avoiding any beta agonists, like dobutamine, dopamine, isoproterenol, or epinephrine. If these measures are inadequate to reduce the severity of SAM, another pump run to improve the SAM is indicated. A further procedure that may improve SAM is a sliding posterior leaflet advancement (sliding plasty), which reduces the anterior-posterior height of the posterior leaflet.

Sliding annuloplasty is currently used as a component of the primary operative procedure on patients who are considered at risk for developing SAM, particularly those with severe myxomatous leaflets with substantial redundancy, which has significantly reduced the incidence of this complication in those patients in whom it has been used.[78,79] If SAM persists despite these maneuvers, the final recourse is mitral prosthetic implantation. Patients in whom SAM is dis-

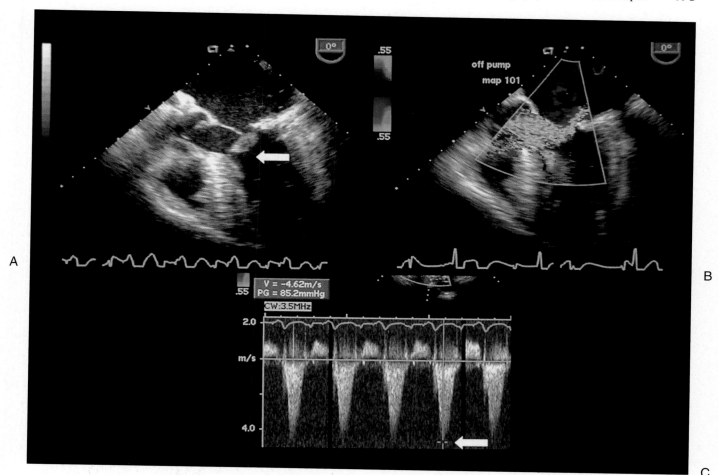

Figure 20–13. Series of images indicating the presence of systolic anterior motion at the end of the first pump run (A, arrow) leading to severe mitral regurgitation (B) and outflow obstruction. The maximal velocity measured in the outflow tract by continuous-wave Doppler (C) from the deep transgastric transesophageal echocardiographic view, was 4.6 m/s, allowing estimation of an outflow tract pressure gradient of approximately 85 mm Hg.

covered by TTE days or longer after mitral valve repair, which are obviously a subset selected to have milder obstruction by successful weaning from bypass and extubation, may be treated medically with negative inotropic agents. Some patients show a late reduction in the LV outflow gradient, but obstruction may remain inducible by exercise, catecholamine infusions, or inhalation of amyl nitrite.[80]

Suture Dehiscence

Occasionally, suture dehiscence leads to significant MR after mitral valve repair. This complication was found by the postpump IOE in 2% of operations in one series.[64] Dehiscence of a suture at the site of the leaflet resection or a suture line of the sliding plasty simulates a leaflet perforation mechanistically. This is now the most common cause of persistent MR after repair, and it is easily repaired on a second pump run. Another rare complication of mitral valve repair that can be

detected by IOE is partial dehiscence of the annuloplasty ring. The annuloplasty ring shows increased mobility and regurgitation may originate outside the ring (Fig. 20–14).

Left Ventricular Systolic Dysfunction

Some reduction in LV function is often detected after mitral valve repair.[81,82] Early dysfunction after weaning from CPB may reflect the transient effects of cardioplegia and the suboptimal metabolic milieu. When dysfunction persists, it is most often global and may reflect the unmasking of LV dysfunction present preoperatively that had been concealed by the effects of increased ventricular preload and decreased afterload. In a minority of instances, a regional wall motion abnormality is detected, despite normal coronary vasculature preoperatively. This abnormality is usually caused by passage of air into a coronary vessel, most commonly a transient wall motion abnormality in the right coro-

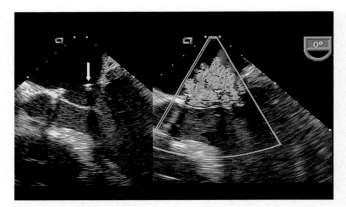

Figure 20–14. Late failure of mitral repair resulting from annular ring dehiscence (arrow, left panel) *leading to severe mitral regurgitation* (right panel).

nary artery (RCA) distribution, which usually but not always resolves without permanent infarction.[20,70] Because of its anterior position, air is more likely to travel to the right coronary artery in a supine patient, causing inferior wall motion abnormalities.

The vast majority (over 80%) of isolated mitral surgeries performed at Cleveland Clinic in the last 6 to 8 years have been done using a hemisternotomy, which is one of the most popular types of less invasive heart surgeries, involving a vertical incision about 8 to 10 cm long. This operation causes less chest trauma, less bleeding, and is associated with more rapid return to work, but it also involves less visual exposure of the heart, a problem largely filled by intraoperative TEE.[17] Air within the LV cavity is readily detected by echocardiography because it is echodense. The presence of large amounts of air on postpump IOE is an indication for increased surgical venting of the heart to prevent coronary embolization. In minimally invasive operations in which smaller incisions are used, surgical venting may be difficult or impossible. In this situation, resumption of CPB may be necessary for a period of time to allow slow resolution of the air. Fortunately, most instances of air embolization of the coronary vessels resolve without significant long-term ventricular dysfunction.

Tricuspid Regurgitation

TR is a common concomitant lesion to MR. More than moderate TR should be treated with a ring annuloplasty at the time of mitral surgery. In all patients, whether tricuspid surgery is done or not, the amount of TR should be rechecked on the postpump IOE.[83] The success of the tricuspid surgery should be checked only after the intravascular volume status has been normalized.[84] Occasionally, TR that did not appear to be significant preoperatively may appear to be more severe on the postpump study and require a further pump run for tricuspid repair.

Mitral Stenosis

In performing a mitral valve repair in a nonrheumatic valve, the surgeon may remove a significant portion of the leaflet or perform an annuloplasty that reduces the size of the mitral annular orifice. Despite these anatomic derangements, it is unusual to have any significant stenosis in degenerative or ischemic mitral valve repair because there is not any fusion of the mitral commissures or narrowing at the subvalvular level. The normal annulus area is 5 to 10 cm², varying with the size of the annuloplasty ring inserted. In contrast, residual stenosis of mild degree is common after rheumatic mitral valve repair because of the thickened leaflets and fusion of subvalvular chordae and commissures. The mitral valve gradient should be measured using CW Doppler after every mitral valve repair. A mean gradient in excess of 5 mm Hg should arouse suspicion of some degree of stenosis of the valve.

Mitral Valve Repair Involving Commissurotomy

Mitral repair with open commissurotomy is decreasingly used, resulting from a progressive decline in the United States of the frequency of rheumatic valvular disease and the recognition that repair of such valves is fraught with recurrence as a result of postoperative progression of the postinflammatory fibrosis. Also balloon valvuloplasty is a more common method of treating patients with isolated mitral stenosis. Nevertheless, mitral repair with open commissurotomy still has a place, especially in patients with moderate or less valve calcification, or combined mitral stenosis and significant MR, especially when nonprosthetic outcomes are desirable, for example, in anticipation of future pregnancy. Before surgery, IOE is used to determine the severity of stenosis as a reference to assess the success of surgery. The severity of mitral stenosis is determined from the CW Doppler recording by planimetering the diastolic velocity envelope, to measure the transmitral pressure gradient, and by measuring the pressure half-time (PHT).[85-87] An epicardial approach using a parasternal short-axis equivalent view may be used to obtain views suitable for planimetry of the mitral orifice itself, but most TEE short-axis views of the mitral valve from the transgastric window are not of sufficient quality for quantitative purposes. The mechanism of the stenosis, whether valvular or subvalvular, should also be determined. A splitability score generated in a manner similar to the transthoracic method used for percutaneous mitral valvuloplasty may help to determine the degree of valvular fibrosis and calcification and whether a valve-sparing procedure is feasible.[88] Because the surgeon can débride the valve under direct vision,

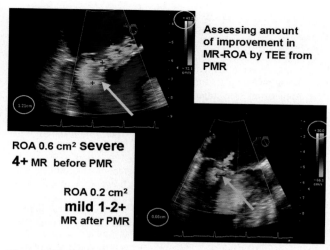

Assessing amount of improvement in MR-ROA by TEE from PMR

ROA 0.6 cm² **severe 4+** MR before PMR

ROA 0.2 cm² **mild 1-2+** MR after PMR

Figure 20–15. Improvement in the amount of mitral regurgitation (MR) in a patient undergoing the percutaneous mitral repair (PMR) is illustrated. In the upper left panel, *the flow convergence zone is measured in a patient with severe prolapse of the posterior leaflet in a midesophageal transesophageal echocardiographic (TEE) view from which the aliasing radius, at a Nyquist of 43 cm/s permitted calculation of a regurgitant orifice area (ROA) of 0.6 cm². After percutaneous edge-to-edge repair,* (lower right), *the MR has been reduced to mild or 1 to 2+ with an ROA of 0.2 cm², based on an aliasing radius of 0.66 cm at a Nyquist of 30 cm/s.*

open commissurotomy is sometimes possible even with a moderately high splitability score of 9 to 11, when a balloon valvuloplasty is not as likely to be effective or durable (see Chapter 21). The presence of MR is also determined and its mechanism determined, which is usually restricted leaflet motion. It is important also to detect left atrial appendage thrombus preoperatively so that the surgeon can remove it.

On the postpump echocardiogram, the mitral valve gradient and area, and MR are again assessed. The presence of residual MR of 2+ or greater, or a mitral valve area of less than 1.5 cm² by pressure half-time is an indication for a further pump run, either to improve the repair or to implant a prosthesis. Frequently, when the patient has atrial fibrillation, a Maze procedure or pulmonary vein ablation will be performed. The left atrial appendage may be ligated in an effort to reduce the embolic risk, although in up to one third of patients, blood may still enter and leave the appendage.[89]

Future Directions

New People

Although not really new, more and more IOE services are staffed primarily by cardiac anesthesiologists, who have acquired the requisite skills. This has reduced the need for dedicated cardiology support in some cardiac ORs, except to consult when specific problems arise.

Online consultation is increasingly feasible with the availability of digital archival and retrieval of images on a common server. New technology has been developed on the echocardiographic machines, including Doppler myocardial imaging, strain and strain rate (SR) assessment, and contrast analysis software. In addition, smaller handheld machines having many of the capabilities of bigger machines are available for use in cardiac ORs, though sophisticated technology is often more applicable for IOE because of the significant diagnostic accuracy that is needed.

New Imaging Tools

Three-dimensional (3D) echocardiography has tremendous potential in the analysis of complex cardiac morphology, including the assessment of lesions in which mitral repair or reconstruction is being considered (see Chapter 14).[90] The complex 3D geometry of some valvular and congenital lesions is easier to display and understand using 3D echocardiography.[91,92] 3D reconstruction may allow more appropriate selection of patients, help determine the most appropriate surgical procedure, and potentially allow the surgeon to map out the reconstruction ahead of time in 3D computer space.[93-95] 3D data yielded incremental information to TEE in up to 25% of patients[96] 3D imaging can reconstruct structures, such as the ROA[97] and the location of mitral valve prolapse (MVP).[98] Real-time 3D echocardiographic acquisition using transesophageal transducers has the potential to further expand echocardiographic abilities intraoperatively. Importantly, 3D echocardiography allows additional slices to be derived at a later time from one stored volumetric data set.

New Valve Procedures

Guidance by imaging is more important when the therapy involved is new or for some reason associated with more risks of mistaken objectives or faulty outcome. For this reason, IOE is an appropriate component of mitral valve operations in which new techniques are used. One such emerging arena is less invasive valve procedures. For example, robotic heart surgery is new field that requires special techniques and technology. Again, robotic valve surgery relies heavily on IEO.[99]

Another innovation involves percutaneous valve procedures, which are done entirely via endovascular access. For example, an edge-to-edge technique that mimics the Alfieri stitch, done via a transseptal technique, also requires intraprocedural TEE guidance[100] (Fig. 20–15). Percutaneous valve replacement has also been developed, though only for the aortic valve so far.[101,102] These procedures are pushing the envelope of therapy for valvular heart disease into cardiac interventional procedures in the catheterization laboratory. Imaging before, during, and after such procures typically involves echocardiography.

KEY POINTS

- IOE is useful before mitral valve repair to determine the mechanism and severity of the MR and after repair to determine the success of surgery.

- The mechanism of MR, discerned from leaflet by two-dimensional echocardiography and the jet direction by color Doppler, allows prediction of the feasibility of repair and the surgical techniques of doing so.

- When residual MR is found on the postpump transesophageal echocardiogram, further repair of the valve during a second pump run often improves the result and has a positive impact on postop survival and freedom from reoperation.

- Guidance by TEE imaging is more essential when the therapy involved is new or associated with more risks of faulty outcome, such as less invasive surgery and transcatheter valve procedures.

REFERENCES

1. Stewart WJ, Thomas JD, Klein AL, et al: Ten year trends in the utilization of 6340 intraoperative echoes. *Circulation* 92(Suppl I):514, 1995.
2. Gussenhoven EJ, van Herwerden LA, Roelandt J, et al: Intraoperative two-dimensional echocardiography in congenital heart disease. *J Am Coll Cardiol* 9:565-572, 1987.
3. Ungerleider RM, Greeley WJ, Sheikh KH, et al: Routine use of intraoperative epicardial echocardiography and Doppler color flow imaging to guide and evaluate repair of congenital heart lesions. *J Thorac Cardiovasc Surg* 100:297-309, 1990.
4. Marwick TH, Stewart WJ, Lever HM, et al: Benefits of intraoperative echocardiography in the surgical management of hypertrophic cardiomyopathy. *J Am Coll Cardiol* 20:1066-1072, 1992.
5. Stewart WJ, Schiavone WA, Salcedo EE, et al: Intraoperative Doppler echocardiography in hypertrophic cardiomyopathy: Correlations with the obstructive gradient. *J Am Coll Cardiol* 10:327-335, 1987.
6. Ribakove GH, Katz ES, Galloway AC, et al: Surgical implications of transesophageal echocardiography to grade the atheromatous aortic arch. *Ann Thorac Surg* 53:758-761, 1992.
7. Wiet SP, Pearce WH, McCarthy WJ, et al: Utility of transesophageal echocardiography in the diagnosis of disease of the thoracic aorta. *J Vasc Surg* 20:613-620, 1994.
8. Bryan AJ, Barzilai BN, Kouchoukos NT: Transesophageal echocardiography and adult cardiac operations. *Ann Thorac Surg* 59:773-779, 1995.
9. Topol EJ, Weiss JL, Guzman PA, et al: Immediate improvement of dysfunctional myocardial segments after coronary revascularization: Detection by intraoperative transesophageal echocardiography. *J Am Coll Cardiol* 4:1123-1134, 1984.
10. Lazar HL, Plehn JF, Schick EM, et al: Effects of coronary revascularization on regional wall motion. *J Thorac Cardiovasc Surg* 98:498-505, 1989.
11. Eisenberg MJ, London MJ, Leung JM, et al: Monitoring for myocardial ischemia during noncardiac surgery. *JAMA* 268:210, 1992.
12. Gewertz BL, Kremser PC, Zarina CK, et al: Transesophageal echocardiographic monitoring of myocardial ischemia during vascular surgery. *J Vasc Surg* 5:607-613, 1987.
13. Harpole DH, Clements FM, Quill T, et al: Right and left ventricular performance during and after abdominal aortic aneurysm repair. *Ann Surg* 209:356-362, 1989.
14. Orihashi K, Hong YW, Chung G, et al: New applications of two-dimensional transesophageal echocardiography in cardiac surgery. *J Cardiothorac Vasc Anesth* 5:33-39, 1991.
15. Barzilai B, Davila-Roman VG, Eaton MH, et al: Transesophageal echocardiography predicts successful withdrawal of ventricular assist devices. *J Thorac Cardiovasc Surg* 104:1410-1416, 1992.
16. Applebaum RM, Cutler WM, Bhardwaj N, et al: Utility of transesophageal echocardiography during port-access minimally invasive cardiac surgery. *Am J Cardiol* 82:183-188, 1998.
17. Secknus MA, Asher CR, Scalia GM, et al: Intraoperative transesophageal echocardiography in minimally invasive cardiac valve surgery. *J Am Soc Echocardiogr* 12:231-236, 1999.
18. Duff HJ, Buda AJ, Kramer R, et al: Detection of entrapped intracardiac air with intraoperative echocardiography. *Am J Cardiol* 46:255-260, 1980.
19. Orihashi K, Matsuura Y, Hamanaka Y, et al: Retained intracardiac air in open heart operations examined by transesophageal echocardiography. *Ann Thorac Surg* 55:1467-1471, 1993.
20. Obarski TP, Loop FD, Cosgrove DM, et al: Frequency of acute myocardial infarction in valve repairs versus valve replacement for pure mitral regurgitation. *Am J Cardiol* 65:887-890, 1990.
21. Topol EJ, Humphrey LS, Borkon AM, et al: Value of intraoperative left ventricular microbubbles detected by transesophageal two-dimensional echocardiography in predicting neurologic outcome after cardiac operations. *Am J Cardiol* 56:773-775, 1985.
22. Chan K: Transesophageal echocardiography for assessing cause of hypotension after cardiac surgery. *Am J Cardiol* 62:1142-1143, 1988.
23. Reichert CL, Visser CA, Koolen JJ, et al: Transesophageal echocardiography in hypotensive patients after cardiac operations. *J Thorac Cardiovasc Surg* 104:321-326, 1992.
24. Sheikh KH, deBruijn NP, Rankin JS, et al: The utility of transesophageal echocardiography and Doppler color flow imaging in patients undergoing cardiac valve surgery. *J Am Coll Cardiol* 15:363-372, 1990.
25. Click RL, Abel MD, Schaff HV: Intraoperative transesophageal echocardiography: 5-year prospective review of impact on surgical management. *Mayo Clinic Proc* 75(3):241-247, 2000.
26. Chaliki HP, Click RL, Abel MD: Comparison of intraoperative transesophageal echocardiographic examinations with the operative findings: A prospective review of 1918 cases. *J Am Soc Echocardiogr* 12:237-240, 1999.
27. Stewart WJ, Currie PJ, Agler DA, Cosgrove DM: Intraoperative epicardial echocardiography: Technique, imaging planes, and use in valve repair for mitral regurgitation. *Dynamic Cardiovasc Imaging* 1:166-173, 1987.
28. Lambert AS, Miller JP, Foster E, et al: The diagnostic validity of digitally captured intraoperative transesophageal echocardiography examinations compared with analog recordings: A pilot study. *J Am Soc Echocardiogr* 12:974-980, 1999.
29. Shanewise JS, Cheung AT, Aronson S, et al: ASE/SCA guidelines for performing a comprehensive intraoperative multiplane transesophageal examination: Recommendations of the American Society of Echocardiography Council for Intraoperative Echocardiography and the Society of Cardiovascular Anesthesiologists Task Force for Certification in Perioperative Transesophageal Echocardiography. *J Am Soc Echocardiogr* 12:884-900, 1999.
30. Urbanowicz JH, Kernoff RS, Oppenheim G, et al: Transesophageal echocardiography and its potential for esophageal damage. *Anesthesiology* 72:40-43, 1990.
31. Helmcke F, Nanda NC, Hsiung MC, et al: Color Doppler assessment of mitral regurgitation with orthogonal planes. *Circulation* 75:175-183, 1987.
32. Schiller NB, Foster E, Redberg RF: Transesophageal echocardiography in the evaluation of mitral regurgitation. The twenty-four signs of severe mitral regurgitation. *Cardiol Clin* 11:399-408, 1993.

33. Chen C, Thomas JD, Anconina J, et al: Impact of impinging wall jet on color Doppler quantification of mitral regurgitation. *Circulation* 84:712-720, 1991.

34. Bargiggia GS, Tronconi L, Sahn DJ, et al: A new method for quantification of mitral regurgitation based on color flow Doppler imaging of flow convergence proximal to regurgitant orifice. *Circulation* 84:1481, 1991.

35. Klein AL, Stewart WJ, Bartlett J, et al: Effects of mitral regurgitation on pulmonary venous flow and left atrial pressure: An intraoperative transesophageal echocardiographic study. *J Am Coll Cardiol* 20:1345-1352, 1992.

36. Stewart WJ, Currie PJ, Salcedo EE, et al: Intraoperative Doppler color flow mapping for decision-making in valve repair for mitral regurgitation. Technique and results in 100 patients. *Circulation* 81:556-566, 1990.

37. Maurer G, Czer LS, Chaux A, et al: Intraoperative Doppler color flow mapping for assessment of valve repair for mitral regurgitation. *Am J Cardiol* 60:333-337, 1987.

38. Sheikh KH, Bengston JR, Rankin JS, et al: Intraoperative transesophageal Doppler color flow imaging used to guide patient selection and operative treatment of ischemic mitral regurgitation. *Circulation* 84:594-604, 1991.

39. Kleinman JP, Czer LS, DeRobertis M, et al: A quantitative comparison of transesophageal and epicardial color Doppler echocardiography in the intraoperative assessment of mitral regurgitation. *Am J Cardiol* 64:1168-1172, 1989.

40. Flachskampf FA, Frieske R, Engelhard B, et al: Comparison of transesophageal Doppler methods with angiography for evaluation of severity of mitral regurgitation. *J Am Soc Echocardiogr* 11:888-892, 1998.

41. Pu M, Griffin BP, Vandervoort PM, et al: The value of assessing pulmonary venous flow velocity for predicting severity of mitral regurgitation: A quantitative assessment integrating left ventricular function. *J Am Soc Echocardiogr* 12:736-743, 1999.

42. Pu M, Griffin BP, Vandervoort PM, et al: Intraoperative validation of mitral inflow determination by transesophageal echocardiography: Comparison of single, biplane and thermodilution techniques. *J Am Coll Cardiol* 26:1047-1053, 1995.

43. Risk SC, D'Ambra MN, Griffin B, et al: Left atrial V waves following mitral valve replacement are not specific for significant mitral regurgitation. *J Cardiothorac Vasc Anesth* 6:3-7, 1992.

44. Goldman ME, Mindich BP, Teichholz LE, et al: Intraoperative contrast echocardiography to evaluate mitral valve operations. *J Am Coll Cardiol* 4:1035-1040, 1984.

45. Vandervoort PM, Rivera JM, Mele D, et al: Application of color Doppler flow mapping to calculate effective orifice area. An in vitro study and initial clinical observations. *Circulation* 88:1150-1156, 1993.

46. Recusani F, Bargiggia GS, Yoganathan AP, et al: A new method for quantification of regurgitant flow rate using color Doppler flow imaging of the flow convergence region proximal to a discrete orifice: An in vitro study. *Circulation* 83:594-604, 1991.

47. Pu M, Vandervoort PM, Griffin BP, et al: Quantification of mitral regurgitation by the proximal flow convergence method using transesophageal echocardiography: Clinical validation of a geometric correction for proximal flow constraint. *Circulation* 92:2169-2177, 1995.

48. Stewart WJ: Choosing the "golden moment" for operation in the era of valve repair fo mitral regurgitation. *ACC Heart House Learning Center Highlights* 10:2-4, 1995.

49. Cosgrove DM, Stewart WJ: Mitral valvuloplasty. *Curr Probl Cardiol* 14:359-415, 1989.

50. Chaudhry FA, Upadya SP, Singh VP, et al: Identifying patients with degenerative mitral regurgitation for mitral valve repair and replacement: a transesophageal echocardiographic study. *J Am Soc Echocardiogr* 17: 988-994, 2004.

51. Stewart WJ, Griffin B, Thomas JD: Multiplane transesophageal echocardiographic evaluation of mitral valve disease. *Am J Card Imaging* 9:121-128, 1995.

52. Fehske W, Grayburn PA, Omran H, et al: Morphology of the mitral valve as displayed by multiplane transesophageal echocardiography. *J Am Soc Echocardiogr* 7:472-479, 1994.

53. Foster GP, Isselbacher EM, Rose GA, et al: Accurate localization of mitral regurgitant defects using multiplane transesophageal echocardiography. *Ann Thorac Surg* 65:1025-1031, 1998.

54. Grewal KS, Malkowski MJ, Kramer CM, et al: Multiplane transesophageal echocardiographic identification of the involved scallop in patients with flail mitral valve leaflet: Intraoperative correlation. *J Am Soc Echocardiogr* 11:966-971, 1998.

55. Stewart WJ, Currie PJ, Salcedo EE, et al: Evaluation of mitral leaflet motion by echocardiography and jet direction by Doppler color flow mapping to determine the mechanism of mitral regurgitation. *J Am Coll Cardiol* 20:1353-1361, 1992.

56. Izumi S, Miyatake K, Beppu S, et al: Mechanism of mitral regurgitation in patients with myocardial infarction: A study using real time two-dimensional Doppler flow imaging and echocardiography. *Circulation* 76:777-785, 1987.

57. Hendren WG, Morris AS, Rosenkranz ER, et al: Mitral valve repair for bacterial endocarditis. *J Thorac Cardiovasc Surg* 103:124-128, 1992.

58. Enriquez-Sarano M, Freeman WK, Tribouilloy CM, et al: Functional anatomy of mitral regurgitation: Accuracy and outcome implications of transesophageal echocardiography. *J Am Coll Cardiol* 34:1129-1136, 1999.

59. Tunick PA, Gindea A, Kronzon I: Effect of aortic valve replacement for aortic stenosis on severity of mitral regurgitation. *Am J Cardiol* 65:1219-1221, 1990.

60. Harris KM, Malenka DJ, Haney MF, et al: Improvement in mitral regurgitation after aortic valve replacement. *Am J Cardiol* 80:741-745, 1997.

61. Reichert SL, Visser CA, Moulijn AC, et al: Intraoperative transesophageal color-coded Doppler echocardiography for evaluation of residual regurgitation after mitral valve repair. *J Thorac Cardiovasc Surg* 100:756-761, 1990.

62. Saiki Y, Kasegawa H, Kawase M, et al: Intraoperative TEE during mitral valve repair: Does it predict early and late postoperative mitral valve dysfunction. *Ann Thorac Surg* 66:1277-1281, 1998.

63. Orszulak TA, Schaff HV, Danielson GK, et al: Results of reoperation for periprosthetic leakage. *Ann Thorac Surg* 35:584-589, 1983.

64. Marwick TH, Stewart WJ, Currie PJ, Cosgrove DM: Mechanisms of failure of mitral valve repair: An echocardiographic study. *Am Heart J* 122:149-156, 1991.

65. Freeman WK, Schaff HV, Khandheria EK, et al: Intraoperative evaluation of mitral valve regurgitation and repair by transesophageal echocardiography: Incidence and significance of systolic anterior motion. *J Am Coll Cardiol* 20:599-609, 1992.

66. Agricola E, Oppizzi M, Maisano F, et al: Detection of mechanisms of immediate failure by transesophageal echocardiography in quadrangular resection mitral valve repair technique for severe mitral regurgitation. *Am J Cardiol* 91(2):175-179, 2003.

67. Gillinov AM, Cosgrove DM, Blackstone EH, et al: Durability of mitral valve repair for degenerative disease. *J Thorac Cardiovasc Surg* 116(5):734-743, 1998.

68. Matsunaga A, Shah PM, Aidan A: Impact of intraoperative echocardiography/surgery team on successful mitral valve repair: A community hospital experience. *J Heart Valve Dis* 14:325-360, 2005.

69. Kongsaerepong V, Shiota M, Gillinov AM, et al: Echocardiographic predictors of successful versus unsuccessful mitral valve repair in ischemic mitral regurgitation. *Am J Cardiol* 98(4):504-508, 2006.

70. Northrup WF 3rd, DuBois KA, Kshettry VR: Morbidity and mortality of a failed attempt at mitral valve repair converted to re-

placement at the same operation. *J Heart Valve Dis* 12(6):700-706, 2003.

71. Isada LR, Stewart WJ, Torelli J, et al: Morbidity and mortality is not affected by a second pump run for initially unsuccessful mitral valve repair [abstract]. *J Am Soc Echocardiogr* 5:312, 1992.

72. Fix J, Isada L, Cosgrove D, et al: Do patients with less than "echo-perfect" results from mitral valve repair by intraoperative echocardiography have a different outcome? *Circulation* 88(5 Pt 2):II39-II48, 1993.

73. Kronzon I, Cohen ML, Winer HE, Colvin SB: Left ventricular outflow obstruction: A complication of mitral valvuloplasty. *J Am Coll Cardiol* 4:825-828, 1984.

74. Kreindel MS, Schiavone WA, Lever HM, Cosgrove DM: Systolic anterior motion of the mitral valve after Carpentier ring valvuloplasty for mitral valve prolapse. *Am J Cardiol* 57:408-412, 1986.

75. Lee KS, Stewart WJ, Lever HM, et al: Mechanism of outflow tract obstruction causing failed mitral valve repair. Anterior displacement of leaflet coaptation. *Circulation* 88(5 Pt 2):II24-II29, 1993.

76. Mihaileanu S, Marino JP, Chauvaud S, et al: Left ventricular outflow obstruction after mitral repair (Carpentier's technique): Proposed mechanism of disease. *Circulation* 1988;78(2 Pt 2):I78-I84, 1988.

77. Maslow AD, Regan MM, Haering JM, et al: Echocardiographic predictors of left ventricular outflow tract obstruction and systolic anterior motion of the mitral valve after mitral valve reconstruction for myxomatous valve disease. *J Am Coll Cardiol* 34:2096-2104, 1999.

78. Perier P, Clausnizer B, Mistarz K: Carpentier "sliding leaflet" technique for repair of the mitral valve: Early results. *Ann Thorac Surg* 57:383-386, 1994.

79. Jebara VA, Mihaileanu S, Acar C, et al: Left ventricular outflow tract obstruction after mitral valve repair. *Circulation* 88(5 Pt 2):II30-II34, 1993.

80. Schiavone WA, Cosgrove DM, Lever HM, et al: Long-term follow-up of patients with left ventricular outflow tract obstruction after Carpentier ring mitral valvuloplasty. *Circulation* 78(3 Pt 2):I60-I65, 1988.

81. Carabello BA: Mitral valve disease. *Curr Probl Cardiol* 18:423-478, 1993.

82. Starling MR, Kirsh MM, Montgomery DG, Gross MD: Impaired left ventricular contractile function in patients with long-term mitral regurgitation and normal ejection fraction. *J Am Coll Cardiol* 22:239-250, 1993.

83. Wong M, Matsumura M, Kutsuzawa S, et al: The value of Doppler echocardiography in the treatment of tricuspid regurgitation in patients with mitral valve replacement. *J Thorac Cardiovasc Surg* 99:1003-1010, 1990.

84. Czer L, Maurer G, Bolger A, et al: Tricuspid valve repair: Operative and follow-up evaluation by Doppler color flow mapping. *J Thorac Cardiovasc Surg* 98:101-110, 1989.

85. Stoddard MF, Prince CR, Ammash NM, et al: Two-dimensional transesophageal echocardiographic determination of mitral valve area in adults with mitral stenosis. *Am Heart J* 127:1348-1353, 1994.

86. Stoddard MF, Prince CR, Tuman WL, et al: Angle of incidence does not affect accuracy of mitral stenosis area calculation by pressure half-time: Application to Doppler transesophageal echocardiography. *Am Heart J* 127:1562-1572, 1994.

87. Poh KK, Hong EC, Yang H, et al: Transesophageal echocardiography during mitral valve repair underestimates mitral valve area by pressure half-time calculation. *Int J Cardiol* 108(2):177-180, 2006.

88. Marwick T, Torelli J, Obarski T, et al: Assessment of the mitral valve splitability score by transthoracic and transesophageal echocardiography. *Am J Cardiol* 68:1106-1107, 1991.

89. Katz ES, Tsiamtsiouris T, Applebaum RM, et al: Surgical left atrial appendage ligation is frequently incomplete: A transesophageal echocardiographic study. *J Am Coll Cardiol* 36:468-471, 2000.

90. Schwartz SL, Cao QL, Azevedo J, Pandian NG: Simulation of intraoperative visualization of cardiac structures and study of dynamic surgical anatomy with real-time three-dimensional echocardiography. *Am J Cardiol* 73:501-507, 1994.

91. Marx GR, Fulton DR, Pandian NG, et al: Delineation of site, relative size and dynamic geometry of atrial septal defects by real-time three-dimensional echocardiography. *J Am Coll Cardiol* 25:482-490, 1995.

92. Levine RA, Handschumacher MD, Sanfilippo AJ, et al: Three-dimensional echocardiographic reconstruction of the mitral valve, with implications for the diagnosis of mitral valve prolapse. *Circulation* 80:589-598, 1989.

93. De Castro S, Salandin V, Cartoni D, et al: Qualitative and quantitative evaluation of mitral valve morphology by intraoperative volume-rendered three-dimensional echocardiography. *J Heart Valve Dis* 11(2):173-180, 2002.

94. Valocik G, Kamp O, Visser CA: Three-dimensional echocardiography in mitral valve disease. *Eur J Echocardiogr* 6(6):443-454, 2005.

95. Delabays A, Jeanrenaud X, Chassot PG, et al: Localization and quantification of mitral valve prolapse using three-dimensional echocardiography. *Eur J Echocardiogr* 5(6):422-942, 2004.

96. Abraham TP, Warner JG Jr, Kon ND, et al: Feasibility, accuracy and incremental value of intraoperative three-dimensional transesophageal echocardiography in valve surgery. *Am J Cardiol* 80:1577-1582, 1997.

97. Breburda CS, Griffin BP, Pu M, et al: Three-dimensional echocardiographic planimetry of maximal regurgitant orifice area in myxomatous mitral regurgitation: Intraoperative comparison with proximal flow convergence. *J Am Coll Cardiol* 32:432-437, 1998.

98. De Castro S, Salandin V, Cartoni D, et al: Qualitative and quantitative evaluation of mitral valve morphology by intraoperative volume-rendered three-dimensional echocardiography. *J Heart Valve Dis* 11(2):173-180, 2002.

99. Sorrell VL, Rajeev AG, Nifong LW, et al: Intraoperative transesophageal echocardiography with a special focus on a patient undergoing advanced robotic-assisted procedures. *Echocardiography* 19(7 Pt 1):583-587, 2002.

100. Silvestry FE, Wiegers SE, Hermann HC, et al: Echocardiographic guidance of percutaneous repair for mitral regurgitation with the Evalve® System: Lessons learned from the first 27 cases (abstr). *J Am Coll Cardiol* 45(3), 2A, 1001-1062.

101. Cribier A, Eltchaninoff H, Tron C, et al: Treatment of calcific aortic stenosis with the percutaneous heart valve: mid-term follow-up from the initial feasibility studies: the French experience. [Journal Article] *J Am Coll of Cardiol* 47(6):1214-1223, 2006.

102. Webb JG, Chandavimol M, Thompson CR, et al: Percutaneous aortic valve implantation retrograde from the femoral artery. *Circulation* 113(6):842-850, 2006.

Chapter 21

Echocardiography in the Patient Undergoing Catheter Balloon Mitral Valvuloplasty: Patient Selection, Hemodynamic Results, Complications, and Long-Term Outcome

BERNARD IUNG, MD • ALEC VAHANIAN, MD

Echocardiography plays a vital role in the assessment of mitral stenosis (MS). As in other heart valve diseases, it has superseded invasive investigations for assessing the severity and consequences of MS. In addition, the possibility to analyze valve anatomy has emerged as a method to improve the choice of the most appropriate intervention and this has been of particular interest with the development of balloon mitral valvuloplasty (BMV). Growing experience with the use of echocardiography and the analysis of a large series reporting results of BMV now enable indications for interventions to be better ascertained. Besides validated approaches, there are also promising research applications and future perspectives, although their implications in clinical practice remain to be substantiated by further studies.

Background

Unlike other valve diseases, the main etiology of MS remains rheumatic heart disease, even in Western countries.[1] The sharp decrease in the incidence of rheumatic fever in Western countries explains the decrease in the prevalence of rheumatic heart valve disease, which has been compensated by the increase of "degenerative" valve diseases.[2] However, MS still accounts for approximately 10% of all native heart valve diseases in Europe.[1] The presentation of MS has changed in Western countries, where it now tends to affect older patients, with more frequent valve calcification, than in countries where rheumatic fever remains endemic.[3]

Besides epidemiological changes, the management of MS has dramatically changed with the development of BMV since its first description in 1984.[4] The possibility to treat MS using a low-risk procedure progressively led to extend indications of interventional treatment. At the same time, technical refinements in ultrasonographic examinations improved the possibility to noninvasively assess the severity of valve disease, its consequences, and to describe the anatomical lesions.

In contrast with Western countries, rheumatic fever remains endemic in developing countries, where the prevalence of rheumatic heart disease is estimated between 1 and 5 per 1000 patients.[5,6] In these countries, MS remains a major health problem, in particular in young patients, and the availability of percutaneous techniques is limited by economical constraints.

Basic Principles and Echocardiographic Approach

The aims of echocardiographic examination in MS can be summarized as follows: diagnosis, evaluation of the severity and consequences of valve lesions, assessment of valve anatomy and of associated diseases.

Diagnosis

Transthoracic echocardiography (TTE) is mandatory for any clinical suspicion of MS. Given the decreased awareness toward MS in Western countries and the difficulties of auscultatory diagnosis, MS may only be diagnosed when TTE is performed to establish the cause of unexplained dyspnea or thromboembolic event.

The diagnosis of rheumatic MS relies mainly on two-dimensional (2D) echocardiography, which shows leaflet thickening and decreased mobility, commissural fusion, and involvement of the subvalvular apparatus, as assessed using parasternal and apical views. The parasternal short-axis view is of particular importance to assess commissural fusion. The same views are used for the detailed anatomical evaluation of the leaflets and subvalvular apparatus. This analysis also enables rheumatic MS to be distinguished from rare congenital or degenerative MS.

Evaluation of Severity

The assessment of the severity of MS is based on the estimation of valve area. Gradient is not a reliable marker of the severity of valve stenosis because it is highly dependent on heart rate (HR) and cardiac output (CO).[7] Different techniques can be used to assess mitral valve area.

- Planimetry of mitral orifice, using the transthoracic parasternal short-axis view, is considered the reference measurement[8] (Fig. 21–1). It is the only direct measurement of valve area and correlates closely with anatomic findings.[9] Planimetry does not involve hypotheses concerning loading conditions, compliance of cardiac chambers, or associated valve disease. However, planimetry requires particular expertise to ensure that the cross-sectional area (CSA) corresponds to the leaflet tips, and it is not always feasible.

- The pressure half-time (PHT) method is frequently used because it is relatively easy to perform, provided the Doppler signal of transmitral flow is of good quality with a well-defined linear slope of the Doppler E wave. However, its validity may be questioned if loading conditions change or if the compliance of cardiac chambers is markedly abnormal. This is particularly the case with associated aortic regurgitation (AR) or immediately after BMV.[10-12]

- The continuity equation is based on the ratio between stroke volume (SV) in the left or right ventricular outflow tract and velocity time integral (VTI) of the mitral flow.[13] Because it combines a

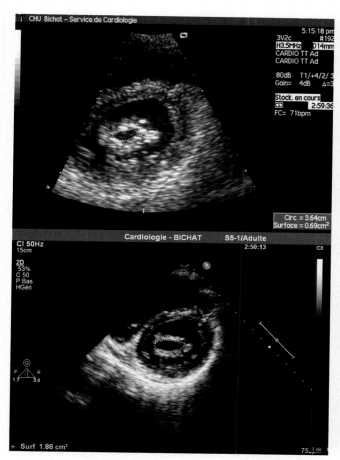

Figure 21–1. *Planimetry of mitral stenosis before and after successful balloon mitral valvuloplasty with opening of both commissures. Transthoracic echocardiography, parasternal short-axis view.* Top, *Before balloon mitral valvuloplasty;* bottom, *after balloon mitral valvuloplasty.*

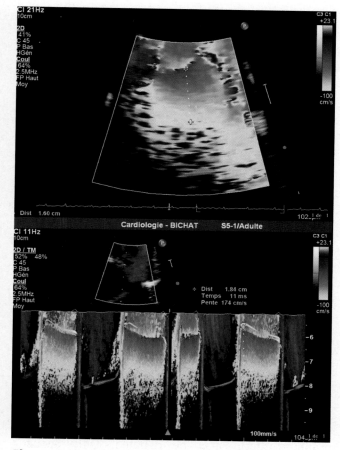

Figure 21–2. *Assessment of mitral valve area using the proximal isovelocity surface.* Top, *two-dimensional echocardiography;* bottom, *color M-mode echocardiography.*

number of different measurements, the risk of error is increased. It is valid only in the absence of significant mitral regurgitation (MR).

- The proximal isovelocity surface area (PISA) method is based on the hemispherical shape of the convergence of mitral flow as shown by color Doppler. This method can be used in the presence of significant MR. However, it is technically demanding and requires multiple measurements. The use of M-mode improves its accuracy, enabling simultaneous measurement of flow and velocity[14] (Fig. 21–2).

Assessment of Consequences

Mean mitral gradient, as assessed by pulsed or continuous-wave Doppler, gives information on the consequences of MS because it is the main determinant of the increase of upstream pressures in left atrium and pulmonary circulation.

Left atrial (LA) enlargement is a result of chronic pressure overload. M-mode measurement may be inac-

curate because enlargement does not follow a spherical pattern in most cases. The use of 2D echocardiographic measurements is preferred to estimate LA area or volume (Fig. 21–3).

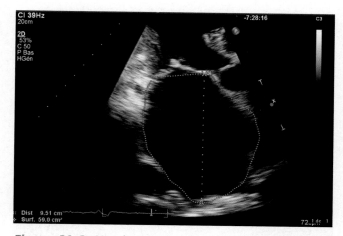

Figure 21–3. *Mitral stenosis with severe antero-posterior enlargement of left atrium. Transthoracic echocardiography, apical view. In this case, the parasternal M-mode measurement underestimates the size of left atrium.*

Systolic pulmonary artery (PA) pressure is estimated from the velocity of Doppler tricuspid flow. Diastolic and mean PA pressures can be derived from pulmonary flow.

Assessment of Valve Anatomy

A detailed analysis of the different components of the mitral valve is necessary not only for diagnosis but also for the choice of the most appropriate intervention:

- Leaflet mobility is particularly well analyzed using the long-axis parasternal view.
- Leaflet thickening is considered significant if 5 mm or greater in thickness.
- Leaflet calcification is suspected in the presence of increased echo brightness.
- The extent of commissural fusion is analyzed using the short-axis parasternal view.
- The impairment of subvalvular apparatus is analyzed from long-axis parasternal and apical views, which show thickening, fusion, or shortening of chordae.

The echocardiographic report should accurately describe the extent and location of each abnormality, in particular in regard to commissural areas.

The definition of calcification using ultrasonographic criteria may be debated. Only acoustic shadowing is specific to calcification alone, whereas localized brightness can also result from fibrosis (Fig. 21–4). For this reason, certain teams require the confirmation of calcification using fluoroscopic examination.[15]

Different scoring systems combine the features of mitral valve anatomy. Their value and limitations in the prediction of the results of BMV and patient selection are addressed further.

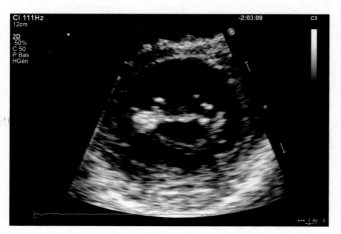

Figure 21–4. Mitral stenosis with a calcified nodule in the postero-medial commissure and a smaller nodule close to the antero-lateral commissure. Parasternal short-axis view.

Mitral Regurgitation

The detection and quantitation of associated MR has important implications for the choice of intervention. Quantitative measurements should be combined and are preferred over methods using color flow mapping of the regurgitant jet in the left atrium.[16] The presence of MR does not alter the validity of the quantitation of MS, except in regard to continuity equation.

Associated Lesions

Dysfunction of the tricuspid valve is frequently associated with MS. It is most often functional tricuspid regurgitation (TR), due to chronically increased PA pressures that result in right ventricular (RV) dilatation and lack of coaptation of tricuspid leaflets, despite normal valve anatomy. There is no consensus for the choice of the optimal method to quantitate TR.[16] Whatever the method used, quantitation of TR is highly dependent on loading conditions. Echocardiographic examination should include the measurement of the tricuspid annulus because severe enlargement may compromise the likelihood of a decrease in regurgitation after isolated correction of MS. Rheumatic tricuspid disease is far less frequent and is characterized by thickening and decreased mobility of tricuspid leaflets. Quantitation of tricuspid stenosis relies on mean gradient.

Associated rheumatic aortic valve disease is quantitated, if required, using standard techniques. Severe aortic stenosis (AS) may be associated with a low gradient because SV is often decreased in MS. Thus, careful quantitation of aortic valve area is needed, using the continuity equation and/or planimetry of the aortic valve with TTE or transesophageal echocardiography (TEE).

Left ventricular (LV) enlargement and systolic dysfunction are unusual in MS and mandate a search for associated valvular regurgitation or coronary artery disease (CAD).

Thromboembolic Complications

The diagnosis of LA thrombosis relies on TEE, which has a much higher sensitivity than TTE, in particular for thrombus located in the left appendage. Echocardiography also plays an important role in risk stratification of thromboembolism. LA enlargement is only one of the numerous risk factors of thromboembolism. LA spontaneous contrast is a stronger predictor of thromboembolic risk in patients with MS.[17]

Use of the Different Echocardiographic Techniques

A comprehensive evaluation of MS can be performed using TTE in most cases; TTE plays also an important role during the procedure to monitor valve opening and to quantitate MR.

In the rare cases, in which the TTE is of poor quality, TEE may be required. However, the main indication for TEE is the detection of LA thrombosis before BMV.

Other than research purposes, the main indication for stress echocardiography is exercise echocardiography in asymptomatic patients.

Technique, Quantitation, and Data Analysis

The respective parts of different features analyzed by echocardiography differ according to whether echocardiography is performed as an initial evaluation or to assess the results of an interventional procedure, immediately or during late follow-up.

Before Balloon Mitral Valvuloplasty

Valve Function

Moderate MS is defined by a valve area between 1 and 1.5 cm^2 and severe MS by a valve area of less than 1 cm^2.[18] The threshold of 1.5 cm^2 is the most relevant in practice because this is the value above which hemodynamics are not affected at rest, and there is a consensus for considering intervention when mitral valve area is less than 1.5 cm^2.[18-20] It is advised to index valve area to body surface area (BSA) to take into account patient's body size. Although no value can be firmly established from the literature, it is generally agreed that MS is significant when index valve area is less than 0.9 to 1 cm^2/m^2 body surface area.[18-20]

The main pitfall when using planimetry is overestimation of valve area because of inappropriate positioning of the measurement plane above the leaflet tips.

The best way to avoid this is to scan slowly from the apex to the base and to select of the narrowest orifice. Technical difficulties inherent to planimetry justify the systematic use of the PHT method, keeping in mind its limitations. In our experience, the most important discrepancies with planimetry are observed in patients older than 60 and in those in atrial fibrillation (AFib), not only after, but also before BMV.[21]

In current practice, 2D planimetry and the PHT method are recommended in the standard evaluation of MS. Other methods are used only if usual measurements are inconclusive or inconsistent with clinical data.

Valve Anatomy

Different approaches have been developed to combine the different anatomical features of MS, aiming to predict the results of BMV, and therefore, to improve patient selection.

The most widely used scoring system is the Wilkins score, in which four components are graded from 1 to 4: leaflet mobility, thickness, calcification, and impairment of subvalvular apparatus[22] (Table 21–1). Another approach relies on a global assessment of mitral valve anatomy, with a classification into three groups according to the best surgical alternative: patients in group 1 are optimal candidates for closed-heart commissurotomy; patients in group 2 are more likely to be candidates for open-heart commissurotomy; and patients in group 3 are usually treated using prosthetic valve replacement[15,23] (Table 21–2). These two scores were developed at the beginning of the development of BMV. Other scoring systems have been described but are not widely used.[24-26]

A common limitation of these two scoring systems is the lack of information on the location of leaflet

TABLE 21–1. Assessment of Mitral Valve Anatomy According to the Wilkins Score

Grade	Mobility	Thickening	Calcification	Subvalvular Thickening
1	Highly mobile valve with only leaflet tips restricted	Leaflets near normal in thickness (4-5 mm)	A single area of increased echo brightness	Minimal thickening just below the mitral leaflets
2	Leaflet midportions and base portions have normal mobility	Midleaflets normal, considerable thickening of margins (5-8 mm)	Scattered areas of brightness confined to leaflet margins	Thickening of chordal structures extending to one of the chordal length
3	Valve continues to move forward in diastole, mainly from the base	Thickening extending through the entire leaflet (5-8 mm)	Brightness extending into the mid portions of the leaflets	Thickening extended to distal third of the chords
4	No or minimal forward movement of the leaflets in diastole	Considerable thickening of all leaflet tissue (>8-10 mm)	Extensive brightness throughout much of the leaflet tissue	Extensive thickening and shortening of all chordal structures extending down to the papillary muscles

The total score is the sum of the four items and ranges between 4 and 16.
From Wilkins GT, Weyman AE, Abascal VM, et al: *Br Heart J* 60:299-308, 1988.

TABLE 21-2. Assessment of Mitral Valve Anatomy According to the Cormier Score

Echocardiographic Group	Mitral Valve Anatomy
Group 1	Pliable noncalcified anterior mitral leaflet and mild subvalvular disease (i.e., thin chordae ≥ 10 mm long)
Group 2	Pliable noncalcified anterior mitral leaflet and severe subvalvular disease (i.e., thickened chordae < 10 mm long)
Group 3	Calcification of mitral valve of any extent, as assessed by fluoroscopy, whatever the state of subvalvular apparatus

From Cormier B, Vahanian A, Michel PL, et al: *Arch Mal Coeur* 82:185-191, 1989; Iung B, Cormier B, Ducimetière P, et al: *Circulation* 94:2124-2130, 1996.

thickening and calcification, specifically in relation to the commissures, which may influence the results of BMV.[27-29] Another drawback of the current scoring systems is that the weight of each abnormality may be debated. In particular, the importance of subvalvular apparatus impairment is probably underestimated.[30]

At the present time, there are no large-scale comparative evaluations of the predictive value of different scoring systems, which could lead to recommend the use of particular one. For the echocardiographer, the best solution is to use a method of analysis with which one is familiar and to include valve anatomy among other clinical and echocardiographic findings.

Evaluation on Exercise

Mean mitral gradient and systolic PA pressure can be recorded in most cases and are the most relevant variables for decision making.[18,19] SV and valve area are more difficult to obtain during exercise, and they are analyzed only for research purposes.

During Balloon Mitral Valvuloplasty

Echocardiography plays also an important role in the catheterization laboratory, in particular with the Inoue technique[31] (Fig. 21-5). The main advantages of the Inoue balloon are its ease of use, partly related to self-positioning, and the possibility to perform stepwise inflations with a progressive increase in balloon diameter. TTE enables valve area, the degree of commissural opening, mean gradient, and MR to be assessed after each balloon inflation, leading the interventional cardiologist to continue balloon inflation to reach a high diameter or to stop the procedure (Fig. 21-6). Planimetry should be used to monitor BMV because the PHT method is not

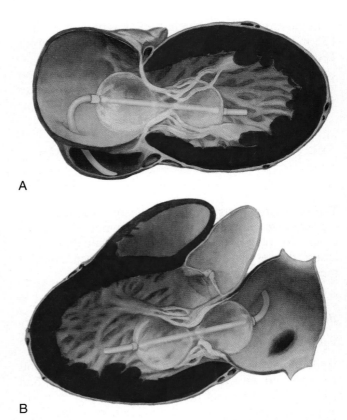

A

B

Figure 21-5. Catheter balloon mitral valvuloplasty using the Inoue balloon. The catheter is inserted through the atrial septum, and the balloon is inflated across the mitral valve. The waist of the balloon is positioned in the mitral orifice and continuing inflation will ensure commissural opening. A, Right anterior oblique view; B, left anterior oblique view.

reliable in this context.[12] Mean gradient is also influenced by changes in loading conditions or heart rate.

Echocardiography is also helpful in the catheterization laboratory to promptly detect pericardial effusion, which is a rare but severe complication of transseptal catheterization.

In rare instances, TEE can be required during BMV, mainly to guide transseptal catheterization in difficult situations. This may be the case in patients with major atrial enlargement, severe thoracic deformations, or situs inversus.[32] Given the discomfort for the patient, the procedure is generally conducted under general anesthesia when TEE is used.

Early after Balloon Mitral Valvuloplasty

Even more than in other situations, planimetry using 2D echocardiography is the reference measurement of mitral valve area immediately after BMV. It enables commissural opening to be visualized; valvular area tracing should include opened commissures. The PHT method is inaccurate in this setting, the possible explanations being acute changes in cardiac chamber compliance or the presence of right-to-left shunt at the site

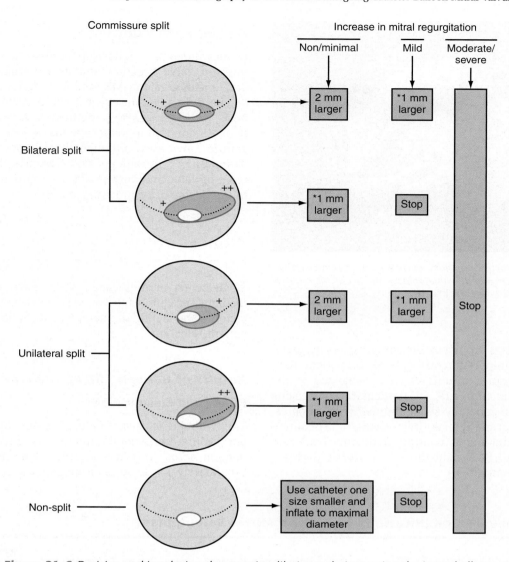

Figure 21-6 *Decision making during the stepwise dilation technique using the Inoue balloon, according to echocardiographic findings after each balloon inflation. The* white area *shows the pre-BMV valve area with the* dark area *indicating the post-BMV valve area. The line of normal leaflet opening is shown by the* dashed line. *+, incomplete split; ++, complete split; *, stop in cases of severely diseased valve or age greater than 65 years. (From Vahanian A, Iung B, Cormier B: Mitral valvuloplasty. In Topol E [ed]:* Textbook of Interventional Cardiology, *4th ed. Philadelphia, WB Saunders, 2003.)*

of the transseptal puncture.[12] However, the PHT method has good specificity, although low sensitivity, to identify good valve opening, which may be helpful in technically difficult examinations.[21]

Although gradient is not a reliable marker of the severity of MS, it should be assessed after BMV because of its predictive value in regard to good late functional results. In patients who had initial pulmonary hypertension, there is a frequent early decrease of PA pressure, although it is generally more pronounced after several months.[33]

In most cases, there is little or no increase in MR after BMV. Moderate MR is often related to incomplete closure of free edges or commissures because of thick-

ening and rigidity.[34,35] In these cases, color Doppler shows central and/or commissural small jets and 2D echocardiography does not suggest a traumatic lesion. If MR is more than moderate, its mechanism should be carefully assessed by looking for traumatic lesions and using TEE if needed. Traumatic MR is mainly caused by a noncommissural leaflet tear and is frequently associated with an absence of commissural opening as shown by surgical or echocardiographic findings.[35,36] Lesions of the subvalvular apparatus are frequent, being mainly rupture of chordae, although partial or total papillary muscle rupture occurs rarely (Fig. 21-7). These lesions cause particularly severe MR in patients with pliable leaflets.

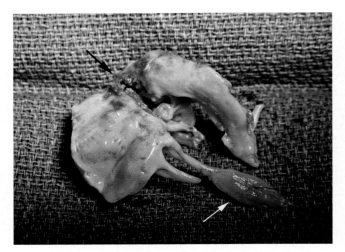

Figure 21–7. Partial papillary muscle rupture (white arrow) *following balloon mitral valvuloplasty on a calcified mitral stenosis (calcification)* (black arrow).

Other findings from postprocedural echocardiography have less important consequences on patient management. Interatrial shunts can be visualized at the transseptal puncture site, in particular when using TEE. These are generally small shunts, which progressively disappear in the majority of cases.[34,37] The intensity of LA spontaneous contrast frequently decreases after successful BMV, and there is a further decrease until the sixth month.[38]

During Follow-Up

Echocardiographic follow-up assesses the usual features of valve function and its consequences: valve area, mean gradient, MR, and systolic PA pressure.

The most frequent event is the occurrence of restenosis, which is generally defined as a valve area less than 1.5 cm² and a greater than 50% loss of the initial gain in valve area, although there is no standardized definition.[31,39] In patients with restenosis, the assessment of valve anatomy should pay particular attention to the degree of commissural fusion.

Clinical Utility

Single-center or multicenter series have analyzed immediate and late results of BMV and enable predictive factors to be identified, thereby contributing to improve patient selection.

Results of Balloon Mitral Valvuloplasty

Failure and Complications

The two main causes of failure are the impossibility of performing transseptal puncture or positioning the balloon across the mitral orifice. Failure rate is approximately 1% in series from experienced teams.[39-43]

TABLE 21–3. Severe Complications of Balloon Mitral Valvuloplasty

	n =	Age (years)	In-hospital Death (%)	Tamponade (%)	Embolic Events (%)	Severe Mitral Regurgitation (%)
NHLBI Registry*[44]	738	54				
n < 25			2	6	4	4
25 ≤ n < 100			1	4	2	3
n ≥ 100			0.3	2	1	3
Chen (1985-1994)*[40]	4,832	37	0.1	0.8	0.5	1.4
Meneveau (1986-1996)[47]	532	54	0.2	1.1	—	3.9
Stefanadis (1988-1996)*[48]	441	44	0.2	0	0	3.4
Hernandez (1989-1995)[39]	620	53	0.5	0.6	—	4.0
Ben Farhat (1987-1998)[41]	654	33	0.5	0.6	1.5	4.6
Arora (1987-2000)[42]	4,850	27	0.2	0.2	0.1	1.4
Palacios (1986-2000)[49]	879	55	0.6	1.0	1.8	9.4
Neumayer (1989-2000)[50]	1,123	57	0.4	0.9	0.9	6.0
Iung (1986-2001)[43]	2,773	47	0.4	0.2	0.4	4.1
Fawzy (1989-2003)[51]	504	31	0	0.8	0.6	1.8

*Multicenter series.
Data from references 39-44, 47-51.

TABLE 21-4. Immediate Results of Balloon Mitral Valvuloplasty: Increase in Mitral Valve Area

	Patients *n* =	Age (years)	Mitral Valve Area (cm²)		Technique
			Before BMV	*After BMV*	
Chen and Cheng[40]	4,832	37	1.1	2.1	Inoue balloon
Meneveau and colleagues[47]	532	54	1.0	1.7	Double or Inoue balloon
Stefanadis and colleagues[48]	441	44	1.0	2.1	Modified single, double, or Inoue balloon (Retrograde)
Bonhoeffer and colleagues[54]	100	31	0.8	2.0	Multi-track balloon
Hernandez and colleagues[39]	561	53	1.0	1.8	Inoue balloon
Eltchaninoff, Koning, Derumeaux, Cribier[55]	500	34	0.9	2.1	Metallic commissurotome
Kang and colleagues[56] (randomized comparison)	152 / 150	42 / 40	0.9 / 0.9	1.8 / 1.9	Inoue balloon / Double balloon
Ben Farhat and colleagues[41]	654	33	1.0	2.1	Inoue or double balloon
Arora and colleagues[42]	4,850	27	0.7	1.9	Inoue or double balloon or metallic commissurotome
Palacios and colleagues[49]	879	55	0.9	1.9	Inoue or double balloon
Neumayer and colleagues[50]	1,123	57	1.1	1.8	Inoue balloon
Iung and colleagues[43]	2,773	47	1.0	1.9	Inoue, single, or double balloon
Fawzy and colleagues[51]	493	31	0.9	2.0	Inoue balloon

BMV, balloon mitral valvuloplasty.
Data from references 39-43, 47-51, 54-56.

Higher rates were reported during early experience, which illustrates the importance of the learning curve.[44-46]

Severe complications are rare and, thus, need to be assessed using large series[39-44,47-51] (Table 21-3). In-hospital death occurs in less than 1% of patients, who are frequently in poor clinical conditions because of advanced age and/or severe hemodynamic impairment. Tamponade is a consequence of perforation by the transseptal needle or metallic guide wires. The risk of thromboembolic events is generally below 2%. Embolism leaving sequelae are mainly caused by fibrinothrombotic clots. They may occur despite systematic screening of LA thrombosis using TEE. Gas embolism caused by balloon rupture is rare with the Inoue balloon. Procedural complications are highly dependent on the experience of the interventional cardiologist, as shown by their relationship with the number of cases performed.[44] Technical simplifications inherent to the Inoue technique contribute to low complication rates, in particular tamponade and partly account for the wide use of this technique.[25]

Severe traumatic MR is the most frequent severe complication of BMV, occurring in between 1% and 10% of cases. Attempts to identify predictive factors did not lead to consistent results, which may be related to the small number of cases analyzed and differences in the methods used to define severe MR.[35,36,52] Severe MR is more frequent in patients with a tight MS and in those with severe impairment of leaflets and subvalvular apparatus, in particular when there is a heterogeneous distribution of leaflets abnormalities.[52,53] However, severe MR remains largely unpredictable in any given patient.[53] Severe acute MR frequently requires surgery within weeks or months but seldom as an emergency.

Immediate Results

After BMV, there is approximately a doubling of mitral valve area in populations with varied characteristics and with different techniques used[39-43,47-51,54-56] (Table 21-4). Series including heart catheterization demonstrated significant decreases in LA and PA pressures and an increase in cardiac output. However, invasive investigations are now unlikely to be performed in routine assessment.

Besides the global assessment of the results, the identification of predictive factors is the most relevant finding for optimizing patient selection. To simplify interpretation and comparison of series, immediate results are also expressed following a binary endpoint, which is most often the association of final valve area

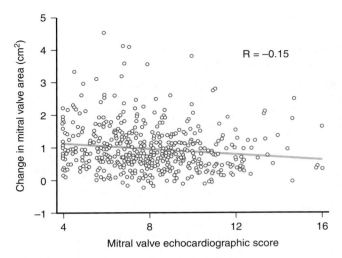

Figure 21–8. *Influence of mitral valve echo score on change in mitral valve area (by cardiac catheterization, cm²) from before to immediately after balloon mitral valvuloplasty. The R value for all points is −0.15. (From the NHLBI balloon valvuloplasty registry participants:* Circulation *85:448-461, 1992.)*

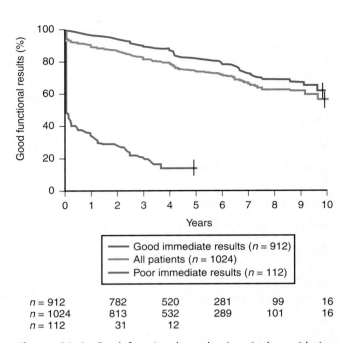

n = 912	782	520	281	99	16
n = 1024	813	532	289	101	16
n = 112	31	12			

Figure 21–9. *Good functional results (survival considering cardiovascular-related deaths with no need for mitral surgery or repeat dilatation and in New York Heart Association functional Class I or II) after balloon mitral valvuloplasty in 1024 patients. (From Iung B, Garbarz E, Michaud P, et al:* Circulation *99:3272-3278, 1999.)*

greater than or equal to 1.5 cm² without MR greater than grade 2/4.

Mitral valve anatomy, as assessed by echocardiography whatever the scoring system used, is a strong predictor of immediate results of BMV.[41,46-51] The discriminant cut-off point of the Wilkins score has been set at 8 according to analyses of immediate results of BMV. However, all scoring systems are of limited predictive value, as shown by the low correlation ($r = -0.15$) between the Wilkins score and final valve area[57] (Fig. 21–8). Large series including patients with diverse presenting characteristics have shown that other factors strongly influence immediate results of BMV.[24,46,57,58] Older age and smaller valve area predict poor immediate results with a similar predictive strength as valve calcification.[46] There are less consistent associations between poor immediate results and previous commissurotomy or baseline MR, which may be related to a differential effect according to other characteristics, as shown by significant interactions. In my experience, the interaction between age and previous commissurotomy means that previous commissurotomy is a factor for poor immediate results only in patients aged over 50 years.[46]

Consistent with these predictors, series that include mostly young patients with favorable valve anatomy report particularly good immediate results.[40-42,51]

Late Results

The assessment of late outcome following BMV is based on clinical endpoints in most series because standardized echocardiographic follow-up raises obvious difficulties when a number of patients are followed over a long time period.

Late results should be interpreted according to the quality of immediate results. The majority of patients with residual stenosis or severe MR after BMV experience early cardiac events. Surgery is required in most cases, and its timing depends largely on comorbidities and the policy of the medical team. Conversely, cardiovascular events seldom occur following successful BMV, and most patients experience sustained functional improvement (Fig. 21–9). Mitral restenosis is the most frequent cause of late clinical deterioration as it was after successful surgical commissurotomy.[39,59-62]

Overall, late results of BMV are satisfying, however, there is a wide range in clinical outcome[39,41,47-49,51,62-65] (Table 21–5). Apparent discrepancies are mainly related to differences in patient characteristics. Series from developing countries include a majority of young patients with favorable anatomical conditions and report high rates of event-free survival. Series from Western countries include older patients who have more diverse characteristics, in particular in regard to valve anatomy, and report less favorable outcome. Series comprising a wide range of patient characteristics enable predictive factors of late results to be identified. As for the prediction of immediate results, valve anatomy is a strong predictive factor of late clinical outcome, but it is only a factor among others[39,41,47-49,51,62-65] (Fig. 21–10). Besides impaired anatomy, baseline predictors of poor late outcome are higher age and characteristics related to the consequences of MS, such as a high functional class and the presence of AFib

TABLE 21–5. Late Results after Balloon Mitral Valvuloplasty

	n =	Age (years)	Follow-up (years)	Event-free Survival (%)
Cohen and colleagues[63]	146	59	5	51*
Dean and colleagues (NHLBI registry)[64]	736	54	4	60*
Orrange and colleagues[65]	132	44	7	65*
Meneveau and colleagues[47]	532	54	7.5	52†
Stefanadis and colleagues[48]	441	44	9	75†
Hernandez and colleagues[39]	561	53	7	69†
Iung and colleagues[62]	1,024	49	10	56†
Ben Farhat and colleagues[41]	654	34	10	72†
Palacios and colleagues[49]	879	55	12	33†
Fawzy and colleagues[51]	493	31	13	74†

*Survival without intervention.
†Survival without intervention and in New York Heart Association Class I or II.
Data from references 39, 41, 47-49, 51, 62-65.

TABLE 21–6. Predictors of Poor Late Functional Results in 912 Patients Who Had Good Immediate Results after Balloon Mitral Valvuloplasty (Valve Area ≥1.5 cm² with No Regurgitation >2/4). Multivariate Analysis

Variable	Subgroups	Relative Risk and 95% Confidence Interval	p
Before Procedure			
Age (years)	<50	1	0.0008
	50-70	1.5 (1.2-2.0)	
	≥70	2.4 (1.4-3.9)	
Functional class (NYHA)	I-II	1	<0.0001
	III-IV	2.7 (1.7-4.4)	
Rhythm	Sinus	1	<0.0001
	AFib	2.0 (1.4-2.7)	
Echocardio-graphic group	1	1	0.003
	2	1.5 (1.1-1.9)	
	3	2.2 (1.3-3.7)	
After Procedure			
Valve area (cm²)	≥2.00	1	0.001
	1.75-2.00	1.4 (1.1-1.7)	
	1.50-1.75	1.9 (1.3-2.8)	
Mean gradient (mm Hg)	≤3	1	<0.0001
	3-6	2.0 (1.6-2.5)	
	≥6	4.0 (2.5-6.2)	
Mitral regurgitation	0-1	1	0.04
	2	1.4 (1.0-2.0)	

AFib, atrial fibrillation; NYHA, New York Heart Association.
From Iung B, Garbarz E, Michaud P, et al: *Circulation* 99:3272-3278, 1999.

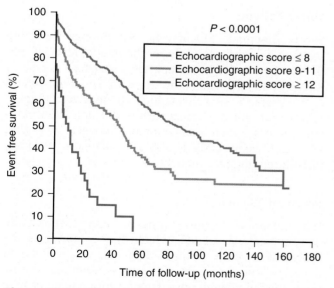

Figure 21–10. Event-free survival (alive and free of mitral valve replacement or redo percutaneous mitral valvuloplasty) according to echocardiographic score. (From Palacios IF, Sanchez PL, Harrell LC, et al: Circulation 105:1465-1471, 2002.)

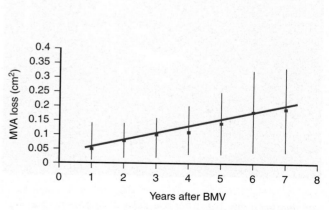

Figure 21–11. Decrease in mitral valve area after balloon mitral valvuloplasty, as a function of time. BMV, balloon mitral valvuloplasty; MVA, mitral valve area. (From Hernandez R, Banuelos C, Alfonso F, et al: Circulation 9:1580-1586, 1999.)

(Table 21–6). These predictors are consistent with previous experience with surgical commissurotomy.[61]

Even in patients with good immediate results, the degree of valve opening has an impact on late outcome.[39,62] Besides postprocedural valve area, gradient is also a strong predictor of late clinical results, suggesting that it provides additional information.[62] The persistence of a high gradient following BMV despite good valve opening can be related to limited valve reserve with a loss of pliability, which is likely to influence late restenosis.

Series with serial echocardiographic examinations show a progressive decrease in mean mitral valve area over time, following a linear pattern[39,59] (Fig. 21–11). The yearly decrease in valve area varies between series, in particular because of differences in patient characteristics, leading to inhomogeneous estimations of restenosis rates.[39,59] Conversely, there is generally no increase in mild-to-moderate MR.[39]

Specific Subgroups

Restenosis after Previous Commissurotomy

In patients with restenosis following prior closed- or open-heart commissurotomy, BMV is feasible and is an interesting alternative to avoid iterative surgery.[66-68] Even if the results are less satisfying than in native valves, a study reported a 48% rate of 8-year good functional results.[69] The possibility to defer surgery by at least 8 years in half of the patients enables prosthesis-related complications to be postponed because surgery consists in prosthetic valve replacement in most patients with restenosis. Analysis of predictive factors suggests that young patients are likely to derive the greatest benefit from BMV for restenosis.[67-69]

Repeat BMV can be performed in selected patients and gives good midterm clinical results, in particular in

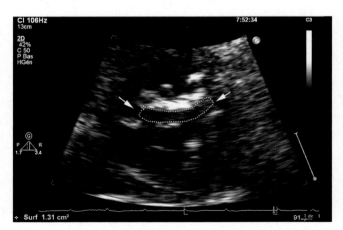

Figure 21–12. Mitral restenosis after previous open-heart commissurotomy. Transthoracic echocardiography, parasternal short-axis view. Both commissures are opened (arrows) and restenosis is a result of rigidity of valvular and subvalvular apparatus. The anterior leaflet is calcified with acoustic shadowing of the posterior leaflet.

young patients with mild or no calcification,[70,71] although its efficacy is less convincing in older patients with calcified valves.[72,73]

Echocardiographic analysis of valve anatomy should carefully look at the extent of commissural refusion. Results of repeat BMV are less satisfying in patients who have incomplete commissural fusion.[73] Whatever the type of initial commissurotomy, BMV should not be considered in case of persistent opening of both commissures (Fig. 21–12).

The Elderly

Theoretically, elderly patients are not good candidates for BMV because they combine predictive factors of poor immediate and late outcome, in particular as a result of old age, frequent valve calcification, AFib, and severe symptoms. Despite unfavorable anatomical conditions, good immediate results are frequently obtained, but subsequent deterioration occurs more rapidly than in younger patients.[74,75] However, these results should be weighed against the alternative of surgery, which is at high risk in this population. Even with unfavorable mitral anatomy, BMV can be considered as a palliative procedure in a number of old patients with severely symptomatic MS.

Echocardiographic examination should confirm the rheumatic etiology and distinguish it from degenerative MS with calcification of the mitral annulus and opened commissures. This disease is frequent in the elderly but seldom causes severe MS. Because there is no commissural fusion in these cases, BMV is not a relevant treatment.

Young Patients

Severe rheumatic MS may be encountered in young patients in countries where rheumatic fever is endemic. Two series have reported consistent results of BMV in patients aged below 20, who were followed up to 12 years.[76,77] Results tended to be better than in adults and late functional results did not differ, with event-free survival rates ranging between 70% and 80% at 10 years. BMV is also a valid treatment of MS in children younger than 12.[78]

Pregnant Women

Hemodynamic changes during pregnancy worsen the clinical tolerance of MS, which may compromise the prognosis of both mother and fetus, in particular at delivery. Therefore, intervention is required during pregnancy in women who remain symptomatic despite medical therapy. BMV can be safely performed during pregnancy and fetal tolerance is good.[79-81] The increase of thromboembolic risk during pregnancy underlines

TABLE 21-7. Contraindications to Balloon Mitral Valvuloplasty

Persistent left atrial thrombosis (including in the left atrial appendage)
More than mild mitral regurgitation
Massive or bicommissural calcification
Severe concomitant aortic valve disease
Severe organic tricuspid stenosis or severe functional regurgitation with enlarged annulus
Severe concomitant coronary artery disease requiring bypass surgery

the need for TEE, which is best performed under anaesthesia just before the procedure to reduce the mother's discomfort.

Implications for Patient Selection

Contraindications

Contraindications to BMV are summarized in Table 21–7. Although cases of BMV using the Inoue balloon have been reported in patients with thrombosis located in the left appendage,[82] the experience remains limited. The potential hazards related to thrombus migration suggest that persistent thrombus of left atrium, even when localized to the LA appendage, is a contraindication in most cases. However, if the patient is in stable condition, the decision should be postponed until after repeat TEE following at least two months of optimal anticoagulant therapy. LA thrombosis has been shown to disappear in approximately one out of four patients after 6 months of anticoagulant therapy, in particular in patients with a small thrombus and low grade LA spontaneous contrast.[83]

More than mild MR, or with a grade greater than 2/4 when using a semiquantitative approach, is a contraindication to BMV. Although no study has validated thresholds based on quantitative echocardiography, this corresponds to an effective regurgitant orifice greater than 20 mm^2 or a regurgitant volume greater than 30 mL/beat. In patients who have borderline MR, BMV is more likely to be considered if valve anatomy is favorable.

Valve calcification is a contraindication to BMV in the rare cases where it is massive or localized in both commissures.

Other contraindications are related to associated heart diseases needing surgical correction. Particular attention should be paid to avoid underestimating the degree of aortic stenosis. Conversely, associated moderate aortic regurgitation without LV dilation is not a contraindication to BMV because progression is slow.[84] Surgery is preferred if there is severe associated organic tricuspid disease or severe functional TR with major enlargement of the tricuspid annulus. In other cases, severe functional TR may decrease after BMV.[85]

Choice of the Procedure

There is now evidence supporting BMV as the procedure of choice in young patients. Young age is frequently associated with favorable valve anatomy, both features being strong predictors of good immediate and late results.[86] Randomized trials conducted in these homogeneous populations show that 3- and 7-year results of BMV are as good as those obtained with open-heart commissurotomy and better than with closed-heart commissurotomy.[87,88] Moreover, the possibility to perform conservative treatment and to repeat it in selected patients is particularly attractive in young patients, including children and adolescents, to avoid iterative surgical interventions. However, a number of good candidates to BMV cannot benefit from the procedure for financial reasons. Young patients with MS are mainly encountered in developing countries that cannot always afford the cost of the balloon. This justifies attempts to lower the cost of the device, such as a multitrack system and the metallic commissurotome.[54,55,89] The possibility to reuse the metallic part of the percutaneous commissurotome significantly lowers the cost of the procedure.

The decision is more difficult in older patients who have frequent impairment of the anatomy of the leaflets and subvalvular apparatus and who represent the majority of patients with MS in Western countries.[1,86] They form a heterogeneous group for whom no randomized studies are available. Patients should not be denied BMV on the only basis of unfavorable valve anatomy, given the low predictive value of valve anatomy alone. Good immediate and midterm results can be obtained in patients with unfavorable mitral anatomy, even with calcified valves.[86,90-93] Patient selection should rely on a global assessment, which can be aided by the use of predictive analyses and derived multivariate models enabling results of BMV to be estimated according to individual patient characteristics.[46,62,69,93,94]

In patients with impaired valve anatomy, BMV can be considered in particular when their other characteristics are favorable, in particular age below 70 years, mitral valve area between 1 and 1.5 cm^2, moderate symptoms (New York Heart Association [NYHA] Class II), and sinus rhythm. Predictive models show a high likelihood of good immediate and late results in these patients.[46,62,69] This enables surgery to be postponed for several years, thereby deferring prosthesis-related complications because the surgical alternative is valve replacement in most of these patients. This is illustrated by the simulation of midterm results of BMV in patients with calcified mitral valves according to the extent of calcification and other characteristics[93] (Fig. 21–13). Conversely, there is a much lower likelihood of sustained improvement in older patients who have unfavorable mitral anatomy, tight stenosis, severe symptoms, and AFib.[62,93] Moreover, the relevance of deferring surgery may be debatable in

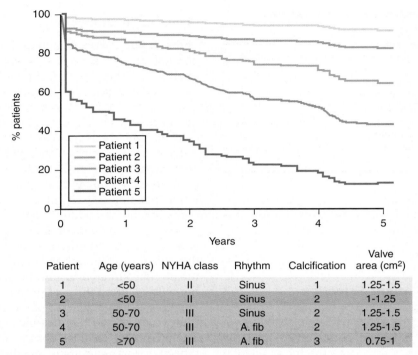

Patient	Age (years)	NYHA class	Rhythm	Calcification	Valve area (cm²)
1	<50	II	Sinus	1	1.25-1.5
2	<50	II	Sinus	2	1-1.25
3	50-70	III	Sinus	2	1.25-1.5
4	50-70	III	A. fib	2	1.25-1.5
5	≥70	III	A. fib	3	0.75-1

Figure 21-13. *Predicted probability of good immediate results (valve area ≥ 1.5 cm² without regurgitation > grade 2/4) and good late functional results (survival with no intervention and in New York Heart Association (NYHA) functional Class I or II) after balloon mitral valvuloplasty in calcified mitral stenosis, according to patient characteristics. The extent of calcification is graded from 1 (small nodule) to 4 (extensive calcification). (From Iung B, Garbarz E, Doutrelant L, et al: Am J Cardiol 85:1308-1314, 2000.)*

this age group. Thus, mitral surgery, often combined with tricuspid repair, can be considered as the first line treatment provided the operative risk is acceptable. The choice between BMV and surgery in these difficult situations should also take into account the local expertise of interventional cardiologists and surgeons and the wishes of the patient.

In Western countries, there is a trend for BMV to be performed in older patients with more severe impairment of valve anatomy.[43] In the Euro Heart Survey on valvular heart disease performed in 2001, surgical commissurotomy accounted for only 4% of the interventions performed for MS, whereas BMV was used in 34% of the patients and prosthetic valve replacement in 62%.[1]

Timing of the Procedure

There is a consensus to advise intervention, whether it is percutaneous or surgical, in patients who have significant MS (valve area < 1.5 cm² or 1 cm²/m² body surface area) and symptoms.[18] Better insights into the prognosis of MS, in particular in regard to thromboembolic risk and the availability of intervention at low risk, lead to consideration of BMV at an earlier stage of the disease. Intervention is not considered in mild MS because the progression of MS is highly variable and risk-benefit analyses does not support prophylactic

BMV.[18,95] However, BMV is now considered more widely in selected patients with significant MS and few or no symptoms, aiming to decrease the risk of thromboembolic events or hemodynamic complications.

The efficacy of BMV has been demonstrated on different markers of the thromboembolic risk in MS: LA spontaneous contrast, LA size and contractility, LA appendage flow velocity, and activation of coagulation in left atrium.[38,96-98] Although the efficacy of BMV on the thromboembolic risk has not been demonstrated by randomized studies, a prospective series showed that the performance of BMV was strongly associated with a decreased thromboembolic risk in patients with MS and AFib.[99]

It is more difficult to evaluate the risk of acute hemodynamic complications in MS, except in particular cases, such as pregnancy. Exercise echocardiography is of potential interest because it provides additional information as compared with baseline evaluation. Guidelines recommend BMV, when anatomical conditions are favorable, if mean mitral gradient is greater than 15 mm Hg or systolic pulmonary artery (PA) pressure is greater than 60 mm Hg at peak exercise.[18,19] However, such thresholds are debatable because their prognostic value has not been validated in large series.

Recommendations on BMV in asymptomatic patients with MS are summarized in Table 21-8.

TABLE 21-8. Recommendations for Balloon Mitral Valvuloplasty in Asymptomatic Patients with Mitral Stenosis

ACC/AHA Guidelines[18]	Recommendations of the Working Group on Valvular Heart Diseases of the ESC[19]
Asymptomatic patients with moderate or severe mitral stenosis (mitral valve area ≤ 1.5 cm²) and valve morphology favorable for percutaneous balloon valvotomy in the absence of left atrial thrombus or moderate to severe mitral regurgitation, who have: —pulmonary hypertension (pulmonary artery systolic pressure > 50 mm Hg at rest or 60 mm Hg with exercise; Class IIa) *or* —new onset of atrial fibrillation (Class IIb)	Selected asymptomatic patients with mitral stenosis (valve area ≤ 1.5 cm² or ≤ 1 cm²/m² body surface area) in the absence of contraindication and: —increased risk of thromboembolic events: prior embolism, dense spontaneous echocardiographic contrast in the left atrium, or recent or paroxysmal atrial fibrillation *or* —risk of hemodynamic decompensation: pulmonary hypertension (systolic pulmonary pressure > 50 mm Hg at rest or 60 mm Hg on exercise), wish for pregnancy, or need for major extracardiac surgery

ACC, American College of Cardiology; AHA, American Heart Association; ESC, European Society of Cardiology.

Research Applications

Stress Echocardiography

Changes in the severity of MS and its consequences can be observed according to changes in hemodynamic conditions, as shown by exercise or pharmacologic stress combined with invasive measurements. They have been replaced by stress echocardiography, which has the advantage of being noninvasive, in particular when performing repeated measurements.

Exercise echocardiography is the most physiological approach. Different series consistently show an increase in mean gradient and systolic PA pressure at submaximal effort or peak effort.[100-103] However, there is variability among patients in the exercise change in stroke volume, mitral gradient, and systolic PA pressure, which does not relate to baseline severity of MS.[101-103] A possible explanation for this heterogenous response comes from differences in the change in valve area with exercise, as measured by the continuity equation. An increase in valve area on exercise is associated with an increase in SV. Conversely, SV does not increase when there is no significant change in valve area during exercise.[103,104] These two different patterns are not related to differences in baseline valve orifice area but to degree of valve deformity and stiffness.[104] Another possible explanation from a study using exercise echocardiography to evaluate atrioventricular (AV) compliance is that systolic PA pressure at rest, and even more so on exercise, is strongly correlated with atrioventricular compliance but not with mitral valve area.[103] Finally, the level of increase in systolic PA pressure on exercise seems to be related to the type of limiting symptoms, whether they are dyspnea of fatigue.[102]

Most of the previous studies used treadmill and were based on postexercise data. An advantage of using semisupine bicycle ergometry is that hemodynamic changes can be assessed for each workload. My preliminary experience suggests that the pattern of increase of mitral gradient is more closely related to the type of limiting symptom rather than the level of mean gradient or systolic PA pressure at peak exercise.[105]

Although dobutamine stress echocardiography (DSE) may seem a less physiological approach in MS than exercise echocardiography, it is also associated with significant increases in mean gradient and systolic PA pressure, as compared with resting values.[106] The only study that which has analyzed so far the relationship between findings from stress echocardiography and clinical outcome was based on dobutamine stress echocardiography.[107] This study of 53 patients showed that mean mitral gradient during dobutamine stress echocardiography was an independent predictor of clinical events during 5-year follow-up, the cut-off value being 18 mm Hg. The incremental prognostic value was particularly marked in patients who had a valve area between 1 and 1.5 cm².[107] Another study using dobutamine stress echocardiography showed greater valve reserve (i.e., a larger increase in valve area with stress) in patients who had had previous commissurotomy as compared with those who had native MS.[108]

Stress echocardiography seems to be a promising approach to refine the knowledge of hemodynamic consequences of MS. However, at the present time, its implications in decision making need to be assessed by further prospective studies. This is particularly needed to validate thresholds of gradient and PA pressure leading to consider intervention in asymptomatic patients with MS.[18,19]

Evaluation of Valve Anatomy

Given the limitations of commonly used scoring systems for the prediction of the results of BMV, alternate approaches have been developed, in particular taking into account the location of valve abnormalities in relation to the commissures. Series have shown that commissural location of valve thickening and calcification influences immediate results of BMV.[27-29] However, no

TABLE 21–9. Echocardiographic Score Proposed by Padial and Colleagues for the Prediction of Severe Mitral Regurgitation

Grade	Anterior Leaflet	Posterior Leaflet	Commissural Calcification	Subvalvular Disease
1	Leaflet near normal (4-5 mm) or with only a thick segment	Leaflet near normal (4-5 mm) or with only a thick segment	Fibrosis and/or calcium in only one commissure	Minimal thickening of chordal structures just below the valve
2	Leaflet fibrotic and/or calcified evenly; no thin area	Leaflet fibrotic and/or calcified evenly; no thin area	Both commissures mildly affected	Thickening of chordae extending up to one third of chordal length
3	Leaflet fibrotic and/or calcified with uneven distribution; thinner segments are mildly thickened (5-8 mm)	Leaflet fibrotic and/or calcified with uneven distribution; thinner segments are mildly thickened (5-8 mm)	Calcium in both commissures, one markedly affected	Thickening to the distal third of the chordae
4	Leaflet fibrotic and/or calcified with uneven distribution; thinner segments are near normal (4-5 mm)	Leaflet fibrotic and/or calcified with uneven distribution; thinner segments are near normal (4-5 mm)	Calcium in both commissures, both markedly affected	Extensive thickening and shortening of all chordae extending down the papillary muscle.

The total score is the sum of the four items and ranges between 4 and 16.
Data from Padial LR, Freitas N, Sagie A, et al: *J Am Coll Cardiol* 27:1225-1231, 1996.

scoring system including these findings has been validated on large series in comparison with commonly used scoring systems. Another scoring system has been developed to predict the occurrence of severe MR, which is the most frequent complication following BMV.[52] It has the advantage of taking into account the heterogeneity of leaflet impairment and the presence of commissural fibrosis or calcification (Table 21–9). Nevertheless, its predictive value on immediate valve opening and late functional results has not been studied, and its usefulness in the prediction of severe MR has not been confirmed in large series.

Besides the location of valvular abnormalities, mechanical properties of valvular tissue probably influence immediate and late results of BMV. Resting atrioventricular compliance is closely related to upstream pressures, however, its impact on late outcome is not known.[109]

Thus, there are different approaches to refine the assessment of valve anatomy, combining more detailed scoring systems and evaluations of valvular mechanical properties. However, more complex analyses raise concerns regarding their applicability in current practice and their reproducibility. Moreover, it will be necessary to demonstrate their incremental predictive value on outcome, as compared with current validated multifactorial approaches.

Potential Limitations and Future Directions

Despite technical refinements, there remain limitations in the feasibility or the relevance of certain echocardiographic analyses in MS.

Although planimetry is considered as the reference measurement, its applicability is reduced by the need for technical expertise to ensure optimal positioning of the measurement plan on the mitral orifice, which may be the cause of significant interobserver variability. Recent reports suggested that real-time three-dimensional (3D) echocardiography is useful in optimizing the positioning of the measurement plan, and therefore, improving reproducibility.[110-111]

Even with experienced operators, planimetry may not be feasible in patients with poor echocardiographic windows and/or in case of severe valve deformity; three-dimensional echocardiography does not seem to give better results in such situations.[111] Other methods of measurements should be used and interpreted taking into account their own limitations.[112] Further studies are needed to confirm preliminary findings on the role of three-dimensional echocardiography in the assessment of commissural opening and the detection of leaflet tear after BMV[113] (Fig. 21–14).

Doppler enables PA pressure to be assessed in most patients. However, it is not possible to reliably assess capillary wedge pressure and thus pulmonary vascular resistance, using ultrasonographic techniques. Pulmonary hypertension is passive in most patients, as a result of an increase in LA pressure with normal pulmonary vascular resistance. However, in certain patients, who frequently have long-standing diseases, pulmonary vascular resistance is increased because of pulmonary vascular disease. The risk of surgery is higher in these patients, and BMV should be favored when feasible because it provides functional improvement and progressive improvement in hemodynamics.[114,115] Estimation of pulmonary vascular resistance, using cardiac catheterization, is useful in patients who present with

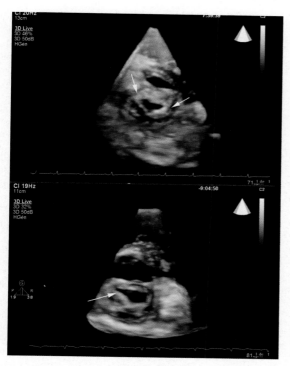

Figure 21–14. *Real-time three-dimensional echocardiography.* Top, *Restenosis with fusion of both commissures* (arrows); bottom, *restenosis with persistent opening of a commissure* (arrow).

severe pulmonary hypertension seeming out of proportion with the degree of MS or pulmonary congestion as assessed by chest X-ray (CXR).

The limitations of anatomical scoring systems for the prediction of immediate and late results of BMV have been reviewed above. Given the multiple determinants of the results of BMV, there is a low likelihood that any echocardiographic scoring system will ensure an optimal prediction of the results of BMV. Combined assessment using multislice computed tomography (CT) to quantitate valve calcification might be an interesting approach.

Future improvements in patient selection will probably come from the incorporation of improved anatomical evaluation using echocardiography and other imaging techniques and other variables, such as stress hemodynamics indices in multivariate models, rather than the optimization of a single scoring system.

Alternate Approaches

Right and left heart cardiac catheterization enables valve area to be evaluated using the Gorlin formula. The Gorlin formula is sometimes considered as the reference method, however, this is mainly for historical reasons. Experimental and clinical data raise concerns regarding the validity of the Gorlin formula in cases of low output and immediately after BMV.[116,117] This ex-

plains why guidelines advise limiting invasive evaluation of the severity of MS to the rare situations in which echocardiography is inconclusive or when there are discrepancies between different measurements and clinical evaluation.[18] Right heart catheterization is indicated in cases of suspected pulmonary vascular hypertension. In current practice, the main indication for invasive investigations is the assessment of associated coronary disease using coronary angiography.[18] However, cardiac catheterization remains frequently performed, in particular as a systematic evaluation associated to coronary angiography, although this is not supported by guidelines.[1,18]

Preliminary reports suggest that magnetic resonance imaging (MRI) is a valid alternate noninvasive method for planimetry of the mitral valve.[118] This could be particularly useful when planimetry using 2D echocardiography is not feasible.

The experience with intracardiac echocardiography is limited. It may be helpful to rule out LA thrombosis in patients who have contraindications to TEE or to monitor transseptal puncture in difficult cases, thereby avoiding the use of TEE under general anesthesia[119,120] (Fig. 21–15). However, the high cost of the single-use device limits its use.

In conclusion, growing experience with BMV enables the validity and the predictive value of echocardiographic findings in MS to be validated. The prediction of the results of BMV is intrinsically multifactorial,

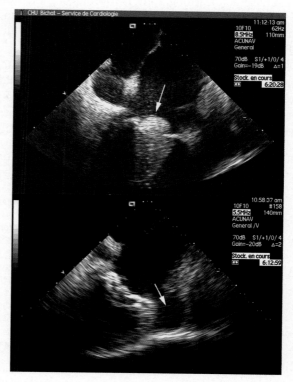

Figure 21–15. *Intracardiac echocardiography during balloon mitral valvuloplasty.* Top, *Inflation of the Inoue balloon* (arrow) *across the mitral valve;* bottom, *visualization of the left atrium and left atrial appendage* (arrow).

which underlines the need for a complete assessment combining clinical and echocardiographic findings. Analyses of the results of BMV in large series or in selected subgroups are helpful in decision making for the choice of the most appropriate procedure and its timing at different stages of the disease.

KEY POINTS

- Planimetry using 2D echocardiography is the reference measurement for valve area.

- The use of cardiac catheterization to evaluate mitral valve area should be limited to the situations in which noninvasive measurements are inconsistent or discordant with clinical findings.

- Patient selection should not overstress the assessment of valve anatomy but take into account a number of clinical and echocardiographic variables, the predictive value of which has been validated in large series.

- BMV should be considered in patients who have MS with unfavorable anatomy, provided their other characteristics, in particular age, are favorable.

- Severe MR is the most frequent complication of BMV. It remains difficult to predict in a given patient.

- The most frequent cause of late functional deterioration after BMV is mitral restenosis, which occurrence follows an approximately linear pattern.

- Exercise echocardiography is a promising method to refine indications for intervention in asymptomatic patients. However, there is still a need for validation through prognostic studies.

- BMV and surgery should not be considered concurrent, but complementary, techniques, which should be used at different times of the evolution of MS.

REFERENCES

1. Iung B, Baron G, Butchart EG, et al: A prospective survey of patients with valvular heart disease in Europe: The Euro Heart Survey on valvular heart disease. *Eur Heart J* 13:1231-1243, 2003.
2. Soler-Soler J, Galve E: Worldwide perspective of valve disease. *Heart* 83:721-725, 2000.
3. Carroll JD, Feldman T: Percutaneous mitral balloon valvotomy and the new demographics of mitral stenosis. *JAMA* 270:1731-1736, 1993.
4. Inoue K, Okawi T, Nakamura T, et al: Clinical application of transvenous mitral commissurotomy by a new balloon catheter. *J Thorac Cardiovasc Surg* 87:394-402, 1984.
5. Bahadur KC, Sharma D, Shresta MP, et al: Prevalence of rheumatic and congenital heart disease in schoolchildren of Kathmandu valley in Nepal. *Indian Heart J* 55:615-618, 2003.
6. Rizvi SFH, Khan MA, Kundi A, et al: Current status of rheumatic heart diseases in rural Pakistan. *Heart* 90:394-399, 2004.
7. Rahimtoola SH, Durairaj A, Mehra A, et al: Current evaluation and management of patients with mitral stenosis. *Circulation* 106:1183-1188, 2002.

8. Palacios I: What is the gold standard to measure mitral valve area postmitral balloon valvuloplasty? *Cathet Cardiovasc Diagn* 33:315-316, 1994.
9. Faletra F, Pezzano A Jr, Fusco R, et al: Measurement of mitral valve area in mitral stenosis: Four echocardiographic methods compared with direct measurement of anatomic orifices. *J Am Coll Cardiol* 28:1190-1197, 1996.
10. Thomas JD, Wilkins GT, Choong CYP, et al: Inaccuracy of mitral pressure half-time immediately after percutaneous mitral valvotomy. Dependence on transmitral gradient and left atrial and ventricular compliance. *Circulation* 78:980-993, 1988.
11. Karp K, Teien D, Bjerle P, Eriksson P: Reassessment of valve area determinations in mitral stenosis by the pressure half-time method: impact of left ventricular stiffness and peak diastolic pressure difference. *J Am Coll Cardiol* 13:594-599, 1989.
12. Chen C, Wang Y, Guo B, Lin Y: Reliability of the Doppler pressure half-time method for assessing effects of percutaneous mitral balloon valvuloplasty. *J Am Coll Cardiol* 13:1309-1313, 1989.
13. Nakatani S, Masuyama T, Kodama K, et al: Value and limitations of Doppler echocardiography in the quantification of stenotic mitral valve area: Comparison of the pressure half-time and the continuity equation methods. *Circulation* 77:78-85, 1988.
14. Messika-Zeitoun D, Yiu SF, Cormier B, et al: Sequential assessment of mitral valve area during diastole using colour M-mode flow convergence analysis: New insights into mitral stenosis physiology. *Eur Heart J* 24:1244-1253, 2003.
15. Cormier B, Vahanian A, Michel PL, et al: Evaluation by two-dimensional and doppler echocardiography of the results of percutaneous mitral valvuloplasty. *Arch Mal Coeur Vaiss* 82:185-191, 1989.
16. Zoghbi WA, Enriquez-Sarano M, Foster E, et al: Recommendations for evaluation of the severity of native valvular regurgitation with two-dimensional and Doppler echocardiography. *J Am Soc Echocardiogr* 16:777-802, 2003.
17. Black IW, Hopkins AP, Lee LC, Walsh WF: Left atrial spontaneous echo contrast: A clinical and echocardiographic analysis. *J Am Coll Cardiol* 18:398-404, 1991.
18. Bonow RO, Carabello B, de Leon AC Jr, et al: ACC/AHA guidelines for the management of patients with valvular heart disease. *J Am Coll Cardiol* 32:1486-1588, 1998.
19. Iung B, Gohlke-Bärwolf C, Tornos P, et al: Recommendations on the management of the asymptomatic patient with valvular heart disease. *Eur Heart J* 23:1253-1266, 2002.
20. Tribouilloy C, De Gevigney G, Acar C, et al: Recommandations de la Société Française de Cardiologie concernant la prise en charge des valvulopathies acquises et des dysfonctions de prothèse valvulaire. *Arch Mal Coeur* 98(suppl):5-61, 2005.
21. Messika-Zeitoun D, Meizels A, Cachier A, et al: Echocardiographic evaluation of the mitral valve area before and after percutaneous mitral commissurotomy; the pressure half-time revisited. *J Am Soc Echocardiogr* 18:1409-1414, 2005.
22. Wilkins GT, Weyman AE, Abascal VM, et al: Percutaneous balloon dilatation of the mitral valve: An analysis of echocardiographic variables related to outcome and the mechanism of dilatation. *Br Heart J* 60:299-308, 1988.
23. Vahanian A, Michel PL, Cormier B, et al: Results of percutaneous mitral commissurotomy in 200 patients. *Am J Cardiol* 63:847-852, 1989.
24. Nobuyoshi M, Hamasaki N, Kimura T, et al: Indications, complications, and short-term clinical outcome of percutaneous transvenous mitral commissurotomy. *Circulation* 80:782-792, 1989.
25. Bassand JP, Schiele F, Bernard Y, et al: The double-balloon and Inoue techniques in percutaneous mitral valvuloplasty: comparative results in a series of 232 cases. *J Am Coll Cardiol* 18:982-989, 1991.
26. Miche E, Bogunovic N, Fassbender D, et al: Predictors of unsuccessful outcome after percutaneous mitral valvotomy including

a new echocardiographic scoring system. *J Heart Valve Dis* 5:430-435, 1996.

27. Fatkin D, Roy P, Morgan JJ, Feneley MP: Percutaneous balloon mitral valvotomy with the Inoue single-balloon catheter: Commissural morphology as a determinant of outcome. *J Am Coll Cardiol* 21:390-397, 1993.

28. Cannan CR, Nishimura RA, Reeder GS, et al: Echocardiographic assessment of commissural calcium: A simple predictor of outcome after percutaneous mitral balloon valvotomy. *J Am Coll Cardiol* 29:175-180, 1997.

29. Sutaria N, Northridge DB, Shaw TRD: Significance of commissural calcification on outcome of mitral balloon valvotomy. *Heart* 84:398-402, 2000.

30. Turgeman Y, Atar S, Rosenfeld T: The subvalvular apparatus in rheumatic mitral stenosis. Methods of assessment and therapeutic implications. *Chest* 124:1929-1936, 2003.

31. Vahanian A, Iung B, Cormier B: Mitral valvuloplasty. In Topol EJ (ed): *Textbook of Interventional Cardiology*, 4th ed. Philadelphia, WB Saunders, 2003, pp. 921-940.

32. Nallet O, Iung B, Cormier B, et al: Specifics of technique in percutaneous mitral commissurotomy in a case of dextrocardia and situs inversus with mitral stenosis. *Cathet Cardiovasc Diagn* 39:85-88, 1996.

33. Fawzy ME, Mimish L, Sivanandam V, et al: Immediate and long-term effect of balloon mitral valvotomy on severe pulmonary hypertension in patients with mitral stenosis. *Am Heart J* 131:89-93, 1996.

34. Porte JM, Cormier B, Iung B, et al: Value of transesophageal echocardiography in the follow-up of successful percutaneous mitral valvotomy. *Arch Mal Coeur* 87:211-218, 1994.

35. Essop MR, Wisenbaugh T, Skoularigis J, et al: Mitral regurgitation following mitral balloon valvotomy. Differing mechanisms for severe versus mild-to-moderate lesions. *Circulation* 84:1669-1679, 1991.

36. Herrmann HC, Lima JAC, Feldman T, et al: Mechanisms and outcome of severe mitral regurgitation after Inoue balloon valvuloplasty. *J Am Coll Cardiol* 22:783-789, 1993.

37. Cequier A, Bonan R, Serra A, et al: Left-to-right atrial shunting after percutaneous mitral valvuloplasty. *Circulation* 81:1190-1197, 1990.

38. Cormier B, Vahanian A, Iung B, et al: Influence of percutaneous mitral commissurotomy on left atrial spontaneous contrast of mitral stenosis. *Am J Cardiol* 71:842-847, 1993.

39. Hernandez R, Banuelos C, Alfonso F, et al: Long-term clinical and echocardiographic follow-up after percutaneous mitral valvuloplasty with the Inoue balloon. *Circulation* 99:1580-1586, 1999.

40. Chen CR, Cheng TO: Percutaneous balloon mitral valvuloplasty by the Inoue technique. A multicenter study of 4832 patients in China. *Am Heart J* 129:1197-1202, 1995.

41. Ben Farhat M, Betbout F, Gamra H, et al: Predictors of long-term event-free survival and of freedom from restenosis after percutaneous balloon mitral commissurotomy. *Am Heart J* 142:1072-1079, 2001.

42. Arora R, Kalra GS, Singh S, et al: Percutaneous transvenous mitral commissurotomy: Immediate and long-term follow-up results. *Catheter Cardiovasc Interv* 55:450-456, 2002.

43. Iung B, Nicoud-Houel A, Fondard O, et al: Temporal trends in percutaneous mitral commissurotomy over a 15-year period. *Eur Heart J* 25:702-708, 2004.

44. Complications and mortality of percutaneous balloon mitral commissurotomy. A report from the National Heart, Lung, and Blood Institute Balloon Valvuloplasty Registry. *Circulation* 85:2014-2024, 1992.

45. Tuzcu EM, Block PC, Palacios IF: Comparison of early versus late experience with percutaneous mitral balloon valvuloplasty. *J Am Coll Cardiol* 17:1121-1124, 1991.

46. Iung B, Cormier B, Ducimetière P, et al: Immediate results of percutaneous mitral commissurotomy: A predictive model on a series of 1514 patients. *Circulation* 94:2124-2130, 1996.

47. Meneveau N, Schiele F, Seronde MF, et al: Predictors of event-free survival after percutaneous mitral commissurotomy. *Heart* 80:359-364, 1998.

48. Stefanadis C, Stratos C, Lambrou S, et al: Retrograde nontransseptal balloon mitral valvuloplasty. Immediate results and intermediate long-term outcome in 441 cases—a multi-centre experience. *J Am Coll Cardiol* 32:1009-1016, 1998.

49. Palacios IF, Sanchez PL, Harrell LC, et al: Which patients benefit from percutaneous mitral balloon valvuloplasty? Prevalvuloplasty and postvalvuloplasty variables that predict long-term outcome. *Circulation* 105:1465-1471, 2002.

50. Neumayer U, Schmidt HK, Fassbender D, et al: Early (three-month) results of percutaneous mitral valvotomy with the Inoue Balloon in 1123 consecutive patients comparing various age groups. *Am J Cardiol* 90:190-193, 2002.

51. Fawzy ME, Hegazy H, Shoukri M, et al: Long-term clinical and echocardiographic results after successful mitral balloon valvotomy and predictors of long-term outcome. *Eur Heart J* 26:1647-1652, 2005.

52. Padial LR, Freitas N, Sagie A, et al: Echocardiography can predict which patients will develop severe mitral regurgitation after percutaneous mitral valvulotomy. *J Am Coll Cardiol* 27:1225-1231, 1996.

53. Iung B, Cormier B, Berdah P, et al: What are the mechanisms of severe mitral regurgitation following percutaneous mitral commissurotomy, and are they related to patient or procedure characteristics? *Circulation* 96 (supp):203(abstract), 1997.

54. Bonhoeffer P, Esteves C, Casal U, et al: Percutaneous mitral valve dilatation with the Multi-Track system. *Catheter Cardiovasc Interv* 48:178-183, 1999.

55. Eltchaninoff H, Koning R, Derumeaux G, Cribier A: Percutaneous mitral commissurotomy by metallic dilator. Multicenter experience with 500 patients. *Arch Mal Coeur Vaiss* 93:685-692, 2000.

56. Kang DH, Park SW, Song JK, et al: Long-term clinical and echocardiographic outcome of percutaneous mitral valvuloplasty. Randomized comparison of Inoue and double-balloon techniques. *J Am Coll Cardiol* 35:169-175, 2000.

57. Multicenter experience with balloon mitral commissurotomy. NHLBI Balloon Valvuloplasty Registry Report on immediate and 30-day follow-up results. The National Heart, Lung, and Blood Institute Balloon Valvuloplasty Registry Participants. *Circulation* 85:448-461, 1992.

58. Herrmann HC, Ramaswamy K, Isner JM, et al: Factors influencing immediate results, complications, and short-term follow-up status after Inoue balloon mitral valvotomy: A North American multicenter study. *Am Heart J* 124:160-166, 1992.

59. Wang A, Krasuski RA, Warner JJ, et al: Serial echocardiographic evaluation of restenosis after successful percutaneous mitral commissurotomy. *J Am Coll Cardiol* 39:328-334, 2002.

60. Heger JJ, Wann LS, Weyman AE, et al: Long-term changes in mitral valve area after successful mitral commissurotomy. *Circulation* 59:443-448, 1979.

61. Hickey MSJ, Blackstone EH, Kirklin JW, Dean LS: Outcome probabilities and life history after surgical mitral commissurotomy: Implications for balloon commissurotomy. *J Am Coll Cardiol* 17:29-42, 1991.

62. Iung B, Garbarz E, Michaud P, et al: Late results of percutaneous mitral commissurotomy in a series of 1024 patients. Analysis of late clinical deterioration: Frequency, anatomical findings, and predictive factors. *Circulation* 99:3272-3278, 1999.

63. Cohen DJ, Kuntz RE, Gordon SPF, et al: Predictors of long-term outcome after percutaneous balloon mitral valvuloplasty. *N Engl J Med* 327:1329-1335, 1992.

64. Dean LS, Mickel M, Bonan R, et al: Four-year follow-up of patients undergoing percutaneous balloon mitral commissurotomy. A report from the National Heart, Lung, and Blood Institute Balloon Valvuloplasty Registry. *J Am Coll Cardiol* 28:1452-1457, 1996.

65. Orrange SE, Kawanishi DT, Lopez BM, et al: Actuarial outcome after catheter balloon commissurotomy in patients with mitral stenosis. *Circulation* 95:382-389, 1997.

66. Davidson CJ, Bashore TM, Mickel M, et al: Balloon mitral commissurotomy after previous surgical commissurotomy. *Circulation* 86:91-99, 1992.

67. Lau KW, Ding ZP, Gao W, et al: Percutaneous balloon mitral valvuloplasty in patients with mitral restenosis after previous surgical commissurotomy. A matched comparative study. *Eur Heart J* 17:1367-1372, 1996.

68. Gupta S, Vora A, Lokhandwalla Y, et al: Percutaneous balloon mitral valvotomy in mitral restenosis. *Eur Heart J* 17:1560-1564, 1996.

69. Iung B, Garbarz E, Michaud P, et al: Percutaneous mitral commissurotomy for restenosis after surgical commissurotomy: Late efficacy and implications for patients selection. *J Am Coll Cardiol* 35:1295-1302, 2000.

70. Fawzy ME, Hassan W, Shoukri M, et al: Immediate and long-term results of mitral balloon valvotomy for restenosis following previous surgical or balloon mitral commissurotomy. *Am J Cardiol* 96:971-975, 2005.

71. Iung B, Garbarz E, Michaud P, et al: Immediate and mid-term results of repeat percutaneous mitral commissurotomy for restenosis following earlier percutaneous mitral commissurotomy. *Eur Heart J* 21:1683-1689, 2000.

72. Pathan AZ, Mahdi NA, Leon MN, et al: Is redo percutaneous mitral balloon valvuloplasty (PMV) indicated in patients with post-PMV mitral restenosis? *J Am Coll Cardiol* 34:49-54, 1999.

73. Turgeman Y, Atar S, Suleiman K, et al: Feasibility, safety and morphologic predictors of outcome of repeat percutaneous balloon mitral commissurotomy. *Am J Cardiol* 95:989-991, 2005.

74. Sutaria N, Elder AT, Shaw TR: Long term outcome of percutaneous mitral balloon valvotomy in patients aged 70 and over. *Heart* 83:433-438, 2000.

75. Iung B, Cormier B, Farah B, et al: Percutaneous mitral commissurotomy in the elderly. *Eur Heart J* 16:1092-1099, 1995.

76. Gamra H, Betbout F, Ben Hamda K, et al: Balloon mitral commissurotomy in juvenile rheumatic mitral stenosis: A ten-year clinical and echocardiographic actuarial results. *Eur Heart J* 24:1349-1356, 2003.

77. Fawzy ME, Stefadouros MA, Hegazy H, et al: Long term clinical and echocardiographic results of mitral balloon valvotomy in children and adolescents. *Heart* 91:743-748, 2005.

78. Kothari SS, Ramakrishnan S, Kumar CK, et al: Immediate-term results of percutaneous transvenous mitral commissurotomy in children less than 12 years of age. *Catheter Cardiovasc Interv* 64:487-490, 2005.

79. Iung B, Cormier B, Elias J, et al: Usefulness of percutaneous balloon commissurotomy for mitral stenosis during pregnancy. *Am J Cardiol* 73:398-400, 1994.

80. Ben Farhat M, Gamra H, Betbout F et al: Percutaneous balloon mitral commissurotomy during pregnancy. *Heart* 77:564-567, 1997.

81. De Souza JAM, Martinez EE, Ambrose JA, et al: Percutaneous balloon mitral valvuloplasty in comparison with open mitral valve commissurotomy during pregnancy. *J Am Coll Cardiol* 37:900-903, 2001.

82. Chen WJ, Chen MF, Liau CS, et al: Safety of percutaneous transvenous balloon mitral commissurotomy in patients with mitral stenosis and thrombus in the left atrial appendage. *Am J Cardiol* 70:117-119, 1992.

83. Silaruks S, Thinkhamrop B, Kiatchoosakun S, et al: Resolution of left atrial thrombus after 6 months of anticoagulation in candidates for percutaneous transvenous mitral commissurotomy. *Ann Intern Med* 140:101-105, 2004.

84. Vaturi M, Porter A, Adler Y, et al: The natural history of aortic valve disease after mitral valve surgery. *J Am Coll Cardiol* 33:2003-2008, 1999.

85. Song JM, Kang DH, Song JK, et al: Outcome of significant functional tricuspid regurgitation after percutaneous mitral valvuloplasty. *Am Heart J* 145:371-376, 2003.

86. Shaw TRD, Sutaria N, Prendergast B: Clinical and haemodynamic profiles of young, middle aged, and elderly patients with mitral stenosis undergoing mitral balloon valvotomy. *Heart* 89:1430-1436, 2003.

87. Reyes VP, Raju BS, Wynne J, et al: Percutaneous balloon valvuloplasty compared with open surgical commissurotomy for mitral stenosis. *N Engl J Med* 331:961-967, 1994.

88. Ben Farhat M, Ayari M, Maatouk F, et al: Percutaneous balloon versus surgical closed and open mitral commissurotomy. Seven-year follow-up results of a randomized trial. *Circulation* 97:245-250, 1998.

89. Cribier A, Eltchaninoff H, Koning R, et al: Percutaneous mechanical mitral commissurotomy with a newly designed metallic valvulotome: immediate results of the initial experience in 153 patients. *Circulation* 99:793-799, 1999.

90. Feldman T, Carroll JD, Isner JM, et al: Effect of valve deformity on results and mitral regurgitation after Inoue balloon commissurotomy. *Circulation* 85:180-187, 1992.

91. Hildick-Smith DJR, Taylor GJ, Shapiro LN: Inoue balloon mitral valvuloplasty: Long-term clinical and echocardiographic follow-up of a predominantly unfavorable population. *Eur Heart J* 21:1691-1698, 2000.

92. Tuzcu EM, Block PC, Griffin B, et al: Percutaneous mitral balloon valvotomy in patients with calcific mitral stenosis: immediate and long-term outcome. *J Am Coll Cardiol* 23:1604-1609, 1994.

93. Iung B, Garbarz E, Doutrelant L, et al: Late results of percutaneous mitral commissurotomy for calcific mitral stenosis. The advantage of an individual assessment for patient selection. *Am J Cardiol* 85:1308-1314, 2000.

94. Vahanian A, Palacios IF: Percutaneous approaches to valvular diseases. *Circulation* 109:1572-1579, 2004.

95. Gordon SP, Douglas PS, Come PC, Manning WJ: Two-dimensional and Doppler echocardiographic determinants of the natural history of mitral valve narrowing in patients with rheumatic mitral stenosis: implications for follow-up. *J Am Coll Cardiol* 19:968-973, 1992.

96. Stefanadis C, Dernellis J, Stratos C, et al: Effects of balloon mitral valvuloplasty on left atrial function in mitral stenosis as assessed by pressure-area relation. *J Am Coll Cardiol* 32:159-168, 1998.

97. Porte JM, Cormier B, Iung B, et al: Early assessment by transesophageal echocardiography of left atrial appendage function following percutaneous mitral commissurotomy. *Am J Cardiol* 77:72-76, 1996.

98. Peverill RE, Harper RW, Gelman J, et al: Determinants of increased regional left atrial coagulation activity in patients with mitral stenosis. *Circulation* 94:331-339, 1996.

99. Chiang CW, Lo SK, Ko YS, et al: Predictors of systemic embolism in patients with mitral stenosis. A prospective study. *Ann Intern Med* 128:885-889, 1998.

100. Leavitt JI, Coats MH, Falk RH: Effects of exercise on transmitral gradient and pulmonary artery pressure in patients with mitral stenosis or a prosthetic mitral valve: A Doppler echocardiographic study. *J Am Coll Cardiol* 17:1520-1526, 1991.

101. Voelker W, Berner A, Regele B, et al: Effect of exercise on valvular resistance in patients with mitral stenosis. *J Am Coll Cardiol* 22:777-782, 1993.

102. Tunick PA, Freedberg RS, Gargiulo A, Kronzon I: Exercise Doppler echocardiography as an aid to clinical decision making in mitral valve disease. *J Am Soc Echocardiogr* 5:225-230, 1992.

103. Schwammenthal E, Vered Z, Agranat O, et al: Impact of atrioventricular compliance on pulmonary artery pressure in mitral stenosis. A exercise echocardiographic study. *Circulation* 102:2378-2384, 2001.

104. Dahan M, Paillole C, Martin D, Gourgon R: Determinants of stroke volume response to exercise in patients with mitral stenosis: A Doppler echocardiographic study. *J Am Coll Cardiol* 21:384-389, 1993.

105. Brochet E, Fondard O, Iung B, et al: Patterns of haemodynamic responses during exercise are related to exercise tolerance in patients with severe mitral stenosis with few or no symptoms. *Circulation* 108 (suppl III):654 (abstract), 2004.

106. Hecker SL, Zabalgoitia M, Ashline P, et al: Comparison of exercise and dobutmaine stress echocardiography in assessing mitral stenosis. *Am J Cardiol* 80:1374-1377, 1997.

107. Reis G, Motta MS, Barbosa MM, et al: Dobutamine stress echocardiography for noninvasive assessment and risk stratification of patients with rheumatic mitral stenosis. *J Am Coll Cardiol* 43:393-401, 2004.

108. Okay T, Deligonul U, Sancaktar O, Kozan O: Contribution of mitral valve reserve capacity to sustained symptomatic improvement after balloon valvulotomy in mitral stenosis: Implications for restenosis. *J Am Coll Cardiol* 22:1691-1696, 1993.

109. Li M, Dery JP, Dumesnil JG, et al: Usefulness of measuring net atrioventricular compliance by Doppler echocardiography in patients with mitral stenosis. *Am J Cardiol* 96:432-435, 2005.

110. Zamorano J, Cordeiro P, Sugeng L, et al: Real-time three-dimensional echocardiography for rheumatic mitral valve stenosis evaluation. An accurate and novel approach. *J Am Coll Cardiol* 43:2091-2096, 2004.

111. Sebag IA, Morgan JG, Handschumacher MD, et al: Usefulness of three-dimensionally guided assessment of mitral stenosis. *Am J Cardiol* 96:1151-1156, 2005.

112. Otto CM, Davis KB, Holmes DR Jr, et al: Methodologic issues in clinical evaluation of stenosis severity in adults undergoing aortic or mitral balloon valvuloplasty. The NHLBI balloon valvuloplasty registry. *Am J Cardiol* 69:1607-1616, 1992.

113. Applebaum RM, Kasliwal RR, Kanojia A, et al: Utility of three-dimensional echocardiography during balloon mitral valvuloplaty. *J Am Coll Cardiol* 32:1405-1409, 1998.

114. Krishnamoorty KM, Dash PK, Radhakrishnan S, Shrivastava S: Response of different grades of pulmonary artery hypertension to balloon mitral valvuloplasty. *Am J Cardiol* 90:1170-1173, 2002.

115. Dev V, Shrivastava S: Time course of changes in pulmonary vascular resistance on mechanism of regression of pulmonary artery hypertension after balloon mitral valvuloplasty. *Am J Cardiol* 67:439-442, 1991.

116. Segal J, Lerner DJ, Miller DC, et al: When should Doppler-determined valve area be better than the Gorlin formula? Variation in hydraulic constants in low flow states. *J Am Coll Cardiol* 9:1294-1305, 1987.

117. Petrossian GA, Tuzcu EM, Ziskind AA, et al: Atrial septal occlusion improves the accuracy of mitral valve area determination following percutaneous mitral balloon valvotomy. *Cathet Cardiovasc Diagn* 22:21-24, 1991.

118. Lin SJ, Brown PA, Watkins MP, et al: Quantification of stenotic mitral valve area with magnetic resonance imaging and comparison with Doppler ultrasound. *J Am Coll Cardiol* 44:133-137, 2004.

119. Cafri C, de la Guardia B, Barasch E, et al: Transseptal puncture guided by intracardiac echocardiography during percutaneous transvenous mitral commissurotomy in patients with distorted anatomy of the fossa ovalis. *Catheter Cardiovasc Interv* 50:463-467, 2000.

120. Green NE, Hansgren AR, Carroll JD: Initial clinical experience with intracardiac echocardiography in guiding balloon mitral valvuloplasty: technique, safety, utility, and limitations. *Catheter Cardiovasc Interv* 63:385-394, 2004.

Chapter 22

Clinical Decision Making in Patients with Endocarditis: The Role of Echocardiography

CHRISTOPHER H. CABELL, MD, MHS

Background

Since the advent of two-dimensional (2D) transthoracic echocardiography (TTE) in the 1970s and high frequency transesophageal echocardiography (TEE) imaging in the 1980s, echocardiography has become a standard diagnostic tool in patients with suspected infective endocarditis (IE). The first report of the use of echocardiography to detect endocarditis was made by Dillon and colleagues in the 1970s.[1] In the late 1980s,

---

This work was supported in part by National Institute of Health grant HL70861 (CHC).

as the technology of TEE imaging became more widely available, Daniel and colleagues described the first experience of the improved diagnostic yield for endocarditis over standard chest wall imaging.[2] Based on these and other studies, it is now well established that echocardiography is the imaging technology of choice for the diagnosis of IE and that echocardiography can detect cardiac involvement in a significant proportion of patients with clinically occult IE.[3] Because IE is a lethal infection that can be difficult to diagnose, clinicians who care for patients at risk for IE often have a low threshold for employing echocardiography. In fact, because of the role that echocardiography plays in both the diagnosis and in understanding the prognosis of patients with IE, it has been suggested that echocardiography is mandatory in all patients when there is suspicion for IE.[4]

This chapter discusses the imaging considerations in patients with suspected and documented IE, implications on the use of echocardiography, the role of echocardiography in understanding prognosis, how echocardiography can be used to assist in therapeutic decision making, and musings on the future of imaging for diseases, such as endocarditis.

Basic Principles and Echocardiographic Approach

Historically, IE has been defined as an infection of the endothelial surfaces within the cardiac chambers. In recent years this definition has been expanded to include an infection on any structure within the heart, including normal endothelial surfaces (e.g., myocardium and valvular structures), prosthetic heart valves (e.g., mechanical, bioprosthetic, homografts, and autografts), and implanted devices (e.g., pacemakers, implantable cardioverter defibrillators, and ventricular assist devices). As the age of the population in industrialized countries continues to increase, it is likely that the latter categories of prosthetic valves and devices will continue to grow substantially.[5,6]

To understand the disease process of IE and how echocardiography has become central to making this diagnosis, it is useful to revisit the way in which the diagnosis has been made historically. In 1885, Sir William Osler, as one of the newest members of the Royal College of Physicians, was asked to give the Gulstonian Lectures. In these three lectures, Osler provided on overview of IE that summarized the current knowledge of the disease at the time.[7-9] In that era, even before the advent of microbiologic techniques that allowed for routine use of blood cultures, it is not surprising that the actual diagnosis of endocarditis was all too often made at the time of postmortem examination. In fact, Osler is quoted as saying "Few diseases present greater difficulties in the way of diagnosis than malignant endocarditis, difficulties which in many cases are practically insurmountable. It is no disparagement to the many skilled physicians who have put their cases upon record to say that, in fully one-half the diagnosis was made postmortem."[9] Despite this difficulty, Osler advocated that the diagnosis of IE could be made based on clinical presentation in certain cases of endocarditis. For instance, he stated that "the existence of fever of an irregular type, and the occurrence of embolism, generally suffice to make the diagnosis clear," a situation that is still true today.

The diagnosis of IE has always hinged on clinical suspicion derived from association with appropriate signs and symptoms and, most importantly, the demonstration of continuous bacteremia. Surprisingly, it was not until the late 1970s that a strict case definition was developed. Pelletier and Petersdorf developed this definition based on a longitudinal experience of caring for patients with IE in Seattle.[10] Although this case definition was highly specific for the diagnosis of IE, it lacked sufficient sensitivity.

The next major diagnostic advance came in 1981 when von Reyn and colleagues[1] published an analysis that provided four diagnostic categories in cases of suspected IE (rejected, possible, probable, and definite).[11] These criteria, based on broader clinical findings, improved both the sensitivity and the specificity of the previous case definition but unfortunately did not incorporate imaging information from the burgeoning field of echocardiography.

In 1994, IE diagnostic criteria were refined further by Durack and colleagues from Duke University Medical Center.[12] These criteria, which have come to be known as the Duke Criteria, incorporated echocardiographic evidence of IE for the first time. These criteria had improved test performance characteristics when compared to previous criteria (Table 22–1) and have been validated subsequently by others.[13-15] Recently, proposed modifi-

TABLE 22–1. Comparison of Diagnostic Criteria in 69 Cases of Pathologically Proven Infective Endocarditis

		Probable	Possible	Rejected	Total (%)
Duke criteria	Definite	32	19	4	55 (80%)
	Possible	3	3	8	14 (20%)
	Reject	0	0	0	0 (0%)
	Total (%)	35 (51%)	22 (32%)	12 (17%)	69 (100%)

From Durack DT, Lukes AS, Bright DK: *Am J Med* 96:200-209, 1994.

TABLE 22-2. The Modified Duke Criteria for Diagnosis of Infective Endocarditis

Major Criteria

a. Microbiologic
  Typical microorganisms isolated from two separate blood cultures, microorganism isolated from persistently positive blood cultures, or single positive blood culture for *Coxiella burnetii* (or phase I IgG antibody titer to *C. burnetii* >1:800)
b. Evidence of endocardial involvement
  New valvular regurgitation or positive echocardiogram (intracardiac mass, periannular abscess, or new dehiscence of prosthetic valve)

Minor Criteria

a. Predisposition to infective endocarditis including:
  Previous infective endocarditis
  Injection drug use
  Prosthetic heart valve
  Mitral valve prolapse
  Cyanotic congenital heart disease
  Other cardiac lesions creating turbulent flow within the intracardiac chambers
b. Fever
c. Vascular phenomena (e.g., embolic event)
d. Immunologic phenomena (e.g., presence of serologic markers, glomerulonephritis, Osler's nodes, or Roth spots)
e. Microbiologic findings not meeting major criteria

Define endocarditis: 2 major criteria *or* 1 major and 3 minor criteria *or* 5 minor criteria.
Possible endocarditis: 1 major plus 1 minor *or* 3 minor criteria.
Adapted from Li JS, Sexton DJ, Mick N, et al: *Clin Infect Dis* 30:633-638, 2000.

TABLE 22-3. Echocardiographic Characteristics of Infective Endocarditis

Lesion	Description
Vegetation	Irregularly shaped, discrete echogenic mass Adherent to, yet distinct from, cardiac surface Oscillation of mass supportive, not mandatory
Abscess	Thickened area or mass within the myocardium or annular region Appearance is non-homogeneous with both echogenic and echolucent characteristics Evidence of flow within area is supportive, not mandatory
Aneurysm	Echolucent space bounded by thin tissue
Fistulae	Connection between two distinct cardiac blood spaces through nonanatomical channel
Leaflet perforation	Defect in body of myocardial valve leaflet with evidence of flow through defect
Valvular dehiscence	Rocking motion of prosthetic valve with excursion >15 degrees in at least one direction

Adapted from Sachdev M, Peterson GE, Jollis JG: *Dis Clin North Am* 16:319-337, 2002.

cations have been published (Table 22-2),[16] but the test performance characteristics of the modified criteria have yet to be fully evaluated by other investigators.

Technical Details, Quantitation, and Data Analysis

Based on the defined role of imaging in the diagnosis of IE, echocardiography has become the central tenant in evaluating patients that have a clinical presentation that raises the concern for IE. There are several findings on echocardiography that provide evidence of IE and include vegetations; evidence of periannular tissue destruction (abscess); aneurysm; fistula; leaflet perforation; and valvular dehiscence (Table 22-3).

Vegetations

Pathologically, a vegetation is a collection of microorganisms embedded in a meshwork of fibrin and other inflammatory cellular material adherent to an endothelial surface within the heart. White blood cells are uncommon, the absence of which has not fully been explained by experimental work.[17] In part, this may be a result of the dense nature of the vegetation tissue, which may restrict the migration of white blood cells to the infected area. In addition, the bacteria are frequently embedded in a nongrowing state deep in the vegetation, which may limit the typical host infection response.

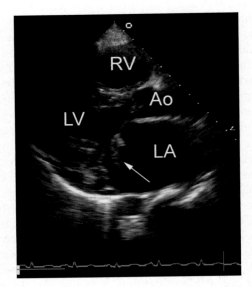

Figure 22-1. Example of a typical vegetation by transthoracic imaging. The arrow points to the vegetation on the anterior leaflet of the mitral valve. Ao, aorta; LA, left atrium; LV, left ventricle; RV, right ventricle.

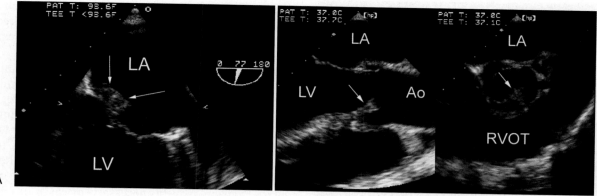

Figure 22–2. *Typical locations of mitral valve and aortic valve vegetations.* A, *Typical vegetation on the mitral valve by TEE. The* arrows *point to the vegetation on the anterior leaflet of the mitral valve.* B, *Typical vegetation on the aortic valve by TEE. In the* left panel, *the TEE long-axis view is shown, whereas in the* right panel, *the short-axis view is shown. The* arrows *point to the vegetation that is located on the right coronary cusp of the aortic valve. Ao, aorta; LA, left atrium; LV, left ventricle; RVOT, right ventricular outflow tract; TEE, transesophageal echocardiography.*

With two-dimensional echocardiographic imaging, the cardiac structures are viewed throughout the cardiac cycle. Vegetations are defined as an irregularly shaped, discrete echogenic masses, which are often oscillating, and located at sites where vegetations typically occur, such as on valves, chordae, or in the path of turbulent jets of blood passing through incompetent valves or septal defects.[1,12] These masses must be adherent to, yet distinct from the endothelial cardiac surface. Mass oscillation, high frequency movement independent from that of intrinsic structures, is supportive but not mandatory for the echocardiographic diagnosis of a vegetation.

Vegetations have the consistency of mid-myocardium (Fig. 22–1) but may also have areas of both echo-lucency and echo-density. Vegetations typically occur on the low pressure side of a high velocity turbulent jet; therefore, with underlying regurgitant valvular disease, vegetations are most often visualized on the atrial aspect of the mitral and tricuspid valves or on the ventricular aspect of the aortic and pulmonic valves (Fig. 22–2).

Although cardiac valves are the most common sites of infection, vegetations may occur in other intracardiac locations. These include nonvalvular surfaces, such as atrial or ventricular surfaces, and on intracardiac devices, such as pacemakers or defibrillators. When a vegetation occurs on a nonvalvular structure, it generally appears at a site of endothelial disruption. If this occurs on a myocardial wall, it is common for this to be at a site where a high velocity jet of blood flow has damaged the endothelial integrity such as an uncorrected restrictive ventricular septal defect or eccentric mitral valve regurgitation jet (Fig. 22–3). In addition to a myocardial wall attachment for a vegetation, other nonvalvular structures include intracardiac devices, such as pacemakers or implantable defibrilla-

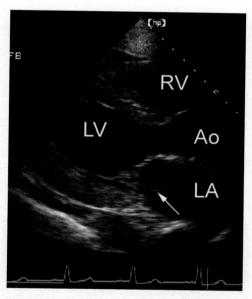

Figure 22–3. *This vegetation* (arrow) *is located on the myocardial wall on the posterior aspect of the left atrium. Ao, aorta; LA, left atrium; LV, left ventricle; RV, right ventricle.*

tors (Fig. 22–4). These devices often have nonuniform endothelialization that allows for the attachment once bacteria are circulating in the bloodstream.

Not all intracardiac mass lesions represent vegetations from IE. For instance, inflammatory disorders, such as systemic lupus erythematosus, can have associated valvular mass lesions that can be difficult to distinguish from vegetations resulting from IE (Fig. 22–5). Termed Libman-Sacks endocarditis,[18] these inflammatory mass lesions are usually less than 1 cm in diameter, vary in shape, have irregular borders, and have heterogeneous echo-densities. These lesions are typically broad based without independent motion or oscillation characteristics, unlike vegetations resulting

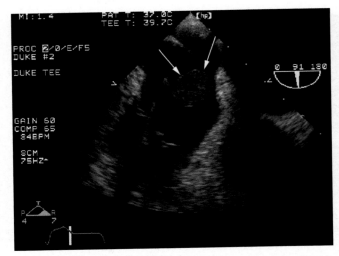

Figure 22-4. *Transesophageal image of a large vegetation (arrows) on a pacemaker wire seen in a TEE view of the right heart. The pacemaker wire can be seen as it traverses the right atrium, through the tricuspid valve, into the right ventricle.*

from IE. In addition, Libman-Sacks lesions are frequently located on the basilar portion of the valve leaflets and are not necessarily located on low velocity surfaces.

In addition to Libman-Sacks inflammatory masses, other mass lesions can occur on the valvular structures. For instance, sterile vegetations (termed murantic endocarditis) may also occur in patients with advanced malignancies (e.g., renal cell carcinoma or melanoma). In addition, myxomatous valves, ruptured chordae unrelated to infection, cardiac tumors, and

degenerative valvular changes may all involve echocardiographic findings that can be misleading. Moreover, normal variants, such as prominent Lambl's excrescences, may mimic IE findings (Fig. 22-6).

Lambl's excrescences were first described in the 1850s as small filiform processes on the aortic valve.[19] In the 1940s, Margerey studied 250 mitral valves and postulated that the mechanism of formation is intimal damage resulting from mechanical trauma at the leaflet coaptation.[20] In general, these lesions appear to be wear-and-tear lesions that originate in the endothelium of the contact margins of a valve, commonly the aortic valve. Excision may be necessary in cases of cryptogenic stroke. Although most Lambl's excrescences can be distinguished from vegetations by their small size and filamentous appearance, larger lesions may be more difficult to discern from vegetations resulting from IE.

Importantly, there are no echocardiographic features of noninfective lesions that can absolutely differentiate them from vegetations resulting from IE. Therefore, it is always paramount to correlate the echocardiographic findings to the clinical presentation and findings to develop a diagnostic and care plan that is optimized for the individual patient.

Periannular Extension of Infection

Periannular extension of infection, or abscess formation, is one of the most serious complications of IE. When this occurs, it marks an indication for surgical therapy. On echocardiography, a myocardial abscess

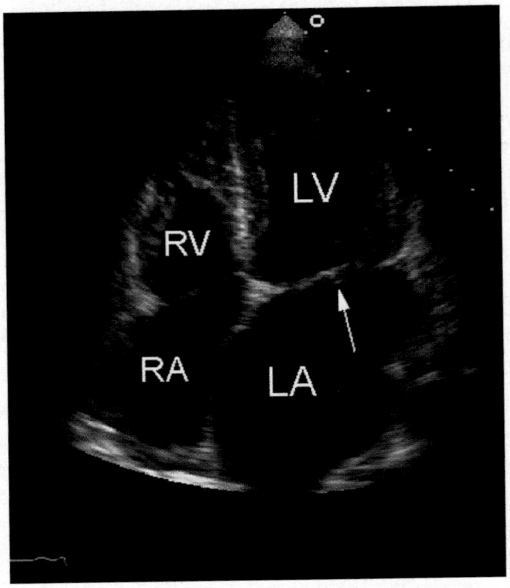

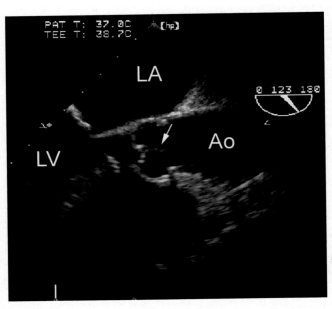

Figure 22-5. *Libman-Sacks endocarditis on the mitral valve seen in a transthoracic apical four-chamber view. The arrow points to the vegetation on the anterior leaflet of the mitral valve. Ao, aorta; LA, left atrium; LV, left ventricle; RV, right ventricle.*

Figure 22-6. *This transesophageal long axis view shows a long filamentous mobile mass on the aortic valve consistent with a Lambl's excrescence (arrow). Ao, aorta; LA, left atrium; LV, left ventricle.*

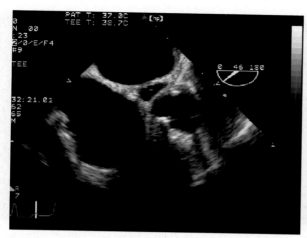

Figure 22–7. *Myocardial abscess with evidence of an echo-cardigraphic free space in a transesophageal short-axis view just posterior to the aortic valve annulus, consistent with myocardial abscess formation.*

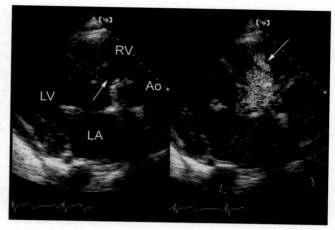

Figure 22–8. *Fistula tract formation due to infective endocarditis in a transthoracic parasternal long-axis view. In the* left panel, *there is evidence of a myocardial abscess between the left ventricular outflow tract and the right ventricle (arrow). In the* right panel, *Doppler examination shows clear evidence of flow communication between cardiac chambers (arrow), in this case between the left ventricular outflow tract and the right ventricle. Ao, aorta; LA, left atrium; LV, left ventricle; RV, right ventricle.*

can be defined as a thickened area or mass in the myocardium or annular region with an appearance that is generally non-homogeneous. If there is evidence of flow within the area, then this is considered to be supportive but not mandatory for the diagnosis of myocardial abscess. An echo-free space suggests that complete liquefaction of the myocardium has occurred (Fig. 22–7).

The most important feature of abscess formation is the substantial morbidity and mortality associated with this complication. For instance, the abscess can extend and rupture creating a fistulous tract between two separate blood pools. In addition, if the abscess extends into the septum the conduction system can be affected leading to heart block. In the literature, abscess formation tends to be more commonly associated with aortic valve IE, particularly those with aortic prosthetic valve IE.[21,22] Moreover, the mortality rate is often high despite surgical intervention.[21] Although TTE imaging can establish the diagnosis of abscess formation, overall the resolution associated with typical TTE imaging in adults is insufficient for the full characterization of most intracardiac abscess cavities.

Fistula Formation

Spread of infection from valvular structures to the surrounding perivalvular tissue results in periannular complications that may place the patient at increased risk of adverse outcomes including heart failure (HF) and death. This is particularly true with aortic valve IE in which aortic abscesses and mycotic pseudoaneurysms involving the sinuses of Valsalva may rupture internally. This leads to the development of aorto-cavitary or aorto-pericardial fistulas. Aorto-cavitary communications create intracardiac shunts, which may result in further clinical deterioration and hemodynamic instability (Fig. 22–8).

Fistula formation resulting from IE is uncommon; therefore there are few published series that allow for a broad understanding of this disease process. Recently, a multicenter study from Spain has provided new information related to this complication. In this case-series, the incidence of fistula formation in patients with IE was 1.6% or 76 fistulas identified in 4681 episodes of IE.[21] The incidence was higher in selected populations; for instance in patients with prosthetic valve IE, the incidence of fistula formation was 3.5%. Not surprisingly, in this series *Staphylococcus aureus* was the most commonly associated microorganism (46%). In addition, despite a high rate of surgery in this population (87%), short-term mortality remained high (41%).

There are a few basic tenants that are critical for the diagnosis and management of IE associated fistula tracts. The first is that suspicion is paramount, and if clinical suspicion warrants, then TEE imaging is justified early in the clinical course. Second, evidence of fistula tract formation represents an indication for urgent surgery before the infection can cause further tissue destruction and possible hemodynamic compromise. Finally, it is critical for the echocardiographer to provide as much information to the surgical team as possible to help in planning the appropriate surgical approach, particularly to the origin and destination of the fistula tract.

Perforation

Perforation of a valvular leaflet is another lesion that may develop if the infective process is allowed to continue unabated (Fig. 22–9). There is little information

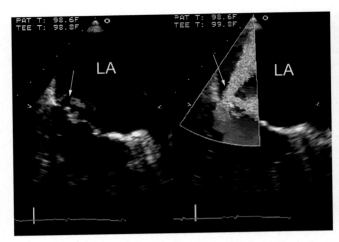

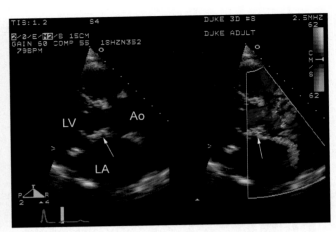

Figure 22–9. Perforation of the mitral valve seen in a transesophageal two-chamber view. The vegetation on the mitral valve is associated with a mitral valve perforation. In the left panel, there is evidence of the perforation on the standard two-dimensionl image (arrow), but this is seen definitively under Doppler evaluation as seen in the right panel (arrow). LA, left atrium.

Figure 22–10. Dehiscence of a prosthetic mitral valve seen in a transthoracic long axis view. The mechanical prosthetic mitral valve is seen with evidence of a perivalvular space (left panel arrow) on standard imaging that is confirmed to allow significant perivalvular regurgitation on Doppler examination (right panel arrow). In addition, on real-time imaging, there was rocking of the prosthetic valve greater than 15 degrees, consistent with prosthetic valvular dehiscence. Ao, aorta; LA, left atrium; LV, left ventricle.

available about the timing of perforation formation, but it is generally accepted that this is either associated with a virulent microorganism, such as *S. aureus,* or occurs when the infection process continues for a substantial amount of time without detection. Once a perforation forms, a significant amount of valvular regurgitation may develop. This mechanical complication may then need surgical repair depending on the hemodynamic status of the patient and the amount of regurgitation present.

New Valvular Regurgitation

The endocarditis process can also involve the mechanical function of the valve to cause significant valvular regurgitation. This can occur with or without the presence of a perforated valve leaflet. This mechanical disruption can occur at the valve leaflets secondary to a physical impairment of proper leaflet coaptation or to the vegetative process. In addition, the mechanical disruption can involve the rupture of the chordae tendineae and possibly a flail leaflet. In this instance, significant valvular regurgitation can develop, leading to a need for urgent surgical repair.

Dehiscence of Prosthetic Valve

Dehiscence of a prosthetic valve resulting from IE is a serious complication in patients with prosthetic valves. Dehiscence is generally defined as a rocking motion of the prosthetic valve greater than 15 degrees in any one plane (Fig. 22–10). This complication may lead to a gross separation of the prosthetic annulus from the native tissue in the most serious cases. Invariably, prosthetic valve dehiscence is associated with significant

perivalvular regurgitation and may be associated with hemodynamic compromise. Dehiscence represents a relative urgent indication for surgical therapy.

Special Considerations in Patients with Infective Endocarditis

Prosthetic Valve Infective Endocarditis

Prosthetic valve endocarditis (PVE) is a special case when it comes to choosing an imaging modality. Although several aspects in which TEE imaging may be superior to standard TTE imaging have been previously mentioned, these discussions have presented data on large groups of patients with IE. In specific patient populations, such as those with PVE, characteristics and limitations of the imaging technique are critical. For instance, in aortic valve PVE, it is difficult to assess the entire annular circumference with either TTE or TEE alone. In addition, in mitral valve PVE, it is likewise difficult to evaluate both the atrial and ventricular aspects of the annulus with a single technique. Importantly, when there is a prosthesis in both the aortic and mitral positions, there is no single echocardiographic technique that allows for adequate evaluation.

Overall, in patients with PVE, it may be beneficial to perform both TTE and TEE studies. In this way, a full evaluation of the infected area can be performed including: the annulus of the valve infected; the function of the valve; abscess formation; presence of a fistula tract; assessment for dehiscence; assessment for perivalvular regurgitation; and full assessment of overall regurgitation.

Right-Sided Infective Endocarditis

Patients with right-sided IE may also represent a special population when it comes to the selection of imaging modalities. For instance, although the tricuspid valve is usually seen well in the standard TTE views, patients with tricuspid valve IE are more likely to be infected with organisms, such as *S. aureus*. In patients with *S. aureus* IE, TEE has superior test characteristics.[23] In addition, the pulmonic valve may not be adequately seen from the standard TTE views. These issues must be taken into context with clinical outcomes data that show that injection drug uses with isolated right-sided IE may be adequately treated with 2 weeks of appropriate antibiotic therapy. Therefore, in this specific clinical scenario, the small risk of TEE may be outweighed by the small likelihood of diagnostic information that will change therapeutic management. In these patients, collaboration between the care team and the echocardiography laboratory is a necessity to develop the appropriate imaging strategy.

Intracardiac Device-Related Infections

Intracardiac devices (e.g., pacemaker and implantable cardioverter defibrillators) have become an integral part of modern cardiovascular medicine. Recently, a steady stream of randomized trials has provided definitive evidence that these devices improve symptoms, rehospitalization, or outcomes in selected patient populations. The growing number of evidence-based indications for cardiac devices coupled with an aging population in the Western world ensures a continued increase in the implantation of cardiac devices in the foreseeable future. Recent evidence from a study of the U.S. Medicare population has shown that the device implantation rate had a relative increase of 42% in the 1990s, but that there was a 124% relative increase in patients with documented device infections during the same time period.[5]

There are several important imaging considerations in patients with suspected intracardiac device infections. For instance, it is imperative to image the device throughout its course in the cardiac chambers. Special attention should be made at the point where the device crosses a valve, such as the tricuspid valve, in that there is likely high velocity regurgitation at this point, establishing the appropriate milieu for infection. In addition, devices that tract from the superior vena cava (SVC) should be imaged as far as possible into the superior vena cava as a result of the fact that device-related infections in this area have been well documented. The diagnosis of an intracardiac device infection has important implications for clinical management. Specifically, it is recommend that systematic extraction of cardiac devices be performed in all patients with documented cardiac device infections.[24,25] This should be followed by a course of intravenous (IV) antibiotics and device implantation at another site during a separate surgical procedure.

Consideration for Multiple Echocardiographic Evaluations

Suspicion of IE and/or complications related to IE are critical in the overall use of echocardiography in the diagnosis and treatment of IE (Table 22–4). If the initial TTE images are negative in a patient in whom there is high suspicion for IE, then TEE imaging should be performed as soon as possible. Likewise, TEE should follow rapidly in patients with a positive TTE for vegetations in which there is significant clinical concern for intracardiac complications, such as abscess formation. In addition, repeat echocardiography is often advisable in cases of initial negative echocardiograms but with ongoing clinical suspicion. For instance, small vegetations may reach detectable size and/or perivalvular extension may become evident on later examinations.

Several studies have shown that multiple echocardiographic evaluations may be useful in determining the prognosis of patients with IE. For instance, Rohmann and colleagues performed serial TEE studies in 83 patients.[26] They found that if a vegetation stayed static or enlarged, then prognosis was much worse than if the vegetation shrank with therapy.

Serial examinations can be taken to extreme. For instance, Vieira and colleagues published data evaluating serial echocardiographic examinations.[27] Over a 3-year period, they evaluated 262 patients with suspected IE referred for echocardiography. They found that repeat echocardiography was frequent; TTEs were repeated at least once in 192 (72.2%) patients, whereas TEEs were repeated in 49 (18.4%) of patients. The average number of TTE examinations was 2.4, but 6 patients had at least 6 TTEs. In a similar fashion, the mean number of TEE examinations was 1.7, although 4 patients had at least 4 TEEs and 1 patient had 5 TEEs. The authors found that although repeated echocardiograms were occasionally helpful, no additional diagnostic information was provided after the second or third echocardiogram (TTE or TEE).

Clinical Utility and Outcome Data

Use of Echocardiography in Patients Suspected of Having Infective Endocarditis

It is now well established that echocardiography is the imaging technology of choice for the diagnosis of IE and that echocardiography can detect cardiac involvement in a significant proportion of patients with clinically occult IE.[3,4] Because IE is a lethal infection that can be difficult to diagnose clinically, clinicians who

TABLE 22–4. Use of Echocardiography during the Diagnosis and Treatment of Endocarditis

Early
Echocardiography as soon as possible (<12 hours after initial evaluation)
TEE preferred; obtain TTE views of any abnormal findings for later comparison
TTE if TEE is not immediately available
TTE may be sufficient in small children

Repeat Echocardiography
TEE after positive TTE as soon as possible in patients at high risk for complications
TEE 7-10 days after initial TEE if suspicion exists without diagnosis of infective endocarditis or with worrisome clinical course during early treatment of infective endocarditis

Intraoperative
Prepump
Identification of vegetations, mechanism of regurgitation, abscesses, fistulas, and pseudoaneurysms
Postpump
Confirmation of successful repair of abnormal findings
Assessment of residual valve dysfunction
Elevated afterload if necessary to avoid underestimating valve insufficiency or presence of residual abnormal flow

Completion of Therapy
Establish new baseline for valve function and morphology and ventricular size and function
TTE usually adequate; TEE or review of intraoperative TEE may be needed for complex anatomy to establish new baseline

TEE, transesophageal echocardiography; TTE, transthoracic echocardiogphy.
Used with permission from Baddour LM, Wilson WR, Bayer A, et al: *Circulation* 111:3167-3184, 2005.

care for patients at risk for IE often have a low threshold for employing echocardiography. In addition, published diagnosis and treatment guidelines advocate the early use of echocardiography to establish the diagnosis of IE. This clinical practice has several implications. Although echocardiography can often provide a rapid diagnosis, its optimal use is predicated on the appropriate pretest probability of disease.[28] Echocardiography is increasingly overused in clinical scenarios with a low (<2% to 3%) pretest probability of disease; its diagnostic utility diminishes in these cases.[29]

To use a diagnostic tool such as echocardiography in an effective manner, it is important to simultaneously include several clinical features including: an appropriate pretest probability of disease (e.g., >2% to 3%); an understanding of the diagnostic technology; and a clinical situation in which the diagnostic test results will likely change the management of the patient. Although there is little empiric data to quantitate the pretest probability of disease, there is a general acceptance that certain clinical characteristics increase the pretest probability of IE significantly (Table 22–5). When focusing on the diagnostic technology, the basic

characteristics of echocardiography must be kept in mind. For instance, in approximately 15% of patients, the sound transmission from the chest wall may be attenuated by a variety of factors (e.g., obesity, lung hyperinflation) such that there is insufficient resolution to make a firm diagnosis. In these situations, TEE may be indicated as a primary imaging modality.

Overuse of Echocardiography

Recent literature has provided evidence that imaging technologies such as echocardiography can be overused in certain clinical scenarios, such as the evaluation of suspected endocarditis. For instance, Kuruppu and colleagues have shown that 53% of echocardiograms could be avoided without loss of diagnostic accuracy by using a simple algorithm in patients with a low pretest probability of disease.[30]

Notably, Greaves and colleagues have shown that the collective absence of five simple clinical criteria indicated a zero probability of a TTE showing evidence of endocarditis.[29] These clinical criteria included: vasculitic/embolic phenomena; presence of central venous access; recent history of injection drug use; presence of prosthetic valve; and positive blood cultures. Collectively, these studies have shown that in patients with very low pretest probability of disease, echocardiography can be used sparingly, and in specific, clinical cases may be avoided without the loss of diagnostic accuracy.

Transthoracic Echocardiography versus Transesophageal Echocardiography

Both TTE and TEE have an important role in the diagnosis and management of patients with suspected IE. It is widely accepted that echocardiography should be performed in all cases of suspected IE (American Heart Association [AHA] Class I recommendation; Level of Evidence A).[4] If the clinical suspicion is relatively low or imaging is likely to be of high quality, then TTE may be sufficient. When imaging is suboptimal or when TTE does not provide definitive evidence, then TEE should

TABLE 22–5. Characteristics Suggestive of Endocarditis

Fever
Organisms grown on blood culture, particularly without a known source of infection
Recent history of injection drug use
Congenital cardiac structural abnormality (e.g., mitral valve prolapse)
Known rheumatic heart disease
Presence of prosthetic valve or intracardiac device
Vasculitic/embolic phenomena

Modified from Greaves K, Patel A, Celermajer D: *Heart* 89:273-275, 2003.

be considered. An approach to the use of echocardiography has been developed by the American Heart Association for patients with suspected IE[31] (Fig. 22–11).

In general, TTE is widely available and can provide rapid important diagnostic information. As discussed previously, there are clinical situations in which TTE imaging alone does not provide adequate resolution to make a firm diagnosis. These situations include chronic obstructive pulmonary disease (COPD), previous thoracic surgery, and morbid obesity. In addition, as previously noted, the presence of prosthetic heart valves creates specific imaging challenges that may necessitate the use of TEE or a combination of TTE and TEE. TEE imaging is typically performed at a higher frequency (6 to 7 MHz) as compared to TTE (2 to 4 MHz). This higher frequency allows for greater spatial resolution of nearby structures including the cardiac valves. Under ideal conditions, TTE can reliably identify structures as small as 5 mm in diameter, whereas TEE can depict structures as small as 1 mm.

Cost-Effectiveness of Diagnostic Imaging Strategies

While certain clinical scenarios may dictate the type and order of diagnostic strategies, there are recent data that help guide this decision making. For example, there is now evidence for both the evaluation of the general patient suspected of having IE and for the patient with catheter associated *S. aureus* bacteremia.

In the general patient in whom there is a suspicion of IE, current guidelines highlight the use of TTE and/ or TEE imaging depending on the clinical scenario. Recently, studies have shown that an initial strategy of TEE imaging is the most cost-effective in the majority of clinical situations. For instance, Heidenreich and colleagues have shown that in suspected endocarditis, a diagnostic strategy that focuses on TEE as the initial imaging modality is more cost-effective than a staged procedure with TTE and is a dominant strategy over empiric antibiotic therapy alone.[28] In this study, trans-

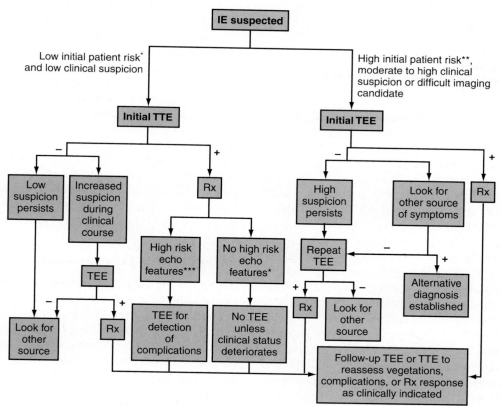

Figure 22–11. *An approach to the diagnostic use of echocardiography.*
*For example, a patient with fever and a previously known heart murmur, heart failure, or other stigmata of infective endocarditis.
**High initial patient risks include prosthetic heart valves, many congenital heart diseases, previous endocarditis, new murmur, heart failure, or other stigmata of endocarditis. Rx indicates antibiotic treatment for endocarditis.
***High-risk echocardiographic features include large and/or mobile vegetations, valvular insufficiency, suggestion of perivalvular extension or secondary ventricular dysfunction.
+, positive for endocarditis; −, no evidence of endocarditis; echo, echocardiographic; IE, infective endocarditis; TEE, transesophageal echocardiography; TTE, transthoracic echocardiography.

esophageal imaging was optimal for patients who had a prior probability of endocarditis that is observed commonly in clinical practice (4% to 60%) with a reduced cost of $18 per person compared with the use of TTE. In contrast, strategies that reserved the use of TEE for patients who had an inadequate transthoracic study provided similar quality adjusted life years but cost modestly more per patient.

In a similar study, Rosen and colleagues[32] set out to determine the cost-effectiveness of TEE in establishing the duration of therapy for catheter-associated bacteremia.[32] In this study, three management strategies were compared:[32] (1) empirical treatment with 4 weeks of antibiotics (long course); (2) empirical treatment with 2 weeks of antibiotic therapy (short course); and (3) TEE-guided therapy. In the case of the TEE strategy, a positive TEE dictated long-course therapy and a negative TEE dictated short-course therapy. The effectiveness of an empiric long-course strategy and a TEE-guided strategy were both superior to empiric short-course therapy. When costs were taken into account, the TEE-guided strategy was superior to the empiric long-course strategy, which cost over $1,500,000 per quality adjusted life year saved.

Echocardiography to Predict Complications and Guide Therapeutic Decision Making

Once the diagnosis of IE has been established, the information from the echocardiographic examination can be used to establish the prognosis and guide future decision making. For instance, echocardiographic findings that establish evidence of infection extension into the perivalvular tissue (e.g., abscess, pseudoaneurysm, and fistula) may indicate a need for urgent surgical consideration. In addition, Doppler data that allow for the assessment of valvular regurgitation and cardiac function can greatly assist the clinician in understanding the current and future hemodynamic status. Finally, there is substantial evidence to support decision making related to the association between vegetation size and risk for thromboembolic complications.

Since the early 1990s, multiple studies have shown a strong association between vegetation size and subsequent thromboembolic risk. For instance, Sanfilippo and colleagues found that the risk of embolization was directly related to vegetation size.[33] In fact, for vegetations greater than 6 mm in size the risk of subsequent embolization was linearly related to an increase in vegetation size (Fig. 22–12). These findings have been verified by several investigators.[34-36] Tischler and Vaitkus conducted a meta-analysis that incorporated 10 studies involving 738 patients with IE.[34] They found that the pooled odds ratio (OR) for risk of embolization was three times higher in patients with large vegetations (>10 mm) com-

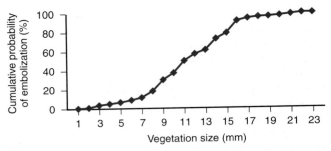

Figure 22–12. Risk of systemic embolization by size of vegetation. (Adapted from Sanfilippo AJ, Picard MH, Newell JB, et al: J Am Coll Cardiol 18:1191-1199, 1991.)

pared to patients with no detectable or small vegetations (OR 2.90, 95% CI [confidence interval] 1.95, 4.02).

Importantly, Di Salvo and colleagues have extended these findings by studying both clinically apparent thromboembolic events and clinically silent embolic events diagnosed by standard imaging in all patients.[36] The investigators found that both vegetation size and mobility were predictive of embolic events. Specifically, 70% of the embolic events were in patients with large (>15 mm) vegetations. In addition, vegetation mobility was also related to embolic risk; in the 73 patients with moderate-severe mobility in the vegetation, 45 (62%) had a subsequent embolic event.

One issue in the interpretation of such findings is the high degree of interobserver variability in recording the specific characteristics of vegetations. For instance, Heinle and colleagues observed that there was a high degree of variability in the interpretation of specific vegetation findings.[37] Specifically, they found only 57% agreement in regard to mobility, 36% in shape, and 40% in the site of attachment. Therefore, in the absence of interobserver consistency, these findings must be used with caution to support decision making.

Perioperative Echocardiography

As with many areas of perioperative management, patients with endocarditis that may require surgical intervention benefit from echocardiographic assessment. Preoperatively, data from echocardiograms can help in surgical planning by delineating the nature and extent of infection, documenting perivalvular extension, determining the mechanisms of valvular dysfunction, and/or regions of myocardial disruption. In addition, certain surgical needs, such as the determination of preoperative estimates of annular size, can be useful in surgical planning.

Intraoperative echocardiography can be used to assess the dysfunctional valves and other valves and contiguous structures. Postcardiopulmonary bypass images are useful to determine the adequacy of the valve repair and/or valve replacement. These images can also be used to document the adequate repair of fistulous tracts and perforation. In addition, afterload augmentation can be used to mimic ambulatory hemodynamics to assess for persistent regurgitation and to ensure the overall adequacy of the surgical correction.

Echocardiography at the Completion of Therapy

Patients with a history of endocarditis represent a high-risk group for future episodes of endocarditis.[38] This is especially true in those patients that have had a surgical repair. Therefore, it is important for the future care of these patients to establish a new baseline for valvular morphology, including the presence of vegetations, ventricular function, and valvular insufficiency once therapy has been completed. At the completion of therapy, TTE may be preferable as a result of a decrease in the need for higher resolution in this follow up stage. Specific focus should include documentation of residual regurgitation and evidence of perivalvular destruction. TEE may be necessary in patients with poor acoustic windows or after extensive surgical repair. Posttreatment echocardiography can guide further medical therapy and the timing of future surgical intervention if necessary.

Research Applications

Real-time three-dimensional echocardiography (RT3DE) has become available with the availability of sophisticated matrix transducers that incorporate computer processing technology that allows simultaneous transmission and data processing. A full matrix array transducer (X4, Phillips Medical Systems, Andover, Mass.), which uses 3000 elements in contrast to the 256 elements of the sparse matrix array probe, has been developed. This new development in transducer technology has resulted in (1) improved side-lobe performance (contrast resolution), (2) higher sensitivity and penetration, and (3) harmonic capabilities, which may be used for both grey scale and contrast imaging.[39]

The benefits of RT3DE are particularly well suited to the study of valvular heart disease, specifically the mitral valve given its complex morphology and the importance of delineating its anatomy precisely. For similar reasons, it is anticipated that RT3DE will likely prove valuable for assessing lesions associated with IE. Although there have been several reports of the use of RT3DE in the evaluation of patients with IE, these have been limited to case reports.[40-42] Based on these initial experiences, it is felt that RT3DE offers promise for improving the morphologic descriptions of vegetation lesions, increasing the detection of perivalvular extension and assisting in presurgical decision making.

Future Directions

IE remains a serious and deadly disease. Despite advances in imaging with echocardiography, IE is a disease that requires a high degree of clinical suspicion to use the best echocardiographic technique at the appropriate time in the clinical course. Notably, echocardiography has become a mainstay in the diagnosis of IE and is emerging as an important prognostic tool. To improve the care of patients with IE, studies should focus on how best to use echocardiography to guide therapeutic decision making. Specifically, empiric evidence is needed to validate risk stratification schemas, often based largely on echocardiographic data that identify patients in need of aggressive and early surgical intervention.

Alternative Approaches

Other types of imaging may be used to support the diagnosis of IE and/or evaluate for potential complications. For instance, chest radiography can be used to provide supporting evidence of IE, such as nodular pulmonary infiltrates in a febrile injection drug user likely signifying right-sided IE with septic pulmonary emboli. In addition, cardiomegaly may indicate chamber enlargement resulting from significant valvular regurgitation, whereas enlarged pulmonary vessels provide evidence for congestive heart failure.

Computed tomography (CT) and magnetic resonance imaging (MRI) have long been used to assess for evidence of thromboembolic complications, such as stroke or visceral embolic events, in patients with IE, but their role in imaging cardiac pathology is less established. For instance, there have only been isolated case reports of the use of computed tomography imaging to diagnosis complications of IE, such as aortic root abscess. In a similar fashion, there have been multiple case reports of the use of magnetic resonance imaging in patients with IE, but no large studies have been performed.

For both computed tomography and magnetic resonance imaging, the enhanced spatial resolution provided by the current imaging modalities and the likely improvements in this resolution over time, provide for the possibility of evaluating cardiac manifestations of the infective process in a more refined way. Enthusiasm for either of these modalities must be tempered by current limitations as a result of temporal resolution. For instance, the length of time currently required to acquire images, the difficulty in evaluating motion, and the presence of motion artifacts are important limitations in a disease such as IE.

KEY POINTS

■ Echocardiography has become the central tenant in evaluating patients that have a clinical suspicion for IE.

■ There are several findings on echocardiography that provide evidence of IE, including vegetations, evidence of periannular tissue destruction, aneurysm, fistula, leaflet perforation, and valvular dehiscence.

■ Vegetations have the consistency of mid-myocardium but also may have areas of echo-lucency and echo-density.

■ Not all intracardiac mass lesions represent vegetations, therefore the differential diagnosis should include Libman-Sacks valvular lesions, murantic lesions, malignancies (primary and secondary), myxomatous changes, ruptured chordae, and degenerative changes, such as Lambl's excrescences.

■ Prosthetic valve endocarditis may require special consideration regarding the choice of the type of imaging and in many cases may require both TTE and TTE.

■ Patients with intracardiac devices represent a risk group for IE that is growing rapidly.

■ If the initial TTE is negative in which there is high degree of clinical suspicion for IE, then TEE should follow rapidly.

■ TEE should be the primary imaging modality of choice for clinical situations in which there is a suspicion for intracardiac complications.

■ Recent data provide evidence that an initial strategy of diagnostic TEE may be cost-effective in most clinical situations.

■ Echocardiography can be used to determined prognosis and guide therapeutic decision making.

REFERENCES

1. Dillon JC, Feigenbaum H, Konecke LL, et al: Echocardiographic manifestations of valvular vegetations. *Am Heart J* 86:698-704, 1973.
2. Daniel WG, Mugge A, Martin RP, et al: Improvement in the diagnosis of abscesses associated with endocarditis by transesophageal echocardiography. *N Engl J Med* 324:795-800, 1991.
3. Pedersen WR, Walker M, Olson JD, et al: Value of transesophageal echocardiography as an adjunct to transthoracic echocardiography in evaluation of native and prosthetic valve endocarditis. *Chest* 100:351-356, 1991.
4. Baddour LM, Wilson WR, Bayer A, et al: Diagnosis, antimicrobial therapy, and management of complications. A statement for healthcare professionals from the committee on rheumatic fever, endocarditis, and Kawasaki disease, Council on cardiovascular disease in the young, and the Councils on clinical cardiology, stroke, and cardiovascular surgery and anesthesia, American Heart Association—executive summary. *Circulation* 111:3167-3184, 2005.
5. Cabell C, Heidenreich P, Chu V, et al: Increasing rates of cardiac device infections among Medicare beneficiaries: 1990-1999. *Am Heart J* 147:582-586, 2004.
6. Fowler VG, Miro JM, Hoen B, et al: Staphylococcus aureus endocarditis: A consequence of medical progress. *JAMA* 293:3012-3021, 2005.
7. Osler W: Gulstonian lectures on malignant endocarditis. Lecture I. *Lancet* 1:415-418, 1885.
8. Osler W. Gulstonian lectures on malignant endocarditis. Lecture II. *Lancet* 1:459-464, 1885.
9. Osler W. Gulstonian lectures on malignant endocarditis. Lecture III. *Lancet* 1:505-508, 1885.
10. Pelletier L, Petersdorf R: Infective endocarditis: A review of 125 cases from the University of Washington Hospitals, 1963-72. *Medicine* 56:287-313, 1977.
11. von Reyn CF, Levy BS, Arbeit RD, et al: Infective endocarditis: Analysis based on strict definitions. *Ann Intern Med* 94:505-518, 1981.
12. Durack DT, Lukes AS, Bright DK: New criteria for diagnosis of infective endocarditis: Utilization of specific echocardiographic findings. *Am J Med* 96:200-209, 1994.
13. Hoen B, Selton-Suty C, Danchin N, et al: Evaluation of the Duke criteria versus the Beth Israel criteria for the diagnosis of infective endocarditis. *Clin Infect Dis* 21:905-909, 1996.
14. Olaison L, Hogevik H: Comparison of the von Reyn and Duke criteria for the diagnosis of infective endocarditis: A critical analysis of 161 episodes. *Scand J Infect Dis* 28:399-406, 1996.
15. Cecchi E, Parrini I, Chinaglia A, et al: New diagnostic criteria for infective endocarditis. A study of sensitivity and specificity. *Eur Heart J* 18:1149-1156, 1997.
16. Li JS, Sexton DJ, Mick N, et al: Proposed modifications to the Duke criteria for the diagnosis of infective endocarditis. *Clin Infect Dis* 30:633-638, 2000.
17. Durack DT, Beeson PB: Experimental bacterial endocarditis. I. Colonization of a sterile vegetation. *Br J Exp Pathol* 53:44-49, 1972.
18. Libman E, Sacks B: A hitherto undescribed form of valvular and mural endocarditis. *Arch Intern Med* 33:701-737, 1924.
19. Lambl V: [Papillare exkreszenzen an der semilunar-klappe der aorta.] *Wien Med Wochenschr* 6:244-247, 1856.
20. Magarey F: On the mode of formation of Lambl's excrescences and their relation to chronic thickening of the mitral valve. *J Pathol Bacteriol* 61:203-208, 1949.
21. Anguera I, Miro JM, Vilacosta I, et al: Aorto-cavitary fistulous tract formation in infective endocarditis: Clinical and echocardiographic features of 76 cases and risk factors for mortality. *Eur Heart J* 26:288-297, 2005.
22. Anguera I, Miro JM, Cabell C, et al: Clinical characteristics and outcome of aortic endocarditis with periannular abscess in the International Collaboration on Endocarditis Merged Database. *Am J Cardiol* 96:976-981, 2005.
23. Fowler VG, Li J, Corey GR, et al: Role of echocardiography in evaluation of patients with Staphylococcus aureus bacteremia. *J Am Coll Cardiol* 30:1072-1078, 1997.
24. Chua JD, Wilkoff BL, Lee I, et al: Diagnosis and management of infections involving implantable electrophysiologic cardiac devices. *Ann Intern Med* 133:604-608, 2000.
25. Chamis A, Peterson GE, Cabell CH, et al: Staphylococcus aureus bacteremia in patients with permanent pacemakers or implantable cardioverter-defibrillators. *Circulation* 104:1029-1033, 2001.
26. Rohmann S, Erbel R, Darius H, et al: Prediction of rapid versus prolonged healing of infective endocarditis by monitoring vegetation size. *J Am Soc Echocardiogr* 4:465-474, 1991.
27. Vieira ML, Grinberg M, Pomerantzeff PM, et al: Repeated echocardiographic examinations of patients with suspected infective endocarditis. *Heart* 90:1020-1024, 2004.
28. Heidenreich P, Masoudi F, Maini B, et al: Echocardiography in patients with suspected endocarditis: A cost effectiveness analysis. *Am J Med* 107:198-208, 1999.
29. Greaves K, Patel A, Celermajer D: Clinical criteria and the appropriate use of transthoracic echocardiography for the exclusion of infective endocarditis. *Heart* 89:273-275, 2003.

30. Kuruppu JC, Corretti M, Mackowiak P, Roghmann MC: Overuse of transthoracic echocardiography in the diagnosis of native valve endocarditis. *Arch Intern Med* 162:1715-1720, 2002.

31. Bayer AS, Bolger AF, Taubert KA, et al: Diagnosis and management of infective endocarditis and its complications. *Circulation* 98:2936-2948, 1998.

32. Rosen AB, Fowler VG, Corey GR, et al: Cost-effectiveness of transesophageal echocardiography to determine the duration of therapy for intravascular catheter-associated Staphylococcus aureus bacteremia. *Ann Intern Med* 130:810-820, 1999.

33. Sanfilippo AJ, Picard MH, Newell JB, et al: Echocardiographic assessment of patients with infectious endocarditis: Prediction of risk for complications. *J Am Coll Cardiol* 18:1191-1199, 1991.

34. Tischler MD, Vaitkus PT: The ability of vegetation size on echocardiography to predict clinical complications: a meta-analysis. *J Am Soc Echocardiogr* 10:562-568, 1997.

35. Cabell CH, Pond KK, Peterson GE, et al: The risk of stroke and death in patients with aortic and mitral valve endocarditis. *Am Heart J* 142:75-80, 2001.

36. Di Salvo G, Habib G, Pergola V, et al: Echocardiography predicts embolic events in infective endocarditis. *J Am Coll Cardiol* 37:1069-1076, 2001.

37. Heinle S, Wilderman N, Harrison JK, et al: Value of transthoracic echocardiography in predicting embolic events in active infective endocarditis. *Am J Cardiol* 74:799-801, 1994.

38. Strom BL, Abrutyn E, Berlin JA, et al: Dental and cardiac risk factors for infective endocarditis. A population-based, case-control study. *Ann Intern Med* 129:761-769, 1998.

39. Sugeng L, Weinert L, Lang RM: Left ventricular assessment using real time three dimensional echocardiography. *Heart* 89:29-36, 2003.

40. Nemes A, Lagrand WK, McGhie JS, ten Cate FJ: Three-dimensional transesophageal echocardiography in the evaluation of aortic valve destruction by endocarditis. *J Am Soc Echocardiogr* 19:355, 2006.

41. Kort S: Real-time 3-dimensional echocardiography for prosthetic valve endocarditis: Initial experience. *J Am Soc Echocardiogr* 19:130-139, 2006.

42. El Muayed M, Burjonroppa SC, Croitoru M: Added accuracy with 3D echocardiographic imaging of valvular vegetations. *Echocardiography* 22:361-362, 2005.

43. Sachdev M, Peterson GE, Jollis JG: Imaging techniques for diagnosis of infective endocarditis. *Infect Dis Clin North Am* 16:319-337, 2002.

Chapter 23

Aortic Stenosis: Echocardiographic Evaluation of Disease Severity, Disease Progression, and the Role of Echocardiography in Clinical Decision Making

RAPHAEL ROSENHEK, MD

The author acknowledges David M. Shavelle, MD, and Catherine M. Otto, MD, the previous authors of this chapter in *The Practice of Clinical Echocardiography*, second edition.

■ Natural History and Progression of Aortic Stenosis

Natural History
Progression of Aortic Stenosis
Risk Stratification
Scheduling Control Intervals
Timing of Surgery in Patients with Nonsevere Aortic Stenosis Undergoing Cardiac Surgery
Aortic Stenosis with Reduced Left Ventricular Function
Assessment of Coronary Artery Disease
Arterial Hypertension

■ Optimizing the Surgical Approach

Evaluation of Patients with Aortic Stenosis Undergoing Noncardiac Surgery
The Role of Echocardiography in Optimizing the Surgical Approach and the Role of Perioperative Echocardiography
The Postoperative Assessment after Aortic Valve Replacement

■ Assessment of the Effects of Aortic Valve Replacement

Aortic stenosis (AS) is the most frequent valvular heart disease. As the population is aging, its incidence is further increasing and is in the range of about 2% to 9% in elderly patients. Aortic sclerosis, the precursor of AS is present in 29% of patients older than 65 years. With the widespread use of echocardiography, AS less frequently remains undiagnosed.

AS is suspected when a typical systolic murmur is heard or when symptoms, such as angina pectoris, exertional dyspnea or syncope, occur.

Not uncommonly, AS is coincidentally diagnosed in patients referred to echocardiography for other reasons. Today, echocardiography has become the most important examination technique for diagnosis and quantification of AS. It also permits the assessment of left ventricular (LV) systolic and diastolic function, of LV hypertrophy, and of other associated valve lesions. For an adequate interpretation, the limitations and pitfalls of the technique have to be considered and will therefore be discussed in this chapter. The prognostic value of these echocardiographic findings will be reviewed together with the natural history and progression of the disease so as to be comprehensively included in an optimized management strategy.

Aortic Stenosis on Two-Dimensional Echocardiography

From a clinical point of view, calcific AS is the most common form of AS, followed by rheumatic stenosis (which is in decline in Western societies) and congeni-

tal stenosis.[1] Roberts and Ko report an incidence of bicuspid aortic valves of 53% in a large series of 933 consecutively excised stenotic aortic valves (Fig. 23–1).[2] These data suggest that congenitally abnormal aortic valves are thus more frequent than currently assumed. Particular care should therefore be applied when describing the echocardiographic morphology of the aortic valve. At more advanced disease stages, congenitally stenotic valves calcify and mechanisms of calcification resemble those observed in calcific AS.

Calcific Aortic Stenosis

Historically, AS was believed to be the result of mechanical deterioration resulting from wear and tear of the aortic valve itself and was therefore termed degenerative. However, it has been recognized that it is an active and progressive disease that is showing a number of parallels with atherosclerotic vascular degeneration, such as inflammation, lipid infiltration, dystrophic calcification, and even ossification.[3-8] Therefore, the term calcific AS is more appropriate. The valve is characterized by thickened and calcified cusps with reduced systolic opening and reduced leaflet motion (Fig. 23–2).

Congenital Aortic Stenosis

Congenitally stenotic aortic valves present as unicuspid, bicuspid, tricuspid, and quadricuspid valves.[9] Bicuspid valves account for the majority of cases of

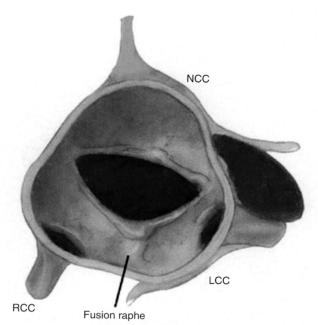

Figure 23–1. Bicuspid aortic stenosis with anterior/posterior orientation and a raphe in a transesophageal echocardiography short-axis view orientation. LCC, left coronary cusp; NCC, noncoronary cusp; RCC, right coronary cusp.

congenital AS. The two valve cups are typically of different size, and the larger cusp often contains a raphe (that represents the fusion-line of two leaflets) (see Fig. 23-1). A prominent raphe may be misleading resulting in diagnosis of a trileaflet aortic valve. Therefore, the opening of the aortic valve should be assessed with particular care in systole. In some cases, definite morphologic attribution might only be possible by transesophageal echocardiography (TEE). Typically the leaflets in bicuspid aortic valves are oriented in an anterior/posterior or right/left manner. Other malformations that are associated with a bicuspid aortic valve and that should not be overlooked include aortic coarctation, a persistent ductus arteriosus, or a ventricular septal defect. Unicuspid valves may present without an identifiable commissure (acommissural) or as a unicommissural valve.

Rheumatic Aortic Stenosis

Rheumatic AS is characterized by commissural fusion and thickening of the leaflet edges and sometimes leaflet retraction (Fig. 23-3). Not all the commissures are necessarily fused. Associated aortic regurgitation (AR) and mitral valve involvement are frequent in rheumatic disease.

Assessment of Aortic Valve Calcification

Aortic valve calcification is best assessed in a short-axis view. In the presence of severe calcification, the differentiation of the underlying AS etiology may be dif-

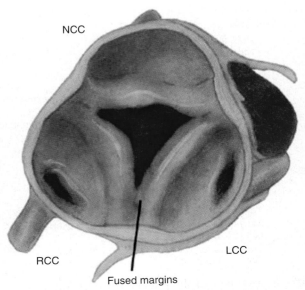

Figure 23-3. Rheumatic aortic stenosis with commissural fusion, thickening of the leaflet edges and leaflet retraction in a transesophageal echocardiography short-axis view orientation. LCC, left coronary cusp; NCC, noncoronary cusp; RCC, right coronary cusp.

ficult. Because of its prognostic importance, the degree of aortic valve calcification should be routinely described. The degree of calcification can be classified as mild (isolated, small spots), moderate (multiple bigger spots), or severe (extensive thickening/calcification of all cusps)[10] (Fig. 23-4).

Aortic Root Involvement

Echocardiography allows an assessment of the aortic annulus size, of the aortic root, and of the ascending aorta. Bicuspid[11] but also unicuspid aortic valves[12] are associated with aortic root dilation in about 50% of the cases. Although the concept of poststenotic dilatation resulting from hemodynamic factors is still accepted, primary tissue abnormalities of the aortic media, which are present in patients with congenitally malformed aortic valves, contribute to further aortic dilation.[11]

Indirect Echocardiographic Findings

Several indirect echocardiographic findings are suggestive of the presence of AS. These include aliasing in the left ventricular outflow tract (LVOT), LV hypertrophy, and an increased aortic velocity when visualization of the valve is suboptimal.

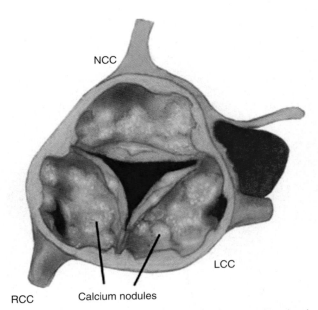

Figure 23-2. Calcific aortic stenosis with thickened and calcified cusps in a transesophageal echocardiography short-axis view orientation. LCC, left coronary cusp; NCC, noncoronary cusp; RCC, right coronary cusp.

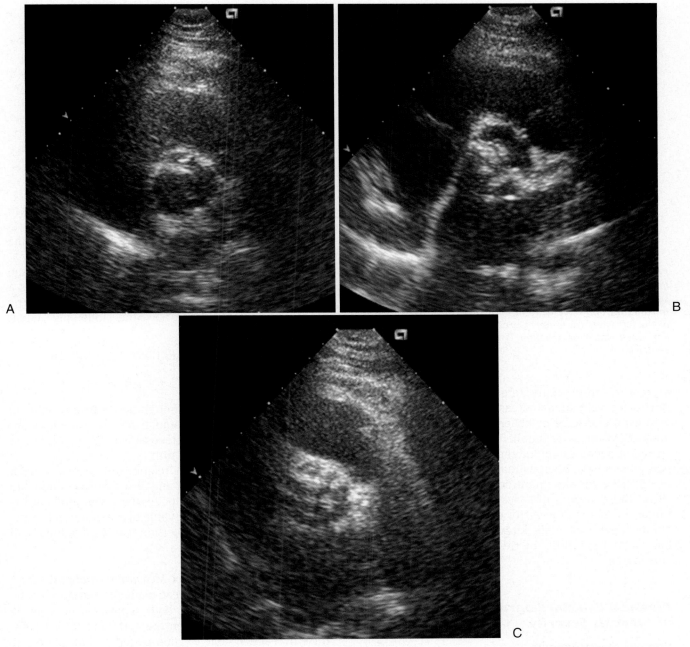

Figure 23-4. A, *Parasternal short-axis view of a mildly calcified stenotic aortic valve showing isolated spots of calcification. B, Parasternal short-axis view of a moderately calcified stenotic aortic valve showing multiple spots of calcification. C, Parasternal short-axis view of a severely calcified stenotic aortic valve showing extensive calcification of all cusps.*

Differential Diagnosis

Whereas valvular AS accounts for most cases of LVOT obstruction, the differential diagnosis of subvalvular stenosis, supravalvular stenosis, or hypertrophic cardiomyopathy needs to be considered.

Furthermore a concomitant subvalvular obstruction, which may be present in addition to valvular AS, should be ruled out.[13]

Quantification of Aortic Stenosis Severity

A normally opening aortic valve is not obstructive to blood flow. It has an opening area of about 3 to 4 cm², and the normal transvalvular flow is laminar with a peak velocity below 2 m/s. When the valve becomes stenotic, and thus obstructive to blood flow,

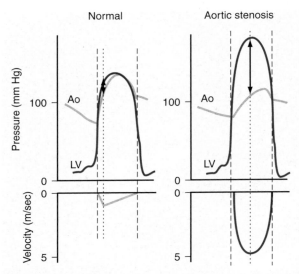

Normal   Aortic stenosis

Figure 23–5. *Relationship of pressures to Doppler velocities in normal and aortic stenosis. Note that the maximum pressure gradient (double-headed arrow) corresponds to the maximum Doppler velocity in both situations, but the timing of the left ventricle to aorta pressure gradient is quite different when valve obstruction is present. Ao, aorta; LV, left ventricle.*

a pressure drop occurs across the valve (Fig. 23–5). Aortic jet velocities increase accordingly, with the greatest increase being observed once the aortic valve area (AVA) becomes smaller than 1 cm², and the obstruction becomes hemodynamically relevant. Several parameters have been validated for the quantification of AS. Whereas the quantification of AS is unequivocal in the majority off cases, the integration of additional measures of severity can be helpful for an accurate diagnosis. Also, knowledge of the theoretical basis and limitations of these measures have to be considered.

Classical Echocardiographic Measures of Stenosis Severity

Doppler Measurements

Transaortic Gradients. *Transvalvular* gradients are derived from velocities using the Bernoulli equation, which is based on the conservation of energy principle in a closed system. In practice, accurate gradient calculations are performed using the simplified Bernoulli equation that ignores viscous losses and the effects of flow acceleration, both of which can generally be neglected in the clinical setting:

$$\Delta P = 4v^2$$

Doppler derived gradients correlate well with invasively measured pressure gradients as has been demonstrated in the experimental and in the clinical setting.[14-26] Furthermore, Doppler gradients also accurately

reflect pressure gradient changes that occur with a change in flow rate.[15,16,27]

The simplified Bernoulli equation ignores the flow velocity proximal to the stenosis, which is an acceptable assumption as long as the transvalvular velocity is significantly greater than the proximal flow velocity. However, if this difference is less accentuated (i.e., in the presence of accelerated flow or less significant stenosis, the use of the following form of the Bernoulli equation is more appropriate, where v_2 and v_1 represent the transvalvular and the proximal flow velocities, respectively:

$$\Delta P = 4(v_2^2 - v_1^2)$$

The peak transaortic pressure gradient corresponds to the maximal difference between the pressure in the aorta and the ventricle. With increasing stenosis severity, the peak of the gradient occurs later during systole.[28]

The mean gradient is calculated by integrating the peak gradient over the duration of systole. There is a linear relationship between peak and mean transaortic gradients that is given by the following equations[20,21,29,30]:

$$\text{Mean } \Delta P = (\text{Max } \Delta P/1.45) - 2.2 \text{ mm Hg}$$

$$\text{Mean } \Delta P = 2.4 \ (V_{max})^3$$

These two equations, though derived from separate patient populations, give similar results. They only apply to native aortic valve stenosis with its typical shape of the velocity curve over time.

Thus there is a direct relationship between peak velocity and peak gradient and also a close relationship between maximum jet velocity and mean gradient explain, emphasizing on the value of maximum jet velocity data alone in clinical decision making in adults with valvular AS.

Comparison with Catheter-Measured Gradients. Doppler mean gradients and mean gradients measured in the catheterization laboratory both represent the average pressure difference between the aorta and the left ventricle over the systolic ejection period and ideally correlate when they are recorded simultaneously in practice.

However, the peak Doppler echocardiographic gradient corresponds to the maximal difference between the aortic and the instantaneous LV pressure.

The peak-to peak gradient corresponds to the difference between peak aortic pressure and peak LV pressure. Because these two peaks do no occur simultaneously, the peak-to-peak gradient does not exist physiologically and also cannot be determined by Doppler echocardiography (Fig. 23–6).

Pitfalls

Technical Considerations. Particular care is required when recording aortic jet velocities in patients with AS. To record the peak velocity, it is of utmost impor-

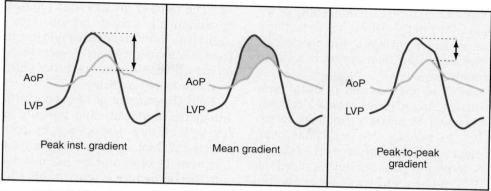

Figure 23–6. *Peak Doppler echocardiographic gradient corresponds to the maximal difference between the aortic and the instantaneous left ventricular pressure (left panel). Mean gradients represent the average pressure difference between the aorta and the left ventricle over the systolic ejection (central panel). The peak-to peak gradient corresponds to the difference between peak aortic pressure and peak left ventricular pressure (right panel). LVP, left ventricular pressure.*

tance to align the Doppler probe with the jet direction. Any such error in alignment leads to an underestimation of the Doppler gradient. Because the exact orientation of the aortic jet cannot be predicted from the two-dimensional (2D) image, multiple transducer positions (i.e., right parasternal, suprasternal, apical, and even subcostal) have to be used to obtain the maximum signal. The use of a small, dedicated continuous-wave (CW) Doppler transducer (pencil probe) is recommended in this setting (Fig. 23–7). For future examinations, the image window used to record the peak transaortic velocity should be mentioned on the examination report. When the rate of hemodynamic progression is determined, measure-

ments recorded from the same window should be compared.

Even with an experienced operator and attention to technical details, there is some degree of measurement variability, as with any clinical measurement. In the absence of interval physiologic changes, the coefficient of variability for recording and measuring aortic jet velocity is 3%,[31] so that a change in jet velocity of more that 0.2 m/s and a change in mean gradient of more than 4 mm Hg are outside the range of measurement variability and indicate actual progression of the disease.

Other Signals. While recording the Doppler signal, care has to be applied not to confound the signal with that of another form of obstruction or another flow

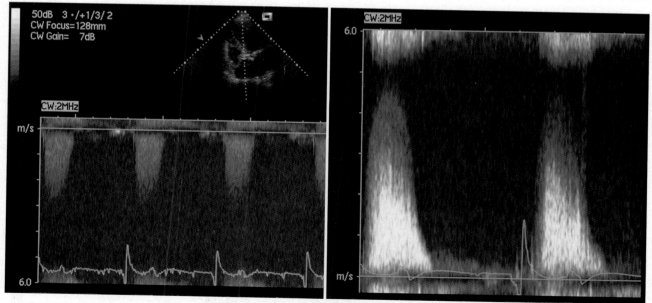

Figure 23–7. *Continuous-wave Doppler tracings of aortic stenosis velocity obtained from an apical (A) and a right parasternal recording using a pencil probe (B) in the same patient. This example emphasizes on the value of using a dedicated continuous wave Doppler transducer and the importance of alignment of the Doppler probe with the aortic jet direction to record the maximal signal.*

signal, such as that of mitral regurgitation (MR) or tricuspid regurgitation (TR). If the patient has atrial fibrillation (AFib), the measurement has to be repeated for several consecutive beats and than averaged so as to obtain a representative result.

Pressure Recovery. The phenomenon of distal pressure recovery explains discrepancies between catheter and Doppler assessment of pressure gradients in patients with AS.[32-37] In valvular AS, a laminar high-velocity jet is present across the narrowed orifice.[38] The minimal cross-sectional area (CSA) of fluid is called the vena contracta (VC); it has a smaller diameter and occurs distal to the anatomic valve orifice. Pressure is lowest and velocity is greatest at the level of the VC.

Distal to the VC, the jet expands and decelerates. Because total energy remains constant according to Bernoulli's law, the reduction in velocity is accompanied by an increase in aortic pressure.

The Doppler gradient corresponds to the peak gradient at the site of the VC and thus is higher than the catheter gradient that is measured farther downstream.

Pressure recovery accounts for some of the discrepancies between Doppler and invasive data reported in the literature. In most cases the observed magnitude of pressure recovery is of about 10 mm Hg, an effect that in most cases does not affect clinical decision making.[34] However, pressure recovery may be significant in the presence of less severe AS and a small ascending aorta.[39] The phenomenon can be predicted from Doppler velocity, AVA, and the size of the ascending aorta.[40] Thus, patients with severe AS and poststenotic aortic root dilation may show less pressure recovery than patients with mild-to-moderate stenosis and a small or normal aortic root dimension. The maximum aortic jet velocity reflects the pressure difference between the left ventricle and the

VC. The Doppler velocity thus represents an important measure that is accurate in most cases. Albeit rare, situations with more pronounced pressure recovery phenomenon are encountered; in these settings, the actual load on the left ventricle may be better reflected by the invasively measured gradient.

Flow Dependence of Measurements. Doppler measurements of velocity and pressure gradient are limited by their flow dependence. In fact, the presence of a high flow rate, such as in hyperdynamic states or in the presence of significant AR, may lead to an overestimation of the true severity of AS. On the other hand, a low flow rate, such as in the presence of a depressed LV function or coexisting MR may lead to an underestimation of AS severity. Furthermore, aortic jet velocity varies in the same patients when there are changes in transaortic flow volume, such as those occurring during exercise. If the patient is not in sinus rhythm—the most common situation being atrial fibrillation—there is a beat-to-beat variability in flow measurements and several consecutive beats have to be averaged (Fig. 23–8).

Altogether, it is therefore important to rely on a flow independent measurement of AS severity. The calculation of aortic valve area represents a measure that is more independent of the transaortic volume flow rate.

Valve Area Calculation

Calcific aortic valve stenosis is characterized by stiff leaflets that open to a variable degree depending on the force applied on the valve. This limits attempts at direct measurement of AVA, a consideration that even applies to the situation where the surgeon applies direct force while inspecting the valve with a finger.

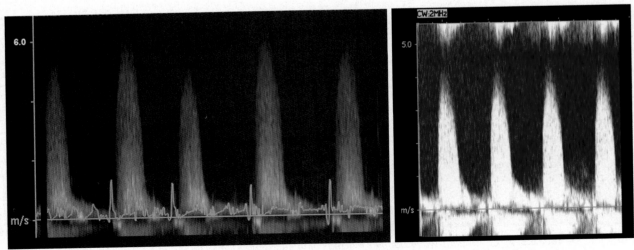

A   B

Figure 23–8. Continuous-wave Doppler tracings of aortic stenosis velocity from a right parasternal approach using a pencil probe in a patient with atrial fibrillation (A) and a patient with sinus rhythm (B). When beat-to-beat variability is present, measurements of consecutive beats have to be averaged.

Continuity Equation. The continuity equation method for the calculation of valve areas has the advantages of being noninvasive and of not containing an empirical constant.[15,17,21,41-44] Using the continuity equation, AVA can be calculated using either peak aortic jet velocities (V) or velocity time integrals:

$$AVA = (V_{LVOT} \times CSA_{LVOT})/V_{AS-JET}$$

in which V_{LVOT} and V_{AS-JET} are the velocities in LVOT and at the level of the stenotic aortic valve, respectively. For the calculation of the CSA of the LVOT, the LVOT diameter is measured from a 2D parasternal long-axis view, parallel and adjacent to the aortic valve plane. The area is then calculated assuming a circular outflow tract.

The LVOT flow velocity is measured from an apical approach using pulsed Doppler ultrasound; and the aortic stenosis jet (AS_{jet}) velocity is measured with continuous-wave Doppler from the echocardiographic window that yields the highest velocity signal (Fig. 23–9). Continuity equation valve area calculations assume accurate recording of the maximum aortic jet velocity, as discussed previously for pressure gradients. However, the largest source of variability in continuity equation valve area calculations lies in the measurement of the outflow tract diameter. The mean interobserver and intraobserver measurement variability is 5% to 8%, resulting in a variability of the calculated valve area of about 0.15 cm^2 for a valve area of 1 cm^2. In an indi-

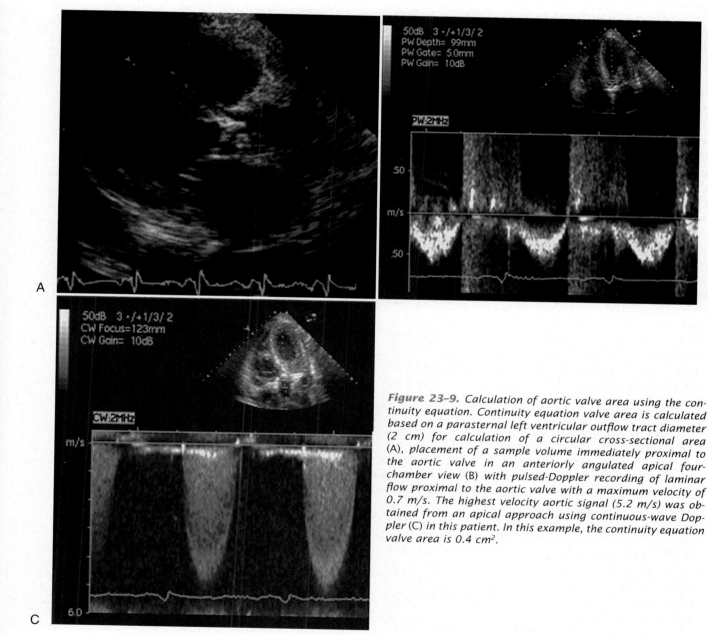

Figure 23–9. Calculation of aortic valve area using the continuity equation. Continuity equation valve area is calculated based on a parasternal left ventricular outflow tract diameter (2 cm) for calculation of a circular cross-sectional area (A), placement of a sample volume immediately proximal to the aortic valve in an anteriorly angulated apical four-chamber view (B) with pulsed-Doppler recording of laminar flow proximal to the aortic valve with a maximum velocity of 0.7 m/s. The highest velocity aortic signal (5.2 m/s) was obtained from an apical approach using continuous-wave Doppler (C) in this patient. In this example, the continuity equation valve area is 0.4 cm^2.

vidual patient, the outflow tract diameter remains relatively constant over time, such that a change in valve area of more than 0.1 cm² most likely represents an actual change in valve area.

An accurate measurement of the transaortic volume flow rate is an essential step for the calculation of the effective aortic valve area (AVA). Theoretically, volume flow rate can be measured at several intracardiac sites (pulmonary artery [PA], mitral annulus, and LVOT). Flow measurements just proximal to the stenotic aortic valve are technically feasible in nearly all adult patients, whereas volume flow rate calculations at other intracardiac sites often are limited by image quality. Furthermore, when coexisting AR is present (which is present to some degree in >80% of adults with valvular AS) volume flow measured across other valves may not equal the volume flow rate across the aortic valve.[31] Thus, in practice, the LVOT is used for measurement of transaortic volume flow rate in nearly all cases.

Volume flow measurement proximal to the stenotic aortic valve assumes that: (1) the CSA of flow is circular in systole and flow fills the anatomic CSA; (2) the pattern of blood flow is laminar with uniform parallel stream lines of flow; (3) CSA and flow velocity are measured at the same site; and (4) the spatial flow velocity profile is relatively flat during ventricular ejection, that is, flow velocities are the same in the center and at the edges of the flowstream. The assumptions of a circular CSA with flow filling the anatomic area have been corroborated by careful short-axis 2D and color flow imaging in animal models and in patients with valvular obstruction.[21] Laminar flow is confirmed by recording a narrow band of velocities throughout ejection on the pulsed Doppler spectral tracing.

For the calculation of the circular CSA of the outflow tract, the LVOT diameter is measured in a 2D parasternal long-axis view, immediately adjacent and parallel to the aortic valve plane in mid-systole. In this view the outflow tract is perpendicular to the ultrasound beam and axial resolution provides a more accurate diameter measurement than the use of apical views. Flow velocity is accurately measured from an apical approach in which the ultrasound beam can be aligned with the direction of the blood flow. To ensure that the diameter and flow measurements are recorded from the *same anatomic site*, both measurements should be made as close to the aortic valve as possible. On the 2D image, the valve leaflet insertions provide an accurate and reproducible landmark, whereas on the Doppler recordings, the aortic valve closing click ensures that the sample volume is adjacent to the aortic valve. Although flow acceleration occurs on the ventricular side of the stenotic aortic valve, this area is spatially small and easily avoided by recognition of spectral broadening on the Doppler velocity tracing.

In theory, the tapering of the outflow tract and the acceleration of blood during systole, both of which re-

sult in blunt flow profiles at the entrance to large vessels, produce a relatively flat spatial flow profile in the outflow tract. A direct examination of the spatial flow profile in the LVOT proximal to the stenotic aortic valve was initially performed with conventional pulsed Doppler by carefully recording flow at sequential sites across the 2D image in both apical long-axis and anteriorly angulated four-chamber views of the outflow tract.[31,45] Another study, using color flow imaging to map the spatial flow profile in 10 patients with AS both before and after aortic valve replacement, showed variable skewing in the spatial flow profile, with highest velocities most often encountered in the region from the center of the outflow tract toward the septum[46] (Fig. 23–10). Also, patients with predominant AS were found to have relatively flat flow profiles, whereas normal subjects and patients with AR had skewed velocity profiles with the highest velocities occurring anteroseptally.[47] For clinical practice, even when the flow profile is skewed to some extent, a reasonably accurate volume flow rate can be calculated if the recorded flow velocity reasonably approximates the spatial and temporal flow velocity in the outflow tract. Such an approximation can most likely be obtained in most patients, when the Doppler sample volume is positioned close the center of the outflow tract in two orthogonal views.

A more pragmatic approach to validating the accuracy of transaortic volume flow measurements is to compare Doppler data to an established standard of reference. This is difficult in clinical studies because most patients with AS have coexisting AR or MR. Even hemodynamically trivial regurgitation will lead to an inaccurate assessment of forward (Fick or thermodilution) and of total (angiographic) cardiac output (CO), thereby inadequately representing the volume flow rate across the aortic valve. In the research setting, transaortic volume flow rate can be measured directly, using an electromagnetic or a transit time flow meter. In both acute and chronic models of valvular AS, Doppler transaortic volume flow rates have been shown to be accu-

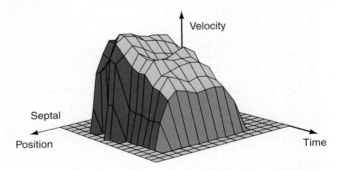

Figure 23–10. *Three-dimensional plot of velocity distribution in left ventricular outflow tract close to the level of aortic annulus. Velocity is plotted against position in the left ventricular outflow tract diameter and against time. There are 20 msec intervals along the time axis and approximately 2 mm between each observation along the diameter axis. (From Wiseth R, Samstad S, Rossvoll O, et al: J Am Soc Echocardiogr 6:279-285, 1993.)*

rate (Table 23–1)[21,27] with a standard error of the estimate of 2 to 4 mL and of 0.25 to 0.5 L/min for stroke volume (SV) and CO, respectively over a wide range of flow rates (Figs. 23–11 and 23–12).

Comparison of Valve Areas Calculated by the Continuity Equation and by the Gorlin Formula. AVAs have been accurately calculated from invasive hemodynamic data using the formula of Gorlin and Gorlin[48]

since its publication in 1951, which thus provided important data for clinical decision making. More recently, Doppler echocardiography has emerged as a noninvasive technique allowing calculation of valve area using the continuity equation.[31,41,43,44,49,50]

Gorlin valve areas have been used as the standard of reference for validation of continuity equation valve areas. The knowledge of the basic principles underlying these equations is important to understand

TABLE 23–1. In Vivo Studies of Simultaneous Invasive and Doppler Volume Flow Measurements from Left Ventricular Outflow Tract at Aortic Annulus in Subjects with and without AS

Model	n	Standard of Reference	Cardiac Output			Stroke Volume			Reference
			r	Range, l/min	SEE, l/min	r	Range, mL	SEE, mL	
Chronic valvular AS (closed-chest and open-chest dogs) altered volume flow rate	75	Transit time-flow	0.86	0.9-6.2	0.50	0.86	9-45	3.6	15
Acute valvular AS (open-chest dogs) altered volume flow rate	52	Electromagnetic flow	0.90	0.9-3.2	0.25	0.88	5-26	2.4	39
Normal (open-chest dogs) altered volume flow rate	33	Roller pump	0.98	0.5-5.0	0.30	—	—	—	151
Patients (no AS)	35	Thermodilution	0.91	2.1-9.5	0.63	0.95	24-87	6.4	152
Patients (no AS)	31	Thermodilution	0.90	1.6-8.4	0.95	—	—	—	153

AS, aortic stenosis.

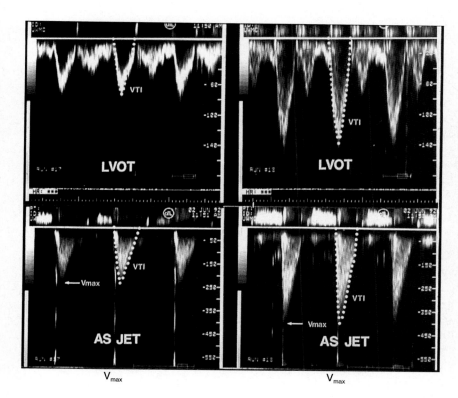

Figure 23–11. Typical Doppler-echo recordings made in one subject at two different volume flow rates. The left ventricular outflow tract (LVOT) velocity profile and velocity time integrals (VTI) (top left) and aortic stenosis (AS JET) velocity (Vmax) and VTI (bottom left) are displayed at one flow rate. Increases in LVOT velocity (top right) and AS JET velocities (bottom right) were observed in the same subject with a dobutamine-induced increase in volume flow rate. (From Burwash IG, Thomas DD, Sadahiro M, et al: Circulation 89:827-835, 1994.)

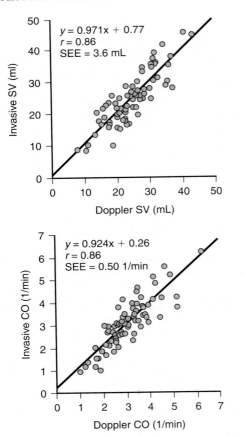

Figure 23–12. *Correlation of simultaneous echocardiographic Doppler and ascending aortic transit time-stroke volume (SV) and cardiac output (CO) during 75 separate interventions. (From Burwash IG, Forbes AD, Sadahiro M, et al: Am J Physiol 265:H1734-H1743, 1993.)*

the different approaches used by these two methods (Fig. 23–13).

According to the formula by Gorlin and Gorlin, AVA is calculated as:

$$AVA = (CO)/(C \times SEP \times \sqrt{\Delta P_{mean}})$$

in which ΔP_{mean} represents the manometrically measured mean pressure gradient, SEP the systolic ejection period, and *C* is a constant.

Accurate pressure gradient measurements depend on careful attention to frequency response, damping, and catheter positioning. The use of a double-lumen catheter or alternatively two separate catheters (with simultaneous measurements obtained in the left ventricle and in the aorta), as opposed to measurement of the femoral artery pressure as a surrogate for the aortic pressure, provide more accurate results. CO should reflect transaortic volume flow rate. While the Fick or thermodilution methods can be used to calculate CO in isolated AS, an angiographically assessed CO is more appropriate in the presence of AR. In the presence of both MR and AR an accurate invasive determination of the transaortic volume flow rate is not possible in the clinical setting.

The Gorlin formula contains an empirically derived constant *(C)*, incorporating the coefficient of contraction, reflecting the difference between the anatomic valve area and the area of the VC, the coefficient of velocity, relating to the conversion of potential to kinetic energy, measurement of pressure in mm Hg, and an empiric correction factor. Both in vitro and in vivo studies suggest that the Gorlin constant may vary with

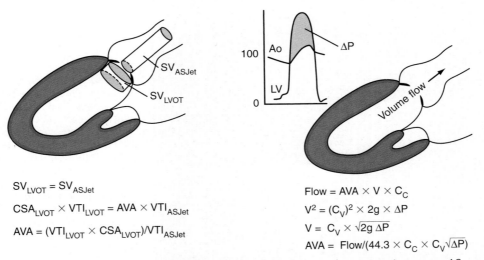

$SV_{LVOT} = SV_{ASJet}$

$CSA_{LVOT} \times VTI_{LVOT} = AVA \times VTI_{ASJet}$

$AVA = (VTI_{LVOT} \times CSA_{LVOT})/VTI_{ASJet}$

Flow $= AVA \times V \times C_C$

$V^2 = (C_V)^2 \times 2g \times \Delta P$

$V = C_V \times \sqrt{2g\,\Delta P}$

$AVA = Flow/(44.3 \times C_C \times C_V\sqrt{\Delta P})$

Figure 23–13. *Comparison of Gorlin and continuity equation valve areas. Ao, aorta; AS$_{JET}$, aortic stenosis jet; AVA, aortic valve area; C$_C$, coefficient of orifice contraction; CSA, cross sectional area; C$_V$, coefficient of velocity; ΔP, pressure gradient; LV, left ventricle; LVOT, left ventricular outflow tract; SV, stroke volume; V, velocity of flow; VTI, velocity time integral.*

changes in volume flow rate, orifice shape, and stenosis severity.[51-55]

When comparing Gorlin and continuity equation valve areas, it is fundamental to bear in mind that they measure different parameters: The Gorlin formula examines the hydraulic load and calculates an anatomic orifice area, whereas the continuity equation describes the physiologic flow area of the VC.[56,57] Thus, one cannot expect these two measurements to yield identical results. Recently, it has been shown that pressure recovery is an important factor contributing to the differences between the two methods.[58] In terms of clinical decision making, their precision, reproducibility, and ability to predict patient outcome are more important than agreement or disagreement. As Gorlin and Gorlin note: "We need not be frustrated when valve areas derived by two different methods are not the same. Rather, we should, like the princes of Serendip, seize upon the difference for what it reveals about the anatomy of the valve orifice as opposed the physiology of the total obstructing valve tract under active pressure and flow conditions."[59]

Definition of the Degree of Severity

In clinical practice, it is important to assess the degree of LV outflow obstruction due to valve narrowing. In this process, the combined information of aortic jet velocity, mean gradient, and valve area should be integrated. The differentiation between severe and nonsevere stenosis is of particular importance because it bears significant consequences for patient management. In the past, severe or critical AS was defined in terms of a specific valve area or valve area index. In many clinical studies, a peak aortic jet velocity greater than 4 m/s is considered to indicate severe AS.[10,60,61] Cut-off values for the effective AVA in the range of 0.8 to 1 cm^2 to define severe AS are encountered in the literature, but the more recent guidelines suggest using a cut-off area 1 cm^2.[62-65] In terms of mean gradient, the ACC/AHA guidelines define severe AS as a mean gradient at least 40 mm Hg, whereas the ESC guidelines suggest a breakpoint of 50 mm Hg for defining severe AS.[62,63] However, a marked overlap in hemodynamic severity between symptomatic and asymptomatic patients has been observed indicating that the critical degree of valve narrowing varies from patient to patient (Fig. 23–14). This finding has been confirmed in prospective studies showing that symptom onset occurs with a jet velocity as low as 3 m/s or may be delayed until the jet velocity is over 5 m/s. Similarly, some patients remain asymptomatic with a valve area less than 0.7 cm^2, whereas others have definite symptoms with a valve area greater than 1 cm^2.

It has also been suggested to index aortic valve area to body surface area (BSA) with a value of 0.6 cm^2/m^2 put forward to define severe AS.[66] However, the distribution of the body surface area is variable, and there is distortion at the extremes of the spectrum, particularly in slim, small people and in obese people. Nevertheless patient stature, build, and predisposition should be considered when determining the degree of AS. Most importantly, the quantification of AS needs to be individualized, particularly when the measured values are in the borderline zone between moderate and severe stenosis. In this regard, consideration of the symptomatic status of the patient is essential.

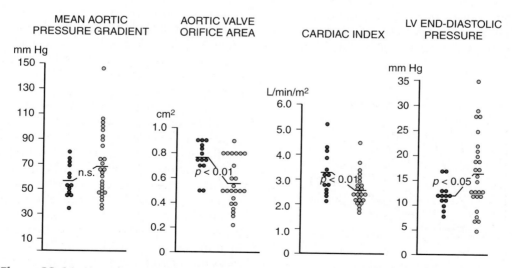

Figure 23–14. *Hemodynamically severe aortic stenosis: mean aortic pressure gradient, valve orifice area, cardiac index, and left ventricular end-diastolic pressure in severely symptomatic* (open circles) *and asymptomatic or mildly symptomatic* (closed circles) *patients. Mean value* (horizontal line) *and statistical difference between both groups are indicated. LV, left ventricular; NS, not significant. (From Turina J, Hess O, Selpucri F, Kayenbeual HP: Eur Heart J 8:471-473, 1987.)*

The differentiation between aortic sclerosis and mild and moderate AS is less critical because the immediate consequences are of a lesser consequence; nevertheless they have relevance for prognosis and timing of follow-up.[60,67,68] Mild AS is usually defined as an aortic valve area greater than 1.5 cm^2 a mean gradient of less than 25 mm Hg or a jet velocity of less than 3 m/s.

Other Measures of Severity

Aortic Valve Resistance

Valve resistance is calculated from invasive or Doppler data as[69,70]:

$$Resistance = (\Delta P_{mean}/Q_{mean}) \times 1333$$

in which ΔP_{mean} represents the mean transaortic pressure gradient in mm Hg, Q_{mean} the mean volume flow rate in mL/s, and 1333 is a conversion factor and resistance is in dyne-s-cm^{-5}. The concept of valve resistance offers the advantage that no empirical constant is involved as compared to the Gorlin formula. Several investigators have observed a curvilinear relationship between valve resistance and valve area (with invasive and Doppler data).[69,70] This observation is supported by the mathematical derivation of the valve area and resistance concepts. In fact, the concepts of valve area and valve resistance are to some extent mutually exclusive. Valve area calculations with the Gorlin formula assume a quadratic relationship between pressure gradient and flow rate. Conversely, the valve resistance concept assumes a linear relationship between these two variables. Most clinical and experimental data support the concept of a quadratic, rather than linear, relationship between pressure gradient and flow rate across a stenotic valve[71] (Fig. 23–15). More complete modeling of the interaction between the left ventricle, the valve, and the peripheral vasculature may enhance

understanding of the hemodynamics of valvular AS.[72] From several studies, it appears that valve resistance is flow dependent, thus not offering a direct advantage over aortic valve area calculations.[73-75] So far, aortic valve resistance has largely been used as a research tool and has not gained wide spread acceptance into clinical practice. This is a result from, on the one hand, the familiarity of most cardiologists with gradients and valve areas and a lack of consensus among studies in terms of added information to conventional measures of severity.[69,76,77]

Aortic Valve Changes during the Cardiac Cycle

AVA changes over the cardiac cycle, with a slower opening and closing motion of the valve in patients with AS, compared to those with normal valves.[78] The rate of change in the AVA during the cardiac cycle has therefore been proposed as an additional measure of AS severity and as a predictor of disease progression.[79] When the rate of change of AVA throughout the ejection phase of the cardiac cycle was expressed as a ratio (AVA ratio), patients with a large AVA ratio were found have more rapid disease progression than those with a lower AVA ratio. This measure may prove useful in patients with valve areas of borderline significance (i.e., about 1 cm^2) by identifying those with a higher probability for rapid disease progression (Fig. 23–16).

Stroke Work Loss

Based on the energy loss concept, the amount of work expended by the left ventricle to keep the aortic valve open during systole compared to the amount of work resulting in effective forward blood flow has been suggested as a potential measure of stenosis severity. This measure would reflect the intrinsic stiffness of the valve leaflets and thus be less dependent on volume flow rate.[80-82] For a stenotic aortic valve, the difference between work calculated from LV pressures and aortic pressures represents the amount of work lost in opening the stiff leaflets. When the aortic valve is normal, this difference is not significant.

Work is calculated by generating a power curve, multiplying instantaneous flow with pressure. Total potential stroke work is calculated by integrating power over the systolic ejection period[82] either using LV (for total work) or aortic (for effective work) pressures. The steady component of work is defined as mean systolic pressure multiplied by SV; pulsatile work is defined as total minus steady work. Stroke work loss then represents the difference between LV and effective work and can be calculated for total, steady, and pulsatile components[80] as:

$$LV\ stroke\ work\ loss = LV\ work - effective\ work$$

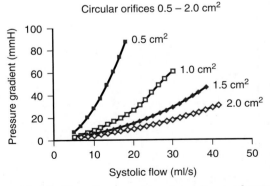

Figure 23–15. Plot of square-law dependence of pressure gradient on flow demonstrated for circular stenoses with orifices from 0.5 to 2.0 cm^2. (From Voelker W, Ruehl H, Nienhaus G, et al: Circulation 91:1196-1204, 1995.)

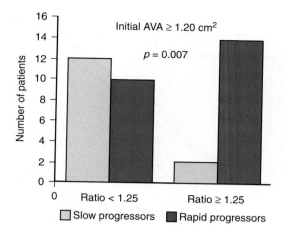

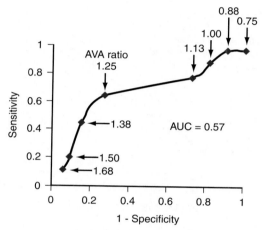

Figure 23–16. Relationship of the change in valve area during the systolic ejection period to the rate of progression of aortic stenosis. The aortic valve area (AVA) ratio was calculated as the aortic valve area during the midpoint of deceleration divided by the valve area during the midpoint of acceleration. A larger AVA ratio indicates stiffer aortic valve leaflets. Rapid progression was defined as a decrease in valve area greater than or equal to 0.20 cm²/year. In patients with a baseline AVA greater than or equal to 1.2 cm², the number of rapid and slow progressors for a ratio less than 1.25 and greater than or equal to 1.25 is shown (top). In patients with a baseline AVA greater than or equal to 1.2 cm², the receiver operating curve for AVA ratio (bottom) indicates the sensitivity and specificity of various AVA ratios for predicting rapid progression of disease. AUC, area under the curve. (From Lester SJ, McElhinney DB, Miller JP, et al: Circulation 101:1947-1952, 2000.)

Because potential work increases with an increasing flow rate, the potential work loss across the stenotic valve is indexed for volume flow rate and expressed as the percent LV stroke work loss.

$$\% \text{ LV stroke work loss} =$$
$$(\text{stroke work loss}/\text{LV stroke work}) \times 100$$

Given that stroke work is the instantaneous product of pressure and flow, and stroke work loss is the differ-

ence of LV work to aortic work, this proposed index of stenosis severity also is likely to vary with volume flow rate if the actual degree of valve opening varies. Note that when the ratio of LV work to aortic work is calculated, the terms for transaortic volume flow rate cancel each other, so that stroke work loss can be determined from Doppler pressure calculations alone. A new index of energy loss, which takes body surface area into account and can be calculated from Doppler derived data, was recently evaluated in an experimental model.[83] The model used fixed stenoses and bioprosthetic valves of two sizes that were evaluated at different flow rates. Using this model, valve area was compared to the energy loss index. In a retrospective analysis of 138 patients with moderate or severe AS, the index and valve area were compared in predicting clinical outcome, defined as death or need for valve replacement. This energy loss index was a significant predictor of clinical outcome with a positive predictive value of 67%.

Planimetry of the Aortic Valve Area

The opening surface of a stenotic aortic valve represents a complex three-dimensional (3D) structure that cannot be reliably assessed with a planar 2D image. The presence of valvular calcification may further limit an accurate delineation of the aortic valve orifice.[84] From a transthoracic approach, the image quality is often insufficient to permit an adequate delineation of the aortic valve orifice. But also TEE is subject to the limitations mentioned previously.

Whereas some investigators have reported favorable correlations between planimetered stenotic orifice areas obtained on multiplane TEE and continuity equation valve areas and/or Gorlin valve areas,[85-88] others have found planimetry of the aortic orifice to be difficult and less accurate than continuity equation valve areas obtained from transthoracic imaging.[89] Such an approach is only needed in a small subset of patients, mostly when transthoracic imaging quality is poor such as in ventilated patients an intensive care unit (ICU) setting.

Also, Doppler TEE has been applied using a transgastric view.[90,91] Aortic valve area as derived from Doppler TEE was similar to that measured by planimetry but could not be obtained in approximately 70% of patients because of failure to adequately align the Doppler beam.[91]

Three-Dimensional Echocardiography

3D echocardiography has largely been used as a research tool but has become widely available in commercial echocardiographic systems. Two small series report the use of this imaging modality to planimeter the inner surface of the aortic valve leaflets in 23 and 48 patients, respectively.[92,93] Measurements were reported to be feasible in the majority of patient with a good correlation of the valve area to that derived by the Gorlin formula. Nevertheless, 3D echocardiography is not an accepted standard for the quantification of AS.

Physiologic Variability in Measures of Stenosis Severity

Exercise Hemodynamics

Exercise testing is contraindicated in symptomatic patients with severe valvular AS due to the high risk of complications.[94] However, exercise testing can be safely performed in asymptomatic patients; a number of studies have provided insight into the relationship between hemodynamic severity and clinical symptoms[74,95-101] (Table 23-2). In asymptomatic patients with AS, exercise results in an appropriate rise in heart rate and CO. The increase in CO with upright exercise is mediated almost entirely by heart rate with little change in SV. However, even though SV remains constant, transaortic volume flow rate is increased as a result from the shortening of the systolic ejection period. Thus, exercise results in an increase in peak aortic jet velocity, with a corresponding increase in the mean transaortic gradient as predicted by the Bernoulli equation.

The continuity equation predicts a linear relationship between maximum volume flow rate (Q_{max}) and maximum jet velocity (V_{max}) for any given valve area.[101] In clinical studies—where normally only two data points can be acquired—the slope of the change in V_{max} relative to Q_{max} parallels the slope predicted by the continuity equation in patients when the valve area remains constant with exercise. If the valve area increases with exercise, the observed slope is greater than that predicted for a fixed valve area.

Changes in Aortic Valve Area with Changes in Volume Flow Rate

The effect of changes in volume flow rate on valve areas calculated using the Gorlin and the continuity equation has been examined in in vitro and animal models[102] and in patients with valvular AS (Fig. 23-17). These studies consistently show an increase in valve area with an increase in transaortic volume flow rate.[74,80,95,97,100,103-106] Although these apparent increases could be the result of some extent to errors inherent to the valve area formulas, the concept that valve area itself, both anatomic and physiologic, varies with transaortic volume flow rate is supported by in vitro

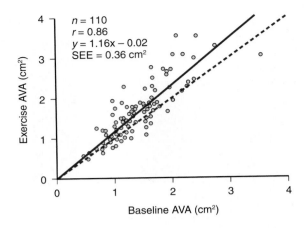

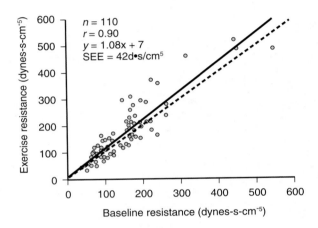

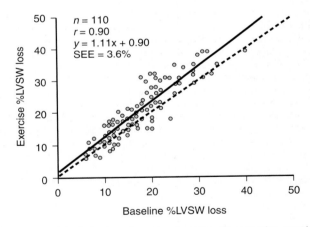

Figure 23-17. Relation of rest and continuity equation aortic valve area (top), aortic valve resistance (middle), and percent left ventricular stroke work loss (bottom) in 110 exercise studies. The slopes of the regression lines (solid line) are greater than the line of identity (dashed line), demonstrating an increase in all three indexes with exercise. AVA, aortic valve area; LVSW, left ventricular stroke work. AVA, aortic valve area; LVSW, left ventricular stroke work. (From Burwash IG, Pearlman AS, Kraft CD, et al: J Am Coll Cardiol 24:1342-1350, 1994.)

TABLE 23–2. Physiologic Changes with Exercise in Adults with Valvular Aortic Stenosis

	Bache/71[97]	Ettinger/72[98]	Otto/92[101]	Martin/92[100]	Burwash/94[103]
N	20	10	28	85	110
Measurements	Invasive	Invasive	Doppler echocardiography	Invasive	Doppler echocardiography
Type of Exercise	Supine bicycle	Supine bicycle	Treadmill	Supine bicycle	Treadmill
HR (bpm)					
Rest	79±3	87±5	71±17	71±2	63±14
Exercise	112±5	109±5	147±28	98±2	104±23
Systolic BP (mm Hg)					
Rest	120±3	118±8	139±15	—	143±22
Exercise	136±3	133±8	155±24	—	163±29
SV (ml)					
Rest	—	—	98±29	—	103±30
Exercise	—	—	89±32	—	96±30
Q_{mean} (ml/s)					
Rest	245±14	—	300±85	275±8	319±80
Exercise	318±21	—	366±159	325±10	400±140
CO (L/min)					
Rest	5.4±0.3	8.6±1.1	6.5±1.7	6.0±0.2	6.3±1.7
Exercise	8.5±0.6	9.2±0.9	10.7±4.4	9.3±0.2	9.9±3.8
ΔP mean (mm Hg)					
Rest	59±4	37±9	39±20	37±2	30±14
Exercise	74±5	38±11	52±26	41±2	41±18
Vmax (m/s)					
Rest	—	—	4.0±0.9	—	3.6±0.8
Exercise	—	—	4.6±1.1	—	4.3±0.8
AVA (cm²)					
Rest	0.8±0.1	1.8±0.3	1.2±0.5	1.1±0.1	1.4±0.5
Exercise	0.9±0.1	1.9±0.3	1.3±0.7	1.3±0.1	1.6±0.7
Valve resistance (dyne-s-cm⁻⁵)					
Rest	—	—	—	191±12	137±81
Exercise	—	—	—	182±12	155±97
Stroke work loss (%)					
Rest	—	—	—	26±1	17±7
Exercise	—	—	—	25±1	20±9
LV-EDP (mm Hg)					
Rest	12±6	15±3	—	—	—
Exercise	20±2	15±4	—	—	—

AVA, aortic valve area; BP, blood pressure; CO, cardiac output; ΔP, pressure gradient; HR, heart rate; LV-EDP, left ventricular end-diastolic pressure; SV, stroke volume; Vmax, peak aortic jet velocity.
Data from references 97, 98, 100, 101, 103.

pulsatile flow model data[71] and video imaging of flow-dependent changes in valve opening.[107] Another recent study confirmed that the effects of flow-rate changes on the valve area are not a result of artifacts but can be explained by an actual increase in leaflet opening with increasing flow rates and to unsteady effects at low flow rates.[108] This finding is in agreement with the observation that even normal aortic valve leaflets open less when volume flow rate is decreased; for example, in patients with a dilated cardiomyopathy.

Change in Other Measures of Stenosis Severity with Change in Volume Flow Rate

Some investigators have suggested that valve resistance is independent of flow rate,[104,109] whereas others have shown changes in valve resistance with changes in volume flow rate both in in vitro models,[71] animal models, and in patients with asymptomatic aortic stenosis.[27,103] In part, the relative stability of valve resistance with changes in flow rate observed in some studies[69,110] may relate to the range of stenosis severity evaluated. As a result of the curvilinear relationship between resistance and valve area, with larger valve areas (right side of curve), resistance changes little even with substantial changes in valve area, whereas with smaller valve areas (left side of curve), large changes in resistance are expected with only small changes in valve area.

Similarly, LV stroke work loss varies with changes in volume flow rate.[71,74,111] Overall, there is an inverse correlation between valve area and both total and steady LV stroke work loss. However, for a specific valve anatomy, work loss increases with an increase in SV despite a concurrent increase in valve area. This suggests that for a given degree of leaflet stiffness, greater opening of the valve is achieved at the expense of greater work loss. Alternatively, because work includes both potential and kinetic energy, a decrease in the percentage of potential work converted to kinetic work would lead to this observation. In studies to date, only potential work has been measured resulting from the conceptual and technical difficulties in measurement of kinetic work. Changes in the effective frictional loss component with changes in volume flow rate also may affect calculated measures of stenosis severity.

Theoretical Considerations

Degenerative calcific aortic valve stenosis is characterized by thickened, stiff leaflets without commissural fusion. Given this anatomic substrate, it is not surprising that the degree of valve opening varies with the amount of force applied to the valve, whether this force is represented by the surgeon's finger, a balloon valvuloplasty catheter, or the rate and volume of blood ejected by the left ventricle. Most investigators to date have found that each proposed measure of stenosis severity, when examined in detail, varies with changes in volume flow rate. These measures include peak LV to aortic pressure gradient, mean transaortic pressure gradient, maximum Doppler aortic jet velocity, Gorlin valve area, continuity equation valve area, LV stroke work loss, and valve resistance. Despite this potential limitation, most clinical decisions can be made with a high degree of reliability using these, albeit imperfect, indices of disease severity. For the quantification of AS

severity, the specific goals of measuring severity, for example being clinical patient management or research applications, must be specified.

The ideal measure of stenosis severity for clinical decision making should reflect disease severity and even more importantly be predictive of clinical outcome, while at the same time having an acceptable intraobserver and interobserver reproducibility. In addition, it should be noninvasive, easy to perform, readily available, and inexpensive. Clearly, Doppler echocardiographic measures of jet velocity and valve area meet these criteria. In the clinical setting, the impetus to derive a flow-independent measure of stenosis severity arises from the relatively unusual clinical situation in which there is coexisting LV systolic dysfunction and an anatomically abnormal aortic valve. Potential approaches to this clinical dilemma are discussed later in this chapter.

For specific research applications additional characteristics are warranted. One research goal is to explain the paradox of the marked overlap in hemodynamic severity between symptomatic and asymptomatic patients with AS. Some patients with hemodynamically severe disease remain asymptomatic, whereas other patients with only moderate valve obstruction develop definite symptoms.[64,65,112] Whether these apparent discrepancies between hemodynamic severity and clinical manifestations of disease are related to other factors (such as diastolic ventricular function[113]) or whether they reflect the inadequacy of available measures of stenosis severity remains unclear.

The assessment of disease progression over time is another important research application. The aim is to define the natural history and potential predictors of outcome of this disease and to assess the effects of potential therapies directed towards preventing or slowing the hemodynamic progression of AS. Determination of hemodynamic progression is also important in the clinical setting.[10] For this purpose, measures of stenosis severity with a high degree of reproducibility over time and between institutions are required.

The Left Ventricular Response to Valvular Aortic Stenosis

Diastolic Function

The initial physiologic response to chronic pressure overload of the left ventricle is impaired early diastolic relaxation as manifested by a prolonged time constant of relaxation (τ), a lengthened isovolumic relaxation time (IVRT), and a reduced early diastolic filling velocity, similar to the changes seen in patients with systemic hypertension.[114-118] Changes in diastolic function typically precede evidence of systolic dysfunction and thus may be present early in the disease course. Although some investigators suggest that Doppler measures of early and late diastolic filling velocities (or rates) may not be sensitive for detection of early diastolic dysfunction,[118] others propose that diastolic parameters can distinguish symptomatic from asymptomatic patients.[113] Tissue Doppler imaging (TDI) has been reported to allow estimation the diastolic performance and LV filling pressures in these patients.[119] Later in the disease course, decreased diastolic compliance plus a rightward shift on the passive diastolic pressure-volume relationship may result in a filling patient characterized by a shortened IVRT, increased early diastolic filling velocity, rapid early deceleration slope, and reduced atrial contribution to diastolic filling, a pattern often referred to as pseudonormalization.[117]

Wall Stress and Concentric Hypertrophy

As the severity of stenosis increases, concentric LV hypertrophy develops in response to the chronic elevation in LV systolic pressure. This increase in myocardial wall thickness allows maintenance of normal wall stress given that wall stress is directly related to chamber pressure and dimension but inversely related to wall thickness. LV hypertrophy is assessed most reliably by calculation of LV mass, although simple chamber dimensions and diastolic wall thickness may be adequate for clinical evaluation in many patients.

In general, the time course of development of LV hypertrophy parallels the course of stenosis severity in most patients. As demonstrated by a reduced coronary vasodilator reserve, LV hypertrophy in patients with AS is associated with abnormalities in coronary microcirculatory function.[120] This microcirculatory dysfunction may not necessarily be explained by the presence of hypertrophy itself but rather by an increased extravascular compression and a reduced diastolic perfusion time.[121] In particular, in this study, changes in coronary microcirculation after aortic valve replacement were not directly related to a regression of LV mass.

In some individuals, the degree of hypertrophy appears out of proportion to the severity of AS. In these cases, other causes for hypertrophy, such as hypertension, coexisting hypertrophic cardiomyopathy, or an infiltrative myocardial process, should be considered. It is particularly important to evaluate these possibilities carefully on 2D imaging because the clinical presentation of hypertrophic cardiomyopathy may be similar to that of valvular AS. The high prevalence of arterial hypertension in patients with AS may explain some of the cases of hypertrophy, in particular when AS is only mild.[122] Genetic factors also play a role in the degree of LV hypertrophy. For example, recent studies found that certain polymorphisms of the angiotensin-converting enzyme (ACE) gene were associated with increased LV hypertrophy.[123,124] Excessive ventricular hypertrophy has also been reported to result in an increased risk of postoperative mortality.[125]

Gender Differences

Several investigators have found significant gender differences in the LV response to the chronic pressure overload of AS.[126] In symptomatic patients referred for aortic valvuloplasty, although women and men had similar valve areas, women had higher transaortic gradients, higher relative wall thicknesses, and a higher prevalence of LV hypertrophy using gender-specific hypertrophy criteria. In addition, women had a lower functional status score for the same degree of aortic valve obstruction.[127] Another study observed higher peak LV pressures, higher ejection fractions (EFs), smaller LV end-diastolic dimensions, and a higher relative wall thickness in women, compared to men, with AS.[128] Although LV mass did not differ in women versus men, LV geometry differed as reflected in a lower circumferential wall stress for a given degree of hypertrophy.

Similar findings were observed in a consecutive series of asymptomatic AS patients.[129] Even though there were no gender differences in AS severity, women reported more functional limitation, had smaller LV end-diastolic and end-systolic volumes, and mass index but had a higher relative wall thickness and fractional shortening compared to men. In addition, women had a shorter treadmill exercise duration and a smaller increase in CO with exercise even though heart rate and blood pressure responses were similar in men and women.[129]

The importance of gender differences in the LV response to chronic pressure overload are illustrated by the observation that after aortic valve replacement in patients with depressed LV systolic function (EF < 45%), women had a greater improvement in ejection fraction at a mean of 1.4 years after valve replacement, although survival was similar between men and women. The ejection fraction increased from 33±8% to 48±15% in women, compared to 32±9% to 42±15% in men ($p < 0.02$).[130]

In summary, the degree of increase in LV mass is variable, in both men and women. However, women tend to have small ventricles with thick walls, low wall stress, and normal or hyperdynamic systolic function. In contrast, men tend to have LV dilation with normal wall thickness, increased wall stress, and depressed systolic function. Polymorphisms in the ACE gene might account for a gender specific modulation of ventricular hypertrophy in AS.[124]

Systolic Dysfunction

LV systolic dysfunction resulting from valvular AS usually occurs late in the course of the disease. Given the high ventricular afterload resulting from the stenotic valve, LV contractility typically remains normal, despite a low ejection fraction. Relief of the high afterload with valve replacement leads to rapid normalization of systolic function in the majority of patients. However, in adult patients, LV systolic dysfunction may be caused by other mechanisms than AS, such as coronary artery or myocardial disease. Under these circumstances, LV function often fails to improve with valve replacement, and the outcome remains poor. In the setting of a moderate aortic valve gradient, distinguishing poor LV systolic function resulting from severe AS from that resulting from concurrent ischemic or myocardial disease with only moderate aortic valve disease remains a difficult dilemma. One approach to this problem is to use a flow independent measure of stenosis severity or to look at the change in stenosis severity with a change in volume flow rate; an alternate approach is to utilize a load-independent measure of LV contractility to evaluate myocardial function. Unfortunately, a load-independent measure of contractility has proven as elusive as a flow-independent measure of stenosis severity.[118,128]

Natural History and Progression of Aortic Stenosis

Natural History

The natural history of AS is characterized by an asymptomatic phase of variable duration, during which the left ventricle is subjected to an increasing outflow ob-

struction and adaptive mechanisms[131-133] (Table 23–3). The occurrence of symptoms clearly presents a change in the natural history of the disease. Patients with congenital AS may become symptomatic in early childhood or adolescence; in particular, patients with unicuspid valves tend to present with early symptoms. Later, at young adult age, these patients may also present with symptoms resulting from restenosis after a surgical valvotomy in childhood. In patients with a congenital bicuspid stenotic aortic valve, surgery is typically performed at an age of 50 to 70 years.[2,134,135] In the elderly patient with degenerative calcific valve disease, symptom onset may already occur at an age of 50 years but typically occurs in at an age of 70 to 90 years.[2]

Rheumatic valvular AS has a variable course with significant aortic valve obstruction (in conjunction with mitral valve involvement) occurring over a wide age range.

Asymptomatic versus Symptomatic Aortic Stenosis and Severe versus Nonsevere Aortic Stenosis

With an aging population, the incidence of calcific aortic valve disease is increasing. Furthermore, with the widespread use of echocardiography, the diagnosis is made even more commonly in asymptomatic patients

TABLE 23–3. Event-Free Survival of Patients with Aortic Stenosis

First Author (Year)	Entry Criteria	Symptom Status	n	Age (yrs)	AS-Severity	Mean Follow-Up	Event-Free Survival
Kelly (1988)[141]	$V_{max} \geq 3.6$ m/s	Asymptomatic Symptomatic	51 39	63±19 72±11	ΔP 68±19 mm Hg ΔP 68±19 mm Hg	15±10 months	90% at 2 yr 60% at 2 yr
Pellikka (1990)[61]	$V_{max} \geq 4$ m/s	Asymptomatic	143	72 (40-94)	V_{max} 4.4 (4-6.4) m/s	20 months	62% at 2 yr
Kennedy (1991)[142]	Moderate AS at cath, no AVR	18% asymptomatic	66	67±10	AVA 0.92±0.13 cm²	35 months	59% at 4 yr
Otto (1997)[60]	Abnormal valve with $V_{max} > 2.6$ m/s	Asymptomatic	123	63±16	$V_{max} < 3.0$ m/s V_{max} 3-4 m/s $V_{max} > 4.0$ m/s	2.5 years	84% at 2 yr 66% at 2 yr 21% at 2 yr
Rosenhek (2000)[10]	Abnormal valve with $V_{max} > 4.0$ m/s	Asymptomatic	128	60±18	V_{max} 5.0±0.7 m/s	22±18 months	67% at 1 yr 56% at 2 yr 33% at 4 yr
Rosenhek (2003)[68]	Abnormal valve with V_{max} 2.5 to 3.9 m/s	Asymptomatic	176	58±19	V_{max} 3.1±0.4 m/s	48±19 months	95% at 1 yr 75% at 2 yr 60% at 5 yr
Pellikka (2005)[150]	Abnormal valve with $V_{max} > 4.0$ m/s	Asymptomatic	622	72±11	V_{max} 4.4±0.4 m/s	5.4±4.0 years	82% at 1 yr 67% at 2 yr 33% at 5 yr

AS, aortic stenosis; AVA, aortic valve area; AVI, aortic valve index; AVR, aortic valve replacement; cath, catheterization; ΔP, pressure gradient; Vmax, maximum aortic jet velocity.
Data from references 10, 60, 61, 68, 141, 142, 150.

as coincidental finding or after suspicion resulting from a systolic murmur. Its spectrum ranges from severe symptomatic stenosis on one side to aortic sclerosis without hemodynamic implications on the other. In between are the asymptomatic patients with severe, moderate, and mild AS. The incidence of AS in the population of advanced age is estimated to be between 2% and 9%, aortic sclerosis is present in up to 25% of patients over 65 years of age.[67,136,137]

The first step in the clinical decision-making process for the timing of intervention in a patient with valvular AS is a careful history as to whether symptoms (angina, exertional dizziness, exercise intolerance, or heart failure) are present or absent. The use of exercise testing may be appropriate in asymptomatic patients and may unmask latent symptoms in up to one third of these apparently asymptomatic patients.[138,139] It has to be emphasized that exercise testing is only appropriate in asymptomatic patients but should definitely not be performed in symptomatic patients. When properly performed, exercise testing in asymptomatic patients with severe AS has been shown to be safe.[138]

Symptomatic Severe Aortic Stenosis

The poor outcome of patients with severe symptomatic AS has been well documented in the past.[132] After the onset of symptoms, the average survival has been reported to be less than 2 to 3 years (Fig. 23–18). This data was derived from studies of patients who refused surgical intervention.[64,65,131,140-143] In patients with severe, symptomatic AS, predictors of survival include

the transaortic gradient or velocity, LV systolic function as assessed qualitatively by echocardiography, age, and gender.[144] Of note, patients with a higher transaortic gradient have a better prognosis, most likely because when severe stenosis is present, a low gradient indicates a low transaortic stroke volume. On the other hand, current results of aortic valve replacement for acquired AS have been shown to be excellent.[64] Valve surgery for relief of stenosis remains the appropriate treatment for symptomatic patients, even the elderly.[145,146] Thus, it has generally been accepted that surgery must be strongly recommended for patients with critical AS who develop symptoms. Only rarely does severe comorbid disease result in an unacceptably high operative morbidity and mortality. Surprisingly, in clinical practice surgery seems to be denied far more frequently than would actually be expected in elderly patients, less so appropriately because of comorbidities but more often inappropriately in patients with LV dysfunction and older age.[147]

Asymptomatic Severe Aortic Stenosis

The management of asymptomatic patients with severe AS remains a matter of controversy. It is important to understand that it has been shown that it is relatively safe to delay surgery until symptoms develop following a watchful waiting strategy.[10] However, there are concerns when patients with AS are following a conservative treatment plan.[148] When treating asymptomatic patients with AS conservatively, the risk of sudden death is one of the major concerns. In three

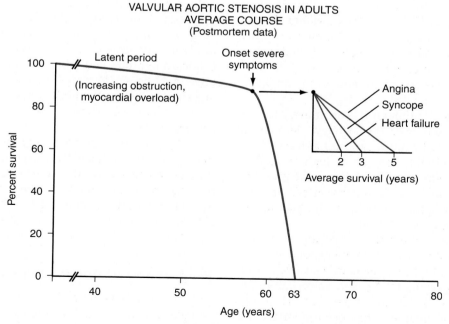

Figure 23–18. *Natural history of aortic stenosis. Poor outcome is indicated by the occurrence of symptoms. (From Ross J Jr, Braunwald E: Circulation Supplement 5:V-61–V-67, 1968.)*

studies in which significant numbers of patients with nonsevere stenosis were included, no sudden death was reported: Otto and colleagues[60] followed 123 patients with an average peak velocity of 3.6 ± 0.6 m/s for 30 months. The two other series with 51[141] and 37 patients[149] had follow-up periods of 1.5 and 2 years, respectively. Only two studies reported the outcome of larger cohorts of patients with exclusively severe stenosis as defined by a peak aortic jet velocity is equal to 4 m/s. Pellikka and colleagues[61] observed two sudden deaths among 113 patients during a mean follow-up of 20 months. Both patients, however, had developed symptoms at least 3 months before death. In a recently published study, which is the largest to date, 11 sudden deaths were observed among 622 patients have been followed for a mean of 5.4 years.[150] Rosenhek and colleagues[10] reported one sudden death that was not preceded by any symptoms among 104 patients followed for 27 months on average. Thus, sudden death may indeed occur even in the absence of preceding symptoms in patients with AS, but this appears to be an uncommon event with a rate of probably less than one percent per year during the asymptomatic phase of the disease. Finally, it has to be considered, that sudden death has even been reported after successful valve replacement with an incidence of about 0.3%, and this risk cannot be entirely eliminated by surgical treatment.[151,152]

Another concern, when conservatively treating patients with severe AS is that they do not report the occurrence of new symptoms promptly and are then subjected to an increased risk of sudden death. The same thoughts apply to symptomatic patients on waiting lists for aortic valve surgery, which are still encountered in some countries with mortality rates of around 14% per year.[153] Operative mortality is also significantly lower, as long as the patients are only mildly symptomatic and when surgery is scheduled in comparison to an increased surgical risk for more symptomatic patients or urgent and even emergent surgery.

On the other hand, although the operative risk has dramatically decreased over the last few decades, it must be considered to be in the range of at least 2% to 3%.[154] Operative mortality may be as high as 10% in the elderly[155] and even markedly higher in the presence of comorbidities, such as coronary artery disease (CAD).[156] In an asymptomatic patient, this risk has to be outweighed by a proven benefit.

After valve replacement with a mechanical or bioprosthetic valve, valve related complications such as thromboembolism, bleeding, endocarditis, valve thrombosis, paravalvular regurgitation, and valve failure occur at a rate of at least 2% to 3% per year. Death directly related to the prosthesis has been reported at a rate of up to 1% per year. The individual course of the disease is highly variable, and some patients have been followed for many years without developing symptoms. Considering that valve replacement does not represent a cure in this disease, general recommendation of early surgery can therefore not be justified.

In particular, an appropriate risk stratification individually selecting those patients who are likely to benefit from early elective surgery is required.

Aortic Sclerosis and Mild-to-Moderate Aortic Stenosis

A number of older studies have reported a relatively benign course of moderate AS, suggesting a stable course of the disease.[64,131,140] These data have led many physicians to believe that mild and moderate AS represent a relatively benign disease, although one study described a poor outcome of moderate AS with 14 deaths attributed to AS among 66 patients followed for 35 months.[142] However, most of these studies date back to catheter era and are limited by small patient numbers and their retrospective nature.[64,131,140,142]

More recent studies have shed a new light on the seriousness of the disease. In a community-based study it was shown that the presence of aortic valve sclerosis is associated with a significantly increased cardiovascular and all-cause mortality in the absence of hemodynamic obstruction to blood flow.[67] Recent studies have also shown that mild-to-moderate AS is not a benign disease with an increased cardiovascular and also an increased noncardiac mortality.[60,68] Thus aortic sclerosis and mild-to-moderate AS have to be viewed as indicators for a poor overall prognosis.

In addition, the prognosis of these patients is also influenced by a progression of the disease. In fact, the progression of aortic sclerosis to AS affects about 16% of patients within a short time period.[157] The interval between observing aortic valve sclerosis on echocardiography and clinical evidence of severe stenosis may be as short as 5 to 10 years. Also the progression to severe, hemodynamically significant stenosis is common and may be more rapid than previously assumed.[68]

As long as the AS is not severe these patients can be managed conservatively. However, knowing that rapid progression to severe AS may occur, it is important to instruct even patients with mild and moderate AS about the typical symptoms of severe AS and the necessity to immediately refer to a physician in case that they appear.

Progression of Aortic Stenosis

Until recently, data on the hemodynamic progression of valvular AS was limited to studies of patients who had undergone two or more cardiac catheterizations.[158-163]

The fact that only patients who did not die or undergo valve replacement after the first catheterization and required a second catheterization for clinical indications are included in these series clearly resulted in a selection bias.

The availability of an accurate, noninvasive method to evaluate hemodynamic severity has allowed larger and more detailed studies on the rate of hemodynamic progression.[10,68,79,112,149,164-168] Also recent intervention studies, designed to assess the effects of statin therapy in halting or delaying the progression of AS provide additional information on hemodynamic progression[169-173] (Table 23-4). Overall, these studies showed an average rate of increase in mean pressure gradient of about 8 mm Hg per year and a decrease in valve area between 0.15 cm^2 per year. In these studies, the average rate of increase in aortic jet maximum velocity ranges from 0.2 to 0.4 m/s/year. However, marked individual variability in the rate of hemodynamic progression was observed (Figs. 23–19 and 23–20). Although Doppler echocardiographic studies have the advantage of larger patient numbers and potentially less selection bias (a repeat echocardiographic study is likely to be requested more often than a repeat cardiac catheterization), many of these studies are retrospective with the data extracted from ongoing clinical databases. Thus, patients with rapid progression, those developing symptoms, or those requiring surgical intervention may be overrepresented. Conversely, repeat studies may not have been performed in clinically stable patients. The results of more recent prospective studies may avoid some of these biases.[10,60,171]

As the disease progresses, increasing obstruction to LV outflow most often is reflected by a decrease in valve area and an increase in jet velocity and pressure gradient. However, if there is a concurrent decrease in transaortic volume flow rate, a decrease in valve area alone may be seen with no change in jet velocity or transaortic gradient. This situation may occur secondary to comorbid disease, such as increasing MR or myocardial infarction but may be a result of a decrease in LV function late in the disease course of isolated AS. On the other hand, an increase in jet velocity and pressure gradient with no change in valve area may be observed if transaortic SV is increased resulting from hyperdynamic states (e.g., anemia, fever, pregnancy) or increasing AR.

Risk Stratification

Clinical Factors and Factors Predicting Hemodynamic Progression

At this point, it is not clear whether the rate of hemodynamic progression in an individual patient is either predictable or "steady." In fact, it is most likely that the

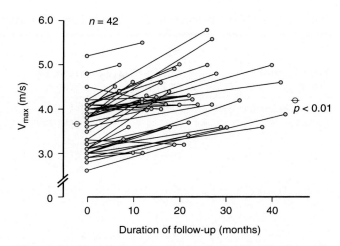

Figure 23–19. Maximal aortic jet velocity (V_{max}) is plotted for the initial and final Doppler studies in 42 asymptomatic patients. Group means are indicated by the symbol ⊖. (From Otto CM, Pearlman AS, Gardner CL: J Am Coll Cardiol 13:545-550, 1989).

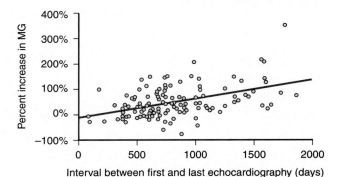

Figure 23–20. Change in mean aortic gradient (MG) in 394 consecutive patients with aortic stenosis represented according to the follow-up duration. Although there was a strong correlation predicting the increase of the gradient over time (r = 0.40; p < 0.0001), interindividual variability of hemodynamic progression can be appreciated. (From Brener SJ, Duffy CI, Thomas JD, Stewart WJ: J Am Coll Cardiol 25:305-310, 1995.)

rate of progression is nonlinear; that is, a fairly slow rate of progression may change to a rapid increase in severity when the opposing forces of LV ejection and leaflet stiffness can no longer be balanced.

Factors that predict the rate of hemodynamic progression in an individual patient have remained elusive. Clearly, valve anatomy is an important factor in disease progressive because most patients with a bicuspid stenotic valve require surgical intervention at a younger age than those with degenerative AS.[135] Gender also is important because the ratio of men to women with AS is approximately 2 to 1. Other factors associated with the rate of disease progression are the

TABLE 23–4. **Hemodynamic Progression of Valvular Aortic Stenosis**

First Author (Year)	Clinical Status at Entry	Type of Study	n	Mean Follow-up (years)	Increase in Mean ΔP (mm Hg/yr)	Increase in V_{max} (m/s/yr)	Decrease in Aortic Valve Area (cm²/yr)
Catheterization Studies							
Bogart (1979)[158]	Two cardiac caths	Retrospective	11	4.9	11.6 (1.2 to 24)	—	0.2 (0.02 to 0.6)
Cheitlin (1979)[159]	Two cardiac caths	Retrospective	29	4	8.4 (−12 to 45)	—	—
Wagner (1982)[163]	Two cardiac caths	Retrospective	50	3.5	"Rapid" (n = 21)	—	0.32±0.20
					"Slow" (n = 29)	—	0.02±0.13
Jonasson (1983)[161]	Calcific AS	Retrospective	26	9	—	—	0.1
Nestico (1983)[162]	Two cardiac caths	Retrospective	29	5.9	0.8 (−8 to 10.4)	—	0.05 (0 to 0.5)
Davies, (1991)[160]	Two cardiac catheters	Retrospective	47	—	6.5 (−10 to 38)	—	—
Echocardiographic Studies							
Otto (1989)[112]	Asymptomatic	Prospective	42	1.7	8 (−7 to 23)	0.36±0.31	0.1 (0 to 0.5)
Roger (1990)[168]	AS on echo	Retrospective	112	2.1	—	0.23±0.37	—
Faggiano (1992)[149]	AS on echo	Prospective	45	1.5	—	0.4±0.3	0.1±0.13 (−0.7 to 0.1)
Peter (1993)[167]	AS on echo	Retrospective	49	2.7	7.2	—	—
Brener (1995)[165]	AS on echo	Retrospective	394	6.3	—	—	0.14
Otto (1997)[60]	Asymptomatic	Prospective	123	2.5	7±7	0.32±0.34	0.12±0.19
Bahler (1999)[164]	AS on echo	Retrospective	91	1.8	2.8	0.2	0.04
Palta (2000)[166]	AS on echo	Retrospective	170	1.9	—	—	0.10±0.27
Rosenhek (2000)[10]	AS on echo with V_{max} > 4.0 m/s	Prospective	128	1.8	Slow / Rapid	0.14±0.18 / 0.45±0.38	—
Rosenhek (2000)[10]	AS on echo with V_{max} 2.5 to 3.9 m/s	Retrospective	176	3.8	—	0.24±0.30	—
Echocardiographic Intervention Studies							
Novaro (2000)[172]	AS on echo with AVA 1.0 to 1.8 cm²	Retrospective	174	1.7	Statin therapy / No statin	— / —	0.06±0.16 / 0.11±0.18
Bellamy (2002)[170]	AS on echo with AVA < 2.0 cm²	Retrospective	156	3.7	Statin therapy / No statin	— / —	0.04±0.15 / 0.09±0.17
Rosenhek (2004)[173]	AS on echo with V_{max} > 2.5 m/s	Retrospective	211	2.0	Statin therapy / No statin	0.1±0.41 / 0.39±0.42	— / —
Cowell (2005)[171]	AS on echo with V_{max} > 2.5 m/s	Prospective	134	2.1	Statin therapy / No statin	0.2±0.21 / 0.2±0.21	0.08±0.11 / 0.08±0.11
Moura (2007)[236]	AS on echo with AVA 1.0 to 1.5 cm²	Prospective	121	1.4	Statin therapy / No statin	0.4±0.38 / 0.24±0.30	0.05±0.12 / 0.1±0.09

AS, aortic stenosis; AVA, aortic valve area; caths, cardiac catheterizations; ΔP, pressure gradient; echo, echocardiography; V_{max}, peak aortic jet velocity.
Data from references 10, 60, 112, 149, 158-168, 170-173, 236.

severity of AS when initially seen (more severe disease leads to symptoms more rapidly than milder disease) and age (older patients have more rapid disease progression than younger patients). Clinical factors, such as elevated serum lipid levels, hypertension, smoking, and diabetes, have been found to be associated with AS.[174] In addition, a recent study found that smoking, hypercholesterolemia, and elevated creatinine and calcium levels were associated with more rapid disease progression.[166] However, further studies are needed to confirm these results. Three recent studies suggest that the amount of aortic valve calcium is an important determinate of disease progression.[10,68,164] These studies found an association between the rate of disease progression and the presence of a calcified aortic valve. Furthermore, these studies confirmed previous observations that the rate of disease progression is highly variable for individual patients.

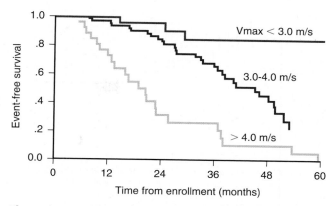

Figure 23–21. *Kaplan-Meier event-free survival of 123 asymptomatic patients with aortic stenosis according to their degree of severity expressed by peak aortic jet velocity (Vmax) (p < 0.0001). (From Otto CM, Burwash IG, Legget ME, et al: Circulation 95:2262-2270, 1997.)*

Predictors of Outcome in Aortic Stenosis

The identification of predictors of outcome is particularly useful in the setting of asymptomatic patients with severe AS. On the one hand, the identification of high risk patients allows an optimized timing of control visits. On the other hand, specific predictors of outcome might define a subgroup of patients that would benefit from early elective surgery while still being asymptomatic.

One of the most important predictors of outcome in patients with AS is stenosis severity. A number of studies have confirmed that the necessity for subsequent aortic valve surgery is directly related with peak aortic jet velocity over the whole spectrum of disease with event rates being lowest in patients with mild stenosis, followed by moderate and severe stenosis[10,60,68] (Fig. 23–21).

Significant calcification, rapid hemodynamic progression, and the presence of CAD also indicate lower rates of event-free survival in patients with mild-to-moderate AS.[68]

In a prospective study including 126 patients with asymptomatic severe AS, the presence of a moderately-to-severely calcified aortic valve was associated with a significantly increased event rate, and 80% of these patients developed symptoms warranting aortic valve replacement or died within 4 years (Fig. 23–22). The combination of a calcified aortic valve with a rapid hemodynamic progression, defined as an increase in peak aortic jet velocity of more than 0.3 m/s within one year, identified a patient group at particularly high-risk with an event rate of 79% within 2 years[10] (Fig. 23–23). The echocardiographic determination of aortic valve calcification has the advantage of being fast and easily obtainable at the moment of the echocardio-

graphic examination. While being a semi-quantitative method, the differentiation between no or mild and moderate-to-severe calcification can be easily performed. The finding that aortic valve calcification is associated with a poor outcome was also confirmed by a study that assessed the degree of aortic valve calcification by electron beam tomography.[175]

Lancellotti and colleagues assessed the value of exercise Doppler echocardiographic measurements in 69 patients with severe asymptomatic AS.[176] In this study, an exercise-induced increase of mean transaortic gradient equal to 18 mm Hg (Fig. 23–24), an abnormal exercise test, and an aortic valve area of less than 0.75 cm^2 were significant predictors of subsequent events on multivariate analysis, and all had an incremental value when occurring together. Still these findings need confirmation in larger studies.

There is also a role for exercise testing in asymptomatic patients with severe AS for risk stratification and in unmasking symptoms. Patients who have a negative exercise test have a relatively good outcome.[138] On the other side, the exercise test is particularly useful in unmasking symptoms (up to 30% of patients) in apparently asymptomatic patients and has the best positive predictive value for active patients younger than 70 years.[139] The occurrence of an ST-segment depression, an abnormal blood pressure response, or the occurrence of arrhythmias during exercise had a lower predictive value in this study.[139]

Finally B-type natriuretic peptide (BNP) levels have been shown to correlate with the symptomatic status in patients with AS; however, it is unclear whether this information is of additional benefit to the physical examination.[177] An elevated BNP level is associated with a poor outcome, both in symptomatic and in asymptomatic patients.[178] Smaller studies have also shown

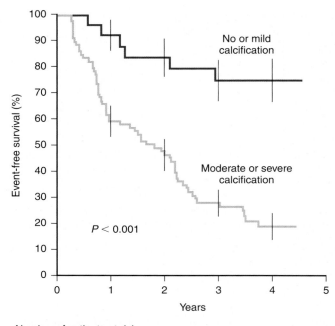

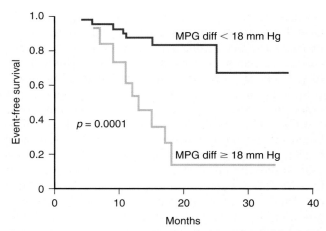

Figure 23–24. *Event-free survival curves according to exercise-induced changes in mean transaortic pressure gradient (MPG) in 69 consecutive patients with severe aortic stenosis. (From Lancellotti P, Lebois F, Simon M, et al:* Circulation *112[Supplement 9]:1377-1382, 2005.)*

Number of patients at risk:

No or mild calcification	25	23	20	17	9
Moderate or severe calcification	101	48	38	21	7

Figure 23–22. *Kaplan-Meier analysis of event-free survival among 25 patients with no or mild aortic valve calcification, as compared with 101 patients with moderate or severe calcification. The vertical bars indicate standard errors. All the subjects in this study had an initial aortic jet velocity of at least 4 m/s (mean 5±0.6 m/s). (From Rosenhek R, Binder T, Porenta G, et al:* New Engl J Med *343:611-617, 2000.)*

that BNP levels might also be useful for prediction of symptom onset but these findings have to be confirmed in larger studies.[179]

Scheduling Control Intervals

One of the main aims of a control examination is to assess the symptomatic status of the AS patient including a meticulous inquiry about any changes in physical condition.

Given the continued uncertainty regarding which factors predict progression in an individual patient, it is prudent to follow patients with aortic valve thickening closely, monitoring for early symptoms of valve obstruction. Periodic echocardiographic examinations also are warranted, particularly for any change in symptoms or functional status. Serial echocardiographic examinations are warranted to assess hemodynamic progression, changes in LV function and hypertrophy. There is no clear consensus with regard to the required follow-up intervals: In any case, they need to be individualized. The peak aortic jet velocity at entry should be considered as it reflects the stage of disease: patients with moderate AS will require earlier control examinations than patients with mild AS. Furthermore, the aforementioned risk factors—in particular the presence of a significantly calcified aortic valve, concurrent CAD, and rapid hemodynamic progression—allow further risk stratification. Serial echocardiographic examinations at yearly intervals are an accepted practice in most patients with moderate or severe AS. However, with rapid progression, shorter control intervals may be advisable, particularly when the aortic valve is calcified. Some of these high-risk patients might require half-yearly control examinations. It is definitely important to instruct even patients with nonsevere AS about the possibility

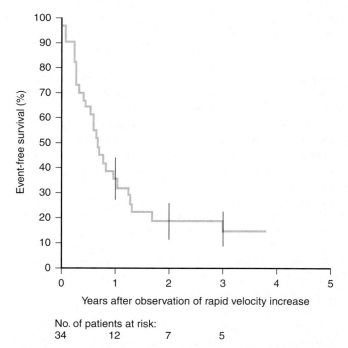

No. of patients at risk:

34	12	7	5

Figure 23–23. *Kaplan-Meier analysis of event-free survival patients with moderately to severely calcified aortic valves and a rapid hemodynamic progression defined by an increase in peak aortic jet velocity of more than 0.3 m/s within 12 months. The vertical bars indicate standard errors. (From Rosenhek R, Binder T, Porenta G, et al:* New Engl J Med *343:611-617, 2000.)*

of hemodynamic progression of their disease and of the importance to promptly report any symptoms. The goals of the follow-up visit are best summarized in an editorial by Catherine Otto titled "Listen to the Patient, Look at the Valve."[180]

Timing of Surgery in Patients with Nonsevere Aortic Stenosis Undergoing Cardiac Surgery

It is clear that a severely stenotic aortic valve should be replaced at the time of cardiac surgery performed for another reason. Uncertainty as to the rate of hemodynamic progression in an individual patient complicates the decision as to whether concurrent aortic valve replacement should be performed in patients in which is not severe who are undergoing coronary artery bypass surgery. Some surgeons recommend prophylactic valve replacement for moderate AS because otherwise reoperation may be needed within 5 years.[181] Definitely, the degree of severity and also risk factors associated with a rapid hemodynamic progression will have to be considered in this decision.[182,183] Furthermore, the combined risks of surgery and prosthesis associated complications have to be weighed against the risks of two separate operations if valve replacement is needed at a later time. For example the presence of a significantly calcified valve in a patient with moderate AS will balance the decision in favor of valve surgery.

Aortic Stenosis with Reduced Left Ventricular Function

The presence of reduced LV function in a patient with AS is generally associated with a poor outcome. However, there is a fundamental differentiation between patients with a high transaortic gradient, despite poor ventricular function, and those with a reduced transaortic gradient in the setting of a low volume flow rate.

AS with LV Dysfunction and a High Transaortic Gradient

It is recognized that patients with severe AS who have the onset of LV systolic dysfunction should undergo aortic valve replacement. These patients benefit from surgery and LV function can generally be expected to improve in this setting.

When LV function is significantly impaired and the duration of dysfunction is unknown, operative risk is significantly higher. However, improvement of LV function and of symptoms has been reported to occur in the majority of patients. Patients with reduced systolic function and a history of a prior myocardial infarction (MI) experience a particularly poor outcome following valve replacement.[184] Also, the presence of

atrial fibrillation predicts a higher operative risk and lower postoperative survival in patients with AS and reduced LV function.[185]

Low-Flow Low-Gradient Aortic Stenosis

The situation of low-flow low-gradient AS is particularly challenging. In this setting it is unclear whether valve opening is restricted as a result of excessive leaflet stiffness or whether there is only limited leaflet motion resulting from a low transaortic SV. Two different research approaches have been proposed to distinguish between severe AS with consequently depressed LV systolic function and nonsevere stenosis with reduced leaflet motion resulting from intrinsic LV dysfunction. These approaches are based either on a flow-independent measure of stenosis severity or a load-independent measure of LV systolic function. Although significant progress has been made with both of these approaches, neither approach has provided a clear answer.

The risk of aortic valve replacement surgery in the setting of low-flow low-gradient AS is high with an operative mortality in the range between 9% and 33%.[186-188]

However, symptomatic improvement and an improvement of LV function can be observed among the patients who survive surgery.[187,188]

If LV systolic dysfunction is a result of AS, improvement is expected after valve replacement. However, if LV dysfunction results from end-stage ischemic disease or a primary cardiomyopathy, little improvement is expected after aortic valve surgery.

Stress echocardiography with low-dose dobutamine (maximal dose 20 μg/kg/min) has been shown to be useful for the evaluation and risk stratification of these patients. In patients with relative or pseudosevere AS, the augmentation of transaortic volume flow rate will result in a significant increase (>0.2 cm^2) in valve area as the flexible leaflets open to a greater extent, while the transaortic gradient increased only slightly. Conversely, when true severe AS is present, valve area will change little due to stiff, rigid valve leaflets that do not respond to an increased flow rate, so that the transaortic gradients will increase significantly.

Another approach is to consider contractile reserve, defined as an increase in SV of 20% or more with dobutamine or exercise.[189] In the presence of contractile reserve, true severe AS can be differentiated from relative AS.[190,191] If the ventricle fails to respond to inotropic stimulation (i.e., no increase in CO), interpretation is more difficult.[104,190,192]

However, a small increase in AVA can be seen in some patients with surgically confirmed severe AS and therefore does not exclude fixed valve disease.[193] The effect of dobutamine infusion leads to a variable increase in transaortic flow rate, and in some patients, a given flow rate might not be reached. In an attempt to standardize these findings, the use of a projected AVA (at a normal flow rate of 250 ml/s), which is determined by plotting (and extrapolating if necessary) the AVA against transvalvular flow at the different stages of the examinations, has been proposed to improve accuracy for distinguishing true severe and pseudosevere AS.[194]

In the largest multicentric study published to date, patients with contractile reserve who underwent surgery had a significantly improved survival in comparison to medically treated patients with contractile reserve[189] (Fig. 23–25). Patients without contractile reserve had a poor overall survival, nevertheless a trend toward slightly improved outcome was seen even for patients without contractile reserve undergoing surgery as compared to those being followed medically. The failure of volume flow rate to increase may be a result of limitation of flow by a severely stenotic valve or may be a result of an unresponsive myocardium. In this study, only 7 out of 136 patients had relative AS. In contrast, in two smaller studies, 8 of 24 and 5 of 12 patients with contractile reserve had relative AS.[190,191] From these studies it also appears that surgery leads to an improved outcome in patients with true severe AS and preserved LV function. A recent study has shown that LV function may even improve in patients surviving aortic valve replacement surgery despite the absence of contractile reserve, suggesting that even in this subgroup of patients, surgery might be beneficial.[195] To optimize the strategy for these patients further studies are mandatory.

Although stress echocardiography may not always give all the expected answers, a pragmatic clinical approach to this patient group that includes looking at the valve, looking at the patient, and at the options might

be helpful. A heavily calcified valve will be an argument in favor of valve replacement whereas thin, flexible leaflets argue against valve surgery. If the risk of surgery is acceptable or if the patient is having surgery for coexisting CAD, the threshold for valve replacement is certainly lower. Assessment of the coronary arteries by angiography is an important part of the workup of these patients. If the risk of valve replacement is excessively high as a result of comorbid disease, medical therapy may be appropriate. If the patient has failed aggressive medical therapy, surgical intervention may be indicated even if the risk is high.

Assessment of Coronary Artery Disease

CAD is frequent in patients with calcific AS. In patients undergoing valve replacement for symptomatic AS, concurrent coronary artery bypass grafting (CABG) is recommended in the presence of significant CAD. If concomitant CAD is present at the time of aortic valve replacement for AS, operative mortality is significantly lower when additional coronary bypass grafting is performed (1.1% to 4.8%) in contrast to when valve replacement is performed alone (4% to 13.2%).[196,197] Also a significantly higher risk of sudden death after valve replacement is encountered when patients with concomitant CAD are not revascularized at the time of surgery.[198] Furthermore, the need of early reoperation for CAD is prevented.

In patients with AS with angina, the prevalence of significant CAD ranges from 40% to 80%, so that a preoperative coronary angiography is definitely needed.

However, even in the absence of angina the prevalence of significant CAD ranges between 0% and 54% (average 16%). The appropriate diagnostic approach to these patients is less clear. Exercise treadmill testing is contraindicated in symptomatic patients with AS. It is of note that even in asymptomatic patients, ST-segment depression during exercise is often nondiagnostic for the presence of CAD and is possibly related to LV hypertrophy.[101,199]

The utility of echocardiographic stress imaging for the diagnosis of CAD in patients with AS has not been extensively evaluated. Studies on the exercise physiology of AS or on the response to inotropic stimulation with dobutamine have focused on Doppler evaluation of AS severity and CO rather than on segmental wall motion abnormalities of the left ventricle.[109] A study including 50 patients with severe AS evaluated the use of adenosine stress echocardiography for the detection of CAD.[200] The sensitivity and specificity of stress echocardiography was 85% and 97%, respectively. In addition, no major complications occurred during the procedure. Clearly, these observations need confirmation in other studies. In our experience, definite exercise-induced reversible segmental wall motion abnormalities have been seen in a few patients with AS in whom subsequent coronary angiog-

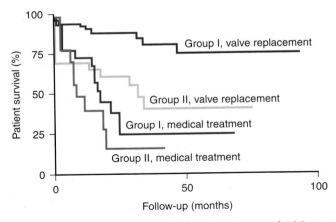

Figure 23–25. *Kaplan-Meier survival estimates of 136 consecutive patients with low-flow low-gradient aortic stenosis. Group I (n = 92) represents patients with contractile reserve determined by low-dose dobutamine echocardiography; Group II represents the group of patients with absent contractile reserve (n = 44). Survival estimates are represented according to contractile reserve and treatment strategy (aortic valve replacement versus medical therapy). (From Monin JL, Quere JP, Monchi M, et al: Circulation 108[3]:319-324, 2003).*

raphy confirmed significant CAD. More often however, no definite wall motion abnormalities are seen, even though subsequent catheterization does show greater than 50% narrowings in the coronary arteries. Whether this lack of sensitivity relates to exercise limitation by AS itself (the ischemic threshold is not reached), to diffuse subendothelial ischemia obscuring segmental abnormalities, or whether the degree of stenosis being treated with bypass grafting is insufficient to cause ischemia remains unclear. Further studies of stress echocardiography in AS patients may clarify this issue.

Exercise tomographic thallium imaging in patients with AS has a sensitivity of 90% and a specificity of 70% for the presence of significant (>50% luminal diameter narrowing) CAD.[201] Similarly, adenosine thallium stress testing in patients with AS has a sensitivity in the range of 88% to 92% and a specificity of only 71% to 72%.[202,203] When combined with a pretest likelihood of disease (based on gender, age, and cardiac risk factors), the posttest likelihood of CAD can be helpful in deciding whether or not coronary angiography is necessary and may result in a reduction in overall costs of patient evaluation.[204]

With advances in imaging quality, multidetector computed tomography (CT) coronary angiography is becoming increasingly available as a noninvasive technique for the assessment of the coronary anatomy. Recently, two small studies including a total of 82 patients with AS have reported negative predictive values of 100% and 99% for this technique to rule out the presence of significant CAD.[205,206] While these findings have to be confirmed in larger studies, this technique might become an alternative to coronary angiography in patients at low to moderate risk for the presence of CAD.

Currently, most clinicians choose to perform coronary angiography because of the low risk of this procedure and the potential impact of the diagnosis on the operative procedure and survival in a specific individual.

Arterial Hypertension

Approximately 40% of patients with AS have concomitant hypertension.[60,68] Patients with AS are a population at high risk for cardiovascular events,[68] thus requiring a thorough adjustment of their risk factors, one of them being arterial hypertension. In addition, the presence of arterial hypertension leads to an increased wall stress of the left ventricle. However, treatment of hypertension needs to be done cautiously in patients with AS.

There is a concern that vasodilators may lead to a reduction of the coronary perfusion pressure. In fact, the use of ACE inhibitors in AS is classically considered to be contraindicated.[207] In this context, the observation that the prescription rates for ACE inhibitors among patients with AS may be as high as 50% may appear surprising.

Although not designed to assess the safety of ACE inhibitor use in patients with AS, the findings of a retrospective study indicate that a significant number of patients with AS seen in daily clinical practice receive treatment with ACE inhibitors because of concomitant arterial hypertension (102 of 211 patients).[173] The observation that a high proportion of patients with documented AS already receive ACE inhibitors is also shared by O'Brien and colleagues.[208] In their series, 30% received an ACE inhibitor.

There are also data suggesting that their use may be safe in AS. O'Brien and colleagues have recently demonstrated that the initiation of ACE inhibitors was safe and well tolerated in a group of 13 patients with mild-to-moderate AS with preserved LV function.[208]

In the SCOPE-AS trial, symptomatic patients with severe AS and normal LV function who were not candidates for surgery, were randomized to treatment with enalapril or placebo.[209] ACE inhibitors were well tolerated in these patients; however, patients with reduced LV functions were prone to develop hypotension.

Finally, Jimenez-Candil and colleagues designed an elegant drug withdrawal study. Twenty patients with moderate-to-severe AS already receiving and ACE inhibitor were included.[210] Both the withdrawal and the careful reintroduction of the drug were well tolerated. While taking the ACE inhibitor, patients had a lower blood pressure and higher transvalvular gradients but kept an unchanged exercise capacity and symptomatic status.

These data suggest ACE inhibitors therapy may be cautiously used in patients with AS. However, it has to be considered, that with an increasing severity of AS, reducing the dosage of antihypertensive might be necessary because hypertension may become less accentuated and even hypotension may develop as a result of further narrowing of the aortic valve.

Optimizing the Surgical Approach

Evaluation of Patients with Aortic Stenosis Undergoing Noncardiac Surgery

Because of the high incidence of AS, the situation where these patients have to undergo noncardiac surgery is increasing. The urgency and importance of the noncardiac operation plays a central role for the management decisions.

In this setting, echocardiography allows assessment of disease severity, monitoring of LV function before, during, and after the procedure and alerting the clinician to the need for invasive hemodynamic monitoring in some cases. Some reports indicate that these patients, even with severe obstruction, can be managed without valve replacement if loading conditions are optimized preoperatively and careful invasive monitoring is continued in the postoperative period.[151,211,212] Other studies describe an increased perioperative mortality in patients with AS with a predictive role of the severity of the stenosis.[213,214] Common postoperative complications include pulmonary edema or congestive heart failure (CHF) associated with tachycardia, which usually resolves quickly with rate control and diuresis. In particular, an increased risk of peri-interventional myocardial infarctions was observed, which can probably be explained by a high incidence of CAD in these patients.[212,214] In an elective setting, the option of performing aortic valve replacement before the noncardiac surgery has to be considered when stenosis is hemodynamically significant. In any case, risk stratification with regard to ruling out significant CAD is advisable.

The Role of Echocardiography in Optimizing the Surgical Approach and the Role of Perioperative Echocardiography

Echocardiography is currently an integral part of many cardiovascular and surgical procedures. Its impact on management in interventional cardiology and surgery are well established.[215] In addition, intraoperative TEE can be helpful in quantifying the severity of valvular lesions that might coexist and thus aid in the decision whether it is necessary to perform surgery on additional valves.

There are numerous reports of incidental findings, such as masses, thrombi, patent foramen ovale (PFO), atrial septal defects, and membranous subaortic stenosis, found during heart surgery.[216-218] The detection of these abnormalities is of importance because surgical management may be required.

In addition, surgical complications, such as LVOT obstruction,[219] pericardial or mediastinal hematoma, or ischemia can be detected. Based on these findings, intraoperative TEE permits immediate assessment of the surgical result and thus facilitates decision making whether immediate correction of the detected problem is required.

Measurement of the aortic annulus and the LVOT diameter with intraoperative TEE allows optimal sizing of aortic valve prostheses.[220,221] If a Ross procedure is attempted, TEE allows assessment of pulmonary valve morphology and function to determine if the valve is suitable as an autograft.[222] Intraoperative TEE also permits exact measurements of the aortic and pulmonary annulus and thus is able to detect a size mismatch.[223]

Paravalvular Regurgitation

Paravalvular leaks are by far the most frequent causes of regurgitation after valve replacement. TEE using color Doppler has a high sensitivity for the detection of paravalvular leaks.[224,225] Paravalvular regurgitation must be distinguished from normal "functional" regurgitation of mechanical prosthetic valves. Quantification of paravalvular regurgitation is performed using color Doppler under off-pump conditions. The degree of valvular regurgitation may be underestimated by intraoperative TEE resulting from the effects of general anesthesia and altered loading conditions.[220,226] Thus, the patient's volume status should be normalized and the peripheral systolic blood pressure and the pulmonary artery systolic pressure must be considered when quantifying mitral and tricuspid regurgitation (TR).

Exact localization of the leak(s) allows the surgeon to rapidly find the defect if correction of the paravalvular regurgitation is necessary.[227]

The Postoperative Assessment after Aortic Valve Replacement

After aortic valve replacement surgery, baseline echocardiographic data should be obtained for each individual patient—ideally after 3 to 4 weeks. The knowledge of baseline data can be helpful when changes in the clinical condition occur. They can be related to possible changes of the Doppler data. Even in the setting of a routine echocardiography examination, interpretation of Doppler data is always easier when baseline data are available for comparison.

Every valve type has its own hemodynamic properties resulting in specific normal values for gradients and valve area. Among bioprosthetic valves, the stentless valves are less obstructive than the stented valves. In addition, modern mechanical valves are less obstructive than older valve types, such as caged-ball valves. Finally, bileaflet valves are characterized by localized high velocities between the two leaflets resulting in high Doppler gradients.[228] In addition, normal values also depend on valve size with smaller valves being significantly more obstructive than larger valves. Thus, precise knowledge of valve type and size is indispensable for an appropriate interpretation of the Doppler data (see Chapters 24, 25, and 26). Once this information is known, the measured values can be compared with published normal values.[229]

Assessment of the Effects of Aortic Valve Replacement

Excellent survival rates after aortic valve replacement have been reported. Structural failure of mechanical valves are rare; however, there is a risk of thromboembolic and bleeding complications.[230] The use of biological prothesis has the advantage of not requiring long-term anticoagulation; however, there is a risk of structural deterioration of the valve that can ultimately lead to the necessity of a reintervention.[231] However, an acceptable operative risk has been reported even for repeat aortic valve replacement surgery.[232]

In the majority of patients, LV hypertrophy regresses after aortic valve replacement.[233] However, in a subgroup of patients, regression of LV hypertrophy does not occur; and these patients have a worse outcome with a higher mortality and an increased risk for the development of congestive heart failure.[234] Finally a residual risk of sudden death in the range of 0.3%/year remains even after aortic valve replacement surgery.[198,235]

KEY POINTS

■ With an aging population and widespread use of echocardiography, AS is increasingly diagnosed.

■ Knowledge of the prognostic implications of the echocardiographic findings in AS is essential for optimal management and should always be put in the clinical context.

■ Echocardiography is the method of choice for the follow-up of patients with AS and allows for:

1. Determination of the etiology stenosis (i.e., calcific, rheumatic, or congenital)
2. Exclusion of other causes of obstruction to LV outflow (i.e., supravalvular AS, subvalvular AS, or hypertrophic obstructive cardiomyopathy)
3. Identification of consequences of AS such as LV hypertrophy, impairment of LV systolic function, presence of diastolic dysfunction and concomitant valve lesions
4. Quantification of stenosis severity using flow dependent (peak aortic jet velocity, mean gradient) and flow independent (AVA assessed by the continuity equation) variables. Pitfalls of aortic stenosis quantification include failure to:
   - Consider the flow dependence of pressure gradients when LV systolic dysfunction or a small LV chamber is present
   - Systematically record aortic jet velocity from multiple ultrasound windows including a right parasternal approach
5. Measurement of hemodynamic progression
6. Risk stratification by integrating the information on stenosis severity, rate of hemodynamic progression, and degree of aortic valve calcification

■ In summary, echocardiography plays a central role in management decisions including surgical indications and scheduling control intervals

REFERENCES

1. Iung B, Baron G, Butchart EG, et al: A prospective survey of patients with valvular heart disease in Europe: The Euro Heart Survey on Valvular Heart Disease. *Eur Heart J* 24:1231-1243, 2003.
2. Roberts WC, Ko JM: Frequency by decades of unicuspid, bicuspid, and tricuspid aortic valves in adults having isolated aortic valve replacement for aortic stenosis, with or without associated aortic regurgitation. *Circulation* 111:920-925, 2005.
3. Mohler ER 3rd, Adam LP, McClelland P, et al: Detection of osteopontin in calcified human aortic valves. *Arterioscler Thromb Vasc Biol* 17:547-552, 1997.
4. Mohler ER 3rd, Gannon F, Reynolds C, et al: Bone formation and inflammation in cardiac valves. *Circulation* 103:1522-1528, 2001.
5. O'Brien KD, Reichenbach DD, Marcovina SM, et al: Apolipoproteins B, (a), and E accumulate in the morphologically early lesion of 'degenerative' valvular aortic stenosis. *Arterioscler Thromb Vasc Biol* 16:523-532, 1996.
6. Otto CM, Kuusisto J, Reichenbach DD, et al: Characterization of the early lesion of 'degenerative' valvular aortic stenosis. Histological and immunohistochemical studies. *Circulation* 90:844-853, 1994.
7. Rajamannan NM, Sangiorgi G, Springett M, et al: Experimental hypercholesterolemia induces apoptosis in the aortic valve. *J Heart Valve Dis* 10:371-374, 2001.
8. Rajamannan NM, Subramaniam M, Rickard D, et al: Human aortic valve calcification is associated with an osteoblast phenotype. *Circulation* 107:2181-2184, 2003.
9. Waller B, Howard J, Fess S: Pathology of aortic valve stenosis and pure aortic regurgitation. A clinical morphologic assessment—Part I. *Clin Cardiol* 17:85-92, 1994.
10. Rosenhek R, Binder T, Porenta G, et al: Predictors of outcome in severe, asymptomatic aortic stenosis. *N Engl J Med* 343:611-617, 2000.
11. Keane MG, Wiegers SE, Plappert T, et al: Bicuspid aortic valves are associated with aortic dilatation out of proportion to coexistent valvular lesions. *Circulation* 102:III35-III39, 2000.
12. Novaro GM, Mishra M, Griffin BP: Incidence and echocardiographic features of congenital unicuspid aortic valve in an adult population. *J Heart Valve Dis* 12:674-678, 2003.
13. Bach DS: Subvalvular left ventricular outflow obstruction for patients undergoing aortic valve replacement for aortic stenosis: Echocardiographic recognition and identification of patients at risk. *J Am Soc Echocardiogr* 18:1155-1162, 2005.
14. Callahan MJ, Tajik AJ, Su-Fan Q, Bove AA: Validation of instantaneous pressure gradients measured by continuous-wave Doppler in experimentally induced aortic stenosis. *Am J Cardiol* 56:989-993, 1985.
15. Currie PJ, Hagler DJ, Seward JB, et al: Instantaneous pressure gradient: a simultaneous Doppler and dual catheter correlative study. *J Am Coll Cardiol* 7:800-806, 1986.
16. Currie PJ, Seward JB, Reeder GS, et al: Continuous-wave Doppler echocardiographic assessment of severity of calcific aortic stenosis: A simultaneous Doppler-catheter correlative study in 100 adult patients. *Circulation* 71:1162-1169, 1985.
17. Galan A, Zoghbi WA, Quinones MA: Determination of severity of valvular aortic stenosis by Doppler echocardiography and relation of findings to clinical outcome and agreement with hemodynamic measurements determined at cardiac catheterization. *Am J Cardiol* 67:1007-1012, 1991.
18. Harrison MR, Gurley JC, Smith MD, et al: A practical application of Doppler echocardiography for the assessment of severity of aortic stenosis. *Am Heart J* 115:622-628, 1988.
19. Hatle L, Angelsen BA, Tromsdal A: Non-invasive assessment of aortic stenosis by Doppler ultrasound. *Br Heart J* 43:284-292, 1980.
20. Hegrenaes L, Hatle L: Aortic stenosis in adults. Non-invasive estimation of pressure differences by continuous wave Doppler echocardiography. *Br Heart J* 54:396-404, 1985.
21. Otto CM, Pearlman AS, Gardner CL, et al: Experimental validation of Doppler echocardiographic measurement of volume flow through the stenotic aortic valve. *Circulation* 78:435-441, 1988.

22. Simpson IA, Houston AB, Sheldon CD, et al: Clinical value of Doppler echocardiography in the assessment of adults with aortic stenosis. *Br Heart J* 53:636-639, 1985.

23. Smith N, McAnulty JH, Rahimtoola SH: Severe aortic stenosis with impaired left ventricular function and clinical heart failure: Results of valve replacement. *Circulation* 58:255-264, 1978.

24. Stamm RB, Martin RP: Quantification of pressure gradients across stenotic valves by Doppler ultrasound. *J Am Coll Cardiol* 2:707-718, 1983.

25. Yeager M, Yock PG, Popp RL: Comparison of Doppler-derived pressure gradient to that determined at cardiac catheterization in adults with aortic valve stenosis: Implications for management. *Am J Cardiol* 57:644-648, 1986.

26. Yoganathan AP, Valdes-Cruz LM, Schmidt-Dohna J, et al: Continuous-wave Doppler velocities and gradients across fixed tunnel obstructions: Studies in vitro and in vivo. *Circulation* 76:657-666, 1987.

27. Burwash IG, Forbes AD, Sadahiro M, et al: Echocardiographic volume flow and stenosis severity measures with changing flow rate in aortic stenosis. *Am J Physiol* 265:H1734-1743, 1993.

28. Hatle L: Noninvasive assessment and differentiation of left ventricular outflow obstruction with Doppler ultrasound. *Circulation* 64:381-387, 1981.

29. Otto CM, Davis KB, Holmes DR Jr, et al: Methodologic issues in clinical evaluation of stenosis severity in adults undergoing aortic or mitral balloon valvuloplasty. The NHLBI Balloon Valvuloplasty Registry. *Am J Cardiol* 69:1607-1616, 1992.

30. Rozenman Y, Gotsman MS: Heart rate influence on the systolic gradient across the stenotic aortic valve: Theoretical evaluation and implications. *Cathet Cardiovasc Diagn* 11:533-538, 1985.

31. Otto CM, Pearlman AS, Comess KA, et al: Determination of the stenotic aortic valve area in adults using Doppler echocardiography. *J Am Coll Cardiol* 7:509-517, 1986.

32. Baumgartner H, Khan S, DeRobertis M, et al: Discrepancies between Doppler and catheter gradients in aortic prosthetic valves in vitro. A manifestation of localized gradients and pressure recovery. *Circulation* 82:1467-1475, 1990.

33. Baumgartner H, Schima H, Tulzer G, Kuhn P: Effect of stenosis geometry on the Doppler-catheter gradient relation in vitro: a manifestation of pressure recovery. *J Am Coll Cardiol* 21:1018-1025, 1993.

34. Laskey WK, Kussmaul WG: Pressure recovery in aortic valve stenosis. *Circulation* 89:116-121, 1994.

35. Levine RA, Cape EG, Yoganathan AP: Pressure recovery distal to stenoses: Expanding clinical applications of engineering principles. *J Am Coll Cardiol* 21:1026-1028, 1993.

36. Levine RA, Jimoh A, Cape EG, et al: Pressure recovery distal to a stenosis: potential cause of gradient "overestimation" by Doppler echocardiography. *J Am Coll Cardiol* 13:706-715, 1989.

37. Voelker W, Reul H, Stelzer T, Schmidt A, Karsch KR: Pressure recovery in aortic stenosis: an in vitro study in a pulsatile flow model. *J Am Coll Cardiol* 20:1585-1593, 1992.

38. Yoganathan AP: Fluid mechanics of aortic stenosis. *Eur Heart J* 9(suppl E):13-17, 1988.

39. Niederberger J, Schima H, Maurer G, Baumgartner H: Importance of pressure recovery for the assessment of aortic stenosis by Doppler ultrasound. Role of aortic size, aortic valve area, and direction of the stenotic jet in vitro. *Circulation* 94:1934-1940, 1996.

40. Baumgartner H, Stefenelli T, Niederberger J, et al: "Overestimation" of catheter gradients by Doppler ultrasound in patients with aortic stenosis: A predictable manifestation of pressure recovery. *J Am Coll Cardiol* 33:1655-1661, 1999.

41. Grayburn PA, Smith MD, Harrison MR, et al: Pivotal role of aortic valve area calculation by the continuity equation for Doppler assessment of aortic stenosis in patients with combined aortic stenosis and regurgitation. *Am J Cardiol* 61:376-381, 1988.

42. Otto CM. The difficulties in assessing patients with moderate aortic stenosis. *Heart* 82:5-6, 1999.

43. Teirstein P, Yeager M, Yock PG, Popp RL: Doppler echocardiographic measurement of aortic valve area in aortic stenosis: A noninvasive application of the Gorlin formula. *J Am Coll Cardiol* 8:1059-1065, 1986.

44. Zoghbi WA, Farmer KL, Soto JG, et al: Accurate noninvasive quantification of stenotic aortic valve area by Doppler echocardiography. *Circulation* 73:452-459, 1986.

45. Otto CM, Pearlman AS: Doppler echocardiography in adults with symptomatic aortic stenosis. Diagnostic utility and cost-effectiveness. *Arch Intern Med* 148:2553-2560, 1988.

46. Wiseth R, Samstad S, Rossvoll O, et al: Cross-sectional left ventricular outflow tract velocities before and after aortic valve replacement: a comparative study with two-dimensional Doppler ultrasound. *J Am Soc Echocardiogr* 6:279-285, 1993.

47. Sjoberg BJ, Ask P, Loyd D, Wranne B: Subaortic flow profiles in aortic valve disease: A two-dimensional color Doppler study. *J Am Soc Echocardiogr* 7:276-285, 1994.

48. Gorlin R, Gorlin SG: Hydraulic formula for calculation of the area of the stenotic mitral valve, other cardiac valves, and central circulatory shunts. I. *Am Heart J* 41:1-29, 1951.

49. Ohlsson J, Wranne B. Noninvasive assessment of valve area in patients with aortic stenosis. *J Am Coll Cardiol* 7:501-508, 1986.

50. Skjaerpe T, Hegrenaes L, Hatle L: Noninvasive estimation of valve area in patients with aortic stenosis by Doppler ultrasound and two-dimensional echocardiography. *Circulation* 72:810-818, 1985.

51. Cannon SR, Richards KL, Crawford M: Hydraulic estimation of stenotic orifice area: A correction of the Gorlin formula. *Circulation* 71:1170-1178, 1985.

52. Cannon SR, Richards KL, Crawford MH, et al: Inadequacy of the Gorlin formula for predicting prosthetic valve area. *Am J Cardiol* 62:113-116, 1988.

53. Clark C: Relation between pressure difference across the aortic valve and left ventricular outflow. *Cardiovasc Res* 12:276-287, 1978.

54. Flachskampf FA, Weyman AE, Guerrero JL, Thomas JD: Influence of orifice geometry and flow rate on effective valve area: An in vitro study. *J Am Coll Cardiol* 15:1173-1180, 1990.

55. Segal J, Lerner DJ, Miller DC, et al: When should Doppler-determined valve area be better than the Gorlin formula? Variation in hydraulic constants in low flow states. *J Am Coll Cardiol* 9:1294-1305, 1987.

56. Dumesnil JG, Yoganathan AP: Theoretical and practical differences between the Gorlin formula and the continuity equation for calculating aortic and mitral valve areas. *Am J Cardiol* 67:1268-1272, 1991.

57. Lemler MS, Valdes-Cruz LM, Shandas RS, Cape EG: Insights into catheter/Doppler discrepancies in congenital aortic stenosis. *Am J Cardiol* 83:1447-1450, 1999.

58. Garcia D, Dumesnil JG, Durand LG, et al: Discrepancies between catheter and Doppler estimates of valve effective orifice area can be predicted from the pressure recovery phenomenon: Practical implications with regard to quantification of aortic stenosis severity. *J Am Coll Cardiol* 41:435-442, 2003.

59. Gorlin R, Gorlin WB: Further reconciliation between pathoanatomy and pathophysiology of stenotic cardiac valves. *J Am Coll Cardiol* 15:1181-1182, 1990.

60. Otto CM, Burwash IG, Legget ME, et al: Prospective study of asymptomatic valvular aortic stenosis. Clinical, echocardiographic, and exercise predictors of outcome. *Circulation* 95:2262-2270, 1997.

61. Pellikka PA, Nishimura RA, Bailey KR, Tajik AJ: The natural history of adults with asymptomatic, hemodynamically significant aortic stenosis. *J Am Coll Cardiol* 15:1012-1017, 1990.

62. Vahanian A, Baumgartner H, Bax J, et al: Guidelines on the management of valvular heart disease: The Task Force on the Management of Valvular Heart Disease of the European Society of Cardiology. *Eur Heart J* 28:230-268, 2007.

63. Bonow RO, Carabello BA, Chatterjee K, et al: ACC/AHA 2006 guidelines for the management of patients with valvular heart disease: A report of the American College of Cardiology/ American Heart Association Task Force on Practice Guidelines (writing Committee to Revise the 1998 guidelines for the management of patients with valvular heart disease) developed in collaboration with the Society of Cardiovascular Anesthesiologists endorsed by the Society for Cardiovascular Angiography and Interventions and the Society of Thoracic Surgeons. *J Am Coll Cardiol* 48:e1-e148, 2006.

64. Horstkotte D, Loogen F: The natural history of aortic valve stenosis. *Eur Heart J* 9(suppl E):57-64, 1988.

65. Turina J, Hess O, Sepulcri F, Krayenbuehl HP: Spontaneous course of aortic valve disease. *Eur Heart J* 8:471-483, 1987.

66. Rahimtoola SH: Perspective on valvular heart disease: An update. *J Am Coll Cardiol* 14:1-23, 1989.

67. Otto CM, Lind BK, Kitzman DW, et al: Association of aortic-valve sclerosis with cardiovascular mortality and morbidity in the elderly. *N Engl J Med* 341:142-147, 1999.

68. Rosenhek R, Klaar U, Schemper M, et al: Mild and moderate aortic stenosis; Natural history and risk stratification by echocardiography. *Eur Heart J* 25:199-205, 2004.

69. Cannon JD Jr, Zile MR, Crawford FA Jr, Carabello BA: Aortic valve resistance as an adjunct to the Gorlin formula in assessing the severity of aortic stenosis in symptomatic patients. *J Am Coll Cardiol* 20:1517-1523, 1992.

70. Fox KM: Efficacy of perindopril in reduction of cardiovascular events among patients with stable coronary artery disease: randomised, double-blind, placebo-controlled, multicentre trial (the EUROPA study). *Lancet* 362:782-788, 2003.

71. Voelker W, Reul H, Nienhaus G, et al: Comparison of valvular resistance, stroke work loss, and Gorlin valve area for quantification of aortic stenosis. An in vitro study in a pulsatile aortic flow model. *Circulation* 91:1196-1204, 1995.

72. Laskey WK, Kussmaul WG, Noordergraaf A: Valvular and systemic arterial hemodynamics in aortic valve stenosis. A model-based approach. *Circulation* 92:1473-1478, 1995.

73. Blais C, Pibarot P, Dumesnil JG, et al: Comparison of valve resistance with effective orifice area regarding flow dependence. *Am J Cardiol* 88:45-52, 2001.

74. Burwash IG, Pearlman AS, Kraft CD, et al: Flow dependence of measures of aortic stenosis severity during exercise. *J Am Coll Cardiol* 24:1342-1350, 1994.

75. Mascherbauer J, Rosenhek R, Bittner B, et al: Doppler echocardiographic assessment of valvular regurgitation severity by measurement of the vena contracta: An in vitro validation study. *J Am Soc Echocardiogr* 18:999-1006, 2005.

76. Antonini-Canterin F, Faggiano P, Zanuttini D, Ribichini F: Is aortic valve resistance more clinically meaningful than valve area in aortic stenosis? *Heart* 82:9-10, 1999.

77. Roger VL, Seward JB, Bailey KR, et al: Aortic valve resistance in aortic stenosis: Doppler echocardiographic study and surgical correlation. *Am Heart J* 134:924-929, 1997.

78. Badano L, Cassottano P, Bertoli D, et al: Changes in effective aortic valve area during ejection in adults with aortic stenosis. *Am J Cardiol* 78:1023-1028, 1996.

79. Lester SJ, McElhinney DB, Miller JP, et al: Rate of change in aortic valve area during a cardiac cycle can predict the rate of hemodynamic progression of aortic stenosis. *Circulation* 101:1947-1952, 2000.

80. Springings DC, Chambers JB, Cochrane T, et al: Ventricular stroke work loss: Validation of a method of quantifying the severity of aortic stenosis and derivation of an orifice formula. *J Am Coll Cardiol* 16:1608-1614, 1990.

81. Tobin JR Jr, Rahimtoola SH, Blundell PE, Swan HJ: Percentage of left ventricular stroke work loss. A simple hemodynamic concept for estimation of severity in valvular aortic stenosis. *Circulation* 35:868-879, 1967.

82. Milnor W: *Cardiac dynamics*, Baltimore, Williams & Wilkins, 1982.

83. Garcia D, Pibarot P, Dumesnil JG, et al: Assessment of aortic valve stenosis severity: A new index based on the energy loss concept. *Circulation* 101:765-771, 2000.

84. Cormier B, Iung B, Porte JM, et al: Value of multiplane transesophageal echocardiography in determining aortic valve area in aortic stenosis. *Am J Cardiol* 77:882-885, 1996.

85. Dittrich HC, McCann HA, Walsh TP, et al: Transesophageal echocardiography in the evaluation of prosthetic and native aortic valves. *Am J Cardiol* 66:758-761, 1990.

86. Hoffmann R, Flachskampf FA, Hanrath P: Planimetry of orifice area in aortic stenosis using multiplane transesophageal echocardiography. *J Am Coll Cardiol* 22:529-534, 1993.

87. Stoddard MF, Arce J, Liddell NE, et al: Two-dimensional transesophageal echocardiographic determination of aortic valve area in adults with aortic stenosis. *Am Heart J* 122:1415-1422, 1991.

88. Tribouilloy C, Shen WF, Peltier M, et al: Quantitation of aortic valve area in aortic stenosis with multiplane transesophageal echocardiography: comparison with monoplane transesophageal approach. *Am Heart J* 128:526-532, 1994.

89. Bernard Y, Meneveau N, Vuillemenot A, et al: Planimetry of aortic valve area using multiplane transoesophageal echocardiography is not a reliable method for assessing severity of aortic stenosis. *Heart* 78:68-73, 1997.

90. Blumberg FC, Pfeifer M, Holmer SR, et al: Quantification of aortic stenosis in mechanically ventilated patients using multiplane transesophageal Doppler echocardiography. *Chest* 114:94-97, 1998.

91. Stoddard MF, Hammons RT, Longaker RA: Doppler transesophageal echocardiographic determination of aortic valve area in adults with aortic stenosis. *Am Heart J* 132:337-342, 1996.

92. Ge S, Warner JG Jr, Abraham TP, et al: Three-dimensional surface area of the aortic valve orifice by three-dimensional echocardiography: Clinical validation of a novel index for assessment of aortic stenosis. *Am Heart J* 136:1042-1050, 1998.

93. Menzel T, Mohr-Kahaly S, Kolsch B, et al: Quantitative assessment of aortic stenosis by three-dimensional echocardiography. *J Am Soc Echocardiogr* 10:215-223, 1997.

94. Faggiano P, Gualeni A, Antonini-Canterin F, et al: Doppler echocardiographic assessment of hemodynamic progression of valvular aortic stenosis over time: Comparison between aortic valve resistance and valve area. *G Ital Cardiol* 29:1131-1136, 1999.

95. Anderson FL, Tsagaris TJ, Tikoff G, et al: Hemodynamic effects of exercise in patients with aortic stenosis. *Am J Med* 46:872-885, 1969.

96. Aronow WS, Harris CN: Treadmill exercise test in aortic stenosis and mitral stenosis. *Chest* 68:507-509, 1975.

97. Bache RJ, Wang Y, Jorgensen CR: Hemodynamic effects of exercise in isolated valvular aortic stenosis. *Circulation* 44:1003-1013, 1971.

98. Ettinger PO, Frank MJ, Levinson GE: Hemodynamics at rest and during exercise in combined aortic stenosis and insufficiency. *Circulation* 45:267-276, 1972.

99. Lee SJ, Jonsson B, Bevegard S, et al: Hemodynamic changes at rest and during exercise in patients with aortic stenosis of varying severity. *Am Heart J* 79:318-331, 1970.

100. Martin TW, Moody JM Jr, Bird JJ, et al: Effect of exercise on indices of valvular aortic stenosis. *Cathet Cardiovasc Diagn* 25:265-271, 1992.

101. Otto CM, Pearlman AS, Kraft CD, et al: Physiologic changes with maximal exercise in asymptomatic valvular aortic stenosis

assessed by Doppler echocardiography. *J Am Coll Cardiol* 20:1160-1167, 1992.

102. Kitabatake A, Fujii K, Tanouchi J, et al: Doppler echocardiographic quantitation of cross-sectional area under various hemodynamic conditions: an experimental validation in a canine model of supravalvular aortic stenosis. *J Am Coll Cardiol* 15:1654-1661, 1990.

103. Burwash IG, Thomas DD, Sadahiro M, et al: Dependence of Gorlin formula and continuity equation valve areas on transvalvular volume flow rate in valvular aortic stenosis. *Circulation* 89:827-835, 1994.

104. Casale PN, Palacios IF, Abascal VM, et al: Effects of dobutamine on Gorlin and continuity equation valve areas and valve resistance in valvular aortic stenosis. *Am J Cardiol* 70:1175-1179, 1992.

105. Cochrane T, Kenyon CJ, Lawford PV, et al: Validation of the orifice formula for estimating effective heart valve opening area. *Clin Phys Physiol Meas* 12:21-37, 1991.

106. Montarello JK, Perakis AC, Rosenthal E, et al: Normal and stenotic human aortic valve opening: in vitro assessment of orifice area changes with flow. *Eur Heart J* 11:484-491, 1990.

107. Chambers JB, Sprigings DC, Cochrane T, et al: Continuity equation and Gorlin formula compared with directly observed orifice area in native and prosthetic aortic valves. *Br Heart J* 67:193-199, 1992.

108. Kadem L, Rieu R, Dumesnil JG, et al: Flow-dependent changes in Doppler-derived aortic valve effective orifice area are real and not due to artifact. *J Am Coll Cardiol* 47:131-137, 2006.

109. Bermejo J, Garcia-Fernandez MA, Torrecilla EG, et al: Effects of dobutamine on Doppler echocardiographic indexes of aortic stenosis. *J Am Coll Cardiol* 28:1206-1213, 1996.

110. Ford LE, Feldman T, Chiu YC, Carroll JD: Hemodynamic resistance as a measure of functional impairment in aortic valvular stenosis. *Circ Res* 66:1-7, 1990.

111. Burwash IG, Dickinson A, Teskey RJ, et al: Aortic valve area discrepancy by Gorlin equation and Doppler echocardiography continuity equation: relationship to flow in patients with valvular aortic stenosis. *Can J Cardiol* 16:985-992, 2000.

112. Otto CM, Pearlman AS, Gardner CL: Hemodynamic progression of aortic stenosis in adults assessed by Doppler echocardiography. *J Am Coll Cardiol* 13:545-550, 1989.

113. Archer SL, Mike DK, Hetland MB, et al: Usefulness of mean aortic valve gradient and left ventricular diastolic filling pattern for distinguishing symptomatic from asymptomatic patients. *Am J Cardiol* 73:275-281, 1994.

114. Gallino RA, Milner MR, Goldstein SA, et al: Left ventricular filling patterns in aortic stenosis in patients older than 65 years of age. *Am J Cardiol* 63:1103-1106, 1989.

115. Hess OM, Ritter M, Schneider J, et al: Diastolic stiffness and myocardial structure in aortic valve disease before and after valve replacement. *Circulation* 69:855-865, 1984.

116. Krayenbuehl HP, Hess OM, Monrad ES, et al: Left ventricular myocardial structure in aortic valve disease before, intermediate, and late after aortic valve replacement. *Circulation* 79:744-755, 1989.

117. Otto CM, Pearlman AS, Amsler LC: Doppler echocardiographic evaluation of left ventricular diastolic filling in isolated valvular aortic stenosis. *Am J Cardiol* 63:313-316, 1989.

118. Villari B, Hess OM, Kaufmann P, et al: Effect of aortic valve stenosis (pressure overload) and regurgitation (volume overload) on left ventricular systolic and diastolic function. *Am J Cardiol* 69:927-934, 1992.

119. Bruch C, Stypmann J, Grude M, et al: Tissue Doppler imaging in patients with moderate to severe aortic valve stenosis: Clinical usefulness and diagnostic accuracy. *Am Heart J* 148:696-702, 2004.

120. Rajappan K, Rimoldi OE, Dutka DP, et al: Mechanisms of coronary microcirculatory dysfunction in patients with aortic steno-

sis and angiographically normal coronary arteries. *Circulation* 105:470-476, 2002.

121. Rajappan K, Rimoldi OE, Camici PG, et al: Functional changes in coronary microcirculation after valve replacement in patients with aortic stenosis. *Circulation* 107:3170-3175, 2003.

122. Chambers J, Takeda S, Rimington H, et al: Determinants of left ventricular mass in aortic stenosis. *J Heart Valve Dis* 13:873-880, 2004.

123. Dellgren G, Eriksson MJ, Blange I, et al: Angiotensin-converting enzyme gene polymorphism influences degree of left ventricular hypertrophy and its regression in patients undergoing operation for aortic stenosis. *Am J Cardiol* 84:909-913, 1999.

124. Orlowska-Baranowska E, Placha G, Gaciong Z, et al: Influence of ACE I/D genotypes on left ventricular hypertrophy in aortic stenosis: Gender-related differences. *J Heart Valve Dis* 13:574-581, 2004.

125. Orsinelli DA, Aurigemma GP, Battista S, et al: Left ventricular hypertrophy and mortality after aortic valve replacement for aortic stenosis. A high risk subgroup identified by preoperative relative wall thickness. *J Am Coll Cardiol* 22:1679-1683, 1993.

126. Carroll JD, Carroll EP, Feldman T, et al: Sex-associated differences in left ventricular function in aortic stenosis of the elderly. *Circulation* 86:1099-1107, 1992.

127. Douglas PS, Otto CM, Mickel MC, et al: Gender differences in left ventricle geometry and function in patients undergoing balloon dilatation of the aortic valve for isolated aortic stenosis. NHLBI Balloon Valvuloplasty Registry. *Br Heart J* 73:548-554, 1995.

128. Aurigemma GP, Silver KH, McLaughlin M, et al: Impact of chamber geometry and gender on left ventricular systolic function in patients >60 years of age with aortic stenosis. *Am J Cardiol* 74:794-798, 1994.

129. Legget ME, Kuusisto J, Healy NL, et al: Gender differences in left ventricular function at rest and with exercise in asymptomatic aortic stenosis. *Am Heart J* 131:94-100, 1996.

130. Morris JJ, Schaff HV, Mullany CJ, et al: Gender differences in left ventricular functional response to aortic valve replacement. *Circulation* 90:II183-II189, 1994.

131. Frank S, Johnson A, Ross J Jr: Natural history of valvular aortic stenosis. *Br Heart J* 35:41-46, 1973.

132. Ross J Jr, Braunwald E: Aortic stenosis. *Circulation* 38:61-67, 1968.

133. Selzer A: Changing aspects of the natural history of valvular aortic stenosis. *N Engl J Med* 317:91-98, 1987.

134. Beppu S, Suzuki S, Matsuda H, et al: Rapidity of progression of aortic stenosis in patients with congenital bicuspid aortic valves. *Am J Cardiol* 71:322-327, 1993.

135. Pachulski RT, Chan KL: Progression of aortic valve dysfunction in 51 adult patients with congenital bicuspid aortic valve: assessment and follow up by Doppler echocardiography. *Br Heart J* 69:237-240, 1993.

136. Aronow WS, Kronzon I: Prevalence and severity of valvular aortic stenosis determined by Doppler echocardiography and its association with echocardiographic and electrocardiographic left ventricular hypertrophy and physical signs of aortic stenosis in elderly patients. *Am J Cardiol* 67:776-777, 1991.

137. Lindroos M, Kupari M, Heikkila J, Tilvis R: Prevalence of aortic valve abnormalities in the elderly: An echocardiographic study of a random population sample. *J Am Coll Cardiol* 21:1220-1225, 1993.

138. Amato MC, Moffa PJ, Werner KE, Ramires JA: Treatment decision in asymptomatic aortic valve stenosis: role of exercise testing. *Heart* 86:381-386, 2001.

139. Das P, Rimington H, Chambers J: Exercise testing to stratify risk in aortic stenosis. *Eur Heart J* 26:1309-1313, 2005.

140. Chizner MA, Pearle DL, deLeon AC Jr: The natural history of aortic stenosis in adults. *Am Heart J* 99:419-424, 1980.

141. Kelly TA, Rothbart RM, Cooper CM, et al: Comparison of outcome of asymptomatic to symptomatic patients older than 20 years of age with valvular aortic stenosis. *Am J Cardiol* 61:123-130, 1988.

142. Kennedy KD, Nishimura RA, Holmes DR Jr, Bailey KR: Natural history of moderate aortic stenosis. *J Am Coll Cardiol* 17:313-319, 1991.

143. O'Keefe JH Jr, Vlietstra RE, Bailey KR, Holmes DR Jr: Natural history of candidates for balloon aortic valvuloplasty. *Mayo Clin Proc* 62:986-991, 1987.

144. Otto CM, Mickel MC, Kennedy JW, et al. Three-year outcome after balloon aortic valvuloplasty. Insights into prognosis of valvular aortic stenosis. *Circulation* 89:642-650, 1994.

145. Aranki SF, Rizzo RJ, Couper GS, et al: Aortic valve replacement in the elderly. Effect of gender and coronary artery disease on operative mortality. *Circulation* 88:II17-II23, 1993.

146. Elayda MA, Hall RJ, Reul RM, et al: Aortic valve replacement in patients 80 years old. Operative risks and long-term results. *Circulation* 88:II11-II16, 1993.

147. Iung B, Cachier A, Baron G, et al: Decision-making in elderly patients with severe aortic stenosis: why are so many denied surgery? *Eur Heart J* 26:2714-2720, 2005.

148. Rosenhek R, Maurer G, Baumgartner H: Should early elective surgery be performed in patients with severe but asymptomatic aortic stenosis? *Eur Heart J* 23:1417-1421, 2002.

149. Faggiano P, Ghizzoni G, Sorgato A, et al: Rate of progression of valvular aortic stenosis in adults. *Am J Cardiol* 70:229-233, 1992.

150. Pellikka PA, Sarano ME, Nishimura RA, et al: Outcome of 622 adults with asymptomatic, hemodynamically significant aortic stenosis during prolonged follow-up. *Circulation* 111:3290-3295, 2005.

151. Easterling TR, Chadwick HS, Otto CM, Benedetti TJ: Aortic stenosis in pregnancy. *Obstet Gynecol* 72:113-118, 1988.

152. Keane JF, Driscoll DJ, Gersony WM, et al: Second natural history study of congenital heart defects. Results of treatment of patients with aortic valvar stenosis. *Circulation* 87:I16-I27, 1993.

153. Lund O, Nielsen TT, Emmertsen K, et al: Mortality and worsening of prognostic profile during waiting time for valve replacement in aortic stenosis. *Thorac Cardiovasc Surg* 44:289-295, 1996.

154. Lindblom D, Lindblom U, Qvist J, Lundstrom H: Long-term relative survival rates after heart valve replacement. *J Am Coll Cardiol* 15:566-573, 1990.

155. Mullany CJ: Aortic valve surgery in the elderly. *Cardiol Rev* 8:333-339, 2000.

156. Kolh P, Lahaye L, Gerard P, Limet R: Aortic valve replacement in the octogenarians: perioperative outcome and clinical follow-up. *Eur J Cardiothorac Surg* 16:68-73, 1999.

157. Cosmi JE, Kort S, Tunick PA, et al: The risk of the development of aortic stenosis in patients with "benign" aortic valve thickening. *Arch Intern Med* 162:2345-2347, 2002.

158. Bogart DB, Murphy BL, Wong BY, et al: Progression of aortic stenosis. *Chest* 76:391-396, 1979.

159. Cheitlin MD, Gertz EW, Brundage BH, et al: Rate of progression of severity of valvular aortic stenosis in the adult. *Am Heart J* 98:689-700, 1979.

160. Davies SW, Gershlick AH, Balcon R: Progression of valvar aortic stenosis: A long-term retrospective study. *Eur Heart J* 12:10-14, 1991.

161. Jonasson R, Jonsson B, Nordlander R, et al: Rate of progression of severity of valvular aortic stenosis. *Acta Med Scand* 213:51-54, 1983.

162. Nestico PF, DePace NL, Kimbiris D, et al: Progression of isolated aortic stenosis: analysis of 29 patients having more than 1 cardiac catheterization. *Am J Cardiol* 52:1054-1058, 1983.

163. Wagner S, Selzer A: Patterns of progression of aortic stenosis: A longitudinal hemodynamic study. *Circulation* 65:709-712, 1982.

164. Bahler RC, Desser DR, Finkelhor RS, et al: Factors leading to progression of valvular aortic stenosis. *Am J Cardiol* 84:1044-1048, 1999.

165. Brener SJ, Duffy CI, Thomas JD, Stewart WJ: Progression of aortic stenosis in 394 patients: Relation to changes in myocardial and mitral valve dysfunction. *J Am Coll Cardiol* 25:305-310, 1995.

166. Palta S, Pai AM, Gill KS, Pai RG: New insights into the progression of aortic stenosis: Implications for secondary prevention. *Circulation* 101:2497-2502, 2000.

167. Peter M, Hoffmann A, Parker C, et al: Progression of aortic stenosis. Role of age and concomitant coronary artery disease. *Chest* 103:1715-1719, 1993.

168. Roger VL, Tajik AJ, Bailey KR, et al: Progression of aortic stenosis in adults: New appraisal using Doppler echocardiography. *Am Heart J* 119:331-338, 1990.

169. Aronow WS, Ahn C, Kronzon I, Goldman ME: Association of coronary risk factors and use of statins with progression of mild valvular aortic stenosis in older persons. *Am J Cardiol* 88:693-695, 2001.

170. Bellamy MF, Pellikka PA, Klarich KW, et al: Association of cholesterol levels, hydroxymethylglutaryl coenzyme-A reductase inhibitor treatment, and progression of aortic stenosis in the community. *J Am Coll Cardiol* 40:1723-1730, 2002.

171. Cowell SJ, Newby DE, Prescott RJ, et al: A Randomized Trial of Intensive Lipid Lowering Therapy in Calcific Aortic Stenosis. *N Engl J Med* 352:2389-2397, 2005.

172. Novaro GM, Tiong IY, Pearce GL, et al: Effect of hydroxymethylglutaryl coenzyme a reductase inhibitors on the progression of calcific aortic stenosis. *Circulation* 104:2205-2209, 2001.

173. Rosenhek R, Rader F, Loho N, et al: Statins but not angiotensin-converting enzyme inhibitors delay progression of aortic stenosis. *Circulation* 110:1291-1295, 2004.

174. Stewart BF, Siscovick D, Lind BK, et al: Clinical factors associated with calcific aortic valve disease. Cardiovascular Health Study. *J Am Coll Cardiol* 29:630-634, 1997.

175. Messika-Zeitoun D, Aubry MC, Detaint D, et al: Evaluation and clinical implications of aortic valve calcification measured by electron-beam computed tomography. *Circulation* 110:356-362, 2004.

176. Lancellotti P, Lebois F, Simon M, et al: Prognostic importance of quantitative exercise Doppler echocardiography in asymptomatic valvular aortic stenosis. *Circulation* 112:I377-I382, 2005.

177. Gerber IL, Stewart RA, Legget ME, et al: Increased plasma natriuretic peptide levels reflect symptom onset in aortic stenosis. *Circulation* 107:1884-1890, 2003.

178. Lim P, Monin JL, Monchi M, et al: Predictors of outcome in patients with severe aortic stenosis and normal left ventricular function: role of B-type natriuretic peptide. *Eur Heart J* 25:2048-2053, 2004.

179. Bergler-Klein J, Klaar U, Heger M, et al: Natriuretic peptides predict symptom-free survival and postoperative outcome in severe aortic stenosis. *Circulation* 109:2302-2308, 2004.

180. Otto CM: Aortic stenosis—listen to the patient, look at the valve. *N Engl J Med* 343:652-654, 2000.

181. Collins JJ Jr, Aranki SF: Management of mild aortic stenosis during coronary artery bypass graft surgery. *J Card Surg* 9:145-147, 1994.

182. Pereira JJ, Balaban K, Lauer MS, et al: Aortic valve replacement in patients with mild or moderate aortic stenosis and coronary bypass surgery. *Am J Med* 118:735-742, 2005.

183. Smith WTt, Ferguson TB Jr, Ryan T, et al: Should coronary artery bypass graft surgery patients with mild or moderate aortic stenosis undergo concomitant aortic valve replacement? A decision analysis approach to the surgical dilemma. *J Am Coll Cardiol* 44:1241-1247, 2004.

184. Powell DE, Tunick PA, Rosenzweig BP, et al: Aortic valve replacement in patients with aortic stenosis and severe left ventricular dysfunction. *Arch Intern Med* 160:1337-1341, 2000.

185. Levy F, Garayalde E, Quere JP, et al: Prognostic value of preoperative atrial fibrillation in patients with aortic stenosis and low ejection fraction having aortic valve replacement. *Am J Cardiol* 98:809-811, 2006.

186. Brogan WC 3rd, Grayburn PA, Lange RA, Hillis LD: Prognosis after valve replacement in patients with severe aortic stenosis and a low transvalvular pressure gradient. *J Am Coll Cardiol* 21:1657-1660, 1993.

187. Connolly HM, Oh JK, Schaff HV, et al: Severe aortic stenosis with low transvalvular gradient and severe left ventricular dysfunction: Result of aortic valve replacement in 52 patients. *Circulation* 101:1940-1946, 2000.

188. Pereira JJ, Lauer MS, Bashir M, et al: Survival after aortic valve replacement for severe aortic stenosis with low transvalvular gradients and severe left ventricular dysfunction. *J Am Coll Cardiol* 39:1356-1363, 2002.

189. Monin JL, Quere JP, Monchi M, et al: Low-gradient aortic stenosis: operative risk stratification and predictors for long-term outcome: A multicenter study using dobutamine stress hemodynamics. *Circulation* 108:319-324, 2003.

190. deFilippi CR, Willett DL, Brickner ME, et al: Usefulness of dobutamine echocardiography in distinguishing severe from non-severe valvular aortic stenosis in patients with depressed left ventricular function and low transvalvular gradients. *Am J Cardiol* 75:191-194, 1995.

191. Schwammenthal E, Vered Z, Moshkowitz Y, et al: Dobutamine echocardiography in patients with aortic stenosis and left ventricular dysfunction: predicting outcome as a function of management strategy. *Chest* 119:1766-1777, 2001.

192. Carabello BA: Do all patients with aortic stenosis and left ventricular dysfunction benefit from aortic valve replacement? *Cathet Cardiovasc Diagn* 17:131-132, 1989.

193. Lin SS, Roger VL, Pascoe R, et al: Dobutamine stress Doppler hemodynamics in patients with aortic stenosis: Feasibility, safety, and surgical correlations. *Am Heart J* 136:1010-1016, 1998.

194. Blais C, Burwash IG, Mundigler G, et al: Projected valve area at normal flow rate improves the assessment of stenosis severity in patients with low-flow, low-gradient aortic stenosis: The multicenter TOPAS (Truly or Pseudo-Severe Aortic Stenosis) study. *Circulation* 113:711-721, 2006.

195. Quere JP, Monin JL, Levy F, et al: Influence of preoperative left ventricular contractile reserve on postoperative ejection fraction in low-gradient aortic stenosis. *Circulation* 113:1738-1744, 2006.

196. Iung B, Drissi MF, Michel PL, et al: Prognosis of valve replacement for aortic stenosis with or without coexisting coronary heart disease: a comparative study. *J Heart Valve Dis* 2:430-439, 1993.

197. Lund O, Nielsen TT, Pilegaard HK, et al: The influence of coronary artery disease and bypass grafting on early and late survival after valve replacement for aortic stenosis. *J Thorac Cardiovasc Surg* 100:327-337, 1990.

198. Czer LS, Gray RJ, Stewart ME, et al: Reduction in sudden late death by concomitant revascularization with aortic valve replacement. *J Thorac Cardiovasc Surg* 95:390-401, 1988.

199. Kveselis DA, Rocchini AP, Rosenthal A, et al: Hemodynamic determinants of exercise-induced ST-segment depression in children with valvular aortic stenosis. *Am J Cardiol* 55:1133-1139, 1985.

200. Patsilinakos SP, Kranidis AI, Antonelis IP, et al: Detection of coronary artery disease in patients with severe aortic stenosis with noninvasive methods. *Angiology* 50:309-317, 1999.

201. Kupari M, Virtanen KS, Turto H, et al: Exclusion of coronary artery disease by exercise thallium-201 tomography in patients with aortic valve stenosis. *Am J Cardiol* 70:635-640, 1992.

202. Samuels B, Kiat H, Friedman JD, Berman DS: Adenosine pharmacologic stress myocardial perfusion tomographic imaging in patients with significant aortic stenosis. Diagnostic efficacy and comparison of clinical, hemodynamic and electrocardiographic variables with 100 age-matched control subjects. *J Am Coll Cardiol* 25:99-106, 1995.

203. Patsilinakos SP, Spanodimos S, Rontoyanni F, et al: Adenosine stress myocardial perfusion tomographic imaging in patients with significant aortic stenosis. *J Nucl Cardiol* 11:20-25, 2004.

204. Georgeson S, Meyer KB, Pauker SG: Decision analysis in clinical cardiology: When is coronary angiography required in aortic stenosis? *J Am Coll Cardiol* 15:751-762, 1990.

205. Gilard M, Cornily JC, Pennec PY, et al: Accuracy of multislice computed tomography in the preoperative assessment of coronary disease in patients with aortic valve stenosis. *J Am Coll Cardiol* 47:2020-2024, 2006.

206. Reant P, Brunot S, Lafitte S, et al: Predictive value of noninvasive coronary angiography with multidetector computed tomography to detect significant coronary stenosis before valve surgery. *Am J Cardiol* 97:1506-1510, 2006.

207. Stewart WJ, Carabello BA: Aortic valve disease. In Topol E (ed): *Textbook of Cardiovascular Medicine.* 3rd ed. Philadelphia, Lippincott Williams & Wilkins, 2007, pp. 366-388.

208. O'Brien KD, Zhao XQ, Shavelle DM, et al: Hemodynamic effects of the angiotensin-converting enzyme inhibitor, ramipril, in patients with mild to moderate aortic stenosis and preserved left ventricular function. *J Investig Med* 52:185-191, 2004.

209. Chockalingam A, Venkatesan S, Subramaniam T, et al: Safety and efficacy of angiotensin-converting enzyme inhibitors in symptomatic severe aortic stenosis: Symptomatic Cardiac Obstruction-Pilot Study of Enalapril in Aortic Stenosis (SCOPE-AS). *Am Heart J* 147:E19, 2004.

210. Jimenez-Candil J, Bermejo J, Yotti R, et al: Effects of angiotensin converting enzyme inhibitors in hypertensive patients with aortic valve stenosis: A drug withdrawal study. *Heart* 91:1311-1318, 2005.

211. O'Keefe JH Jr, Shub C, Rettke SR: Risk of noncardiac surgical procedures in patients with aortic stenosis. *Mayo Clin Proc* 64:400-405, 1989.

212. Zahid M, Sonel AF, Saba S, Good CB: Perioperative risk of noncardiac surgery associated with aortic stenosis. *Am J Cardiol* 96:436-438, 2005.

213. Torsher LC, Shub C, Rettke SR, Brown DL: Risk of patients with severe aortic stenosis undergoing noncardiac surgery. *Am J Cardiol* 81:448-452, 1998.

214. Kertai MD, Bountioukos M, Boersma E, et al: Aortic stenosis: An underestimated risk factor for perioperative complications in patients undergoing noncardiac surgery. *Am J Med* 116:8-13, 2004.

215. Click RL, Abel MD, Schaff HV: Intraoperative transesophageal echocardiography: 5-year prospective review of impact on surgical management. *Mayo Clin Proc* 75:241-247, 2000.

216. Leslie D, Hall TS, Goldstein S, Shindler D: Mural left atrial thrombus: A hidden danger accompanying cardiac surgery. *J Cardiovasc Surg (Torino)* 39:649-650, 1998.

217. Liu F, Ge J, Kupferwasser I, et al: Has transesophageal echocardiography changed the approach to patients with suspected or known infective endocarditis? *Echocardiography* 12:637-650, 1995.

218. Nakao T, Hollinger I, Attai L, Oka Y: Incidental finding of papillary fibroelastoma on the atrial septum. *Cardiovasc Surg* 2:423-424, 1994.

219. Gillham MJ, Tousignant CP: Diagnosis by intraoperative transesophageal echocardiography of acute thrombosis of mechanical aortic valve prosthesis associated with the use of biological glue. *Anesth Analg* 92:1123-1125, 2001.

220. Czer LS, Maurer G, Bolger AF, et al: Intraoperative evaluation of mitral regurgitation by Doppler color flow mapping. *Circulation* 76:III108-III116, 1987.

221. Guarracino F, Zussa C, Polesel E, et al: Influence of transesophageal echocardiography on intraoperative decision making for

toronto stentless prosthetic valve implantation. *J Heart Valve Dis* 10:31-34, 2001.

222. Nowrangi SK, Connolly HM, Freeman WK, Click RL: Impact of intraoperative transesophageal echocardiography among patients undergoing aortic valve replacement for aortic stenosis. *J Am Soc Echocardiogr* 14:863-866, 2001.

223. Andrade A, Vargas-Barron J, Romero-Cardenas A, et al: Transthoracic and transesophageal echocardiographic study of pulmonary autograft valve in aortic position. *Echocardiography* 11:221-226, 1994.

224. Grahame-Clarke C, Pugsley WB, Swanton RH: Supravalvar aortic stenosis: Unexpected findings at surgery. *Heart* 79:627-628, 1998.

225. Maurer G, Czer LS: Intraoperative color Doppler assessment in valve repair surgery. *Echocardiography* 8:263-271, 1991.

226. Maurer G, Siegel RJ, Czer LS: The use of color flow mapping for intraoperative assessment of valve repair. *Circulation* 84:I250-I258, 1991.

227. Grewal KS, Malkowski MJ, Piracha AR, et al: Effect of general anesthesia on the severity of mitral regurgitation by transesophageal echocardiography. *Am J Cardiol* 85:199-203, 2000.

228. Chafizadeh ER, Zoghbi WA: Doppler echocardiographic assessment of the St. Jude Medical prosthetic valve in the aortic position using the continuity equation. *Circulation* 83:213-223, 1991.

229. Rosenhek R, Binder T, Maurer G, Baumgartner H: Normal values for Doppler echocardiographic assessment of heart valve prostheses. *J Am Soc Echocardiogr* 16:1116-1127, 2003.

230. Emery RW, Erickson CA, Arom KV, et al: Replacement of the aortic valve in patients under 50 years of age: Long-term follow-up of the St. Jude Medical prosthesis. *Ann Thorac Surg* 75:1815-1819, 2003.

231. Hammermeister K, Sethi GK, Henderson WG, et al: Outcomes 15 years after valve replacement with a mechanical versus a bioprosthetic valve: Final report of the Veterans Affairs randomized trial. *J Am Coll Cardiol* 36:1152-1158, 2000.

232. Potter DD, Sundt TM 3rd, Zehr KJ, et al: Operative risk of reoperative aortic valve replacement. *J Thorac Cardiovasc Surg* 129:94-103, 2005.

233. Lund O, Emmertsen K, Dorup I, et al: Regression of left ventricular hypertrophy during 10 years after valve replacement for aortic stenosis is related to the preoperative risk profile. *Eur Heart J* 24:1437-1446, 2003.

234. Lessick J, Mutlak D, Markiewicz W, Reisner SA: Failure of left ventricular hypertrophy to regress after surgery for aortic valve stenosis. *Echocardiography* 19:359-366, 2002.

235. Gohlke-Barwolf C, Peters K, Petersen J, et al: Influence of aortic valve replacement on sudden death in patients with pure aortic stenosis. *Eur Heart J* 9(suppl E):139-141, 1988.

236. Moura LM, Ramos SF, Zamorano JL, et al: Rosuvastatin affecting aortic valve endothelium to slow the progression of aortic stenosis. *J Am Coll Cardiol* 49:544-561, 2007.

Chapter 24

Fluid Dynamics
of Prosthetic Valves

AJIT P. YOGANATHAN, PhD • BRANDON R. TRAVIS, PhD

The work reported from the authors' laboratory has been supported by grants from the Food and Drug Administration, the American Heart Association, and the Heart Valve Industry and generous gifts from Tom and Shirley Gurley and the Lilla Boz Foundation.

Doppler echocardiography has made noninvasive examination of prosthetic heart valve function a clinical reality. Unfortunately, there are still many imperfections in echocardiographic examinations as a result of acoustic shadowing, reflections caused by implanted valves, and limitations in ultrasound (US) technology. Despite these limitations, a number of important parameters can be calculated or estimated to aid in the assessment of prosthetic heart valve function and performance. Once a valve has been implanted, its function is governed primarily by its hemodynamic characteristics. To understand the hemodynamic performance of prosthetic heart valves, it is necessary to have a solid background in the physical laws that govern their function. Therefore, the purpose of this chapter is to introduce cardiologists to the governing principles of fluid dynamics, relevant formulations used in prosthetic valve assessment, and fluid mechanical characteristics of specific prosthetic heart valves.

Principles of Fluid Dynamics

Conservation of Mass

Conservation of mass, or continuity, is a mass balance over the boundaries of a volume. This volume can be made to coincide with a section of an artery, with the

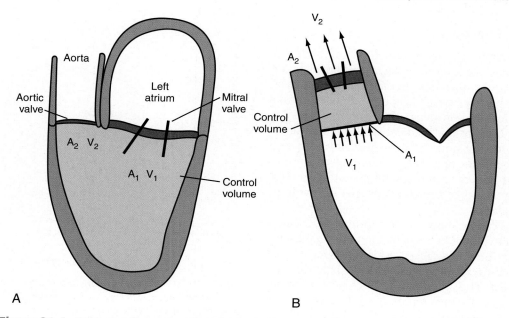

Figure 24–1. *Control volumes used for determining* (A) *mitral and* (B) *aortic valve area with conservation of mass. V_1 and V_2 represent average velocity of the blood flowing over areas A_1 and A_2.*

left ventricle or with the surface of a blood cell, and may be made to move over time as well. Such a volume is called a control volume, and its boundaries are usually chosen to give information regarding an unknown flow rate, average velocity, or surface area flow into or out of the volume based on more easily measurable quantities. Examples of control volumes useful for determining aortic and mitral valve areas with conservation of mass are shown in Figure 24–1.

Barring a nuclear reaction, mass can be neither created nor destroyed. Because nuclear reactions do not occur in cardiovascular applications, conservation of mass within the control volume can be expressed in words as:

$$\text{rate of mass accumulation} = \qquad (1)$$
$$\text{rate of mass input} - \text{rate of mass output}$$

In cardiovascular applications, an important simplification to Equation 1 can be made: the density of blood is constant. Because mass is the product of density and volume, mass conservation can be expressed as volume conservation:

$$\text{rate of volume accumulation} = \qquad (2)$$
$$\text{rate of volume input} - \text{rate of volume output}$$

In mathematical variables, this is:

$$\frac{(V_f - V_i)}{t} = Q_{in} = Q_{out} \qquad (3)$$

In which Q_{in} is the total flow rate into the control volume, Q_{out} is the total flow rate out of the control vol-

ume, V_i is the size of the control volume at the beginning of the observation, and V_f is the size of the control volume after an observation time t. It is important to recognize that Q_{in} and Q_{out} are the total flow rate into and out of the control volume. There can be multiple inputs and outputs (say, from branching vessels). For example, in a control volume with three inputs and outputs:

$$Q_{in} = (Q_{in(1)} + Q_{in(2)} + Q_{in(3)}) \qquad (4)$$
$$Q_{out} = (Q_{out(1)} + Q_{out(2)} + Q_{out(3)}) \qquad (5)$$

Conservation of mass becomes:

$$\frac{1}{t}(V_f - V_i) = \qquad (6)$$
$$(Q_{in(1)} + Q_{in(2)} + Q_{in(3)}) - (Q_{out(1)} + Q_{out(2)} + Q_{out(2)})$$

Equation 3 is true for control volumes that change with time, such as the volume of the left ventricle. An additional simplification can be made if the volume does not change with time. In this case, the left-hand side of Equation 3 is zero, and conservation of mass can be expressed as:

$$Q_{in} = Q_{out} \qquad (7)$$

This is approximately true in most blood vessels. Often, flow rate in circular, nonbranching vessels can be decomposed into an average axial velocity and a cross-sectional area (CSA). In this situation, conservation of mass can be used to define unknown average velocities or CSAs into or out of the control volume:

$$\bar{v}_{in}A_{in} = \bar{v}_{out}A_{out} \qquad (8)$$

Mechanical Energy

Mechanical energy can be described as the ability to accelerate a mass of material over a certain distance. Energy per unit volume has the same dimensions as pressure. It is perhaps best to report energy in cardiovascular applications on a per unit volume basis because the majority of the medical field is accustomed to working with the units of pressure. However, it is important to consider pressure as one of several forms of mechanical energy. Although they share the same units, pressure and mechanical energy per unit volume are not equivalent.

Pressure *(p)* can be shown to be a form of mechanical energy per unit volume by recognizing that it represents a force *(F_p)* per unit area *(A)*. If a force moving a mass over a distance *(d)*, it performs work, expending pressure energy *(E_p)*. The area that the force acts on multiplied by the same distance represents a volume *(V)*:

$$\frac{E_p}{V} = \frac{F_p d}{Ad} = \frac{F_p}{A} = p \tag{9}$$

Pressure is not the only form of mechanical energy in the circulation. Acceleration due to gravity *(g)* creates another form of mechanical energy per unit volume. A mass *(m)* accelerating due to gravity creates a force *(F_g)*. If this force moves the mass over a vertical distance *(h)*, it too performs work and expends gravitational energy *(E_g)*. The energy per unit volume is obtained by substituting density *(ρ)* for mass per unit volume.

$$\frac{E_g}{V} = \frac{F_g h}{V} = \frac{mgh}{V} = \rho gh \tag{10}$$

Finally, mechanical energy per unit volume exists in the circulation in the form of kinetic energy or energy of movement. If a mass *(m)* is moving at a velocity *(v)*, it contains kinetic energy, equivalent to half the product of the mass and the square of the velocity of the mass:

$$\frac{E_k}{V} = \frac{\frac{1}{2}mv^2}{V} = \frac{1}{2}\rho v^2 \tag{11}$$

Again, the energy per unit volume is obtained by substituting density for mass per unit volume. Thus, there are three forms of mechanical energy in the circulation. Pressure is the primary form of mechanical energy per unit volume in the healthy arterial circulation. In diseased or venous circulations, however, gravity and kinetic energy play a significant role in the movement of flow.

The primary source of mechanical energy in the circulation is the work performed by the left ventricle. Contraction of the ventricle creates an increase in pressure inside the ventricle. As Equations 9 infers, subsequent movement of a volume of fluid by this pressure results in the generation of mechanical energy. The energy generated by the ventricle during one cardiac

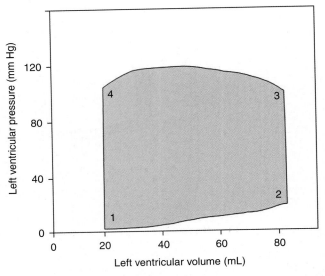

Figure 24–2. Pressure-volume diagram for the left ventricle. The shaded area represents the energy given to the flow by one stroke of the ventricle.

cycle is illustrated in Figure 24–2. This diagram represents the pressure and volume within the ventricle during the course of one cardiac cycle. The curve between points 1 and 2 represents the period of diastolic filling, where the mitral valve is open and the ventricle fills. The mitral valve shuts at point 2, and the period of isovolumic contraction begins. Between points 2 and 3, the volume of blood in the ventricle remains constant, but the pressure rises considerably. The aortic valve opens at point 3. This starts the period of systolic ejection, in which blood is moved by the ventricle into the aorta. At point 4, the aortic valve closes, and the period of isovolumic relaxation begins. During this period, the ventricular volume again remains constant, but the pressure falls. The fall in pressure returns the ventricle to its state at point 1. The energy generated by the ventricle during one cardiac cycle is equivalent to integral of the pressure-volume diagram (the shaded area in Fig. 24–2). The energy per unit volume generated by the ventricle is equivalent to the integral of the pressure diagram divided by the stroke volume (SV). This is roughly equivalent to the average increase in left ventricular (LV) pressure from diastole to systole. The ventricle thus creates energy in the form of pressure, but this energy is converted to gravitational and kinetic energy elsewhere in the circulation.

Bernoulli's Equation

Pressure, gravitational, and kinetic energies in the circulation can be freely converted from one to another without energy loss. Bernoulli's equation for steady flow illustrates this. Bernoulli's equation for steady flow relates the relative amounts of pressure, gravitational, and kinetic energy per unit volume between two spatial locations along a path of a flow (locations 1 and

2, where location 2 is downstream of location 1), assuming that no energy is lost:

$$\frac{1}{2}\rho v_1^2 + \rho g h_1 + p_1 = \frac{1}{2}\rho v_2^2 + \rho g h_2 + p_2 \qquad (12)$$

Bernoulli's equation for steady flow states the total mechanical energy per unit volume at locations 1 and 2 is the same but can exist in different forms. It shows that a decrease in pressure from location 1 to location 2 may be balanced from an increase in either fluid velocity or height without loss of energy. A pressure drop is therefore not mechanical energy loss if it is accompanied by increases in either gravitational or kinetic energy. These energies can be converted back to pressure energy later.

Additional variables can be added to Bernoulli's equation for steady flow to account for the effects of unsteady flow and mechanical energy loss:

$$\frac{1}{2}\rho v_1^2 + \rho g h_1 + p_1 = \qquad (13)$$
$$\frac{1}{2}\rho v_2^2 + \rho g h_2 + p_2 + \int_1^2 \rho \frac{\partial v}{\partial t} ds + \Phi$$

in which s represents the distance of the path between locations 1 and 2 and Φ represents loss of mechanical energy per unit volume. The added terms represents the contribution of temporal acceleration of the fluid to the flow energy and the conversion of mechanical energy to heat, respectively, between locations 1 and 2.

Mechanisms of Mechanical Energy Loss

Mechanical energy can be converted to heat through friction between blood moving at different velocities and the vessel walls. Such heat cannot be again converted to mechanical energy, and therefore this energy is said to be lost. As shown by Equation 13, mechanical energy loss per unit volume can be expressed as:

$$\Phi = (p_1 - p_2) + \qquad (14)$$
$$\frac{1}{2}\rho(v_1^2 - v_2^2) + \rho g(h_1 - h_2) - \int_1^2 \rho \frac{\partial v}{\partial t} ds$$

Such frictional losses take one of three forms: viscous losses, turbulent losses, and flow separation losses. All such losses are a result of the fluid interaction with the solid boundary of the vessel wall. Additional energy can be effectively lost in the circulation as result of valvular leakage. These forms of energy loss are described in the following sections.

Viscous Losses

As a result of frictional forces, fluid immediately adjacent to a solid boundary moves with the same velocity as the boundary. In the case of a stationary vessel, this means that fluid immediately adjacent to the ves-

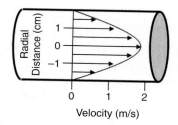

Figure 24-3. *Variations in velocity with respect to radial distance in a blood vessel. These variations are a result of viscous forces.*

sel wall does not move, no matter how fast the surrounding flow is moving. As one moves away from the solid boundary, the velocity increases. This leads to differences in fluid velocity with respect to radial distance within the vessel (Fig. 24-3). Fluid viscosity, the tendency of the fluid components or molecules to "stick" to each other, creates friction between the fluid components in close proximity if they move at different velocities. This is the mechanism of viscous energy loss. Viscous losses are proportional to flow rate. This type of energy loss is unavoidable but can be reduced notably in vessel flow by slight increases in radius. This is why vasodilators are effective in relieving LV workload.

Turbulent Losses

Turbulent losses usually do not occur in the circulation but can be greater in magnitude than viscous losses when they do. Turbulence is characterized by random spatial and temporal differences in the direction and magnitude of fluid velocity. It is a result of the inertia of the flow being too great for frictional forces to stabilize its movement. A useful analogy to turbulent flow is a car approaching a curve in the road. As the car turns, it undergoes a change in inertia in the direction of the curve. As long as the car maintains a low velocity relative to the friction that its tires generate in holding it to the road, the car follows the path of movement of its tires. If it does not, the frictional forces cannot hold the car to the road, and it slides across the pavement. This sliding greatly increases the friction between the tires and the road, resulting in large kinetic energy conversion to heat. This is similar to what happens in a turbulent flow. In a straight vessel, changes in inertia are initiated by small irregularities, or roughness, in the surface of the vessel. If these changes become large enough, viscous forces can no longer dampen them, and they propagate changes in inertia elsewhere in the flow. Friction between fluid components in close proximity moving at different velocities eventually converts this random kinetic energy to heat. Like in the case of the tendency for a car to skid, tendency for turbulence in a fluid flow depends on the geometry of the path that the fluid must travel and the ratio of inertial to frictional forces in the flow. The inertial force of a moving flow is the force required to bring the flow to rest, whereas the frictional force of such a flow is created by viscous shear stress acting on solid surfaces. In vessel flow, this ratio is approximated by the Reynolds number:

$$N_{Re} = \frac{D\bar{v}\rho}{\mu} \qquad (15)$$

in which D is the inner diameter of the vessel, v is the average velocity of the flow, ρ is the fluid density, and μ is the fluid viscosity. Flow through a straight pipe transitions to turbulence at Reynolds numbers of approximately 2000 and becomes fully turbulent at Reynolds numbers of approximately 6000.[1] Flow through small, circular orifices creates a phenomenon known as a free jet. For steady free jet flows, which are inherently more unstable than pipe flows, the critical Reynolds number is approximately 1000, with fully turbulent flow occurring at Reynolds numbers greater than 3000.[2,3] In pulsatile flow, the transition to turbulence depends on the ratio of local acceleration to frictional forces, or the Womersley number:

$$N_{Wo} = \frac{D}{2}\sqrt{\frac{\rho\omega}{\mu}} \qquad (16)$$

and the Reynolds number and chamber geometry.[4,5] The critical Reynolds numbers for the transition to turbulence in pulsatile flow is much higher than the corresponding numbers in steady flow. Estimates of transition to turbulence in the ascending aorta by Yoganathan and colleagues (based on work by Nerem and Seed[6]) indicated that the critical Reynolds number for transition is approximately 8000.[7] Turbulent losses are in general proportional to the square of the flow rate. Such losses can be eliminated by reducing the Reynolds number below the value at which the flow transitions to turbulence. Turbulent losses can also be eliminated or reduced by removing sharp corners and bends from a flow geometry because these can cause the flow to destabilize at lower Reynolds numbers. Finally, turbulent losses can be reduced by smoothening solid surfaces.

Flow Separation Losses

Flow separation occurs when the slow moving flow near a solid boundary reverses its direction. In the circulation, such reversal always occurs either after the passage of the pressure wave form the heart or after the flow has experienced a sudden expansion. In both such situations, the flow experiences a deceleration. Bernoulli's equation shows that in the absence of differences in gravitational energy, sudden decel-

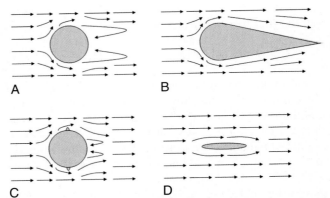

Figure 24–4. A shows flow separation distal to a sphere that may be thought of as the ball portion of a ball-and-cage heart valve. A considerable area of flow separation can be observed in the downstream flow. In B the ball has been converted into a teardrop shape, and flow separation is prevented by making the flow expansion gradual. In C the downstream portion of the ball has a protrusion that causes turbulence in the flow, reducing the area of flow separation. In D the ball replaced by a disc shape typical of a tilting disc valve, which is oriented parallel to the incoming flow direction, again reducing the area of flow separation.

eration (a decrease in kinetic energy) is accompanied by a sudden rise in downstream pressure. If such a rise occurs, it can overcome the inertia of the slow moving flow near the vessel wall and reverse its direction. A substantial amount of energy may be required to reinitiate the forward movement of reversed flow. This is energy loss resulting from flow separation. Recirculating or vortical flows are characteristic of the region downstream of flow separation. Figure 24–4A illustrates flow reversal caused by an expansion distal to a ball valve. Like turbulence, flow separation originates from changes in fluid momentum, and energy loss from separation is generally proportional to the square of the flow rate. Flow separation losses are heavily dependent on the ratio of smaller to larger radius during the flow expansion. Such losses can be reduced or eliminated by ensuring that all flow expansion is gradual (Fig. 24–4B), initiating turbulence in the flow (Fig. 24–4C), or orienting oblique obstructions parallel to the incoming flow direction (Fig. 24–4D). Gradual expansion allows the low velocity fluid near the vessel wall to mix with the higher velocity fluid closer to the vessel center as the pressure gradient increases. This mixing gives forward momentum to the low velocity fluid, preventing its separation. Turbulence accelerates the rate of mixing between low and higher velocity fluid, permitting more abrupt flow expansions without separation. Orienting oblique flow obstructions parallel to the incoming flow direction reduces the area over which flow is likely to separate.

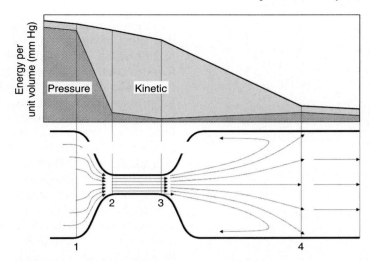

Figure 24–5. Schematic of pressure and kinetic energy loss and conversion as flow traverses a stenosis. The flow undergoes contraction from location 1 to location 2. The throat of the stenosis lies between locations 2 and 3, and the flow suddenly expands from location 3 to location 4.

Valvular Leakage

To compensate for the regurgitant flow, the ventricle must reverse the momentum of this flow and pump it again through the circulation. The additional energy required to perform this action while maintaining the required net forward flow rate represents an important form of energy loss. As can be expected, this form of energy loss is heavily dependent on the regurgitant volume and can be minimized by reducing the magnitude of this volume.

Mechanical Energy Conversion and Loss in a Stenosis

To show how mechanical energy may be changed from one form to another or lost, it is perhaps best to refer to an illustration depicting the changes in mechanical energy across an aortic stenosis (AS). Such an illustration is shown in Figure 24–5. This figure shows the conversion and losses in total, pressure, and kinetic energies as blood flow traverses the contraction, throat, and expansion sections of the stenosis.

The first section of the stenosis, from 1 to 2, is a flow contraction. Because the continuity equation states that the velocity at 2 must be higher than that at 1, kinetic energy increases from 1 to 2. This increase in kinetic energy occurs at the expense of a large amount of pressure energy. A relatively small amount of total energy is actually lost in the flow contraction. Most of the lost energy in flow contraction is a result of from viscous losses. There may, however, be a small amount of flow separation immediately following especially abrupt contractions. Flow separation occurs because the momentum of the flow causes it to continue to converge for a short period after the anatomic contraction (see Fig. 24–5). Such abrupt contractions have considerably more energy loss than gradual ones.

The second section of the stenosis, from 2 to 3, represents a throat of constant CSA. In this section, the continuity equation states that the velocity at 2 and 3 are the same. Therefore, there is no loss in kinetic energy; the total energy lost in this section is completely pressure energy. It is worth noting that only in nonbranching vessels of constant CSA is pressure gradient equivalent to total energy loss per unit volume and that usually only a small amount of total energy is lost in the stenosis throat. This energy loss is viscous in nature if the flow is laminar and completely turbulent in nature if the flow has enough momentum to enable its transition to turbulence.

Finally, in the expansion section of the stenosis, from 3 to 4, a large amount of total energy is lost. All of this lost energy is kinetic in nature, which explains why the Doppler gradient correlate so strongly with total mechanical energy loss. However, the Doppler gradient does not completely specify total energy loss because a portion of the kinetic energy is converted into pressure. This is the cause of the pressure recovery phenomenon. Pressure recovery is most significant in stenoses in which the flow expansion is either small or gradual in nature. Figure 24–6 illustrates the difference between gradual and sudden and small and large flow expansions. The expansion section of the stenosis illustrates why pressure gradients can be misleading in the estimation of the lost driving force for flow. Although the pressure increased in the expansion section, the total energy loss was very large.

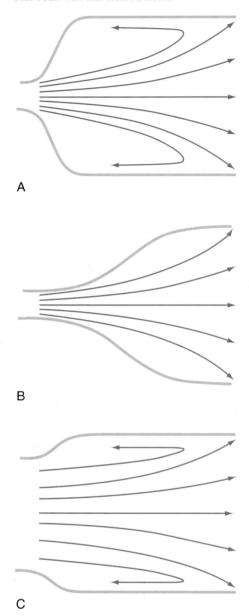

A

B

C

Figure 24–6. *Flow expansions. A, Sudden and large; B, gradual and large; and C, sudden and small.*

Applications of Fluid Dynamics to Prosthetic Heart Valves

Pressure Drop

Pressure drop across a heart valve is commonly used to estimate the amount of energy lost by the flow in traversing the valve. Such pressure drops can be directly measured with invasive catheter techniques. Equation 14 shows that the pressure drop across a heart valve is equivalent to energy loss per unit volume if changes in the kinetic energy, gravitational energy, and local acceleration of the flow can be neglected. Because of

Equation 8, changes in kinetic energy are negligible if diameters of the vessels are the same at the locations of the upstream and downstream pressure measurements and if the downstream measurements are obtained at a location far enough from the valve to allow for pressure recovery. Changes in gravitational energy are negligible if the patient is supine because there is little to no height difference between upstream and downstream measurement locations. Changes in local acceleration of the flow are negligible if measurements are obtained during peak flow rate across the valve (often called the peak gradient) or if measurements are averaged over the forward flow portion of the valve cycle (often called the mean gradient). Pressure drop is also often reported in terms of a peak-to-peak gradient, in which changes in local acceleration are likely close to negligible. Differences between peak and peak-to-peak gradients are shown in Figure 24–7.

Doppler Gradient

Although energy lost by the flow in traversing the valve can be estimated more directly with catheterization, such losses are now typically estimated noninvasively with the help of echocardiography, when such equipment is available. Such estimation is based on the observation that in a narrow stenosis with an abrupt expansion, nearly all the pressure that is converted to kinetic energy as the flow contracts (see Figure 24–5) is lost when it expands again. A simplified form of Equation 14 is used to estimate the amount of pressure converted to kinetic energy as the flow contracts from well upstream of the valve to the point of maximum flow contraction:

$$\Delta p = 4(v_{max}^2 - v_{ups}^2) \qquad (17)$$

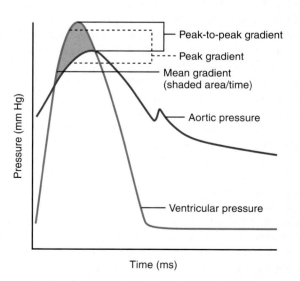

Figure 24–7. *Mean, peak, and peak-to-peak pressure differences across an aortic valve.*

in which Δp is the pressure drop ($p_1 - p_2$) during the flow contraction in mm Hg, v_{ups} is the velocity upstream of the contraction during forward flow in cm/s, and v_{max} is the velocity at the point of maximum flow contraction during forward flow in cm/s. The constant 4 is used to account for the density of blood and unit conversions. This simplification assumes that mechanical energy loss and changes in gravitational energy and local acceleration are negligible as the flow contracts. As shown in Figure 24–5, if a contraction is gradual, it contributes little mechanical energy loss. Justification of the latter assumptions was given in the discussion of pressure drop.

The conversion from pressure to kinetic energy within the flow contraction of Figure 24–5 is therefore the quantity measured when estimating pressure gradient with Doppler echocardiography. Because some of the pressure that is converted to kinetic energy is recovered as the flow expands, the Doppler gradient does not necessarily measure energy lost by the flow. In sudden expansion from a narrow orifice, the conversion of pressure to kinetic energy is correlated quite strongly to total mechanical energy loss. However, pressure recovery can be expected to cause problems in the estimation of pressure gradient in patients with prosthetic valves because these valves usually present only a small degree of stenosis.

Another problem in the use of Doppler US in pressure gradient estimation is the placement of the transducer relative to the axis of the jet issuing from the stenosis. If the transducer is placed obliquely with respect to the jet axis, the measured velocity will underestimate the true velocity of the jet.[7] Because the errors resulting from pressure recovery and oblique transducer placement tend to offset each other, Doppler US can at times match pressure measurements obtained from catheterization quite precisely. However, this is somewhat of a chance occurrence and should be regarded as the exception rather than the rule.

Additional complications in the use of Doppler gradient to evaluate the total energy loss across mechanical prostheses arise because these valves have more than one orifice and because the resistance that each orifice offers to flow can be different. Velocity measurements made in the one orifice are therefore not representative of the gradient in either pressure or total energy as flow traverses the valve. This is a particular problem with bileaflet prostheses,[8] because the central orifice of most current designs of these prostheses creates considerably more resistance to flow than the two lateral orifices. The difference between Doppler and catheter gradients has been so notable for mechanical prostheses that empirically derived correction factors, dependent on valve design, have been suggested to the Food and Drug Administration (FDA).[9] Some studies

claim that there is negligible difference between pressure gradients measured with catheter and Doppler, particularly with regard to mean gradients.[10] However, because of its potential problems, the use of Doppler to evaluate the performance of mechanical prostheses should be approached with caution, and Doppler measurements from the same orifice are desirable if they are to be compared.

Often, Equation 17 is simplified further by assuming that upstream velocity is small relative to the maximum velocity within the contraction:

$$\Delta p = 4v_{max}^2 \tag{18}$$

This simplification should be performed with caution because in most new generation prosthetic valves the upstream velocity is *not* small relative to the maximum velocity.

Effective Orifice Area

Evaluation of valve performance by pressure drop and Doppler gradient are heavily dependent on the flow rate across the valve. Effective orifice area (EOA) does not vary considerably with flow rate, and therefore can be applied as an evaluation of valve performance independent of cardiac output (CO) and heart rate (HR).

EOA does not represent the anatomic orifice area; it instead represents the CSA of the jet issuing from the valve at the point of its largest contraction. The size of the EOA depends on the nature of the contraction and the size of the orifice itself. For this reason, a sudden contraction may have a smaller effective orifice area than a gradual contraction, even though the two orifices have identical anatomic orifice areas (Fig. 24–8).

When echocardiography equipment is available, EOA is typically estimated by applying Equation 8 to echocardiography measurements of the upstream vessel area (A_{ups}), the temporal average of the velocity upstream of the contraction during forward flow and

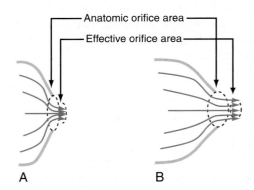

Figure 24–8. *Orifices with identical anatomic areas but different effective orifice areas. Sudden flow contractions result in small effective orifice areas.*

the temporal average of the velocity at the point of maximum flow contraction during forward flow:

$$EOA = \frac{A_{ups}V_{ups}}{V_{max}} \quad (19)$$

When echocardiography is unavailable, the Gorlin formula can be used to estimate EOA. The Gorlin formula is a combination of Equations 8 and 18:

$$EOA = \frac{Q}{51.6\sqrt{\Delta p}} \quad (20)$$

In which EOA is in cm^2, Q is the temporal average of the flow rate during forward flow in cm^3/s and Δp is the average pressure drop across the valve during forward flow in mm Hg. The constant 51.6 is used to account for the density of blood and unit conversions. In the application of Equation 20, two subtleties should be kept in mind. The first of these is that for an accurate estimation of the EOA, the pressure gradient term in Equation 20 should be the Doppler gradient. When the Gorlin formula is used with catheter measurements, Equation 20 can be expected to overestimate effective orifice area as a result of the pressure recovery phenomenon. However, the catheter formulation, dubbed the energy loss coefficient, may be useful as a separate entity in evaluating the severity of aortic stenosis. The second subtlety is that all variables in Equation 20 are averages during the systolic period. Instantaneous values of pressure and flow rate cannot be used in Equation 20 unless taken at peak flow rate. This is because the Gorlin formula is derived using Bernoulli's equation for steady flow and is therefore invalid in situations in which there is a large net temporal acceleration or deceleration in the flow. Averages over the entire cycle may not be relevant either, especially if aortic regurgitation occurs concurrently.[11] Most techniques for estimation of forward flow rate that do not involve echocardiography (Fick's method, thermal dilution, and dye dilution) are averages over the entire cardiac cycle (Q_{net}). If no regurgitation is present, these methods can be used to estimate the average forward flow rate during systole. However, if aortic regurgitation is present, direct application of Gorlin's formula will result in an underestimation in EOA:

$$Q = \frac{Q_{net}}{(1-RF)} \quad (21)$$

in which *RF* represents the regurgitant fraction of the aortic valve.

A measure of a valve's resistance to forward flow that is based on EOA is the performance index. This is the ratio of effective orifice area to the valve sewing ring area:

$$PI = \frac{EOA}{A_{sew}} \quad (22)$$

and provides a measure of how well a valve design utilizes its total mounting area, the area the flow would experience without the valve. Whereas EOA is dependent on valve size, performance index effectively normalizes effective orifice area for valve size.

Regurgitant Volume

Pressure drop, Doppler gradient, and EOA give quantitative estimates of the energy lost by the flow in traversing a valve during forward flow. Flow energy can also be lost as a result of leakage across the valve when the pressure gradient across the valve reverses. A small amount of flow leaks across the valve during valve closure. In addition, mechanical prosthetic valves are unable to form tight seals when closed, and regurgitant jets are present in these valves under normal conditions. Normal regurgitant flow is characterized by a closing volume during valve closure and leakage after closure. These parameters are illustrated in Figure 24–9. The regurgitant volume is the total volume of fluid through the valve per beat as a result of the retrograde flow. It is equal to the sum of the closing volume and the leakage volume. The closing volume is the volume of fluid flowing retrograde through the valve during valve closure. Any fluid volume accumulation after valve closure results from leakage and is referred to as the leakage volume.

Regurgitant volume of prosthetic valves is governed by valve type, size, and position. Bioprostheses have a small closing volume but do not leak if functioning properly. Bileaflet mechanical designs tend to have greater regurgitant volume than tilting disc designs.[12] Larger valves leak more than smaller ones. Regurgitant volume is most problematic in positions in which the pressure gradient during closure and leakage is high and in which the duration of leakage is long. Energy

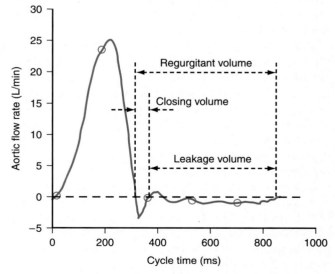

Figure 24–9. *Regurgitant, closing, and leakage volumes across an aortic valve.*

losses resulting from regurgitant flow can exceed forward flow energy losses in large mitral prostheses.[12] Although prosthetic valves normally exhibit a small amount of regurgitant flow, they can cause substantial regurgitation when they malfunction. To distinguish normal from abnormal valve function, it is important to differentiate between normal regurgitant volume and additional regurgitation resulting from disease. Most means of quantifying regurgitant volume use some form of a control volume and conservation of mass.

Perhaps the most commonly used example is the proximal isovelocity surface area, or PISA, method[13-16] of estimating regurgitant volume. The principle of the PISA technique is based on the fact that a fluid enters a regurgitant orifice must accelerate to reach a peak velocity at the throat of the orifice. If the orifice is circular, this acceleration region should be axisymmetric about the center of the orifice (Fig. 24–10). Thus, upstream of the regurgitant orifice, a series of hemispherical isovelocity contours can be defined within the flow field. Equation 7 states that for a control volume that does not change in size, the same amount of fluid that enters the volume must exit it as well. If the control volume is constructed to coincide with a hemispherical contour and the regurgitant orifice:

$$RV = 2\pi r^2 v_{ups} t \tag{23}$$

in which v_{ups} the temporal average of the velocity at a radial distance r upstream of the regurgitant orifice during forward flow and t represents the time during which regurgitation takes place during a single beat. The expression $2\pi r^2$ in this equation represents the surface area of the hemispherical shell surrounding the control volume.

The most serious limitation of the PISA technique is its assumption that isovelocity contours around regurgitant orifices are hemispherical in shape. This assumption has been reported to function quite well for estimating regurgitant volume in patients with functional mitral regurgitation from natural valves. However, it is likely invalid for patients with mechanical prostheses. Such valves have several asymmetric regurgitant orifices, some of which are partially surrounded by solid boundaries.

Novel Energy Loss Parameters

As Figure 24–5 infers, much more mechanical energy is lost in flow expansion than in flow contraction or in the throat regions of prosthetic valves. This is particularly true in tissue valves, resulting from gradual nature of the flow contraction and the small throat region. The localization of energy loss to the flow expansion region simplifies the problem considerably by allowing energy losses occurring in aortic valve stenoses to be modeled by an abrupt expansion. The total energy loss per unit volume across an abrupt expansion can be derived using Equation 8, Equation 14, and a form of conservation of momentum[17]:

$$\Phi = 4v_{max}^2 \left(1 - \left(\frac{EOA}{A_{aorta}}\right)\right)^2 \tag{24}$$

in which Φ is in mm Hg and v_{max} is the temporal average of the velocity at the point of maximum flow contraction in cm/s. Equation 24, like recovered pressure, is thus a strong function of the EOA and the CSA of the aorta. As this area ratio approaches zero, the energy loss per unit volume in the expansion approaches the Doppler gradient. Thus, in cases of severe valvular stenosis, the Doppler gradient is equivalent to mechanical energy loss per unit volume. The advantage of using Equation 24 rather than pressure drop or Doppler gradient is that Equation 24 allows the estimation of energy lost by the flow in traversing the valve by noninvasive echocardiography while compensating for pressure recovery. In using this formulation in the aorta, the CSA of the expansion should be taken as the CSA of the aorta at the sinotubular junction because the separated flow disappears after the flow has traversed the sinuses of Valsalva.

The energy loss in Equation 24, like pressure drop and Doppler gradient, is dependent on flow rate. It is desirable to have a parameter that is closely related to energy loss but relatively independent of flow rate for the evaluation of prosthesis function. Such a parameter can be derived by substituting Equation 24 for the Dop-

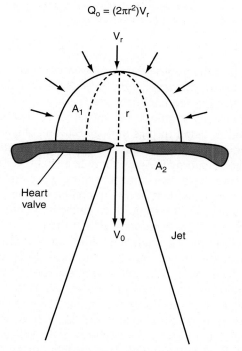

$$Q_o = (2\pi r^2)V_r$$

Figure 24–10. *Proximal isovelocity surface area schematic. V_r is the velocity on a hemispheric shell defined by radius r and surface area A_1. A_2 is the regurgitant orifice area, and V_o is the peak jet velocity.*

pler gradient in Equation 20. This parameter has been dubbed the energy loss coefficient[18]:

$$ELCo = \frac{A_{aorta}EOA}{(A_{aorta} - EOA)} \quad (25)$$

In which EOA is measured by echocardiography, using either Equation 19 or Equation 20. The energy loss coefficient is equivalent to Equation 20 if Δp in Equation 20 is measured with pressure transducers that are placed far enough downstream to account for energy recovery. The advantage of using the energy loss coefficient rather than EOA is that the energy loss coefficient is based on recovered pressure.

Hemodynamics of Native Valves

To effectively analyze flow through prosthetic heart valves in the mitral or aortic positions, it is important to understand the conditions under which natural valves function. Figure 24–9 illustrates typical pressure and flow waveforms for healthy individuals at both the aortic and the mitral valves. During systole, the pressure difference required to drive the blood through the aortic valve is on the order of a few millimeters of mercury. Diastolic pressure differences across the aortic valve are much larger than systolic, the pressure usually being about 80 millimeters of mercury. The valve closes near the end of the deceleration phase of systole with little reverse flow. The blood flow through the mitral valve is biphasic during diastole, as shown in Figure 24–11. The first peak, the E-wave, results from ventricular relaxation, whereas the second peak, the A-wave, is caused by contraction of the left atrium. This means that all valves in the mitral position open and close twice during each cardiac cycle. It is also evident that all cardiac valves are closed during both isovolumic contraction and isovolumic relaxation.

Measurements of the velocity profile just distal to the aortic valve have been performed with Doppler echocardiography in normal subjects.[19] The peak systolic velocity is 1.35±0.35 m/s, and the velocity profile at the level of the aortic valve annulus is relatively flat. However there is usually a slight skew toward the septal wall (less than 10% of the center line velocity) caused by the orientation of the aortic valve relative to the long axis of the left ventricle. This skew in the velocity profile has been shown by many experimental techniques, including hot film anemometry,[20,21] Doppler US,[22] and magnetic resonance imaging (MRI).[23]

The flow patterns distal to the aortic valve also play an important role in proper valve function. During systole, vortices form behind each leaflet in the sinus region. In vitro studies have attempted to relate these vortices to effective valve closure.[24,25] It has been

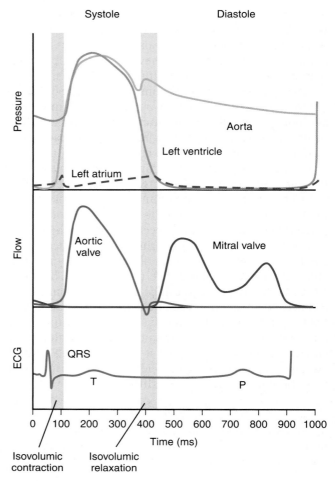

Figure 24–11. *Pressure and flow waveforms for the left-sided heart. ECG, electrocardiogram.*

shown that the ventricular vortices are unnecessary for valve closure; however, they do ensure that the valve closes quickly, reducing leakage.[26]

The velocity profile at the mitral valve has been determined in detail in pigs and should be comparable to the velocity profile in humans because of the similarity in cardiac anatomy.[27] Again there is a slight skew to the profile, but there does not seem to be a preferred orientation. It is dependent on the particular geometry of the mitral valve, the diastolic flow patterns within the left ventricle, and the location at which the pulsed Doppler sample volume is placed. When the sample volume was placed at the mitral annulus, the peak early diastolic velocity was 63.6±16.1 cm/s, whereas the late diastolic peak velocity was 53.7±10.8 cm/s. When the sample volume was at the tip of the mitral valve leaflets, the peak early diastolic velocity was 82.9±30.8 cm/s and the peak late diastolic velocity was 39.6±14.2 cm/s.

Vortices develop in the left ventricle during diastole, as blood enters through the mitral valve. Bellhouse[28] proposed that the vortices helped to close the mitral valve at the end of diastole. Later work has shown that the vortices play a role in early closing of the mitral valve but late closure is dominated by LV pressure.[29]

Because of the restrictive area of prosthetic valves, the peak velocities are usually higher, and the spatial velocity profiles are dramatically different from those in natural valves. The shear stresses in prosthetic valves will also be much larger because of the higher velocities and turbulence. The magnitude of the shear stress varies greatly depending on the type of prosthetic valves. It is important to note the differences and similarities between valve types in terms of shear stress magnitudes, peak velocities, and flow patterns so that an effective assessment of prosthetic valve function can be performed.

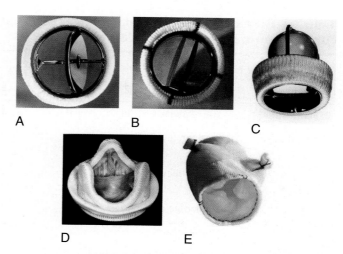

Figure 24–12. *Major types of prosthetic heart valves.* A, *Tilting disc;* B, *bileaflet;* C, *ball;* D, *stented bioprosthesis; and* E, *stentless bioprosthesis.*

Hemodynamics of Specific Prosthesis Designs

Prosthetic heart valves have been successfully used in heart valve replacement over the past 40 years. Currently, heart valve prostheses can be classified into two primary categories, mechanical and biological. Mechanical valves in current clinical use are comprised of three basic designs or classifications: ball and cage, tilting disc and bileaflet. The biological valves can be further classified into three categories: stented, unstented, and homograft valves. Figure 24–12 shows examples of each type of prosthesis.

Although significant progress has been made in the development of better prostheses through new materials and more physiologic valve designs, several problems associated with prosthetic valves have not been eliminated. Existing problems that can be related to the valve hemodynamics or local fluid mechanics are (1) thrombosis and thromboembolism, (2) hemolysis, (3) tissue overgrowth, (4) damage to endothelial lining, and (5) regurgitation. The presence of high shear stresses can lead to damage of formed blood elements, platelet activation, and initiation of biochemical processes affecting coagulation. Lethal damage to red cells can occur with fluid shear stresses as low as 800 dynes/cm[2].[30] However, these levels can be significantly lower, 10 to 100 dynes/cm[2], in the presence of foreign surfaces, such as presented by a valve prostheses.[31,32] In addition, platelet activation and damage have been shown to occur in shear stresses ranging from 100 to 500 dynes/cm[2].[33] The residence time of the cell in the damaging fluid environment is a significant factor in determining lethal stress levels that further complicates the mechanism for damage. Additionally, regions of flow separation and stagnation form local environments suitable for accumulation and growth of thrombi and fibrous/pannous tissue.[34] The fluid mechanic performance of prosthetic heart valves is often assessed through in vitro testing to determine transvalvular pressure drops, regurgitant volumes

(closure and leakage), distal and proximal velocity fields, and the locations and levels of turbulent stresses. The relationship between valve fluid mechanics and development of problematic function has been studied by numerous investigators over the past two decades. In vitro studies have concentrated on quantifying local fluid stress levels through flow measurement techniques, such as laser Doppler anemometry, hot film anemometry, and US velocimetry. Table 24–1 summarizes the peak velocity and turbulent shear stress levels for many of the 27 mm aortic valves in clinical use, whereas EOA and performance indices for such valves are provided in Tables 24–2 and 24–3.

The fluid mechanics of the various prosthetic valve designs will be discussed in this section. Comparisons between the many valve designs within each classification of prostheses will be left to the many references dealing with the assessment of individual valves. Both antegrade and retrograde flow fields will be described. All flow characteristics will be referenced from in vitro experiments conducted in our laboratory unless otherwise specified. In most citations, the data will be representative of 25 or 27 mm aortic prostheses tested under physiologic pulsatile flow conditions providing a CO of 5 to 6 L/min and a heart rate of 70 beats per minute. Exact test conditions (valve size, CO, heart rate, pressures) will be noted for each citation.

Mechanical Valves

The three major mechanical valve designs or classes are the tilting disc, bileaflet, and ball and cage. These valves differ primarily in the type and function of the occluder. Although these different designs influence the valvular fluid mechanics, all three designs share common flow structures, such as well-defined jet flows, wakes with some degree of flow reversal, and

TABLE 24-1. Peak Systolic Velocity and Turbulent Shear Stress Levels for Common 27 mm Aortic Valve Prostheses*

Valve Type	Valve	Measurement Location	Peak Velocity (cm/s)	Peak Turbulent Shear Stress (dynes/cm²)
Ball-and-cage	Starr-Edwards 1260	12 mm downstream	220	1850
Tilting disc	Björk-Shiley Convexo-concave	7 mm downstream 11 mm downstream	200 200	3400 1800
	Björk-Shiley Monostrut	8 mm downstream 11 mm downstream	200 200	1250 800
	Medtronic-Hall	13 mm downstream	200	1500
	Omnicarbon	14 mm downstream	225	2000
Bileaflet	St. Jude Medical Standard	13 mm downstream	210	1500
	Duramedics	13 mm downstream	210	2300
	CarboMedics	12 mm downstream	228	1520
Stented bioprosthesis	Carpentier-Edwards Porcine 2625	15 mm downstream	370	4500
	Carpentier-Edwards Porcine 2650	15 mm downstream	200	2000
	Carpentier-Edwards Pericardial 2900	17 mm downstream	180	1000
	Hancock MO Porcine 250	10 mm downstream	330	2900
	Hancock II Porcine 410	18 mm downstream	260	2500
	Ionescu-Shiley Standard Pericardial	27 mm downstream	230	2500
	Hancock Pericardial	18 mm downstream	170	2100
Nonstented bioprosthesis	Medtronic Freestyle†	Leaflet tips 10 mm from tips	125 100	— —
	TSPV†	Leaflet tips 10 mm from tips	150 125	— —

*Heart rate 70 beats per minute; cardiac output 5 L/min; 120/80 mm Hg aortic pressure.
†Data obtained from in vitro Doppler ultrasound measurements.

turbulent shear layers. The antegrade flow and regurgitant flow characteristics for each valve design will be discussed separately in the following sections. EOA and performance indices for several prosthetic valve designs in clinical use today are provided in Tables 23-2 and 23-3. Because the design of a valve can strongly influence the local fluid dynamics, a brief discussion of the pertinent design features of each class of valve will be provided.

Tilting Disc Valves

The tilting disc valve has one occluder (disc) generally of a circular cross section. The disc is often mounted such that it is free to rotate about a pivot axis, typically displaced from the disc diameter. Metal struts are used to secure the disc within the valve housing and control

its range of motion. Numerous design variations of the tilting disc valve exist. These designs vary in the pivot mechanism or strut design, the range of disc motion allowed, or in the geometry of the disc, which can range from flat to curved. Typically, the occluder opens to angles between 60 and 80 degrees with respect to the valve annulus.

The tilting disc valve is characterized by two orifices separated by the occluder. The major orifice is the larger open area formed between the disc pivot axis and the housing, as the disc swings distally to the open position. This orifice is free of blockage as a result of mounting struts and causes little resistance to transvalvular flow. As the disc opens, the remaining part of the disc, on the other side of the pivot axis, swings in the proximal direction forming the minor orifice. Mounting struts, which can vary from one to two depending on

TABLE 24–2. In Vitro Hemodynamic Data for Common Aortic Valve Prostheses*

Valve Type	Valve	Size	Regurgitant Volume (mL/beat)	EOA† (cm²)	PI
Ball-and-cage	Starr-Edwards 1260	27	5.5	1.75	0.30
		25	4.3	1.62	0.33
		21	2.5	1.23	0.36
Tilting disc	Björk-Shiley Convexo-concave	27	8.5	2.59	0.45
		25	7.3	2.37	0.48
		21	5.5	1.54	0.45
	Björk-Shiley Monostrut	27	9.2	3.34	0.58
		25	7.6	2.62	0.53
		23	6.9	2.00	0.48
		21	5.9	1.45	0.42
		19	5.5	1.07	0.38
	Medtronic-Hall	27	9.6	3.64	0.64
		25	8.4	3.07	0.62
		23	7.3	2.26	0.54
		20	6.2	1.74	0.51
Bileaflet	St. Jude Standard	27	10.8	4.09	0.71
		25	9.9	3.23	0.66
		23	8.3	2.24	0.54
		21	6.8	1.81	0.52
		19	6.8	1.21	0.43
	St. Jude Regent	29	13.5	4.98	0.75
		27	12.3	4.40	0.77
		25	11.2	3.97	0.81
		23	10.3	3.47	0.83
		21	9.0	2.81	0.81
		19	7.6	2.06	0.73
		17	6.3	1.56	0.69
	CarboMedics	27	7.5	3.75	0.65
		25	6.1	3.14	0.64
		23	6.51	2.28	0.55
		21	3.4	1.66	0.48
		19	3.0	1.12	0.40
Stented bioprosthesis	Carpentier-Edwards Porcine 2625	27	<3	1.95	0.34
		25	<2	1.52	0.31
		21	<2	1.28	0.37
	Carpentier-Edwards Porcine 2650	27	<2	2.74	0.48
		25	<2	2.36	0.48
		21	<2	1.38	0.40
		19	<2	1.17	0.41
	Carpentier-Edwards Pericardial 2900	27	<3	3.70	0.64
		25	<2	3.25	0.66
		21	<2	1.88	0.54
		19	<2	1.56	0.55
	Hancock Porcine 242	27	<3	2.14	0.37
		25	<2	1.93	0.39
		23	<2	1.73	0.42
		21	<2	1.31	0.38
		19	<2	1.15	0.41

*Heart rate 70 beats per minute; cardiac output 5 L/min, typical; 120/80 mm Hg aortic pressure.
†EOA computed from Equation 8.
EOA, effective orifice area; PI, performance index.

Continued

TABLE 24–2. **In Vitro Hemodynamic Data for Common Aortic Valve Prostheses—cont'd**

Valve Type	Valve	Size	Regurgitant Volume (mL/beat)	EOA† (cm²)	PI
Stented bioprosthesis— cont'd	Hancock MO Porcine 250	25	<2	2.16	0.44
		23	<2	1.94	0.47
		21	<2	1.43	0.41
		19	<2	1.22	0.43
	Hancock II Porcine 410	27	<2	2.36	0.41
		25	<2	2.10	0.43
		23	<2	1.81	0.44
		21	<2	1.48	0.43
	Ionescu-Shiley Standard Pericardial	27	<3	2.35	0.41
	Medtronic Mosaic Porcine	29	<3	3.15	0.48
		27	<2	2.81	0.49
		25	<2	2.11	0.43
		23	<2	1.74	0.42
		21	<1	1.54	0.44
	CarboMedics Mitroflow Pericardial	29	<4	3.71	0.56
		23	<3	2.12	0.51
		19	<2	1.34	0.47
Nonstented bioprosthesis	Medtronic Freestyle Porcine	27	<4	3.75	0.65
		25	<4	3.41	0.69
		23	<3	2.69	0.65
		21	<2	2.17	0.63
		19	<2	1.84	0.65

valve design, typically span the minor orifice. As a result of the upstream protrusion of the disc into the minor orifice tract and the presence of the mounting struts, a slight obstruction of flow is encountered. At least one tilting disc designs, the Omni-Carbon, incorporate pivots rather than mounting struts.

Antegrade Flow. Figure 24–13 illustrates the antegrade flow patterns of the Medtronic-Hall tilting disc valve. The antegrade flow is characterized by a major orifice jet and a minor orifice jet. The major orifice jet is spatially larger than the minor orifice jet. It is semicircular in cross section with peak systolic velocities of approximately 2 m/s in the aortic position. Under comparable flow conditions, most tilting disc valves exhibit similar major orifice jet structures and peak velocity magnitudes.

The spatial structure of the minor jet varies depending on the number of struts used to secure the disc. In single strut designs, such as the Bjork-Shiley monostrut and the Medtronic-Hall tilting disc, the minor orifice jet appears as two jets separated by a well-defined wake behind the strut. The flow on each side of the strut is nearly symmetric with similar spatial structure and velocity magnitude. The Omni-Carbon valve has a minor orifice jet similar in magnitude to the Bjork-Shiley

but lacks the wake because it does not have a strut. Valves with two struts display a minor orifice jet structure consisting of a strong central jet bounded by two weaker jets. The adjacent weaker jets are separated from the central jets by the wakes of the struts. Their velocity magnitude is roughly 30% to 40% of the velocity magnitude of the central jet. The peak velocities of the minor orifice jet are typically of the same magnitude or slightly less than the peak velocity in the major orifice jet in nearly all tilting disc designs.

Wake regions are observed behind the valve struts and disc. These wake regions are areas of flow separation with significant velocity defect and nearly stagnant flow. Wake regions persist for 10 to 20 mm downstream of the valve annulus. As a result of the opening angle of the disc, the major and minor orifice jets are directed toward the wall on the major orifice side of the valve, following the occluder. In the aortic position, this results in a region of separated flow in the sinuses located below or near the minor jet at peak systole. As a result of the strong major orifice jet and the orientation of the disc with respect to the flow, strong secondary flow structures are encountered downstream of the valve. These secondary flows form a pair of counter-rotating vortices or helical motions. The vortices are generated by the high momentum fluid in the major jet

TABLE 24–3. In Vitro Hemodynamic Data for Common Mitral Valve Prostheses*

Valve Type	Valve	Size	Regurgitant Volume (mL/beat)	EOA† (cm²)	PI
Ball-and-cage	Starr-Edwards 1260	30	—	1.99	0.28
		28	—	1.66	0.27
		26	—	1.56	0.29
Tilting disc	Björk-Shiley Standard	31	—	3.40	0.45
		29	6.7	2.79	0.42
		25	—	2.15	0.44
	Björk-Shiley Convexo-concave	29	10.1	2.96	0.45
		27	8.3	2.28	0.40
		25	—	2.03	0.41
	Medtronic-Hall	31	10.0	3.53	0.47
		29	10.0	3.53	0.53
		27	8.9	2.73	0.47
		25	7.2	2.23	0.45
Bileaflet	St. Jude Medical Standard	31	13.1	3.67	0.48
		29	10.9	3.40	0.51
		27	9.7	2.81	0.49
Stented bioprosthesis	Hancock Porcine 342	35	<4	2.72	0.28
		33	<4	2.54	0.30
		31	<4	2.36	0.31
		29	<4	2.11	0.32
		27	<2	1.77	0.31
		25	<2	1.63	0.33
	Hancock II Porcine	33	<4	2.66	0.31
		31	<3	2.29	0.30
		29	<3	2.05	0.31
		27	<2	1.78	0.31
		25	<2	1.59	0.32
	Carpentier-Edwards Porcine 6650	27	<2	2.03	0.35
	Carpentier-Edwards Porcine 6900	27	<2	2.68	0.47
	Carpentier-Edwards Porcine 6625	31	<4	2.58	0.39
	Edwards SAV	33	—	1.60	—
		31	—	1.58	—
		29	—	1.56	—
		27	—	1.32	—
		25	—	1.20	—
	Edwards Perimount	33	—	2.80	—
		31	—	2.76	—
		29	—	2.70	—
		27	—	1.92	—
		25	—	1.76	—
	Ionescu-Shiley Standard Pericardial	31	<5	3.00	0.40
		27	<2	1.77	0.31
		25	<2	1.61	0.33

*Heart rate 70 beats per minute; cardiac output 5 L/min, typical.
†EOA computed from Equation 8.
EOA, effective orifice area; PI, performance index.

Continued

TABLE 24-3. In Vitro Hemodynamic Data for Common Mitral Valve Prostheses—cont'd

Valve Type	Valve	Size	Regurgitant Volume (mL/beat)	EOA† (cm²)	PI
Stented bioprosthesis—cont'd	Mosaic Porcine	33	<4	2.38	0.28
		31	<3	2.26	0.30
		29	<3	2.02	0.31
		27	<2	1.71	0.30
		25	<2	1.55	0.32
	St. Jude Biocor Pericardial	31	—	2.53	—
		29	—	1.48	—
		33	—	2.04	—
		29	—	1.96	—
Nonstented bioprosthesis	Mitral Valve Allograft‡	25	—	3.38	0.69
		23	—	1.80	0.43

‡In vitro measurements at 5 L/min.

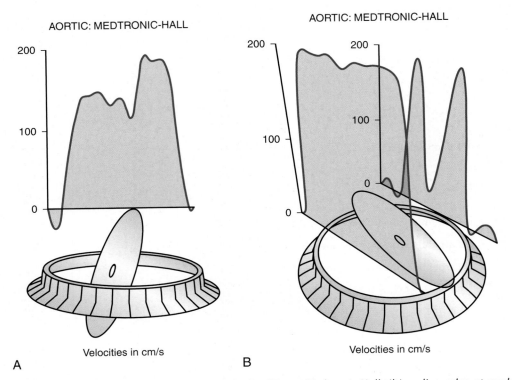

AORTIC: MEDTRONIC-HALL

Velocities in cm/s

A

AORTIC: MEDTRONIC-HALL

Velocities in cm/s

B

Figure 24-13. *Velocity profiles downstream of a 27-mm Medtronic-Hall tilting disc valve at peak systole. A, Centerline 15 mm downstream; B, traversing major and minor orifices 13 mm downstream.*

wrapping around the sides of the disc and flowing into the low momentum, separated flow regions immediately behind the disc. Flow over the disc generates vortex shedding similar to that observed with flow over a delta wing airfoil.

Normal Regurgitant Flow. The tilting disc design shows slightly lower regurgitant volumes than the bi-leaflet design resulting from both reduced closing and leakage volumes. Ranges for the regurgitant volume of the tilting disc valve vary from approximately 5.5 mL/beat for 19 and 20 mm valves to 9 mL/beat for the 29 mm sizes. Tables 24-2 and 24-3 list the regurgitant volumes for several prosthetic valve designs.

The leakage flow of mechanical valves is often in the form of small scale regurgitant jets. In the tilting disc design, these jets emanate from small gaps around the perimeter of the valve between the disc and the valve housing. Baldwin and colleagues[35] measured the gap width of a Bjork-Shiley monostrut valve with Delrin rings and obtained widths of approximately 75 μm, which varied non-uniformly around the valve perimeter. These leakage jets were believed to be advantageous as a result of the potential for washing of the perimeter of the valve housing during closure. However, recent studies have shown that the regurgitant jets are of a significant velocity magnitude, ranging from 2 to 5 m/s, and turbulent stresses may be several times greater than in the antegrade flow field.

Orientation. The orientation of the tilting disc valve in the mitral position has been studied in vivo by Jones and colleagues.[36] These authors made comparisons of the orientations of the major orifice jet of tilting disc valves with respect to the LV geometry. The studies indicated that the preferred orientation for tilting disc valves in the mitral position is with the major orifice oriented toward the LV free wall, as opposed to the septum. Greater intraventricular turbulence was observed with a septal orientation of the major orifice compared to a free wall orientation. Orientation of the major orifice toward the septal wall produced large areas of velocity reversal, directed against the minor orifice. In contrast, free wall orientation of the major orifice produced more physiologic LV flow patterns. These results have been corroborated in in vitro flow visualization studies conducted in our laboratory, under physiological flow conditions in an anatomically correct LV model.[37]

Studies by Travis and colleagues[38] and Kleine and colleagues[39] have examined the effects of valve orientation on forward flow hemodynamics through mechanical prostheses in the aortic position. Travis and colleagues studied the effects of valve orientation on fluid mechanical energy loss and transvalvular pressure drop in angled in vitro models of the aortic inflow tract. This studies have shown that orientation of the disc such that it is parallel to the proximal flow direction when the valve is in the open position minimizes energy loss and pressure drop for the tilting disc valve. Kleine and colleagues used an in vivo pig model to examine the effects of prosthesis orientation on turbulent stresses. These researchers found a minimum in turbulent stress magnitude with orientation of the major orifice to the right posterior aortic wall, which is the area of highest velocities during ejection.

Bileaflet Valves

The bileaflet design is characterized by two semicircular leaflets typically made of pyrolytic carbon that are hinged to the valve housing. The leaflets divide the flow into three regions, two lateral orifices and a central orifice. Many subtle differences exist between bileaflet valves to improve their hemodynamics. Hinge design variations are employed to control opening angle and influence the local fluid mechanics, washout, and flow patterns generated in the hinge, which may affect leaflet function and pressure drop. The ATS valve pivot, for example, is inverted relative to other designs to provide improved pivot washout. Bileaflet valves have comparable or smaller pressure drops and comparable or larger EOAs than comparably sized tilting disc designs, and their large opening angles are likely one of the reasons for this. Nonetheless, there is variation in opening angle between 75 and 90 degrees among the different bileaflet valve designs. Curvature is at times incorporated into bileaflet valve design. The leaflets of the Sorin Bicarbon valve have curvature to ensure equal distribution of flow across the three orifices. Finally, the housing can be altered to improve fluid dynamics. The St. Jude Medical Regent valve features a thinner housing thickness than other designs to increase EOA of the valve. The On-X design enhances the EOA through a housing that ensures that flow expansion and contraction near the valve are more gradual than other designs.

Antegrade Flow Fields. The antegrade flow fields of bileaflet designs are characterized by three jets. Two jets emanate from the lateral orifices and one from the central orifice as illustrated in Figure 24–14. Greater forward flow emerges from the lateral orifices than from the central orifice in most valve designs. The cross section of the lateral jets tends to be of a crescent shape, whereas the central jet is nearly planar in cross section. Wakes generated from the leaflets separate the three jets and persist for several centimeters downstream. The triple jet pattern is also discernible in two-dimensional color flow maps using color Doppler US techniques as illustrated in Figure 24–15. This color Doppler flow map was obtained in pulsatile flow in vitro studies of a 31-mm St. Jude bileaflet valve in the mitral position.

The central jet loses its coherence after 2 to 3 cm as the lateral jets grow and merge into the central flow region. However, the lateral jets do maintain their coherence and relatively high velocity magnitude over a greater distance. The flow is initially well ordered during the early acceleration phase and becomes turbulent before peak systole. Separated regions with flow reversal are generally observed around the perimeter of the housing. The separated regions tend to be asymmetric around the valve with larger spatial dimensions near the hinges than adjacent to the lateral jets.

Normal Regurgitant Flow. Retrograde flow characteristics for the bileaflet design are similar to those for the tilting disc valve. Regurgitant volume characteristics are summarized in Tables 24–2 and 24–3. The bileaflet design shows slightly larger regurgitant volumes than the tilting disc valve. Leakage flow through the bileaflet

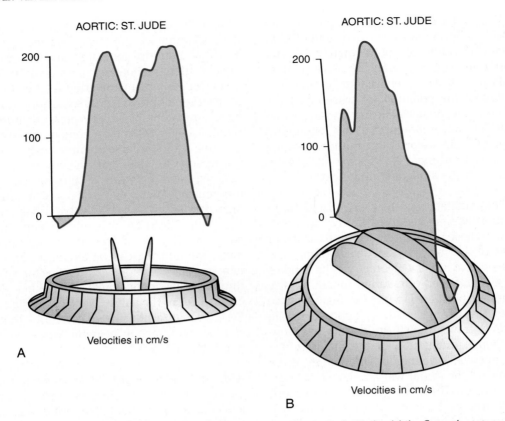

AORTIC: ST. JUDE

AORTIC: ST. JUDE

Velocities in cm/s

Velocities in cm/s

A

B

Figure 24–14. *Velocity profiles downstream of a 27-mm St. Jude Medical bileaflet valve at peak systole. A, Centerline 13 mm downstream; B, traversing lateral and central orifices 13 mm downstream.*

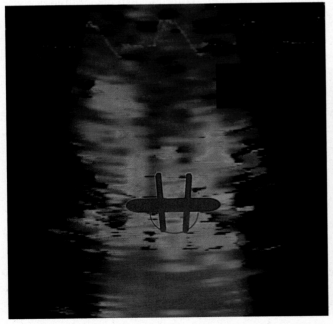

Figure 24–15. *Two-dimensional color-Doppler flow mapping of the downstream triple jet flow fields of a bileaflet valve design under physiologic pulsatile flow conditions.*

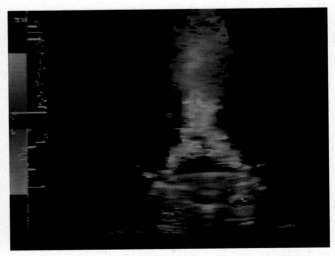

Figure 24–16. *Two-dimensional color-Doppler flow mapping of the leakage jet flow fields of a bileaflet valve design under physiologic pulsatile flow conditions.*

valve design occurs primarily through the pivots (Fig. 24–16). In addition, leakage is also observed around the periphery and from the gap between the two leaflets. Velocity and turbulence measurements, obtained both within the pivots and 1 mm upstream of the valve housing in the aortic position, indicate that the major jets persist through nearly all of diastole. The mean velocity magnitudes in the jets are on the order of 2 to 3 m/s with turbulent shear stress levels exceeding 3000 dynes/cm^2.

Orientation. The bileaflet valve is mounted in one of two orientations in the mitral position. The first position is the "anatomic position," with the leaflet hinge plane of the valve oriented in a direction perpendicular to the plane of the aortic outflow and mitral inflow tracts. The leaflets pivot in a similar plane as that of the native mitral valve leaflets. The second position is the "antianatomic position." The valve is mounted such that the leaflet hinge plane is rotated 90 degrees from the anatomic position. The orientation of the St. Jude bileaflet valve in the mitral position has been studied in in vitro flow visualization experiments conducted in our laboratory. The results of these studies indicate that the antianatomic position provides better flow patterns along the posterior wall of the ventricle. Potentially better lateral flow expansion in the plane perpendicular to the plane of the aortic outflow and mitral inflow tracts is also observed. However, the anatomic position provides adequate flow patterns within the left ventricle with slightly narrower lateral expansion of the inflow jets.

Van Rijk-Zwikker and colleagues[40] investigated the effects of orientation of the CarboMedics bileaflet valve in in vivo pig studies. Two-dimensional echocardiographic and color Doppler measurements were analyzed to determine the influence of valve orientation on valve function and the transvalvular flow patterns within the left ventricle. The 90-degree, antianatomical orientation was found to be superior to the anatomical orientation of the valve. The anatomical orientation resulted in diastolic backflow directed toward the valve, which may lead to asymmetric motion of the valve leaflets. The antianatomical position produced diastolic backflow patterns that enter the left ventricular outflow tract (LVOT). Minimal interference with the function of the leaflets is expected from these flow patterns.

The studies of Travis and colleagues[38] and Kleine colleagues[39] examined the effects of aortic bileaflet valve orientation and tilting disc valve orientation on forward flow hemodynamics. Travis and colleagues found that orienting the leaflets of the open valve parallel to the proximal flow direction resulted in decreases in energy losses and pressure drops in vitro. Kleine and colleagues found that turbulence created by a bileaflet valves was minimal when one of the lateral orifices faces the right posterior wall of the aorta.

Ball Valve

The ball-and-cage valve is characterized by a silicone ball mounted into a wire cage, as illustrated in Figure 24–12. The only ball-and-cage valve in use today is the Starr-Edwards 1260. The cage is constructed from three wire struts separated by 120 degrees. The struts emanate from the valve housing and converge at the distal end of the valve, called the apex of the cage. The ball is free to travel along the cage, typically over a 1-cm to 2-cm distance. Ball-and-cage valves have much larger pressure drops and smaller EOAs than comparably sized tilting disc and bileaflet valves, mostly as a result of the large separation region behind the ball.

Antegrade Flow Fields. The flow fields of these valves consist of annular jets that emerge from around the occluder or poppet. In the aortic position, the jets are initially directed toward the wall of the aorta where they impact and then follow the contour of the aortic wall. Peak systolic velocities in the aorta are comparable to those encountered in the other valve designs, approximately 2 m/s at peak systole. The annular jets show rapid development early in systole during the acceleration phase of flow. A gradual divergence and growth of the jet is observed with increasing displacement downstream, where the jet maintains its structure over a considerable axial distance. Velocity profiles at peak systole are shown in Figure 24–17, 30 mm down-

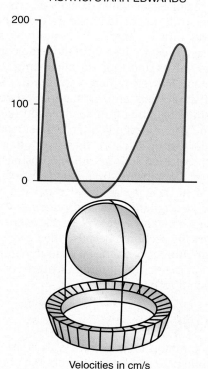

AORTIC: STARR-EDWARDS

Velocities in cm/s

Figure 24–17. *Centerline velocity profile 30 mm downstream of a 27-mm Starr-Edwards ball-and-cage valve at peak systole.*

stream of the valve. Large mean velocity gradients are observed alongside the annular jet, with values exceeding 1500 per second. The flow field in the mitral position is similar to the jet structure in the aortic position. However, the jet peak velocities are lower, the jet decays more rapidly, and greater lateral expansion of the jet occurs in the ventricle.

The ball generates a large wake in the central part of the flow field that starts in early systole and grows into a region of reverse flow lasting from peak to end-systole. The lateral extent of this region of reverse flow is on the order of 8 to 10 mm distal to apex of the cage. Peak reverse velocities can be as high as 20 to 25 cm/s. These regions of large separation are responsible for the thrombogenecity of these valves.[41] The ball in these types of valves is often observed to fluctuate at the apex, which is most likely a result of flow instabilities within the wake or vortex shedding from the ball. This phenomenon increases the lateral extent of the wake and produces an increase in the relative velocity between the ball and the model wall and an increase in pressure drop across the prosthesis.

Normal Regurgitant Flow. The normal regurgitant flow of the ball and cage design is composed mainly of the closing volume flow. The seating of the ball valve is generally good with little or no leakage flow.

Bioprostheses

The three major tissue valve designs or classes are the stented xenograft, unstented xenograft, and homograft. These valves differ primarily in tissue type and structure. Tissue valves are less thrombogenic compared to mechanical valves and thus do not require anticoagulant treatment. However, these valves suffer from calcification of the leaflets and/or material fatigue leading to valve failure resulting from leaflet rupture or tearing. Calcification of the tissue is often a precursor to leaflet rupture and tearing because these are often observed adjacent to calcified lesions. All bioprosthesis designs share the characteristics of flexible leaflets, a single orifice, and no leakage after valve closure. The antegrade flow, regurgitant flow, and pressure drop characteristics for each valve type will be discussed separately in the following sections. Because the design of a valve can strongly influence the local fluid dynamics, a brief discussion of the pertinent design features of each class of valve will also be provided.

Stented Valves

The most common bioprosthetic valves are composed of three biological leaflets made from the porcine aortic valve or bovine pericardium. They are constructed similarly to the natural aortic valve. The annular ring is cloth covered and molded to function similarly to the aortic annulus. Metal or polymeric stents provide support to the leaflets at their commissures in the stented design, whereas the leaflet commissures in nonstented aortic valves must be attached to the native aorta for support. The clinically available designs vary mainly in the support structure and in the leaflet material and fixation media. However, all trileaflet bioprostheses open to a centrally located orifice with respect to the valve annulus and mimic the open geometry of the normal aortic valve but with a smaller orifice area.

All stented porcine tissue valves are mildly stenotic compared to the natural valve in large sizes and moderately to severely stenotic in the small sizes. Porcine valves in small sizes exhibit a higher degree of stenosis than comparably sized mechanical valves. This stenotic behavior is results in part from the construction of the leaflets, the stiffness of the fixed tissue, and the man-made commissures. The presence of the stents also acts to restrict the motion of the leaflets somewhat during opening. The new generation of stented pericardial valves (Carpentier-Edwards and MitroFlow) has pressure drop characteristics comparable to the St. Jude Standard and Medtronic-Hall mechanical valve designs in all sizes.

Antegrade Flow Fields

All stented bioprosthetic valves have central jet type flow fields as illustrated in Figure 24–18. The newer generation porcine valves and most pericardial valves create flatter velocity profiles then earlier porcine valve designs. This results in more evenly distributed down-

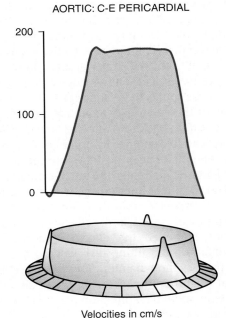

AORTIC: C-E PERICARDIAL

Velocities in cm/s

Figure 24–18. Centerline velocity profile 17 mm downstream of a 27-mm Carpentier-Edwards pericardial valve at peak systole.

stream flow fields and lower turbulent shear stress levels. Early designs, such as the Carpentier-Edwards porcine model 2625 and the Hancock I porcine valves, generated asymmetric jet profiles. The jets were directed slightly away from the stent in a plane that bisected one leaflet and the stent opposite that leaflet. Peak aortic velocities exceed 3 m/s at peak systole for normal flow conditions.

The newer porcine designs, such as the Carpentier-Edwards porcine 2650 and the pericardial valves, produce jets that are wider and have more blunted profiles. These jets exhibit a more axisymmetric velocity profile with large mean velocity gradients (viscous stresses) alongside the jets. Peak velocities range from 2 to 3 m/s under normal flow conditions in the aortic position. These jets still show a slight laterally directed motion similar to the older porcine valve designs but not as pronounced. In in vitro experiments, stagnant flow can be observed throughout systole between the outflow surfaces of the valve leaflets and the flow model wall. In earlier valve designs, these stagnation regions were larger and exhibited regions of flow reversal. Stented bioprosthesis stagnant regions can be amplified in conditions of low CO in which one of the three leaflets may fail to open fully. Flow stasis can lead to deposition of thrombogenic elements on the outflow surfaces of the leaflets.

Normal Regurgitant Flow

All tissue valves exhibit some degree of regurgitant flow in the closing volume. Leakage volume is essentially zero in properly functioning valves. However, the closing volumes are generally lower than in the mechanical prostheses. This results from more rapid closure of the valve leaflets for tissue valves compared to the occluders of the mechanical valve designs. Regurgitant volumes are on the order of 1 mL/beat for most tissue valves. However, the Ionescu-Shiley pericardial valve has closing volumes ranging from 2.5 to 6.5 mL/beat, depending on valve size and position (aortic or mitral). Typical values of the regurgitant volumes for several bioprosthetic valves are given in Tables 24–2 and 24–3. Regurgitant jets are normally nonexistent, and the presence of such a jet indicates valve incompetence.

Nonstented Valves

Nonstented aortic valve prostheses have been fashioned from porcine, bovine, and equine tissue. Some valves, such as the Medtronic Freestyle, include the natural valve and some length of the intact aorta. In these valves, the right and left coronary arteries are ligated with short remnants to aid in reimplantation of the patient's coronaries. Others, such as the Sorin Pericarbon Freedom, are fabricated from sheets of tissue and implanted below the coronaries. In vitro testing of nonstented aortic bioprostheses requires a compliant test chamber capable of simulating the human aortic root.

As a result of the added complexity of the unstented design and the increased factors governing selection and style, optimal flow performance of these valves both in vitro and in vivo is dependent on the type of valve configuration used for a particular patient geometry and on the proper sizing of the valve. Improper selection of style and size can compromise hemodynamic performance of the valve. In vitro tests of the Medtronic Freestyle valve indicate that the EOA can be optimized by the use of a valve one size larger than the size of the simulated aorta. Thus a 23-mm valve should be used in a 21-mm size aorta. Total root or an inclusion cylinder valve geometry technique showed better EOA results than partially or fully scalloped valve configurations.

Unstented valves typically have comparable pressure drops to similar sized mechanical prostheses[42-44] and lower pressure drops than similar sized stented valves. An example of this can be seen in comparing the Medtronic Freestyle and Mosaic porcine valves. These valves have the same exact tissue and tissue treatment processes. However, the effective orifice area of a 23-mm Freestyle valve was found to be similar to that of a 27-mm Mosaic valve. Thus, removal of stents results in less forward flow obstruction and significantly improves overall hemodynamic performance.

During the past few years, several investigators have begun testing and using mitral valve heterografts.[45] These mitral heterografts typically use fixed valves with or without intact papillary muscles. These new mitral replacements can be considered to be nonstented bioprostheses. While no mitral valve replacements are currently approved in the United States, one design is in clinical trials in Europe. This valve, the St. Jude Quattro valve, is fashioned from pericardium and offers reasonable hemodynamics. Intermediate term clinical results of this valve are promising. Mitral heterografts have the potential for better hemodynamic performance, reduced thrombogenesis, and improved LV function.

Antegrade Flow Fields

Doppler results for a 27-mm Medtronic Freestyle valve[42] indicate that the flow accelerates uniformly through the valve with an apparent uniform and flat profile downstream of the valve. Doppler measured peak velocities at the leaflet tips ranged from 75 to 125 cm/s at COs from 3 to 5 per minute. The peak velocities decreased to a range of 60 to 100 cm/s at 5 to 10 mm from the leaflet tips over the same range of COs. There is no appearance of a jet with steep velocity gradients, as is observed in stented bioprostheses. Similar results were obtained from US Doppler measurements conducted with a 29-mm St. Jude Medical Toronto SPV valve design, and can be expected from other designs as well.

Normal Regurgitant Flow

The nonstented aortic valves exhibit regurgitant volumes that are comparable to closing volumes of valves exhibiting similar EOAs. Good coaptation is observed with little or no leakage.

Nonstented mitral valve heterografts tested in our laboratory exhibited comparable closing volumes to unfixed natural valves tested in the same flow loop. Good coaptation was observed with no leakage. The function of mitral heterografts is strongly dependent on the implantation technique. This is expected when considering the complicated function of the mitral complex compared to the aortic valve.

Homograft Valves

Homograft valves are cryopreserved human valves and have been used for more than two decades in the aortic position. With the advent of improvements in surgical techniques and viable mitral heterografts, a mitral homograft is also a possibility. Aortic homografts are typically implanted as a complete valve, annulus, and aortic section. As a result, the effective annulus area is reduced from the original aortic valve annulus before replacement. Mitral homografts consist of intact mitral valves with annulus, papillary muscles, and chordae tendineae. Homografts have lower pressure drops and larger EOAs relative to mechanical and stented valves.

Antegrade Flow Fields

The flow field characteristics of the homograft aortic valves are similar to those of the natural valve, although peak velocities are slightly higher as a result of the reduced EOAs resulting from the smaller area of the outflow tract. However, peak velocities are smaller than those observed in other prosthetic designs for comparably sized valves. The aortic homograft shows excellent hemodynamics over the entire size range in contrast to the stented bioprostheses, which show increased stenosis in the smaller valve sizes.

Studies conducted in our lab indicate that sheep allograft mitral valves and untreated normal mitral valves have excellent hemodynamics compared to stented valves.[46] The unfixed mitral valves exhibit both qualitatively and quantitatively similar forward flow characteristics to those observed clinically for normal human mitral valves.

Normal Regurgitant Flow

As with other bioprosthetic valves, the homograft valves exhibit small closing volumes. Properly functioning homograft valves should exhibit little or no re-gurgitation as a result of leakage. The mitral homografts show the same dependency of implantation technique on overall hemodynamics. Proper implantation of the valve complex including proper alignment of the papillary muscles with the valve annulus will result in superior function with no regurgitation other than normal closing volume.

Future Directions

We foresee that the future directions in prosthetic valve research will follow several courses: development of polymeric prostheses; tissue engineering bioprosthetic valves, invention of novel tissue fixation techniques; improving designs of mechanical valves; improving in vitro, computational, and animal testing protocols; and development of noninvasive diagnostic capabilities. Polymeric prostheses may offer patients a durable alternative to mechanical and bioprostheses with little tendency for calcification or thromboembolic complications. The goal of tissue engineering research is to grow living human aortic valves in the laboratory, preferably using the patient's own tissue. Potential advantages involve total acceptance of the living tissue, with hemodynamic and cellular function similar to the normal human aortic valve resulting in a lifetime equal to that of native valves. Tissue xenografts are currently fixed in glutaraldehyde, which stiffens the compliance of the valve material and hinders hemodynamic performance. Other fixative techniques may improve hemodynamic performance or increase the functional lifetime of xenografts. For mechanical valves, the focus will be on reducing their thrombogenic properties. This could possibly be accomplished by development of biocompatible surface coatings and materials or by changing valve geometry to improve closure and leakage flow through these valves. A first step in this research should be in improved understanding of blood element damage, thromboembolic events, and thrombus formation. In vitro evaluation techniques and in vivo diagnostic techniques for bulk flow hemodynamics will focus more closely on mechanical energy loss, and more attention will be devoted to the small-scale, local hemodynamics that may give rise to thromboembolic complications.

KEY POINTS

- Application of conservation of mass to a control volume allows the calculation of unknown flow rates, average velocities, or surface areas into or out of the volume based on measurable quantities.

- Mechanical energy per unit volume is a measure of the work available to drive flow.

■ Pressure as one of several forms of mechanical energy, but there are others (kinetic and gravitational). These forms can be freely converted from one to another without loss. Pressure loss and mechanical energy loss per unit volume are not equivalent because pressure can be recovered from a fall in either gravitational or kinetic energy.

■ Effective means of reducing mechanical energy loss in the circulation include ensuring any expansions in flow occur gradually, ensuring bends and corners in the flow path are not sudden or sharp and increasing vessel radius.

■ The Doppler gradient measures the conversion of pressure to kinetic energy in flow across a valvular prosthesis. It does not measure mechanical energy loss, although it can be closely related to it.

■ The EOA of a valvular prosthesis represents the CSA of a flow at its smallest contraction. It is equal to or smaller than the anatomic orifice area.

■ Mechanical energy losses occur as a result of regurgitant flow and forward flow. Losses resulting from regurgitant flow can be greater than losses resulting from forward flow in large, mitral mechanical prostheses.

REFERENCES

1. Batchelor G: *An Introduction to Fluid Dynamics.* Cambridge, Cambridge University Press, 1994.
2. Blevins R: *Applied Fluid Dynamics Handbook.* New York, Van Nostrand Reinhold Company, 1984.
3. McNaughton K, Sinclair C: Submerged jets in short cylindrical flow vessels. *J Fluid Mech* 25:367-375, 1966.
4. Sarpkaya T: Experimental determination of the critical Reynolds number for pulsating Poiseuille flow. *J Basic Engineering* September:589-598, 1966.
5. Yellin E: Laminar-turbulent transition process in pulsatile flow. *Circ Res* 19:791-804, 1966.
6. Nerem R, Seed W: An in vivo study of aortic flow disturbances. *Cardiovasc Res* 6:1-4, 1972.
7. Yoganathan AP, Recusani F, Valdez-Cruz L, et al: Oblique flow vectors from dispersing jets produce the velocity overestimation on angle corrected continuous wave Doppler studies: *in vitro* laser Doppler investigations. *Circulation* 76(suppl IV):355-355, 1987.
8. Mascherbauer J, Schima H, Maurer G, Baumgartner H: Doppler assessment of mechanical aortic valve prostheses: effect of valve design and size of the aorta. *J Heart Valve Dis* 13(5):823-830, 2004.
9. Stewart SF, Herman BA, Nell DM, and Retta SM. Effects of valve characteristics on the accuracy of the Bernoulli equation: a survey of data submitted to the U.S. FDA. *J Heart Valve Dis* 13(3):461-466, 2004.
10. Knebel F, Gliech V, Walde T, et al: High concordance of invasive and echocardiographic mean pressure gradients in patients with a mechanical aortic valve prosthesis. *J Heart Valve Dis* 14(3):332-337, 2005.
11. Scotten L, Walker D, Dutton J: Modified Gorlin equation for the diagnosis of mixed aortic valve pathology. *J Heart Valve Dis* 11:360-368, 2002.
12. Strüber M, Campbell A, Richard G, Laas J: Hydrodynamic function of tilting disc prostheses and bileaflet valves in double valve replacement. *Eur J Cardiothor Surg* 10:422-427, 1996.
13. Recusani F, Bargigga G, Yoganathan A, et al: A new method for quantification of regurgitant flow rate using color Doppler flow imaging of the flow convergence region proximal to a discrete orifice. An in vitro study. *Circulation* 83:594-604, 1991.
14. Utsunomiya T, Ogawa T, Doshi R, et al: Doppler color flow "proximal isovelocity surface area" method for estimating volume flow rate: Effects of orifice shape and machine factors. *J Am Coll Cardiol* 17:1103-1111, 1991.
15. Utsunomiya T, Ogawa T, Tang H, et al: Doppler color flow mapping of the proximal isovelocity surface area: A new method for measuring volume flow rate across a narrowed orifice. *J Am Soc Echocardiogr* 4:338-348, 1991.
16. Utsunomiya T, Doshi R, Patel D, et al: Regurgitant volume estimation in patients with mitral regurgitation: initial studies using the color Doppler "proximal isovelocity surface area" method. *Echocardiography* 9:63-70, 1991.
17. Garcia D, Pibarot P, Dumesnil JG, et al: Assessment of aortic valve stenosis severity: A new index based on the energy loss concept. *Circulation* 101(7):765-771, 2000.
18. Garcia D, Dumesnil JG, Durand L, et al: Discrepancies between catheter and Doppler estimates of valve effective orifice area can be predicted from the pressure recovery phenomenon. *J Am Coll Cardiol* 41(3):435-442, 2003.
19. Rossvoll O, Samstad S, Torp H, et al: The velocity distribution in the aortic annulus in normal subjects: A quantitative analysis of two-dimensional Doppler flow maps. *J Am Soc Echocardiogr* 4:367-378, 1991.
20. Paulsen P, Hasenkam J: Three-dimensional visualization of velocity profiles in the ascending aorta in dogs, measured with a hot film anemometer. *J Biomech* 16:201-210, 1983.
21. Paulsen P, DMSc: Copenhagen, 1989.
23. Kilner P, Yang G, Mohiaddin R, et al: Helical and retrograde secondary flow patterns in the aortic arch studied by three-directional magnetic resonance velocity mapping. *Circulation* 88:2235-2247, 1993.
24. Bellhouse B: Velocity and pressure distributions in the aortic valve. *J Fluid Mech* 37:587-600, 1969.
25. Bellhouse B, Bellhouse F: Fluid mechanics of model normal and stenosed aortic valves. *Circ Res* 25:693-704, 1969.
26. Reul H, Talukdar N: In Hwang N, Gross D, Patel D (eds): *Quantitative Cardiovascular Studies Clinical and Research Applications of Engineering Principles.* Baltimore: University Park Press, 1979, pp. 527-564.
27. Kim W, Bisgaard T, Nielsen S, et al: Two-dimensional mitral flow velocity profiles in pig models using epicardial Doppler echocardiography. *J Am Coll Cardiol* 24:532-545, 1994.
28. Bellhouse B: Fluid mechanics of a model mitral valve and left ventricle. *Circ Res* 6:199-210, 1972.
29. Reul J, Talukder N, Müller E: Fluid mechanics of the natural mitral valve. *J Biomech* 14:361-372, 1981.
30. Lu PC, Lai HC, Liu JS: A reevaluation and discussion on the threshold limit for hemolysis in a turbulent shear flow. *J Biomech* 34(10):1361-1364, 2001.
31. Mohandas H, Hockmuth RM, Spaeth EE: Adhesion of red cells to foreign surfaces in the presence of flow. *J Biomed Mater Res* 8:119-136, 1974.
32. Blackshear PL: Hemolysis at prosthetic surfaces. *Chemistry of Biosurfaces* 2:523-561, 1972.
33. Klaus S, Korfer S, Mottaghy K, et al: In vitro blood damage by high shear flow: human versus porcine blood. *Int J Artif Organs* 25(4):306-312, 2002.
34. Yoganathan AP, Wick TM, Reul H: Influence of flow characteristics on thrombus formation. In Butchart EG, Bodnar E (eds): *Thrombosis, Embolism and Bleeding* London, ICR Publishers, 1992, pp. 123-148.
35. Baldwin JT, Deutsch S, Geselowitz DB, Tarbell JM: LDA measurements of mean velocity and Reynolds stress fields within an artificial heart ventricle. *J Biomech Eng* 116:190-200, 1994.

36. Jones M, McMillan S, Eidbo E, et al: Evaluation of prosthetic heart valves by Doppler flow imaging. *Echocardiography* 3:513-525, 1986.

37. Lefebvre X: Georgia Institute of Technology, 1992.

38. Travis B, Heinrich R, Ensley A, et al: The hemodynamic effects of mechanical prosthetic valve type and orientation on fluid mechanical energy loss and pressure drop in *in vitro* models of ventricular hypertrophy. *J Heart Valve Dis* 7(3):345-354, 1998.

39. Kleine P, Perthel M, Nygaard H, et al: Medtronic Hall versus St. Jude Medical mechanical aortic valve: downstream turbulences with respect to rotation in pigs. *J Heart Valve Dis* 7(5):548-555, 1998.

40. Van Rijk-Zwikker G, Delemarre B, Huysmans H: The orientation of the bi-leaflet Carbomedics valve in the mitral position determines left ventricular spatial flow patterns. *Eur J Cardiothor Surg* 1996;10(7):513-520, 1996.

41. Yoganathan AP, Raemar HH, Corcoran WH, et al: The Starr-Edwards aortic ball valve: flow characteristics, thrombus formation and tissue overgrowth. *Artif Organs* 5:6-17, 1981.

42. Yoganathan AP, Eberhardt CE, Walker PG: Hydrodynamic performance of the Medtronic Freestyle aortic root bioprosthesis. *J Heart Valve Dis* 3:571-580, 1994.

43. Nagy Z, Fisher J, Walker P, Watterson K: The effect of sizing on the *in vitro* hydrodynamic characteristics and leaflet motion of the Toronto SPV stentless valve. *J Thorac Cardiovasc Surg* 117(1):92-98, 1999.

44. Erikson M, Brodin L, Dellgren G, Radegran K: Rest and exercise hemodynamics of an extended stentless aortic bioprosthesis. *J Heart Valve Dis* 6(6):653-660, 1997.

45. Vrandecic M, Gontijo BF, Fantini FA, et al: Anatomically complete heterograft mitral valve substitute: surgical technique and immediate results. *J Heart Valve Dis* 1:254-259, 1992.

46. Vetter HO, Yoganathan AP, Fontaine AA, et al: Hydrodynamic characteristics of a new stentless mitral valve allograft: In vitro results, In Leipschs D (ed): *3rd International Symposium on Biofluid Mechanics.* Munich, Germany, VDI-Verlag GmbH Publishers, 1994, pp. 287-294.

Chapter 25

Echocardiographic Recognition and Quantitation of Prosthetic Valve Dysfunction

MIGUEL ZABALGOITIA, MD

Thirty years ago, prosthetic valves were limited to the ball-and-cage mechanism; since then, single and double tilting discs and several stented and stentless biologic devices have been introduced. Each of these valves has individual ultrasonic and hemodynamic characteristics depending on their size and functional mechanism (see Chapter 24), making the role of the echocardiographer and sonographer understandably more complex.

Doppler echocardiography is the imaging modality of choice in evaluating patients with suspected prosthetic valve dysfunction because it provides structure

TABLE 25–1. Classification of Prosthetic Heart Valves

Mechanical
Ball and cage (Starr-Edwards)
Single tilting disc (Medtronic-Hall, Omnicarbon)
Double tilting disc (St. Jude Medical, CarboMedics, ATS, On-X)

Biological
Heterograft stented (Hancock I and II, Carpentier-Edwards porcine and pericardium bovine)
Heterograft stentless for aortic valve (Toronto SPV, Medtronic Freestyle, and CryoLife-O'Brien)
Heterograft stentless for pulmonic valve (CryoLife-Ross)
Homografts (aortic, pulmonic, and mitral)

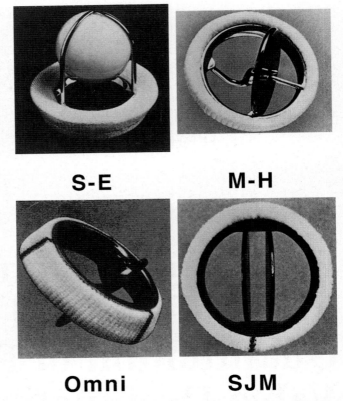

S-E   **M-H**

Omni   **SJM**

Figure 25–1. Mechanical heart valves. Starr-Edwards (S-E), Medtronic-Hall (M-H), Omnicarbon (OC), and St. Jude Medical (SJM).

and function information of the device, native valves, and ventricular myocardium.[1-3] Nowadays, multiplane transesophageal echocardiography (TEE) is routinely done because of the superior anatomical and functional information.[4-6] Three-dimensional (3D) echocardiography still is an evolving technology with a potential use in patients with prosthetic heart valves, particularly biological devices.

Prosthetic Heart Valve Classification

Prosthetic heart valves are divided into mechanical and biological. Table 25–1 lists the most common prosthetic heart valves currently used in clinical practice.

Mechanical Valves

Ball-and-Cage

The first successful valve replacement used a ball-and-cage design,[7,8] and after several modifications, only the Starr-Edwards valve has endured. It consists of a Silastic ball with a circular sewing ring and a cage formed by metal arches located around the sewing ring (Fig. 25–1). The silicone rubber ball retracts toward the apex of the cage as antegrade blood flows through the valve orifice and between the ball and the stents.[9] The Starr-Edwards valve has significant thromboembolic potential, particularly in the mitral position and in small ventricles requiring aggressive anticoagulation.

Single Tilting Disc

A single tilting disc consists of a circular sewing ring with a circular disc eccentrically attached by lateral or central metal struts. Björk-Shiley, Medtronic-Hall, OmniScience, and Omnicarbon are representative from this group. The Björk-Shiley valve was intro-

duced in 1969[10]; however, when engineering changes were made to correct problems of thrombosis, a fracture in the strut resulted on their newer concave-convex disk model, and the valve was taken off the United States market.

The Medtronic Hall central pivoting-disk valve introduced in 1977 has an opening angle of 70 degrees producing regurgitation volumes of less than 5% without compromising forward flow. The large opening angle and slim disk occluder along with a thinner sewing ring provide improved hemodynamics with comparably larger effective orifice areas (EOAs) and lower mean pressure gradients (see Fig. 25–1).

A potential hemodynamic disadvantage of the OmniScience valve is the incomplete disk opening ranging between 45 and 76 degrees, depending on valve size, orientation during implantation, and anticoagulation status. A subsequent generation is the Omnicarbon monoleaflet released in 2001. The housing material is made of pyrolytic carbon instead of titanium. As a result, the incidence of thromboembolism, valvular thrombosis, and reoperations has significantly decreased. For all tilting-disk valves, meticulous surgical technique is important because retained leaflets or chordae can cause subvalvular interference and leakage.

Double Tilting Disc

Bileaflet valves have two semicircular pyrolytic carbon discs attached to the valve ring by two small midline hinges. St. Jude Medical, CarboMedics, Advancing the Standard ATS bileaflet and the On-X are the prototypes of this group (see Fig. 25–1). The bileaflet design, introduced by St. Jude Medical in 1977, significantly improved hemodynamics compared to older valves with less blood stagnation, more complete leaflets opening, and reduced incidence of thromboembolism. The St. Jude Medical is the most widely used mechanical valve at present because of its excellent hemodynamics and ease to insert. The ATS prosthesis has been in clinical use in this country since 2000. Similar to the Carbomedics, the ATS valve is a low-profile bileaflet prosthesis with a pyrolytic housing and leaflets with an opening angle up to 85 degrees. Valve noise, a bothersome problem for some patients, is also reduced. The sewing cuff is mounted to a titanium ring, which enables the surgeon to rotate the valve orifice during implantation. The bileaflet valve most recently approved by the Food and Drug Administration (FDA) (2002) is the On-X valve. Instead of silicon-alloyed pyrolytic carbon, as in other mechanical valves, the On-X is made only of pyrolytic carbon allowing increased orifice length and a flared inlet that reduces transvalvular gradient. Early clinical results are promising with little hemolysis.

Mechanical valves are extremely durable with overall actuarial survival rates of 94%±2% at 10 years.[11-13] Primary structural abnormalities are rare,[14-16] and most valve malfunctions are caused by perivalvular leak and thrombosis. Chronic anticoagulation is required in all patients with mechanical valves to prevent valve thrombosis and embolic events. With adequate anticoagulation, the rate of thrombosis is 0.6% to 1.8% per patient-year for bileaflet valves.[11,17,18]

Biological (Tissue) Valves

Stented Bioprostheses

Stented bioprostheses are preferred in patients over age 70 in sinus rhythm because these valves deteriorate more slowly in older subjects. In addition, some elderly patients may not outlive their mechanical valves. The single most attractive advantage of bioprostheses is that in most cases, anticoagulation is not needed; however, the increased risk of reoperation is a high price to pay for the reduced risk of bleeding through avoiding anticoagulation.

Stented bioprosthesis are divided based on their material source into porcine (Hancock I, Hancock II, Carpentier-Edwards, and the mosaic) and pericardial (Carpentier-Edwards). Porcine cusps are treated with glutaraldehyde to reduce antigenicity, but they are less

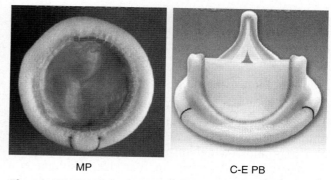

MP   C-E PB

Figure 25–2. Biological heart valves. Mosaic Porcine (MP) and Carpentier-Edwards Pericardial Bovine (C-E PB).

pliable than human valves.[19] The Carpentier-Edwards porcine valve has a stent made from a single piece of wire, and the three cusps are mounted above the sewing ring, allowing a larger orifice area (Fig. 25–2). Both porcine bioprostheses have a similar macroscopic appearance, but they are easily recognized by their radiographic features: Hancock appears as a circular ring whereas Carpentier-Edwards appears as a crown. The primary mechanical failure is a major problem with 15% to 20% deterioration at 10 years, more noticeable in younger subjects. In addition, durability of porcine valves is less in the mitral than in aortic position probably as a result of higher ventricular systolic pressures as compared with the lower diastolic pressures.

The Carpentier-Edwards pericardial valve uses bovine pericardium to fabricate a trileaflet valve that is cut, fitted, and sewn onto a flexible cobalt, chromium, nickel alloy (Elgiloy) wire frame for stress reduction. The tissue is preserved with glutaralderhyde at no pressure, and the leaflets are treated with the calcium mitigation agent *XenoLogiX*. Long-term durability for the Carpentier-Edwards pericardial valve is strong, and compared to third-generation porcine valves, valve-related complications are similar.

A major advantage of bioprosthetic valves is their low rate of thromboembolism (1.6% per patient-year) in the absence of chronic anticoagulation;[20] however, stented heterograft valves are subject to progressive calcific degeneration and failure typically after 6 to 8 years.[21-26] Calcific degeneration is faster in children, young adults, and in patients with abnormal calcium metabolism.[27,28] In several large series, the rate of degeneration for porcine valves was 3.3% per patient-year, and a freedom from valve failure rate for aortic valves was 78% and for mitral valves 69%.[20,29,30] After 10 years, the rate of deterioration accelerates abruptly with freedom from valve failure rates of 49% for aortic and 32% for mitral.[29] Using the porcine bioprosthesis in patients over 70 years of age, a 90% freedom from valve replacement at 12 to 15 years has been reported.[30,31] This finding may be related to a decreased rate of degeneration in the elderly or an increased rate of death from other than valve-related causes. The newer porcine and bovine pericardial valves are bioengineered at low-pressure (or no-pressure) fixation, antimineralization processes, attached to a low-profile, semiflexible stents.

Stentless Bioprostheses

Stentless bioprostheses are expected to improve hemodynamics and long-term durability while retaining the fundamental advantages of tissue valves. The absence of a stent and sewing cuff make it possible to implant a larger valve for a given annular size, resulting in a greater EOA. A nonstented bioprosthesis uses the patient's own aortic root as the stent, absorbing the stress induced during the cardiac cycle. Stentless bioprostheses include the Toronto SPV,[32,33] Medtronic Freestyle,[34-37] and CryoLife-O'Brien.[38-40] There are several variations within the same valve, depending on the patient's needs and the surgeon's preference. These variations include the full root technique with reimplantation of the coronary arteries, the root inclusion technique with preservation of the native coronary arteries, or the subcoronary technique. Figure 25–3 depicts a subcoronary implantation. Removal of the stent appears to eliminate much of the stress that promotes calcification and valve deterioration. Stentless valves are manufactured from intact porcine aortic valves processed at low fixation pressures. Some (i.e., Medtronic Freestyle) are treated with the anticalcificant amino-oleic acid, which may further decrease calcific deposits. The addition of a layer of polyester fabric around the graft adds support and aids implantation.[41,42]

Stentless valves have been used primarily in the aortic position in men older than 60 years of age. The reported operative mortality rate is 3% to 6%,[43,44] but it may reflect patient selection. Postoperative complications at 12 months appear to be low, with endocarditis reported at 1% to 2%, thromboembolism at 2% to 3%, and hemorrhage at 1.5%.[41,43,44] Primary structural failure is low, and the reported survival rates have been 91% at 6 years.[44,45]

The CryoLife-Ross valve is a pulmonary stentless valve made of three noncoronary porcine cusps used to correct congenital defects involving the pulmonic valve, and they can also be used during the Ross procedure.

Homografts

Homografts are antibiotic-sterilized, cryogenically-preserved valves harvested from cadaveric human hearts. Their major advantages are resistance to infection, lack of need for anticoagulation, and excellent hemodynamic profile, most notably in smaller aortic root sizes.[46,47] As illustrated in Figure 25–4, homografts have been developed for aortic, pulmonic, and even for mitral valves. The homograft preparation and the meticulous and highly skilled freehand surgical techniques at implantation have limited their use. Typically, homo-

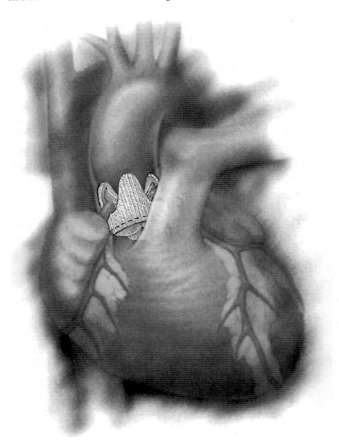

Figure 25–3. Drawing of a nonstented aortic valve (Toronto SPV) at the subcoronary position. (Courtesy of St. Jude Medical, Inc., St. Paul, Minn. All rights reserved. Copyright © 2001 St. Jude Medical, Inc. Toronto SPV is a registered trademark of St. Jude Medical, Inc.)

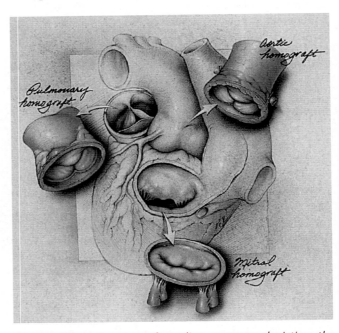

Figure 25–4. Drawing of cardiac anatomy depicting the availability of homografts for the pulmonary, aortic, and mitral valves. (Courtesy of CryoLife, Kennesaw, Ga.)

grafts are inserted without a stent, using the patient's natural fibrous annular tissue for support.

Ross Procedure

The pulmonic autograft (or Ross I procedure to differentiate it from Ross II procedure in which the pulmonary autograft is inserted in the mitral position) was first described in 1967. The Ross I procedure consists of replacing the abnormal aortic valve with the native pulmonic valve of the same patient, then placing a stentless homograft or porcine bioprosthesis in the pulmonic position. The operation is technically demanding; the pulmonic valve is removed with healthy tissue above and below valve insertion requiring reconstruction of the right ventricular outflow tract (RVOT). In addition, the coronary arteries are reimplanted into the pulmonary artery (PA) trunk that serves as the new aortic root. Although the Ross I procedure involves two valve operations to correct one diseased valve, it provides optimal hemodynamics and echocardiographic performance and low valve-related complications.[48] The main long-term problem with this operation has been degeneration and failure of the right-sided valve caused by obstruction in the distal segment of the homograft conduit.[49,50] Early autograft failure (<6 months) most often is the result of technical errors or persistent endocarditis, and late failures generally result from aortic annulus dilation, endocarditis, or valve degeneration.[51,52]

Fundamental Principles Pertaining to Prostheses

Modified Bernoulli Equation

Blood flow velocity through an orifice is related to the pressure difference between two chambers as described by the Bernoulli principle. In prosthetic heart valves, the modified Bernoulli equation is used to convert flow velocity (m/s) to pressure gradient (mm Hg) in a similar way as that used in native valves:

$$\text{Pressure gradient} = 4 \bullet (V_{MAX})^2$$

in which V_{MAX} is the maximal (peak) velocity across the valve. It is important to recognize that the modified Bernoulli equation neglects the effects of acceleration and viscous losses, and yet it has proved to be accurate when compared with simultaneous catheter-derived pressure gradients.[53-58] When the left ventricular outflow tract (LVOT) velocity (V_1) is greater than 1 m/s, such as in aortic regurgitation (AR), V_1 should be subtracted from V_{MAX}. Maximal instantaneous and mean gradients should be calculated for aortic valves and mean gradient for mitral valves. One must remember that a relatively high gradient in the setting of anemia, tachycardia, or sepsis does not necessarily indicate

stenosis; conversely, an upper normal limits gradient in patients with severe left ventricular (LV) dysfunction may indicate significant stenosis.

Pressure Recovery

Valve gradients that appear as overestimation when compared to catheter-derived gradients may result from distal pressure recovery. This hemodynamic concept refers to the conversion of kinetic energy present at the valve level to pressure energy distal to the valve.[59,60] When flow passes through the prosthesis, components of velocity and momentum are directed centrally, causing the flow stream to contract distally for a short distance. This point of maximal constriction is called vena contracta (VC) and occurs distally from the location of the prosthesis. The amount of recovered energy depends on how smooth is the transition of flow between the valve and the downstream conduit. As the jet expands and decelerates beyond the VC, the associated turbulence results in an increase in aortic pressure or pressure recovery. Under these circumstances, when the aortic pressure is measured in the upper ascending aorta (distal to the VC), the pressure difference between the left ventricle and the aorta is less than the aortic pressure measured at the VC. The degree of pressure recovery may be as high as 10 mm Hg in small St. Jude Medical valves challenged under physiologic flow rates. The magnitude of pressure recovery is greater with larger valve areas and smaller aortic roots; therefore, patients with severe prosthetic stenosis and poststenotic root dilation may show less pressure recovery than those with mild to moderate stenosis and normal aortic root diameter.

Pressure recovery and VC are important hemodynamic principles to bear in mind when Doppler- and catheter-derived pressure gradients are being compared. Because continuous-wave (CW) Doppler measures velocity at the level of the VC (physiologic variable) and catheterization measures the difference between left ventricle and the fully recovered static pressure in the aorta, catheter-derived data must be interpreted with caution. Failure of the invasive technique to record the pressure gradient at the VC level may explain some of the reported discrepancies.[61]

Continuity Equation

An important limitation of Doppler velocities (and pressure gradients derived thereof) is that they are flow volume rate-dependent. When transvalvular flow is decreased, such as in patients with significant left ventricular systolic dysfunction, Doppler velocities may only be moderately elevated despite severe stenosis. Thus, comparisons may be confounded by interval changes in flow volume rate. For these reasons, estimation of valve areas, in addition to mean gradients, should be routinely calculated and reported.

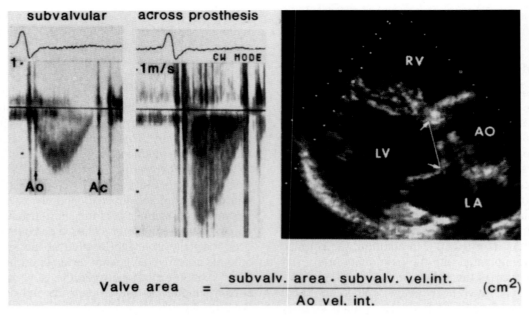

Figure 25–5. *Effective orifice area (EOA) calculation for an aortic valve prosthesis. The left panel corresponds to the outflow tract (subvalvular) velocity, also known as V_1. The middle panel corresponds to the prosthesis velocity, also known as V_2. The right panel corresponds to the parasternal long-axis view, showing the outflow tract diameter (arrows). Ac, aortic closure; AO, aorta; Ao, aortic opening; LA, left atrium; LV, left ventricle; RV, right ventricle; subvalve, subvalvular; vel. int., velocity integral.*

The equation of continuity can be used to estimate aortic and mitral valve areas (MVAs). Figure 25–5 illustrates how to apply the continuity equation in aortic prostheses:

$$EOA_{AORTIC} = (CSA_{LVOT} \times VTI_{LVOT})/VTI_{TRANSPROSTHESIS}$$

Where, CSA_{LVOT} is the cross-sectional area (CSA) of the outflow tract measured just underneath the prosthesis from the parasternal long-axis view. VTI_{LVOT} is the velocity time integral (VTI) proximal to the leaflets/occluder as seen from an apical five-chamber view using pulsed wave Doppler. Care should be exercised in locating the sample volume adjacent to the prosthesis from the apical five-chamber view while avoiding the region of subvalvular acceleration. The Doppler wave form should be smooth with minimal spectral broadening and a well-defined peak. $VTI_{TRANSPROSTHESIS}$ is the velocity time integral across the prosthesis using CW Doppler. Because the direction of the jet may be eccentric, apical, suprasternal, and right parasternal, windows should be carefully examined to detect the highest velocity signal.

Continuity equation valve areas have been compared with invasive data for bioprosthetic[62-64] and mechanical valves.[65,66] The largest source of variability is the reliable LVOT measurement. When this diameter is difficult to obtain from the precordial window, TEE offers an excellent alternative.[67]

For mitral valve area, the continuity equation is as follows:

$$EOA_{MITRAL} = (CSA_{LVOT} \times VTI_{LVOT})/VTI_{TRANSPROSTHESIS}$$

where, CSA_{LVOT} is cross-sectional aortic valve area measured from the LVOT dimension from the parasternal long-axis view, VTI_{LVOT} is velocity time integral at the LVOT, and $VTI_{TRANSPROSTHESIS}$ is velocity time integral across the mitral prosthesis.[68] Because the continuity equation is based on the principle of conservation of mass, it assumes that flow across the mitral prosthesis and that across a second valve are equal. Thus, in patients with more than mild mitral regurgitation (MR), the preferred method is the pressure half-time (PHT). In the presence of AR, the pulmonic area and flow can be used in lieu of the aortic. The limiting step in using the pulmonic valve is the reproducible RVOT diameter from the precordial approach. An important advantage of the continuity equation is its relative independence from valvular gradient and chamber compliance.[69] However, data acquisition for the continuity equation is more cumbersome than the PHT.

Doppler Velocity Index

The Doppler velocity index (DVI) is a dimensionless ratio of LVOT to prosthesis velocities, and expressed as:

$$DVI = V_{LVOT}/V_{TRANSPROSTHESIS}$$

Because it is independent of valve size, this index can be helpful when the cross-sectional area of the outflow tract cannot be obtained. Because the velocity proximal to the valve is subtracted from that across the prosthesis, the patient serves as his or her own control, with flow being the main dependent factor. The higher the index, the larger the area; the lower the index, the smaller the area. Index values calculated from 25 patients with normally functioning St. Jude Medical aortic valves were 0.39, range 0.28 to 0.55. In a small group of patients with severe stenosis of St. Jude Medical aortic valves requiring reoperation, the DVI was 0.19±0.05, range 0.12 to 0.27, which was significantly different from normal values at the 0.05 level.[70]

Valve Resistance

Resistance is the quotient of gradient and flow (R = ΔP/Q). This concept suggested by Ford, Feldman, Chiu, and Carroll[71] is an alternative to the Gorlin formula in assessing severity of native aortic stenosis (AS). It can be calculated from echocardiographic Doppler data as follows:

$$\text{Resistance} = 1.33\ \Delta P\ (ET/SV)$$

in which ΔP is the mean pressure gradient in mm Hg, ET is the ejection time in seconds, and SV is the stroke volume in mL per minute. The ratio of mm Hg to mL per minute is converted to dyne-sec-cm[5] when multiplied by 1.33. In conditions characterized by variation of flow, valve resistance remained more constant than the Gorlin estimated area. However, one must recognize that most valve resistance data have been derived from native valve stenosis and not from prostheses; no information is available during changing flow conditions, such as exercise. In addition, there is virtually no clinical data of valve resistance in prosthetic mitral valves.

Saad and colleagues[70] studied two groups with prosthetic aortic malfunction (predominant stenosis versus predominant regurgitation). EOA (continuity equation), DVI, and valve resistance were all helpful in separating the groups. It is unclear, however, whether valve resistance per se added clinically significant information beyond that derived by valve area and DVI. An important role of valve resistance in artificial valves may be in patients with small aortic valve areas, relatively low flow velocities, and severe LV systolic dysfunction, to differentiate severe prosthetic valve stenosis from a low cardiac output (CO) state, which has been shown to be useful in patients with native AS.[72]

Pressure Half-Time

The PHT is the time required for the peak velocity to decline by a factor of 1 divided by the square root of 2, and it can be helpful in separating normal from obstructed prostheses. The PHT is determined from the Doppler spectral display of the prosthetic mitral inflow. This method has been used to calculate the EOA of mitral and tricuspid valve prostheses based on the inverse relationship between PHT and valve area using the experimentally derived constant of 220,[73] originally derived for native rheumatic mitral stenosis (MS).

$$\text{EOA (cm}^2) = 220/\text{PHT (msec)}$$

The PHT is commonly regarded as a flow-independent measure. However, it is dependent on several factors, including atrial and ventricular compliance, ventricular stiffness, atrioventricular (AV) pressure gradient, and of course, the actual EOA. In addition, it is important to remember that this method might be unreliable whenever inadequate spectral signal is obtained, such as in patients with concomitant severe AR, atrioventricular block, and atrial tachycardia. It is my practice to restrain from reporting the MVA under these circumstances based on the principle that no data is better than bad data, which may lead to disastrous consequences.

Despite of these limitations, the PHT formula has been validated with invasive techniques producing good correlation. Kapur and colleagues[74] compared prosthetic mitral valve areas derived by PHT with those by the Gorlin formula in 32 patients and found correlations of 0.94 and 0.79 for bioprosthetic and mechanical valves, respectively. In contrast, Wilkins and colleagues,[54] using simultaneous catheterization and Doppler techniques in 11 patients with mitral prosthesis, found poor correlation. The continuity equation is an excellent alternative to the PHT to calculate mitral valve area.[75]

Leakage Backflow

Mechanical valves have a normal regurgitant volume known as leakage backflow that occurs when the valve occluder has already been seated and blood leaks into the proximal chamber between and around the occluder assembly. In theory, this built-in regurgitation prevents stasis and thrombus formation by a "washing" mechanism. Real-time, beat-to-beat characterization of color-flow Doppler is of great value in assessing leakage backflow. These jets are short, narrow, symmetrical (bileaflet valves), and nonaliasing velocities in a homogeneous color-red or blue, depending on transducer location (assuming Nyquist limit >0.53 m/s).[76,77]

Regurgitant jet size is influenced by severity, pressure gradient, and technical aspects, such as gain setting. Abnormal jets are longer, wider, larger, asymmetrical across the valve midline, frequently eccentric ("hugging the wall"), extending far into the receiving chamber, and display a mosaic pattern reflecting high-velocity, turbulent flow. A jet with an unusual angle (i.e., one anteriorly directed toward the atrial appendage) is also typical of a paravalvular leak. Figure 25–6 depicts the typical appearance of a normal backflow in a bileaflet mitral valve (Fig. 25–6A). In contrast, a larger, wider, eccentric jet "hugging" the left atrial lateral wall of severe perivalvular regurgitation is seen (Fig. 25–6B). Table 25–2 highlights the differences between physiologic leakage backflow and pathologic regurgitant jets.

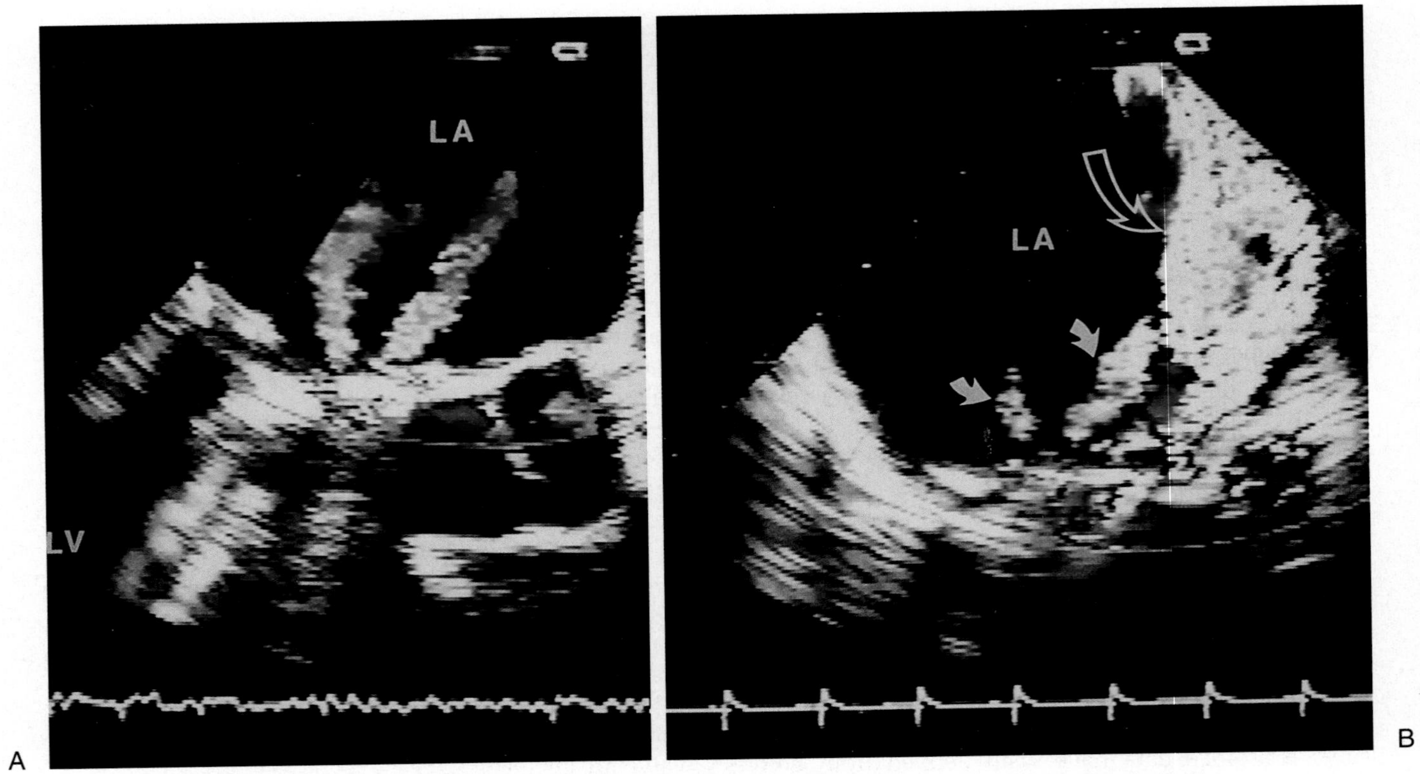

Figure 25–6. *Transesophageal echocardiography longitudinal views of a normal CarboMedics valve in the mitral position (A). Two symmetrical regurgitant backflow jets are seen within the left atrium (LA). These jets are low velocity, non-aliased, and encoded in red. In contrast, a pathologic periprosthetic leak is seen in an abnormal valve (B). The jet is high velocity, mosaic in color, and eccentric, and it encircles the left atrial wall (open arrow). The normal regurgitant backflow jets (solid arrows) are also seen. See Table 25–2 for differentiation of physiologic versus pathologic jets. LV, left ventricle.*

TABLE 25–2. Physiologic versus Pathologic Regurgitation of Mechanical Prosthesis

Jet Feature	Physiologic Leakage	Pathologic Regurgitation
Size	Short and narrow	Large and wide
Symmetry	Symmetrical (bileaflet valves)	Asymmetrical
Aliasing	No (low velocity)	Yes (high velocity)
Eccentricity	No	Yes

Echocardiography of Normal Prosthetic Valve Function

The same principles used in native valves are applicable to artificial valves. The size and type of the valve determine the range of flow velocities and is in essence what separates normal from abnormal valve function. The report must include the patient's identifiers, reason for the study, date of implant, follow-up time, type and size of valve, expected upper normal limits, and method used to calculate hemodynamics, i.e., PHT versus continuity equation. Rhythm should be included in the report because the preceding cycle affects measurements. An average of five representative signals should be reported in atrial fibrillation (AFib) or atrial flutter; however, if the patient has a rapid ventricular response, refrain from valve calculations. Ideally, serial comparisons should be done using same method, machine, and if possible, sonographer. Echocardiography has some limitations related to reverberations and shadowing from the interface between ultrasound (US) and material composing the valve.[78] Intense reverberations projected behind the prosthesis can mask normal structures or instead create artifacts. Table 25–3 describes common limitations and technical errors or pitfalls and suggestions on how to overcome or minimize their impact.

A complete examination should include estimation of pressure gradients and valve area, degree of normal or abnormal regurgitation, LV size and function, native valve structure and function, and calculation of the PA systolic pressures. M-mode recording may assist in evaluating disc or leaflet excursion, whereas color

TABLE 25–3. Echocardiography of Prosthetic Valves: Pitfalls

Technical Limitations	Suggestions
Acoustic shadowing	Use window where region of interest is not obscured by the valve's artifact; consider TEE
Failure to detect peak velocity	Image from multiple windows
Underestimation or overestimation of valve gradient or effective orifice area	Include proximal velocity in continuity equation if >1 m/s Consider pressure recovery Use mean valve gradient, not peak-to-peak or maximal instantaneous gradient
Unexpected high gradient or small effective orifice area	Consider high cardiac output setting (i.e., tachycardia, anemia, or sepsis) Calculate Doppler velocity index and valve resistance Consider prosthesis-patient mismatch Consider valve thrombosis or pannus formation

TEE, transesophageal echocardiography.

TABLE 25–4. Recommended Follow-Up in Patients with Prosthetic Heart Valves

Patient Category	Recommendation
Early Postoperative Any type of valve	Baseline study in all patients
Follow-Up *Stented bioprosthesis* Clinically normal	Every 2 years for the first 6 years, then every year for 4 years, then every 6 months
Patient-prosthesis mismatch	Once a year
Chronic renal failure	Once a year
Stentless bioprosthesis and homografts Clinically normal	Every 2 or 3 years
Mechanical valves Clinically normal	Every 2 or 3 years
Patient-prosthesis mismatch	Once a year

M-mode in timing regurgitant jets. Two-dimensional (2D) imaging should identify sewing ring and occluder mechanism. The ball or disc is often indistinctly imaged because of echocardiographic reverberations. The cusps of normal biological valves should be thin with an unrestricted motion.

A helpful and frequently overlooked practice is the comparison with prior studies. The importance of a timely baseline postoperative study cannot be overemphasized. It is our practice to perform a transthoracic study prior to hospital discharge, or in the patient's first outpatient visit (<30 days), because this establishes the baseline gradients and area, the postoperative ventricular function, and the systolic PA pressures for that particular patient. The need for such study despite the fact that a TEE might have used at the time of implantation needs to be remembered. This anatomic and hemodynamic profile is subsequently used whenever prosthetic dysfunction becomes a concern. How often routine follow-up studies should be performed is controversial. In my practice, the first follow-up is in a year and then I follow the recommendations listed in Table 25–4. Follow-up for stentless bioprostheses and homografts should be different from stented bioprostheses because the former's deterioration rates seem to be lower. Tables 25–5 and 25–6 provide the normal range of in vivo velocities for mechanical and bioprosthetic valves in the aortic and mitral positions, respectively.

Echocardiographic Features by Valve Type

Ball-and-Cage

Flow through a normally functioning ball-and-cage valve is turbulent resulting from the high-profile ball at the center of the blood path and by the eddies created as flow circulates retrogradely (Fig. 25–7). Consequently, when compared with single and double tilting disc valves, the hemodynamic performance of the ball-and-cage valve is less, with higher pressure gradients. Color flow in a normal ball-and-cage valve includes low-velocity closure backflow (2 to 5 mL per beat).[9,79] In the mitral position, the cage projects deep into the left ventricle; thus, it is unwise to implant this valve in small ventricles, where the cage may contact the ventricular wall or cause outflow tract obstruction.

Single Tilting Disc

During implantation of the Medtronic-Hall in the mitral position, the larger orifice should be oriented posteriorly when using the larger valve sizes to minimize potential for disk impingement. Smaller valves (27 mm or less) should be oriented with the larger orifice anteriorly to optimize hemodynamics. Figure 25–8 illustrates a single tilting disc valve in the mitral position. The left panel is the typical antegrade flow through the major and minor orifices in the correct orientation (major orifice toward the lateral aspect, away from the outflow tract) as opposed to the incorrect orientation seen on right panel. Typical flow velocity of a single tilting disc valve is around 2 m/s. Flow through the minor orifice consists of two jets separated by a well-defined wake behind the tilting disc but with a velocity similar to the major orifice. Color flow includes a small amount of normal

TABLE 25–5. Normal Doppler Values for Aortic Prostheses

Type	Peak Velocity (m/s)	Mean Gradient (mm Hg)	Area Mean (cm²)	Area Range (cm²)
Starr-Edwards	3.1±0.5	24±4	*	*
Björk-Shiley	2.5±0.6	14±5	*	*
St. Jude Medical	3.0±0.8	11±6	*	*
Medtronic-Hall	2.6±0.3	12±3	*	*
OmniScience	2.8±0.4	14±3	*	*
Hancock	2.4±0.4	11±2	1.8	1.4-2.3
Carpentier-Edwards	2.4±0.5	14±6	1.8	1.2-3.1
Aortic Homograft	1.8±0.4	7±3	2.2	1.7-3.1
Toronto SPV†	2.2±0.4	3±4	2.2	2.0-2.8
Freestyle†	2.2±0.4	3±4	2.2	2.0-2.8
O'Brien†	2.2±0.4	3±4	2.2	2.0-2.8

*Insufficient data available.
†Stentless bioprostheses.

TABLE 25–6. Normal Doppler Values for Mitral Prostheses

Type	Peak Velocity (m/s)	Mean Gradient (mm Hg)	Area Mean (cm²)	Area Range (cm²)
Starr-Edwards	1.8±0.4	4.6±2.4	2.1	1.2-2.5
Björk-Shiley	1.6±0.3	5.0±2.0	2.4	1.6-3.7
St. Jude Medical	1.6±0.3	5.0±2.0	2.9	1.8-4.4
Medtronic-Hall	1.7±0.3	3.1±0.9	2.4	1.5-3.9
OmniScience	1.8±0.3	3.3±0.9	1.9	1.6-3.1
Hancock	1.5±0.3	4.3±2.1	1.7	1.3-2.7
Carpentier-Edwards	1.8±0.2	6.5±2.1	2.5	1.6-3.5
Homograft	1.8±0.4	6.4±3.0	2.2	1.9-2.9

backflow (5 to 9 mL per beat), originated from small gaps around the perimeter of the valve.[80,81] Hixson and colleagues[76] have reported that the Medtronic-Hall valve has a large central regurgitant backflow that can extend back into the left atrium with aliasing, whereas the peripheral jets are nonaliasing, low-velocity flow.

Double Tilting Disc

The bileaflet tilting disk valve has three separate orifices, a central rectangular-shaped and two larger semicircular orifices. The true gradient is the contribution of the three orifices; however, when the flow velocity of the central orifice is detected by the CW beam, an overestimation may occur because the central orifice is smaller with higher velocity. Flow dynamics vary widely depending upon the valve size. For instance, a St. Jude valve of 29 mm has a peak flow velocity less than 2.5 m/s, whereas a 19 mm may have a peak velocity of 4.5 m/s; yet in both instances, the valve function is intrinsically normal.

Figure 25–9 illustrates the anatomic orientation of a bileaflet valve in the mitral position during diastole and normal mitral inflow. Blood flow is near-laminar with a path similar to the laminar flow of the native valve. In the opening position, the hemidiscs appear as parallel lines with a short angle between them. Imaging of the normal valve includes the sewing ring and two distinct echoes in the opening position and a wide obtuse angle in the closing position. Identification of the two hemidiscs may be problematic with the transthoracic echocardiography (TTE) approach, particularly in the aortic position, a problem that can be resolved with multiplane TEE.

In normally functioning bileaflet valves, color demonstrates a small amount of normal backflow (5 to 10 mL

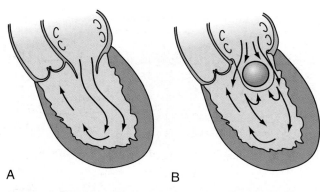

Figure 25-7. A, *Normal diastolic intracavitary flow pattern. B, Disturbed antegrade flow across a ball-and-cage valve. Note the high-profile ball located in the center of the bloodstream, creating turbulence and eddying as flow changes direction.*

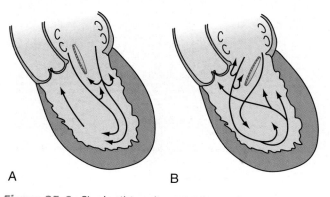

Figure 25-8. *Single tilting disc mitral prosthesis. A, Correct anatomic disc orientation, allowing the major orifice flow to be directed away from the left ventricular outflow tract. B, Incorrect anatomic disc orientation, in which the major orifice flow is directed toward the left ventricular outflow tract, creating turbulence.*

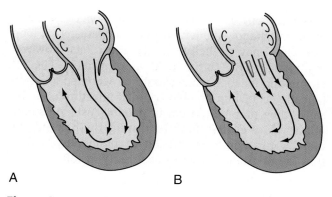

Figure 25-9. *Double tilting disc mitral valve. A, Normal mitral inflow. B, Mitral inflow across a double tilting disc valve, with flow passing through three separate orifices, creating a near-normal flow pattern.*

per beat) designed to decrease the risk of thrombosis by a "wash out" mechanism. TEE visualization of the bileaflet valve depends on the image orientation in the parallel or perpendicular position of the discs. In the parallel position, the discs appear in profile as two lines. Color may reveal up to three distinct jets: two at the

edges of the valve directed upward and outward, and one centrally directed straight up. In the perpendicular position, the leaflets reflect dense reverberations into the ventricular cavity and color shows a semicircular flare on the atrial aspect.[76,77] The CarboMedics is a newer version of bileaflet mechanism with recessed pivots that may result in larger regurgitant jets.[82]

Stented Bioprostheses

The cross-sectional appearance of porcine valves is of three cusps and three struts with an echogenic sewing ring. Normal flow pattern is a bell-shaped central flow with a relatively flat profile. Peak velocities commonly found in the aortic position are around 2.5 m/s and in the mitral position, 1.7 m/s. Mild backflow in normal bioprostheses is less common than in mechanical valves, reported in less than 10% of the cases.[83]

Stentless Valves

Careful measurement of the patient's sinotubular junction is an important contribution of US in choosing the size of the valve.[84] After implantation, the prosthesis can be indistinguishable from a normal native aortic valve; the increased echogenicity in the annular region may be the only hint.[85] Reported hemodynamics are encouraging with nearly natural transvalvular gradients resulting in significant reduction in afterload and wall stress.[45] Ventricular reverse remodeling through regression of cardiac hypertrophy is an important predictor of survival after valve replacement, hypertrophy regression as early as 6 months after valve replacement has been reported.[86]

Homografts

Preoperative or intraoperative TEE measurement of the aortic annulus has been used to select the correct homograft size.[47] The 2D imaging of the stentless homograft is similar to the native aortic valve, with increased echoes at the level of the annulus resulting from the retaining sutures as the only hint of a new valve. Homograft failure commonly results from progressive aortic insufficiency; valve stenosis is rare.[87,88] In the Ross procedure I, TEE plays an important role in providing accurate measurement of the RVOT. In addition, color flow Doppler of the LVOT and RVOT provides essential information regarding aortic and pulmonic regurgitation, respectively.

Valved Conduits and Composite Grafts

Valved conduits have been used most often in the repair of congenital heart disease. Reestablishing flow from the right heart to the PA is often performed with a bioprosthesis. Echocardiographic evaluation should include the anatomic relation of the valve conduit to the heart, and flow velocity through the proximal and distal ends of the conduit as stenosis can occur anywhere along the conduit. The extracardiac course of the conduit can result in variable angles and directions of flow; therefore, colored flow Doppler is helpful in defining the location of high-velocity turbulent flow. Additional views from the subcostal, subclavian, and right parasternal windows may be necessary to align the Doppler beam with the direction of the flow.

Composite grafts for left-sided valves are most commonly seen in patients with aortic valve and aortic root diseases, such as connective tissue disorders (e.g., Marfan syndrome), leading to aortic aneurysm or dissection. Complications include pseudoaneurysm of the ascending aorta caused by dehiscence, which can occur at the annulus, at the distal anastomosis with the native aorta, or at the coronary artery reimplantation site.[89] Serial TTE is essential for follow-up; however, only TEE can provide with appropriate views of the ascending aorta.

Echocardiographic Features by Valve Position

Aortic

In general, M-mode and 2D from the precordial approach have low yield for detecting prosthetic aortic dysfunction. Thus, aortic valve dysfunction heavily depends on a careful Doppler examination. The peak gradient obtained by Doppler closely correlates with the maximal instantaneous gradient derived by catheterization. The mean gradient obtained with either technique correlates closely with each other. When Doppler and fluid-filled pressure gradients are recorded at the same time, the degree of concordance is superb.[53,54,74] Burstow and colleagues[53] found excellent correlation for the mean gradient (tissue valves, $r = 0.93$; mechanical valves, $r = 0.96$) when data were recorded simultaneously; however, when they were not simultaneous, the correlations fell slightly (tissue valves, $r = 0.85$; mechanical valves, $r = 0.87$). Values derived with the continuity equation have correlated well with prosthesis size.[90]

Peak velocities as high as 3.5 to 4 m/s have been recorded in normally functioning prosthetic mechanical aortic valves. These high-flow velocities exist briefly at valve opening; however, the mean gradient usually falls within the normal range. Therefore, the mean gradient, not the peak gradient, should be used in making clinical decisions. If the mean pressure gradient is abnormally elevated, prosthetic valve stenosis should be suspected and TEE considered.

Mitral

The mean Doppler and catheterization gradients correlate well when both data are recorded simultaneously. As illustrated in Figure 25–10, the mean gradient is the average of multiple gradient calculations across the Doppler spectral envelope.

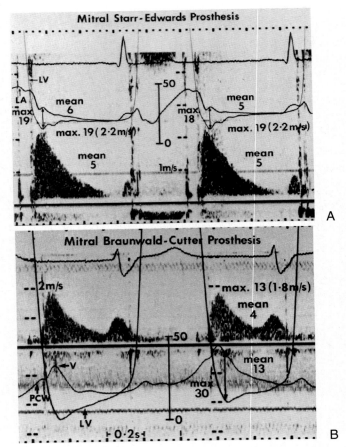

Figure 25–10. *Simultaneous catheterization and Doppler recordings in a Starr-Edwards prosthesis (A) and a Braunwald-Cutter prosthesis (B) in the mitral position. Note the excellent pressure gradient correlations. (From Burstow DJ, Nishimura RA, Bailey KR, et al: Circulation 80:504-514, 1989.)*

Assessment of MR is often difficult because reverberations shadow the left atrium. The parasternal long-axis view may be helpful in eccentric jets; however, multiplanar TEE is the method of choice. The left atrium and its appendage should be searched for spontaneous echocardiographic contrast and thrombus because they may be present in patients with prosthetic mitral valves even if they are in sinus rhythm and normal LV function.[91] Evaluation of pulmonary venous flow is important in assessing severity of MR.

Tricuspid

Data with tricuspid valve prostheses are far more limited. In many respects evaluation is similar to mitral prostheses. The valve should be imaged from all available views (parasternal short-axis, parasternal right ventricular inflow, apical four-chamber, and subcostal). Bioprostheses are preferred over mechanical valves because of their high thrombogenic potential in this position. Severe tricuspid regurgitation (TR) is frequently caused by annular dilation; thus, rings are nowadays preferred over prosthetic valves to correct significant tricuspid regurgitation. TEE plays an important role by differentiating annular dilation from intrinsic leaflet abnormality as the origin of the regurgitation.

Pulmonic

Prostheses in this position are relatively uncommon because percutaneous balloon valvuloplasty is an effective procedure in hemodynamically significant stenosis.[92] When a surgical intervention is needed, valvotomy is frequently used to palliate the valve, later in life a bioprosthesis can be used. As with the native pulmonic valve, the bioprosthesis is best seen from the parasternal short-axis and subcostal views. The more commonly used TEE views include the basal short-axis and the longitudinal views, which may be helpful in choosing the appropriate homograft size. Color flow Doppler examination within the RVOT is important to document residual regurgitation.

Echocardiography of Prosthetic Valve Dysfunction

For mechanical valves, cinefluoroscopy renders a means to evaluate the actual valve motion. It is indicated whenever valve thrombosis is suspected. One needs to determine the valve's rotational orientation by positioning the imaging intensifier in a view perpendicular to the valve plane. The fluoroscopic side view renders important information in determining the closing angle degree. To achieve the side view, the image intensifier should be moved longitudinally 90 degrees and rotated transversely to a position in line with the valve leaflets. For the St. Jude Medical valve, the opening angle between the two parallel lines should be 10 degrees (Fig. 25–11A). In the closing position, the two lines form a wide obtuse angle in the form of a "V" (Fig. 25–11B); for valves less than 25 mm, the angle should be 120 degrees, and for valves greater than 27 mm it should be 130 degrees. In the typical case of thrombosis of a double tilting disc prosthesis, only one leaflet may be moving, indicating leaflet entrapment. Figure 25–12 shows still frames recorded during cinefluoroscopy in a patient with valve thrombosis and entrapment.

Primary Mechanical Failure

Dysfunction from an intrinsic valve problem is known as primary mechanical failure. The Starr-Edwards valve had a rare intrinsic complication called ball variance, in which changes of the ball structure resulted in emboli either from ball material or thrombi from the cracked ball.[93] Figure 25–13 illustrates an example of ball variance with a crack seen across the midportion of the ball and a large thrombus trapped between the ball and the cage. Disc embolization from single or double tilting disc valves is extremely rare. The older Björk-Shiley version had several reported cases of fractured struts resulting in disc embolization.

For bioprosthesis, the most important primary mechanical failure is the calcific degeneration characterized by restricted cusp motion leading to stenosis or cusp tears leading to regurgitation and mixed lesions.[94,95] The probability of structural failure with currently available porcine valves begins after 8 years and reaches over 60% at 15 years. The appearance of a new murmur or new heart failure symptoms should prompt to an urgent TTE and TEE. Structural valve degeneration is the main reason for reoperations in these patients. Flail cusp owing to leaflet tears is associated with severe regurgitation; therefore, detection of a flail cusp has important clinical implications. Figures 25–14A and B illustrate the TEE at the midesophageal level of a patient with a flail cusp in a bioprosthesis and the explanted device.

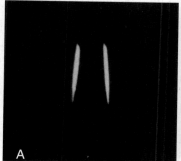
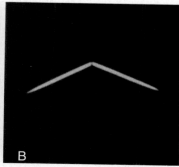
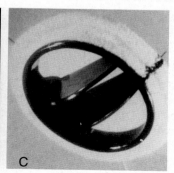

Figure 25–11. Radiographic side view of a bileaflet valve. In the opening position (A), the two discs form a 10-degree angle, whereas in the closing position (B), they form a 120-degree (<25 mm) or 130-degree (<27 mm) angle, depending on valve size. C, Photograph of a bileaflet mechanical valve in the opening position.

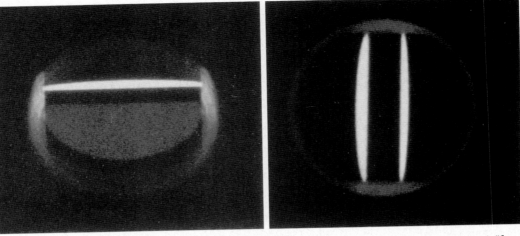

Figure 25–12. *Radiographic representation of a bileaflet valve in the opening position. A, A "frozen" leaflet. By cinefluoroscopy, only one leaflet moves during the cardiac cycle. B, Normal appearance as rotated 90 degrees.*

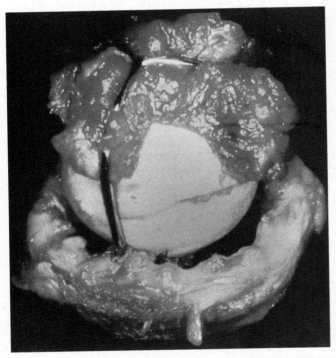

Figure 25–13. *Pathologic specimen showing ball variance in a Starr-Edwards valve. Notice the crack seen across the midportion of the ball and a large thrombus entrapped between the ball and the cage.*

A musical or "cooing" sound has been reported with pulsed Doppler in patients with perforated or torn leaflets, which result in a striated, "shuddering" appearance to the signal, referred to as harmonics.[96,97] Leaflet thickening in the absence of endocarditis most likely represents milder degrees of calcific degeneration; however, a thickened and often irregular appearance can also be seen in endocarditis. In patients with "fibrocalcific" changes on their cusps, the differentiation between calcific degeneration and endocarditis should be based on the clinical context.

Thrombosis

Thrombosis occurs almost exclusively in mechanical valves, leading to predominant stenosis with or without regurgitation. Figure 25–15 illustrates a thrombosed mitral Beall valve (disc-in-cage) in a patient presenting in pulmonary edema. The onset of symptoms may be gradual or sudden, and its incidence does not vary significantly among different mechanical valves, except in the tricuspid position. The low flow rate through the right-sided chambers is the likely factor for thrombosis rates as high as 20%,[98] limiting the use of mechanical valves in this position. Echocardiography should focus on determining the range of occluder motion. Several views should be used to determine the plane of maximal excursion. Bileaflet valves present a unique problem as thrombosis can affect only one hemidisc (see Fig. 25–12).

TEE is a sensitive tool for diagnosing valve thrombosis and efficacy of thrombolytic therapy.[99,100] Although reoperation is frequently recommended in these patients, thrombolysis has been used many times in critically ill patients, who are not otherwise good candidates for reoperation. Emergent surgery for acute valve thrombosis has a perioperative mortality of 30% to 40%, the risk is linked to the preoperative New York Heart Association (NYHA) class, LV systolic function, urgency of operation, and concomitant coronary artery disease (CAD).[101,102] Thrombolytic therapy is a logical alternative to surgery in high-risk patients, TEE the ideal method to image, and Doppler the mode of choice to assess serial hemodynamic changes postthrombolysis.

Numerous reports of the use of thrombolytics in acutely thrombosed mechanical valves have been

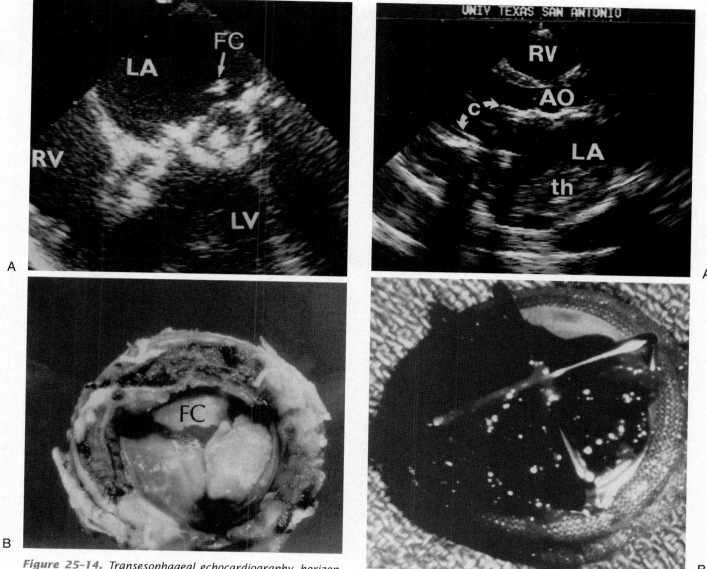

Figure 25-14. *Transesophageal echocardiography, horizontal four-chamber view, demonstrating a flail cusp (FC) in a mitral stented bioprosthesis (A). The patient presented to the hospital with progressive dyspnea on exertion, orthopnea, and fatigue. Ten years earlier, his mitral valve was replaced with a Hancock bioprosthesis. B, The excised valve with one of the cusps flailed and the other two with signs of degeneration. LA, left atrium; LV, left ventricle; RA, right atrium.*

Figure 25-15. *Prosthetic valve thrombosis in a Beall valve. A, Parasternal long-axis view from a patient with a disc-in-cage prosthesis (c) in the mitral position. A large thrombus (th) is noted in the posterior left atrial (LA) wall. B, The excised valve with a large thrombus obstructing the disc motion. AO, aorta; RV, right ventricle.*

published.[103-107] Tong and colleagues[107] reported an international registry of 107 patients with valve thrombosis who underwent thrombolytic therapy and TEE. The hemodynamic success rate was 85% and was similar across valves. However, the overall complications were nearly 18% with a death rate of 5.6%. In clinically stable patients with stuck leaflets and no high-risk thrombi, thrombolysis is highly successful and safe, both in the primary episode and in recurrence. The best thrombolytic regimen is yet to be established, but streptokinase has been the drug most commonly used. For patients with large thrombus, valve replacement is clearly indicated unless the surgical risk is prohibitive.

Thromboembolism

Is perhaps the most common complication of both biological and mechanical mitral prostheses. Chronic atrial fibrillation increases the risk of thromboembolism. In general, the better the valve hemodynamics, the lower the risk of thromboemboli. The incidence of thromboemboli in currently available bileaflet valves and tilting-disk valves is similar to that of bioprosthetic valves—about 1.5% to 2% per patient-year.[108-110] Thromboembolism in patients with mitral valve replacement is lower in those with a small left atrium, sinus rhythm, and normal CO. Thrombosis of a mechanical valve, once a feared complication of tilting-disk valves, is now relatively rare unless anticoagulation is stopped for a period of time.

An interesting observation described with TEE is fibrin strands,[111] commonly located on the atrial aspect of mitral prostheses or on the ventricular aspect of aortic prostheses. As illustrated in Figure 25–16, their appearance is that of thin structures a few millimeters in length, moving independently from the leaflets. Fibrin strands should be distinguished from vegetations or

thrombi by their chaotic movement in and out of the imaging plane. They are more commonly seen on mechanical valves, but they also have been reported on tissue valves, and they have been associated with a higher incidence of embolic events. In a study by Isada, Torelli, Stewart, and Klein[112] fibrin strands were found in 15 (18%) of 83 prosthetic mitral valve patients, and of those 15 patients, 8 (53%) had embolic events compared with 12 (18%) of 68 without strands. In contrast, fibrin strands have also been detected in otherwise normal prosthetic valves. In summary, the clinical significance of fibrin strands is unknown.

Endocarditis

The incidence of prosthetic endocarditis is usually higher during the initial 6 months after surgery. In a recent study evaluating echocardiographic findings and their relation to morbidity and mortality,[113] the presence of an infected prosthetic valve was a major risk factor for death. Five of 11 deaths related to endocarditis occurred in patients with prosthetic valves. The annual rate for late prosthetic endocarditis is estimated at 0.5% per year. According to the Veterans Cooperative[108] and the Edinburgh study,[110] there is no significant difference of between mechanical and stented bioprosthesis; however, when compared with native valves, prosthetic valve endocarditis is more likely to be associated with ring abscess, conduction abnormalities, and a worse prognosis.[114]

The diagnosis should be suspected if heart failure symptoms or a new murmur appear in the setting of sepsis. The most frequent organisms are *Streptococcus* and *Staphylococcus;* the latter is usually hospital acquired. A number of patients with bioprosthetic endocarditis can be "cured" of low-potency organisms such as *Streptococcus.* However, it is less likely that antibiotics alone can sterilize more virulent valve infections, i.e., *Staphylococcus.* Surgical indications for prosthetic valve endocarditis are persistent sepsis despite antibiotics, persistent or worsening heart failure, large perivalvular leak, or repetitive septic emboli. The size of the vegetation per se is not a surgical indication; however, large vegetations (>10 mm in length) tend to emboli more often than smaller vegetations and thus, it may help in setting the case to surgical colleagues in conjunction with other supporting arguments.[115,116]

Vegetations typically appear as irregular masses of echoes attached to the valve components commonly moving with the blood path. On tissue valves vegetations usually result in leaflet destruction, whereas on mechanical valves they may interfere with the occluder mechanism, resulting in stenosis, regurgitation, or both. Figure 25–17 shows a midesophageal TEE in a septic patient with a stented bioprosthesis in the aortic position. Differentiation from thrombus may be difficult. A

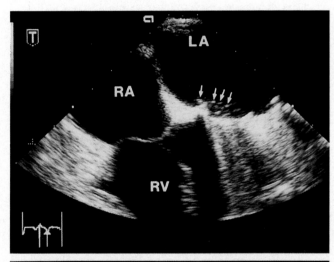

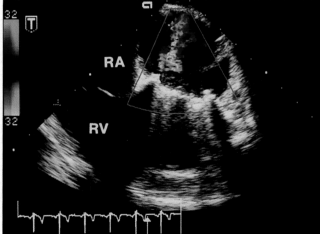

Figure 25–16. Transesophageal echocardiography, horizontal four-chamber view, demonstrating fibrin strands (arrows) on the atrial side of a St. Jude Medical prosthesis (top). Chaotic movement of these structures in and out of the imaging plane characterizes real-time imaging. Mild mitral regurgitation is noted in the medial aspect of the prosthesis. LA, left atrium; RA, right atrium; RV, right ventricle.

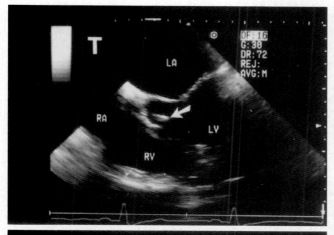

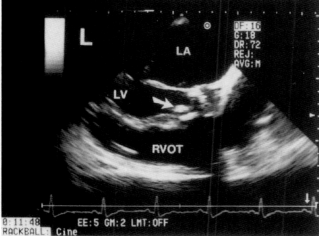

Figure 25–17. Transesophageal echocardiography at the midesophageal level from the transverse (T) and longitudinal (L) views in a septic patient with a stented bioprosthesis in the aortic position. A large echodense mass in the left ventricular outflow tract is clearly seen (arrows). LA, left atrium; LV, left ventricle; RA, right atrium, RVOT, right ventricular outflow tract.

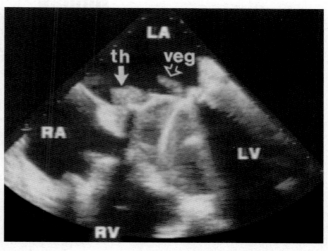

Figure 25–18. Transesophageal echocardiography at the midesophageal level from the transverse view in a septic patient with a St. Jude Medical valve in the mitral position and a stented bioprosthesis in the tricuspid position. A large vegetation (veg) and a thrombus (th) are clearly identified within the left atrium. LV, left ventricle; RA, right atrium; RV, right ventricle.

hint is that endocarditis tend to be associated with regurgitant lesions, whereas thrombosis with stenotic lesions. Either condition, however, can be seen as mobile echocardiographic dense masses. Thus, separation should be based on the clinical grounds and bacteriologic results. Rarely, both complications may be present in the same valve. Figure 25–18 corresponds to a midesophageal view in a septic patient with a St. Jude Medical valve in the mitral position and a bioprosthesis in the tricuspid position. A large vegetation and a thrombus can be seen on the atrial aspect of the mitral valve.

Early and accurate identification of septic complications in patients with prosthetic valves have a significant impact on the decision-making process. TEE has dramatically improved the accuracy in detecting vegetations, abscesses, and other associated complications.[117,118] Studies comparing TTE and TEE have included both native and prosthetic valves in their

analysis. Table 25–7 lists studies comparing the two modalities in which patients with prosthetic valves were included. Although prosthetic valves are not analyzed separately, the data clearly favors TEE as a superior diagnostic modality; therefore, TEE should be performed routinely in patients with suspected prosthetic valve endocarditis, most notably in those who fail to improve despite appropriate antibiotics.

Development of a perivalvular abscess is associated with a grave prognosis and indicates the need for aggressive medical and surgical therapies. Clinical findings suggestive of an abscess include persistent sepsis despite antibiotics, new or worsening heart failure symptoms, and development of first-degree atrioventricular block or incomplete right bundle branch block (RBBB). Figure 25–19 illustrates a range of possible outcomes of a prosthetic valve abscess. Rupture may occur into adjacent structures, including the pericardial sac creating cardiac tamponade; however, a rather common outcome is a perivalvular dehiscence with a tunnel communicating the aorta with the LVOT and consequently significant perivalvular regurgitation. Under those circumstances, emergent (or semi-emergent) surgery may be a lifesaving procedure.

Echocardiographic findings of perivalvular abscess include valve rocking, periaortic root thickening, or perivalvular echolucency.[119] As noted in Table 25–8, identification of an abscess is difficult from the precordial approach; therefore, TEE is mandatory when this complication is suspected. In addition, fistulous tracts connecting the perivalvular space with adjacent structures can be imaged and tracked down with color-flow Doppler over imposed to the 2D imaging.

TABLE 25–7. Sensitivity and Specificity of Transthoracic Echocardiography versus Transesophageal Echocardiography for Vegetations and Abscesses in Patients with Endocarditis

Reference	No. of Patients	No. of Patients with PVE	TTE Sens (%)	TTE Spec (%)	TEE Sens (%)	TEE Spec (%)
Mugge, Daniel, Frank, Litchtlen[115]*	105	25	58	‡	90	‡
Taams and colleagues[116]*	33	12	36	100	100	100
Daniel and colleagues[117]†	118	34	28	99	87	95

*Identification of vegetations.
†Identification of abscesses.
‡Insufficient data available, but smaller studies have reported specificity of TEE at 100%.
PVE, prosthetic valve endocarditis; TEE, transesophageal echocardiography; TTE, transthoracic echocardiography.
Data from references 115-117.

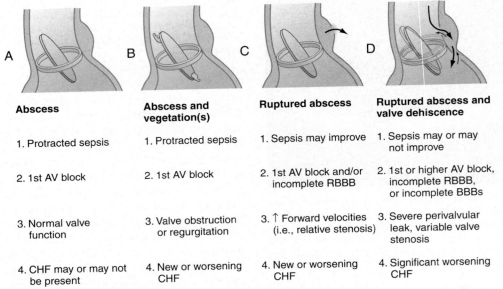

Figure 25–19. A to D, Clinical, electrocardiographic, and echocardiographic characteristics in septic complications of mechanical valves. AV, atrioventricular; CHF, congestive heart failure; RBBB, right bundle branch block.

Figure 25–20 represents the midesophageal and upper esophageal images in a septic, critically ill patient with a St. Jude Medical aortic prosthesis who presented to the emergency department with acute aortic insufficiency and pulmonary edema; a large perivalvular abscess is clearly noted.

Patient-Prosthesis Mismatch

Patient-prosthesis mismatch is present when the EOA of the inserted prosthesis is too small in relation to the patients' body surface area (BSA).[120] A given valve area acceptable for a small relatively inactive subject may be inadequate for a larger physically active individual. Its main hemodynamic consequence is the generation of higher than expected gradients through a normally functioning valve. Patient-prosthesis mismatch is commonly seen in the following clinical settings: (1) Patients with small aortic annulus sizes, particularly women; (2) patients in whom aortic valve replacement was performed because of native stenosis as opposed to regurgitation; and (3) young patients who outgrow their initially inserted prosthesis. In general, one must insert the largest valve size that can possibly fit that individual. As noted previously, a normally functioning 19-mm St. Jude valve in the aortic position may generate peak flow velocities up to 4.5 m/s, representing a mean gradient in excess of 40 mm Hg. Not surprisingly such individual may fail to improve and may feel even worse. The long-term implications of this condition are

TABLE 25–8. Prosthetic Valve Exercise Doppler Hemodynamics

	No.	Valve Sizes (mm)	Mean Gradient (mm Hg)		
			Rest	Exercise*	Increase (%)
Aortic Position					
Carpentier-Edwards	4	21	15±3	21±3	70
Medtronic-Hall	14	21	15±4	24±6	80
Medtronic-Hall	14	21-27	9±4	15±6	83
St. Jude Medical	17	21-27	11±4	18±7	81
Mitral Position					
Björk-Shiley	11	25-31	4.9±1.8	10.3±2.9	100
Starr-Edwards	6	28-32	4.6±1.2	12.6±4.1	130
St. Jude Medical	17	26-32	2.5±1.4	5.1±3.5	102
Medtronic-Hall	15	26-32	3.0±1.1	7.0±2.9	116

*Exercise protocols used were symptom-limited treadmill and upright or supine bicycle.

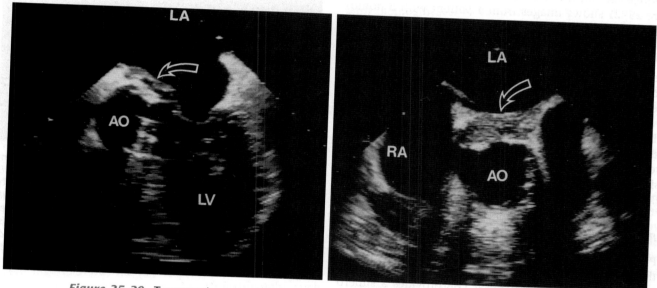

A   B

Figure 25–20. Transesophageal echocardiography in a septic patient with a St. Jude Medical aortic valve. A, Partial dehiscence and a large abscess cavity (arrow). B, Cross-sectional view of the same pathology. The abscess cavity is composed of echodense and echolucent material (arrow). AO, aorta; LA, left atrium; LV, left ventricle; RA, right atrium.

now known and include persistence of symptoms that prompted for the operation, higher complication rates (particularly bleeding), and higher mortality rates.[121]

After successful aortic valve replacement, regression of cardiac hypertrophy is expected and commonly detected by serial echocardiography. Failure to regress the LV mass index at 6 months may be an indication that residual stenosis is present.[121,122] In some patients, inadequate hemodynamics may be apparent only at higher CO settings (i.e., exercise). For patients with exertional symptoms suggesting high valve resistances without evidence of a primary valve dysfunction, stress echocardiography (treadmill or bicycle) should be considered. The diagnosis of patient-prosthesis mismatch requires exclusion of an intrinsic valve dysfunction, which further emphasizes the need for a baseline postoperative study.

Patient-prosthesis mismatch can also be seen in the mitral position. Dumesnil's group has found that the indexed EOA of mitral prostheses should be no less than 1.2 to 1.3 cm^2/m^2 to avoid abnormally elevated transmitral gradients resulting in persistently elevated PA pressures.[123] Prevention of patient-prosthesis mismatch in the mitral position is a challenge because

examination in these patients.

Prosthetic Mitral Regurgitation

The approach to prosthetic MR severity ideally integrates multiple parameters rather than a single measurement. This helps to minimize the effects of technical errors inherent to each method. It is also important to distinguish between amount of MR and its hemodynamic consequences. For example, a relatively modest regurgitant volume occurring suddenly into a small,

colleagues proposed a number of mec... on in vitro models.[129] Figure 25–22 corresponds to a 53-year-old man who underwent mitral valve replacement with a Medtronic-Hall valve 6 months before this study. Patient was admitted with shortness of breath, severe, unexplained anemia (hemoglobin 6.7 g/dL), and reticulocytosis. A grade II/VI systolic ejection murmur was noted along the left sternal border thought to be the result of "normal" turbulence created by the prosthesis exacerbated by the anemia. However, prominent V-waves were noted on neck ex-

there is no alternative technique to implant a larger valve. Consequently, surgical colleagues should implant the device with the largest EOA available.

Prosthetic Aortic Stenosis

The initial suspicion of prosthetic valve stenosis may be the incidental finding of abnormally high flow velocities detected during a routine Doppler examination. One must bear in mind that high-flow velocities

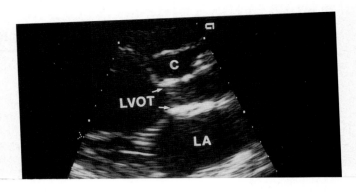

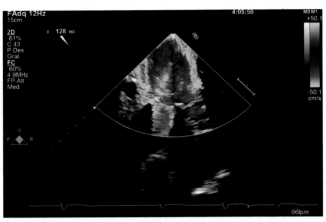

Figure 25–22. *Fifty-three-year-old man underwent mitral valve replacement (Medtronic-Hall valve) 6 months before being admitted with shortness of breath and severe, unexplained anemia (hemoglobin 6.7 g/dL), and reticulocytosis. A grade II/VI systolic ejection murmur was noted along the left sternal border thought to be a result of turbulent flow by the prosthesis exacerbated by the anemia. However, prominent V-waves were noted on neck examination. Transthoracic echocardiography was suboptimal in part as a result of metallic reverberations within the left atrium. Transesophageal echocardiography demonstrated a large eccentric perivalvular leak "hugging" left atrial wall (Coanda effect). These findings were consistent with severe mitral regurgitation resulting from a dehiscent valve; patient underwent a successful reoperation.*

amination. TTE was suboptimal in part as a result of metallic reverberations within the left atrium; TEE demonstrated a large eccentric perivalvular leak "hugging" the left atrial wall, phenomenon known as Coanda effect.[130] These findings were consistent with severe MR resulting from a dehiscent valve; patient underwent a successful reoperation.

Prosthetic valve dehiscence, a separation of the sewing ring from the native fibrous ring, is caused by detachment of the retaining sutures. Careful TEE annular evaluation at the midesophageal and transgastric levels can reveal a dropout of echoes; when color Doppler is over imposed, an eccentric jet may become obvious. Detection of valve dehiscence is important because it usually means severe regurgitation requiring surgical repair or replacement. Figure 25–23 is a set of TEE images illustrating a patient with a Hancock bioprosthesis in the mitral position with dehiscence and severe eccentric regurgitation.

The morphology of the pulmonary vein Doppler waveform is dependent on both regurgitant volume and left atrial properties. Pulmonary vein flow characteristics have been useful in assessing severity of native mitral valve regurgitation. Typically, there is loss of the systolic wave amplitude and eventually reversal of systolic flow as the severity increases. However, in vivo models suggest that pulmonary venous flow reversal is more likely in acute MR than in chronic MR, because the atrium is less compliant and has a smaller initial volume. In addition, characterization of the pulmonary

vein flow in prosthetic MR is lacking, and extrapolation of data from native valves has not been documented.

Stress Echocardiography in Assessing Prosthetic Valve Function

In patients with suspected prosthetic valve dysfunction, one may encounter symptomatic patients in whom the 2D and Doppler imaging indicates normal valve function at rest. Under these circumstances, exercise echocardiography may elicit abnormal hemodynamics indicating valve dysfunction or patient-prosthesis mismatch. In my laboratory, I prefer supine bicycle ergometry over treadmill because serial hemodynamic data can be obtained at different exercise stages. Normal hemodynamics with stress in these patients excludes valve dysfunction as the cause of the patient's symptoms. Valve gradient, valve area, degree of regurgitation, and systolic PA pressure can all be calculated at rest and at peak stress (or immediately afterward). Despite its potential, relatively few stress echocardiographic studies in patients with suspected prosthetic dysfunction have been published.[56,131-134] Table 25–8 summarizes data available regarding valve gradients at rest and exercise.

Dobutamine provides an excellent alternative for evaluating valve hemodynamics when the patient is unable or unwilling to undergo treadmill or bicycle ergometry.[135] In my laboratory, I use a protocol similar to that for ischemic heart disease; that is, I attempt to reach 85% to 90%, of the maximal predicted heart rate according. I start with dobutamine at 10 μg/kg per minute and increase every 3 minutes to 20, 30, and 40 μg/kg per minute. If the Doppler signal intensity of tricuspid regurgitation is weak because of trivial or mild regurgitation, I may use a small amount of diluted Definity to enhance signal intensity, allowing estimation of systolic PA pressure. In patients with single tilting disc prostheses in the aortic position, peak and mean gradients are higher with the dobutamine stress echocardiography (DSE) compared with symptom-limited treadmill exercise.[135]

Evaluation of patients with decreased LV systolic function and possible prosthetic AS is problematic. In 25 adults with native aortic valve stenosis (area = 0.5 cm²/m²), mean gradient less than 30 mm Hg, and ventricular dysfunction (ejection fraction = 0.45), deFilippi and colleagues[136] performed echocardiography at baseline and at peak dobutamine stress to distinguish severe fixed AS from flow-dependent (relative) stenosis. Three hemodynamic subsets were identified: (1) fixed AS with increased CO and transvalvular gradient and no change in valve area; (2) relative AS with increased valve area but no change in gradient; and (3) lack of contractile reserve with indeterminate stenosis because of inability to increase CO. Theoretically, a similar

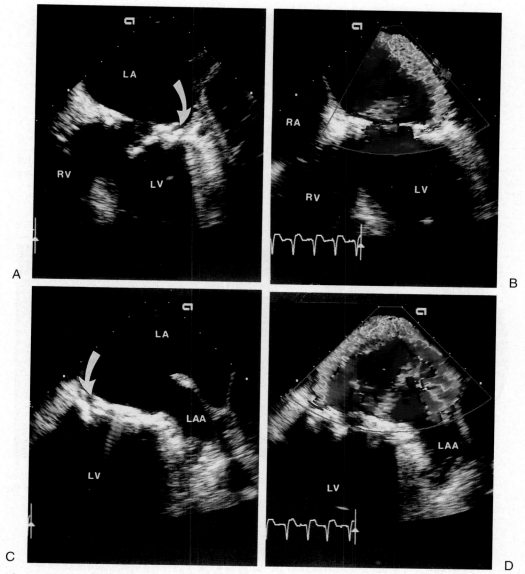

Figure 25–23. *Transesophageal echocardiography showing dehiscence in a stented mitral bioprosthesis with perivalvular regurgitation. A and C, The dehiscent site (arrows) is seen as a dropout of echoes at the annular attachment. B and D, Eccentric severe paravalvular regurgitation is seen through the dehiscence. LA, left atrium; LAA, left atrial appendage; LV, left ventricle; RA, right atrium; RV, right ventricle.*

study may be applicable, although not proved, in patients with severe ventricular dysfunction and prosthetic stenosis of undetermined severity.

Three-Dimensional Echocardiography in Assessing Prosthetic Valve Function

Current echocardiographic approaches for EOA are based on flow characteristics, which depend on several factors in addition to the actual orifice area, including ventricular compliance, systolic function, and loading conditions. A classic problem arises when a patient with mechanical aortic valve has high flow velocities detected in a routine Doppler examination. Is this a normal finding? Is this pannus formation and thus, some stenosis? Is this a patient-prosthesis mismatch?

3D echocardiography involves the acquisition and display of cardiac structures in three spatial dimensions allowing visualization and analysis as they move in time and space. Figure 25–24 illustrates a commonly used rotational scanning mechanism in which the transducer is rotated at 3-degree increments up to 180 degrees. Dynamic 3D imaging may provide a more realistic representation of prosthetic morphology than 2D images. Recent advances in US equipment, digital storage, and display have made 3D clinically feasible; however, the clinical potential of 3D imaging has just begun to be

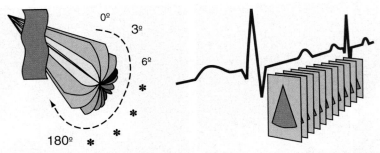

Figure 25–24. Left, *The rotational mechanism for acquisition of two-dimensional images at three-degree intervals from 0 to 180 degrees.* Right, *The two-dimensional images are piled up one after another, gated by the electrocardiogram.*

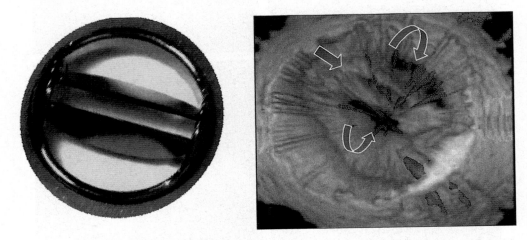

Figure 25–25. *Three-dimensional reconstruction of a St. Jude Medical valve in the mitral position as seen from the left atrium or "surgeon's view." The semicircular orifices* (curved arrows) *and the rectangular orifice* (straight arrow) *are seen.*

recognized. Figure 25–25 depicts a 3D reconstruction of a St. Jude Medical valve performed in my laboratory. The two hemicircular lateral orifices and the central rectangular orifice are clearly indicated.

Mitral annular rings have been reconstructed with 3D technology. Dall'Agata and colleagues[137] used TEE to analyze mitral valve rings in 19 consecutive patients who underwent annuloplasty. Fifteen patients received a Cosgrove-Edwards (flexible) ring and four a Carpentier (rigid) ring. Imaging acquisition used the rotational technique immediately after operation and considered adequate in 17 of them. The authors were able to differentiate values from end-systolic to end-diastolic orifice areas (4.2 ± 1.5 cm^2 versus 4.8 ± 1.5 cm^2; $P < 0.0001$) in the Cosgrove-Edwards ring and no significant change in the Carpentier ring.[137]

In the near future, advances in real-time 3D imaging (not reconstruction), the spatial distribution of prosthetic valve flow, i.e., regurgitation, will be readily available, enhancing measurements of flow convergence, VC, and quantitation of prosthetic valve function.

KEY POINTS

■ Echocardiography is the method of choice to assess prosthetic valve function. The size and type of valve determine the range of flow velocities and is in essence what separates normal from abnormal valve function.

■ Baseline Doppler echocardiography should be performed soon after valve implantation.

■ With the exception of homografts and stentless valves, all prosthetic heart valves are inherently stenotic.

■ TEE is an obligatory complement in assessing prosthetic valve dysfunction.

■ Failure of the catheter technique to record pressure gradients at the VC may explain some of the discrepancies between Doppler- and catheter-derived pressure gradients.

■ In patient-prosthesis mismatch, the prosthesis is structurally normal but with a significantly greater degree of stenosis than expected for the valve type and size.

■ The most attractive advantage of bioprostheses is that in most cases anticoagulation is not needed; however, the increased risk of reoperation is a high price to pay for the reduced risk of bleeding through avoiding anticoagulation.

■ Primary mechanical failure is valve dysfunction from an intrinsic problem, such as calcific degeneration in bioprostheses.

■ Thrombolytic therapy is a logical alternative to surgery in high-risk patients, TEE the ideal method to image lysis.

■ Exercise echocardiography may elicit abnormal hemodynamics indicating valve dysfunction.

REFERENCES

1. Nanda NC, Cooper JW, Mahan EF, Fan PH: Echocardiographic assessment of prosthetic valves. *Circulation* 84(suppl I):I228-I239, 1991.
2. Zabalgoitia M: Echocardiographic assessment of prosthetic heart valves. *Curr Probl Cardiol* 17:267-325, 1992.
3. Wilkins GT, Flachskampf FA, Weyman AE: Echo-Doppler assessment of prosthetic heart valves. In Weyman AE (ed): *Principles and Practice of Echocardiography.* Philadelphia, Lea & Febiger, 1994, pp. 1198-1230.
4. Herrera CJ, Chaudhry FA, Mehlman DJ, et al: Value and limitations of transesophageal echocardiography in evaluating prosthetic or bioprosthetic valve dysfunction. *Am J Cardiol* 69:697-699, 1992.
5. Zabalgoitia M: *Echocardiography of prosthetic heart valves.* Austin, Tex, RG Landes Co, 1994.
6. Peterson GE, Brickner ME, Reimold SC: Transesophageal echocardiography: Clinical indications and applications. *Circulation* 107:2398-2402, 2003.
7. Harken D, Soroff HS, Taylor WJ: Partial and complete prosthesis in aortic insufficiency. *J Thorac Cardiovasc Surg* 40:744, 1960.
8. Starr A, Edwards M: Mitral replacement: Clinical experience with a ball valve prosthesis. *Ann Surg* 154:726-740, 1961.
9. Alton ME, Pasierski TJ, Orsinelli DA, et al: Comparison of transthoracic and transesophageal echocardiography in evaluation of 47 Starr-Edwards prosthetic valves. *J Am Coll Cardiol* 20:1503-1511, 1992.
10. Björk VO: A new tilting disc valve prosthesis. *Scand J Thorac Cardiovasc Surg* 3:1-10, 1969.
11. Tatoulis J, Chaiyaroj S, Smith JA: Aortic valve replacement in patients 50 years old or younger with the St. Jude Medical valve: 14-year experience. *J Heart Valve Dis* 5:491-497, 1996.
12. Godje OL, Fischlein T, Adelhard K, et al: Thirty-year results of Starr-Edwards prostheses in the aortic and mitral position. *Ann Thorac Surg* 63:613-619, 1997.
13. Orszulak TA, Schaff HV, Puga FJ, et al: Event status of the Starr-Edwards aortic valve to 20 years: A benchmark for comparison. *Ann Thorac Surg* 63:620-626, 1997.
14. Joob AW, Kron IL, Carddock GB, et al: A decade of experience with the Model 103 and 104 Beall valve prostheses. *J Thorac Cardiovasc Surg* 89:444-447, 1985.
15. Conti VR, Nishimura A, Coughlin TR, Farrell RW: Indications for replacement of the Beall 103 and 104 disc valves. *Ann Thorac Surg* 42:315-320, 1986.
16. Grunkemeier GL, Starr A, Rahimtoola SH: Prosthetic heart valve performance: Long term follow-up. *Curr Probl Cardiol* 17:331-406, 1992.
17. Thevenet A, Albat B: Long-term follow up of 292 patients after valve replacement with the Omnicarbon prosthetic valves. *J Heart Valve Dis* 4:634-639, 1995.
18. Nitter-Hauge S, Abdelnoor M, Svennevig JL: Fifteen-year experience with the Medtronic-Hall valve prosthesis: A follow-up study of 1104 consecutive patients. *Circulation* 94(suppl II):105-108, 1996.
19. Thomson F, Barret-Boyes BG: The gluteraldehyde treated heterograft valve. Some engineering observations. *J Thorac Cardiovasc Surg* 74:317-321, 1977.
20. Jamieson WR, Munro Ai, Miyagishima RT, et al: Carpentier-Edwards standard porcine bioprosthesis: Clinical performance to seventeen years. *Ann Thorac Surg* 60:999-1006, 1995.
21. Goffin YA, Deuvaert F, Wellens F, et al: Normally and abnormally functioning left-sided porcine bioprosthetic valves after long-term implantation in patients: Distinct spectra of histologic and histochemical changes. *J Am Coll Cardiol* 4:324-332, 1984.
22. Magilligan DJ Jr, Lewis JW, Jara FM, et al: Spontaneous degeneration of porcine bioprosthetic valves. *Ann Thorac Surg* 30:259-266, 1980.
23. Oyer PE, Miller DC, Stinson EB, et al: Clinical durability of the Hancock porcine bioprosthetic valve. *J Thorac Cardiovasc Surg* 80:824-833, 1980.
24. Cohn LH, Mudge GH, Pratter F, Collins JJ: Five to eight year follow-up of patients undergoing porcine heart valve replacement. *N Engl J Med* 304:258-262, 1981.
25. Gallo, I, Ruiz B, Nistal F, Duran CM: Degeneration of porcine bioprosthetic cardiac valves: Incidence of primary tissue failures among 938 bioprostheses at risk. *Am J Cardiol* 53:1061-1065, 1984.
26. Schoen FJ: Pathology of bioprostheses and other tissue heart valve replacements. In Silver MD (ed): *Cardiovascular pathology.* New York, Churchill Livingstone, 1991, pp. 1547-1606.
27. Sanders SP, Levy RJ, Freed MD, et al: Use of Hancock porcine xenografts in children and adolescents. *Am J Cardiol* 46:429-438, 1980.
28. Dunn JM: Porcine valve durability in children. *Ann Thorac Surg* 32:357-368, 1981.
29. Fann JI, Miller DC, Moore KA, et al: Twenty-year clinical experience with porcine bioprostheses. *Ann Thorac Surg* 62:1301-1311, 1996.
30. Jones EL, Weintraub WS, Craver JM, et al: Ten-year experience with the porcine bioprosthetic valve: Interrelationship of valve survival and patient survival in 1,050 valve replacements. *Ann Thorac Surg* 49:370-384, 1990.
31. Cohn LH, Collins JJ, Disesa VJ, et al: Fifteen-year experience with 1678 Hancock porcine bioprosthetic heart valve replacements. *Ann Surg* 210:435-443, 1989.
32. David TE, Bos J, Rakowski H: Aortic valve replacement with the Toronto SPV bioprosthesis. *J Heart Valve Dis* 1:244-248, 1992.
33. David TE, Ropchan GC, Butany JW: Aortic valve replacement with stentless porcine bioprosthesis. *J Cardiovasc Surg* 3:501-505, 1988.
34. Kon ND, Westaby S, Amarasena N, et al: Comparison of implantation techniques using Freestyle stentless porcine aortic valve. *Ann Thorac Surg* 59:857-862, 1995.
35. Westaby S, Amarasena N, Long V, et al: Time-related hemodynamic changes after aortic valve replacement with the Freestyle stentless xenograft. *Ann Thorac Surg* 60:1633-1638, 1995.
36. Westaby S, Amarasena N, Ormerod O, et al: Aortic valve replacement with the Freestyle stentless xenograft. *Ann Thorac Surg* 60(suppl 2):S422-S427, 1995.
37. Yoganathan AP, Eberhardt CE, Walker PG: Hydrodynamic performance of the Medtronic Freestyle aortic root bioprosthesis. *J Heart Valve Dis* 3:571-580, 1994.
38. O'Brien MF: Composite stentless xenograft for aortic valve replacement: Clinical evaluation of function. *Ann Thorac Surg* 60(suppl 2):S406-S409, 1995.

39. O'Brien MF: The Cryolife-O'Brien composite aortic stentless xenograft: Surgical technique of implantation. *Ann Thorac Surg* 60(suppl 2):S410-S413, 1995.

40. Hvass U, Chatel D, Ouroudji M, et al: The O'Brien-Angell stentless valve: Early results of 100 implants. *Eur J Cardiothorac Surg* 8:384-387, 1994.

41. del Rizzo DF, Goldman BS, David TE: Aortic valve replacement with a stentless porcine bioprosthesis: Multicentre trial. Canadian investigators of the Toronto SPV valve trial. *Can J Cardiol* 11:597-603, 1995.

42. Jin XY, Gibson DG, Yacoub MH, Pepper JR: Perioperative assessment of aortic homograft, Toronto stentless valve, and stented valve in the aortic position. *Ann Thorac Surg* 60(suppl 2):S395-S401, 1995.

43. Mohr FW, Walther T, Baryalei M, et al: The Toronto SPV bioprosthesis: One-year results in 100 patients. *Ann Thorac Surg* 60:171-175, 1995.

44. Dossche K, Vanermen H, Daenen W, et al: Hemodynamic performance of the PRIMA Edwards stentless aortic xenograft: Early results of a multicenter clinical trial. *Thorac Cardiovasc Surg* 44:11-14, 1996.

45. Goldman BS, del Rizzo D, Christakis GT, et al: Aortic valve replacement with a stentless porcine bioprosthesis. *Isr J Med Sci* 32:846-848, 1996.

46. Barrat-Boyes BG, Roche AH, Whitlock RM: Six-year review of the results of freehand aortic valve replacement using an antibiotic sterilized homograft valve. *Circulation* 55:353-361, 1997.

47. Jaffe WM, Coverdale A, Roche AH, et al: Doppler echocardiography in the assessment of the homograft aortic valve. *Am J Cardiol* 63:1466-1470, 1989.

48. Moidl R, Simon P, Auschauer C, et al: Does the Ross operation fulfill the objective performance criteria established for new prosthetic heart valves? *J Heart Valve Dis* 9:190-194, 2000.

49. Robles A, Vaughan M, Lau JK, et al: Long-term assessment of aortic valve replacement with autologous pulmonary valve. *Ann Thorac Surg* 39:238-242, 1985.

50. Oury JH, Eddy AC, Cleveland JC: The Ross procedure: A progress report. *J Heart Valve Dis* 3:361-364, 1994.

51. Bodnar E, Wain WH, Martelli V, Ross DN: Long-term performance of homograft and autograft valves. *Artif Organs* 4:20-23, 1980.

52. Elkins RC, Lane MM, McCue C: Pulmonary autograft reoperation: Incidence and management. *Ann Thorac Surg* 62:450-455, 1996.

53. Burstow DJ, Nishimura RA, Bailey KR, et al: Continuous wave Doppler echocardiographic measurements of prosthetic valve gradients. A simultaneous Doppler-catheter correlative study. *Circulation* 80:504-514, 1989.

54. Wilkins GT, Gillam LD, Kritzer GL, et al: Validation of continuous-wave Doppler echocardiographic measurements of mitral and tricuspid prosthetic valve gradients: A simultaneous Doppler-catheter study. *Circulation* 74:786-795, 1986.

55. Leavitt JI, Coats MH, Falk RH: Effects of exercise on transmitral gradient and pulmonary artery pressure in patients with mitral stenosis or a prosthetic mitral valve: A Doppler echocardiographic study. *J Am Coll Cardiol* 17:1520-1526, 1991.

56. van den Brink RB, Verheul HA, Visser CA, et al: Value of exercise Doppler echocardiography in patients with prosthetic or bioprosthetic cardiac valves. *Am J Cardiol* 69:367-372, 1992.

57. Stewart SFC, Nast EP, Arabia FA, et al: Errors in pressure gradient measurement by continuous wave Doppler ultrasound: Type, size and age effects in bioprosthetic aortic valves. *J Am Coll Cardiol* 18:769-779, 1991.

58. Cape EG, Jones M, Yamada I, et al: Turbulant/viscous interactions control Doppler/catheter pressure discrepancies in aortic stenosis. *Circulation* 94:2975-2981, 1996.

59. Vandervoort PM, Greenberg NL, Pu M, Powell KA, et al: Pressure recovery in bileaflet heart valve prostheses. *Circulation* 92:3464-3472, 1995.

60. Voelker W, Reul H, Stelzer T, et al: Pressure recovery in aortic stenosis: An in vitro study in a pulsatile flow model. *J Am Coll Cardiol* 20:1585-1593, 1992.

61. Chambers JB: Is pressure recovery an important cause of "Doppler aortic stenosis" with no gradient at cardiac catheterization? *Heart* 76;381-383, 1996.

62. Rothbart RM, Castriz JL, Harding LV, et al: Determination of aortic valve area by two-dimensional and Doppler echocardiography in patients with normal and stenostic bioprosthetic valves. *J Am Coll Cardiol* 15:817-824, 1990.

63. Dumesnil JG, Honos GN, Lemieux M, Beauchemin J: Validation and applications of indexed aortic prosthetic valve areas calculated by Doppler echocardiography. *J Am Coll Cardiol* 16:637-643, 1990.

64. Chambers JB, Cochrane T, Black MM, Jackson G: The Gorlin formula validated against directly observed orifice area in porcine mitral bioprostheses. *J Am Coll Cardiol* 13:1561-1571, 1989.

65. Chafizadeh ER, Zoghbi WA: Doppler echocardiographic assessment of the St. Jude Medical prosthetic valve in the aortic position using the continuity equation. *Circulation* 83:213-223, 1991.

66. Baumgartner H, Khan S, DeRobertis M, et al: Effect of prosthetic aortic valve design on the Doppler-catheter gradient correlation: An in-vitro study of normal St. Jude, Medtronic-Hall, Starr-Edwards and Hancock valves. *J Am Coll Cardiol* 19:324-332, 1992.

67. Zabalgoitia M, Herrera CJ, Chaudry FA, et al: Improvement in the diagnosis of bioprosthetic valve dysfunction by transesophageal echocardiography. *J Heart Valve Dis* 2:595-603, 1993.

68. Dumesnil JG, Honos GN, Lemieux M, Beauchemin J: Validation and applications of mitral prosthetic valvular areas by Doppler echocardiography. *Am J Cardiol* 65:1443-1448, 1990.

69. Burwash IG, Thomas DD, Sadahiro M, et al: Dependence of Gorlin formula and continuity equation valve areas on transvalvular volume flow rate in valvular aortic stenosis. *Circulation* 89:827-835, 1994.

70. Saad RM, Barbetseas J, Olmos L, et al: Application of the continuity equation and valve resistance to the evaluation of St. Jude Medical prosthetic aortic valve dysfunction. *Am J Cardiol* 80:1239-1242, 1997.

71. Ford LE, Feldman T, Chiu YC, Carroll JD: Hemodynamic resistance as a measure of functional impairment in aortic valvular stenosis. *Circ Res* 66:1-7, 1990.

72. Cannon JD, Zile MR, Crawford FA, Carabello BA: Aortic valve resistance as an adjunct to the Gorlin formula in assessing the severity of aortic stenosis in symptomatic patients. *J Am Coll Cardiol* 20:1517-1523, 1992.

73. Hatle L, Angelson B: *Doppler Ultrasound in Cardiology: Physical Principles and Clinical Applications,* 2nd ed. Philadelphia, Lea & Febiger, 1982, pp. 82-83.

74. Kapur KK, Fan P, Nanda NC, et al: Doppler color flow mapping in the evaluation of prosthetic mitral and aortic valve function. *J Am Coll Cardiol* 13:1561-1571, 1989.

75. Dumesnil JG, Honos GN, Lemieux M, Beauchemin J: Validation and application of mitral prosthetic valvular areas calculated by Doppler echocardiography. *Am J Cardiol* 65:1443-1448, 1990.

76. Hixson CS, Smith MD, Mattson MD, et al: Comparison of transesophageal color flow Doppler imaging of normal mitral regurgitant jets in St. Jude Medical and Medtronic-Hall prostheses. *J Am Soc Echocardiogr* 5:57-62, 1992.

77. Lange HW, Olson JD, Pederson WR, et al: Transesophageal color Doppler echocardiography of the normal St Jude Medical mitral valve prosthesis. *Am Heart J* 122:489-494, 1991.

78. Zabalgoitia M, Garcia M: Pitfalls in the echo-Doppler diagnosis of prosthetic valve disorders. *Echocardiography* 10:203-212, 1993.

79. Yoganathan AP, Heinrich RS, Fontaine AA: Fluid dynamics of prosthetic valves. In Otto CM (ed): *The Practice of Clinical Echocardiography.* Philadelphia, WB Saunders, 1997, pp. 773-796.

80. Baldwin JT, Deutsch S, Geselowitz DB, Tarbell JM: Measurements of mean velocity and Reynolds stress fields within an artificial heart ventricle. *J Biomech Eng* 116:190-200, 1994.

81. Kohler J, Wirtz R, Fehske W: In vitro steady leakage jet formation of technical heart valve prostheses: A photo video optical and color Doppler study. In Liepschs D (ed): *Third International Symposium on Biofluid Mechanics.* Munich, Germany, VDI-Verlag GmbH Publishers, 1994, pp. 315-323.

82. Chambers J, Cross J, Deverall P, Sowton E: Echocardiographic description of the Carbomedics bileaflet prosthetic heart valve. *J Am Coll Cardiol* 21:398-405, 1993.

83. Reisner SA, Meltzer RS: Normal values of prosthetic valve Doppler echocardiographic parameters: A review. *J Am Soc Echocardiogr* 1:201-210, 1988.

84. Barratt Boyes BG, Christie GW, Raudkivi PJ: The stentless bioprosthesis: Surgical challenges and implications for long-term durability. *Eur J Cardiothorac Surg* 6(suppl 1):S39-S42, 1992.

85. Walther T, Falk V, Autschbach R, et al: Hemodynamic assessment of the stentless Toronto SPV bioprosthesis by echocardiograhy. *J Heart Valve Dis* 3:657-665, 1994.

86. Jin XY, Pepper JR, Gibson DG: Effects of incoordination on left ventricular force-velocity relation in aortic stenosis. *Heart* 76:495-501, 1996.

87. Bartzokis T, St Goar F, DiBiase A, et al: Freehand allograft aortic valve replacement and aortic root replacement. *J Thorac Cardiovasc Surg* 101:545-554, 1991.

88. Barratt-Boyes BG, Roche AH, Subramanyan RS, et al: Long-term follow-up of patients with the antibiotic-sterilized aortic homograft valve inserted freehand in the aortic position. *Circulation* 75:768-777, 1987.

89. Barbetseas J, Crawford ES, Safi HJ, et al: Doppler echocardiographic evaluation of pseudoaneurysms complicating composite grafts of the ascending aorta. *Circulation* 85:212-222, 1992.

90. Chafizadeh ER, Zoghbi WA: Doppler echocardiographic assessment of the St. Jude Medical prosthetic valve in the aortic position using the continuity equation. *Circulation* 83:213-223, 1991.

91. Reisner SA, Rinkevich D, Markiewicz W, et al: Spontaneous echocardiographic contrast with the carbomedics mitral valve prosthesis. *Am J Cardiol* 70:1497-1499, 1992.

92. Kan JS, White RJ, Mitchell SE: Percutaneous balloon valvuloplasty: A new method for treating congenital pulmonary valve stenosis. *N Engl J Med* 307:540, 1982.

93. Grunkemeier GL, Starr A: Late ball variance with the Model 1000 Starr-Edwards aortic valve prosthesis: Risk analysis and strategy of operative management. *J Thorac Cardiovasc Surg* 91:918-923, 1986.

94. Bansal RC, Morrison DL, Jacobson JG: Echocardiography of porcine aortic prosthesis with flail leaflets due to degeneration and calcification. *Am Heart J* 107:591-593, 1984.

95. Cipriano PR, Billingham ME, Oyer PE, et al: Calcification of porcine prosthetic heart valves: A radiographic and light microscopic study. *Circulation* 66:1100-1104, 1982.

96. Alam M, Rosman HS, Lakier JB, et al: Doppler and echocardiographic features of normal and dysfunctioning bioprosthetic valves. *J Am Coll Cardiol* 10:851-858, 1987.

97. Kinney EL, Machado H, Cortada X: Cooing intracardiac sound in a perforated porcine mitral valve detected by pulsed Doppler echocardiography. *Am Heart J* 112:420-423, 1986.

98. Barzilai B, Eisen HJ, Saffitz JE, Perez JE: Detection of thrombotic obstruction of a Björk-Shiley prosthesis by Doppler echocardiography. *Am Heart J* 112:1088-1090, 1988.

99. Lanzieri M, Michaelson S, Cohen IS: Transesophageal echocardiography in the diagnosis of mitral bioprosthetic obstruction. *Crit Care Med* 19:979-981, 1991.

100. Dzavik V, Cohen G, Chan KL: Role of transesophageal echocardiography in the diagnosis and management of prosthetic valve thrombosis. *J Am Coll Cardiol* 18:1829-1833, 1991.

101. Young E, Shapiro SM, French WJ, Ginzton LE: Use of transesophageal echocardiography during thrombolysis with tissue plasminogen activator of a thrombosed prosthetic mitral valve. *J Am Soc Echocardiogr* 5:153-158, 1992.

102. Husebye DG, Pluth JR, Piehler JM, et al: Reoperation of prosthetic heart valves: An analysis of risk factors in 552 patients. *J Thorac Cardiovasc Surg* 86:543-552, 1983.

103. Witchitz S, Veyrat C, Moisson P, et al: Fibrinolytic treatment of thrombus on prosthetic valves. *Br Heart J* 44:545-554, 1980.

104. Lorient Roudaut MF, Ledain L, Roudaut R, Boisseau MR: Thrombolytic treatment of acute thrombotic obstruction with disk valve prostheses: Experience with 26 cases. *Semin Thromb Hemost* 13:201-205, 1987.

105. Shapira Y, Herz I, Vatury M, et al: Thrombolysis is an effective and safe therapy in stuck bileaflet mitral valves in the absence of high-risk thrombi. *J Am Coll Cardiol* 35:1874-1880, 2000.

106. Özkan M, Kaymaz C, Kirma C, et al: Intravenous thrombolytic treatment of mechanical prosthetic valve thrombosis: A study using serial transesophageal echocardiography. *J Am Coll Cardiol* 35:1881-1889, 2000.

107. Tong AT, Roudaut R, Özkan M, et al: Transesophageal echocardiography improves risk assessment of thrombolysis of prosthetic valve thrombosis: results of the international PRO-TEE registry. *J Am Coll Cardiol* 43:77-84, 2004.

108. Bloomfield P, Wheatley DJ, Prescott RJ, Miller HC: Twelve-year comparison of a Björk-Shiley mechanical heart with a porcine bioprosthesis. *N Engl J Med* 324:573-579, 1991.

109. Cannegieter SC, Rosendaal FR, Briet E: Thromboembolic and bleeding complications in patients with mechanical heart valve prostheses. *Circulation* 89:635-641, 1994.

110. Hammermeister KE, Henderson WG, Burchfiel CM, et al: Comparison of outcome after valve replacement with a bioprosthesis versus a mechanical prosthesis: Initial 5 year results of a randomized trial. *J Am Coll Cardiol* 10:719-732, 1987.

111. Stoddard MF, Dawkins PR, Longaker RA: Mobile strands are frequently attached to the St. Jude Medical mitral valve prosthesis as assessed by two-dimensional transesophageal echocardiography. *Am Heart J* 124:671-674, 1992.

112. Isada LR, Torelli JN, Stewart WJ, Klein AL: Detection of fibrous strands on prosthetic mitral valves with transesophageal echocardiography: Another potential embolic source. *J Am Soc Echocardiogr* 7:641-651, 1994.

113. Jaffe WM, Morgan DE, Pearlman AS, Otto CM: Infective endocarditis, 1983-88: Echocardiographic findings and factors influencing morbidity and mortality. *J Am Coll Cardiol* 15:1227-1233, 1990.

114. Sanfilippo AJ, Picard MH, Newell JB, et al: Echocardiographic assessment of patients with infectious endocarditis: Prediction of risk for complications. *J Am Coll Cardiol* 18:1191-1199, 1991.

115. Mugge A, Daniel WG, Frank G, Lichtlen PR: Echocardiography in infective endocarditis: Reassessment of prognostic implications of vegetation size determined by the transthoracic and the transesophageal approach. *J Am Coll Cardiol* 14:631-638, 1989.

116. Taams MA, Gussenhoven EJ, Bos E, et al: Enhanced morphological diagnosis in endocarditis by transesophageal echocardiography. *Br Heart J* 63:109-113, 1990.

117. Daniel WG, Mugge A, Martin RP, et al: Improvement in the diagnosis of abscesses associated with endocarditis by transesophageal echocardiography. *N Engl J Med* 324:795-800, 1991.

118. Yvorchuk KJ, Chan KL: Application of transthoracic and transesophageal echocardiography in the diagnosis and management

of infective endocarditis. *J Am Soc Echocardiogr* 14:294-308, 1994.

119. Ellis SG, Goldstein J, Popp RL: Detection of endocarditis-associated perivalvular abscesses by two-dimensional echocardiography. *J Am Coll Cardiol* 5:647-653, 1985.
120. Rahimtoola SH: The problem of valve prosthesis-patient mismatch. *Circulation* 58:20-24, 1978.
121. Pibarot P, Dumesnil JG: Prosthesis-patient mismatch: definition, clinical impact, and prevention: *Heart* 92:1022-1029, 2006.
122. Tasca G, Bruelli F, Cirillo M, et al: Impact of the improvement of valve area achieved with aortic valve replacement on the regression of left ventricular hypertrophy in patients with pure aortic stenosis. *Ann Thorac Surg* 79:1291-1296, 2005.
123. Li M, Dumesnil JG, Mathieu P, et al: Impact of valve prosthesis-patient mismatch on pulmonary arterial pressure after mitral valve replacement. *J Am Coll Cardiol* 45:1034-1040, 2005.
124. Von Dohlen TW, Gross CM, Rogers WB: Conventional and color Doppler assessment of prosthetic cardiac valves. In Nanda NC (ed): *Doppler Echocardiography*. Philadelphia, Lea & Febiger, 1993, pp. 160-174.
125. Perry GJ, Helmcke F, Nanda NC, et al: Evaluation of aortic insufficiency by Doppler color-flow mapping. *J Am Coll Cardiol* 9:952-959, 1987.
126. Yoshida K, Yoshikawa J, Akasaka T, et al: Value of acceleration flow signals proximal to the leaking orifice in assessing the severity of prosthetic mitral valve regurgitation. *J Am Coll Cardiol* 19:333-338, 1992.
127. Cohen GI, Davison MB, Klein AL, et al: A comparison of flow convergence with other transthoracic echocardiographic indexes of prosthetic mitral regurgitation. *J Am Soc Echocardiogr* 5:620-627, 1992.
128. Nellessen U, Maysuyama T, Appleton CP, et al: Mitral prosthesis malfunction. Comparative Doppler echocardiographic studies of mitral prostheses before and after replacement. *Circulation* 79:330-336, 1989.
129. Garcia M, Vandervoot P, Stewart WJ, et al: Mechanisms of hemolysis with mitral prosthetic regurgitation study using transesophageal echocardiography and fluid dynamic simulation. *J Am Coll Cardiol* 27:399-406, 1996.
130. Chao K, Moises VA, Shandas R, et al: Influence of the Coanda effect on color Doppler jet area and color encoding. In vitro studies using color Doppler flow mapping. *Circulation* 85:333-341, 1992.
131. Tatineni S, Barner HB, Pearson AC: Rest and exercise evaluation of St. Jude Medical and Medtronic-Hall prostheses. *Circulation* 80(suppl I):16-23, 1989.
132. Wiseth R, Levang OW, Tangen G: Exercise hemodynamics in small (<21mm) aortic valve prostheses assessed by Doppler echocardiography. *Am Heart J* 125:138-146, 1993.
133. Reisner SA, Lichtenberg GS, Shapiro JR, et al: Exercise Doppler echocardiography in patients with mitral prosthetic valves. *Am Heart J* 118:755-759, 1989.
134. Halbe DW, Woodruff RC, Ojile MC, et al: Non-invasive exercise-evaluation of St. Jude and Medtronic-Hall prosthetic heart valves. *Circulation* 78(suppl II):16-23, 1988.
135. Zabalgoitia M, Kopec K, Abochamh DA, et al: Usefulness of dobutamine echocardiography in the hemodynamic assessment of mechanical prostheses in the aortic valve position. *Am J Cardiol* 80:523-526, 1997.
136. deFilippi CR, Willett DL, Brickner E, et al: Usefulness of dobutamine echocardiography in distinguishing severe from nonsevere valvular aortic stenosis in patients with depressed left ventricular function and low transvalvular gradients. *Am J Cardiol* 75:191-194, 1995.
137. Dall'Agata A, Taams MA, Fioretti PM, et al: Cosgrove-Edwards mitral ring dynamics measured with transesophageal three-dimensional echocardiography. *Ann Thorac Surg* 65:485-490, 1998.

Chapter 26

Echocardiographic Recognition of Unusual Complications after Surgery on the Great Vessels and Cardiac Valves

WILLIAM A. ZOGHBI, MD

The author would like to thank Mrs. JoAnn Rabb for her expert secretarial assistance.

The past three decades have witnessed an unprecedented evolution of the surgical approach to diseases of the aorta and cardiac valves. Concurrent with these developments, echocardiography and particularly Doppler techniques have been refined, allowing a better definition of cardiac structures and flow dynamics. Furthermore, transesophageal echocardiography (TEE) has improved the diagnostic capabilities of ultrasound (US) techniques by providing superior imaging of the aorta and cardiac structures, thus increasing the diagnostic impact of echocardiography in patients with diseases of the aorta and cardiac valves.

A variety of complications may occur early or late in the postoperative period in patients undergoing surgery on the great vessels and cardiac valves. These range from infectious complications, thrombosis, obstruction, or dehiscence of prosthetic material to progression of the underlying disease disorder, particularly in diseases of the aorta. The general recognition of diseases of the aorta and of the infectious complications and dysfunction of prosthetic valves have been addressed in detail (Chapters 24 and 25). The current chapter will focus predominantly on unusual complications following surgery on the aorta and/or cardiac valves and the role of echocardiographic techniques in the assessment of these complications.

Unusual Complications following Surgery on the Aorta

Pseudoaneurysms of Composite Aortic Grafts

Clinical Setting

In patients with aortic aneurysm or dissection of the aortic root involving the aortic sinuses and aortic valve not amenable to repair, replacement of the aortic root with a composite graft is now widely accepted.[1-10] Since its first description in 1968 by Bentall and Debono[1] and with more recent modifications of the procedure,[5,6,10-13] this surgical approach has significantly prolonged the life expectancy of patients affected with annuloaortic ectasia.[5,9,14] Knowledge of this surgical procedure, its variations, and complications is crucial for the echocardiographer. This is particularly important because echocardiography with Doppler has emerged as a powerful diagnostic modality in the assessment of function and complications of composite aortic grafts.

The original Bentall procedure consists of replacement of the aortic root and valve with a composite aortic graft (ascending aortic graft and prosthetic aortic valve).[1] The coronary arteries are reimplanted onto the graft, and the aorta is wrapped around the graft to improve hemostasis.[1-4,15] The development of pseudoaneurysm of the ascending aorta is one of the complications of aortic grafts. This occurs secondary to dehiscence of the suture line at the aortic annulus, coronary ostia, or distal graft anastomosis. Using the original Bentall procedure, this potentially lethal complication has been reported to occur in 7% to 25% of patients with composite grafts.[3,16-19] Several modifications of the original method have been proposed to decrease the incidence of pseudoaneurysm formation.[2,5,6,11-13] In 1981, Cabrol and colleagues[2] modified the operation by introducing a second tube graft connecting both coronary ostia and the main ascending aortic graft (Fig. 26–1). In 1991, Kouchoukos and colleagues[5] showed that the "open or button technique" for reimplantation of the coronary arteries leads to a lower incidence of pseudoaneurysms. At present, with the aforementioned modifications, the

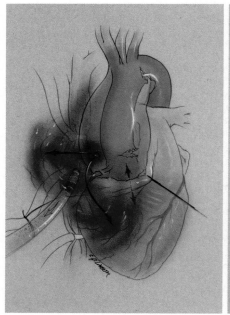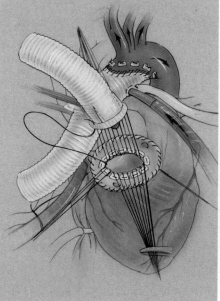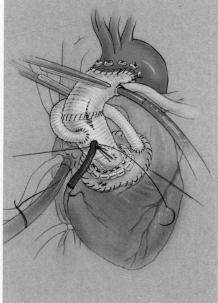

Figure 26–1. Illustration of the surgical reconstruction of the aortic root in a patient with ruptured aortic dissection using a composite aortic graft (modified Cabrol technique). The native aortic root is excised and replaced with a composite graft. A tube graft connects the aortic graft to the left main coronary artery. A vein graft (dark blue) was used in this case to bypass a stenosed right coronary artery. (Courtesy of Dr. Hazim J. Safi.)

incidence of pseudoaneurysm formation has decreased to less than 6%.[5,7-9,12,19-24]

The clinical symptoms associated with pseudoaneurysm formation are variable. Whereas some patients have nonspecific symptoms or may be completely asymptomatic, others may be severely limited with dyspnea and fatigue. With the possibility of aortic rupture, early diagnosis of aortic pseudoaneurysm is essential. Echocardiography with Doppler and particularly TEE have had a significant impact in the detection and evaluation of patients with pseudoaneurysms of composite grafts.[18,25-32]

Echocardiographic and Doppler Findings

A normal composite aortic graft is visualized with echocardiography as an echo-dense ascending aortic root with a prosthetic valve in the aortic position. The maximal diameter of the composite graft depends on its size. In 27 patients with normal composite grafts evaluated in my institution, the diameter of the ascending aorta ranged between 3.2 and 5 cm (mean of 4.2 cm).[18] In patients who underwent wrapping of the graft with the native aorta, a small echo-free space between the graft and the wall of the aorta is seen in the majority of patients (80%) and is usually small, ranging between 0 and 1.4 cm (mean 0.6 cm).[18] In all cases of normal composite graft, Doppler examination showed no evidence of flow in this small echo-free space nor the presence of more than trivial aortic insufficiency.[33]

In patients with pseudoaneurysm formation, echocardiography can provide important diagnostic information as to the presence of the pseudoaneurysm and to the site of dehiscence of the surgical anastomosis.[18,34-36] The identification of an enlarged ascending aorta with an echo-free space around the aortic graft should prompt investigation for the presence of a pseudoaneurysm. Other considerations include a hematoma without pseudoaneurysm, or depending on the clinical setting, the presence of graft infection with abscess formation. The space around the graft may contain variable amounts of echo-dense debris or thrombus. A pseudoaneurysm is diagnosed as an enlarged ascending aorta with an echo-free space between the aortic graft and the wall of the aorta along with the demonstration of flow into the echo-free space[18,34,35] (Fig. 26-2). In a series of patients with pseudoaneurysms diagnosed in my institution,[18] the maximal diameter of

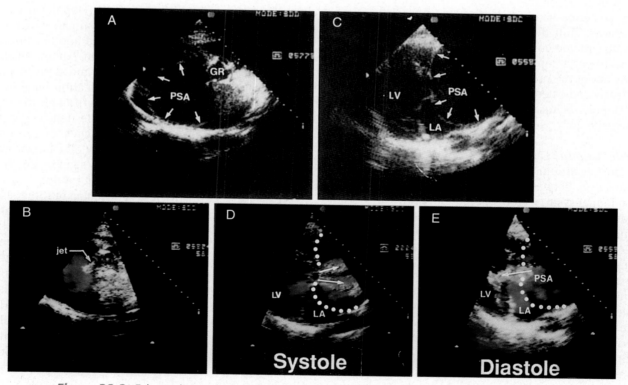

Figure 26-2. *Echocardiographic and Doppler findings using transthoracic echocardiograph in a patient with a large pseudoaneurysm of the ascending aorta complicating a composite graft. The dehiscence was at the aortic annulus anastomosis. A and C show the extent of the pseudoaneurysm (arrows). The origin and extent of the systolic jet into the pseudoaneurysm are shown in B and D. During diastole, blood converges from the pseudoaneurysm toward the aortic annulus and enters the left ventricle (white arrow, E), through the dehiscence, mimicking aortic insufficiency. The corresponding angiographic findings are shown in Figure 26-9. GR, aortic graft; LA, left atrium; LV, left ventricle; PSA, pseudoaneurysm. (From Barbetseas J, Crawford ES, Safi HJ, et al: Circulation 85:212-222, 1992. Reproduced with permission of the American Heart Association.)*

the ascending aorta ranged between 6 and 14 cm. The maximal echo-free space between the aortic graft and the wall of the ascending aorta ranged between 2 and 7 cm. This space may be eccentric or concentric around the graft. Although the majority of reported cases of pseudoaneurysms have more than 2 cm of echo-free space surrounding the graft, the demonstration of flow into the space outside the graft is essential for the diagnosis, irrespective of the size of the echo-free space.

Once a pseudoaneurysm is suspected, special attention is directed to imaging the ascending aorta, aortic root, the plane of the prosthetic valve, and coronary ostia from the left and right parasternal and suprasternal windows. In cases of pseudoaneurysms, color flow Doppler imaging frequently demonstrates evidence of pulsatile flow jet into the echo-free space between the graft and the wall of the ascending aorta (see Fig. 26–2). This finding confirms the entity of pseudoaneurysm as opposed to the mere presence of blood or fluid collection around the graft (Fig. 26–3). In some patients however, it is my experience that transthoracic color flow examination may not identify flow in the echo-free space. In these cases, transesophageal examination clearly demonstrates flow into the pseudoaneurysm (Fig. 26–4). This stems from the lower resolution and sensitivity of surface echocardiography combined with posterior shadowing from the graft and aortic prosthesis. Transthoracic echocardiography (TTE) and TEE do provide complementary information regarding the status of a composite aortic graft. If any suspicion arises about the presence of a pseudoaneurysm, a TEE is clearly indicated. The following is a description of the Doppler echocardiographic findings observed with composite graft pseudoaneurysms.

Aortic Annulus Dehiscence. In cases of dehiscence at the aortic annulus anastomosis, with ensuing communication between the left ventricle (LV) and the pseudoaneurysm, color Doppler identifies a systolic jet arising from the paraprosthetic valve area, directed cranially into the pseudoaneurysm (see Figs. 26–2 and 26–4). Because the jet is frequently eccentric, the imaging plane showing the flow jet in the long axis of the aortic root is usually lateral or medial to the plane showing the aortic graft. Thus the flow jet and aortic graft may not be seen in the same longitudinal plane (see Fig. 26–2). The short axis at the level of the prosthetic aortic valve demonstrates the jet arising in the paravalvular area and oriented into the pseudoaneurysm. Further cranial short-axis levels demonstrate the orientation of the jet in the pseudoaneurysm in relation to the aortic graft. These considerations apply for both TTE and TEE imaging (see Fig. 26–2 and 26–4). Overall, detection of the dehiscence and flow into the pseudoaneurysm is much easier with TEE than with TTE.

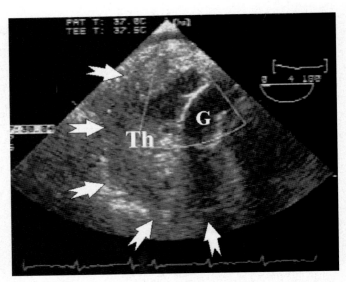

Figure 26–3. *Transesophageal horizontal plane demonstrating a large hematoma (arrows) surrounding a composite aortic graft (G) in a patient early after operation. There was no flow detected around the graft by Doppler echocardiography at any level. The hematoma was secondary to postoperative bleeding complications. Th, thrombus.*

In the majority of cases with dehiscence at the aortic annulus, continuous-wave (CW) Doppler from the apical window demonstrates two distinct systolic jets: one through the prosthetic valve and another through the left ventricular-pseudoaneurysm communication (Fig. 26–5). The maximal velocity and derived pressure gradient through the communication have been, in my experience, higher than those through the prosthesis.[18] The systolic jet through the dehiscence frequently starts before the opening click of the prosthetic valve, and its duration is usually longer than the ejection time through the valve (see Fig. 26–5). In all cases of dehiscence of the aortic annulus, a diastolic jet is seen in the left ventricular outflow simulating valvular aortic insufficiency. In these cases, concomitant aortic insufficiency arising from within the valve cannot usually be excluded with confidence. However, with TEE, the mechanism of regurgitation can be much better defined. CW Doppler recording of these diastolic jets also may mimic severe aortic insufficiency by having a short pressure half-time (PHT). In few cases, an abrupt termination of diastolic flow before the prosthetic aortic valve click and at the time of onset of early systolic flow through the communication supports that this regurgitation is not through the aortic valve (see Fig. 26–5).

Coronary Artery Dehiscence. Coronary artery dehiscence is diagnosed by color flow Doppler as a jet directed into the pseudoaneurysm arising from the level of the coronary ostia or coronary anastomosis. This is

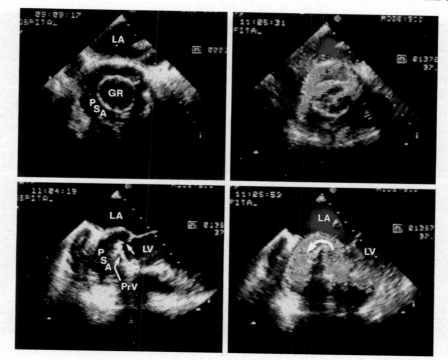

Figure 26–4. Transesophageal echocardiographic frames and corresponding color-Doppler systolic frames in a patient with composite graft pseudoaneurysm. The transthoracic examination in this patient did not demonstrate flow in the pseudoaneurysm. The upper panels are at the level of the ascending aorta and the lower panels at the prosthetic aortic valve level. The dehiscence at the aortic annulus is depicted by a straight arrow. Color-flow Doppler demonstrates flow into the pseudoaneurysm. GR, aortic graft; LA, left atrium; LV, left ventricle; PrV, prosthetic valve; PSA, pseudoaneurysm. (From Barbetseas J, Crawford ES, Safi HJ, et al: Circulation 85:212-222, 1992. Reproduced with permission from the American Heart Association.)

Prosthetic Aortic Valve LV - PSA Communication

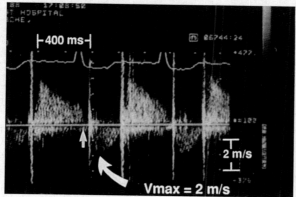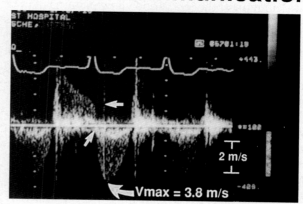

Figure 26–5. Continuous-wave Doppler from the apical window of the case shown in Figure 26–2 with aortic annulus dehiscence. Recordings are obtained from the same position on the chest wall, with minor change in angulation. Compared to the systolic jet velocity through the prosthetic aortic valve, the systolic jet through the ventricular-pseudoaneurysm communication has a higher maximal velocity (Vmax), is of longer duration, and starts (oblique arrow) before the first click of the prosthetic valve (horizontal arrow). The diastolic regurgitant jet into the left ventricle has a steep deceleration slope and ends before the first systolic aortic valve click (straight arrow in upper panel), at the time of onset of systolic flow into the pseudoaneurysm. (From Barbetseas J, Crawford ES, Safi HJ, et al: Circulation 85:212-222, 1992. Reproduced with permission from the American Heart Association.)

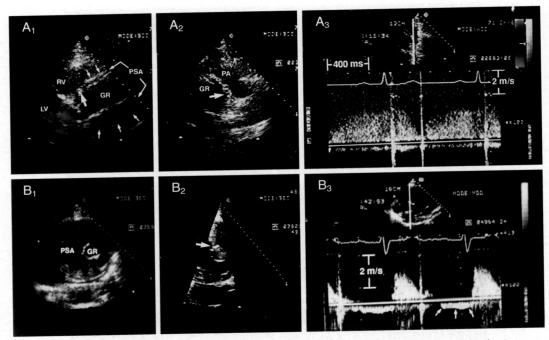

Figure 26–6. *Examples of different velocity patterns observed by continuous-wave Doppler in two patients with coronary artery dehiscence. In patient A (upper panels), the color jet arising from the left main dehiscence is depicted in the parasternal long (A_1) and short axis (A_2) by a large arrow. In this patient with concomitant aortic annulus dehiscence, continuous-wave Doppler (A_3) shows increased systolic and diastolic velocities directed from the graft into the pseudoaneurysm. Patient B (lower panels) has a sole dehiscence at the right coronary anastomosis depicted in short axis (B_1 and B_2). Continuous-wave Doppler recording (B_3) shows flow directed from the graft into the pseudoaneurysm in systole and flow reversal from the pseudoaneurysm into the graft in diastole (small arrows). GR, graft; LA, left atrium; LV, left ventricle; PA, pulmonary artery; PSA, pseudoaneurysm; RV, right ventricle. (From Barbetseas J, Crawford ES, Safi HJ, et al: Circulation 85:212-222, 1992. Reproduced with permission from the American Heart Association.)*

usually easier to define in patients in which the pseudoaneurysm is large because of the more defined spatial distribution of the jet. Various flow patterns may be recorded as shown on Figure 26–6. Whether the flow is predominantly systolic into the pseudoaneurysm or systolic and diastolic depends on several factors, which include the compliance of the pseudoaneurysm and whether a communication exists between the pseudoaneurysm and the LV.

Compression of the Composite Graft or Adjacent Structures. Compression of the graft may occur because of hematoma or pseudoaneurysm formation.[29] This is most commonly observed with aortic annulus dehiscence. With two-dimensional (2D) echocardiography, pulsatile compression of the graft can be seen during systole (Fig. 26–7), most likely because of the high pressure surrounding the graft and possible Venturi phenomenon in the graft. Using CW Doppler, a high systolic velocity jet can be recorded, similar to findings in an obstructed prosthetic aortic valve. Differentiation of the two entities may be difficult. However, visualization of the pulsatile compression of the graft provides a good assessment of the underlying condition.

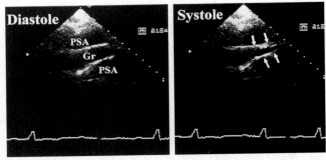

Figure 26–7. *Right parasternal transthoracic echocardiographic images of composite graft pseudoaneurysm demonstrating systolic compression of the graft by the pseudoaneurysm. Gr, graft; PSA, pseudoaneurysm.*

If the pseudoaneurysm is extensive, it may compress adjacent structures. Compression of the pulmonary artery (PA) with resultant PA stenosis has been reported as a complication of a large pseudoaneurysm.[36]

Role of Transesophageal Echocardiography

The use of TEE is clearly advantageous in the overall definition of complications of composite aortic grafts.[18,29,32,34-37] For delineation of pseudoaneurysms, the aortic suture ring is clearly visualized with TEE, enhancing the evaluation of dehiscence at this level with both echocardiography and Doppler techniques. Furthermore, the anastomosis of the coronary arteries to the aortic graft is better assessed. Evaluation of flow in the potential space between the graft and native rapped-around aorta or fibrous tissue—in the case of excision of the native aorta—is improved. Dehiscence at the distal anastomosis of the aortic graft to the aortic arch remains difficult to assess because of limitations of imaging in this area. This type of dehiscence, however, is the least frequent and is rare to occur alone.

In cases of pseudoaneurysm formation secondary to endocarditis, TEE may detect vegetations that can further substantiate the diagnosis (Fig. 26–8). However, in the absence of such a finding, exclusion of an infected graft by echocardiography—or for that matter by any structural imaging alone—is difficult. Because of shadowing anteriorly from the prosthetic valve and graft, an optimum assessment of the aortic root in composite grafts involves combined transthoracic and transesophageal studies. In cases of suspected pseudoaneurysm formation, whereby a collection of blood or thrombus is seen around the graft without demonstration of flow by TTE or other imaging modalities, a transesophageal study is crucial in providing the diagnosis.[18]

Other Imaging Modalities

Several diagnostic modalities have been suggested to screen for the development of pseudoaneurysm after composite graft surgery including chest X-ray (CXR), computed tomography (CT), digital subtraction angiography, and more recently magnetic resonance imaging (MRI).[3,17,38,39] Although chest X-ray may alert to this possibility, its sensitivity and specificity for the diagnosis is poor. CT and MRI are currently recommended diagnostic imaging modalities for the serial evaluation of composite grafts and progression of the underlying disease to other segments of the aorta.[10] As to the diagnosis of pseudoaneurysm, CT scanning or MRI can provide the diagnosis of blood or fluid collection around the graft. However, whether this represents a mere collection of fluid around the graft or the result of communication with the ventricle, coronary arteries or aorta may not be adequately differentiated.

Aortography was initially the most widely used method for diagnosis of pseudoaneurysms as a primary diagnostic modality and later for further evaluation of fluid collection around the composite graft on CT, MRI, or echocardiography.[39] Aortography is still an excellent modality to diagnose dehiscence of the composite graft at the coronary artery anastomosis and distal graft (Fig. 26–9). However, in cases of isolated dehiscence of the

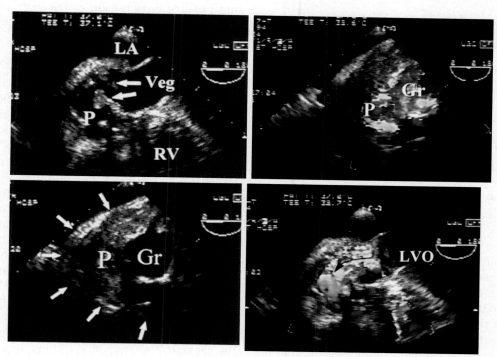

Figure 26–8. *Transesophageal echocardiographic frames and corresponding color Doppler systolic frames in a patient with endocarditis and composite graft pseudoaneurysm secondary to aortic annulus dehiscence. The upper panels are at the level of the prosthetic valve and the lower panels at the level of the left main coronary artery. Two large vegetations are depicted by arrows near the site of dehiscence. Systolic flow into the pseudoaneurysm is shown. P, pseudoaneurysm; Gr, graft; LA, left atrium; LVO, left ventricular outflow; LA, left atrium; P, pseudoaneurysm; RV, right ventricle; Veg, vegetations.*

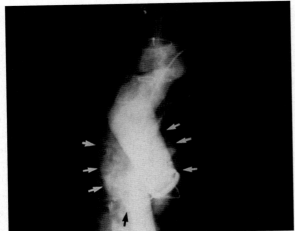

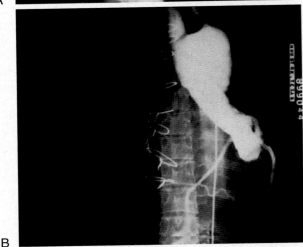

Figure 26–9. Aortograms of thoracic aorta in two patients with pseudoaneurysm complicating composite aortic graft. A, The pseudoaneurysm around the ascending graft is opacified and is delineated by arrows. B, *The aortogram of the patient whose echocardiographic images are in Figure 26–2. In this case with single aortic annulus dehiscence, the large pseudoaneurysm is not opacified. (From Barbetseas J, Crawford ES, Safi HJ, et al: Circulation 85:212-222, 1992. Reproduced with permission from the American Heart Association.)*

graft at the aortic annulus anastomosis, aortography has been found to completely miss the diagnosis of pseudoaneurysm.[18,29] This is explained by the fact that in these cases, the pseudoaneurysm communicates only with the LV; an aortic root contrast injection would therefore not opacify the LV or the pseudoaneurysm. An example of such a case is presented in Figures 26–2 and 26–9. Echocardiography in these cases is superior to aortography in the detection of pseudoaneurysms. Because in the majority of these cases, the prosthetic aortic valve is not crossed at catheterization, opacification of the pseudoaneurysm necessitates a left ventriculogram using the transeptal technique or the levo phase of a pulmonary angiogram. In cases with concomitant dehiscence at the coronary or distal graft anastomosis, or those with coexisting aortic insufficiency, the pseudoaneurysm may be opacified with aortography.[18]

Complications of Aortic Allografts for Replacement of the Aortic Valve and Aortic Root

Clinical Setting

Allograft or homograft replacement of the aortic root has also provided an effective therapy for diseases of the aortic root and the aortic valve.[40-43] Three general techniques for insertion have been used: subcoronary valve implantation, a mini root implantation or inclusion root implantation, and aortic root replacement. Compared to composite graft replacement of the aortic root, the use of an allograft is particularly helpful in recurrent complications of the aortic root, especially in the presence of infection. Aortic allografts have been therefore predominantly performed in patients with destruction of the aortic root with endocarditis, in congenitally narrowed or hypoplastic aortic roots, in patients with complications involving previous root replacement, such as heavy calcifications, and in those who have contraindications to anticoagulation. Among the most common reported complications of aortic allografts are calcifications of the root, aortic regurgitation (AR), or infectious complications primarily in patients whose underlying indication for aortic root replacement was endocarditis. Similar to composite aortic grafts, problems with anastomotic sites, such as dehiscence with pseudoaneurysm formation, problems with coronary artery anastomosis, and possible compression of the graft, are among unusual complications of aortic root homografts.[41,43-45]

Echocardiographic and Doppler Findings

There is a paucity of data on the echocardiographic findings in aortic root allografts.[45,46] Examination of a normal aortic root allograft, especially early after surgery, may be difficult to differentiate from a native aortic root. However, late after surgery, calcifications of the homograft are common and are detected by echocardiography as increased echogenicity in the aortic root. If leaflet degeneration occurs, variable degrees of aortic insufficiency with or without aortic stenosis may be present. In a recent study, paravalvular aortic insufficiency and eccentric jets were more common in patients with subcoronary aortic allograft implantation (41%) than with root replacement (11%).[46] Some unusual complications may affect the allograft. These have occurred early in the postoperative period and can be detected with intraoperative TEE. Recently, cases have been described with complications related to anastomosis of the coronary arteries with the allograft.[44] Aliasing by color flow was detected along with ischemia in the distribution of the involved anastomosis (left main or right coronary artery). Other reported complications include dehiscence of the homograft with resultant pseudoaneurysm formation. Compression of the graft by the pseudoaneurysm may occur, simulating valve stenosis[45] (Fig. 26–10). With more extensive experi-

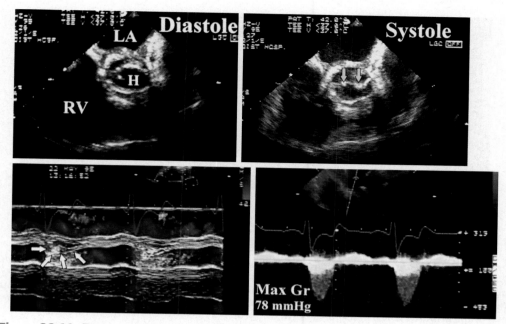

Figure 26–10. Transesophageal echocardiographic findings in a patient with systolic compression of aortic homograft secondary to dehiscence at the aortic annulus anastomosis. The upper panels display the dynamic compression of the homograft in short axis. Color M-mode at the same level shows the systolic compression of the graft (white arrows) and systolic flow in both the pseudoaneurysm (above the arrows) and homograft. Continuous-wave Doppler recording from the transgastric view depicts the high gradient through the obstruction. The aortic valve was normal. Gr, gradient; H, aortic homograft; LA, left atrium; RV, right ventricle. (From Nagueh SF, Bozkurt B, Li GA, et al: Am Heart J 132:1070-1073, 1996. Reproduced with permission of the American Heart Journal.)

ence of cardiac imaging in these patients, the spectrum of complications and the role of echocardiography and other imaging modalities in patients undergoing aortic allograft surgery will be better defined.

Replacement of the Aorta with an "Elephant Trunk" Procedure

In patients with extensive aortic aneurysmal disease or dissection involving the ascending aorta, arch, and descending aorta, replacement of the aortic arch and various extent of the aorta can be a major undertaking. Borst and colleagues[47] described a dual-staged technique whereby the ascending aorta and arch are replaced first, leaving a segment of the distal tubular graft in the descending thoracic aorta. Borst coined the name "elephant trunk" technique for this procedure.[47] At a second stage, the distal aorta is repaired beyond the subclavian artery. Since its original description, few modifications to the technique have been applied.[6,48,49] After the first stage of the operation, imaging the descending aorta with TEE shows the free position of the distal tubular graft in the descending aneurysm, with blood flow detected in the graft emptying into the aneurysm (Fig. 26–11). This finding at this stage is normal and should not be mistaken for dehiscence of the graft. Following a successful first stage of the procedure, the most serious and usually fatal complication is

rupture of the remaining descending thoracic aneurysm while awaiting the second stage of the surgery. I have observed an unusual interim complication of severe hemolytic anemia following the first stage, which resolved after the second stage of the repair. The intravascular hemolysis was the result of insertion of the distal graft into the false lumen during the first operation. Because insertion of the graft into the descending aorta during the first stage of the surgery is performed blindly, some surgeons currently use intraoperative TEE to assess the position of the inserted graft in the descending aorta.

Other Complications

Progression of aortic disease with further aneurysm formation and/or dissection in additional segments of the aorta is the most common cause for reoperation in patients with diseases of the aorta.[19,50-52] Monitoring progression of aortic disease after the initial surgery is crucial in the overall management of these patients and affects prognosis. In addition to the complications mentioned, rupture of the great vessels with fistula formation, although infrequent, can occur as a complication of aortic dissection or aneurysm. Communication between the aorta and PA is clinically suspected by the findings of a continuous murmur, similar to patent ductus arteriosus or the presence of heart failure. Echocardiographic

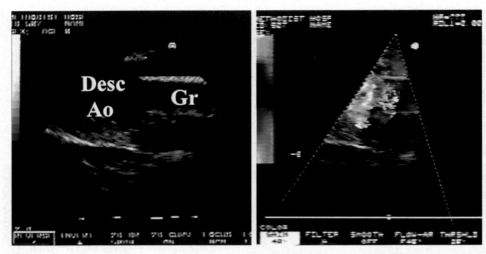

Figure 26-11. Transesophageal imaging of the descending aorta (longitudinal plane) in a patient with aortic aneurysm involving the arch and descending aorta following a successful first stage of an "elephant trunk" procedure. The free distal end of the tubular graft is seen in the descending thoracic aneurysm. Color-flow Doppler shows flow into the descending aorta arising from the distal end of the graft. Desc Ao, descending aorta; Gr, graft.

findings depend on the size of the shunt and may include volume overload of the LV and elevated pulmonary pressures. Doppler echocardiographic findings are those of continuous flow into the PA from the aorta.

Unusual Complications following Valve Surgery

Left Ventricular Pseudoaneurysm after Mitral Valve Replacement

Clinical Setting

Rupture of the LV with pseudoaneurysm formation is a rare but serious complication after mitral valve replacement. Overall, the incidence appears to range from 0.5% to 2% in isolated or combined mitral valve procedures.[53-57] Rupture of the LV may occur immediately after surgery presenting with hemodynamic collapse or may present in the delayed postoperative period as a false aneurysm of the LV. Several anatomic characteristics have been described predisposing to rupture of the ventricle, such as heavy mitral or annular calcifications, the operative procedure itself, the number of previous surgical procedures, or other hemodynamic considerations. However, often no clear cause for the pseudoaneurysm formation can be found.[58] The clinical presentation of pseudoaneurysm formation is variable. In the early postoperative period, it can present as poor postoperative progress, chest pain, heart failure, or as development of a new murmur.[54,55,59] Late postoperative presentation may be similar or may be totally asymptomatic. In unusual cases, the pseudoaneurysm can compress the coronary arteries leading to ischemia or myocardial hibernation.[60]

Echocardiographic and Doppler Findings

Echocardiographic techniques play a significant role in the diagnosis of left ventricular pseudoaneurysm.[61,62] A pseudoaneurysm, in contrast to a true aneurysm, is visualized as a saccular or globular chamber communicating with the LV through a narrow and abrupt discontinuity in the ventricular myocardium. Over the past few years, the important role of Doppler echocardiography in the diagnosis of pseudoaneurysms has been increasingly appreciated. The demonstration of flow into the pseudoaneurysm by pulsed and color flow Doppler substantiates the diagnosis and may at times be the only clue for its presence in cases in which the origin of the pseudoaneurysm cannot be visualized.[63-65] Doppler echocardiography is crucial in differentiating a pseudoaneurysm from other etiologies, such as pericardial cysts, loculated pericardial effusion, or hematoma, especially in cases in which communication of the cavity with the LV is not seen. As with true left ventricular aneurysm, a pseudoaneurysm demonstrates akinesis or dyskinesis during ventricular systole. Characteristic Doppler patterns can be seen with systolic filling and diastolic emptying of the pseudoaneurysm.[66] In patients with sinus rhythm, filling of the pseudoaneurysm during atrial contraction can also be seen. With the availability of intravenous (IV) contrast echocardiographic agents that can cross the pulmonary circulation,[67] the administration of contrast can be of important diagnostic value in these situations by identifying whether such a communication exists with the LV and by localizing its site. This is particularly helpful when the communication with the ventricle is rather large and blood velocity in the cavity is too low to be clearly detected with Doppler.

The location of the pseudoaneurysm can be variable in relation to the prosthetic valve. Although TTE can demonstrate its presence and characteristic features, the pseudoaneurysm may be frequently missed because of technical difficulties and imaging in the far field. TEE is currently the echocardiographic method of choice in patients with suspected left ventricular pseudoaneurysms complicating mitral valve replacement.[66,68-70] An example of a pseudoaneurysm complicating mitral valve replacement demonstrated by TEE and missed by TTE is shown on Figure 26–12.

Other Imaging Modalities

Nonsurgical detection of pseudoaneurysm has previously been dependent on left ventriculography. Angiography is still important in the diagnosis of pseudoaneurysms in patients in whom the TTE may be difficult and also provides a spatial distribution of the pseudoaneurysm (see Fig. 26–12). Because of its tomographic nature, TEE can further add to left ventricular angiography in pinpointing the site of origin of the pseudoaneurysm and its relation to adjacent structures for later surgical correction.[71] The intraoperative use of TEE in surgical repair of these cases can also be crucial when the repair involves areas close to

the coronaries, in the assessment of ventricular function immediately postoperatively, and to indirectly detect whether injury occurred in the area of the coronary vessels with the evaluation of regional myocardial function.[66] It is generally agreed that management of patients with pseudoaneurysm formation of the LV necessitates surgical intervention because of the risk of rupture and potential sudden death. Although this has been carried out almost uniformly in the reported literature, some authors have advocated continued follow-up in asymptomatic patients.[70]

Left Atrial Dissection after Mitral Valve Replacement

Clinical Setting

Dissection of the left atrium with resultant pseudoaneurysm formation is a rare complication of mitral valve replacement.[72-78] Predisposing factors for this unusual complication are similar to those for left ventricular pseudoaneurysms and include mitral annulus calcifications, external cardiac massage, friable atrial tissue, preexisting pericardial adhesions, and techni-

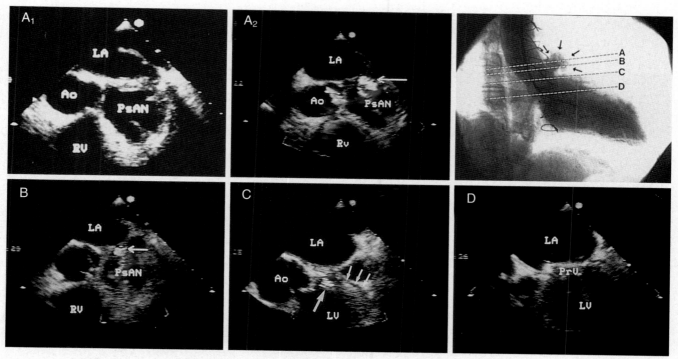

Figure 26–12. *Transverse transesophageal echocardiographic planes at four levels (A-D) are shown along with contrast left ventriculography in the right oblique view demonstrating opacification of a left ventricular pseudoaneurysm complicating mitral valve replacement. The approximate location of the transverse echocardiographic planes are schematically shown on the angiogram. A_1 and A_2, The maximal extent of the pseudoaneurysm and respective color flow demonstrating flow in the cavity. B and C, The neck of the pseudoaneurysm by color Doppler and its proximity and impingement on the proximal circumflex artery (C, arrows). The most caudal plane (D) is at the level of the prosthetic valve, which is normal. Ao, aorta; LA, left atrium; LV, left ventricle; PsAN, pseudoaneurysm; RV, right ventricle. (From Baker WB, Klein MS, Reardon MJ, Zoghbi WA: J Am Soc Echocardiogr 6:548-552, 1993. Reproduced with permission from the American Society of Echocardiography.)*

cal considerations during surgery. Clinical presentation is variable, ranging from detection in the operating room (OR) with TEE to the presence of a systolic murmur of mitral regurgitation (MR) to heart failure or an asymptomatic state. Surgical correction is recommended for symptomatic cases or those with severe left atrial compression. Spontaneous healing has been reported in only one case in the literature.[74] Internal drainage of the false lumen into the right atrium has been recently proposed in cases where the dehiscence at the mitral annuls is small.[75]

Echocardiographic and Doppler Findings

On echocardiography, a cavity formation is seen within the left atrium, with a linear echocardiographic density consisting of the dissection of the atrial wall. This is best delineated with TEE[75,76] (Fig. 26–13). Paraprosthetic valve regurgitation is usually seen, with flow by Doppler entering into the false lumen through the communication.[76] Recording of the jet with CW Doppler provides various degrees of velocity and duration of flow, depending on the size of the communication, and compliance of the false lumen.

Pseudoaneurysm of the Ascending Aorta after Aortic Valve Replacement

Clinical Setting

False aneurysm of the ascending aorta is a rare but serious complication of aortic valve replacement. Potential contributing factors to this complication include leaking aortotomy suture lines, needle punctures for de-airing procedures after surgery, postoperative endocarditis, or friability of the aortic wall.[79-82] Clinical presentation is quite variable, from an asymptomatic incidental finding on chest X-ray or echocardiography to atypical chest discomfort or dyspnea or a continuous murmur because of further complications of fistula formation with adjacent cardiac chambers.[79-82] Surgical repair is generally recommended because these pseudoaneurysm have a high propensity for rupture.

Echocardiographic and Doppler Findings

Echocardiography shows a typical pseudoaneurysmal cavity arising from the ascending aorta, in the vicinity of the prosthetic aortic valve. Usually the aorta is of normal size and the neck of the pseudoaneurysm is small and may be difficult to appreciate on TTE. TEE

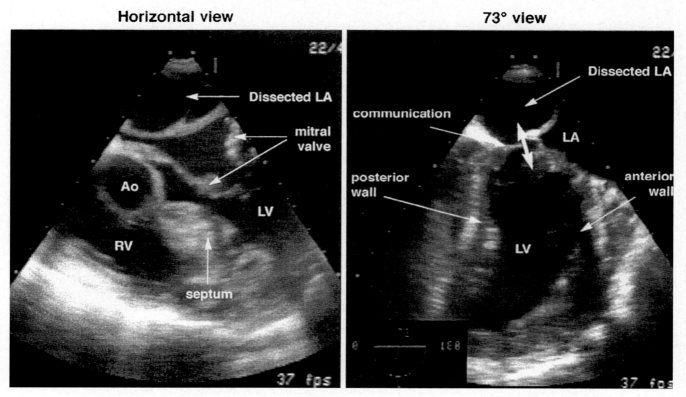

Figure 26–13. Dissection of the left atrium demonstrated with intraoperative transesophageal echocardiography after mitral valve surgery. Ao, aorta; LA, left atrium; LV, left ventricle; RV, right ventricle. (Reproduced with permission from Genoni M, Jenni R, Schmid ER, et al: Ann Thorac Surg 68:1394-1396, 1999.)

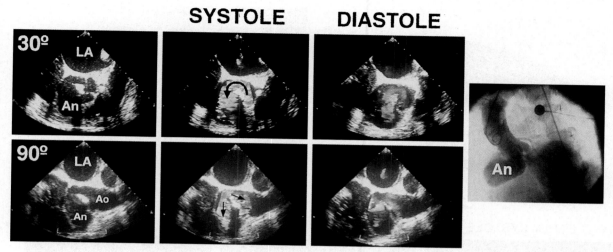

SYSTOLE   **DIASTOLE**

Figure 26–14. *Echocardiographic and Doppler images of an aortic pseudoaneurysm obtained with transesophageal echocardiography in the 30-degree and 90-degree planes. Flow is seen entering the pseudoaneurysm in systole and emptying in diastole. The corresponding aortogram delineates the extent of the pseudoaneurysm. An, pseudoaneurysm; Ao, aorta; LA, left atrium.*

enhances imaging and definition of the pseudoaneurysm that could be lined with thrombus. Color Doppler identifies flow into the cavity in systole, emptying in diastole (Fig. 26–14). In a typical aortic pseudoaneurysm, there is no associated aortic insufficiency or continuous flow seen in the cavity. However, in case of further complications of the pseudoaneurysm, a continuous flow could be detected, the site of rupture into the right atrium or right ventricle.[81,82]

Similar to other pseudoaneurysms of the aorta, aortography, CT or MRI can also delineate the pseudoaneurysm (see Fig. 26–14).

Pseudoaneurysm of the Mitral-Aortic Intervalvular Fibrosa

Clinical Setting

The region of the mitral-aortic continuity or mitral-aortic intervalvular fibrosa (MAIVF) contains mostly fibrous, relatively avascular tissue. Because of its composition, the MAIVF is the weakest segment of the aortic ring[83] and has been noted to be prone to infection and more sensitive to trauma. The roof of the MAIVF is formed of pericardium, and its ventricular side is the posterior portion of the left ventricular outflow tract (LVOT). Dehiscence in the MAIVF region, secondary to infection, trauma, or even surgical manipulation, may result in the formation of an abscess or a pouch between the medial wall of the left atrium and the aorta. An intervalvular pseudoaneurysm ensues when the abscess or pouch communicates with the LVOT.[84-87] Figure 26–15 shows an example of an MAIVF pseudoaneurysm. The majority of pseudoaneurysms in the MAIVF region are secondary to infection and are more common in patients with prosthetic valves.[88]

Other etiologies include trauma, surgical trauma, and congenital pseudoaneurysms.[88-90] The importance of detection of these pseudoaneurysms lies in the potential complications, which may include rupture into the left atrium or aorta resulting in MR or AR, respectively, or even rupture into the pericardial space with ensuing cardiac tamponade and death.[84,87,89]

It is difficult to determine the incidence of MAIVF pseudoaneurysms. Before TEE, few reports have surfaced at pathology or during angiography. With the advent of TEE, the most sensitive technique for evaluation of these lesions, MAIVF pseudoaneurysms was detected in 9% of patients undergoing TEE for suspected aortic valve and/or ring disease.[88] The clinical presentation is variable but most commonly is that of endocarditis, congestive heart failure (CHF), valvular regurgitation, or an asymptomatic state, without an antecedent history of endocarditis. Because of the location of the pseudoaneurysm between the left atrium and aorta and its origin in the left ventricular outflow, it is not readily identified at surgery and may be missed. Thus, accurate detection and delineation of MAIVF pseudoaneurysms and differentiation from ring abscesses is important in overall patient management and in the guidance of surgical correction.

Echocardiographic and Doppler Findings

TTE has been used for the diagnosis of aortic root complications.[91,92] Its sensitivity however has been recently shown to be limited in the evaluation of posterior lesions, particularly in the presence of prosthetic aortic valves. TEE, on the other hand, substantially improves the diagnosis of such lesions.[93,94] In a series from my institution, TTE detected 43% of a total of 23 lesions affecting the aortic root, whereas TEE identified 90% of

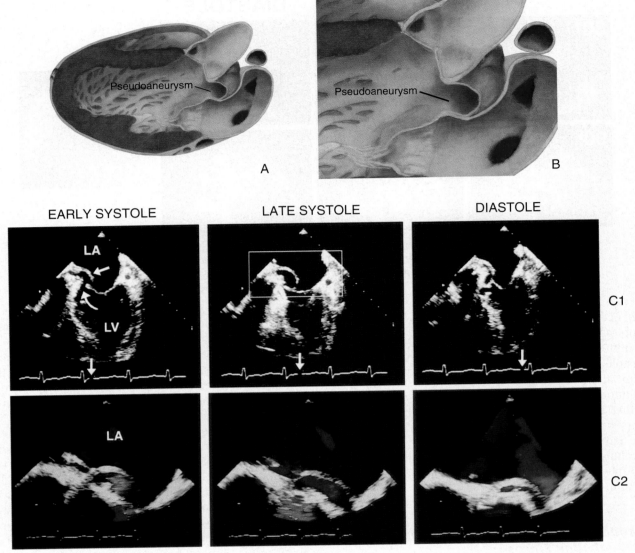

Figure 26–15. *A three-dimensional schematic rendition of a pseudoaneurysm of the mitral-aortic intervalvular fibrosa communicating with the left ventricular outflow tract (A and B) along with transesophageal images from a patient with mitral-aortic intervalvular fibrosa pseudoaneurysm. The transesophageal images show the pulsatility and flow patterns in the mitral-aortic intervalvular fibrosa during the cardiac cycle. C1, The straight arrow points to the pseudoaneurysm, whereas the curved arrow shows the communication with the left ventricular outflow. The pseudoaneurysm begins to expand during early systole, remains distended in late systole, and collapses during diastole. C2, Magnified color Doppler views of the area within the outlined box. During early systole, the pseudoaneurysm fills showing high, aliased velocities. This is followed by low, nonaliased velocities during the remainder of systole while the pseudoaneurysm remains expanded (middle bottom panel). During diastole, the pseudoaneurysm empties and collapses. LA, left atrium; LV, left ventricle.*

the lesions.[88] However, the importance of TTE in detecting anterior ring abscesses cannot be ignored, particularly in the presence of prosthetic aortic valves, where TEE may have significant limitations because of shadowing of the prosthesis in the region of the anterior aortic ring. Thus combined TTE and TEE would allow a comprehensive evaluation of the aortic root and is strongly recommended.

In contrast to aortic ring abscesses, intervalvular pseudoaneurysms exhibit a characteristic dynamic feature during the cardiac cycle. A marked pulsatility is observed in the majority of MAIVF pseudoaneurysms, with expansion during early systole and collapse in diastole[88] (see Fig. 26–15). This is explained by the fact that the pressure in the pseudoaneurysm reflects left ventricular pressure and that a large portion of the pseudoaneurysm is surrounded by the left atrium. Thus, when left ventricular pressure decreases in diastole and reaches a point when atrial pressure exceeds left ventricular pressure, the pseudoaneurysm empties into the LV and collapses, whereas it fills and expands in systole. This dynamic behavior is indeed the first clue as to the presence of an MAIVF pseudoaneurysm. In contrast, aortic ring abscesses located anteriorly or posteriorly in the aortic root do not exhibit this marked pulsatility. This may be explained by several factors. In walled-off abscesses without detectable flow, pulsatility is not expected. In ring abscesses with systolic and diastolic flow, the site of paraprosthetic aortic insufficiency, the higher pressure throughout the cardiac cycle in these cavities compared to adjacent chambers explains this phenomenon. Although collapsibility is an indirect evidence for the presence of an MAIVF pseudoaneurysm, confirmation of this diagnosis requires visualization of the neck of the pseudoaneurysm in the left ventricular outflow. This communication can rarely be seen by TTE.[88] However, it is usually well visualized with TEE. In my experience, the size of the neck has ranged between 0.5 and 2.1 cm in diameter. In cases where there is still doubt about whether the cavity communicates with the aorta or LV, the administration of intravenous contrast agents that cross the pulmonary circulation can help resolve this issue.

Color Doppler imaging is essential in the evaluation of MAIVF pseudoaneurysms. Its application helps assess whether rupture of this cavity into adjacent chambers has occurred and define its communication. The following are characteristic Doppler features in ruptured and unruptured MAIVF pseudoaneurysms. In the case of unruptured pseudoaneurysms, Doppler evaluation is usually less impressive. Only a brief duration of flow into the pseudoaneurysm occurs during early systole (20 to 60 msec) at which time equalization of pressure between the pseudoaneurysm and LV occurs and no further flow is detected by Doppler[88] (see Fig. 26–15). During diastole, a brief period of flow exiting from the pseudoaneurysm may be seen but can frequently be missed because of its low velocity. In contrast, in pseudoaneurysms that have ruptured either into the left atrium or aorta, an intense color flow signal can be seen during the cardiac cycle. In cases of rupture into the left atrium, color Doppler shows holosystolic, intense flow signal in the pseudoaneurysm and eccentric "mitral" regurgitation through the perforation of the pseudoaneurysm; the latter acting as a conduit for blood flow from the LV to the left atrium (Fig. 26–16). The use of color Doppler actually facilitates the identification of the rupture site of the pseudoaneurysm by tracking the origin of the regurgitant jet. The ruptured site is usually rarely seen by TTE but can be suspected by the presence of eccentric MR arising close to the aortic root. Similar to unruptured pseudoaneurysms, those communicating with the left atrium show systolic expansion and diastolic collapse (see Fig. 26–16). In cases in which rupture of the pseudoaneurysm occurs into the aorta, with or without concomitant dehiscence of the prosthetic aortic valve, aortic insufficiency is detected (Fig. 26–17). In systole, color Doppler shows antegrade flow from the ventricle through both the pseudoaneurysm and the prosthetic aortic valve. In diastole, retrograde flow of "aortic" insufficiency is seen directed from the aortic root into the pseudoaneurysm and into the ventricle.

Other Imaging Modalities

Cine angiography has been until recently the standard for diagnosing aortic root lesions.[95] However, with the advent of echocardiography with Doppler and more recently TEE, these techniques have rivaled the invasive diagnostic modality. Regarding MAIVF pseudoaneurysms, few cases have been described with angiography.[86,96,97] The pulsatility described previously is also

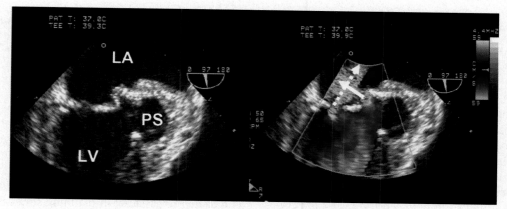

Figure 26–16. Two-dimensional and color-flow transesophageal echocardiographic images of a complicated mitral-aortic intervalvular fibrosa pseudoaneurysm with rupture into the left atrium in the setting of endocarditis after aortic valve replacement. The direction of the jet into the left atrium from the ruptured pseudoaneurysm is shown by the solid arrow. The broken arrow shows the jet of native mitral regurgitation. LA, left atrium; LV, left ventricle; PS, pseudoaneurysm of the mitral aortic intervalvular fibrosa.

SYSTOLE   DIASTOLE

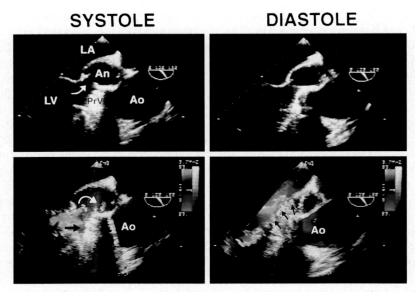

Figure 26–17. *Two-dimensional and color-Doppler frames during omniplane transesophageal examination at an angulation of 120 showing a ruptured mitral-aortic intervalvular fibrosa pseudoaneurysm into the aorta. During systole, blood flows into the pseudoaneurysm and from the pseudoaneurysm into the aorta through small fenestrations (white arrow). The black arrow points to the normal flow direction through the prosthesis. During diastole, blood regurgitates into the left ventricle through the pseudoaneurysm (black arrows). An, pseudoaneurysm; Ao, aorta; LA, left atrium; LV, left ventricle; PrV, prosthetic aortic valve. (From Afridi I, Apostolidou MA, Saad RM, Zoghbi WA: J Am Coll Cardiol 25:137-145, 1995. Reproduced with permission from the American College of Cardiology.)*

Systole   Diastole

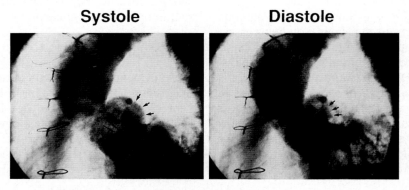

Figure 26–18. *Left anterior oblique view during aortography in a patient with mitral-aortic intervalvular fibrosa pseudoaneurysm and aortic insufficiency. The mitral-aortic intervalvular fibrosa pseudoaneurysm is delineated by arrows and shows pulsatility during the cardiac cycle. (From Afridi I, Apostolidou MA, Saad RM, Zoghbi WA: J Am Coll Cardiol 25:137-145, 1995. Reproduced with permission from the American College of Cardiology.)*

seen on angiography (Fig. 26–18). In a case series in which patients underwent both diagnostic modalities, MAIVF pseudoaneurysms were more frequently detected by TEE than by aortography.[88] Only two of nine pseudoaneurysms were identified by aortography, both of which had associated aortic insufficiency (Fig. 26–19). The direct communication between the LVOT and pseudoaneurysm explains the need for a ventricular injection of dye to detect this abnormality. This finding is similar to that described above for pseudoaneurysms of composite aortic grafts with a single dehiscence at the aortic annulus anastomosis. Thus in patients without aortic

insufficiency, demonstration of the pseudoaneurysm with angiography requires left ventriculography through a transeptal technique. Compared with angiography, TEE more clearly delineates the origin of the intervalvular pseudoaneurysms and their communication elucidating the etiology of concomitant MR or aortic insufficiency and therefore assisting in planning surgical repair.[88]

Patients with cavitary lesions complicating aortic valve disease (particularly prosthetic valves) require extensive surgical intervention including aortic root replacement in some cases. Because of the risk of possible rupture into the pericardium, surgical correction

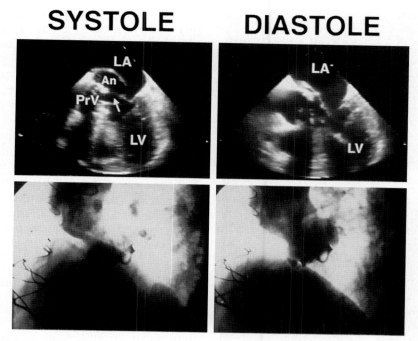

Figure 26–19. *Example of a patient with an unruptured mitral-aortic intervalvular fibrosa pseudoaneurysm diagnosed with transesophageal echocardiography and missed at aortography.* Top, *Transesophageal echocardiographic transverse planes showing the mitral-aortic intervalvular fibrosa pseudoaneurysm expanding during systole* (left) *and collapsing during diastole* (right). *The arrow points to the communication between the pseudoaneurysm and left ventricular outflow region.* Bottom, *Aortogram during systole and diastole in the same patient appears normal. An, mitral-aortic intervalvular fibrosa pseudoaneurysm; LA, left atrium; LV, left ventricle; PrV, prosthetic aortic valve. (From Afridi I, Apostolidou MA, Saad RM, Zoghbi WA: J Am Coll Cardiol 25:137-145, 1995. Reproduced with permission from the American College of Cardiology.)*

of MAIVF pseudoaneurysm is warranted in the majority of cases. Although the natural history of uncomplicated pseudoaneurysm is unclear, surgical repair was performed in the majority of cases reported. In patients not undergoing immediate operation, TEE may be useful to identify serial changes in the pseudoaneurysm or development of rupture into adjacent chambers, which may help plan appropriate therapy.

Intracardiac Fistulae following Valve Replacement or Aortic Root Reconstruction

Clinical Setting

Intracardiac fistula formation is an uncommon complication following valve replacement surgery. Several types of fistulae may occur following mitral valve replacement including left ventricular to right atrial communications and left ventricular to coronary sinus fistulae.[98-101] These complications are mostly attributed to excessive debridement and operative injury to the mitral annulus during surgery. However, concomitant endocarditis may be an underlying mechanism in late postoperative cases. More recently, LVOT to right atrial fistula has been described as a rare complication in

patients undergoing aortic root reconstruction surgery, sparing the native aortic valve[102] (Fig. 26–20).

In the early postoperative period, the clinical presentation may include a new systolic murmur, findings of high cardiac output (CO), or a high oxygen saturation in the PA. This condition may be often misdiagnosed as remnant tricuspid regurgitation (TR) or periprosthetic valve regurgitation.

On the other hand, fistula formation following aortic valve replacement, between the aorta and cardiac chambers, such as left or right atrium or right ventricle is usually secondary to infectious causes but could also be in the setting of a ruptured pseudoaneurysm.[81,82] Findings in these conditions are similar to those of rupture of sinus of Valsalva including a continuous murmur.

Echocardiographic and Doppler Findings

A left ventricular to right atrial fistula mimics tricuspid insufficiency and its differentiation from the latter may be difficult. Few direct and indirect clues may raise the suspicion for this diagnosis. In contrast to the majority of tricuspid insufficiency jets, which are directed toward the interatrial septum, the jet from the fistula by color Doppler arises near the crux of the heart and is

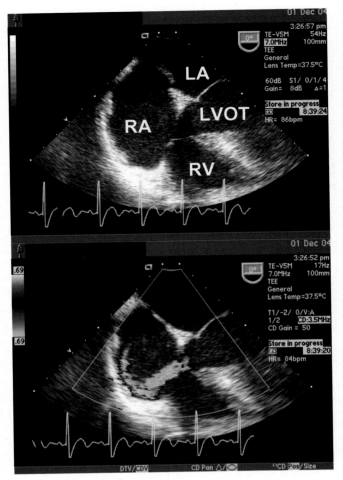

Figure 26–20. Two-dimensional and color-Doppler transesophageal echocardiographic images showing a fistula between the left ventricular outflow tract and the right atrium following repair of the aorta, with left to right shunting during systole. LA, left atrium; LVOT, left ventricular outflow tract; RA, right atrium; RV, right ventricle. (Reproduced with permission from Ramasubbu K, Coselli J, Zoghbi WA: J Am Soc Echocardiogr 19:469, 2006.)

usually directed centrally or towards the free wall of the right atrium (see Fig. 26–20). Unconventional imaging planes to assess the origin of the jet may provide visualization of proximal velocity acceleration on the left ventricular side raising suspicion of the diagnosis. Recording of jet velocity by CW Doppler will invariably lead to registering a high velocity jet, similar to MR. If there is concomitant MR, the jet velocities are almost equal. This will lead to an overestimation of PA pressure when using the modified Bernoulli equation. However, a close examination of right ventricular function, septal motion, pulmonary flow velocity contour, and, pulmonary insufficiency jet, if available, may reveal a discordance between findings of normal pressure by these indices and that derived from the "tricuspid insufficiency" jet, raising suspicion of the diagnosis. Further confirmation may be carried out with TEE aiming at better definition of the origin of the jet.

In the case of left ventricular to coronary sinus fistula, a high velocity intense color jet is seen in the coronary sinus, which in these cases, is usually dilated. The differential diagnosis includes a coronary artery to coronary sinus fistula, where in contrast, a continuous flow occurs.[103] On the other hand, fistula formation between the aorta and cardiac chambers through a periprosthetic aortic valve abscess rupture is diagnosed as a continuous systolic and diastolic jet into the respective chamber, with a continuous and intense recording by CW Doppler of high velocity reflecting the high pressure difference between aorta and the communicating chamber. In the aforementioned conditions, the most often used alternative diagnostic modality is contrast cineangiography demonstrating the communications.

Pulmonary Valve Autotransplantation: The Ross Operation

In 1967, Ross described the use of autologous pulmonary valve to replace the diseased aortic valve. The procedure, presently known as the Ross operation, consists of implantation of the patient's own pulmonary valve within the aortic root and replacement of the pulmonary valve with either an aortic or pulmonary allograft. This procedure is performed predominantly in young adult patients and children with aortic valve disease and offers the advantage of valve viability and potential for growth in young patients, elimination of the need for long-term anticoagulation in addition to longer durability compared to aortic allografts and bioprosthetic valves in this age group.[104,105] Among complications of the Ross operation are the potential for aortic insufficiency because of malalignment of the pulmonic valve in the aortic position and valve degeneration, late after surgery. Replacement of the aortic root with a pulmonary root autograft was later proposed.[106-108] The potential advantage of this procedure compared to simple pulmonary valve autograft is the more optimal alignment and function of the valve leaflets because the sinuses of Valsalva are also transplanted. More experience with the procedure has been acquired.[43,109-113] Progressive annular dilatation of the pulmonary autograft and aortic insufficiency, however, have also been observed after implantation in the aortic position[114-118] with possible aneurysmal or pseudoaneurysmal formation.[119,120] Progressive stenosis of the allograft in the pulmonary position is infrequently reported.[108,117,121] Freedom from reoperation on the pulmonary autograft has ranged between 75% and 88% at 10 years,[116,117] whereas freedom from reoperation on the pulmonary allograft was 86%.[116] Reoperation on the pulmonary allograft may be necessary in up to 20% of patients at 20 years.[43]

Echocardiographic techniques are ideally suited for the follow-up and the detection of complications in patients with pulmonary valve or pulmonary root autografts.[108,114-117,119-123] In the majority of cases, TTE with Doppler is sufficient to evaluate the aortic root and the presence and severity of aortic insufficiency. In suspected complications, TEE improves the definition of aortic root pathology.[119] Similarly, echocardiography can provide serial assessment of allograft function in the pulmonary position. Stenosis at the distal anastomosis has been recently reported with Doppler echocardiography, requiring reoperation in few patients.[120,121] TEE may be needed to evaluate complex lesions or the mechanism of postoperative complications.

Summary

Surgical techniques have grown in potential, complexity, and impact over the years, allowing correction of several valvular disorders and complex diseases of the aorta. Complications arising from these surgeries are varied and usually involve dehiscence or trauma at the site of surgery with unusual communications, infectious complications, and fistula formation. Echocardiography with Doppler, combining transthoracic and transesophageal techniques, is well suited to identify and localize these complications for guidance of surgical repair and improved patient management and outcome.

KEY POINTS

- Unusual complications after surgery on the cardiac valves or aorta include, among others, pseudoaneurysm formation, dissection of adjacent structures, and intracardiac fistulae.

- TEE with Doppler complements TTE in identifying the surgical complications and characteristic flow patterns.

- Pseudoaneurysm formation complicating composite aortic grafts may arise from dehiscence at the aortic annulus, at the anastomosis of the coronary arteries, and less frequently, at the distal aortic anastomosis. Dehiscence at the aortic annulus may mimic AR.

- Mitral valve replacement may infrequently be complicated by pseudoaneurysm formation of the LV or dissection of the left atrium.

- Pseudoaneurysm formation of the ascending aorta may complicate aortic valve replacement.

- The mitral aortic intravalvular fibrosa (MAIVF) is most susceptible to infection or trauma, which can lead to abscess or pseudoaneurysm formation.

- In contrast to abscess formation, pseudoaneurysm in MAIVF is characteristically pulsatile, communicates most often with the LVOT and has a brief transient flow pattern.

- Rupture of MAIVF into the left atrium leads to MR, whereas rupture into the aorta results in "AR"; the pseudoaneurysm in both situations acts as a conduit for the regurgitant flow.

- Intracardiac fistulae can occur after valve replacement and have been described recently after aortic root reconstruction. The LV-to-right atrial fistula may simulate the presence of a ventricular septal defect or tricuspid regurgitation.

- Echocardiography with Doppler is ideally suited to follow patients after a Ross procedure and evaluate possible complications of aneurysmal or pseudoaneurysmal dilatation of the pulmonary autograft, AR, or development of stenosis of the pulmonary allograft.

REFERENCES

1. Bentall H, Debono BA: A technique for complete replacement of the ascending aorta. *Thorax* 23:338-339, 1968.
2. Cabrol C, Pavie A, Gandjbakhch I, et al: Complete replacement of the ascending aorta with reimplantation of the coronary arteries: New surgical approach. *J Thorac Cardiovasc Surg* 81:309-315, 1981.
3. Kouchoukos NT, Marshall WG Jr, Wedige-Stecher TA: Eleven-year experience with composite graft replacement of the ascending aorta and aortic valve. *J Thorac Cardiovasc Surg* 92:691-705, 1986.
4. Crawford ES, Coselli JS, Svensson LG, et al: Diffuse aneurysmal disease (chronic aortic dissection, Marfan, and mega aorta syndromes) and multiple aneurysm. Treatment by subtotal and total aortic replacement emphasizing the elephant trunk operation. *Ann Surg* 211:521-537, 1990.
5. Kouchoukos NT, Wareing TH, Murphy SF, Perrillo JB: Sixteen-year experience with aortic root replacement. Results of 172 operations. *Ann Surg* 214:308-318, 1991.
6. Svensson LG: Rationale and technique for replacement of the ascending aorta, arch, and distal aorta using a modified elephant trunk procedure. *J Card Surg* 7:301-312, 1992.
7. Lewis CT, Cooley DA, Murphy MC, et al: Surgical repair of aortic root aneurysms in 280 patients. *Ann Thorac Surg* 53:38-45, 1992.
8. Gott VL, Cameron DE, Pyeritz RE, et al: Composite graft repair of Marfan aneurysm of the ascending aorta: results in 150 patients. *J Card Surg* 9:482-489, 1994.
9. Finkbohner R, Johnston D, Crawford ES, et al: Marfan syndrome. Long-term survival and complications after aortic aneurysm repair. *Circulation* 91:728-733, 1995.
10. Gott VL, Greene PS, Alejo DE, et al: Replacement of the aortic root in patients with Marfan's syndrome. *N Engl J Med* 340:1307-1313, 1999.
11. Cabrol C, Gandjbakhch I, Cham B: [Aneurysms of the ascending aorta; total replacement with reimplantation of the coronary arteries (author's transl)]. *Nouv Presse Med* 7:363-365, 1978.
12. Coselli JS, Crawford ES: Composite valve-graft replacement of aortic root using separate Dacron tube for coronary artery reattachment. *Ann Thorac Surg* 47:558-565, 1989.
13. Kawazoe K, Eishi K, Kawashima Y: New modified Bentall procedure: Carrel patch and inclusion technique. *Ann Thorac Surg* 55:1578-1579, 1993.

14. Crawford ES, Svensson LG, Coselli JS, et al: Surgical treatment of aneurysm and/or dissection of the ascending aorta, transverse aortic arch, and ascending aorta and transverse aortic arch. Factors influencing survival in 717 patients. *J Thorac Cardiovasc Surg* 98:659-673, 1989.

15. Taniguchi K, Nakano S, Matsuda H, et al: Long-term survival and complications after composite graft replacement for ascending aortic aneurysm associated with aortic regurgitation. *Circulation* 84:III31-III39, 1991.

16. Donaldson RM, Ross DN: Composite graft replacement for the treatment of aneurysms of the ascending aorta associated with aortic valvular disease. *Circulation* 66:I116-I121, 1982.

17. Marvasti MA, Parker FB Jr, Randall PA, Witwer GA: Composite graft replacement of the ascending aorta and aortic valve. Late follow-up with intra-arterial digital subtraction angiography. *J Thorac Cardiovasc Surg* 95:924-928, 1988.

18. Barbetseas J, Crawford ES, Safi HJ, et al: Doppler echocardiographic evaluation of pseudoaneurysms complicating composite grafts of the ascending aorta. *Circulation* 85:212-222, 1992.

19. Carrel T, Pasic M, Jenni R, et al: Reoperations after operation on the thoracic aorta: Etiology, surgical techniques, and prevention. *Ann Thorac Surg* 56:259-268, 1993.

20. Dossche KM, Schepens MA, Morshuis WJ, et al: A 23-year experience with composite valve graft replacement of the aortic root. *Ann Thorac Surg* 67:1070-1077, 1999.

21. Luciani GB, Casali G, Barozzi L, Mazzucco A: Aortic root replacement with the Carboseal composite graft: 7-year experience with the first 100 implants. *Ann Thorac Surg* 68:2258-2262, 1999.

22. Cabrol C, Pavie A, Mesnildrey P, et al: Long-term results with total replacement of the ascending aorta and reimplantation of the coronary arteries. *J Thorac Cardiovasc Surg* 91:17-25, 1986.

23. Panos A, Amahzoune B, Robin J, et al: Influence of technique of coronary artery implantation on long-term results in composite aortic root replacement. *Ann Thorac Surg* 72:1497-1501, 2001.

24. Svensson LG, Crawford ES, Hess KR, et al: Composite valve graft replacement of the proximal aorta: Comparison of techniques in 348 patients. *Ann Thorac Surg* 54:427-437, 1992.

25. Wendel CH, Cornman CR, Dianzumba SB: Diagnosis of pseudoaneurysm of the ascending aorta by pulsed Doppler cross sectional echocardiography. *Br Heart J* 53:567-570, 1985.

26. Rice MJ, McDonald RW, Reller MD: Diagnosis of coronary artery dehiscence and pseudoaneurysm formation in postoperative Marfan patient by color flow Doppler echocardiography. *J Clin Ultrasound* 17:359-365, 1989.

27. Hoadley SD, Hartshorne MF: Noninvasive diagnosis of pseudoaneurysm of the ascending aorta. *J Clin Ultrasound* 15:325-332, 1987.

28. Shioi K, Nagata Y, Tsuchioka H: Usefulness of echocardiography in the long-term follow-up study after surgical treatment of annuloaortic ectasia. *Jpn J Surg* 18:636-640, 1988.

29. Rosenzweig BP, Donahue T, Attubato M, et al: Left ventricle-to-ascending aorta communication complicating composite graft repair undetected by aortography: Diagnosis by transesophageal echocardiography. *J Am Soc Echocardiogr* 4:639-644, 1991.

30. Lasorda DM, Power TP, Dianzumba SB, Incorvati RL: Diagnosis of aortic pseudoaneurysm by echocardiography. *Clin Cardiol* 15:773-776, 1992.

31. Mautner SL, Mautner GC, Curry CL, Roberts WC: Massive perigraft aortic aneurysm late after composite graft replacement of the ascending aorta and aortic valve in the Marfan syndrome. *Am J Cardiol* 71:624-627, 1993.

32. Sakai K, Nakamura K, Ishizuka N, et al: Echocardiographic findings and clinical features of left ventricular pseudoaneurysm after mitral valve replacement. *Am J Cardiol* 124:975-982, 1992.

33. Zoghbi WA, Enriquez-Sarano M, Foster E, et al: Recommendations for evaluation of the severity of native valvular regurgitation with two-dimensional and Doppler echocardiography. *J Am Soc Echocardiogr* 16:777-802, 2003.

34. Morocutti G, Di CA, Fontanelli A, et al: [The usefulness of transesophageal echocardiography in the follow-up of patients operated on for replacement of the ascending aorta with a tubular-valvular prosthesis (Cabrol's intervention)]. *G Ital Cardiol* 25:183-192, 1995.

35. Davis G, Millner R, Roberts D: Transesophageal echocardiographic detection of complications after Cabrol's procedure. *J Am Soc Echocardiogr* 10:375-376, 1997.

36. Van Camp G, De MJ, Daenen W, et al: Pulmonary stenosis caused by extrinsic compression of an aortic pseudoaneurysm of a composite aortic graft. *J Am Soc Echocardiogr* 12:997-1000, 1999.

37. Ishizuka N, Sakai K, Nakagawa M, et al: [Clinical significance of transesophageal echocardiography for evaluation of patients after Bentall's operation: detection of graft failure]. *J Cardiol* 25:139-146, 1995.

38. Pucillo AL, Schechter AG, Moggio RA, et al: Postoperative evaluation of ascending aortic prosthetic conduits by magnetic resonance imaging. *Chest* 97:106-110, 1990.

39. Nath PH, Zollikofer C, Castaneda-Zuniga WR, et al: Radiological evaluation of composite aortic grafts. *Radiology* 131:43-51, 1979.

40. Gula G, Pomerance A, Bennet M, Yacoub MH: Homograft replacement of aortic valve and ascending aorta in a patient with non-specific giant cell aortitis. *Br Heart J* 39:581-585, 1977.

41. Belcher P, Ross D: Aortic root replacement—20 years experience of the use of homografts. *Thorac Cardiovasc Surg* 39:117-122, 1991.

42. Ross DN, McKay R: Aortic root replacement. In Stark J, Pacifico AD (ed): *Reoperations in cardiac surgery*, New York: Springer-Verlag, 1989, pp. 259-270.

43. Kouchoukos NT: Aortic allografts and pulmonary autografts for replacement of the aortic valve and aortic root. *Ann Thorac Surg* 67:1846-1848, 1999.

44. Koh TW, Ferdinand FD, Jin XY, et al: Coronary artery problems during homograft aortic valve replacement: role of transesophageal echocardiography. *Ann Thorac Surg* 64:533-535, 1997.

45. Nagueh SF, Bozkurt B, Li GA, et al: Progressive dehiscence and dynamic compression of an aortic root homograft: detection and characterization by transesophageal echocardiography. *Am Heart J* 132:1070-1073, 1996.

46. Willems TP, van Herwerden LA, Taams MA, et al: Aortic allograft implantation techniques: pathomorphology and regurgitant jet patterns by Doppler echocardiographic studies. *Ann Thorac Surg* 66:412-416, 1998.

47. Borst HG, Walterbusch G, Schaps D: Extensive aortic replacement using "elephant trunk" prosthesis. *Thorac Cardiovasc Surg* 31:37-40, 1983.

48. Griepp RB, Stinson EB, Hollingsworth JF, Buehler D: Prosthetic replacement of the aortic arch. *J Thorac Cardiovasc Surg* 70:1051-1063, 1975.

49. Coselli JS, Buket S, Djukanovic B: Aortic arch operation: current treatment and results. *Ann Thorac Surg* 59:19-26, 1995.

50. Crawford ES, Crawford JL, Safi HJ, Coselli JS: Redo operations for recurrent aneurysmal disease of the ascending aorta and transverse aortic arch. *Ann Thorac Surg* 40:439-455, 1985.

51. Crawford ES, Crawford JL, Safi HJ: Reoperations for thoracic and thoracoabdominal aneurysms. In Stark J, Pacifico AD (ed): *Reoperations in cardiac surgery*, New York, Springer-Verlag, 1989, pp. 361-381.

52. Lawrie GM, Earle N, DeBakey ME: Long-term fate of the aortic root and aortic valve after ascending aneurysm surgery. *Ann Surg* 217:711-720, 1993.

53. Roberts WC, Morrow AG: Causes of early postoperative death following cardiac valve replacement. Clinico-pathologic correla-

tions in 64 patients studied at necropsy. *J Thorac Cardiovasc Surg* 54:422-437, 1967.

54. Bjork VO, Henze A, Rodriguez L: Left ventricular rupture as a complication of mitral valve replacement. *J Thorac Cardiovasc Surg* 73:14-22, 1977.

55. Karlson KJ, Ashraf MM, Berger RL: Rupture of left ventricle following mitral valve replacement. *Ann Thorac Surg* 46:590-597, 1988.

56. Yoshida K, Ohshima H, Murakami F, et al. Left ventricular free wall rupture following mitral valve replacement. *Ann Thorac Cardiovasc Surg* 4:336-339, 1998.

57. Cheng LC, Chiu CS, Lee JW: Left ventricular rupture after mitral valve replacement. *J Cardiovasc Surg (Torino)* 40:339-342, 1999.

58. Sobczyk WL, Jones JW, McManus BM: Clinically occult "false-on-true" left ventricular aneurysm: Association with late sudden death following mitral valve replacement. *Am Heart J* 112:1090-1092, 1986.

59. Azariades M, Lennox SC: Rupture of the posterior wall of the left ventricle after mitral valve replacement: Etiological and technical considerations. *Ann Thorac Surg* 46:491-494, 1988.

60. Baker WB, Klein MS, Reardon MJ, et al: Reversible cardiac dysfunction (hibernation) from ischemia due to compression of the coronary arteries by a pseudoaneurysm. *N Engl J Med* 1991, 325:1858-1861, 1991.

61. Catherwood E, Mintz GS, Kotler MN, et al: Two-dimensional echocardiographic recognition of left ventricular pseudoaneurysm. *Circulation* 62:294-303, 1980.

62. Roelandt JR, Sutherland GR, Yoshida K, Yoshikawa J: Improved diagnosis and characterization of left ventricular pseudoaneurysm by Doppler color flow imaging. *J Am Coll Cardiol* 12:807-811, 1988.

63. Kupari M, Verkkala K, Maamies T, Hartel G: Value of combined cross sectional and Doppler echocardiography in the detection of left ventricular pseudoaneurysm after mitral valve replacement. *Br Heart J* 58:52-56, 1987.

64. Olalla JJ, Vazquez de Prada JA, et al: Color Doppler diagnosis of left ventricular pseudoaneurysm. *Chest* 94:443-444, 1988.

65. Alam M, Rosman HS, Lewis JW, Brymer JF: Color Doppler features of left ventricular pseudoaneurysm. *Chest* 95:231-232, 1989.

66. Baker WB, Klein MS, Reardon MJ, Zoghbi WA: Left ventricular pseudoaneurysm complicating mitral valve replacement: Transesophageal echocardiographic diagnosis and impact on management. *J Am Soc Echocardiogr* 6:548-552, 1993.

67. Mulvagh SL, DeMaria AN, Feinstein SB, et al. Contrast echocardiography: current and future applications. *J Am Soc Echocardiogr* 13:331-342, 2000.

68. Alam M, Glick C, Garcia R, Lewis JW Jr: Transesophageal echocardiographic features of left ventricular pseudoaneurysm resulting after mitral valve replacement surgery. *Am Heart J* 123:226-228, 1992.

69. Esakof DD, Vannan MA, Pandian NG, et al: Visualization of left ventricular pseudoaneurysm with panoramic transesophageal echocardiography. *J Am Soc Echocardiogr* 7:174-178, 1994.

70. Sakai K, Nakamura K, Ishizuka N, et al: Echocardiographic findings and clinical features of left ventricular pseudoaneurysm after mitral valve replacement. *Am Heart J* 124:975-982, 1992.

71. Ono M, Wolf RK: Left ventricular pseudoaneurysm late after mitral valve replacement. *Ann Thorac Surg* 73:1303-1305, 2002.

72. Lukacs L, Kassai I, Lengyel M: Dissection of the atrial wall after mitral valve replacement. *Tex Heart Inst J* 23:62-64, 1996.

73. Ballal R, Nanda NC, Sanyal R: Intraoperative transesophageal echocardiographic diagnosis of left atrial pseudoaneurysm. *Am Heart J* 123:217-218, 1992.

74. Barretta G, Bui F, Bidi G, et al: Transesophageal echocardiogram diagnosis of postoperative left atrial pseudoaneurysm with spontaneous healing. *Echocardiography* 14:61-64, 1997.

75. Genoni M, Jenni R, Schmid ER, et al: Treatment of left atrial dissection after mitral repair: internal drainage. *Ann Thorac Surg* 68:1394-1396, 1999.

76. Idir M, Deville C, Roudaut R: Delayed left atrial wall dissection after mitral valve replacement. *Echocardiography* 17:259-261, 2000.

77. Gallego P, Oliver JM, Gonzalez A, et al: Left atrial dissection: pathogenesis, clinical course, and transesophageal echocardiographic recognition. *J Am Soc Echocardiogr* 14:813-820, 2001.

78. Heidt MC, Menon AK, Roth P, et al: Left atrial dissection after mitral operation mimicking severe mitral regurgitation. *J Thorac Cardiovasc Surg* 127:596-597, 2004.

79. Eliot RS, Levy MJ, Lillehei CW, Edwards JE: False aneurysm of the ascending aorta following needle puncture and cross-clamping. *J Thorac Cardiovasc Surg* 47:248-253, 1964.

80. Baba N, McKissick TL: Mycotic false aneurysm of the aorta following aortic valvular prosthesis; A case report. *Circulation* 31:575-578, 1965.

81. Aoyagi S, Akashi H, Kawara T, et al: False aneurysm of the ascending aorta with fistula to the right atrium. Noninvasive diagnosis by computed tomographic scan and two-dimensional echocardiography with successful repair. *Thorac Cardiovasc Surg* 42:58-60, 1994.

82. Roy D, Saba S, Grinberg I, et al: Aorto-right ventricular fistula: a late complication of aortic valve replacement. *Tex Heart Inst J* 26:140-142, 1999.

83. Allwork SP: The anatomical basis of infection of the aortic root. *Thorac Cardiovasc Surg* 34:143-148, 1986.

84. Chesler E, Korns ME, Porter GE, et al: False aneurysm of the left ventricle secondary to bacterial endocarditis with perforation of the mitral-aortic intervalvular fibrosa. *Circulation* 37:518-523, 1968.

85. Edwards JE, Burchell HB: The pathological anatomy of deficiencies between the aortic root and the heart, including aortic sinus aneurysms. *Thorax* 12:125-139, 1957.

86. Layman TE, January LE: Mycotic left ventricular aneurysm involving the fibrous atrioventricular body. *Am J Cardiol* 20:423-427, 1967.

87. Qizilbash AH, Schwartz CJ: False aneurysm of left ventricle due to perforation of mitral-aortic intervalvular fibrosa with rupture and cardiac tamponade. Rare complication of infective endocarditis. *Am J Cardiol* 32:110-113, 1973.

88. Afridi I, Apostolidou MA, Saad RM, Zoghbi WA: Pseudoaneurysms of the mitral-aortic intervalvular fibrosa: Dynamic characterization using transesophageal echocardiographic and Doppler techniques. *J Am Coll Cardiol* 25:137-145, 1995.

89. Taliercio CP, Oh JK, Summerer MH, et al: Traumatic left ventricular false aneurysm with significant regurgitation from left ventricular outflow tract to left atrium: Delineation by two-dimensional and color flow Doppler echocardiography. *J Am Soc Echocardiogr* 1:354-358, 1988.

90. Chesler E, Joffe N, Schamroth L, Meyers A: Annular subvalvular left ventricular aneurysms in the South African Bantu. *Circulation* 32:43-51, 1965.

91. Russo G, Tamburino C, Greco G, et al: Echocardiographic detection of aortic valve ring abscesses. *J Ultrasound Med* 9:319-323, 1990.

92. Saner HE, Asinger RW, Homans DC, et al: Two-dimensional echocardiographic identification of complicated aortic root endocarditis: Implications for surgery. *J Am Coll Cardiol* 10:859-868, 1987.

93. Daniel WG, Mugge A, Martin RP, et al: Improvement in the diagnosis of abscesses associated with endocarditis by transesophageal echocardiography. *N Engl J Med* 324:795-800, 1991.

94. Bansal RC, Graham BM, Jutzy KR, et al: Left ventricular outflow tract to left atrial communication secondary to rupture of mitral-aortic intervalvular fibrosa in infective endocarditis: Diagnosis by transesophageal echocardiography and color flow imaging. *J Am Coll Cardiol* 15:499-504, 1990.

95. Miller SW, Dinsmore RE: Aortic root abscess resulting from endocarditis: spectrum of angiographic findings. *Radiology* 153:357-361, 1984.

96. Waldhausen JA, Petry EL, Kurlander GJ: Successful repair of subvalvular annular aneurysm of the left ventricle. *N Engl J Med* 275:984-987, 1966.

97. Reid CL, McKay C, Kawanishi DT, et al: False aneurysm of mitral-aortic intervalvular fibrosa: Diagnosis by 2-dimensional contrast echocardiography at cardiac catheterization. *Am J Cardiol* 51:1801-1802, 1983.

98. Miller DC, Schapira JN, Stinson EB, Shumway NE: Left ventricular-coronary sinus fistula following repeated mitral valve replacements. *J Thorac Cardiovasc Surg* 76:43-45, 1978.

99. Rogers AG, Rossi NP: Left ventricular-coronary sinus fistula after mitral valve replacement. *J Thorac Cardiovasc Surg* 94:637-638, 1987.

100. Yee GW, Naasz C, Hatle L, et al: Doppler diagnosis of left ventricle to coronary sinus fistula: an unusual complication of mitral valve replacement. *J Am Soc Echocardiogr* 1:458-462, 1988.

101. Watanabe A, Kazui T, Tsukamoto M, Komatsu S: Left ventricular pseudoaneurysm and intracardiac fistulas after replacement of mitral valve prosthesis. *Ann Thorac Surg* 55:1236-1239, 1993.

102. Ramasubbu K, Coselli J, Zoghbi WA: Unusual complication of aortic root reconstruction with sparing of the aortic valve: Left ventricular outflow tract to right atrial fistula. *J Am Soc Echocardiogr* 19:469, 2006.

103. Lowry RW, Young JB, Kleiman NS, Zoghbi WA: Transesophageal echocardiographic demonstration of right coronary artery-to-coronary sinus fistula in a heart transplant recipient. *J Am Soc Echocardiogr* 6:449-452, 1993.

104. Ross DN: Replacement of aortic and mitral valves with a pulmonary autograft. *Lancet* 2:956-958, 1967.

105. Ross D: Pulmonary valve autotransplantation (the Ross operation). *J Card Surg* 3:313-319, 1988.

106. Gerosa G, McKay R, Davies J, Ross DN: Comparison of the aortic homograft and the pulmonary autograft for aortic valve or root replacement in children. *J Thorac Cardiovasc Surg* 102:51-60, 1991.

107. Sievers HH, Leyh R, Loose R, et al: Time course of dimension and function of the autologous pulmonary root in the aortic position. *J Thorac Cardiovasc Surg* 105:775-780, 1993.

108. Kouchoukos NT, vila-Roman VG, Spray TL, et al: Replacement of the aortic root with a pulmonary autograft in children and young adults with aortic-valve disease. *N Engl J Med* 330:1-6, 1994.

109. Santini F, Dyke C, Edwards S, et al: Pulmonary autograft versus homograft replacement of the aortic valve: A prospective randomized trial. *J Thorac Cardiovasc Surg* 113:894-899, 1997.

110. Oury JH, Hiro SP, Maxwell JM, et al: The Ross Procedure: current registry results. *Ann Thorac Surg* 66:S162-S165, 1998.

111. Niwaya K, Knott-Craig CJ, Santangelo K, et al: Advantage of autograft and homograft valve replacement for complex aortic valve endocarditis. *Ann Thorac Surg* 67:1603-1608, 1999.

112. Dossche KM, de la Riviere AB, Morshuis WJ, et al: Aortic root replacement with the pulmonary autograft: An invariably competent aortic valve? *Ann Thorac Surg* 68:1302-1307, 1999.

113. Knott-Craig CJ, Elkins RC, Santangelo KL, et al: Aortic valve replacement: comparison of late survival between autografts and homografts. *Ann Thorac Surg* 69:1327-1332, 2000.

114. Savoye C, Auffray JL, Hubert E, et al: Echocardiographic follow-up after Ross procedure in 100 patients. *Am J Cardiol* 85:854-857, 2000.

115. Hokken RB, Bogers AJ, Taams MA, et al: Does the pulmonary autograft in the aortic position in adults increase in diameter? An echocardiographic study. *J Thorac Cardiovasc Surg* 113:667-674, 1997.

116. Kouchoukos NT, Masetti P, Nickerson NJ, et al: The Ross procedure: long-term clinical and echocardiographic follow-up. *Ann Thorac Surg* 78:773-781, 2004.

117. Luciani GB, Favaro A, Casali G, et al: Ross operation in the young: a ten-year experience. *Ann Thorac Surg* 80:2271-2277, 2005.

118. Schmidtke C, Bechtel M, Hueppe M, Sievers HH: Time course of aortic valve function and root dimensions after subcoronary ross procedure for bicuspid versus tricuspid aortic valve disease. *Circulation* 104:I21-I24, 2001.

119. Shahid MS, Al-Halees Z, Khan SM, Pieters FA: Aneurysms complicating pulmonary autograft procedure for aortic valve replacement. *Ann Thorac Surg* 68:1842-1843, 1999.

120. Takkenberg JJ, Zondervan PE, van Herwerden LA: Progressive pulmonary autograft root dilatation and failure after Ross procedure. *Ann Thorac Surg* 67:551-553, 1999.

121. Clarke GB, Salley RK, Sapin PM, et al: Echocardiographic assessment of valvular function in patients undergoing replacement of the aortic valve with a pulmonary autograft. *J Am Soc Echocardiogr* 8:353, 1995.

122. Pacifico AD, Kirklin JK, McGiffin DC, Matter GJ, et al: The Ross operation—early echocardiographic comparison of different operative techniques. *J Heart Valve Dis* 3:365-370, 1994.

123. Joyce F, Tingleff J, Aagaard J, Pettersson G: The Ross operation in the treatment of native and prosthetic aortic valve endocarditis. *J Heart Valve Dis* 3:371-376, 1994.

Part Five

Cardiomyopathies and Pericardial Disease

Chapter 27

Doppler Echocardiography in Heart Failure and Cardiac Resynchronization

MARTIN ST. JOHN SUTTON, MD

Basic Principles

Definition of Heart Failure

Heart failure (HF) is a clinical syndrome characterized by fatigue, shortness of breath, exercise intolerance, and fluid retention with lower extremity and/or pulmonary edema. HF may be primarily the result of either abnormal myocardial excitation-contraction coupling (systolic failure) or to abnormal relaxation and increased myocardial passive stiffness (diastolic failure). The symptomatic presentations of systolic and diastolic heart failure (DHF) are indistinguishable clinically, but the two etiologies can be differentiated with Doppler echocardiography by differences in left ventricular (LV) architecture and function. Distinction between systolic and DHF is important because their respective treatments and prognoses are widely different. Historically DHF has been regarded as a more benign form of HF than systolic HF. However, the annual mortality from DHF is between 5% and 15%, and the readmission rate for new onset DHF approaches 50% within the first 6 months.[1-4]

A proportion of patients with systolic HF have markedly abnormal diastolic myocardial function, and patients with primary DHF may subsequently develop systolic dysfunction. Thus, there is no absolute separation between systolic and DHF because of the degree of overlap that exists and the frequent transition from initially diastolic to systolic HF manifest in patients with ischemic heart disease.

Systolic HF may be defined, in the simplest terms, as the inability of the heart to supply the metabolic requirements of the body tissues. In systolic HF, myocardial shortening is impaired, and results in a shift of the length-tension relationship to the right of the normal pressure-volume relationship (Fig. 27–1). Similar abnormal relationships between LV pressure and LV cavity area have been demonstrated by simultaneous echocardiography and micromanometer tipped catheter recordings of LV pressure.[5]

DHF may be defined in general terms as the inability of the heart to receive blood from the body tissues at normal filling pressures.[4] In DHF, the myocardial passive/resting length-tension relationship is displaced upward and leftward of the normal relationship (see Fig. 27–1), so that significant increases in LV diastolic pressure may occur with little or no detectable change in volume.[6] Thus myocardial relaxation is delayed or incomplete at the time of minimum LV diastolic pressure[6] as a result of impaired or delayed cytosolic calcium sequestration by the sarcoplasmic reticulum resulting in increased passive myocardial stiffness. Both

the active (systolic) and the passive (diastolic) mechanisms of HF are initially reversible. However, if the abnormal length-tension or pressure-volume relationships become chronic and persist unaltered over the long term, adverse changes in LV architecture and function become irreversible.

The abnormal pressure-volume relations in systolic HF result in LV dilatation that induces a stretch-activated increase in collagen synthesis and myocardial collagen content that alters the material properties of the extracellular matrix. The enhanced extracellular collagen matrix increases myocardial stiffness that serves as a counterbalance to the distending forces and attenuates the progressive deterioration in ventricular function and development of HF. This pattern of remodeling is known as "eccentric remodeling" and typifies systolic HF. A chronically abnormal resting end-systolic pressure-volume relationship is also associated with a hypertrophic response in which normal LV cavity size or volume are maintained, wall thickness is increased, and ejection performance preserved. This latter form of "concentric remodeling" results in increased diastolic stiffness and incomplete or slowed relaxation that is characteristic of DHF. The time-dependent changes in LV architecture and function resulting in systolic and/or DHF in individual patients or cohorts of patients can be quantified by Doppler echocardiography (Fig. 27–2).

The purpose of this chapter is to demonstrate how Doppler echocardiography can be used to confirm the clinical diagnosis of HF, determine the etiology of HF, and distinguish systolic from DHF. Another equally important purpose of this chapter is to show how Doppler echocardiography can be used to assess the efficacy of new treatments for HF and guide the selection of pharmacologic and/or devices for optimal therapy.

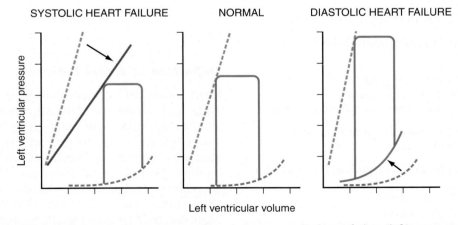

Figure 27–1. Left ventricular pressure-volume loops in systolic heart failure (left), a normal control (center), and diastolic heart failure (right). In systolic heart failure, there is a decrease in the slope of the end-systolic pressure-volume relationship (decreased left ventricular contractility), whereas in diastolic heart failure the pressure-volume loop is shifted up and to the left (increased stiffness). (From Aurigemma GP, Zile MR, Gaasch WH: Circulation 113:296-304, 2006.)

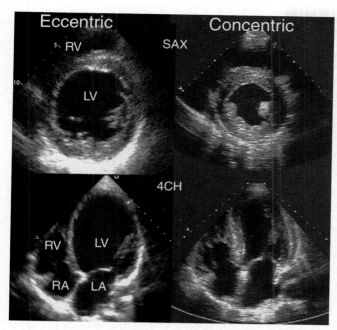

Figure 27–2. *Short-axis* (top left) *and apical four-chamber view* (bottom left) *of a patient with "eccentric" hypertrophy. This is the result of a primary volume overload with a compensatory increase in wall thickness that fails to match the increase in cavity radius. On the right, short-axis* (top) *and apical four-chamber view* (bottom) *of a patient with "concentric" hypertrophy. This is the result of a primary pressure overload with an increase in wall thickness without significant change in cavity radius. LA, left atrium; LV, left ventricle; RA, right atrium; RV, right ventricle; SAX, short-axis view; 4CH, four-chamber view.*

Prevalence of Heart Failure: The Size of the Problem

There are approximately 22 million people with chronic HF worldwide. Five million HF patients reside in the United States where there are between five and six hundred thousand new cases diagnosed each year.[7] A large proportion of the new HF patients each year are diagnosed by noninvasive imaging with Doppler echo-

cardiography. Systolic HF is approximately twice as prevalent as DHF and portends a much worse prognosis.[8] HF is also the most commonly documented hospital discharge diagnosis in patients older than 65 years. As the population lives longer, the expectation is that HF will become even more prevalent.

Currently between 6% and 10% of subjects older than 65 years have HF, and the prevalence of HF increases with advancing age. By the year 2038, the predicted population of persons older than 75 years of age in the United States will exceed 50 million.[9] The costs of the diagnostic related group (DRG) for HF in the United States alone have already exceeded $28 billion per year. These striking population statistics not surprisingly have resulted in HF becoming a high priority health care policy initiative.

Etiology of Heart Failure

There are many different etiologies of left and right HF and their individual prevalence varies geographically. In West Africa, restrictive cardiomyopathy is the predominant etiology of HF. In Central and South America, HF is most frequently associated with chronic infection by Trypanosoma cruzi. By contrast, in Europe, the United States, and Canada, atherosclerotic coronary artery disease (CAD) and myocardial infarction (MI), resulting in acute loss of contracting myocytes, are by far the most common etiology, accounting for more than two thirds of all cases of chronic HF.[10] These three widely different etiologies of HF have their own individual structural and functional stigmata that can be easily recognized by Doppler echocardiography (Fig. 27–3). Other major causes of HF can also be diagnosed echocardiographically and include chronic pressure overload from systemic hypertension; pressure or volume overload from valvular heart disease; and primary dilated cardiomyopathy (DCM), hypertrophic cardiomyopathy (HCM), and restrictive cardiomyopathies resulting from genetically determined structural abnor-

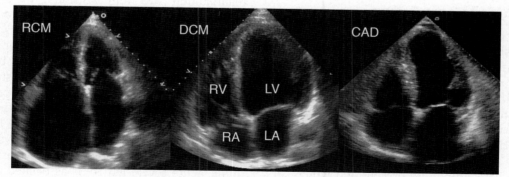

Figure 27–3. *Apical four-chamber view of a patient with restrictive cardiomyopathy* (left) *showing a small left ventricle and a biatrial dilatation; apical four-chamber view of a dilated cardiomyopathy* (center) *with a dilated left ventricle; and an apical four-chamber view of a patient with coronary artery disease* (right) *showing apical dilatation. CAD, coronary artery disease; DCM, dilated cardiomyopathy; LA, left atrium; LV, left ventricle; RA, right atrium; RCM, restrictive cardiomyopathy; RV, right ventricle.*

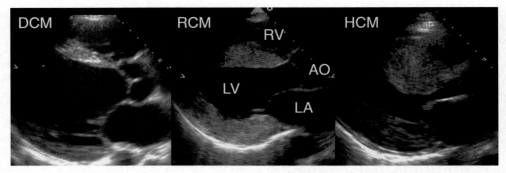

Figure 27–4. *Parasternal long axis of a patient with dilated cardiomyopathy demonstrates an increase in the internal diameter of the left ventricle with normal wall thickness* (left); *parasternal long axis of a patient with amyloid restrictive cardiomyopathy* (center) *(the walls are thick and highly echo reflective, and the left ventricular diameter is normal); and parasternal long axis of a hypertrophic cardiomyopathy with asymmetrical septal hypertrophy* (right) *(the upper interventricular septum measures 4 cm) and a small left ventricle. AO, aorta; DCM, dilated cardiomyopathy; HCM, hypertrophic cardiomyopathy; LA, left atrium; LV, left ventricle; RCM, restrictive cardiomyopathy; RV, right ventricle.*

malities of the sarcomeric contractile proteins or infiltrative diseases involving the extracellular matrix. In addition, an infrequent cause of HF cardiac toxins, such as chronic excessive ingestion of alcohol or chemotherapeutic agents, such as cytoxan and doxorubicin, in high dosage for treatment of primary malignant solid and liquid tumors. Some of these conditions express consistent phenotypes that are pathognomic and easily diagnosed with Doppler echocardiography, for example the typical findings of restrictive cardiomyopathic features of cardiac amyloid, HCM, and DCM (Fig. 27–4). However, it is not well understood which factors trigger one patient with hypertension to develop systolic HF and another with equally matched LV loading conditions to develop DHF.

Doppler Echocardiographic Diagnosis

Acute Left-Sided Heart Failure

The diagnosis of HF is made based on the clinical history and physical examination. Although the history and examination may provide insight into the etiology and duration of HF, identification of the diagnostic structural and functional abnormalities requires early noninvasive imaging of the heart and great vessels. The single most useful diagnostic test in the evaluation of patients with HF is Doppler echocardiography to determine whether abnormalities of the myocardium, heart valves, or the pericardium are present and which cardiac chambers are involved.[11] In patients with new-onset HF, the American College of Cardiology/American Heart Association (ACC/AHA) practice guidelines recommend an initial Doppler echocardiographic algo-

rithm to address three issues. The first issue is to establish whether the LV ejection fraction (EF) is normal or decreased. The second issue is to determine whether LV structure is normal or abnormal, that is whether the LV is dilated, hypertrophied, or of normal size. The third issue is to assess whether other structural abnormalities, such as valvular heart disease, pericardial disease, right ventricular (RV) abnormalities, or chronic pulmonary disease, could account for the clinical presentation of HF.

Common causes of acute onset of LV systolic HF include (1) acute myocardial infarction (AMI), (2) postinfarction complications, (i.e., rupture of a papillary muscle causing acute severe mitral regurgitation [MR] or rupture of the interventricular septum causing a large left to right shunt), (3) sudden onset of severe MR from degenerative myxomatous mitral valve disease with prolapse resulting from chordal rupture and a flail mitral leaflet or acute severe MR from valve rupture as a result of endocarditis (4) acute severe aortic regurgitation (AR) from avulsion of the aortic valve as a result of endocarditis, (5) acute severe AR resulting from type A aortic dissection; (6) acute myocarditis, (7) exposure to oncologic cardiotoxic chemotherapeutic agents (doxorubicin or cytoxan before bone marrow transplantation), or (8) sudden acute destabilization of previously unrecognized chronic severe end-stage DCM. All of these conditions except for the latter, present with either sudden massive increase in LV loading conditions, acute loss of contracting myocytes, or severe injury to a full complement of working myocardium. Acute severe left HF is associated with inability to modulate stroke volume (SV) beat to beat, so that the only means of augmenting cardiac output (CO) is by increasing heart rate (HR). Doppler echocardiography cannot only distinguish between these different etiologies of acute HF but can also often be used to direct optimal management.

Acute myocardial infarction is usually diagnosed by history and confirmed by electrocardiogram (ECG) changes and elevated cardiac enzymes. Echocardiography early after myocardial contraction infarction demonstrates normal LV size with decreased function and a variable sized regional wall motion abnormality resulting from subjacent noncontracting myocytes and preserved wall thickness, before infarct expansion is completed. Sudden exacerbation of HF in the early peri-infarction period as a result of the rupture of the interventricular septum can be detected and differentiated from acute severe MR resulting from papillary muscle dysfunction or rupture, which cannot reliably be differentiated clinically. These structural changes can be localized by color flow Doppler, their severity quantified as mitral regurgitant volume, the ratio of pulmonary blood flow and systemic blood flow (Qp/Qs), and the magnitude of shunt flow through the ventricular septal defect (VSD).

The remaining causes of acute HF are usually readily recognized by Doppler transthoracic echocardiography (TTE) but may require transesophageal echocardiography (TEE) to diagnose endovascular infections causing perforation or avulsion of the native mitral or aortic valves. TTE and often TEE are required to document the presence of acute severe MR associated with degenerative mitral valve disease resulting from rupture of redundant chordae causing flail leaflets that fail to coapt. The thickened yet excessively mobile prolapsing myxomatous leaflets of degenerative mitral valve disease are easy to recognize especially when redundant, ruptured minor chordae are present. Acute left HF resulting from the use of high doses of oncologic agents results in severe global dysfunction, which has a temporal cause-and-effect relationship to drug administration. In acute HF resulting from doxorubicin, TTE shows that LV end-diastolic size is normal, whereas the end-systolic size is increased so that resting sinus tachycardia is a prerequisite for maintaining resting cardiac output.

Chronic Left-Sided Heart Failure

The common causes of chronic left HF in Europe and the United States include CAD and MI, hypertensive heart disease, valvular heart disease, and cardiomyopathies. These different patho-etiologies in their late stages progress down a final common pathway to left-sided systolic HF that is characterized by structural and functional changes, which are amenable to echocardiographic imaging. One finding that is almost universal in chronic systolic HF is the presence of LV dilatation, which can be quantified echocardiographically either as a cavity diameter at end-diastole and end-systole or

as end-diastolic and end-systolic volumes using the modified Simpson's rule. The importance of LV volumes is their predictive value for adverse clinical outcome. Two-dimensional (2D) TTE has shown that the progressive LV dilatation occurs by a disproportionately greater increase in LV short-axis diameter than in LV long-axis length as exemplified by idiopathic DCM (Fig. 27–5). This consistent pattern of differential increase in the LV short axis confers a mechanically disadvantageous shape that is more spherical than the normal prolate ellipse configuration. The change in LV cavity shape results in the maximum minor axis diameter moving from the base of the LV to almost midway from the base to the apex along the long axis of the LV cavity. This change in LV shape is readily discernible by imaging of the left ventricle in apical two-chamber and apical four-chamber views (Fig. 27–6). As the left ventricle remodels to a larger volume, contractile function deteriorates because the increase in LV volume is discrepantly faster than the increase in LV mass. In contrast, in normal subjects the end-diastolic mass to volume relationship is virtually constant in normotensive hearts from infancy through old age.

There are three important sequelae of abnormal LV size and shape. First, is the increase in loading conditions with the disproportionately greater increase in cavity volume than the increase in LV mass that is associ-

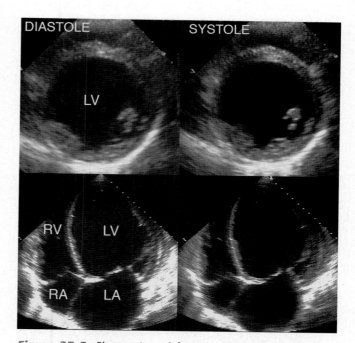

Figure 27–5. *Short-axis and four-chamber view of a dilated cardiomyopathy at end-diastole* (left) *and a short axis and four-chamber view of a dilated cardiomyopathy at end-systole* (right). *Note the greater increase of the minor axis in the short-axis views compared to the left ventricular long-axis diameter in the four-chamber views. LA, left atrium; LV, left ventricle; RA, right atrium; RV, right ventricle.*

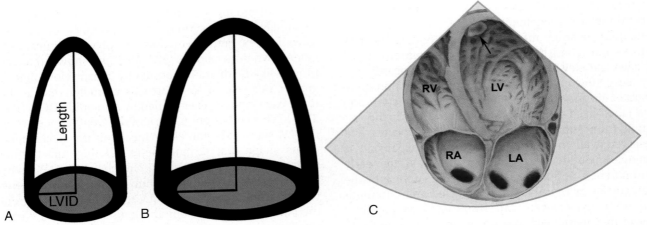

Figure 27–6. Schematic representation of a normal left ventricular shape (A), a spherical left ventricular shape as a result of a greater increase of the minor diameter than the left ventricular length (B), and the typical appearance of dilated cardiomyopathy in an apical four-chamber view (C). In addition to four-chamber enlargement with biventricular systolic dysfunction, there is increased sphericity of the left venticular and an apical thrombus (arrow). LA, left atrium; LV, left ventricle; LVID, left ventricular internal diameter; RA, right atrium; RV, right ventricle.

ated with progressive decrease in contractile function. Second, the LV dilatation combined with the decreased contractile function results in slow flow velocities within the LV especially toward the apex that predisposes to thrombus formation. Thrombus forms within the left-sided heart chambers especially in the apex of the LV cavity if there are subjacent wall motion abnormalities as in ischemic DCM. Thrombus may also occur in the left atrial appendage as a result of low flow velocities, of which is a potential source of systemic embolism (Fig. 27–7). Thrombus formation may be subtle and require echocardiographic imaging in orthogonal planes of the LV long-axis or serial short-axis views with a high frequency transducer. When doubt remains as to the presence of LV thrombus after these image acquisitions, echocardiographic contrast studies are recommended because the consequences of systemic thromboembolism are so devastating. The morphologic features of the LV thrombus that correlate with increased embolic potential include mobility, convex surface, and large size.

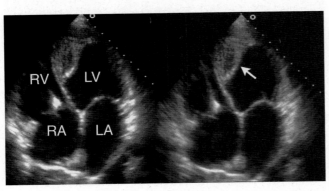

Figure 27–7. Transthoracic apical four-chamber view in diastole (left) and systole (right), showing a voluminous intraventricular sessile thrombus (arrow) is visualized along the apex and the septum in an area of akinesis. LA, left atrium; LV, left ventricle; RA, right atrium; RV, right ventricle.

The third important consequence of LV dilatation and change in LV shape in the genesis of systolic HF is enlargement of the mitral annulus and distortion of the mitral valve and subvalve geometry. The greater spatial separation of the two papillary muscles caused by LV dilatation increases the angle they subtend to the midpoint of the plane of the mitral annulus, which without any lengthening of the chordae, reduces the area of leaflet coaptation resulting in varying severity of MR even though the individual components of the mitral valve are normal (Fig. 27–8). The anatomic relationships between the various components of the mitral valve apparatus are best appreciated with real-time three-dimensional (3D) echocardiography in the short-axis and apical long-axis or four-chamber views (Fig. 27–9).

A different yet frequent cause of MR in patients with HF relates to the presence of provocable ischemia in patients with advanced CAD. Serial quantitative Doppler echocardiographic studies of ischemic MR demonstrate its important adverse impact on both short-term and long-term survival (Fig. 27–10). MR is significantly more common and more severe in the eccentric remodeling that occurs in systolic HF than in concentric remodeling in DHF, in which LV cavity size is usually normal.

The severity of MR can be semi-quantified by two-dimensional TTE as the ratio of color flow Doppler mapping of the mitral regurgitant jet area averaged from orthogonal views and indexed to left atrial area. MR severity can also be quantified as the effective regurgitant orifice area (EROA), regurgitant volume using proximal isovelocity area (PISA) technique, or from the diameter of the vena contracta (see Chapter 18). The significance of MR in systolic HF is that it results in an additional incremental increase in load when loading conditions are already increased.

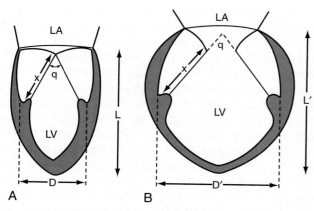

Figure 27–8. Schematic demonstrating the possible mechanism of mitral regurgitation. Left ventricular dilatation as a result of volume overload results in the left ventricle becoming more spherical (A and B). The mitral valve ring circumference increases. The angle subtended by the papillary muscles to the mitral annulus increases, but there is no elongation of the mitral valve leaflets or chordae, which results in incomplete cusp coaptation and mitral regurgitation. D and D´, cavity diameters; L and L´, cavity lengths; LA, left atrium; LV, left ventricle; x, chordal length. (From St. John Sutton M, Plappert T: In St. John Sutton M, Oldershaw P: Textbook of Echocardiography and Doppler in Adults and Children, 2nd ed. Cambridge, Mass, 1996.)

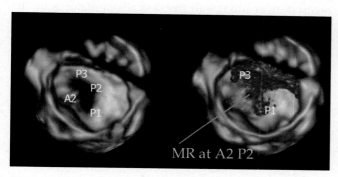

Figure 27–9. Mitral valve visualized by three-dimensional transesophageal echocardiography (right) and with color Doppler (left) showing mitral regurgitation. A2, middle anterior mitral valve scallop; P1, P2, and P3, posterior mitral valve scallops.

In ischemic cardiomyopathy, posteroinferior infarction involving the inferomedial papillary muscle may restrict the timing, extent, and velocity of shortening causing moderate to severe MR. The onset of hemodynamically important MR late in the development of systolic HF may so increase the load on the left ventricle as to escalate further deterioration in contractile function (Fig. 27–11). Ischemic MR causing flash pulmonary edema may not be apparent at rest but be triggered by transient increases in afterload associated with physical exertion in the presence of an intrinsically normal mitral valve. Ischemic MR has a grave prognosis that correlates closely with the quantitative assessment of MR by Doppler echocardiography in terms of regurgitant volume and effective regurgitant orifice area (Figs. 27–12 and 27–13).

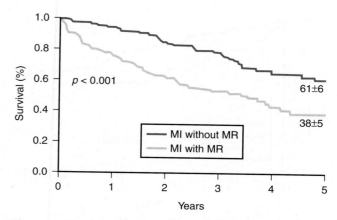

Figure 27–10. Survival (± SE) after diagnosis of myocardial infarction (MI) according to the presence of mitral regurgitation (MR). SE, standard error. (From Grigioni F, Enriquez-Sarano M, Zehr KJ, et al: Circulation 103:1759-1764, 2001.)

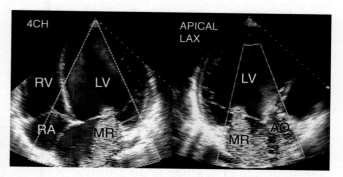

Figure 27–11. Transthoracic apical four-chamber view (left) and apical long-axis view (right) demonstrating MR by color Doppler. Regurgitant flow in the left atrium during systole is consistent with posteriorly directed severe mitral regurgitation. LAX, long-axis view; LV, left ventricle; MR, mitral regurgitation; RA, right atrium; RV, right ventricle; 4CH, four-chamber view.

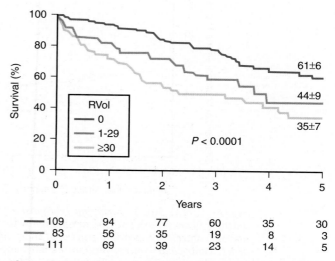

── 109	94	77	60	35	30
── 83	56	35	19	8	3
── 111	69	39	23	14	5

Figure 27–12. Survival after diagnosis according to degree of ischemic mitral regurgitation as graded by regurgitant volume (RVol) equal to 30 ml/beat or less than 30 mL/beat. (From Grigioni F, Enriquez-Sarano M, Zehr KJ, et al: Circulation 103:1759-1764, 2001.)

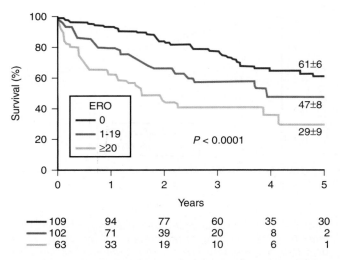

Figure 27–13. *Survival after diagnosis according to degree of ischemic mitral regurgitation graded by effective regurgitant orifice (ERO) area equal to 20 mm² or less than 20 mm². (From Grigioni F, Enriquez-Sarano M, Zehr KJ, et al:* Circulation *103:1759-1764, 2001.)*

Left Ventricular Remodeling in Heart Failure

LV remodeling is a dynamic process that includes progressive LV dilatation, distortion of LV shape, disruption of mitral valve geometry, development of MR, and deterioration in LV function to HF. This type of remodeling is known as eccentric remodeling. These structural and functional changes and the transition to HF have been characterized by Doppler echocardiography.

LV remodeling is triggered by an imbalance between myocardial wall stress and the normal restraining forces exerted by the viscoelastic collagen matrix. Increased wall stress activates cell surface mechanoreceptors (integrins) that in turn activate myocardial matrix metalloproteinases (MMPs) downstream in the mechanotransduction cascade. MMPs are a family of endoproteinases that degrade the extracellular collagen matrix thereby facilitating LV dilatation until a new equilibrium is established between collagen degradation and collagen synthesis that stabilizes LV size and function. Progressive LV dilatation leads to chronically elevated wall stress, which if unchecked leads to development of HF. Thus LV dilatation begets increased wall stress that begets further LV dilatation. LV dilatation results in an increase in loading conditions that can be assessed as meridional and circumferential wall stresses from echocardiographic measurements of LV cavity radius, length, wall thickness, and cuff systolic blood pressure (SBP) can be used to represent LV peak pressure. There is a strong inverse relationship between end-systolic wall stress and LV cavity emptying measured as EF, fractional shortening or velocity of circumferential shortening, such that the greater the load (wall stress) the lower the systolic performance. Increased myocardial wall stress is also a major stimulus for ventricular hypertrophy mediated by the angiotensin I receptor. When the hypertrophic response is insufficient to normalize wall stress, LV function and geometry deteriorate progressively (Fig. 27–14).

Insight into the structural and functional eccentric remodeling process and transition from stable LV function to systolic HF has been demonstrated by Doppler echocardiography in a number of post-MI and HF clinical trials.[12,13] Finite element analysis of regional LV

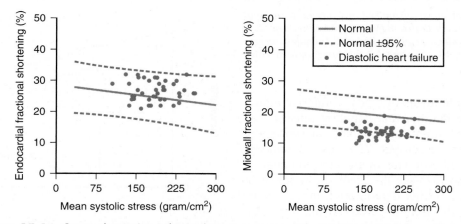

Figure 27–14. *Stress-shortening relationships in patients with diastolic heart failure. Data from diastolic heart failure patients are plotted with reference to the mean ±95% prediction interval for normal controls. Endocardial fractional shortening is plotted against mean systolic stress (an index of left ventricular contractility) in the* left *panel. All of the diastolic heart failure coordinates fall within the normal range. Midwall fractional shortening is plotted against mean systolic stress (an index of myocardial contractility) in the* right *panel. Two thirds of the diastolic heart failure coordinates fall within the normal range. (From Aurigemma GP, Zile MR, Gaasch WH:* Circulation *113:296-304, 2006.)*

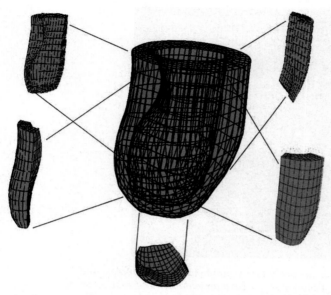

Figure 27-15. *Finite element mesh (2500-element) of patient with anterior myocardial infarction demonstrating the five subdivided regions of the left ventricle (apex, anterior wall, inferior wall, posterior wall, and septum) that make up finished model. Finite element mesh is generated by subdivision of the structure into eight-node "brick" elements. Each model is five elements thick; location of individual elements is similar anatomically for all elements. (From Solomon SD, Aikawa Y, Martini MS, et al: J Am Soc Echocardiogr 11:938-947, 1998.)*

wall stress in experimental animal studies post-MI has shown that in regions of increased wall stress, such as the infarct zone, MMP activity is greatly elevated compared to adjacent or remote myocardium facilitating collagen degradation and LV dilatation (Fig. 27–15). Similar relationships have been demonstrated in animals post-MI with sonomicrometry crystals between strain, regional systolic shortening and activation of MMPs, tissue inhibitors of metalloproteinases (TIMPs), and signaling factors that control the dynamic equilibrium between collagen synthesis and collagen degradation that determines the degree of ventricular remodeling versus the success of myocardial repair.[14,15] The combination of myocardial biochemistry and echocardiographic imaging with the ability to measure regional strain in animal models may elucidate some of the fundamental etiologic mechanisms of HF.

Systolic versus Diastolic Heart Failure

There is currently no consensus regarding criteria for the diagnosis of DHF except for the combination of clinical HF and an LV EF cut-off point equal to 50% to distinguish LV diastolic from systolic HF. There is controversy with regard to nomenclature—DHF versus HF

with normal EF (HFNEF). There is also concern as to whether Doppler indices provide sufficiently specific information about intrinsic passive diastolic properties of the myocardium and whether the information derived from LV filling dynamics equate with intrinsic myocardial diastolic dysfunction.[16] Other investigators have indicated that DHF can be confidently diagnosed by the combined presence of impaired relaxation, decreased compliance, and increased LV filling pressures.[17]

DHF has been less well characterized than systolic HF, but it has become clear over the last decade that LV diastolic dysfunction is responsible for from 30% to 50% of all patients with the clinical symptoms and signs of HF and has an annual mortality of 5% to 15%. Patients with DHF are similar to patients with systolic HF with regard to impaired quality of life, exercise capacity, demographic profiling, and neurohormonal activation. Neurohormonal activation in DHF is similar to systolic failure with regard to norepinephrine levels, but plasma levels of brain natriuretic peptide and atrial natriuretic peptides are consistently greater in systolic HF.[3]

Diastolic dysfunction often precedes the onset of systolic dysfunction in hypertensive heart disease and in CAD, which are the most common etiologies of clinical HF. Factors that determine which patients go on to develop DHF rather than systolic HF are largely unknown. Furthermore, DHF may transition into systolic failure in its terminal stages, confounding the arbitrary division of HF into systolic or diastolic etiologies.

DHF occurs more commonly in elderly women, more than 75% of whom have a history of hypertension and approximately 40% have left ventricular hypertrophy (LVH) defined as a LV mass greater than 125 g/m². The structural and functional concentric pattern of LV remodeling in DHF is characterized echocardiographically by normal or near-normal LV enddiastolic volume and cavity shape, increased absolute and relative wall thicknesses (wall thickness/LV cavity radius), increased LV mass/volume ratio resulting from a disproportionately greater increase in LV mass than volume and preserved EF (>50%). More specific Doppler echocardiographic findings in chronic DHF include abnormal LV filling patterns (larger A wave velocity, a normal E wave deceleration time [DT]), prolonged isovolumic relaxation time (IVRT), which is the period between aortic valve closure and mitral valve opening, decreased propagation velocity in the LV inflow tract, abnormal myocardial diastolic velocities by tissue Doppler imaging (TDI). Tissue Doppler imaging myocardial velocities and myocardial displacement reported in small cohorts of patients with indisputable DHF are normal in more than 50%.[18-22] Furthermore, not all of the more specific Doppler echocardiographic parameters listed are abnormal in every patient with DHF.

Detection of diastolic dysfunction is important because it is associated with a fivefold increase in mortal-

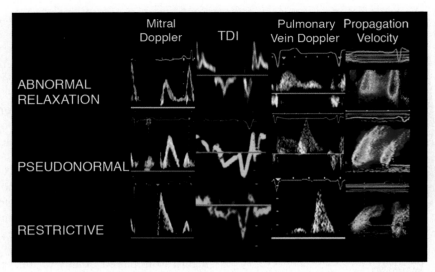

Figure 27–16. Pulsed-wave Doppler, tissue Doppler imaging (TDI), pulmonary vein Doppler, and propagation velocity (Vp) in abnormal relaxation, pseudonormal cardiomyopathy, and restrictive cardiomyopathy.

ity.[23] The transition from diastolic dysfunction to DHF can be followed echocardiographically and is accompanied by further escalation in mortality.

The earliest sign of diastolic dysfunction is impairment of relaxation resulting from slowing of the rate of LV diastolic pressure decay (see Chapter 11). This early evidence for diastolic dysfunction can be detected noninvasively by prolongation of IVRT that can be measured as the time period between aortic valve closure and mitral valve opening. IVRT can be measured with the echocardiographic transducer at the apex of the heart angled to record both aortic and mitral valve leaflet motion recorded at a sweep speed of 100 mm/s.

Slowed and prolonged myocardial relaxation is also detectable as altered mitral inflow velocities with a decreased peak velocity during passive filling (E wave), an increased E wave DT, and an augmented peak velocity during active atrial systolic contraction (A wave) with a shortened duration (Fig. 27–16). As the duration of the peak A wave of the mitral inflow shortens, so the duration of the flow reversal in the pulmonary venous velocity profile increases and finally exceeds the mitral peak A wave duration. Slowed or delayed LV relaxation can be diagnosed by TDI as reduced and delayed E′, velocity of the mitral annulus most frequently obtained from the septum and lateral walls with the transducer at the LV apex. A transmitral A wave that is of shorter duration than a pulmonary venous A wave predicts a LV end-diastolic pressure of greater than 15 mm Hg.

The mitral diastolic flow propagation velocity (Vp) recorded with color flow Doppler at the LV inflow correlates with tau (τ) and decreases progressively with increasing LV diastolic dysfunction. LV filling pressure or pulmonary capillary wedge pressure (PCWP) can be derived from the DT of the E wave of the mitral inflow and a value of less than 140 ms indicates a mitral inflow velocity profile consistent with restrictive physiology.

Alternatively, LV diastolic pressure can be estimated from the ratio of E/E′ over a wide range of filling pressures and LV EFs.[24] Chronic LV diastolic dysfunction may transition to HF, and in doing so, the mitral inflow, pulmonary venous, and TDI flow velocity profiles change from a pattern of impaired relaxation, that is reversible, to a restrictive physiology that may become irreversible (Fig. 27–17). Thus, DHF can be diagnosed in symptomatic patients with normal LV size and EF and evidence for abnormal relaxation, diminished compliance, and increased LV diastolic filling pressure.[17]

Cardiac amyloid exemplifies the changes in cardiac architecture, LV diastolic function and preservation of systolic function until late in the course of the disease. The LV cavity is typically of normal size; wall thickness is moderately to severely increased by deposition of noncontractile proteinaceous material in the myocardial interstitium between the myofilaments. This protein deposition alters the material properties of the myocardium causing increased chamber stiffness and abnormal mitral inflow velocity pattern consistent with restrictive physiology. The DT is dramatically shortened, and the A wave of the mitral inflow is abbreviated and of low amplitude. Shortening of the E wave deceleration time in cardiac amyloid is strongly predictive of clinical outcome.[25] In addition, the pulmonary venous velocity spectra demonstrate attenuation of the systolic wave, and there is usually marked reduction in the E′ wave of the tissue Doppler spectra from the basal septum and the lateral wall. These abnormal Doppler echocardiographic findings progress from the time of diagnosis to the restrictive physiology in the final stages of the disease (see Fig. 27–17).

HCM (Fig. 27–18) may present with DHF with supranormal systolic function and an EF greater than 70%. The LV cavity is small or normal with severe LV hypertrophy often with asymmetric septal hypertrophy

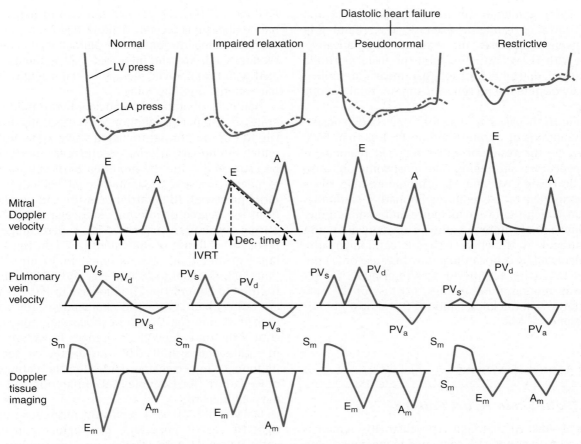

Figure 27–17. *Left ventricular (LV) and left atrial (LA) pressures during diastole, transmitral Doppler LV inflow velocity, pulmonary vein Doppler velocity, and Doppler tissue velocity. A, velocity of left ventricular filling contributed by atrial contraction; PAm, myocardial velocity during filling produced by atrial contraction; Dec. time, e-wave deceleration time; E, early left ventricular filling velocity; Em, myocardial velocity during early filling; IVRT, isovolumic relaxation time; PVa, pulmonary vein velocity resulting from atrial contraction; PVd, diastolic pulmonary vein velocity; Sm, myocardial velocity during systole; Vs, systolic pulmonary vein velocity. (From Zile MR, Brutsaert DL:* Circulation *105:1387-1393, 2002.)*

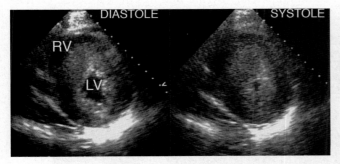

Figure 27–18. *Short-axis view in diastole* (left) *and systole* (right) *of a patient with severe hypertrophic cardiomyopathy. LV, left ventricle; RV, right ventricle.*

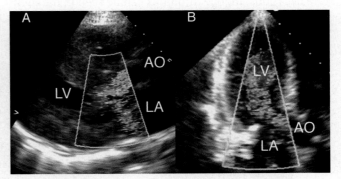

Figure 27–19. A, *Parasternal long axis;* B, *apical long axis with an obstruction in the left ventricular outflow tract as demonstrated by color flow Doppler by the onset of turbulence. AO, aorta; LA, left atrium; LV, left ventricle.*

(ASH) or concentric hypertrophy typical of concentric remodeling with or without a resting or provocable left ventricular outflow tract (LVOT) obstruction. In those with resting obstruction, there are two echocardiographic features that assist in the diagnosis, systolic anterior motion (SAM) of the mitral valve, which narrows the LVOT and is the site of obstruction demon-

strated by color flow Doppler by the onset of turbulence (Fig. 27–19). The second echocardiographic finding is the early systolic closure of the aortic valve that occurs at the end of ejection and may occur within the first half of systolic ejection. The peak and mean systolic LVOT gradients can be measured at rest and after Valsalva or isometric exercise, (i.e., hand grip which usually increases the gradients dramatically). Patients with HCM and HF exhibit the usual portfolio of abnormal diastolic function parameters described previously despite the presence of supranormal systolic function.

Systolic HF is easier to diagnose than DHF, consisting of symptoms of dyspnea and an EF less than 50% that may be the result of either reduced regional or global myocardial shortening. The most common cause of systolic HF is CAD and MI. Chronic systolic HF is best exemplified by ischemic or idiopathic cardiomyopathy in which the LV architecture and systolic function follow a final common pathway of cavity dilatation and contractile dysfunction. Ischemic cardiomyopathy can be detected by echocardiography because of (1) the enlarged LV cavity, (2) the EF less than 40%, (3) regional wall motion abnormalities, (4) loss of the normal uniform wall thickness, and (5) the almost ubiquitous presence of MR.

Right Heart Failure

Acute Right-Sided Heart Failure

Acute right-sided HF and right ventricular (RV) remodeling may occur over hours as compared to the time course of weeks to months in chronic RV failure. A sudden increase in RV afterload resulting from major pulmonary embolism causes acute RV dilatation and usually severe reduction in systolic contractile function with hemodynamic compromise. This constellation of findings can be demonstrated with Doppler echocardiography and the pathoetiologic mechanism ascertained (Fig. 27–20). On rare occasions, mobile thrombus can be seen in the right-sided heart chambers or proximal pulmonary arteries by TTE or TEE (Fig. 27–21). RV function in major pulmonary embolism is severely depressed globally but usually recovers if reperfusion of the pulmonary circulation is reestablished, and the increased load is rapidly attenuated with thrombolytic therapy or acute surgical pulmonary arterial thrombectomy.

Acute RV dilatation is associated with mild to moderate tricuspid regurgitation (TR) resulting from disruption of the normal tricuspid valve apparatus, from which pulmonary arterial systolic pressure (PASP) can be estimated using the modified Bernoulli formula (4 × peak [tricuspid regurgitation jet velocity^2] + right atrial pressure). Right atrial pressure can be estimated from the degree of inferior vena cava (IVC) collapse during respiration expressed as a percentage. Complete IVC collapse is equivalent to 5 mm Hg; IVC collapse greater than 50% is equal to 10 mm Hg; less than 50% is equal to 15 mm Hg; and 0% IVC collapse is equal to 20 mm Hg. The increase in PASP is moderate rather than severe and characteristically does not exceed 55 mm Hg. Doppler echocardiography demonstrates the time-dependent changes in RV remodeling in right-sided systolic HF, the degree of secondary pulmonary hypertension, and often the pathoetiology of RV failure (for example in RV infarction and pulmonary embolism).

Isolated RV MI is a relatively rare cause of acute right HF that is important to recognize and institute early treatment with intravenous (IV) fluid resuscitation and coronary reperfusion. The characteristic hallmark for echocardiographic diagnosis is unequivocal echocardiographic evidence of RV segmental wall motion abnormality. Usually RV infarction is an extension of an inferoposterior LV MI resulting from proximal occlusion of a dominant right coronary artery (RCA). The diagnosis of RV infarction is usually established echocardiographically by the findings of associated LV posteroinferior hypokinesis or akinesis with decreased

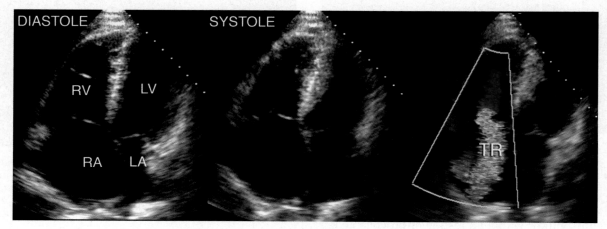

Figure 27–20. *Apical four-chamber view of a patient with acute right ventricular strain at end-diastole* (left), *demonstrating a dilated, overloaded right ventricle. The right atrium is also dilated and the interauricular septum bulges to the left in end-systole* (center) *and color Doppler* (right), *revealing severe tricuspid regurgitation. Acute right ventricular strain was the result of a large pulmonary embolism. The pulmonary pressure was 52 mm Hg. LA, left atrium; LV, left ventricle; RA, right atrium; RV, right ventricle; TR, tricuspid regurgitation.*

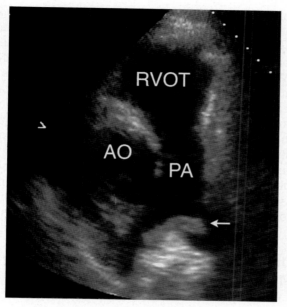

Figure 27-21. Parasternal view of the main pulmonary artery in long-axis view showing a thrombus (arrow) at the pulmonary artery bifurcation. Ao, aorta, PA, pulmonary artery; RVOT, right ventricular outflow tract.

wall thickness resulting from stretching of the infarct region and discrepantly more severe RV dilatation and dysfunction than accounted for by the extent of RV segmental akinesis or hypokinesis (Fig. 27–22).

Chronic Right Ventricular Failure

In chronic systolic right HF, the right ventricle dilates in response to chronically increased loading conditions when hypertrophy can no longer normalize the increase in wall stress. RV hypertrophy may be concentric or eccentric depending on the nature of the stimulus (i.e., whether from pressure or volume overload respectively). As the loading conditions increase, whether a result of pressure or volume overload, the interventricular septum bulges into the LVOT and the

RV shape changes to a more spherical configuration (Fig. 27–23). RV diastolic pressure exceeds that in the left ventricle and may result in abnormal LV diastolic filling and intracardiac shunting from right to left via a patent foramen ovale (PFO) if present. Tricuspid regurgitation develops as the tricuspid subvalve geometry is disrupted by chamber dilatation and accelerates the deterioration in RV function. As RV failure progresses, the RV continues to enlarge and forms the apex of the heart, the left ventricle rotates posteriorly, septal motion becomes reversed and contractile function deteriorates (see Fig. 27–23). Echocardiographic measurements of RV size and function assessed as end-systolic dimension and percent fractional area change in the apical four-chamber or subcostal four-chamber views are important predictors of adverse cardiovascular events in patients with left-sided HF.[15]

The configuration and internal architecture of the right ventricle is not designed to generate or sustain chronically elevated systolic pressures. When RV systolic pressure exceeds 40 mm Hg, tricuspid regurgitation supervenes, which further escalates the already increased loading conditions, and is associated with further RV dilatation, such that a vicious cycle occurs that culminates in right HF. Echocardiography plays a key role not only in detecting right HF but also in differentiating acute from chronic right HF in terms of LV cavity architecture and function (Fig. 27–24). Patients with adult congenital heart disease present with RV rather than LV failure resulting from development of severe pulmonary hypertension from intracardiac shunts or with RV dysfunction when the right ventricle is the systemic ventricle. Echocardiography is not only important in confirming the presence of chronic RV failure but has the additional role of elucidating the abnormal intracardiac anatomy.

Recently M-mode echocardiographic measurements of the tricuspid annular plane systolic excursion (TAPSE) that reflect RV long-axis shortening have been shown to correlate with RV ejection function and predict clinical outcome.[26]

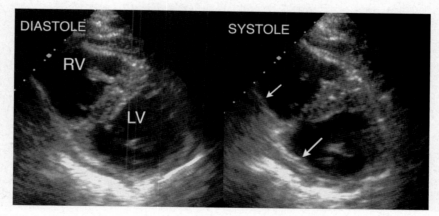

Figure 27-22. Parasternal short axis of a patient with right ventricular infarct in diastole (left) and systole (right). The arrows indicate contiguous posterior myocardial infarction with right ventricular involvement. LV, left ventricle; RV, right ventricle.

Right Heart Failure and Ventricular Remodeling

Until recently, few attempts were made to study RV remodeling because the unusual shape of the right ventricle is difficult to represent by a simple or compound geometric algorithm, which enables reproducible assessment of RV volumes and RVEF. RV remodeling is usually the result of LV disease transmitted to the right-sided heart chambers via the pulmonary venous circulation and the vasoreactive pulmonary arterioles. The pulmonary arterioles react to chronic pressure and

volume overload by developing medial hypertrophy that increases pulmonary vascular resistance and in turn results in pulmonary arterial hypertension. Pulmonary hypertension or increased RV afterload induces RV hypertrophy that may temporarily normalize the increased afterload and preserve near normal RV cavity geometry and function for a prolonged period of time. However, unchecked RV afterload excess from chronic pulmonary hypertension causes progressive RV remodeling with dilatation and continuing hypertrophy in similar fashion to that occurring in the left ventricle. If the maximal hypertrophic response is insufficient to balance the increased afterload, progressive RV dilatation and deterioration in function to HF ensues.

Doppler Echocardiography in the Medical Treatment of Heart Failure

The primary aims in the treatment of chronic systolic HF are to provide symptomatic relief, improve quality of life, and ideally increase longevity. These aims may be achieved in part by preventing progressive LV dilatation and promoting reverse remodeling and improvement in ventricular function. The first-line treatment strategy in chronic systolic HF is to reduce LV loading conditions and to block neurohormonal activation with pharmacologic agents that in turn attenuate LV remodeling. Doppler echocardiography is an ideal method for tracking changes in LV volumes, shape, and function associated with medical and surgical treatments, which has been used successfully in numerous chronic HF trials.

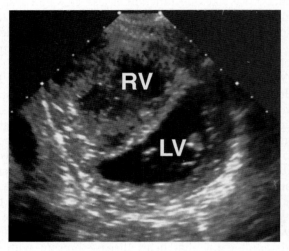

Figure 27–23. Parasternal short axis of a patient with right ventricular hypertrophy. The right ventricular walls are thickened and the interventricular septum exhibits paradoxical motion consistent with severe chronic pulmonary hypertension. LV, left ventricle; RV, right ventricle.

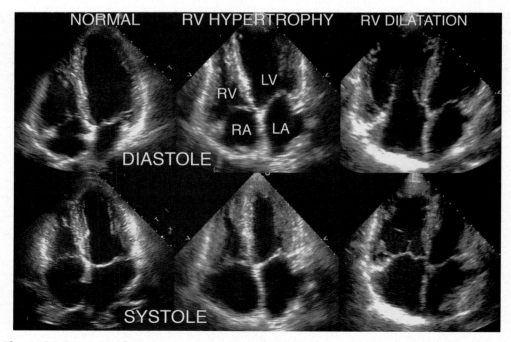

Figure 27–24. Apical four-chamber view of a normal right ventricle (left), right ventricular hypertrophy (center), and right ventricular dilatation (right). LA, left atrium; LV, left ventricle; RA, right atrium; RV, right ventricle.

Contemporary management of acute HF is most frequently medical and involves three fundamental principles. The first is aimed at maintaining systemic blood pressure for organ perfusion by increasing contractile performance (myocardial systolic shortening) with IV catecholamines in hemodynamically compromised patients. The second medical strategy is to reduce LV loading conditions with vasodilator therapy, such as nitrates and hydrallazine. The third medical treatment strategy involves the combination of blocking neurohormonal activation and reducing LV loading conditions with β-adrenergic receptor blockers plus angiotensin receptor blockers (ARBs) or angiotensin converting enzyme (ACE) inhibitors and aldosterone antagonists.

Echocardiography has played a pivotal role in multiple randomized clinical trials in demonstrating the efficacy of pharmacologic interventions by limiting the progressive LV dilatation that typifies the natural history of systolic HF. For example, neurohormonal blockade limits remodeling by reducing load that triggers the biochemical cascade that initiates the remodeling process to HF.

Echocardiography in patients with acute HF from MI provides unique information that is unattainable safely by any other imaging techniques, and it allows early risk stratification and optimal individualized therapy. Numerous clinical post-MI or HF trials have shown unequivocally that echocardiographic measurements of LV volumes, EF, infarct size, and RV systolic shortening predict adverse cardiovascular events, including death, onset of HF, and recurrent MI at both short-term and long-term follow-up.[27] The prevalence of these adverse cardiovascular events increased directly with LV dilatation assessed by echocardiography. Prevention of LV dilatation and remodeling with ACE inhibitors reduced the recurrence rate of HF. Echocardiographically determined LV volumes and percentage change in systolic cavity area are powerful predictors of ventricular arrhythmias from early post-MI through 2-year follow-up (Fig. 27–25).

In the Survival and Ventricular Enlargement (SAVE)[12] trial, serial echocardiographic measurements of LV size and function were obtained in 499 patients with EF less than or equal to or less than 40%. Quantitative echocardiography demonstrated that the beneficial effects on clinical outcome of ACE inhibitors in infarct-related HF are mediated by attenuation of LV dilatation, structural, and functional remodeling.[28] Logistic regression analysis of baseline demographics for predictors of survival in the SAVE trial showed that echocardiographic LV end-systolic size was the single most powerful predictor of survival post-MI, even more than EF.[22] Similar controlled trials of β-adrenergic receptor blocking agents in chronic systolic HF have used quantitative echocardiography to document their efficacy and establish their use in the contemporary optimal management of chronic HF. Thus, quantitative TTE has shown that ACE inhibitors and β-adrenergic receptor blockers confer unequivocal benefit on clinical outcome in HF.

A number of placebo-controlled, randomized clinical trials of acute HF post-MI have enabled Doppler echocardiography to characterize the natural and unnatural histories of the LV remodeling process and how these structural and functional changes transition from acute to chronic HF.

Echocardiography and Mechanical Therapies for Heart Failure

Surgical treatment also has an important role in the management of acute HF and similar to medical treatment is based on two strategies. First, augmentation of CO either with intraaortic balloon counterpulsation, left ventricular assist device (LVAD) and/or right ventricular assist device (RVAD) (Fig. 27–26), or acute heart transplantation. Second, by reducing the acute elevation in LV loading conditions by mitral valve re-

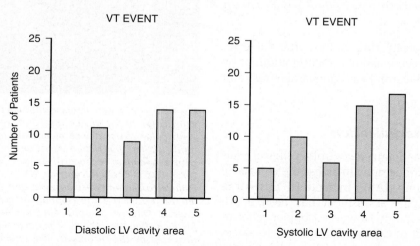

Figure 27–25. Relation between left ventricular diastolic and systolic cavity area and ventricular tachycardia early after myocardial infarction in patients with left ventricular dysfunction and ejection fraction less than or equal to 40%. LV, left ventricular; VT, ventricular tachycardia.

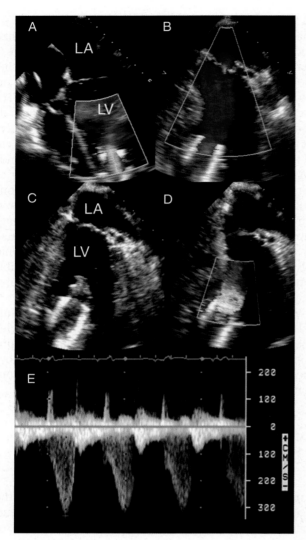

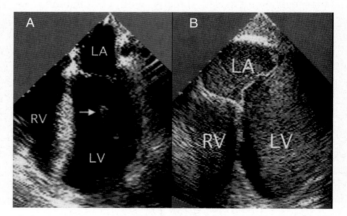

Figure 27-26. *Transesophageal views of a patient with a left ventricular assist device. The canula is visible at the left ventricular apex (A and B). A thrombus can be seen on left ventricular assist device canula with a color flow Doppler showing the obstruction (C and D). Spectral Doppler showing a systolic gradient across the left ventricular assist device draining canula indicating partial obstruction by thrombus (E). LA, left atrium; LV, left ventricle.*

pair with an annuloplasty ring or by aortic valve replacement for acute severe valvular regurgitation, or by deployment of an epicardial or endocardial restraint devices.[29]

Intraaortic Counterpulsation

There have been no randomized controlled clinical trials using Doppler echocardiography to assess the efficacy of intraaortic balloon pump (IABP) in acute HF post-MI in which echocardiographic assessment has been a primary or secondary endpoint. However, Doppler echocardiographic assessment of CO is used routinely to assess the impact of IABP. Forward stroke volume can be estimated as the product of the cross-sectional area (CSA) of the flow stream calculated from echocardiographic mea-

surements of the LVOT diameter, assuming the cross section is circular and the time velocity integral (TVI) recorded from the LVOT. These noninvasive Doppler echocardiographic measurements are critically important before and immediately after deployment of an IABP and during weaning from IABP support. Accurate and reliable serial measurements of CO can be made as counterpulsation to native heart rate is downgraded from 1:1 to 1:2 and 1:3. Stable COs show when withdrawal of IABP can be achieved safely.

Ventricular Assist Devices

Placement of LVADs for severe acute HF or acute decompensation of chronic HF has becoming increasingly frequent.[30] Echocardiographic screening for significant aortic regurgitation and LV apical thrombus before insertion is important to avoid systemic embolization during insertion of the LV cannula (Fig. 27-27). Following insertion of a LVAD, which may provide pulsatile or nonpulsatile flow, the settings of the LVAD pump are routinely evaluated by Doppler echocardiography over a range of flows. LV output is assessed by aligning the continuous-wave Doppler parallel to the direction of blood flow through the sump drain at the LV apex and estimating stroke output as the product of the time velocity integral and the cross-sectional area of the outlet cannula (see Fig. 27-26). Doppler echocardiographic assessment of LV outputs is reliable and correlate closely with LVAD flow rates. When there is divergence between the two estimates of flow, the

Figure 27-27. *Refractory right heart failure 3 days after left ventricular assist device insertion, requiring emergent right ventricular assist device placement in a patient with persistently low left ventricular assist device flows. A, Intraoperative transesophageal echocardiography shows a small mobile thrombus in the left ventricle (LV) in the four-chamber view. Failure to regain consciousness and progressive hypotension led to a repeat transesophageal echocardiography 2 days later. B, This transesophageal view demonstrates almost complete cardiac thrombosis. The normal geometry of the heart is distorted by the thrombus. The patient died from stroke and multiorgan failure on the following day. LA, left atrium; RV, right ventricle. (From Reilly MP, Wiegers SE, Cucchiara AJ, et al: Am J Cardiol 86:1156-1159, A10, 2000.)*

Doppler flow is invariably less, and if this occurs across a range of flow settings, it should suggest partial obstruction of the LV outlet usually by thrombus forming within or protruding into the LV apical cannula.[31] Partial occlusion of the LV outlet cannula is identified by the presence of flow acceleration by color flow Doppler map and a gradient across the LV apical outflow cannula (see Fig. 27–27). LVADs in patients are mostly used as short-term therapy to unload and rest the LV to promote restitution of function or as a bridge to heart transplantation. Recently long-term or destination LVAD therapy has been instituted for patients requiring obligatory mechanical support whom for a variety of reasons are not suitable candidates for orthotopic heart transplantation. These patients require regular corroboration between the pump flows and Doppler echocardiographic estimates of flow.

Surgical Valve Repair or Replacement

Other surgical interventions for acute HF that aim to reduce systolic loading conditions include mitral valve repair or replacement for acute severe MR from chordal rupture resulting in a flail leaflet or papillary muscle rupture following MI. Similar reduction in afterload is the aim in patients presenting with acute severe aortic regurgitation either from aortic valve endocarditis or from acute type A aortic dissection. In addition to establishing these individual diagnoses with either TTE or TEE, assessment of baseline echocardiographic EF and LV size are the major determinants of survival and clinical outcome. Furthermore, Doppler echocardiography has been used to compare LV architecture (LV volumes and mass) and function (EF) preoperatively and postoperatively to determine whether any favorable structural changes have occurred that might explain the symptomatic improvement that occurs after successful surgery.

Restraint Devices in Chronic Heart Failure

Prevention of LV dilatation and remodeling is the physiologic principle underlying the use of myocardial restraint devices. Early experimental animal studies showed that LV dilatation could be prevented and LV function preserved by placing a nondistensible material on the epicardium overlying a subsequent MI.[32] The first device that underwent clinical trial was an epicardial mesh that enveloped the whole heart (ACORN) and was tested in patients with New York Heart Association (NYHA) Symptom Class III/IV with LV dilatation and end-stage LV dysfunction. In this study population, serial Doppler echocardiograms in all patients showed that the device prevented further progressive LV enlargement without evidence for constriction and in a proportion of patients was associated with symptomatic improvement and increased EF.[33] Two further

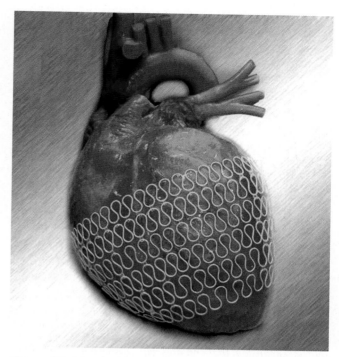

Figure 27–28. *The Paracor Ventricular Support System comprises an implant and a delivery system. The implant is preloaded into the delivery system which is used to place the implant onto the heart. The implant, which is made of Nitinol wire coated with silicone tubing, is placed over the epicardial surface (Courtesy of Paracor, Heart Net System).*

clinical trials are currently in progress in patients with a NYHA Class III/IV systolic HF designation using quantitative serial echocardiography and change in LV volumes as endpoints. One trial is testing an epicardial restraint device (Paracor) that is introduced via a stab wound and limited thoracotomy and envelops the heart (Fig. 27–28). The other clinical trial tests the more recent development of a device (Parachute) to limit or prevent LV dilatation resulting from myocardial infarct expansion that is positioned on the LV apical endocardium via retrograde femoral arterial catheterization. The results of these ongoing clinical trials using Doppler echocardiographic endpoints will determine whether these devices have a role in the treatment of chronic systolic HF or should be deployed early in nonreperfusable expanding MI (Fig. 27–29).

Volume Reduction Surgery in Chronic Heart Failure

Surgical reduction in LV size in patients with LV dilatation and severe dysfunction was attempted over the last decade to improve LV function by reducing LV load (Fig. 27–30). The rationale for this therapy was founded on the interaction between myocardial wall stress and myocardial contractile function. Successful LV volume reduction by excising a section of myocardium and reattaching the free LV margins decreases wall stress by reducing LV cavity radius and preserves wall thickness

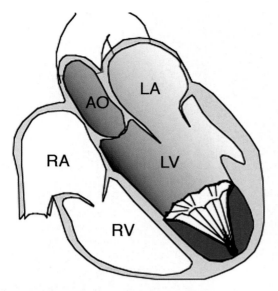

Figure 27–29. Schematic representation of the implantable ventricular partitioning device (VPD) that delivers a partitioning membrane within the compromised ventricle. The VPD isolates the dysfunctional region of the ventricle preventing infarct expansion that initiates left ventricular remodeling, and preventing increases in both chamber volume and myocardial stress and improves hemodynamics (Parachute). AO, aorta; LA, left atrium; LV, left ventricle; RA, right atrium; RV, right ventricle. (Courtesy of Cardiokinetics.)

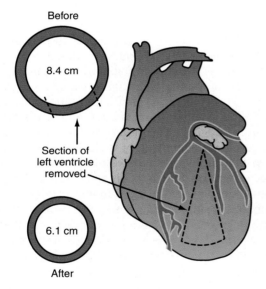

Figure 27–30. Batista procedure: A portion of the left ventricle is removed to reduce left ventricular volume and thereby reduce wall stress back toward normal. The remaining edges of the left ventricle are then sewn together, returning the chamber to its normal size. (From McCarthy M: Lancet 349:855, 1997).

unchanged without inducing too much incremental myocardial damage by the surgery. If removal of myocardium reduced systolic wall stress or redistributed wall stress more uniformly, then contractile function (LVEF) should theoretically improve if the material properties of the myocardium did not change. This LV volume reduction procedure in carefully selected patients was accompanied by amelioration of symptoms and improved LV function. This surgery is rarely performed now for two reasons. First, removal of myocardium appears counterintuitive, and second because LVADs can be used as destination therapy particularly in patients who are not heart transplant candidates.

Cardiac Resynchronization Therapy in Chronic Heart Failure

Cardiac resynchronization therapy (CRT) is an established therapy for patients with NYHA III/IV HR, prolonged QRS duration (>130 ms) and LV dyssynchrony.[18-20] Prolonged QRS duration occurs in 30% to 50% of patients with HF and correlates directly with mortality so that increase in QRS duration is associated with increased mortality.[21] The specific aim of CRT in HF is to alleviate symptoms and reverse LV remodeling. This is achieved by optimizing atrioventricular conduction, prolonging LV filling time, and synchronizing RV and LV contraction by minimizing interventricular and intraventricular mechanical delay.

Symptomatic benefit and improved exercise capacity have been consistent findings in CRT trials in the majority (65%) of patients[19,20,34-36] already receiving optimal medical HF therapy. Doppler echocardiography has played a crucial role in elucidating the mechanism of reverse structural and functional LV remodeling with CRT. Doppler echocardiography has also been used to identify patients likely to respond to CRT before device implantation. The combination of an internal cardiac defibrillator (ICD) with CRT affords further survival benefit[35] by protecting against sudden death.

Recently, large CRT trials[19,20,34-36] have used serial Doppler echocardiography to characterize reverse LV structural and functional remodeling and have shown how quickly it occurs and for how long reverse remodeling is sustained.[36] These trials have used echocardiography as secondary endpoints and demonstrated that CRT results in significant decrease in LV end-diastolic and end-systolic diameters and LV volumes as early as 1 month[36-38] compared to control patients. Further reduction in LV volumes occurs by 6 months (Fig. 27–31) and these changes are sustained at least until 18 months.[28,39,40] The reduction in LV volumes with CRT results in a decrease in LV load or wall stress, which is a powerful stimulus for regression of LV mass. LV mass decreased significantly by 6 months but this occurred at a slower rate than the reduction in LV volume.

Serial echocardiographic studies have clearly shown that the sustained reductions in LV volume and mass with CRT result in alterations in LV architecture and restoration of mitral annular and subvalve geometry toward normal. Changes in the geometry of the mitral valve apparatus are associated with decreased MR. In

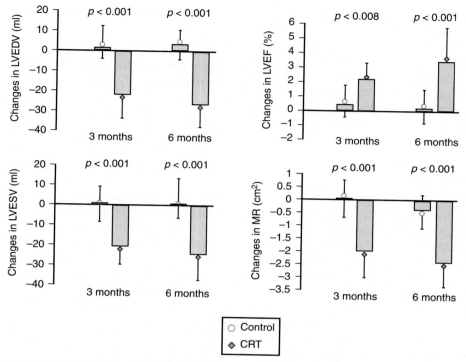

Figure 27–31. *Median change (with 95% confidence intervals) in left ventricular end-diastolic volume* (top left), *left ventricular end-systolic volume* (bottom left), *left ventricular ejection fraction* (top right), *and mitral regurgitation* (bottom right) *at 3 and 6 months after randomization in the control group* (circles) *and the cardiac resynchronization therapy group* (diamonds). *CRT, cardiac resynchronization therapy; LVEDV, left ventricular end diastolic volume; LVEF, left ventricular ejection fraction; LVESV, left ventricular end systolic volume; MR, mitral regurgitation.*

the MIRACLE study, the severity of MR decreased significantly by 3 months, and this was maintained at 6 and 12 months (see Fig. 27–31). The initial decrease in MR precedes the reduction in LV volume[41] and may be the result of restoration of the temporal coordination of mechanical activation of the papillary muscles allowing for increased area of mitral leaflet coaptation.[42] The favorable changes in LV load, architecture and decrease in MR are associated with progressive increase in LV EF at 3 and 6 months from baseline (see Fig. 27–31). Continuous CRT is required to sustain reverse LV remodeling.[41] Cessation of CRT results in abolition of the LV volume reduction achieved, deterioration in LV EF to baseline values, and return of MR within 1 week.[41]

Changes in Diastolic Ventricular Function with Cardiac Resynchronization Therapy

CRT studies have been conducted exclusively in patients with advanced systolic HF, but Doppler echocardiography has demonstrated concomitant improvements in diastolic function.[43] CRT prolongs the duration of LV filling, separates the rapid filling phase from atrial systolic contraction, shortens interventricular mechanical delay (IVMD) and coordinates ventricular contraction and relaxation (see Fig. 27–3). The prolonged LV

diastolic filling time induced by CRT is not associated with changes in transmitral peak flow velocities during passive filling (E wave), during atrial contraction (peak A-wave), E/A ratio, or IVRT. The E wave DT and the myocardial performance index improve by 3 months and improve further by 12 months.[43,44] However, patients with restrictive LV filling characterized by a short DT and peak E wave velocity greater than 1 m/s exhibit little or no response to CRT.

Historically, exercise capacity in systolic HF has not correlated with changes in LV volumes or EF. However, in MIRACLE the symptomatic benefits with CRT occurred predominantly in those patients with the greatest structural and functional LV remodeling quantified by Doppler echocardiography.[43]

Responders and Nonresponders to Resynchronization Therapy

The proportion of NYHA III/IV patients with HF that respond to CRT by exhibiting LV reverse remodeling measured by Doppler echocardiography and symptomatic improvement is similar in patients with ischemic and nonischemic HF. Reduction in LV volumes, decrease in severity of MR, and increase in LVEF are consistently two to three times greater in nonischemic than ischemic HF.[43,44] However, despite the twofold to threefold difference in LV volume reduction in the nonischemic patients at 6 months, both ischemic and nonischemic HF have similar improvement in symptoms and exercise capacity. After adjusting for differences in baseline demographics (including age, gender, EF, LV volumes), the beneficial reduction in LV volumes seen at 6 months had regressed by 12 months in the patients with ischemic HF[44] and was sustained in the nonischemic patients.

Predictors of Optimal Response to Resynchronization Therapy

LV reverse remodeling with CRT does not occur in all patients with HF with QRS duration greater than 130 ms. Between 65% to 75% of all such patients exhibit reverse LV remodeling assessed by Doppler echocardiography, and the reasons for this shortfall are not clear. There are no baseline clinical demographics that distinguish responders from nonresponders to CRT or predict an optimal response before device implantation. A number of possible mechanisms have been proposed. Suboptimal placement of the RV or LV electrodes, especially in ischemic HF in which myocardial scar is subjacent to the LV electrode or when electrode placement is constrained by the anatomy of the coronary sinus may explain failure of response to CRT in some patients and is being assessed currently in two randomized trials. Baseline clinical demographics, QRS duration, echocardiographic measures of LV size, or end-systolic volume, which are normally powerful predictors of clinical outcome, do not reliably predict response to CRT. What appears to be fundamental for a good response to CRT is the presence of regional LV dyssynchrony, which was initially assessed as QRS prolongation. LV mechanical dyssynchrony rather than a prolonged QRS duration is a prerequisite for response to CRT and may be absent despite a prolonged QRS duration.

New Techniques for Detection of Left Ventricular Dyssynchrony

Progress has been achieved in detecting the presence of LV mechanical dyssynchrony. New noninvasive imaging technology has recently been developed to detect and semi-quantify regional (spatial) and temporal LV mechanical dyssynchrony to identify responders to CRT before device placement.[45,46] In the normal heart electrical activation results in synchronous regional long-axis and short-axis contraction. The concentric inward motion can be appreciated visually in LV short-axis echoes or by myocardial tracking with velocity vector imaging (Fig. 27–32) or speckle tracking techniques. LV dyssynchrony is the result of premature regional contraction before ejection or delayed regional contraction disrupting the normal coordinated sequence of contraction and resulting in reduction in EF. The time interval or delay between maximal posterior excursion of the septum and peak anterior excursion of the posterior LV wall by M-mode echocardiography has been used to identify dyssynchrony, defined as a time delay greater than 130 ms.[47] This method is restricted to two opposing walls of the LV and measurement of this time delay may not be possible when the septum is infarcted and does not thicken or move posteriorly in the normal direction. Several Doppler echocardiographic methodologies have been advocated for the diagnosis of dyssynchrony.

The most frequently used Doppler tissue imaging method for detecting LV dyssynchrony (Fig. 27–33) is measurement of the time interval from the onset of the QRS to the peak myocardial systolic velocities in several locations: the basal and middle wall segments of

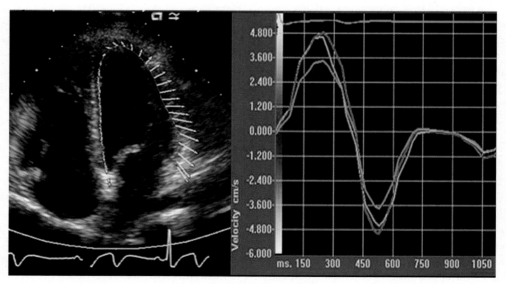

Figure 27–32. *Myocardial tracking in the apical four-chamber view from a normal volunteer. Velocity Vector Imaging (Siemens Medical Solutions).*

Tissue Doppler Imaging

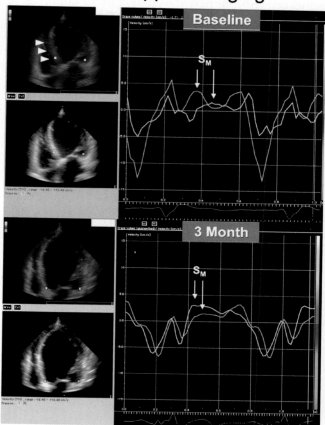

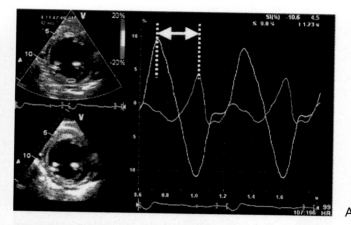

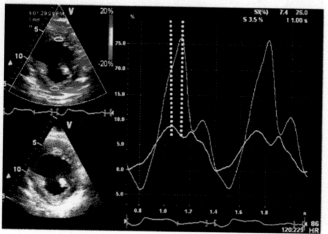

Figure 27-33. Regional myocardial velocity curves obtained by tissue Doppler imaging at the basal septal (yellow) and basal lateral (green) segments. In the color two-dimensional pictures, movement of the myocardium toward the probe (during contraction) is shown in red, whereas movement away from the probe is shown in blue. This patient with left bundle branch block had systolic paradoxical septal motion resulting in significant delay in peak systolic mitral annular motion (S_M) in the septal relative to the lateral wall (arrowheads). Three months after biventricular pacing therapy, systolic synchrony was achieved, as reflected by the superimposition of the myocardial velocity curves and the uniformity of red color in the two-dimensional echocardiography. (From Yu CM, Chau E, Sanderson JE, et al: Circulation 105:438-445, 2002.)

Figure 27-34. Radial strain imaging in a patient with a favorable acute response to cardiac resynchronization therapy. A, Baseline time-strain plots show early anteroseptal peak strain (yellow) followed by late posterior wall peak strain (turquoise), resulting in a large degree of dyssynchrony (arrow). B, Time-strain plots after cardiac resynchronization therapy in the same patient demonstrating an immediate improvement in dyssynchrony. (From Dohi K, Suffoletto MS, Schwartzman D, et al: Am J Cardiol 96:112-116, 2005.)

opposing walls in the apical four-chamber, apical two-chamber, and apical long-axis views. Timing is measured from color-coded or pulsed-tissue Doppler endocardial displacement. Strain and strain rate imaging (Fig. 27-34) allow assessment of peak displacement and/or peak strain respectively throughout the entire left ventricle. LV dyssynchrony can be detected throughout the left ventricle as regional variation in the relative timing of contraction greater than the normal ranges using cut points calculated from mean and standard deviation in normal subjects. These parameters are more robust estimates of LV dyssynchrony than measurement of the QRS duration.

Real-time three-dimensional echocardiography using the conventional 16-segment model of the left ventricle can demonstrate LV dyssynchrony by the regional variation in the timing of acquisition of minimal systolic and maximal diastolic volumes for each of the 16 segments before device implantation (Fig. 27-35). In addition, following resynchronization therapy, restoration of coordinated contraction occurs with minimal differences in the timing of onset of contraction and peak shortening among the 16 segments regions.

Orthotopic Heart Transplantation

Finally, orthotopic heart transplantation is a therapeutic option in patients with acute or chronic HF that is refractory to medical therapy requiring LVAD and sometimes biventricular assist device (BIVAD) therapy as a bridge to heart transplantation. The dramatic changes in LV and RV structure and function of the transplanted heart have been well characterized by Doppler echocardiogra-

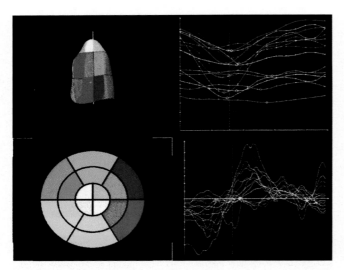

Figure 27–35. Real-time three-dimensional full volume analysis of regional left ventricular function showing (top left) the reconstructed left ventricular cast and the bulls-eye display (bottom left) of the 16 segments. Changes in regional volume (color-matched) for each of the 16 segments is displayed in the upper right. The anteroseptal and septal segments (light blue and green) show poor function and significant delay in achieving a minimum volume compared to other segments. A first derivative display of the regional volume curves is shown in the lower right panel and also demonstrates significant dispersion in the timing of minimal regional volume (indicated by the zero crossing points). (From Bax JJ, Abraham T, Barold SS, et al: J Am Coll Cardiol 46:2153-2167, 2005.)

phy[48] and are described in the chapter on heart transplantation for which reason it will not be described here (see Chapter 31). Doppler echocardiography is of great importance in selecting candidates for transplantation and serial follow-up for detection of myocardial rejection and accelerated graft atherosclerosis expressed as periodic alterations in LV function.

Summary

In summary, a number of new forms of therapy have emerged recently for prevention of HF and treatment of HF in which Doppler echocardiography will continue to play a vital role in patient selection for individual therapies and following the responses to these therapies. CRT is now an effective therapy in the majority of patients with advanced congestive heart failure who are refractory to optimal medical therapy that improves symptoms, exercise capacity, and quality of life. The beneficial clinical outcomes associated with CRT are sustained at least to 18 months has been unequivocally shown by Doppler echocardiography. What remains to be elucidated is the recognition of patients who will have an optimal response to

CRT before device implantation, which will be achieved with the new developments in noninvasive imaging technologies. Evaluation of restraint devices continues to rely on quantitative Doppler echocardiographic rather than any other diagnostic imaging modality in randomized controlled trials. Similar to surgical interventions and devices, new pharmaceutical agents will be required to do more than provide symptom relief either by preventing development of HF or reverse rather than just attenuate the remodeling process. The efficacy of all these therapies will likely be evaluated by quantitative Doppler echocardiography.

KEY POINTS

- Echocardiography is the single most useful diagnostic test in evaluation of patients with HF.
- Echocardiography has shown that, in chronic systolic HF, LV remodeling leads to a change in cavity shape because of the greater increase in the short-axis diameter than in LV long-axis diameter. As a result, the LV loses its ellipsoidal shape and becomes more spherical.
- There are three important sequelae to the abnormal LV size and shape:
  - Decrease in contractile function.
  - Predisposition to thrombus formation.
  - Enlargement of the mitral annulus and distortion of the mitral valve and subvalvular geometry.
- Echocardiography plays a vital role in detecting right-sided HF and differentiating acute from chronic right-sided HF in terms of RV cavity architecture and function.
- CRT aims to reverse LV remodeling by optimizing atrioventricular conduction, prolonging LV filling time, and synchronizing RV and LV contraction.
- CRT is an established therapy for patients with NYHA III/IV HF, prolonged QRS duration (> 130 ms), and LV dyssynchrony.
- CRT studies have been conducted exclusively in patients with advanced systolic HF, but Doppler echocardiography has demonstrated concomitant improvements in diastolic function.
- One third of patients with HF and QRS duration greater than 130 ms do not respond to CRT therapy.
- LV mechanical dyssynchrony rather than a prolonged QRS duration is a prerequisite for response to CRT and may be absent despite prolonged QRS duration.
- New parameters, such as strain and strain rate, are more robust estimates of LV dyssynchrony than QRS duration.

REFERENCES

1. Aurigemma GP, Gaasch WH: Clinical practice. Diastolic heart failure. *N Engl J Med* 351:1097-1105, 2004.
2. Owan TE, Hodge DO, Herges RM, et al: Trends in prevalence and outcome of heart failure with preserved ejection fraction. *N Engl J Med* 355:251-259, 2006.
3. Kitzman DW, Little WC, Brubaker PH, et al: Pathophysiological characterization of isolated diastolic heart failure in comparison to systolic heart failure. *JAMA* 288:2144-2150, 2002.
4. Zile MR, Brutsaert DL: New concepts in diastolic dysfunction and diastolic heart failure: Part I: diagnosis, prognosis, and measurements of diastolic function. *Circulation* 105:1387-1393, 2002.
5. Gorcsan J 3rd, Gasior TA, Mandarino WA, et al: Assessment of the immediate effects of cardiopulmonary bypass on left ventricular performance by on-line pressure-area relations. *Circulation* 89:180-190, 1994.
6. Zile MR, Baicu CF, Gaasch WH: Diastolic heart failure—abnormalities in active relaxation and passive stiffness of the left ventricle. *N Engl J Med* 350:1953-1959, 2004.
7. Thom T, Haase N, Rosamond W, et al: Heart disease and stroke statistics—2006 update: A report from the American Heart Association Statistics Committee and Stroke Statistics Subcommittee. *Circulation* 113:e85-e151, 2006.
8. Vasan RS, Larson MG, Benjamin EJ, et al: Congestive heart failure in subjects with normal versus reduced left ventricular ejection fraction: Prevalence and mortality in a population-based cohort. *J Am Coll Cardiol* 33:1948-1955, 1999.
9. Detaint D, Sundt TM, Nkomo VT, et al: Surgical correction of mitral regurgitation in the elderly: Outcomes and recent improvements. *Circulation* 114:265-272, 2006.
10. Gheorghiade M, Bonow RO: Chronic heart failure in the United States: A manifestation of coronary artery disease. *Circulation* 97:282-289, 1998.
11. Hunt SA, Abraham WT, Chin MH, et al: ACC/AHA 2005 Guideline Update for the Diagnosis and Management of Chronic Heart Failure in the Adult: A report of the American College of Cardiology/American Heart Association Task Force on Practice Guidelines (Writing Committee to Update the 2001 Guidelines for the Evaluation and Management of Heart Failure): developed in collaboration with the American College of Chest Physicians and the International Society for Heart and Lung Transplantation: endorsed by the Heart Rhythm Society. *Circulation* 112:e154-e235, 2005.
12. Pfeffer MA, Braunwald E, Moye LA, et al: Effect of captopril on mortality and morbidity in patients with left ventricular dysfunction after myocardial infarction. Results of the survival and ventricular enlargement trial. The SAVE Investigators. *N Engl J Med* 327:669-677, 1992.
13. Effect of enalapril on mortality and the development of heart failure in asymptomatic patients with reduced left ventricular ejection fractions. The SOLVD Investigators. *N Engl J Med* 327:685-691, 1992.
14. Jackson BM, Gorman JH 3rd, Salgo IS, et al: Border zone geometry increases wall stress after myocardial infarction: Contrast echocardiographic assessment. *Am J Physiol Heart Circ Physiol* 284:H475-H479, 2003.
15. Solomon SD, Aikawa Y, Martini MS, et al: Assessment of regional left ventricular wall stress after myocardial infarction by echocardiography-based structural analysis. *J Am Soc Echocardiogr* 11:938-947, 1998.
16. Maurer MS, Spevack D, Burkhoff D, Kronzon I: Diastolic dysfunction: can it be diagnosed by Doppler echocardiography? *J Am Coll Cardiol* 44:1543-1549, 2004.
17. Oh JK, Hatle L, Tajik AJ, Little WC: Diastolic heart failure can be diagnosed by comprehensive two-dimensional and Doppler echocardiography. *J Am Coll Cardiol* 47:500-506, 2006.
18. Stellbrink C, Breithardt OA, Franke A, et al: Impact of cardiac resynchronization therapy using hemodynamically optimized pacing on left ventricular remodeling in patients with congestive heart failure and ventricular conduction disturbances. *J Am Coll Cardiol* 38:1957-1965, 2001.
19. Abraham WT, Fisher WG, Smith AL, et al: Multicenter InSync Randomized Clinical Evaluation. Cardiac resynchronization in chronic heart failure. *N Engl J Med* 346:1845-1853, 2002.
20. Cazeau S, Leclercq C, Lavergne T, et al: Effects of multisite biventricular pacing in patients with heart failure and intraventricular conduction delay. *N Engl J Med* 344:873-880, 2001.
21. Shamim W, Francis DP, Yousufuddin M, et al: Intraventricular conduction delay: a prognostic marker in chronic heart failure. *Int J Cardiol* 70:171-178, 1999.
22. St John Sutton M, Lee D, Rouleau JL, et al: Left ventricular remodeling and ventricular arrhythmias after myocardial infarction. *Circulation* 107:2577-2582, 2003.
23. Redfield MM, Jacobsen SJ, Burnett JC Jr, et al: Burden of systolic and diastolic ventricular dysfunction in the community: Appreciating the scope of the heart failure epidemic. *JAMA* 289:194-202, 2003.
24. Nagueh SF, Middleton KJ, Kopelen HA, et al: Doppler tissue imaging: A noninvasive technique for evaluation of left ventricular relaxation and estimation of filling pressures. *J Am Coll Cardiol* 30:1527-1533, 1997.
25. Klein AL, Hatle LK, Taliercio CP, et al: Prognostic significance of Doppler measures of diastolic function in cardiac amyloidosis. A Doppler echocardiography study. *Circulation* 83:808-816, 1991.
26. Forfia PR, Fisher MR, Mathai SC, et al: Tricuspid annular displacement predicts survival in pulmonary hypertension. *Am J Respir Crit Care Med* 174:1034-1041, 2006.
27. Zornoff LA, Skali H, Pfeffer MA, et al: Right ventricular dysfunction and risk of heart failure and mortality after myocardial infarction. *J Am Coll Cardiol* 39:1450-1455, 2002.
28. St John Sutton M, Pfeffer MA, Plappert T, et al: Quantitative two-dimensional echocardiographic measurements are major predictors of adverse cardiovascular events after acute myocardial infarction. The protective effects of captopril. *Circulation* 89:68-75, 1994.
29. Acker MA, Bolling S, Shemin R, et al: Mitral valve surgery in heart failure: Insights from the Acorn clinical trial. *J Thorac Cardiovasc Surg* 132:568-577, 577.e1-577.e4, 2006.
30. Birks EJ, Tansley PD, Hardy J, et al: Left ventricular assist device and drug therapy for the reversal of heart failure. *N Engl J Med* 355:1873-1884, 2006.
31. Reilly MP, Wiegers SE, Cucchiara AJ, et al: Frequency, risk factors, and clinical outcomes of left ventricular assist device-associated ventricular thrombus. *Am J Cardiol* 86:1156-1159, A10, 2000.
32. Kelley ST, Malekan R, Gorman JH 3rd, et al: Restraining infarct expansion preserves left ventricular geometry and function after acute anteroapical infarction. *Circulation* 99:135-142, 1999.
33. Blom AS, Mukherjee R, Pilla JJ, et al: Cardiac support device modifies left ventricular geometry and myocardial structure after myocardial infarction. *Circulation* 112:1274-1283, 2005.
34. Young JB, Abraham WT, Smith AL, et al: Combined cardiac resynchronization and implantable cardioversion defibrillation in advanced chronic heart failure: The MIRACLE ICD Trial. *JAMA* 289:2685-2694, 2003.
35. Bristow MR, Saxon LA, Boehmer J, et al: Cardiac-resynchronization therapy with or without an implantable defibrillator in advanced chronic heart failure. *N Engl J Med* 350:2140-2150, 2004.
36. Cleland JG, Daubert JC, Erdmann E, et al: The effect of cardiac resynchronization on morbidity and mortality in heart failure. *N Engl J Med* 352:1539-1549, 2005.

37. Linde C, Leclercq C, Rex S, et al: Long-term benefits of biventricular pacing in congestive heart failure: Results from the MUltisite STimulation in cardiomyopathy (MUSTIC) study. *J Am Coll Cardiol* 40:111-118, 2002.

38. Molhoek SG, Bax JJ, van Erven L, et al: Comparison of benefits from cardiac resynchronization therapy in patients with ischemic cardiomyopathy versus idiopathic dilated cardiomyopathy. *Am J Cardiol* 93:860-863, 2004.

39. Chuang ML, Hibberd MG, Salton CJ, et al: Importance of imaging method over imaging modality in noninvasive determination of left ventricular volumes and ejection fraction: Assessment by two- and three-dimensional echocardiography and magnetic resonance imaging. *J Am Coll Cardiol* 35:477-484, 2000.

40. Burns RJ, Gibbons RJ, Yi Q, et al: The relationships of left ventricular ejection fraction, end-systolic volume index and infarct size to six-month mortality after hospital discharge following myocardial infarction treated by thrombolysis. *J Am Coll Cardiol* 39:30-36, 2002.

41. Yu CM, Chau E, Sanderson JE, et al: Tissue Doppler echocardiographic evidence of reverse remodeling and improved synchronicity by simultaneously delaying regional contraction after biventricular pacing therapy in heart failure. *Circulation* 105:438-445, 2002.

42. Kanzaki H, Bazaz R, Schwartzman D, et al: A mechanism for immediate reduction in mitral regurgitation after cardiac resynchronization therapy: insights from mechanical activation strain mapping. *J Am Coll Cardiol* 44:1619-1625, 2004.

43. St John Sutton MG, Plappert T, Abraham WT, et al: Effect of cardiac resynchronization therapy on left ventricular size and function in chronic heart failure. *Circulation* 107:1985-1990, 2003.

44. Sutton MG, Plappert T, Hilpisch KE, et al: Sustained reverse left ventricular structural remodeling with cardiac resynchronization at one year is a function of etiology: Quantitative Doppler echocardiographic evidence from the Multicenter InSync Randomized Clinical Evaluation (MIRACLE). *Circulation* 113:266-272, 2006.

45. Bax JJ, Abraham T, Barold SS, et al: Cardiac resynchronization therapy: Part 1—issues before device implantation. *J Am Coll Cardiol* 46:2153-2167, 2005.

46. Bax JJ, Abraham T, Barold SS, et al: Cardiac resynchronization therapy: Part 2—issues during and after device implantation and unresolved questions. *J Am Coll Cardiol* 46:2168-2182, 2005.

47. Pitzalis MV, Iacoviello M, Romito R, et al: Ventricular asynchrony predicts a better outcome in patients with chronic heart failure receiving cardiac resynchronization therapy. *J Am Coll Cardiol* 45:65-69, 2005.

48. Bhatia SJ, Kirshenbaum JM, Shemin RJ, et al: Time course of resolution of pulmonary hypertension and right ventricular remodeling after orthotopic cardiac transplantation. *Circulation* 76:819-826, 1987.

Chapter 28

Echocardiography in the Evaluation and Management of Patients with Hypertrophic Cardiomyopathy

ANNA WOO, MD • E. DOUGLAS WIGLE, MD • HARRY RAKOWSKI, MD

Hypertrophic cardiomyopathy (HCM) has unique clinical, echocardiographic, and hemodynamic features.[1] Since the modern description of HCM five decades ago,[2,3] there have been significant advances in its diagnosis, the understanding of its complex pathophysiology, and the evolution of its management.[1] HCM is defined as a hypertrophied, nondilated left ventricle (LV) in the absence of another cardiac or systemic disease that is capable of producing the magnitude of wall thickening[4] (Fig. 28–1). Echocardiography has played a crucial role in determining the pathophysiology of HCM, quantitating its morphologic and hemodynamic severity, and assessing the acute and chronic responses to various therapies.[5]

Echocardiographic studies have also provided invaluable insight into the epidemiology,[6] inheritance,[7] and prognosis[8] of HCM. The ability to perform serial

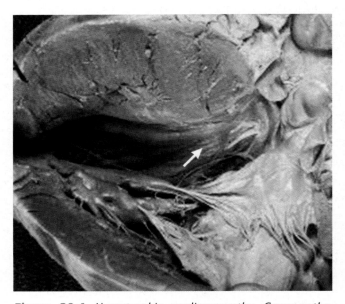

Figure 28–1. Hypertrophic cardiomyopathy. Gross pathologic specimen of the heart from a patient with hypertrophic cardiomyopathy and left ventricular outflow tract obstruction who died suddenly. Note the asymmetric hypertrophy with a markedly thickened interventricular septum and the narrow outflow tract between the basal septum and anterior mitral leaflet, which is thickened and fibrosed from repeated mitral leaflet-septal contact (arrow).

noninvasive studies makes echocardiography the modality of choice in the screening,[7,9] diagnosis,[4] and serial monitoring of patients with this condition. In recent years, the role of echocardiography in this disorder has extended to intraprocedural decision making, with the use of intraoperative transesophageal echocardiography (TEE) during surgical myectomy[10] and the application of myocardial contrast echocardiography (MCE) in the guidance of septal ethanol ablation.[11,12]

Epidemiology

HCM was initially felt to be a rare disorder affecting young adults.[3] However, modern studies using echocardiography in the evaluation of subjects suggest a much higher prevalence of this condition. The Coronary Artery Risk Development in Adults (CARDIA) study, a prospective study of 4111 apparently healthy young adults from a general population, detected HCM by echocardiographic examination in 0.17% of subjects.[6] There was a similar prevalence of HCM in a large study of 33,735 young athletes undergoing preparticipation medical screening in Italy, with a total of 22 cases (0.07%) identified from this cohort.[9] The reported incidence of HCM has ranged from an incidence of 0.4/100,000 person-years from 1980 to 1981 in Western Denmark[13] to 2.5/100,000 person-years between the years 1975 and 1984 in Olmsted County, Minnesota.[14] Recent studies of the incidence of HCM in children have reported an annual incidence of 0.42/100,000 in the United States[15] and 0.32/100,000 children in Australia.[16]

Molecular Genetics

HCM is a genetic disorder with an autosomal dominant pattern of inheritance. This condition is felt to arise from a genetic defect involving one of the genes encoding proteins of the cardiac sarcomeric apparatus[17,18]: (1) β-myosin heavy chain (MYH7), (2) myosin binding protein C (MYBPC3), (3) troponin T (TNNT2), (4) troponin I (TNNI3), (5) α-tropomyosin (TPM1), (6) ventricular myosin regulatory light chain (MYL2), (7) ventricular myosin essential light chain (MYL3), (8) α-cardiac actin (ACTC), (9) α-myosin heavy chain (MYH6), or (10) titin (TTN). The initial genetic defect was described in the late 1980s.[19] Since then, more than 400 different mutations have been associated with HCM.[4]

The extent to which the underlying genotype influences the phenotype of this condition remains unclear. Some studies have suggested that patients with MYH7 mutations have a greater degree and an earlier onset of hypertrophy compared to patients with non-MYH7 defects.[20,21] No significant differences were found in the degree of hypertrophy among patients with different mutations of the MYH7 gene.[22,23] In contrast, mutations of the MYBPC gene have been associated with delayed penetrance.[20,24] However, one large study found no difference in the degree or onset of hypertrophy when comparing patients with mutations involving the thick filament, thin filament, or MYBPC genes.[25]

Diagnosis

Diagnostic Criteria

The diagnosis of HCM is based on the demonstration of left ventricular hypertrophy (LVH) in the absence of other causes, such as systemic hypertension or aortic stenosis (AS)[4] (Fig. 28–2). M-mode echocardiography assumed an early role in the diagnosis of HCM.[26,27] The echocardiographic finding of asymmetric septal hypertrophy (ASH),

defined as a septal to posterior wall thickness ratio of greater than or equal to 1.3, is strongly associated with HCM[28] (Fig. 28–3). The septum is typically at least 15 mm in thickness.[1,28,29] Other findings associated with obstructive HCM, such as systolic anterior motion (SAM),[26] have been detected in other conditions and are not considered pathognomonic for HCM.[29] The diagnosis of HCM is made in children when left ventricular wall measurements are more than two standard deviations above the mean (corrected for age and body surface area).[30] Approximately 25% of patients have obstructive HCM, which has traditionally been defined as a left ventricular outflow tract (LVOT) gradient of at least 30 mm Hg.[31]

Family Screening for Hypertrophic Cardiomyopathy

The first-degree relatives of patients with HCM should be screened for this condition.[1,32] Screening methods for family members include a history and physical examination, 12-lead electrocardiography, and echocardiography. Echocardiography is the most widely ac-

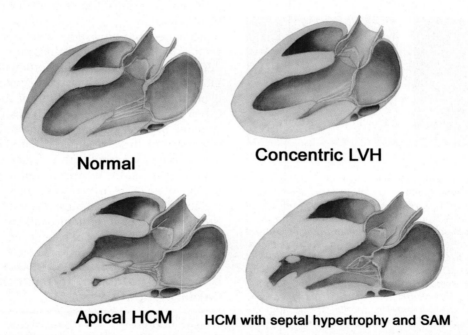

Normal   **Concentric LVH**

Apical HCM   **HCM with septal hypertrophy and SAM**

Figure 28–2. Diagrammatic representation of the various forms of left ventricular hypertrophy, as viewed from sagittal sections of the heart. These cross-sectional images would be analogous to the images obtained in the transthoracic parasternal long-axis views. Upper left panel, Normal wall thickness in a normal subject. The left ventricular and left atrial cavity sizes are normal. Upper right panel, Concentric pattern of left ventricular hypertrophy (LVH) with similar increases in the wall thickness of the interventricular septum and the left ventricular free wall. The left ventricular cavity is small. This is the predominant form of hypertrophy in patients with systemic hypertension or valvular aortic stenosis. Lower left panel, In contrast, patients with apical hypertrophic cardiomyopathy have hypertrophy predominantly of the apical segments. Note that the basal interventricular septum is spared from hypertrophy and the distal left ventricular cavity is small. Patients with apical hypertrophic cardiomyopathy have near obliteration of the distal left ventricular cavity during systole. Lower right panel, The more common form of hypertrophic cardiomyopathy involves asymmetric hypertrophy of the interventricular septum. The left ventricular free wall is normal or minimally thickened. Patients with the obstructive form of hypertrophic cardiomyopathy typically have a narrow left ventricular outflow tract, an anteriorly displaced mitral apparatus, and systolic anterior motion of the anterior mitral leaflet. HCM, hypertrophic cardiomyopathy; SAM, systolic anterior motion.

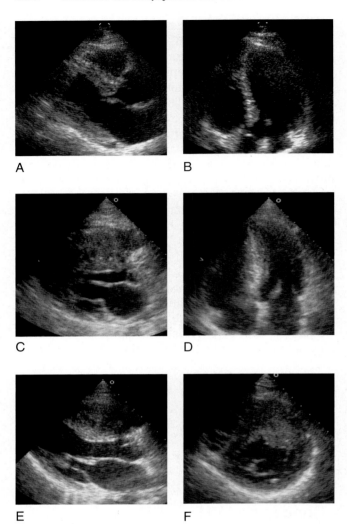

Figure 28–3. Spectrum of asymmetric septal hypertrophy in three patients with hypertrophic cardiomyopathy. Two-dimensional echocardiographic parasternal long-axis (A) and apical four-chamber (B) views from a 30-year-old patient with focal hypertrophy of the basal septum. The basal anterior septum measured 15 mm, whereas all other left ventricular wall segments were normal in thickness. Parasternal long-axis (C) and apical four-chamber (D) views of a 36-year-old patient with massive septal hypertrophy (maximal thickness of 35 mm) involving the entire interventricular septum (from base to apex). There was no systolic anterior motion or left ventricular outflow tract gradient at rest. Parasternal long-axis (E) and parasternal short-axis (basal level) (F) views of a 25-year-old woman with nonobstructive hypertrophic cardiomyopathy. The septal hypertrophy involved the basal and midventricular levels and extended to the anterior wall. Maximal wall thickness was 32 mm at the basal anterior wall.

cepted screening test for HCM. Genetic testing is not widely available and is generally limited to research laboratories.[1] Screening for HCM is recommended by at least 12 years of age (or earlier if a child is symptomatic, engaged in competitive sports, or has a malignant family history of premature death attributed to HCM).[32] Serial evaluations are then performed every 12 to 18 months until physical maturity is achieved (generally between ages 18 to 21). Because HCM may present

in late adulthood, screening is recommended at 5-year intervals during adulthood.[32]

Genetic studies have demonstrated that genotype-positive subjects may have minimal or no hypertrophy evident on echocardiography.[20,23,24,32] Recent studies have shown that tissue Doppler imaging (TDI) is a reliable method for the early detection of patients who are genotype positive before the onset of hypertrophy.[33,34] Reduced systolic and diastolic tissue Doppler velocities have a high sensitivity and high specificity in identifying mutation carriers (Table 28–1). Moreover, serial echocardiographic assessments of patients who are genotype-positive and initially phenotype-negative showed further reductions in tissue Doppler velocities and the development of hypertrophy during subsequent follow-up.[35]

Differential Diagnosis

Other Causes of Increased Wall Thickness

There are multiple potential other causes for the echocardiographic abnormalities seen in HCM[36,37] (Table 28–2). HCM caused by a genetic defect of the cardiac sarcomeric proteins needs to be distinguished from one of the congenital malformations or syndromes (e.g., Noonan's, LEOPARD syndrome). Disproportionate hypertrophy of the ventricular septum may occur with right ventricular hypertrophy and D-transposition of the great arteries.[38] Other nongenetic causes of LVH include athlete's heart, systemic hypertension, and aortic stenosis. Hypertrophy secondary to these disorders is usually concentric but may also be associated with a degree of focal septal hypertrophy or SAM.[29] Increased wall thickness not attributable to myocyte hypertrophy may be secondary to metabolic disorders (storage diseases or hypothyroidism[39]) or infiltrative cardiomyopathies[40] (Fig. 28–4). The increased wall thickness of patients with metabolic disor-

TABLE 28-1. Test Characteristics of Tissue Doppler Findings in Hypertrophic Cardiomyopathy

Tissue Doppler	Sensitivity	Specificity
S_a (lateral) < 13 cm/s	100%	93%
S_a (septal) < 12 cm/s	100%	90%
E_a (lateral) < 14 cm/s	100%	90%
E_a (septal) < 13 cm/s	100%	90%
Average E_a (from 4 corners) ≤ 13.5 cm/s	75%	86%
Average E_a < 15 cm/s + EF ≥ 68%	44%	100%

E_a, tissue Doppler early diastolic velocity; EF, ejection fraction; S_a, tissue Doppler systolic velocity.
Data in rows 1-4 from reference 33* and rows 5-6 from reference 34.**

TABLE 28–2. Differential Diagnosis of Hypertrophic Cardiomyopathy on Echocardiography

Syndromic Hypertrophic Cardiomyopathy
Noonan's syndrome
LEOPARD syndrome
Friedreich's ataxia

Disproportionate Ventricular Septal Hypertrophy
Right ventricular hypertrophy
D-transposition of the great arteries

Other Causes of Left Ventricular Hypertrophy
Athlete's heart
Systemic hypertension
Aortic valve stenosis (and fixed subvalvular and
   supravalvular stenosis)

Metabolic Disease
Fabry's disease
Glycogen storage disease
Mucopolysaccharide storage disorders
Hypothyroidism

Infiltrative Cardiomyopathy
Amyloidosis
Sarcoidosis

LEOPARD stands for Lentigines, ECG abnormalities, Ocular hypertelorism, Pulmonary stenosis, Abnormal genitalia, Retardation of growth, Deafness.

ders or infiltrative cardiomyopathies typically occurs in a concentric pattern but may occasionally manifest as disproportionate septal thickening.

Storage Diseases

Storage diseases should be considered in the work-up of patients with unexplained increased left ventricular wall thickness. Fabry's disease was detected in 7 out of 230 patients with LVH (3% prevalence). All of these patients had a concentric pattern of LVH.[41] In male patients with the diagnosis of HCM, Fabry's disease was detected in 6% of patients diagnosed at greater than or equal to 40 years and in 1% diagnosed at less than 40 years.[42] The pattern of hypertrophy was concentric in five patients and asymmetric in one patient.

Glycogen storage diseases may also mimic HCM. Mutations of the AMP-protein kinase γ_2 (PRKAG2) gene cause a glycogen storage cardiomyopathy, mutations of the lysosome-associated membrane protein 2 (LAMP2) gene cause Danon's disease, and mutations of the acid α-1,4-glucosidase gene cause Pompe's disease.[43] In a cohort of 75 patients with unexplained hypertrophy, 40 patients (53%) were identified with sarcomeric protein gene defects, 1 patient (1%) had a PRKAG2 defect, and 2 patients (3%) had LAMP2 muta-

tions.[43] In another cohort of 24 patients with increased wall thickness and ventricular preexcitation, mutations of the PRKAG2 and LAMP2 genes were detected in 7 (29%) and 4 (17%) patients, respectively. None of these patients had the genetic defects causing Fabry's or Pompe's disease.[43] Finally, a recent study of 1862 subjects from the Framingham Heart Study (of which 50 subjects had unexplained hypertrophy) identified sarcomere protein or storage disease gene mutations in 0.5% of the cohort: eight patients had mutations of the sarcomeric proteins, and one patient had a mutation of the α-galactosidase gene (causing Fabry's disease).[44]

Athlete's Heart

The clinical and echocardiographic differentiation between HCM and athlete's heart may be difficult.[45,46] The left ventricular wall thickness may be greater than or equal to 13 mm (up to 15 to 16 mm) in 2% of elite athletes, raising the possibility of underlying HCM. The left ventricular end-diastolic cavity may be enlarged (>55 mm) in more than one third of elite athletes.[45] The diagnosis of HCM is favored over the diagnosis of athlete's heart in the presence of the following: (1) a family history of HCM, (2) bizarre electrocardiographic patterns, (3) asymmetric hypertrophy (or other unusual pattern of LVH), (4) a small left ventricular cavity size (<45 mm), (5) left atrial enlargement, and (6) an abnormal left ventricular filling pattern.[46] Finally, deconditioning may assist in the differentiation of athlete's heart versus HCM: Deconditioning may lead to significant reductions in wall thickness and cavity size in athlete's heart.[47,48] The distinction between athlete's heart and pathologic hypertrophy may be less of an issue in women because the left ventricular wall thickness of elite female athletes is in the range of 6 to 12 mm, which does not exceed normal age-adjusted limits for wall thickness.[49]

Septal Hypertrophy in the Elderly

It may be difficult to distinguish between elderly patients with HCM and those with hypertensive heart disease.[50] Elderly subjects may develop a sigmoid-shaped septum as an age-related phenomenon.[51] Terms that have been used to describe this finding are sigmoid septum, septal bulge, or discrete upper septal hypertrophy. It is controversial whether this finding should be considered a subtype of HCM or whether it represents a benign anatomic variant.[52,53] Other findings on echocardiographic examination that are more compatible with a septal bulge rather than HCM of the elderly include focal hypertrophy limited to less than 3 cm length of the basal anterior septum, protrusion of the focal hypertrophy into the LVOT, a normal left ventricular end-diastolic diameter, and the absence of other characteristic echocardiographic findings of HCM.[52] Echocardiographic and clinical features of HCM in the elderly are discussed in this chapter.

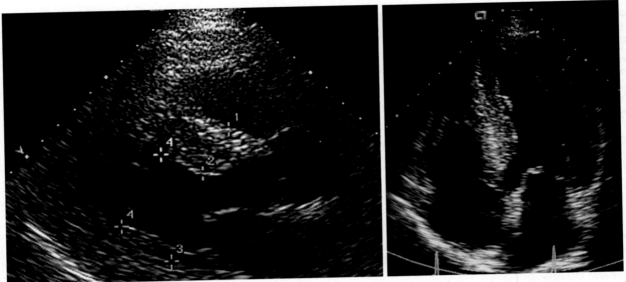

Figure 28–4. Two-dimensional echocardiographic parasternal long-axis (left) *and apical four-chamber* (right) *views from a 55-year-old man referred for evaluation of suspected hypertrophic cardiomyopathy. Echocardiographic evaluation revealed a diffuse increase in left ventricular wall thickness: The basal anterior septum measured 23 mm, and the posterior wall measured 20 mm. There was no systolic anterior motion or left ventricular outflow tract obstruction. Additional investigations showed mild renal insufficiency and a low α-galactosidase level. Endomyocardial biopsy confirmed the diagnosis of Fabry's disease.*

Evaluation by Echocardiography

Left Ventricular Hypertrophy: Severity, Distribution, and Patterns of Hypertrophy

Two-dimensional (2D) echocardiography greatly increased the ability to detect the full extent, distribution, and severity of myocardial hypertrophy.[54-56] Comprehensive echocardiographic assessment requires imaging of the LV from several transthoracic windows, including the parasternal long-axis view, serial parasternal short-axis views, and the apical windows (Fig. 28–5). Measurements of the wall segments are obtained from cross-sectional parasternal short-axis views and are made at three levels: basal (at the level of the mitral valve), midventricular level (at the level of the papillary muscles), and apical.[5] A 10-point scoring system to quantify the extent of left ventricular hypertrophy in HCM has been developed[56,57] (Table 28–3).

HCM has also been classified into four morphologic subtypes[55] (Table 28–4). A minority of patients had involvement of the anterior septum alone (type I). Panseptal hypertrophy, with involvement of both the anterior and posterior septum, was detected in 20% of patients (type II). More than half of the patients with HCM had extension of hypertrophy to the anterolateral wall (type III). All other patterns of hypertrophy (type IV), such as isolated posteroseptal, apical septal, or lone anterolateral wall involvement, constituted 18% of the study cohort.

Technical Factors and Echocardiographic Pitfalls

Echocardiographic studies have demonstrated changes in the acoustic texture of the myocardium in patients with HCM.[54,58] There may be increased ultrasonic reflectivity of the left ventricular walls, especially the interventricular septum. Diffuse bright echoes may be seen throughout the myocardium and may give a ground-glass appearance.

There are other important technical considerations in the echocardiographic assessment of HCM.[36] Oblique cuts of the LV can spuriously produce the appearance of asymmetric septal hypertrophy and overestimate wall thickness.[59] 2D echocardiographic studies have demonstrated that hypertrophy can be quite localized or eccentric in distribution.[5,60] More atypical forms of HCM, such as isolated lateral wall hypertrophy or asymmetric apical hypertrophy, may be missed from standard parasternal long-axis views because the septum and anterior wall appear normal in thickness and there is no systolic anterior motion of the mitral valve. The diagnosis of apical HCM by echocardiography may be missed in patients with difficult or subop-

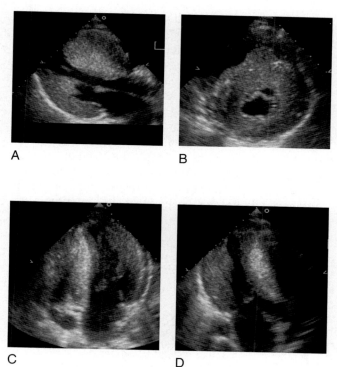

Figure 28–5. *Optimal echocardiographic evaluation of the degree, extent, and distribution of hypertrophy in hypertrophic cardiomyopathy requires imaging from multiple transthoracic windows. Parasternal long-axis view (A), parasternal short-axis view at the basal level (B), apical four-chamber view (C), and apical long-axis view (D) in an 18-year-old patient with hypertrophic cardiomyopathy and left ventricular outflow tract obstruction. Massive hypertrophy was detected with a maximal septal thickness of 34 mm, extension of hypertrophy to the apical level, and anterolateral wall involvement. The patient had New York Heart Association Class III symptoms, severe systolic anterior motion (D), and a resting left ventricular outflow tract gradient of 107 mm Hg and was referred for surgical myectomy.*

timal apical windows or if the apical segments are foreshortened.

Left Ventricular Outflow Tract Obstruction

Pathophysiology of Left Ventricular Outflow Tract Obstruction

M-mode echocardiographic studies demonstrated narrowing of the LVOT,[61] SAM of the mitral valve,[26,29] midsystolic notching of the aortic valve[62] and established the important role of echocardiography in the assessment of LVOT obstruction in patients with HCM.[63] Advances in 2D echocardiography and Doppler techniques provide additional insights into the mechanisms responsible for dynamic outflow tract obstruction[5] as

TABLE 28–3. Extent of Hypertrophy according to Echocardiographic Point Score

Extent of Hypertrophy	Points
Septal Thickness, mm (Basal Third of Septum)	
15-19	1
20-24	2
25-29	3
>30	4
Extension to papillary muscles (basal two thirds of septum)	2
Extension to apex (total septal involvement)	2
Anterolateral wall extension	2
Maximum total	10

From Wigle ED, Sasson Z, Henderson M, et al: *Prog Cardiovasc Dis* 28:1-83, 1985.

TABLE 28–4. Morphological Classification of Hypertrophic Cardiomyopathy

Maron Type	Distribution of Hypertrophy	Percentage of Cases
I	Isolated anterior septum	10
II	Panseptal (anterior and posterior septum) without free wall involvement	20
III	Septum and anterolateral free wall	52
IV	Regions other than basal anterior septum	18

From Maron BJ, Gottdiener JS, Epstein SE: *Am J Cardiol* 48:418-428, 1981. With permission from Excerpta Medica Inc.

summarized in Table 28–5. Morphologic features of HCM that contribute to LVOT obstruction include narrowing of the outflow tract by ventricular septal hypertrophy,[64] intrinsic abnormalities of the mitral leaflets,[65-67] anterior displacement of the mitral apparatus,[54,63,65] and anterior malposition of the papillary muscles.[68]

There is a close relationship between the extent of LVH and the presence of LVOT obstruction. Resting LVOT obstruction is associated with a higher hypertrophy point score.[57] The mitral leaflets in HCM are typically elongated.[66] These mitral leaflets coapt abnormally in the body of the leaflets, rather than at the tip.[65,66] Patients with enlarged mitral valves have typical SAM, characterized by the presence of a sharp,

TABLE 28-5. Factors Contributing to Dynamic Left Ventricular Outflow Tract Obstruction

Narrowing of Left Ventricular Outflow Tract
Septal hypertrophy
Anterior displacement of mitral apparatus
Anterior displacement of papillary muscles

Hydrodynamic Forces (Venturi and Drag Forces) Causing Systolic Anterior Motion
Rapid early left ventricular ejection
Elongated mitral leaflets

right-angled bend of the distal half of the anterior mitral leaflet and contact of the distal and central portions of the anterior mitral leaflet with the septum. In contrast, patients with normal-sized mitral valves have atypical SAM, involving greater portions of the body of the anterior mitral leaflet and related chordae tendineae and with little bending of the anterior mitral leaflet.[67] The degree of anterior displacement of the mitral apparatus has been related to the degree of obstruction.[54,63,65] Furthermore, in HCM, the papillary muscle tips are displaced anteriorly and toward one another. This results in a decrease in the relative tension on the chordae tendineae to the body of the anterior mitral

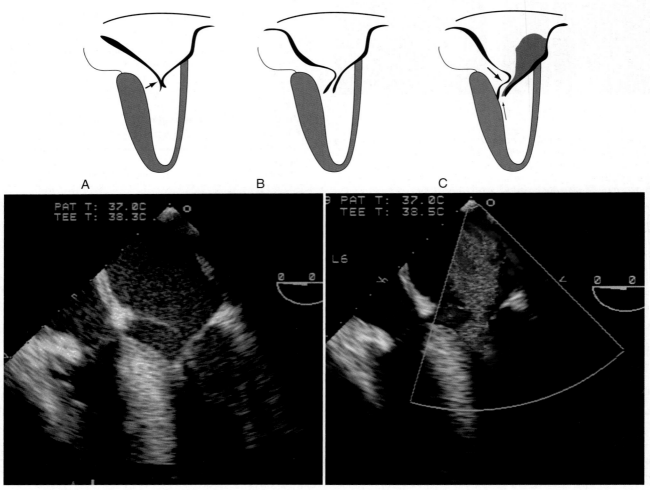

Figure 28–6. *Schematic diagram of a transesophageal echocardiogram (frontal long-axis plane) demonstrating the anterior and basal motion of the anterior mitral leaflet leading to leaflet-septal contact and failure of leaflet coaptation in mid-systole. At the onset of systole (A), the coaptation point (thick arrow) is in the body of the mitral leaflets. During early systole (B) and midsystole (C), there is anterior and basal movement of the residual length of the anterior mitral leaflet (thick arrow) with septal contact and failure of leaflet coaptation. The interleaflet gap (thin arrow) results in a posteriorly directed jet of mitral regurgitation into the left atrial cavity (purple area). Corresponding two-dimensional transesophageal views (D and E) with color flow imaging in a patient with obstructive hypertrophic cardiomyopathy show septal hypertrophy, anterior motion of the anterior mitral leaflet, and color turbulence in the outflow tract with the posteriorly directed mitral regurgitation. (A to C from Grigg LE, Wigle ED, Williams WG, et al: J Am Coll Cardiol 20:42-52, 1990. Reprinted with permission from the American College of Cardiology.)*

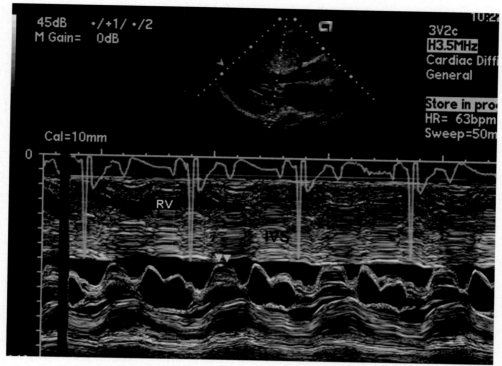

Figure 28–7. *M-mode echocardiographic recording in the parasternal long-axis view obtained at the level of the mitral leaflet tips in a young patient with symptomatic obstructive hypertrophic cardiomyopathy. This tracing demonstrates increased septal thickness, prolonged contact of the anterior mitral leaflet with the septum during systole, and severe systolic anterior motion (double arrowheads). Continuous-wave Doppler assessment of the left ventricular outflow tract revealed a resting left ventricular outflow tract gradient of greater than 100 mm Hg. In addition, the right ventricular cavity is narrowed due to hypertrophy of the septum and the right ventricular free wall. IVS, interventricular septum; RV, right ventricle.*

leaflet, producing relative chordal slack in the central and anterior leaflet portions.[66,69] Reduced chordal tension is more likely when the distance from the papillary muscle tips to the mitral leaflets is decreased by a combination of hypertrophy at the base of the papillary muscles and increased leaflet length.

Mitral Leaflet Systolic Anterior Motion

Although the nature of the hydrodynamic forces on the anterior mitral leaflet remains controversial, it is believed that the anterior leaflet distal to the site of coaptation is subjected to Venturi[54,70] or drag forces.[69] Therefore, SAM occurs, and the tip of the anterior mitral leaflet typically develops a sharp anterior and superior angulation, leading to mitral leaflet-septal contact in early to midsystole (Fig. 28–6). There is a significant relationship between the development of SAM and the onset of the obstructive pressure gradient, which was demonstrated in patients undergoing simultaneous cardiac catheterization and M-mode echocardiographic studies[71] (Fig. 28–7). The presence of mitral leaflet-septal contact occurs almost simultaneously with the onset of the pressure gradient.

M-mode, 2D, and Doppler echocardiography are established noninvasive techniques in the assessment of the degree of LVOT obstruction in patients with HCM. An M-mode echocardiographic study classified the degree of SAM into three categories: (1) mild (SAM septal distance >10 mm), (2) moderate (SAM septal distance <10 mm or brief mitral leaflet-septal contact), and (3) severe (prolonged SAM septal contact, lasting more than 30% of echocardiographic systole).[29] There is a linear relationship between the time of onset of SAM and the severity of LVOT obstruction.[72]

Doppler Assessment of Outflow Tract Obstruction in Hypertrophic Cardiomyopathy

Pulsed-wave (PW) and continuous-wave (CW) Doppler have been used to determine the pressure gradient across the LVOT in patients with HCM. Pulsed-wave Doppler signals can be recorded sequentially from the left ventricular apex to the outflow tract. The peak velocity increases as the sample volume approaches the site of mitral leaflet-septal contact.[5] CW Doppler assessment from an apical approach with the beam directed across the LVOT can be used to determine the peak velocity (V) at the site of obstruction. Patients with outflow tract obstruction have a characteristic spectral profile with an asymmetric leftward concave

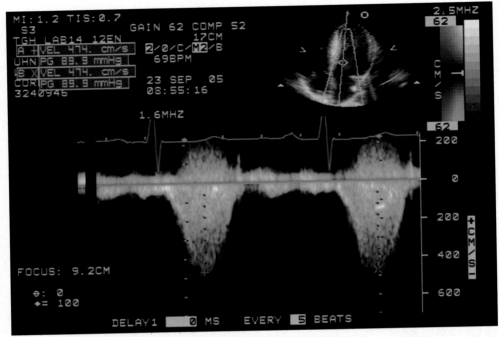

Figure 28–8. Continuous-wave Doppler recordings of the left ventricular outflow tract in a young patient with severely symptomatic obstructive hypertrophic cardiomyopathy. Echocardiographic evaluation revealed severe systolic anterior motion and posteriorly directed mitral regurgitation. The spectral profile has a characteristic dagger-shaped configuration. The peak velocity in the outflow tract is 4.7 m/s, which corresponds to a peak left ventricular outflow tract gradient of 90 mm Hg based on the modified Bernoulli equation.

shape.[73] This results from a relative rapid initial rise in velocity followed by a more gradual increase in the outflow tract velocity to cause a peak in late systole, leading to a dagger-shaped configuration[74] (Fig. 28–8). The peak gradient *(ΔP)* can be estimated using the modified Bernoulli equation:

$$\Delta P = 4V^2$$

There is an excellent correlation between the pressure gradient determined by CW Doppler measurements and by high-fidelity micromanometer recordings during cardiac catheterization.[75] Color flow mapping has been used to characterize the level of obstruction, either in the LVOT or in the midventricle.[76]

Technical Aspects of Doppler Evaluation in Hypertrophic Cardiomyopathy

There are important technical considerations in the performance and interpretation of Doppler studies in patients with HCM. It was not possible to obtain a discernible signal from the LVOT in 16% of patients in one study comparing CW Doppler echocardiography to cardiac catheterization.[73] This inability to acquire a clear spectral display from the outflow tract may be secondary to inadequate transthoracic windows or distortion of left ventricular geometry. In addition, it is imperative to distinguish the high velocity systolic signal coming from the outflow tract from the signal of mitral regurgitation (MR). The spectral profile of MR is characterized by an

earlier onset, a more abrupt initial increase in velocity, and a higher peak velocity than that of an outflow tract signal. Systolic jets with a peak velocity of greater than 5.5 m/s (gradient >120 mm Hg) are most likely secondary to MR rather than LVOT obstruction.[73] Further differentiation of these two jets can be accomplished by orienting the transducer more medially and anteriorly and away from the mitral regurgitant jet. Nevertheless, there may still be contamination of the high-velocity signal of outflow tract obstruction from the jet of MR (Fig. 28–9). This pitfall is particularly more common in patients with concomitant intrinsic mitral valve disease and a more centrally directed jet of MR. Despite optimal imaging, adjustments in instrument settings, and consideration of the differences in the timing and contour of these systolic jets, the distinction between these different Doppler signals may occasionally still be difficult.[77]

Mitral Regurgitation in Hypertrophic Cardiomyopathy

Anterior mitral leaflet-septal contact results in failure of coaptation with the posterior mitral leaflet, creating a funnel-shaped gap through which MR can develop, predominantly in midsystole to late systole.[10] Patients with obstructive HCM and no independent mitral valve disease typically have a posteriorly directed jet of MR.[10,78] MR associated with obstructive HCM has been shown to

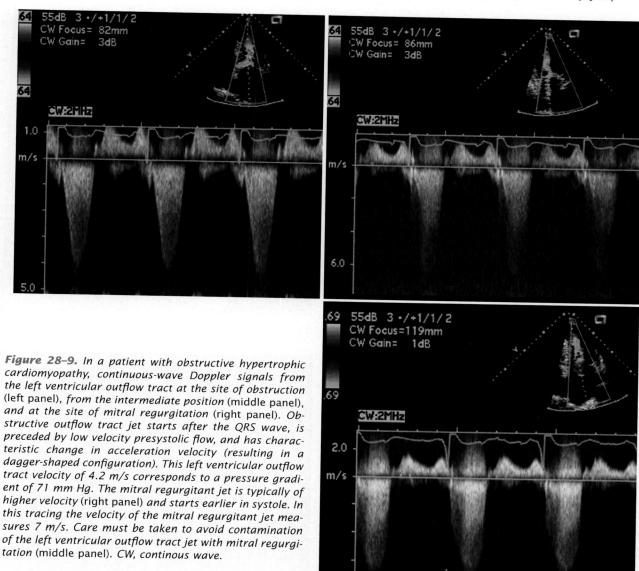

Figure 28–9. *In a patient with obstructive hypertrophic cardiomyopathy, continuous-wave Doppler signals from the left ventricular outflow tract at the site of obstruction* (left panel), *from the intermediate position* (middle panel), *and at the site of mitral regurgitation* (right panel). *Obstructive outflow tract jet starts after the QRS wave, is preceded by low velocity presystolic flow, and has characteristic change in acceleration velocity (resulting in a dagger-shaped configuration). This left ventricular outflow tract velocity of 4.2 m/s corresponds to a pressure gradient of 71 mm Hg. The mitral regurgitant jet is typically of higher velocity* (right panel) *and starts earlier in systole. In this tracing the velocity of the mitral regurgitant jet measures 7 m/s. Care must be taken to avoid contamination of the left ventricular outflow tract jet with mitral regurgitation* (middle panel). *CW, continous wave.*

be related to the degree of anterior leaflet SAM and to the length and mobility of the posterior leaflet, which determine the size of the interleaflet gap and the degree of midsystolic coaptation of the mitral leaflets.[79] These findings were corroborated by an intraoperative TEE study of 104 patients, which demonstrated a significant correlation between the degree of MR, as assessed by color jet area and pulmonary venous flow pattern, and the degree of LVOT obstruction.[78] The presence of a non-posterior jet of MR suggests intrinsic mitral valve leaflet disease independent of SAM.

Independent mitral valve lesions can be identified by echocardiography and are usually related to mitral valve prolapse, ruptured chordae, mitral annular calcification, anomalous insertion of a papillary muscle into the anterior mitral leaflet,[80] or leaflet trauma. Repeated mitral leaflet-septal contact is associated with fibrosis

and thickening of the anterior mitral leaflet (and with subaortic septal endocardial fibrosis and thickening, previously described as a septal "callus").[54] Myectomy alone is generally successful in relieving posteriorly directed MR, without the requirement for associated mitral valve replacement.[78]

Atypical Forms of Hypertrophic Cardiomyopathy

Asymmetric Apical Hypertrophic Cardiomyopathy

Asymmetric apical HCM was initially reported by Japanese investigators in the 1970s.[81,82] This unusual variant of HCM has subsequently been described in

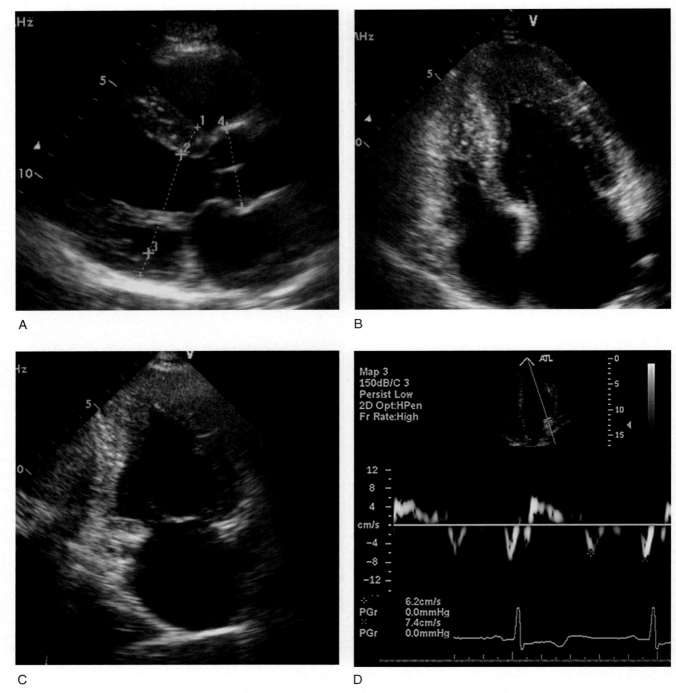

Figure 28–10. *Two-dimensional echocardiographic and tissue Doppler recordings from two patients with asymmetric apical hypertrophic cardiomyopathy. A, Parasternal long-axis view demonstrating minimal hypertrophy of the basal septal and posterior wall segments (13 mm and 11 mm, respectively). B and C, Apical four-chamber and apical two-chamber views show increased thickness of the apical segments (apicoseptal, apicolateral, apicoanterior, and apicoinferior walls) and spade-shaped configuration of the left ventricle at end-diastole. D, Tissue Doppler tracing from the lateral corner of the mitral annulus in a different patient with apical hypertrophic cardiomyopathy demonstrates reduced tissue Doppler early diastolic velocities (Ea), consistent with impaired left ventricular relaxation and increased left ventricular filling pressures.*

non-Asian populations.[83] The striking features of patients with apical hypertrophy include the presence of giant negative T waves (≥10 mm) in the precordial electrocardiographic leads and an "ace of spades" configuration to the left ventricle (Fig. 28–10). The

diagnosis may be missed if acoustic windows are suboptimal and endocardial definition is poor. Contrast echocardiography may be useful in identifying cases of apical hypertrophy.[84] Echocardiography plays an important role in the assessment of the degree and extent of hypertrophy at the apex and the development of such complications as impaired diastolic filling, apical infarction and aneurysm formation (which may result in ventricular tachycardia), and left atrial enlargement (which predisposes to atrial fibrillation). The long-term prognosis of patients with apical HCM is generally excellent.[83]

Midventricular Obstruction

The midventricular form of obstructive HCM, initially described in 1976,[85] is an uncommon variant of this condition. The features of this condition include an hourglass-shaped left ventricular cavity, midventricular obliteration in systole, a distinct apical chamber, color turbulence at the midventricle, and a systolic pressure gradient at the midventricular level[56,76,86] (Fig. 28–11). The combination of color flow mapping, PW, and CW Doppler techniques are useful in localizing the level and severity of obstruction.[76]

Latent Obstructive Hypertrophic Cardiomyopathy

The LVOT obstruction of HCM is dynamic and may be quite variable. Some patients may have latent (or provocable) LVOT obstruction, defined as a resting LVOT gradient less than 30 mm Hg and a provocable LVOT gradient of at least 30 mm Hg. The echocardiographic features of patients with latent LVOT obstruction include a proximal septal bulge, a narrow LVOT diameter (not greater than 2 cm), and a more oblique angle (≥35 degrees) between the ejection flow and the mitral valve.[87] The evaluation of patients with latent LVOT obstruction has traditionally involved performing provocative maneuvers in the cardiac catheterization laboratory (e.g., amyl nitrite inhalation, following a premature ventricular beat, isoproterenol infusion).[56] In the echocardiography laboratory, a provocable LVOT gradient can be elicited following a Valsalva maneuver, amyl nitrite inhalation, upright or supine exercise, or dobutamine infusion.[1,5] Exercise echocardiography can be performed safely in patients with HCM: major complications occurred in only 1 out of 263 patients (0.4%) undergoing treadmill exercise testing.[88] The magnitude of the pressure gradient has been shown to increase almost twofold with upright bicycle exercise.[89] The outflow tract gradients obtained after exercise may be different from those measured after amyl nitrite inhalation and may more accurately reflect patients' symptoms.[90]

Hypertrophic Cardiomyopathy of the Elderly

HCM of the elderly is a subset of this condition with some distinguishing clinical and echocardiographic features.[91,92] The pattern of hypertrophy tends to be focal and localized to the basal anterior or posterior interventricular septum.[93] Elderly patients with HCM tend to have a milder degree of hypertrophy. The shape

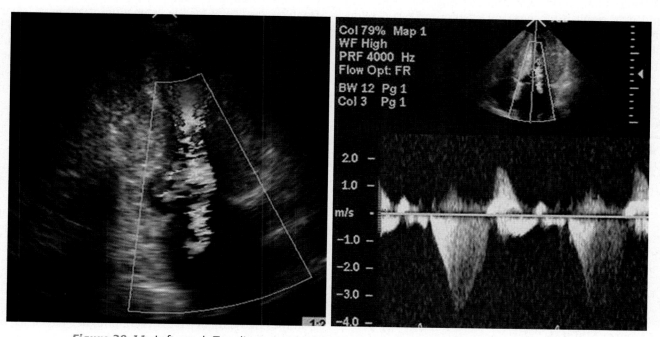

Figure 28–11. Left panel, *Two-dimensional echocardiographic apical two-chamber view with color-Doppler imaging in a patient with hypertrophic cardiomyopathy and midventricular obstruction. There is color turbulence in the midventricular region and a small apical cavity during systole.* Right panel, *Continuous-wave Doppler recording through the area of color turbulence in the midventricular region shows a Doppler spectral pattern similar to that obtained with left ventricular outflow tract obstruction. In this example, the midventricular velocity measures 3.6 m/s, corresponding to a midventricular gradient of 52 mm Hg.*

of the left ventricular cavity in elderly patients is typically ovoid with normal septal curvature. In contrast, younger patients tend to have a crescent-shaped left ventricular cavity and an abnormal convexity to the septum characterized as a reversal of septal curvature.[94] Concomitant mitral annular calcification is a common feature of HCM in the elderly.[95]

The mechanisms leading to LVOT obstruction in HCM of the elderly are different from those seen in younger patients. Elderly patients have a relatively small heart and distorted geometry of the LVOT.[96] Mitral annular calcification results in anterior displacement of the mitral apparatus, narrowing of the outflow tract, and less angulation of the mitral leaflets. Outflow tract obstruction, either at rest or with provocation, is associated with the majority of patients with HCM of the elderly.[94] Furthermore, the presence of mitral annular calcification distorts the mitral annulus and may lead to an independent jet of MR, which is often centrally directed and distinct from the posteriorly directed mitral regurgitant jet caused by systolic anterior motion.

Evaluation of Diastolic Function in Hypertrophic Cardiomyopathy

Factors Contributing to Impaired Diastolic Function in Hypertrophic Cardiomyopathy

Diastolic filling of the left ventricle is impaired in HCM and may result in dyspnea on exertion, elevated filling pressures, and progressive left atrial enlargement. Table 28–6 outlines the factors that contribute to diastolic filling in HCM.[5,56,97] Impaired relaxation of the left ventricle

TABLE 28–6. Factors Affecting Diastolic Function in Hypertrophic Cardiomyopathy

Relaxation
Loads
  Contraction load
    Subaortic stenosis
  Relaxation loads
    Late systolic loading
    End-systolic deformation (restoring forces)
    Coronary filling
    Ventricular filling
Inactivation
  Myocardial calcium overload
Nonuniformity of load and inactivation (nonuniformity of contraction and relaxation)

Chamber Stiffness
Myocardial mass
Left ventricular volume
Myocardial stiffness (fibrosis)

Adapted from Wigle ED, Sasson Z, Henderson M, et al: *Prog Cardiovasc Dis* 28:1-83, 1985; Rakowski H, Sasson Z, Wigle ED: *J Am Soc Echocardiogr* 1:31-47, 1988.

is secondary to increased contraction load, decreased relaxation loads, decreased inactivation, and increased nonuniformity.[56] The early contraction load of outflow tract obstruction impairs and delays the onset of relaxation. The major relaxation loads, coronary and ventricular filling, are decreased. Calcium overload secondary to hypertrophy or ischemia leads to myofibril inactivation of actin-myosin cross-bridges. Relaxation is further impaired by the nonuniformity of load and inactivation in different segments of the LV. Chamber stiffness is directly proportional to the myocardial mass and the degree of myocardial fibrosis and is inversely proportional to the left ventricular chamber volume.[56]

Techniques for the Assessment of Diastolic Function

Impaired left ventricular relaxation is the predominant diastolic abnormality identified in patients with HCM.[98] The mitral inflow pattern typically demonstrates a prolonged isovolumic relaxation time (IVRT), reduced early rapid filling (E), a prolonged deceleration time (DT), and increased atrial filling (A). However, mitral inflow and pulmonary venous flow assessments may not be sensitive for the detection of elevated filling pressures.[99,100] Unlike patients with left ventricular systolic dysfunction, studies of simultaneous echocardiographic and invasive hemodynamic assessments showed no significant correlation between filling pressures and various mitral inflow or pulmonary venous flow parameters.[99,100] Two echocardiographic techniques, color M-mode and tissue Doppler, are useful for the estimation of left ventricular filling pressures in patients with HCM. There is a good correlation between left ventricular filling pressures and the ratios of mitral inflow E velocity/flow propagation velocity (V_P) and mitral inflow E velocity/tissue Doppler early diastolic annular velocity (Ea)[100] (Fig. 28–12).

Tissue Doppler Imaging

In addition to the assessment of left ventricular filling pressures, tissue Doppler can provide important insights in the evaluation of patients with HCM. Reduced tissue Doppler early diastolic velocities have been detected in patients who are genotype-positive without LVH, suggesting that diastolic abnormalities may precede the onset of hypertrophy.[33-35] Early diastolic velocities at the lateral and septal annulus are lower in patients with HCM compared to control subjects.[101] The E/Ea ratio was found to correlate inversely with peak oxygen consumption.[101] Patients with higher left atrial volumes had a higher E/Ea ratio, a higher incidence of diastolic filling abnormalities, and a higher incidence of serious cardiovascular events.[102] In addition, tissue Doppler has been used to monitor the response to invasive therapies. A significant increase in Ea, suggestive of improved left ventricular relaxation, was demonstrated in patients 6 months following septal ethanol

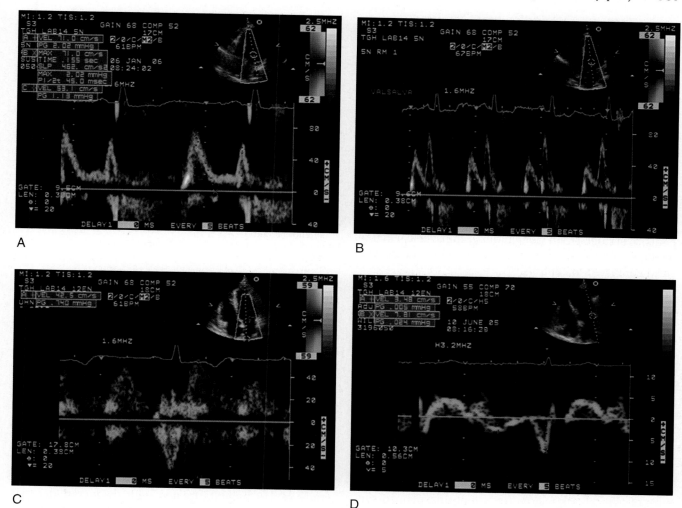

Figure 28–12. *Echocardiographic Doppler evaluation of diastolic function in patients with hypertrophic cardiomyopathy. A, Pulsed-wave Doppler recording at mitral leaflet tip in a patient with hypertrophic cardiomyopathy demonstrates a normal mitral inflow pattern. B, However, following the Valsalva maneuver, impaired left ventricular relaxation is unmasked, consistent with pseudo-normalization of the mitral inflow pattern and abnormal diastolic filling. C, Pulsed-wave Doppler recording from the right upper pulmonary vein of a different patient reveals an increased pulmonary venous A wave (PVa) velocity of 0.43 m/s, compatible with a noncompliant left ventricle. D, Tissue Doppler imaging from the lateral corner of the mitral annulus of a different patient with hypertrophic cardiomyopathy shows a markedly reduced early diastolic velocity, indicative of impaired left ventricular relaxation. The E/Ea ratio of this patient was elevated, which was also suggestive of high left ventricular filling pressures.*

ablation.[103] Similar improvements in diastolic function (as assessed by tissue Doppler and color M-mode Doppler) were demonstrated in patients who underwent septal ethanol ablation or myectomy.[104]

Asynchronous Relaxation in Hypertrophic Cardiomyopathy

The inhomogeneity of relaxation seen in patients with HCM may result in left ventricular intracavitary flow during isovolumic relaxation. Asynchronous relaxation in patients with asymmetric septal hypertrophy leads to earlier relaxation of the apex. Blood flow from the left ventricular base to apex is detected during isovolumic relaxation and has been termed intra-

cavitary *IVRT flow.*[105] In contrast, patients with asymmetric apical HCM may have intracavitary apex-to-base flow, previously described as a paradoxic jet flow, with earlier relaxation of proximal left ventricular segments.[106]

Strain Imaging in Hypertrophic Cardiomyopathy

Myocardial strain imaging allows for the assessment of regional myocardial function. Patients with HCM have reduced myocardial Doppler systolic strain at the ventricular septum.[107] Strain imaging has been shown to be useful in differentiating HCM (nonobstructive form) from hypertensive LVH: One study of 34 patients with LVH (20 patients with biopsy-proven HCM and 14 patients with hypertensive LVH) demonstrated that the septal to posterior wall thickness ratio (>1.3) and systolic strain (ϵ_{sys}) were the two parameters that were useful in distinguishing between these two disorders.[108] The ϵ_{sys} cutoff value of -10.6% discriminated between HCM and hypertensive heart disease with a sensitivity of 85%, specificity of 100%, and predictive accuracy of 91%. The combination of the septal to posterior wall thickness ratio and ϵ_{sys} discriminated HCM from hypertensive heart disease with a predictive accuracy of 96%.[108] These results are supported by observations made with 2D strain. All components of systolic strain (longitudinal, transverse, circumferential, and radial strain) are decreased in patients with HCM compared to controls.[109]

Prognostication by Echocardiography

Echocardiography is increasingly providing important information regarding the long-term prognosis of patients with HCM. Spirito and colleagues determined that the maximal left ventricular wall thickness was an independent risk factor for sudden death.[8] However, other studies have not found the maximum wall thickness either to be associated with cardiovascular mortality[110] or to be a better predictor of sudden death than the presence of clinical risk factors (recurrent unexplained syncope, family history of recurrent early sudden death, nonsustained ventricular tachycardia, and abnormal blood pressure response to exercise).[111] Furthermore, although a wall thickness of greater than or equal to 30 mm was associated with a greater risk of sudden death,[8] the positive predictive accuracy of this echocardiographic finding was low.[111,112] The presence of resting LVOT obstruction has also been associated with increased mortality.[31] Finally, left atrial enlargement has been found to be a significant predictor of atrial fibrillation (AFib) in patients with HCM[113] and of long-term survival in patients following surgical myectomy.[114]

Medical Therapy

Medical management in HCM is optimized by monitoring the response to therapy with serial echocardiographic and Doppler studies[5] (Table 28-7). The three different classes of pharmacologic agents used for the treatment of obstructive HCM are beta-blockers, disopyramide, and calcium channel blockers. The mechanism of benefit of these agents is felt to be a decrease in myocardial contractility, which results in decreased left ventricular ejection velocity, the delayed onset of

TABLE 28-7. Echocardiographic and Doppler Assessment of Effects on Therapy

Decreased or Abolished Obstruction
Decrease in or abolition of SAM
Decreased LVOT velocity
Disappearance of closure systolic aortic valve notching
Decrease in or abolition of mitral regurgitation

Improved Diastolic Function
More rapid time to peak filling
Longer diastasis
Increased LV filling during early diastole
Lower atrial LV filling velocity

LV, left ventricular; LVOT, left ventricular outflow tract; SAM, systolic anterior motion.
Adapted from Rakowski H, Sasson Z, Wigle ED: *J Am Soc Echocardiogr* 1:31-47, 1988.

mitral leaflet SAM, and consequently, decreased outflow tract obstruction and MR. In addition, beta-blockers and calcium channel blockers relieve myocardial ischemia and reduce the heart rate (HR), which prolongs diastole and relaxation and increases passive ventricular filling.[1] However, verapamil should be used with caution in patients with obstructive HCM because it can lead to vasodilation and worsening outflow tract obstruction.[56,115] Disopyramide is a type Ia antiarrhythmic agent with significant negative inotropic properties.[56,116] Cardiac symptoms and the magnitude of the LVOT gradient are significantly improved following the institution of disopyramide. In one multicenter study of 118 patients treated with disopyramide, two thirds of patients were maintained with disopyramide without the need for an invasive intervention.[117]

Dual-Chamber Pacing

Dual-chamber (DDD) atrioventricular pacing reduces LVOT obstruction by inducing both acute and chronic changes.[118,119] Pacing from the right ventricular apex may cause paradoxic or diminished inward movement of the ventricular septum and asynchronous late activation at the basal septum, which may contribute to widening of the LVOT and decreased myocardial contractility. Initial studies had suggested significant symptomatic improvement and left ventricular mass regression with DDD pacing.[120] However, the results of multiple subsequent studies have been less encouraging. Randomized crossover studies of DDD pacing (treatment arm) versus sham pacing (control arm) have shown an incomplete reduction in the LVOT gradient, no significant decrease in left ventricular wall thickness, and no significant increase in peak myocardial oxygen consumption (VO_2) during follow-up.[121-124] The perceived decline in symptoms following pacemaker implantation may, in part, be the result of a placebo effect.[121] These findings were corroborated by a nonrandomized study comparing DDD pacing and septal myectomy, which showed a significantly greater improvement in the functional class, oxygen consumption, and LVOT gradient in the patients who underwent surgery.[125]

Septal Ethanol Ablation

Septal ethanol ablation is an interventional technique that consists of the selective injection of ethanol into a septal perforator branch of the left anterior descending (LAD) artery.[126] This leads to occlusion of the septal branch and localized infarction of the hypertrophied interventricular septum. The targeted infarction results in focal thinning of the septum, widening of the LVOT, and relief of LVOT obstruction.[127] The initial clinical experience with septal ethanol ablation was reported in the 1990s.[126] The selection of the appropriate septal branch to be injected was determined by assessing the reduction in the LVOT gradient following transient occlusion of the targeted vessel by a balloon catheter. However, a vital development in this technique was the use of intraprocedural echocardiography. MCE with transthoracic imaging has become essential for the guidance and monitoring of septal ethanol ablation.[11,12,128]

Myocardial Contrast Echocardiography during Septal Ethanol Ablation

The intraarterial injection of an echo-enhancing agent allows for the specific localization of the vascular beds perfused by individual septal perforator branches of the left anterior descending artery. The vascular territory targeted by contrast echocardiography is the region of contact of the anterior mitral leaflet with the basal septum, which leads to LVOT obstruction. The site of leaflet-septal contact is typically adjacent to the zone of flow acceleration and color turbulence in the LVOT[12] (Fig. 28–13). Contrast agents that have been used during septal ethanol ablation have included sonicated human albumin (Albunex), Levovist, and Optison.[129] Following the injection of the contrast agent the segments of the interventricular septum supplied by the septal branch become opacified. The spatial extent of myocardial opacification can be determined from multiple transthoracic windows. The contrast effect of ethanol has the same distribution as that of the contrast agent, and intraarterial ethanol injection frequently results in increased echogenicity and reflectivity.[11]

Improved Outcomes with Contrast Echocardiography

Intraprocedural contrast echocardiography results in improved outcomes compared with the strategy of target vessel selection by probatory balloon occlusion.[12] The use of contrast echocardiography was associated with a shorter intervention time, a smaller amount of injected ethanol, a smaller infarct, and a significantly higher number of patients with greater than 50% gradient reduction (92% versus 70%). The superiority of this echocardiographic approach persisted at 3-month follow-up, both in terms of improvements in the functional class and in the magnitude of the LVOT gradient.[12]

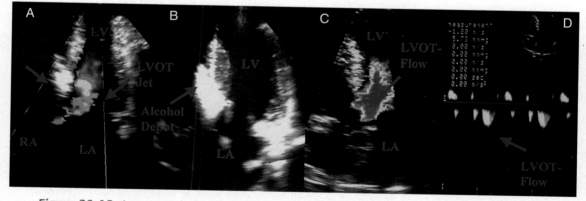

Figure 28–13. *Intraprocedural myocardial contrast echocardiography during septal ethanol ablation. A, Following injection of echocardiographic contrast agent into the first septal perforator of the left anterior descending artery, a contrast depot is identified in the region of the basal septum by transthoracic two-dimensional apical imaging. This opacified area overlies the region of anterior mitral leaflet-septal contact, is adjacent to the site of left ventricular outflow tract turbulence, and is the targeted region of interest. B, Following alcohol injection into the first septal branch, an alcohol depot is identified in the same region as the area of contrast depot. Alcohol injection results in further increased echogenicity of the basal septum. C, Repeat transthoracic apical view with color flow imaging in a patient 3 months following septal ethanol ablation. There is now laminar flow in the left ventricular outflow tract. D, Continuous-wave Doppler recording showing a nonsignificant resting gradient of 6 mm Hg across the left ventricular outflow tract. LA, left atrium; LV, left ventricle; LVOT, left ventricular outflow tract. (From Faber L, Ziemssen P, Seggewiss H: J Am Soc Echocardiogr 13:1074-1079, 2000.)*

Contrast echocardiography is invaluable in detecting contrast opacification in regions remote from the site of mitral leaflet-septal contact. Echocardiographic guidance with a contrast agent can determine whether the selected septal branch supplies other territories such as the left ventricular free wall or apex, right ventricular free wall, or a papillary muscle[128,130,131] (Fig. 28–14). Contrast enhancement in nonseptal sites necessitates the selection of another vessel to be injected or abandonment of the procedure. Studies have shown that 7% to 11% of all procedures have been altered based on information obtained by contrast echocardiography.[128,131]

Furthermore, the size of the induced-infarct, as determined by planimetry of the contrast-enhanced region, can provide incremental information regarding outcomes following septal ethanol ablation.[132] The finding of a larger septal infarction risk area has been associated with a higher risk of cardiovascular complications after the procedure (primarily pacemaker and defibrillator implantation), without necessarily improving the clinical and hemodynamic results of septal ethanol ablation.[132] In summary, MCE optimizes septal ethanol ablation by permitting the targeted delivery of ethanol, limiting the induced infarction to the culprit region of mitral leaflet-septal contact, and by minimizing procedural complications.

Clinical Results following Septal Ethanol Ablation

Studies from multiple experienced centers have demonstrated that septal ethanol ablation can effectively reduce the LVOT gradient in patients with obstructive HCM.[133-136] Subsequent studies beyond 1 year following this procedure have shown ongoing symptomatic improvement.[137,138] Septal ethanol ablation results in an acute deterioration of basal septal function and a delay in left ventricular ejection.[127] There is a gradual and continued decrease in the degree of LVOT obstruction,[134,136] with thinning of the infarcted septal segment and enlargement of the outflow tract[139] (Fig. 28–15). The long-term risk of late ventricular arrhythmias following induced infarction in patients with HCM remains unclear, although studies thus far have not demonstrated an increased risk of ventricular arrhythmias or of sudden death.[135,138] Echocardiographic and Doppler studies are beneficial in the serial noninvasive follow-up of patients following septal ethanol ablation. Multiple studies have documented significant progressive reductions in basal septal thickness and the resting and provocable LVOT gradients.[134,136,140] These developments have been associated with favorable changes in the geometry of the LVOT.[127,139] In addition to the alleviation of LVOT obstruction and septal remodeling, improvements in left ventricular diastolic function have been demonstrated 6 months following this procedure.[103] These changes in diastolic function, as assessed by tissue and color M-mode Doppler, were sustained at 2 years of follow-up.[141]

Surgical Myectomy

Septal myotomy or myectomy has been performed for the past four decades for the management of severe obstructive HCM refractory to maximally tolerated medical therapy. Septal myectomy acutely relieves outflow tract obstruction by widening of the LVOT, which leads to decreased SAM of the mitral valve and de-

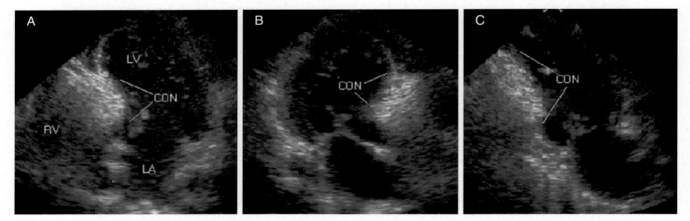

Figure 28–14. Intraprocedural myocardial contrast echocardiography during septal ethanol ablation is essential for guiding the targeted delivery of ethanol. Following intraarterial injection of echocardiographic contrast agent (CON), transthoracic imaging from the apical four-chamber view (A) and the apical three-chamber view (B) demonstrates opacification of the basal and midposterior and anterior interventricular septum. C, However, the apical two-chamber view reveals contrast opacification of the inferior wall. The selected vessel was not felt to be suitable for the injection of ethanol. No other septal perforator branches were identified. The procedure was abandoned and the patient was subsequently referred for surgical myectomy. LA, left atrium; LV, left ventricle; RV, right ventricle.

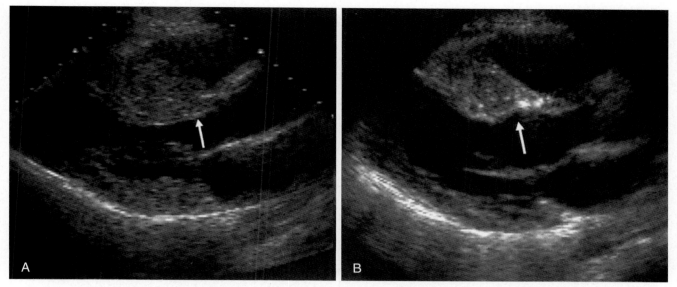

Figure 28–15. *Serial transthoracic echocardiograms in a 25-year-old patient before and 2 years following septal ethanol ablation for drug-refractory symptomatic obstructive hypertrophic cardiomyopathy. A, Parasternal long-axis view obtained before the procedure demonstrates prominent septal hypertrophy (arrow) and resting systolic anterior motion. B, During follow-up 2 years post-septal ethanol ablation, there is striking localized thinning of the anterior septum (arrow), resolution of systolic anterior motion and a resting outflow tract gradient of 6 mm Hg.*

creased dynamic outflow tract obstruction. Echocardiography is useful in the identification of patients suitable for surgical myectomy. The preoperative echocardiographic characteristics predictive of symptomatic benefit from surgical myectomy include asymmetric hypertrophy, severe SAM of the mitral leaflet(s), and a prolonged IVRT.[142] In addition, echocardiography plays an important role in detecting additional lesions requiring surgical management. Comprehensive preoperative echocardiographic imaging in patients referred for surgical myectomy includes the evaluation of independent mitral valve disease, concomitant aortic valve disease, and the assessment of additional levels of obstruction (midventricular or right ventricular outflow tract).[10]

Intraoperative Echocardiography

Surgical myectomy is performed from the transaortic approach and is technically challenging given the limited exposure and visualization of the hypertrophied septum. Before the introduction of intraoperative echocardiography the extent and degree of septal hypertrophy was estimated by surgical palpation[143] and by preoperative transthoracic echocardiographic studies. A vital development in the surgical management of obstructive HCM has been the use of TEE imaging. Intraoperative echocardiography guides the surgical intervention(s), assesses immediate results, and excludes important complications.[10,144] Intraoperative TEE allows for detailed delineation of the depth, width, and length of the required myectomy, the degree of SAM and LVOT obstruction, and the quantitation and mechanism(s) of MR.[10,78] Imaging from multiple TEE

and transgastric views using a multiplane transducer allows for the careful assessment of the thickness of the anterior and posterior portions of the interventricular septum. The length of septal hypertrophy is measured from the base of the right coronary cusp of the aortic valve (Fig. 28–16). The targeted length of resection is 1 cm below the point of anterior mitral leaflet-septal contact. The LVOT gradient can be measured by transgastric imaging in the long-axis view with the CW Doppler beam aligned parallel to the LVOT. Following surgical excision of the basal septum, repeat echocardiographic imaging permits the instantaneous evaluation of the adequacy of the myectomy[10,144] (Fig. 28–17). Intraoperative echocardiography can determine if there is significant residual outflow tract obstruction or hemodynamically important residual MR. In addition, intraoperative echocardiography allows for the immediate detection of such operative complications as a ventricular septal defect[145] and left ventricular dysfunction.[10] The value of intraoperative echocardiography was demonstrated in one study, which showed that intraoperative TEE detected unexpected findings in 17% of cases before cardiopulmonary bypass and in 7% of cases after cardiopulmonary bypass. Intraoperative echocardiography prompted further surgical procedures in 4% of cases.[146]

Outcomes following Myectomy

Studies of the results of surgical myectomy from experienced tertiary referral centers have shown excellent early and long-term postoperative outcomes.[114,147-149] Potential complications following myectomy include

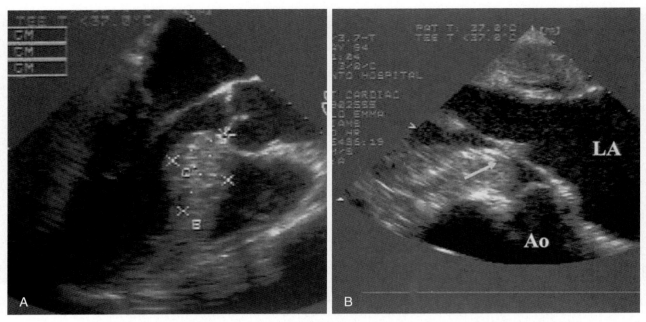

Figure 28-16. A, *Intraoperative transesophageal echocardiogram in the long-axis plane in a patient referred for myectomy. The depth, width, and length of the hypertrophied septum (measured from the base of the right coronary cusp of the aortic valve) and the point of anterior leaflet-septal contact are obtained to guide the resection.* B, *Transgastric views of the mitral valve and left ventricular outflow tract permit detailed examination of the morphology of the mitral leaflets, the point of leaflet-septal contact* (arrow) *and the assessment of systolic anterior motion. Ao, aorta; LA, left atrium.*

heart block, ventricular septal defect, aortic regurgitation, and arrhythmias. Aortic regurgitation is felt to be mainly secondary to the loss of aortic annular support following myectomy.[150] Echocardiographic studies performed at rest and with provocative maneuvers are important in the serial monitoring of patients following myectomy. Multiple studies have documented a significant reduction or abolition of the resting outflow tract gradient in the majority of patients following myectomy, resulting in substantial and lasting symptomatic improvement.[114,147-149,151]

Comparison of Treatment Strategies for Obstructive Hypertrophic Cardiomyopathy

Multiple therapeutic options are currently available in the management of patients with obstructive HCM. Pharmacologic agents have variable effects in reducing the outflow tract gradient and in improving diastolic function. Patients with drug-refractory symptoms are candidates for DDD pacing, septal ethanol ablation, or surgical myectomy. The initial enthusiasm for DDD pacing as a treatment modality for LVOT obstruction has declined considerably. In terms of the outcomes of septal ethanol ablation compared with myectomy, there have been five nonrandomized studies that have compared these two treatment strategies.[152-156] No signifi-

cant differences in cardiac mortality during early and midterm follow-up were identified. Patients who underwent septal ethanol ablation were more likely to develop atrioventricular block and require permanent pacing.[152-155] All these studies showed similar improvements in the functional class and in the resting LVOT gradients following both procedures[152-156] (Table 28-8). The greatest difference in the resting gradients between the two treatment groups occurred at 3 months after the procedure, when patients with septal ethanol ablation were more likely to have a larger resting outflow tract gradient.[153] This divergence likely emerged because myectomy offers immediate relief of the LVOT gradient whereas the effect on the gradient with septal ethanol ablation is more gradual, with the maximal reduction in the gradient occurring at greater than 1 year after the procedure.[134,138] In addition, the long-term benefits of myectomy have been well demonstrated, whereas the long-term sequelae of septal ethanol ablation have yet to be determined.[157-159] Conditions that favor the selection of myectomy over septal ethanol ablation include the presence of coexisting disease (e.g., coronary artery disease, intrinsic disease of the mitral valve or submitral apparatus), the presence of coronary anatomy not amenable to septal ethanol ablation, the requirement for an acute reduction in the LVOT gradient, or the presence of extreme septal hypertrophy.[158]

Septal ethanol ablation and surgical myectomy are challenging techniques. Importantly, both procedures

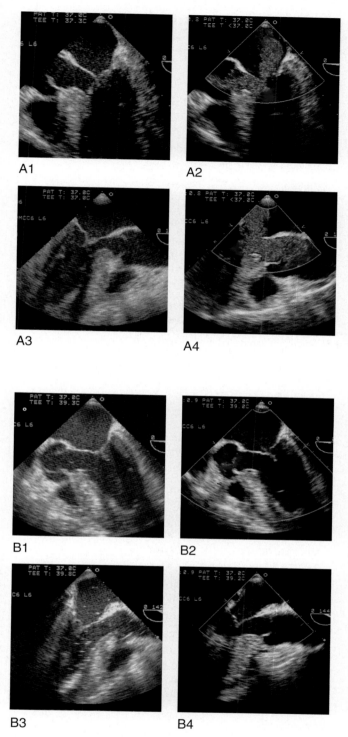

A1

A2

A3

A4

B1

B2

B3

B4

Figure 28–17. *Intraoperative transesophageal echocardiogram before and after myectomy in a patient with obstructive hypertrophic cardiomyopathy and no independent mitral valve disease. A, Preoperative transesophageal study. A1, Transesophageal two-dimensional systolic frame in the four-chamber view demonstrating anterior leaflet-septal contact with failure of mitral leaflet coaptation. A2, Same frame with Doppler color flow imaging demonstrating turbulent left ventricular outflow and a large jet of posteriorly directed mitral regurgitation arising from the gap between the two mitral leaflets. A3, Two-dimensional systolic frame in the long-axis view highlights the septal hypertrophy at the basal level and the anterior leaflet systolic anterior motion. A4, Same frame with Doppler color flow imaging showing the left ventricular outflow tract obstruction and the single jet of posteriorly directed regurgitation. These intraoperative transesophageal findings suggest that the mitral regurgitation will resolve with myectomy alone (with no requirement for mitral valve surgery). B, Postoperative transesophageal study following surgical resection of basal septum (and no additional interventions on the mitral valve). Transesophageal two-dimensional systolic frame in the four-chamber view (B1) and long-axis view (B3) now demonstrate a widened left ventricular outflow tract and abolition of systolic anterior motion of the anterior mitral leaflet. Same frames with color flow imaging in the four-chamber view (B2) and long-axis view (B4) show no significant turbulence in the outflow tract and resolution of the mitral regurgitation.*

need to be performed at centers with both technical and echocardiographic expertise.[158] Comprehensive preprocedural echocardiographic assessment is essential for identifying patients with additional lesions that require surgical correction. The success of both septal ethanol ablation and myectomy depends on experienced intraprocedural echocardiographic guidance, with MCE during septal ethanol ablation and TEE during myectomy. Intraprocedural echocardiographic guidance is indispensable for the identification of the culprit septal segments requiring chemical or surgical reduction, the immediate assessment of the LVOT gradient in response to septal infarction or myectomy, and the monitoring of potential complications.[10,129]

TABLE 28–8. Studies Comparing Left Ventricular Outflow Tract Gradients following Septal Ethanol Ablation and Myectomy

Study	N	Rest Septal Ethanol Ablation LVOT Gradient (mm Hg)		Rest Surgical Myectomy LVOT Gradient (mm Hg)		Follow-up Time	p Value
		Pre	Post	Pre	Post		
Qin and colleagues[153]	51	64±39	24±19	62±43	11±6	3 months	$p < 0.01$
Nagueh and colleagues[152]	82	76±23	8±15	78±30	4±7	1 year	NS
Firoozi and colleagues[154]	44	91±18	21±12	83±23	17±12	1 year	$p = 0.48$
Ralph-Edwards and colleagues[155]	102	74±36	15	64±27	5	1.8±1.1 years (SEA) 2.3±1.5 years (myectomy)	$p < 0.001$
van der Lee and colleagues[156]	72	101±34	23±19	100±20	17±14	1 year	NS

Data shown are the group mean and standard deviation (mean ± standard deviation) left ventricular outflow tract (LVOT) gradients at rest and before (pre) and after (post) the procedure.
NS, not significant; SEA, septal alcohol ablation.
Data from references 152-156.

KEY POINTS

■ The diagnostic feature of HCM on echocardiography is the finding of asymmetric septal hypertrophy, defined as a septal to posterior wall ratio of greater than or equal to 1.3. The maximal wall thickness is typically greater than or equal to 15 mm.

■ Because there may be delayed penetrance of HCM, which has an autosomal dominant pattern of inheritance, serial screening (every 5 years) throughout adulthood is advised for first-degree.

■ The differential diagnosis of HCM is broad and other causes of increased left ventricular wall thickness should be considered (e.g., hypertensive heart disease, athlete's heart), storage diseases (e.g., Fabry's, glycogen storage diseases), and infiltrative cardiomyopathies (e.g., amyloidosis).

■ 2D echocardiography with imaging from several transthoracic windows is used to determine the extent, distribution, and severity of LVH.

■ The pathophysiology of LVOT obstruction involves narrowing of the LVOT (as a result of septal hypertrophy, intrinsic abnormalities of the mitral leaflets, anterior displacement of the mitral apparatus) and hydrodynamic forces causing SAM.

■ The LVOT gradient can be measured with CW Doppler, where the pressure gradient is equal to $4V^2$ (V is LVOT velocity). The Doppler spectral profile is typically a late-peaking, "dagger-shaped" configuration.

■ Subtypes of HCM that can be distinguished by echocardiography are asymmetric apical HCM, midventricular obstruction, latent obstructive HCM, and HCM of the elderly.

■ Diastolic function in patients with HCM can be assessed with tissue Doppler imaging and color M-mode Doppler. The E/Ea ratio correlates well with left ventricular filling pressures.

■ Septal ethanol ablation should be performed with MCE guidance, which allows for the targeted delivery of ethanol to the basal septum, avoids infarction of nonseptal sites, and minimizes complications.

■ Intraoperative TEE during surgical myectomy provides detailed visualization of the septum and the mitral apparatus to guide the surgical resection and permits immediate assessment of the degree of residual outflow tract obstruction and MR.

REFERENCES

1. Maron BJ, McKenna WJ, Danielson GK, et al: Task Force on Clinical Expert Consensus Documents. American College of Cardiology; Committee for Practice Guidelines. European Society of Cardiology. American College of Cardiology/European Society of Cardiology clinical expert consensus document on hypertrophic cardiomyopathy. A report of the American College of Cardiology Foundation Task Force on Clinical Expert Consensus Documents and the European Society of Cardiology Committee for Practice Guidelines. *J Am Coll Cardiol* 42:1687-1713, 2003.
2. Brock RC: Functional obstruction of the left ventricle. *Guys Hosp Rep* 106:221-238, 1957.
3. Teare RD: Asymmetrical hypertrophy of the heart in young adults. *Br Heart J* 20:1-8, 1958.

4. Maron BJ, Towbin JA, Thiene G, et al: Contemporary definitions and classification of the cardiomyopathies: An American Heart Association Scientific Statement from the Council on Clinical Cardiology, Heart Failure and Transplantation Committee; Quality of Care and Outcomes Research and Functional Genomics and Translational Biology Interdisciplinary Working Groups; and Council on Epidemiology and Prevention. *Circulation* 113:1807-1816, 2006.

5. Rakowski H, Sasson Z, Wigle ED: Echocardiographic and Doppler assessment of hypertrophic cardiomyopathy. *J Am Soc Echocardiogr* 1:31-47, 1988.

6. Maron BJ, Gardin JM, Flack JM, et al: Prevalence of hypertrophic cardiomyopathy in a general population of young adults: Echocardiographic analysis of 4111 subjects in the CARDIA study. *Circulation* 92:785-789, 1995.

7. Clark CE, Henry WL, Epstein SE: Familial prevalence and genetic transmission of idiopathic hypertrophic subaortic stenosis. *N Engl J Med* 289:709-714, 1973.

8. Spirito P, Belone P, Harris KM, et al: Magnitude of left ventricular hypertrophy and risk of sudden death in hypertrophic cardiomyopathy. *N Engl J Med* 324:1778-1785, 2000.

9. Corrado D, Basso C, Schiavon M, Thiene G: Screening for hypertrophic cardiomyopathy in young athletes. *N Engl J Med* 339:364-369, 1998.

10. Grigg LE, Wigle ED, Williams WG, et al: Transesophageal Doppler echocardiography in obstructive hypertrophic cardiomyopathy: Clarification of pathophysiology and importance in intraoperative decision making. *J Am Coll Cardiol* 20:42-52, 1992.

11. Nagueh SF, Lakkis NM, He ZX, et al: Role of myocardial contrast echocardiography during nonsurgical septal reduction therapy for hypertrophic obstructive cardiomyopathy. *J Am Coll Cardiol* 32:225-229, 1998.

12. Faber L, Seggewiss H, Gleichmann U. Percutaneous transluminal septal myocardial ablation in hypertrophic obstructive cardiomyopathy: Results with respect to intraprocedural myocardial contrast echocardiography. *Circulation* 98:2415-2421, 1998.

13. Bagger JP, Baandrup U, Rasmussen K, et al: Cardiomyopathy in Western Denmark. *Br Heart J* 52:327-331, 1984.

14. Codd MB, Sugure DD, Gersh BJ, Melton LJ III: Epidemiology of idiopathic dilated and hypertrophic cardiomyopathy. A population-based study in Olmsted County, Minesota, 1975-1984. *Circulation* 80:564-572, 1989.

15. Lipshultz SE, Sleeper LA, Towbin JA, et al: The incidence of pediatric cardiomyopathy in two regions of the United States. *N Engl J Med* 348:1647-1655, 2003.

16. Nugent AW, Daubeney PEF, Chondros P, et al: The epidemiology of childhood cardiomyopathy in Australia. *N Engl J Med* 348:1639-1646, 2003.

17. Seidman C: Hypertrophic cardiomyopathy: from man to mouse. *J Clin Invest* 106:S9-S13, 2000.

18. Marian AJ: Clinical and molecular genetic aspects of hypertrophic cardiomyopathy. *Curr Cardiol Reviews* 1:53-63, 2005.

19. Jarcho JA, McKenna W, Pare JAP, et al: Mapping a gene for familial hypertrophic cardiomyopathy to chromosome 14q1. *N Engl J Med* 321:1372-1378, 1989.

20. Niimura H, Bachinski LL, Sangwatanaroj S, et al: Mutations in the gene for cardiac myosin-binding protein C and late-onset familial hypertrophic cardiomyopathy. *N Engl J Med* 338:1248-1257, 1998.

21. Van Driest SL, Jaeger MA, Ommen SR, et al: Comprehensive analysis of the beta-myosin heavy chain gene in 389 unrelated patients with hypertrophic cardiomyopathy. *J Am Coll Cardiol* 44:602-610, 2004.

22. Solomon SD, Wolff S, Watkins H, et al: Left ventricular hypertrophy and morphology in familial hypertrophic cardiomyopathy associated with mutations of the beta-myosin heavy chain gene. *J Am Coll Cardiol* 22:498-505, 1993.

23. Woo A, Rakowski H, Liew JC, et al: Mutations of the beta myosin heavy chain gene in hypertrophic cardiomyopathy: Critical functional sites determine prognosis. *Heart* 89:1179-1185, 2003.

24. Maron BJ, Niimura H, Casey SA, et al: Development of left ventricular hypertrophy in adults with hypertrophic cardiomyopathy caused by cardiac myosin-binding protein C gene mutations. *J Am Coll Cardiol* 38:315-321, 2001.

25. Van Driest SL, Vasile VC, Ommen SR, et al: Myosin binding protein C mutations and compound heterozygosity in hypertrophic cardiomyopathy. *J Am Coll Cardiol* 44:1903-1910, 2004.

26. Shah PM, Gramiak R, Kramer DH: Ultrasound localization of left ventricular outflow obstruction in hypertrophic obstructive cardiomyopathy. *Circulation* 40:3-11, 1969.

27. Popp RL, Harrison DC: Ultrasound in the diagnosis and evaluation of therapy of idiopathic hypertrophic subaortic stenosis. *Circulation* 40:905-914, 1969.

28. Henry WL, Clark CE, Epstein SE: Asymmetric septal hypertrophy: echocardiographic identification of the pathognomonic anatomic abnormality of IHSS. *Circulation* 47:225-233, 1973.

29. Gilbert BW, Pollick C, Adelman AG, Wigle ED: Hypertrophic cardiomyopathy: Subclassification by M-mode echocardiography. *Am J Cardiol* 45:861-872, 1980.

30. Humez FU, Houston AB, Watson J, et al: Age and body surface area related normal upper and lower limits of M mode echocardiographic measurements and left ventricular volume and mass from infancy to early adulthood. *Br Heart J* 7:276-280, 1994.

31. Maron MS, Olivotto I, Betocchi S, et al: Effect of left ventricular outflow tract obstruction on clinical outcome in hypertrophic cardiomyopathy. *N Engl J Med* 348:295-303, 2003.

32. Maron BJ, Seidman JG, Seidman CE: Proposal for contemporary screening strategies for families with hypertrophic cardiomyopathy. *J Am Coll Cardiol* 44:2125-2132, 2004.

33. Nagueh SF, Bachinski LL, Meyer D, et al: Tissue Doppler imaging consistently detects myocardial abnormalities in patients with hypertrophic cardiomyopathy and provides a novel means for an early diagnosis before and independently of hypertrophy. *Circulation* 104:128-130, 3002.

34. Ho CY, Sweitzer NK, McDonough B, et al: Tissue Doppler imaging predicts the development of hypertrophic cardiomyopathy in subjects with subclinical disease. *Circulation* 105:2992-2997, 2002.

35. Nagueh SF, McFalls J, Meyer D, et al: Assessment of diastolic function with Doppler tissue imaging to predict genotype in preclinical hypertrophic cardiomyopathy. *Circulation* 108:395-398, 2003.

36. Prasad K, Atherton J, Smith GC, et al: Echocardiographic pitfalls in the diagnosis of hypertrophic cardiomyopathy. *Heart* 82(Suppl III):III-8-III-15, 1999.

37. Elliott P, McKenna WJ: Hypertrophic cardiomyopathy. *Lancet* 363:1881-1891, 2004.

38. Riggs T, Hirschfeld S, Rajai H: The pediatric spectrum of dynamic left ventricular obstruction. *Am Heart J* 99:301-309, 1980.

39. Santos AD, Miller RP, Mathew PK, et al: Echocardiographic characterization of the reversible cardiomyopathy of hypothyroidism. *Am J Med* 68:675-682, 1980.

40. Klein AL, Oh JK, Miller FA, et al: Two-dimensional and Doppler echocardiographic assessment of infiltrative cardiomyopathy. *J Am Soc Echocardiogr* 1:48-59, 1988.

41. Nakao S, Takenaka T, Maeda M, et al: An atypical variant of Fabry's disease in men with left ventricular hypertrophy. *N Engl J Med* 333:288-293, 1995.

42. Sachdev B, Takenaka T, Teraguchi H, et al: Prevalence of Anderson-Fabry disease in male pts with late onset hypertrophic cardiomyopathy. *Circulation* 105:1407-1411, 2002.

43. Arad M, Maron BJ, Gorham JM, et al: Glycogen storage diseases presenting as hypertrophic cardiomyopathy. *N Engl J Med* 352:362-372, 2005.

44. Morita H, Larson MG, Barr SC, et al: Single-gene mutations and increased left ventricular wall thickness in the community: the Framingham Heart Study. *Circulation* 113:2697-2705, 2006.

45. Pellicia A, Maron BJ, Spataro A, et al: The upper limit of physiological cardiac hypertrophy in highly trained elite athletes. *N Engl J Med* 324:295-301, 1991.

46. Maron BJ, Pelliccia A, Spirito P: Cardiac disease in young trained athletes: Insights into methods for distinguishing athlete's heart from structural heart disease, with particular emphasis on hypertrophic cardiomyopathy. *Circulation* 91:1596-1601, 1995.

47. Maron B, Pelliccia A, Spataro A, Granata M: Reduction in left ventricular wall thickness after deconditioning in highly trained Olympic athletes. *Br Heart J* 69:125-128, 1993.

48. Pelliccia A, Maron BJ, De Luca R, et al: Remodeling of left ventricular hypertrophy in elite athletes after long-term deconditioning. *Circulation* 105:944-949, 2002.

49. Pellicia A, Maron BJ, Culasso F, et al: Athlete's heart in women. *JAMA* 276:211-215, 1996.

50. Karam R, Lever HM, Healy BP: Hypertensive hypertrophic cardiomyopathy or hypertrophic cardiomyopathy with hypertension? A study of 78 patients. *J Am Coll Cardiol* 13:580-584, 1989.

51. Dalldorf FG, Willis PW IV: Angled aorta ("sigmoid septum") as a cause of hypertrophic stenosis. *Hum Pathol* 16:457-462, 1985.

52. Krasnow N: Subaortic septal bulge simulates hypertrophic cardiomyopathy by angulation of the septum with age, independent of focal hypertrophy: an echocardiographic study. *J Am Soc Echocardiogr* 10:545-555, 1997.

53. Belenkie I, MacDonald RPR, Smith ER: Localized septal hypertrophy: Part of the spectrum of hypertrophic cardiomyopathy or an incidental echocardiographic finding? *Am Heart J* 115:385-390, 1988.

54. Martin RP, Rakowski H, French J, Popp RL: Idiopathic hypertrophic subaortic stenosis viewed by wide-angle, phased-array echocardiography. *Circulation* 59:1206-1217, 1979.

55. Maron BJ, Gottdiener JS, Epstein SE: Patterns and significance of distribution of left ventricular hypertrophy in hypertrophic cardiomyopathy. *Am J Cardiol* 48:418-428, 1981.

56. Wigle ED, Sasson Z, Henderson M, et al: Hypertrophic cardiomyopathy. The importance of the site and extent of hypertrophy. A review. *Prog Cardiovasc Dis* 28:1-83, 1985.

57. Rakowski H, Fulop J, Wigle ED: The role of echocardiography in the assessment of hypertrophic cardiomyopathy. *Postgrad Med J* 62:557-561, 1986.

58. Bhandari AK, Nanda NC: Myocardial texture characterization by two-dimensional echocardiography. *Am J Cardiol* 51:817-825, 1983.

59. Fowles RE, Martin RP, Popp RL: Apparent asymmetric septal hypertrophy due to angled interventricular septum. *Am J Cardiol* 46:386-392, 1980.

60. Klues HG, Schiffers A, Maron BJ: Phenotypic spectrum and patterns of left ventricular hypertrophy in hypertrophic cardiomyopathy: morphologic observations and significance as assessed by two dimensional echocardiography in 600 patients. *J Am Coll Cardiol* 26:1699-1708, 1995.

61. Henry WL, Clark CE, Glancy DL, Epstein SE: Echocardiographic measurement of the left ventricular outflow gradient in idiopathic hypertrophic subaortic stenosis. *N Engl J Med* 288:989-993, 1973.

62. Boughner D, Schuld RL, Persaud JA: Hypertrophic obstructive cardiomyopathy: assessment by echocardiographic and Doppler ultrasound techniques. *Br Heart J* 37:917-923, 1975.

63. Henry WL, Clark CE, Griffith JM, Epstein SE: Mechanism of left ventricular outflow obstruction in patients with obstructive asymmetric septal hypertrophy (idiopathic subaortic stenosis). *Am J Cardiol* 35:337-345, 1975.

64. Spirito P, Maron BJ: Significance of left ventricular outflow tract cross-sectional area in hypertrophic cardiomyopathy: a two-dimensional echocardiographic assessment. *Circulation* 67:1100-1108, 1983.

65. Shah PM, Taylor RD, Wong M: Abnormal mitral valve coaptation in hypertrophic obstructive cardiomyopathy: Proposed role in systolic anterior motion of mitral valve. *Am J Cardiol* 48:258-262, 1981.

66. Jaing L, Levine RA, King ME, Weyman AE: An integrated mechanism for systolic anterior motion of the mitral valve in hypertrophic cardiomyopathy based on echocardiographic observations. *Am Heart J* 113:663-644, 1987.

67. Klues HG, Roberts WC, Maron BJ: Morphologic determinants of echocardiographic patterns of mitral valve systolic anterior motion in obstructive hypertrophic cardiomyopathy. *Circulation* 87:1570-1579, 1993.

68. Reis R, Bolton MR, King JF, et al: Anterior-superior displacement of papillary muscles producing obstruction and mitral regurgitation in idiopathic hypertrophic subaortic stenosis. *Circulation* 49-50(Suppl):181-188, 1974.

69. Sherrid MV, Chu CK, Delia E, et al: An echocardiographic study of the fluid mechanics of obstruction in hypertrophic cardiomyopathy. *J Am Coll Cardiol* 22:816-825, 1993.

70. Wigle ED, Adelman AG, Silver MD: Pathophysiological considerations in muscular subaortic stenosis. In GEW Wolstenholme, M O'Connor: Hypertrophic obstructive cardiomyopathy, Ciba Foundation Study Group, No. 37, J and A Churchill Ltd, London, 1971, p. 63.

71. Pollick C, Morgan CD, Gilbert BW, et al: Muscular subaortic stenosis: The temporal relationship between systolic anterior motion of the anterior mitral leaflet and the pressure gradient. *Circulation* 66:1087-1094, 1982.

72. Pollick C, Rakowski H, Wigle ED: Muscular subaortic stenosis: the quantitative relationship between systolic anterior motion and the pressure gradient. *Circulation* 69:43-49, 1984.

73. Panza JA, Petrone RK, Fananapazir L, Maron BJ: Utility of continuous wave Doppler echocardiography in the noninvasive assessment of left ventricular outflow tract pressure gradient in patients with hypertrophic cardiomyopathy. *J Am Coll Cardiol* 19:91-99, 1992.

74. Bryg RJ, Pearson AC, Williams GA, Labovitz AJ: Left ventricular systolic and diastolic flow abnormalities determined by Doppler echocardiography in obstructive hypertrophic cardiomyopathy. *Am J Cardiol* 59:925-931, 1987.

75. Sasson Z, Yock PG, Hatle LK, et al: Doppler echocardiographic determination of the pressure gradient in hypertrophic cardiomyopathy. *J Am Coll Cardiol* 11:752-756, 1988.

76. Schwammenthal E, Block M, Schwartzkopff B, et al: Prediction of the site and severity of obstruction in hypertrophic cardiomyopathy by color flow mapping and continuous wave Doppler echocardiography. *J Am Coll Cardiol* 20:964-972, 1992.

77. Yock PG, Hatle L, Popp RL: Patterns and timing of Doppler-detected intracavitary and aortic flow in hypertrophic cardiomyopathy. *J Am Coll Cardiol* 8:1047-1058, 1986.

78. Yu E, Omran AS, Wigle ED, et al: Mitral regurgitation in hypertrophic obstructive cardiomyopathy: relationship to obstruction and relief with myectomy. *J Am Coll Cardiol* 36:2219-2225, 2000.

79. Schwammenthal E, Nakatani S, He S, et al: Mechanism of mitral regurgitation in hypertrophic cardiomyopathy. *Circulation* 98:856-865, 1988.

80. Klues HG, Roberts WC, Maron BJ: Anomalous insertion of papillary muscle directly into anterior mitral leaflet in hypertrophic cardiomyopathy: Significance in producing left ventricular outflow obstruction. *Circulation* 84:1188-1197, 1991.

81. Sakamoto T, Tei C, Muramaya M, et al: Giant negative T wave inversion as a manifestation of asymmetric apical hypertrophy (AAH) of the left ventricle. Echocardiographic and ultrasonocardiotomographic study. *Jpn Heart J* 17:611-629, 1976.

82. Yamaguchi H, Ishimura T, Nishiyama S, et al: Hypertrophic nonobstructive cardiomyopathy with giant negative T-waves (apical hypertrophy): ventriculographic and echocardiographic features in 30 patients. *Am J Cardiol* 44:401-412, 1979.

83. Eriksson MJ, Sonnenberg B, Woo A, et al: Long-term outcome in patients with apical hypertrophic cardiomyopathy. *J Am Coll Cardiol* 39:638-645, 2002.

84. Thanigaraj S, Perez JE: Apical hypertrophic cardiomyopathy: echocardiographic diagnosis with the use of intravenous con-

trast image enhancement. *J Am Soc Echocardiogr* 13:146-149, 2000.

85. Falicov RE, Resnekov L, Bharati S, Lev M: Midventricular obstruction: a variant of obstructive cardiomyopathy. *Am J Cardiol* 37:432-437, 1976.

86. Kuhn H, Mercier J, Köhler E, et al: Differential diagnosis of hypertrophic cardiomyopathies: typical (subaortic) hypertrophic cardiomyopathy, atypical (mid-ventricular) hypertrophic obstructive cardiomyopathy and hypertrophic non-obstructive cardiomyopathy. *Eur Heart J* 4(Suppl F):93-104, 1983.

87. Nakatani S, Marwick TH, Lever HM, Thomas JD: Resting echocardiographic features of latent left ventricular outflow obstruction in hypertrophic cardiomyopathy. *Am J Cardiol* 78:662-667, 1996.

88. Drinko JK, Nash PJ, Lever HM, Asher CR: Safety of stress testing in patients with hypertrophic cardiomyopathy. *Am J Cardiol* 93:1443-1444, 2004.

89. Schwammenthal E, Schwartzkopff B, Block M, et al: Doppler echocardiographic assessment of the pressure gradient during bicycle ergometry in hypertrophic cardiomyopathy. *Am J Cardiol* 69:1623-1628, 1992.

90. Marwick TH, Nakatani S, Haluska B, et al: Provocation of latent left ventricular outflow tract gradients with amyl nitrite and exercise in hypertrophic cardiomyopathy. *Am J Cardiol* 75:805-809, 1995.

91. Whiting RB, Powell JW, Dinsmore RE, Sanders C: Idiopathic hypertrophic subaortic stenosis in the elderly. *N Engl J Med* 285:196-200, 1971.

92. Lewis JF, Maron BJ: Clinical and morphologic expression hypertrophic cardiomyopathy in patients ≥65 years of age. *Am J Cardiol* 73:1105-1111, 1994.

93. Chikamori T, Doi Y, Yonazawa Y, et al: Comparison of clinical features of patients >60 years of age to those <40 years of age with hypertrophic cardiomyopathy. *Am J Cardiol* 66:875-877, 1990.

94. Lever HM, Karam RF, Currie PJ, Healy B: Hypertrophic cardiomyopathy in the elderly. Distinction from the young based on cardiac shape. *Circulation* 79:580-589, 1989.

95. Mohamed HE, Roberts WC: Frequency and significance of mitral annular calcium in hypertrophic cardiomyopathy: Analysis of 200 necropsy patients. *Am J Cardiol* 60:877-884, 1987.

96. Rakowski H, Freedman D, Wigle ED: Echocardiographic evaluation of hypertrophic cardiomyopathy in the elderly. *Cardiol Elderly* 3:415-422, 1995.

97. Louie E, Edwards L: Hypertrophic cardiomyopathy. *Prog Cardiovasc Dis* 34:275-308, 1994.

98. Maron BJ, Spirito P, Green KJ, et al: Noninvasive assessment of left ventricular diastolic function by pulsed Doppler echocardiography in patients with hypertrophic cardiomyopathy. *J Am Coll Cardiol* 10:733-742, 1987.

99. Nishimura RA, Appleton CP, Redfield MM, et al: Noninvasive Doppler echocardiographic evaluation of left ventricular filling pressures in patients with cardiomyopathies: A simultaneous Doppler echocardiographic and cardiac catheterization study. *J Am Coll Cardiol* 28:1226-1233, 1996.

100. Nagueh SF, Lakkis NM, Middleton KJ, et al: Doppler estimation of left ventricular filling pressures in patients with hypertrophic cardiomyopathy. *Circulation* 99:254-261, 1999.

101. Matsumura Y, Elliott PM, Virdee MS, et al: Left ventricular diastolic function assessed using Doppler tissue imaging in patients with hypertrophic cardiomyopathy: relation to symptoms and exercise capacity. *Heart* 87:247-251, 2002.

102. Yang H, Woo A, Monakier D, et al: Enlarged left atrial volume in hypertrophic cardiomyopathy: a marker for disease severity. *J Am Soc Echocardiogr* 18:1074-1082, 2005.

103. Nagueh SF, Lakkis NM, Middleton KJ, et al: Changes in left ventricular diastolic function 6 months after nonsurgical septal reduction therapy for hypertrophic obstructive cardiomyopathy. *Circulation* 99:344-347, 1999.

104. Sitges M, Shiota T, Lever HM, et al: Comparison of left ventricular diastolic function in obstructive hypertrophic cardiomyopathy in patients undergoing percutaneous septal alcohol ablation versus surgical myotomy/myectomy. *Am J Cardiol* 91:817-821, 2003.

105. Sasson Z, Hatle L, Appleton CP, et al: Intraventricular flow during isovolumic relaxation: Description and characterization by Doppler echocardiography. *J Am Coll Cardiol* 10:539-546, 1987.

106. Nakamura T, Matsubara K, Jurukawa K, et al: Diastolic paradoxic jet flow in patients with hypertrophic cardiomyopathy: Evidence of concealed apical asynergy with cavity obliteration. *J Am Coll Cardiol* 19:516-524, 1992.

107. Yang H, Sun JP, Lever HM, et al: Use of strain imaging in detecting segmental dysfunction in patients with hypertrophic cardiomyopathy. *J Am Soc Echocardiogr* 16:233-239, 2003.

108. Kato TS, Noda A, Izawa H, et al: Discrimination of nonobstructive hypertrophic cardiomyopathy from hypertensive left ventricular hypertrophy on the basis of strain rate imaging by tissue Doppler ultrasonography. *Circulation* 110:3808-3814, 2004.

109. Serri K, Reant P, Lafitte M, et al: Global and regional myocardial function quantification by two-dimensional strain: application in hypertrophic cardiomyopathy. *J Am Coll Cardiol* 47:1175-1181, 2006.

110. Olivotto I, Gistri R, Petrone P, et al: Maximum left ventricular thickness and risk of sudden death in patients with hypertrophic cardiomyopathy. *J Am Coll Cardiol* 41:315-321, 2003.

111. Elliott P, Blanes JRG, Mahon NG, et al: Relation between severity of left-ventricular hypertrophy and prognosis in patients with hypertrophic cardiomyopathy. *Lancet* 357:420-424, 2001.

112. McKenna WJ, Behr ER: Hypertrophic cardiomyopathy: management, risk stratification, and prevention of sudden death. *Heart* 87:169-176, 2002.

113. Olivotto I, Cecchi F, Casey SA, et al: Impact of atrial fibrillation on the clinical course of hypertrophic cardiomyopathy. *Circulation* 104:2517-2524, 2001.

114. Woo A, Williams WG, Choi R, et al: Clinical and echocardiographic determinants of long-term survival following surgical myectomy in obstructive hypertrophic cardiomyopathy. *Circulation* 111:2033-2041, 2005.

115. Epstein SE, Rosing DR: Verapamil: Its potential for causing serious complications in patients with hypertrophic cardiomyopathy. *Circulation* 64:437-441, 1981.

116. Pollick C: Muscular subaortic stenosis. Hemodynamic and clinical improvement after disopyramide. *N Engl J Med* 307:997-999, 1982.

117. Sherrid M, Barac I, McKenna WJ, et al: Multicenter study of the efficacy and safety of disopyramide in obstructive hypertrophic cardiomyopathy. *J Am Coll Cardiol* 45:1251-1258, 2005.

118. Fananapazir L, Cannon RO, Tripodi D, Panza JA: Impact of dual-chamber permanent pacing in patients with obstructive hypertrophic cardiomyopathy with symptoms refractory to verapamil and β-adrenergic blocker therapy. *Circulation* 85:2149-2161, 1992.

119. Slade AKB, Sadoul N, Shapiro L, et al: DDD Pacing in hypertrophic cardiomyopathy: A multicentre clinical experience. *Heart* 75:44-49, 1996.

120. Fananapazir L, Epstein ND, Curiel RV, et al: Long-term results of dual-chamber (DDD) pacing in obstructive hypertrophic cardiomyopathy: Evidence for progressive symptomatic and hemodynamic improvement and reduction of left ventricular hypertrophy. *Circulation* 90:2731-2742, 1994.

121. Nishimura RA, Trusty JM, Hayes DL, et al: Dual-chamber pacing for patients with hypertrophic obstructive cardiomyopathy: A prospective randomized, double-blind cross-over study. *J Am Coll Cardiol* 29:435-441, 1997.

122. Kappenberger L, Linde C, Daubert C, et al: Pacing in hypertrophic obstructive cardiomyopathy. A randomized crossover study. *Eur Heart J* 18:1249-1256, 1997.

123. Maron BJ, Nishimura RA, McKenna WJ, et al: Assessment of permanent dual-chamber pacing as a treatment for drug-

refractory symptomatic patients with obstructive hypertrophic cardiomyopathy. A randomized, double-blind, cross-over study (M-PATHY). *Circulation* 99:2927-2933, 1999.

124. Sorajja P, Elliott PM, McKenna WJ: Pacing in hypertrophic cardiomyopathy. *Cardiol Clin* 18:67-79, 2000.

125. Ommen SR, Nishimura RA, Squires RW, et al: Comparison of dual-chamber pacing versus septal myectomy for the treatment of patients with hypertrophic obstructive cardiomyopathy. *J Am Coll Cardiol* 34:191-196, 1999.

126. Sigwart U: Non-surgical myocardial reduction for hypertrophic obstructive cardiomyopathy. *Lancet* 346:211-214, 1995.

127. Flores-Ramirez R, Lakkis NM, Middleton KJ, et al: Echocardiographic insights into the mechanisms of relief of left ventricular outflow tract obstruction after nonsurgical septal reduction therapy in patients with hypertrophic obstructive cardiomyopathy. *J Am Coll Cardiol* 37:208-214, 2001.

128. Faber L, Ziemssen P, Seggewiss H: Targeting percutaneous transluminal septal ablation for hypertrophic obstructive cardiomyopathy by intraprocedural echocardiographic monitoring. *J Am Soc Echocardiogr* 13:1074-1079, 2000.

129. Monakier D, Woo A, Vannan MA, Rakowski H: Myocardial contrast echocardiography in chronic ischemic and nonischemic cardiomyopathies. *Cardiol Clin* 22:269-282, 2004.

130. Monakier D, Horlick E, Ross J, et al: Intra-coronary myocardial contrast echocardiography in a patient with drug refractory hypertrophic obstructive cardiomyopathy revealing extensive myocardium at risk for infarction with alcohol septal ablation. *J Invasive Cardiol* 16:482-484, 2004.

131. Faber L, Seggewiss H, Welge D, et al: Echo-guided percutaneous septal ablation for symptomatic hypertrophic obstructive cardiomyopathy: 7 years of experience. *Eur J Echocardiogr* 5:347-355, 2004.

132. Monakier D, Woo A, Puri T, et al: Usefulness of myocardial contrast echocardiographic quantification of risk area for predicting postprocedural complications in patients undergoing septal ethanol ablation for obstructive hypertrophic cardiomyopathy. *Am J Cardiol* 94:1515-1522, 2004.

133. Lakkis NM, Nagueh SF, Kleiman NS, et al: Echocardiography-guided ethanol septal reduction for hypertrophic obstructive cardiomyopathy. *Circulation* 98:1750-1755, 1998.

134. Seggewiss H, Faber L, Gleichmann U: Percutaneous transluminal septal ablation in hypertrophic obstructive cardiomyopathy. *Thorac Cardiovasc Surg* 47:94-100, 1999.

135. Gietzen FH, Leuner CJ, Raute-Kreinsen U, et al: Acute and long-term results after transcoronary ablation of septal hypertrophy (TASH): Catheter interventional treatment for hypertrophic obstructive cardiomyopathy. *Eur Heart J* 20:1342-1354, 1999.

136. Bhagwadeen R, Woo A, Ross J, et al: Septal ethanol ablation for hypertrophic obstructive cardiomyopathy: Early and intermediate results of a Canadian referral centre. *Can J Cardiol* 19:912-917, 2003.

137. Faber L, Meissner A, Ziemssen P, Seggewiss H: Percutaneous transluminal septal myocardial ablation for hypertrophic obstructive cardiomyopathy: Long term follow up of the first series of 25 patients. *Heart* 83:326-331, 2000.

138. Fernandes VL, Nagueh SF, Wang W, et al: A prospective follow-up of alcohol septal ablation for symptomatic hypertrophic obstructive cardiomyopathy—the Baylor experience. 1996-2002. *Clin Cardiol* 28:124-130, 2005.

139. Schulz-Menger J, Strohm O, Waigand J, et al: The value of magnetic resonance imaging of the left ventricular outflow tract in patients with hypertrophic obstructive cardiomyopathy after septal artery embolization. *Circulation* 101:1764-1766, 2000.

140. Mazur W, Nagueh SF, Lakkis NM, et al: Regression of left ventricular hypertrophy after nonsurgical septal reduction therapy for hypertrophic obstructive cardiomyopathy. *Circulation* 103:1492-1496, 2001.

141. Jassal DS, Neilan T, Fifer MA, et al: Sustained improvements in left ventricular diastolic function after alcohol septal ablation for hypertrophic obstructive cardiomyopathy. *Eur Heart J* 27:1805-1810, 2006.

142. McCully RB, Nishimura RA, Bailey KR, et al: Hypertrophic obstructive cardiomyopathy: preoperative echocardiographic predictors of outcome after septal myectomy. *J Am Coll Cardiol* 27:1491-1496, 1996.

143. Morrow AG: Hypertrophic subaortic stenosis. Operative methods utilized to relieve left ventricular outflow obstruction. *J Thorac Cardiovasc Surg* 76:423-430, 1978.

144. Marwick TH, Stewart WJ, Lever HM, et al: Benefits of intraoperative echocardiography in the surgical management of hypertrophic cardiomyopathy. *J Am Coll Cardiol* 20:1066-1072, 1992.

145. Siegman IL, Maron BJ, Permut LC, et al: Operative treatment in hypertrophic subaortic stenosis. Techniques, and the results of pre and postoperative assessments in 83 patients. *Circulation* 52:88-102, 1975.

146. Ommen S, Park SH, Click RL, et al: Impact of intraoperative transesophageal echocardiography in the surgical management of hypertrophic cardiomyopathy. *Am J Cardiol* 90:1022-1024, 2002.

147. Heric B, Lytle BW, Miller DP, et al: Surgical management of hypertrophic obstructive cardiomyopathy: early and late results. *J Thorac Cardiovasc Surg* 110:195-208, 1995.

148. Robbins RC, Stinson EB: Long-term results of left ventricular myotomy and myectomy for obstructive hypertrophic cardiomyopathy. *J Thorac Cardiovasc Surg* 11:586-594, 1996.

149. McCully RB, Nishimura RA, Tajik AJ, et al: Extent of clinical improvement after surgical treatment of hypertrophic cardiomyopathy. *Circulation* 94:467-471, 1996.

150. Sasson Z, Prieur T, Skrobik Y, et al: Aortic regurgitation: A common complication after surgery for hypertrophic obstructive cardiomyopathy. *J Am Coll Cardiol* 13:63-67, 1989.

151. Maron BJ, Merrill WH, Freier PA, et al: Long-term clinical course and symptomatic status of patients after operation for hypertrophic subaortic stenosis. *Circulation* 57:1205-1213, 1978.

152. Nagueh SF, Ommen SR, Lakkis NM, et al: Comparison of ethanol septal reduction therapy with surgical myectomy for the treatment of hypertrophic obstructive cardiomyopathy. *J Am Coll Cardiol* 38:1701-1706, 2001.

153. Qin JX, Shiota T, Lever HM, et al: Outcome of patients with hypertrophic obstructive cardiomyopathy after percutaneous transluminal septal myocardial ablation and septal myectomy surgery. *J Am Coll Cardiol* 38:1994-2000, 2001.

154. Firoozi S, Elliott PM, Sharma S, et al: Septal myotomy-myectomy and transcoronary septal alcohol ablation in hypertrophic obstructive cardiomyopathy: a comparison of clinical, haemodynamic and exercise outcomes. *Eur Heart J* 23:1617-1624, 2002.

155. Ralph-Edwards A, Woo A, McCrindle BW, et al: Hypertrophic obstructive cardiomyopathy: comparison of outcomes after myectomy or alcohol ablation adjusted by propensity score. *J Thorac Cardiovasc Surg* 129:351-358, 2005.

156. van der Lee C, ten Cate FJ, Geleijnse ML, et al: Percutaneous versus surgical treatment for patients with hypertrophic obstructive cardiomyopathy and enlarged anterior mitral valve leaflets. *Circulation* 112:482-488, 2005.

157. Wigle ED, Schwartz L, Woo A, Rakowski H: To ablate or to operate: that is the question! *J Am Coll Cardiol* 38:1707-1710, 2001.

158. Maron BJ, Dearani JA, Ommen SR, et al: The case for surgery in obstructive hypertrophic cardiomyopathy. *J Am Coll Cardiol* 44:2044-2053, 2004.

159. Knight CJ: Alcohol septal ablation for obstructive hypertrophic cardiomyopathy. *Heart* 92:1339-1344, 2006.

Chapter 29

Restrictive Cardiomyopathy: Diagnosis and Prognostic Implications

TASNEEM Z. NAQVI, MD

The author acknowledges Maran Thamilarasan, MD, and Allan L. Klein, MD, the previous authors of this chapter in *The Practice of Clinical Echocardiography,* second edition.

Identification and Causes of Restrictive Cardiomyopathy

Restrictive cardiomyopathy is an idiopathic or systemic myocardial disorder characterized by a primary abnormality of diastolic function in the presence of normal or mildly abnormal systolic dysfunction. Primary diastolic dysfunction that is a characteristic of this disease leads to abnormal ventricular filling, resulting in an increase in ventricular end-diastolic pressure and dilated atria. The biventricular volumes are either reduced or normal.[1] Patients commonly have congestive failure with fatigue, exercise intolerance, right-sided or left-sided heart failure (HF), and atrial fibrillation (AFib).[2,3] An elevated jugular venous pressure with an x and prominent y descent, y descent only (late-stage), and Kussmaul's sign may be present, although pulsus paradoxus is always absent. Depending on the stage of disease, an S4 (early) or S3 (late) may be present. Restriction can be isolated to either ventricle or show biventricular involvement.[4] The prognosis of restrictive cardiomyopathies is generally poor, except for those with reversible causes, such as hemochromatosis. Doppler echocardiography plays a vital role in the diagnosis

TABLE 29–1. Classification of Restrictive Cardiomyopathy

Noninfiltrative	Idiopathic[88] *Scleroderma*[213,214]

Infiltrative	Amyloid heart disease[215-217]
	 Immunoglobulin amyloidosis[218,219]
	 Familial amyloidosis[220]
	 Senile systemic amyloidosis,[221,222]
	    secondary amyloidosis,[223]
	      sarcoid,[224,225] Gaucher's,[226]
	    Hurlers[227]

Storage disease	Hemochromatosis,[228] glycogen storage disease,[229] Fabry's disease[230]

Endomyocardial	Endomyocardial fibrosis[231,232]
	 Hypereosinophilic syndrome[233]
	 Carcinoid[234,235]
	 Scleroderma,[179] Ehlers Danlos
	    syndrome,[180,181] systemic lupus
	    erythematosus[179]
	 Metastatic malignancy[236,237]
	 Radiation[238]
	 Anthracycline toxicity[239,240]
	 Drugs causing fibrous endocarditis[241]
	    (anthracycles, serotonin, methyser-
	    gide[242]), ergotamine, mercurial
	    agents, busulfan, chloroquine[243]

and management of this disease entity. Table 29–1 shows the classification of restrictive cardiomyopathy.

Pathophysiology

Restrictive cardiomyopathy is defined as a disease characterized by primary abnormality of diastolic function with normal left ventricular (LV) volumes and systolic function until late stages of the disease when systolic function impairment is also seen. Before restrictive filling of this disease occurs, several stages of abnormal myocardial relaxation may be seen. In the early phase of diastolic dysfunction, LV relaxation is impaired (Fig. 29–1), and the duration of LV relaxation is prolonged into mid or late diastole, causing a slower decline in LV pressure. This impaired LV relaxation is manifest as decreased mitral annular early E velocity. With normal LV and left atrial (LA) compliance, however, LA and LV pressures remain normal. A small E wave, prolonged isovolumic relaxation time (IVRT) and deceleration time (DT), and a reversal of E/A ratio result from high residual atrial preload and normal LA contractility. In patients with advanced disease, increased myocardial stiffness results in further impairment in myocardial relaxation (Fig. 29–2) and is manifest as further diminution of mitral annular early diastolic velocity. A decrease in chamber compliance during diastolic filling leads to an increase in LV end diastolic pressure. The resulting

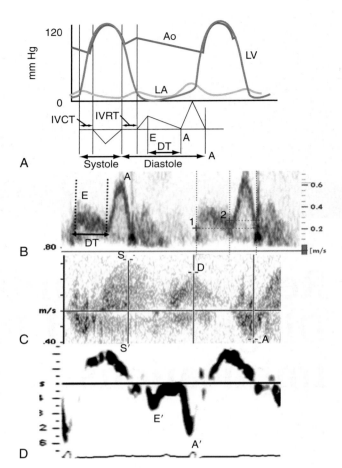

Figure 29–1. *Left ventricular, left atrial, and aortic pressure tracings (A), mitral inflow pulsed-wave Doppler (B), pulmonary vein pulsed-wave Doppler (C) and mitral annular tissue Doppler through cardiac cycle in subject with delayed left ventricular relaxation (D). Mitral inflow velocities were obtained by placing the pulsed-wave Doppler sample volume between the tips of the mitral leaflets and Doppler tissue imaging by placing the pulsed-wave Doppler sample volume at the lateral mitral annulus. Large black horizontal arrows depict the duration of ventricular systole and ventricular diastole. Ventricular relaxation continues to occur in the latter third of diastole causing an E and A ratio less than 1 and prolonged mitral inflow deceleration time. The pulmonary vein flow pattern is systolic dominant, and there is significant pulmonary vein atrial reversal. Ao, aorta; D, diastolic; DT, deceleration time; dur, duration; E and A, mitral inflow early and late diastolic filling velocities; E′ and A′, mitral annular early and late diastolic filling velocities; IVCT, isovolumic contraction time; IVRT, isovolumic relaxation time; L, left atrium; LV, left ventricle; S and D, pulmonary vein systolic and diastolic filling velocities. (B and D from Naqvi TZ: Rev Cardiovasc Med 4[2]:81-99, 2003.)*

increase in LA pressure overrides the effects of impaired LV relaxation,[5,6] causing a pseudonormal mitral inflow that hides the underlying abnormality of LV relaxation.[7] With severe abnormalities of ventricular compliance, advanced diastolic dysfunction develops, characterized by a markedly increased E velocity. DT becomes short from rapid equalization of atrioventricular (AV) pressure soon after early diastolic filling in a noncompliant ventricle. Because of poor LA func-

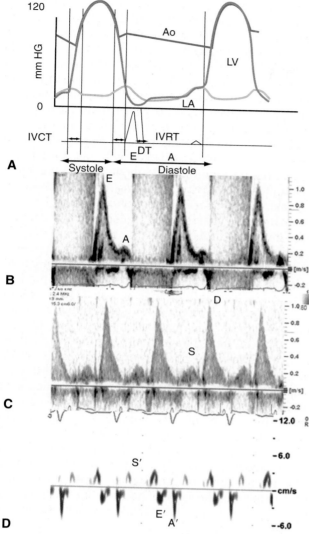

Figure 29–2. *Left ventricular, left atrial, and aortic pressure tracings (A), mitral inflow pulsed Doppler (B), pulmonary vein pulsed Doppler (C), and mitral annular tissue Doppler (D) in a subject with restrictive cardiomyopathy showing abnormal left ventricular relaxation, abnormal left atrial and left ventricular compliance, and elevated left atrial filling pressure. Mitral inflow velocities were obtained by placing the pulsed-wave Doppler sample volume between the tips of the mitral leaflets and Doppler tissue imaging by placing the pulsed-wave Doppler sample volume at the lateral mitral annulus. Large black horizontal arrows depict the duration of ventricular systole and ventricular diastole. Early diastolic left ventricular filling occurs as a result of the pressure gradient between left atrium and left ventricle. Filling beyond the first third of diastole is halted as a result of an increase in left ventricular diastolic pressure. Atrial contraction usually leads to a small filling A wave and marked pulmonary vein atrial reversal. However, in this advanced case, an atrial pump failure has occurred so there is no significant atrial reversal wave despite a small mitral inflow A wave. Pulmonary vein pulsed-wave Doppler shows reversal of the normal S to D ratio with a shortened pulmonary vein D wave deceleration time. Ao, aorta; D, diastolic; DT, deceleration time; dur, duration; E and A, mitral inflow early and late diastolic filling velocities; E' and A', mitral annular early and late diastolic filling velocities; IVCT, isovolumic contraction time; IVRT, isovolumic relaxation time; L, left atrium; LV, left ventricle; S, systolic; S and D, pulmonary vein systolic and diastolic filling veloci-*

tion and limited late diastolic AV pressure gradient from an elevated LV diastolic pressure, A wave amplitude becomes small. Initially, this restrictive mitral inflow pattern is reversible on preload reduction with the Valsalva maneuver or nitroglycerin or diuretic administration. Finally, an irreversible restrictive pattern develops with no significant change with preload reduction. As LA pressure increases, antegrade pulmonary vein systolic flow decreases and the diastolic wave becomes more prominent. The DT of the D wave also becomes shorter, by the same mechanism as mitral inflow E wave DT. With abnormal LV relaxation and compliance, an increase in left ventricular end-diastolic pressure (LVEDP) leads to minimal AV filling on atrial contraction and a prominent and prolonged pulmonary vein A-wave reversal that becomes greater than the mitral inflow A-velocity duration. Finally, impairment of LA contraction resulting from mechanical atrial failure leads to a decrease in amplitude and duration of the pulmonary vein A wave.[8]

Echocardiographic and Doppler Features

Imaging

Echocardiographic assessment for restrictive cardiomyopathy includes a comprehensive evaluation using all echocardiographic modalities.[9,10] Diagnosis of restrictive cardiomyopathy requires appropriate data acquisition using spectral and color Doppler imaging methods. Following is an outline of the method of Doppler data acquisition.

Doppler Recordings

Mitral Inflow Pulsed-Wave Doppler

The pulsed-wave (PW) sample volume is placed between the tips of the mitral leaflets ensuring parallel alignment of the Doppler beam with blood flow. In dilated hearts, AV flow is often directed toward the lateral wall requiring a shift in ultrasound (US) probe angle in the apical four-chamber view to ensure parallel Doppler beam alignment.

Pulmonary Vein Pulsed-Wave Doppler Imaging

Pulmonary vein Doppler is obtained by placing a color flow-guided 2-mm- to 3-mm Doppler PW sample volume from an apical four-chamber position, 1 to 3 cm deep within the right superior pulmonary vein whose flow is most nearly parallel to the ultrasound beam.[11-14] In comparison with the sample volume position used for antegrade flow velocities, the sharpest reverse flow velocity envelope at atrial contraction is often obtained at a position slightly further into the pulmonary vein.

If the Doppler signal is weak or the velocity envelope is incomplete, the use of a larger sample volume size (4 to 5 mm), modified apical transducer position, higher Doppler gain, or reimaging with the patient in a supine position may be attempted to improve the spectral quality. Sometimes better signals are obtained from apical two-chamber or three-chamber views.[15]

Mitral Annular Tissue Doppler Imaging

The tissue Doppler imaging (TDI) PW sample volume is placed at the lateral corner of the mitral annulus and subsequently at the medial (or septal) corner in the apical four-chamber view. The apical four-chamber view is selected because, in contrast with the parasternal window, the velocities are not influenced by anteroposterior translation and Doppler beam alignment is parallel to myocardial or annular motion. To prevent the sample volume from falling outside the mitral annulus during cardiac cycles, the sample volume is set to 5 mm × 8 mm. Because movement of the heart associated with respiration may still change the position of the PW Doppler sample volume in relation to the mitral annulus, a live two-dimensional (2D) view should be obtained from time to time to confirm correct sample volume placement. In patients with excessive respiratory excursion of the annulus, recording these velocities during held breathing can eliminate respiratory movements. Filters are set to exclude high-frequency signals, gain is set at a low level, and the Nyquist limit is adjusted to a velocity range of 15 to 30 cm/s to eliminate the signals produced by transmitral flow and gains are minimal. The resulting velocities are recorded for 5 to 10 cardiac cycles. A recording sweep speed of 100 to 200 mm/s is recommended for measurements of flow duration, whereas peak velocities should be measured at sweep speed of at least 100 mm/s.

Color M-Mode Velocity Propagation

Color Doppler imaging is first used to obtain the orientation of LV inflow in the apical four-chamber view. Normal mitral inflow is directed toward the mid to distal portion of the posterolateral wall of the left ventricle, approximately 20 degrees lateral to the LV apex.[16] With LV dilation, mitral inflow is directed progressively more laterally and posteriorly. Due to these varying intraventricular flow patterns, placement of M-mode cursor for the assessment of flow propagation should be guided by color Doppler ultrasonography. To maximize frame rate, the color sector is kept as narrow as possible and still include the mitral annulus and the LV apex. Zoom function is used to enlarge the image and sweep speed is maximized. The velocity scale is set so that aliasing velocity is 0.5 to 0.7 m/s. A color M-mode Doppler cursor is then aligned through the center of the

mitral ring to the apex, ensuring a minimum angle of incidence (typically less than 20 degrees of ultrasound beam alignment to flow direction) to minimize errors in measurement of peak velocity. The color scale of the velocity filter may be reduced (with a high-pass filter of 12 cm/s) to emphasize low-velocity flow, particularly in patients with poor LV function. The transducer angulation is adjusted and 2D gain is reduced to ensure that a homogenous color flow is seen within the entire LV cavity without dropouts as much as possible. Movement of the heart associated with respiration may change the position of the M-mode sample volume in relation to the LV cavity. Recording these velocities during held breathing or only at end-expiratory phase can eliminate these effects. After a good signal is obtained with multiple cardiac cycle, the sweep speed is adjusted to 100 to 200 mm/s (or the highest possible) during data acquisition. Investigators have proposed different methods of measuring velocity of propagation. These include measurement of: (1) the leading edge of the propagation wave[17] (the segment beginning with the onset of flow in the LV inlet and ending as far as possible into the LV chamber), (2) the temporal difference between the point of maximal velocity at the mitral level and at the apex,[18] (3) the slope of the first aliasing velocity from the mitral tips to a position 4 cm distal to them[19] (Fig. 29–3), and (4) the slope of a line connecting two points, the point of maximal velocity around the mitral orifice and the point at which this velocity decreases to 70% of its initial value.[20] A modified approach involves baseline shift until a distinct color border (blue within red) is obtained and then measurement of the slope of its most linear component past the valve leaflets. Propagation velocity values are expressed in cm/s.

Findings

Specific echocardiographic features of restrictive cardiomyopathy are summarized in Table 29–2. Features include biatrial enlargement (Fig. 29–4), marked concentric left ventricular hypertrophy (LVH) (Figs. 29–4 and 29–5) in the absence of a known cause, moderate AV valvular regurgitation (Fig. 29–6), increased pulmonary artery (PA) systolic (Fig. 29–7) and end diastolic pressure (Fig. 29–8) and increased LA (see Figs. 29–2 and 29–7) and right atrial filling (see Fig. 29–8) pressures and restrictive filling physiology on Doppler.

Mitral Inflow Pulsed-Wave Doppler. Diastolic features of restrictive cardiomyopathy show a spectrum of findings of increasing abnormality diastolic function beginning from a normal diastolic function to abnormal relaxation (see Fig. 29–1) and finally to a progressively abnormal chamber compliance leading to an increase in LA and LV filling pressures (see Fig. 29–2). In the early stages of the disease, mitral inflow filling pattern

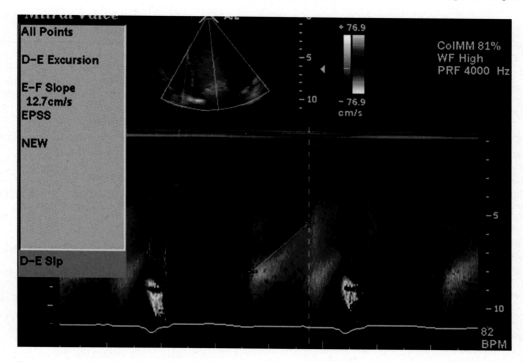

Figure 29–3. *A markedly reduced velocity of E wave propagation (Vp 13 cm/s) on color M-mode in a patient with cardiac amyloid indicating markedly abnormal left ventricular relaxation. (From Naqvi TZ: Rev Cardiovasc Med 4[2]:81-99, 2003.)*

shows an abnormal relaxation pattern characterized by E and A ratio of less than 1, a prolonged mitral inflow E wave DT and a prolonged isovolumic relaxation time (see Fig. 29–1). As the disease progresses and LA and LV diastolic compliance abnormality sets in, a pseudonormal phase is seen on mitral inflow that can reverse to an abnormal relaxation pattern on Valsalva maneuver.[21] With severe abnormalities of ventricular compliance, advanced diastolic dysfunction develops, characterized by a markedly increased E velocity. DT becomes short from rapid equalization of left atrial and ventricular pressures soon after early diastolic filling in a noncompliant ventricle (see Fig. 29–2). A wave amplitude is reduced because of poor LA function and because the elevated left atrial pressure results in a decreased late diastolic left atrial to ventricular pressure gradient. Initially, this restrictive mitral inflow pattern is reversible on preload reduction with the Valsalva maneuver, nitroglycerin, or diuretic administration. Finally, an irreversible restrictive pattern develops with no significant change with preload reduction. Due to a marked increase in LVEDP, diastolic mitral regurgitation (MR) may be seen especially in the presence of first-degree heart block.

Pulmonary Vein Pulsed-Wave Doppler. In the early stages of the disease, pulmonary vein flow may show a systolic dominant pattern with pulmonary vein systolic (S) to diastolic (D) ratio greater than 1 (see Fig. 29–1). Atrial reversal may be normal in the early stages, and

then, as LA compliance abnormality sets in, A wave velocity and duration (dur) progressively increase (see Fig. 29–2). As the compliance abnormality increases, decreased S and increased D waves on pulmonary vein Doppler tracing are seen (see Fig. 29–2). As a result of the combination of decreased LA compliance, increased mean LA pressure[22] and LV pressure,[23] the pulmonary vein S wave becomes blunted. The presence of significant MR may further blunt the S wave as a result of competition between MR and pulmonary vein flow at the atrial inflow chamber.[24] In the presence of AFib, marked blunting of the pulmonary vein S wave with or without MR is the rule. The pulmonary vein D wave, which results from the pulmonary vein-LA pressure gradient created during AV filling in early LV diastole, is dependent on the same factors that influence the early mitral velocity and its DT. Hence in advanced stages of the disease, a tall D wave with a shortened DT is seen. With abnormal LV relaxation and compliance, an increase in LVEDP leads to minimal AV filling on atrial contraction and a prominent and prolonged pulmonary vein A-wave reversal that becomes greater than the mitral inflow atrial duration. Finally, impairment of LA contraction resulting from mechanical atrial failure leads to a decrease in amplitude and duration of the pulmonary vein A wave[25] (see Fig. 29–2).

Tissue Doppler of Mitral Annulus. Unlike load dependence of mitral and pulmonary vein PW Doppler flow patterns, TDI of the septal and lateral mitral an-

TABLE 29-2. Echocardiographic Features of Restrictive Cardiomyopathy

M-Mode and Color M-Mode

Lack of septal bounce
Square root sign in the IVS and PW motion[244]
Myocardial hypertrophy
Decreased velocity of flow propagation

Two-Dimensional Findings

Preserved LV volumes
Preserved LV systolic function (early stages)
Biatrial enlargement
Myocardial hypertrophy without known cause
Myocardial speckling may be present
Atrial septal thickening
Homogenous atrioventricular valve thickening
May show small pericardial effusion
Occasionally ventricular thrombi or apical mass despite normal underlying wall motion

Transmitral Pulsed Doppler

Large E wave, small A wave; E:A ratio > 2; short DT <150 ms; short IVRT <60 ms; no significant change in mitral E wave, deceleration time, or isovolumic relaxation time with phases of respiration[245-248]
Abnormal relaxation pattern with E:A ratio <1 and prolonged deceleration time in early stages followed by pseudonormal and reversible restrictive before irreversible restrictive pattern
No significant respiratory variation

Transtricuspid Pulsed Doppler

Restrictive filling; increased E/A ratio and short deceleration time. With inspiration, there is further shortening of the deceleration time and minimal change in E:A ratio

Pulmonary Vein

Dilated pulmonary veins
Diastolic dominant pattern and S:D ratio <0.5
Prominent atrial reversal velocity with pulmonary vein atrial a-dur > mitral inflow a-dur
No change in D wave with respiration

C Mitral Regurgitation

May show diastolic MR
To evaluate dP/dt and left atrial filling pressure (systolic blood pressure − 4[mitral regurgitant velocity]^2)

CW Tricuspid Regurgitation

To evaluate pulmonary artery systolic pressure (4 × tricuspid insufficiency jet^2 [cm/s])

C Pulmonary Regurgitation

Pulmonary artery diastolic pressure (4 × pulmonary insufficiency jet^2 [cm/s]) plus right atrial pressure

Color Doppler Findings

Mitral and tricuspid regurgitation due to leaflet or papillary muscle involvement
Tricuspid regurgitation may be secondary to pulmonary hypertension
Diastolic mitral regurgitation as a result of increased left ventricular end-diastolic pressure[248]

Mitral Annulus Tissue Doppler Imaging

E/E' ratio to assess left ventricular filling pressure. In restrictive cardiomyopathy E' is usually <8 cm/s and E/E' is >15 as a result of elevated filling pressure[249]

Tricuspid Annulus Tissue Doppler Imaging

To assess right ventricular function[250,251]
To evaluate right atrial pressure[252]

Color M-Mode Examination

Velocity of flow propagation (Vp) is usually <45 cm/s in restrictive cardiomyopathy; E/Vp is >1.5 and can be used to assess left ventricular filling pressure[253]

Hepatic Vein and Hepatic Flow

Dilated hepatic veins, S:D ratio less than 0.5
Prominent atrial and ventricular reversals which increase with inspiration

Inferior Vena Cava

Dilated with reduced respiratory variation

CW, continuous wave Doppler; dP/dt, rate of LV pressure rise; DT, deceleration time; IVRT, isovolumetric relaxation time; LV, left ventricular; PW, posterior wall.

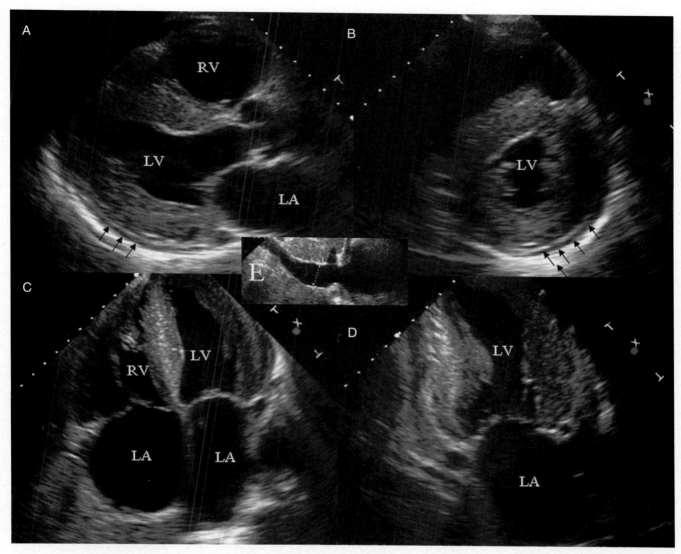

Figure 29–4. A, Parsternal long-axis view; B, short-axis view; C, apical four-chamber view; D, apical two-chamber view; and E, subcostal view in a patient with cardiac amyloidosis. A, Marked generalized hypertrophy is shown in all views. Note ground glass appearance of myocardium, biatrial and right ventricular enlargement, and small pericardial effusion (black arrows) as well dilated inferior vena cava in panel D indicating elevated right atrial pressure. LA, left atrium; LV, left ventricle; RA, right atrium; RV, right ventricle.

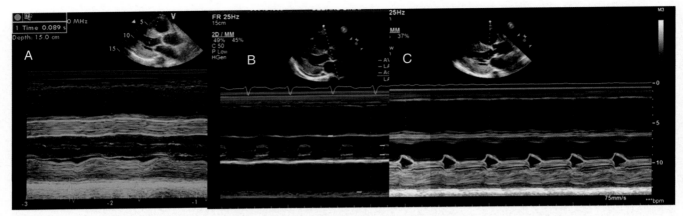

Figure 29–5. A, *Parasternal long-axis M-mode showing dilated right ventricle and normal sized left ventricle and marked increase in left ventricular wall thickness in a patient with senile cardiac amyloidosis;* B, *M-mode at aortic valve level showing deceased systolic opening time of aortic valve as well markedly reduced excursion of aortic root indicating reduced cardiac output and reduced atrial mechanical function;* C, *reduced diastolic opening time of mitral valve consistent with reduced cardiac output.*

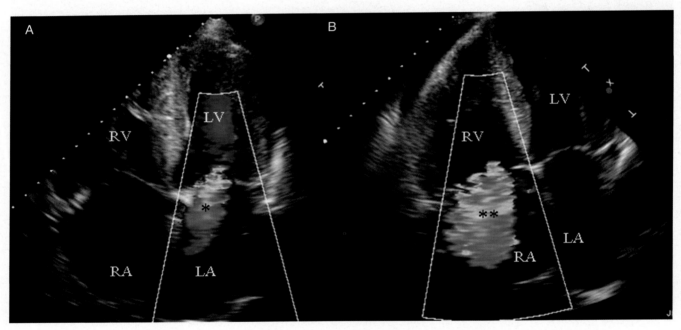

Figure 29–6. A, *Mild to moderate mitral regurgitation;* B, *moderate tricuspid regurgitation in a patient with cardiac amyloidosis. LA, left atrium; LV, left ventricle; RA, right atrium; RV, right ventricle.*

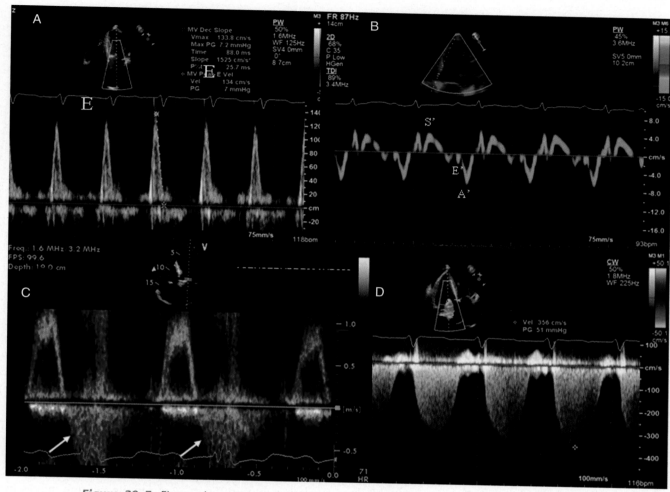

Figure 29–7. *Figure shows Doppler characteristics of patients with restrictive cardiomyopathy. A, Restrictive mitral inflow and presence of atrial fibrillation. B, Mitral annular tissue Doppler showing markedly decreased myocardial diastolic velocities (E' and A'); C, Diastolic mitral regurgitation (white arrows) especially in the presence of prolonged PR interval; and D, Increased pulmonary artery systolic pressure (RV-RA gradient of 3.56 m/s corresponding to a pressure gradient of 51 mm Hg in this case example).*

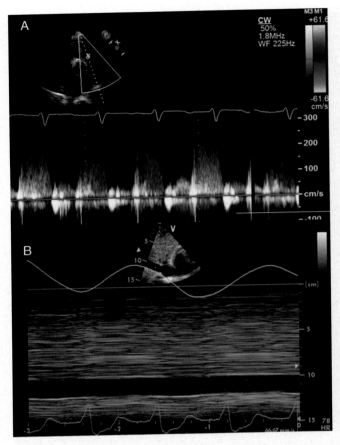

Figure 29–8. Increased pulmonary artery end-diastolic pressure based on increased pulmonary artery–right ventricular end-diastolic velocity of 2 to 2.3 meter per second (A). This corresponds to a gradient of 16 to 21 mm Hg. Increased right atrial pressure is evident from a dilated inferior vena cava with minimum decrease in size with respiration (shown by green respirogram in B), consistent with right atrial pressure of approximately 20 to 25 mm Hg (B). This estimates pulmonary artery diastolic pressure as 36 to 40 mm Hg.

nulus that interrogates myocardial tissue motion directly, allows more reliable and direct quantitation of myocardial relaxation.[26-28] With progressively increasing stages of the disease, the myocardial early motion wave shows a progressive decline in its amplitude so that the ratio of mitral inflow E wave and mitral annular E′ wave increases progressively (see Figs. 29–1 and 29–2). A markedly diminished velocity of diastolic motion is observed in patients with advanced restrictive cardiomyopathy. In fact, decreased TDI velocities are used as a diagnostic method of differentiating between constrictive pericarditis (in which TDI velocities of mitral annulus are preserved) and restrictive cardiomyopathy[29] (Fig. 29–9). A decrease in right ventricular (RV) systolic and diastolic velocities reflects a global impairment in myocardial relaxation (Fig. 29–10).

Color M-Mode. Using the slope of the first aliasing contour (see Fig. 29–3), patients with restrictive cardiomyopathy show a significantly slower than the constriction group. A slope of 100 cm/s provides the best separation between constrictive pericarditis and restrictive cardiomyopathy. In the constrictive group, the maximal velocity reaches the apex almost instantaneously compared with a significant delay in the restrictive group. Figure 29–3 shows an example of the apical time delay in a patient with restrictive cardiomyopathy.

Limitations and Pitfalls

Effect of the incidence angle, amplitude of the reflected echoes, scattering, sweep speed, Nyquist limit, low wall filters are important considerations for Doppler imaging.[30] Common pitfalls in obtaining good pulmonary vein signals may be related to depth of imaging which may in turn be machine or patient related. Inadequate sample size and its placement, lack of signal updating in real time, excessive gain, high filter settings, atrial wall motion artifact, and excessive respiratory excursion causing displacement of Doppler sample volume are other common sources of an inadequate pulmonary vein Doppler signal. TDI sample volume should be placed at the junction of the annulus with the myocardial base. A large sample volume and excessive Doppler gain result in spectral broadening of the velocity envelope that makes measurement of the variables of flow velocity and flow duration more difficult. The sample volume moves in relation to the myocardial wall dynamics in such a way that the selected region of interest of the ventricular myocardium under analysis is not always the same; this causes motion artifacts superimposed on the PW Doppler images. Because of the physiologic beat-to-beat variability of the PW TDI data, an averaged value from a few cardiac cycles should be obtained. Velocity of flow propagation cannot be measured when a linear wave front for early filling is not available in patients with poor echogenicity. In patients with a significantly dilated left ventricle, in which the mitral inflow progresses along the posterolateral wall, parallel alignment of M-mode cursor to blood flow may be difficult and result in falsely low propagation speed. Images are technically inadequate when there is a lack of continuity in the blood column or apical blood flow is not present in the color M-mode picture. When using the aliasing boundary method, it may be difficult to display a clear aliasing boundary when the peak early filling velocity is decreased to less than 25 cm/s. In this case, baseline shift to alias at 75% of peak E-wave velocity should be used. In small ventricles, color M-mode may not accurately reflect LV relaxation properties and may overestimate ventricular relaxation, such as often oc-

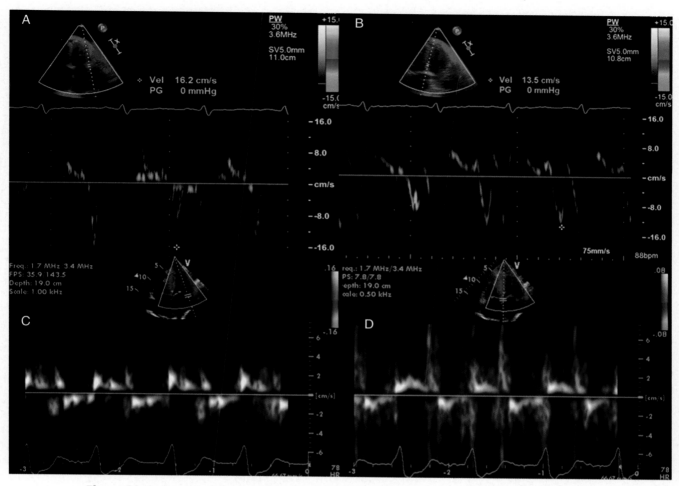

Figure 29–9. A *and* B *show tissue Doppler velocities at the lateral* (A) *and septal* (B) *mitral annulus in a 71-year-old patient with constrictive pericarditis and* C *and* D *show tissue Doppler velocities at the lateral* (C) *and septal* (D) *mitral annulus in a 84-year-old patient with senile cardiac amyloidosis. Note increased diastolic velocities for age in patient with constriction and markedly decreased systolic and diastolic velocities in the patient with restriction.*

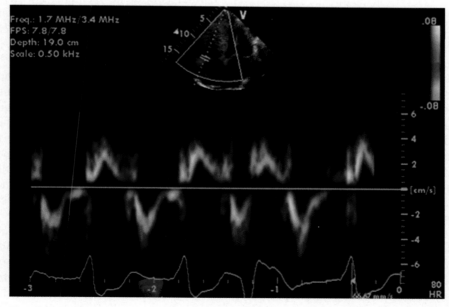

Figure 29–10. *Reduced systolic and diastolic tissue Doppler tricuspid annular velocities in a patient with cardiac amyloidosis.*

curs in patients with restrictive cardiomyopathy. In addition, this parameter may be normal, at least theoretically, in patients with a pseudonormal or restrictive pattern than in those with isolated relaxation abnormality if atrial function is intact and LV size is preserved.

Specific Restrictive Cardiomyopathies

Restrictive cardiomyopathies can be classified as shown in Table 29–1. Echocardiography plays an important role in the characterization of infiltrative cardiomyopathies.[31] Some characteristic echocardiographic features of relatively common restrictive cardiomyopathies are described here, although none is particularly sensitive or specific for the underlying etiology. In most cases, careful consideration of the clinical context and endomyocardial biopsy may be required. Infiltrative processes and metabolic storage diseases, including amyloidosis, hemochromatosis, sarcoidosis, Fabry's disease, and glycogen storage diseases, are the most frequent causes of restrictive cardiomyopathies. Less common forms of restrictive cardiomyopathies include endocardial fibrosis associated with the hypereosinophilic syndrome (Loeffler's cardiomyopathy) and idiopathic restrictive cardiomyopathy.

Amyloidosis

This is the most commonly encountered and recognized cause of restrictive cardiac disease.

Definition

Four different types of amyloidosis have been described according to the underlying disease:

1. *Immunoglobulin amyloidosis:* Immunoglobulin light chain amyloidosis (AL) constitutes about 85% of all newly diagnosed cases of amyloidosis and is the most common cause of cardiac amyloidosis. It includes primary amyloidosis, multiple myeloma, and other plasma cell dyscrasias, such as B-cell lymphoma and Waldenström macroglobulinemia.[32] The building block of the amyloid fibril is an immunoglobulin light chain protein. Primary amyloidosis is a plasma cell disorder in which approximately 5% to 10% of bone marrow plasma cells have clonal dominance of a light chain isotype.[33] There is predominance of lambda versus kappa free light chains (3:1) in primary AL amyloidosis; in comparison, other plasma cell dyscrasias, such as multiple myeloma, usually have a lambda-to-kappa ratio of 1:2. Common presenting features include ne-

phrotic syndrome, sensorimotor peripheral neuropathy, hepatomegaly, splenomegaly, and, less often, macroglossia.[34,35]

2. *Familial amyloidosis:* Familial amyloidosis, or hereditary amyloidosis, is less common than primary amyloidosis and is caused by an autosomal-dominant mutation, most frequently in the transthyretin gene. Common features include peripheral neuropathy, renal impairment, autonomic dysfunction with mainly gastrointestinal (GI) symptoms, and cardiomyopathy.[36] Macroglossia does not occur, and renal involvement is less prevalent than it is in AL amyloidosis.

3. *Senile systemic amyloidosis:* Senile systemic amyloidosis affects approximately 25% of patients over the age of 80 and is derived from normal transthyretin.[37] This type of amyloidosis mainly involves the atria (91%) and less often is isolated in the aorta or involves the entire heart.[38,39] Senile cardiac amyloidosis is not always a benign condition and can result in HF, AFib, and other conduction disturbances.[40,41]

4. *Secondary amyloidosis:* Secondary amyloidosis is characterized by reactive amyloid fibrils, which are acute-phase reactants produced in response to systemic inflammation, such as tuberculosis, leprosy, rheumatoid arthritis, familial Mediterranean fever, inflammatory bowel syndrome, chronic lung diseases, and chronic infections.

Cardiac Features

Restrictive cardiomyopathy is the main finding in cardiac amyloidosis. There is replacement of normal myocardial contractile elements by deposits of amyloid, leading to alterations in cellular metabolism, calcium transport, receptor regulation, and cellular edema. Injury can also occur from circulating light chains in the absence of amyloid fibril formation.[42] Amyloid myocardium becomes firm, rubbery, and noncompliant.[43] Involvement of the cardiac conduction system can lead to fibrosis of sinoatrial and AV nodes and involvement of infra His fibers leading to various types of heart block and arrhythmias.[44] Another cardiac manifestation can be cor pulmonale resulting from amyloid infiltration of pulmonary vasculature, causing significant pulmonary hypertension.[45] An infarction pattern in the absence of epicardial coronary disease can result from amyloid deposition in the microvasculature.[46]

Cardiac involvement occurs in about 50% of patients with immunoglobulin amyloidosis; the primary presentation is with congestive heart failure (CHF) in about 25% of these patients. Cardiac involvement is less common in other forms of primary amyloidosis and least common in secondary amyloidosis. Specific echocardiographic features occur in two thirds of patients, including thickening of the LV walls with low voltages on electrocardiography, increased myocardial reflectivity (the speckled, granular, or ground glass pattern), biatrial enlargement, thickening of the interatrial septum, thickening of mitral and tricuspid valves, mitral and tricuspid regurgitation (TR), presence of a small-to-moderate pericardial effusion and various abnormalities in diastolic filling and filling pressures as described previously (see Figs. 29–4 through 29–10). Significant LVH and wall motion abnormalities may be seen in patients with secondary amyloidosis.[48] The differential diagnosis of amyloidosis includes hypertrophic cardiomyopathy (HCM) and other infiltrative cardiomyopathies. Decreased LV function strongly suggests absence of hypertrophic cardiomyopathy.

Endomyocardial biopsy remains the definitive diagnostic method for cardiac amyloidosis.[49] Transthoracic echocardiography (TTE) has played a major role in the evaluation of amyloid deposition in the heart and is the procedure of choice for the noninvasive diagnosis of cardiac amyloid.[47-50] Increased myocardial echogenicity (granular sparkling) is useful for diagnosing cardiac amyloidosis especially in the presence of increased atrial thickness, specificity of this finding can reach 100%,[47] however this feature is evident only in the advanced stages of the disease and has not found to be helpful in diagnosis in some reports.[51] In recent studies novel parameters, such as TDI and myocardial strain rate, have been investigated for earlier diagnosis of cardiac amyloid, however further studies are needed to define prognostic relevance of these parameters.[52,53] If the combined clinical and echocardiographic picture suggests amyloidosis,[54] then immunocharacterization of the underlying amyloid protein can be obtained less invasively from extracardiac tissue sites.[55] If amyloid deposition is found in noncardiac biopsy sites along with a characteristic appearance on echocardiography, an endomyocardial biopsy is usually not necessary. These sites include the tongue, subcutaneous fat pads, kidneys, bone marrow, gastric mucosa, and less commonly, rectal mucosa.

Other Diagnostic Approaches. A number of modalities besides echocardiography help arrive at a diagnosis of restrictive cardiomyopathy. These are listed in Table 29–3.

Circulating free immunoglobulin light chains are found in over 98% of patients with primary amyloidosis and are used to determine prognosis and response to chemotherapy.[56] Serum levels of cardiac troponin (in response to myocardial injury) and pro-brain natriuretic peptide[57] (released in response to myocardial stress) are independent predictors of survival in patients with primary amyloidosis. Immunocharacterization of the underlying amyloid protein can be obtained by extracardiac tissue sites.[58] However endomyocardial biopsy remains the definitive diagnostic method for cardiac amyloidosis. Interstitial eosinophilic amyloid deposits can be seen on eosin hematoxylin staining. Congo red staining will produce an apple-green birefringence under polarized light and is the most specific stain for amyloid. The characteristic fibrillar pattern of the amyloid deposits can be seen by electron microscopy and immunohistochemical staining can then be used to determine the type of amyloid deposit.[59] Combining a subcutaneous fat pad biopsy and Congo red staining of bone marrow has yielded a tissue diagnosis in 90% of patients with amyloidosis.[60] Electrocardiography shows a low voltage in up to 50% of patients with cardiac amyloidosis and in conjunction with LVH on echocardiography should raise the suspicion for cardiac amyloidosis.[61]

Nuclear scintigraphy with ^{99}Tc pyrophosphate[62] or indium-labeled serum amyloid protein can detect extensive cardiac involvement of cardiac amyloidosis.[63] Tc pyrophosphate scan is positive in familial and senile amyloidosis with a 100% accuracy for diagnosis. A negative scan is 100% specific to exclude the diagnosis of primary amyloidosis.[62] Serum amyloid P (SAP) component is a normal circulating plasma protein that is deposited on amyloid fibrils because of its specific binding affinity for these fibrils. Scintigraphy after the injection of ^{123}I-SAP can be used for diagnosing, locating, and monitoring the extent of systemic amyloidosis.[64,65]

Global delayed endocardial gadolinium enhancement along with reduced subendocardial to blood T1 difference on magnetic resonance imaging (MRI) has been reported to be accurate in advanced stages of cardiac amyloidosis,[66] however utility of MRI in early stages of the disease has not been evaluated.[67]

Natural History

Onset of congestive HF is associated with a poor prognosis often less than 6 months. The prognosis varies according to the type of amyloidosis, the stage of the disease, and the age of the patient at the time of diagnosis. Primary amyloidosis has the worst prognosis, which is exacerbated by multisystem involvement and cardiac involvement in particular.[68] A marked increase in wall thickness, specifically mean LV and RV wall thickness of greater than 15 mm and 7 mm, respectively,[69] reduced LV systolic function,[69] shortened DT of less than 150 ms,[70] and increased early diastolic filling velocity to atrial filling ratio,[70] have all been proposed as predictors of cardiac death, but it has been suggested that a Doppler-derived index of combined systolic and diastolic myocardial performance (known as the Tei index) is a more useful predictor of clinical outcome.[71] In a large prospective follow-up study of 208 patients, fractional shortening and LV wall thickness or TEI index did not predict outcome, whereas mitral inflow E/A ratio and DT predicted cardiac death. This

TABLE 29–3. Other Approaches in the Diagnosis of Restrictive Cardiomyopathies

Diagnostic Modalities	Findings	Limitations
2D or Doppler echocardiography	LV hypertrophy Restrictive filling	Comorbidities of advanced age and coexisting hypertension renders LV hypertrophy nonspecific May be late findings with limited impact on guiding treatment or affecting prognosis Nonreproducible measurements make regression difficult to follow[254] Does not provide etiologic information in amyloidosis[255]
Systemic markers	Light chains, serum amyloid p component, Troponin and Pro B-type natriuretic peptide	Most useful in primary amyloidosis
Biopsy Tongue, subcutaneous fat pads, kidneys, bone marrow, gastric mucosa, rectal mucosa, and endomyocardial	May reveal specific cause of restrictive cardiomyopathy Eosinophilic interstitial deposits on H&E, apple-green birefringence on Congo red staining and fibrillar protein on EM in cardiac amyloid	Procedural risk Uncertainty about sampling error limits use in monitoring disease
Cardiac catheterization	Dip and plateau in diastolic pressure curve RV systolic pressure usually >50 mm Hg LV end-diastolic pressure often more than 5 mm Hg > RV end-diastolic pressure RV end-diastolic pressure < one third of RV systolic pressure	—
Computed tomography imaging	Pericardium of normal thickness	—
Magnetic resonance imaging	High spatial resolution and tissue contrast definition. Global subendocardial late gadolinium enhancement in advanced stage cardiac amyloid and diminished T1 difference between myocardium and blood provides high (97%) accuracy in advanced stage of cardiac amyloidosis	Utility in early stages of the disease has not been evaluated
Nuclear scintigraphy with ^{99}Tc pyrophosphate or indium-labeled systemic amyloid protein scan	Tc pyrophosphate scan differentiates between immunoglobulin light chain and transthyretin related familial and senile amyloidosis. Strong uptake in transthyretin-related amyloidosis with accuracy of 100% Indium cardiac uptake in primary and multi-organ uptake in systemic amyloidosis	—

2D, two dimensional; EM, electron microscopy; H&E, hemotoxylin and eosin stain; LV, left ventricular; RV, right ventricular.

study found that the myocardial integrated back scatter of the posterior wall was the best predictor of cardiac and overall death.[72] Another marker of poor prognostic is RV dilation.[73] Histologically, the worst prognosis is associated with the presence of nodular deposits, thick perimyocytic layers of amyloid, and small myocyte diameters on endomyocardial biopsy.[74] The overall median survival after diagnosis is less than 2 years in most studies. Syncope indicates a poor prognosis as well and is often a precursor of sudden cardiac death.[75]

In secondary amyloidosis, the underlying chronic disease affects the prognosis. Hereditary amyloidoses vary in prognosis according to the specific mutation.[76]

In addition, heart rate variability assessed by Holter monitoring was found to be a possible predictor of mortality in patients with both primary and secondary amyloidosis involving the heart.[77] Impaired LV systolic function is more common in primary than other forms of amyloidosis,[78] which also carries a worse prognosis compared to secondary amyloidosis.

Treatment

The use of high-dose melphalan with rescue autologous peripheral blood stem cell transplantation has resulted in reversal of the clinical manifestations of AL amyloidosis in a significant proportion of patients who survived the procedure.[79-83]

Idiopathic Restrictive Cardiomyopathy

Definition

Idiopathic restrictive cardiomyopathy occurs predominantly in elderly women. It is a rare entity distinguished from the other forms of restrictive cardiomyopathy by the presence of normal ventricular wall thickness. There have been found a few reports of mutations in idiopathic restrictive cardiomyopathy, implicating the desmin and cardiac troponin I genes.[84] Linkage of genes to a region on chromosome 10 has been in autosomal dominant restrictive cardiomyopathy in a family.[85] Idiopathic restricted cardiomyopathy accounts for 2% to 5% of all cardiomyopathies in children.[86] Biatrial enlargement and none or minimal hypertrophy are evident, as in the idiopathic restrictive cardiomyopathy of the adult (Fig. 29–11).

Cardiac Features

Typical features include marked biatrial enlargement and AFib in the absence of valvular heart disease, hypertension, or ischemic heart disease. The diagnosis of idiopathic cardiomyopathy is based on the exclusion of connective tissue disease, carcinoid syndrome, amyloidosis, hemochromatosis, eosinophilic syndrome, malignancy, radiation exposure, cardiotoxic drug exposure, or history of alcohol abuse. Interstitial fibrosis is the predominant histologic finding. LV systolic function is preserved in over two thirds of patients. Compared to cardiac amyloidosis, long-axis function as measured by TDI is often preserved in these patients.[87] AFib is common.[88] Endomyocardial biopsy shows mild to severe interstitial fibrosis and mild myocyte hypertrophy.[88] The interstitial fibrosis found in this condition only rarely interferes with the shortening of myocardial fiber bundles but is sufficient to prevent ventricular dilation and thereby limit diastolic stretch.

Natural History

Idiopathic restrictive cardiomyopathy is characterized by increased mortality—with 5- and 10-year survivals of 64% and 37%, respectively. LA dimension greater than 60 mm is associated with a poor prognosis.[88] The disease carries an even worse prognosis in children with a median survival of 2 years.[89] The strongest predictor of survival in children with idiopathic restrictive cardiomyopathy is the extent of increase in LA to aortic ratio at presentation followed by pulmonary capillary wedge pressure (PCWP) and LVEDP. Symptoms at the time of presentation do not predict outcome.[89]

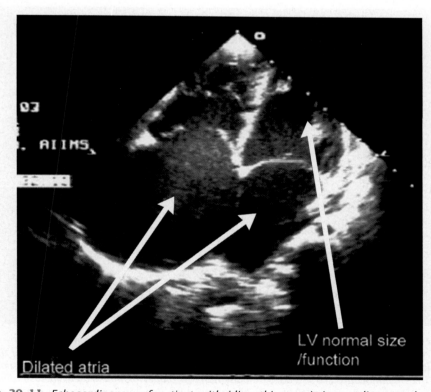

Figure 29–11. Echocardiogram of patient with idiopathic restrictive cardiomyopathy, showing normal sized ventricles with normal systolic function and enlarged left and right atria. LV, left ventricle. (From Seth S, Thatai D, Sharma S, et al: Eur J Heart Fail 6[6]:723-729, 2004).

Hypereosinophilic Syndrome and Endomyocardial Fibrosis

Definition

Idiopathic hypereosinophilic syndrome is a leuko-proliferative disorder characterized by idiopathic sustained peripheral blood eosinophilia ($> 1.5 \times 10^9/l$) and multi-organ dysfunction caused by infiltration of eosinophils. Cardiac dysfunction is the most common cause of morbidity and mortality. Endocardial fibrosis and myocardial inflammation cause HF and ventricular mural thrombus formation.

Cardiac Features

Dyspnea, ascites, peripheral edema, and right-sided HF are common clinical manifestations of the disease in patients with biventricular involvement. Increased endocardial thickness suggestive of fibrosis with restricted leaflet motion of the mitral valve is seen in Loeffler endocarditis and endomyocardial fibrosis.[90] This disease is characterized by fibrosis of the endocardium and of the myocardium of the inlet region and LV apex. Involvement of the papillary muscles leads to regurgitation of mitral and tricuspid valves. Progressive shrinkage of the LV cavity occurs.[91] Ventriculography may show a polylobulated LV silhouette with linear calcific shadows at the "amputated" apex giving an appearance of a clenched fist[92] or a hissing snake.[93]

Echocardiographic findings include Merlon sign (basal hypercontractility), which contrasts with the abnormal apex.[94] M-mode echocardiography typically shows the square root sign in the diastolic motion septum and posterior wall. On 2D echocardiography, there is inversion of the normal-sized relationship between the atria and ventricles with obliterated ventricles and dilated atria. Marked biatrial enlargement is seen when both sides of the heart are involved. The apex of the involved ventricle shows layered thrombus in the early stages, which is later obliterated by fibrosis. Different grades of pericardial effusion are also found. Echocardiography seems to be the only noninvasive method that can detect endomyocardial disease in its early stages.[95,96] Peripheral eosinophilia along with increased cardiac troponin T without other known etiology, which decreases after treatment, has been proposed to be an early marker of disease even before echocardiographic manifestations appear.[97]

There are three stages in hypereosinophilic syndrome: necrotic, thrombotic, and fibrotic. Common echocardiographic findings in the thrombotic stage are mural thrombus with apical cavity obliteration and thickening of the myocardium (Fig. 29–12). AV valves are often involved in the fibrotic process with subsequent valvular regurgitation. A restrictive pattern is typical of the late stage of the disease. There is minimal change in mitral and tricuspid velocities as found in healthy patients, which differentiates endomyocardial

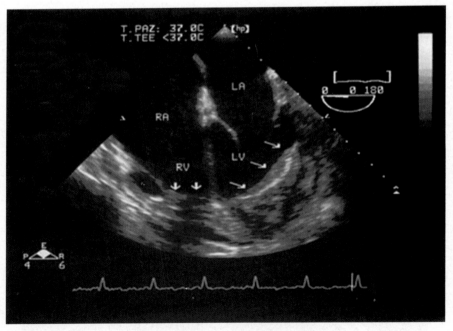

Figure 29–12. Cardiac involvement in idiopathic hypereosinophilic syndrome A 38-year-old man was referred for dyspnea. Transthoracic and transesophageal echocardiography revealed the presence of deposits at the apex of the left and right ventricle (arrows). Routine blood tests showed an increased eosinophil count ($18 \times 109/l$). A bone marrow biopsy demonstrated an eosinophilic myeloproliferative disease. The patient was diagnosed with hypereosinophilic syndrome, in which cardiac involvement is common. The patient was treated with alpha interferon plus oral methylprednisolone. (From Lorenzoni R, Cortigiani L, Melosi A: Heart 87[6]:553, 2002.)

fibrosis from constrictive pericarditis. Furthermore, a restrictive pattern is observed on both AV valves when both sides are involved with a markedly short tricuspid DT. Pulmonary veins show markedly diastolic D wave and a broad reversal A wave (the latter present a low velocity when the wall of the left atrium is diseased) caused by an increased LVEDP to the same extent throughout the respiratory cycle. Hepatic veins show a markedly deep diastolic forward wave throughout the respiratory cycle and a marked reversal with inspiration. Fibrous thickening of the endocardium, made up of collagen without elastic fibers, and sometimes organized thrombus is seen on endomyocardial biopsy. Normal thickness of mitral and tricuspid valve leaflets despite severe regurgitation, involvement of papillary muscles, obliteration of LV apex, and normal-sized to small-sized ventricle in the presence of severe valvular regurgitation distinguishes this condition from rheumatic heart disease. Patients who present with right-sided endocardial fibrosis may have clinical features that may be confused with constrictive pericarditis. Presence of normal pericardial thickness, obliteration of RV apex, and markedly dilated right atrium distinguishes it from constrictive pericarditis. Obliteration of LV apex during both systole and diastole distinguishes endomyocardial fibrosis from apical hypertrophic cardiomyopathy in which obliteration only occurs in systole. The presence of a normal-sized ventricle in the presence of gross cardiomegaly on chest X-ray (CXR) and normal-sized and normal LV systolic function distinguishes it from dilated cardiomyopathy (DCM). Gigantic right atrium and apical obliteration of RV apex may suggest Ebstein's anomaly, however normal attachment of tricuspid leaflets and focal involvement of RV inflow and outflow regions distinguishes right-sided endocardial fibrosis from Ebstein's anomaly.

Natural History and Outcome Data

Early institution of alpha-interferon and steroids and favorable response to treatment may halt the fibrotic process and improve symptoms and prognosis in these patients.

Hemochromatosis

Reversible restrictive cardiomyopathy has been described as a rare clinical feature of hemochromatosis.[98,99] An early echocardiographic study in patients with cardiac hemochromatosis secondary to transfusion in patients with anemia described LVH as characteristic of this disorder,[100] however a subsequent echocardiographic study that examined echocardiographic features of patients with primary hemochromatosis compared to normal subjects found that hypertrophy is not a feature of hemochromatosis cardiomyopathy.[101] Most of the echocardiographic studies in fact report a

DCM with hemochromatosis.[102] A recent study found increased wall thickness that was reversible after iron chelation therapy.[103] Perhaps increased thickness is an early feature of the disease with progression to DCM in later stages.

Sarcoidosis

Definition

Sarcoidosis is a granulomatous disease of unknown etiology that has a predilection for certain ethnic groups, such as African Americans, and pulmonary sarcoid is often the first manifestation of the disease.[104] In a comparative study of cardiac sarcoidosis in Japanese, African Americans, and whites, the incidence of cardiac sarcoid granulomas was 67.8%, 21.2%, and 13.7%, respectively.[105] Endomyocardial biopsy may assist in making a diagnosis with the finding of noncaseating granulomas. The histological diagnostic rate of cardiac sarcoidosis using endomyocardial biopsy has a low sensitivity of 19.2%[106] as a result of a patchy distribution of the pathology and predilection of granulomas for the cephalad portion of the septum that is less accessible to biopsy.

Cardiac Features

Cardiac involvement occurs in 25% of patients with systemic sarcoidosis but is clinically silent in the majority of patients.[107] There have been many reports describing echocardiographic features of cardiac sarcoidosis.[108-117] Diastolic dysfunction is not uncommon in patients with pulmonary sarcoid without any cardiac involvement.[118] Wall motion abnormalities, LV aneurysm, systolic dysfunction, DCM, conduction abnormalities, arrhythmias, and pericardial effusion are more common manifestations of cardiac sarcoidosis.[119] Sarcoid is an important diagnostic consideration in scar-related ventricular tachycardia.[120] Sudden death may be the first manifestation of cardiac sarcoidosis.[121] Sarcoid can be misdiagnosed as idiopathic or arrhythmogenic RV cardiomyopathy. Restrictive cardiomyopathy is more unusual and diagnosis of sarcoid restrictive cardiomyopathy may be made after characteristic findings of noncaseating granulomas on endomyocardial biopsy.[122] To date, no single cardiac investigation has been shown to reliably predict cardiac involvement. Sarcoid lesions are more prominent in the upper portions of the interventricular septum. Valantine's group[123] reported that thinning and the wall motion abnormalities at the base of the intraventricular septum characterize the presence of cardiac sarcoidosis. These findings occur in approximately 10% of patients. Asymmetric septal hypertrophy, recorded in 10% patients, may have had a similar origin.[109] Such abnormalities in the upper portion of the intraventricular septum may be considered a reliable diagnostic element of cardiac sarcoidosis, even though there is no further evidence of other organ involvement. One report found that over 50% of patients with cardiac sarcoidosis had diastolic dysfunction and preserved systolic function.[124] Some patients show thickening of the basal region of the heart.[125] One report described normal LV systolic function, marked biatrial enlargement, severe tricuspid regurgitation and marked thickening of biatrial walls, appendages and interatrial septum.[126] It may be considered that when thickening is present, the sarcoid lesions may be of a progressive nature, which is manifested with interstitial edema resulting from exudative or activate granuloma formation. In the advanced stages of disease, interstitial fibrosis may progress, and thus thinning of the ventricular wall may occur. As a result of low yield on endomyocardial biopsy,[106] the diagnosis is often made with a combination of electrocardiography, Holter monitoring, echocardiography, myocardial perfusion imaging, and, most recently MRI.[127] Radionuclide scanning with thallium 201[128] or sestamibi[129] may show abnormal defects that reverse with dipyridamole,[130] but the clinical value and significance of these findings is still uncertain. One report found that Holter monitoring was associated with a sensitivity of 67% and a specificity of 80% for identification of cardiac involvement in patients with systemic sarcoidosis.[131] The plasma brain natriuretic peptide level is considered to be a useful noninvasive biomarker for identifying a possible cardiac involvement in the sarcoidosis patients with a preserved ejection fraction.[132]

Natural History

Unlike isolated pulmonary disease, cardiac involvement implies a poor prognosis. Patients with sarcoidosis are at increased risk of sudden death. Owing to the progress in antiarrhythmic drugs and pacemaker implantation, the primary cause of death in cardiac sarcoidosis has changed from sudden death to congestive HF.[133]

Outcome Data

For symptomatic patients, medical therapy may include a trial of steroids and immunosuppressive therapy. An excellent response can be achieved with steroid therapy in the early acute inflammatory stage. Monoclonal antibodies against tumor necrosis factor may be employed in refractory cases. Heart block warrants a permanent pacemaker, whereas ventricular tachyarrhythmias are typically amiodarone-unresponsive, requiring implantation of an implantable cardioverter defibrillator. Heart transplantation is a suitable option for patients with end-stage disease.

Storage Disorders

Gaucher's Disease

Definition. Gaucher disease, the most common lysosomal storage disorder[134] is the result of inherited deficiency of the lysosomal enzyme glucocerebrosidase.[135] Clinically, three phenotypes have been delineated on the basis of the presence and severity of central nervous system involvement[136]: Type 1 (nonneuropathic adult form), type 2 (acute neuronopathic form diagnosed classically in several months old infants), and type 3 (subacute neuronopathic juvenile form). Partial deficiency of acid beta-glucosidase is associated with parenchymal disease of the liver, spleen, and bone marrow with concomitant anemia and thrombocytopenia in nonneuropathic, type 1 Gaucher's disease. Severe deficiency of glucocerebrosidase caused by severe mutations is additionally associated with neurological manifestations in the less common type 2 and type 3 subtypes.[137] The perinatal lethal form is rare and prominent features of the severe perinatal form are hepatosplenomegaly, associated with hydrops fetalis, generalized ichthyosis and facial dysmorphy.[138]

Cardiac Features. Echocardiographic features of this disease in the nonneuropathic (adult) form, include increase in LV mass with a septal muscular prominence, areas of apical akinesis, and pericardial changes.[139] Ascending aortic and aortic and mitral valve calcification has been described in a family.[140]

Natural History and Outcome. Enzyme replacement therapy in type I Gaucher's disease regresses hepatosplenomegaly, anemia, thrombocytopenia, bone fractures and bone crisis, whereas neurologic abnormalities and interstitial fibrosis do not respond to treatment.[141,142]

Glycogen Storage Disorder

Pompe's Disease

Definition. Pompe's disease occurs as a result of a α-1,4 glucosidase deficiency, characterized by progressive deposition of glycogen in all tissues.[143] The disease has an autosomal recessive inheritance with a predicted frequency of 1:40,000. Pompe's disease is associated with elevation of muscle enzymes creatine phosphokinase, lactate dehydrogenase, alanine aminotransferase, and aspartate aminotransferase in 90% to 95% of cases and is confirmed by measurement of α-glucosidase deficiency in leukocytes, fibroblasts, or in muscle tissue. The classic infantile form of the disease occurs in infants shortly after birth and is characterized by generalized hypotonia, failure to thrive, and cardiorespiratory failure. Muscular abnormalities and respiratory difficulties are the most common manifestations followed by cardiac manifestations, pain, epilepsy, fatigue, feeding problems, underweight, macroglossia, abnormal speech, hepatosplenomegaly, abnormal mental development, and hyperparathyroidism.[144]

Cardiac Features. One review of 225 patients with adult onset Pompe's disease found echocardiographic evidence of hypertrophic cardiomyopathy in 5% of patients, cor pulmonale in 2%, and other cardiac abnormalities in another 4% of patients.[138] Cardiac hypertrophy was only found in subjects younger than 1 year. Echocardiographic features include severe thickening of the interventricular septum, free wall, and posterior LV wall[145,146] with a tumor-like appearance of the papillary muscles, a small LV cavity, and poor LV function.[147,148] Case reports of apical hypertrophy causing artifacts on myocardial perfusion imaging and restrictive cardiomyopathy have been described.[149] Normal motion of the intraventricular septum and mitral valve leaflets and midsystolic closure of the aortic valve have been noted.[150] The combination of echocardiographic and electrocardiographic findings is helpful in the clinical diagnosis and recognition of the severity of cardiac involvement of this disease.

Natural History. Patients with infantile form of disease usually die within the first year of life. The nonclassic or late-onset form of the disease may occur at any age in childhood or adulthood. It presents predominantly as a slowly progressive proximal myopathy (in 95% of patients), with or without respiratory difficulties (in 44%).[144,151]

Outcome Data. Patients with later onset of disease have better prognosis.[144] Respiratory failure is the most common cause of death. Beneficial effects of recombinant human α-glucosidase have been reported both in patients with the classic infantile form[152] and in patients with the nonclassic or late-onset form of the disease.[153] Enzyme replacement therapy regresses cardiac hypertrophy, improves HF symptoms, skeletal muscle weakness, and respiratory failure, whereas lower motor neuron disease is unresponsive to treatment.[154]

Fabry's Disease

Definition. This is a rare X-linked recessive sphingolipidosis results from the defective activity of the lysosomal enzyme alpha-galactosidase A.[155] Accordingly, hemizygous males have the most severe form of the disease and heterozygous females usually have a more benign presentation.[156] The enzymatic defect in this lysosomal storage disease leads to the accumulation of globotriaosylceramide in several organs including the skin, kidney, nervous system, cornea, and the heart.

Cardiac Features. Cardiac involvement in Fabry's disease may occur in conjunction with involvement of other organs or the disease may manifest only with cardiac involvement. Electrocardiogram features include a short PR interval, abnormalities of conduction and LVH.[157] Echocardiographic findings include aortic root dilatation, generalized asymmetric increase in myocardial wall

thickness, myocardial dysfunction, ultimately dilated cardiac chambers, and valve dysfunction, especially of the mitral valve.[158,159] The increased ventricular wall thickness is the consequence of the deposition of globotriaosylceramide in cardiomyocytes and cellular hypertrophy. In female patients, the features are usually subclinical, however greater than half of heterozygous females may have cardiac hypertrophy on echocardiogram.[160] Endomyocardial biopsy or measurement of plasma α−galactosidase-A activity are definitive diagnostic tests. Sarcoplasmic vacuolization is the classic finding on light microscopy of hematoxylin and eosin stained tissue. On electron microscopy, concentric lamellar bodies are noted in the sarcoplasm of myocardial cells. In two recent studies, Fabry's disease was diagnosed in 3% to 4% of men with concentric LVH.[161,162] Asymmetric septal hypertrophy may be present in as many as four percent of patients with Fabry's disease.[162]

Natural History. LV systolic function progressively deteriorates in untreated patients with Fabry's disease. A large cross-sectional study of a patient cohort from the Anderson Fabry's disease clinical and genetic register showed that the median cumulative survival was 50 years ($n = 51$), which represents an approximately 20 year reduction of life span. Steep decline in survival occurs after age 35. Neuropathic pain (77%), sensorineural deafness (78%), renal failure (30%), cerebrovascular complications (24%), and low body mass index resulting from gastrointestinal complications were common.[163]

Outcomes Data. Recently the availability of enzyme replacement therapy has been shown to result in clearing of vascular endothelial deposits of globotriaosylceramide.[164] Improvement in LV mass and systolic function has also been reported with enzyme replacement treatment.[165]

Drug-Induced Restrictive Cardiomyopathy

Fibrous thickening of LV endocardium with features of restrictive cardiomyopathy occur in anthracycline cardiotoxicity. Ultrastructural abnormalities of the myocytes with myofibrillar loss and cytoplasmic vacuolation are seen both in anthracycline and chloroquine cardiotoxicity. Both restrictive features (Fig. 29–13) and concentric LVH (Fig. 29–14) have been shown to be reversible on chloroquine withdrawal. Methysergide cardiotoxicity involves encasing of heart valves with fibrous tissue causing valvular regurgitation.

Postradiation Cardiomyopathy

Definition

Radiation induced heart disease with its clinical manifestations is becoming a growing problem. Its prevalence is increasing, keeping pace with the increased survival

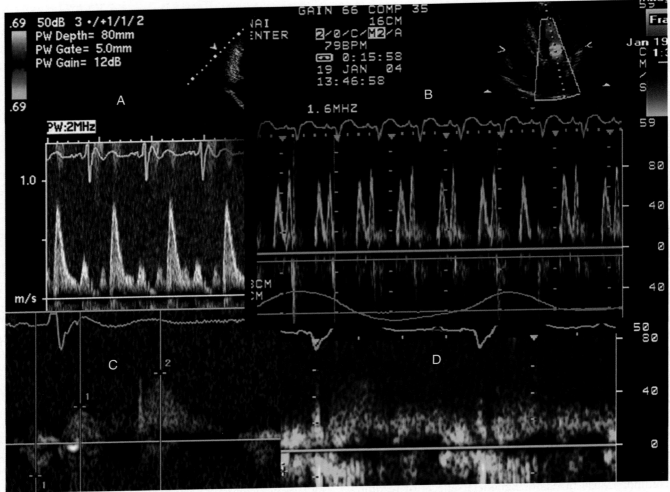

Figure 29–13. *Mitral inflow (A) and pulmonary vein inflow (C) before choloroquine withdrawal and after 7 months of chloroquine withdrawal (B and D). Restrictive mitral and pulmonary vein pulsed-wave Doppler changed to an abnormal relaxation pattern post chloroquine withdrawal. (C and D from Naqvi TZ, Luthringer D, Marchevsky A, et al: J Am Soc Echocardiogr 18[4]:383-387, 2005.)*

of many malignancies.[166] The majority of patients with radiation induced heart disease is constituted by Hodgkin's disease survivors, followed by non-Hodgkin's disease, esophageal carcinoma, thymoma, lung cancer, breast cancer, and metastatic seminoma. Pericardial disease is the most well-known expression of radiation induced heart disease present clinically in 60% to 70% of patients receiving mediastinal irradiation.[166,167] The manifestations include acute pericarditis, pericardial effusion with or without tamponade, and constrictive pericarditis. Almost all of patients who develop radiation induced heart disease develop a pericardial effusion with relative sinus tachycardia 3 to 4 weeks post-radiation, which may be transient. 6 to 12 months after radiation, late damage is manifest as massive pericardial effusion followed by myocardial damage and coronary sclerosis depending on field and radiation dose. The mean time of presentation for constrictive pericarditis is 48 months. Follow-up of the irradiated patients by echo-

cardiography, especially those who received more than 5000 Rad to the heart area is advisable.[168,169] Appropriate cardiac shielding and minimum possible radiation dose are preventive measures.

Cardiac Features

Published observations on the effect of radiation of LV function differ. Gustavsson and colleagues[170] found a decrease of LV shortening in 44% of patients and a decrease in LV end-diastolic dimension in 28% of patients and evidence of diastolic dysfunction in 50% of patients. Others found decrease in LV systolic function in one third of patients and borderline value in another third,[171] whereas others[172,173] found no effect on LV function. The most conspicuous change is diffuse interstitial fibrosis seen chiefly in the right ventricle, presumably because of the commonly used anterior radiation fields leading to congestive HF, typically as a result

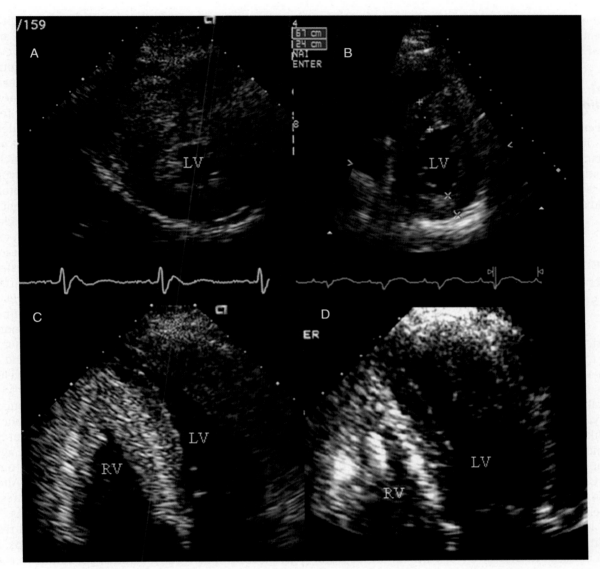

Figure 29–14. *Parasternal short-axis and apical four-chamber views in a 61-year-old Caucasian female with history of treatment with chloroquine for 20 years for systemic lupus erythematosus. A and C are images obtained before, and B and D are images obtained 10 months after discontinuation of chloroquine. Marked concentric left ventricular hypertrophy is shown in A and C, which regresses after chloroquine withdrawal. LV, left ventricle; RV, right ventricle. (A and B from Naqvi TZ, Luthringer D, Marchevsky A, et al:* J Am Soc Echocardiogr *18[4]:383-387, 2005.)*

of a restrictive cardiomyopathy. In an autopsy series, the endocardium was thickened, from fibrous proliferation with some increase in elastic fibers mainly in the right ventricle in 12 of 16 patients making the ventricular muscle less compliant and necessitating higher filling pressures to maintain stroke volume.[174] One series found cardiac involvement in 12 of 108 patients post irradiation for Hodgkin's disease. Chronic pericardial disease and coronary artery disease were the most frequent manifestations.[175] Coronary artery obstructive disease frequently involves ostial coronary segments and the left main and risk appears greater in those with

known risk factors for coronary artery disease.[176,177] All patients undergoing chest irradiation require serial cardiac evaluation. Important risk factors of radiation induced heart disease are previous chemotherapy, radiation exposure exceeding 4000 Rad, administration next to the heart, and on the left side of the chest. Doxorubicin treatment in children for acute lymphoblastic leukemia was found associated with chronic progressive cardiac dysfunction at 12-year follow-up and restrictive cardiomyopathy characterized by reduced cardiac mass, decreased LV dimension, and reduced wall thickness along with reduced LV systolic function. Although seen more commonly after high dose doxorubicin treatment, cardiomyopathy was seen even after low dose of doxorubicin treatment.[178]

Other Causes of Restrictive Cardiomyopathy

Connective tissue diseases, such as scleroderma, systemic lupus erythematosis,[179] and pseudoxanthoma elasticum,[180] may produce features of restrictive cardiomyopathy. Calcified endocardial bands may be seen in those with restrictive cardiomyopathy as a result of pseudoxanthoma elasticum.[181]

Differentiating between Restrictive Cardiomyopathy and Constrictive Pericarditis

Constrictive pericarditis and restrictive cardiomyopathy ought to be considered in any patient with disproportionate degree of right-sided HF in the setting of a normal or mildly depressed LV systolic function and normal valvular function. History of prior pericarditis, surgery, and radiation make diagnosis of constriction more likely. Pericardial calcification on chest X-ray and thickened pericardium on computed tomography (CT) scan are diagnostic findings of constriction. In some cases, CT may have difficulty differentiating pericardial fluid from thickened pericardial tissue. MRI provides comprehensive images of the pericardium and is superior to both CT and echocardiography with respect to its ability to characterize pericardial effusions and pericardial masses. Therefore, CT or MRI should be used when findings at echocardiography are nondiagnostic.[182] Sensitivity of transthoracic 2D echocardiogram in determining thickened pericardium is low. Although transesophageal echocardiography provides high sensitivity, it is invasive and used less often used for this purpose. Pericardial thickness of 3 mm or more on transesophageal echocardiography is highly suggestive of constrictive pericarditis.[183]

However, in about 18% of patients with surgical proven constriction, pericardial thickness may not be increased on noninvasive imaging as a result of the patchy nature of pericardial involvement on histopathology.[184] Surgical pericardiectomy has an excellent outcome, especially in the early phases of diagnosis.[185] Outcome is best for patients with idiopathic pericarditis followed by postoperative constriction.[186] Both constrictive pericarditis and restrictive cardiomyopathy are associated with increased intracardiac filling pressures, however, stiff pericardium versus stiff ventricle differentiate the two conditions and produce specific echocardiographic signs. The most important

pathophysiology of constrictive pericarditis is dissociation of intrathoracic and intracardiac pressure and increased ventricular interdependence. Negative chest pressure during inspiration is thus not transmitted to the cardiac chambers causing a decrease in transmitral gradient during the inspiratory phase secondary to a higher decrease in pulmonary venous pressure relative to LV diastolic pressure. Ventricular interdependence is increased in constrictive pericarditis as a result of lack of transmission of intrathoracic forces from thickened pericardium but absent in restrictive cardiomyopathy because of involvement of the ventricular septum. In constrictive pericarditis, there is abrupt diastolic shift in the ventricular septum toward the left ventricle during inspiration and toward the right ventricle in expiration.[187] Doppler echocardiography demonstrates exaggerated interventricular interdependence in constrictive pericarditis by showing marked respiratory variations in mitral (Fig. 29–15) and tricuspid flow Doppler (Fig. 29–16). Characteristic respiratory variations in Doppler flow velocities in patients with constriction not seen in patients with restriction include greater than 25% expiratory increase in mitral E velocity and expiratory decrease in hepatic vein diastolic flow velocity; greater than 25% increase in diastolic flow reversals compared with inspiratory velocity; greater respiratory variation in pulmonary venous flows; and systolic flow velocity lower than diastolic velocity throughout respiration.[188,189] In some patients who have been aggressively diuresed, volume loading helps to bring out the specific features of constrictive pericarditis.[190] Alternatively preload reduction helps to bring out the respiratory variation in volume overloaded patients.[191] In some patients, there may be features of mixed restrictive cardiomyopathy and constrictive pericarditis, such as those with active myocarditis, postradiation cardiomyopathy, or other forms of cardiomyopathy. In patients with clinical and echocardiographic Doppler features of restrictive cardiomyopathy, constriction still must be excluded.

If pericardial thickness is normal on CT or MRI, biochemical tests to determine the etiology of restrictive cardiomyopathy, such as serum or urine protein electrophoresis, iron studies and so on, should be performed followed by endomyocardial biopsy. This will confirm the specific etiology of restrictive cardiomyopathy in about 39% of patients.[192] A number of studies have reported specific two-dimensional and Doppler features that help differentiate restrictive cardiomyopathy from constrictive pericarditis.[193-202] Given that pericardectomy can cure constrictive pericarditis and that inappropriate surgical exploration is undesirable in restrictive cardiomyopathy, differentiation of these two entities is important. Echocardiographic features differentiating the restrictive cardiomyopathy from constrictive pericarditis conditions are listed in Table 29–4.

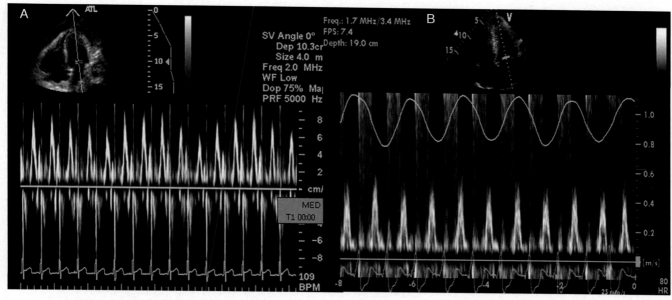

Figure 29-15. *Mitral inflow pulsed-wave Doppler in a patient with constriction (A) and in a patient with cardiac amyloidosis (B). Note marked respiratory changes with decrease in mitral inflow velocities during inspiration and increase during expiration in the patient with constriction and no significant respiratory change in the patient with cardiac amyloidosis.*

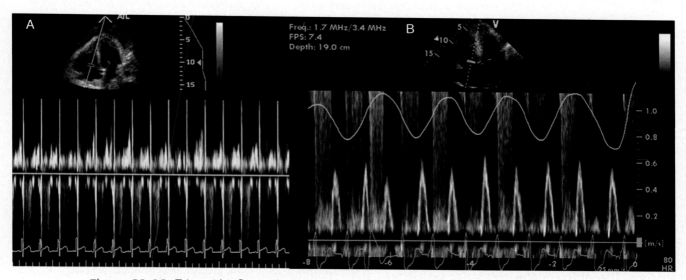

Figure 29-16. *Tricuspid inflow pulsed-wave Doppler in a patient with constriction (A) and in a patient with cardiac amyloidosis (B). Note marked respiratory changes with increase in velocities during inspiration and decrease during expiration in the patient with constriction and no significant respiratory change in the patient with cardiac amyloidosis.*

Early diastolic mitral annular velocity (E') by tissue Doppler echocardiography can be used to differentiate constrictive pericarditis from restrictive cardiomyopathy.[203,204] Patients with constrictive pericarditis had a significantly higher E' at septal annulus than those with primary restrictive cardiomyopathy or cardiac amyloidosis (12.3 versus 5.1 cm/s, $p < 0.001$)[203] (see Fig. 29–16). Specifically an E' cut-off value equal to 8 cm/s is able to distinguish the two conditions with a high sensitivity and specificity (95% sensitivity and 96% specificity). Even in patients who do not manifest the diagnostic sign of greater than 25% variation of mitral inflow with inspiration in patients with constriction mitral annular E' velocity remains normal and helps differentiate constrictive pericarditis from restrictive restrictive cardiomyopathy.[205] Occasionally when pericardial calcification and tethering involves the mitral annulus,[206] E' velocities may be reduced in constrictive pericarditis.

TABLE 29–4. Echocardiographic Features of Restrictive Cardiomyopathy and Constrictive Pericarditis

	Restrictive Cardiomyopathy	Constrictive Pericarditis
Pericardium	Normal	Thickened
Left ventricle	Small May show systolic dysfunction No septal bounce	Small Usually intact, may be abnormal particularly post-CABG or radiation Septal bounce
Atria	Usually dilated	Usually nondilated
Mitral inflow	Increased E:A ratio, short DT No significant respiratory variation of E velocity Diastolic MR	Increased E:A ratio, short DT >25% expiratory increase in E velocity Diastolic MR
Pulmonary vein inflow	Decreased (0.5) S:D ratio Prominent atrial reversal No significant respiratory change	S:D ratio = 1 Decrease in S and D* wave with inspiration
Tricuspid inflow	Mild respiratory variation	>25% inspiration increase in E wave and TR velocity
Inferior vena cava	Dilated	Dilated
Hepatic veins	Blunted S and D ratio >25% increase in atrial reversal in expiration	Inspiration minimal increase in S and D velocity, exp: decreased diastolic flow and increased in reversals compared to inspiration
Peak pulmonary artery pressure	>40 mm Hg	<40 mm Hg
Color M-mode	Decreased Vp <25 cm/s	Normal or increased >100 cm/s
Mitral annular Doppler	Low velocity <8 cm/s	High velocity ≥8 cm/s

*One study found significantly greater decrease of D wave only with respiration in constriction.[258]
CABG, coronary artery bypass graft; DT, deceleration time; MR, mitral regurgitation; TR, tricuspid regurgitation; Vp, velocity flow of propagation.
Adapted from Kushwaha S, Fallon JT, Fuster V: *N Eng J Med* 336:267-276, 1997; Asher CR, Klein AL: *Cardiol Rev* 10:218-229, 2002; Goldstein JA: *Curr Probl Cardiol* 29:503-567, 2004.

Similar to an increased E′ mitral annular velocity, preserved diastolic function in patients with constriction is manifest by a rapid propagation slope on color M-mode of greater than 100 cm/s.[207] Myocardial velocity gradient which is reduced in patients with restriction also differentiates restrictive restrictive cardiomyopathy from constrictive pericarditis.[208] Doppler imaging of the apex and strain rate imaging may help confirm constriction.[209] Even if mitral and pulmonary vein inflow are not diagnostic, TDI and color M-mode are able to correctly differentiate patients with constrictive pericarditis from those with restrictive cardiomyopathy.[203,204]

These echocardiographic findings are usually not diagnostic, and catheterization is often necessary for performing hemodynamic evaluation and obtaining endomyocardial biopsy specimens. Following three criteria have been proposed to differentiate the two conditions: (1) Equalization (less than 5 mm Hg difference between RV end-diastolic pressure and LVEDP) favors constriction[210]; (2) constriction is more often associated with modest elevations of RV systolic pressure (<50 mm Hg), whereas in restriction RV systolic pressures frequently exceed 50 mm Hg[211]; (3) constriction is associated with RV end-diastolic pressure exceeding one third the RV systolic pressure, whereas in restriction the ratio is characteristically less than one third.[211] In one study that evaluated the value of these hemodynamic criteria the predictive accuracy of difference between RV end-diastolic pressures and LVEDP, RV systolic pressure, and the ratio of RV end-diastolic pressure to RV systolic pressure were 85%, 70%, and 76%, respectively.[212]

Summary

Restrictive cardiomyopathy is a disease entity characterized by primarily by an abnormality in diastolic filling and normal or mildly reduced LV systolic function. It can result from multiple etiologies, the most common of which is amyloidosis. Irrespective of its etiology the echocardiographic hallmark of disease is hypertrophy and restriction in diastolic filling from a generalized myocardial process. Echocardiography plays a cornerstone role in the diagnosis and management of restrictive cardiomyopathy.

KEY POINTS

■ Primary abnormality in restrictive cardiomyopathy involves diastolic dysfunction and increase in LVEDP and LA filling pressures. LV systolic function is usually preserved until late stages of the disease. Patients may be asymptomatic in early stages and present with signs and symptoms of right-sided HF, left-sided HF, and low cardiac output.

■ 2D, M-mode and Doppler echocardiography remains the most useful clinical tool for diagnosis of patients with restrictive cardiomyopathy and cardiac catheterization findings, nuclear imaging and MRI are adjunctive diagnostic modalities. Tissue diagnosis remains the gold standard for the diagnosis of infiltrative cardiomyopathies but carries a low sensitivity.

■ Small LV cavity with LVH, valvular and interatrial septal thickening along with a granular sparkling texture and low voltage on electrocardiogram are hallmarks of cardiac amyloidosis.

■ Mitral inflow E/A ratio greater than 2, short DT (<150 ms), decreased pulmonary vein S/D ratio with blunted S, a large D wave with prominent atrial reversal, decreased tissue Doppler diastolic mitral annular velocity of less than 8 cm/s, slow M-mode propagation with increased peak pulmonary artery systolic pressure and right atrial pressure are classic echocardiographic findings of restrictive cardiomyopathy in the absence of known coronary artery disease and hypertension.

■ A combination of diagnostic tests are often needed to differentiate restrictive cardiomyopathy with constrictive pericarditis, however with TDI differentiation can be made with more certainty.

■ Prognosis of restrictive cardiomyopathy is highly variable depending on underlying etiology.

■ Restrictive cardiomyopathy should be considered in a patient post–chest radiation who presents with HF of unknown etiology.

■ Atrial arrhythmias and marked biatrial enlargement in the absence of valvular and myocardial disease are the most common presenting features in idiopathic restrictive cardiomyopathy in the elderly.

■ Drug-induced cardiomyopathy and infiltrative cardiomyopathy in several storage disorders may be reversible on withdrawal of the culprit agent or by enzyme replacement therapy.

REFERENCES

1. Richardson P, McKenna W, Bristow M, et al: Report of the 1995 World Health organization/International Society and Federation of Cardiology Task Force on the Definition and Classification of Cardiomyopathies. *Circulation* 93:841-842, 1996.
2. Child JS, Perloff JK: The restrictive cardiomyopathies. *Cardiol Clin* 6:289-316, 1988.
3. Benotti JR, Grossman W, Cohn PF: Clinical profile of restrictive cardiomyopathy. *Circulation* 61:1206-1212, 1980.
4. Guadalajara J, Vera-Delgado A, Gaspar-Hernandez J, et al: Echocardiographic aspects of restrictive cardiomyopathy: their relation with pathophysiology. *Echocardiography* 15:297-311, 1998.
5. Ishida Y, Meisner JS, Tsujioka K, et al: Left ventricular filling dynamics: Influence of left ventricular relaxation and left atrial pressure. *Circulation* 74:187-196, 1986.
6. Choong CY, Harrmann HC, Weyman AE, Fifer MA: Preload dependency of Doppler-derived indices of left ventricular diastolic function in humans. *J Am Coll Cardiol* 10:800-808, 1987.
7. Courtois M, Vered Z, Barzilai B, et al: The transmitral pressure-flow velocity relation: Effect of abrupt preload reduction. *Circulation* 78:1459-1468, 1988.
8. Plehn JF, Southworth J, Cornwell GG III: Brief report: Atrial systolic failure in primary amyloidosis. *N Engl J Med* 327:1570-1573, 1992.
9. Tam JW, Shaikh N, Sutherland E: Echocardiographic assessment of patients with hypertrophic and restrictive cardiomyopathy: imaging and echocardiography. *Curr Opin Cardiol* 17:470-477, 2002.
10. Thamilarasan M, Klein AL: Restrictive cardiomyopathy: Diagnostic and prognostic implications. In Otto CM (ed): *The practice of clinical echocardiography*, ed 2, Philadelphia, WB Saunders; 2002, pp. 613-638.
11. Oh JK, Appleton CP, Hatle LK, et al: The noninvasive assessment of left ventricular diastolic function with two-dimensional and Doppler echocardiography. *J Am Soc Echocardiogr* 10:246-270, 1997.
12. Appleton CP, Jensen JL, Hatle LK, Oh JK: Doppler evaluation of left and right ventricular diastolic function a technical guide for obtaining optimal flow velocity recordings. *J Am Soc Echocardiogr* 10:271-292, 1997.
13. Klein AL, Tajik AJ: Doppler assessment of pulmonary venous flow in healthy subjects and patients with heart disease. *J Am Soc Echocardiogr* 4:379-392, 1991.
14. Meijburg HWJ, Visser CA. Pulmonary venous flow as assessed by Doppler echocardiography. *Echocardiography* 12:425-440, 1995.
15. Jensen JL, Williams FE, Beilby BJ, et al: Feasibility of obtaining pulmonary venous flow velocity in cardiac patients using transthoracic pulsed wave Doppler technique. *J Am Soc Echocardiogr* 10:60-66, 1997.
16. Yamamoto K, Masuyama T, Tanouchi J, et al: Intraventricular dispersion of early diastolic filling: A new marker of left ventricular diastolic dysfunction. *Am Heart J* 129:291-299, 1995.
17. Brun P, Tribouilloy C, Duval AM, et al: Left ventricular flow propagation during early filling is related to wall relaxation: A color M mode Doppler analysis. *J Am Coll Cardiol* 20:420-432, 1992.
18. Stugaard M, Smiseth DA, Risoe C, Ihlen H: Intraventricular early diastolic filling during acute myocardial ischemia: Assessment by multigated color M-mode Doppler echocardiography. *Circulation* 88:2705, 1993.
19. Garcia MJ, Ares MA, Asher C, et al: An index of early left ventricular filling that combined with pulsed Doppler peak E velocity may estimate capillary wedge pressure. *J Am Coll Cardiol* 29:448-554, 1997.

20. Takatsuji H, Mikami T, Urasawa K, et al: A new approach for evaluation of left ventricular diastolic function: Spatial and temporal analysis of left ventricular filling flow propagation by color M-mode Doppler echocardiography. *J Am Coll Cardiol* 27:365-371, 1996.

21. Courtois M, Vered Z, Barzilai B, et al: The transmitral pressure-flow velocity relation: effect of abrupt preload reduction. *Circulation* 78:1459-1468, 1988.

22. Appleton CP, Gonzalez MS, Basnight MA: Relationship of left atrial pressure and pulmonary venous flow velocities: Importance of baseline mitral and pulmonary venous flow patterns studied in lightly sedated dogs. *J Am Soc Echocardiogr* 7:264-275, 1994.

23. Nishimura RA, Abel MD, Hatle LK, Tajik AJ: Relation of pulmonary vein to mitral vein flow velocities by transesophageal Doppler echocardiography: Effect of different loading conditions. *Circulation* 81:1488-1497, 1990.

24. Keren G, Sherez J, Megidish R, et al: Pulmonary venous flow pattern—its relationship to cardiac dynamics: A pulsed Doppler echocardiographic study. *Circulation* 71:1105-1112, 1985.

25. Plehn JF, Southworth J, Cornwell GG III: Brief report: Atrial systolic failure in primary amyloidosis. *N Engl J Med* 327:1570-1573, 1992.

26. Oki T, Tabata T, Yamada H, et al: Clinical application of pulsed Doppler tissue imaging for assessing abnormal left ventricular relaxation. *Am J Cardiol* 79:921-928, 1997.

27. Nagueh SF, Middleton KJ, Kopelen HA, et al: Doppler tissue imaging: a noninvasive technique for evaluation of left ventricular relaxation and estimation of filling pressures. *J Am Coll Cardiol* 30:1527-1533, 1997.

28. Farias CA, Rodriguez L, Garcia MJ, et al: Assessment of diastolic function by tissue Doppler echocardiography: comparison with standard transmitral and pulmonary venous flow. *J Am Soc Echocardiogr* 12:609-617, 1999.

29. Garcia MJ, Rodriguez L, Ares M, et al: Differentiation of constrictive pericarditis from restrictive cardiomyopathy: Assessment of left ventricular diastolic velocities in longitudinal axis by Doppler tissue imaging. *J Am Coll Cardiol* 27:108-114, 1996.

30. Klein AL, Oh JK, Miller FA, et al: Two-dimensional and Doppler echocardiographic assessment of infiltrative cardiomyopathy. *J Am Soc Echocardiogr* 1:48-59, 1988.

31. Weyman A: Principles of color flow imaging. In: Weyman A (ed): *Principles and practice of echocardiography*, Philadelphia, Lea & Febiger, 1994, pp. 218-233.

32. Benson MD: Amyloidosis. In Scriver CR (ed): *The metabolic and molecular bases of inherited disease*, ed 8, vol 1, New York, McGraw-Hill; 2001, pp. 5345-5348.

33. Falk RH, Comenzo RL, Skinner M: The systemic amyloidoses. *N Engl J Med* 337:898-909, 1997.

34. Kyle RA: Amyloidosis. *Circulation* 91:1269-1271, 1995.

35. Kyle RA, Gertz MA: Primary systemic amyloidosis: clinical and laboratory features in 474 cases. *Semin Hematol* 32:45-59, 1995.

36. Dubrey SW, Davidoff R, Skinner M, et al: Progression of ventricular wall thickening after liver transplantation for familial amyloidosis. *Transplantation* 64:74-80, 1997.

37. Westermark P, Sletten K, Johansson B, Cornwell GG III: Fibril in senile systemic amyloidosis is derived from normal transthyretin. *Proc Natl Acad Sci U S A* 87:2843-2845, 1990.

38. Kawamura S, Takahashi M, Ishihara T, Uchino F: Incidence and distribution of isolated atrial amyloid: histologic and immunohistochemical studies of 100 aging hearts. *Pathol Int* 45:335-342, 1995.

39. Olson LJ, Gertz MA, Edwards WD, et al: Senile cardiac amyloidosis with myocardial dysfunction. Diagnosis by endomyocardial biopsy and immunohistochemistry. *N Engl J Med* 317:738-742, 1987.

40. Pitkanen P, Westermark P, Cornwell GG III: Senile systemic amyloidosis. *Am J Pathol* 117:391-399, 1984.

41. Kyle RA, Spittell PC, Gertz MA, e al: The premortem recognition of systemic senile amyloidosis with cardiac involvement. *Am J Med* 101:395-400, 1996.

42. Hofer JF, Wimmer G: Severe heart failure from light chain cardiomyopathy (cardiac amyloidosis). *Z Kardiol* 92:90-95, 2003.

43. Kushwaha SS, Fallon JT, Fuster V: Restrictive cardiomyopathy. *N Engl J Med* 336:267-276, 1997.

44. Reisinger J, Dubrey SW, Lavalley M, et al: Electrophysiologic abnormalities in AL (primary) amyloidosis with cardiac involvement. *J Am Coll Cardiol* 30:1046-1051, 1997.

45. Dingli D, Utz JP, Gertz MA: Pulmonary hypertension in patients with amyloidosis. *Chest* 120:1735-1738, 2001.

46. Neben-Wittich MA, Wittich CM, Mueller PS, et al: Obstructive intramural coronary amyloidosis and myocardial ischemia are common in primary amyloidosis. *Am J Med* 118:1287, 2005.

47. Falk R, Plehn J, Deering T, et al: Sensitivity and specificity of the echocardiographic features of cardiac amyloidosis. *Am J Cardiol* 59:418-422, 1987.

48. Dubrey SW, Cha K, Simms RW, et al: Electrocardiography and Doppler echocardiography in secondary (AA) amyloidosis. *Am J Cardiol* 77:313-315, 1996.

49. Falk RH, Rubinow A, Cohen AS: Cardiac arrhythmias in systemic amyloidosis: correlation with echocardiographic abnormalities. *J Am Coll Cardiol* 3:107-113, 1984.

50. Klein AL, Oh JK, Miller FA, et al: Two-dimensional and Doppler echocardiographic assessment of infiltrative cardiomyopathy. *J Am Soc Echocardiogr* 1:48-59, 1988.

51. Dubrey SW, Cha K, Anderson J, et al: The clinical features of immunoglobulin light-chain (AL) amyloidosis with heart involvement. *Q J Med* 91:141-157, 1998.

52. Oki T, Tanaka H, Yamada H, et al: Diagnosis of cardiac amyloidosis based on the myocardial velocity profile in the hypertrophied left ventricular wall. *Am J Cardiol* 93:864-869, 2004.

53. Sallach JA, Klein AL: Tissue Doppler imaging in the evaluation of patients with cardiac amyloidosis. *Curr Opin Cardiol* 19:464-471, 2004.

54. Kyle RA, Greipp PR: Amyloidosis: clinical and laboratory features in 229 cases. *Mayo Clin Proc* 58:665-683, 1983.

55. Arbustini E, Verga L, Concardi M, et al: Electron and immunoelectron microscopy of abdominal fat identifies and characterizes amyloid fibrils in suspected cardiac amyloidosis. *Amyloid* 9:108-114, 2002.

56. Lachmann HJ, Gallimore R, Gillmore JD, et al: Outcome in systemic AL amyloidosis in relation to changes in concentration of circulating free immunoglobulin light chains following chemotherapy. *Br J Haematol* 122:78-84, 2003.

57. Palladini G, Campana C, Klersy C, et al: Serum N-terminal pro-brain natriuretic peptide is a sensitive marker of myocardial dysfunction in AL amyloidosis. *Circulation* 107:2440-2445, 2003.

58. Arbustini E, Verga L, Concardi M, et al: Electron and immunoelectron microscopy of abdominal fat identifies and characterizes amyloid fibrils in suspected cardiac amyloidosis. *Amyloid* 9:108-114, 2002.

59. Falk RH, Rubinow A, Cohen AS: Cardiac arrhythmias in systemic amyloidosis: Correlation with echocardiographic abnormalities. *J Am Coll Cardiol* 3:107-113, 1984.

60. Gertz MA, Lacy MQ, Dispenzieri A: Amyloidosis; recognition, confirmation, prognosis, and therapy. *Mayo Clin Proc* 74:490-494, 1999.

61. Dubrey SW, Cha K, Simms RW, et al: Electrocardiography and Doppler echocardiography in secondary (AA) amyloidosis. *Am J Cardiol* 77:313-315, 1996.

62. Perugini E, Guidalotti PL, Salvi F, et al: Noninvasive etiologic diagnosis of cardiac amyloidosis using 99mTc-3,3-diphosphono-1,2-propanodicarboxylic acid scintigraphy. *J Am Coll Cardiol* 46:1076-1084, 2005.

63. Tanaka M, Hongo M, Kinoshita O, et al: Iodine-123 metaiodobenzylguanidine scintigraphic assessment of myocardial sympathetic innervation in patients with familial amyloid polyneuropathy. *J Am Coll Cardiol* 29:168-174, 1997.

64. Hawkins PN, Pepys MB: Imaging amyloidosis with radiolabelled SAP. *Eur J Nucl Med* 22:595-599, 1995.

65. Hawkins PN, Lavender JP, Pepys MB: Evaluation of systemic amyloidosis by scintigraphy with 123I-labeled serum amyloid P component. *N Engl J Med* 323:508-513, 1990.

66. Maceira AM, Joshi J, Prasad SK, et al: Cardiovascular Magnetic Resonance in Cardiac Amyloidosis. *Circulation* 111:186-193, 2005.

67. Kwong RY, Falk RH: Cardiovascular magnetic resonance in cardiac amyloidosis. *Circulation* 111:122-124, 2005.

68. Kyle RA, Gertz MA: Primary systemic amyloidosis: clinical and laboratory features in 474 cases. *Semin Hematol* 32:45-59, 1995.

69. Cueto-Garcia L, Reeder GS, Kyle RA, et al: Echocardiographic findings in systemic amyloidosis: spectrum of cardiac involvement and relation to survival. *J Am Coll Cardiol* 6:737-743, 1985.

70. Klein AL, Hatle LK, Taliercio CP, et al: Prognostic significance of Doppler measures of diastolic function in cardiac amyloidosis: A Doppler echocardiography study. *Circulation* 83:808-816, 1991.

71. Tei C, Dujardin KS, Hodge DO, et al: Doppler index combining systolic and diastolic myocardial performance: Clinical value in cardiac amyloidosis. *J Am Coll Cardiol* 28:658-664, 1996.

72. Koyama J, Ray-Sequin PA, Falk RH: Prognostic significance of ultrasound myocardial tissue characterization in patients with cardiac amyloidosis. *Circulation* 106:556-561, 2002.

73. Patel AR, Dubrey SW, Mendes LA, et al: Right ventricular dilation in primary amyloidosis: An independent predictor of survival. *Am J Cardiol* 80:486-492, 1997.

74. Arbustini E, Merlini G, Gavazzi A, et al: Cardiac immunocyte-derived (AL) amyloidosis: an endomyocardial biopsy study in 11 patients. *Am Heart J* 130:528-536, 1995.

75. Chamarthi B, Dubrey SW, Cha K, et al: Features and prognosis of exertional syncope in light-chain associated AL cardiac amyloidosis. *Am J Cardiol* 80:1242-1245, 1997.

76. Dubrey SW, Cha K, Anderson J, et al: The clinical features of immunoglobulin light-chain (L) amyloidosis with heart involvement. *Q J Med* 91:141-157, 1998.

77. Reyners AK, Hazenberg BP, Reitsma WD, et al: Heart rate variability as a predictor of mortality in patients with AA and AL amyloidosis. *Eur Heart J* 23:157-161, 2002.

78. Mogenson J, Kubo T, Duque M, et al: Idiopathic restrictive cardiomyopathy is part of the clinical expression of cardiac troponin I mutations. *J Clin Invest* 111:209-216, 2003.

79. Comenzo RL, Vosburgh E, Falk RH, et al: Dose-intensive melphalan with blood stem-cell support for the treatment of AL (amyloid light-chain) amyloidosis: survival and responses in 25 patients. *Blood* 91:3662-3670, 1998.

80. Comenzo RL, Gertz MA: Autologous stem cell transplantation for primary systemic amyloidosis. *Blood* 99:4276-4282, 2002.

81. Gertz MA, Lacy MQ, Gastineau DA, et al: Blood stem cell transplantation as therapy for primary systemic amyloidosis (AL). *Bone Marrow Transplant* 26:963-969, 2000.

82. Gillmore JD, Davies J, Iqbal A, et al: Allogeneic bone marrow transplantation for systemic AL amyloidosis. *Br J Haematol* 100:226-228, 1998.

83. Moreau P, Leblond V, Bourquelot P, et al: Prognostic factors for survival and response after high-dose therapy and autologous stem cell transplantation in systemic AL amyloidosis: A report on 21 patients. *Br J Haematol* 101:766-769, 1998.

84. Hofer JF, Wimmer G: Severe heart failure from light chain cardiomyopathy (cardiac amyloidosis). *Z Kardiol* 92:90-95, 2003.

85. Zhang J, Kumar A, Kaplan L, et al: Genetic linkage of a novel autosomal dominant restrictive cardiomyopathy locus. *J Med Genet* 42:663-665, 2005.

86. Lipschutz SE, Sleeper LA, Towbin JA, et al: The incidence of pediatric cardio-myopathy in two regions of the United States. *N Engl J Med* 348:1647-1655, 2003.

87. Enrica Perugini E, Rapezzi C, Reggiani LB, et al: Comparison of ventricular long-axis function in patients with cardiac amyloidosis versus idiopathic restrictive cardiomyopathy. *Am J Cardiol* 95:146-149, 2005.

88. Ammash NM, Seward JB, Bailey KR, et al: Clinical profile and outcome of idiopathic restrictive cardiomyopathy. *Circulation* 101:2490-2496, 2000.

89. Russo LM, Webber SA: Idiopathic restrictive cardiomyopathy in children. *Heart* 91:1199-1202, 2005.

90. Garcia-Pascual J, Gonzalez-Gallarza R, Jimenez M, et al: Loffler's syndrome: Pulmonary vein and transmitral Doppler flow analysis by transesophageal echocardiography-report of a case. *J Am Soc Echocardiogr* 13:690-692, 2000.

91. Hassan WM, Fawzy ME, Al Helaly S, et al: Pitfalls in diagnosis and clinical, echocardiographic, and hemodynamic findings in endomyocardial fibrosis. A 25-year experience. *Chest* 128:3985-3992, 2005.

92. Namboodiri KKN, Bohora S: Clenched fist appearance in endomyocardial fibrosis. *Heart* 92:720, 2006.

93. Pieroni M, Chimenti C, Frustaci A: 'Hissing snake' left ventricle thrombotic phase of hypereosinophilic endomyocardial disease. *Eur Heart J* 27:778, 2006.

94. Berensztein C, Pineiro D, Marcotegui M, et al: Usefulness of echocardiography and Doppler echocardiography in endomyocardial fibrosis. *J Am Soc Echocardiogr* 13:385-392, 2000.

95. Davies J, Gibson DG, Foale R, et al: Echocardiographic features of eosionophilic endomyocardial disease. *Br Heart J* 48:434-440, 1982.

96. Zientek DM, King DL, Dewan SJ, et al: Hypereosinophilic syndrome with rapid progression of cardiac involvement and early echocardiographic abnormalities. *Am Heart J* 130:1295-1298, 1995.

97. Sato Y, Taniguchi R, Yamada T, et al: Measurement of serum concentrations of cardiac troponin T in patients with hypereosinophilic syndrome: A sensitive non-invasive marker of cardiac disorder. *Intern Med* 39:350, 2000.

98. Cutler DJ, Isner JM, Bracey AW, et al: Hemochromatosis heart disease: An unemphasized cause of potentially reversible restrictive cardiomyopathy. *Am J Med* 60:923-928, 1980.

99. Barriales Alvarez V, Simarro Garcia C, Suarez Suarez E, et al: [Restrictive cardiac involvement in a patient with dyserythropoietic anemia and secondary hemochromatosis.] *Rev Esp Cardiol* 49:618-620, 1996.

100. Borer JS, Henry WL, Epstein SE: Echocardiographic observations in patients with systemic infiltrative disease involving the heart. *Am J Cardiol* 39:184-188, 1977.

101. Olson LJ, Baldus WP, Tajik AJ: Echocardiographic features of idiopathic hemochromatosis. *Am J Cardiol* 60:885-889, 1987.

102. Candell-Riera J, Lu L, Se L, et al: Cardiac hemochromotosis: Beneficial effects of iron removal therapy; an echocardiographic study. *Am J Cardiol* 52:824-829, 1983.

103. Cecchetti G, Binda A, Piperno A, et al: Cardiac alterations in 36 consecutive patients with idiopathic haemochromatosis: polygraphic and echocardiographic evaluation. *Eur Heart J* 12:224-230, 1991.

104. Silverman KJ, Hutchins GM, Bulkley BH: Cardiac sarcoid: A clinicopathologic study of 84 unselected patients with systemic sarcoidosis. *Circulation* 58:1204-1211, 1978.

105. Iwai K, Sekiguti M, Hosoda Y, et al: Racial difference in cardiac sarcoidosis incidence observed at autopsy. *Sarcoidosis* 11:26-31, 1994.

106. Uemura A, Morimoto S, Hiramitsu S, et al: Histologic diagnostic rate of cardiac sarcoidosis: Evaluation endomyocardial biopsies. *Am Heart J* 138:299-302, 1999.

107. Silverman KJ, Hutchins GM, Bulkley BH: Cardiac sarcoid: a clinicopathologic study of 84 unselected patients with systemic sarcoidosis. *Circulation* 58:1204-1211, 1978.

108. Cepin D, McDonough M, James F. Cardiac sarcoidosis. A case with unusual manifestation. *Arch Intern Med* 143:142-144, 1983.

109. Gregor P, Widimsky P, Sladkova T, et al: Echocardiography in sarcoidosis. *Jpn Heart J* 25:499-508, 1984.

110. Lewin RF, Mor R, Spitzer S, et al: Echocardiographic evaluation of patients with systemic sarcoidosis. *Am Heart J* 110:116-122, 1985.

111. Walsh TK, Vacek JL, Bellinger RL: Sarcoidosis mimicking cor triatriatum. Echolucency of adenopathy due to sarcoidosis. *Am J Med* 78:501-505, 1985.

112. Rubinstein I, Fisman EZ, Rosenblum Y, et al: Left ventricular exercise echocardiographic abnormalities in patients with sarcoidosis without ischemic heart disease. *Isr J Med Sci* 22:865-872, 1986.

113. Friart A, Philippart C, Bruart J: Echocardiography in systemic sarcoidosis. *Lancet* 1:513, 1987.

114. Angomachalelis N, Hourzamanis A: Diagnostic significance of two-dimensional echocardiography in sarcoid infiltrative cardiomyopathy. In Grassi C, Rizzato G, Pozzi E, (eds): *Sarcoidosis and other granulomatous disorders.* Amsterdam, Elsevier Science, 1988, pp. 503-504.

115. Burstow DJ, Tajik AJ, Bailey KR, et al: Two-dimensional echocardiographic findings in systemic sarcoidosis. *Am J Cardiol* 63:478-482, 1989.

116. Bower SP, Thomson A: Two dimensional echocardiography and left ventriculography in cardiac sarcoidosis. *Aus NZ J Med* 19:724-726, 1989.

117. Ohmori F, Tachibana T: Two-dimensional echocardiographic assessment of systemic sarcoidosis. *Sarcoidosis* 9(Suppl 1):241-244, 1992.

118. Fahy GJ, Marwick T, McCreery CJ, et al: Doppler echocardiographic detection of left ventricular diastolic dysfunction in patients with pulmonary sarcoidosis. *Chest* 109:62-66, 1996.

119. Silverman KJ, Hutchins GM, Bulkley BH: Cardiac sarcoid: a clinicopathologic study of 84 unselected patients with systemic sarcoidosis. *Circulation* 58:1204-1211, 1987.

120. Koplan BA, Soejima K, Baughman K, et al: Refractory ventricular tachycardia secondary to cardiac sarcoid: electrophysiologic characteristics, mapping, and ablation. *Heart Rhythm* 3:924-929, 2006.

121. Furushima H, Chinushi M, Sugiura H, et al: Ventricular tachyarrhythmia associated with cardiac sarcoidosis: its mechanism and outcome. *Clin Cardiol* 27:217-222, 2004.

122. Ratner SJ, Fenoglio JJ Jr, Ursell PC: Utility of endomyocardial biopsy in the diagnosis of cardiac sarcoidosis. *Chest* 90:528-533, 1986.

123. Valantine HA, Tazelaar HD, Macoviak J, et al: Cardiac sarcoidosis: Response to steroids and transplantation. *J Heart Transplant* 6:244-250, 1987.

124. Skold CM, Larsen FF, Rasmussen E, et al: Determination of cardiac involvement in sarcoidosis by magnetic resonance imaging and Doppler echocardiography. *J Intern Med* 252:465-471, 2002.

125. Sekiguchi M, Yazaki Y, Isobe M, Hiroe M: Cardiac sarcoidosis: Diagnostic, prognostic, and therapeutic considerations. *Cardiovasc Drugs Ther* 10:495-510, 1996.

126. Hourigan LA, Burstow DJ, Pohlner P, et al: Transesophageal echocardiographic abnormalities in a case of cardiac sarcoidosis. *J Am Soc Echocardiogr* 14:399-402, 2001.

127. Smedema JP, Snoep G, van Kroonenburgh MP, et al: The additional value of gadolinium-enhanced MRI to standard assessment for cardiac involvement in patients with pulmonary sarcoidosis. *Chest* 128:1629-1637, 2005.

128. Hirose Y, Ishida Y, Hayashida K, et al: Myocardial involvement in patients with sarcoidosis: an analysis of 75 patients. *Clin Nucl Med* 19:522-526, 1994.

129. Le Guludec D, Menad F, Faraggi M, et al: Myocardial sarcoidosis: Clinical value of technetium-99m sestamibi tomoscintigraphy. *Chest* 106:1675-1682, 1994.

130. Tellier P, Paycha F, Antony I, et al: Reversibility by dipyridamole of thallium-201 myocardial scan defects in patients with sarcoidosis. *Am J Med* 85:189-193, 1988.

131. Suzuki T, Kanda T, Kubota S, et al: Holter monitoring as a noninvasive indicator of cardiac involvement in sarcoidosis. *Chest* 106:1021-1024, 1994.

132. Date T, Shinozaki T, Yamakawa M, et al: Elevated plasma brain natriuretic peptide level in cardiac sarcoidosis patients with preserved ejection fraction. *Cardiology* 107:277-280, 2006.

133. Yazaki Y, Hongo M, Hiroyoshi Y, et al: Cardiac sarcoidosis in Japan: Treatment and prognosis. In Sekignchi M, Richardson PJ (eds): *Prognosis and Treatment of Cardiomyopathy and Myocarditis,* Tokyo, University of Tokyo Press, 1994, pp. 351-353.

134. Alizad A, Seward JB: Echocardiographic features of genetic diseases: Part 2. Storage disease. *J Am Soc Echocardiogr* 13:164-170, 2000.

135. Brady RO, Kanfer JN, Shapiro, D: Metabolism of glucocerebrosides. II. Evidence of an enzymatic deficiency in Gaucher's disease. *Biochem Biophys Res Commun* 18:221-225, 1965.

136. Beutler E, Grabowski GA: Gaucher disease. In Scriver CR, Sly WS, Childs B, et al (eds): *The metabolic and molecular bases of inherited disease,* vol. III, New York, McGraw-Hill, 2001, pp. 3635-3668.

137. Germain DP: Gaucher's disease: a paradigm for interventional genetics. *Clin Genet* 65:77-86, 2004.

138. Mignot C, Gelot A, Bessieres B, et al: Perinatal-lethal Gaucher disease, *Am J Med Genet* 120A:338-344, 2003.

139. Saraclar M, Atalay S, Kocak N, Ozkutlu S: Gaucher's disease with mitral and aortic involvement: echocardiographic findings. *Pediatr Cardiol* 13:56-58, 1992.

140. Chabas A, Cormand B, Grinberg D, et al: Unusual expression of Gaucher's disease: cardiovascular calcifications in three sibs homozygous for the D409H mutation. *J Med Genet* 32:740-742, 1995.

141. Brady RO, Tallman JF, Johnson WG, et al: Replacement therapy for inherited enzyme deficiency: use of purified ceramidetrihexosidase in Fabry's disease. *N Engl J Med* 289:9-14, 1973.

142. Brady RO, Pentchev PG, Gal AE, et al: Replacement therapy for inherited enzyme deficiency: use of purified glucocerebrosidase in Gaucher's disease. *N Engl J Med* 291:989-993, 1974.

143. Garber AJ: Heritable disorders of carbohydrate metabolism. In Stein JH (ed): *Internal medicine,* ed 3, Boston, Little, Brown and Company, 1990, pp. 2273-2278.

144. Winkel LP, Hagemans ML, van Doorn PA, et al: The natural course of non-classic Pompe's disease; a review of 225 published cases. *J Neurol* 252:875-884, 2005.

145. De Dominicis E, Finocchi G, Vincenzi M, et al: Echocardiographic and pulsed Doppler features in glycogen storage disease type II of the heart (Pompe's disease). *Acta Cardiol* 46:107-114, 1991.

146. Gussenhoven WJ, Busch HF, Kleijer WJ, de Villeneuve VH: Echocardiographic features in the cardiac type of glycogen storage disease II. *Eur Heart J* 4:41-43, 1983.

147. Lorber A, Luder AS: Very early presentation of Pompe's disease and its cross-sectional echocardiographic features. *Int J Cardiol* 16:311-314, 1987.

148. Shapir Y, Roguin N: Echocardiographic findings in Pompe's disease with left ventricular obstruction. *Clin Cardiol* 8:181-185, 1985.

149. Shi H, Cotton J, Starsiak MD, et al: Apical hypertrophy caused by glycogen storage disease creating artifacts in myocardial perfusion imaging. *Clin Nucl Med* 31:229-231, 2006.

150. Seward JB, Tajik AJ, Edwards WD, Hagler DJ: *Two-dimensional echocardiographic atlas*, Vol 1. *Congenital heart disease*. New York, Springer-Verlag, 1987, p. 385.

151. van der Beek NA, Hagemans ML, van der Ploeg AT, et al: Pompe disease (glycogen storage disease type II): Clinical features and enzyme replacement therapy. *Acta Neurol Belg* 106:82-86, 2006.

152. Klinge L, Straub V, Neudorf U, Voit T: Enzyme replacement therapy in classical infantile pompe disease: Results of a ten-month follow-up study. *Neuropediatrics* 36:6-11, 2005.

153. Winkel LP, Van den Hout JM, Kamphoven JH, et al: Enzyme replacement therapy in late-onset Pompe's disease: a three-year follow-up. *Ann Neurol* 55:495-502, 2004.

154. Amalifitano A, Bengur AR, Morse RP, et al: Recombinant human acid alpha-glucosidase enzyme therapy for infantile glycogen storage disease type II: Results of a phase I/II clinical trial. *Genet Med* 3:132-138, 2001.

155. Brady RO, Gal AE, Bradley RM, et al: Enzymatic defect in Fabry's disease: Ceramidetrihexosidase deficency. *N Engl J Med* 276:1163-1167, 1967.

156. Desnick RJ, Ioannou YA, Eng CM: Alpha galactosidase A deficiency: Fabry disease. In Scriver CR, Beaudet AL, Sly WS, Valle D (eds): *The metabolic and molecular bases of inherited disease*, ed 8, vol 3. New York, McGraw-Hill, 2001, pp. 3733-3774.

157. Mehta J, Tuna N, Moller JH, et al: Electrocardiographic and vectorcardiographic abnormalities in Fabry's disease. *Am Heart J* 93:699-705, 1977.

158. Pierpont MEM, Moller JH: Cardiac manifestations of systemic disease. In Adams FH, Emmanouilides GC, Riemenschneider TA (eds): *Moss' heart disease in infants, children, and adolescents*, ed 4, Baltimore, Williams & Wilkins, 1989, pp. 778-801.

159. Towbin JA, Roberts R: Cardiovascular diseases due to genetic abnormalities. In Schlant RC, Alexander RW (eds): *The Heart Arteries and Veins*, ed 8, New York, McGraw-Hill, 1994, pp. 1725-1759.

160. Kampmann C, Baehner F, Whybra C, et al: Cardiac manifestations of Anderson-Fabry disease in heterozygous females. *J Am Coll Cardiol* 40:1668-1674, 2002.

161. Nakao S, Takenaka T, Maeda M, et al: An atypical variant of Fabry's disease in men with left ventricular hypertrophy. *N Engl J Med* 333:288-293, 1995.

162. Sachdev B, Takenaka T, Teraguchi H, et al: Prevalence of Anderson-Fabry disease in male patients with late onset hypertrophic cardiomyopathy. *Circulation* 105:1407-1411, 2002.

163. MacDermot KD, Homes A, Miners AH: Anderson-Fabry disease: clinical manifestations and impact of disease in a cohort of 98 hemizygous males. *J Med Genet* 38:750-760, 2001.

164. Eng CM, Guffon N, Wilcox WR, et al: Safety and efficacy of recombinant human alpha galactosidase A replacement in Fabry disease. *N Engl J Med* 345:9-16, 2001.

165. Weidemann F, Breunig F, Beer M, et al: Improvement of cardiac function during enzyme replacement therapy in patients with Fabry disease: a prospective strain rate imaging study. *Circulation* 108:1299-1301, 2003.

166. Fajardo LF, Stewart JR, Cohn KE: Morphology of radiation-induced heart disease. *Arch Pathol* 86:512-519, 1968.

167. Veinot JP, Edwards WD: Pathology of radiation-induced heart disease: A surgical and autopsy study of 27 cases. *Hum Pathol* 27:766-773, 1996.

168. Vallebona A: Cardiac damage following therapeutic chest irradiation. Importance, evaluation and treatment. *Minerva Cardioangiol* 48:79-87, 2000.

169. Akaike A, Kogure T, Oyama K, Oda M: Damage to the heart from tumor irradiation in the thorax—an echocardiographic study. *Radiologe* 25:430-436, 1985.

170. Gustavsson A, Eskilsson T, Landberg T, et al: Late cardiac effects after mantle radiotherapy in patients with Hodgkin's disease. *Ann Oncol* 1:355-363, 1990.

171. Gomez GA, Park JJ, Panahon A, et al: Heart size and function after radiation therapy to the mediastinum in patients with Hodgkin's disease. *Cancer Treatm Rep* 67:1099-1103, 1983.

172. Green DM, Gingell RL, Pearce J, et al: The effect of mediastinal irradiation on cardiac function of patients treated during childhood and adolescence for Hodgkin's disease. *J Clin Oncol* 5:239-245, 1987.

173. Morgan GW, Freeman AP, McLean RG, et al: Late cardiac, thyroid, and pulmonary sequelae of mantle radiotherapy for Hodgkin's disease. *Int J Radiat Oncol Biol Phys* 11:1925-1931, 1985.

174. Brosius FC, Waller BF, Roberts WC: Analysis of 16 young (aged 15 to 33 years) necropsy patients who received over 3500 rads to the heart. *Am J Med* 70:519-530, 1981.

175. Piovaccari G, Ferretti RM, Prati F, et al: Cardiac disease after chest irradiation for Hodgkin's disease: Incidence in 108 patients with long follow-up. *Int J Cardiol* 49:39-43, 1995.

176. King V, Constine LS, Clark D, et al: Symptomatic coronary artery disease after mantle irradiation for Hodgkin's disease. *Int J Radiol Oncol Biol Phys* 36:881-889, 1996.

177. Glanzmann C, Kaufmann P, Jenni R, et al: Cardiac risk after mediastinal irradiation for Hodgkin's disease. *Radiother Oncol* 46:51-62, 1998.

178. Lipshultz SE, Lipsitz SR, Sallan SE, et al: Chronic progressive cardiac dysfunction years after doxorubicin therapy for childhood acute lymphoblastic leukemia. *J Clin Oncol* 23:2629-2636, 2005.

179. Branea I, Stanciu L, Tomescu M, et al: The value of echocardiography in the early diagnosis of myocardial impairment due to connective tissue diseases. *Med Interne* 24:197-205, 1986.

180. Navarro-Lopez F, Llorian A, Ferrer-Roca O, et al: Restrictive cardiomyopathy in pseudoxanthoma elasticum. *Chest* 78:113-115, 1980.

181. Challenor VF, Conway N, Monro JL: The surgical treatment of restrictive cardiomyopathy in pseudoxanthoma elasticum. *Br Heart J* 59:266-269, 1988.

182. Wang ZJ, Reddy GP, Gotway MB, et al: CT and MR imaging of pericardial disease. *Radiographics* 23:S167-S180, 2003.

183. Ling L, Oh J, Tei C: Pericardial thickness measured with transesophageal echocardiography: Feasibility and potential clinical usefulness. *J Am Coll Cardiol* 29:1317-1323, 1997.

184. Talreja DR, Edwards WD, Danielson GK, et al: Constrictive pericarditis in 26 patients with histologically normal pericardial thickness. *Circulation* 108:1852-1857, 2003.

185. McCaughan BC, Schaff HV, Piehler JM, et al: Early and late results of pericardiectomy for constrictive pericarditis. *J Thorac Cardiovasc Surg* 89:340-350, 1985.

186. Bertog SC, Thambidorai SK, Parakh K, et al: Constrictive pericarditis: etiology and cause-specific survival after pericardiectomy. *J Am Coll Cardiol* 43:1445-1452, 2004.

187. Hancock E: Differential diagnosis of restrictive cardiomyopathy and constrictive pericarditis. *Heart* 86:343-349, 2001.

188. Hatle L, Appleton C, Popp R: Differentiation of constrictive pericarditis and restrictive cardiomyopathy by Doppler echocardiography. *Circulation* 79:357-370, 1989.

189. Klein AL, Cohen GI, Pietrolungo JF: Differentiation of constrictive pericarditis from restrictive cardiomyopathy by Doppler transesophageal echocardiographic measurements of respiratory variations in pulmonary venous flow. *J Am Coll Cardiol* 22:1935-1943, 1993.

190. Abdalla IA, Murray RD, Lee JC, et al: Does rapid volume loading during transesophageal echocardiography differentiate constrictive pericarditis from restrictive cardiomyopathy? *Echocardiography* 19:125-134, 2002.

191. Oh JK, Tajik AJ, Appleton CP, et al: Preload reduction to unmask the characteristic Doppler feature of constrictive pericarditis. A new observation. *Circulation* 95:796-799, 1997.

192. Schoenfeld M, Supple E, Dec W, et al: Restrictive cardiomyopathy versus constrictive pericarditis: Role of endomyocardial biopsy in avoiding unnecessary thoracotomy. *Circulation* 75:1012-1017, 1987.

193. Vaitkus P, Kussmaul WG: Constrictive pericarditis versus restrictive cardiomyopathy a reappraisal and update of diagnostic criteria, *Am Heart J* 122:1431-1441, 1991.

194. Rajagopalan N, Garcia M, Rodriguez L, et al: Comparison of new Doppler echocardiographic methods to differentiate constrictive pericardial heart disease and restrictive cardiomyopathy. *Am J Cardiol* 87:86-94, 2001.

195. Hatle L, Appleton C, Popp R: Differentiation of constrictive pericarditis and restrictive cardiomyopathy by Doppler echocardiography. *Circulation* 79:357-370, 1989.

196. Mancuso L, D'Agostino A, Pitrolo F, et al: Constrictive pericarditis versus restrictive cardiomyopathy: The role of Doppler echocardiography in differential diagnosis. *Int J Cardiol* 31:319-327, 1991.

197. Klein A, Cohen G, Pietrolungo J, et al: Differentiation of constrictive pericarditis from restrictive cardiomyopathy by Doppler transesophageal echocardiographic measurement of respiratory variations in pulmonary venous flow. *J Am Coll Cardiol* 22:1935-1943, 1993.

198. Palka P, Lange A, Donnelly E, et al: Differentiation between restrictive cardiomyopathy and constrictive pericarditis by early diastolic Doppler myocardial velocity gradient at the posterior wall. *Circulation* 102:655-662, 2000.

199. Klodas E, Nishimura R, Appleton C, et al: Doppler evaluation of patient with constrictive pericarditis: Use of tricuspid regurgitation velocity curves to determine enhanced ventricular interaction. *J Am Coll Cardiol* 28:652-657, 1996.

200. Ha JW, Oh J, Ling L, et al: Annulus paradoxus: transmitral flow velocity to mitral annular velocity ratio is inversely proportional to pulmonary capillary wedge pressure in patients with constrictive pericarditis. *Circulation* 104:976-978, 2001.

201. Klodas E, Nishimura RA, Appleton CP, et al: Doppler evaluation of patients with constrictive pericarditis use of tricuspid regurgitation velocity curves to determine enhanced ventricular interaction, *J Am Coll Cardiol* 28:652-657, 1996.

202. Goldstein JA: Cardiac tamponade, constrictive pericarditis, and restrictive cardiomyopathy. *Curr Prob Cardiol* 29:503-506, 2004.

203. Ha JW, Ommen SR, Tajik AJ, et al: Differentiation of constrictive pericarditis from restrictive cardiomyopathy using mitral annular velocity by tissue Doppler echocardiography. *Am J Cardiol* 94:316-319, 2004.

204. Garcia MJ, Rodriguez L, Ares M, et al: Differentiation of constrictive pericarditis from restrictive cardiomyopathy: Assessment of left ventricular diastolic velocities in longitudinal axis by Doppler tissue imaging. *J Am Coll Cardiol* 27:108-114, 1996.

205. Ha JW, Oh JK, Ommen SR, et al: Diagnostic value of mitral annular velocity for constrictive pericarditis in the absence of respiratory variation in mitral inflow velocity. *J Am Soc Echocardiogr* 15:1468-1471, 2002.

206. Arnold MF, Voight JU, Kukulski T, et al: Does atrioventricular ring motion always distinguish constriction from restriction? A Doppler myocardial imaging study. *J Am Soc Echocardiogr* 14:391-395, 2001.

207. Rajagopalan N, Garcia MJ, Rodriguez L, et al: Comparison of new Doppler echocardiographic methods to differentiate constrictive pericardial heart disease and restrictive cardiomyopathy. *Am J Cardiol* 87:86-94, 2001.

208. Palka P, Lange A, Donnelly JE, Nihoyannopoulos P: Differentiation between restrictive cardiomyopathy and constrictive pericarditis by early diastolic Doppler myocardial velocity gradient at the posterior wall. *Circulation* 102:655-662, 2000.

209. Sengupta PP, Mohan JC, Pandian NG: Tissue Doppler echocardiography: Principles and applications. *Indian Heart J* 54:368-378, 2002.

210. Wood P: Chronic constrictive pericarditis. *Am J Cardiol* 7:48-61, 1961.

211. Yu PN, Lovejoy FW, Joos HA, et al: Right auricular and ventricular pressure patterns in constrictive pericarditis. *Circulation* 7:102-107, 1953.

212. Vaitkus PT, Kussmaul WG: Constrictive pericarditis versus restrictive cardiomyopathy: A reappraisal and update of diagnostic criteria. *Am Heart J* 122:1431-1441, 1991.

213. Branea I, Stanciu L, Tomescu M, et al: The value of echocardiography in the early diagnosis of myocardial impairment due to connective tissue diseases. *Med Interne* 24:197-205, 1986.

214. Schurle DR, Evans RW, Cohlmia JB, Lin J: Restrictive cardiomyopathy in scleroderma. *J Kans Med Soc* 85:49-50, 1984.

215. Chew C, Ziady GM, Raphael MJ, Oakley CM: The functional defect in amyloid heart disease: The "stiff heart" syndrome. *Am J Cardiol* 36:438-444, 1975.

216. Cueto-Garcia L, Tajik AJ, Kyle RA, et al: Serial echocardiographic observations in patients with primary systemic amyloidosis: An introduction to the concept of early (asymptomatic) amyloid infiltration of the heart. *Mayo Clin Proc* 59:589-597, 1984.

217. Moyssakis I, Triposkiadis F, Rallidid L, et al: Echocardiographic features of primary, secondary and familial amyloidosis. *Eur J Clin Invest* 29:484-489, 1999.

218. Hofer JF, Wimmer G: Severe heart failure from light chain cardiomyopathy (cardiac amyloidosis). *Z Kardiol* 92:90-95, 2003.

219. Reisinger J, Dubrey SW, Lavalley M, et al: Electrophysiologic abnormalities in AL (primary) amyloidosis with cardiac involvement. *J Am Coll Cardiol* 30:1046-1051, 1997.

220. Gertz MA, Kyle RA, Thibodeau SN: Familial amyloidosis: A study of 52 North American-born patients examined during a 30-year period. *Mayo Clin Proc* 67:428-440, 1992.

221. Olson LJ, Gertz MA, Edwards WD, et al: Senile cardiac amyloidosis with myocardial dysfunction. Diagnosis by endomyocardial biopsy and immunohistochemistry. *N Engl J Med* 317:738-742, 1987.

222. Kawamura S, Takahashi M, Ishihara T, Uchino F: Incidence and distribution of isolated atrial amyloid: Histologic and immunohistochemical studies of 100 aging hearts. *Pathol Int* 45:335-342, 1995.

223. Dubrey SW, Cha K, Simms RW, et al: Electrocardiography and Doppler echocardiography in secondary (AA) amyloidosis. *Am J Cardiol* 77:313-315, 1996.

224. Matsui Y, Iwai K, Tachibana T, et al: Clinicopathological study of fatal myocardial sarcoidosis. *Ann N Y Acad Sci* 278:455-469, 1976.

225. Perry A, Vuitch F: Causes of death in patients with sarcoidosis: a morphologic study of 38 autopsies with clinicopathologic correlations. *Arch Pathol Lab Med* 119:167-172, 1995.

226. Smith RL, Hutchins GM, Sack GH Jr, Ridolfi RL: Unusual cardiac, renal and pulmonary involvement in Gaucher's disease: Interstitial glucocerebroside accumulation, pulmonary hypertension and fatal bone marrow embolization. *Am J Med* 65:352-360, 1978.

227. Renteria VG, Ferrans VJ, Roberts WC: The heart in the Hurler syndrome: Gross, histologic and ultrastructural observations in five necropsy cases. *Am J Cardiol* 38:487-501, 1976.

228. Furth PA, Futterweit W, Gorlin R: Refractory biventricular heart failure in secondary hemochromatosis. *Am J Med Sci* 290:209-213, 1985.

229. Olson LJ, Reeder GS, Noller KL, et al: Cardiac involvement in glycogen storage disease III: morphologic and biochemical characterization with endomyocardial biopsy. *Am J Cardiol* 53:980-981, 1984.

230. Hillsley RE, Hernandez E, Steenbergen C, et al: Inherited restrictive cardiomyopathy in a 74-year-old woman: a case of Fabry's disease. *Am Heart J* 129:199-202, 1995.

231. Chew CY, Ziady GM, Raphael MJ, et al: Primary restrictive cardiomyopathy: non-tropical endomyocardial fibrosis and hypereosinophilic heart disease. *Br Heart J* 39:399-413, 1977.

232. Fawzy ME, Ziady G, Halim M, et al: Endomyocardial fibrosis: report of eight cases. *J Am Coll Cardiol* 5:983-988, 1985.

233. Olsen EG, Spry CJ: Relation between eosinophilia and endomyocardial disease. *Prog Cardiovasc Dis* 27:241-254, 1985.

234. Lundin L, Norheim I, Landelius J, et al: Carcinoid heart disease: relationship of circulating vasoactive substances to ultrasound-detectable cardiac abnormalities. *Circulation* 77:264-269, 1988.

235. Pellikka PA, Tajik AJ, Khandheria BK, et al: Carcinoid heart disease: Clinical and echocardiographic spectrum in 74 patients. *Circulation* 87:1188-1196, 1993.

236. Roberts WC, Glancy DL, DeVita VT Jr: Heart in malignant lymphoma (Hodgkin's disease, lymphosarcoma, reticulum cell sarcoma and mycosis fungoides): A study of 196 autopsy cases. *Am J Cardiol* 22:85-107, 1968.

237. Stark RM, Perloff JH, Glick HJ, et al: Clinical recognition and management of cardiac metastatic disease: Observations in a unique case of alveolar soft-part sarcoma. *Am J Med* 63:653-659, 1977.

238. Gottdiener JS, Katin MJ, Borer JS, et al: Late cardiac effects of therapeutic mediastinal irradiation: Assessment by echocardiography and radionuclide angiography. *N Engl J Med* 308:569-572, 1983.

239. Mortensen SA, Olsen HS, Baandrup U. Chronic anthracycline cardiotoxicity: Haemodynamic and histopathological manifestations suggesting a restrictive endomyocardial disease. *Br Heart J* 55:274-282, 1965.

240. Bu'Lock FA, Mott MG, Oakhill A, Martin RP: Left ventricular diastolic function after anthracycline chemotherapy in childhood: relation with systolic function, symptoms, and pathophysiology. *Br Heart J* 73:340-350, 1995.

241. Billingham ME: Pharmacotoxic myocardial disease: an endomyocardial study. *Heart Vessels* Suppl 1:278-282, 1985.

242. Mason JW, Billingham ME, Friedman JP: Methysergide-induced heart disease: A case of multivalvular and myocardial fibrosis. *Circulation* 56:889-890, 1977.

243. Naqvi TZ, Luthringer D, Marchevsky A, et al: Chloroquine induced cardiomyopathy—echocardiographic features. *J Am Soc Echocardiogr* 18:383-387, 2005.

244. Berensztein C, Pineiro D, Marcotegui M, et al: Usefulness of echocardiography and Doppler echocardiography in endomyocardial fibrosis. *J Am Soc Echocardiogr* 13:385-392, 2000.

245. Asher CR, Klein AL: Diastolic heart failure: restrictive cardiomyopathy, constrictive pericarditis, and cardiac tamponade: clinical and echocardiographic evaluation. *Cardiol Rev* 10:218-229, 2002.

246. Klein AL, Hatle LK, Taliercio CP, et al: Prognostic significance of Doppler measures of diastolic function in cardiac amyloidosis: A Doppler echocardiography study. *Circulation* 83:808-816, 1991.

247. Klein AL, Hatle LK, Burstow DJ, et al: Doppler characterization of left ventricular diastolic function in cardiac amyloidosis. *J Am Coll Cardiol* 13:1017-1026, 1989.

248. Oh J, Appleton C, Hatle L, et al: The noninvasive assessment of left ventricular diastolic function with two-dimensional and Doppler echocardiography. *J Am Soc Echocardiogr* 10:246-270, 1997.

249. Garcia M, Thomas J, Klein A: New Doppler echocardiographic applications for the study of diastolic function. *J Am Coll Cardiol* 32:865-875, 1998.

250. Meluzin J, Spinarova L, Bakala J, et al: Pulsed Doppler tissue imaging of the velocity of tricuspid annular systolic motion; a new, rapid, and non-invasive method of evaluating right ventricular systolic function. *Eur Heart J* 22:340-348, 2001.

251. Miller D, Farah MG, Liner A, et al: The relation between quantitative right ventricular ejection fraction and indices of tricuspid annular motion and myocardial performance. *J Am Soc Echocardiogr* 17:443-447, 2004.

252. Lanzarini L, Fontana A, Lucca E, et al: Noninvasive estimation of both systolic and diastolic pulmonary artery pressure from Doppler analysis of tricuspid regurgitant velocity spectrum in patients with chronic heart failure. *Am Heart J* 144:1087-1094, 2002.

253. Garcia M, Thomas J, Klein A: New Doppler echocardiographic applications for the study of diastolic function. *J Am Coll Cardiol* 32:865-875, 1998.

254. Koyama J, Ray-Sequin PA, Falk RH: Longitudinal myocardial function assessed by tissue velocity, strain, and strain rate tissue Doppler echocardiography in patients with AL (primary) cardiac amyloidosis. *Circulation* 107:2446-2452, 2003.

255. Lachmann HJ, Booth DR, Booth SE, et al: Misdiagnosis of hereditary amyloidosis as AL (primary) amyloidosis. *N Engl J Med* 346:1786-1791, 2002.

256. Kushwaha S, Fallon JT, Fuster V: Restrictive cardiomyopathy. *N Eng J Med* 336:267-276, 1997.

257. Goldstein JA: Cardiac tamponde, constrictive pericarditis, and restrictive cardiomyopathy. *Curr Probl Cardiol* 29:503-567, 2004.

258. Rajagopalan N, Garcia MJ, Rodriguez L, et al: Comparison of new Doppler echocardiographic methods to differentiate constrictive pericardial heart disease and restrictive cardiomyopathy. *Am J Cardiol* 87:86-94, 2001.

Chapter 30

Pericardial Disease

BRAD I. MUNT, MD • ROBERT R. MOSS, MD • CHRISTOPHER R. THOMPSON, MD

The authors would like to thank their cardiac sonographers, R. P. Gilles, K. Perry, V. L. Echelli, C. L. Jones, M. L. Hughes, and T. N. Chipp, for providing the images and advice on the chapter; and their spouses, Stephanie and Annabelle, for their ongoing support.

Basic Principles

Anatomy of the Pericardium

The pericardium consists of two layers that surround the heart and proximal segments of the aorta, pulmonary artery (PA), pulmonary veins, and venae cavae. The outermost layer is a thick fibrous structure, which blends with the adventitia of the aorta and pulmonary arteries to provide firm support for the heart. This layer has supporting ligamentous attachments to the diaphragm, sternum, and vertebrae.[1,2] The inner layer is a serous membrane consisting of a single layer of mesothelial cells, which directly overlies the epicardial fat to form the visceral pericardium. This membrane reflects back on itself to line the inside of the fibrous layer and forms the parietal pericardium. The pericardial space is enclosed between the two layers of serous pericardium. This space is limited superiorly by the attachments of the fibrous pericardium to the great arteries. It is limited posteriorly by reflections of the pericardium as the pulmonary veins and venae cavae enter the atria. These reflections result in the formation of two blind-ending tunnels or sinuses. The oblique sinus lies behind the left atrium (LA) and is limited superiorly by the pericardial reflection to the upper pulmonary veins, laterally by the reflections of the pericardium around the left pulmonary veins and medially by the reflections of the pericardium around the right pulmonary veins and venae cavae. The transverse sinus lies above the pulmonary vein reflection and is bounded anteriorly by the great arteries and posteriorly by the left atrial roof (Figs. 30-1, 30-2, and 30-3). The main arterial supply of the pericardium is from a branch of the internal thoracic artery, the pericardiophrenic artery. Venous drainage is by the pericardiophrenic veins, which drain into the brachiocephalic veins. The phrenic nerve provides sensory innervation; the sympathetic trunks provide vasomotor innervation.

Pericardial Fluid

The pericardial space normally contains 10 to 50 mL of fluid that lubricates the contact between the two serosal layers of the pericardium.[3] This fluid is an ultrafiltrate of plasma and contains proteins, electrolytes, and phospholipids. It is believed to be formed in the visceral pericardium. The pericardial space drains via the thoracic and right lymphatic ducts. Any condition obstructing lymphatic flow or raising central venous pressure will lead to accumulation of pericardial fluid. Fluid will also accumulate in conditions increasing the normal pericardial permeability. The normal pericardium has a relatively small capacitance volume; acute accumulation of fluid will result in small increases in pericardial pressure until the capacitance has been exceeded. With additional increase in pericardial volume, a rapid rise in pericardial pressure and progressive hemodynamic disturbances will ensue[4] (Fig. 30-4).

Functions of the Pericardium

The pericardium serves to reduce friction between the heart and the surrounding mediastinal structures and provides a barrier against the local spread of infection or malignancy to the heart.[2] However, by the nature of the pericardium, in that it is a semirigid layer completely enclosing the heart, it serves to distribute the pressure within the pericardial space to the cardiac structures enclosed within the pericardium. It also mediates ventricular coupling or interaction.[5] Understanding the role of the pericardium in pressure modulation and ventricular interaction is important to appreciate the hemodynamic effects and therefore the echocardiographic features of compressive pericardial disease.

Pericardial Pressure

Over a century ago, Bernard concluded that the pericardium significantly constrained cardiac filling.[6] The concept of transmural pressure (the intracavity end-diastolic pressure [EDP] minus the pericardial pressure) subsequently evolved to take into account this pericardial restraint. This concept is extremely important because transmural pressure is likely to be a closer representation of preload than the intracavity end-diastolic pressure. However, controversy exists as to the magnitude of this constraint because of difficulties in the accurate determination of pericardial pressure. Using a balloon to measure pericardial pressure, pericardial pressure approximates right atrial and right ventricular (RV) end diastolic pressure. Others contend that balloon-based measurement techniques overestimate pericardial pressure and therefore underestimate true transmural pressure.[7]

Despite the incomplete understanding of true pericardial (and therefore transmural) pressure, the influences of pericardial restraint and pericardial pressure are important to bear in mind when assessing ventricular filling and function.

Pericardial Restraint and Ventricular Interaction

Because the pericardium is a relatively stiff structure, intrapericardial pressure rises rapidly as intrapericardial volume is increased acutely.[8] This increase in intrapericardial pressure may occur because of an accumulation of pericardial fluid or an increase in the volume of any intracardiac structure; particularly an increase in RV volume (see Fig. 30-4). Shirato and colleagues showed that acute volume loading in dogs with an intact pericardium caused a reduction in left ventricular (LV) compliance.[9] This is because an increase in intrapericardial volume (as a result of an increase in right-sided chamber volumes) increases intrapericardial pressure restraining LV filling. The opposite effects were seen with reductions in cardiac volume using nitroprusside. These effects were abolished by pericardectomy. Other experimental models of acute RV pressure/volume loading have yielded similar results.[10] Examples of ventricular interaction under different loading conditions effects have been seen in human studies.[11] It is interesting to speculate that as the human pericardium is much thicker than the canine pericardium; pericardial influence in humans may be even more pronounced.

The restraining effects of the pericardium are much less apparent in the chronic volume overloaded state because pericardial compliance and surface area are able to increase under chronic strain conditions[8] (see Fig. 30-4).

An increase in pericardial pressure resulting from pericardial fluid accumulation will also reduce transmural filling pressure and shift ventricular pressure/volume

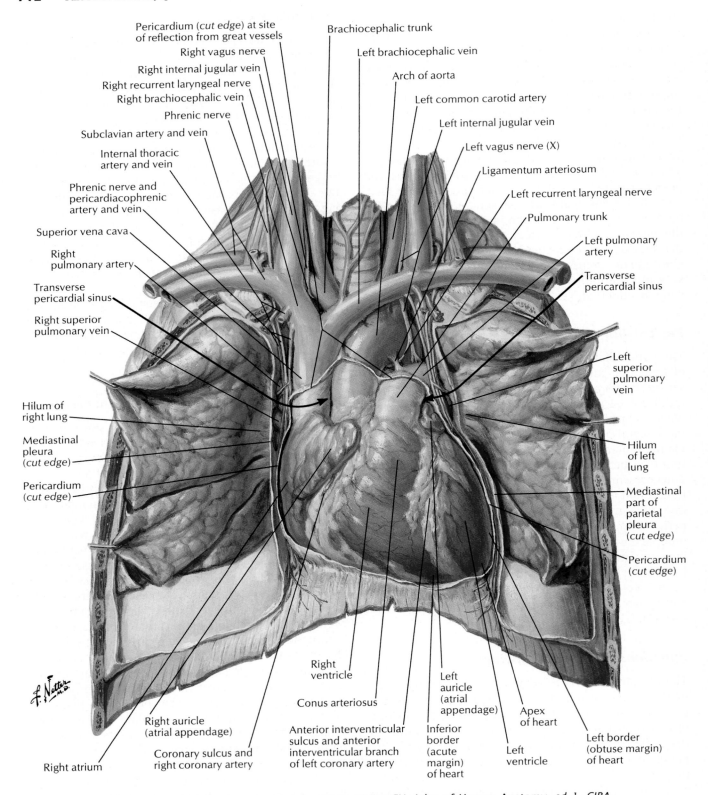

Figure 30–1. *Heart: anterior exposure. (From Netter FH:* Atlas of Human Anatomy, *ed 1, CIBA-GEIGY Pharmaceutical, 1989.)*

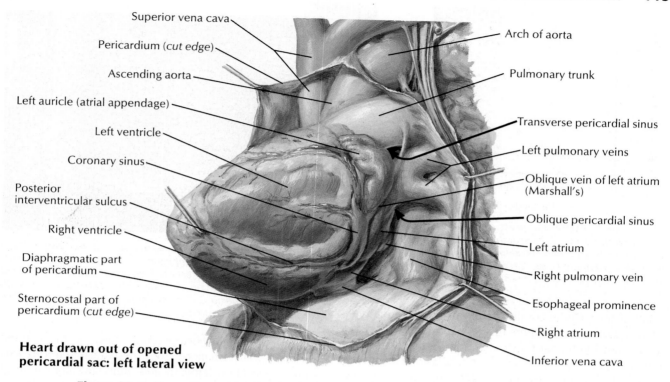

Superior vena cava

Pericardium (cut edge)

Ascending aorta

Left auricle (atrial appendage)

Left ventricle

Coronary sinus

Posterior interventricular sulcus

Right ventricle

Diaphragmatic part of pericardium

Sternocostal part of pericardium (cut edge)

Arch of aorta

Pulmonary trunk

Transverse pericardial sinus

Left pulmonary veins

Oblique vein of left atrium (Marshall's)

Oblique pericardial sinus

Left atrium

Right pulmonary vein

Esophageal prominence

Right atrium

Inferior vena cava

Heart drawn out of opened pericardial sac: left lateral view

Figure 30–2. *Heart drawn out of opened pericardial sac: left lateral view. (From Netter FH: Atlas of Human Anatomy, ed 1, CIBA-GEIGY Pharmaceutical, 1989.)*

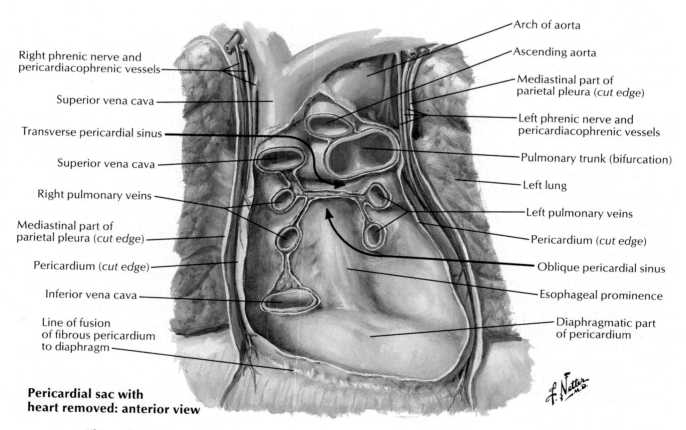

Right phrenic nerve and pericardiacophrenic vessels

Superior vena cava

Transverse pericardial sinus

Superior vena cava

Right pulmonary veins

Mediastinal part of parietal pleura (cut edge)

Pericardium (cut edge)

Inferior vena cava

Line of fusion of fibrous pericardium to diaphragm

Arch of aorta

Ascending aorta

Mediastinal part of parietal pleura (cut edge)

Left phrenic nerve and pericardiacophrenic vessels

Pulmonary trunk (bifurcation)

Left lung

Left pulmonary veins

Pericardium (cut edge)

Oblique pericardial sinus

Esophageal prominence

Diaphragmatic part of pericardium

Pericardial sac with heart removed: anterior view

Figure 30–3. *Pericardial sac with heart removed: anterior view. (From Netter FH: Atlas of Human Anatomy, ed 1, CIBA-GEIGY Pharmaceutical, 1989.)*

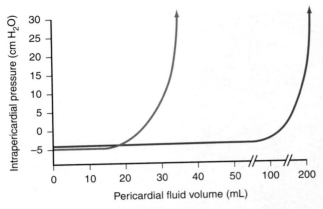

Figure 30–4. *Pericardial pressure-volume relationships in a patient with normal pericardial anatomy* (red line) *and a patient who has gradually developed a pericardial effusion* (blue line). *(From Edmunds HL:* Cardiac Surgery in the Adult, *New York, McGraw-Hill, 1997, p. 1305).*

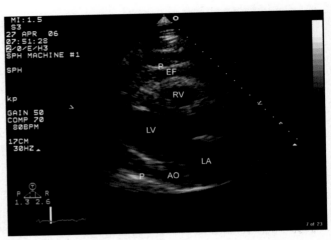

Figure 30–5. *Parasternal long-axis view of the normal pericardium. The pericardium appears as a bright echogenic structure anteriorly and posteriorly. Epicardial fat is appreciated between the pericardium and the right ventricular free wall. AO, descending aorta; EF, epicardial fat; LA, left atrium; P, pericardium; RV, right ventricle.*

relationships. Under conditions of raised pericardial volume and pressure or where the pericardium is stiff, there is enhanced potential for the left and right ventricles to interact and influence each other's diastolic behavior. Ventricular interaction can be either in series (i.e., the output of the right ventricle influencing LV venous return and consequently, filling of the left ventricle), or in parallel, in which ventricular filling characteristics are changed by the side-by-side nature of the ventricles within a constrained pericardial volume. An understanding of the effects of ventricular interdependence is key to understanding the hemodynamic, and therefore, echocardiographic features of compressive pericardial disease, such as tamponade or constriction.

Echocardiographic Examination of the Pericardium

The pericardium covers the entire external surface of the heart, and therefore is visualized from all standardized echocardiographic acoustic windows. Echocardiographically, the pericardium appears as a thin, usually single echogenic structure that is more obvious posteriorly than anteriorly (Fig. 30–5). Normal pericardial thickness measures 1 mm or less. Normal pericardial fluid volume is minimal, and therefore the pericardial space is not appreciated in most normal subjects. Occasionally a small amount of physiological pericardial fluid may be seen in the posterior pericardial space, especially in younger patients with good imaging characteristics (Figs. 30–6 and 30–7). The majority of pericardial processes are evident in the parasternal long-axis view.[12,13] This is because the majority of pericardial processes result in diffuse pericardial involvement and pericardial fluid tends to accumulate in the oblique sinus initially. As well, complete or partial absence of the pericardium results in marked cardiac displacement or left atrial appendage herniation or enlargement,[14] and pericardial cysts are usually located

at the left or right costophrenic angle.[15,16] All of these areas are well visualized from the parasternal long-axis view, especially if leftward and rightward angulation of the transducer is performed. An important exception is postsurgical pericardial effusions. Therefore, in the nonsurgical patient, in whom the clinical suspicion of a primary pericardial disease is low, a normal parasternal long-axis view has been promoted to adequate to rule out pericardial pathology. Unfortunately, in a recent series of patients who underwent pericardiocentesis for tamponade,[17] the diagnosis of pericardial effusion was not initially considered in 44% of patients before echocardiography, and an alternative working diagnosis was thought to be more likely in a further 36%. As the diagnosis of pericardial tamponade may often not be considered clinically, we advocate that the pericardial space be studied in all standard echocardiographic acoustic windows as part of the standard echocardiographic examination, with special attention in all postoperative patients.

There is a relatively poor correlation between measurements of pericardial thickness by transthoracic echocardiography (TTE) and pathological examination.[18] Although a good correlation has been suggested between transesophageal echocardiographically (TEE) derived pericardial thickness and computed tomography (CT),[19] we still prefer computed tomography or magnetic resonance imaging (MRI) to evaluate the pericardium for thickening. These techniques allow for a more comprehensive visualization of the entire pericardium.

Visualization of the RV and right atrial free walls, often with high frame rate M-mode or two-dimensional (2D) recordings of motion are required to determine the hemodynamic significance of pericardial effusions. As well, pulsed-wave (PW) Doppler recordings of RV and LV inflow, with respiratory tracking and multiple complexes recorded are needed as a minimum.

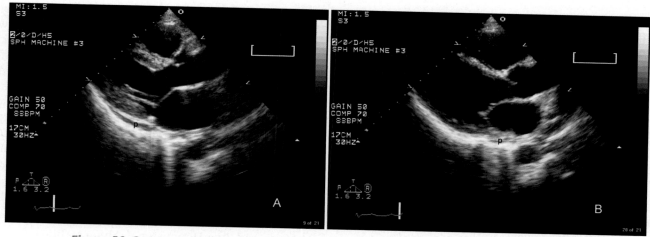

Figure 30–6. *Parasternal long-axis two-dimensional view of a patient with a physiological amount of pericardial fluid. In systole, (A) an echolucent space is seen in the area of the oblique sinus posterior to the left atrium and ventricle. The echolucent space is almost completely obliterated in diastole (B). p, oblique sinus of the pericardial space.*

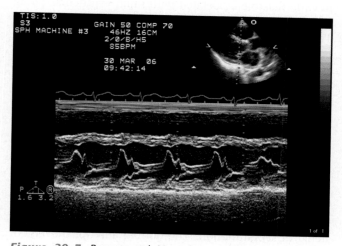

Figure 30–7. *Parasternal M-mode recording at the mitral valve level of a patient with a physiological amount of pericardial fluid. The echolucent space posterior to the left ventricle is more prominent during systole than diastole.*

We strongly advocate that all patients with pericardial effusions undergo an initial full, detailed, echocardiographic examination to rule out conditions that may affect echocardiographic indicators of hemodynamically significant pericardial fluid (such as atrial septal defects, RV hypertrophy), and detect coexisting cardiac conditions (Table 30–1). Follow-up examinations may be of a more directed, limited nature.

Constrictive Pericarditis

A variety of disorders can cause pericardial inflammation and may cause subsequent thickening, fibrosis, and calcification (Table 30–2). Pericardial thickening

TABLE 30–1. Echocardiographic Imaging Protocol in Suspected Pericardial Disease

1. Full two-dimensional examination with emphasis on the location, volume, and characteristics of the pericardial fluid and the characteristics of the pericardium. Views of right atrium and right ventricular free walls are especially important. When recording digital images, extended loops (up to 10 beats may be required) to be recorded to capture changes related to the respiratory cycle.
2. M-mode examination with attention to imaging the right ventricular free wall.
3. Pulsed-wave Doppler assessment of tricuspid, mitral inflow, pulmonary vein flow, and hepatic vein flow. Superior vena cava flow to be imaged is selected patients. Long loops with respiratory tracking are recorded to appreciate respiratory changes in Doppler velocities.
4. Tissue Doppler recordings of medial and lateral annulus, with systolic and diastolic waves shown.
5. Careful imaging of the inferior vena cava and associated changes with respiration.
6. In postoperative patients a detailed search for localized fluid collections and any resulting localized chamber compression.

results in impaired cardiac filling and characteristic echocardiographic signs.

Pathophysiology

The thickened, fibrotic pericardium constricts the heart and reduces operative chamber compliance. Consequently, diastolic filling is impeded and the end-diastolic cardiac volume is determined by the pericardial volume. Early diastolic filling is usually not impaired (in fact may be supranormal), whereas mid-diastolic and late-diastolic filling is impaired.

TABLE 30-2. Causes of Pericardial Inflammation

Idiopathic

Infectious Diseases
Bacterial (including tuberculosis, *Chlamydia*, borreliosis, treponema pallidum, hemophilus, meningococcus, pneumococcus, gonococcus)
Fungal (including *Candida*, histoplasmosis)
Viral (including coxsackie A9, B1-4, echo B, mumps, Epstein Barr, cytomegalovirus, Varicella, rubella, HIV, parvo B19)
Parasitic (including toxoplasma, echinococcus, entamoeba histolytica)

Trauma
Blunt or penetrating trauma
Cardiac surgery

Connective Tissue Disorders
Including rheumatoid arthritis, systemic lupus erythematosus, systemic sclerosis, Reiter syndrome

Neoplasia
Primary benign or malignant pericardial tumors
Secondary (including lung, breast, gastric, colon leukemia, melanoma)

Metabolic Disorders
Including renal failure, hypothyroidism, Addison disease

Miscellaneous
Mediastinal irradiation
Pulmonary asbestosis

The pericardial thickening usually involves the whole pericardial surface (although the degree of thickening can vary) and leads to elevation and equalization of diastolic pressures in all four cardiac chambers, especially at end-diastole. In early diastole, ventricular filling occurs at a more rapid rate than normal because of elevated atrial pressures and a cardiac volume that is less than the limiting volume of the pericardium. However, once the pericardial volume is reached, filling halts abruptly, and there is little further increase in total chamber volume. This limitation to filling in mid and late diastole leads to M-mode, 2D, and Doppler abnormalities and to the typical square root sign seen with invasive hemodynamic measurement.[20]

The thickened pericardium partially isolates the heart from the normal respiratory swings in intrathoracic pressure. However, respiratory fluctuations in pulmonary venous pressure still occur (because portions of the pulmonary veins lie outside the pericardium), and a fall in pulmonary venous pressure with inspiration leads to a fall in the driving pressure across the mitral valve. This prolongs the isovolumic relaxation time, reduces early diastolic transmitral flow velocity, and prolongs the deceleration time

(DT).[21] These changes are an exaggeration of changes seen in normal patients; respiratory variations in flow are not characteristic of patients with restrictive cardiomyopathy. The pericardial limitation to filling also serves to exaggerate normal ventricular coupling. A reduction in LV filling with inspiration allows a compensatory increase in right-sided heart filling. These respiratory fluctuations in left-sided and right-sided heart filling cause characteristic changes in mitral and tricuspid Doppler inflow patterns, ventricular dimensions, and aortic and pulmonary peak velocities.

Echocardiographic Diagnosis

M-Mode and Two-Dimensional Abnormalities

The abrupt cessation of flow in mid diastole results in flattening of the motion of the posterior LV wall in mid and late diastole. This follows relatively normal motion in early diastole associated with rapid ventricular filling and is the M-mode equivalent of the square root sign. This sign is relatively sensitive, being reported in 85% of patients with constriction. However, it is also seen in 20% of normal subjects.[22] Abnormalities of interventricular septal motion are common in constriction. Septal position is influenced by pressure gradients between the left and right ventricles, and changes in septal position with respiration are exacerbated by the constricting effect of the rigid pericardium. Both parasternal M-mode and 2D echocardiography can demonstrate marked movement of the septum posteriorly with inspiration and the anteriorly with expiration, and consequent respiratory changes in LV and RV volumes.[23] A further M-mode sign seen with constriction is a "double component" of septal motion. The normal anterior movement of the septum after atrial systole is preceded by brief posterior displacement. This results from a transient increase in the RV pressure above that of the left ventricle with the onset of right atrial systole. A second posterior septal movement occurs in early diastole as LV pressure decays more quickly than RV pressure. This second posterior septal movement is an exaggeration of the normal diastolic posterior septal movement that occurs at this time in the cardiac cycle. Abrupt cessation of LV filling may sometimes be appreciated on 2D imaging as a perceptible 'checking' of LV diastolic expansion.

Premature pulmonary valve opening also occurs and can be appreciated using M-mode echocardiography. The abnormally elevated filling pressure associated with constriction leads to RV diastolic pressure exceeding pulmonary artery diastolic pressure in mid diastole and consequent premature pulmonary valve opening.

Pericardial thickening and calcification can be appreciated using M-mode and 2D modalities although the sensitivity and specificity have been questioned. Early reports of M-mode sensitivity of almost 100% in diagnosing pericardial thickening,[24] or diagnosing constrictive pericarditis from other findings[25] have not been confirmed in later studies.[22,26-28] A systematic overestimation of true thickness using transthoracic echocardiography was found in dogs with experimental constrictive pericarditis.[18] These difficulties have been attributed to technical difficulties such as gain settings and resolution, and to fibrosis obscuring cardiac boundaries. Patchy pericardial thickening may also cause diagnostic difficulties. A more recent study found that transesophageal echocardiography (TEE) was more accurate, with a sensitivity of 95% and specificity of 86% in the detection of thickened pericardium (using CT scanning as the gold standard).[19] It is important to note that surgically verified constriction has been noted in patients with normal pericardial thickness.[29] Adhesion or tethering of the pericardium to the heart or surrounding anatomical structures by pericardial adhesions may be appreciated on 2D imaging, especially in the subcostal view.

The inferior vena cava is also typically dilated with blunting of the normal respiratory variation in its diameter.[30] This is, however, a nonspecific sign and is frequently seen in other conditions with elevated right atrial pressures.

Despite all of these signs, no single or combination of M-mode or 2D echocardiographic feature is diagnostic of constrictive pericarditis. The diagnosis therefore requires a careful integration of the results of M-mode, Doppler, and 2D imaging and a consideration of the clinical context.

Doppler Flow Abnormalities

In keeping with rapid early diastolic flow, the LV (mitral) inflow pattern typically shows a high E wave velocity, short deceleration time, and a low A wave velocity. However, this pattern reflects elevated left atrial pressure and therefore is not specific to pericardial constriction. Of much more use is the change in LV (mitral) and RV (tricuspid) inflow patterns seen with respiration because these appear to be much more reliable in diagnosing constriction. Several studies[21,31] have reported that in patients with pericardial constriction there is: (1) prolongation of the LV isovolumic relaxation time by greater than 25% with inspiration in all patients with constriction, whereas normals changed by less than 5%; (2) reduction of greater than 25% in peak early LV inflow (E wave) velocity with inspiration in all patients compared with less than 5% in normals; (3) larger expiratory decreases in RV inflow velocity than in normals; (4) a 14% reduction in aortic velocity with inspiration versus a 4% reduction in normals; (5) a 16% increase in pulmonary artery velocity with inspiration as compared to 5% in normals; (6) changes in all parameters were greatest in the first beat following inspiration as compared to changes two or three beats later in those patients with pulmonary disease; (7) an absence of these significant respiratory fluctua-

tions after successful pericardectomy. In modern series, approximately 60% of patients have complete normalization of cardiac physiology post-pericardectomy.[32,33] There is a greater normalization of values in patients post-pericardectomy who become asymptomatic versus those who remain symptomatic.[34]

Respiratory fluctuations in mitral inflow velocity are not always present. One study suggested normal respiratory fluctuations in 12% of patients with proven constriction.[31] The authors speculated that the mechanism was a markedly elevated left atrial pressure forcing mitral valve opening to occur on a steeper part of the LV curve, thus masking inspiratory changes in inflow velocity and isovolumic relaxation time.[31] This was supported in a subsequent study that showed that in patients with constriction, but with blunted respiratory changes, preload reduction unmasked the characteristic respiratory variation.[35]

The increased flow through the right-sided heart (with the resultant increase in RV volume and pressure) with inspiration in patients with constriction alters tricuspid regurgitation (TR) jet parameters. Increased RV preload increases the cavity pressure, increasing the regurgitation velocity and velocity time integral (VTI). Klodas and colleagues[36] showed that in patients with constrictive pericarditis, there was a 13% increase in tricuspid regurgitation velocity with inspiration, as compared to an 8% drop in jet velocity in normal patients.

Abnormalities of pulmonary and hepatic vein flow have also been described in association with constrictive pericarditis. The predominant forward hepatic vein flow in constriction is typically during early diastole. This is the result of an elevated right atrial pressure inhibiting inflow during systole and driving flow across a high early diastolic trans-tricuspid gradient.[31] However, this pattern is not uniform and systolic forward flow can also predominate. Augmentation of right-sided heart filling during inspiration increases hepatic forward flow, and expiration causes a marked increase in flow reversal with atrial systole, and a decrease or paradoxical reversal of flow in early diastole. In a series of patients with surgically proven constrictive pericarditis, echocardiographic criteria based on respiratory variations in mitral and hepatic vein flow correctly diagnosed constriction in 22 of 25 patients.[31] This data leads us to currently use Doppler flow abnormalities, especially fluctuations with respiration, as our primary echocardiographic criteria in the evaluation of patients in which constrictive pericarditis is in the differential diagnosis.

Pulmonary vein flow abnormalities described in association with constrictive pericarditis include a reduction in systolic wave and diastolic wave velocities and a reduction in the systolic to diastolic ratio.[31] As with mitral inflow, these patterns are a reflection of diastolic dysfunction and elevated filling pressures and are not specific to constriction. However, respiratory fluctuations in pulmonary venous flow have also been reported in constriction and used to differentiate constriction from restriction and from normal subjects.[37] Doppler interrogation of superior vena cava (SVC) flow has been used to differentiate pericardial constriction from other entities, such as chronic obstructive pulmonary disease (COPD), in which ventricular interaction is enhanced and in which significant variation in mitral and tricuspid inflow velocities may be seen. In COPD, significant increases in SVC flow velocity will be noted with inspiration. In constrictive pericarditis, minimal or no increase in superior vena caval flow velocity with inspiration is noted.[38]

Doppler Tissue Imaging Abnormalities

In patients with pericardial constriction, the velocity of early diastolic posterior LV wall motion has been shown to be increased, consistent with rapid early filling, and the time from aortic valve closure to peak LV wall velocity appears to be shortened.[39] Abnormalities of septal motion were also demonstrated by tissue Doppler imaging (TDI) consistent with the M-mode abnormalities described previously.

TDI may be useful in differentiating pericardial constriction from restriction, with myocardial relaxation velocities (reflecting intrinsic myocardial disease), being significantly lower in restriction than in constriction.[40] As well, the early diastolic tissue Doppler wave (E') in patients with constriction was found to be higher than in normal controls. An E' velocity 2 cm/s greater than predicted for age could differentiate patients with constriction from controls with a sensitivity of 76% and a specificity of 82%.[41] Recent work has pointed to some limitations that exist in the use of TDI to differentiate constriction from restriction,[42] and the two disease states can coexist in the same patients, especially after radiation therapy.[43]

The echocardiographic evaluation of pericardial constriction remains challenging task. Important diagnostic pitfalls may arise when localized constriction leads to an atypical hemodynamic picture. Arrhythmias, especially atrial fibrillation (AFib) may make the interpretation of Doppler velocities difficult. The diagnosis of pericardial constriction relies of the integration of information acquired from high quality 2D M-mode and Doppler imaging with a good understanding of the underlying clinical picture. On occasion, hemodynamic evaluation in an experienced cardiac catheterization lab will still be required.

Pericardial Effusion

The pericardial space normally contains 10 to 50 mL of fluid that serves to lubricate the contact between the two serosal layers of the pericardium.[3] This fluid is an ultrafiltrate of plasma and contains proteins, electrolytes, and phospholipids. It is believed to originate in the visceral pericardium. A wide variety of conditions, broadly divided into inflammatory, neoplastic, endocrine, and traumatic, can lead to an increase in pericardial fluid (see Table 30–2). This results in separation of the parietal pericardium from the visceral pericardium and fluid accumulation in this physiological potential space. Clinically, the consequences of this pericardial effusion are alterations in the physiology of cardiac function as the intrapericardial pressure progressively increases. This reduces true (transmural) intracardiac filling pressures. Because right-sided pressures tend to be lower than left-sided pressure, direct effects of the pericardial fluid are usually first seen in right-sided chambers.[44]

M-Mode and Two-Dimensional Echocardiography

Echocardiographic Appearance of Pericardial Fluid and other Common Disorders Simulating Pericardial Effusion

The hallmark of a pericardial effusion is visualization of echolucent material with properties consistent with fluid in the pericardial space. If pericardial anatomy is relatively normal prior before fluid accumulation, fluid will first accumulate in the oblique sinus posterior to the left ventricle[12] (see Fig. 30–3) and is best viewed in the parasternal long-axis view. Once approximately 100 mL of fluid has accumulated in the pericardium, the fluid will tend to become circumferential filling the entire pericardial space.

It is important to differentiate normal anatomic variants and nonpericardial processes from pericardial fluid.

Left-sided pleural effusions can appear posterior to the heart. The echocardiographic hallmark separating pericardial from pleural effusions is that pericardial fluid will track anterior to the proximal descending thoracic aorta, whereas pleural effusions will not (Fig. 30–8). As well, large amounts of pericardial fluid will tend to be located circumferentially around the heart, whereas large left pleural effusions will remain predominantly posterior. Visualization of partially atelectatic lung in the fluid cavity can also aid in the diagnosis of a pleural effusion (Fig. 30–9).

Epicardial fat also leads to an echolucent space in the area of the pericardium (Fig. 30–10). However, epicardial fat tends to occur anteriorly. Using standard imaging settings, epicardial fat will have echogenicity between that of the blood pool and myocardium[45,46] and tends to have a characteristic speckled appearance, whereas pericardial effusion has echogenicity closer to the blood pool. Epicardial fat is more common in older individuals (prevalence <1% in subjects 20 to 30 years old to >15% for those >80 years old)

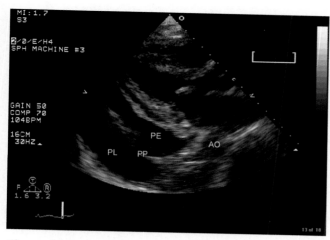

Figure 30–8. *Parasternal long-axis two-dimensional view of a patient with both a pericardial and pleural effusion. AO, descending thoracic aorta (off axis); PE, pericardial fluid; PL, pleural fluid; PP, parietal pericardium.*

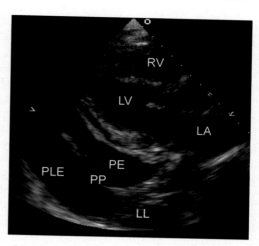

Figure 30–10. *Parasternal long-axis view showing both a pericardial and pleural effusion. The pericardial effusion is predominantly posterior. A portion of atelectatic lung is seen. The parietal pericardium is seen delineating the pericardial from the pleural fluid. LA, left atrium; LL, lung; LV, left ventricle; PE, pericardial effusion; PLE, pleural effusion; PP, parietal pericardium; RV, right ventricle.*

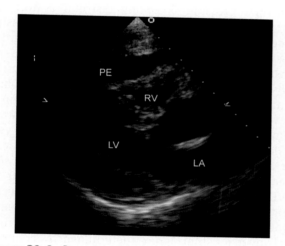

Figure 30–9. *Parasternal long-axis view of a moderate, predominantly anterior pericardial effusion. There is right ventricular diastolic collapse. LA, left atrium; LV, left ventricle; PE, pericardial effusion; RV, right ventricle.*

Clinical Considerations

A common clinical scenario is a request for determination of the presence or absence of pericardial effusion, and if present, a determination of the effusion size and hemodynamic effect. It must be remembered that an incompletely understood complex interaction of factors leads to the ultimate physiological consequences of pericardial effusion and influences the hemodynamic effects in a given patient. These include the pericardial pressure/volume relationship, the rapidity of fluid accumulation, underlying cardiac pathology (particularly hypertrophy and shunts), and systemic volume status.[49] A combination of clinical experience and animal experimentation have led to the following clinically useful observations, small acute pericardial effusions (occurring most commonly postintervention or traumatically) can lead to dramatic physiological effects, whereas moderate-sized or even large-sized pericardial effusions that accumulate slowly can be hemodynamically well tolerated.[8] Localized cardiac compression may lead to dramatic hemodynamic consequences without producing classical echocardiographic indications of "tamponade."[50-52]

and is also more common in subjects who are female, obese, hypertensive, and who have higher glucose and low-density lipoprotein (LDL) levels.[47]

Factors Affecting the Appearance of Pericardial Effusions

The echogenicity of the pericardial fluid can be influenced by features intrinsic to the fluid (e.g., fluid composition including protein content, hemorrhage, chyle, cholesterol, or bacteria) or related to the same process that leads to the fluid (e.g., tumor infiltration of the pericardium). In general, as the protein or cellular content of the fluid increases, so does its echogenicity. However, characterization of the exact fluid composition from its echocardiographic appearance is not possible.[48]

Pericardial Tamponade

Two-Dimensional Echocardiographic Findings

Right Ventricular Compression, Inversion, or Collapse

Perhaps the most useful echocardiographic indicator of a hemodynamically significant pericardial effusion is RV diastolic collapse. Echocardiographically, this is seen on M-mode or 2D recordings as a persistent inward motion of the RV free wall during diastole (Fig. 30–11). By the time this is noted in experimental preparations, there is already a significant reduction (approximately 20%) in forward cardiac output (CO) and elevation in heart rate (HR) without a change in mean arterial pressure (MAP).[53] There is no precise relationship between the duration or degree of RV diastolic collapse and the degree of elevation of intrapericardial pressure or the severity of the hemodynamic effect of the pericardial fluid.[54] Clinically, one can appreciates all degrees of this phenomenon, from a barely perceptible dip, only appreciated with high frame rate recordings, to complete collapse and obliteration of the right ventricle throughout diastole.

Increases in RV intracavitary volume,[55,56] RV pressure,[57] and increased chamber stiffness will all reduce the amount of RV diastolic collapse for any given increase in intrapericardial pressure. Clinically this may be manifested in patients with pulmonary hypertension, RV hypertrophy, left to right shunts (especially atrial septal defects), or RV ischemia not manifesting RV diastolic collapse despite significant elevations of pericardial pressure[55-57] (see Fig. 30–12).

Because the sensitivity and specificity and therefore the negative and positive predictive value of RV diastolic collapse depend on the definition of tamponade (Table 30–3), we use a clinical approach to this finding. In a patient with clinical findings of tamponade, we would interpret RV diastolic collapse to indicate a significant hemodynamic contribution of the effusion to the patient's clinical state and require immediate therapy to remove pericardial fluid. In a patient without clinical tamponade, we would interpret RV diastolic

collapse to indicate intrapericardial pressure at or above RV diastolic pressure and a potential existing for relatively acute hemodynamic deterioration. Although not viewing this as an indication for immediate pericardial fluid removal, urgent action is indicated to reverse any factors worsening the hemodynamic effect of the effusion.

Large pleural effusions can cause RV diastolic collapse.[58] In our experience, this has not lead to confusion as to the diagnosis. If we encounter a patient with tamponade physiology and a large pleural effusion, who also has a pericardial effusion, we drain the pleural effusion first and then clinically and echocardiographically reassess the patient for their hemodynamic status.

Right Atrial Compression, Inversion, or Collapse

Right atrial pressures are lower than RV pressures throughout most of the cardiac cycle. Because intrapericardial pressure is evenly distributed over the heart, one would surmise that right atrial compression would occur before RV compression as pericardial pressure is raised. This is borne out in imaging studies in which the right atrium and ventricle are continuously imaged during pericardiocentesis.[44] Subsequently, right atrial inversion, which tends to begin in late ventricular diastole (just before or at the p wave if sinus rhythm is present) but persists into early ventricular systole, is an extremely sensitive sign of cardiac tamponade[59] (Fig. 30–12). However, it is less specific than RV diastolic collapse (see Table 30–3). The depth of right atrial collapse bears an imprecise relationship to the intrapericardial pressure or hemodynamic effect of the fluid.[50,60] Conversely, the right atrial inversion time index (determined by counting the total number of frames showing atrial inversion divided by the total number of frames in the cycle), has been reported to have a high sensitivity and specificity for the presence of clinical cardiac tamponade[60] (see Table 30–3). It should be noted that respiration, and although less well studied, the same factors that interfere with RV diastolic collapse may diminish right atrial collapse. Ventricular pacing has also been reported to affect the accuracy of this sign.[60]

Left Atrial Compression, Inversion, or Collapse

Normally, mean left atrial pressure is higher than right atrial pressure. Therefore, one would speculate that left atrial compression, inversion, or collapse would be less sensitive but more specific than right atrial findings for tamponade. This has been borne out in studies[59] (see Table 30–3). Left atrial collapse may be useful in settings of abnormally high right-sided pressures (e.g., pulmonary embolism) and may be the only sign of tamponade in the postoperative patient.[52]

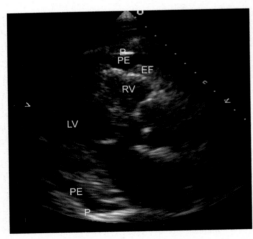

Figure 30–11. *Parasternal long-axis view in end systole of a small, circumferential pericardial effusion with epicardial fat. The pericardial fluid is seen anteriorly and posteriorly between the parietal and visceral pericardium. The epicardial fat is seen lying between the right ventricular wall and the visceral pericardium. EF, epicardial (pericardial) fat; LV, left ventricle; P, pericardium; PE, pericardial effusion; RV, right ventricle.*

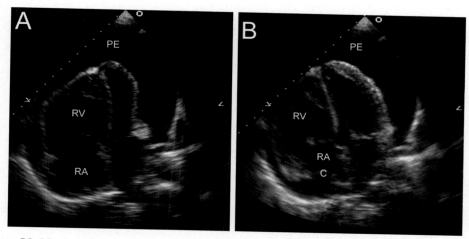

Figure 30–12. *Apical view of a large pericardial effusion.* Top panel (A) *is in ventricular systole; the right atrium and ventricle are dilated but right atrial contour appears relatively normal.* Bottom panel (B) *is in early ventricular diastole; marked right atrial collapse is seen. The patient has a connective tissue disease resulting in pulmonary arterial hypertension with elevation of pulmonary artery systolic pressure to 70 mm Hg. Therefore, right ventricular diastolic collapse is not seen. C, collapsed segment of right atrial wall; PE, pericardial effusion; RA, right atrium; RV, right ventricle.*

Phasic Respiratory Changes and Plethora of the Inferior Vena Cava

Decreased phasic respiratory changes and plethora of the inferior vena cava have been reported in tamponade.[30] It is well recognized that multiple other conditions can lead to this finding, and therefore it has a high sensitivity but low specificity for tamponade[30] (see Table 30–3).

Other M-Mode and Two-Dimensional Features of Altered Pericardial Pressure

Other features suggested in the echocardiographic literature to indicate the presence of a hemodynamic effect of tamponade are predominantly related to the increases in right-sided flow and the enhanced ventricular interaction that occurs with raises in intrapericardial pressures. These include decreased mitral valve opening with inspiration (with a resultant decrease in the excursion of the anterior leaflet and diminished ejection fraction [EF] slope)[61,62] and increases in right-sided and decreases in left-sided heart sizes with inspiration.[63] In general, we feel these physiological phenomenon are better assessed in the modern era with Doppler flow recordings than with M-mode or 2D recordings.

Doppler Echocardiography

The determination of variations in intracardiac flows with respiration, specifically using pulsed-wave Doppler, has proven to aid clinical decision making in patients with pericardial effusions. During inspiration, normally intrathoracic, intrapericardial, and intracardiac pressures decrease in unison and to a similar extent. There is normally a small augmentation of right-sided transvalvular flows and a decrease in left-sided transvalvular flows accompanying inspiration.[64] The explanation for this is a combination of increased venous return secondary to decreased intrathoracic pressure, a fall in pulmonary vascular impedance, and ventricular interaction. With accumulation of pericardial fluid, there is a blunting of transmission of pressure changes from the intrathoracic compartment to the intrapericardial compartment.[64] As portions of the pulmonary veins are intrathoracic (but extra pericardial), the pulmonary venous pressure falls with inspiration; however, the fall in pericardial pressure is blunted, resulting in a fall in driving pressure filling the left atrium and therefore a reduction in LV filling.[64] Respiratory augmentation remains intact on the right side and RV filling increases during inspiration.[65] As pericardial fluid volume increases, available pericardial space becomes limited, enhancing the potential for ventricular interaction (Fig. 30–13). The disparate patterns of left-sided and right-sided filling with respiration are amplified by ventricular interaction. A summary of the magnitude and direction of flow disturbance in intracardiac flows are presented in Table 30–4. The magnitude of this flow disturbance is greater, and statistical separation of values from normal occurs earlier, with right-sided flows than left-sided flows. Although most literature has concentrated on changes in transvalvular flow velocities, there is also a decrease in LV ejection time and LV inflow duration.[65] The combination of a decrease in both of these quantities results in an increase in LV isovolumic relaxation time as measured by echocardiography with inspiration.[65]

TABLE 30-3. Sensitivity, Specificity, Negative, and Positive Predictive Values of Echocardiographic Features of Pericardial Tamponade

Author	Year	Echocardiographic Sign Evaluated	Patients	Definition of Tamponade	Sensitivity	Specificity	PPV	NPV
Armstrong and colleagues[125]	1982	Right ventricular diastolic collapse, M-mode, (posterior movement of the right ventricular free wall in early and mid diastole as timed from the ECG)	86 (17 tamponade)	Presence of a moderate to large pericardial effusion, at least two of the following: (1) elevated venous pressure, (2) systemic hypotension, (3) pulsus paradoxus and resolution of signs after pericardiocentesis	76	84	54	93
Armstrong and colleagues[125]	1982	Right ventricular diastolic collapse, 2D (any indentation of the right ventricular free wall during diastole)	41 (10 tamponade)	Same as above	100	87	71	100
Engel, Hon, Fowler, Plummer[126]	1982	Right ventricular diastolic collapse, M-mode (persistent posterior motion of the right ventricular free wall greater than 50 ms after mitral valve opening)	37 (21 tamponade)	Pulsus paradoxus >10 mm Hg, elevated systemic venous pressure, and resolution of signs with pericardiocentesis	81	94	89	80
Gillam and colleagues[60]	1983	Right atrial collapse (inversion of the right atrial free wall at any point of the cardiac cycle)	123 (19 tamponade)	Two or more of the following: (1) elevated jugular venous pressure, (2) relative hypotension, (3) pulsus paradoxus >10 mm Hg and resolution of the symptoms with pericardiocentesis	100	82	50	100
Gillam and colleagues[60]	1983	Right atrial diastolic collapse (right atrial inversion time index >0.34 [defined as the number of video fields demonstrating right atrial inversion divided by the total number of fields per cardiac cycle])	36 (18 tamponade)	Same as above	94	100	100	95
Kronzon, Cohen, Winer[59]	1983	Right atrial collapse, 2D (any reduction in right atrial size during diastole)	29 (9 tamponade)	Clinical with relief after pericardiocentesis	100	85	75	100

First author, year	Echocardiographic sign	Criteria for tamponade	No. of patients	Sensitivity	Specificity	PPV	NPV
Kronzon, Cohen, Winer[59], 1983	Left atrial collapse, 2D (posterior left atrial wall motion of at least 10 mm in diastole)	Same as above	29 (9 tamponade)	54	95	83	83
Singh and colleagues[44], 1984	Right ventricular diastolic collapse, 2D (persistent inward motion of the right ventricular endocardial surface after opening of the mitral valve)	Equalization of right atrial, pulmonary capillary wedge, and intrapericardial pressures and elevation of these pressures to >10 mm Hg	16 (12 tamponade)	92	100	100	80
Singh and colleagues[44], 1984	Right atrial collapse, 2D (right atrial free wall appears to be inverted at any point during the cardiac cycle)	Same as above	12 (8 tamponade)	63	100	100	57
Singh and colleagues[44], 1986	Right ventricular diastolic collapse, 2D (persistent inward motion of the right ventricular endocardial surface after mitral valve opening)	Equalization of the intrapericardial, right atrial, and pulmonary wedge pressures with elevations of these pressures to >10 mm Hg	21 (16 tamponade)	93	100	100	83
Himelman, Kircher, Rockey, Schiller[30], 1988	Inferior vena cava plethora, 2D (a decrease in proximal vena cava diameter by <50% after a deep inspiration)	Either of the following: (1) elevation (mean >12 mm Hg) and equalization (≤5 mm Hg) of diastolic filling pressures; (2) systolic blood pressure <100 mm Hg that increased by >20 mm Hg after pericardiocentesis	115 (33 tamponade)	97	40	40	97
Himelman, Kircher, Rockey, Schiller[30], 1988	Right atrial collapse, 2D (dynamic inversion of the right atrial wall occurring in late diastole or early systole)	Same as above	115 (33 tamponade)	55	66	39	78
Himelman, Kircher, Rockey, Schiller[30], 1988	Right ventricular diastolic collapse, 2D (early diastolic inversion of the right ventricular free wall that varied with respiration)	Same as above	115 (33 tamponade)	48	68	38	77

Some of the values in the table differ from those reported in the original studies, as data from patients with "equivocal" tamponade have not been used. Sensitivity (true positives/true positives + false negatives) and specificity (true negatives/true negatives + false positives).
ECG, electrocardiogram; NPV, negative predictive value (true negatives/true negatives + false negatives); PPV, positive predictive value (true positives/true positives + false positives); 2D, two-dimensional.
Data from references 30, 44, 59, 60, 125, 126.

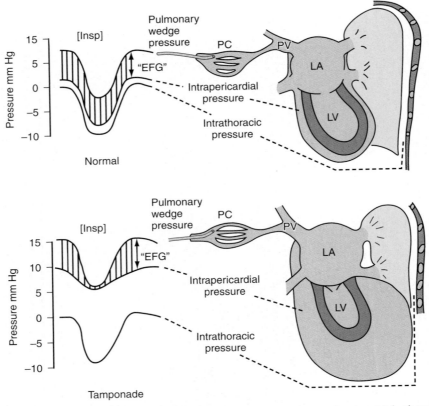

Figure 30–13. *The top half of the figure represents the normal situation in which changes in intrathoracic pressure are transmitted to both the pericardial sac and the pulmonary veins. The effective filling gradient (EFG) changes only slightly during respiration. The bottom half of the figure represents cardiac tamponade in which changes in intrathoracic pressure are transmitted to the pulmonary veins but not to the pericardial sac. The EFG falls during inspiration. Insp, inspiration; LA, left atrium; LV, left ventricle; PC, pulmonary capillaries; PV, pulmonary veins. (From Bunnell IL, Holand JF, Griffith GT, Greene DG: Am J Med 25:640-646, 1960).*

Although increased respiratory variation in mitral and tricuspid inflow velocities is an early predictor of tamponade physiology in the setting of pericardial effusion, the relationship of the magnitude of this change to the severity of tamponade has been questioned.[66] Others have noted a quantitative relationship between rise in pericardial pressure and the degree of respiratory variation in inflow velocities.[67]

The venae cavae and pulmonary veins are less enclosed by the pericardium and therefore less influenced by pericardial forces. Therefore more subtle flow disturbances are seen in these structures.[68]

Clinically, we depend primarily on LV and RV inflow variations with respiration. We find they are the most easily obtainable in patients with dyspnea, who, as a result of orthopnea, are reluctant to lay flat.

The Role of Echocardiography in Patient Management

It is important to recognize that significance falls in cardiac output and increases in filling pressures occur bore the appearance of clinical tamponade (which we

define as a fall in mean arterial pressure and a pulsus paradoxus greater than10 mm Hg as a result of raised pericardial pressure).[53] As well, the clinical transformation from stable to unstable can occur abruptly with small changes in any of the factors that influence the hemodynamic effect of a given pericardial effusion. Therefore, echocardiography has come to play a pivotal role in the management of patients with pericardial effusion, as some echocardiographic findings will occur when intrapericardial pressure is elevated but before clinical compromise. It must be appreciated that the physiological effects of an increasing pericardial effusion lie on a continuum, and therefore any separation into distinct stages is arbitrary. However, clinically we find it useful to divide patients with pericardial effusions echocardiographically into three hemodynamic categories. First, those without echocardiographic evidence of hemodynamic compromise, (no RV collapse, no right or left atrial collapse, physiological changes in intracardiac flows with inspiration) we describe as "no evidence of hemodynamic effect" on the echocardiographic report). Second, those with any degree of RV diastolic collapse, prolonged (>35% of the cardiac cy-

TABLE 30-4. Respiratory Variation in Intracardiac Flows Reported in Normal Subjects, Pericardial Effusion without Tamponade, Tamponade, and Postpericardiocentesis

Author	Year	Subjects	Normal		Tamponade		Effusion without Tamponade	
			Inspiration	Expiration	Inspiration	Expiration	Inspiration	Expiration
Pandian and colleagues[127]	1985	9 dogs (at baseline, effusion without tamponade, and with tamponade) 3 patients (all with tamponade)						
Mitral mean flow velocity			↓10±2%		↓42±3%		↓12±1%	
Tricuspid mean flow velocity			↑17±2%		↑117±19%		↑17±3%	

			Normal		Tamponade		Postpericardiocentesis	
			Inspiration	Expiration	Inspiration	Expiration	Inspiration	Expiration
Leeman, Riley, Carl, Come[128]	1987	19 (11 tamponade)						
Mitral TVI			↓8%		↓35%		↓3%	
Tricuspid TVI			↑9%		↑80%		↑11%	
Aortic TVI			↓3%		↓33%		↓7%	
Pulmonary TVI			↑9%		↑86%		↑11%	
Appleton, Hatle, Popp[65]	1988	27 (7 tamponade)						
Mitral E velocity (cm/s)			82±17	85±18	39±12	68±19	71±12	77±13
Tricuspid E velocity (cm/s)			64±10	56±9	60±6	30±9	60±9	50±8
Aortic velocity (cm/s)			109±9	113±9	80±22	107±26	103±22	107±22
IVRT (ms)			74±15	72±14	117±39	64±20	69±15	67±17

E, early diastolic filling wave of the left (mitral) or right (tricuspid) ventricle; IVRT, isovolumetric relaxation time; TVI, time velocity integral.
Data from references 65, 127, 128.

cle) right atrial collapse, or marked (>25% LV or >50% RV early filling [E] velocity changes with inspiration), we report as showing "echocardiographic indications of "tamponade". Tamponade is in quotation marks to acknowledge our understanding that tamponade is a clinical syndrome. Thirdly, we report patients that fit into neither of the aforementioned categories as having "echocardiographic indicators of elevated pericardial pressure without echocardiographic features of 'tamponade.'" These rules are applicable to patients with relatively normal pericardial and cardiac physiology. However, it cannot be overemphasized that with localized cardiac compression or abnormal physiological states, hemodynamic compromise may be present as a result of elevated pericardial pressure without any classic M-mode, 2D or Doppler echocardiographic indicators of raised intrapericardial pressure.[50-52]

Tissue Doppler Findings in Pericardial Effusion with Tamponade

In eight patients with pericardial effusion and tamponade, E' was reported to be lower than age-matched and sex-matched control subjects, and unlike LV inflow (E wave), velocity did not show respiratory variation. E' values returned to normal after pericardiocentesis.[41]

Determination of Pericardial Fluid Volume

While 2D (using a prolate ellipse model)[69] and especially three-dimensional (3D) echocardiography[70] has the ability to determine the volume of a pericardial effusion, we find our referring physicians prefer characterization of the effusion as minimal, small, moderate, or large in size. For circumferential pericardial effusions, we characterize any pericardial effusion with less than 5 mm of pericardial separation in diastole (corresponding to a fluid volume of 50 to 100 mL) as minimal, 5 to 10 mm of separation as small (corresponding to a fluid volume of 100 to 250 mL), 10 to 20 mm of separation as moderate (corresponding to a fluid volume of 250 to 500 mL), and greater than 20 mm separation as large (corresponding to a fluid volume of >500 mL). We also routinely report (for any moderate or large effusion or any effusion with a hemodynamic effect) the location of the fluid, loculations, the presence of an appropriate approach for percutaneous drainage, and our estimation of the risk of complications from percutaneous intervention.

Localized and Loculated Pericardial Fluid Collections

In some cases, loculation or combinations of localized with more generalized cardiac compression can occur rendering both the diagnosis and potential contribution of the pericardial process to cardiac pathology difficult. In our experience and in the experience of others,[50-52] this is especially problematical post–cardiac surgery. In these instances, it is not possible to rely on the absence of traditional echocardiographic markers of hemodynamic effect of the fluid to rule out a contribution of the pericardial fluid. A careful search for localized chamber compression, echogenic structures suggesting collections of blood inside or adjacent to the pericardial space, and nontraditional markers of hemodynamic perturbations, such as LV or left atrial diastolic collapse,[71] must be performed. Transesophageal echocardiography often adds incremental information.[72-74] If doubt remains as to the presence or hemodynamic effect of a collection, alternative-imaging techniques, catheter-based hemodynamic monitoring with volume manipulation or even surgical exploration may be required for both diagnostic and therapeutic purposes.[52] Often the most important role of the echocardiogram is to rule out other cardiac causes of the patient's clinical state.

Echocardiographically Guided Pericardiocentesis

Before the advent of 2D echocardiography, percutaneous pericardiocentesis was viewed with trepidation by even the most experienced clinicians. In cardiac catheterization laboratories, with the procedure performed under continuous fluoroscopic, electrocardiographic, and hemodynamic monitoring, experienced clinicians in large volume centers achieved success rates of 86% in obtaining fluid, with death rates of 4%, and a further 4% risk of other major complications.[75] In contrast, echocardiographically guided series have indicated success rates of greater than 99%, no deaths, and total complication rates of three percent to five percent (pneumothorax, hemothorax, subsequent purulent pericarditis, or transient ventricular tachycardia).[76-78]

Multiple techniques exist for echocardiographically guided pericardiocentesis,[78-80] and the best technique in an individual case depends on the amount and location of the pericardial fluid, the clinical status of the patient, and the operator's experience. In all but emergency situations, we prefer to perform the procedure in our coronary care unit (CCU), under continuous echocardiographic, electrocardiographic, noninvasive or invasive blood pressure, and oximetric monitoring. Pericardiocentesis is not indicated as definitive therapy in patients with pericardial effusions as a result aortic dissection, a direct puncture wound, or ruptured ventricular aneurysm in which surgical drainage with suppression of bleeding is needed. The steps we employ for nonemergency echocardiographically guided pericardiocentesis are outlined here:

1. The patient's echocardiogram is reviewed to determine the amount and location of pericardial fluid, the presence of loculations, the possible percutaneous approaches, and any underlying cardiac pathology.

2. The patient's chart is reviewed, and if needed, a history taken and a directed physical examination performed. We determine the clinical effects of the pericardial effusion, the presence of any bleeding diathesis or anticoagulant drugs, and underlying general medical or specific cardiac issues that could modify our approach (e.g., avoidance of areas documented to have adhesions or allergies).

3. Lab tests are ordered or reviewed. As a minimum we suggest a hemoglobin, platelet count, electrolytes, creatinine, international normalized ratio (INR) and activated partial thromboplastin time (APTT). Any coagulopathy, significant anemia, or electrolyte disturbance (especially hypokalemia) should be corrected.

4. Informed consent is obtained, a large-bore peripheral intravenous (IV) line is placed, a noninvasive blood pressure cuff (if an arterial line is not present) is applied and readings taken every 2 minutes. Oxygen saturation monitoring and oxygen by nasal prongs is placed.

5. If an echocardiographer is performing the study, we prefer to image the patient ourselves to obtain a "feel" for the correct approach. We choose the approach that provides the most direct route to the largest collection of fluid, as far removed from vital structures as possible. Special attention should be made to avoid the internal thoracic arteries (located 0.5 to 2 cm lateral to the sternal edge). We then mark a proposed entry point (with a permanent marker or indent the skin with the top of a syringe cap) and then re-image from this location to determine the depth to the fluid, the depth to the nearest cardiac structure, and the correct angle. The angulation of the transducer in three-dimensional space is noted; this provides an invaluable reference in subsequent direction of the pericardiocentesis needle. We find it useful to form a mental map by drawing an imaginary line along the direction of the transducer and then noting its intersection with a remote anatomical structure, such as the point of the left shoulder or tip of the scapula. This helps us to replicate the transducer orientation, and hence ensures that when the pericardiocentesis needle is placed, it is reliably directed toward the pericardial effusion. We then determine if an acoustic window is available, remote to the proposed puncture site (that will not interfere with the sterility of the procedure,) to directly visualize the procedure. If so, we have sonographers image from this window while the procedure is performed. If not, we cover the imaging probe with a sterile cover and have it available for the physician performing the procedure to use if needed.

6. We then prepare and drape the patient and open a commercial pericardiocentesis kit. If the effusion is at a depth greater than 5 cm from the surface, or if there is less than 2 cm of fluid between the pericardium and any cardiac structure at the proposed puncture site, we prepare a three-way stopcock device for injection of echo-contrast. This is done by connecting two, 10-mL Luer lock syringes, one syringe filled with 5 mL of sterile saline agitated with 0.25 to 0.5 mL of air (similar to the set up used for a peripheral venous contrast study). We perform the procedure in a sterile gown and gloves.

7. The skin (including an area for an eventual suture) and subcutaneous tissue along the proposed approach are then thoroughly anesthetized with 1% or 2% lidocaine using a small (19 to 25 gauge) needle. We use a needle, if possible, that is long enough to reach the pericardial fluid but not any cardiac structures. Adequate local anesthetic is a must. The needle is advanced along the previ-

ously determined pathway until the pericardial fluid is reached, or the predetermined appropriate length of the needle is inserted.

8. We then attach a needle (that we have confirmed will accommodate the guide wire) to a 10-mL Luer lock syringe with 5 mL of 1% lidocaine. Under direct imaging if possible, the needle is advanced until pericardial fluid is obtained, or a depth of needle is inserted that could contact a cardiac structure (i.e., if the pericardial fluid is 4 cm from the skin surface at the entry point and there is 2 cm of fluid in this area, we would limit our insertion to <6 cm). Constant aspiration during the advancement of the needle followed by a slight pause for injection should be performed to ensure that a plug of tissue or clot is not occluding the needle tip. A small amount of additional lidocaine may need to be injected during the needle advancement. There is a characteristic "feel" to the needles contact with pericardium and its puncture. Resulting from the tomographic nature of 2D imaging and the high reflectivity of the pericardial puncture needle, care must be taken to avoid misinterpretation of the image during the procedure. In particular the tip of the pericardiocentesis needle and its course may be difficult to identify with imaging from a remote acoustic window. Indentation of the pericardium by the needle may be noted just before pericardial puncture, which is occasionally helpful. Direct visualization does not substitute for clinical judgment or allow one to continue insertion of the needle to depths where cardiac puncture can occur.

9. Once the pericardium is entered (Fig. 30–14), there should be free flow of fluid into the syringe. If there is any doubt as to the structure punctured and in all cases of small effusions, we confirm the position of the needle with the injection of 0.5 to 1.0 mL of agitated saline through the needles (using the three-way stopcock configuration described previously). Visualization of the contrast only in the pericardial space confirms the needle position (see Fig. 30–14). A "J" guide wire is introduced, once again under direct vision, into the pericardial space. The needle is withdrawn, a small "nick" is placed in the skin at the wire's entry point, and dilators are employed. A pigtail catheter is placed over the wire into the pericardial space, the guide wire removed, and a 50-mL Luer lock syringe attached to withdraw fluid for analysis. Once the majority of the fluid has been removed, we attach a suction drainage device to the pigtail and suture the pigtail in place. If a large amount of fluid is present, the process can be made quicker by incorporating a three-way stopcock into the circuit and

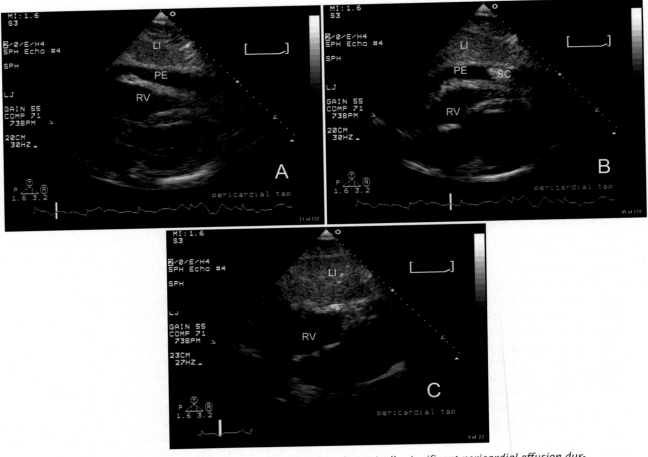

Figure 30–14. *Subcostal view of a small but hemodynamically significant pericardial effusion during a pericardiocentesis. Panel A demonstrates the effusion. Panel B is after injection of approximately 0.1 mL of agitated saline through the pericardiocentesis needle to confirm position in the pericardial space. Panel C shows the shaft of the pigtail catheter (at the arrow head, two discrete parallel echogenic lines reflecting the catheter walls with the echo-free area representing the catheter lumen) lying in the pericardial space after the majority of fluid has been drained. LI, liver; PE, pericardial effusion; RV, right ventricle; SC, saline contrast.*

using the side port to expel the fluid once the syringe is full.

If it is clear we are in the pericardial space after the initial puncture, we often omit the stage of contrast injection into the pericardium. In these cases, we advance the needle an additional 1 to 2 mm after the initial pericardial puncture, remove the 10-mL syringe and attach a 50-mL Luer lock syringe to withdraw fluid for analysis. The needle in the pericardial space must not be allowed to advance to depths where a cardiac structure could be punctured. The 50-mL Luer lock syringe is removed and the guide wire advanced.

Care should be taken to keep the proximal 5 to 10 cm of the external pigtail sterile in case repositioning is required.

Analysis of pericardial should be ordered according to the clinical setting, as the yield of routine tests appears to be low.[81-83]

Following diagnostic pericardiocentesis, the pericardial drain may be removed after the pericardial fluid has been fully aspirated, however, in most cases we leave the catheter in situ for 12 to 36 hours. Intermittent echocardiographic reevaluation of the pericardial fluid volume throughout the aspiration procedure is useful to assess the degree of remaining pericardial fluid.

10. The puncture site is treated with an iodine-based antibacterial and the site is covered with an occlusive dressing. Once drainage from the catheter ceases we reimage the patient and remove the catheter once only a minimal amount of fluid remains. Analgesia is given as required to eliminate the discomfort, usually mild, from the indwelling catheter.

To remove the catheter, we give the patient a small dose of intravenous sedation and analgesia if possible, disconnect the pigtail from the drainage device and remove the dressing. We then cut the suture, attach a 10- to 50-mL Luer lock syringe (depending on the amount of residual effusion) to the pigtail, and withdraw at a rate of 2 to 4 cm/s while applying gentle suction on the system with the syringe. To reposition the catheter, we give the patient a small dose of intravenous sedation and analgesia if possible, and with sterile technique, disconnect the pigtail from the drainage device, remove the dressing, cut the suture, attach a 10-mL Luer lock syringe to the pigtail, or withdraw the catheter up to 5 cm while applying gentle suction on the system with the syringe. Advancing the catheter usually requires reintroducing a guide wire and risks inserting a nonsterile portion of the catheter into the patient.

In an emergency situation, the physicians at our institution still prefer to have echocardiographic confirmation of an effusion, if at all possible. When effusions are found, they use the information obtained to guide the percutaneous approach. Most often, this occurs during percutaneous interventions. This so-called "rescue pericardiocentesis" is successful in relieving tamponade in 99% of cases and may be the only and definitive therapy in 82% of cases.[77] Often the patient will be prepared and draped by the time the echocardiographic machine and echocardiographer arrive at the catheterization lab. Usually, the interventional cardiologist performs the pericardiocentesis with the echocardiographer imaging and guiding.

Outpatient echocardiographically guided pericardiocentesis[84] and percutaneous pericardial biopsy,[85] and the creation of pericardial windows with balloon techniques[86-88] and sclerotherapy[89] have been described. Imaging probes that allow needle insertion in the center of the imaging plane are available.[90]

Acute Pericarditis

Acute pericarditis is usually a self-limiting syndrome with a paucity of echocardiographic findings. On occasion however, acute pericarditis may be complicated by effusion, myocarditis, transient or chronic pericardial constriction, constrictive effusive pericarditis, or cardiac tamponade.

An echocardiogram is often ordered in patients in whom acute pericarditis is suspected. No echocardiographic feature is pathognomonic of the disease. Patients with uncomplicated viral pericarditis will have a normal echocardiogram. The value of echocardiogra-

phy in acute pericarditis lies in its unique ability to detect complications, at times aid in the diagnosis of the underlying etiology, or detecting other cardiac processes that may account for the patient's clinical presentation. Complications acutely include pericardial effusion with or without hemodynamic effect, myopericarditis, or ventricular systolic or diastolic dysfunction. A transient constrictive phase during acute pericarditis has been described,[91,92] and acute pericarditis may on occasion progress to overt constrictive pericarditis. The echocardiogram may visualize tumor (Fig. 30–15) or a regional wall motion abnormality suggesting previous myocardial infarction (MI) as an underlying etiology. A myriad of other cardiac diagnosis can mimic acute pericarditis, and the echocardiogram may be useful in this regard (e.g., detecting a vegetation and mitral regurgitation (MR) in a patient with fever and a new auscultatory finding).

We occasionally find echocardiography useful in patients presenting with chest pain (especially of <12 hours duration in which thrombolysis may be indicated) and electrocardiogram (ECG) changes in which the differential diagnosis includes an acute coronary syndrome (ACS) and pericarditis. The finding of a regional wall motion abnormality in an anatomic distribution without pericardial effusion suggests therapy toward an acute coronary syndrome is warranted. The finding of a pericardial effusion without a regional wall motion abnormality suggests pericarditis is more likely. Unfortunately, not even these findings are absolute, and thrombolytic therapy has been administered to patients in whom, in retrospect, the real diagnosis was pericarditis.[93] In practice most of these patients now proceed to diagnostic coronary angiography.

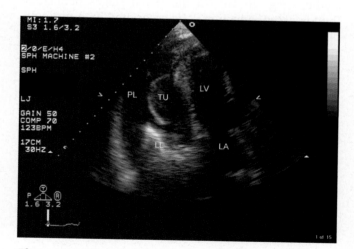

Figure 30–15. *Apical long-axis view of a large mass attached to the pericardium in a patient with lung cancer. There is associated pleural effusion seen in this view (note the collapsed lung in the fluid). A small amount of pericardial fluid was seen from in other views. LA, left atrium; LL, lung; LV, left ventricle; PL, pleural effusion; TU, tumor.*

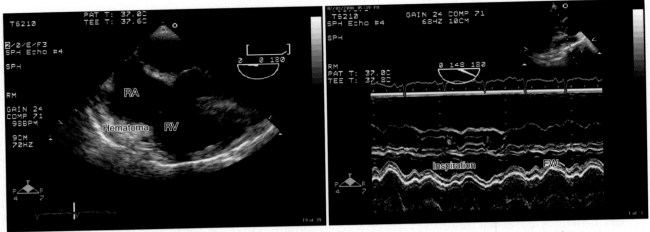

Figure 30–16. *Transesophageal echocardiography in a patient 10 days post–cardiac transplant. Panel A shows hemopericardium in relation to the right atrium and right ventricle, especially in the posterior atrioventricular groove area. This is a common site for hemopericardium following cardiac surgery. Panel B shows M-mode imaging of the right ventricular free wall and septum. Significant variation in the right ventricular dimension is noted with respiration indicating enhanced ventricular interaction. In the clinical context, the echocardiographic findings were suggestive of effusive constriction. FW, right ventricular free wall; RA, right atrium; RV, right ventricle.*

Effusive Constrictive Pericarditis

Effusive constrictive pericarditis is a syndrome characterized by pericardial constriction by the visceral pericardium in the presence of a pericardial effusion. The hallmark of effusive constrictive pericarditis is persistence of constrictive physiology following the removal of the pericardial fluid.[94] The hemodynamic findings may share common features of both pericardial tamponade and constriction. In our experience, effusive constriction may be seen after pericardial hematoma complicating cardiac surgery or following acute pericarditis (Fig. 30–16). In the initial stages pericardial fluid is noted, which may be associated with fibrinous or organizing material and adhesions in the pericardial space. 2D M-mode and Doppler signs of raised pericardial pressure may be present. The diagnosis of effusive constriction may be suspected echocardiographically if septal motion is abnormal or if venous expiratory flow reversals are present.[95] The natural history of this condition is not well defined, however progress to chronic constriction is not inevitable.[95]

Pericardial Effusion as an Incidental Finding at Echocardiography

Occasionally a pericardial effusion will be noted as an incidental finding in an echocardiogram requested for an indication not likely to be related to pericardial disease. The question is then raised as to whether diagnostic pericardiocentesis is indicated. Although pericardiocentesis of chronic effusions will result in resolution in 50% of cases,[96] our practice is to perform pericardiocentesis only if important hemodynamic effect is present, as we believe the diagnostic yield to be low. A careful search needs to be made for underlying disease likely to result in pericardial effusion (see Table 30–2). Follow-up echocardiography is imperative.

Congenital Disorders of the Pericardium

Congenital Absence of the Pericardium

Congenital absence of the pericardium is a rare clinical entity found in approximately 1 in 10,000 autopsies. Partial left-sided absence of the pericardium is most common (two thirds of reported cases) with right-sided absence occurring in the majority of the rest. Complete absence of the pericardium is reported rarely. Most patients are asymptomatic.[97] Reported symptoms in the literature include paroxysmal stabbing chest pain (largely nonexertional), heart murmur, an abnormal chest X-ray (CXR) and rarely incarceration of the left atrium or ventricle (in isolated partial left-sided absence).[14] The echocardiographic features of congenital absence of the pericardium include unusual echocardiographic windows, cardiac hypermotility, abnormal ventricular septal motion, and abnormal swinging motion of the heart.[98] At least one, and usually two, of these findings are reported in all patients with complete absence of the pericardium.[98] In patients with partial absence, displacement and enlargement of a cardiac structure as it herniates through the pericardium may be noted. This finding has potential significance as case reports exist of coronary artery obstruction,[99,102] left atrial strangulation,[103,104] herniation of the left atrium causing syncope,[105] or herniation of the left or right ventricle causing mitral or tricuspid regurgitation.[106,107] Although a diagnosis of complete absence of the pericardium may be established with a combination of clinical presentation, chest radiography and echocardiography, partial absence of the pericardium often requires ancillary imaging techniques to fully delineate the nature and extent of the defect. In this regard, magnetic resonance imaging has proven to be especially useful.[14,108,109] Reports of combined congenital pericardial and diaphragmatic defects also exist.[107] Pericardioplasty with synthetic materials or bovine pericardium, with amputation of the atrial appendage if strangulation is imminent has been described.[14]

Pericardial Cysts

Pericardial cysts are congenital, benign intrathoracic lesions thought to be remnants of a defect in embryologic development of the pericardium. Prenatal diagnosis has been reported.[110] They usually involve the left or right costophrenic angle although they may be found adjacent to any cardiac structure.[15,111,112] Rarely, hydatid pericardial cysts[113] or a cardiac hemangioma[114] may have echocardiographic features mimicking pericardial cysts. Reported complications of pericardial cysts include cardiac tamponade,[115,116] hemorrhage,[117] or erosion of cardiac structures.[111,112,118] The echocardiographic hallmark of a pericardial cyst is a round or oval echo-free structure, related to one of the cardiac chambers, from which it is separated by a definite wall of echoes.[119,120] The presence of internal echoes suggesting a more solid structure should alert the clinician to the possibility of a less benign process. A report exists of a pericardial cyst that was not diagnosed on transthoracic echocardiography being apparent on a transesophageal study.[121] Differentiation of benign pericardial cysts from other cardiac pathology appears important because numerous therapeutic, relatively noninvasive treatments exist for benign pericardial cysts. These include videoscopic resection,[122] ethanol sclerosis,[123] or needle aspiration and drainage.[16,124]

KEY POINTS

■ An understanding of the effects of ventricular interdependence is key to understanding the hemodynamic and therefore echocardiographic features of compressive pericardial disease, such as tamponade or constriction.

■ No one echocardiographic sign is diagnostic of pericardial constriction. The diagnosis of pericardial constriction requires a careful integration of the results of M-mode Doppler and 2D imaging and a consideration of the clinical context.

■ Echocardiography is pivotal to management strategy and decision making in pericardial effusion.

■ Traditional echocardiographic markers of cardiac tamponade may be absent in patients with localized pericardial effusions, especially in the postcardiac surgery setting.

■ The presence of diastolic collapse of the free wall of the right ventricle is a specific but not sensitive sign of pericardial tamponade.

■ Percutaneous drainage of pericardial fluid may be safely performed with echocardiographic guidance.

■ When an acute hemopericardium occurs, for instance in the setting of interventional cardiologic procedures, rapid and serious hemodynamic disturbance may ensue, despite the accumulation of a relatively small amount of fluid in the pericardial space.

■ In acute pericarditis, the echocardiographic examination is commonly normal.

■ The hallmark of effusive constrictive pericarditis is persistence of constrictive physiology following the removal of the pericardial fluid.

■ In complex pericardial disease, or when echocardiographic images are suboptimal, integration of echocardiographic findings with findings from other imaging modalities may be required.

REFERENCES

1. Holt J: The normal pericardium. *Am J Cardiol* 26:455-465, 1970.
2. Hoit B: Pericardial heart disease. *Curr Probl Cardiol* 22:353-400, 1997.
3. Spodick D: The normal and diseased pericardium: Current concepts of pericardial physiology, diagnosis and treatment. *J Am Coll Cardiol* 1:240-251, 1983.
4. Goldstein J: Cardiac tamponade, constrictive pericarditis, and restrictive cardiomyopathy. *Curr Probl Cardiol* 2004;29:⁹503-67.
5. Baker A, Dani R, Smith E, et al: Quantitative assessment of independent contributions of pericardium and septum to direct ventricular interaction. *Am J Physiol* 275(2 Pt 2):H476-H483, 1998.
6. Bernard H: The functions of the pericardium. *J Physiology* 22:43, 1898.
7. Slinker BK, Ditchey RV, Bell SP, Le Winter MM: Right heart pressure does not equal pericardial pressure in the potassium chloride-arrested canine heart in situ. *Circulation* 76:357-362, 1987.
8. Freeman G, Le WM: Pericardial adaptations during chronic cardiac dilation in dogs. *Circ Res* 54:294-300, 1984.
9. Shirato K, Shabetai R, Bhargava V, et al: Alteration of the left ventricular diastolic pressure-segment length relation produced

by the pericardium. Effects of cardiac distension and afterload reduction in conscious dogs. *Circulation* 57:1191-1198, 1978.

10. Belenkie I, Dani R, Smith E, Tyberg J: The importance of pericardial constraint in experimental pulmonary embolism and volume loading. *Am Heart J* 123:733-742, 1992.

11. Atherton J, Moore T, Lele S, et al: Diastolic ventricular interaction in chronic heart failure [see comments]. *Lancet* 349:1720-1724, 1997.

12. Martin R, Rakowski H, French J, Popp R: Localization of pericardial effusion with wide angle phased array echocardiography. *Am J Cardiol* 42:904-912, 1978.

13. Martin R, Bowden R, Filly K, Popp R: Intrapericardial abnormalities in patients with pericardial effusion. Findings by two-dimensional echocardiography. *Circulation* 61:568-572, 1980.

14. Gatzoulis M, Munk M, Merchant N, et al: Isolated congenital absence of the pericardium: clinical presentation, diagnosis, and management. *Ann Thorac Surg* 69:1209-1215, 2000.

15. Salyer D, Salyer W, Eggleston J: Benign developmental cysts of the mediastinum. *Arch Pathol Lab Med* 101:136-139, 1977.

16. Volpino P, De CA, Bononi M, et al: [Pericardial cysts. Report on 9 treated cases]. *G Chir* 18:811-814, 1997.

17. Larose E, Ducharme A, Mercier L, et al: Prolonged distress and clinical deterioration before pericardial drainage in patients with cardiac tamponade. *Can J Cardiol* 16:331-336, 2000.

18. Pandian N, Skorton D, Kieso R, Kerber R: Diagnosis of constrictive pericarditis by two-dimensional echocardiography: studies in a new experimental model and in patients. *J Am Coll Cardiol* 4:1164-1173, 1984.

19. Ling L, Oh J, Tei C, et al: Pericardial thickness measured with transesophageal echocardiography: Feasibility and potential clinical usefulness. *J Am Coll Cardiol* 29:1317-1323, 1997.

20. Kern M, Aguirre F: Interpretation of cardiac pathophysiology from pressure waveform analysis: pericardial compressive hemodynamics, Part III. *Cathet Cardiovasc Diagn* 26:152-158, 1992.

21. Hatle L, Appleton C, Popp R: Differentiation of constrictive pericarditis and restrictive cardiomyopathy by Doppler echocardiography [see comments]. *Circulation* 79:357-370, 1989.

22. Voelkel A, Pietro D, Folland E, et al: Echocardiographic features of constrictive pericarditis. *Circulation* 58:871-875, 1978.

23. Gibson T, Grossman W, McLaurin L, et al: An echocardiographic study of the interventricular septum in constrictive pericarditis. *Br Heart J* 38:738-743, 1976.

24. Chandraratna P, Aronow W, Imaizumi T: Role of echocardiography in detecting the anatomic and physiologic abnormalities of constrictive pericarditis. *Am J Med Sci* 283:141-146, 1982.

25. Janos G, Arjunan K, Meyer R, et al: Differentiation of constrictive pericarditis and restrictive cardiomyopathy using digitized echocardiography. *J Am Coll Cardiol* 1(2 Pt 1):541-549, 1983.

26. Hinds S, Reisner S, Amico A, Meltzer R: Diagnosis of pericardial abnormalities by 2D-echo: A pathology-echocardiography correlation in 85 patients. *Am Heart J* 123:143-150, 1992.

27. Morgan J, Raposo L, Clague J, et al: Restrictive cardiomyopathy and constrictive pericarditis: Non-invasive distinction by digitised M mode echocardiography. *Br Heart J* 61:29-37, 1989.

28. Engel P, Fowler N, Tei C, et al: M-mode echocardiography in constrictive pericarditis. *J Am Coll Cardiol* 6:471-474, 1985.

29. Talreja D, Edwards W, Danielson G, et al: Constrictive pericarditis in 26 patients with histologically normal pericardial thickness. *Circulation* 108:1852-1857, 2003.

30. Himelman RB, Kircher B, Rockey DC, Schiller NB: Inferior vena cava plethora with blunted respiratory response: A sensitive echocardiographic sign of cardiac tamponade. *J Am Coll Cardiol* 12:1470-1477, 1988.

31. Oh J, Hatle L, Seward J, et al. Diagnostic role of Doppler echocardiography in constrictive pericarditis [see comments]. *J Am Coll Cardiol* 23:154-162, 1994.

32. Senni M, Redfield M, Ling L, et al: Left ventricular systolic and diastolic function after pericardiectomy in patients with constrictive pericarditis: Doppler echocardiographic findings and correlation with clinical status. *J Am Coll Cardiol* 33:1182-1188, 1999.

33. De VP, Baumgartner W, Casale A, et al: Current indications, risks, and outcome after pericardiectomy. *Ann Thorac Surg* 52:219-224, 1991.

34. Sun J, Abdalla I, Yang X, et al: Respiratory variation of mitral and pulmonary venous Doppler flow velocities in constrictive pericarditis before and after pericardiectomy. *J Am Soc Echocardiogr* 14:1119-1126, 2001.

35. Oh J, Tajik A, Appleton C, et al: Preload reduction to unmask the characteristic Doppler features of constrictive pericarditis. A new observation [see comments]. *Circulation* 95:796-799, 1997.

36. Klodas E, Nishimura R, Appleton C, et al: Doppler evaluation of patients with constrictive pericarditis: Use of tricuspid regurgitation velocity curves to determine enhanced ventricular interaction [see comments]. *J Am Coll Cardiol* 28:652-657, 1996.

37. Klein A, Cohen G, Pietrolungo J, et al: Differentiation of constrictive pericarditis from restrictive cardiomyopathy by Doppler transesophageal echocardiographic measurements of respiratory variations in pulmonary venous flow. *J Am Coll Cardiol* 22:1935-1943, 1993.

38. Boonyaratavej S, Oh J, Tajik A, et al: Comparison of mitral inflow and superior vena cava Doppler velocities in chronic obstructive pulmonary disease and constrictive pericarditis. *J Am Coll Cardiol* 32:2043-2048, 1998.

39. Oki T, Tabata T, Yamada H, et al: Right and left ventricular wall motion velocities as diagnostic indicators of constrictive pericarditis. *Am J Cardiol* 81:465-470, 1998.

40. Garcia MJ, Rodriguez L, Ares M, et al: Differentiation of constrictive pericarditis from restrictive cardiomyopathy: Assessment of left ventricular diastolic velocities in longitudinal axis by Doppler tissue imaging. *J Am Coll Cardiol* 27:108-114, 1996.

41. Sohn D, Kim Y, Kim H, et al: Unique features of early diastolic mitral annulus velocity in constrictive pericarditis. *J Am Soc Echocardiogr* 17:222-226, 2004.

42. Sengupta P, Mohan J, Mehta V, et al: Accuracy and pitfalls of early diastolic motion of the mitral annulus for diagnosing constrictive pericarditis by tissue Doppler imaging. *Am J Cardiol* 93:886-890, 2004.

43. Yamada H, Tabata T, Jaffer S, et al: Clinical features of mixed physiology of constriction and restriction: Echocardiographic characteristics and clinical outcome. *Eur J Echocardiogr* Apr 15 2006 [epub ahead of print].

44. Singh S, Wann LS, Schuchard GH, et al: Right ventricular and right atrial collapse in patients with cardiac tamponade—a combined echocardiographic and hemodynamic study. *Circulation* 70:966-971, 1984.

45. Rifkin R, Isner J, Carter B, Bankoff M: Combined posteroanterior subepicardial fat simulating the echocardiographic diagnosis of pericardial effusion. *J Am Coll Cardiol* 3:1333-1339, 1984.

46. Wada T, Honda M, Matsuyama S: Extra echo spaces: ultrasonography and computerized tomography correlations. *Br Heart J* 47:430-438, 1982.

47. Savage D, Garrison R, Brand F, et al: Prevalence and correlates of posterior extra echocardiographic spaces in a free-living population based sample (the Framingham study). *Am J Cardiol* 51:1207-1212, 1983.

48. Lopez-Sendon J, Garcia-Fernandez M, Coma-Canella I, et al: Identification of blood in the pericardial cavity in dogs by two-dimensional echocardiography. *Am J Cardiol* 53:1194-1197, 1984.

49. Reddy P, Curtiss E, O'Toole J, Shaver J: Cardiac tamponade: Hemodynamic observations in man. *Circulation* 58:265-272, 1978.

50. Kronzon I, Cohen ML, Winer HE: Cardiac tamponade by loculated pericardial hematoma: Limitations of M-mode echocardiography. *J Am Coll Cardiol* 1:913-915, 1983.

51. Duvernoy O, Larsson S, Persson K, et al: Pericardial effusion and pericardial compartments after open heart surgery. An analysis by computed tomography and echocardiography. *Acta Radiol* 31:41-46, 1990.

52. Chuttani K, Tischler M, Pandian N, et al: Diagnosis of cardiac tamponade after cardiac surgery: Relative value of clinical, echocardiographic, and hemodynamic signs. *Am Heart J* 127 (4 Pt 1):913-918, 1994.

53. Leimgruber PP, Klopfenstein HS, Wann LS, Brooks HL: The hemodynamic derangement associated with right ventricular diastolic collapse in cardiac tamponade: An experimental echocardiographic study. *Circulation* 68:612-620, 1983.

54. Gaffney F, Keller A, Peshock R, et al: Pathophysiologic mechanisms of cardiac tamponade and pulsus alternans shown by echocardiography. *Am J Cardiol* 53:1662-1666, 1984.

55. Cogswell TL, Bernath GA, Wann LS, et al: Effects of intravascular volume state on the value of pulsus paradoxus and right ventricular diastolic collapse in predicting cardiac tamponade. *Circulation* 72:1076-1080, 1985.

56. Klopfenstein HS, Cogswell TL, Bernath GA, et al: Alterations in intravascular volume affect the relation between right ventricular diastolic collapse and the hemodynamic severity of cardiac tamponade. *J Am Coll Cardiol* 6:1057-1063, 1985.

57. Cogswell TL, Bernath GA, Keelan MH Jr, et al: The shift in the relationship between intrapericardial fluid pressure and volume induced by acute left ventricular pressure overload during cardiac tamponade. *Circulation* 74:173-180, 1986.

58. Kaplan L, Epstein S, Schwartz S, et al: Clinical, echocardiographic, and hemodynamic evidence of cardiac tamponade caused by large pleural effusions. *Am J Respir Crit Care Med* 151(3 Pt 1):904-908, 1995.

59. Kronzon I, Cohen ML, Winer HE: Diastolic atrial compression: A sensitive echocardiographic sign of cardiac tamponade. *J Am Coll Cardiol* 2:770-775, 1983.

60. Gillam L, Guyer D, Gibson T, et al: Hydrodynamic compression of the right atrium: A new echocardiographic sign of cardiac tamponade. *Circulation* 68:294-301, 1983.

61. D'Cruz I, Cohen H, Prabhu R, Glick G: Diagnosis of cardiac tamponade by echocardiography: Changes in mitral valve motion and ventricular dimensions, with special reference to paradoxical pulse. *Circulation* 52:460-465, 1975.

62. Vignola P, Pohost G, Curfman G, Myers G: Correlation of echocardiographic and clinical findings in patients with pericardial effusion. *Am J Cardiol* 37:701-707, 1976.

63. Settle H, Adolph R, Fowler N, et al: Echocardiographic study of cardiac tamponade. *Circulation* 56:951-959, 1977.

64. Sharp J, Bunnell I, Holland J, et al: Hemodynamics during induced cardiac tamponade in man. *Am J Med* 29:640-646, 1960.

65. Appleton C, Hatle L, Popp R: Cardiac tamponade and pericardial effusion: Respiratory variation in transvalvular flow velocities studied by Doppler echocardiography. *J Am Coll Cardiol* 11:1020-1030, 1988.

66. Gonzalez M, Basnight M, Appleton C: Experimental pericardial effusion: Relation of abnormal respiratory variation in mitral flow velocity to hemodynamics and diastolic right heart collapse. *J Am Coll Cardiol* 17:239-248, 1991.

67. Picard M, Sanfilippo A, Newell J, et al: Quantitative relation between increased intrapericardial pressure and Doppler flow velocities during experimental cardiac tamponade. *J Am Coll Cardiol* 18:234-242, 1991.

68. Nishimura R, Housmans P, Hatle L, Tajik A: Assessment of diastolic function of the heart: background and current applications of Doppler echocardiography. Part I. Physiologic and pathophysiologic features. *Mayo Clin Proc* 64:71-81, 1989.

69. D'Cruz I, Hoffman P: A new cross sectional echocardiographic method for estimating the volume of large pericardial effusions. *Br Heart J* 66:448-451, 1991.

70. Vazquez dPJ, Jiang L, Handschumacher M, et al: Quantification of pericardial effusions by three-dimensional echocardiography. *J Am Coll Cardiol* 24:254-259, 1994.

71. Chuttani K, Pandian N, Mohanty P, et al: Left ventricular diastolic collapse. An echocardiographic sign of regional cardiac tamponade. *Circulation* 83:1999-2006, 1991.

72. Kochar G, Jacobs L, Kotler M: Right atrial compression in postoperative cardiac patients: detection by transesophageal echocardiography. *J Am Coll Cardiol* 16:511-516, 1990.

73. Jadhav P, Asirvatham S, Craven P, et al: Unusual presentation of late regional cardiac tamponade after aortic surgery. *Am J Card Imaging* 10:204-206, 1996.

74. Brooker R, Farah M: Postoperative left atrial compression diagnosed by transesophageal echocardiography. *J Cardiothorac Vasc Anesth* 9:304-307, 1995.

75. Krikorian J, Hancock E: Pericardiocentesis. *Am J Med* 65:808-814, 1978.

76. Callahan J, Seward J, Nishimura R, et al: Two-dimensional echocardiographically guided pericardiocentesis: experience in 117 consecutive patients. *Am J Cardiol* 55:476-479, 1985.

77. Tsang T, Freeman W, Barnes M, et al: Rescue echocardiographically guided pericardiocentesis for cardiac perforation complicating catheter-based procedures. The Mayo Clinic experience. *J Am Coll Cardiol* 32:1345-1350, 1998.

78. Salem K, Mulji A, Lonn E: Echocardiographically guided pericardiocentesis—the gold standard for the management of pericardial effusion and cardiac tamponade. *Can J Cardiol* 15:1251-1255, 1999.

79. Pandian N, Brockway B, Simonetti J, et al: Pericardiocentesis under two-dimensional echocardiographic guidance in loculated pericardial effusion. *Ann Thorac Surg* 45:99-100, 1988.

80. Tsang T, Freeman W, Sinak L, Seward J: Echocardiographically guided pericardiocentesis: Evolution and state-of-the-art technique. *Mayo Clin Proc* 73:647-652, 1998.

81. Mueller X, Tevaearai H, Hurni M, et al: Etiologic diagnosis of pericardial disease: The value of routine tests during surgical procedures. *J Am Coll Surg* 184:645-649, 1997.

82. Koh K, In H, Lee K, et al: New scoring system using tumor markers in diagnosing patients with moderate pericardial effusions. *Int J Cardiol* 61:5-13, 1997.

83. Edwards N: The diagnostic value of pericardial fluid pH determination. *J Am Anim Hosp Assoc* 32:63-67, 1996.

84. Ziskind A, Rodriguez S, Lemmon C, Burstein S: Percutaneous pericardial biopsy as an adjunctive technique for the diagnosis of pericardial disease. *Am J Cardiol* 74:288-291, 1994.

85. Uthaman B, Endrys J, Abushaban L, et al: Percutaneous pericardial biopsy: Technique, efficacy, safety, and value in the management of pericardial effusion in children and adolescents. *Pediatr Cardiol* 18:414-418, 1997.

86. Kouvaras G, Polydorou A, Hatziantoniou G: Percutaneous balloon pericardiotomy for management of cardiac tamponade in a patient with lung cancer and large pericardial effusion. *Acta Cardiol* 49:549-553, 1994.

87. Iaffaldano RA, Jones P, Lewis BE, et al: Percutaneous balloon pericardiotomy: A double-balloon technique. *Cathet Cardiovasc Diagn* 36:79-81, 1995.

88. Law DA, Haque R, Jain A: Percutaneous balloon pericardiotomy: Non-surgical treatment for patients with cardiac tamponade. *W V Med J* 93:310-312, 1997.

89. Girardi L, Ginsberg R, Burt M: Pericardiocentesis and intrapericardial sclerosis: Effective therapy for malignant pericardial effusions. *Ann Thorac Surg* 64:1422-1427; discussion 1427-1428, 1997.

90. Hanaki Y, Kamiya H, Todoroki H, et al: New two-dimensional, echocardiographically directed pericardiocentesis in cardiac tamponade. *Crit Care Med* 18:750-753, 1990.

91. Oh J, Hatle L, Mulvagh S, Tajik A: Transient constrictive pericarditis: Diagnosis by two-dimensional Doppler echocardiography. *Mayo Clin Proc* 68:1158-1164, 1993.

92. Haley J, Tajik A, Danielson G, et al: Transient constrictive pericarditis: Causes and natural history. *J Am Coll Cardiol* 43:271-275, 2004.

93. Millaire A, de GP, Decoulx E, et al: Outcome after thrombolytic therapy of nine cases of myopericarditis misdiagnosed as myocardial infarction. *Eur Heart J* 16:333-338, 1995.

94. Hancock E: Subacute effusive-constrictive pericarditis. *Circulation* 43:183-192, 1971.

95. Sagrista-Sauleda J, Angel J, Sanchez A, et al: Effusive-constrictive pericarditis. *N Engl J Med* 350:469-475, 2004.

96. Sagrista-Sauleda J, Angel J, Permanyer-Miralda G, Soler-Soler J: Long-term follow-up of idiopathic chronic pericardial effusion. *N Engl J Med* 341:2054-2059, 1999.

97. Maisch B, Seferovic P, Ristic A, et al: Guidelines on the diagnosis and management of pericardial diseases executive summary; The Task force on the diagnosis and management of pericardial diseases of the European society of cardiology. *Eur Heart J* 25:587-610, 2004.

98. Connolly H, Click R, Schattenberg T, et al: Congenital absence of the pericardium: echocardiography as a diagnostic tool. *J Am Soc Echocardiogr* 8:87-92, 1995.

99. Amiri A, Weber C, Schlosser V, Meinertz T: Coronary artery disease in a patient with a congenital pericardial defect. *Thorac Cardiovasc Surg* 37:379-381, 1989.

100. Rees A, Risher W, McFadden P, et al: Partial congenital defect of the left pericardium: Angiographic diagnosis and treatment by thoracoscopic pericardiectomy: case report. *Cathet Cardiovasc Diagn* 28:231-234, 1993.

101. Larsen R, Behar V, Brazer S, et al: Chest pain presenting as ischemic heart disease. Congenital absence of the pericardium. *N C Med J* 55:306-308, 1994.

102. Saito R, Hotta F: Congenital pericardial defect associated with cardiac incarceration: Case report. *Am Heart J* 100(6 Pt 1):866-870, 1980.

103. Vanderheyden M, De SJ, Nellens P, et al: Herniation of the left atrial appendage due to partial congenital absence of the left pericardium. *Acta Clin Belg* 51:91-93, 1996.

104. Finet G, Bozio A, Frieh J, et al: Herniation of the left atrial appendage through a congenital partial pericardial defect. *Eur Heart J* 12:1148-1149, 1991.

105. Hoorntje J, Mooyaart E, Meuzelaar K: Left atrial herniation through a partial pericardial defect: a rare cause of syncope. *Pacing Clin Electrophysiol* 12:1841-1845, 1989.

106. Reginao E, Speroni F, Riccardi M, et al: Post-traumatic mitral regurgitation and ventricular septal defect in absence of left pericardium. *Thorac Cardiovasc Surg* 28:213-217, 1980.

107. Tosson R, Korbmacher B, Schulte H: Combined congenital pericardial and diaphragmatic defects: A case report. *Cardiovasc Surg* 4:57-59, 1996.

108. Croisille P, Revel D: Magnetic resonance imaging of cardiac and pericardial disease. *J Belge Radiol* 80:133-136, 1997.

109. Gassner I, Judmaier W, Fink C, et al: Diagnosis of congenital pericardial defects, including a pathognomic sign for dangerous apical ventricular herniation, on magnetic resonance imaging. *Br Heart J* 74:60-66, 1995.

110. Lewis K, Sherer D, Goncalves L, et al: Mid-trimester prenatal sonographic diagnosis of a pericardial cyst. *Prenat Diagn* 16:549-553, 1996.

111. Chopra P, Duke D, Pellett J, Rahko P: Pericardial cyst with partial erosion of the right ventricular wall. *Ann Thorac Surg* 51:840-841, 1991.

112. Williamson B, Spotnitz W, Gay S, Parekh S: Pericardial cyst. A rare mass abutting the aorta. *J Comput Tomogr* 12:264-266, 1988.

113. Gurlek A, Dagalp Z, Ozyurda U: A case of multiple pericardial hydatid cysts. *Int J Cardiol* 36:366-368, 1992.

114. Landolphi D, Belkin R, Hjemdahl-Monsen C, La FR: Cardiac cavernous hemangioma mimicking pericardial cyst: Atypical echocardiographic appearance of a rare cardiac tumor. *J Am Soc Echocardiogr* 10:579-581, 1997.

115. Bandeira F, De SV, Moriguti J, et al: Cardiac tamponade: An unusual complication of pericardial cyst. *J Am Soc Echocardiogr* 9:108-112, 1996.

116. Bava G, Magliani L, Bertoli D, et al: Complicated pericardial cyst: Atypical anatomy and clinical course. *Clin Cardiol* 21:862-864, 1998.

117. Borges A, Gellert K, Dietel M, et al: Acute right-sided heart failure due to hemorrhage into a pericardial cyst [see comments]. *Ann Thorac Surg* 63:845-847, 1997.

118. Mastroroberto P, Chello M, Bevacqua E, Marchese A: Pericardial cyst with partial erosion of the superior vena cava. An unusual case. *J Cardiovasc Surg (Torino)* 37:323-324, 1996.

119. Pezzano A, Belloni A, Faletra F, et al: Value of two-dimensional echocardiography in the diagnosis of pericardial cysts. *Eur Heart J* 4:238-246, 1983.

120. Bini R, Nath P, Ceballos R, et al: Pericardial cyst diagnosed by two-dimensional echocardiography and computed tomography in a newborn. *Pediatr Cardiol* 8:47-50, 1987.

121. Padder F, Conrad A, Manzar K, et al: Echocardiographic diagnosis of pericardial cyst. *Am J Med Sci* 313:191-192, 1997.

122. Ferguson M: Thoracoscopic management of pericardial disease. *Semin Thorac Cardiovasc Surg* 5:310-315, 1993.

123. Kinoshita Y, Shimada T, Murakami Y, et al: Ethanol sclerosis can be a safe and useful treatment for pericardial cyst. *Clin Cardiol* 19:833-835, 1996.

124. Rice T: Benign neoplasms and cysts of the mediastinum. *Semin Thorac Cardiovasc Surg* 4:25-33, 1992.

125. Armstrong WF, Schilt BF, Helper DJ, et al: Diastolic collapse of the right ventricle with cardiac tamponade: an echocardiographic study. *Circulation* 65:1491-1496, 1982.

126. Engel PJ, Hon H, Fowler NO, Plummer S: Echocardiographic study of right ventricular wall motion in cardiac tamponade. *Am J Cardiol* 50:1018-1021, 1982.

127. Pandian N, Wang S, McInerney K, et al: Doppler echocardiography in cardiac tamponade: Abnormalities in tricuspid and mitral inflow responce to respiration in experimental and clinical tamponade. *J Am Coll Cardiol* 5:485, 1985.

128. Leeman D, Riley M, Carl L, Come P: Doppler echocardiography in cardiac tamponade: A exaggerated respiratory variation in transvalvular blood flow velocity integrals. *J Am Coll Cardiol* 9:17A, 1987.

Chapter 31

End-Stage Heart Failure: Ventricular Assist Devices and the Posttransplant Patient

AUDREY H. WU, MD, MPH

Background

Improving medical management and advances in surgical techniques have increased the numbers of patients surviving with severe heart failure (HF). Cardiac transplantation remains the treatment of choice for end-stage HF. More than 3000 cardiac transplants are performed worldwide annually. At the time of transplantation, roughly half of cardiac transplant recipients are treated with inotropic agents, whereas almost one quarter require some form of mechanical circulatory support, primarily in the form of a left ventricular assist device (LVAD); these are significant increases compared to the patient population only 5 years ago, when 34% were on inotropic support and 15% were on mechanical support (11% on LVAD support). Mortality rate is greatest in the first 6 months following transplantation, with 1-year survival after cardiac transplantation being about 83%. Survival has steadily improved since the early 1980s, despite the increasingly high-risk profile of the recipient population. Graft failure accounts for a significant proportion of deaths in the first year following transplantation, whereas after five years, allograft vasculopathy (transplant coronary disease) and late graft failure (likely a result of allograft vasculopathy) together account for one third of deaths.[1]

However given the scarcity of suitable donor organs, many patients die while awaiting transplantation. In addition, a significant proportion of patients with end-stage HF cannot be listed for cardiac transplantation resulting from contraindications such as age or concurrent severe noncardiac medical condition. Implantation of a LVAD is increasingly used to treat patients with severe HF, primarily as a bridge to cardiac transplantation but also as long-term definitive therapy ("destination therapy") or in a small proportion of patients as a bridge to recovery of myocardial function. Survival during mechanical device support has been reported to be 83% at 1 month and 50% at 1 year.[2]

For the cardiac transplant recipient, echocardiography is a valuable tool in assisting surveillance for allograft rejection and transplant vasculopathy. For the patient with a LVAD, echocardiography assists in monitoring native cardiac function, device function, and troubleshooting device problems.

Normal Structure and Function of the Transplanted Heart

Transplant Technique and Atrial Structure and Function

With the traditional biatrial technique for cardiac transplantation, bilateral atrial cuffs from the recipient are retained for direct anastomosis of the cardiac allograft to recipient atrial cuffs. Although providing some operative technical advantages, this approach resulted in large atrial cavities with long suture lines, which resulted in abnormal atrial geometry and function, which in turn have been implicated as contributors to mitral and tricuspid valve abnormalities and atrial thrombus formation.[3] The bicaval technique, using separate caval and pulmonary vein anastomoses, was developed to circumvent these problems.

This technique did not become popular until the late 1980s and is currently the most widely employed technique.[4] In two different series comparing patients transplanted with biatrial versus bicaval techniques, half of biatrial-technique patients had spontaneous echocardiographic contrast present, up to one quarter had atrial thrombi present by echocardiography, and roughly 15% had systemic embolism (including stroke, mesenteric ischemia, and lower limb ischemia), whereas none of the patients transplanted with the bicaval technique demonstrated spontaneous echocardiographic contrast or atrial thrombi, and none experienced a systemic embolic event.[5,6] In one series, left atrial diameter averaged 58±6 versus 42±4 mm ($p = 0.0006$) for biatrial versus bicaval techniques, respectively.[5] In addition to more normal atrial size and geometry, the bicaval technique results in more physiologic atrial function. Both atrial transport (ratio of late diastolic to total diastolic transmitral flow velocity integrals) and atrial ejection force (0.5 × ρ [density of blood or 1.06 g/cm^3] × mitral orifice area × peak A velocity squared)[7] are significantly higher in patients who underwent cardiac transplantation using the bicaval technique versus those who were transplanted using the biatrial technique and have been found to be comparable to that of normal controls.[8] Although the contribution of atrial function to overall cardiac function is likely trivial during normal allograft functioning, more physiologic atrial function may support better cardiac function in the setting of ventricular dysfunction, such as during acute rejection.

The remainder of this chapter will assume use of the bicaval technique (Figs. 31–1 and 31–2).

Physiology of the Cardiac Allograft

Although cardiac transplantation confers improved survival, functional capacity, and quality of life on patients with end-stage HF, physiology of the transplanted heart is not normal. Hemodynamics are abnormal immediately after cardiac transplantation and are characterized by elevated filling pressures associated with impaired relaxation. This hemodynamic profile improves over the initial few weeks to months after transplantation, may continue to normalize over years but may also persist to a subtle degree.[9,10] Restrictive physiology early after transplantation may be the result of a combination of ischemic myocardial injury, recipient pulmonary hypertension, and volume overload, whereas persistent restrictive physiology may be attributed to donor-recipient size mismatch, ischemic fibrosis, or increased afterload as a result of systemic hypertension. Because it is denervated, the cardiac allograft has an altered response to exercise, characterized by a slower early rise in heart rate (HR) and an overall blunted chronotropic response, with increases in car-

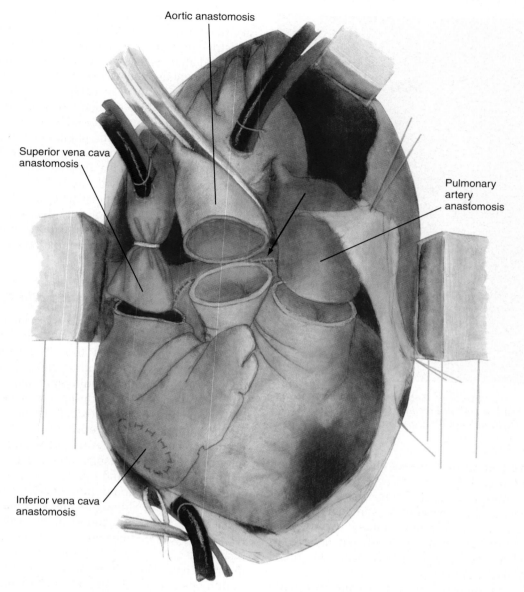

Aortic anastomosis

Superior vena cava
anastomosis

Pulmonary
artery
anastomosis

Inferior vena cava
anastomosis

Figure 31–1. Nearly completed heart transplant (bicaval technique), showing allograft-recipient anastomoses.

diac output (CO) primarily the result of increases in stroke volume (SV) rather than heart rate.[11]

Ventricular Systolic and Diastolic Function

Early after transplantation, left ventricular (LV) mass and end-diastolic volume (EDV) increase, and these changes may or may not persist for years, without adverse consequences to systolic function.[12,13] In the absence of complications causing graft dysfunction, allograft ventricular systolic function generally remains normal for many years. One long-term observational study of a cohort of 65 cardiac transplant recipients demonstrated normal mean ejection fraction (EF) of 62.8±7.3% and fractional shortening of 35.4±10.3%

as long as 10 to 15 years after transplantation. This series also found left ventricular hypertrophy (LVH) as a common finding particularly late after transplantation, with calculated LV mass in males of 263.8±111.4 g and in females of 373.0±181.1 g.[14]

Although systolic ventricular function remains largely normal, diastolic function is abnormal early after transplantation, the effects of which are frequently compounded by postoperative volume overload. A restrictive filling pattern may persist to some degree chronically in some patients, or reemerge during episodes of acute rejection. Early after transplantation, a restrictive filling pattern is observed, characterized by shorter isovolumic relaxation time (IVRT; 65±18 msec) and pressure half-time (PHT; 39±8 msec), and higher early diastolic filling velocity (E; 0.77±0.20 m/s), with gradual evolution to a

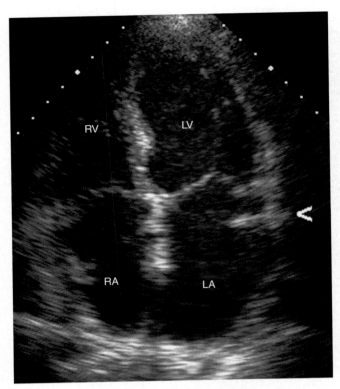

Figure 31–2. Appearance of biatrial technique heart transplant. Arrowhead, atrial suture line; LA, left atrium; LV, left ventricle; RA, right atrium; RV, right ventricle.

nonrestrictive pattern by 6 weeks after transplantation (IVRT 95 ± 17 msec, PHT 48 ± 11 msec, E 0.63 ± 0.12 m/s) in one series. Various clinical factors, such as preoperative pulmonary systolic pressures or pulmonary vascular resistance, duration of cardiopulmonary bypass, total ischemia time, or age of donor heart, did not significantly correlate with parameters of restrictive filling early after transplantation.[15]

Diastolic abnormalities persist beyond the early postoperative period in a small proportion of patients. In a series of 64 cardiac transplant recipients 1 year or more posttransplant (mean 5 years, range 1 to 13 years posttransplant) undergoing routine annual hemodynamic evaluation, 10 (15%) demonstrated a pattern of right ventricular (RV) and LV filling consistent with restrictive-constrictive physiology, with a characteristic dip-and-plateau hemodynamic tracing in early diastole. In general, transplant recipients with constrictive-restrictive hemodynamics had higher right-sided and left-sided filling pressures, shorter LV IVRTs and PHTs and higher M_1:M_2 (early:peak mitral flow velocity) and T_1:T_2 (early:peak tricuspid valve flow velocity). Transplant recipients with constrictive-restrictive physiology had significantly more previous rejection episodes and a greater proportion had HF symptoms. Five of the ten patients with constrictive-restrictive physiology had acute rejection diagnosed at the time of the biopsy per-

formed concurrent with echocardiography, whereas all six diagnoses of rejection occurred in patients with constrictive-restrictive physiology.[16] It has also been observed that persistence of restrictive filling pattern (in one study defined as 15% decrease in IVRT or PHT or 20% increase in peak early mitral inflow velocity) up to 6 months after cardiac transplantation is associated with significantly reduced actuarial survival. Patients with greater than the population mean of studies showing diastolic dysfunction in the first 6 months after transplantation had a 70% 3-year survival versus 92% for the group with less than the population mean.[17] The etiology of persistent diastolic dysfunction after transplantation is not fully defined but likely includes cumulative immune-mediated injury, fibrosis related to immune or nonimmune damage, and transplant vasculopathy (Fig. 31–3).

Right Ventricular Structure and Function

Several factors uniquely impact RV structure and function in the transplant patient. A significant proportion of patients with severe HF have pulmonary hypertension as a result of longstanding elevated left-sided filling pressures. Significant pulmonary hypertension is in fact a contraindication to cardiac transplantation given the risk of fulminant right-sided HF in the cardiac allograft. Pulmonary hypertension generally improves to normal or near-normal levels in the weeks to months following cardiac transplantation. The evolution of right-sided structure and function after transplantation parallels the resolution of pulmonary hypertension and volume overload, although some RV enlargement may persist long term. In a cohort of 24 cardiac transplant recipients, RV enlargement was present on echocardiography immediately postoperatively (RV end-diastolic diameter 3.29 ± 0.45 cm), increased up to 1 month postoperatively and returned to immediate postoperative levels by 1 year. All patients initially demonstrated end-diastolic flattening of the interventricular septum, a pattern consistent with RV volume and pressure overload that persisted in less than half of patients 1 year after transplantation.[18] Although one series found tricuspid regurgitation (TR) of varying degrees present in over 60% of transplant recipients in the postoperative period and roughly one third in the same group of patients 1 year after transplant,[18] the incidence of right-sided heart abnormalities and TR appear to increase during longer term follow up.[14] Among patients 10 to 15 years after transplantation, many demonstrate right atrial and RV enlargement (right atrium 40.7 ± 11.8 mm, right ventricle 37.4 ± 8.3 mm in one series) and a significant proportion (70% in one series) have at least mild TR.[14] Despite the abnormalities in right-sided heart size and function, clinical signs and symptoms of HF are generally absent.[14]

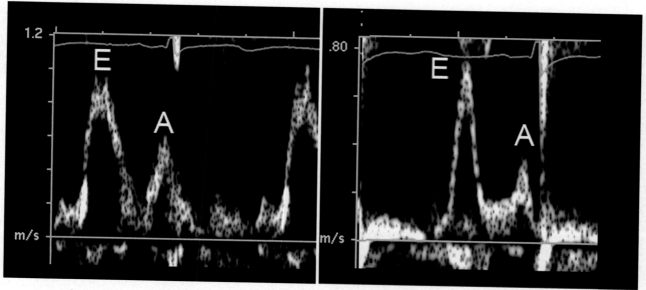

Figure 31–3. Mitral valve inflow velocities showing a normal E/A ratio and normal deceleration slope with normal diastolic function (A) compared to a pattern of "restrictive" filling with an increased E velocity with a steep deceleration slope and a reduced a velocity (B). A, late transmitral flow velocity; E, early transmitral flow velocity.

Severity of TR—likely a marker of RV dysfunction—noted on intraoperative transesophageal echocardiogram (TEE) appears to correlate with poor late survival. In one series of 181 patients, 20% of donor hearts at the time of transplantation had at least mild TR, which correlated strongly with presence of RV dysfunction, as defined by RV free wall hypokinesis and dilatation. Five-year survival in this series was 85% for patients with mild or no intraoperative TR, versus 57% for those with mild to severe TR.[19] It has not been established whether prophylactic donor tricuspid valve annuloplasty would improve long-term survival.

Structure and Function of the Transplanted Heart during Acute Rejection

Changes in Systolic and Diastolic Function

Allograft rejection remains a significant limitation of cardiac transplantation. Acute cardiac allograft rejection is usually characterized by lymphocytic infiltration with or without myocyte necrosis, termed *cellular rejection*.[20] A rarer, less well-understood type of rejection, termed *vascular rejection*, involves endothelial cell activation and complement deposition primarily involving the allograft vasculature.[21] Echocardiographic abnormalities of the cardiac allograft during rejection may include changes in systolic and diastolic function and increases in LV wall thickness or mass. Currently, the

gold standard for diagnosing rejection is by endomyocardial biopsy, although this technique is limited by the risks inherent to an invasive procedure and by sampling error. An ideal method to screen for rejection would be noninvasive and simple to perform; thus echocardiography has been frequently studied as a tool to evaluate for rejection.

Although gross systolic dysfunction is relatively easy to detect by echocardiography, only a small fraction of rejection episodes manifest with a decline in EF. New onset systolic dysfunction in the setting of acute rejection is generally a late finding and indicates higher-grade rejection, which is associated with hemodynamic compromise and clinical symptoms. The vast majority of rejection episodes are not associated with systolic impairment, and significant changes in systolic function parameters, such as peak aortic velocity, ejection time, and end-systolic volume during acute rejection, are generally lacking. Abnormalities of diastolic filling are the earliest alterations to manifest in acute rejection.[22,23] Rejection of increasing severity has been associated with a progressive shortening of IVRT and PHT and with an increase in peak early mitral flow velocity (M_1), although the latter has not been a consistent finding.[22-24] One study found that with a cutoff of 20% decrease in PHT as indicative of acute rejection, with sensitivity and specificity approaching 90%.[24] Measures of diastolic dysfunction generally return to baseline values after treatment of acute rejection with immunosuppression.[24]

Defined as the sum of isovolumic contraction time (IVCT) and IVRT divided by ejection time, the myocar-

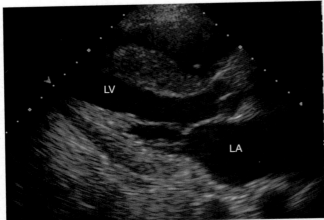

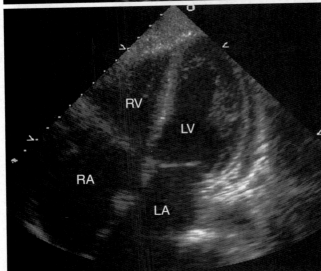

Figure 31–4. Increase in ventricular wall thickness in the setting of vascular rejection seen in a parasternal long-axis view (A) and apical four-chamber view (B). This 27-year-old woman was 1 year status post–cardiac transplantation for peripartum cardiomyopathy with interval development of significant left ventricular wall thickness and new diagnosis of hemodynamically significant vascular rejection confirmed with immunofluorescence examination of endomyocardial biopsy. LA, left atrium; LV, left ventricle; RA, right atrium; RV, right ventricle.

dial performance index is a single composite measurement of systolic and diastolic myocardial function.[25] Myocardial performance index is not affected by alterations in heart rate, systemic blood pressure, preload or afterload.[26] Until recently, cardiac rejection was graded on biopsy as 0, 1A, 1B, 2, 3A, 3B (now simplified to 0, 1, 2, 3, 4 scale) in order of increasing severity of rejection. In one series of 24 patients, myocardial performance index was significantly higher for 1B rejection (0.75±0.20 verus 0.60±0.13 for no rejection, grade 0). Using a cutoff value of 0.69 had a modest sensitivity and specificity of 67% to discriminate between no and mild rejection.[27] However another group found no significant utility in using myocardial performance index

to diagnose acute rejection. Concurrent decreases in IVRT and increases in isovolumic contraction time, indicating development of abnormalities in diastolic and systolic function, respectively, with acute rejection resulted in an overall neutral effect on the myocardial performance index.[28]

Changes in Left Ventricular Mass or Wall Thickness

Although older reports have suggested LV mass increases in the setting of acute cellular rejection,[29] this has not been a consistent finding[30] and change in LV wall thickness alone has not proven to be a sensitive enough marker to diagnose cellular rejection.[31] Increased LV mass in the setting of rejection may be the result of increased interstitial edema or vascular leakage of fibrin.[32] Significant increase in LV mass has been described during episodes of vascular rejection. In a series of 41 cardiac transplant patients, LV mass increased from a baseline of 109±17 g to 151±17 g during vascular rejection ($N = 14$), although it did not significantly change during cellular rejection (95±7 g versus 104±7 g). Concurrently LV wall thickness increased by nearly 20% during vascular rejection (1.3±0.1 cm at baseline versus 1.6±0.1 cm)[33] (Fig. 31–4).

Tissue Doppler

Traditional Doppler-derived parameters of diastolic function, such as transmitral Doppler flow analysis, is influenced by variables other than ventricular diastolic function, such as ventricular loading conditions, and in transplant patients specifically, the cardiac allograft may develop baseline diastolic filling abnormalities unrelated to acute rejection.[16] Tissue Doppler imaging (TDI) is a technique for assessing LV diastolic function, involving measurements of tissue contraction and relaxation velocities. Although early (E_M) and late (A_M) diastolic mitral annular motion velocity have been found to be significantly decreased in cardiac transplant patients experiencing acute severe rejection (grade 3A or higher), receiver operator curve (ROC) analysis identifying an ideal cutoff of A_{DTI} less than 8.7 cm/s demonstrated a sensitivity of 82% and a poor specificity of 53% for detecting severe rejection.[34] However specificity is not significantly improved when both systolic and diastolic tissue Doppler parameters are used. The combined peak systolic and peak diastolic velocity (peak-to-peak amplitude) of the tissue Doppler mitral annular waveforms was significantly lower in patients experiencing any rejection (grade 1B or greater). ROC analysis showed high sensitivity and negative predictive value but a relatively modest specificity.[35] Although it appears that tissue Doppler measurements are sensitive for detecting various degrees of acute rejection and for excluding rejection if measurements fall below ROC determined cutoffs, they do not appear to be robust tools in differentiating impaired contraction or relaxation resulting from acute rejection rather than other causes. This poor specificity reflects confounding by the background diastolic filling abnormalities inherent to transplant physiology, which makes detection of early diastolic dysfunction as a result of acute rejection difficult.

Echocardiographic Guidance for Endomyocardial Biopsy

Endomyocardial biopsy remains the gold standard for diagnosing allograft rejection and following response to immunosuppressive treatment for rejection. The usual approach for introduction of the biopsy catheter is via the right internal jugular vein or less frequently, the left internal jugular vein or right femoral vein. Traditionally, fluoroscopy has been employed to guide the biopsy catheter tip to the intraventricular septum to obtain biopsies. This technique does have a number of drawbacks, including radiation exposure to the operator and patient and limited portability. Echocardiography has been successfully used to guide endomyocardial biopsies with the added benefits of lack of radiation exposure, portability, and provision of information on cardiac structure and function. Complication rates using echocardiography for biopsies are extremely low and comparable to that for fluoroscopic guided biopsies (<0.5% of all biopsies attempts).[36,37] The development of severe TR in the cardiac allograft, sometimes requiring surgical tricuspid valve repair or replacement, is correlated with the total number of biopsies performed, presumably as a result of inadvertent damage to the tricuspid valve apparatus by the biopsy catheter as it passes into the right ventricle.[38] Although measures, such as use of a long sheath to introduce the bioptome directly into the right ventricle, lessen the risk of developing TR, it has not been definitively established whether the routine use of echocardiography to guide biopsies would lessen this risk.

Pericardial Effusion

Although pericardial effusion occurs frequently after cardiac surgery, the significance and natural history of pericardial effusion after cardiac transplantation is not well defined. Early, postoperative effusions likely carry different clinical implications than effusions occurring or persisting late beyond the immediate postoperative period. One single center series of 241 patients undergoing orthotopic cardiac transplantation found 21% developed significant pericardial effusions in the postoperative period, although hospital length of stay and long-term survival were not associated with presence

or absence of effusion.[39] In another series of 203 patients, 9% developed moderate-sized to large-sized pericardial effusions, with slightly less than half requiring pericardiocentesis, and of those, roughly one third ultimately requiring pericardiectomy. There was no significant correlation between presence of effusion and occurrence of rejection.[40] Pericardial effusion occurring more than 1 month after transplantation carries less favorable implications. One series found a significant correlation between late pericardial effusion and number and severity of acute rejection episodes.[41] Increase in effusion size may be associated with acute rejection.[42] Pericardial fluid is usually sterile, although given these patients' altered immunity, infection should generally be considered as a possible cause.[42]

Transplant Vasculopathy

Pathophysiology and Natural History

Transplant or cardiac allograft vasculopathy is an entity distinct from native coronary disease of the nontransplanted heart and is one of the primary factors limiting the long-term functioning and life span of the allograft. Transplant vasculopathy is an accelerated form of intimal hyperplasia, likely resulting from both immune and nonimmune mechanisms. A classic finding is diffuse "pruning" of the smaller distal coronary vasculature, although discrete stenoses characteristic of native coronary disease may develop as well. In addition to transplant-specific, immunologic risk factors, typical risk factors for native coronary disease, such as dyslipidemia and hypertension, also impact the development of cardiac allograft vasculopathy. Distinct from the de novo development of allograft vasculopathy, there is also some component of atherosclerosis already present in the donor allograft, progression of which does not appear to be correlated with development of de novo vasculopathy.[43] In comparison to native coronary atherosclerosis, the time course for development of cardiac allograft vasculopathy is accelerated and accounts for a significant proportion of deaths 5 years after transplantation.[1] Angiographic identification of transplant vasculopathy is associated with a fivefold greater risk of cardiac events, such as myocardial infarction (MI), HF, and sudden death.[44] As a result of cardiac denervation, clinical symptoms from cardiac allograft vasculopathy are frequently late and atypical, if at all. Coronary angiography has proven to be fairly insensitive in detecting cardiac allograft vasculopathy, but with the addition of coronary intravascular ultrasound (IVUS) is sensitive. The current role for echocardiography in cardiac allograft surveillance includes IVUS in conjunction with coronary angiography and imaging in conjunction with stress testing.

Coronary Angiography with Intravascular Ultrasound

Coronary angiography is relatively insensitive in detecting early transplant vasculopathy; up to three quarters of patients with intimal thickening by IVUS have normal coronary angiograms.[45,46] Coronary angiography, which defines the luminal silhouette of the coronary artery, is not able to detect the often diffuse and concentric intimal hyperplasia that characterizes allograft vasculopathy. Because IVUS images vascular wall morphology, it has emerged as the gold standard for detecting transplant vasculopathy, particularly in its early stages. Extent of vasculopathy can be quantified according to intimal thickness and circumferential extent and also by change in measures of plaque burden over time. IVUS findings of allograft vasculopathy can be classified as minimal (intimal thickness <0.3 mm, circumferential involvement <180 degrees), mild (intimal thickness >0.3 mm, circumferential involvement >180 degrees), moderate (intimal thickness 0.3 to 0.5 mm, or intimal thickness >0.5 mm and circumferential involvement <180 degrees), or severe (intimal thickness >1 mm, or intimal thickness >0.5 mm and circumferential involvement >180 degrees).[45] Severity of transplant vasculopathy progresses over time, most notably in the first 2 years after transplantation, whereas calcification of plaques occurs to a significant extent predominately beyond 5 years after transplantation.[47] Early changes by IVUS during the first posttransplant year correlate with long-term prognosis. Changes in the allograft vasculature in the first year after transplantation likely reflect the cumulative result of multiple insults, such as donor explosive brain death, early rejection, and cytomegalovirus infection, which influence the recipient's immune response to the allograft and thus the likelihood of developing vasculopathy.[48,49] Progression of maximal intimal thickening of greater than or equal to 0.5 mm in the first year after transplantation is associated with a significantly higher risk of development of angiographic disease, nonfatal major adverse cardiac events, and death or graft loss in long-term follow up[50,51] (Fig. 31–5).

Dobutamine Stress Echocardiography

Dobutamine stress echocardiography (DSE) has proven to be a valuable tool for detecting cardiac allograft vasculopathy and yielding prognostic information. Using intracoronary IVUS as the gold standard, DSE is highly sensitive and specific in detecting cardiac allograft vasculopathy, defined characteristically in one study as angiographic changes of luminal irregularities with vessel lumen diameter reduction less than 30% or IVUS showing intimal thickness less than 0.3 mm and circumferential extent equal to 180 degrees. Two-dimensional (2D) DSE alone had a 72% sensitivity and 88% specificity, and after combination with M-mode analysis, sensitivity was 85% and specificity was 82%. Compared with tests with abnormal findings, normal findings at rest and even more so with DSE was associated with a lower risk for cardiac events, including myocardial infarction, HF, retransplantation, cardiac death, or interventional revascularization of coronary stenosis. In one series of 117 patients followed over

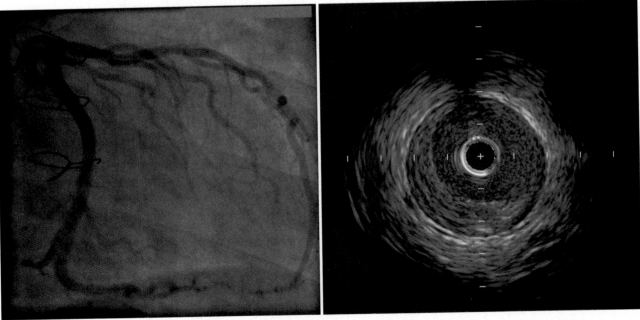

Figure 31–5. The coronary angiogram (A) in this posttransplant patient appears to show no significant narrowing of the lumen. However an intravascular ultrasound image in the mid-left anterior descending coronary (B) shows a significant atherosclerotic plaque.

TABLE 31-1. Example of Routine Surveillance Studies after Cardiac Transplantation in Patient without Complications

Endomyocardial Biopsy

First year—weeks 1-4, 6, 8, 12, 16, 20, 24; months 8, 10, 12
Second year—first 6 months: every 2 to 3 months; second
  6 months: every 3 to 6 months
Third year and indefinitely—every 6 months

Echocardiography

Postoperative and annually

Transplant Vasculopathy

Coronary angiography with intravascular ultrasound at
  1 year
Then alternating noninvasive stress testing with coronary
  angiography with intravascular ultrasound (IVUS)
  annually

Note there is variation in practice between institutions.

3500 patient-months, 4% of those with normal resting studies versus 25% of those with abnormal resting studies experienced a cardiac event, whereas no patient with normal stress study versus 24% of those with abnormal stress studies experienced a cardiac event.[52] Other studies examining patients several years following transplant also confirm the value of DSE in predicting future cardiac events or death[53] (Table 31–1).

Ventricular Assist Devices

Clinical Use and Device Types

The use of LVADs for treatment of end-stage HF, either as a bridge to transplantation or as destination therapy, is becoming more common as patients survive longer with severe HF as a result of advances in medical and device therapy, improving surgical technique, and persistent donor organ shortage. In a small proportion of patients, LVADs are used as a bridge to recovery of cardiac function. In the Randomized Evaluation of Mechanical Assistance for the Treatment of Congestive Heart Failure (REMATCH) trial, implantation of a LVAD significantly improved survival compared to optimal medical management (52% versus 25% at 1 year, 23% versus 8% at 2 years) in a population of patients with end-stage HF who were not candidates for cardiac transplantation but were a severely ill subset of patients with already severe end-stage disease. The majority of morbidity and mortality associated with LVADs stems from device infections and failures.[54] Survival of patients bridged to cardiac transplantation with a LVAD was superior to that of patients bridged with inotropes, both for survival to transplantation and survival after transplan-

tation, despite the early perioperative mortality associated with the LVAD implantation surgery. This survival benefit likely reflects improved knowledge of appropriate selection criteria for device placement and for patients having the opportunity for recovery of end-organ dysfunction and rehabilitation before transplantation.[55]

LVADs can be classified as extracorporeal or intracorporeal devices and as providing pulsatile or axial flow. The advantage of extracorporeal devices include relative ease of implantation, ability to be used for left-sided and/or right-sided support, and ability to be implanted in smaller patients because the pump is extracorporeal. The disadvantages include the necessity for patients to remain in the hospital as a result of the large-bore external vascular cannulae and the large and complex controllers. The pump for intraperitoneal devices is usually implanted preperitoneal. The inflow valve conduit drains the left ventricle at the apex, whereas the outflow valve conduit enters the ascending aorta. Valves in the inflow and outflow conduits are generally bioprosthetic. The advantage of intracorporeal devices is that because the pump mechanism is intracorporeal, the patient is able to move about freely, and in fact, there is an extensive and successful outpatient experience with several types of extracorporeal devices. A few models do not require anticoagulation. Disadvantages include infection risk in models with a percutaneous driveline and minimum body size requirement given the necessity of implanting the pump intracorporeal. Recently, totally implantable pumps have been developed and are currently being evaluated in clinical trials. The newest generation of LVADs includes axial flow pumps, the advantages of which include simpler mechanics, small size, and lack of valves.

Although certain devices are also available for RV circulatory support in the case of RV failure, by far the more common use for ventricular assist devices is for left-sided circulatory support. This chapter exclusively discusses ventricular assist devices as LVADs (Fig. 31–6).

Preoperative and Intraoperative Assessment before and during Left Ventricular Assist Device Implantation

Preexisting anatomic and physiologic abnormalities can potentially lead to complications related to LVAD implantation. A patent foramen ovale (PFO) may result in right-to-left shunting and systemic hypoxia or paradoxical embolus as the LVAD unloads the left ventricle and left-sided filling pressures are markedly reduced.[56] This abnormality can readily be diagnosed on echocardiography with injection of agitated saline as a contrast agent. Aortic atheroma burden is well assessed by transesophageal echocardiography and should be taken into account in the context of anastomosis site for the outflow can-

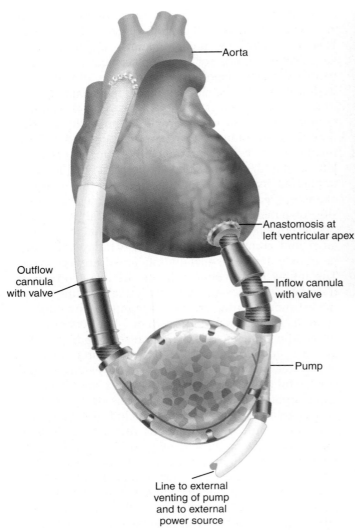

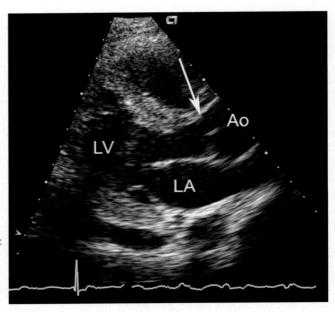

Figure 31-7. Parasternal long-axis view in a 24-year-old woman with acute myocarditis after placement of a left ventricular assist device. The aortic valve remains closed and the mitral valve remains partially open throughout the cardiac cycle. In real time, there is little endocardial motion or wall thickening. Ao, aorta; LA, left atrium; LV left ventricle.

Figure 31-6. Implanted left ventricular assist device (in this example, a Thoratec HM VXE), showing positions of inflow and outflow cannulae. (Redrawn with permission from Thoratec Corporation.)

nula. Aortic valve regurgitation may be worsened after LVAD implantation because of the resultant subphysiologic LV intracardiac pressures. The regurgitant volume increases device preload and inappropriately causes progressively increasing LVAD rates and flows. Prophylactic aortic valve repair or replacement for aortic valve regurgitation severity greater than mild is generally performed. Mitral and TR usually improve after LVAD initiation, resulting from unloading of the left ventricle and generally do not require specific corrective therapy.

Intraoperative transesophageal echocardiography is used to monitor de-airing of the pump before full activation, confirm inlet cannula position, and monitor RV and LV morphology and function. Appropriate LVAD functioning is highly dependent on adequate RV function, which generates adequate filling of the left-sided heart and which in turn ensures adequate device preload. Based on echocardiographic measurements, sys-

tolic RV fractional area change can be calculated, using the formula ([end-diastolic area − end-systolic area]/end-diastolic area) × 100. Although in general, the RV fractional area change of patients with end-stage HF being considered for a LVAD ranges from 20% to 30%, patients with a RV fractional area change less than 20% are at risk for developing acute right-sided HF on LVAD implantation resulting from continued unloading of the left-sided heart with simultaneous insufficient emptying of the right ventricle as a result of inadequate RV function. Finally, the inlet cannula orifice should be central in the apical cavity. If significant angulation of the cannula is present, obstruction can occur[57] (Figs. 31-7, 31-8, and 31-9).

LV thrombus is a known complication of LVADs, but the incidence has significantly declined with improvements in device design, with current estimates ranging about 10% to 15%.[56,58] Intracavitary thrombus may be detected at the LV apex or the left atrium, particularly when the patient has a history of atrial fibrillation (AFib). Although risk of stroke is higher in the setting of a documented intracardiac thrombus, in one series it did not appear to affect likelihood of successful transplantation.[58]

Changes in Cardiac Structure after Left Ventricular Assist Device Implantation

Changes in LV structure and function are apparent soon after implantation of a LVAD as a result of unloading of the left ventricle.

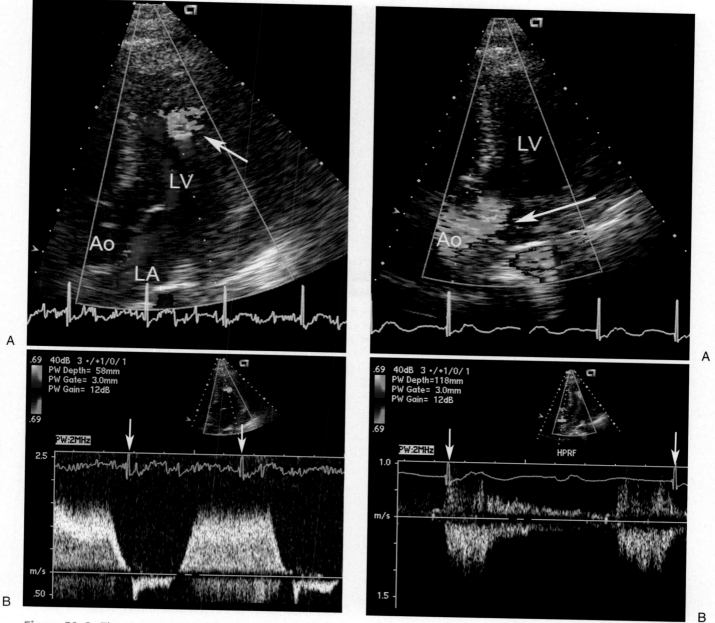

Figure 31–8. *The position of the left ventricular assist device inflow cannula in the left ventricular apex is seen (arrow) using color Doppler (A) from the apical view in the same patient as in Figure 31–7. Pulsed Doppler shows normal low velocity phasic inflow into the assist device but the timing of inflow is related to the pump timing and not to the patient's QRS on the electrocardiogram (B, arrow). Ao, aorta; LA, left atrium; LV, left ventricle.*

Figure 31–9. *The outflow from the left ventricular assist device into the aorta (arrow) is seen from an apical view using color Doppler (A) in the same patient as in Figure 31–7. Pulsed Doppler (B) shows an ejection type velocity curve, however timing of flow is not related to the patient's QRS complex (arrows). Ao, aorta; LV, left ventricle.*

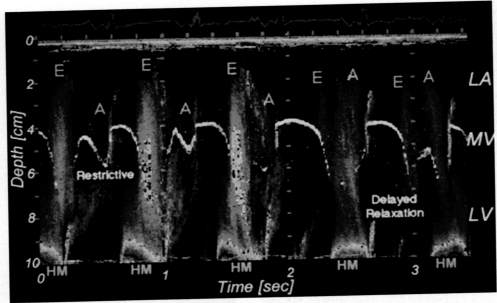

Figure 31–10. Color M-mode echocardiogram showing the spatial (vertical axis, calibration = 1 cm) and temporal (horizontal axis, calibration = 200 ms) distribution of flow from the left atrium (LA) (top) through the mitral valve (MV) (middle) into the left ventricular assist device cannula at the ventricular apex (bottom). The variable timing of the left ventricular assist device filling relative to mitral valve opening changes the transmitral filling pattern from one of restriction to delayed relaxation. LV, left ventricle. (From Nakatani S, Thomas JD, Savage RM, et al: J Am Coll Cardiol 30:1292, 1997.)

In almost all patients, the aortic valve no longer opens or opens infrequently, indicating significant LV afterload reduction by the device. LV and left atrial chamber size decrease and wall thickness increases as a result of decompression of the left ventricle immediately after implantation. In one series of 19 patients supported with LVAD, a mean of 68±33 days LV diastolic diameter decreased from 63±15 mm at baseline to 41±9 mm shortly after pump implantation, whereas intraventricular septum increased from 10±2 mm to 14±2 mm. Long-term follow up in this series demonstrated that chamber size and wall thickness did not change significantly from measurements obtained immediately after pump implantation. Histologic examination of the myocardium demonstrates reduction in measures of myocyte damage and increased fibrosis, likely related to healing necrosis.[59] A later series of 31 patients supported with LVAD for a longer period (mean 137 days; range 31 to 505 days) found similar changes in LV size and also found significant improvement in native cardiac function as assessed by EF (0.11±0.05 to 0.22±0.17) and hemodynamics (cardiac index increased from 1.96±0.52 L/min/m² to 2.93±0.73 L/min/m²; pulmonary capillary wedge pressure (PCWP) decreased from 24.18±6.27 mm Hg to 14.48±3.01 mm Hg).[60]

Improvements in diastolic function also occur with ventricular unloading. Patients with end-stage HF typically have a restrictive filling pattern, manifesting as a single, higher-than-normal mitral inflow wave with a short filling time (<200 msec) and little or no late

filling. Improvements in diastolic filling parameters improve soon after device implantation, reflecting a decline in LV filling pressure and improved LV relaxation.[61,62] In a series of eight patients undergoing LVAD implantation, intraoperative transesophageal echocardiography before and after device implantation showed a rapid beat to beat variation in transmitral flow velocity patterns, but when values from 10 consecutive beats are used, the overall filling pattern tended to normalize, with significantly decreased early filling (87±31 cm/s to 64±26 cm/s), increased late filling (8±11 cm/s to 32±23 cm/s), and prolonged deceleration time (DT) of early filling (112±40 ms to 160±44 msec). This beat-to-beat variation in transmitral flow pattern occurs as a result of acute change in ventricular loading conditions that result when there is asynchronous native cardiac systole and diastole versus device filling, which in the automatic mode occurs when roughly 90% of the pump chamber fills with blood, regardless of what is occurring simultaneously in the native cardiac cycle[62] (Fig. 31–10).

Diagnosing Left Ventricular Assist Device Malfunction

In addition to confirming normal functioning of the device, transthoracic echocardiography can identify several common types of LVAD malfunction, including inflow and outflow valve regurgitation, obstruction or distortion of inflow and outflow cannulae, and acquired disease of the native aortic valve. Inflow valve regurgitation is the most common mechanical cause of LVAD dysfunction and may be caused by a tear or dehiscence of the bioprosthetic inlet valve. Under normal operating conditions, intracavitary flow is laminar and unidirectional. On two-dimensional echocardiography, inflow valve regurgitation manifests as turbulent flow originating from the inflow cannula during LVAD ejection. Pulsed Doppler at the inflow cannula demonstrates significant variability of the inflow cannula regurgitation flow relative to the native cardiac cycle. When the LVAD ejects during native LV diastole, the relatively low intracavitary pressure allows for a greater volume of inflow valve regurgitation, manifesting as higher velocity, denser regurgitant waveforms on pulsed Doppler. The reverse holds true for LVAD ejection during native LV systole. Because of partial redirecting of total LVAD output to regurgitant flow, outflow graft velocities, velocity time integral (VTI), and stroke volume are significantly reduced in the setting of inflow valve regurgitation. In one series, normal peak velocity averaged 2.12 ± 0.39 m/s, velocity time integral 35.9 ± 7.9 cm, and outflow graft stroke volume (calculated as outflow graft diameter area $\times$ velocity time integral) 76.5 ± 15.1 mL. Among patients with inflow valve regurgitation, outflow graft peak velocity averaged 1.60 ± 0.30 m/s, velocity time integral 23.7 ± 3.7 cm, and stroke volume 51.1 ± 7.4 mL. Furthermore, with a normally functioning LVAD, LV diastolic dimensions are normal or reduced (49 ± 10 mm) as a result of effective unloading of the left ventricle, whereas in the setting of inflow valve regurgitation the left ventricle is significantly dilated (61 ± 6 mm) as a result the regurgitant flow back into the left ventricle from the device. For the same reason, the native aortic valve rarely opens during normal functioning of the LVAD but opens more frequently in the setting of inflow valve regurgitation (Fig. 31–11). Inflow valve obstruction is diagnosed when the usual laminar diastolic flow into the inflow cannula is intermittently interrupted on pulsed Doppler of the apical cannula[63] (Figs. 31–12, 31–13, and 31–14).

Assessing Myocardial Recovery

Long-term pressure and volume unloading of the left ventricle with a LVAD leads to favorable reverse remodeling of chronic ventricular dilation[64] and improvements at the cellular level, including reduced myocyte hypertrophy and apoptosis.[65,66] Despite this, only a small proportion of patients on LVADs will manifest myocardial recovery to the degree that device explantation is possible. Estimates for successful explantation are about five percent, with the vast majority of patients being supported for less than 3 months.[2,67] Long-term survival approached 80% at 5 years after LVAD removal in one series.[68] Clinical parameters suggesting higher likeli-

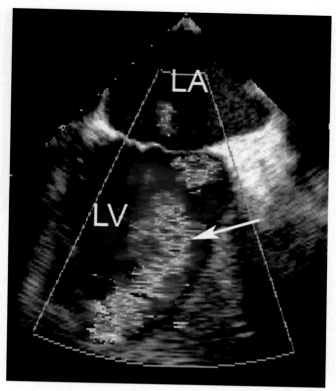

Figure 31–11. *Color flow Doppler showing regurgitation of the left ventricular assist device in a transesophageal four-chamber view. The turbulence in the left ventricle (arrow) is regurgitation from the assist device inflow cannula located in the left ventricular apex. LA, left atrium; LV, left ventricle.*

hood of myocardial recovery include ability to exercise to a peak oxygen consumption (VO$_2$max) of greater than 20 mL/kg/min or peak cardiac output greater than 10 L/min, whereas echocardiographic parameters of such include consistent aortic valve opening, normal shortening fraction, and absence of marked LV dilation.[67] Various protocols for weaning LVAD support and identifying appropriate candidates for explantation exist, and protocols continue to be developed and refined as experience with these devices grows. A combination of cardiac structural and functional assessment with noninvasive imaging, hemodynamics measured invasively, and determination of overall cardiovascular functional capacity through exercise testing (usually cardiopulmonary exercise testing) is typically used to gauge myocardial recovery and chances for weaning.

DSE is a commonly used modality to assess extent of myocardial recovery on LVAD support. In several series the protocol for dobutamine infusion is typical for standard testing (initiating at 5 μg/kg/min and titrating every 5 minutes up to 40 μg/kg/min) and is performed with LVAD support at a minimum (low flow). In a series of 16 LVAD patients, DSE with simultaneous invasive hemodynamic measurements discriminated between patients who underwent successful weaning and explantation and those who could not.

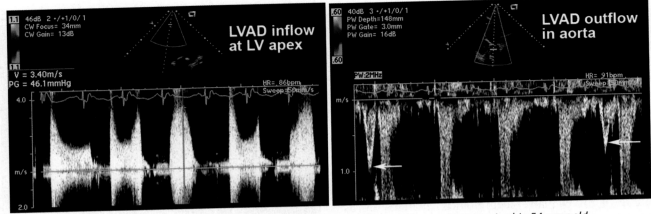

Figure 31-12. *Doppler recordings of apical inflow (A) show an unusual pattern in this 54-year-old woman with a chronic left ventricular assist device (LVAD) for severe heart failure resulting from a cardiomyopathy. On some beats, the velocity is as high as 4 m/s, consistent with a left ventricular (LV) systolic pressure of at least 64 mm Hg and obstruction of the inflow cannula. The flow into the aorta (B) shows intermittent antegrade flow across the aortic valve (arrows) in addition to the LVAD flow signals.*

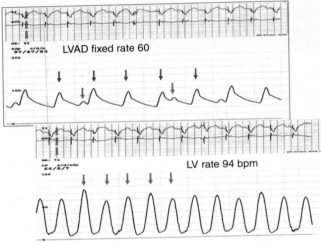

Figure 31-13. *Cardiac catheterization in the same patient as Figure 31-12 shows the left ventricular assist device (LVAD) pressure waveform in the aorta (top) at the LVAD set rate of 60 per minute (blue arrows) with superimposed lower pressure peaks (red arrows) resulting from spontaneous ventricular contraction. Left ventricular (LV) pressure recordings (bottom) show a variable LV systolic pressure in the 60 mm Hg range due to ventricular contraction (red arrows) after each QRS complex. Only the higher pressure beats result in aortic valve opening.*

Compared to patients who did not undergo explantation, patients who did had greater increase in LV dP/dt (1090±70 mm Hg to 1291±26 mm Hg versus 1280±144 mm Hg to 2670±254 mm Hg, respectively; $p = 0.02$) and EF (27±12% to 27±11% versus 30±7% to 48±9%, respectively; $p < 0.01$), and LV end-systolic dimension significantly decreased (3.35 ± 0.7 cm to 4.63±0.6 cm versus 4.33±0.6 cm to 3.43±0.9 cm, respectively; $p < 0.001$) at peak dobutamine infusion. On hemodynamic monitoring, patients who underwent explantation had greater increases in cardiac index (2.1±0.4 L/min/m²

to 3.1±0.3 L/min/m² versus 2.5±0.5 L/min/m² to 4.9±1.3 L/min/m², respectively; $p = 0.02$). All nine patients who demonstrated favorable responses to dobutamine underwent LVAD explantation, and six survived more than 12 months.[69]

Examination of cardiac performance on reduced pump support may also assist in assessing myocardial recovery and identifying potential candidates for device explantation. Off-pump echocardiographic parameters of LV EF greater than or equal to 45% and LV diastolic diameter less than or equal to 55 mm during weaning surveillance and HF duration less than 5 years before LVAD implantation have been found predictive of successful explantation and freedom from recurrent HF symptoms after explantation in one series. However sphericity index, LV end-diastolic relative wall thickness (2 × posterior wall thickness/LV diastolic diameter), and Doppler indices of diastolic function (E/A ratio, E deceleration time, or IVRT) did not significantly predict freedom from HF recurrence after LVAD removal.[68] In one series of 18 LVAD patients, the 6 patients who experienced myocardial recovery and underwent successful LVAD explantation showed better LV chamber dynamics on echocardiography during low flow LVAD support compared to those patients who did not undergo explantation—LV size increased to a lesser degree; stroke area ([end-diastolic area at mid-LV short-axis plane at papillary muscle level] − [end-systolic area]) increased rather than decreased, and fractional area change ([stroke area]/[end-diastolic area] × 100%) remained stable rather than decreased. Patients who underwent successful explantation also maintained blood pressure rather than showing decline during low flow LVAD support.[70] Preload-adjusted maximal power, a relatively load-independent index, was also

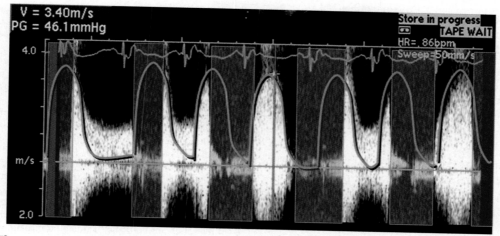

Figure 31–14. *The probable left ventricular (LV) pressure curve* (green) *and the timing of flow into the left ventricular assist device (LVAD)* (noncolored areas between pink bars) *show how the combination of LV contraction and flow into the LVAD result in the Doppler velocity curves. Obstruction of inflow into the LVAD at connection between the LV apex and conduit was confirmed at subsequent surgery.*

TABLE 31–2. Example of Routine Surveillance Diagnostic Studies after Left Ventricular Assist Device Implantation in Patient without Complications

Every 6 Months

Chest X-ray
Echocardiogram
Right-sided heart catheterization
Cardiopulmonary exercise test
Gated-rest nuclear medicine myocardial perfusion scan
  (using agent such as technetium Tc-99 tetrofosmin) to
  quantify biventricular volumes, regional and global func-
  tion, and ejection fraction

In Addition, If Evidence for Myocardial Recovery Present and Considering Left Ventricular Assist Device Explantation

Dobutamine stress echocardiogram

Note there is variation between institutions.

used by this group to gauge myocardial recovery. Measurements were obtained during unassisted beats during LVAD support. LV power is the product of instantaneous pressure and flow. Rate of volume change (dV/dt) can be used as a surrogate for flow, and rate of change of LV cross-sectional area (CSA: dA/dt) obtained by echocardiographic automatic border detection can be substituted for dV/dt. Power was divided by a correction factor for reducing preload sensitivity, (end-diastolic area)$^{3/2}$.[71] Preload adjusted maximal power was the most discriminative variable between patients who underwent successful explantation (6.7 ± 2.4 mW/cm^4) versus those who did not (1.2 ± 1.2 mW/cm^4, $p < 0.005$)[70] (Table 31–2).

KEY POINTS

■ Currently the bicaval technique of cardiac transplantation is more widely used than the older bi-atrial technique, with resultant lesser appearance of biatrial enlargement seen on echocardiography and better structural and functional preservation of the donor atria.

■ The transplanted heart in general demonstrates preserved systolic size and function long term in the absence of acute rejection.

■ Diastolic dysfunction is prominent in the early postoperative period after cardiac transplantation, likely related to ischemic injury during procurement, transport, and transplantation surgery. Persistence of a restrictive filling pattern chronically is associated with poor prognosis.

■ Although only a small fraction of acute rejection episodes are associated with gross systolic dysfunction on echocardiography, systolic dysfunction generally indicates higher-grade rejection with hemodynamic compromise.

■ Abnormalities in diastolic filling are the earliest manifestations of acute rejection, although some studies have also observed increases in LV wall thickness, particularly in the setting of vascular rejection.

■ Transplant vasculopathy is an accelerated intimal hyperplasia of the allograft vasculature that ultimately limits the long-term life span of the allograft in a significant proportion of cardiac transplant patients. Because it is a diffuse process, standard coronary angiography is generally not sensitive enough for diagnosis; adjunctive IVUS is generally needed. Transplant vasculopathy can also be detected by noninvasive modalities, such as DSE.

■ Preoperative or intraoperative evaluation for LVAD implantation includes evaluation for patent foramen ovale or atrial septal defect, aortic insufficiency, and RV dysfunction.

■ After LVAD implantation, LV chamber size decreases acutely and chronically, accompanied by evidence for improved diastolic function and histologic evidence of reduction in myocyte damage and necrosis.

■ Echocardiography can detect several types of LVAD malfunctioning, including inflow and outflow valve regurgitation, obstruction or distortion of inflow or outflow cannulae, or acquired disease of the native aortic valve.

■ DSE can be used to assess myocardial recovery while on LVAD support.

REFERENCES

1. Taylor DO, Edwards LB, Boucek MM, et al: Registry of the International Society for Heart and Lung Transplantation: twenty-second official adult heart transplant report–2005. *J Heart Lung Transplant* 24:945-955, 2005.
2. Deng MC, Edwards LB, Hertz MI, et al: Mechanical circulatory support device database of the International Society for Heart and Lung Transplantation: third annual report–2005. *J Heart Lung Transplant* 24:1182-1187, 2005.
3. Angermann CE, Spes CH, Tammen A, et al: Anatomic characteristics and valvular function of the transplanted heart: transthoracic versus transesophageal echocardiographic findings. *J Heart Transplant* 9:331-338, 1990.
4. Aziz TM, Burgess MI, El-Gamel A, et al: Orthotopic cardiac transplantation technique: a survey of current practice. *Ann Thorac Surg* 68:1242-1246, 1999.
5. Bouchart F, Derumeaux G, Mouton-Schleifer D, et al: Conventional and total orthotopic cardiac transplantation: a comparative clinical and echocardiographic study. *Eur J Cardiothorac Surg* 12:555-559, 1997.
6. Riberi A, Ambrosi P, Habib G, et al: Systemic embolism: a serious complication after cardiac transplantation avoidable by bicaval technique. *Eur J Cardiothorac Surg* 19:307-312, 2001.
7. Manning WJ, Silverman DI, Katz SE, Douglas PS: Atrial ejection force: a noninvasive assessment of atrial systolic function. *J Am Coll Cardiol* 22:221-225, 1993.
8. Freimark D, Czer LSC, Aleksic I, et al: Improved left atrial transport and function with orthotopic heart transplantation by bicaval and pulmonary venous anastomoses. *Am Heart J* 130:121-126, 1995.
9. Corcos T, Tamburino C, Leger P, et al: Early and late hemodynamic evaluation after cardiac transplantation: A study of 28 cases. *J Am Coll Cardiol* 11:264-269, 1988.
10. Greenberg ML, Uretsky BF, Reddy S, et al: Long-term hemodynamic follow-up of cardiac transplant patients treated with cyclosporine and prednisone. *Circulation* 3:487-494, 1985.
11. Cotts WG, Oren RM: Function of the transplanted heart: Unique physiology and therapeutic implications. *Am J Med Sci* 314:164-172, 1997.
12. Antunes ML, Spotnitz HM, Clark MB, et al: Long-term function of human cardiac allografts assessed by two-dimensional echocardiography. *J Thorac Cardiovasc Surg* 98:275-284, 1989.
13. Tischler MD, Lee RT, Plappert T, et al: Serial assessment of left ventricular function and mass after orthotopic heart transplantation: A 4-year longitudinal study. *J Am Coll Cardiol* 19:60-66, 1992.
14. Wilhemi M, Pethig K, Wilhemi M, et al: Heart transplantation: echocardiographic assessment of morphology and function after more than 10 years of follow-up. *Ann Thorac Surg* 74:1075-1079, 2002.
15. St Goar FG, Gibbons R, Schnittger I, et al: Left ventricular diastolic function: Doppler echocardiographic changes soon after cardiac transplantation. *Circulation* 82:872-878, 1990.
16. Valantine HA, Appleton CP, Hatle LK, et al: A hemodynamic and Doppler echocardiographic study of ventricular function in long-term cardiac allograft recipients. *Circulation* 79:66-75, 1989.
17. Ross HJ, Gullestad L, Hunt SA, et al: Early Doppler echocardiographic dysfunction is associated with an increased mortality after orthothopic cardiac transplantation. *Circulation* 94(9 Suppl):II289-II293, 1996.
18. Bhatia SJS, Kirshenbaum JM, Shemin RJ, et al: Time course of resolution of pulmonary hypertension and right ventricular remodeling after orthotopic cardiac transplantation. *Circulation* 76:819-826, 1987.
19. Anderson CA, Shernan SK, Leacche M, et al: Severity of intraoperative tricuspid regurgitation predicts poor late survival following cardiac transplantation. *Ann Thorac Surg* 78:1635-1643, 2004.
20. Billingham ME, Cary NR, Hammond ME, et al: A working formulation for the standardization of nomenclature in the diagnosis of heart and lung rejection: Heart Rejection Study Group. *J Heart Transplant* 9:587-593, 1990.
21. Ensley RD, Hammond EH, Renlund DG, et al: Clinical manifestations of vascular rejection in cardiac transplantation. *Transplant Proc* 23:1130-1132, 1991.
22. Valantine HA, Fowler MB, Hunt SA, et al: Changes in Doppler echocardiographic indexes of left ventricular function as potential markers of acute cardiac rejection. *Circulation* 76:V86-V92, 1987.
23. Amende I, Simon R, Seegers A, et al: Diastolic dysfunction during acute cardiac allograft rejection. *Circulation* 81(2 Suppl):III66-III70, 1990.
24. Desruennes M, Corcos T, Cabrol A, et al: Doppler echocardiography for the diagnosis of acute cardiac allograft rejection. *J Am Coll Cardiol* 12:63-70, 1988.
25. Tei C: New non-invasive index for combined systolic and diastolic ventricular function. *J Cardiol* 26:135-136, 1995.
26. Tei C, Ling LH, Hodge DO, et al: New index of combined systolic and diastolic myocardial performance: a simple and reproducible measure of cardiac function—a study in normals and dilated cardiomyopathy. *J Cardiol* 26:357-366, 1995.
27. Toumanidis ST, Papadopoulou ES, Saridakis NS, et al: Evaluation of myocardial performance index to predict mild rejection in cardiac transplantation. *Clin Cardiol* 27:352-358, 2004.
28. Burgess MI, Bright-Thomas RJ, Yonan N, Ray SG: Can the index of myocardial performance be used to detect acute cellular rejection after heart transplantation? *Am J Cardiol* 92:308-311, 2003.
29. Sagar KB, Hastillo A, Walfgang TC, Lower RR, Hess ML: Left ventricular mass by M-mode echocardiography in cardiac transplant patients with acute rejection. *Circulation* 64(2 Pt 2):II217-II220, 1981.
30. Mannaerts HF, Balk AH, Simoons ML, et al: Changes in left ventricular function and wall thickness in heart transplant recipients and their relation to acute rejection: An assessment by digitized M mode echocardiography. *Br Heart J* 68:356-364, 1992.

31. Ciliberto GR, Mascarello M, Gronda E, et al: Acute rejection after heart transplantation: noninvasive echocardiographic evaluation. *J Am Coll Cardiol* 23:1156-1161, 1994.

32. Hammond EH, Yowell RL, Nunoda S, et al: Vascular (humoral) rejection in heart transplantation: pathologic observations and clinical implications. *J Heart Transplant* 8:430-443, 1989.

33. Gill EA, Borrego C, Bray BE, et al: Left ventricular mass increases during cardiac allograft vascular rejection. *J Am Coll Cardiol* 25:922-926, 1995.

34. Stengel S-M, Allemann Y, Zimmerli M, et al: Doppler tissue imaging for assessing left ventricular diastolic dysfunction in heart transplant recipients. *Heart* 86:432-437, 2001.

35. Mankand S, Murali S, Kormos RL, et al: Evaluation of the potential role of color-coded tissue Doppler echocardiography in the detection of allograft rejection in heart transplant recipients. *Am Heart J* 138:721-730, 1999.

36. Miller LW, Labovitz AJ, McBride LA, et al: Echocardiography-guided endomyocardial biopsy: A 5-year experience. *Circulation* 78(5 Pt 2):II99-102, 1988.

37. Bedanova H, Necas J, Petrikovits E, et al: Echo-guided endomyocardial biopsy in heart transplant recipients. *Transpl Int* 17:622-625, 2004.

38. Nguyen V, Cantarovich M, Cecere R, Gianetti N: Tricuspid regurgitation after cardiac transplantation: How many biopsies are too many? *J Heart Lung Transplant* 24:S227-S231, 2005.

39. Quin JA, Taurianinen MP, Huber LM, et al: Predictors of pericardial effusion after orthotopic heart transplantation. *J Thorac Cardiovasc Surg* 124:979-983, 2002.

40. Hauptman PJ, Couper GS, Aranki SF, et al: Pericardial effusions after cardiac transplantation. *J Am Coll Cardiol* 23:1625-1629, 1994.

41. Ciliberto GR, Anjos MC, Gronda E, et al: Significance of pericardial effusion after heart transplantation. *Am J Cardiol* 76:297-300, 1995.

42. Valantine HA, Hunt SA, Gibbons R, et al: Increasing pericardial effusion in cardiac transplant recipients. *Circulation* 79:603-609, 1989.

43. Kapadia SR, Nissen SE, Ziada KM, et al: Development of transplantation vasculopathy and progression of donor-transmitted atherosclerosis: Comparison by serial intravascular ultrasound imaging. *Circulation* 98:2672-2678, 1998.

44. Uretsky BF, Murali S, Reddy PS, et al: Development of coronary artery disease in cardiac transplant patients receiving immunosuppressive therapy with cyclosporine and prednisone. *Circulation* 76:827-834, 1987.

45. St. Goar FG, Pinto FJ, Alderman EL, et al: Intracoronary ultrasound in cardiac transplant recipients. *Circulation* 85:979-987, 1992.

46. Pinto FJ, Chenzbraun A, Botas J, et al: Feasibility of serial intracoronary ultrasound imaging for assessment of progression of intimal proliferation in cardiac transplant recipients. *Circulation* 90:2348-2355, 1994.

47. Rickenbacher PR, Pinto FJ, Chenzbraun A, et al: Incidence and severity of transplant coronary artery disease early and up to 15 years after transplantation as detected by intravascular ultrasound. *J Am Coll Cardiol* 25:171-177, 1995.

48. Mehra MR, Prasad A, Uber PA, et al: The impact of explosive brain death on the genesis of cardiac allograft vasculopathy: An intravascular ultrasound study. *J Heart Lung Transplant* 19:522-528, 2000.

49. Kobashigawa JA, Miller L, Yeung A, et al: Does acute rejection correlate with the development of transplant coronary artery disease? A multicenter study using intravascular ultrasound. *J Heart Lung Transplant* 22:58-69, 2003.

50. Tuzcu EM, Kapadia SR, Sachar R, et al: Intravascular ultrasound evidence of angiographically silent progression in coronary atherosclerosis predicts long-term morbidity and mortality after cardiac transplantation. *J Am Coll Cardiol* 45:1538-1542, 2005.

51. Kobashigawa JA, Tobis JA, Starling RA, et al: Multicenter intravascular ultrasound validation study among heart transplant recipients: Outcomes after five years. *J Am Coll Cardiol* 45:1532-1537, 2005.

52. Spes CH, Klauss V, Mudra H, et al: Diagnostic and prognostic value of serial dobutamine stress echocardiography for noninvasive assessment of cardiac allograft vasculopathy. *Circulation* 100:509-515, 1999.

53. Bacal F, Moreira F, Souza G, et al: Dobutamine stress echocardiography predicts cardiac events or death in asymptomatic patients long-term after heart transplantation: 4-year prospective evaluation. *J Heart Lung Transplant* 23:1238-1244, 2004.

54. Rose EA, Gelijns AC, Moskowitz AJ, et al: Long-term use of a left ventricular assist device for end-stage heart failure. *N Engl J Med* 345:1453-1463, 2001.

55. Aaronson KD, Eppinger MJ, Dyke DB, et al: Left ventricular assist device therapy improves utilization of donor hearts. *J Am Coll Cardiol* 39:1247-1254, 2002.

56. Shapiro GC, Leibowitz DW, Oz MC, et al: Diagnosis of patent foramen ovale with transesophageal echocardiography in a patient supported with a left ventricular assist device. *J Heart Lung Transplant* 14:594-597, 1995.

57. Scalia GM, McCarthy PM, Savage RM, et al: Clinical utility of echocardiography in the management of implantable ventricular assist devices. *J Am Soc Echocardiogr* 13:754-763, 2000.

58. Reilly MP, Wiegers SE, Cucchiara AJ, et al: Frequency, risk factors, and clinical outcomes of left ventricular assist device-associated ventricular thrombus. *Am J Cardiol* 86:1156-1159, 2000.

59. Nakatani S, McCarthy PM, Kottke-Marchant K, et al: Left ventricular echocardiographic and histologic changes: Impact of chronic unloading by an implantable ventricular assist device. *J Am Coll Cardiol* 27:894-901, 1996.

60. Frazier OH, Benedict CR, Radovancevic B, et al: Improved left ventricular function after chronic left ventricular unloading. *Ann Thorac Surg* 62:675-682, 1996.

61. Westaby S, Jin XY, Katsumata T, et al: Mechanical support in dilated cardiomyopathy: signs of early left ventricular recovery. *Ann Thorac Surg* 64:1303-1308, 1997.

62. Nakatani S, Thomas JD, Wandervoort PM, et al: Left ventricular diastolic filling with an implantable ventricular assist device: beat to beat variability with overall improvement. *J Am Coll Cardiol* 30:1288-1294, 1997.

63. Horton SC, Khodaverdian R, Chatelain P, et al: Left ventricular assist device malfunction: an approach to diagnosis by echocardiography. *J Am Coll Cardiol* 45:1435-1440, 2005.

64. Levin HR, Oz MC, Chen JM, et al: Reversal of chronic ventricular dilation in patients with end-stage cardiomyopathy by prolonged mechanical unloading. *Circulation* 91:2717-2720, 1995.

65. Zafeiridis A, Jeevanandam V, Houser SR, Margulies KB: Regression of cellular hypertrophy after left ventricular assist device support. *Circulation* 98:656-662, 1998.

66. Patten RD, Denofrio D, El-Zaru M, et al: Ventricular assist device therapy normalizes inducible nitric oxide synthase expression and reduces cardiomyocyte apoptosis in the failing human heart. *J Am Coll Cardiol* 45:1419-1424, 2005.

67. Mancini DM, Beniaminovitz A, Levin H, et al: Low incidence of myocardial recovery after left ventricular assist device implantation in patients with chronic heart failure. *Circulation* 98:2383-2399, 1998.

68. Dandel M, Weng Y, Siniawski H, et al: Long-term results in patients with idiopathic dilated cardiomyopathy after weaning from left ventricular assist devices. *Circulation* 112(Suppl I):I37-I45, 2005.

69. Khan T, Delgado RM, Radovancevic B, et al: Dobutamine stress echocardiography predicts myocardial improvement in patients supported by left ventricular assist devices (LVADs): hemodynamic and histologic evidence of improvement before LVAD explantation. *J Heart Lung Transplant* 22:137-146, 2003.

70. Gorcsan J, Severyn D, Murali S, Kormos RL: Non-invasive assessment of myocardial recovery on chronic left ventricular assist device: Results associated with successful device removal. *J Heart Lung Transplant* 22:1304-1313, 2003.

71. Mandarino WA, Pinsky MR, Gorcsan J: Assessment of left ventricular contractile state by preload-adjusted maximal power using echocardiographic automated border detection. *J Am Coll Cardiol* 31:861-868, 1998.

Part Six

The Pregnant Patient

Role of Echocardiography in the Diagnosis and Management of Heart Disease in Pregnancy

KAREN K. STOUT, MD

The author acknowledges Catherine M. Otto, MD, Thomas R. Easterling, MD, and Thomas J. Benedetti, MD, the previous authors of this chapter in *The Practice of Clinical Echocardiography*, second edition.

Echocardiography is often requested in pregnant women to evaluate preexisting heart disease or to assess women with cardiac symptoms or abnormal findings on physical examination. Many healthy women experience symptoms of fatigue, decreased exercise tolerance, or dyspnea during pregnancy. Clinical examination may be nondiagnostic, prompting a request for echocardiographic evaluation. Although a "flow murmur" is present in most pregnant women, this normal finding cannot always be clinically distinguished from a pathologic murmur. Diagnostic testing can differentiate between the normal alterations in cardiovascular physiology and anatomy resulting from pregnancy and from pathologic findings.

In pregnant patients with known cardiac disease, expected findings (and appropriate normal reference values) may be different from those in nongravid patients. Echocardiography may be used to monitor cardiovascular function during pregnancy and the peripartum period. In pregnant patients with concurrent systemic disease or with preeclampsia, echocardiography can provide important insights into the effect of the disease process on cardiovascular physiology and can assist in management of individual patients.

In this chapter, the normal hemodynamic and echocardiographic changes during pregnancy are reviewed and the role of echocardiography in management of pregnant women with known or suspected cardiac disease is summarized.

Normal Hemodynamic and Echocardiographic Changes with Pregnancy

Normal Hemodynamic Changes

During normal pregnancy, plasma volume, erythrocyte volume, and cardiac output (CO) increase substantially over baseline values (Table 32-1 and Fig. 32-1). Many original studies of hemodynamic changes during pregnancy were based on right-sided heart catheterization with Fick or thermodilution CO data. These studies included small numbers of patients with evaluation of limited points during pregnancy.[1,2] More recent use of Doppler CO measurement techniques has greatly increased our understanding of the magnitude and timing of CO changes during pregnancy.[2-4]

CO increases during pregnancy by as much as 45% over baseline values.[4-7] Noninvasive Doppler measurements consistently show a definite rise in CO that occurs as early as 10 weeks of gestation. Some studies suggest that maximum CO is reached at 24 weeks of gestation with no further increase in later pregnancy (Fig. 32-2). Other studies (Fig. 32-3 and Fig. 32-4) show a continued increase in CO throughout pregnancy, with higher stroke volume (SV) accounting for much of

TABLE 32-1. Normal Anatomic and Hemodynamic Changes of Pregnancy

Anatomic	
Aortic root	Slight increase in diameter (2-3 mm)
Left ventricle	Slight increase in end-diastolic dimension and slight decrease in end-systolic dimension
Left atrium	Slight increase in size
Hemodynamic	
Cardiac output	Increased beginning in first trimester; maximum increase (at term) of 45% over baseline value
Stroke volume	Increased
Heart rate	Increased by 25%-30%
Blood pressure	Unchanged
Systemic vascular resistance	Decreased
Pulmonary artery pressure	Unchanged
Left ventricular end-diastolic pressure	Unchanged

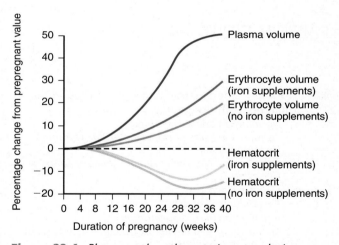

Figure 32-1. *Plasma and erythrocyte increase during pregnancy. (From Pitkin PM:* Clin Obstet Gynecol *19:489-513, 1976.)*

the first-trimester increase, followed by a continued elevation in heart rate (HR; and thus CO) in the last two trimesters. On average, HR increases 25% to 30% over baseline values during pregnancy[8] (Fig. 32-5).

The underlying etiology of increased CO with pregnancy is presumably hormonal, but the exact mechanism remains unclear.[9] Vasodilation may be mediated by nitric oxide[10] and hormones, such as relaxin.[11] An increase in venous tone during pregnancy contributes

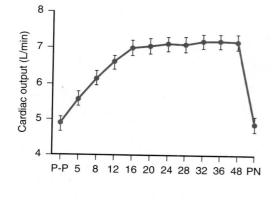

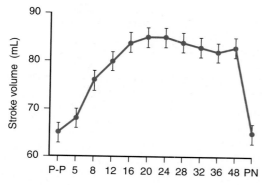

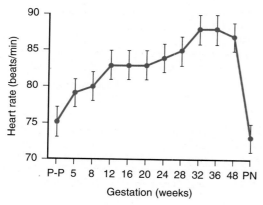

Figure 32–2. *Increase in cardiac output from the nonpregnant state throughout pregnancy. P-P, prepregnancy; PN, postnatal. (From Hunter S, Robson SC: Br Heart J 68:540-543, 1992.)*

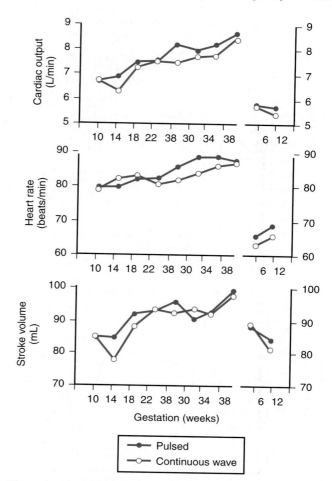

Figure 32–3. *Hemodynamic changes during pregnancy and postpartum. (From Mabie WC, DiSessa TG, Crocher LG, et al: Am J Obstet Gynecol 170:849-856, 1994.)*

to preload augmentation.[4] In addition, decreased aortic stiffness reduces afterload.[6] Arterial capacitance increases during pregnancy, accounting for the decrease in total peripheral resistance.[12] This fall in systemic vascular resistance (SVR) allows blood pressure to rise only slightly despite increased SV (see Fig. 32–5). Some studies suggest that pregnancy is associated with an increased ventricular wall stress.[13] However, this view is challenged by other studies demonstrating a 30% decrease in wall stress.[4,14] Left ventricular (LV) contractility may to be depressed in pregnancy, based on mea-

surement of the afterload adjusted velocity of circumferential fiber shortening.[13,14] LV systolic performance is maintained, despite this possible decrease in contractility, as a result of the altered loading conditions of pregnancy. However other studies suggest that there is no change in ventricular contractility.[1,12] Pulmonary pressures remain normal during pregnancy,[15] suggesting a similar decrease in pulmonary vascular resistance (PVR) to balance the increased blood volume. Diastolic filling pressures in both the right-sided and left-sided heart also remain normal in pregnancy.[16]

Technical Aspects of Doppler Cardiac Output Measurements

Doppler measurement of CO in pregnancy is based on the same principles as in nonpregnant patients. SV (SV) is calculated from the cross-sectional area (CSA) of flow multiplied by the velocity time integral (VTI) of flow at that site:

$$SV = CSA \times VTI$$

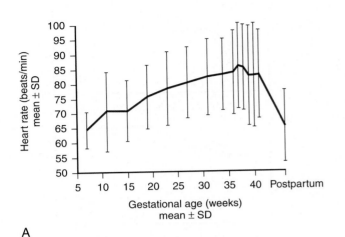

HEART RATE - NORMAL PREGNANCY

A

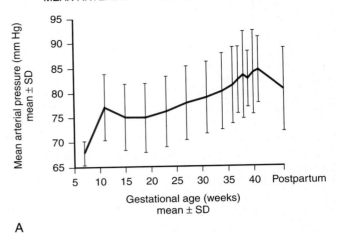

MEAN ARTERIAL PRESSURE - NORMAL PREGNANCY

A

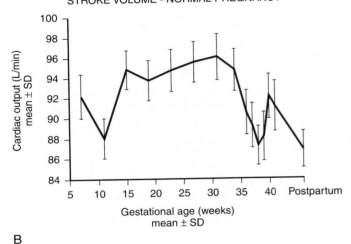

STROKE VOLUME - NORMAL PREGNANCY

B

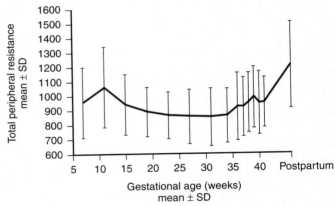

TOTAL PERIPHERAL RESISTANCE - NORMAL PREGNANCY

B

Figure 32–5. Sequential changes in mean arterial pressure (A) and a total peripheral resistance (B) in 89 women with no cardiac disease and a normal pregnancy. SD, standard deviation. *(Data from Easterling TR, Benedetti TJ, Schmucker BC, Millard SP: Obstet Gynecol 76:1061-1069, 1990.)*

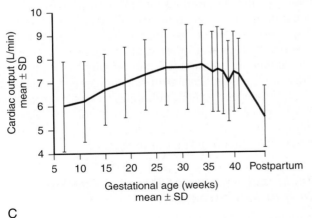

CARDIAC OUTPUT - NORMAL PREGNANCY

C

Figure 32–4. Serial changes in heart rate (A), *stroke volume* (B), *and cardiac output* (C) *recorded using Doppler echocardiography in a series of 89 women with no cardiac disease and a normal pregnancy. SD, standard deviation. (Data from Easterling TR, Benedetti TJ, Schmucker BC, Millard SP: Obstet Gynecol 76:1061-1069, 1990.)*

Typically, CSA is assumed to be circular and is calculated from a two-dimensional (2D) echocardiographic diameter measurement recorded with the ultrasound (US) beam perpendicular to the flow diameter. The velocity time integral is measured by either pulsed-wave (PW) or continuous-wave (CW) Doppler ultrasound, with the Doppler beam aligned parallel to the flow stream. As in nonpregnant patients, it is critical that (1) diameter is measured accurately, (2) the Doppler beam is aligned parallel to the direction of blood flow, and (3) diameter and velocity data are obtained almost simultaneously from the same intracardiac site. In addition, this method assumes that flow is laminar with a relatively flat (or blunt) flow-velocity profile and that flow fills the anatomic CSA. Although these assumptions appear to be warranted in nonpregnant patients according to numerous studies validating this approach,[17] the potential effect of the altered flow conditions during pregnancy warrants reevaluation. Specific concerns in pregnant patients include the possibility that the flow profile may not be blunt or may be asymmetric given the higher flow volumes. Possible changes in cross-sectional flow areas during pregnancy may also affect these measurements.

Validation of CO measurements in pregnancy has been performed by several groups of investigators using either of two basic Doppler approaches (Table 32–2). Some investigators have applied the technique of measuring ascending aortic flow with a continuous wave Doppler probe from a suprasternal approach.[18,19] The CSA of flow is calculated from a carefully recorded A-mode aortic diameter (Fig. 32–6) measured at the sinotubular junction, the narrowest segment of the aorta

TABLE 32–2. Validation of Doppler Cardiac Output Measurements in Pregnancy

Author	n	Gestational Age	Doppler Method	Standard of Reference	r	Regression Equation (L/min)	SEE (L/min)
Easterling[18]	23	Third trimester	CWD	TD	0.93	Dop = 1.07 TD - 0.58	—
			A-mode AO	—	—	—	—
Robson[24]	15	Nonpregnant	PD asc Ao	Fick	0.93	Fick = 1.0 Dop + 0.8	0.4
			2D Ao-leaflets	—	—	—	—
Robson[24]	40	Pregnant	Ao	Doppler	—	—	—
		Nonpregnant	MV versus PA	MV	0.96	Ao = 1.02 MV - 0.96	0.37
			—	PA	0.96	Ao = 0.97 PA + 0.40	0.47
			—	—	0.97	MV = 0.92 PA + 0.62	0.34
Lee[19a]	16	Pregnant	LVOT	TD	0.94	TD = 0.74 LVOT + 1.91	0.64

Ao, aorta; asc, ascending; CWD, continuous-wave Doppler; Dop, Doppler; LVOT, left ventricular outflow tract; MV, mitral valve; PA, pulmonary artery; PD, pulsed Doppler; SEE, standard error of estimate; TD, thermodilution; 2D, two-dimensional.

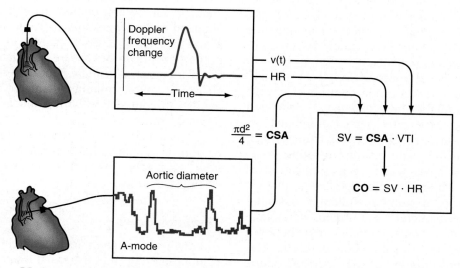

Figure 32–6. Doppler measurement of cardiac output based on a continuous-wave Doppler recording of the velocity time integral (VTI) in the ascending aorta, heart rate (HR), and an A-mode aortic diameter (D) for calculation of cross-sectional area (CSA) at the sinotubular junction. Stroke volume (SV) and cardiac output (CO) are calculated as shown. (From Easterling TR, Watts HD, Schmucker BC, Benedetti TJ: Obstet Gynecol 69:845-850, 1987. Reprinted with permission from The American College of Obstetricians and Gynecologists.)

because the highest flow velocity (as obtained with continuous wave Doppler) will correspond to the smallest flow area. Doppler COs calculated with this method correlated well with simultaneous thermodilution COs in pregnant women undergoing right-sided heart catheterization for clinical indications.[18] Of note, serial studies in pregnant women suggest that aortic root diameter increases during pregnancy,[20,21] so that repeat aortic diameter measurements are needed at each time point. This contrasts with the situation in nonpregnant adults in whom both left ventricular outflow tract (LVOT) and aortic diameters tend to remain relatively constant over time.

Other investigators have measured CO in pregnant women using standard clinical cardiac ultrasound systems.[5,22-24] LVOT diameter is measured from a 2D parasternal long-axis view; LVOT flow is recorded via an apical approach using pulsed Doppler echocardiography, with the sample volume positioned just proximal to the aortic valve plane.[25] This method correlates well with simultaneous Fick COs in nonpregnant patients.[17] In a group of pregnant women, internal consistency between Doppler COs measured from diameter and flow data across the aortic, mitral, and pulmonic valves was demonstrated.[26]

Reproducibility, in addition to accuracy, is critical for the application of these methods in following individual patients during the course of pregnancy. Several studies suggest that both these methods can be performed reproducibly with an acceptable degree of recording and measurement variability in pregnant patients, with a coefficient of variation of 5 percent to 8 percent.[18,26] Although there is still concern that these methods have been validated against invasive standards in only small numbers of pregnant women, the data should still accurately reflect hemodynamic changes over time (if not absolute values) both in individuals and in groups of patients.

Compared with the 2D/pulsed Doppler approach, the advantage of the A-mode/continuous wave method is that a smaller, less expensive, dedicated instrument can be used for CO measurements. Although optimal results require careful data acquisition, focused education and training of appropriate individuals allows more widespread application of this technique. Potential disadvantages include (1) the possibility of a nonperpendicular measurement of aortic root diameter (resulting in overestimation of CO), (2) a nonparallel intercept angle between the Doppler beam and the direction of aortic flow (resulting in underestimation of CO), and (3) failure to recognize abnormal aortic flow conditions (e.g., aortic stenosis [AS] or aortic regurgitation [AR]) that invalidate the Doppler method. When any of these problems are suspected, a standard clinical echocardiographic examination should be performed to resolve the difficulty.

M-Mode and Two-Dimensional Echocardiographic Changes

The increased CO of pregnancy is reflected in changes in LV dimensions, volumes, and geometry (Table 32–3). M-mode studies show that LV end-diastolic dimension increases slightly (by 2 to 3 mm on average) and end-systolic dimension is unchanged, so that there is a slight increase in fractional shortening during pregnancy.[19,26-28] The change in LV diastolic dimension correlates with increased preload caused by changes in systemic venous tone.[29] LV wall thickness also increases slightly, with a corresponding increase in calculated LV mass. Similar changes in right ventricular (RV) dimensions have been noted.

With 2D echocardiography, a slight increase in end-diastolic volume and in ejection fraction (EF) is seen, with little change in end-systolic volume.[6,21,27,28,30,31] These findings are consistent with the altered loading conditions of an increased end-diastolic volume and decreased SVR and do not imply an increase in LV contractility. There are conflicting data on the changes in contractility with pregnancy.[4,14,16,27] There have been few studies evaluating LV geometry in normal pregnancy; however no dramatic changes in ventricular shape have been observed.

Several investigators have found consistent increases in aortic and LVOT diameters during pregnancy, with the magnitude of this change averaging 1 to 2 mm.[19,32] Even this small average change is significant for accurate CO calculations, and given the wide range of values, some individuals have more pronounced changes in outflow tract geometry.

Left atrial anteroposterior dimension increases by about 4 mm. When compared with echocardiograms obtained several weeks postpartum, the maximal atrial size is seen at term.[21] Changes in atrial dimension in the peripartum period are associated with changes in serum atrial natriuretic peptide levels.[33] A small increase in mitral annulus diameter has been documented in conjunction with a much larger change in tricuspid annulus diameter.[21]

A small pericardial effusion is seen on echocardiography is as many as 25% of normal pregnant women, with a higher prevalence in women with preeclampsia.[33]

Doppler Flows

Although enlargement in annular diameters partially compensate for the increased transvalvular volume flow of pregnancy, higher transvalvular flow velocities are also seen[23] (Table 32–4). Both the maximum aortic and LVOT flow velocity rises by approximately 0.3 m/s compared with the nongravid state. Less dramatic changes in transmitral velocities are seen with an increase in early (E) velocity of only 0 to 0.1 m/s and an

TABLE 32–3. Normal Echocardiographic Measurements in Pregnancy (Maximum Changes)

Measurement	Modality	Mean ± SD	Gestational Age	Comparison Value	Time of Comparison	Reference
Aortic root	M-mode	30±12	Third trimester	28±3	2 months pp	Sadaniantz and colleagues[21]
	A-mode	25±2	Term	24±4	10 weeks	Easterling and colleagues[20]
LVOT (cm²)	2D area	3.5±0.3	Term	3.2±0.3	2 months pp	Vered and colleagues[189]
LA dimension (mm)	2D	38±4	Term	34±5	2 months pp	Vered and colleagues[189]
	M-mode	36	Term	31	Preconception	Sadaniantz and colleagues[21]
	M-mode	37	Term	33	24 weeks pp	Robson and colleagues[28]
LV EDD (mm)	M-mode	47±4	Term	48±4	12 weeks pp	Mabie and colleagues[6]
	M-mode	46±3	24 to 32 weeks	43±3	Nonpregnant controls	Rubler, Damani, Pinto[192]
	M-mode	51±3	Third tri	50±4	2 months pp	Sadaniantz and colleagues[21]
	M-mode	48	Third tri	45	Preconception	Robson and colleagues[25]
	M-mode	49	Term	47	24 weeks pp	Robson and colleagues[28]
	2D	52±4	Term	50±3	2 months pp	Vered and colleagues[189]
LV ESD (mm)	M-mode	32	Term	32	24 weeks pp	Robson and colleagues[28]
	M-mode	29±3	Term	30±2	Nonpregnant controls	Rubler, Damani, Pinto[192]
	2D	33±4	Term	34±5	2 months pp	Vered and colleagues[189]
PWT (mm)	M-mode	10±1	Term	9±1	12 weeks pp	Mabie and colleagues[6]
	M-mode	7±1	Third tri	6±1	2 months pp	Sadaniantz and colleagues[21]
	2D	8±1	Term	7±1	2 months pp	Vered and colleagues[189]
LV mass (gm)	M-mode	175±37	Term	135±25	12 weeks pp	Mabie and colleagues[6]
	M-mode	203	Term	157	24 weeks pp	Robson and colleagues[28]
	M-mode	183	Term	120	Preconception	Robson and colleagues[25]
	M-mode	186±39	Term	151±34	2 months pp	Vered and colleagues[189]
FS (%)	M-mode	40±7	Term	33±7	12 weeks pp	Mabie and colleagues[6]
	M-mode	30±5	Term	35±5	2 months pp	Vered and colleagues[189]
LV EDV (mL)	2D	108±14	Term	102±13	2 months pp	Vered and colleagues[189]
LV ESV (mL)	2D	44±10	Term	44±7	2 months pp	Vered and colleagues[189]
EF (%)	2D	60±4	Term	57±4	2 months pp	Vered and colleagues[189]
RV (mm)	M-mode	20±1	Third tri	18±1	2 months pp	Sadaniantz and colleagues[21]
	M-mode	19±3	24 to 32 weeks	15±2	Nonpregnant controls	Rubler, Damani, Pinto[192]
Mitral annulus (mm)	2D	24±5	Third tri	21±4	2 months pp	Sadaniantz and colleagues[21]
Tricuspid annulus (mm)	2D	27±3	Third tri	18±3	2 months pp	Sadaniantz and colleagues[21]

EDD, end-diastolic dimension; EDV, end-diastolic volume; ESD, end-systolic dimension; ESV, end-systolic volume; EF, ejection fraction; FS, fractional shortening; LA, left atrial; LV, left ventricular; LVOT, left ventricular outflow tract; pp, postpartum; PWT, posterior wall thickness; RV, right ventricular; tri, trimester; 2D, two-dimensional.
Data from references 6, 20, 21, 25, 28, 189, 192.

TABLE 32–4. Normal Doppler Flow Velocities in Pregnancy

Measurement	Modality	Value	Gestational Age	Comparison Value	Time of Comparison	Reference
Aorta (m/s)	CWD	1.4±0.2	Term	1.1±0.2	12 weeks pp	Mabie and colleagues[6]
LVOT (m/s)	PD	1.3±0.1	Term	1.0±0.1	12 weeks pp	Mabie and colleagues[6]
Mitral E (m/s)	MV-tips	0.7±0.2	Third tri	0.8±0.1	2 months pp	Sadaniantz and colleagues[21]
		0.9±0.1	6 to 12 weeks	0.8±0.1	12 weeks pp	Mabie and colleagues[6]
Mitral A (m/s)	MV-tips	0.6±0.1	Third tri	0.5±0.1	2 months pp	Sadaniantz and colleagues[21]
		0.6±0.1	24 to 27 weeks	0.5±0.1	12 weeks pp	Mabie and colleagues[6]
E/A	MV-tips	1.5±0.2	Term	1.8±0.2	12 weeks pp	Mabie and colleagues[6]
		1.3±0.3	Third tri	1.6±0.4	2 months pp	Sadaniantz and colleagues[21]
Heart rate (bpm)		84±10	Third tri	70±16	2 months pp	Sadaniantz and colleagues[21]
		89±15	32 to 35 weeks	69±12	12 weeks pp	Mabie and colleagues[6]
		87	Term	69	24 weeks pp	Robson and colleagues[28]
		77±10	Term	70±7	2 months pp	Vered and colleagues[189]
Cardiac output (L/min)		6.5±1.5	Term	4.3±0.6	2 months pp	Vered and colleagues[189]
		7.6	Term	5.0	24 weeks pp	Robson and colleagues[28]

CWD, continuous-wave Doppler; LVOT, left ventricular outflow tract; MV, mitral valve; PD, pulsed Doppler; pp, postpartum; tri, trimester.
Data from references 6, 21, 28, 189.

increase in atrial (A) velocity of only 0.1 to 0.2 m/s. However the relative increase in E and A velocities being unequal, the E/A ratio changes from the normal pattern in young women (higher E than A with an E/A ratio of >1.5) to a pattern of equalized or reversed E/A velocities (E/A ratio of <1) later in pregnancy. Peak pulmonary venous a-wave velocity but not duration also increases during pregnancy.[6]

Postpartum Changes

Interestingly, the estimated magnitude of changes in hemodynamics and cardiac anatomy during pregnancy depends on whether the values obtained during pregnancy are compared to postpartum values or to values obtained in the same patient before pregnancy. It is often difficult to obtain data in the prepregnant time period (because women typically present to the physician after the onset of pregnancy), but a few studies have followed women prospectively starting from preconception. These studies found hemodynamic and anatomic changes of greater magnitude than studies that compared values obtained during pregnancy with postpartum data. This suggests that at least some of the changes of pregnancy may persist into the postpartum period or may be permanent. Although in the postpartum period hemodynamic and anatomic changes return rapidly toward baseline over 6 to 12 weeks (see

Fig. 32–6),[5,25] the postpartum baseline may be different from the prepartum baseline. Specifically, aortic and LV dimensions, although remaining within normal adult limits, may remain larger than the prepregnant values in that individual. Analysis of this data is complicated by the small number of subjects studied, the possibly confounding effects of breastfeeding or other factors and by the measurement variability of the techniques. Further studies are needed because if there are significant, persistent changes after pregnancy, perhaps adult normal values not only should be indexed for body size and gender but also should consider parity.

Normal Valvular Regurgitation

As in nonpregnant patients, a small degrees of valvular regurgitation is often found on Doppler echocardiography.[5,29,34] It is unlikely that these small regurgitant leaks are audible on auscultation or account for the presence of a murmur in pregnant patients. Early studies suggested an unusually high prevalence of tricuspid regurgitation (TR) in pregnant women.[29] With the recognition of the extremely high prevalence of small amounts of tricuspid, mitral, and pulmonic regurgitation in normal individuals, it is now apparent that the prevalence of physiologic degrees of valvular regurgitation in pregnant women is similar to that in nonpregnant normal adults.

Similarity of Hemodynamic Changes with Exercise and during Pregnancy

Many of the hemodynamic changes of pregnancy are similar to the normal changes seen with exercise. The increase in HR and CO and decrease in SVR are analogous to changes seen at a moderate level of physical exertion. In addition, the changes in cardiac anatomy seen with pregnancy are similar to those seen with repetitive activity in physically conditioned individuals. Specifically, the increases in LV end-diastolic dimensions, volume, and LV mass, with normal diastolic filling patterns, are analogous to the changes seen with regular physical activity in nonpregnant women and in men. Presumably, these changes represent a similar hemodynamic response to chronic elevation in volume flow rate. In contrast, the increase in aortic root dimension observed in pregnant women by several groups of investigators has not been seen with physical conditioning, suggesting that the mechanism of this effect is related to physical changes in the vessel wall, possibly mediated by hormonal effects.

Doppler Echocardiographic Evaluation of Hemodynamics in Pregnancy

Positional Hemodynamic Changes

Doppler echocardiography can readily evaluate the effect of positional changes on hemodynamics. Orthostatic changes from sitting to standing positions are similar to the changes seen in nonpregnant individuals, with no significant differences between early and late pregnancy.[31] When a pregnant patient changes from a supine to a standing position, HR increases, SV and CO decrease, and SVR rises, maintaining mean arterial pressure (MAP). During pregnancy, the supine position is associated with compression of the inferior vena cava (IVC) by the gravid uterus, resulting in a decrease in venous return to the right atrium and a decline in SV and CO.[23] This supine decrease in CO can be reversed (or prevented) by placing the patient in a left lateral decubitus position. Accordingly, diagnostic echocardiographic studies should be performed with the pregnant patient in a left lateral decubitus position whenever possible. If optimal imaging requires a supine position, the length of time the patient is positioned on her back should be limited.

Peripartum Period

Dramatic changes in loading conditions occur in the peripartum period related to the effects of (1) uterine contractions, (2) the pain associated with labor and delivery, (3) anesthetic medications, (4) the immediate blood loss associated with delivery (Fig. 32–7), (5) and the delivery of the placenta. Although these physiologic

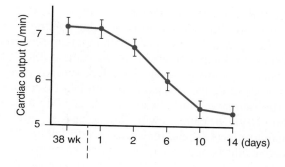

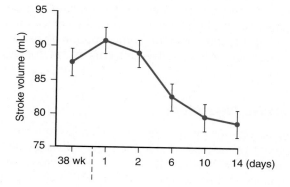

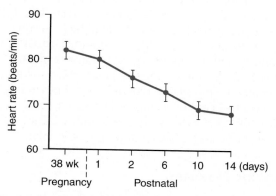

Figure 32–7. Changes in heart rate and cardiac output after normal delivery. (From Hunter S, Robson SC: Br Heart J 68:540–543, 1992.)

changes are well tolerated by healthy women, they can result in acute decompensation in women with underlying heart disease.

During labor, uterine contractions result in an acute increase in both HR and intravascular volume as uterine blood is forced into the circulation. The magnitude of CO rise during contractions increases as labor progresses, with an augmentation of as much as 20% in CO with each contraction.[35,36] There are also mild increases in pulmonary and LV pressures, which may be accentuated in patients with decreased LV compliance (e.g., those with AS or left ventricular hypertrophy [LVH]). Despite the acute blood loss associated with delivery, SV and CO actually rise after delivery of the placenta (by about 10%)[25] and remain elevated for about 24 hours.[25,35] Over the next several days to 2 weeks, CO declines by about 25% to 30% compared with the immediately prepartum value, related to a decrease in both HR and intravascular volume.

Volume changes associated with cesarean section and delivery are greater than those associated with vaginal delivery, so there is rarely hemodynamic advantage to this mode of delivery in patients with heart disease.[37]

The hemodynamic effects of pain include increased HR and SVR. In patients with cardiac disease, the hemodynamic effects of pain may lead to a decline in CO. The negative effects of pain can be eliminated by appropriate anesthesia. However, anesthesia-related changes in preload and afterload also affect cardiac function, especially in patients with heart disease. Thus, the choice of anesthetic agent and route of administration depends on the specific cardiovascular concerns in an individual patient.[37]

Exercise Physiology

Exercise physiology in pregnant women is similar to nonpregnant women except that the basal values are altered by pregnancy. Resting HR and SV are elevated during pregnancy. With exercise, HR and CO rise appropriately.[38,39] Exercise in pregnant women at 32 weeks gestation was associated with a higher exercise HR, higher maximal oxygen consumption, and high atrio-venous oxygen difference compared to 3 months postpartum.[40]

Conditioned pregnant women have a greater CO than sedentary women for any given HR, as is seen in nonpregnant, physically conditioned individuals.[41-45] However, the cardiovascular effects of aerobic conditioning are most evident during strenuous (not during mild or moderate) exercise in pregnant women.[46]

Systemic Diseases

Doppler echocardiography is a useful tool for examining the hemodynamic changes associated with systemic diseases in pregnant patients. For example, in hyperthyroid pregnant women, elevated CO and decreased SVR can be documented, and the resolution of these changes with therapy can be monitored.[47] Echocardiographic evaluation of the effects of beta-agonist tocolysis,[48] pheochromocytoma,[49] sickle cell disease,[50] and renal artery stenosis[51] have also been reported.

Pregnancy-Induced Hypertension and Preeclampsia

Hemodynamics

There are four hypertensive conditions in pregnancy: preeclampsia, chronic hypertension, chronic hypertension with superimposed preeclampsia, and gestational hypertension.[52]

Preeclampsia is defined as systolic blood pressure greater than or equal to 140 mm Hg or diastolic blood pressure greater than or equal to 90 mm Hg and proteinuria greater than 0.3 g per 24 hours, developing after the 20th week of pregnancy in a previously normotensive woman. Eclampsia is the onset of seizures in a woman with preeclampsia. Gestational hypertension is hypertension after the 20th week of pregnancy in a previously normotensive woman, without proteinuria or signs of preeclampsia. Gestational hypertension may progress to preeclampsia but frequently resolves after delivery and has a more benign course than preeclampsia.[53] In a prospective study of 400 primigravida women, gestational hypertension developed in 24 and preeclampsia in 20 women.[54] Chronic hypertension is defined as systolic blood pressure greater than or equal to 140 mm Hg or diastolic blood pressure greater than or equal to 90 mm Hg that antedated pregnancy, developed prior to 20 weeks of gestation, or persists longer than 12 weeks postpartum. If proteinuria develops after 20 weeks gestation in a woman with chronic hypertension, she is diagnosed with preeclampsia. Preeclampsia in a woman with preexisting hypertension and proteinuria is diagnosed if she develops severe hypertension (systolic >160 mm Hg or diastolic >110 mm Hg) in the last half of pregnancy.

The hemodynamics of preeclampsia and gestational hypertension are complex. There is a growing body of literature regarding the pathophysiology of preeclampsia.[22,44,55-57] Preeclampsia may be a heterogeneous disease with different hemodynamic subsets.[58] Investigators have identified that early in the disease course, CO is elevated and later in the course, elevated SVR is seen associated with decreased CO and clinical decompensation.[54] For any given CO, mean arterial pressure is elevated in preeclamptic in comparison with normotensive pregnant women[54,57,59] (Fig. 32–8). Central venous, pul-

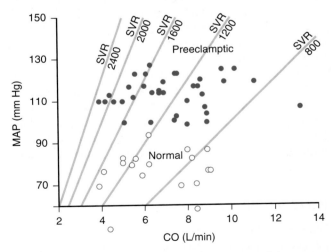

Figure 32–8. *Cardiac output (CO), mean arterial pressure (MAP), and systemic vascular resistance (SVR) in 35 preeclamptic patients and 18 normotensive patients. (From Easterling TR, Watts HD, Schmucker BC, Benedetti TJ: Obstet Gynecol 69:845-850, 1987. Reprinted with permission from The American College of Obstetricians and Gynecologists.)*

monary capillary wedge pressures (PCWPs) and pulmonary artery (PA) pressures tend to be normal. The exception is decompensated patients with pulmonary edema, in whom central venous and pulmonary wedge pressures can be discrepant to the point that invasive hemodynamic monitoring is needed. However because serum oncotic pressure is reduced even more than normal in preeclamptic pregnant patients, interstitial fluid in the lungs and pulmonary edema can occur at relatively low left atrial and pulmonary wedge pressures.

Echocardiographic Findings

In the few studies that have compared cardiac structure in preeclamptic versus normotensive pregnant patients, there have been few or no differences in LV dimensions, volumes, fractional shortening, or LV mass (Table 32–5). Aortic root dimension appears to be slightly greater in preeclamptic than in normotensive pregnant patients and tends to be inversely related to total peripheral resistance.[20]

Impact on Prognosis and Treatment Plans

The use of Doppler CO measurements and calculation of SVR in patients with pregnancy-induced hypertension and preeclampsia to tailor medical therapy is controversial. Some authors have described medication choice based on whether the patient has an elevated CO or elevated SVR.[60] For example, hypertension related to a high CO might respond to beta-blocker therapy, whereas elevated SVR might respond to vasodilator therapy. Importantly, maternal hemodynamics affect fetal growth: High-resistance hypertension is associated with lower birthweights.[61]

Investigators identified women at risk of preeclampsia based on an elevated CO (>7.4 L/min by Doppler echocardiogram) before 24 weeks gestation. In a subsequent double-blind, randomized trial of women with an elevated CO early in pregnancy, atenolol decreased the incidence of preelampsia (1/28 versus 5/28, $p = 0.04$) but increased the risk of a low birth weight infant ($p = 0.02$).[62]

Heart Disease in Pregnancy

Given the low prevalence of heart disease in women of childbearing age in the general population, few pregnant women have significant heart disease. Despite this low prevalence, heart disease is a leading cause of maternal morbidity and mortality. The prevalence of specific types of heart disease in pregnancy reflects both the geographic distribution of these diseases and the patterns of health care in the overall population.[61,63-65] For example, in the U.S. and Europe, the prevalence of rheumatic valvular disease in young

TABLE 32–5. Echocardiographic Findings in Preeclampsia

Author	Normal Pregnant Women	Women with PIH	p Value
EDD (mm)			
Kuzniar and colleagues[a]	51.4±2.2	49.2±3.4	0.01
Thompson and colleagues[b]	45±2.3	44±5.1	NS
Veille and colleagues[c]	50±4	48±4	NS
ESD (mm)			
Kuzniar and colleagues[a]	33.8±2.6	32.3±3.8	NS
Thompson and colleagues[b]	28.7±1.9	29.8±4.7	NS
EDV (mL)			
Kuzniar and colleagues[a]	128.5±14.4	115.2±18.8	0.01
ESV (mL)			
Kuzniar and colleagues[a]	46.9	42.5	NS
FS (%)			
Kuzniar and colleagues[a]	35±3	35±4	NS
Thompson and colleagues[b]	36±5	34±4	NS
Veille and colleagues[c]	32±4	37±7	<0.02
Ao-Root			
Easterling and colleagues[d]	25±0.2	27.3±1	0.01
LV Mass			
Thompson and colleagues[b]	147±12	157±16	<0.01
Veille and colleagues[c]	105±14	117±20	<0.05

Ao, aorta; EDD, end-diastolic dimension; EDV, end-diastolic volume; ESD, end-systolic dimension; ESV, end-systolic volume; EF, ejection fraction; FS, fractional shortening; LV, left ventricular; PIH, pregnancy-induced hypertension.
[a]Kuzniar J, Piela A, Skret A: *Am J Obstet Gynecol* 146:400-405, 1983 (25 normals, 42 PIH).
[b]Thompson JA, Hays PM, Sagar KB, Cruikshank DP: *Am J Obstet Gynecol* 155:994-999, 1986 (11 normals, 14 PIH).
[c]Veille JC, Hosenpud JD, Morton MJ: *Am J Obstet Gynecol* 150:443-449, 1984 (17 normals, 23 PIH).
[d]Easterling TR, Benedetti TJ, Schmucker BC, Carlson K, Millard SP: *Obstet Gynecol* 78:1073-1077, 1991 (89 normals, 9 PIH).

women is decreasing, whereas that of surgically treated congenital heart disease (CHD) with survival to adulthood is increasing.

Although the incidence of significant heart disease is low, suspected cardiac disease is a common reason for echocardiographic evaluation of pregnant women. The most common symptoms and signs prompting a suspicion of cardiac disease are (1) evaluation of a murmur; (2) evaluation of cardiac symptoms, such as congestive heart failure (CHF); and (3) a history of preexisting heart disease. It is important that the normal hemodynamic changes of pregnancy be distinguished from pathologic abnormalities when these patients are evaluated.

The echocardiographic diagnosis of significant heart disease in a pregnant woman can affect patient management in several ways.[61,64-66] First, the cardiac diagnosis may have important prognostic implications (morbidity and mortality) for both mother and fetus. Second, special or more intensive monitoring of the mother or fetus may be needed during pregnancy or in the peripartum period. Third, surgical or medical intervention may be needed either during or after pregnancy. Finally, the risk of CHD in the fetus may be increased, suggesting the need for fetal echocardiographic evaluation.

Pulmonary Vascular Disease

Elevated PA pressures may be the result of primary pulmonary hypertension, pulmonary emboli, chronic lung disease, left-sided heart disease or CHD with systemic to pulmonary shunting. Elevated pulmonary pressures of any cause are associated with poor maternal and fetal outcomes.

Initial concerns regarding the risk of pulmonary hypertension in pregnancy were raised by studies of women with Eisenmenger syndrome. Eisenmenger syndrome develops when a left-to-right shunt causes equalization of pulmonary and SVR resulting right-to-left shunting and cyanosis.[67] Women with Eisenmenger syndrome have cyanosis, arterial oxygen desaturation, and polycythemia. One of the largest single center studies reported 70 pregnancies in 44 women with a maternal mortality of 52%. Over half of pregnancies delivered prematurely and neonatal mortality was nearly 30%.[68] In a review of pulmonary vascular disease in pregnancy, 73 women with Eisenmenger syndrome had a maternal mortality of 36%, 27 with primary pulmonary hypertension had a mortality of 30%, and 25 with secondary pulmonary hypertension had a maternal mortality of 56%.[69] The neonatal survival was 88% in all groups with all maternal deaths occurring within 35 days after delivery. Effective therapies for these conditions during pregnancy are not currently available, although small case reports describe pregnancies in patients receiving epoprostenol, sildenafil, or nitric oxide.[70-74] Despite the appeal of novel pulmonary vasodilators, maternal death is nonetheless reported following pregnancy treated with these medications.[75-77]

Doppler echocardiographic measurement of pulmonary pressures allows identification of women with pulmonary hypertension, quantitation of disease severity, and evaluation of the response to therapy.[76,78] Doppler data is limited to assessment of pressures not vascular resistance and therefore may incompletely assess the extent of the underlying pathology.

Congenital Heart Disease

Acyanotic Patients with No Prior Surgical Procedures[80]

The most common congenital defect newly diagnosed during pregnancy is an atrial septal defect (ASD). These patients are usually asymptomatic but have a prominent "flow murmur" prompting a request for echocardiography. 2D echocardiographic and Doppler diagnosis of ASDs in pregnancy is straightforward (Fig 32–9). Contrast echocardiography is not needed for detection of significant interatrial shunt and should be avoided to minimize embolic risks. Given the increased CO and ventricular volumes of pregnancy, evaluation of the shunt ratio can be problematic in borderline cases (Fig. 32–10). At least in theory the decreased SVR of pregnancy might result in increased systemic blood flow without affecting pulmonary blood flow, decreasing the pulmonic to systemic shunt ratio, and underestimating the true magnitude of the ASD. However, accurate definition of the shunt ratio is not necessary during pregnancy because pregnancy is well tolerated if pulmonary pressures are normal, regardless of the size of the left-to-right shunt.[81]

Ventricular septal defects (VSD) in acyanotic adults are typically small and associated with a loud systolic murmur. On Doppler examination a high-velocity jet from left to right ventricle is seen with normal chamber dimensions and function. This lesion is also well tolerated, except for an increased risk of endocarditis, and further evaluation or treatment is rarely needed. Pregnancy does not significantly alter the echocardiographic findings. Large unrestrictive VSDs are uncommon in adulthood and almost always associated with Eisenmenger syndrome.

Occasionally, a patient with a previously undiagnosed patent ductus arteriosus becomes noticeable during pregnancy. The classic continuous machinery-like murmur may or may not be appreciated on auscultation if the murmur is soft. When a patent ductus arteriosus is not suspected a priori, the findings of left atrial or LV enlargement in excess of the expected changes of pregnancy, diastolic flow reversal in the descending thoracic aorta in the absence of significant aortic regurgitation or unexplained pulmonary hypertension should prompt a careful search for this possible diagnosis. On 2D imaging, the patent ductus is often difficult to visualize in adults, so that a directed Doppler examination is essential when this diagnosis is suspected. Diastolic flow reversal in the PA is seen with both color flow imaging and pulsed Doppler techniques. The hemodynamic impact of a patent ductus arteriosus is similar to that of a VSD and is also associated with Eisenmenger syndrome when large.

Other types of unoperated acyanotic CHD seen in pregnant patients include mild pulmonic stenosis and Ebstein's anomaly of the tricuspid valve. Both are well tolerated, provided there is no associated cyanosis.[82] Ebstein's anomaly may occur as an isolated anomaly with varying degrees of tricuspid regurgitation or may be associated with an ASD. The regurgitant jet may be directed at the atrial septum and in combination with impaired diastolic function may cause right-to-left shunting and cyanosis. In women with acyanotic Ebstein's anomaly, pregnancy is well tolerated.[83,84] Despite varying degrees of tricuspid regurgitation, no maternal deaths, strokes, heart failure (HF), or arrhythmias were reported in 111 pregnancies in 44 women with Ebstein's anomaly.[85]

Congenitally corrected transposition of the great arteries (CCTGA), also known as L-transposition with ventricular inversion (Fig. 32–11), is most often is associated with a normal physiologic pattern of blood flow through the heart and may first be recognized during pregnancy. Although there is physiologic blood flow through the heart, the anatomic right ventricle is the systemic ventricle, and the tricuspid valve is the systemic atrioventricular valve. Associated defects are common, including VSDs, pulmonic stenosis, complete heart block, and regurgitation of the systemic atrioventricular valve, at times the result of Ebstein's anomaly of the tricuspid valve.

Outcome during pregnancy depends on the associated defects and systemic ventricular function in patients with CCTGA. Published summaries in a total of 87 women with 118 pregnancies demonstrated a live birth rate of 83%.[82,86,87] Complications during pregnancy included congestive heart failure, increased cyanosis, endocarditis, stroke, and myocardial infarction (MI). Although there is little data regarding the fate of the systemic right ventricle following pregnancy in CCTGA, studies of the systemic right ventricle in patients with transposition of the great arteries corrected with an atrial level switch (Mustard or Senning repair) may provide some insight. A study with longitudinal echocardiographic data of 16 women with 24 pregnancies demonstrated decline in systemic RV dysfunction during pregnancy in four patients (25%) with return to baseline in only one of those patients.[88] Patients with systemic right ventricles, including CCTGA, should have echocardiographic assessment during and after pregnancy.

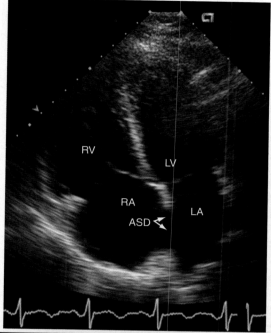

A

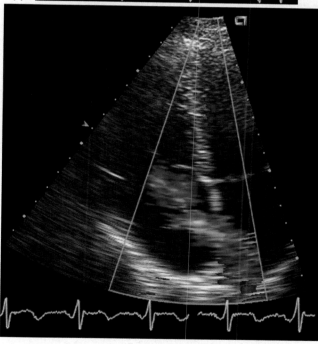

B

Figure 32–9. A G_1P_0 24-year-old woman at 14 weeks' gestation is referred for echocardiography in evaluation of palpitations and a murmur. Key findings from an apical four-chamber view included a secundum atrial septal defect (ASD) by two-dimensional (A) imaging, left to right shunt by color Doppler (B), and right ventricular and right atrial enlargement (A). Also found were normal pulmonary pressures, and a 1.8:1 estimated left to right shunt (see Figure 32–10 for method of shunt calculation). She was asymptomatic aside from the palpitations and went on to have an uneventful pregnancy with closure of her ASD via a percutaneous approach 4 months after delivery. LA, left atrium; LV, left ventricle; RA, right atrium; RV, right ventricle.

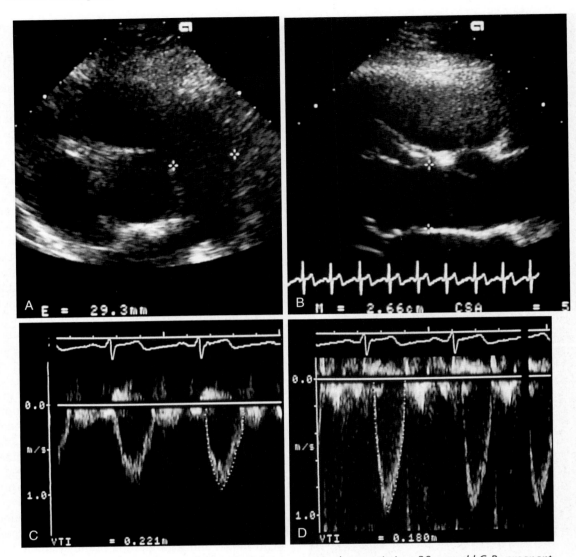

Figure 32–10. *Calculation of the pulmonic to systemic shunt ratio in a 26-year-old G_1P_0 pregnant woman with an atrial septal defect. The pulmonic flow rate is calculated as the product of the pulmonary artery (PA) cross-sectional area using a parasternal pulmonary artery diameter measurement (A) and the velocity time integral (VTI) in the pulmonary artery recorded with pulsed Doppler (C). Systemic flow is calculated as the product of the cross-sectional area of the left ventricular (LV) outflow tract using a parasternal long-axis diameter measurement (B), and the velocity time-integral in the left ventricular outflow tract recorded from an apical approach using pulsed Doppler (D). In this example, the calculated Qp/Qs was 1.5 to 1. Ao, aorta; LVOT, left ventricular outflow tract; RVOT, right ventricular outflow tract.*

Acyanotic Patients with Prior Surgical Procedures

As medical therapy and cardiac surgery for CHD have advanced, the number of patients reaching adulthood has markedly increased. The majority of patients with complex CHD will have had at least one surgical repair in childhood. Additionally, the favored surgical repair of certain defects, such as transposition of the great arteries, has evolved over time and results in different anatomy and physiology depending on the era in which the patient was repaired. When these patients become pregnant, echocardiographic evalua-

tion can detect any residual structural or functional cardiac abnormalities, evaluate for long-term complications of the surgical procedure, and optimize patient management during pregnancy and in the peripartum period. Data on maternal and fetal outcomes in these patient populations is based on case series, with many series including multiple congenital abnormalities. As a consequence, although our understanding of pregnancy in CHD is increasing, recommendations based on large clinical trials are not available and recommendations must be tailored on an individual basis.

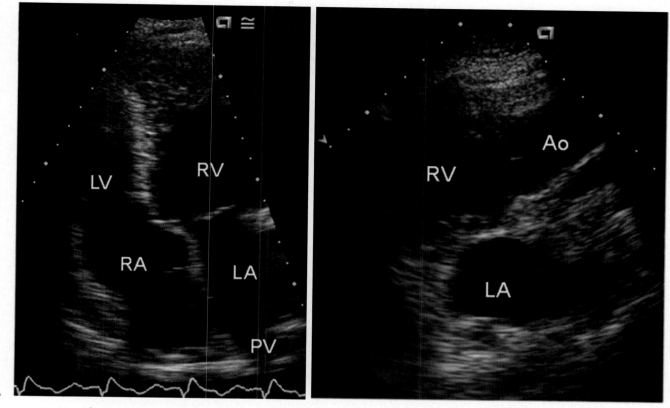

Figure 32–11. *A 34-year old G₃P₃ woman with a history of congenitally corrected transposition of the great vessels returns for routine follow-up. Her pregnancies had all been uneventful, and she has done well since her last delivery 2 years ago with minimal decrease in ventricular function. She required a pacemaker for complete heart block 1 year ago. On echocardiography, apical views demonstrate a hypertrophied anatomic right ventricle that is rightward of the anatomic left ventricle (A). An anterior aorta, typical of transposition of the great vessels is seen on parasternal images (B). Ao, aorta; AV, aortic valve: LA, left atrium; LV, left ventricle; PV, pulmonary vein; RA, right atrium; RV, right ventricle.*

In patients with previous surgical procedures that completely correct the congenital abnormality, outcome in pregnancy is similar to that in normal women. For example, closure of an uncomplicated ASD, VSD, or patent ductus arteriosus ligation often result in normal cardiac anatomy and function, with a corresponding normal echocardiographic examination.[81] When mild abnormalities remain after corrective surgery for CHD, maternal outcome is also likely to be similar to that in women without heart disease, with the proviso that the echocardiographic examination should be directed toward potential residual abnormalities or late complications. With complex CHD and palliative or partially corrective surgical procedures, residual or recurrent anatomic/functional cardiac abnormalities occur commonly, resulting in an increased maternal risk. Echocardiographic evaluation is especially valuable in these patients both before pregnancy to assess the potential risk and during pregnancy to monitor cardiovascular function. In pregnant patients with complex CHD, arrhythmias are a frequent cause of morbidity and mortality.[89]

Tetralogy of Fallot. Patients with surgical repair of tetralogy of Fallot (TOF) often have pulmonary insufficiency, recurrent or residual right ventricular outflow tract (RVOT) obstruction, VSD, or aneurysm of the right ventricular outflow tract[90] (Fig. 32–12). Multiple series of pregnancies in patients with TOF have been reported, and the two largest describe 92 women with 175 pregnancies. Cardiac complications included arrhythmias and symptomatic HF, which occurred in 8% of women and 4.5% of pregnancies.[91,92] There were no reported maternal deaths, but fetal complications included a high rate of spontaneous abortion. In one study, the risk of maternal and fetal complications was associated with LV dysfunction, severe pulmonary hypertension, and severe pulmonary insufficiency and RV dilation.[92]

An echocardiographic evaluation of LV size and function during pregnancy in patients with TOF followed 11 women with 17 pregnancies. An increase in LV end-diastolic diameter was noted in controls but not seen in patients with TOF. A progressive increase in the Tei index as the pregnancy progressed was seen in pa-

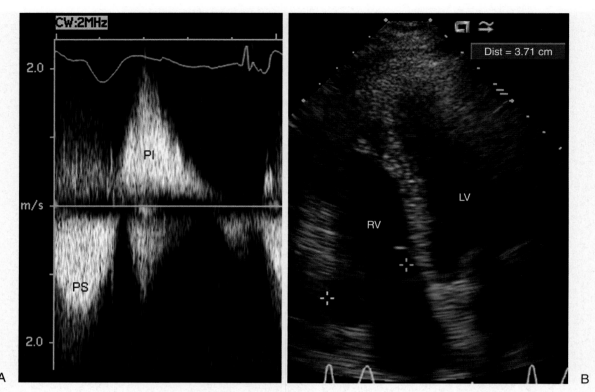

Figure 32–12. *A G_0P_0 25-year-old woman with tetralogy of Fallot presents for preconception counseling. She underwent initial Blalock-Taussig shunt palliation as an infant and subsequent complete repair with takedown of the Blalock-Taussig shunt at age 4. She is asymptomatic. An echocardiogram and cardiopulmonary exercise test are obtained. Key findings on echocardiography include significant pulmonary insufficiency (A), mild pulmonary stenosis (A), mild to moderate right ventricular enlargement (B), and normal biventricular[189] systolic function. Exercise testing demonstrated a mild reduction in exercise capacity. She was advised that pregnancy was likely to be well tolerated and regular reassessment of her cardiac status during pregnancy was recommended. LV, left ventricle; PI, pulmonary insufficiency; PS, pulmonary stenosis; RV, right ventricle.*

tients with TOF. Although this returned to normal postpartum, the progressive increase in Tei index was not seen in normal women.[93] This suggests some of the normal echocardiographic findings in women without heart disease may not manifest in patients with CHD.

Coarctation of the Aorta. Patients with a previous aortic coarctation repair may have residual or recurrent stenosis[94,95] (Fig. 32–13). Even in the absence of restenosis, these patients are at risk for late systemic hypertension, which may present initially as exercise-induced hypertension.[96] Women with a repaired coarctation and a residual gradient less than 20 mm Hg can have successful pregnancies with one study reporting 29 births for 36 pregnancies.[88] A study of 50 women with coarctation found no significant maternal cardiovascular complications in 118 pregnancies. Thirty percent of women were hypertensive during pregnancy, and of those, 75% had a hemodynamically significant coarctation. The rate of spontaneous abortion and preeclampsia was similar to that of the general population.[97] Both studies and other case reports suggest that

hypertension during pregnancy is more common and needs to be controlled. Additionally, aneurysm in the area of prior repair or in the ascending aorta can be seen in patients with coarctation. These patients represent a higher risk group and consideration to aneurysm repair before pregnancy may be warranted. Echocardiographic evaluation may be insufficient to fully evaluate for aortic aneurysm in these patients and other imaging modalities, such as magnetic resonance imaging (MRI) or computed tomography (CT) may be needed.[98]

Fontan Repair. Following the initial description by Fontan[99] of surgical atriopulmonary connection to alleviate cyanosis in tricuspid atresia, modifications of the original repair have evolved, as have the underlying defects treated with a Fontan type repair. The goal of the repair is to alleviate cyanosis in congenital defects that result in essentially single ventricle physiology. In this circulation, there is not a subpulmonic ventricle. Survival after Fontan repair is now 60% at 10 years, so that some women undergoing this procedure will reach

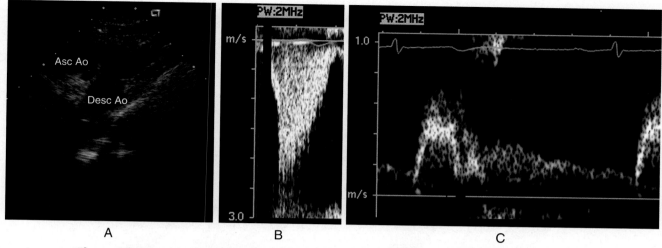

Figure 32–13. *A G₁P₀ 19-year-old woman underwent coarctation repair at age 6 months with subsequent repair of recoarctation at age 2 years. She has a known mild residual coarctation and is now 7 weeks pregnant. By clinical examination, her right arm blood pressure is normal and she has a 10 mm Hg gradient by blood pressure measurements in the arms and legs. Key findings on echocardiography include narrowing by two-dimensions in the aortic arch (A), a peak velocity by continuous-wave Doppler of 2.3 m/s (B), and evidence of diastolic runoff in the abdominal aorta (C). Continuous-wave Doppler is often an inaccurate measure of coarctation severity when using the Bernoulli equation; however the finding of continuous forward flow is a better predictor of coarctation severity.[190,191] Further evaluation with computed tomography or gadolinium magnetic resonance aortic imaging at 7 weeks gestation was not felt warranted, given the patient's normal blood pressure and attendant risks of radiation and gadolinium. She was followed closely during her pregnancy, and although her blood pressure and gradient increased minimally, fetal growth remained normal and she delivered a healthy girl by assisted vaginal delivery. Asc Ao, ascending aorta; Desc ao, descending aorta.*

childbearing age and may become pregnant.[89] Maternal survival has been documented, but fetal outcome is uncertain.[100] In a series of 33 pregnancies in women with a Fontan repair, there were only 15 (45%) live births, however, there were no significant maternal complications and no deaths.[101] Another study of 38 women with Fontan repair identified 6 women with 10 pregnancies. They found a 50% spontaneous abortion rate, and of the four completed pregnancies, 50% of women had cardiac complications during the pregnancy including atrial arrhythmias and decline in New York Heart Association (NYHA) class. Fetal outcome of the live births was uniformly complicated, with all live infants delivered prematurely or small for gestational age, and there was one neonatal death.[102]

Based on the limited data available, women with Fontan repairs may carry pregnancies to term. Maternal complications are generally related to supraventricular arrhythmias, especially in women with atriopulmonary anastomoses. However the high rate of fetal loss and neonatal complications should be considered when counseling these patients.

Transposition of the Great Arteries. Complete transposition of the great vessels (Fig. 32–14*A*) requires surgical repair in childhood for survival and resolution of cyanosis. Initial repairs redirected blood flow at the

atrial level, such that systemic venous return was directed to the left ventricle and then the PA and pulmonary venous return was directed to the right ventricle and then the aorta (see Fig. 44–2). In the early and mid 1960s, Mustard and Senning each described a different surgical approach to atrial level switch procedures that bear their names.[103,104] By redirecting blood flow at the atrial level, these repairs leave the morphologic right ventricle as the systemic ventricle.

Pregnancy in patients with a previous Mustard or Senning interatrial baffle repair (Fig. 32–15) for transposition of the great arteries has been reported in multiple series. The largest single series of 28 women with 69 pregnancies found a decline in NYHA class during pregnancy in approximately one third of pregnancies.[105] Multiple series have demonstrated a decline in systemic ventricular function that is permanent in some cases.[88,105,106] No maternal deaths were reported, but there was an increased rate of spontaneous abortion. In a study of asymptomatic patients who had excellent baseline prepregnancy functional status, none had significant maternal complications.[106] Specifically, none had significant baffle leaks or obstruction, significant systemic atrioventricular (AV) valve regurgitation, or systemic ventricular systolic dysfunction.

The available data suggests that in patients with significant functional cardiac abnormalities, maternal

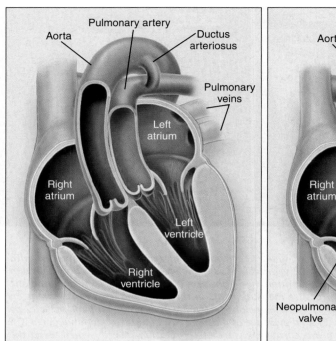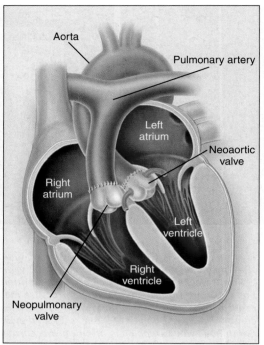

Figure 32–14. Sketches of complete transposition of the great vessels (A) and an arterial switch repair (B). (From Brickner EM, Hillis LD, Lange RA: New Engl J Med 342:334-342, 2000.)

outcome is dependent on the specific underlying abnormalities (e.g., patients with systemic ventricular dysfunction are at risk for HF during pregnancy). Thus echocardiographic evaluation is directed toward evaluation of the interatrial baffle (which may require transesophageal imaging), evaluation of systemic and venous ventricular function, detection and quantitation of systemic atrioventricular (tricuspid) valve regurgitation, and assessment of any other residual or acquired abnormalities.

Patients with transposition of the great arteries and VSD may undergo a Rastelli repair, which baffles LV flow to the aorta through the VSD and uses a RV to PA conduit.[107] There is little data on pregnancy in the setting of Rastelli repair of transposition of the great arteries, and a series of 6 patients reports a 50% incidence of progressive LVOT obstruction during pregnancy.[108] Echocardiographic evaluation of these patients must focus on LVOT obstruction, and dysfunction of the right ventricle to PA conduit.

Currently, the preferred correction of transposition of the great arteries is the arterial switch operation as described by Jatene[109] and later modified by LeCompte[109a] (see Fig. 32–14B). As this operation did not replace the Mustard and Senning repair until the early 1990s, the first patients with the arterial switch repair are just entering their reproductive years. Because the left ventricle is the systemic ventricle, the anticipated problems relate less to ventricular function than issues related to the surgical repair, including ostial coronary stenoses, supravalvular and branch pulmonary stenosis, and su-

praaortic stenosis. There is one case report of a successful pregnancy in a patient with an arterial switch repair.[110]

Cyanotic Heart Disease

Eisenmenger's physiology (Fig. 32–16) is characterized by equalization of pulmonary and systemic vascular pressures in association with a large systemic to pulmonary communication, such as a VSD or atrioventricular canal defect.[111] During pregnancy and in the peripartum period, the decrease in SVR, in the setting of irreversible pulmonary hypertension, can result in increased right-to-left shunting and decreased pulmonary blood flow, with subsequent cardiovascular collapse resulting from hypoxia and hypotension.[112,113] Death usually occurs in the peripartum period including cases reported 3 to 4 weeks postpartum. Maternal mortality is extremely high (between 30% and 70% in different series) and only 15% of infants are born at term, so pregnancy should be avoided in these patients.[67,114]

PA systolic pressure may be difficult to estimate in patients with Eisenmenger physiology as a result of inadequate tricuspid regurgitation jet. The presence of pulmonary hypertension must therefore be inferred from findings of a large, nonrestrictive intracardiac communication or large systemic artery to PA shunt, such as a patient ductus arteriosus, a short time to peak velocity in the PA, midsystolic notching on the pulmonic valve M-mode, and the pattern of ventricular

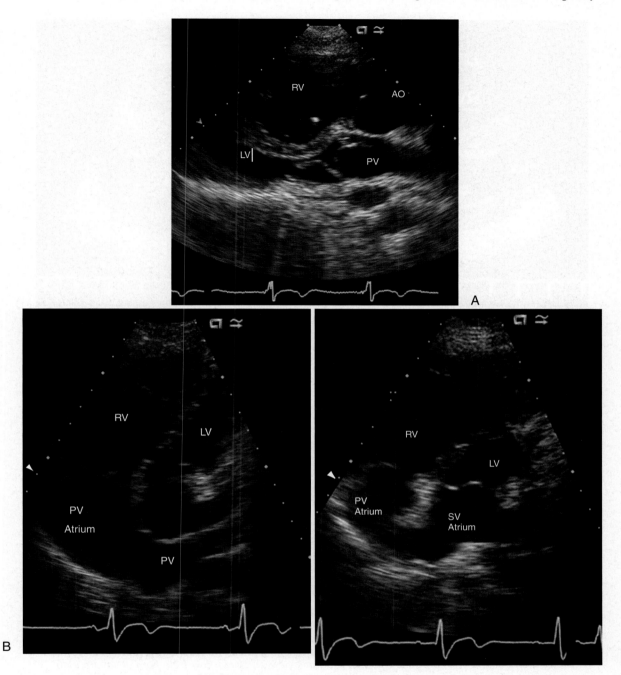

Figure 32–15. A 28-year-old woman G_2P_1 with a history of transposition of the great vessels who underwent a Mustard repair in infancy presents at 10 weeks' gestation. Before pregnancy she was asymptomatic with normal exercise tolerance. Echocardiography demonstrated significant right ventricular enlargement with mildly reduced systolic function. Longstanding well tolerated subpulmonic obstruction, in part as a result systolic anterior motion of the mitral apparatus was evident in parasternal views (A). The systemic and pulmonary venous return were unobstructed by two-dimensional (B and C), color-flow, and pulsed-wave Doppler. No baffle leaks were identified. Longstanding mild tricuspid regurgitation was present. Her pregnancy was uneventful, and she delivered a healthy girl by an assisted vaginal delivery. Ventricular function remained unchanged following delivery. AO, aorta; LV, left ventricle; PV, pulmonary vein; RV, right ventricle; SV, systemic ventricle.

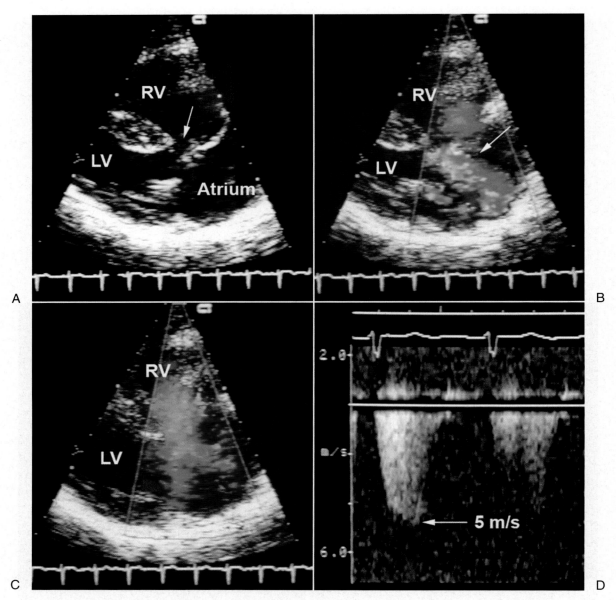

Figure 32–16. *Endocardial cushion defect with a large ventricular septal defect, atrial septal defect, and Eisenmenger's physiology in a 19-year-old G_1P_0 pregnant woman with no previous cardiac diagnosis. A modified four-chamber view (A) shows the atrial and ventricular septal defects (arrow) and the common atrioventricular valve. Color flow imaging (B) shows severe atrioventricular valve regurgitation (arrow). A diastolic frame in the same view (C) shows flow from both atria into both ventricles. The tricuspid regurgitant jet velocity (D) is elevated to 5 m/s, confirming severe pulmonary hypertension. Despite relatively stable hemodynamics during pregnancy and delivery with careful hemodynamic monitoring, the patient had abrupt hemodynamic collapse 48 hours postpartum and died. LV, left ventricle; RV, right ventricle.*

septal motion. If severe pulmonary hypertension is not clearly established, other confirmatory diagnostic tests should be considered in view of the grave prognosis associated with this condition. Rarely, a patient with previously unevaluated CHD is diagnosed during pregnancy with Eisenmenger's physiology.

Cyanotic CHD without Eisenmenger's physiology also connotes high maternal mortality and morbidity.[112,113,115] In 822 pregnancies in 416 cyanotic women, the rate of maternal cardiovascular complications was 32%, with one maternal death. Fetal outcome was also suboptimal; only 43% of pregnancies resulted in live births, 37% of which were premature. Factors that predict a poor outcome include functional status before pregnancy, arterial oxygen saturation, and blood hemoglobin. Other studies suggest that maternal outcome is also strongly related to the degree of RV pressure overload.[116,117] Thus echocardiographic evaluation should include estimates of pulmonary systolic pressure and definition of the anatomic abnormalities and ventricular function.

For CHD with decreased pulmonary blood flow that cannot be physiologically repaired, palliative shunts to increase pulmonary blood flow are often used. These patients are cyanotic resulting from intracardiac shunting and decreased pulmonary blood flow, rather than from pulmonary hypertension and Eisenmenger syndrome. Little data exists on pregnancy in these patients, however in a series of 41 pregnancies in 15 women with cyanosis after partial repair for complex pulmonary atresia, there were only eight healthy children. Although there were no maternal deaths in this series or in a smaller study, maternal complications were high including pulmonary embolism, HF, and arrhythmias.[102,103,116,117]

Valvular Heart Disease in the Pregnant Patient

Valvular Stenosis

In a pregnant patient, stenosis of a semilunar valve is usually the result of a congenitally abnormal valve.[104] Mild to moderate stenosis of the pulmonic valve is well tolerated, whereas severe pulmonic stenosis is rare in adults. In contrast to patients with pulmonic valve stenosis, those with aortic valve stenosis, even if asymptomatic before pregnancy, may decompensate during pregnancy. In clinical series, the majority of pregnant patients with AS have bicuspid valves.[118] Patients with a previous surgical commissurotomy may have significant restenosis[119]; one study estimated that about 20% of such patients require reoperation at a mean interval of 13 (range 3 to 26) years after the initial procedure.[120] Thus depending on the patient's age at the initial commissurotomy, restenosis may be diagnosed during pregnancy.

As SV increases across the stenotic valve with pregnancy, an increase in the pressure gradient measured by Doppler echocardiography is seen. Calculation of valve area with the continuity equation still provides accurate assessment of stenosis severity (Fig. 32–17). Some patients may become symptomatic during pregnancy as a result of increased metabolic demands in the setting of a limited ability to increase SV across the valve.[119,121] These patients may develop angina or dyspnea during pregnancy even though they were asymptomatic before pregnancy. Reduced diastolic ventricular compliance secondary to left ventricular hypertrophy can also lead to congestive heart failure. Even when patients with AS remain physiologically compensated during pregnancy, any superimposed hemodynamic alteration can lead to acute decompensation. For example, the high CO and HR associated with an infection or anemia may result in acute pulmonary edema resulting from a combination of an increased valve gradient and a shortened diastolic filling time.

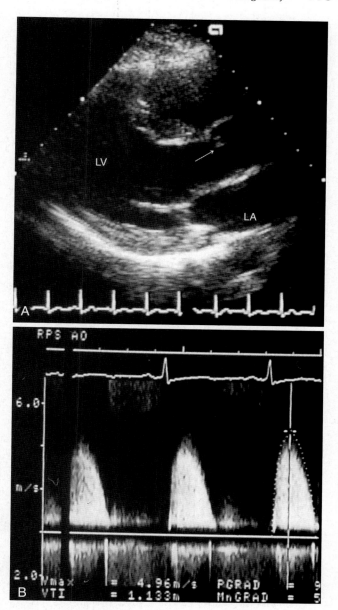

Figure 32–17. Aortic valvular aortic stenosis in a 25-year-old G_1P_0 pregnant woman who underwent an aortic valve commissurotomy 10 years previously. The parasternal long-axis view shows a congenitally abnormal aortic valve (arrow) with reduced systolic opening. The maximum jet across the aortic valve, recorded with continuous-wave Doppler from a high right parasternal position, shows a maximum velocity of 5 m/s. There was mild to moderate coexisting aortic regurgitation. Aortic valve area, calculated by the continuity equation, was 1 cm^2. This patient was managed with placement of a pulmonary artery catheter and arterial line at the time of delivery. Because of fetal presentation, she underwent a cesarean section with epidural anesthesia, which was tolerated well.

The role of echocardiography in pregnant patients with AS is to accurately delineate disease severity so that monitoring and therapy during pregnancy and in the peripartum period can be optimized (Fig. 32–18). In some patients the severity of stenosis may worsen during pregnancy, possibly related to the hormonal and metabolic changes. Most pregnant women with AS can be managed medically, but balloon aortic valvuloplasty or valve replacement during pregnancy has been required in rare cases.[121-125] A series of 39 patients with 49 pregnancies divided groups based on stenosis severity. The mild to moderate stenosis group had no maternal complications, whereas pulmonary edema or arrhythmias occurred in 10% of pregnancies complicated severe AS. Interestingly, fetal complications, such as small for gestational age and prematurity, were found in both groups of patients, but more often in the mild to moderate stenosis group. Patients with severe stenosis were more likely to require valve replacement in the peripartum period than those with mild-moderate AS.[118]

Rheumatic mitral valve stenosis is often diagnosed during pregnancy (Fig. 32-19). If mitral stenosis (MS) is moderate in severity or if disease progression has been gradual, the patient may not have noted symptoms or exercise limitation before the pregnancy. Early in pregnancy the increased transmitral volume flow rate and the shortened diastolic filling time resulting from the increase in HR result in further elevation of left atrial pressures. This may result in pulmonary edema, depending on the severity of mitral valve obstruction. Because it is often difficult to appreciate the diastolic murmur of MS in pregnant dyspneic patients, MS should be considered in the differential diagnosis of all pregnant patients with HF or pulmonary congestion. Echocardiography reliably differentiates MS from other causes of HF (e.g., cardiomyopathy or diastolic dysfunction) and will distinguish cardiac from noncardiac causes of respiratory distress. Echocardiographic measures of MS severity, including 2D valve area, Doppler gradients, and pressure half-time (PHT) valve area, remain valid in pregnancy, so that echocardiographic evaluation allows optimization of patient monitoring and therapy.

Usually, patients can be managed medically during pregnancy using beta-blockers to improve diastolic filling, even with severe MS, although decompensation may require invasive monitoring in an intensive care unit setting.[126] In some severe cases, maternal or fetal complications may necessitate mechanical relief of stenosis during pregnancy, preferably with percutaneous balloon valvuloplasty.[127,128] Concerns regarding balloon angioplasty and pregnancy include both maternal risks of the procedure and the effects of radiation exposure on the fetus. One group reported 5-year follow-up of 22 women who underwent valvuloplasty during pregnancy at a mean gestation of 25 weeks. They demonstrated excellent maternal outcomes and

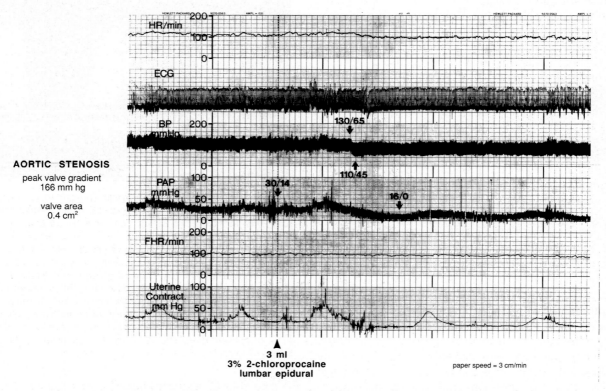

Figure 32-18. Hemodynamic responses in a patient with severe valvular aortic stenosis showing increased vascular return associated with uterine contractions. BP, blood pressure; ECG, electrocardiogram; FHR, fetal heart rate; HR, heart rate; PAP, pulmonary artery pressure. (From Easterling TR, Chadwick HS, Otto CM, Benedetti TJ: Obstet Gynecol 72:113-118, 1988. Reprinted with permission from The American College of Obstetricians and Gynecologists.)

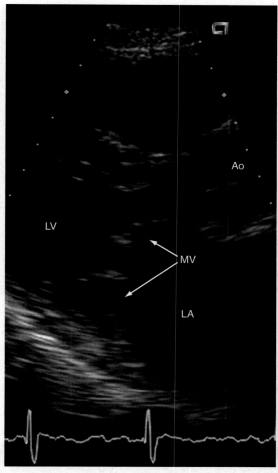

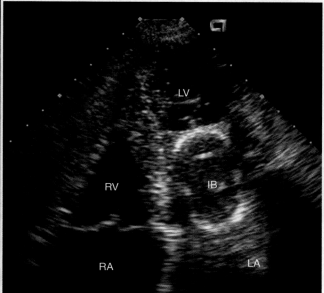

Figure 32–19. *A 35-year-old G_2P_1 woman presented with respiratory distress at 26 weeks' gestation. She was found to be in atrial fibrillation and echocardiography demonstrated severe rheumatic mitral stenosis. Two-dimensional imaging is shown from a parasternal view (A). Despite efforts at medical stabilization, she remained in pulmonary edema. Balloon mitral valvuloplasty was performed using an Inoue balloon, seen from an apical view (B), and she symptomatically improved. She delivered at 35 weeks and required intravenous diuretics in the 48 hours after delivery to alleviate pulmonary edema. She subsequently recovered uneventfully. Ao, aorta; IB, Inoue balloon; LA, left atrium; LV, left ventricle; RA, right atrium; RV, right ventricle.*

no evidence of any clinical abnormalities in the children.[129] Echocardiography clearly plays a valuable role in assessing the likelihood of complications and the expected result of percutaneous mitral valvuloplasty.[130-132] Echocardiographic monitoring also minimizes fluoroscopy time.[133,134]

Valvular Regurgitation

Pathologic valvular regurgitation in pregnancy may be the result of a congenital abnormality (bicuspid aortic valve), previous bacterial endocarditis, rheumatic disease, or myxomatous valve disease (Fig. 32–20) or may be associated with more complex CHD (Fig. 32–21). Standard 2D and Doppler echocardiographic methods for detection and evaluation of valvular regurgitation are applicable in the pregnant patient. Physiologically, it is plausible that pregnancy may result in a decrease in regurgitant severity as a result the pregnancy related afterload reduction. This potentially beneficial physiologic effect may be counterbalanced, to some extent, by the hormonal and vascular changes of pregnancy. Increased aortic root dimensions may increase aortic re-

gurgitant severity, whereas increased laxity of valve tissues may lead to an increase in mitral regurgitant severity.

Valvular regurgitation is well tolerated during pregnancy by some patients. Others develop signs and symptoms of congestive heart failure with pulmonary congestion, decreased exercise tolerance, orthopnea, and paroxysmal nocturnal dyspnea. Decompensation can occur in patients with chronic valvular regurgitation because of either (1) the increased CO demands of pregnancy or (2) worsening of the underlying valvular abnormality (e.g., chordal rupture in a patient with myxomatous mitral valve disease). Echocardiographic evaluation can distinguish between these possibilities and optimize therapy in the decompensated patient.

Quantitation of valvular regurgitant severity and evaluation of LV systolic function may be confounded by the anatomic and hemodynamic changes of pregnancy. In patients with severe AR or mitral regurgitation (MR), decreased SVR resulting from pregnancy can result in an apparent decrease in regurgitant severity and improvement in LV systolic function. In these patients, surgical intervention may be inappropriately

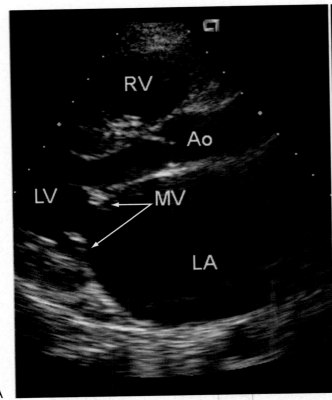

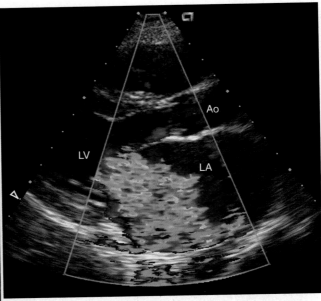

Figure 32–20. *A 34-year-old G₃P₂ woman presented at 28 weeks' gestation with dyspnea with minimal exertion. Failure of coaptation is seen on two-dimensional imaging (A) and color Doppler shows severe mitral regurgitation (B). She was managed with diuretics and bedrest and delivered a healthy baby boy. After delivery she underwent mitral valve repair. Ao, aorta; LA, left atrium; LV, left ventricle; MV, mitral valve; RV, right ventricle.*

Figure 32–21. *Cleft mitral valve and atrial septal defect in a pregnant patient with a cardiac murmur. A modified four-chamber view (A) shows the atrial septal defect in an ostium primum position (arrow), with color flow imaging (C) showing a prominent flow stream across this region. A parasternal short-axis view (B) shows a cleft anterior mitral valve leaflet (arrows), and color flow imaging in a long-axis view (D) shows mild to moderate mitral regurgitation. Ao, aorta; LA, left atrium; LV, left ventricle; RV, right ventricle; RA, right atrium.*

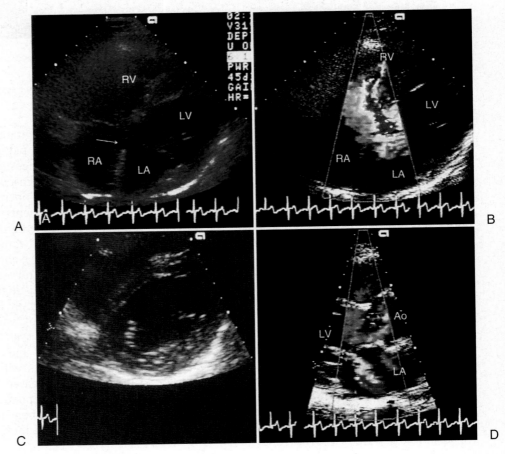

delayed. Conversely, LV dimensions may be slightly larger than in the nonpregnant state, resulting in misdiagnosis in a patient with only moderate regurgitation. In either case, postpartum reevaluation of regurgitant severity and ventricular function will provide accurate data for clinical decision making.

Prosthetic Heart Valves

The outcome of pregnancy is significantly affected by the presence of a prosthetic heart valve.[135-138] With mechanical valves, the risks of valve thrombosis (8% to 9%), embolic events (3% to 5%), serious bleeding (5%), HF (28%), and maternal death (4% to 8%) are high,[139] even with careful monitoring of anticoagulation. With a bioprosthetic valve, there is less risk of maternal death (0% to 5%), but accelerated valve degeneration during pregnancy may occur and results in a high rate of HF (35%) and urgent repeat replacement of the valve in the early postpartum period (35%).[136] The effect of pregnancy in accelerating valve degeneration is controversial. Initial studies made the observation that women with prosthetic heart valves and more than one pregnancy have a lower 10-year graft survival rate for bioprosthetic valves (17%) than women with only one pregnancy (55%).[140] However, another study demonstrated no change in durability of bovine pericardial valves in women who bore children compared with a population that did not.[141] An evaluation of women who underwent pulmonary allograft replacement in the setting of a Ross repair for aortic valve disease did not demonstrate valvular degeneration of the pulmonic allograft.[142]

Echocardiography plays a critical role in identifying valve dysfunction and in assessing valve degeneration during pregnancy (Fig. 32–22). Assessment of prosthetic valves in women who are pregnant may be confounded by the normal hemodynamic changes of pregnancy. The increased HR and SV affect Doppler evaluation of velocities and pressure gradients across prosthetic valves. Thus the volume flow rate should be taken into consideration when evaluating prosthetic valves in pregnant women. The alterations in loading conditions may also affect the accuracy of the pressure half-time method.[143] Ideally, a baseline Doppler echocardiographic study in the prepartum period or early in pregnancy can be used to accurately assess changes later in pregnancy.

Cardiomyopathies in the Pregnant Patient

The risk of pregnancy in a patient with a known cardiomyopathy is related to the severity of the underlying disease.[144] In familial types of cardiomyopathy, including hypertrophic (Fig. 32–23) and some forms

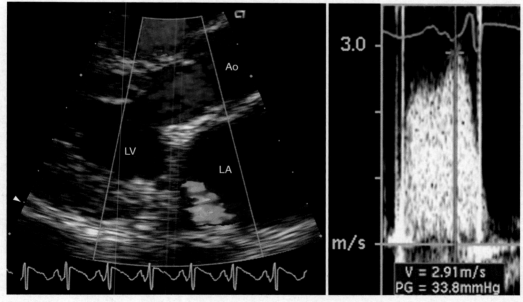

Figure 32–22. A 24-year-old G_1P_0 woman with a St. Jude's mitral prosthesis placed at age 20 presented at 12 weeks' gestation with dyspnea and exertional chest pain. Her anticoagulation had been subtherapeutic and echocardiography demonstrated more than the expected amount of mitral insufficiency (A) for this type of prosthesis by color Doppler and a peak gradient of 33 mm Hg and mean gradient of 20 mm Hg (B) by pulsed and continuous-wave Doppler. Despite aggressive anticoagulation and medical therapy, she did not improve. After discussion of the relative risks and benefits of thrombolytic therapy versus surgery, she was taken to the operating room for emergent valve replacement. She recovered uneventfully, however the fetus did not survive. A subsequent pregnancy managed with therapeutic anticoagulation was uneventful, and she delivered a healthy baby. Ao, aorta; LA, left atrium; LV, left ventricle; MR, mitral regurgitation.

of dilated cardiomyopathy, the genetic implications of the diagnosis also need to be taken into consideration. Echocardiography is used to confirm or exclude the diagnosis in patients considering pregnancy who are at risk for an inherited cardiomyopathy and to assess disease severity in patients with a known cardiomyopathy.[145]

Peripartum cardiomyopathy[144,146] was initially defined as HF presenting in the last month of pregnancy within 6 months of delivery, without other reason for cardiomyopathy.[147] More recently authors have suggested that the definition include LV dysfunction with an echocardiographic ejection fraction of less than 45%.[148] Others argue that the disease can be found earlier in pregnancy and that the "traditional" presentations represent a spectrum of disease that includes those patients with the earlier onset cardiomyopathy. The diagnosis typically is established by echocardiography in the appropriate clinical setting. Despite overall improvement in therapy of HF, the mortality of peripartum cardiomyopathy remains greater than 20%.[149] The

risk to women in subsequent pregnancies is high, particularly if the ejection fraction did not return to normal (Fig. 32–24). Echocardiographic monitoring of disease severity, especially LV systolic function, helps optimize patient management.

Pregnancy in patients after cardiac transplantation has described.[150,151] In one series of 29 organ recipients (26 heart and 3 heart-lung), 21% of women experienced a rejection episode during pregnancy, although only 3% had graft loss within 2 years of delivery. Fetal outcomes were notable for an 18% spontaneous abortion rate, higher than expected in the general population. Of liveborn infants, 40% were premature and 40% were low birthweight.[152] As medical therapy for transplant patients evolves and the population requiring transplant includes more young women as a result of the increase in adults with CHD, one would expect an increase in the number of women bearing children following cardiac transplantation. Echocardiography can be used to evaluate for evidence of rejection during and after pregnancy.

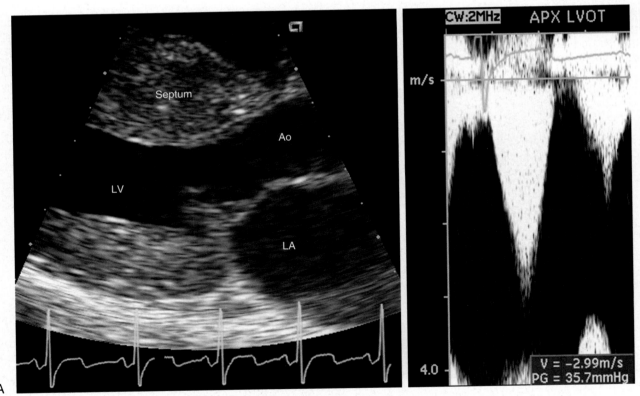

Figure 32–23. *A 21-year-old G_1P_0 woman with hypertrophic cardiomyopathy was seen throughout pregnancy. Before pregnancy, she had minimal symptoms of chest pain and exertional dyspnea. Echocardiography demonstrated marked septal hypertrophy with posterior hypertrophy (A). Post-PVC peak gradient is approximately 3.0 m/s (B) and is stable from prior studies. Pulmonary pressures are normal. Her symptoms worsened during pregnancy but were controlled with diuretics and continued beta-blockers. She had an uneventful delivery and subsequently returned to her prepregnancy baseline. Ao, aorta; LA, left atrium; LV, left ventricle; PVC, premature ventricular contraction.*

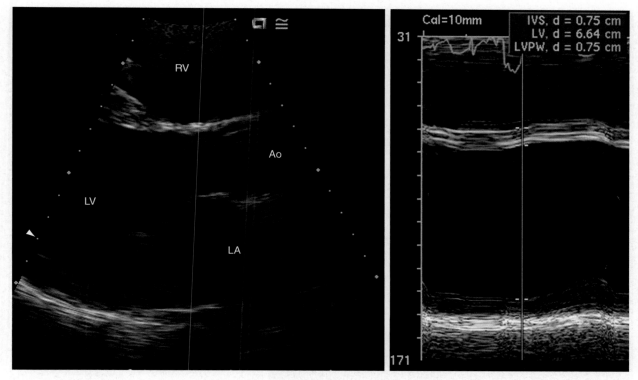

Figure 32–24. *A 32-year-old G_1P_1 woman with a history of peripartum cardiomyopathy returns to clinic for preconception counseling. She developed heart failure symptoms in the week following delivery and had marked ventricular enlargement and dysfunction. She was treated medically and improved to baseline New York Heart Association class II symptoms. Echocardiogram is shown with two-dimensional and M-mode demonstration of marked left ventricular enlargement with and left ventricular end-diastolic diameter of 6.6 cm. Ejection fraction was 32%. She was advised that pregnancy posed a significant risk of death or cardiac decompensation and elected not to pursue another pregnancy. Ao, aorta; LA, left atrium; LV, left ventricle; RV, right ventricle.*

Other Heart Diseases in Pregnancy

Marfan Syndrome

Pregnancy in patients with Marfan syndrome is associated with an increased risk of aortic dissection (Fig. 32–25). The mechanism of aortic dissection in pregnant women with Marfan syndrome presumably relates to (1) the underlying defect in aortic wall structure, (2) normal structural changes in the aortic wall with pregnancy, and (3) the increased SV and LV dP/dt of pregnancy. Gestational hypertension may further aggravate the risk of dissection.[153]

As is the case with many cardiac disorders in pregnancy, there are difficulties in gleaning appropriate care recommendations based on the available literature. Initial series suggested a high risk of dissection: Of 32 women with Marfan syndrome and at least one pregnancy, 20 (63%) suffered an acute aortic dissection and 16 (50%) died during pregnancy.[154] Subsequent series suggested a maternal mortality rate of only one percent, especially when aortic diameter is only mildly increased.[155-159] However, in a study of 91 pregnancies in 36 women with Marfan syndrome, 4 of 36 (11%) had dissection related to pregnancy and 2 others required aortic surgery following delivery for a total aortic complication rate of 17%.[160]

As in nonpregnant patients, risk of aortic dissection increases with the degree of aortic dilation. Several studies have demonstrated an increase in the risk of dissection in women with aortic diameter greater than 4 cm.[157,158] One study evaluated 61 women, of whom 23 had had 31 pregnancies with known aortic root dimensions,[159] in this group, there were no complications in women with aortic diameters of 25 to 45 mm, with the only complication in a woman with a prior dissection. In addition to absolute diameter, change in aortic size during pregnancy has also been identified as a risk for dissection. Some patients with Marfan syndrome suffer aortic dissection with only mildly increased aortic root dimensions,[160,161] although a case report describes a woman with an aortic diameter of 8 cm who did not dissect during pregnancy.[162]

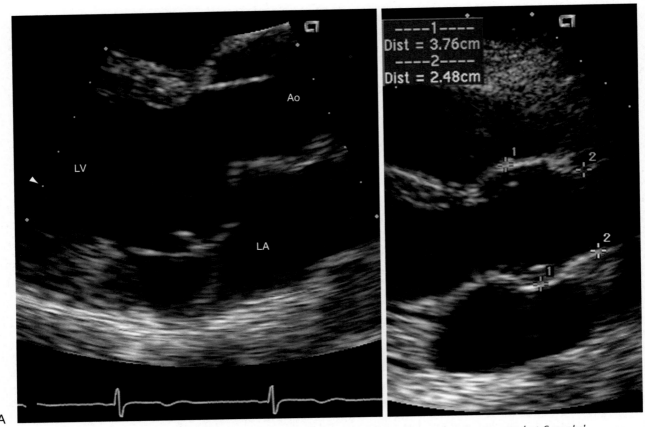

A

B

Figure 32–25. *A 23-year-old G₁P₀ woman with a history of Marfan syndrome presented at 6 weeks' gestation. She had a history of myxomatous mitral valve disease (A) without regurgitation and stable mild aortic enlargement with a maximal dimension of approximately 3.8 cm at the sinuses of Valsalva (B). She was followed through pregnancy with serial echocardiograms with stable aortic dimensions. She had an assisted vaginal delivery and delivered a healthy baby girl who was noted to have some features suggestive of Marfan syndrome. Ao, aorta; LA, left atrium; LV, left ventricle.*

Echocardiography is extremely valuable in the pre-conceptual assessment of women with Marfan syndrome, as several authors have recommended prophylactic aortic root replacement when pregnancy is planned, if aortic root dilation is present.[163,164] Echocardiographic monitoring during pregnancy allows risk stratification by assessing both initial aortic diameter and progression in size increase over time. With careful echocardiographic evaluation of aortic root dimensions and geometry, review of the patient's family history and consultation between the cardiologist and geneticist,[165] women with Marfan syndrome can be counseled about the potential risks before pregnancy, especially because the risk of dissection during pregnancy appears to be directly related to the degree of aortic root dilation. Treatment with beta-blocked[166,167] and careful peripartum anesthetic management[168] may improve the prognosis in pregnant patients with Marfan syndrome. Successful surgical repair during pregnancy of aortic dissection in Marfan syndrome has been reported.[169]

Aortic Dissection

There is an increased risk of aortic dissection during pregnancy, even in women without Marfan syndrome. Patients with connective tissue disorders, such as Ehlers-Danlos syndrome are at higher risk, as are women with bicuspid aortic valve and dilated aortic root,[157] Turner syndrome,[170] and severe hypertension. Echocardiography is often the initial diagnostic test requested in these patients. Prompt recognition and surgical intervention can be lifesaving.[171]

Ischemic Heart Disease

Acute coronary events and MI are rare in pregnancy, resulting from the low prevalence of coronary artery disease (CAD) in women of childbearing age. In women aged 15 to 44 years, the incidence of MI unrelated to pregnancy is 5 per 100,000 women years and the rate of cerebrovascular events is 10.7 per 100,000 women years.[172] However, coronary dissection and thromboembolic events are unusual causes of MI disproportionately represented in pregnancy. A literature review of 125 cases of MI in pregnancy found the highest incidence in multigravida women over age 33 years. MI tended to occur in the third trimester, often during labor and delivery.[173] Forty-three percent of the MIs were the result of atherosclerosis, 21% were thrombotic without evidence of underlying atherosclerosis, 16% were the result of coronary dissection, and in 29% coronary anatomy was normal, suggesting the possibility of coronary spasm.[172]

Another study identified 859 MIs related to pregnancy, which was a case event rate of 6.2 per 100,000. The case fatality rate was 5.1%, demonstrating that although rare, MI related to pregnancy carries a significant risk of mortality. In this study, classic risk factors for coronary artery disease, including hypertension, diabetes mellitus, and smoking, were significant risk factors. Additionally, the risk was 30 times higher for women older than 40 years of age compared with women younger than 20 years of age.[174] As women delay childbirth, the incidence of MI in pregnancy may rise.[175]

The usual criteria for MI apply in pregnancy and the purpureum, with the exception of myoglobin and creatinine kinase myocardial band (CK-MB), which may increase twofold in normal women within 30 minutes of delivery.[176] Troponin I is a more accurate marker in this setting. Segmental wall motion abnormalities on echocardiography should raise the possibility of ischemic heart disease.

Data regarding therapy of MI is limited during pregnancy. Thrombolytic therapy is contraindicated in pregnancy and the early postpartum period so the optimal clinical approach to revascularization is percutaneous balloon angioplasty with or without placement of an intracoronary stent, although coronary bypass grafting surgery during pregnancy also has been described.[177-180] The use of clopidogrel can complicate delivery, therefore stent selection is based on the anticipated delivery date and duration of clopidogrel therapy to protect from stent thrombosis.[181] Little is known about the risk of subsequent pregnancy for women with a pregnancy complicated by MI.

Echocardiographic Monitoring in Pregnant Patients

In addition to monitoring disease severity and cardiovascular hemodynamics in pregnant patients, both transthoracic echocardiography (TTE) and transesophageal[133] echocardiography (TEE) have been used to monitor diagnostic and therapeutic procedures. One of the advantages of echocardiographic monitoring during pregnancy is the avoidance of exposure to ionizing radiation. Echocardiographic monitoring in pregnant women has been reported for electrophysiologic testing,[140] pacer implantation,[182] and percutaneous balloon mitral valvuloplasty.[183]

Common Clinical Presentations during Pregnancy

Pulmonary Edema and Heart Failure in the Third Trimester and Peripartum Period

In the pregnant patient with acute respiratory distress, the initial differential diagnosis is cardiac and noncardiac causes, such as acute pulmonary embolism, pneumonia, or an acute viral syndrome. An echocardiographic study in these situations helps demonstrate normal cardiac anatomy and function, allowing attention to be focused on potential noncardiac causes of the illness. Conversely, a cardiac etiology can be quickly identified and evaluated, permitting appropriate therapeutic interventions.

Of the cardiac conditions presenting with pulmonary edema in the third trimester or in the peripartum period (Table 32–6), the most prevalent are mitral valve stenosis and peripartum cardiomyopathy. On physical examination the diastolic rumbling murmur of MS is difficult to appreciate and the patient herself is often unaware of a heart condition. The added hemodynamic burden of pregnancy may result in a previously asymptomatic patient being diagnosed with "sudden" and "unexplained" pulmonary edema. It is not unusual for the echocardiogram (ordered for other reasons) to be the first clue that valvular obstruction is present.

Peripartum cardiomyopathy may present with the insidious onset of HF symptoms or may be more abrupt in onset. In the latter case, it is likely that the patient has unrecognized HF symptoms that can be elicited in retrospect. The degree of LV systolic dysfunction is variable. Typically, clinical symptoms are first noted between 1 month ante-partum and 1 month postpartum.[144,184] Echocardiographically, peripartum cardiomyopathy is indistinguishable from other forms of dilated cardiomyopathy.

Evaluation of the Pregnant Patient with a Cardiac Murmur

A systolic murmur is a common finding during pregnancy, being reported in as many as 80% of women in some series.[185] This murmur typically is a "flow" murmur resulting from the increased volume flow rate of pregnancy. Depending on its location and timing, it most often originates from the pulmonic valve, al-

TABLE 32–6. Respiratory Distress in Pregnancy: Echocardiographic Differential Diagnosis

Pathophysiology	Examples
Cardiac	
↓ Left ventricular (or systemic ventricle) systolic function	Peripartum cardiomyopathy
	Congenital heart disease
	Dilated cardiomyopathy
Left ventricular diastolic function	Hypertension
	Aortic stenosis
Left ventricular pressure overload	Aortic stenosis
	Hypertension
Impaired cardiac filling	Mitral stenosis
	Pericardial disease
Left ventricular (or systemic ventricle) volume overload	Aortic regurgitation
	Mitral regurgitation
	Tricuspid regurgitation in systemic right ventricle
↓ Pulmonary blood flow	Eisenmenger's physiology
	Palliative systemic to pulmonary shunts
Noncardiac	
Capillary "leak"	Preeclampsia
	Adult respiratory distress syndrome
Infection	Pneumonia
	Viral syndrome
Pulmonary vascular obstruction	Pulmonary embolus

From Vered Z, Poler SM, Gibson P, et al: *Clin Cardiol* 14:327-334, 1991.

though some flow murmurs of pregnancy may be the result high flow across the aortic valve. With the normal murmur of pregnancy, Doppler echocardiography shows no abnormal flow patterns, although antegrade velocities are increased, as expected in pregnancy.

One study of 103 women with no previous cardiac history referred for evaluation of a murmur during pregnancy found that 79% had a benign murmur on physical examination, and all of these individuals had normal results on Doppler echocardiography.[185] Benign ejection murmurs were soft and midsystolic. Even in the 14% with a loud or long ejection murmur, most had normal Doppler study results, with abnormalities seen in only three patients (one mitral valve prolapse with mild mitral regurgitation, one nonobstructive hypertrophic cardiomyopathy, one bicuspid aortic valve). In contrast, in the 7% of patients with a pansystolic, late systolic, or diastolic murmur, all had abnormal echocardiographic results. This group included three VSDs, one large ASD, one ASD in conjunction with rheumatic mitral regurgitation, one mitral valve prolapse, and one nonobstructive hypertrophic cardiomyopathy.

Although it is likely that the prevalence of specific cardiac diagnoses will vary with the population, this series clearly demonstrates the importance of careful patient selection in requesting echocardiography for evaluation of a murmur in pregnancy. To minimize the inappropriate use of echocardiography in pregnant women, one approach is to limit echocardiographic evaluation to pregnant women with a murmur only if they have (1) a history of underlying heart disease, (2) definite cardiac symptoms, (3) a grade 3/6 or greater systolic murmur, or (4) a diastolic murmur. Use of these criteria will avoid unnecessary echocardiography.

Conversely, it is critically important to perform an echocardiographic examination in patients with pathologic or possibly pathologic murmurs. Many cases of previously undiagnosed CHD, valvular stenosis, and valvular regurgitation are recognized during pregnancy. In addition to the prognostic information obtained by having the correct cardiac diagnosis, the echocardiographic data resulted in significant changes in patient management. Such changes included recommendation of endocarditis prophylaxis at delivery for structural heart disease, surgical closure of an ASD postpartum, and genetic counseling in patients with inherited diseases in the study described previously.[185]

Like other clinical guidelines, these criteria are not absolute, and given the negligible risk of echocardiography, it is preferable to err on the side of performing echocardiographic studies in normal women than to miss a case of significant heart disease in a pregnant patient. When a pathologic murmur is present, it is incumbent on the echocardiographer to make sure the referring physician is aware of the significance of this finding and to ensure appropriate assessment of maternal and fetal risk. In view of the multidisciplinary nature of care for pregnant women with heart disease and the impact of maternal heart disease on both mother and fetus, referral to a maternal-fetal specialist in a high-risk obstetrics clinic is needed for optimal care, particularly in patients with hemodynamically significant lesions. This consideration also applies to non-pregnant women with heart disease in whom appropriate counseling regarding the risks of pregnancy and contraceptive options is needed either to avoid unnecessary anxiety and delay in starting a family (if the maternal-fetal risk is low) or to avoid a high-risk complicated pregnancy (when the maternal-fetal risk is high). The echocardiographer often initiates communication with the maternal-fetal specialist.

Mitral Valve Prolapse

Because a diagnosis of mitral valve prolapse is common in young women, concern is often raised that this diagnosis may affect the risk or management of pregnancy. Some series report a history of mitral valve prolapse in as many as 1.2% of all pregnancies.[186] No echocardiographic changes regarding the presence or degree of mitral prolapse[159] and no increase in maternal risk have been seen in pregnant patients with this diagnosis.[187,188] Many of these women have only minor abnormalities of leaflet anatomy or motion without significant valvular dysfunction. Thus echocardiography plays an important role in reassuring both patient and referring physician that the risk of pregnancy is not affected by this diagnosis and that the management of pregnancy and the peripartum period can be considered routine, other than the need for endocarditis prophylaxis. In the patient with significant functional mitral valve disease—myxomatous leaflets and mitral regurgitation—echocardiography allows assessment of the degree of regurgitation and the LV response to chronic volume overload.

Palpitations and Arrhythmias in Pregnancy

Most women experience an increased awareness of their heartbeat with occasional premature ventricular and atrial beats during pregnancy. Significant arrhythmias, associated with hypotension, dizziness, or shortness of breath, most often occur in patients with known underlying heart disease or a history of arrhythmias. The onset of symptomatic arrhythmia during pregnancy warrants echocardiographic evaluation, as in the nonpregnant patient, to evaluate for structural heart disease.

Limitations of Echocardiography and Alternative Approaches

Echocardiography often provides all the information needed for patient management in pregnant women with heart disease, but in some situations other diagnostic approaches or imaging modalities may be needed. If transthoracic imaging is inadequate because of poor ultrasound tissue penetration, transesophageal echocardiography is appropriate and can be safely performed during pregnancy. Other useful imaging procedures in patients with CHD and valvular heart disease include radionuclide ventriculography, magnetic resonance imaging, computed tomographic imaging, and angiographic evaluation in the catheterization laboratory. In pregnant patients the use of ionizing radiation with some of these techniques needs to be considered in the overall risk-benefit analysis of whether evaluation is needed during pregnancy or can be safely postponed to the postpartum period.

When direct and repeated measurements of pulmonary pressures, LV filling pressures, and CO are needed, invasive monitoring with an indwelling right-sided heart catheter is the procedure of choice. In patients with significant heart disease, invasive monitoring may be needed in the peripartum period to allow maintenance of optimal loading conditions under the changing volume and hemodynamic conditions of labor, delivery, and anesthesia.

Future Directions

Current data on the management of pregnancy in women with heart disease, particularly those with surgically treated CHD, are limited. The increasingly successful medical and surgical therapies for CHD, connective tissue disorders, HF, combined with an increasing number of women delaying pregnancy will likely increase the number of women for whom cardiac disease is a significant issue during pregnancy. It must be hoped that, if careful records of management and maternal-fetal outcome are kept the knowledge base will increase in this area. In any future studies, echocardiographic evaluation is likely to play a critical role in diagnosis, assessment of disease severity, and patient monitoring.

KEY POINTS

- Hemodynamic changes of pregnancy include increased CO, increased HR, decreased SVR, and increased blood volume.
- Normal echocardiographic changes of pregnancy include an increased LV end-diastolic dimension with preserved systolic dimension, slight increase in aortic and LVOT diameters, and increased left atrial size.
- The most common cardiac conditions seen in pregnancy are valvular heart disease and CHD.

■ Residual cardiac defects after surgical treatment of CHD may increase the risk of pregnancy including:

Severe pulmonary regurgitation in patients with TOF

Systemic ventricular systolic dysfunction after an interatrial baffle repair for transposition of the great arteries

■ There is a higher risk of maternal and fetal complications with pregnancy in patients with:

Eisenmenger syndrome or severe pulmonary hypertension

Severe left-sided valvular stenosis (AS or MS)

Decreased systemic ventricular function (ejection fraction <40%)

Cyanotic heart disease including palliated complex CHD and Fontan repairs

Mechanical valve prostheses

Marfan syndrome, especially with a dilated ascending aorta

■ Echocardiography before planned pregnancy is recommended in all women with CHD or valvular heart disease to assess prognosis, consider repair of any high risk lesions, and optimize medical management.

REFERENCES

1. Cole P, St. John Sutton M: Cardiovascular physiology in pregnancy. In: Douglas PS (ed): *Cardiovascular Health and Disease in Women*, Philadelphia, WB Saunders, 1993, pp. 305-328.
2. Capeless EL, Clapp JF: Cardiovascular changes in early phase of pregnancy. *Am J Obstet Gynecol* 161:1449-1453, 1989.
3. Edouard DA, Pannier BM, London GM, et al: Venous and arterial behavior during normal pregnancy. *Am J Physiol* 274: H1605-H1612, 1998.
4. Gilson GJ, Samaan S, Crawford MH, et al: Changes in hemodynamics, ventricular remodeling, and ventricular contractility during normal pregnancy: A longitudinal study. *Obstet Gynecol* 89:957-962, 1997.
5. Hunter S, Robson SC: Adaptation of the maternal heart in pregnancy. *Br Heart J* 68:540-543, 1992.
6. Mabie WC, DiSessa TG, Crocker LG, et al: A longitudinal study of cardiac output in normal human pregnancy. *Am J Obstet Gynecol* 170:849-856, 1994.
7. Easterling TR, Benedetti TJ: Measurement of cardiac output by impedance technique. *Am J Obstet Gynecol* 163:1104-1106, 1990.
8. Mesa A, Jessurun C, Hernandez A, et al: Left ventricular diastolic function in normal human pregnancy. *Circulation* 99:511-517, 1999.
9. Duvekot JJ, Cheriex EC, Pieters FA, et al: Early pregnancy changes in hemodynamics and volume homeostasis are consecutive adjustments triggered by a primary fall in systemic vascular tone. *Am J Obstet Gynecol* 169:1382-1392, 1993.
10. Soubassi L, Haidopoulos D, Sindos M, et al: Pregnancy outcome in women with pre-existing lupus nephritis. *J Obstet Gynaecol* 24:630-634, 2004.
11. Carbillon L, Challier JC, Uzan S: Hemodynamical changes on the maternal side of the placental circulation in normal and complicated pregnancies. *Placenta* 25:834, 2004.
12. Poppas A, Shroff SG, Korcarz CE, et al: Serial assessment of the cardiovascular system in normal pregnancy: Role of arterial compliance and pulsatile arterial load. *Circulation* 95:2407-2415, 1997.
13. Mone SM, Sanders SP, Colan SD: Control mechanisms for physiological hypertrophy of pregnancy. *Circulation* 94:667-672, 1996.
14. Geva T, Mauer MB, Striker L, et al: Effects of physiologic load of pregnancy on left ventricular contractility and remodeling. *Am Heart J* 133:53-59, 1997.
15. Robson SC, Hunter S, Boys RJ, et al: Serial changes in pulmonary haemodynamics during human pregnancy: A non-invasive study using Doppler echocardiography. *Clin Sci (Lond)* 80:113-117, 1991.
16. Clark SL, Cotton DB, Lee W, et al: Central hemodynamic assessment of normal term pregnancy. *Am J Obstet Gynecol* 161:1439-1442, 1989.
17. Otto CM: *Textbook of Clinical Echocardiography*, 2nd ed., Philadelphia, Saunders, 2000.
18. Easterling TR, Carlson KL, Schmucker BC, et al: Measurement of cardiac output in pregnancy by Doppler technique. *Am J Perinatol* 7:220-222, 1990.
19. Easterling TR, Benedetti TJ: Techniques differ in use of Doppler ultrasonography. *Am J Obstet Gynecol* 161:1748-1749, 1989.
19a. Lee W, Rokey K, Cotton DB: Noninvasive maternal stroke volume and cardiac output determinations by pulsed Doppler echocardiography. *Am J Obstet Gynecol* 158(3 Pt 1):505-510, 1988.
20. Easterling TR, Benedetti TJ, Schmucker BC, et al: Maternal hemodynamics and aortic diameter in normal and hypertensive pregnancies. *Obstet Gynecol* 78:1073-1077, 1991.
21. Sadaniantz A, Kocheril AG, Emaus SP, et al: Cardiovascular changes in pregnancy evaluated by two-dimensional and Doppler echocardiography. *J Am Soc Echocardiogr* 5:253-258, 1992.
22. Cotton DB, Lee W, Huhta JC, et al: Hemodynamic profile of severe pregnancy-induced hypertension. *Am J Obstet Gynecol* 158:523-529, 1988.
23. McLennan FM, Haites NE, Rawles JM: Stroke and minute distance in pregnancy: a longitudinal study using Doppler ultrasound. *Br J Obstet Gynaecol* 94:499-506, 1987.
24. Robson SC, Dunlop W, Moore M, et al: Combined Doppler and echocardiographic measurement of cardiac output: theory and application in pregnancy. *Br J Obstet Gynaecol* 94:1014-1027, 1987.
25. Robson SC, Hunter S, Boys RJ, et al: Hemodynamic changes during twin pregnancy. A Doppler and M-mode echocardiographic study. *Am J Obstet Gynecol* 161:1273-1278, 1989.
26. Robson SC, Boys RJ, Hunter S: Doppler echocardiographic estimation of cardiac output: analysis of temporal variability. *Eur Heart J* 9:313-318, 1988.
27. Rubler S, Schneebaum R, Hammer N: Systolic time intervals in pregnancy and the postpartum period. *Am Heart J* 86:182-188, 1973.
28. Robson SC, Hunter S, Moore M, et al: Haemodynamic changes during the puerperium: A Doppler and M-mode echocardiographic study. *Br J Obstet Gynaecol* 94:1028-1039, 1987.
29. Laird-Meeter K, van de Ley G, Bom TH, et al: Cardiocirculatory adjustments during pregnancy—an echocardiographic study. *Clin Cardiol* 2:328-332, 1979.
30. Easterling TR, Schmucker BC, Benedetti TJ: The hemodynamic effects of orthostatic stress during pregnancy. *Obstet Gynecol* 72:550-552, 1988.
31. Hart MV, Morton MJ, Hosenpud JD, et al: Aortic function during normal human pregnancy. *Am J Obstet Gynecol* 154:887-891, 1986.
32. Pouta AM, Rasanen JP, Airaksinen KE, et al: Changes in maternal heart dimensions and plasma atrial natriuretic peptide levels in the early puerperium of normal and pre-eclamptic pregnancies. *Br J Obstet Gynaecol* 103:988-992, 1996.

33. Campos O, Andrade JL, Bocanegra J, et al: Physiologic multivalvular regurgitation during pregnancy: A longitudinal Doppler echocardiographic study. *Int J Cardiol* 40:265-272, 1993.

34. Limacher MC, Ware JA, O'Meara ME, et al: Tricuspid regurgitation during pregnancy: two-dimensional and pulsed Doppler echocardiographic observations. *Am J Cardiol* 55:1059-1062, 1985.

35. Robson SC, Dunlop W, Boys RJ, et al: Cardiac output during labour. *Br Med J (Clin Res Ed)* 295:1169-1172, 1987.

36. Lee W, Rokey R, Miller J, et al: Maternal hemodynamic effects of uterine contractions by M-mode and pulsed-Doppler echocardiography. *Am J Obstet Gynecol* 161:974-977, 1989.

37. Strickland RA, Oliver WC, Jr, Chantigian RC, et al: Anesthesia, cardiopulmonary bypass, and the pregnant patient. *Mayo Clin Proc* 66:411-429, 1991.

38. Veille JC, Hellerstein HK, Bacevice AE Jr: Maternal left ventricular performance during bicycle exercise. *Am J Cardiol* 69:1506-1508, 1992.

39. Sady MA, Haydon BB, Sady SP, et al: Cardiovascular response to maximal cycle exercise during pregnancy and at two and seven months postpartum. *Am J Obstet Gynecol* 162:1181-1185, 1990.

40. Khodiguian N, Jaque-Fortunato SV, Wiswell RA, et al: A comparison of cross-sectional and longitudinal methods of assessing the influence of pregnancy on cardiac function during exercise. *Semin Perinatol* 20:232-241, 1996.

41. Pivarnik JM, Ayres NA, Mauer MB, et al: Effects of maternal aerobic fitness on cardiorespiratory responses to exercise. *Med Sci Sports Exerc* 25:993-998, 1993.

42. Pivarnik JM, Lee W, Clark SL, et al: Cardiac output responses of primigravid women during exercise determined by the direct Fick technique. *Obstet Gynecol* 75:954-959, 1990.

43. Van Hook JW, Gill P, Easterling TR, et al: The hemodynamic effects of isometric exercise during late normal pregnancy. *Am J Obstet Gynecol* 169:870-873, 1993.

44. Sibai BM, Mabie WC: Hemodynamics of preeclampsia. *Clin Perinatol* 18:727-747, 1991.

45. Guzman CA, Caplan R: Cardiorespiratory response to exercise during pregnancy. *Am J Obstet Gynecol* 108:600-605, 1970.

46. Wolfe LA, Preston RJ, Burggraf GW, et al: Effects of pregnancy and chronic exercise on maternal cardiac structure and function. *Can J Physiol Pharmacol* 77:909-917, 1999.

47. Easterling TR, Schmucker BC, Carlson KL, et al: Maternal hemodynamics in pregnancies complicated by hyperthyroidism. *Obstet Gynecol* 78:348-352, 1991.

48. Finley J, Katz M, Rojas-Perez M, et al: Cardiovascular consequences of beta-agonist tocolysis: An echocardiographic study. *Obstet Gynecol* 64:787-791, 1984.

49. Easterling TR, Carlson K, Benedetti TJ, et al: Hemodynamics associated with the diagnosis and treatment of pheochromocytoma in pregnancy. *Am J Perinatol* 9:464-466, 1992.

50. Veille JC, Hanson R: Left ventricular systolic and diastolic function in pregnant patients with sickle cell disease. *Am J Obstet Gynecol* 170:107-110, 1994.

51. Easterling TR, Brateng D, Goldman ML, et al: Renal vascular hypertension during pregnancy. *Obstet Gynecol* 78:921-925, 1991.

52. Roberts JM, Pearson G, Cutler J, et al: Summary of the NHLBI working group on research on hypertension during pregnancy. *Hypertension* 41:437-445, 2003.

53. Clinical Management Guidelines for Obstetrician-Gynecologists: Diagnosis and management of preeclampsia and eclampsia. *Obstet Gynecol* 99:159-167, 2002.

54. Bosio PM, McKenna PJ, Conroy R, et al: Maternal central hemodynamics in hypertensive disorders of pregnancy. *Obstet Gynecol* 94:978-984, 1999.

55. Broughton Pipkin F, Rubin PC: Pre-eclampsia—the 'disease of theories'. *Br Med Bull* 50:381-396, 1994.

56. Easterling TR: The maternal hemodynamics of preeclampsia. *Clin Obstet Gynecol* 35:375-386, 1992.

57. Easterling TR, Benedetti TJ, Schmucker BC, et al: Maternal hemodynamics in normal and preeclamptic pregnancies: a longitudinal study. *Obstet Gynecol* 76:1061-1069, 1990.

58. Easterling TR, Watts DH, Schmucker BC, et al: Measurement of cardiac output during pregnancy: validation of Doppler technique and clinical observations in preeclampsia. *Obstet Gynecol* 69:845-850, 1987.

59. Easterling TR, Benedetti TJ, Carlson KC, et al: The effect of maternal hemodynamics on fetal growth in hypertensive pregnancies. *Am J Obstet Gynecol* 165:902-906, 1991.

60. Easterling TR, Benedetti TJ, Schmucker BC, et al: Antihypertensive therapy in pregnancy directed by noninvasive hemodynamic monitoring. *Am J Perinatol* 6:86-89, 1989.

61. Easterling TR, Brateng D, Schmucker, et al: Prevention of preeclampsia: A randomized trial of atenolol in hyperdynamic patients before onset of hypertension. *Obstet Gynecol* 93:725-733, 1999.

62. Rutherford JD, Hands ME: Pregnancy with preexisting heart disease. In: Douglas PS (ed): *Cardiovascular Health and Disease in Women*, Philadelphia, WB Saunders, 1993, pp. 329-336.

63. Clark SL: Cardiac disease in pregnancy. *Crit Care Clin* 7:777-797, 1991.

64. Oakley CM: Cardiovascular disease in pregnancy. *Can J Cardiol* 6(Suppl B):3B-9B, 1990.

65. James KB: Heart disease arising during pregnancy. In Douglas PS (ed): *Cardiovascular health and disease in women*, Philadelphia, WB Saunders, 1993, pp. 337-359.

66. Hess DB, Hess LW: Management of cardiovascular disease in pregnancy. *Obstet Gynecol Clin North Am* 19:679-695, 1992.

67. Vongpatanasin W, Brickner ME, Hillis LD, et al: The Eisenmenger syndrome in adults. *Ann Intern Med* 128:745-755, 1998.

68. Gleicher N, Midwall J, Hochberger D, et al: Eisenmenger's syndrome and pregnancy. *Obstet Gynecol Surv* 34:721-741, 1979.

69. Weiss BM, Zemp L, Seifert B, et al: Outcome of pulmonary vascular disease in pregnancy: A systematic overview from 1978 through 1996. *J Am Coll Cardiol* 31:1650-1657, 1998.

70. Bendayan D, Hod M, Oron G, et al: Pregnancy outcome in patients with pulmonary arterial hypertension receiving prostacyclin therapy. *Obstet Gynecol* 106:1206-1210, 2005.

71. Geohas C, McLaughlin VV: Successful management of pregnancy in a patient with Eisenmenger syndrome with epoprostenol. *Chest* 124:1170-1173, 2003.

72. Lacassie HJ, Germain AM, Valdes G, et al: Management of Eisenmenger syndrome in pregnancy with sildenafil and L-arginine. *Obstet Gynecol* 103:1118-1120, 2004.

73. Lam GK, Stafford RE, Thorp J, et al: Inhaled nitric oxide for primary pulmonary hypertension in pregnancy. *Obstetr Gynecol* 98:895-898, 2001.

74. Decoene C, Bourzoufi K, Moreau D, et al: Use of inhaled nitric oxide for emergency Cesarean section in a woman with unexpected primary pulmonary hypertension : [L'inhalation d'oxyde nitrique pour la cesarienne d'urgence associee a une hypertension pulmonaire primitive inattendue]. *Can J Anaesth* 48:584-587, 2001.

75. Monnery L, Nanson J, Charlton G: Primary pulmonary hypertension in pregnancy: A role for novel vasodilators. *Br J Anesth* 87:295-298, 2001.

76. Lust KM, Boots RJ, Dooris M, et al: Management of labor in Eisenmenger syndrome with inhaled nitric oxide. *Am J Obstet Gynecol* 181:419-423, 1999.

77. Goodwin TM, Gherman RB, Hameed A, et al: Favorable response of Eisenmenger syndrome to inhaled nitric oxide during pregnancy. *Am J Obstet Gynecol* 180:64-67, 1999.

78. Easterling TR, Ralph DD, Schmucker BC: Pulmonary hypertension in pregnancy: treatment with pulmonary vasodilators. *Obstet Gynecol* 93:494-498, 1999.

79. Pitkin RM, Perloff JK, Koos BJ, et al: Pregnancy and congenital heart disease. *Ann Intern Med* 112:445-454, 1990.

80. Zuber M, Gautschi N, Oechslin E, et al: Outcome of pregnancy in women with congenital shunt lesions. *Heart* 81:271-275, 1999.

81. Horvath KA, Burke RP, Collins JJ Jr, et al: Surgical treatment of adult atrial septal defect: early and long-term results. *J Am Coll Cardiol* 20:1156-1159, 1992.

82. Lundstrom U, Bull C, Wyse RK, et al: The natural and "unnatural" history of congenitally corrected transposition. *Am J Cardiol* 65:1222-1229, 1990.

83. Donnelly JE, Brown JM, Radford DJ: Pregnancy outcome and Ebstein's anomaly. *Br Heart J* 66:368-371, 1991.

84. Celermajer DS, Bull C, Till JA, et al: Ebstein's anomaly: presentation and outcome from fetus to adult. *J Am Coll Cardiol* 23:170-176, 1994.

85. Connolly HM, Warnes CA: Ebstein's anomaly: outcome of pregnancy. *J Am Coll Cardiol* 23:1194-1198, 1994.

86. Therrien J, Barnes I, Somerville J: Outcome of pregnancy in patients with congenitally corrected transposition of the great arteries. *Am J Cardiol* 84:820-824, 1999.

87. Connolly HM, Grogan M, Warnes CA: Pregnancy among women with congenitally corrected transposition of great arteries. *J Am Coll Cardiol* 33:1692-1695, 1999.

88. Guedes A, Mercier L-A, Leduc L, et al: Impact of pregnancy on the systemic right ventricle after a Mustard operation for transposition of the great arteries. *J Am Coll Cardiol* 44:433-437, 2004.

89. Driscoll DJ, Offord KP, Feldt RH, et al: Five- to fifteen-year follow-up after Fontan operation. *Circulation* 85:469-496, 1992.

90. Murphy JG, Gersh BJ, Mair DD, et al: Long-term outcome in patients undergoing surgical repair of tetralogy of Fallot. *N Engl J Med* 329:593-599, 1993.

91. Meijer JM, Pieper PG, Drenthen W, et al: Pregnancy, fertility, and recurrence risk in corrected tetralogy of Fallot. *Heart* 91:801-805, 2005.

92. Veldtman GR, Connolly HM, Grogan M, et al: Outcomes of pregnancy in women with tetralogy of fallot. *J Am Coll Cardiol* 44:174-180, 2004.

93. Hidaka Y, Akagi T, Himeno W, et al: Left ventricular performance during pregnancy in patients with repaired tetralogy of Fallot: Prospective evaluation using the Tei index. *Circ J* 67:682-686, 2003.

94. Kupferminc MJ, Lessing JB, Jaffa A, et al: Fetomaternal blood flow measurements and management of combined coarctation and aneurysm of the thoracic aorta in pregnancy. *Acta Obstet Gynecol Scand* 72:398-402, 1993.

95. Cohen M, Fuster V, Steele PM, et al: Coarctation of the aorta. Long-term follow-up and prediction of outcome after surgical correction. *Circulation* 80:840-845, 1989.

96. Kimball TR, Reynolds JM, Mays WA, et al: Persistent hyperdynamic cardiovascular state at rest and during exercise in children after successful repair of coarctation of the aorta. *J Am Coll Cardiol* 24:194-200, 1994.

97. Beauchesne LM, Connolly HM, Ammash NM, et al: Coarctation of the aorta: Outcome of pregnancy. *J Am Coll Cardiol* 38:1728-1733, 2001.

98. Therrien J, Thorne SA, Wright A, et al: Repaired coarctation: a cost-effective approach to identify complications in adults. *J Am Coll Cardiol* 35:997-1002, 2000.

99. Fontan F, Baudet E: Surgical repair of tricuspid atresia. *Thorax* 26:240-248, 1971.

100. Hess DB, Hess LW, Heath BJ, et al: Pregnancy after Fontan repair of tricuspid atresia. *South Med J* 84:532-534, 1991.

101. Canobbio MM, Mair DD, van der Velde M, et al: Pregnancy outcomes after the Fontan repair. *J Am Coll Cardiol* 28:763-767, 1996.

102. Drenthen W, Pieper PG, Roos-Hesselink JW, et al: Pregnancy and delivery in women after Fontan palliation. *Heart* 92:1290-1294, 2006.

103. Mustard WT: Progress in the total correction of complete transposition of the great vessels. *Vasc Dis* 3:177-179, 1966.

104. Senning A: Surgical treatment of transposition of the great vessels. *Mal Cardiovasc* 6:421-433, 1965.

105. Drenthen W, Pieper PG, Ploeg M, et al: Risk of complications during pregnancy after Senning or Mustard (atrial) repair of complete transposition of the great arteries. *Eur Heart J* 26:2588-2595, 2005.

106. Genoni M, Jenni R, Hoerstrup SP, et al: Pregnancy after atrial repair for transposition of the great arteries. *Heart* 81:276-277, 1999.

107. Rastelli GC, McGoon DC, Wallace RB: Anatomic correction of transposition of the great arteries with ventricular septal defect and subpulmonary stenosis. *J Thorac Cardiovasc Surg* 58:545-552, 1969.

108. Radford DJ, Stafford G: Pregnancy and the Rastelli operation. *Aust N Z J Obstet Gynaecol* 45:243-247, 2005.

109. Jatene AD, Fontes VF, Paulista PP, et al: Anatomic correction of transposition of the great vessels. *J Thorac Cardiovasc Surg* 72:364-370, 1976.

109a. LeCompte Y, Zannini L, Hazan E, et al: Anatomic correction of the transposition of the great arteries. *J Thorac Cardiovasc Surg* 82(4):629-631, 1981.

110. Ploeg M, Drenthen W, van Dijk A, et al: Successful pregnancy after an arterial switch procedure for complete transposition of the great arteries. *Bjog* 113:243-244, 2006.

111. Hopkins WE, Waggoner AD: Right and left ventricular area and function determined by two-dimensional echocardiography in adults with the Eisenmenger syndrome from a variety of congenital anomalies. *Am J Cardiol* 72:90-94, 1993.

112. Presbitero P, Somerville J, Stone S, et al: Pregnancy in cyanotic congenital heart disease. Outcome of mother and fetus. *Circulation* 89:2673-2676, 1994.

113. Weiss BM, Atanassoff PG: Cyanotic congenital heart disease and pregnancy: Natural selection, pulmonary hypertension, and anesthesia. *J Clin Anesth* 5:332-341, 1993.

114. Yentis SM, Steer PJ, Plaat F. Eisenmenger's syndrome in pregnancy: Maternal and fetal mortality in the 1990s. *Br J Obstet Gynaecol* 105:921-922, 1998.

115. Caruso A, de Carolis S, Ferrazzani S, et al: Pregnancy outcome in women with cardiac valve prosthesis. *Eur J Obstet Gynecol Reprod Biol* 54:7-11, 1994.

116. Neumayer U, Somerville J: Outcome of pregnancies in patients with complex pulmonary atresia. *Heart* 78:16-21, 1997.

117. Connolly HM, Warnes CA: Outcome of pregnancy in patients with complex pulmonic valve atresia. *Am J Cardiol* 79:519-521, 1997.

118. Silversides CK, Colman JM, Sermer M, et al: Early and intermediate-term outcomes of pregnancy with congenital aortic stenosis. *Am J Cardiol* 91:1386-1389, 2003.

119. Lao TT, Sermer M, MaGee L, et al: Congenital aortic stenosis and pregnancy—a reappraisal. *Am J Obstet Gynecol* 169:540-545, 1993.

120. Horstkotte D, Loogen F: The natural history of aortic valve stenosis. *Eur Heart J* 9(Suppl E):57-64, 1988.

121. Easterling TR, Chadwick HS, Otto CM, et al: Aortic stenosis in pregnancy. *Obstet Gynecol* 72:113-118, 1988.

122. Lao TT, Adelman AG, Sermer M, et al: Balloon valvuloplasty for congenital aortic stenosis in pregnancy. *Br J Obstet Gynaecol* 100:1141-1142, 1993.

123. Brian JE Jr, Seifen AB, Clark RB, et al: Aortic stenosis, cesarean delivery, and epidural anesthesia. *J Clin Anesth* 5:154-157, 1993.

124. Sreeram N, Kitchiner D, Williams D, et al: Balloon dilatation of the aortic valve after previous surgical valvotomy: immediate and follow up results. *Br Heart J* 71:558-560, 1994.

125. Ben-Ami M, Battino S, Rosenfeld T, et al: Aortic valve replacement during pregnancy. A case report and review of the literature. *Acta Obstet Gynecol Scand* 69:651-653, 1990.

126. al Kasab SM, Sabag T, al Zaibag M, et al: Beta-adrenergic receptor blockade in the management of pregnant women with mitral stenosis. *Am J Obstet Gynecol* 163:37-40, 1990.

127. Ben Farhat M, Gamra H, Betbout F, et al: Percutaneous balloon mitral commissurotomy during pregnancy. *Heart* 77:564-567, 1997.

128. Gupta A, Lokhandwala YY, Satoskar PR, et al: Balloon mitral valvotomy in pregnancy: maternal and fetal outcomes. *J Am Coll Surg* 187:409-415, 1998.

129. Mangione JA, Lourenco RM, dos Santos ES, et al: Long-term follow-up of pregnant women after percutaneous mitral valvuloplasty. *Catheter Cardiovasc Interv* 50:413-417, 2000.

130. Patel JJ, Mitha AS, Hassen F, et al: Percutaneous balloon mitral valvotomy in pregnant patients with tight pliable mitral stenosis. *Am Heart J* 125:1106-1109, 1993.

131. Ribeiro PA, Fawzy ME, Awad M, et al: Balloon valvotomy for pregnant patients with severe pliable mitral stenosis using the Inoue technique with total abdominal and pelvic shielding. *Am Heart J* 124:1558-1562, 1992.

132. Ruzyllo W, Dabrowski M, Woroszylska M, et al: Percutaneous mitral commissurotomy with the Inoue balloon for severe mitral stenosis during pregnancy. *J Heart Valve Dis* 1:209-212, 1992.

133. Stoddard MF, Longaker RA, Vuocolo LM, et al: Transesophageal echocardiography in the pregnant patient. *Am Heart J* 124:785-787, 1992.

134. Gangbar EW, Watson KR, Howard RJ, et al: Mitral balloon valvuloplasty in pregnancy: Advantages of a unique balloon. *Cathet Cardiovasc Diagn* 25:313-316, 1992.

135. Pavankumar P, Venugopal P, Kaul U, et al: Pregnancy in patients with prosthetic cardiac valve. A 10-year experience. *Scand J Thorac Cardiovasc Surg* 22:19-22, 1988.

136. Sbarouni E, Oakley CM: Outcome of pregnancy in women with valve prostheses. *Br Heart J* 71:196-201, 1994.

137. Johnson JW, Longmate JA, Frentzen B: Excessive maternal weight and pregnancy outcome. *Am J Obstet Gynecol* 167:353-370; discussion 370-352, 1992.

138. Badduke BR, Jamieson WR, Miyagishima RT, et al: Pregnancy and childbearing in a population with biologic valvular prostheses. *J Thorac Cardiovasc Surg* 102:179-186, 1991.

139. Waller BF: *Pathology of the Heart and Great Vessels*, New York, Churchill Livingstone, 1988.

140. Lee CN, Wu CC, Lin PY, et al: Pregnancy following cardiac prosthetic valve replacement. *Obstet Gynecol* 83:353-356, 1994.

141. Salazar E, Espinola N, Roman L, et al: Effect of pregnancy on the duration of bovine pericardial bioprostheses. *Am Heart J* 137:714-720, 1999.

142. Dore A, Somerville J: Pregnancy in patients with pulmonary autograft valve replacement. *Eur Heart J* 18:1659-1662, 1997.

143. Rokey R, Hsu HW, Moise KJ Jr, et al: Inaccurate noninvasive mitral valve area calculation during pregnancy. *Obstet Gynecol* 84:950-955, 1994.

144. Homans DC: Peripartum cardiomyopathy. *N Engl J Med* 312:1432-1437, 1985.

145. Mabie WC, Hackman BB, Sibai BM: Pulmonary edema associated with pregnancy: echocardiographic insights and implications for treatment. *Obstet Gynecol* 81:227-234, 1993.

146. Nwosu EC, Burke MF: Cardiomyopathy of pregnancy. *Br J Obstet Gynaecol* 100:1145-1147, 1993.

147. Demakis JG, Rahimtoola SH: Peripartum cardiomyopathy. *Circulation* 44:964-968, 1971.

148. Hibbard JU, Lindheimer M, Lang RM: A modified definition for peripartum cardiomyopathy and prognosis based on echocardiography. *Obstetr Gynecol* 94:311-316, 1999.

149. Elkayam U, Tummala PP, Rao K, et al: Maternal and fetal outcomes of subsequent pregnancies in women with peripartum cardiomyopathy. *N Engl J Med* 344:1567-1571, 2001.

150. Carvalho AC, Almeida D, Cohen M, et al: Successful pregnancy, delivery and puerperium in a heart transplant patient with previous peripartum cardiomyopathy. *Eur Heart J* 13:1589-1591, 1992.

151. Scott JR, Wagoner LE, Olsen SL, et al: Pregnancy in heart transplant recipients: Management and outcome. *Obstet Gynecol* 82:324-327, 1993.

152. Cowan SW, Coscia LC, Philips LZ, et al: Pregnancy outcomes in female heart and heart-lung transplant recipients. *Transplant Proceed* 34:1855-1856, 2002.

153. Chow SL: Acute aortic dissection in a patient with Marfan's syndrome complicated by gestational hypertension. *Med J Aust* 159:760-762, 1993.

154. Pyeritz RE: Maternal and fetal complications of pregnancy in the Marfan syndrome. *Am J Med* 71:784-790, 1981.

155. Pyeritz RE: The Marfan syndrome. *Am Fam Physician* 34:83-94, 1986.

156. Rosenblum NG, Grossman AR, Gabbe SG, et al: Failure of serial echocardiographic studies to predict aortic dissection in a pregnant patient with Marfan's syndrome. *Am J Obstet Gynecol* 146:470-471, 1983.

157. Immer FF, Bansi AG, Immer-Bansi AS, et al: Aortic dissection in pregnancy: Analysis of risk factors and outcome. *Ann Thorac Surg* 76:309-314, 2003.

158. Lind J, Wallenburg HCS: The Marfan syndrome and pregnancy: A retrospective study in a Dutch population. *Eur J Obstet Gynecol Reprod Biol* 98:28-35, 2001.

159. Meijboom LJ, Drenthen W, Pieper PG, et al: Obstetric complications in Marfan syndrome. *Int J Cardiol* 110:53-59, 2006.

160. Lipscomb KJ, Smith JC, Clarke B, et al: Outcome of pregnancy in women with Marfan's syndrome. *Br J Obstet Gynaecol* 104:201-206, 1997.

161. Legget ME, Unger TA, O'Sullivan CK, et al: Aortic root complications in Marfan's syndrome: Identification of a lower risk group. *Heart* 75:389-395, 1996.

162. Mayet J, Steer P, Somerville J: Marfan syndrome, aortic dilatation, and pregnancy. *Obstet Gynecol* 92:713, 1998.

163. Treasure T: Elective replacement of the aortic root in Marfan's syndrome. *Br Heart J* 69:101-103, 1993.

164. Gott VL, Greene PS, Alejo DE, et al: Replacement of the aortic root in patients with Marfan's syndrome. *N Engl J Med* 340:1307-1313, 1999.

165. Pereira L, Levran O, Ramirez F, et al: A molecular approach to the stratification of cardiovascular risk in families with Marfan's syndrome. *N Engl J Med* 331:148-153, 1994.

166. Shores J, Berger KR, Murphy EA, et al: Progression of aortic dilatation and the benefit of long-term beta-adrenergic blockade in Marfan's syndrome. *N Engl J Med* 330:1335-1341, 1994.

167. Roman MJ, Rosen SE, Kramer-Fox R, et al: Prognostic significance of the pattern of aortic root dilation in the Marfan syndrome. *J Am Coll Cardiol* 22:1470-1476, 1993.

168. Gordon CF 3rd, Johnson MD: Anesthetic management of the pregnant patient with Marfan syndrome. *J Clin Anesth* 5:248-251, 1993.

169. Cola LM, Lavin JP Jr: Pregnancy complicated by Marfan's syndrome with aortic arch dissection, subsequent aortic arch replacement and triple coronary artery bypass grafts. *J Reprod Med* 30:685-688, 1985.

170. The Practice Committee of the American Society for Reproductive M: Increased maternal cardiovascular mortality associated with pregnancy in women with Turner syndrome. *Fertil Steril* 83:1074-1075, 2005.

171. Snir E, Levinsky L, Salomon J, et al: Dissecting aortic aneurysm in pregnant women without Marfan disease. *Surg Gynecol Obstet* 167:463-465, 1988.

172. Petitti DB, Sidney S, Quesenberry CP Jr, et al: Incidence of stroke and myocardial infarction in women of reproductive age. *Stroke* 28:280-283, 1997.

173. Roth A, Elkayam U: Acute myocardial infarction associated with pregnancy. *Ann Intern Med* 125:751-762, 1996.

174. James AH, Jamison MG, Biswas MS, et al: Acute myocardial infarction in pregnancy: A United States population-based study. *Circulation* 113:1564-1571, 2006.

175. Sullebarger JT, Fontanet HL, Matar FA, et al: Percutaneous coronary intervention for myocardial infarction during pregnancy: a new trend? *J Invasive Cardiol* 15:725-728, 2003.

176. Shivvers SA, Wians FH Jr, Keffer JH, et al: Maternal cardiac troponin I levels during normal labor and delivery. *Am J Obstet Gynecol* 180:122, 1999.

177. Eickman FM: Acute coronary artery angioplasty during pregnancy. *Cathet Cardiovasc Diagn* 38:369-372, 1996.

178. Ascarelli MH, Grider AR, Hsu HW: Acute myocardial infarction during pregnancy managed with immediate percutaneous transluminal coronary angioplasty. *Obstet Gynecol* 88:655-657, 1996.

179. Webber MD, Halligan RE, Schumacher JA: Acute infarction, intracoronary thrombolysis, and primary PTCA in pregnancy. *Cathet Cardiovasc Diagn* 42:38-43, 1997.

180. Garry D, Leikin E, Fleisher AG, et al: Acute myocardial infarction in pregnancy with subsequent medical and surgical management. *Obstet Gynecol* 87:802-804, 1996.

181. Dwyer BK, Taylor L, Fuller A, et al: Percutaneous transluminal coronary angioplasty and stent placement in pregnancy. *Obstet Gynecol* 106:1162-1164, 2005.

182. Jordaens LJ, Vandenbogaerde JF, Van de Bruaene P, et al: Transesophageal echocardiography for insertion of a physiological pacemaker in early pregnancy. *Pacing Clin Electrophysiol* 13:955-957, 1990.

183. Kultursay H, Turkoglu C, Akin M, et al: Mitral balloon valvuloplasty with transesophageal echocardiography without using fluoroscopy. *Cathet Cardiovasc Diagn* 27:317-321, 1992.

184. Carvalho A, Brandao A, Martinez EE, et al: Prognosis in peripartum cardiomyopathy. *Am J Cardiol* 64:540-542, 1989.

185. Mishra M, Chambers JB, Jackson G: Murmurs in pregnancy: An audit of echocardiography. *Bmj* 304:1413-1414, 1992.

186. Rayburn WF, LeMire MS, Bird JL, et al: Mitral valve prolapse. Echocardiographic changes during pregnancy. *J Reprod Med* 32:185-187, 1987.

187. Jana N, Vasishta K, Khunnu B, et al: Pregnancy in association with mitral valve prolapse. *Asia Oceania J Obstet Gynaecol* 19:61-65, 1993.

188. Tang LC, Chan SY, Wong VC, et al: Pregnancy in patients with mitral valve prolapse. *Int J Gynaecol Obstet* 23:217-221, 1985.

189. Vered Z, Poler SM, Gibson P, et al: Noninvasive detection of the morphologic and hemodynamic changes during normal pregnancy. *Clin Cardiol* 14:327-334, 1991.

190. Carvalho JS, Redington AN, Shinebourne EA, et al: Continuous wave Doppler echocardiography and coarctation of the aorta: gradients and flow patterns in the assessment of severity. *Br Heart J* 64:133-137, 1990.

191. Tan JL, Babu-Narayan SV, Henein MY, et al: Doppler echocardiographic profile and indexes in the evaluation of aortic coarctation in patients before and after stenting. *J Am Coll Cardiol* 46:1045-1053, 2005.

192. Rubler S, Damani PM, Pinto ER: Cardiac size and performance during pregnancy estimated with echocardiography. *Am J Cardiol* 40:534-540, 1977.

Part Seven

Vascular and Systemic Diseases

Chapter 33

Aortic Dissection and Trauma: Value and Limitations of Echocardiography

HUSAM H. FARAH, MD • ANN F. BOLGER, MD

The mortality of acute aortic dissection escalates hourly,[1] reaching 50% by 48 hours. Immediate diagnosis and therapy are critical for survival. Two thousand new cases of acute dissection are reported in the United States per year[2]; the true incidence, including the large numbers of patients who die from unrecognized dissection, has been estimated at more that 10,000 per year.[3] Further, 10% to 30% of acute dissections occurring in the hospital may be misdiagnosed. It is a great clinical challenge that patient's symptoms may be nonspecific or even misleading. Aortic dissection must be included in the differential diagnosis of chest pain in many patients at risk for dissection and also when simultaneous acute involvement of multiple organ systems does not have a ready explanation. Acute dissection of the aorta can share many of the features of acute myocardial infarction (AMI): pain (related to the dissection itself or to myocardial ischemia), electrocardiographic abnormalities consistent with ischemia (resulting from involvement of the coronary ostia in proximal dissection),[4] and elevated serum creatinine kinase levels.[5]

True myocardial ischemia is a potential component of the syndrome of aortic dissection; Hirst and colleagues[6] found involvement of the coronary arteries on pathologic examination in 39 of 505 cases of acute dissection (7.7%). Confusion of acute dissection with myocardial infarction (MI) not only delays appropriate treatment but also may lead to disastrous consequences if thrombolytics are administered.[7] Thrombolysis impedes compensatory thrombosis of the false channel and promotes uncontrollable hemorrhage in the event of aortic rupture. Given that the incidence of aortic dissection is far less than that of myocardial infarction and that ST segment elevation is a relatively rare finding in patients with aortic dissection, electrocardiogram (ECG) changes without physical findings suggesting dissection will rarely mislead clinicians toward thrombolysis.[8] Maintenance of a high suspicion for dissection must be paired with highly reliable tests to avoid such infrequent but catastrophic misdiagnoses.

The optimal diagnostic test for acute aortic dissection, therefore, must be accurate, safe, and immediately applicable in a broad range of medical environments. The limited sensitivity of echocardiography for dissection from the transthoracic approach has been greatly improved by transesophageal approaches; transesophageal examinations can be performed within minutes in the emergency department (ED), operating room (OR), or intensive care unit (ICU) and provide high-quality images of the thoracic aorta and of other cardiac and vascular structures at risk. The advantages and limitations of echocardiographic techniques in the management of patients with aortic dissection have been carefully investigated at many centers and support their critical role in the diagnosis, repair, and follow-up of aortic dissection.

Pathophysiology of Aortic Dissection

Anatomy and Histology

The diameter of the aorta decreases distally in a tapering fashion, from a size of less than 2.1 cm/m^2 in the ascending aorta to less than 1.6 cm/m^2 at the level of the aortic arch.[9] The size of aorta increases with age during childhood at a rate 1 to 2 mm/year; aging is associated with a loss of compliance and increased wall stiffness.

The aortic wall comprises three layers: the intima, which is a single layer of vascular endothelium; the media, with concentric layers of smooth muscle cells, collagen, elastin, and extracellular matrix proteoglycans; and the peripheral adventitia, consisting of loose connective tissue that anchors the aorta in surrounding tissues. The vaso vasorum, which perfuses the aortic wall, is contained within the adventitia. Of the three layers of the aortic wall, the structure of the media dominates the wall's mechanical properties.[10] Medial smooth muscle directly influences wall stiffness by contraction. In addition, smooth muscle cells are the major source of the extracellular matrix components. These include the elastin fibers, which can be stretched to 300% of their resting length without rupturing[11] and are important contributors to the normal pulsatile behavior of the vessel. Elastin is less important to the overall strength of the aorta than collagen, however, which is both stiffer and much stronger than elastin.

The components of the media vary from vessel to vessel and change with age. In the aortas of older patients, the elastin content decreases and collagen increases, resulting in increased vascular stiffness.[12] The mechanical properties of the vasculature are also almost always disturbed in cases of systemic hypertension.[13]

Mechanical and Shear Stresses

The aortic wall is subjected to mechanical stresses of several forms. Stress, which is expressed as force per unit area, may occur in radial, circumferential, or longitudinal directions. The normal intima bears little of the aorta's stress load. It is exposed to shear stresses, however, which are forces applied parallel to the vessel wall as a result of the viscous effects of blood flow. The amount of these shear stresses varies with the distribution of velocity across the vessel lumen and with local vessel geometry.

Circumferential stress predominantly affects the media. This type of stress (δ) increases with the radial pressure from the aortic lumen (P) and the aortic radius (r), and decreases with increasing wall thickness (h):

$$\delta = Pr/2h$$

The danger of aortic dilation can therefore be understood: In dilated, thin-walled aortas, the circumferential stresses may be increased many times above normal. In addition, the geometry of the dilating aorta changes progressively from the normal cylinder to an ellipsoidal or even spherical shape. This slowly increases the circumferential stress but quickly exacerbates longitudinal stress. Most atraumatic aortic tears are caused by longitudinal stress, which explains why they are generally transverse in orientation.[14] The ascending aorta experiences additional longitudinal stress owing to the motion of the aortic annulus. Finally, dilated or aneurysmal vessels demonstrate marked stiffness, in part because of loss of elastin.[15] Combined aortic dilation, wall thinning, and shape change sets the stage for intimal rupture and the initiation of dissection.

Intimal or medial abnormalities of the aorta increase the resistance to both shear and circumferential stresses. Stress failures of both types may play a role in aortic dissection. Circumferential stress failure can occur when the stresses caused by intraluminal pressure are greatly magnified in the thin fibrous cap of an atheromatous lesion. If the lesion fractures and a small crack develops, the circumferential stress will cause it to extend through the wall.[10] Shear stress failure is the result of inhomogeneity in the properties of the vessel wall. Even under normal conditions, mural stresses are greater on the inner than on the outer wall.[16] In the presence of atherosclerosis, incremental variations in the shear resistance between contiguous regions of diseased and normal wall occur. The progression of aortic dissection probably represents an example of shear failure, where the interface between two such aortic segments with different stiffness leads to separation of medial and intimal layers; the two layers slide relative to one another as the "glue" of the extracellular matrix cannot withstand the shear stress.[10]

Once initiated, dissections behave like a two-ply tube. The intima and the internal elastic lamina of the media form the inner layer, whereas the outer layer consists of the external elastic lamina and the adventitia. A velocity-dependent shear force will then further separate the two layers, creating a false lumen separated from the true lumen by the intima and internal elastic lamina. Experimentally, it has been demonstrated that the work per unit area of tissue required to propagate a tear in the aorta is small (15.9 ± 0.9 mJ cm^{-2}), and independent of the depth of the tear.[16]

Increasing recognition of intramural hematoma as one of the acute aortic syndromes has expanded the understanding of the precursors of dissection. In the case of hematoma formation, the inciting event is hemorrhage into the media from the vaso vasorum. This lesion may expand and rupture into the aortic lumen, creating what is recognized as an entry tear and allowing progression of the intimal detachment along the arterial tree. In other cases, the hematoma is contained but creates a risk of external rupture.

These concepts of shear and tensile failure are the basis for understanding why different patient populations are at increased risk for aortic dissection. Medial elastic tissue degeneration resulting from hereditary defects of the arterial wall creates the substrate for dissection in patients with Marfan syndrome, Turner's syndrome,[17] Noonan's disease, Ehlers-Danlos syndrome, and osteogenesis imperfecta.[14,18] In these patients and in other groups, dilation of the aorta is an important source of tensile failure and a precursor to dissection.

Both wall abnormalities (shear failure) and increased wall stress (tensile failure) as a result of dilation are important in nonhereditary risk groups. Dissection occurring in hypertensive patients is generally based on high blood pressure, moderate aortic dilation, and medial muscular degeneration predisposing the internal layer to tear.[14] The contribution of shear stress in those patients is infrequent and unpredictable.

Risk Factors for Aortic Dissection

Hypertension and atherosclerosis are the predominant conditions that result in dissection. More infrequently, pregnancy, inflammatory disorders, such as giant cell arteritis and Takayasu Disease, or congenital collagen disorders, such as Marfan syndrome, Turner's syndrome or Ehlers-Danlos syndrome, are etiologic. Bicuspid aortic valve or aortic coarctation are other congenital causes.

Cocaine use, trauma, and iatrogenic disruption of the arterial structures during surgery or cardiac catheterization can also be the initiator[19-25] (Table 33-1).

Atherosclerosis

Atherosclerosis is a highly prevalent disorder whose generalized and focal manifestations can predispose to dissection. True aortic aneurysms are a result of atherosclerotic degeneration of the media and progress to involve all three layers of the vessel wall and to gradual dilation. Increasing risk accompanies enlarged diameters, rapid expansion, or symptoms. Formation of laminar thrombus within the aneurysm does not decrease the wall stress. The 1-year survival rate in patients with thoracic aortic aneurysms is less than 60%, and the 5-year survival rate approximately 20%. Up to 14% of patients presenting with dissection in the International Registry of Acute Aortic Dissection had preexisting aortic aneurysm.[26]

Trauma

Dissection may occur in external, accidental trauma and be difficult to assess in the setting of major multisystem injuries. The region most prone to traumatic

TABLE 33–1. Patient Populations at Risk for Aortic Dissection

Genetic Disorders (Medial Abnormalities)
Marfan syndrome
Turner's syndrome
Noonan's disease
Ehlers-Danlos syndrome
Osteogenesis imperfecta

Congenital Disorders
Aortic coarctation
Unicuspid or bicuspid aortic valve

Degenerative Disorders
Hypertension
Atherosclerotic vascular disease
  Aortic ulcer
  Aortic aneurysm
Non-Marfan syndrome cystic medial necrosis

Traumatic Causes
Deceleration injury
Penetrating injury
Heimlich maneuver

Postprocedural Causes
Cardiac surgery
  Cannulation
  Cross-clamping
  Aortic valve replacement
Angioplasty
  Coronary
  Renal

Inflammatory Disorders
Syphilis
Giant cell arteritis

Other Conditions
Pregnancy
Weightlifting
Cocaine use
Discontinuation of beta-blockers
Polycystic kidney disease

injury is the aortic isthmus, in which relative tethering by the spinal arteries and ligamentum arteriosum resists abrupt deceleration more than the more mobile transverse arch.[27] Other vulnerable sites include the origin of the innominate artery, particularly with vertical forces from falls, and the ascending aorta above the sinus of Valsalva.[28] Traumatic injuries to the aorta may result in intimal tears, recognizable on transesophageal echocardiography (TEE) as mobile flaps. Thrombus may be seen protruding into the lumen; in other cases, intramural hematoma without apparent intimal discontinuity is seen. Although minor lesions, such as minimal hematomas, may regress spontaneously, the prognosis of significant aortic trauma is grave. Without repair, there is 30% mortality within the first 24 hours. Within 1 week, mortality is greater than 50%.[29] Prompt recognition is therefore critical to patient outcome. TEE has been shown to be safe and highly sensitive for aortic trauma after motor vehicle accidents, equivalent to angiography and more expeditiously applied.[30] TEE

may also detect other signs of cardiac trauma, including wall motion abnormalities, pericardial effusion, and valvular regurgitation. When the suspicion of aortic rupture in the territory of the transverse arch remains high, computed tomography (CT) may provide better images of those territories.

Other sources of trauma include the Heimlich maneuver for respiratory obstruction and cardiovascular procedures. Operative sources of tears in the aorta include cannulation sites for cardiopulmonary bypass (CPB), aortic transections for valve or aortic segment replacement, and proximal anastomotic sites for coronary bypass grafts.[31,32] Uncommonly, aortic catheterization for angiography may traumatize an atherosclerotic region and prompt dissection.[33] Angioplasty procedures of coronary or renal vessels can also initiate the process.[34] A history of these procedures may be important in alerting the clinician to the possibility of dissection in these patients.

Cocaine

Cocaine stimulates central neural sympathetic outflow and blocks reuptake of catecholamines in the synaptic clefts. The resulting intense vasoconstriction, prothrombosis and increase in heart rate (HR), blood pressure, and myocardial contractility increase the risk of aortic dissection. In one series, 14 out of 38 cases of aortic dissection were associated with cocaine use during the preceding 24 hours (average, 2 hours). The proportion of types A and B dissection was similar to noncocaine users.[35]

Pregnancy

Although aortic dissection is mostly a disease of middle-aged or elderly males, women and children can also experience dissection. It has been claimed that half of all aortic dissections occurring in women younger than 40 years of age are associated with pregnancy, particularly during the third trimester or the postpartum period.[36-38] This has been disputed by Oskoui and Lindsay,[39] who reviewed their own experience and published a series of 1253 dissections in consecutive patients (868 males and 385 females), with no cases occurring in pregnancy. They concluded that most women experiencing aortic dissection in pregnancy had other risk factors, such as hypertension or Marfan syndrome, and that the apparent association could result from selective reporting and coincidental occurrence of dissection with the common condition of pregnancy.

The most up-to-date information on acute aortic dissection in women from the International Registry of Acute Aortic Dissection implies that dissection generally affects women at a more advanced age than men and that they fare worse than their male counterparts with respect to rupture, hypotension, and surgical mortality.[26]

Genetic Diseases

Of the genetic causes of aortic medial disease and aortic dissection, Marfan syndrome is the most common and best studied. Although a clinical diagnosis, Marfan syndrome may be confirmed by linkage to the dominantly inherited gene MFS-1 on 15q21 or by determination of the specific family mutation.[40] Histologic examination of the aortic wall in Marfan syndrome patients reveals fragmentation of aortic components, especially the elastic fibers[41] and abnormal accumulation of collagenous and mucoid materials in the media.[42] Fragmentation of elastin-associated microfibrils also occurs in aortic valve leaflets.[43] The disruption and loss of elastic tissue of the media is attributed to a deficiency of fibrillin, a microfibrillar protein that scaffolds the elastic lamellae in the aortic wall.[44,45] These changes are greatest in the ascending aorta, which is subject to the greatest pulsatile expansion and therefore the highest stress in systole.[14] The alterations in aortic wall components are associated with abnormal functional properties: Aortic elasticity is abnormal in patients with Marfan syndrome, irrespective of the aortic diameter.[46] A comparative study of aortic wall dynamics between patients with Marfan syndrome and normal controls confirmed that in both groups stiffness of the wall increases with age and aortic diameter, but at all ages the Marfan syndrome group exhibits a stiffer aorta for a given diameter than controls.[47] Furthermore, patients with Marfan syndrome have large ascending aortic diameters but not abdominal aortic size after correction for body surface area (BSA).[46] Dissection occurs in patients with Marfan syndrome because of this dilation in combination with wall weakness; mural stress increases dramatically with increasing radius and becomes self-perpetuating.[14]

Echocardiographic evidence of aortic root dilation is present in 60% to 80% of patients with Marfan syndrome[48] (Fig. 33–1). In one series, aortic dilation was generalized in 51% and localized in 28%.[49] Localized dilation did not appear to represent an earlier stage of aortic involvement because the patient ages in both groups were identical, as was the duration of follow-up. It could not be determined whether generalized dilation reflected more severe underlying cystic medial necrosis from different specific mutations in fibrillin. Generalized dilation, however, was associated with higher rates of expansion and aortic regurgitation (AR). In patients with Marfan syndrome, AR has been associated with decreased survival.[25] The existence of mitral valve prolapse (MVP) does not appear to be an independent predictor of outcome. The clinical course of patients with Marfan syndrome with respect to progressive aortic dilation and dissection is variable;[50] in-

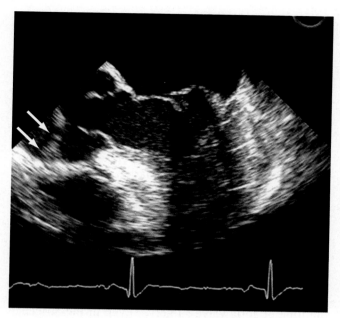

Figure 33–1. *Type A aortic dissection* (arrows *indicate intimal flap) in a patient with Marfan syndrome on transesophageal imaging. Enlargement of the proximal aortic root and prolapse of the posterior mitral valve leaflet are also noted.*

creased risk has been associated with older age,[49,50] male gender, aortic root diameters exceeding 60 mm,[51] aortic growth rate[49,50] and a family history of dissection.[52] In one study, two groups of patients with Marfan syndrome were identified according to the speed of their aortic root dilatation.[53] The speed of dilatation was not related to the use of beta-blockers or the family history. The fast growing group had significantly more type A dissection and more elective root replacement, compared to subjects with slower dilatation. Of great concern is the observation that aortic dissection can occur in patients with Marfan syndrome even in the absence of aortic root dilation.[54]

Medical management of patients with Marfan syndrome with aortic dilatation involves beta-blockers and observation of aortic root diameter to determine timing of elective surgery aimed at preventing aortic dissection. Long-term fatality rates are improved with prophylactic aortic root replacement; 5-year survival approximating 97% for elective surgery versus only 51% with emergency surgery for dissection.[55] Operative mortality in experienced centers for elective surgery in patients with Marfan syndrome is low (1.3% to 1.5% 30-day mortality versus 11.7% for emergency surgery).[56,57] In patients with normal aortic valve leaflets, elective aortic valve sparing surgery may provide better clinical outcomes than aortic root replacement.[58] Although in this retrospective review, those undergoing aortic root replacement with aortic valve replacement had more cardiac comorbidities than the group in which valve-sparing surgery was possible. The size of aneurysm often determines the feasibility of valve-sparing surgery, hence, some centers recommend elective surgery when the aortic root reaches 50 mm.

Bicuspid Aortic Valve

Bicuspid aortic valve is the most common congenital heart anomaly, with a prevalence of 1% to 2%. It has been estimated that patients with bicuspid valves have a ninefold increase in the risk of dissection compared to those with normal valves, and up to a 5% lifetime risk of dissection.[59] As with Marfan syndrome, aortic histology in patients with bicuspid aortic valve demonstrates cystic medial necrosis, with significantly increased expression of matrix metalloproteinase (MMP) 2 and MMP 9. It is important to remember that replacement of the malformed valve does not correct progressive aortic root dilatation or the elevated risk of dissection; aortic valve and ascending aorta replacement is indicated when the aortic diameter exceeds 45 mm at the time of aoric valve surgery.[60] Even in the abscence of indications for valve surgery, ascending aorta replacement is recommended when diameter exceeds 50 mm or has a rapid rate of dilation.

Familial Aortic Dissection

Twenty percent of patients with aortic dissection have a first-degree relative with a history of thoracic aneurysm or aortic aneurysm. The inherited risk for dissection appears to follow an autosomal dominant pattern, and surveillance of family members is warranted.[60]

Spectrum of Aortic Dissection

The primary entry tear that initiates aortic dissection is usually transverse and involves more than half of the circumference of the aorta. In 65% of cases it occurs within 3 cm of the coronary ostia. Ten percent of tears occur in the descending thoracic aorta and another 10% in the arch. Primary tears are rare in the abdominal aorta.[61] Whatever the location of the initial tear, dissections may extend caudally, proximally, or occasionally in both directions.

Anatomic Classification

There are several widely used classification systems for dissection (Table 33–2). The DeBakey classification divides dissections with involvement of the ascending aorta into type I, which extends into the transverse arch and distal aorta, and type II, which is confined to the ascending aorta. DeBakey type III dissections involve the descending aorta only.[62] The Stanford classification[63] was developed from a functional approach based on whether the ascending aorta is involved, re-

TABLE 33–2. Nomenclature of Aortic Dissection

Dissection Type	Classification
Ascending aorta involved	Stanford type A DeBakey I DeBakey II University of Alabama "ascending"[56] Massachusetts General Hospital "proximal"[57]
Ascending aorta not involved	Stanford type B DeBakey III University of Alabama "descending"[56] Massachusetts General Hospital "distal"[57]

gardless of the site of primary intimal tear and irrespective of the extent of distal propagation. This reflects clinical observations that the biologic behavior of the dissection, the clinical prognosis, and how the patient should be managed pivot almost exclusively on whether the ascending aorta is involved.[64-66] This system of nomenclature describes type A dissections as any with involvement of the ascending aorta (including DeBakey types I and II), and type B dissections as dissection limited to the descending aorta (DeBakey type III).

The clinical classification schemes described above do not emphasize the location of the primary entry tear or the extent of the distal propagation of the dissection. These two factors are of less prognostic value and can be technically difficult to determine.[67,68] When identification of the entry site is possible, the culprit primary intimal tear is more easily resected. Although successful resection of the primary tear does not appear to affect early or late survival rates, it may decrease the incidence of late reoperation.[69]

Some cases of aortic dissection will present with multiple "primary" tears. Two separate dissections in the same patient may be more common than previously reported. Roberts and Roberts[70] reported that 3 of 40 necropsy patients had separate proximal and distal thoracic dissections. Although all fatal events were caused by rupture of the acute proximal dissections, a separate distal dissection may still pose a risk for late complications, and therefore recognizing two separate dissections may have important implications regarding follow-up and therapy.[71] Multiple distal "exit" tears, which decompress the false lumen, are extremely common.

Time Course

Dissections are also differentiated with respect to their time course. Acute dissections are detected within 2 weeks of the onset of initial symptoms. Chronic dissections present more than 2 weeks after onset.[66,72] This division is arbitrary; it may primarily reflect the fact that the majority of type A dissection patients will die within 2 weeks if untreated. Chronic dissections may be detected because of symptoms or be an incidental finding. They are differentiated from aortic aneurysms by the presence of an intimal flap and false lumen. These may not be easy to recognize when the false lumen is largely thrombosed. Pronounced atherosclerotic changes may be present in the false lumen in chronic dissections, even when the true lumen walls appear normal and hyperlipidemia is absent.[73]

Sequelae

The concomitant sequelae of aortic dissection are many and varied. Obstruction of branch vessels may explain acute myocardial ischemia and infarction of cerebral, spinal, bowel, and renal territories. Aortic valve dehiscence with regurgitation, cardiac tamponade from retrograde extension into the pericardium, and frank aortic rupture are all highly morbid consequences.

Echocardiography in Aortic Dissection

Time is of the essence when aortic dissection is suspected, and the entire thoracic aorta must be visualized. Transthoracic echocardiography (TTE) is immediately available, and in some cases of proximal dissection it may visualize the ascending aortic intimal flap and false lumen, or a flap in the descending aorta may be visible from the suprasternal or subcostal windows (Figs. 33–2 and 33–3). Other clues to dissection available from transthoracic approaches include pericardial effusion with or without tamponade, AR with or without leaflet dehiscence, aortic root dilation, or regional wall motion abnormalities. Given the variable occurrence of any of these abnormalities, it is not surprising that the sensitivity of transthoracic echocardiography has been limited (Table 33–3).

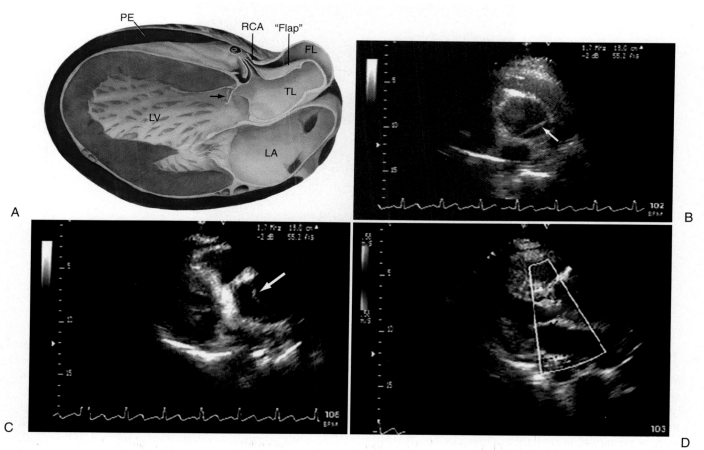

Figure 33–2. *Illustration of the complications of aortic dissection (A). The intimal flap is seen in the ascending aorta separating the true lumen (TL) from the false lumen (FL). The flap may extend into the right coronary artery (RCA) resulting in myocardial ischemia, may rupture into the pericardial space with a hemorrhagic pericardial effusion (PE) and tamponade physiology or may disrupt the valve leaflet attachment with a flail leaflet (small arrow) and aortic regurgitation. Conventional transthoracic views are often the first clue to the diagnosis of aortic dissection. Parasternal short (B) views demonstrate the intimal flap in the proximal aortic root (arrow). Long-axis views show the mobile flap (C) and the associated aortic regurgitation (D).*

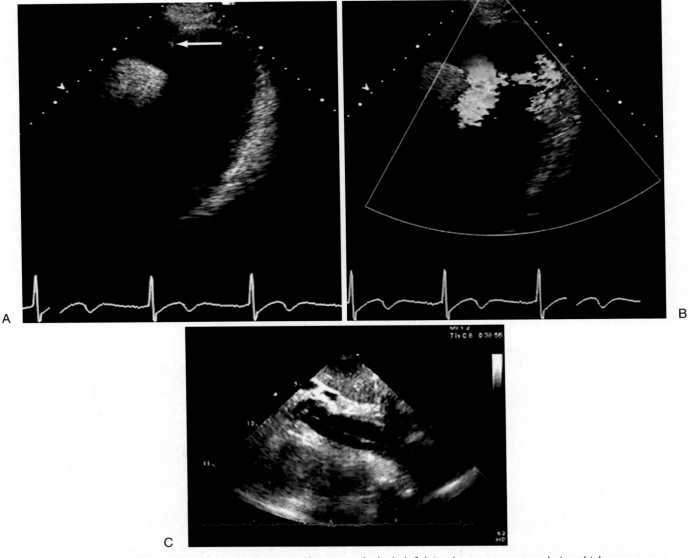

Figure 33–3. *Transthoracic views can be particularly helpful in the transverse arch in which transesophageal echocardiographic views may be suboptimal. Suprasternal views of the transverse and descending aorta demonstrate the intimal flap* (A, arrow) *and an entry tear with systolic flow from the true lumen into the false lumen* (B). *Subcostal views offer another important vantage point for the descending aorta* (C).

Transesophageal Imaging

Multiple studies have documented that the specificity and sensitivity of TEE in the range of 98% and 99%, respectively. The recognized blind spot of TEE, involving the distal ascending aorta and superior aspect of the arch, is an important limitation, especially because entry tears in this region are important to clinical management. The goal of imaging the entire thoracic aorta may therefore require a combination of modalities and approaches, including transthoracic views (often from the suprasternal notch), transesophageal windows, and often direct epiaortic or epicardial views at the time of surgery.

TEE has many discrete advantages in the diagnosis of acute aortic dissection, the most important of which

is its documented accuracy. Erbel and colleagues[74] reporting for the European Cooperative Study Group for Echocardiography on a series of 164 patients suspected of acute dissection, demonstrated sensitivity and specificity rates of 99% and 98%, respectively. Another large study by Nienaber and colleagues[75] compared TEE with magnetic resonance imaging (MRI). Both TEE and MRI had perfect sensitivity; the 100% specificity of MRI exceeded the 68% specificity of TEE. The authors suggested that limited visualization of common ascending aorta pathology of the TEE might have accounted for the higher rate of false-positive studies. In that study strict criteria for diagnosing dissection were not applied (see later discussion); more stringent criteria could minimize false-positive results. Transthoracic

TABLE 33–3. Imaging Modalities for Aortic Dissection

Modality	Sensitivity	Specificity	Positive Predictive Value	Negative Predictive Value	Accuracy
TTE[67]	77	93	—	—	—
TTE[66]	59	83	—	—	—
TTE[65]	83	63	80	70	75
TEE[66]	98	77	—	—	—
TEE[1]	98	97	98	97	97
TEE[65]	100	68	82	100	87
Aortography[64]	88	94	96	84	—
Aortography[1]	88	97	97	85	91
MRI[65]	100	100	100	100	100
MRI[66]	98	98	—	—	—
CT[83]	83	100	100	86	—
CT[124]	100	100	—	—	100

CT, Computed tomography; MRI, magnetic resonance imaging; TEE, transesophageal echocardiography; TTE, transthoracic echocardiography.

echocardiography from the suprasternal notch provides additional views of this vulnerable area. The sequential use of TEE and CT, aortography, or MRI is clearly extremely powerful in clarifying suspicious or clinically incongruous results.[76,77]

TEE provides additional information about left ventricular (LV) and right ventricular (RV) wall motion and global function, and aortic and mitral valve competence. Importantly, with acute type A dissections, TEE is able to detect and determine the severity and mechanism of aortic valve regurgitation[78] and may influence the decision to replace or repair the valve.

An important advantage of TEE in cases of dissection is its rapid and safe performance in a wide range of clinical environments, including emergency departments, intensive care units, and the operating room. TEE requires minimal patient preparation, avoids the contrast and X-ray exposure associated with CT and angiography, and eliminates the time delays and practical encumbrances of MRI. Choice of a "best test" must always take into account the individual center's track record with each modality and access issues.

Safety of Transesophageal Echocardiography

Safety of transesophageal examinations depends on adequate patient preparation with respect to pain, anxiety, and airway protection. Careful monitoring of the electrocardiogram and blood pressure is critical to avoiding adverse affects of TEE. In a study of 54 ambulatory patients, TEE was accompanied by an increase in systolic pressure in 77% of patients. This elevation was moderate (average increase of 16 mm Hg) in most patients, but some patients had acute increases of as much as 51 mm Hg.[79] Abrupt increases of blood pressure must clearly be avoided in any patient suspected of dissection. Serial blood pressure monitoring, pulse oximetry, intravenous (IV) sedation, topical anesthesia, and control of blood pressure with intravenous vasodilators and beta-blockers, if needed, are important to patient safety. With these precautions, the majority of patients can undergo esophageal intubation with minimal distress and good hemodynamic stability. Despite this, there has been a reported case of aortic rupture occurring during TEE in a patient with an acute dissection, which might have been elicited by retching and elevated blood pressure.[80] Other commonly reported adverse events during transesophageal studies that must be anticipated and avoided are nonsustained atrial and ventricular arrhythmias, excessive vagotonia with transient atrioventricular (AV) block, and arterial hypoxemia.[81]

Diagnostic Features

The diagnosis of aortic dissection is most secure when specific criteria are met. Identification of an intimal flap, seen as a mobile, linear echo within the vascular lumen and flow in the true and false channels on either side of the flap are highly sensitive features of dissection. The motion of the intimal flap toward the false lumen during systole may be a helpful feature (Fig. 33–4). A thickening of the aortic wall in excess of

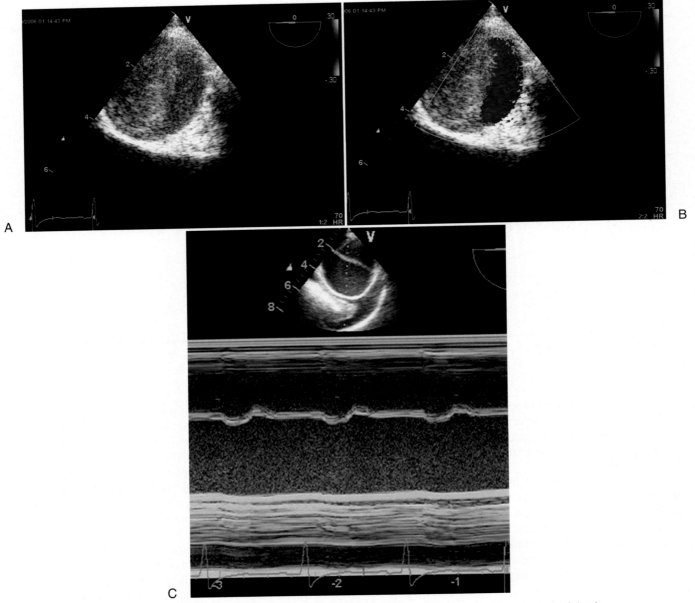

Figure 33-4. *Transesophageal views of the descending aorta demonstrate the true and false lumens. This intimal flap is difficult to see because of thrombosis in the false lumen (A). Color Doppler confirms systolic flow in the true lumen (B). M-mode can also be used to demonstrate the characteristic bowing of the intimal flap toward the false lumen during systole (C).*

15 mm has also been used as a sign of dissection, suggesting thrombosis of a false channel, which makes the intimal flap difficult to recognize.[82] Strict adherence to these criteria can avoid confusion from imaging artifacts and manifestations of other types of disease and minimize false-positive results.[83] This is particularly important because most patients suspected of having an aortic dissection have evidence of vascular disease involving the thoracic aorta. In one series of 40 patients evaluated for dissection, abnormal aortic findings (including atherosclerotic plaques, intravascular and extravascular masses, thrombi, and dilation) were found in 16 of 17 patients in whom aortic dissection and coronary artery disease (CAD) were excluded as explanations for their chest pain.[84] Other underlying aortic abnormalities such as coarctation or prior surgical repair, may affect clinical management, but they are also important potential sources of misdiagnosis.

Doppler Findings

Color Doppler flow imaging during TEE is an excellent descriptor of aortic flow patterns with acute dissection. Flow in the false channel is variable and complicated;

the true lumen, which is often dwarfed by the false channel, is identified by forward systolic flow. With large proximal entry tears, flow in the nearby segments of the false lumen may have the same direction and timing as the true lumen flow and may reverse in diastole.[85,86] With smaller or more distal tears, false lumen flow is less similar to true lumen flow: It may be directed in the opposite direction, and peak velocity may occur later in the cardiac cycle, representing delay of flow into the false lumen. Many areas will show extremely slow, swirling flow with spontaneous echocardiographic contrast or partial thrombosis. These segments tend to be remote from large entry or exit sites in which high velocity flow keeps these changes from occurring. Finally, areas of complete thrombosis are also seen, and care must be taken to ascertain that the hematoma is entirely intravascular and not actually the result of adventitial rupture, pseudoaneurysm formation, or intramural hematoma.

Multiple communications between the true and false lumens are often identified on careful scanning of the entire thoracic aorta. Some will represent entry sites with flow from the true toward the false channel, and others will be exit sites or have bidirectional flow (Fig. 33–5). Exit tears, where flow reenters the true lumen from the false lumen, may occur at one or multiple

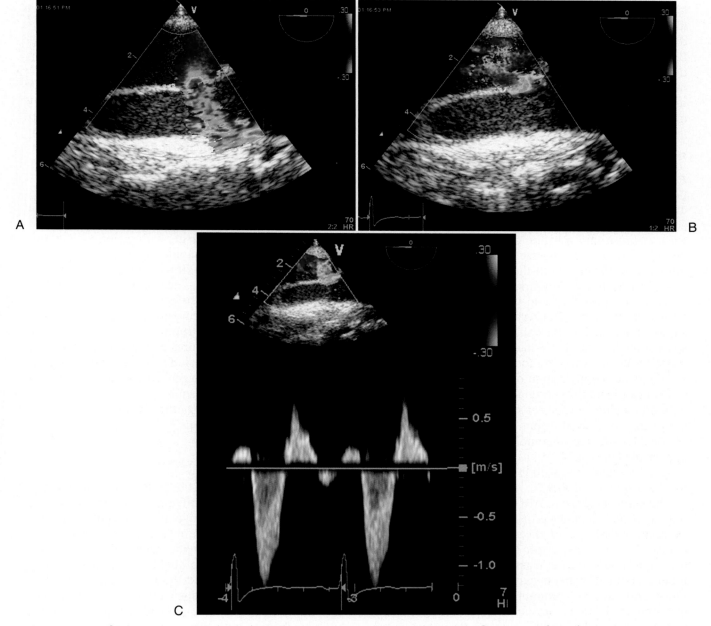

Figure 33–5. *Entry tear in the transverse aortic arch.* A, *During systole, flow crosses from the true lumen into the false lumen.* B, *During diastole, flow reverses as the false lumen decompresses.* C, *The alternating direction and timing of flow can be confirmed with spectral Doppler.*

sites. The exact location of a given tear can be estimated from the depth of probe insertion from the incisors, an arbitrary but convenient reference point. Recording this information at the time of the procedure and on the written report not only is helpful in the surgical correction of dissection but also is extremely important for comparison with postoperative follow-up TEE studies, where many of the original tears may still be detectable.

Identification of the primary entry site must be deduced from location, size, and flow patterns. In some cases the primary tear cannot clearly be assigned to any one tear, either because of multiple tears as described previously or in some cases because of the TEE "blind spot." Adachi and colleagues[87] were able to identify the entry site in 50 of 57 patients with acute dissection. They were more successful in this with type B dissections (90%) than with type A (83%). As mentioned previously, identification of the primary tear is mostly important because ensuring that the surgical repair resects the primary entry site may decrease the incidence of late reoperation.

Intramural Hematoma

A small number of aortic dissections, estimated at three percent to five percent, occur without apparent intimal disruption.[6,88] The pathologic process in these cases of aortic intramural hematoma (AIH) is rupture of the vasa vasorum into a region of medial degeneration or possibly rupture of atherosclerotic plaque without an intimal tear. Patients with this form of disease tend to be older (mean age, 70 years, versus 56 years for communicating dissection) and have frequently had long-term hypertension. Transesophageal images demonstrate a thickened aortic wall with intramural echo-free spaces, an increased distance from the TEE probe to the inner aortic wall, and focal distortion of the transverse circular configuration of the aorta.

Echocardiographic criteria have been proposed for AIH, and include a crescent-shaped or circular thickening of the aortic wall 7 mm or more in thickness, extending 1 to 20 cm longitudinally, without an intimal flap or evidence of flow in the thickened aortic wall. TEE has a sensitivity of 100% and a specificity of 91% for the diagnosis of AIH.[89]

The clinical course of AIH is similar to aortic dissection with high incidence of aortic dilatation resulting from the expansion of the false lumen, pleural and pericardial effusions, aortic regurgitation, aortic rupture, and progression to classical dissection. The early prognosis in AIH patients may be slightly better than in those with acute "communicating" dissections; this may reflect the tendency for the noncommunicating medial space to heal with complete thrombus formation.[90] Many AIH progress to typical dissection (in 33%) or to rupture (in 27%), however, and therefore

usually require surgical rather than medical management.[91]

About half of the patients progress despite medical treatment, and predictors of disease progression include involvement of the ascending aorta, a maximum aortic diameter greater or equal to 50 mm, persistent pain, progressive thickening of the aortic wall, or expanding aortic diameter. The treatment of AIH is similar to aortic dissection; if the AIH is located in the ascending aorta, early surgical intervention with aortic graft replacement is often recommended. Mortality after surgery ranges from 10% to 50% at 30 days.[92-94] Another strategy that has been advocated is initial medical therapy with aggressive antihypertensive treatment and frequent imaging follow up, with elective surgery for patients who develop complications.[95]

Early prognosis in those patients was somewhat better than in those with acute "communicating" dissections; this may reflect the tendency for the noncommunicating medial space to heal with complete thrombus formation.[90] These intramural hematomas may progress to typical dissection (in 33%) or to rupture (in 27%), and therefore usually require surgical rather than medical management.[91]

Penetrating Ulcer

Ulceration of an atheromatous plaque into the internal elastic lamina of the aorta creates a penetrating atheromatous ulcer (PAU).[96] Patients with penetrating atheromatous ulcer are typically older, have more cardiovascular risk factors, and diffuse atherosclerosis. The ulcers are predominately located in the descending aorta where atherosclerosis tends to be more severe. They can progress to aneurysm formation, intramural hematoma, dissection, or rupture.

Echocardiographic features of penetrating atheromatous ulcers of the aorta include a crater-like out pouching of the aorta with jagged edges, associated with complex atheromatous plaque.

Controversy remains regarding medical versus surgical therapy for these lesions.[97,98]

Complications of Dissection

An important goal of echocardiographic imaging in aortic dissection is identifying associated complications. Type A dissections may produce acute AR resulting from annular dilation or disruption of leaflet suspension. TEE can provide detailed morphologic information regarding the quality of the leaflet tissue and the mechanism of AR; these can help in the decision regarding valve resuspension versus replacement. Pericardial effusion and tamponade are manifestations of aortic rupture with dissection and are often readily identified on transthoracic views (Fig. 33-6). The Doppler manifestations of pericardial tamponade may be

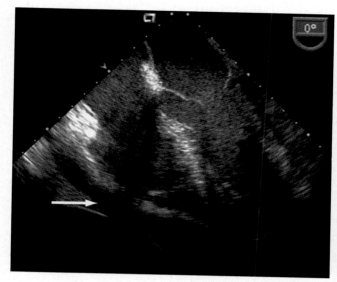

Figure 33–6. *A four-chamber transesophageal echocardiographic view during contrast injection (Optison) shows contrast in the left ventricular cavity but not in the small pericardial effusion (arrow), which was unassociated with tamponade physiology.*

best obtained from external apical views and may obviate preoperative TEE in the interest of moving the patient emergently to the operating room. Other rupture syndromes can occur at different sites. Uncontained rupture into the mediastinum or pleural space causes sudden death. Some ruptures are contained by the aortic adventitia, resulting in pseudoaneurysm formation or hematoma (Fig. 33–7). In these cases TEE can detect the intimal breach and the extension of the hematoma into the surrounding tissues. An important proviso is to image the aorta at an adequate imaging depth so that such a hematoma can be recognized. These extravasations can be missed if the imaging field is restricted to the expected aortic contours; disastrous consequences can ensue if the site of the extravasation is not corrected along with the proximal aortic repair. Contrast may be useful in ruling out extravasation (Fig. 33–8).

Coronary Artery Involvement

Involvement of coronary arteries by aortic dissection is an important issue, and one that raises the question of whether preoperative coronary angiography is mandatory. Involvement of one or both coronary arteries by acute aortic dissection has been estimated to occur in 10% to 20% of cases[99] (Fig. 33–9). In a series of 34 aortic dissection patients, Ballal and colleagues[100] detected coronary involvement with TEE in six of seven surgically documented dissected coronaries. Of note, electrocardiogram changes were demonstrated in only two of the six patients with coronary involvement. Adequate views of the ostia and proximal vessel were obtained for 88% of left main arteries and 50% of right

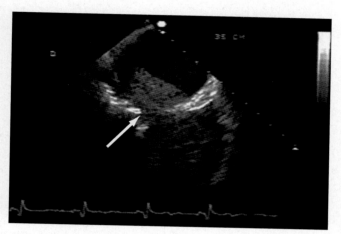

Figure 33–7. *Transesophageal view of the descending aorta shows a large thrombus in the aortic lumen. There is a discontinuity of the posterior aortic wall (arrow) underlying the thrombus and extension of clot into the periaortic tissues. This was confirmed to be a descending thoracic aortic rupture on subsequent surgery.*

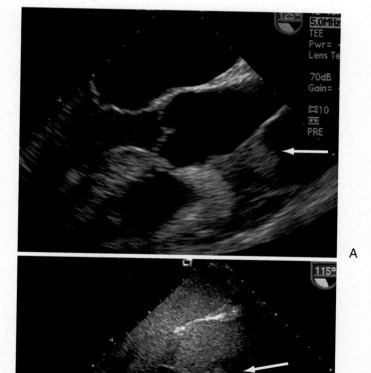

Figure 33–8. *A transesophageal echocardiographic view of the ascending aorta suggests an intimal flap with possible lumen rupture. Contrast injection (A) (Optison) does not confirm extravasation outside the aorta (B, arrow).*

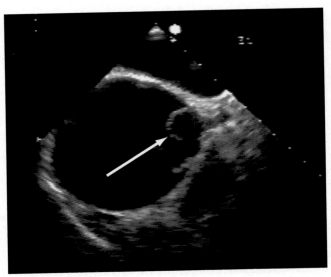

Figure 33–9. *A short-axis transesophageal echocardiographic view of the aortic root demonstrates an intimal flap in proximity to the left coronary ostium* (arrow).

coronary arteries overall. Visualization of the ostia and proximal coronaries continues to improve as variable imaging plane TEE probes are used and higher frequencies become available.

A separate but related issue is whether concomitant coronary artery disease, independent of coronary dissection, is an important consideration that should prompt routine angiography. Given the underlying vascular disease that affects many patients with dissection, it is not surprising that coronary disease has been found in up to 43% of patients with aortic dissection. The benefits of addressing potentially important coronary stenoses must be weighed against the risk of delays and aortic manipulation during acute dissection and adjusted for the patient's baseline likelihood of coronary disease. A series of 122 patients from the Cleveland Clinic found no difference in the in-hospital mortality between patients who had emergency coronary arteriography before dissection repair and those who did not. Three fourths of all coronary artery bypass graft (CABG) procedures performed in that series were done because of coronary dissection rather than obstruction resulting from coronary artery disease.[101]

Surgical Considerations

The planning of surgical correction of aortic dissection is heavily influenced by many of the features discussed previously. The extent of the dissection, the location of primary tears, and concomitant valvular regurgitation and coronary disease are all critically

TABLE 33–4. Operative Uses of Transesophageal Echocardiography in Aortic Dissection

Precardiopulmonary Bypass Assessment
Aorta*
  Intimal flap
  Entry tear
  Intramural hematoma
  Aortic rupture
  Aortic pseudoaneurysm
  Distal extent of extension
  Additional tears
  False lumen flow patterns, including thrombus
  Branch vessel involvement
    Coronary situs and dissection
    Involvement of origins of great vessels
  Underlying pathology
    Atheromatous disease
    Coarctation
    Sites of previous repairs
  Cannulation and cross clamp sites
Aortic valve
  Regurgitation
  Suitability for repair versus replacement
  Sizing for allograft replacement
Mitral valve
  Regurgitation
  Suitability for repair versus replacement
Left and right ventricle
  Wall motion abnormalities
Pericardium
  Effusion

Postcardiopulmonary Bypass Assessment
Aorta*
  Confirm competency of proximal anastomosis
  Establish baseline for false lumen flow and distal tears
Aortic valve
  Confirm competency of repaired valve
Mitral valve
  Confirm competency
Left and right ventricle
  Wall motion
Intraaortic balloon*
  Confirm position in true lumen

*Epicardial and/or epiaortic scanning may be important in fully defining these features.

important to the surgical team. In addition, safe cannulation sites, aortic valve repair strategies, need for coronary reimplantation with root replacement, and confirmation of adequate CPB and even intraaortic balloon function can all be addressed with intraoperative ultrasound (US) (Table 33–4). Transesophageal imaging during surgery has the advantage of being unobtrusive (at least for the surgeon, if not for the anesthesiologist) and is commonly also used as an accurate monitor of left ventricular wall motion and volume status. The long-term outcomes for surgery are promising; a recent review found 96% and 90% survival at 1 and 3 years, respectively, after surgery for type A dissection.[102]

Intraoperative Echocardiographic Monitoring

An additional tool for completing the scan of the aorta is intraoperative imaging from the epicardium or surface of the aorta. The unlimited number of acoustic windows from this approach allows careful interrogation of the aortic root, origins of the great vessels, cardiac valves, and left ventricular wall motion (Fig. 33–10). The transesophageal blind spots in the ascending aorta and transverse arch can be thoroughly inspected from the epicardium, and potential aortic cannulation sites can be evaluated from the exterior aortic surface. Epicardial views give much greater freedom of visualization and measurement of the aortic valve and allow precise annular sizing before CPB to expedite selection of the valvular prosthesis. The position of the coronary ostia relative to the dissection and the annulus can be defined precisely with epicardial views, which may also aid in surgical decisions regarding valve-graft conduit placement or coronary ostial reimplantation.

The amount of time required for imaging in the surgical field can be limited to a few minutes, but this requires an experienced team with a surgeon or cardiologist familiar with the epicardial techniques and views. The combination of epicardial and transesophageal techniques ensures that a high-quality ultrasound image is acquired of all segments of the aorta above the diaphragm and eliminates any uncertainty regarding involvement of the ascending aorta. Post-CPB images from the epicardium can also be extremely helpful in reassessing proximal tears and interrogating suture lines between aorta and conduit.

Transesophageal views at the conclusion of cardiac surgery confirm aortic valve or prosthetic valve competency and allow prompt reinstitution of support if sig-

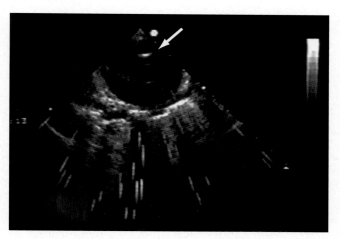

Figure 33–11. Intraaortic balloon pump position can be confirmed with transesophageal echocardiography. The intraaortic balloon pump can be seen properly positioned in the anterior true lumen (arrow).

nificant aortic regurgitation demands surgical revision. Intraaortic balloon pump (IABP) position can be assessed with TEE (Fig. 33–11); accidental placement of the balloon in the false lumen can be disastrous if not immediately recognized.[103] Finally, postoperative TEE images of the graft and native aorta create a baseline for subsequent follow-up studies.

Aortic Regurgitation

Aortic valve regurgitation complicating aortic dissection has negative effects on outcome and may dictate important issues in surgical approach. Preservation of the native aortic valve is possible in 86% of type A dissection with excellent results.[104] If the aortic annulus is abnormal as a result of Marfan syndrome or annulo-aortic ectasia, aortic valve replacement is preferred because of the limited long-term durability of aortic valve reconstruction in these patients. Initiation of cardioplegia for CPB usually depends on a competent aortic valve to allow antegrade perfusion of the coronaries; in the presence of significant AR, therefore, individual ostial cannulation or coronary sinus retroperfusion may be indicated. The specific causes of AR are also important.[78] Normal-appearing leaflets with a prolapsing cusp owing to avulsion of the leaflet base may be amenable to aortic repair with resuspension. Other cases may require aortic valve replacement. The specific involvement of the adjacent aortic root is also critical and may require a variable extent of prosthetic conduit. In some cases, human aortic allografts are used, which have the advantage of supplying both natural aortic valve and root.

In proximal aortic involvement, the position and involvement of the coronary ostia are important. Ostial reimplantation may be necessary; coronary bypass grafting may be unavoidable if the coronaries are dissected. Coronaries may be reattached by direct reim-

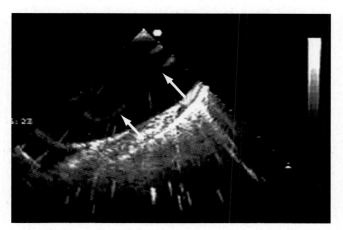

Figure 33–10. Intraoperative epiaortic view of the transverse aortic arch in a patient with acute proximal aortic dissection. The intima is widely dissected and highly mobile (arrows). Note the linear streaking artifact from electrocautery.

plantation with or without a surrounding button of aortic tissue, reattached to a piece of prosthetic conduit, or completely bypassed with saphenous vein or internal mammary artery grafts.

Mitral Regurgitation

Mitral regurgitation (MR) is a different example of a valvular abnormality associated with aortic dissection. New regurgitation may result from wall motion abnormalities induced by coronary involvement in the dissection, or from acute left ventricular dilation induced by AR. In other cases MR is part of the underlying disorder, as is the case with Marfan syndrome with mitral valve prolapse. Identification of the etiologic factors in the MR (e.g., leaflet degeneration, ventricular dilation, papillary muscle ischemia) will influence the need for repair or prosthetic replacement. Confirmation of results on early post-CPB images is important, especially when the decision is made to leave the mitral valve alone despite some regurgitation in hopes that correction of acute ischemia or dilation will remedy it.

Perfusion of Distal Vascular Beds

In the throes of acute aortic dissection, organs may be perfused by either the true or the false lumen flow. Organ underperfusion may occur if flow to the source lumen is compromised. During surgery, malperfusion may be caused by flow reversal when CPB is established by cannulation of the femoral artery, with obliteration of major communication between the two lumens from cross clamping or with repair of the dissection itself. Neustein and colleagues[105] describe a case in which femoral CPB compressed the true lumen and created severe malperfusion once the dissection was repaired. Perfusion through the new ascending aortic graft allowed immediate reinstitution of forward flow.

Follow-up of Patients after Repair of Aortic Dissection

Persistent Intimal Flaps

Despite successful surgical repair of aortic dissection, the aorta retains many abnormalities of structure and flow. Distal to the repair, the intimal flap and false lumen persist. The false lumen may thrombose, or it may retain flow along with entry and exit flow through multiple fenestrations (Fig. 33–12). One study detected persistent flap and false lumen in 100% of patients postrepair by MRI.[106] Persistent flow in the false lumen can be detected with TEE in the majority of patients

after surgical repair. Mohr-Kahaly and colleagues[86] found persistence of the false lumen in 71% of their postoperative patients at a follow-up interval of 1 to 41 months and in 82% of their patients treated medically.[86] Dinsmore and Willerson[107] have suggested that long-term survival is poorer in patients with persistent flow in the false lumen. Thrombosis of the false channel seems to be protective, a "natural buttress against future or further extension of the dissection" (p. 570). TEE confirms that sites without communications develop low-velocity flow and thrombus, whereas "healing" changes are less likely to occur in regions with significant tears and persistent flow. TEE also demonstrates aggressive atherosclerotic changes and calcification of the "neointima" lining the false channel.

Progression of Disease

Patients with previous dissection may develop progressive abnormalities of both operated and nonoperated aortic segments. Of original dissections, 25% to 40% will enlarge over time, and the rate and extent of enlargement are primary factors driving the need for reoperation.[99] In addition, dilation of noncontiguous, nonoperated aortic segments develops in 17% of patients with prior acute type A dissections. Early recognition of this progressive downstream aortic pathology allows reoperation in hopes of preventing rupture or redissection.[108] The concern regarding disease progression commits these patients to routine follow-up studies indefinitely.

Pseudoaneurysm Formation

Pseudoaneurysms form in 7% to 25% of patients with composite grafts, such as a Bentall procedure, secondary to hemorrhage at a suture line dehiscence.[109] Blood between the graft and aortic wall can create supravalvular aortic stenosis (AS).[110] Both of these complications can be detected and completely delineated by TEE,[111] CT, angiography, and MRI.[112,113] Color flow Doppler will demonstrate blood flow into the echo-free space between the graft and the aortic wall. Other postoperative complications include endocarditis and development of a sinus of Valsalva aneurysm.[114]

Recurrent Disease

Because the symptoms of acute redissection or expansion of a chronic dissection are nonspecific, the ability to reassess rapidly and compare the current findings with previous images is extremely important. Younger patients, those with Marfan syndrome, and those with primary tears involving the transverse arch are particularly prone to progression of their disease.[115] Because TEE may not be able to reproducibly measure the true

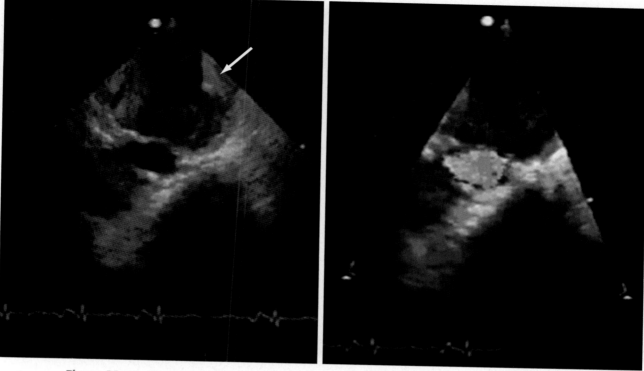

Figure 33–12. Transesophageal echocardiogram of the descending thoracic aorta in a patient with acute aortic dissection demonstrates a small true lumen (A) that can be identified using color Doppler during systole (B). The large false lumen contains both thrombus (arrow) and sludge-like flow.

transverse diameter of an ectatic aorta, suspicion of chronic expansion usually requires additional confirmatory tests such as CT or MRI. Excellent definition of the intimal flap, false channel thrombi and flow patterns, and consistent reference landmarks for serial sizing over time makes MRI a highly reliable method. When recurrent chest pain or hemodynamic instability suggests acute redissection, TEE can rapidly define the new pathologic abnormality and its extent. Changes from baseline postoperative or postdissection images can be extremely helpful in clarifying the etiologic site and event.

Limitations of Transesophageal Echocardiography

False-Negative Results

The interposition of the trachea between the esophagus and the heart creates a blind spot that obscures portions of the distal ascending aorta, superior transverse arch, and origins of the great vessels. As a result, a dissection limited to these areas could be missed by transesophageal imaging alone. This is of concern because the clinical behavior and therapeutic approach to the

patient depends largely on whether the proximal aorta is involved in the dissection. The occurrence of this extremely limited type of dissection must be rare because the incidence of false-negative studies has been minimal in large series.[73] In addition, large series have not confirmed a positive angiographic or CT result when the initial TEE result was negative. The involvement of the great vessels may not modify the surgical approach and can be assessed at operation.[116] The combination of transesophageal imaging with transthoracic imaging from suprasternal and parasternal windows yields a much more thorough assessment of the arch. CT, MRI, or angiography can also be used to assess this area when there is persistent clinical suspicion of a dissection that is not detectable by TEE.

False-Positive Results

The path of ultrasound through the esophageal wall and surrounding tissues may generate near-field artifacts that are often disconcertingly linear and run parallel to the aortic wall, mimicking an intimal flap. In patients with severe atherosclerotic disease, calcification in the wall can present similar artifacts and shadows (Fig. 33–13). Abrupt aortic dilation can create a "shelf," which can resemble a flap as well. Determin-

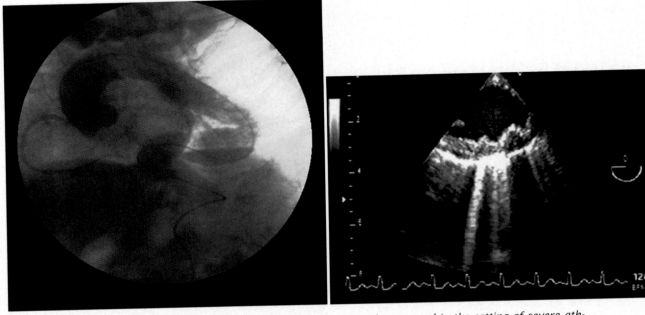

Figure 33–13. Imaging artifacts and difficult views can be expected in the setting of severe atherosclerosis (A) and aortic tortuosity and/or ectasia (B). Complementary methods, such as computed tomography and magnetic resonance imaging, may assist in difficult cases with low confidence images.

ing that these do not represent true intimal flaps depends on recognizing the minimal mobility of these "structures" and the homogeneity of flow on both sides of the line. The ability to change to a second imaging plane, as is possible with biplane or multiple-plane TEE probes, is extremely helpful in resolving the issue of artifactual "flaps."[83,117] Multiple-plane imaging also allows better visualization of the proximal ascending aorta, in which atherosclerosis and ectasia can be misinterpreted as dissection.[74]

Aneurysmal dilation of the aorta is another source of false-positive TEE studies for dissection.[118] Flow in aneurysmal areas is often low-velocity and swirling, similar to the flow in false channels. The absence of an intimal flap is important in avoiding misdiagnosis in this situation. The possibility that the intimal flap is not seen because the false channel has thrombosed must be excluded by carefully scanning up and down the aorta from the abnormal site. An intimal layer identified proximally or distally may be followed back to the suspicious dilated segment to suggest dissection.

Alternative Approaches to the Diagnosis of Dissection

Echocardiography is only one of several diagnostic tests for acute aortic syndromes (Fig. 33–14). The choice of one over the other and the clinical confidence in positive or negative results, needs to be gauged relative to the test's performance (see Table 33–3). A recent meta-analysis of 16 studies involving a total of 1139 patients reviewed the reliability of TEE, helical CT, and MRI.[119] The sensitivity and specificity of the three modalities were equivalent. After stratifying the patients for pretest likelihood of dissection (high-risk features included typical tearing chest pain in the back, hypotension, and pulse disparities) the positive likelihood ratio was highest for MRI, suggesting that this is the most powerful modality to confirm dissection in a patient with a high pretest likelihood of dissection. Helical CT had the lowest negative likelihood ratio of the three tests, suggesting that it is best at ruling out dissection in patients at lower risk. Angiography is a time-honored diagnostic method for aortic dissection that may identify the intimal flap and false lumen and coronary and great vessel involvement. Its sensitivity and specificity for dissection (88% and 94%, respectively[120]) are limited by false lumen thrombosis, intramural hematomas, and equal flow in true and false lumens.[121,122] The last case is also an important limitation for CT studies, in which differential flow may not be detectable even with dynamic CT imaging.[123] Ongoing improvements with multidetector, helical CT methods have improved the CT performance compared to early methods with lesser spatial and temporal resolution in assessing patients for aortic dissection.[124] Nevertheless, despite CT's high specificity (up to 100% in some series), a negative CT result in the presence of high clinical suspicion of dissection requires a second confirmatory test. This is also true for clinically discordant results from TEE or MRI as well.

Extremely slow, swirling flow within a segment of the false channel may not be completely differentiated

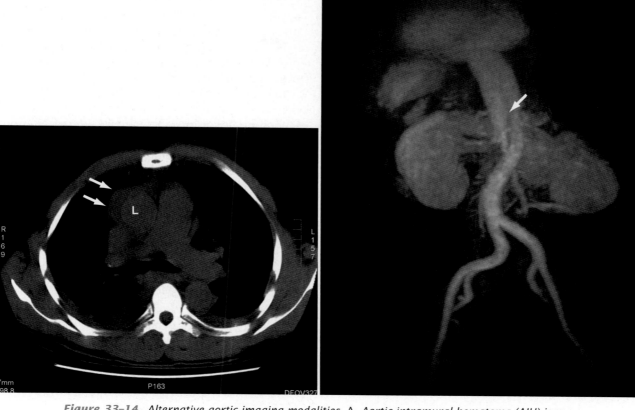

Figure 33–14. Alternative aortic imaging modalities. A, Aortic intramural hematoma (AIH) is recognized as a crescent-shaped thickening of the aortic wall without communication to the true lumen (L) of the aorta. Modern helical computed tomography methods demonstrate aortic intramural hematoma well (arrows), but with attendant radiation and contrast exposure. B, Gadolinium-enhance magnetic resonance angiography (MRA) can be used to create three-dimensional images of the aorta and branches. Follow-up of patients after acute dissection requires careful comparison of aortic dimensions; MRA is particularly useful for this. This demonstrates a chronic dissection (arrow indicates the intimal flap) that extends to the level of the renal arteries.

from thrombus by MRI.[125] The excellent definition of the important components of aortic dissection by MRI have resulted in its excellent sensitivity, however, which approaches 100%.[126] The pragmatic issues of imaging acutely ill patients with needs for hemodynamic monitoring or infusion of medications or those at risk for hemodynamic collapse continue to make TEE preferable in many acute settings. As mentioned previously, MRI may be the procedure of choice for the follow-up of patients with repaired or chronic dissections.

Research Applications and Future Directions

TEE images provide excellent spatial resolution, and in combination with the high temporal resolution of M-mode methods they allow investigation of aortic dis-

tensibility in normal patients, in patients at risk for vascular disease, and after repair of aneurysms or dissection. These types of methods have documented decreases in elastic aortic properties after aortic surgery, which predispose patients to redissection.[127] Two-dimensional (2D) echocardiographic assessments of aortic distensibility have been shown to estimate changes in aortic mechanical properties resulting from increasing age;[128] Doppler estimates of pulse wave velocity are also being investigated as measures of aortic compliance.[129] Animal models for validation of these parameters include chronic models of accelerated atherogenesis and acute aortic ischemia and decreased distensibility generated by removal of the vasa vasorum.[130] Multidimensional TEE images continue to inform regarding diagnosis and surgical planning (Fig. 33–15).

High-frequency ultrasonic integrated backscatter methods are also being applied to the aortic wall. Recchia and colleagues[131] detected sixfold decreases in backscatter and 15-fold decreases in anisotropy, sug-

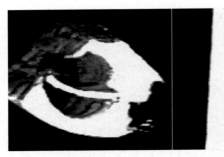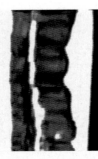

Figure 33–15. Three-dimensional constructed views of the aorta in short-axis (left) and long-axis (right) orientations demonstrate the intimal flap separating true and false lumens.

gesting marked disorganization of the three-dimensional (3D) aortic architecture in the aortas of patients with Marfan syndrome compared to normal patients.[131] These types of functional and structural investigations may improve the recognition of aortic disease of many stages and refine our prediction of risk of dissection.

TEE is playing an important role in the placement of stents for treatment of type B dissections. TEE offers the best detection and delineation of endo-leaks and is an important addition to angiography and intravascular ultrasound (IVUS) at the time of stent placement and at follow up.[132]

Summary

The grim prognosis of patients with undetected acute aortic dissection demands a rapid, highly sensitive, and efficient diagnostic approach. Transesophageal imaging has excellent sensitivity for aortic dissection, its multiple complications, and its imitators. Intraoperatively, TEE or epicardial imaging identifies surgically relevant features of aortic valve damage and ventricular function. Postoperative or chronic dissection patients can be followed with TEE, and serious events, such as expansion or re-dissection, can be quickly defined when symptoms of recurrent pain appear. Echocardiography is already established as a mainstay in the emergent diagnosis, treatment, and follow-up of patients with acute and chronic aortic dissection, and new technologies and applications will continue to expand its role in the future.

KEY POINTS

■ The immediate management and prognosis of aortic dissection and intramural hematoma hinge on whether the ascending aorta is involved.

■ Any dissection involving the ascending aorta is type A—irrespective of the site of the entry tear or direction of propagation.

■ Mortality of type A aortic dissection is one percent per hour for the first 48 hours.

■ TEE, MRI, and CT have similar clinical performance in assessing aortic regurgitation:

To rule our aortic dissection in a patient with low pretest probability, CT may be best but requires contrast and radiation exposure.

To confirm aortic dissection in a patient with high pretest probability, MRI may be best but is often inappropriate for unstable patients.

TEE can rapidly diagnose dissection and identify high-risk features, including pericardial effusion, aortic regurgitation, and wall motion abnormalities.

■ Aortic intramural hematoma (AIH) has the same prognosis and urgency as aortic dissection.

■ Aortic dissection can occur without significant root enlargement in a patient with Marfan syndrome.

■ Patients with bicuspid aortic valve remain at risk for progressive aortic dilation and dissection even after aortic valve replacement.

■ After surgery for dissection, the intimal flap and false lumen usually persist distal to the graft, and multiple entry and exit tears may be seen.

REFERENCES

1. Chirillo F, Marchiori MC, Andriolo L, et al: Outcome of 290 patients with aortic dissection: A 12 year multicentre experience. *Eur Heart J* 11:311-319, 1990.
2. Demos TC, Posniak HV, Marsan RE: CT of aortic dissection. *Semin Roentgenol* 24:22-37, 1989.
3. Lilienfeld DE, Gunderson PD, Sprafka JM, et al: Epidemiology of aortic aneurysms: 1. Mortality trends in the United States, 1951-1981. *Arteriosclerosis* 7:637-643, 1987.
4. Satler FL, Levine S, Kent KM, et al: Aortic dissection masquerading as acute myocardial infarction: Implication for thrombolytics therapy without cardiac catheterization. *Am J Cardiol* 54:1134-1145, 1984.
5. Davidson E, Weinberger I, Rotenberg Z, et al: Elevated serum creatinine kinase levels: An early diagnostic sign of acute dissection of the aorta. *Arch Intern Med* 148:2184-2186, 1988.
6. Hirst AE, Johns VJ, Kime SW: Dissecting aneurysm of the aorta. A review of 505 cases. *Medicine* 37:217-279, 1958.
7. Butler J, Davies AH, Westaby S: Streptokinase in acute aortic dissection. *Br Med J* 300:517-519, 1990.
8. Weiss P, Weiss I, Zuber M, Ritz R: How many patients with acute dissection of the thoracic aorta would erroneously receive thrombolytics therapy based on the electrocardiographic findings on admission? *Am J Cardiol* 72:1329-1330, 1993.
9. Erbel R, Eggebrecht H: Aortic dimensions and the risk of dissection. *Heart* 92:137-142, 2006.
10. Lee RT, Kamm RD: Vascular mechanics for the cardiologist. *J Am Coll Cardiol* 23:1289-1295, 1994.
11. Mukherjee DP, Kagan HM, Jordan RE, Franzblau C: Effect of hydrophobic elastin ligands on the stress-strain properties of elastin fibers. *Connect Tissue Res* 4:177-179, 1976.
12. Buntin CM, Silver FH: Noninvasive assessment of mechanical properties of peripheral arteries. *Ann Biomed Eng* 18:549-566, 1990.

13. Dzau VJ, Safar ME: Large conduit arteries in hypertension: role of the vascular renin-angiotensin system. *Circulation* 77:947-954, 1988.

14. Robicsek F, Thubrikar MJ: Hemodynamic considerations regarding the mechanism and prevention of aortic dissection. *Ann Thorac Surg* 58:1247-1253, 1994.

15. MacSweeney ST, Young G, Greenhalgh RM, Powell JT: Mechanical properties of the aneurysmal aorta. *Br J Surg* 79:1281-1284, 1992.

16. Carson MW, Roach MR: The strength of the aortic media and its role in the propagation of aortic dissection. *J Biomech* 23:579-588, 1990.

17. Rubin K: Aortic dissection and rupture in Turner syndrome. *J Pediatr* 122:670, 1993.

18. Ashraf SS, Shaukat N, Masood M, et al: Type I aortic dissection in a patient with osteogenesis imperfecta. *Eur J Cardiothorac Surg* 7:665-666, 1993.

19. Biagini A, Maffei S, Baroni M, et al: Familiar clustering of aortic dissection in polycystic kidney disease. *Am J Cardiol* 72:741-742, 1993.

20. Schor JS, Horowitz MD, Livingstone AS: Recreational weight-lifting and aortic dissection: Case report. *J Vasc Surg* 17:774-776, 1993.

21. Chauvel C, Cohen A, Albo C, et al: Aortic dissection and cardiovascular syphilis: Report of an observation with transesophageal echocardiography and anatomopathologic findings. *J Am Soc Echocardiogr* 7:419-421, 1994.

22. Eber B, Tscheliessnigg KH, Anelli-Monti M, et al: Aortic dissection due to discontinuation of beta-blocker therapy. *Cardiology* 83:128-131, 1993.

23. Evans JM, Bowles CA, Bjornsson J, et al: Thoracic aortic aneurysm and rupture in giant cell arteritis. A descriptive study of 41 cases. *Arthritis Rheum* 37:1539-1547, 1994.

24. Gersbach P, Lang H, Kipfer B, et al: Impending rupture of the ascending aorta due to giant cell arteritis. *Eur J Cardiothorac Surg* 7:667-670, 1993.

25. Marsalese DL, Moodie DS, Lytle BW, et al: Cystic medial necrosis of the aorta in patients without Marfan's syndrome: Surgical outcome and long-term follow-up. *J Am Coll Cardiol* 16:68-73, 1990.

26. Nienaber CA, Fattori R, Mehta RH, et al: Gender-related differences in acute aortic dissection. *Circulation* 109:3014-3021, 2004.

27. Pretre R, Chilcott M: Blunt trauma to the heart and great vessels. *N Engl J Med* 336:626-632, 1997.

28. Vlahakes GJ, Warren RL: Traumatic rupture of the aorta. *N Engl J Med* 332:389-390, 1995.

29. Parmley LF, Mattingly TW, Manion WC, et al: Nonpenetrating traumatic injury of the aorta. *Circulation* 17:1086-1101, 1958.

30. Smith MD, Cassidy JM, Souther S, et al: Transesophageal echocardiography in the diagnosis of traumatic rupture of the aorta. *N Engl J Med* 332:356-362, 1995.

31. Pieters FA, Widdershoven JW, Gerardy AC, et al: Risk of aortic dissection after aortic valve replacement. *Am J Cardiol* 72:1043-1047, 1993.

32. Katz ES, Tunick PA, Colvin SB, et al: Aortic dissection complicating cardiac surgery: Diagnosis by intraoperative biplane transesophageal echocardiography. *J Am Soc Echocardiogr* 6:217-222, 1993.

33. Sakamoto I, Hayashi K, Matsunaga N, et al: Aortic dissection caused by angiographic procedures. *Radiology* 191:467-471, 1994.

34. Dorsey DM, Rose SC: Extensive aortic and renal artery dissection following percutaneous transluminal angioplasty. *J Vasc Interv Radiol* 4:493-495, 1993.

35. Hsue PY, Salinas CL, Bolger AF, et al: Acute aortic dissection related to crack cocaine. *Circulation* 105:1592-1595, 2002.

36. Braunwald E: *Heart disease*, Philadelphia, WB Saunders, 1992, pp. 1536-1551.

37. Nolte JE, Rutherford RB, Nawaz S, et al: Arterial dissections associated with pregnancy. *J Vasc Surg* 21:515-520, 1995.

38. Roberts WC: Aortic dissection: Anatomy, consequences and causes. *Am Heart J* 101:195-241, 1981.

39. Oskoui R, Lindsay J Jr: Aortic dissection in women less than 40 years of age and the unimportance of pregnancy. *Am J Cardiol* 73:821-823, 1994.

40. Child AH: Marfan syndrome-current medical and genetic knowledge: How to treat and when. *J Card Surg* 12(2 Suppl):131-135, 1997.

41. McDonald GR, Schaff HV, Pyeritz RE, et al: Surgical management of patients with Marfan syndrome and dilatation of the ascending aorta. *J Thorac Cardiovasc Surg* 81:180-186, 1981.

42. Murdoch JL, Walker BA, Halpern BL, et al: Life expectancy and causes of death in the Marfan syndrome. *N Engl J Med* 286:804-808, 1972.

43. Gott VL, Laschinger JC, Cameron DE, et al: The Marfan syndrome and the cardiovascular surgeon. *Eur J Cardiothorac Surg* 10:149-158, 1996.

44. Pyeritz RE, McKusick VA: The Marfan syndrome diagnosis and management. *N Engl J Med* 300:772-777, 1979.

45. Hollister DW, Godfrey M, Sakai LY, Pyeritz RE: Immunohistologic abnormalities of the microfibrillar-fiber system in the Marfan syndrome. *N Engl J Med* 323:152-159, 1990.

46. Hirata K, Triposkiadis F, Sparks E, et al: The Marfan syndrome: Abnormal aortic elastic properties. *J Am Coll Cardiol* 18:57-63, 1991.

47. Jeremy RW, Huang H, Hwa J, et al: Relation between age, arterial distensibility, and aortic dilatation in the Marfan syndrome. *Am J Cardiol* 74:369-373, 1994.

48. Come PC, Fortuin NJ, White RI, McKusick VA: Echocardiographic assessment of cardiovascular abnormalities in the Marfan syndrome. Comparison with clinical findings and with roentgenographic estimation of aortic root size. *Am J Med* 74:465-474, 1983.

49. Roman MJ, Rosen SE, Kramer-Fox R, Devereux RB: Prognostic significance of the pattern of aortic root dilation in the Marfan syndrome. *J Am Coll Cardiol* 22:1470-1476, 1993.

50. Legget ME, Unger TA, O'Sullivan CK, et al: Aortic root complications in the Marfan's syndrome: Identification of a lower risk group. *Heart* 75:389-395, 1996.

51. Gott VL, Pyeritz RE, Magovern GJ Jr, et al: Surgical treatment of aneurysms of the ascending aorta in the Marfan syndrome. Results of composite-graft repair in 50 patients. *N Engl J Med* 314:1070-1074, 1986.

52. Pyeritz RE: Predictors of dissection of the ascending aorta in Marfan syndrome (abstr). *Circulation* 84(Suppl II):II-351, 1991.

53. Meijboom LJ, Timmermans J, Zwinderman AH, et al: Aortic root growth in men and women with the Marfan's syndrome. *Am J Cardiol* 96:1441-1444, 2005.

54. Roberts WC, Honig HS: The spectrum of cardiovascular disease in the Marfan syndrome: A clinicomorphologic study of 18 necropsy patients and comparison to 151 previously reported necropsy patients. *Am Heart J* 104:115-135, 1982.

55. Groenink M, Lohuis TA, Tijssen JG, et al: Survival and complication free survival in Marfan's syndrome: implications of current guidelines. *Heart* 82:499-504, 1999.

56. Gott VL, Greene PS, Alejo DE, et al: Replacement of the aortic root in patients with Marfan's syndrome. *N Engl J Med* 340:1307-1313, 1999.

57. Coselli JS, LeMaire SA, Buket S: Marfan syndrome: the variability and outcome of operative management. *J Vasc Surg* 21:432-443, 1995.

58. Tambeur L, David TE, Unger M, et al: Results of surgery for aortic root aneurysm in patients with the Marfan syndrome. *Eur J Cardiothorac Surg* 17:415-419, 2000.

59. Erbel R, Eggebrecht H: Aortic dimensions and the risk of dissection. *Heart* 92:137-142, 2006.

60. Gleason TG. Heritable disorders predisposing to aortic dissection. *Semin Thorac Cardiovasc Surg* 17:274-281, 2005.

61. Svensson LG, Labib SB: Aortic dissection and aortic aneurysm surgery. *Curr Opin Cardiol* 9:191-199, 1994.

62. DeBakey ME, McCollum CH, Crawford ES, et al: Dissection and dissecting aneurysms of the aorta: Twenty year follow-up of five hundred twenty seven patients treated surgically. *Surgery* 92:1118-1134, 1982.

63. Daily PO, Trueblood HW, Stinson EB, et al: Management of acute aortic dissections. *Ann Thorac Surg* 10:237-247, 1970.

64. Miller DC: Surgical management of aortic dissections: Indications, perioperative management, and long term results. In: Doroghazi RM, Slater EE (eds): *Aortic Dissection*, New York, McGraw-Hill, 1983, pp. 193-243.

65. Applebaum A, Karp RB, Kirklin JW: Ascending vs. descending aortic dissections. *Ann Surg* 183:296, 1976.

66. DeSanctis RW, Doroghazi RM, Austen WG, Bucklet MJ: Aortic dissection. *N Engl J Med* 317:1060-1067, 1987.

67. Miller DC: Acute dissection of the descending thoracic aorta. *Chest Surg Clin North Am* 2:347-378, 1992.

68. Dinsmore RE, Willerson JT: Dissecting aneurysms of the aorta. Angiographic features affecting prognosis. *Radiology* 105:567, 1972.

69. Miller DC: Improved follow-up for patients with chronic dissections. *Semin Thorac Cardiovasc Surg* 3:270-276, 1991.

70. Roberts CS, Roberts WC: Aortic dissection with the entrance tear in the descending thoracic aorta: analysis of 40 necropsy patients. *Ann Surg* 213:356-368, 1991.

71. Duch PM, Chandrasekaran K, Karalis DG, Ross JJ Jr: Improved diagnosis of coexisting types II and III aortic dissection with multiplane transesophageal echocardiography. *Am Heart J* 127:699-701, 1994.

72. Slater EE: Aortic dissection: Presentation and diagnosis. In: Doroghazi RM, Slater EE (eds): *Aortic Dissection*, New York, McGraw-Hill, 1983, pp. 61-70.

73. Grossman CM, Dagostino AN: Advanced atherosclerosis in false channels of chronic aortic dissection. *Lancet* 342:1428-1429, 1993.

74. Erbel R, Engberding R, Daniel W, et al: Echocardiography in diagnosis of aortic dissection. *Lancet* 1:457-461, 1989.

75. Nienaber CA, Spielmann RP, von Kodolitsch Y, et al: Diagnosis of thoracic aortic dissection: Magnetic resonance imaging versus transesophageal echocardiography. *Circulation* 85:434-447, 1992.

76. Nienaber CA, von Kodolitsch Y, Nicolas V, et al: The diagnosis of thoracic aortic dissection by noninvasive imaging procedures. *N Engl J Med* 328:1-9, 1993.

77. Victor MF, Mintz GS, Kotler MN, et al: Two-dimensional echocardiographic diagnosis of aortic dissection. *Am J Cardiol* 48:1155-1159, 1981.

78. Movsowitz HD, Levine RA, Hilgenberg AD, et al: Transesophageal echocardiographic description of the mechanisms of aortic regurgitation in acute type A aortic dissection: Implications for aortic valve repair. *J Am Coll Cardiol* 36:884-890, 2000.

79. Geibel A, Kasper W, Behroz A, et al: Risk of transesophageal echocardiography in awake patients with cardiac diseases. *Am J Cardiol* 62:337-339, 1988.

80. Silvey SV, Stroughton TL, Pearl W, et al: Rupture of the outer partition of aortic dissection during transesophageal echocardiography. *Am J Cardiol* 68:286-287, 1991.

81. Pearson AC, Castello R, Labovitz AJ: Safety and utility of transesophageal echocardiography in the critically ill patient. *Am Heart J* 119:1083-1089, 1990.

82. Iliceto S, Nanda NC, Rizzon P, et al: Color Doppler evaluation of aortic dissection. *Circulation* 75:748-755, 1987.

83. Appelbe AF, Walker PG, Yeoh JK, et al: Clinical significance and origin of artifacts in transesophageal echocardiography of the thoracic aorta. *J Am Coll Cardiol* 21:754-760, 1993.

84. Chan KL: Usefulness of transesophageal echocardiography in the diagnosis of conditions mimicking aortic dissection. *Am Heart J* 122:495-504, 1991.

85. Erbel R, Mohr-Kahaly S, Rennollet H, et al: Diagnosis of aortic dissection: The value of transesophageal echocardiography. *Thorac Cardiovasc Surg* 35:126-133, 1987.

86. Mohr-Kahaly S, Erbel R, Rennollet H, et al: Ambulatory follow-up of aortic dissection by transesophageal two-dimensional and color-coded Doppler echocardiography. *Circulation* 80:24-33, 1989.

87. Adachi H, Kyo S, Takamoto S, et al: Early diagnosis and surgical intervention of acute aortic dissection by transesophageal color flow mapping. *Circulation* 82(Suppl 4):19-23, 1990.

88. Eichelberger JP: Aortic dissection without intimal tear: Case report and findings on transesophageal echocardiography. *J Am Soc Echocardiogr* 7:82-86, 1994.

89. Willens HJ, Kessler KM: Transesophageal echocardiography in the diagnosis of diseases of the thoracic aorta: part 1. Aortic dissection, aortic intramural hematoma, and penetrating atherosclerotic ulcer of the aorta. *Chest* 116:1772-1779, 1999.

90. Erbel R, Oelert H, Meyer J, et al: Effect of medical and surgical therapy on aortic dissection evaluated by transesophageal echocardiography. Implications for prognosis and therapy. The European Cooperative Study Group on Echocardiography. *Circulation* 87:1604-1615, 1993.

91. Robbins RC, McManus RP, Mitchell RS, et al: Management of patients with intramural hematoma of the thoracic aorta. *Circulation* 88:II1-II10, 1993.

92. Nienaber CA, Sievers HH: Intramural hematoma in acute aortic syndrome: More than one variant of dissection? *Circulation* 106:284-285, 2002.

93. Dake MD: Aortic intramural haematoma: Current therapeutic strategy. *Heart* 90:375-378, 2004.

94. Evangelista A, Mukherjee D, Mehta RH, et al: Acute intramural hematoma of the aorta: a mystery in evolution. *Circulation* 111:1063-1070, 2005.

95. Song JK, Kim HS, Kang DH, et al: Different clinical features of aortic intramural hematoma versus dissection involving the ascending aorta. *J Am Coll Cardiol* 37:1604-1610, 2001.

96. Stanson AW, Kazmier FJ, Hollier LH, et al: Penetrating atherosclerotic ulcers of the thoracic aorta: Natural history and clinicopathologic correlations. *Ann Vasc Surg* 1:15-23, 1986.

97. Cooke JP, Kazimer FJ, Orszulak TA: The penetrating aortic ulcer: Pathology, diagnosis and management. *Mayo Clin Proc* 63:718-725, 1988.

98. Harris JA, Bis KG, Glover JL, et al: Penetrating atherosclerotic ulcers of the aorta. *J Vasc Surg* 19:90-98, 1994.

99. Crawford ES: The diagnosis and management of aortic dissection. *J Am Med Assoc* 264:2537-2541, 1990.

100. Ballal RS, Nanda NC, Gatewood R, et al: Usefulness of transesophageal echocardiography in assessment of aortic dissection. *Circulation* 84:1903-1914, 1991.

101. Penn MS, Smedira N, Lytle B, et al: Does coronary angiography before emergency aortic surgery affect in-hospital mortality? *J Am Coll Cardiol* 35:889-894, 2000.

102. Tsai TT, Evangelista A, Nienaber CA, et al: Long-term survival in patients presenting with type A acute aortic dissection: Insights from the International Registry of Acute Aortic Dissection (IRAD). *Circulation* 114:I350-I356, 2006.

103. Nakatani S, Beppu S, Tanaka N, et al: Application of abdominal and transesophageal echocardiography as a guide for insertion of intraaortic balloon pump in aortic dissection. *Am J Cardiol* 64:1082-1083, 1989.

104. Mazzucotelli JP, Deleuze PH, Baufreton C, et al: Preservation of the aortic valve in acute aortic dissection: Long-term echocardiographic assessment and clinical outcome. *Ann Thorac Surg* 55:1513-1517, 1993.

105. Neustein SM, Lansman SL, Quintana CS, et al: Transesophageal Doppler echocardiographic monitoring for malperfusion during aortic dissection repair. *Ann Thorac Surg* 56:358-361, 1993.

106. Laissy JP, Blanc F, Soyer P, et al: Thoracic aortic dissection: Diagnosis with transesophageal echocardiography versus MR imaging. *Radiology* 194:331-336, 1995.

107. Dinsmore RE, Willerson JT: Dissecting aneurysms of the aorta. Angiographic features affecting prognosis. *Radiology* 105:567-572, 1972.

108. Heinemann M, Laas J, Karck M, Borst HG: Thoracic aortic aneurysms after acute type A aortic dissection: Necessity for follow-up. *Ann Thorac Surg* 49:580-584, 1990.

109. Barbetseas J, Crawford S, Safi HJ, et al: Doppler echocardiographic evaluation of pseudoaneurysms complicating composite grafts of the ascending aorta. *Circulation* 85:212-222, 1992.

110. Vilacosta I, Camino A, San Roman JA, et al: Supravalvular aortic stenosis after replacement of the ascending aorta. *Am J Cardiol* 70:1505-1507, 1992.

111. San Roman JA, Vilacosta I, Castillo JA, et al: Role of transesophageal echocardiography in the assessment of patients with composite aortic grafts for therapy in acute aortic dissection. *Am J Cardiol* 73:519-521, 1994.

112. Nath PH, Zollikofer C, Castaneda-Zuniga WR, et al: Radiological evaluation of composite aortic grafts. *Radiology* 131:43-51, 1979.

113. Pucillo AL, Schechter AG, Moggio RA, et al: Postoperative evaluation of ascending aortic prosthetic conduits by magnetic resonance imaging. *Chest* 97:106-110, 1990.

114. Simon P, Owen AN, Moidl R, et al: Sinus of Valsalva aneurysm: A late complication after repair of ascending aortic dissection. *Thorac Cardiovasc Surg* 42:29-31, 1994.

115. Haverich A, Miller DC, Scott WC, et al: Acute and chronic aortic dissections-determinant of long-term outcome for operative survivors. *Circulation* 72(Suppl 2):22-34, 1985.

116. Chan KL: Impact of transesophageal echocardiography on the treatment of patients with aortic dissection. *Chest* 101:406-410, 1992.

117. Adachi H, Omoto R, Kyo S, et al: Emergency surgical intervention of acute aortic dissection with the rapid diagnosis by transesophageal echocardiography. *Circulation* 84(Suppl 3):14-19, 1991.

118. Alter P, Herzum M, Maisch B: Echocardiographic findings mimicking type A aortic dissection. *Herz* 31:153-155, 2006.

119. Shiga T, Wajima Z, Apfel CC, et al: Diagnostic accuracy of transesophageal echocardiography, helical computed tomography, and magnetic resonance imaging for suspected thoracic aortic dissection: Systematic review and meta-analysis. *Arch Intern Med* 166:1350-1356, 2006.

120. Erbel R, Engberding R, Daniel W, et al: Echocardiography in diagnosis of aortic dissection *Lancet* 1:457-461, 1989.

121. Cigarroa JE, Isselbacher EM, DeSanctis RW, Eagle KA: Diagnostic imaging in the evaluation of suspected aortic dissection. Old standards and new directions. *N Engl J Med* 328:35-43, 1993.

122. Bansal RC, Chandrasekaran K, Ayala K, Smith DC: Frequency and explanation of false negative diagnosis of aortic dissection by aortography and transesophageal echocardiography. *J Am Coll Cardiol* 25:1393-1401, 1995.

123. Mugge A, Daniel WG, Laas J, et al: False-negative diagnosis of proximal aortic dissection by computed tomography or angiography and possible explanations based on transesophageal echocardiographic findings. *Am J Cardiol* 65:527-529, 1990.

124. Yoshida S, Akiba H, Tamakawa M, et al: Thoracic involvement of type A aortic dissection and intramural hematoma: diagnostic accuracy-comparison of emergency helical CT and surgical findings. *Radiology* 228:430-435, 2003.

125. Barzilai B, Waggoner AD: Diagnosis of aortic dissection with transesophageal echocardiography. *Cardiology* 91:73-83, 1991.

126. Laissy JP, Blanc F, Soyer P, et al: Thoracic aortic dissection: Diagnosis with transesophageal echocardiography versus MR imaging. *Radiology* 194:331-336, 1995.

127. Imawaki S, Maeta H, Shiraishi Y, et al: Decrease in aortic distensibility after an extended aortic reconstruction for Marfan's syndrome as a cause of postoperative acute aortic dissection DeBakey type I: A report of two cases. *Surgery Today* 23:1010-1013, 1993.

128. Lacombe F, Dart A, Dewar E, et al: Arterial elastic properties in man: A comparison of echo-Doppler indices of aortic stiffness. *Eur Heart J* 13:1040-1045, 1992.

129. Lehmann ED, Hopkins KD, Gosling RG: Aortic compliance measurements using Doppler ultrasound: In vivo biochemical correlates. *Ultrasound Med Biol* 19:683-710, 1993.

130. Stefanadis CI, Karayannacos PE, Boudoulas HK, et al: Medial necrosis and acute alterations in aortic distensibility following removal of the vasa vasorum of canine ascending aorta. *Cardiovasc Res* 27:951-956, 1993.

131. Recchia D, Sharkey AM, Bosner MS, et al: Sensitive detection of abnormal aortic architecture in Marfan syndrome with high-frequency ultrasonic tissue characterization. *Circulation* 91:1036-1043, 1995.

132. Koschyk DH, Nienaber CA, Knap M, et al: How to guide stent-graft implantation in type B aortic dissection? Comparison of angiography, transesophageal echocardiography, and intravascular ultrasound. *Circulation* 112:I260-I264, 2005.

Chapter 34

Hypertension: Impact of Echocardiographic Data on the Mechanism of Hypertension, Treatment, Options, Prognosis, and Assessment of Therapy

JOHN S. GOTTDIENER, MD

It has long been appreciated that hypertension has important structural and functional effects on the heart. In 1867, the great French physician, Auguste Laennec described a relationship between cardiac hypertrophy and characteristics of the arterial circulation in noting[1]: "When affecting the left ventricle, I have seen its parietes more than an inch thick...the septum between the two ventricles becomes also notably thickened in the disease of the left ventricle...Symptoms are—a strong full pulse, strong and obvious pulsation of the heart..." Subsequently, the noted English clinician, Thomas Janeway, described congestive heart failure (CHF) as the manifestation of hypertensive cardiovascular disease.[2] Later, the relation between hypertension and hypertrophy of the left ventricle was established in observations linking cardiac findings to the then new technique of indirect blood pressure (BP) measurement with sphygmomanometry. Although left ventricular hypertrophy (LVH) was quickly associated with CHF, the relation of hypertension to cardiovascular morbidity and death is, in fact, complex. Many patients with hypertension do not have isolated hypertension. Rather, there is a complex interplay between hypertension, atherosclerotic disease, diabetes, and abnormal lipid metabolism. Nonetheless, clinical and epidemiologic studies have convincingly demonstrated the independent predictive value of echocardiographically measured LVH for cardiovascular morbidity and mortality[3-5] and surrogate arrhythmic endpoints.[6-8]

Research studies using echocardiography have provided valuable insights into the cardiovascular pathophysiology of hypertension. Moreover, hypertension affects over 20%[9] of the U.S. population (60% of blacks >60 years of age), and it is tempting to apply echocardiography routinely in clinical practice to define cardiac pathophysiology in individual patients. However, while echocardiography is unquestionably informative, its routine use in all patients with hypertension could impose enormous costs, which may not be justified by clinical benefit. These are all compelling reasons to review the role of echocardiography in the evaluation of patients with hypertension.

Cardiac Changes in Hypertension: Pathologic Findings

Pathologic findings in hypertension (Fig. 34–1) have included increased left ventricular (LV) wall thickness, increased cardiac weight, perivascular and myocardial fibrosis, and increased myocyte diameter.[10] Diabetes mellitus, which combines with hypertension in producing greater risk for CHF[11] and myocardial infarction (MI)[12] than would occur with either disease alone, also exacerbates the pathological effects of hypertension to a greater extent than would occur with either disease alone. Comparing autopsy findings in patients with hypertension, diabetes, and those with both diseases, it was found[10] that heart weight and fibrosis was greatest in diabetic hypertensive hearts. Moreover, findings of CHF were associated with the degree of myocardial fibrosis.

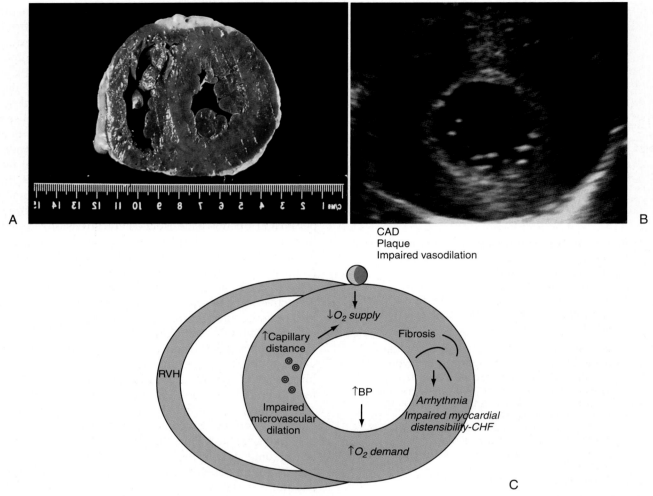

Figure 34-1. *Cross-sectional slice through left ventricle from a patient with severe hypertension showing marked symmetric increased thickness of left ventricular septal and free walls (A) with normal sized cavity (i.e., concentric left ventricular hypertrophy). Short-axis echocardiographic view of another patient (B) shows similar findings. Anatomic relations of some of the pathophysiology of left ventricular hypertrophy are illustrated in schematic (C). CAD, coronary artery disease; CHF, congestive heart failure; O$_2$, oxygen; RVH, right ventricular hypertrophy.*

Echocardiographic Studies in Hypertension

Prevalence of Left Ventricular Hypertrophy in Hypertension

The reported prevalence of LVH in hypertension[13-18] varies greatly, from about 10% to 60%, in part reflecting differences in study population (e.g., obesity, severity of hypertension) and criteria for LVH. In one of the earliest echocardiographic studies of LVH in hypertension, 51% of hypertensive participants (average systolic BP 150±20 mm Hg in treated participants) in the Framingham cohort had LVH as defined by values of LV mass exceeding the 95% prediction interval derived from normotensive participants. Subsequently, investigators at Cornell[14] using cutoff values for LV mass of 110 g/m^2 (body surface area [BSA]) in men and 134 g/m^2 in women, found that 12% of borderline hypertensives and 20% of mild hypertensives had LVH. In the Treatment of Mild Hypertension Study[15] in which the mean systolic BP was 140±12 mm Hg the prevalence of LVH (Cornell criteria) was 13% in men and 20% in women. However, using criteria that adjust for height rather than BSA, and hence are more sensitive in the presence of obesity, the prevalence of LVH rose to 24% in men and 45% in women. Black participants did not have greater LV mass or prevalence of LVH than white participants. In the Hypertension Genetic Epidemiology Network (HyperGen) study,[17] which evaluated hypertensive (many on treatment with average BP 131/75 in overweight, 140/76 in obese subjects) members of sibships (≥two siblings with hypertension) the prevalence of LVH (Cornell criteria) was 14% in obese versus 19% in nonobese subjects. However, when body size was adjusted for by height[2,7] the prevalence of LVH in nonobese versus obese subjects reversed to 20% and 32%, respectively. In a Veterans Affairs study[16] of 692 men with hypertension of somewhat greater severity than some other studies discussed here (average BP 150/100 mm Hg), 63% met Framingham criteria and 46% met Cornell criteria for LVH. One study,[18] which evaluated the relationship between hypertension control and LVH prevalence (Cornell criteria) in over 2000 participants, found a prevalence of 14% in untreated patients (average BP 148±16 mm Hg), 19% in controlled hypertension (average systolic BP 128±8 mm Hg) and 29% in uncontrolled patients (average systolic BP 158±19 mm Hg).

In patients who are entering renal dialysis, the prevalence of LVH is particularly high, about 70% to 80%.[19-22] This may be related to the presence of multiple comorbidities in addition to hypertension, such as diabetes, volume overload, anemia, and secondary hyperparathyroidism.

Concentric versus Eccentric Hypertrophy

Because of the strong clinical relationship between CHF and hypertension, there had been a presumption that CHF resulted from an end-stage hypertensive cardiomyopathy characterized by a poorly contractile, dilated left ventricle. However, this has not been proven in human hypertension uncomplicated by coronary artery disease (CAD) or hypertension. In studies of cardiac anatomy and function in hypertensive subjects using echocardiography, concentric LVH (Fig. 34–2) had been considered the usual cardiac finding.[15,16,23-27] In such patients, systolic function as measured by ejection phase indices, such as fractional shortening or ejection fraction (EF), has usually been normal or actually enhanced. However, most clinical echocardiography studies have used previously treated patients with hypertension. Studies of population-based cohorts have usually included a mix of subjects without previously treated hypertension and those with hypertension who may have been treated for unknown duration with incompletely identified medications. In studies, which evaluated newly identified patients who had never received antihypertensive drugs,[18,28] an increase in relative wall thickness (variably defined as relative wall thickness = 0.40 to 0.45), without increases in LV weight sufficient to exceed the partition value defining LV hypertrophy (i.e., concentric remodeling) or eccentric hypertrophy have been more common than concentric LVH. However, there a substantial numbers of obese hypertensive patients who may have nondilated eccentric LVH in which LV mass is increased, but neither LV cavity is not dilated and relative wall thickness is not increased.[16]

Disproportionate Septal Thickening

Echocardiography studies have shown disproportionate septal thickening (DST) in 6% to 18% of patients,[29,30] suggesting overlap of the cardiac manifestations of hypertension with those of hypertrophic cardiomyopathy (HCM) where asymmetric septal hypertrophy (ASH) is a prominent feature. However, the echocardiographic findings in most patients with hypertensive hypertrophy differ substantially from those of HCM.[31,32] Moreover early M-mode studies showing disproportionate

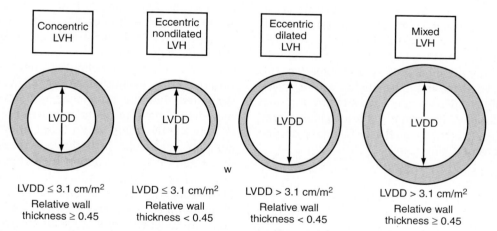

Figure 34–2. Left ventricular architecture characterized by relation of wall thickness to cavity size. LVDD, left ventricular diastolic cavity dimension in diastole; LVDDI, left ventricular diastolic cavity dimension after indexing for body surface area; LVH, left ventricular hypertrophy. (From Gottdiener JS, Reda DJ, Materson BJ, et al: J Am Coll Cardiol 24:1492-1498, 1994. With permission from the American College of Cardiology. Based on data from Savage DD, Garrison AR, Kannel WB: Circulation 75:126-133, 1987.)

septal thickening or asymmetric septal hypertrophy in hypertension may have used septal measurements, which were exaggerated by inclusion of right ventricular (RV) muscular structures, such as the moderator band, crista supraventricularis and even trabeculations. Because RV muscle is commonly thickened in patients with hypertensive LVH,[33-35] it is possible that inclusion of RV muscular structures may have contributed to the apparent thickness of the midanterior ventricular septum in older studies using M-mode without two-dimensional (2D) guidance. Even using 2D guidance to acquire echocardiographic data, measurement of the M-mode interfaces without inspection of the simultaneously acquired 2D images can still lead to incorrect choices of M-mode interfaces. Nonetheless, one 2D echocardiographic study[36] of patients with hypertension and unusually thickened LV walls did find patterns of hypertrophy, which overlapped those in patients with HCM.

Hypertensive Hypertrophic Cardiomyopathy of the Elderly

Although hypertensive HCM of the elderly[37] has been used to describe substantial increases in LV wall thickness, exaggerated systolic function and impairment of diastolic LV filling, particularly in elderly women, is seen and the echocardiogram (ECG) in such patients differs substantially from that in patients with HCM. However, (proportion of wall thickness to ventricular cavity size) that description more than 20 years ago by Topol and colleagues[37] of marked increase in relative wall thickness, small cavity size, and systolic hyperfunction is consistent with more recent observations of inappropriate hypertrophy, that is hypertrophy in excess of that which would be predicted by the loading conditions of the ventricle.[38] Specifically, such patients have lower than normal wall stress, exaggerated systolic function, small LV cavity, and marked increases in relative wall thickness. Notably, data from the Framingham study[39] also found a similar pattern of cardiac hypertrophy in elderly women, but not men, with systolic hypertension; and others[40] have suggested that patients with exaggerated hypertrophic responses may have a neurohormonal drive to hypertrophy. Importantly, these patients may fail to decrease, or actually increase, LV mass despite adequate BP lowering with drugs.

Left Ventricular Hypertrophy and Risk

A principal use of echocardiography in cardiovascular epidemiologic studies has been the identification of LVH, a discrete variable based on selection of a partition value of LV mass. As surrogate endpoints of risk,

abnormalities of diastolic,[41-50] electrophysiologic,[6,8,51,52] systolic,[53-58] and endothelial functions[59] have been associated with the presence of LVH or inappropriate LV mass.[60] The importance of LVH, in itself, in the morbidity of hypertensive disease has been underscored by the number of electrocardiographic and echocardiographic studies which have convincingly demonstrated its importance as an independent predictor of morbidity and mortality[3,52,61-63] Not only does LVH as a dichotomous variable predict adverse outcome, but the magnitude of LV mass as a continuous variable is also associated with cardiovascular risk, even with values for LV mass within the normal range. In the Framingham Heart Study, it was shown[64] that for each 50 g/m increase in LV mass (corrected for height) that there was a relative risk for mortality of 1.73, even in subjects free of clinically apparent cardiovascular disease. It was also demonstrated that this risk was independent of BP, age, antihypertensive treatment, and other cardiovascular risk factors. In addition to expressing increases in LV mass as that which exceeds the LV mass predicted by allometric body size, one can also consider the amount of LV mass that is in excess of that in association with body size and hemodynamic load. The close relation between body size and LV mass in infancy and childhood decreases with age, possibly resulting from an increasing impact of hemodynamic factors on LV mass.[38] The amount of LV mass, which exceeds that which can be accounted for by body size and by hemodynamic load, has been termed *inappropriate LV mass.* Excess LV mass has shown prognostic value for cardiovascular events over and above that of traditional LV mass and predicts risk even in the absence of LVH defined in usual ways.[65]

Additionally, the pattern of LVH and the magnitude of increase in LV mass is of importance in predicting the risk of LVH for cardiovascular morbidity (Fig. 34–3). It has been reported[61] that individuals with a higher relative wall thickness at any value of LV mass, including values below the partition value for LVH (i.e., concentric remodeling)[61,66] have greater risk of cardiovascular events. However, a recent study[67] has suggested that the prognostic importance concentric remodeling may not be independent of LV mass.

Importantly, there is an association of LVH with complex ventricular arrhythmia, a possible precursor of sudden death in hypertensive patients, even in patients without coronary artery disease on angiography.[8] In patients with reversible myocardial perfusion defects on thallium scintigraphy, both LVH and inducible ischemia are independently associated with ventricular arrhythmia.[51] Research has also suggested that regression of LVH may be associated with reduction of arrhythmia[68] and improvement in electrophysiologic characteristics, such as QT dispersion,[69] associated with arrhythmic risk.

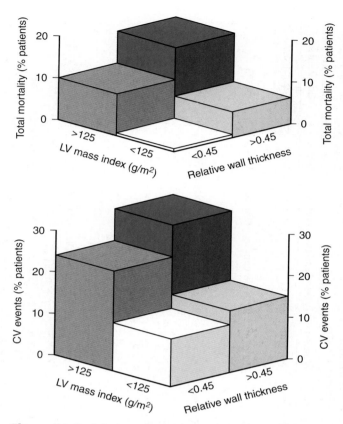

Figure 34–3. Relation of left ventricular (LV) architecture, left ventricular hypertrophy, and outcome. Increased mortality (top) and morbidity (bottom) are associated with increased relative wall thickness (>0.45) even in the absence of increased left ventricular mass (<125 g/m²), that is, concentric remodeling. CV, cardiovascular. (From Koren MJ, Devereaux RB, Casale PN: Ann Intern Med 114:345-352, 1991, with permission.)

Although there is comorbidity between hypertension, LVH, and coronary artery disease, LVH is nonetheless associated with an increase in mortality even in the absence of coronary disease on angiography.[62]

Relationships of Left Ventricular Mass to Body Size: What Is Normal?

The heart is no exception from other body organs, in that its size is proportionate to that of the body.[70] Numerous studies of population cohorts have demonstrated the relationship between echocardiographic measurements, height, and weight.[71-76] Moreover echocardiographic dimensions and LV mass decrease with starvation[70,77,78] and increase with refeeding.[77,79]

Hence to assess whether individual echocardiographic dimensions, including derived LV mass, differ from normal values, some sort of adjustment for body size is desirable. One commonly used adjust-

ment is to divide (normalize) LV mass by BSA. However, echocardiographic studies of normal subjects from infancy through old age[71,72] have shown that cardiac dimensions are not linearly related to BSA. Moreover, variance in body weight may reflect more than allometric (physiological growth) factors. Specifically, obesity both increases BP[80,81] and is a strong stimulus for LVH[82,83] greater than BP itself.[16,84] Therefore, normalization of LV mass by BSA, which is computed using body weight, tends to flatten the contribution of obesity to LV mass and LVH.[82] For that reason, independent groups of investigators have suggested using height for allometric indexation. The Framingham group[82] has developed norms for LV mass indexed by height alone, whereas studies from the Cornell group[85] have suggested that indexation is better accomplished by dividing by height to the power of 1.7.

Although advancing age has been associated with increases in LV mass,[72,86,87] this association may be the result of concomitant disease rather than affect of aging per se.[87,88] Effects of gender[72,89] on LV mass are somewhat problematic. Echocardiographic studies have shown greater LV mass in men than women.[71,72,90,91] However, it is uncertain whether the differences in LV mass represent an independent effect of gender or if the effect of gender differences on lean body weight, itself, is an important descriptor of LV mass.[74,88] Greater lean body weight in men may account for greater LV mass in men than in women.[88] The effect of gender on LV mass seems to be minor even taking total body weight into account.[72-74]

Hence the determination of abnormal LV mass in individual patients or groups of patients undergoing clinical echocardiographic evaluation may be complicated by uncertainty as to what is abnormal. Nonetheless, LV mass has generally been "corrected" for body size (height or BSA) and presented as gender-specific values. Table 34–1 summarizes normal values for LV mass using these various approaches.

Demographic and Physiologic Descriptors of Left Ventricular Hypertrophy in Hypertension

Although elevated BP is considered to be an important factor promoting increase in LV mass and LVH, it has become clear that only a portion of the observed variance in LV mass is accounted for by BP. Other clinical descriptors,[15,49,75,82,83,87,92-98] which have been implicated as contributing to LVH, include obesity, age, race, dietary sodium intake, insulin resistance, and other neurohormonal factors including adrenergic factors and the renin-angiotensin system (Table 34–2).

TABLE 34–1. Normal Values for Left Ventricular Mass

Source	Population				Left Ventricular Mass Average		Left Ventricular Mass Upper Limits		Basis for Upper Limits	Method	Body-Size Indexation Units	Measurement Convention
	Year	Men	Women	Age (Yr)	Men	Women	Men	Women				
Gardin and colleagues	1980	78	58	20-97	160±25 g*	107±17 g/m²	210 g*	140 g/m²	95% CL	M-mode	None	ASE§(Troy)
Devereux and colleagues[88] (Cornell)	1981	106	120	39±13 (18-72)	89±21	69±19	136 g/m²	112 g/m²	97th percentile	M-mode	BSA	Penn§
Devereux and colleagues[88] (Cornell)	1981	106	120	39±13 (18-72)	89±21	69±19	136 g/m²	112 g/m²	97th percentile	M-mode	BSA	Penn§
Hammond and colleagues[14] (Cornell)	1984	83	77	44±13	155±50 g (Penn) 193±55 g (ASE) 84±23 g/m² (Penn)	—	134 g/m²	110 g/m²	Comparison with hypertensive population: LV determination	M-mode	BSA	Penn
Byrd and colleagues[b]	1985	44	40	35±10 (23-58)	148±26 g 76±13 g/m²	108±21 g 66±11 g/m²	200 g 102 g/m²	150 g 88 g/m²	95th percentile	2D echo	BSA	Truncated Ellipsoid
Levy and colleagues[91] (Framingham)	1987	347	50	43±12	208±43 g (ASE) 177±41 g (Penn)	145±7 g (ASE) 118±24 g (Penn)	294 g 163 g/m 150 g/m²	198 g 121 g/m 120 g/m²	M + 2SD	M-mode	Height/BSA	ASE

Study	Year	No.	No.	Age				CV risk at 10 years			
Koren and colleagues[61] (Cornell)	1991	167‡	86‡	47±13	—		125 g/m²	125 g/m²	M-mode	BSA	Penn
DeSimone and colleagues[85]	1992	137	91	39±14	155±34 g	117±28 g	173 g	223 g	M-mode	None	Penn
					89±19 g/m	72±17 g/m	106 g/m	127 g/m	M-mode	Height	Penn
					35±8 g/m²·⁷	32±8 g/m²·⁷	48 g/m²·⁷	51 g/m²·⁷	M-mode	Height²·⁷	Penn
					89±16 g/m²	73±16 g/m²	105 g/m²	117 g/m²	M-mode	BSA	Penn
Kutch and colleagues[c]	2000	213	291	42±12	97±21 g/m	71±18 g/m	107 g/m	139 g/m	M-mode	Height	ASE
					37±8 g/m²·⁷	31 ± 8 g/m²·⁷	47 g/m²·⁷	53 g/m²·⁷	M-mode	Height²·⁷	ASE
					89±18 g/m²	70±17 g/m²	104 g/m²	135 g/m²	M-mode	BSA	ASE
					2.91±.59 g/kg	2.71±0.70 g/kg	4.11 g/kg	4.09 g/kg	M-mode	FFM	ASE
Cardiovascular Health Study[d¶]	2001	651	1066	72±5 (65-98)	166±45 g	127±35 g	197 g	256 g	M-mode	None	Penn
					96±27 g/m	80±2 g/m	124 g/m	150 g/m	M-mode	Height	Penn
					37±11 g/m²·⁷	36±10 g/m²·⁷	56 g/m²·⁷	59 g/m²·⁷	M-mode	Height²·⁷	Penn
					87±24 g/m²	77±19 g/m²	115 g/m²	135 g/m²	M-mode	BSA	Penn

*For purposes of comparison, values approximated from nomogram assuming age 60 years and body surface area 1.5 m². Predicted means and 95% CL are approximated from published nomogram.

†Cardiovascular risk at 4.8 years follow-up.

‡Population including subjects with hypertension.

§$1.05\,([LVDD + PW + VS]^3 - [LVDD]^3)$; $1.04\,([LVDD + PW + VS]^3 - [LVDD]^3) - 14\ g$

¶Personal communication; healthy subgroup—excludes hypertension, prevalent coronary artery disease, or prevalent congestive heart failure.

ASE, American Society of Echocardiography; BSA, body surface area; Cornell, Cornell measurement convention (inner edges and posterior wall; CL, confidence limits; CV, cardiovascular; FFM, fat free mass; Framingham, Framingham measurement convention; H, height; LVDD, left ventricle diastolic dimension; LVH, left ventricular hypertrophy; Penn, University of Pennsylvania measurement convention; PW, posterior wall thickness; VS, ventricular septum thickness.

aGardin J, Henry W, Savage D, et al: J Clin Ultrasound 7:439-447, 1979.
bByrd BF, Wahr D, Wang YS, et al: J Am Coll Cardiol 6:1021-1025, 1984.
cKuch B, Hense HW, Gneiting B, et al: Circulation 102:405-410, 2000, with permission.
dCardiovascular Health Study, Gottdiener J (personal communication).

Data from references 14, 61, 85, 88, 91.

TABLE 34–2. Factors That Affect Left Ventricular Mass

Demographic and Physiologic Variables

Age
Race
Gender
Body size

Hemodynamic Workload

Blood pressure
Vascular resistance or impedance
LV inotropy and geometry
Stress
    Exercise
    Physiologic

Nonhemodynamic Factors

Renin-angiotensin system
Parathyroid hormone
Genetic susceptibility
Growth hormones
Salt intake

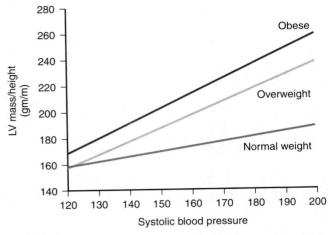

Figure 34–4. *Effect of obesity on relation between systolic blood pressure and left ventricular (LV) mass. Body weight categories are the same as in Figure 32–3. (From Gottdiener JS, Reda DJ, Materson BJ, et al: J Am Coll Cardiol 24:1492-1498, 1994. With permission from the American College of Cardiology.)*

Obesity and Left Ventricular Hypertrophy

In one study of normal subjects and patients with hypertension,[93] obesity was associated with eccentric LVH consequent to LV cavity dilatation, and LV mass was not higher in lean hypertensives than in lean normotensive subjects. Hammond and colleagues[74] also found that increased LV mass with obesity was a consequence of LV cavity dilatation but not increased wall thickness. In the Framingham Heart Study,[82,83] which used echocardiography in a large population-based cohort, obesity measured by body mass index (BMI) or by skinfold thickness was associated with substantial increases in the prevalence of LVH in men. Although both hypertension and obesity were independently associated with LV mass and wall thickness, the associations were additive but not synergistic. Liebson and colleagues[15] noted that in patients with mild hypertension and virtual absence of LVH on ECG, that body weight and body mass index were important predictors of LV wall thickness, LV mass, and hypertrophy on ECG. However, eccentric dilated hypertrophy was the most common pattern (52%) of LVH, followed by concentric LVH (33%).

In a study[16] of 692 male veterans with mild-moderate hypertension and high prevalence (63% using Framingham criteria) of LVH, both LV wall thickness and LV cavity volume were greater in obese and overweight hypertensive men, than in those of normal weight. Moreover, despite the importance of obesity in the cohort, even lean hypertensives with mild-moderate hypertension had a high prevalence of LVH in contrast to a previous study.[93] Also relative wall thickness was equally increased in all adiposity groups. Hence concentric hypertrophy is common even in obese men with mild-moderate hypertension. Moreover it was found that obesity amplified the slope relationship of systolic BP with LV mass (Fig. 34–4). Hence there appears to be a synergistic effect of obesity and hypertension on LV mass and hypertrophy.

However, in the Strong Heart Study, a population-based study of cardiovascular risk in American Indians, it was found[99] that LV mass was only marginally related to adipose mass, in contrast to having a stronger relationship with fat free mass.

Increases in LV mass in obesity might be a compensatory mechanism for increased workload. In a recent study of American Indian adolescents[100] from the Strong Heart Study, obese and overweight participants both had greater LV diameter, mass, and prevalence of LVH (34% and 12%, respectively) than those with normal weight (LVH = 4%). However, there was a fourfold higher probability of obese adolescents having LV mass exceeding values compensatory for their cardiac workload, and this excess LV mass was associated with lower EF, myocardial contractility, and greater force developed by left atrium to complete LV filling.

Age and Left Ventricular Hypertrophy

Studies have differed in their findings on the independence of the relationship between age and LV mass.[15,75,83,87,96] Research[15,94] has found that in patients with established hypertension, the relationship of LV mass to age is not independent of BP. Moreover, in the Cardiovascular Health Study, an epidemiologic study of almost 6000 community-based men and women older than 65 years of age, Gardin and colleagues[101] found that after adjustment for other covariates, age was only weakly associated with LV mass.

Although elderly normotensive subjects do not have higher LV mass than do younger subjects,[102] wall thickness is greater, and the Doppler ratio of early to late diastolic filling (E/A ratio) is decreased. In the Systolic Hypertension in the Elderly Program (SHEP) study,[43] elderly subjects with isolated systolic hypertension had greater LV mass and relative wall thickness than age-matched normotensive control subjects.

Race and Left Ventricular Hypertrophy

The prevalence and severity of hypertension is greater in blacks than whites[103,104] and ECG studies have suggested a greater prevalence of LVH (Fig. 34–5) as well.[105,106] However, using echocardiographic LV hypertrophy as a reference standard, Lee and colleagues[106] found that the specificity of ECG criteria for LVH, not adjusted for race, is lower for blacks than whites.

An early echocardiographic study of a relatively small number of black and white hypertensives[107] found greater LV mass in blacks consequent to greater LV cavity size. However, possible racial differences in obesity, which is known to increase LV volume, were not controlled. Other studies have failed to show higher LV mass in blacks,[15,16,94,95,108] including one in which the ECG prevalence of LVH was twofold to sixfold greater in blacks based on the ECG criteria used.[109] However, blacks did have greater septal wall, posterior wall, and relative wall thickness than whites in this and other studies.[94,95]

In the Jackson Heart Study[110] the prevalence of LVH (Framingham criteria) was as high as 83% in black women with diabetes, hypertension, and obesity and

as low as 28% (still substantial) in black men without any of those risk factors. In contrast, the population-based prevalence of LVH in adults in the Framingham heart study,[83] which had relatively few black participants but included hypertension and obesity, was 16% in men and 19% in women.

Left Ventricular Mass and Hemodynamic Workload

Previously, increases in LV mass, noted in 20% to 60% of subjects with mild-moderate hypertension[16,24,74,83] were considered to be passively related to increase in the cardiac workload imposed by hypertension. Usually, BP or systemic resistance, derived in part from BP, has been used to quantify hemodynamic workload. However, an increasing body of research has shown that while the relation between casual BP and LV mass is significant, the magnitude of that relation is relatively small. Although this relation may be improved somewhat using ambulatory BP recording for 24 hours, the correspondence with LV mass is still relatively weak.[111-114] Although systolic BP averaged over 30 years[115] is also a better predictor of LV mass and wall thickness than casual systolic BP, the variance of LV mass is still largely related to factors other than BP. Even using 20-year average systolic BP, the correlation coefficient with LV mass divided by height was 0.27 compared with 0.23 for index systolic pressure. Of the three structural components on the echocardiogram used to calculate LV mass (septal wall thickness, posterior wall thickness, and LV diastolic cavity dimension), wall thicknesses, but not LV diastolic cavity dimension, were statistically correlated with systolic BP.

Besides patients with hypertension, LVH may exist in subjects normotensive by usual criteria.[26,116] Several animal studies have shown a dissociation between LV mass and BP.[117,118] In the spontaneously hypertensive rat (SHR), a genetic model of hypertension in which both hypertension and LVH occur spontaneously, LV mass increases before increases in BP.[119] Of note, this model also demonstrated enhanced hemodynamic reactivity to environmental stresses, similar to that noted in human subjects with hypertension.[120] It has also been shown that subhypertensive doses of norepinephrine result in LVH despite a failure to elevate BP.[121]

A genetic contribution to LVH is suggested by the finding of increased LV mass in normotensive children of hypertensive parents.[122,123] Of interest, the finding of relatively high LV mass in normotensive children is predictive of the subsequent development of sustained hypertension.[124] Hence although BP and LV mass may be covariables, elevation of BP may not be the primary etiologic factor for LVH.

The poor relation between BP and LV mass does not necessarily indicate the absence of hemodynamic stim-

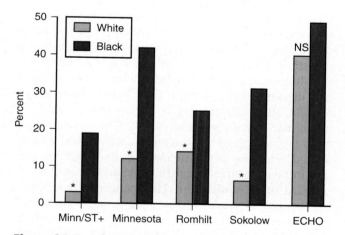

Figure 34–5. *Influence of race on prevalence of left ventricular hypertrophy (LVH): Echocardiographic (ECHO) versus various electrocardiographic criteria (Minnesota codes, Romhilt-Estes, Sokolow). Despite statistically insignificant difference in LVH prevalence on echocardiogram, markedly greater prevalence of LVH is present on electrocardiogram in black men with established hypertension with all criteria used (P < 0.05 all comparisons). (Based on data from Gottdiener JS, Reda DJ, Materson BJ, et al:* J Am Coll Cardiol *24:1492-1498, 1994.)*

uli to LV muscle hypertrophy. In an elegant study using echocardiography to express LV hemodynamic load in hypertension patients as "total load" (product of systolic BP and endocardial surface area) and as "peak meridional force" (product of systolic BP and LV cross-sectional area [CSA]), Ganau and colleagues[125] found better correlation of LV mass with total load and with peak meridional force than with systolic BP.

It is important to note that in echocardiographic studies comparing various measures of LV afterload and preload with LV mass, there is the danger of tautologic colinearity. That is, the use of a common parameter to derive the dependent variable and one or more independent variables, could mathematically force highly significant relationships. For example, if LV diastolic dimension were to be used in the previous study to derive LV cross-sectional area, endocardial surface area, and LV mass, one would expect LV mass to be correlated with hemodynamic load simply because of arithmetic linkage. Tautologic colinearity was avoided in the study of Ganau and colleagues[125] by calculating LV mass from M-mode echocardiograms, which were measured independently from the 2D echocardiograms used to calculate hemodynamic load. Nonetheless, M-mode or 2D calculation of LV mass uses a model in which a solid geometric shape of the LV cavity (prolate ellipse of revolution for example) is subtracted from a larger one of the outer, epicardial, LV volume to derive a shell, which expresses the volume of LV muscle. Hence the linear LV diastolic dimension (used in the calculation of LV mass) obtained by passing the M-mode cursor through the center of the LV cross-sectional image, and the area of that image (used to calculate hemodynamic load) might still be expected to link LV mass and hemodynamic load, unless LV wall thickness actually decreased with increasing preload to maintain LV mass at a constant value.

Because the LV wall thickness, even in hypertension patients, is usually much less (approximately 8 to 14 mm) than the LV diastolic dimension (approximately 40 to 55 mm), a constant measurement error might be expected to lead to much greater proportional error in the measurement of the LV wall thickness than the LV cavity dimension. This would decrease the ability to measure true differences in wall thickness (type II statistical error) despite preservation of the ability to measure true difference in LV cavity dimension. Therefore, one might be concerned that measurement of LV mass might be unduly dependent on LV diastolic dimension and thereby bias studies of hemodynamic load—LV mass relationships toward an association of LV mass with preload. However, echocardiographic studies in normal subjects[126] have demonstrated that decreases in LV cavity size during dobutamine infusion, consequent to the drugs effects on LV preload, are accompanied by measurable increases in diastolic wall thickness sufficient to maintain calculated LV mass at a constant value.

Hence it seems likely that increases in LV cavity size with volume loading of the LV should be accompanied by compensatory decrease in LV wall thickness, unless the volume overload in fact serves as a hemodynamic stimulus to LVH. The findings of Framingham, cited previously, which found no relationship between LV diastolic dimension and systolic BP but a significant relationship between systolic BP and wall thickness, are consistent with the data of the Cornell group in suggesting that hemodynamic stress is a stimulus to hypertrophy. Combining the findings, increased afterload manifested by elevations of systolic BP results in increases of LV wall thickness. In some patients, compensatory decreases in LV preload are sufficient to maintain LV mass at normal values (concentric remodeling). In others, volume overload prevents this response resulting in increases in LV mass, which are disproportionate to the pressure overload.

Stress Reactivity, Behavior, and Left Ventricular Hypertrophy

Given the absence of hypertension at rest in some individuals with LVH, it is reasonable to consider possible association of marked pressor response to physical or mental activity to LVH.

Exercise Stress

The presence of LVH on echocardiogram in normotensive men has been documented[116] in normotensive men who had systolic BP response of 210 mm Hg or greater to upright treadmill exercise. Because elevation of systolic or diastolic BP above predicted normal ranges with exercise may indicate a propensity to the future development of sustained hypertension, the purpose of this study was to determine if LVH could occur even in the absence of sustained hypertension. Echocardiography disclosed LVH in more than half of men with a systolic BP of 210 mm Hg or greater but in only one individual with a lower exercise BP. The increase in LV mass in association with exercise reactivity was characterized primarily by an increase in the posterior wall and intraventricular septal thicknesses rather than an increase in LV dimension. This pattern of concentric hypertrophy is similar to that seen in individuals with established hypertension. Additionally, the subjects with enhanced exercise BP reactivity also had greater left atrial (LA) size consistent with an adverse effect of the increased LV mass on LV filling, even in the absence of symptoms or hypertensive disease. Of note, there was a linear relation between the maximum systolic BP achieved during exercise and the LV mass index. When the 64% prevalence of LVH in these normotensive men with exaggerated BP response to exercise is extrapolated to the estimated 6.3% prevalence of this BP response in healthy men, the estimate of LVH prevalence in a population of healthy men would be approximately 4%. This is comparable to the value of 3.1% detected in normotensive subjects by Hammond and colleagues[14]

Studying 60 normotensive men with exaggerated systolic BP response to exercise, identified by screening 582 normotensive men, Polonia and colleagues[127] found LVH on echocardiogram in 52%, most of whom had eccentric hypertrophy and normal diastolic LV function on Doppler. This was in contrast to their patients with established hypertension who had predominantly concentric LVH and abnormal diastolic function. Of interest, 24-hour urinary metanephrines and 24-hour average systolic and diastolic BPs were also higher in the men with exaggerated systolic BP response to exercise stress than in control subjects, despite only marginally higher casual BP. Supporting the relationship between exercise pressor reactivity and LV mass in normotensive subjects was the presence of significant correlation between LV mass and peak exercise BP, but not BP during milder levels of physical activity ordinarily performed by these sedentary subjects.

In 189 normotensive subjects with exaggerated systolic BP response to exercise in the Framingham cohort, Lauer and colleagues[128] found significantly higher LV mass and prevalence of LVH in normotensive men and women than in control subjects without exaggerated systolic BP response to exercise. Adjustment of LV mass/height for age, resting systolic BP, and body mass index reduced but did not eliminate the difference in LV mass/height. However, the differences in average LV mass indexed by height were small, and after adjustment for the above covariables, there was no difference in prevalence of LVH.

As described subsequently, cardiac magnetic resonance imaging (MRI) may have better reproducibility than echocardiogram for measurement of LV mass. In a study[129] using cardiac MRI in 43 women and 34 men, aged 55 to 75 years, without evidence of cardiovascular disease, maximal systolic BP was the strongest correlate of LV mass among resting and exercise hemodynamic measures and was independently associated with LV mass after adjustment for lean body mass and gender.

Consistent with the hypothesis that exercise pressor reactivity is a predictor rather than a consequence of increased LV mass are findings from the Muscatine Study of normal children[124] that subsequent magnitude of LV mass was predicted by exercise but not resting BP.

Psychologic Reactivity to Stress

Psychologic reactivity to stress refers to hemodynamic and neuroendocrine changes produced in response to behavioral stress.[130] Because the magnitude of such changes usually cannot be inferred from resting (baseline) measures of these variables, reactivity measurements often contribute unique information on the physiologic functioning of the individual.

Several sources suggest LV mass in man correlates better with BP during mental challenge than during resting conditions. Devereux and colleagues[131] showed that the strongest correlations of LV mass and LV wall thickness with BP occurred during workplace activity. Furthermore, it was demonstrated that a measure of psychologic job strain[132] correlated with increased LV mass in working men. These studies suggest that LV mass either reflects the integrated effects of daily hemodynamic load on the heart, best indicated by BP recorded during work stress, or that the response of BP to work stress is a marker for a common pathophysiologic substrate underlying LVH.

The notion that psychologic stress may produce LVH in the absence of sustained hypertension is supported by the studies of Julius and colleagues.[133] Hindquarter compression in dogs produced transient, neurogenic elevation of peripheral arterial resistance and mean BP (average of 25 mm Hg). Although sustained elevations of BP did not occur, concentric LVH nonetheless was evident as early as 3 weeks, progressing to a 28% increase over baseline values at 9 weeks. Additionally, studying cynomolgus monkeys, Kaplan and colleagues[134] found an association between increased cardiac reactivity to psychologic stress and cardiac mass, but only in animals with resting BP greater than the sample median.

Studies of the relationship between psychologic reactivity and LV mass in humans have had mixed results. One study[135] found that BP reactivity to mental stress was predictive of subsequent increase in LV mass among borderline hypertensives during a 2-year follow-up. Moreover, Manuck,[136] studying normotensive young men, noted an association between LV mass indexed by BSA and diastolic BP response to mental stress tasks. Similar to the study cited previously in monkeys, the association of pressor reactivity and LV mass was present only in individuals in whom resting BP exceed the sample median.

Rostrup and colleagues[137] found healthy young men in the upper 99th percentile of BP had greater pressor and chronotropic responses to mental stress, but not cold pressor, than controls. However, no association was found between reactivity and either LV wall thickness or LV mass. In another study[138] of normal individuals there was a relation of LV mass (not adjusted for body size) to the magnitude of increase in systolic BP with cold pressor ($r = 0.35$, $p = 0.05$), with exercise ($r = 0.39$, $p = 0.03$), and with body weight ($r = 0.60$, $p < 0.001$). Moreover, LV mass was associated with higher degrees of morning psychologic activation and subjects with high anxiety levels had greater LV mass than those with lower levels.

In obese individuals with mild to moderate hypertension it was shown that systolic BP responses to mirror tracing task and to cold pressor were associated with LV mass, even after adjustments for obesity and resting BP.[139] In a Finnish epidemiology study[140] of risk factors for cardiovascular disease, the "anticipatory" systolic BP recorded before performing bicycle exercise was associated with LV mass in younger middle aged men. However, another study found no relationship of LV mass with mental stress BP but did note an association with concentric remodeling[141]

Failure of the expected diurnal decrease in systolic and diastolic BPs during nighttime hours may also be associated with a higher LV mass at any level of casual or 24-hour BP.[142] Rather than representing a greater hemodynamic stress because of persistently elevated systolic BP during nighttime hours, the observed relation between nocturnal pressure to decrease an enhanced LV mass response to hypertension may, in fact, represent a role of diurnal BP variation as a marker of sympathetic or other neurohumoral pathophysiology. Measurements of beat-by-beat variability of BP may also be important predictors of target organ damage.

Other Factors

It is surprising that whereas in vitro and in vivo animal models demonstrate an excellent relationship between LVH and mechanically imposed afterload, there is poor correspondence of BP to LVH in patients with hypertension. However, not only do BP measurements fail to provide an accurate measure of integrated BP over time in any given subject, but systolic BP is an incomplete measure of the actual impedance to LV ejection. Additionally, impedance to ejection is not the only hemodynamic stressor experienced by the left ventricle. Theoretic and experimental observations in humans have indicated that, in fact, inotropic properties of the left ventricle, LV geometry, and BP are important in describing ideal LV mass.[125] Nonetheless, nonhemodynamic factors remain an important consideration in the pathogenesis of LVH in human hypertension. Such considerations have included neurohumoral factors, genetic susceptibility, neurobehavioral aspects, diet—particularly salt intake and the interaction of hypertension with other pathologic processes, such as atherosclerosis and diabetes mellitus. However, it remains unproven that humoral factors mediate right ventricular hypertrophy and LVH in response to hemodynamic overload of the ventricle and that elevation of BP and cardiac hypertrophy are, in fact, secondary responses to a primary neuroendocrine disorder. Supporting a role of the adrenergic system as the mediator of cardiac hypertrophy has been the finding that subhypertensive doses of norepinephrine are capable of inducing LVH.[121]

Additionally, it has been demonstrated that serum from animals with LVH may induce hypertrophy of cardiac myocyte in vitro.[143] Additionally, a correlation in human hypertensives between LV muscle mass and plasma catecholamine concentration has been described.[144] However, research has suggested that regional rather than systemic sympathetic activation may influence LVH in hypertension. Schlaich and colleagues[145] used radiotracer dilution methods to measure total body, renal and cardiac norepinephrine spillover, and microneurography to record muscle sympathetic nerve activity. Total body and renal norepinephrine spillover were increased in hypertensives with and without LVH. However, muscle sympathetic nerve activity and cardiac norepinephrine spillover were increased only in patients with LVH. Moreover, there was a linear relation between cardiac norepinephrine spillover and LV mass index. Additional support for a neurohumoral stimulus for LVH, independent of BP, has been the findings of several studies that cardiac hypertrophy in humans and in animals may not be reversed by vasodilators, such as hydralazine and minoxidil, or by diuretics despite BP reduction equal to that produced by drugs which do regress LVH, such as alphamethyldopa or calcium inhibitor drugs.[146-149] This failure to regress LVH has been considered to result from reflex adrenergic or renin-angiotensin activation. However, it should be noted that virtually every antihypertensive drug has been shown in at least some studies to produce regression of LVH in hypertension patients. Additionally, there is a complex interaction of direct and reflex effects of drugs, involving not only BP reduction but also renal and endocrine responses. LV mass may be affected by reflex changes in heart rate (HR) and consequently, preload. Hence increased LV cavity size, which accompanies the bradycardia produced by beta-blocker drugs, may be expected to limit, or even abolish, reductions of LV mass, which might be expected with BP reduction, despite decreases in LV wall thickness.[150]

Renin-Angiotensin System Relation to Left Ventricular Hypertrophy

Because angiotensin I and angiotensin II may stimulate myocardial protein synthesis[151,152] and the renin-angiotensin system has been established as playing a role in some forms of hypertension, it is reasonable to suspect a direct link between the angiotensin-renin system and myocardial hypertrophy. Animal studies of regression of LVH in the spontaneously hypertensive rat have documented a parallel reduction of plasma renin activity and LV mass in animals treated with propranolol or alphamethyldopa, but an increase in both parameters in animals treated with minoxidil producing similar BP reduction.[146] Although these studies were not sufficient to demonstrate a direct link between angiotensin and LVH, angiotensin-converting enzyme (ACE) inhibiting drugs have prevented the development of cardiac hypertrophy in both spontaneously hypertensive rats[153] and in salt-sensitive and salt-resistant Dahl rats.[153,154] Additionally, ACE inhibitors have consistently produced reductions of LV mass in clinical studies. Further, drugs which elevate plasma renin activity (hydralazine, diuretics) seem to less consistently induce regression of LVH than do drugs which inhibit renin activity.[155] However, echocardiographic studies in patients with high renin versus low renin forms of hypertension have failed to show differences of LV mass.[55] Even though the relation between renin-angiotensin activation and LV mass is uncertain, it appears that LV performance in hypertensive subjects is worse in high renin subgroups.[156] Of note, high renin profile has also been associated with a greater risk of MI in patients with hypertension.[157] While the mechanisms for these associations remain uncertain, it has been well documented that angiotensin has potent vasoconstrictive effects. Hence these patients may have altered coronary reactivity with a propensity toward infarction and accelerated atherosclerosis perhaps related to smooth muscle hyperplasia.[158,159]

Parathyroid Hormone and Left Ventricular Hypertrophy

There are important relationships between intracellular calcium metabolism and myocardial protein synthesis. Moreover, in primary hyperparathyroidism, LVH is almost invariably present,[160,161] and LV mass decreases after parathyroidectomy even without change in BP.[162] Several studies have described the role of intracellular calcium both as a mediator of myocardial trophic stimuli and in the induction of proto-oncogenes, which direct protein synthesis.[159] Although calcium metabolism is regulated in part by parathyroid function, it has not been established that parathyroid gland abnormality plays a role in the relation between intracellular calcium, myocardial protein synthesis or arteriolar smooth muscle contraction and resistance. However, relations between parathyroid function, parathyroid hormone and hypertension have been described in some studies,[163,164] whereas hypercalcemia, per se, has not been associated with LVH, parathormone levels have been.[118,165]

Left Ventricular Hypertrophy and Salt Intake

Although the role between salt intake, salt excretion, and BP in hypertension has been well appreciated, relations between LV mass and sodium metabolism independent of BP have been less well studied. Experimental studies have indicated a role for sodium intake in LVH. Despite failure to reverse hypertension, sodium restriction in rats with induced renal hypertension may produce reductions in heart weight.[166] In a clinical study, sodium excretion predicted not only increased LV mass increase consequent to increase in LV volume as might be expected with sodium-related volume overload but was also a strong predictor of increased posterior wall thickness and relative wall thickness. In fact, it was the strongest predictor of all other nonhemodynamic determinants including body mass index, hematocrit, and serum epinephrine.[167] However, further work is needed to determine the independence of sodium intake from systolic BP in the induction of LVH in hypertension patients.

Left Ventricular Hypertrophy and Myocardial Infarction

It has been recognized in epidemiologic studies that patients with hypertension and LVH suffer a worse outcome with acute myocardial infarction (AMI) than might otherwise be expected.[168] Although this may be related to acceleration of atherosclerosis by hypertension, the presence of LVH may increase the extent of myocardial necrosis.[169,170] This may occur from both increased oxygen demand of hypertrophic myocardium and decreased oxygen supply consequent to impaired subendocardial perfusion. Hence the echocardiographic finding of LVH in patients with known ischemic coronary disease should indicate particular risk for increased morbidity and mortality following MI.

Left Ventricular Mass as Predictor of Subsequent Hypertension

Although ventricular hypertrophy seems to be a consequence of hypertension, the reverse may also be true, that is, hypertension may be of cardiogenic origin. Longitudinal evaluation of young hypertensive patients[171] has shown initially normal systemic vascular resistance (SVR) with normal or increased cardiac output (CO), but gradual decline in cardiac output and increase in systemic resistance during two decades of follow-up. The predictive value of echocardiographic LV mass for subsequent elevation of BP in initially normotensive individuals has been established in children[124,172] and adults.[173-175]

Hypertensive Heart Disease

Left Ventricular Hypertrophy and Systolic Function

The hypertrophic response to pressure and volume overload has been considered adaptive because an increase in functioning muscle mass seemingly preserves cardiac function despite increasing hemodynamic load.

With mechanical pressure overload, the cardiac response is characterized primarily by an increase in LV wall thickness. This increase in wall thickness can moderate or even prevent an increased afterload according to the Laplace relation:

$$\text{Tension} = PR/2h$$

in which P is LV systolic pressure, R is the internal radius, and h is diastolic wall thickness.

Presumably, at some point, LVH becomes maladaptive and systolic failure occurs. However, cardiac hypertrophy is often accompanied by alterations of myocardial perfusion even before systolic failure. Such alterations include subendocardial ischemia, decreased coronary flow reserve and increased minimal coronary vascular resistance. However, mechanical pressure overload models of LVH may not be entirely pertinent to essential hypertension in which the pathogenesis of both hypertension and LVH may be considerably more complex than increased systemic resistance.

Echocardiographic studies of LV function at rest in hypertension patients generally disclose normal or even increased[16,53-55,176,177] EF despite the presence of LVH. However, it has been suggested[56] that exaggerated LV function in some patients may be the result of unloading of the left ventricle by marked decreases in end-systolic stress from excessive increases in LV wall thickness. Rather than being a favorable prognostic feature, supranormal EF was associated with greater peripheral target organ damage than patients with lesser hypertrophy and lower (but still normal) EF.

It is important to note, however, that both fractional shortening, obtained readily from end-diastolic and end-systolic cavity measurements of the LV chamber minor axis between endocardial surfaces and EF derived from the same parameters are affected by loading conditions of the LV. Hence, according to the Laplace equation, where wall tension describes afterload, either a decrease in cavity size, increase in wall thickness, or decrease in systolic BP can decrease afterload and result in normal or even increased fractional shortening, despite the presence of myocardial dysfunction. One approach to determine the presence of myocardial dysfunction has been to assess LV contraction in relation to afterload.[178] In comparing groups of patients, graphic plots of fractional shortening against end-systolic stress have been useful in describing LV function, which is relatively independent of afterload. LV dysfunction in individual patients can be determined by plotting the patients' values against those obtained in normal subjects. Using this approach,[56] patients with supranormal EF at rest in fact had normal contractility when fractional shortening was adjusted for end-systolic stress. In contrast, increased resting inotropy was found in 22% of patients with hypertension with normal EF at rest.

Even assessment of fractional shortening in relation to afterload is problematic. Conventional measurement of fractional shortening measures chamber and not myocardial dynamics. Moreover, assessment of chamber dynamics may overestimate myocardial function, particularly in the presence of increased LV wall thickness.[57,58,179,180] There are several explanations for this. End-systolic stress at the endocardium does not extend across the thickness of the LV wall from endocardium to epicardium. Moreover, transmural thickening is not uniform during systole; the inner, or endocardial, half of the LV wall thickens more than the outer, or epicardial, half resulting in a relative epicardial movement of the midwall during systole. Additionally, it is probably physiologically inappropriate to use meridional stress, which acts longitudinally from apex to base, to adjust for fractional shortening, which largely represents circumferential muscle fiber contraction at right angles to the vector for stress.[180] Furthermore, endocardial muscle fibers are oriented longitudinally. Hence systolic contraction of the minor axis (fractional shortening) is actually produced by midwall muscle fibers (Fig. 34–6), which are circumferentially oriented.[181,182] It has therefore been suggested that assessment of myocardial contractility using the relation of systolic shortening to end-systolic stress is better accomplished with fractional shortening obtained at the midwall[58,179,180,183] with care to adjust for nonuniform transmural thickening of the LV wall. Using this approach in the catheterization laboratory, Shimizu and colleagues[57] found that fractional shortening obtained by their modified midwall method was lower in patients with hypertension with LVH than in controls or hypertension patients without LVH. In contrast, endocardial fractional shortening and fractional shortening calculated by a midwall method, which did not correct for nonuniform transmural thickening, did not differ between the three groups.

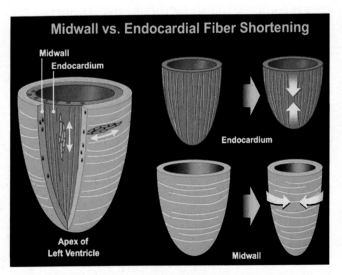

Figure 34–6. Schematic showing apex to base orientation of endocardial myocardial muscle fiber shortening, versus circumferential shortening of midwall fibers.

Fortunately, cardiac catheterization is not required to measure modified midwall fractional shortening-end-systolic stress relationships. Using 2D-guided M-mode echocardiography to assess midwall fractional shortening, De Simone and colleagues[58] reanalyzed those fractional shortening to end-systolic stress relationships,[56] which previously demonstrated enhanced inotropy in 22% of patients with normal EF at rest and found that only 5% of patients now exceeded the 95th percentile for normal myocardial function (Fig. 34–7). Moreover, the proportion with subnormal function increased from 1.5% to 16.5%.

One potential limitation to the use of M-mode echocardiography to assess myocardial function is the possibility that decreased midwall fiber shortening in the short-axis plane may be compensated by increased shortening in the plane of the long axis. However, studies by Aurigemma and colleagues[180] using both 2D and M-mode echocardiography to measure myocardial shortening in both orthogonal planes also demonstrated depressed myocardial function in hypertensive LVH despite preservation of endocardial fractional shortening.

Another way to evaluate LV function has been to study the response of the left ventricle to stress. Studies of LV function during exercise stress, using radionuclide ventriculography, have demonstrated impaired LV functional reserve in some patients with hypertension,[184,185] which may be dependent on the presence of LVH.[186]

Although it remains unknown whether hypertensive LVH can in and of itself lead to a cardiomyopathy with severely decreased LV EF, a study[187] of community-based elderly individuals showed an independent relationship between high baseline LV mass and subsequent development of subnormal EF.

Diastolic Function

The importance of diastolic function in hypertension and LVH is underscored by epidemiologic studies showing that despite the presence of CHF, systolic function is commonly preserved, particularly in elderly individuals[188-192] and that abnormalities of diastolic function may predict the development of heart failure.[192]

Numerous echocardiographic studies have shown alteration of diastolic LV filling in hypertension with and without LVH.[41,44-46,49,193-197] Importantly, it has been shown in experimental animals that abnormalities of diastolic function may accompany increases in either the fibrous[198] or muscular components[199] of hypertrophy. Additionally, LVH may be associated with diastolic dysfunction in the absence of elevated systolic pressure.[48]

LV diastolic function in hypertension has been most commonly assessed using Doppler flow velocity recording of the inflow tract and tissue velocity recording of mitral anular velocity and by color M mode propagation velocity of mitral inflow and pulmonary vein velocities. The techniques of diastolic assessment are reviewed elsewhere in this volume.

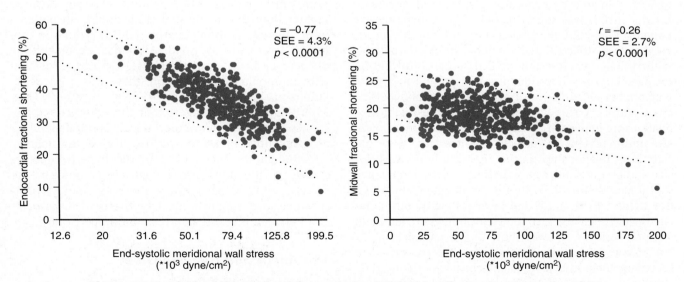

Figure 34–7. *Afterload-independent left ventricular (LV) function displayed as a relation of LV midwall* (right) *or endocardial* (left) *fractional shortening to end-systolic stress in hypertensive patients. When endocardial fractional shortening is used, many patients are above the 95% confidence interval of the normal relation* (parallel dotted lines), *suggesting enhanced contractility. With midwall fractional shortening, few patients exceed the confidence limits while many are below them, which is consistent with depressed contractility. SEE, standard error of estimate. (From De Simone G, Devereaux RB, Roman MJ, et al: J Am Coll Cardiol 23:1444-1451, 1994. With permission from the American College of Cardiology.)*

Complicating the use of Doppler for evaluation of diastolic function in patients with hypertension has been the sensitivity of Doppler parameters are sensitive to loading conditions of the ventricle, LA pressure, heart rate, and passive and active diastolic properties of the LV chamber and myocardium.[200-202] Additionally, compensatory reflex changes, which are autonomically mediated, may moderate the effects of loading on diastolic filling patterns. In normal subjects studied over a short time interval,[201,202] autonomic blockade with propranolol and atropine substantially altered the effects of decreases in preload (passive tilt) and increases in afterload (handgrip) on Doppler diastolic filling patterns.

The most common form of diastolic dysfunction in uncomplicated hypertension is impaired relaxation (grade 1 diastolic dysfunction), found in 20% of patients[50] and is associated with concentric LV geometry. The presence of abnormal mitral filling pattern has been associated with a particularly high risk of developing CHF in community-based elderly,[192] and a high E/A ratio has been found to predict cardiac and all cause mortality in American Indians,[203] a population at particular risk for obesity, hypertension, and diabetes.

Left Atrial Size

Although most echocardiographic studies in hypertension have focused on structural and functional alterations of the left ventricle, effects on the left atrium are also important. LA size is of clinical relevance for the occurrence of atrial fibrillation (AFib), stroke, and CHF.[204,205] In an early echocardiographic study increased LA dimension was found in only 5% of hypertensive patients[176] and LA dimension was only weakly correlated with systolic BP and LV mass. In elderly patients with systolic hypertension studied as part of SHEP, LA enlargement on echocardiogram was present in 51% of patients but also in 30% of age-matched, nonhypertensive controls.[43] This is consistent with the established relationship between LA size and age in both normotensive and hypertensive subjects.[176] There were weak but significant relationships in the SHEP study between LA size and LV mass indexed by BSA ($r = 0.20$) and relative wall thickness ($r = 0.31$). In the Framingham study of a free living cohort,[206] BP and LV mass were both correlated with LA enlargement on echocardiogram, although on multivariable analysis most of the variance in LA dimension was explained by LV mass. The prevalence of LA enlargement in hypertension is heavily influenced by obesity. In a study of Veterans with mild to moderate hypertension,[207] the prevalence of LA enlargement was 56% in obese, 42% in overweight, and 25% in normal weight men with hypertension. In the Losartan Intervention For Endpoint Reduction in Hypertension (LIFE) trial,[208] the prevalence of LA enlargement in hypertensive patients with ECG LVH was 56% in women and 38% in men. Multiple comorbidities including obesity, mitral regurgitation, atrial fibrillation, and echocardiographic LVH influenced LA size.

Although most studies have used single LA dimension to assess LA size evidence suggests that estimation of LA volume from 2D[209] or three-dimensional (3D) echocardiography may be a more sensitive and accurate[210-212] method.

Right Ventricular Hypertrophy

Although extensive studies have been reported on the relation between LVH and systemic arterial pressure overload, relatively little attention has been focused on the anatomic response of the right ventricle in patients with increased impedance to LV ejection. Because RV pressure overload does not ordinarily accompany arterial hypertension, determination of the presence of RV hypertrophy in patients with systemic hypertension[35] can be considered a test of the hypothesis that ventricular hypertrophy may be dissociated from pressure overload. One study performed 2D echocardiographic targeted M-mode echocardiography in patients with systemic overload of the LV (systemic hypertension and aortic stenosis [AS]) to determine the prevalence of increased RV wall thickness and its association with the clinical and hemodynamic descriptors in patients with echocardiographic evidence of increased LV wall thickness.[33] It was found that the average RV wall thickness in hypertensive patients of (7 + 2 mm) and in patients with aortic stenosis (6 + 2 mm) was significantly greater than that in normal subjects and in patients with dilated cardiomyopathy (DCM) who did not have LV pressure overload. Although the magnitude of increase in RV wall thickness was not associated with pulmonary hypertension, there was a linear relationship between LV and RV wall thickness (Fig. 34–8). These data suggest that the hypertrophic response of cardiac ventricular muscle is not dependent on a sustained pressure overload of that ventricle.

Although the mechanism of the hypertrophic response of the nonstressed ventricle is unclear, the presence of RV hypertrophy in the absence of RV pressure overload supports the hypothesis of disassociation between pressure overload and hypertrophy.

The Aorta and Hypertension

Clinicians have long been aware with the association between hypertension, aortic dilation, and aortic regurgitation. In a study of 3366 hypertensive patients,[213] the prevalence of aortic dilation (aortic diameter >40 mm in men and 38 mm in women) was 8.5% in men and 3.1% in women. In comparison to hypertensive patients with-

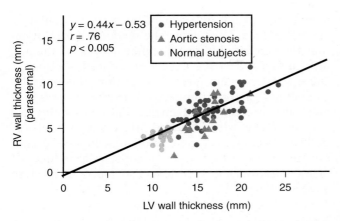

Figure 34–8. *Relationship between right ventricular* (RV) *and left ventricular* (LV) *wall thickness in patients with LV pressure overload. (From Gottdiener JS, Gay JA, Maron BJ, Fletcher RD: J Am Coll Cardiol 6:550-555, 1985. With permission from the American College of Cardiology.)*

out aortic dilation, those with aortic dilation had greater diastolic BP, were older, and were more likely to have metabolic syndrome, diabetes, LVH, and increased carotid intima-media thickness. The prevalence of aortic dilation (at the level of the sinuses of Valsalva) was 4.6% in the Hypergen study, which evaluated 2096 hypertensive and 361 normotensive subjects. Aortic root diameter was particularly high in hypertensives with inadequate BP control and was associated with age, male gender, increased LV mass, aortic valve sclerosis, and regional LV wall motion abnormality. The presence of aortic regurgitation was as expected associated with larger aortic root diameter. In another large study of hypertensive patients[214] with ECG evidence of LVH, the prevalence of aortic root dilation was 10%. Aortic root dilation was associated with higher LV mass, eccentric geometric pattern of LVH, and lower LV contractility.

In addition to the association of aortic root dilation with markers of cardiovascular risk, findings of the Cardiovascular Health Study[215] indicate that aortic root size is predictive of incident cardiovascular disease outcomes. Even with adjustment for other known risk factors, increased aortic root diameter was associated with increased risk for incident heart failure, stroke, and total mortality.

Effects of Antihypertensive Therapy on the Heart

Left Ventricular Mass

Although antihypertensive therapy has been shown to reduce LV mass and the prevalence of LV hypertrophy,[216,217] some studies[146,149,218,219] indicate that not all

drugs are equally effective in reducing LV mass, even with comparable reduction of BP. In particular, it has been suggested that diuretics and vasodilators may be ineffective in decreasing LV mass because of their failure to inhibit neurohumoral mechanisms responsible for LVH.[146] However, much of the literature[216] on LV mass regression has been based on uncontrolled, short-term, and nonrandomized studies with only one or two therapeutic limbs and relatively small numbers of patients. Moreover, the influence of covariates other than drug selection known to affect LV mass,[5,16] such as obesity, the magnitude of weight loss, the extent of systolic BP reduction, race, plasma renin, sodium excretion, and physical activity have often not been evaluated.

Although thiazide diuretics are effective and inexpensive drugs for the therapy of mild-moderate hypertension, some studies[220-225] have suggested that diuretics are either completely ineffective for reduction of LV mass or produce only small decreases in LV mass, disproportionate to their effects on BP. Moreover, studies in animals and in humans[155,221,226-228] have provided a physiological basis for ineffective regression of LVH with diuretics, in contrast to that produced by other drugs. Although beta-blockers, ACE inhibitors, calcium blockers, and centrally acting alpha blockers reduce BP and interfere with postulated neurohormonal mechanisms of hypertrophy, diuretics and peripheral vasodilators either produce no inhibition of these mechanisms or actually result in their reflex activation.[229] Therefore, despite reduction of BP, diuretics and peripheral vasodilators might be expected to be associated with no decrease, or even increases in LV mass.

Despite these considerations, a meta-analysis[230] suggested that diuretics can in fact produce decreases in LV mass.[231-235] Although many studies of LV mass reduction have been criticized for methodologic limitations,[220] including short duration, lack of controls, small sample sizes, and uncertain blinding, the Treatment of Mild Hypertension Study (TOMHS), avoided these methodologic shortcomings. TOMHS was a double-blind, placebo-controlled trial of 844 patients with mild hypertension and low prevalence of LVH, randomized to nutritional-hygienic intervention in combination with one of five classes of active antihypertensive drugs or placebo. Echocardiographic evaluation over 4 years showed decreased LV mass for all treatment groups including placebo and chlorthalidone. However, LV mass decreased more than placebo only in the chlorthalidone treatment group ($p = 0.03$) based on longitudinal analyses adjusted for baseline LV mass.[236]

The Veterans Affairs Trial of Monotherapy in Mild-Moderate Hypertension was a placebo-controlled, titration trial of monotherapy, employing six active drugs and placebo to test the comparative efficacy of different classes of drugs for the lowering of diastolic BP.[237] One objective of this study was to use echocardiography to assess the response of LV mass and its structural components over the 2-year period of antihypertensive monotherapy. Because the mechanisms responsible for LV hypertrophy and presumably its regression are multifactorial,[16] the echocardiographic data were analyzed with adjustment for potentially contributory factors in addition to drug selection, such as body weight, the magnitude of BP reduction, race, and age using appropriate statistical methods.[150] Patients with mild to moderate hypertension (diastolic BP 95 to 109 mm Hg) were randomly allocated to treatment with atenolol, captopril, clonidine, diltiazem, hydrochlorothiazide, prazosin, or placebo in a double-blinded trial in which medications were titrated to achieve a goal diastolic BP of 90 mm Hg. At 2 years, only hydrochlorothiazide was associated with reduction of LV mass. The effect of hydrochlorothiazide persisted even after adjustment for covariates and was the result of decreased wall thickness. LV mass increased with atenolol. Presently, the efficacy of different monotherapy choices for reduction of LV mass is of less interest given the common use of multiple drug regimens to treat hypertension.

Nonpharmacologic treatment of hypertension has also been associated with reduction of LV mass. In one study,[238] a greater trend in LV mass reduction was seen with weight loss than with drug therapy of hypertension, despite better reduction of BP with drugs. Additionally, McMahon and colleagues[239] demonstrated greater reduction of LV mass with weight reduction than with metoprolol. Moreover, salt restriction has also been associated with reduction of LV mass on echocardiogram.[240,241] Although exercise has been successful in reducing BP in patients with hypertension, it has been associated with increased LV mass on echocardiography,[242] secondary to increased LV cavity size with no change in wall thickness. This pattern of increase in LV mass, accompanied by preservation of diastolic LV function was considered consistent with physiologic hypertrophy.

Left Ventricular Systolic Function

Loss of contractile protein with LV mass reduction during antihypertensive therapy might, in principle, have adverse effects on LV systolic function, particularly if increases in BP toward initial levels or higher were to occur without "protection" from the previously elevated LV mass. However, clinical studies, which have evaluated ejection phase indices of LV function with echocardiography,[89,150,193,216,243] have not demonstrated adverse effects of LV mass reduction on systolic function during or after antihypertensive therapy. Studies employing ejection phase indices, such as velocity of circumferential fiber shortening, fractional shortening, and EF might not have be capable of de-

tecting myocardial impairment because these indices are highly load dependent. The tendency for LV function to increase during the initial stages of therapy may in fact reflect the effects of reduced afterload.[89] Other studies which measured relationships of endocardial fractional shortening to end-systolic stress may have also overestimated myocardial contractility for reasons previously discussed. However, a study of midwall fractional shortening relationships with end-systolic stress in patients with substantial reductions of LV mass during treatment also failed to disclose adverse effects.[244]

Diastolic Function

Conceivably, reduction of LV mass might be associated with adverse effects on diastolic LV function. This could occur if reduction of LV mass occurred without reduction in connective tissue mass. Then, with reduction of total LV mass, a relative increase in the collagen to LV weight ratio could result in decreased diastolic distensibility of the left ventricle.

However, studies using Doppler echocardiography have failed to disclose worsened diastolic function with LVH regression.[194,216,245,246] Indeed, some studies have shown improvement in diastolic indices of LV filling on Doppler.[194,245]

Regression of Left Ventricular Fibrosis

Fibrosis may account for a substantial portion of the effects of LVH on diastolic function. Hence it is important to know if reduction of LV mass includes regression in collagen and muscle. All hypertensive agents may not be equally effective in regression of the increased myocardial fibrosis, which accounts for part of the LV hypertrophic response to hypertension. In a rat model of LVH reduction of BP and LV mass zofenopril, nifedipine, and labetalol given in equipotent doses for reduction of BP all produced regression of LVH, whereas only nifedipine and zofenopril regressed myocardial fibrosis.[247] In a human study[248] using endomyocardial biopsy to compare the effects of lisinopril with hydrochlorothiazide, ACE inhibition with lisinopril was associated with regression of fibrosis and improvement in diastolic function, whereas hydrochlorothiazide was not. Notably, regression of LV mass occurred with diuretic but not with ACE inhibitor, possibly related to previous optimal BP control in all patients in combination with added reduction of preload in association with diuretic.

Effect of Left Ventricular Mass Reduction on Cardiovascular Risk

Although reduction of LV mass with treatment of hypertension does not produce adverse effects on surrogate measures of outcome, such as LV function, there are no prospective controlled trials that test the hypothesis that reduction of LV mass is beneficial independently of reduction of BP and the selected therapy. However, in an analysis of a cohort of hypertensive patients receiving drug therapy, Verdecchia and colleagues[249] showed that regression of LVH was associated with reduction in clinical events independently of the magnitude of BP decrease. Moreover, in the Framingham study[250] reduction of ECG features of LVH were also independently associated with reduced risk for cardiovascular disease. In a prospective study of hypertension patients with ECG LVH[251] achievement of lower LV mass after treatment was associated with a reduced rate of a composite endpoint (cardiovascular death, MI, stroke) independent of drug assignment or magnitude of BP lowering. It remains uncertain whether treatment targeted to reduction of LV mass, rather than to maximum reduction of BP, would improve mortality and morbidity of hypertension.

Echocardiographic Methods and Technical Considerations in the Evaluation of Hypertension

Echocardiography has become the technique of choice for clinical cardiac structure and function assessment of LVH. It has also found extensive application in research studies documenting effects of antihypertensive therapy. Although it is performance dependent, it is unlikely in the near future to be replaced by newer technologies such as rapid computed tomography (CT) scan or MRI. Images obtained by echocardiography provide near tomographic planes of the heart in real time thus allowing combined assessment of LV mass, architecture, and motion. Moreover information provided by Doppler on intracardiac blood flow velocity and tissue velocity adds substantially to the power of this technique in the assessment of systolic and diastolic function in hypertension. In addition, echocardiographic assessment of LA size and aortic dimension are of importance.

Technical Limitations of Echocardiography

Although echocardiography provides information on cardiac function and structure unavailable by any other means and is free of known risks or significant discomfort, the technique confers substantial technical problems in data acquisition and interpretation. Hence to optimize accuracy and reproducibility, careful methodology needs to be applied in training, acquisition, and interpretation of echocardiographic data. The reader is referred to a recent guidelines publication from the American Society of Echocardiography[252] on recommendations for optimizing the use of echocardiography in clinical research.

All LV mass algorithms, obtain a "shell" volume of the LV muscle by subtracting the LV volume from that volume enclosed by the LV epicardial-pericardial interface.[253] LV mass is then calculated by multiplying the shell volume by myocardial (1.04 g/mL).

A commonly used, well-validated[254] method, for calculation of LV mass uses a formula that is derived from modeling the LV as a prolate ellipse of revolution: LV mass $=0.8 \times (1.04[Dd + PW + VS])^3 - (Dd)^3 + 0.6g$; in which Dd is diastolic dimension, PW is posterior wall thickness, and VS is septal thickness. The three linear dimensions in this formula may be obtained from 2D-guided M-mode echocardiogram or directly from correctly aligned parasternal views.[255,256] However, even small errors in these measurements, when cubed, can create large errors in LV mass. However, with care in obtaining accurate primary dimension measurements in an experienced core laboratory, good reproducibility of LV mass can be obtained.[255]

LV mass can also be calculated from planimetered dimensions of 2D images obtained during real-time transthoracic imaging[257] employing area length or truncated ellipsoid formalae.[258]

However, the linear dimensions obtained from M-mode echocardiogram or directly from 2D images may fail to adequately represent true cardiac chamber volume if there are distortions in cardiac geometry. Although area measurements from 2D echocardiographic still frames provide greater image sampling of cardiac structures than "ice pick" M-mode dimensions, still frames (even of technically optimal studies) suffer from image degradation, with generally greater uncertainty in identification of cardiac borders than with M-mode echo. With either means of echocardiographic display, the use of primary echocardiographic data to obtain cardiac volumes requires using mathematical algorithms that rely on assumptions of cardiac geometry.

Under some circumstances, any geometric model of LV volume (see Fig. 34–2) may not be true to actual LV geometry. For example, the "bullet" formula for LV volumes (V = 5/6 AL; A = LV short axis area; L = LV long axis) assumes a "bullet" shape of the LV, which does not exist in the case of LV aneurysm. Here, use of Simpson's Rule (method of discs), which uses integral calculus to segment an irregular LV contour into multiple cylinders, is preferable. However, a technical trade-off is incurred as apical views of the LV must be used. These views, which image the LV endocardium in lateral (poor) resolution, generally result in overestimation of LV cavity volume, in contrast to the parasternal short-axis view required by the bullet formula, which images the LV endocardium mostly in axial (good) resolution.

Use of any model mandates meticulous alignment of the ultrasound (US) beam in reference to the proper anatomic axes. Variations of angulation of the manually directed echocardiographic sector between serial examinations will result in variability of primary echocardiographic measurements. It is easy to improperly align the echocardiographic sector (Fig. 34–9) or to properly place the M-mode cursor during 2D targeted recording (Fig. 34–10) of the LV potentially resulting in large errors in LV mass measurement.

Although one may select the algorithm appropriate to each subject and use it on subsequent examinations, intervening clinical events, such as apical MI, may make this difficult. Hence the sources of variability in echocardiographic studies separated by several years may be substantial.

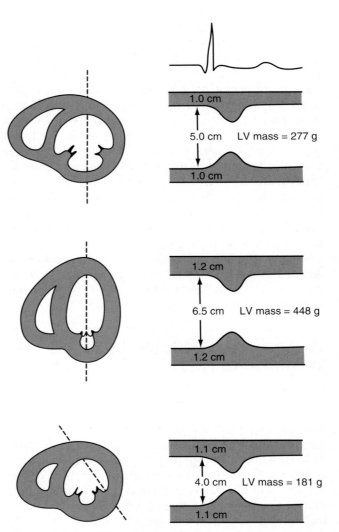

Figure 34–10. Effects of beam angulation errors on two-dimensional targeted M-mode measurements of left ventricular (LV) mass.

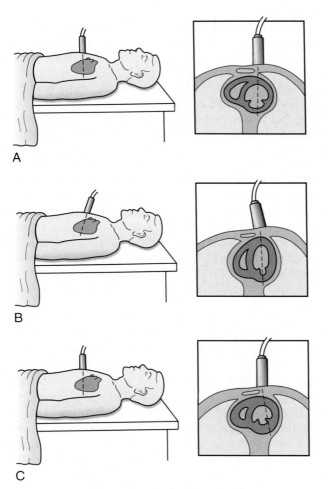

Figure 34–9. Distortion produced in parasternal short-axis images by inappropriate angulation of the echocardiographic beam (B and C) through the heart. A, Correct angulation and nondistorted, orthogonal short axis.

Two-Dimensional Targeted M-Mode versus Two-Dimensional Echocardiographic Measurement of Left Ventricular Mass

Controversy exists as to specific measurement techniques used to determine LV mass, with some investigators[14] suggesting that enhanced reproducibility and accuracy may be obtained using planimetry of 2D echocardiographic still frames, whereas probably a larger experience has been obtained with the use of the M-mode and then subsequently, 2D targeted M-mode recordings.[15-17] Although both approaches have their merits, large quantities of normal and diseased population data, have been obtained using 2D targeted M-mode recordings. The principal advantage of 2D targeted M-mode recording is that it allows more certain identification of interfaces defining the endocardial and epicardial margins of the LV posterior wall, providing ready calculation of LV mass based on certain geometric assumptions. A theoretic disadvantage is imposed by the selection of essentially three measurements for LV mass calculation although, in fact, the distribution of muscle mass in the left ventricle is neither homogeneous nor conforms exactly to the geometric models used. Although 2D echocardiography, by providing multiple planes of image with essentially full visualization of LV walls and cavity, offers theoretic advantages for computation of LV mass, many of these advantages are lost by the uncertainty imposed on measurements by the generally vague cardiac borders seen on still frame images. Additionally, subtle differences in regional LV wall thickness, which can be appreciated qualitatively, are difficult to measure on 2D echocardiography because of resolution difficulties, principally in lateral and azimuthal image planes.

Distorted Left Ventricular Geometry and Left Ventricular Volume Measurement

In cases in which echocardiograms that show distorted LV geometry may not meet the assumptions necessary for the measurement of cardiac volumes using 2D targeted M-mode echocardiography, 2D echocardiography may provide improved accuracy and reproducibility of LV mass measurement. In addition, a good quality 2D or M mode images from the parasternal location may not be obtainable in all patients. However, some of these may have adequate 2D echocardiographic images obtainable from an apical echocardiographic window.

Critique of Algorithms for Left Ventricular Mass Measurement

Although 2D echoes obtained from the apical window provide more complete interrogation of the LV than parasternal images, lateral resolution limitations of apical images require that wall thickness be measured from parasternal short-axis images. However, because the position of the echocardiographic transducer on the chest wall is relatively fixed, the circular cross-sectional image obtainable from this window cannot be iterated from base to apex to create a LV shell volume, which would represent LV mass. Hence, even 2D algorithms for estimation of LV mass use the parasternal window echocardiographic images to calculate an average LV wall thickness, which can then be applied to either bullet or apical window disc method algorithms for LV volumes, to obtain LV mass.

Unfortunately, however, LV wall thickness is not uniform even in normal ventricles, and following MI, substantial segmental thinning of the LV wall can occur. Hence problems in the estimation of LV mass imposed by distorted LV geometry following MI are not completely solved by substituting 2D echocardiographic for 2D targeted M-mode methods.

Three-Dimensional Echocardiography

3D echocardiography may have the advantage of quantifying LV volumes and LV mass, without having to rely on geometric assumptions to model the LV. Using a polyhedral surface reconstruction method investigators[259,260] have demonstrated the feasibility of measuring LV mass with 3D echocardiogram.

In an in vitro validation study in which excised sheep and pig left ventricles were imaged in a water bath using 3D echocardiography, the correspondence of echocardiographic LV mass to LV weight was excellent ($r = 0.995$; standard error of the estimate [SEE] = 2.91 g). Moreover, in normal human subjects LV mass on 3D echocardiography was more closely related ($r = 0.90$) to that determined on MRI than LV mass measured by either 2D echocardiographic bullet formula ($r = 0.71$) or 2D guided M-mode echocardiography ($r = 0.73$). Additionally, interobserver variability was better with 3D echocardiography than with other echocardiographic techniques. In a comparison study of 3D echocardiography, using a magnetic tracking system with cardiac MRI, Chuang and colleagues[261] found correlations of MRI with 2D echocardiography for measurement of LV mass in 45 patients of 0.84 to 0.92 based on the 2D method used. The standard error of the estimate was at best 22.5 g (22.5 to 30.8). In contrast, the correlation with 3D echocardiography was 0.99 and the standard error of estimate was only 6.9 g. Moreover, interobserver variation for 3D echocardiography was 7.6% compared with 17.7% for 2D echocardiography.

A limitation of 3D echocardiogram for measurement of LV mass has been the extensive amount of time required for off-line analyses, even with real-time 3D acquisition, which is faster than 2D echocardiogram. Newer techniques for volumetric analysis of 3D echocardiogram, however, are being developed which permit semi-automation of edge detection and volume calculation.[262]

Additionally 3D echocardiogram is promising for measurement of LA volume.[210,263,264] Increasingly it has been appreciated that LA volume is an important marker of diastolic function over time and is associated with hypertension, heart failure, and cardiovascular risk.[209,265,266]

The Use of Echocardiography in Epidemiologic Studies and Clinical Trials

There may be a significant learning curve present in recording technically adequate echocardiographic studies, particularly in subjects over the age of 60 years. In the

Framingham report describing M-mode echocardiograms performed in over 6000 subjects aged 17 to 90, the ability to record acceptable quality echocardiograms in subjects older than 60 years rose from a minimum of 28% during the first 5 months of the study to a maximum of 74% to 81% during studies 2 years later.[267] In the Cardiovascular Health Study, a large epidemiologic evaluation of nearly 6000 community-based participants older than 60 years of age, the "yield" for M-mode measurements of LV mass was only 67%. Moreover, older subjects within the Cardiovascular Health Study cohort were less likely to have measurable and interpretable studies than younger subjects. Hence echocardiography "drop-outs" were not randomly distributed within the cohort leading to the possibility of bias in data interpretation. However, the yield of measurable studies for LV mass in clinical trials has been reported to be as high as 91% to 98%,[268] using correctly aligned images with either 2D targeted M-mode or direct measurement of LV wall thickness and cavity dimensions.

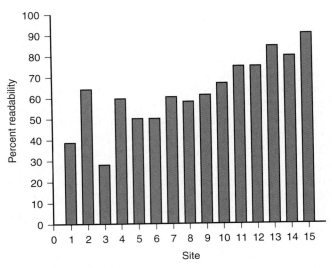

Figure 34–11. *Differences in technical adequacy ("readability") of echocardiograms for estimation of left ventricular mass in multicenter clinical trial of hypertension therapy.*

Differences between Field Centers

In previous large echocardiography trials major differences in echocardiographic quality have existed between field centers. For example, in a 15-center Veterans Affairs trial of antihypertensive monotherapy, the percent of readable echocardiograms for LV mass varied from approximately 30% to 85% (Fig. 34–11). This was not the result of differences between centers in the proportion of easy or difficult patients. Although the use of suboptimal equipment in some cases contributed to poor studies, the intercenter differences were mostly because of variation in technical performance. Importantly, extensive previous clinical experience in echocardiography was no guarantee of high quality echocardiograms for research purposes.

Training of Cardiac Sonographers

Echocardiography is a performance art. Cardiac sonographers, including experienced and clinically capable individuals, have been trained to use subtle eye-hand coordination to obtain optimum images pertinent to clinical diagnosis. Although the examination generally contains common structured and repetitive elements, a good sonographer will focus her or his study on clinical questions, which have been previously identified on the order form, or modify the examination technique to develop and fine tune findings as they are encountered during the echocardiographic examination. Unfortunately many of the habits of experienced sonographers, which are useful in clinical practice, are counterproductive in obtaining studies suitable for the estimation of LV mass. For example, sonographers will commonly seek to obtain a panoramic view of the aorta, left atrium, and left ventricle in the parasternal long-axis view. Although this image may be esthetically pleasing and clinically

informative, it usually results in angulation of the LV long axis such that targeted M-mode recordings of the LV at the tips of the mitral valve record elongated LV dimensions, which can easily be 10 mm greater than the true value. Cubing this error, as is done in the computation of LV mass from the 2D targeted M-mode recording results in enormous error. Moreover, the 2D parasternal short-axis cross-sectional images would be elliptical instead of circular. Hence 2D echocardiographic calculation of LV mass using these distorted parasternal short-axis images would also produce substantial error.

Reliability of Echocardiography for Measurement of Left Ventricular Mass

The use of echocardiography in the management of hypertension is dependent on the accuracy of echocardiography in detection of clinically important abnormality (e.g., LVH, LV systolic and diastolic dysfunction). Equally important in a chronic disease like hypertension is the ability of the test to reliably measure serial changes in quantitative parameters of disease. Hence, if therapy is targeted to regression of increased LV mass, echocardiography must be able to detect increases in LV mass associated with increased risk or decreases in LV mass of the magnitude that would occur with effective antihypertensive therapy.

In one study[269] of the temporal variability of echocardiography for measurement of LV mass and function in patients with hypertension, the width of the confidence interval (CI) for LV mass was 59 g. Decreases in LV mass in clinical trials[230] have generally been substantially smaller.

More recent studies of test-retest reliability also have shown substantial variability. In one study[270] of 261 subjects who had repeat echocardiograms in 16 centers, with central reading, the test-retest variability was 65 g, similar to that in the previously discussed study. Even in another study[271] in which a single highly experienced reader evaluated and corrected virtually all of the readings, 95% test-retest reliability was still ±35 g. Hence, changes in LV mass greater than that value would be required to infer either worsening or improvement of LV mass in an individual patient.

Although measurement of LV mass with 2D echocardiography may be more reproducible than 2D targeted M-mode in normal subjects and patients with distorted LV contour,[272] it has not been demonstrated that it is sufficiently reproducible for the clinical measurement of sequential change in LV mass in hypertensive patients of varying echogenicity.

Left Ventricular Hypertrophy Regression or Regression to the Mean?

Given the large confidence width for measurement of LV mass, one could argue that serial echocardiography during treatment should be reserved for patients with markedly increased LV mass. A decrease in LV mass with treatment that exceeds test-retest variability could then be taken to represent a true therapeutic effect. However, selecting patients with values for LV mass of any given value above (or for that matter, below) the population mean can result in subsequent determinations reflecting regression to the mean. Therefore, values higher than "true" values for LV mass on an initial determination tend to decrease on subsequent measurement (Fig. 34–12). Hence given the large measurement variability, any treatment choice is likely to show

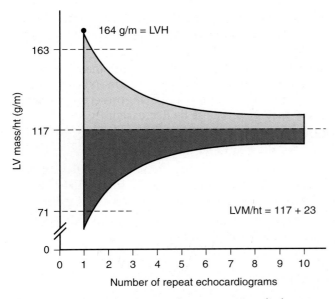

Figure 34–12. Regression to the mean as applied to measurement of left ventricular (LV) mass when only patients exceeding a given partition value are selected for follow-up examination. Ht, height; LVH, left ventricular hypertrophy; LVM, left ventricular mass. (From Gottdiener J: J Am Soc Echocardiogr 9:585-590, 1996.)

benefit if only patients with particularly high values for LV mass are selected. Of course, patients with particularly low values for LV mass are likely to show "worsening," that is, increase in LV mass, with subsequent measurement.

Clinical Use of Echocardiography in Patients with Hypertension

The value of echocardiography as a research tool in hypertension is uncontested. Although it has been suggested that treatment choices in individual patients should be guided by echocardiographic findings,[273] the value of echocardiography in the clinical management of hypertension is unproved.

Potential Impact on Clinical Management

The benefits of echocardiography depend on its value in affecting treatment decisions and in early identification and intervention in patients at risk who would not otherwise be treated (Table 34–3). Moreover, demonstration of value requires that the impact of echocardiography on clinical decisions is accompanied by improvement in patient outcome. Importantly, any consideration of the usefulness of echocardiography is contingent on its reliability for assessment of target measures, such as LV mass. However, little information is available on the impact of echocardiographic data on physician behavior or on patient outcomes in hypertension.

Before formulating strategies for using echocardiography in the management of hypertension, it is helpful to specifically consider which echocardiographic assessments are likely to be of value and then consider clinical situations in which the findings of those assessments might influence clinical decision making. For example, pertinent echocardiographic assessments might include quantitation of LV mass, determining the presence or absence of LVH, assessment of LV architecture (e.g., relative wall thickness, concentric remodeling), and measurement of LV systolic and diastolic function. Because of the comorbidity of hypertension and coronary artery disease, assessment of regional wall motion abnormality also is an appropriate goal of echocardiography in the evaluation of patients with hypertension. Another targeted echocardiographic assessment in elderly patients with hypertension is age-related degenerative valvular disease, principally aortic stenosis, which may have clinical interactions with hypertensive LVH. Also, inappropriately small LV cavity size and markedly thickened LV walls (hypertensive HCM) may contribute to orthostatic hypotension in older patients, particularly with usage of diuretics or vasodilators. Hence echocardiography may be of particular importance in the management of hypertension in the elderly.

TABLE 34-3. Hypothetical Impact of Echocardiography on Clinical Management

Clinical Subset	Echocardiographic Target	Finding	Possible Impact
Established hypertension	LV mass or LVH	No LVH Unequivocal Persistent LVH with therapy	Diuretics and vasodilators OK Neurohormonal blockade (ACE inhibitors); ? calcium blockers Change drugs
Borderline hypertension; "white-coat" hypertension	LV mass or LVH	No LVH Equivocal or mild LVH Unequivocal LVH	Follow closely Nutritional Rx Drug Rx
Hemodynamic profile	Cardiac output and total peripheral resistance	High output–low resistance High resistance–low output	Beta-blocker, diuretics, calcium blockers ACE inhibitors, vasodilators
High risk for coronary artery disease	RWMA	RWMA present RWMA and ↓ LV function	Prior infarct—? stress test ? Angiography; drug selection—"antiischemic" antihypertensive drugs
Hypertension in the elderly	Valvular disease, LV architecture LV outflow tract dynamic gradient	Mitral annular calcification Aortic stenosis ↑↑ relative wall thickness, small LV cavity, LV outflow tract obstruction	Avoid vasodilators, diuretics; ? avoid calcium blockers Avoid diuretics; avoid vasodilators; ? beta blockers

ACE, angiotensin converting enzyme; LV, left ventricular; LVH, left ventricular hypertrophy; Rx, therapy; RWMA, regional wall motion abnormality.

Another way to look at the potential application of echocardiography in clinical hypertension is to consider how the findings might effect management of certain clinical subsets or hemodynamic profiles. Table 34–3 summarizes this potential strategy. The results of assessment of LV mass and architecture, according to this schema, could have clinical impact on management choices in established hypertension, "white coat hypertension," and borderline hypertension. For example, marginally elevated BP, or intermittently elevated BP in the physician's office in the presence of concentric remodeling or clear-cut LVH, might result in drug therapy with agents believed to be effective for reduction of LV mass. In contrast, the absence of cardiac abnormality might suggest the feasibility of close follow-up, perhaps coupled with nutritional-hygienic management (e.g., weight loss, exercise, salt restriction).

KEY POINTS

■ Echocardiography shows many of the effects of hypertension on the heart, including LVH, LA enlargement, aortic dilation, and some of the effects of comorbidities (e.g., atherosclerosis), such as segmental LV wall motion abnormality.

■ LVH on echocardiography is an important predictor of cardiovascular risk.

■ Reduction of LVH is associated with reduction of risk.

■ Despite the foregoing, the use of echocardiography in clinical practice to monitor effects of antihypertensive treatment on LV mass, LVH, and direct therapy accordingly is not supported by current data.

■ LV mass or geometry is affected by factors other than BP, including body weight, obesity, age, and race.

■ The relation between LV mass and hypertension is bidirectional, that is, both are predicted by the other.

■ Hypertension is associated with diastolic heart failure. However, whereas ejection phase indices (e.g., EF) of LV performance are preserved contractility may nonetheless be decreased.

■ Cardiac effects of hypertension involve all chambers of the heart and the aorta.

■ Virtually all regimens, which are effective for treating hypertension, have in some study, been shown to associated with reduction of LV mass.

■ Reduction of LV mass does not produce impairment of diastolic or systolic LV function.

REFERENCES

1. Laennec R: *Of Hypertrophia, or Simple Enlargement of the Heart, A Treatise on the Diseases of the Chest*, Philadelphia, James Webster, 1823.
2. Janeway TC: A clinical study of hypertensive cardiovascular disease. *Arch Intern Med* 12:755, 1913.

3. Casale PN, Devereux RB, Milner M: Value of echocardiographic measurement of left ventricular mass in predicting cardiovascular morbid events in hypertensive men. *Ann Intern Med* 105:173-178, 1986.

4. Drizel T, Dannenberg AL, Engel A: *Blood pressure levels in persons 18-74 years of age in 1978-80 and trends in blood pressure from 1960 to 1980 in the United States,* NCHS Series II #234, Washington, DC: US Government Printing Office, 1986.

5. Rowland M, Roberta J: *Blood pressure levels and hypertension in persons ages 6-74 years: United States, 1976-1980,* National Center for Health Statistics, 1993.

6. McLenachan JM, Dargie HJ: Ventricular arrhythmias in hypertensive left ventricular hypertrophy: Relationship to coronary artery disease, left ventricular dysfunction, and myocardial fibrosis. *Am J Hypertens* 3:735-740, 1990.

7. Levy D, Anderson KM, Savage DD: Risk of ventricular arrhythmias in left ventricular hypertrophy: The Framingham Heart Study. *Am J Cardiol* 60:560-565, 1987.

8. Ghali JK, Kadakia S, Cooper RS, Liao YL: Impact of left ventricular hypertrophy on ventricular arrhythmias in the absence of coronary artery disease. *J Am Coll Cardiol* 17:1277-1282, 1991.

9. Burt VL, Whelton P, Roccella EJ, et al: Prevalence of hypertension in the US adult population. Results from the Third National Health and Nutrition Examination Survey, 1988-1991. *Hypertension* 25:305-313, 1995.

10. van Hoeven KH, Factor SM: A comparison of the pathological spectrum of hypertensive, diabetic, and hypertensive-diabetic heart disease. *Circulation* 82:850-855, 1990.

11. Stearns S, Schlesinger MJ, Rudy A: Incidence and clinical significance of coronary artery disease in diabetes mellitus. *Arch Int Med* 80:463-474, 1947.

12. Assman G, Schulte H: The prospective cardiovascular munster (PROCAM) study: Prevalence of hyperlipidemia in persons with hypertension and/or diabetes mellitus and the relationship to coronary artery disease. *Am Heart J* 116:1713-1724, 1980.

13. Savage DD, Drayer JI, Henry WL, et al: Echocardiographic assessment of cardiac anatomy and function in hypertensive subjects. *Circulation* 59:623-632, 1979.

14. Hammond IW, Devereux RB, Aldermann MA: The prevalence and correlates of echocardiographic left ventricular hypertrophy among employed patients with uncomplicated hypertension. *J Am Coll Cardiol* 7:639-650, 1986.

15. Liebson PR, Grandits G, Prineas R, et al: Echocardiographic correlates of left ventricular structure among 844 mildly hypertensive men and women in the treatment of mild hypertension study (TOMHS). *Circulation* 87:476-486, 1993.

16. Gottdiener JS, Reda DJ, Materson BJ, et al: Importance of obesity, race and age to the cardiac structural and functional effects of hypertension. *J Am Coll Cardiol* 24:1492-1498, 1994.

17. Palmieri V, De Simone G, Arnett DK, et al: Relation of various degrees of body mass index in patients with systemic hypertension to left ventricular mass, cardiac output, and peripheral resistance (The Hypertension Genetic Epidemiology Network Study). *Am J Cardiol* 88:1163-1168, 2001.

18. Mancia G, Carugo S, Grassi G, et al: Prevalence of left ventricular hypertrophy in hypertensive patients without and with blood pressure control: Data from the PAMELA population. *Pressioni Arteriose Monitorate E Loro Associazioni. Hypertension* 39:744-749, 2002.

19. Montanaro D, Gropuzzo M, Tulissi P, et al: Effects of successful renal transplantation on left ventricular mass. *Transplant Proc* 37:2485-2487, 2005.

20. Ayus JC, Go AS, Valderrabano F, et al: Effects of erythropoietin on left ventricular hypertrophy in adults with severe chronic renal failure and hemoglobin <10 g/dL. *Kidney Int* 68:788-795, 2005.

21. Yildiz A, Oflaz H, Pusuroglu H, et al: Left ventricular hypertrophy and endothelial dysfunction in chronic hemodialysis patients. *Am J Kidney Dis* 41:616-623, 2003.

22. Ventura JE, Tavella N, Romero C, et al: Aortic valve calcification is an independent factor of left ventricular hypertrophy in patients on maintenance haemodialysis. *Nephrol Dial Transplant* 17:1795-1801, 2002.

23. Liebson PR, Grandits GA, Dianzumba S, et al: Comparison of five antihypertensive monotherapies and placebo for change in left ventricular mass in patients receiving nutritional-hygienic therapy in the Treatment of Mild Hypertension Study (TOMHS). *Circulation* 91:698-706, 1995.

24. Devereux RB, Pickering TG, Alderman MG: Left ventricular hypertrophy in hypertension: Prevalence and relationship to pathophysiologic variables. *Hypertension* 9(suppl 2):II-53-II-59, 1987.

25. Liebson PR, Savage DD: Echocardiography in hypertension: A Review: I. Left ventricular wall mass, standardization and ventricular function. *Echocardiography* 3:181, 1986.

26. Savage DD, Garrison AR, Kannel WB: The spectrum of left ventricular hypertrophy in a general population sample: The Framingham Study. *Circulation* 75:I-26-I-33, 1987.

27. Drayer JIM, Gardin JM, Weber MA: Echocardiographic left ventricular hypertrophy in hypertension. *Chest* 84:217, 1983.

28. Ganau A, Devereux RB, Roman MJ, et al: Patterns of left ventricular hypertrophy and geometric remodeling in essential hypertension. *J Am Coll Cardiol* 19:1550-1558, 1992.

29. Savage DD, Devereux RB, Sachs I, Laragh JH: Disporportionate ventricular septal thickness in hypertensive patients. *J Cardiovasc Ultrasonography* 1:79-85, 1982.

30. Shapiro LM, Kleinebenne A, McKenna WJ: The distribution of left ventricular hypertrophy in hypertensive cardiomyopathy: Comparison to athletes and hypertensives. *Eur Heart J* 6:967-974, 1985.

31. Maron BJ, Gottdiener JS, Epstein SE: Patterns and significance of the distribution of left ventricular hypertrophy in hypertrophic cardiomyopathy: A wide angle 2-dimensional study of 125 patients. *Am J Cardiol* 48:418-427, 1981.

32. Maron BJ, Gottdiener JS, Epstein SE: Echocardiographic identification of patterns of left ventricular hypertrophy in hypertrophic cardiomyopathy. In Kaltenbach M, Epstein SE, (eds): *Hypertrophic Cardiomyopathy,* Berlin, Springer-Verlag, 1982.

33. Gottdiener JS, Gay JA, Maron BJ, Fletcher RD: Increased right ventricular wall thickness in left ventricular pressure overload: Echocardiographic determination of hypertrophic response of the non-stressed ventricle. *J Am Coll Cardiol* 6:550-555, 1985.

34. Pool PE, Piggott WJ, Seagren SC, Skelton CL: Augmented right ventricular function in systemic hypertension-induced hypertrophy. *Cardiovasc Res* 10:124-128, 1976.

35. Rubler S, Halperin MS, Dolgin M, et al: Right ventricular wall thickness in left ventricular hypertrophy: An echocardiographic study. *J Cardiovasc Ultrasonography* 2:63-68, 1983.

36. Lewis JF, Mauer BJ: Diversity of patterns of hypertrophy in patients with systemic hypertension and marked left ventricular wall thickness. *Am J Cardiol* 65:874-881, 1990.

37. Topol EJ, Traill TA, Fortuin NJ: Hypertensive hypertrophic cardiomyopathy of the elderly. *N Engl J Med* 312:277-283, 1985.

38. De Simone G, Devereux RB, Kimball TR, et al: Interaction between body size and cardiac workload: influence on left ventricular mass during body growth and adulthood. *Hypertension* 31:1077-1082, 1998.

39. Krumholz HM, Larson M, Levy D: Sex differences in cardiac adaptation to isolated systolic hypertension. *Am J Cardiol* 72:310-313, 1993.

40. Sugishita Y, Iida K, Yukisada K, Ito I: Cardiac determinants of regression of left ventricular hypertrophy in essential hypertension with antihypertensive treatment. *J Am Coll Cardiol* 15:665-671, 1990.

41. Papademetriou V, Gottdiener JS, Fletcher RD, Freis ED: Diastolic left ventricular function and left ventricular hypertrophy in patients with borderline or mild hypertension. Echocardiographic assessment by computer-assisted analysis. *Am J Cardiol* 56:546-550, 1985.

42. Gottdiener JS: Left ventricular mass, diastolic dysfunction and hypertension. In Leonard J, (ed): *Advances in Internal Medicine*, 38th ed, St. Louis, Mosby Year Book, Inc., 1993, pp. 31-56.

43. Pearson AC, Gudipati C, Nagelhout D, et al: Echocardiographic evaluation of cardiac structure and function in elderly subjects with isolated systolic hypertension [see comments]. *J Am Coll Cardiol* 17:422-430, 1991.

44. Ren JF, Pancholy SB, Iskandrian AS, et al: Doppler echocardiographic evaluation of the spectrum of left ventricular diastolic dysfunction in essential hypertension. *Am Heart J* 127:906-913, 1994.

45. Kramer PH, Djalaly A, Poehlmann H: Abnormal diastolic left ventricular posterior wall motion in left ventricular hypertrophy. *Am Heart J* 106:1066-1069, 1983.

46. Gardin JM, Drayer JIM, Weber M: Doppler echocardiographic assessment of left ventricular systolic and diastolic function in mild hypertension. *Hypertension* 9(suppl 2):2, 1987.

47. Cuocolo A, Sax FL, Brush JE: Left ventricular hypertrophy and impaired diastolic filling in essential hypertension; Diastolic mechanisms for systolic dysfunction during exercise. *Circ Res* 81:978-986, 1990.

48. Buda AJ, Li Y, Brant D: Changes in left ventricular diastolic filling during the development of LVH in a unique canine model. *Am Heart J* 121:1759-1767, 1991.

49. Egan B, Fitzpatrick MA, Juni J, et al: Importance of overweight in studies of left ventricular hypertrophy and diastolic function in mild systemic hypertension. *Am J Cardiol* 64:752-755, 1989.

50. De Simone G, Kitzman DW, Chinali M, et al: Left ventricular concentric geometry is associated with impaired relaxation in hypertension: the HyperGEN study. *Eur Heart J* 26:1039-1045, 2005.

51. Szlachcic J, Tubau JF, O'Kelly B: What is the role of silent coronary artery disease and left ventricular hypertrophy in the genesis of ventricular arrhythmias in men with essential hypertension? *J Am Coll Cardiol* 19:803-808, 1992.

52. Messerli FH, Ventura HO, Elizardi DJ: Hypertension and sudden death: Increased ventricular ectopic activity in left ventricular hypertrophy. *Am J Med* 77:18-22, 1984.

53. Liebson P: Echocardiographic assessment of the left ventricle in hypertension: Perspectives on epidemiologic studies and clinical trials. *J Vasc Biol Med* 4:285-310, 1993.

54. Liebson PR, Savage DD: Echocardiography in hypertension: A review. II. Echocardiographic studies of the effects of antihypertensive agents on left ventricular wall mass and function. *Echocardiography* 4:215-249, 1987.

55. Devereux RB, Savage DD, Drayer JIM: Left ventricular hypertrophy and function in high-, normal-, and low-renin forms of essential hypertension. *Hypertension* 4:524-531, 1982.

56. Blake J, Devereux RB, Herrold EM, et al: Relation of concentric left ventricular hypertrophy and extracardiac target organ damage to supranormal left ventricular performance in established essential hypertension. *Am J Cardiol* 62:246-252, 1988.

57. Shimizu G, Hirota Y, Kita Y, et al: Left ventricular midwall mechanics in systemic arterial hypertension. Myocardial function is depressed in pressure-overload hypertrophy. *Circulation* 83:1676-1684, 1991.

58. De Simone G, Devereux RB, Roman MJ, et al: Assessment of left ventricular function by the midwall fractional shortening/end-systolic stress relation in human hypertension *J Am Coll Cardiol* 23:1444-1451, 1994.

59. Palmieri V, Storto G, Arezzi E, et al: Relations of left ventricular mass and systolic function to endothelial function and coronary flow reserve in healthy, new discovered hypertensive subjects. *J Hum Hypertens* 19:941-950, 2005.

60. De Simone G, Kitzman DW, Palmieri V, et al: Association of inappropriate left ventricular mass with systolic and diastolic dysfunction: The HyperGEN study. *Am J Hypertens* 17:828-833, 2004.

61. Koren MJ, Devereux RB, Casale PN: Relation of left ventricular mass and geometry to morbidity and mortality in uncomplicated essential hypertension. *Ann Intern Med* 114:345-352, 1991.

62. Ghali JK, Liao Y, Simmons B, et al: The prognostic role of left ventricular hypertrophy in patients with or without coronary artery disease. *Ann Intern Med* 117:831-836, 1992.

63. Devereux RB, Roman MJ, O'Grady MJ, et al: Differences in echocardiographic findings and systemic hemodynamics among non-diabetic American Indians in different regions. The strong heart study [In Process Citation]. *Ann Epidemiol* 10:324-332, 2000.

64. Levy D, Garrison RJ, Savage DD, et al: Prognostic implications of echocardiographically determined left ventricular mass in the Framingham Heart Study. *N Engl J Med* 322:1561-1566, 1990.

65. De Simone G, Verdecchia P, Pede S, et al: Prognosis of inappropriate left ventricular mass in hypertension: the MAVI Study. *Hypertension* 40:470-476, 2002.

66. Verdecchia P, Schillaci G, Borgioni C, et al: Adverse prognosis significance of concentric remodeling of the left ventricle in hypertensive patients with normal left ventricular mass. *J Am Coll Cardiol* 25:871-878, 1995.

67. Krumholz HM, Larson M, Levy D: Prognosis of left ventricular geometric patterns in the Framingham Heart Study. *J Am Coll Cardiol* 25:879-884, 1995.

68. Papademetriou V, Narayan P, Kokkinos P: Effects of diltiazem, metoprolol, enalapril and hydrochlorothiazide on frequency of ventricular premature complexes. *Am J Cardiol* 73:242-246, 1994.

69. Karpanou EA, Vyssoulis GP, Psichogios A, et al: Regression of left ventricular hypertrophy results in improvement of QT dispersion in patients with hypertension. *Am Heart J* 136:765-768, 1998.

70. Keys A, Brozek J, Henschel A, et al: *The Biology of Human Starvation*, vol I, Minneapolis, University of Minnesota Press, 1950, p. 185.

71. Henry WL, Ware J, Gardin JM, et al: Echocardiographic measurements in normal subjects from infancy to old age. *Circulation* 62:1054-1061, 1980.

72. Gardin JM, Savage DD, Ware JH, Henry WL: Effect of age, sex and body surface area on echocardiographic left ventricular wall mass in normal subjects. *Hypertension* 9:II-36-II-39, 1987.

73. Kupari M, Koskinen P, Virolainen J: Correlates of left ventricular mass in a population sample aged 36 to 37 years. Focus on lifestyle and salt intake. *Circulation* 89:1041-1050, 1994.

74. Hammond IW, Devereux RB, Alderman MH, Laragh JH: Relation of blood pressure and body build to left ventricular mass in normotensive and hypertensive employed adults. *J Am Coll Cardiol* 12:996-1004, 1988.

75. Savage DD, Levy D, Dannenberg AL, et al: Association of echocardiographic left ventricular mass with body size, blood pressure and physical activity (the Framingham Study). *Am J Cardiol* 65:371-376, 1990.

76. Gutgesell HP, Rembold CM: Growth of the human heart relative to body surface area. *Am J Cardiol* 65:662-668, 1990.

77. Gottdiener JS, Gross HA, Henry WL, et al: Effects of self-induced starvation on cardiac size and function in anorexia nervosa. *Circulation* 58:425-433, 1978.

78. De Simone G, Scalfi L, Galderisi M, et al: Cardiac abnormalities in young women with anorexia nervosa. *Br Heart J* 71:287-292, 1994.

79. St. John Sutton MG, Plappert T, et al: Effects of reduced left ventricular mass on chamber architecture, load, and function: A study of anorexia nervosa. *Circulation* 72:991-1000, 1985.

80. Havlik RJ, Hubert HB, Fabsitz RR, Feinleib M: Weight and hypertension. *Ann Intern Med* 98:855-859, 1983.

81. Kannel WB, Brand N, Skinner JJ Jr, et al: The relation of adiposity to blood pressure and development of hypertension. *Ann Intern Med* 67:48-49, 1967.

82. Lauer MS, Anderson KM, Kannel WB, Levy D: Separate and joint influences of obesity and mild hypertension of left ventricular mass and geometry: The Framingham Heart Study. *J Am Coll Cardiol* 19:130-134, 1992.

83. Levy D, Anderson KM, Savage DD, et al: Echocardiographically detected left ventricular hypertrophy: Prevalence and risk factors. The Framingham Heart Study. *Ann Intern Med* 108:7-13, 1988.

84. De Simone G, Devereux RB, Roman MJ, et al: Relation of obesity and gender to left ventricular hypertrophy in normotensive and hypertensive adults. *Hypertension* 23:600-606, 1994.

85. De Simone G, Daniels SR, Devereux RB, et al: Left ventricular mass and body size in normotensive children and adults: Assessment of allometric relations and impact of overweight. *J Am Coll Cardiol* 20:1251-1260, 1992.

86. Thurston CL, Randich A: Acute increases in arterial blood pressure produced by occlusion of the abdominal aorta induces antinociception: preipheral and central substrates. *Brain Res* 519:12-22, 1990.

87. Dannenberg AL, Levy D, Garrison RJ: Impact of age on echocardiographic left ventricular mass in a healthy population (the Framingham Study). *Am J Cardiol* 64:1066-1068, 1989.

88. Devereux RB, Lutas EM, Casale RN, et al: Standardization of M-mode echocardiographic left ventricular anatomic measurements. *J Am Coll Cardiol* 4:1222-1230, 1984.

89. Khatri IM, Gottdiener JS, Notargiacomo AV, Freis E: The effect of therapy on left ventricular function in hypertension. *Clin Sci* 59:435s-439s, 1980.

90. Marcus R, Krause L, Weder AB, et al: Sex-specific determinants of increased left ventricular mass in the Tecumseh Blood Pressure Study. *Circulation* 90:928-936, 1994.

91. Levy D, Savage DD, Garrison RJ, et al: Echocardiographic criteria for left ventricular hypertrophy: The Framingham Heart Study. *Am J Cardiol* 59:956-960, 1987.

92. Messerli FH, Nunez BD, Ventura HO, Snyder DW: Overweight and sudden death: Increased ventricular ectopy in cardiopathy of obesity. *Arch Intern Med* 147:1725-1728, 1987.

93. Messerli FH, Sungaard-Riise K, Reisin ED, et al: Dimorphic cardiac adaptation to obesity and arterial hypertension. *Ann Intern Med* 99:757-761, 1983.

94. Hammond IW, Alderman MH, Devereux RB, et al: Contrast in cardiac anatomy and function between black and white patients with hypertension. *J Natl Med Assoc* 76:247-255, 1984.

95. Chaturvedi N, Athanassopoulos G, McKeigue PM, et al: Echocardiographic measures of left ventricular structure and their relation with rest and ambulatory blood pressure in blacks and whites in the United Kingdom. *J Am Coll Cardiol* 24:1499-1505, 1994.

96. Koren MJ, Mensah GA, Blake J, et al: Comparison of left ventricular mass and geometry in black and white patients with essential hypertension. *Am J Hypertens* 6:815-823, 1993.

97. Sasson Z, Rasooly Y, Bhesania T, Rasooly I: Insulin resistance is an important determinant of left ventricular mass in the obese. *Circulation* 88:1431-1436, 1993.

98. Dahlof B: Factors involved in the pathogenesis of hypertensive cardiovascular hypertrophy. A review. *Drugs* 35 (Suppl 5):6-26, 1988.

99. Bella JN, Devereux RB, Roman MJ, et al: Relations of left ventricular mass to fat-free and adipose body mass: The strong heart study. The Strong Heart Study Investigators. *Circulation* 98:2538-2544, 1998.

100. Chinali M, De Simone G, Roman MJ, et al: Impact of obesity on cardiac geometry and function in a population of adolescents: the Strong Heart Study. *J Am Coll Cardiol* 47:2267-2273, 2006.

101. Gardin JM, Siscovick D, Anton-Culver H, et al: Sex, age, and disease affect echocardiographic left ventricular mass and systolic function in the free-living elderly. The cardiovascular health study. *Circulation* 91:1739-1748, 1995.

102. Pearson AC, Gudipati CV, Labovitz AJ: Effects of aging on left ventricular structure and function. *Am Heart J* 121:871-875, 1991.

103. Hypertension Detection and Follow-Up Program Cooperative Group (HDFP): Race, education and prevalence of hypertension. *Am J Epidemiol* 106:351-361, 1977.

104. Freis ED: Age, race, sex and other indices of risk in hypertension. *Am J Med* 55:275-280, 1973.

105. Kannel WB, Dannenberg AL: Prevalence and natural history of electrocardiographic left ventricular hypertrophy. In Messerli FH (ed): *The heart and hypertension*, New York: York Medical Books, 1987, pp. 53-62.

106. Lee DK, Marantz PR, Devereux RB, et al: Left ventricular hypertrophy in black and white hypertensives. Standard electrocardiographic criteria overestimate racial differences in prevalence. *J Am Med Assoc* 267:3294-3299, 1992.

107. Dunn FG, Oigman W, Sungaard-Riise K: Racial differences in cardiac adaptation to essential hypertension determined by echocardiographic indexes. *J Am Coll Cardiol* 5:1348-1351, 1983.

108. Savage DD, Henry WL, Mitchell JR, et al: Echocardiographic comparison of black and white hypertensive subjects. *J Am Med Assoc* 71:709-712, 1979.

109. Massie BM, Der E, Gottdiener JS, et al: Contrasting effects of demographic factors on ECG and echocardiographic indices of left ventricular hypertrophy. *Circulation* 90:I-26, 1994.

110. Arnett DK, Skelton TN, Liebson PR, et al: Comparison of M-mode echocardiographic left ventricular mass measured using digital and strip chart readings: The Atherosclerosis Risk in Communities (ARIC) study. *Cardiovasc Ultrasound* 1:8, 2003.

111. Drayer JIM, Gardin JM, Brewer DD, Weber MA: Disparate relationships between blood pressure and left ventricular mass in patients with and without left ventricular hypertrophy. *Hypertension* 9(Suppl 2):II-61-II-64, 1987.

112. Verdecchia P, Schillaci G, Boldrini F, et al: Sex, cardiac hypertrophy and diurnal blood pressure variations in essential hypertension. *J Hypertens* 10:683-692, 1992.

113. Gottdiener JS, Wakeford CW, Asgharnejad M, et al: Relation between blood pressure, blood pressure variability and LV mass in hypertension: Interaction of sex and race. *Am J Hypertens* 5(5 Pt 2):24A, 1992.

114. Parati G, Pomidossi G, Albini F, et al: Relationship of 24-hour blood pressure mean and variability to severity of target-organ damage in hypertension. *J Hypertens* 5:93-98, 1987.

115. Lauer MS, Anderson KM, Levy D: Influence of contemporary versus 30-year blood pressure levels on left ventricular mass and geometry: The Framingham Heart Study [see comments]. *J Am Coll Cardiol* 18:1287-1294, 1991.

116. Gottdiener JS, Brown J, Zoltick J, Fletcher RD: Identification of left ventricular hypertrophy in normotensive men with an exaggerated blood pressure response to exercise. *Ann Intern Med* 112:161-166, 1990.

117. Pasquini JA, Gottdiener JS, Cutler DJ, Fletcher RD: Myocarditis with transient left ventricular apical dyskinesis. *Am Heart J* 109:371-372, 1985.

118. Bauwens FR, Duprez DA, DeBuyzere ML: Influence of the arterial blood pressure and nonhemodynamic factors on left ventricular hypertrophy in moderate essential hypertension. *Am J Cardiol* 68:925-929, 1991.

119. Yamori Y, Mori C, Nishio T: Cardiac hypertrophy in early hypertension. *Am J Cardiol* 4:964-969, 1979.

120. Folkow B: Central neurohormonal mechanism in spontaneously hypertensive rats as compared with human essential hypertension. *Clin Sci Mol Med* 48:205-214, 1975.

121. Laks MM, Morady F: Norepinephrine—the myocardial hypertrophy hormone? *Am Heart J* 91:674-675, 1976.

122. DeLeonardis V, SeScalzi M, Falchetti A: Echocardiographic evaluation of children with and without family history of essential hypertension. *Am J Hypertens* 1:305-308, 1988.

123. Nielson JR, Oxhoj H: Echocardiographic variables in progeny of hypertensive and normotensive parents. *Acta Med Scand Suppl* 693:61-64, 1985.

124. Mahoney LT, Scheiken RM, Clarke WT: Left ventricular mass and exercise responses predict future blood pressure: The Muscatine study. *Hypertension* 12:206-213, 1988.

125. Ganau A, Devereux RB, Pickering TG, et al: Relation of left ventricular hemodynamic load and contractile performance to left ventricular mass in hypertension. *Circulation* 81:25-36, 1990.

126. Hausnerova E, Gottdiener JS, Hecht GM, et al: Increased diastolic left ventricular wall thickness during dobutamine stress echocardiography: Effect on afterload. *Circulation* 90:391, 1994.

127. Polonia J, Martins L, Bravo-Faria F, et al: Higher left ventricle mass in normotensives with exaggerated blood pressure responses to exercise associated with higher ambulatory blood pressure load and sympathetic activity. *Eur Heart J* 13(Suppl A):30-36, 1992.

128. Lauer MS, Levy D, Anderson KM, Plehn JF: Is there a relationship between exercise systolic blood pressure response and left ventricular mass? The Framingham Heart Study. *Ann Intern Med* 116:203-210, 1992.

129. Sung J, Ouyang P, Silber HA, et al: Exercise blood pressure response is related to left ventricular mass. *J Hum Hypertens* 17:333-338, 2003.

130. Krantz DS, Manuck SB: Acute psychophysiologic reactivity and risk or cardiovascular disease: A review and methodologic critique. *Psychol Bull* 96:435-464, 1984.

131. Devereux RB, Pickering TG, Harshfield GA: Left ventricular hypertrophy in patients with hypertension: Importance of blood pressure response to regularly recurring stress. *Circulation* 68:470-476, 1983.

132. Schnall PL, Pieper G, Schwartz JE: The relationship between "job strain," workplace diastolic blood pressure, and left ventricular mass index: Results of a case-control study. *J Am Med Assoc* 263:1929-1935, 1990.

133. Julius S, Li Y, Brant D: Neurogenic pressor episodes fail to cause hypertension, but do induce hypertrophy. *Hypertension* 13:422-425, 1989.

134. Kaplan JR, Manuck SB, Adams MR, et al: Nonhuman primates as a model for evaluation behavioral influences on atherosclerosis, and cardiac structure and function. In Shapiro AP, Baum A (eds): *Perspectives on Behavioral Medication,* Hillsdale, NJ, Lawrence Erlbaum Associates, Inc, 1991, pp. 105-129.

135. Spence JD, Bass M, Robinson H, et al: Prospective study of ambulatory monitoring and echocardiography in borderline hypertension. *Clin Invest Med* 14:241-250, 1991.

136. Manuck SB: Cardiovascular reactivity in cardiovascular disease: "Once more unto the breach." *Int J Behav Med* 1:4-31, 1994.

137. Rostrup M, Smith G, Bjornstad H, et al: Left ventricular mass and cardiovascular reactivity in young men. *Hypertension* 23: I168-I171, 1994.

138. Gottdiener JS, Hecht GM, Patterson SM, et al: Relation between behavior, hemodynamic reactivity, and LV mass. *Circulation* 88(Suppl I):168, 1993.

139. Sherwood A, Gullette EC, Hinderliter AL, et al: Relationship of clinic, ambulatory, and laboratory stress blood pressure to left ventricular mass in overweight men and women with high blood pressure. *Psychosom Med* 64:247-257, 2002.

140. Kamarck TW, Eranen J, Jennings JR, et al: Anticipatory blood pressure responses to exercise are associated with left ventricular mass in Finnish men: Kuopio Ischemic Heart Disease Risk Factor Study. *Circulation* 102:1394-1399, 2000.

141. al'Absi M, Devereux RB, Rao DC, et al: Blood pressure stress reactivity and left ventricular mass in a random community sample of African-American and Caucasian men and women. *Am J Cardiol* 97:240-244, 2006.

142. Verdecchia P, Schillaci G, Guerrieri M, et al: Circadian blood pressure changes and left ventricular hypertrophy in essential hypertension. *Circulation* 81:528-536, 1990.

143. Simpson P, McGrath S, Savion S: Myocyte hypertrophy in neonatal heart cultures and its regulation by serum and by catecholamines. *Circ Res* 51:787-801, 1982.

144. Corea L, Bentivoglio M, Berdecchia P: Plasma norepinephrine in left ventricular hypertrophy in systemic hypertension. *Am J Cardiol* 53:1299-1301 1984.

145. Schlaich MP, Kaye DM, Lambert E, et al: Relation between cardiac sympathetic activity and hypertensive left ventricular hypertrophy. *Circulation* 108:560-565, 2003.

146. Tarazi RC, Sen S, Fouad FM, Wicker P: Regression of myocardial hypertrophy: Conditions and sequelae of reversal in hypertensive heart disease. In Alpert NR (ed): *Perspectives in cardiovascular research,* 7th ed, New York, Raven Press, 1983, p. 637.

147. Sen S, Tarazi RC, Bumpus FM: Cardiac hypertrophy and antihypertensive therapy. *Cardiovasc Res* 11:427-433, 1977.

148. Sharma JN, Fernandez PG, Kim BK: Cardiac regression and blood pressure control in the Dahl rat treated with either enalapril maleate (MK 421, an angiotensin-converting enzyme inhibitor) or hydrochlorothiazide. *J Hypertens* 1:251-256, 1983.

149. Schulman SP, Weiss JL, Becker LC, et al: The effects of antihypertensive therapy on left ventricular mass in elderly patients. *N Eng J Med* 322:1350-1356, 1990.

150. Gottdiener JS, Reda DJ, Massie BM, et al: Effect of single-drug therapy on reduction of left ventricular mass in mild to moderate hypertension: Comparison of six antihypertensive agents. The department of Veterans Affairs cooperative study group on antihypertensive agents. *Circulation* 95:2007-2014, 1997.

151. Robertson AL Jr, Khairallah PA: Angiotensin II: Rapid localization in nuclei of smooth and cardiac muscle. *Science* 172:1138-1139, 1971.

152. Roth RH, Hughes J: Acceleration of protein biosynthesis by angiotensins correlation with angiotensin's effect on catecholamine biosynthesis. *Biochem Pharmacol* 21:3182-3187, 1972.

153. Sen S, Bumpus FM: Collagen synthesis in development and reversal of cardiac hypertrophy in spontaneously hypertensive rats. *Am J Cardiol* 44:954-958, 1979.

154. Fernandez PG, Snedden W, Idikio H: The reversal of left ventricular hypertrophy with control of blood pressure in experimental hypertension. *Scand J Clin Lab Invest* 44:711-716, 1984.

155. Devereux RB, Pennert K, Cody RJ: Relation of renin-angiotensin system activity to left ventricular hypertrophy and function in experimental and human hypertension. *J Clin Hypertens* 13:87-103, 1987.

156. Vensel LA, Devereux RB, Pickering TG: Cardiac structure and function in renovascular hypertension produced by unilateral and bilateral renal artery stenosis. *Am J Cardiol* 58:575-582, 1986.

157. Alderman MH, Madhavan S, Ooi WL: Association of the renin-sodium profile with the risk of myocardial infarction in patients with hypertension. *N Eng J Med* 324:1098-1104, 1991.

158. Meyer P: Similarities in cellular proliferative mechanisms in hypertension and neoplasia. In Laragh JH, Brenner BM (eds): *Hypertension: Pathophysiology, Diagnosis and Management,* New York, Raven Press, 1990, pp. 541-545.

159. Marban E, Koretsune Y: Cell calcium, oncogenes, and hypertrophy. *Hypertension* 15:652-658, 1990.

160. Stefenelli T, Abela C, Frank H, et al: Cardiac abnormalities in patients with primary hyperparathyroidism: Implications for follow-up. *J Clin Endocrinol Metab* 82:106-112, 1997.

161. Symons C, Fortune F, Greenbaum RA, Dandona P: Cardiac hypertrophy, hypertrophic cardiomyopathy, and hyperparathyroidism—an association. *Br Heart J* 54:539-542, 1985.

162. Piovesan A, Molineri N, Casasso F, et al: Left ventricular hypertrophy in primary hyperparathyroidism. Effects of successful parathyroidectomy. *Clin Endocrinol (Oxf)* 50:321-328, 1999.

163. McCarron DA, Pingree PA, Rubin RJ: Enhanced parathyroid function in essential hypertension: A homeostatic response to urinary calcium leak. *Hypertension* 2:162-168, 1980.

164. Grobbee DE, Hacking WHL, Birkenhager JC: Raised plasma intact parathyroid hormone concentration in young people with mildly raised blood pressure. *Br Med J Clin Res* 296:814-816, 1988.

165. Ha SK, Park HS, Kim SJ, et al: Prevalence and patterns of left ventricular hypertrophy in patients with predialysis chronic renal failure. *J Korean Med Sci* 13:488-494, 1998.

166. Lindpainter K, Sen S: Role of sodium in hypertensive cardiac hypertrophy. *Circ Res* 57:610, 1985.

167. Schmeider RE, Messerli FH, Garavaglia GE: Dietary salt intake: A determinant of cardiac involvement in essential hypertension. *Circulation* 78:951-956, 1988.

168. Kannel WB: Role of blood pressure in cardiovascular morbidity and mortality. *Prog Cardiovasc Dis* 17:5-24, 1974.

169. Marcus ML: Effects of cardiac hypertrophy on the coronary circulation. In Marcus ML (ed): *The Coronary Circulation in Health and Disease*, New York, McGraw-Hill, 1983.

170. Dellsperger KC, Clothier JL, Hartnett JA: Acceleration of the wavefront of myocardial necrosis by chronic hypertension and left ventricular hypertrophy in dogs. *Circ Res* 63:87-96, 1988.

171. Lund-Johansen P: Central haemodynamics in essential hypertension at rest and during exercise: A 20-year follow-up study. *J Hypertens* 7:S52, 1989.

172. Himmelmann A, Svensson A, Sigstrom L, Hansson L: Predictors of blood pressure and left ventricular mass in the young: The hypertension in pregnancy offspring study. *Am J Hypertens* 7:381-389, 1994.

173. De Simone G, Devereux RB, Roman MJ, et al: Echocardiographic left ventricular mass and electrolyte intake predict arterial hypertension. *Ann Intern Med* 114:202-209, 1991.

174. Iso H, Kiyama M, Doi M, et al: Left ventricular mass and subsequent blood pressure changes among middle-aged men in rural and urban Japanese populations. *Circulation* 89:1717-1724, 1994.

175. Post WS, Larson MG, Levy D: Impact of left ventricular structure on the incidence of hypertension (The Framingham Heart Study). *Circulation* 90:179-185, 1994.

176. Savage DD, Drayer JIM, Henry WL, et al: Echocardiographic assessment of cardiac anatomy and function in hypertensive subjects. *Circulation* 59:623-630, 1979.

177. Abi-samra R, Fouad FM, Tarazi RC: Determinants of left ventricular hypertrophy and function in hypertensive patients: An echocardiographic study. *Am J Med* 75:26-33, 1983.

178. Borow KN, Green LH, Grossman W, Braunwald E: Left ventricular end-systolic stress-shortening and stress length relations in humans. Normal values and sensitivity to inotropic state. *Am J Cardiol* 50:1301-1308, 1982.

179. Shimizu G, Zile MR, Blaustein AS, Gaasch WH: Left ventricular chamber filling and midwall fiber lengthening in patients with left ventricular hypertrophy: overestimation of fiber velocities by conventional midwall measurements. *Circulation* 71:266-272, 1985.

180. Aurigemma GP, Silver KH, Priest MA, Gaasch WH: Geometric changes allow normal ejection fraction despite depressed myocardial shortening in hypertensive left ventricular hypertrophy. *J Am Coll Cardiol* 26:195-202, 1995.

181. Greenbaum R, Ho S, Gibson D: Left ventricular fibre architecture in man. *Br Heart J* 45:248-263, 1981.

182. Streeter D, Spotnitz H, Patel D: Fiber orientation in the canine left ventricle during diastole and systole. *Circ Res* 24:339-346, 1969.

183. Shimizu G, Hirota Y, Kawamura K: Empiric determination of the transition from concentric hypertrophy to congestive heart failure in essential hypertension. *J Am Coll Cardiol* 25:888-894, 1995.

184. Wasserman AG, Katz RJ, Varghee PJ: Exercise radionuclide ventriculographic responses in hypertensive patients with chest pain. *N Eng J Med* 311:1276-1280, 1984.

185. Borer JS, Jason M, Devereux RB, et al: Function of the hypertrophied left ventricle at rest and during exercise; hypertension and aortic stenosis. *Am J Med* 75:34-39, 1983.

186. Tubau JF, Szlachcic J, Braun S, Massie BM: Impaired left ventricular functional reserve in hypertensive patients with left ventricular hypertrophy. *Hypertension* 14:1-8, 1989.

187. Drazner MH, Rame JE, Marino EK, et al: Increased left ventricular mass is a risk factor for the development of a depressed left ventricular ejection fraction within five years: The Cardiovascular Health Study. *J Am Coll Cardiol* 43:2207-2215, 2004.

188. Vasan RS, Benjamin EJ, Levy D: Prevalence, clinical features and prognosis of diastolic heart failure: An epidemiologic perspective. *J Am Coll Cardiol* 26:1565-1574, 1995.

189. Kitzman DW, Gardin JM, Gottdiener JS, et al: Importance of heart failure with preserved systolic function in patients > or = 65 years of age. CHS Research Group. Cardiovascular Health Study. *Am J Cardiol* 87:413-419, 2001.

190. Gottdiener JS, Arnold AM, Aurigemma GP, et al: Predictors of congestive heart failure in the elderly: the Cardiovascular Health Study. *J Am Coll Cardiol* 35:1628-1637, 2000.

191. Vasan RS, Benjamin EJ, Levy D: Congestive heart failure with normal left ventricular systolic function. Clinical approaches to the diagnosis and treatment of diastolic heart failure. *Arch Intern Med* 156:146-157, 1996.

192. Aurigemma GP, Gottdiener JS, Shemanski L, et al: Predictive value of systolic and diastolic function for incident congestive heart failure in the elderly: The Cardiovascular Health Study. *J Am Coll Cardiol* 37:1042-1048, 2001.

193. Phillips RA, Ardeljan M, Shimabukuro S: Normalization of left ventricular mass and associated changes in neurohormones and atrial natriuretic peptide after 1 year of sustained nifedipine therapy for severe hypertension. *J Am Coll Cardiol* 17:1595-1602, 1991.

194. Trimarco B, DeLuca N, Rosiello G: Improvement of diastolic function after reversal of left ventricular hypertrophy induced by long-term antihypertensive treatment with tertatolol. *Am J Cardiol* 64:745-751, 1989.

195. Pearson AC, Labovitz AJ, Mrosek D, et al: Assessment of diastolic function in normal and hypertrophied hearts: comparison of Doppler echocardiography and M-mode echocardiography. *Am Heart J* 113:1417-1425, 1987.

196. Kuwajima I, Miyao M, Uno A, et al: Diagnostic value of electrocardiography and echocardiography for white coat hypertension in the elderly. *Am J Cardiol* 73:1232-1234, 1994.

197. Modena MG, Mattioli AV, Parato VM, Mattioli G: Effect of antihypertensive treatment with nitrendipine on left ventricular mass and diastolic filling in patients with mild to moderate hypertension. *J Cardiovasc Pharmacol* 19:148-153, 1992.

198. Doering CW, Jalil JE, Janicki JS, et al: Collagen network remodelling and diastolic stiffness of the rat left ventricle with pressure overload hypertrophy. *Cardiovasc Res* 22:686-695, 1988.

199. Douglas PS, Tallant B: Hypertrophy, fibrosis and diastolic dysfunction in early canine experimental hypertension. *J Am Coll Cardiol* 17:530-536, 1991.

200. Thomas JD, Weyman AE: Echocardiographic Doppler evaluation of left ventricular diastolic function. *Circulation* 84:977-990, 1991.

201. Kmetzo JJ, Plotnick GD, Gottdiener JS: Effect of postural changes and isometric exercise on Doppler derived measurements of diastolic function in normal subjects. *Chest* 100:357-363, 1991.

202. Plotnick GD, Kmetzo JJ, Gottdiener JS: Effect of autonomic blockade, postural changes, and isometric exercise on Doppler indices of diastolic left ventricular function. *Am J Cardiol* 67:1284-1290, 1991.

203. Brilla CG, Janicki JS, Weber KT: Impaired diastolic function and coronary reserve in genetic hypertension. Role of interstitial fibrosis and medial thickening of intramyocardial coronary arteries. *Circ Res* 69:107-115, 1991.

204. Gustafsson C, Britton M, Brolund F, et al: Echocardiographic findings and the increased risk of stroke in nonvalvular atrial fibrillation. *Cardiology* 81:189-195, 1992.

205. The Stroke Prevention in Atrial Fibrillation Investigators: Predictors of thromboembolism in atrial fibrillation: II. Echocardiographic features of patients at risk. *Ann Intern Med* 116:6-12, 1992.

206. Vaziri SM, Lauer MS, Larson MG, et al: Influence of blood pressure on LA size. *Hypertension* 25:1155-1160, 1995.

207. Gottdiener JS, Reda DJ, Williams DW, Materson BJ: LA size in hypertensive men: Influence of obesity, race and age. Department of Veterans Affairs Cooperative Study Group on Antihypertensive Agents. *J Am Coll Cardiol* 29:651-658, 1997.

208. Gerdts E, Oikarinen L, Palmieri V, et al: Correlates of LA size in hypertensive patients with left ventricular hypertrophy: The Losartan Intervention For Endpoint Reduction in Hypertension (LIFE) Study. *Hypertension* 39:739-743, 2002.

209. Tsang TS, Abhayaratna WP, Barnes ME, et al: Prediction of cardiovascular outcomes with LA size: is volume superior to area or diameter? *J Am Coll Cardiol* 47:1018-1023, 2006.

210. Keller AM, Gopal AS, King DL: Left and right atrial volume by freehand three-dimensional echocardiography: In vivo validation using magnetic resonance imaging. *Eur J Echocardiogr* 1:55-65, 2000.

211. Khankirawatana B, Khankirawatana S, Lof J, Porter TR: LA volume determination by three-dimensional echocardiography reconstruction: validation and application of a simplified technique. *J Am Soc Echocardiogr* 15:1051-1056, 2002.

212. Gottdiener JS: LA size: renewed interest in an old echocardiographic measurement. *Am Heart J* 147:195-196, 2004.

213. Cuspidi C, Meani S, Fusi V, et al: Prevalence and correlates of aortic root dilatation in patients with essential hypertension: relationship with cardiac and extracardiac target organ damage. *J Hypertens* 24:573-580, 2006.

214. Bella JN, Wachtell K, Boman K, et al: Relation of left ventricular geometry and function to aortic root dilatation in patients with systemic hypertension and left ventricular hypertrophy (the LIFE study). *Am J Cardiol* 89:337-341, 2002.

215. Gardin JM, Arnold AM, Polak J, et al: Usefulness of aortic root dimension in persons > or = 65 years of age in predicting heart failure, stroke, cardiovascular mortality, all-cause mortality and acute myocardial infarction (from the Cardiovascular Health Study). *Am J Cardiol* 97:270-275, 2006.

216. Liebson PR: Clinical studies of drug reversal of hypertensive left ventricular hypertrophy. *Am J Hypertens* 3:512-517, 1990.

217. Trimarco B, Wikstrand J: Regression of cardiovascular structural changes by antihypertensive treatment. Functional consequences and time course of reversal as judged from clinical studies. *Hypertension* 6(suppl 3):III-150, 1984.

218. Sen S: Regression of cardiac hypertrophy. Experimental animal model. *Am J Med* 75(suppl 3A):87, 1983.

219. Fouad-Tarazi F, Liebson PR: Echocardiographic studies of regression of left ventricular hypertrophy in hypertension. *Hypertension* 4(Suppl 2):65-68, 1987.

220. Massie BM: Effect of diuretic therapy on hypertensive left ventricular hypertrophy. *Eur Heart J* 13 (Suppl G):53-60, 1992.

221. Pfeffer MA, Pfeffer JM: Reversing cardiac hypertrophy in hypertension. *N Engl M Med* 322:1388-1390, 1987.

222. Devereux RB, Savage DD, Sachs I, Laragh JH: Effect of blood pressure control on left ventricular hypertrophy and function in hypertension. *Circulation* 62(suppl 3):36, 1980.

223. Wollam GL, Hall WD, Porter VD, et al: Time course of regression of left ventricular hypertrophy in treated hypertensive patients. *Am J Med* 26:100-110, 1983.

224. Drayer JIM, Gardin JM, Weber MA, Aronow WS: Changes in ventricular septal thickness during diuretic therapy. *Clin Pharmac Therap* 32:283-288, 1982.

225. Giles TD, Sander GE, Roffidal LC, et al: Comparison of nitrendipine and hydrochlorothiazide for systemic hypertension. *Am J Cardiol* 60:103-106, 1987.

226. Pfeffer MA, Pfeffer JM: Pharmacologic regression of cardiac hypertrophy in experimental hypertension. *J Cardiovasc Pharmacol* 6(suppl 6):S865, 1984.

227. Pegram BL, Ishise S, Frohlich ED: Effects of methyldopa, clonidine and hydralazine on cardiac mass and haemodynamics in Wistar Kyoto and spontaneously hypertensive rats. *Cardiovasc Res* 16:40, 1982.

228. Plotnick GD, Fisher ML, Wohl B: Improvement in depressed cardiac function in hypertensive patients during pindolol treatment. *Am J Cardiol* 76:25, 1984.

229. Burnier M, Brunner HR: Neurohormonal consequences of diuretics in different cardiovascular syndromes. *Eur Heart J* 13(Suppl G):28-33, 1992.

230. Dahlof B, Pennert K, Hansson L: Reversal of left ventricular hypertrophy in hypertensive patients: A metaanalysis of 109 treatment studies. *Am J Hypertens* 5:95-110, 1992.

231. Reichek N, Franklin BB, Chandler T, et al: Reversal of left ventricular hypertrophy by antihypertensive therapy. *Eur Heart J* 3:165-169, 1982.

232. Cherchi A, Sau F, Seguro C: Regression of left ventricular hypertrophy after treatment of hypertension by chlorthalidone for one year and other diuretics for two years. *J Hypertens* 1(suppl 2):278-280, 1983.

233. Ferrara LA, De Simone G, Mancini M, et al: Changes in left ventricular mass during a double-blind study with chlorthalidone and slow-release nifedipine. *Eur J Clin Pharmacol* 27:525-528, 1984.

234. Mace PJE, Littler WA, Glover DR, et al: Regression of left ventricular hypertrophy in hypertension: Comparative effects of three different drugs. *J Cardiovasc Pharmacol* 7:S52-S55, 1985.

235. Sami M, Haichin R: Regression of left ventricular hypertrophy in hypertension with indapamide. *Am Heart J* 122:1215-1218, 1991.

236. Neaton JD, Grimm RJ Jr, Prineas RJ, et al: Treatment of mild hypertension study. Final results. Treatment of Mild Hypertension Study Research Group. *J Am Med Assoc* 270:713-724, 1993.

237. Materson BJ, Reda DJ, Cushman WC, et al: Single-drug therapy for hypertension in men. A comparison of six antihypertensive agents with placebo. The Department of Veterans Affairs Cooperative Study Group on Antihypertensive Agents. *N Engl J Med* 328:914-921, 1993.

238. Fagerberg B, Berglund A, Andersson OK, et al: Cardiovascular effects of weight reduction versus antihypertensive drug treatment: A comparative, randomized, 1-year study of obese men with mild hypertension. *J Hypertens* 9:431-439, 1991.

239. McMahon SW, Wilcken D, Macdonald GJ: The effect of weight reduction on left ventricular mass. *N Eng J Med* 314:334-339, 1986.

240. Ferrara LA, De Simone G, Pasanisi F, Mancini M: Left ventricular mass reduction during salt depletion in arterial hypertension. *Hypertension* 6:755-759, 1984.

241. Jula AM, Karanko HM: Effects on left ventricular hypertrophy of long-term nonpharmacological treatment with sodium restric-

tion in mild-to-moderate essential hypertension. *Circulation* 89:1023-1031, 1994.

242. Kelemen MH, Effron MB, Valenti SA, Stewart KJ: Exercise training combined with antihypertensive drug therapy: effects on lipids, blood pressure, and left ventricular mass. *J Am Med Assoc* 263:2766-2771, 1990.

243. Oren S, Messerli FH, Grossman E, et al: Immediate and short-term cardiovascular effects of fosinopril, a new angiotensin-converting enzyme inhibitor, in patients with essential hypertension. *J Am Coll Cardiol* 17:1183-1187, 1991.

244. Aurigemma GP, Gottdiener JS, Gaasch WH, et al: Ventricular and myocardial function following regression of hypertensive left ventricular hypertrophy. *J Am Coll Cardiol* (Special Issue) February:251A, 1995.

245. Muiesan ML, Agabiti-Rosei E, Romanelli G: Improved left ventricular systolic and diastolic function after regression of cardiac hypertrophy, treatment withdrawal, and redevelopment of hypertension. *J Cardiovasc Pharmacol* 17(suppl 2):S179-S181, 1991.

246. Gottdiener JS: Measuring diastolic function. *J Am Coll Cardiol* 18:83-84, 1991.

247. Brilla CG: Regression of myocardial fibrosis in hypertensive heart disease: Diverse effects of various antihypertensive drugs. *Cardiovasc Res* 46:324-331, 2000.

248. Brilla CG, Funck RC, Rupp H: Lisinopril-mediated regression of myocardial fibrosis in patients with hypertensive heart disease [see comments]. *Circulation* 102:1388-1393, 2000.

249. Verdecchia P, Schillaci G, Borgioni C, et al: Prognostic significance of serial changes in left ventricular mass in essential hypertension. *Circulation* 97:48-54, 1998.

250. Levy D, Salomon M, D'Agostino RB, et al: Prognostic implications of baseline electrocardiographic features and their serial changes in subjects with left ventricular hypertrophy. *Circulation* 90:1786-1793, 1994.

251. Devereux RB, Wachtell K, Gerdts E, et al: Prognostic significance of left ventricular mass change during treatment of hypertension. *J Am Med Assoc* 292:2350-2356, 2004.

252. Gottdiener JS, Bednarz J, Devereux R, et al: American Society of Echocardiography recommendations for use of echocardiography in clinical trials. *J Am Soc Echocardiogr* 17:1086-1119, 2004.

253. Lang RM, Bierig M, Devereux RB, et al: Recommendations for chamber quantification: A report from the American Society of Echocardiography's Guidelines and Standards Committee and the Chamber Quantification Writing Group, developed in conjunction with the European Association of Echocardiography, a branch of the European Society of Cardiology. *J Am Soc Echocardiogr* 18:1440-1463, 2005.

254. Devereux RB, Alonso DR, Lutas EM, et al: Echocardiographic assessment of left ventricular hypertrophy comparison to necropsy findings. *Am J Cardiol* 57:450-458, 1986.

255. Palmieri V, Dahlof B, De Q, V, et al: Reliability of echocardiographic assessment of left ventricular structure and function: The PRESERVE study. Prospective Randomized Study Evaluating Regression of Ventricular Enlargement. *J Am Coll Cardiol* 34:1625-1632, 1999.

256. Devereux RB, Roman MJ, Paranicas M, et al: Impact of diabetes on cardiac structure and function: the strong heart study. *Circulation* 101:2271-2276, 2000.

257. Schiller NB, Shah PM, Crawford M, et al: Recommendations for quantitation of the left ventricle by two-dimensional echocardiography. American Society of Echocardiography committee on standards, subcommittee on quantitation of two-dimensional echocardiograms. *J Am Soc Echocardiogr* 2:358-367, 1989.

258. Park SH, Shub C, Nobrega TP, et al: Two-dimensional echocardiographic calculation of left ventricular mass as recommended by the American Society of Echocardiography: Correlation with autopsy and M-mode echocardiography. *J Am Soc Echocardiogr* 9:119-128, 1996.

259. King DL, Gopal AS, Keller AM, et al: Three-dimensional echocardiography. Advances for measurement of ventricular volume and mass. *Hypertension* 23:I172-I179, 1994.

260. Gopal AS, Keller AM, Shen Z, et al: Three-dimensional echocardiography: in vitro and in vivo validation of left ventricular mass and comparison with conventional echocardiographic methods [see comments]. *J Am Coll Cardiol* 24:504-513, 1994.

261. Chuang ML, Beaudin RA, Riley MF, et al: Three-dimensional echocardiographic measurement of left ventricular mass: comparison with magnetic resonance imaging and two-dimensional echocardiographic determinations in man. *Int J Cardiovasc Imaging* 16:347-357, 2000.

262. Caiani EG, Corsi C, Sugeng L, et al: Improved quantification of left ventricular mass based on endocardial and epicardial surface detection with real time three dimensional echocardiography. *Heart* 92:213-219, 2006.

263. Jenkins C, Bricknell K, Marwick TH: Use of real-time three-dimensional echocardiography to measure LA volume: comparison with other echocardiographic techniques. *J Am Soc Echocardiogr* 18:991-997, 2005.

264. Rodevan O, Bjornerheim R, Ljosland M, et al: LA volumes assessed by three- and two-dimensional echocardiography compared to MRI estimates. *Int J Card Imaging* 15:397-410, 1999.

265. Kizer JR, Bella JN, Palmieri V, et al: LA diameter as an independent predictor of first clinical cardiovascular events in middle-aged and elderly adults: the Strong Heart Study (SHS). *Am Heart J* 151:412-418, 2006.

266. Gottdiener JS, Kitzman DW, Aurigemma GP, et al: LA volume, geometry, and function in systolic and diastolic heart failure of persons > or = 65 years of age (the cardiovascular health study). *Am J Cardiol* 97:83-89, 2006.

267. Savage DD, Garrison RJ, Kannel WB, et al: Considerations in the use of echocardiography in epidemiology; The Framingham study. *Hypertension* 9(suppl II):II40-II44, 1987.

268. Devereux RB, Dahlof B, Gerdts E, et al: Regression of hypertensive left ventricular hypertrophy by losartan compared with atenolol: the Losartan Intervention for Endpoint Reduction in Hypertension (LIFE) trial. *Circulation* 110:1456-1462, 2004.

269. Gottdiener JS, Livengood SV, Meyer PS, Chase GA: Should echocardiography be performed to assess effects of antihypertensive therapy? Test-retest reliability of echocardiography for measurement of left ventricular mass and function. *J Am Coll Cardiol* 25:424-430, 1995.

270. De Simone G, Muiesan ML, Ganau A, et al: Reliability and limitations of echocardiographic measurement of left ventricular mass for risk stratification and follow-up in single patients: The RES trial. Working Group on Heart and Hypertension of the Italian Society of Hypertension. Reliability of M-mode Echocardiographic Studies. *J Hypertens* 17:1955-1963, 1999.

271. Palmieri V, Dahlof B, DeQuattro V, et al: Reliability of echocardiographic assessment of left ventricular structure and function: The PRESERVE study. Prospective Randomized Study Evaluating Regression of Ventricular Enlargement. *J Am Coll Cardiol* 34:1625-1632, 1999.

272. Himelman RB, Cassidy MM, Landzberg JS, Schiller NB: Reproducibility of quantitative two-dimensional echocardiography. *Am Heart J* 115:425-431, 1988.

273. De Simone G, Ganau A, Verdecchia P, Devereux RB: Echocardiography in arterial hypertension: when, why and how? *J Hypertens* 12:1129-1136, 1994.

Echocardiographic Findings in Acute and Chronic Respiratory Disease

PAUL R. FORFIA, MD • SUSAN E. WIEGERS, MD

Basic Principles

The importance of the right ventricle in maintaining normal circulatory homeostasis was not initially appreciated because early studies demonstrated that extensive thermal destruction of the right ventricular (RV) free wall did not lead to a significant increase in central venous pressure (CVP) or systemic hypotension.[1,2] However, when the damaged right ventricle was coupled to an increased afterload, rapid cardiovascular collapse ensued.[3,4] Almost 30 years later, the serious clinical consequences of RV infarction were described.[5] The clinical and physiologic significance of RV function

The authors acknowledge Selwyn P. Wong, MD, and Catherine M. Otto, MD, the previous authors of this chapter in *The Practice of Clinical Echocardiography*, second edition.

and the consequences of altered ventricular-arterial coupling have been further delineated by recognition of the hemodynamic and clinical impact of right-sided cardiac dysfunction in acute and chronic respiratory disease.[6-8]

Central to patient evaluation in these processes is the echocardiographic examination. This chapter will address the echocardiographic evaluation of right-sided cardiac function. In particular, an emphasis will be placed on the recognition of the three characteristic findings of RV dysfunction; RV enlargement, right-to-left heart disproportion, and RV systolic dysfunction. The integration of the echocardiographic assessment into the diagnosis and treatment of these disorders will also be reviewed.

Right-Sided Heart Anatomy and Blood Supply

The right atrium forms the right-sided heart border, lying superior, posterior, and rightward of the right ventricle, anchoring to the superior surface of the fibrous tricuspid valve (TV) annulus. The internal wall of the right atrium is comprised of a smooth posterior aspect, with fenestrations superoposteriorly and inferiorly that drain the superior and inferior vena cava (IVC). The coronary sinus (CS) drains into the posterior wall of the right atrium, with its opening located between the opening of the IVC and the atrioventricular (AV) orifice. The anterior aspect of the right atrium has a rough internal surface related to the presence of ridge-like pectinate muscle. The interatrial septum forms the posteromedial wall of the right atrium and contains the fossa ovalis lying between the caval orifices.

The TV is comprised of anterior, septal, and posterior leaflets, all of which fasten to the inferior surface of the TV ring. The annular insertion of the TV is approximately 2 mm more apical than the mitral valve. The anterior and posterior TV leaflets attach to the anterior papillary muscle, which is by far the largest and most prominent of the three papillary muscles. The anterior papillary muscle emanates from the anterior wall of the right ventricle and fuses with the moderator band, hinging the anterior papillary muscle to the interventricular septum. Chordae from the posterior and septal leaflets attach to smaller, multiple posterior papillary muscles, which arise from the inferior wall of the right ventricle. The septal papillary muscles arise from the interventricular septum and are smaller and more numerous than the posterior papillary muscles, with chordal attachments to the anterior and septal leaflets of the TV.

The right ventricle forms the majority of the anterior surface of the heart and nearly the entire inferior cardiac border. The right ventricle is comprised of two embryologically distinct regions, the inflow (sinus) portion and a funnel-shaped outflow portion (conus or infundibulum). The body of the right ventricle is formed by the RV free wall and interventricular septum. The RV free wall anchors into the anterior and posterior aspects of the interventricular septum, with its radius of curvature approximating that of a large sphere. The interventricular septum is convexed toward the RV cavity, imparting a crescentic shape to the right ventricle in cross section. The interior of the RV is heavily trabeculated and contains the muscular moderator band traversing from the interventricular septum to the anterior free wall. These features, along with the more apical annular insertion of the TV are useful clinically in discerning the morphologic right from the left ventricle, for example in patients with transposition of the great arteries.

The inflow and outflow portions of the RV are separated by a U-shaped muscular ridge known as the crista supraventricularis, which originates along the tricuspid annulus, extends to the interventricular septum, and bridges across the RV cavity by way of the moderator band to attach to the anterior wall of the RV and anterior papillary muscle. Investigators have hypothesized that the crista functions as a contractile strut, permitting systolic interventricular septal motion to simultaneously narrow the TV annulus and pull the RV free wall toward the septum, promoting TV competence and RV contraction. This structure, coupled with interlacing epicardial muscle fibers that extend from right ventricle to left ventricle form the anatomical basis for systolic ventricular interdependence.[9,10] Under normal circumstances, left ventricular (LV) contraction accounts for an estimated 30% of pressure generation in the right ventricle through the transmission of systolic forces from the left ventricle to the right ventricle.[10] The damaged right ventricle is able to continue to generate tension because the normally contracting left ventricle 'pulls' the damaged RV free wall toward the septum. Experimental animal studies have shown that damage to the right ventricle alone did not adversely affect central venous or systemic arterial pressure, but when a portion of the LV was also damaged via cautery, the animals rapidly succumbed to shock.[11]

The infundibulum is the smooth walled, funnel-shaped outflow portion of the right ventricle, which tapers in a superior and leftward direction to the pulmonic valve. Thus the right ventricle has a complex geometry, with the RV inflow geometry approximating a pyramid with its base at the valve orifice, and its three sides formed by the anterior and posterior free walls and interventricular septum. The outflow portion is cylindrical and tapered like a spout.

The right coronary artery supplies the vast majority of the RV free wall, save a small anterior portion of the right ventricle supplied by branches of the left anterior descending (LAD) coronary artery. The moderator band artery arises from the first septal perforating branch of the left anterior descending artery. In less than 10% of hearts, posterolateral branches of the left circumflex coronary artery supply a portion of the posterior RV free wall. The conus artery, arising from a separate coronary ostia is 30% of cases, supplies the infundibulum. Although coronary blood flow to the left ventricle occurs predominantly in diastole, RV coronary blood flow occurs equally in systole and diastole as a result of the lower intramural compressive forces exerted during RV systole.[12] RV stroke work is approximately one fourth LV stroke work, and RV coronary blood flow is comparatively lower with lower oxygen extraction across the RV myocardium compared to the left ventricle. Thus the right ventricle is far more tolerant of ischemia because of this oxygen extraction reserve along with lower oxygen demand and redundant blood supply. Recovery of RV function is the rule rather than the exception following RV infarction. However, in the presence of increased RV systolic pressure and hypertrophy, the distribution of phasic coronary blood flow to the right ventricle and left ventricle are similar, with the majority of perfusion occurring in diastole.[13] In these conditions, the RV is much less tolerant of ischemia.[14]

Physiology of the Right Ventricle

The primary role of the right ventricle is to deliver oxygen-poor, carbon dioxide-rich blood to the gas exchange membranes of the pulmonary circulation. The right ventricle necessarily generates the identical cardiac output (CO) as the left ventricle but does so with one-sixth the muscle mass of the left ventricle. This is possible as a result of the striking difference in circulatory load imposed by the pulmonary versus systemic vasculature.

Anatomically, the pulmonary circulation is more symmetrical (as opposed to the upper and lower body asymmetry of the systemic circulation), with much shorter path lengths along vascular segments. The walls of the large pulmonary arteries (PAs) are relatively thin, with no well-developed arterioles in the pulmonary circulation. Functionally, this translates to a pulse pressure that is one half, and a mean arterial pressure (MAP) that is one sixth that of the systemic circulation, despite an identical stroke volume (SV) and CO generated by the right ventricle. Through comparison of pulmonary and aortic input impedance spectra, one can appreciate that pulmonary arterial resistance is approximately one tenth systemic, with greater large artery distensibility and lower pulmonary artery pulse wave velocity, along with roughly one third the degree of arterial wave reflection relative to the systemic circulation. In health, a transpulmonary gradient of only 5 mm Hg is required to drive blood flow across the pulmonary circulation, permitting the right ventricle to function as a low-pressure, high-flow pump.

RV systolic function, like LV systolic function, is influenced by changes in preload, afterload, and the intrinsic contractility of the ventricle. The right ventricle generates a comparatively lower systolic pressure, which peaks early in systole and drops off rapidly through the remainder of systole. PA flow however, continues throughout systole despite falling RV systolic pressure, indicating that flow through the latter portion of systole is the result of blood flow inertia created by early RV ejection into a low impedance pulmonary circulation. In contrast, LV systolic pressure plateaus through most of systole as a result of earlier arrival of arterial reflected waves in the systemic circulation and aortic flow falls sharply immediately after peak LV pressure. Also, isovolumic RV contraction is quite brief as compared to the LV.[15,16]

RV contraction occurs in a peristalsis-like fashion, with initial activation of the RV inflow region followed 30 to 40 ms later by contraction of the conus region. Conus contraction contributes less than 15% of RV SV.[17] The contraction pattern of the body of the right ventricle also differs from the left ventricle. Whereas the left ventricle shortens symmetrically in the transverse and longitudinal planes, differences in muscle fiber orientation dictate that RV systolic shortening occurs predominantly in the longitudinal plane, with only a small proportion of RV contraction occurring as a result of transverse free wall motion.[9] The relative importance of these two planes of RV contraction has been a matter of debate. RV longitudinal shortening closely correlates with RV ejection fraction (EF), whereas transverse RV shortening does not.[18] Longitudinal, but not circumferential regional RV stroke work, correlates with global RV stroke work, challenging the notion that RV contraction is primarily dictated by transverse RV free wall motion.[19] Thus, RV contraction perhaps more closely resembles a piston than a bellows, which has important implications on the strategies we apply to quantifying RV systolic function noninvasively.

Diastolic function of the right ventricle also differs from the left ventricle. The thin walls of the right ventricle and its convexed interventricular septum are relatively distensible, allowing large changes in RV volume with only small changes in RV diastolic pressure. This is illustrated by the fact that RV end-diastolic volume is typically 20% to 30% greater than LV end-diastolic volume, despite lower end-diastolic pressure. As a result, the RV EF is typically 35% to 45%, yet generates the identical SV as the left ventricle.[20] The right ventricle is more tolerant of volume overload states than the left ventricle, augmenting its SV while maintaining a normal end-diastolic pressure.

Echocardiographic Examination of the Right Ventricle

Transthoracic Imaging

Given its complex geometry, the entire right ventricle cannot be assessed from a single view. Full assessment of RV size, function, and hemodynamics is important in any complete study and requires special attention.

Historically, the first assessment of RV size was made from the parasternal position with M-mode (Fig. 35–1). The RV diameter obtained at this level is actually that of the high right ventricular outflow tract (RVOT) and not of the body of the right ventricle. The left lateral decubitus position can increase RV diameter by up to 40% in this view. Two-dimensional (2D) imaging in the parasternal long axis again visualizes only the high RV outflow tract and cannot be used for a definitive assessment of RV size. However, the normal RV end-diastolic dimension is less than 60% of the LV end-diastolic dimension. The orthogonal parasternal short-axis view of the right ventricle demonstrates the crescentic shape of the right ventricle as it wraps around the left ventricular cavity (Fig. 35–2). RV dilatation is constrained by the sternum and so the expansion of the right ventricle both laterally and medially is more clearly seen in the short-axis view. Although valuable for initial assessment of RV size, given the asymmetric nature of RV contraction, these views cannot be used for assessment of RV systolic function. The parasternal RV inflow view (Fig. 35–3), obtained by medial and inferior angulation of the transducer from the parasternal long-axis view, allows visual assessment of more of the RV free wall motion, but the imaging plane can be highly variable and is again unreliable in assessing systolic function. This is the only standard view in which the posterior leaflet of the TV is seen, the other leaflet being the anterior leaflet. Color Dopp-

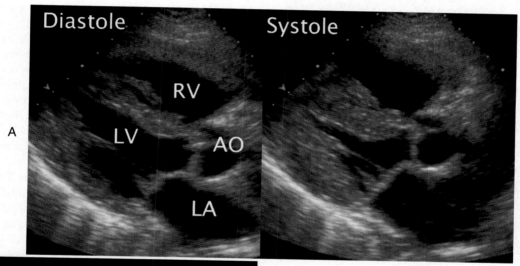

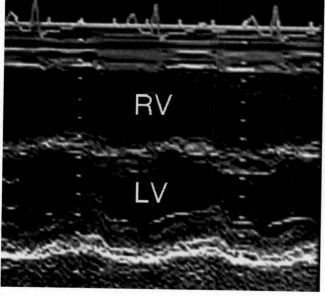

Figure 35–1. *A, Parasternal long-axis view in systole and diastole. The high right ventricular outflow (RV) is seen in diastolic and systolic frames. This patient had normal right ventricular systolic function. The change in right ventricular diameters in this view is not a reliable assessment of right ventricular function. B, M-mode from the parasternal position in a different patient with RV enlargement. The right ventricular end-diastolic diameter approximates the left ventricular end-diastolic diameter, indicating a dilated right ventricle, in this case resulting from an atrial septal defect with significant left to right shunt. Ao, aorta; LA, left atrium; LV, left ventricle.*

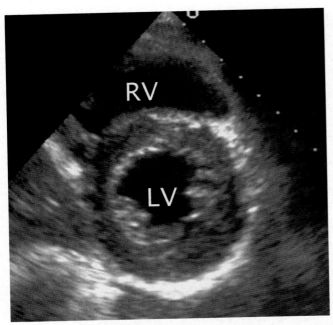

Figure 35–2. Parasternal short axis at the level of the papillary muscles in diastole. The right ventricle (RV) tapers around the interventricular septum, forming a crescent. LV, left ventricle.

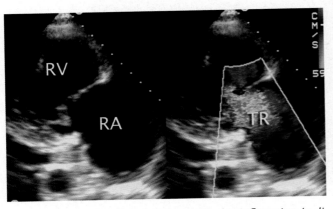

Figure 35–3. Parasternal right ventricular inflow view in diastole. The right ventricle (RV) and right atrium (RA) are enlarged. The posterior and anterior leaflets of the tricuspid valve are imaged in this view. A moderate size pericardial effusion is imaged posterior to the right ventricular wall. The right hand image demonstrates the color Doppler jet of tricuspid regurgitation (TR). The high velocity, turbulent jet has a wide vena contracta consistent with at least moderate TR with increased pulmonary artery pressure. Color and continuous-wave Doppler in the apical four-chamber view is required for further assessment. The RV appears enlarged in systole, which suggests significant dysfunction, but this also requires confirmation in the apical four-chamber view.

ler will demonstrate tricuspid regurgitation (TR), if present but the maximum velocity of the jet is rarely obtained from this view. The ostium of the IVC and the CS are seen in the far field.

The infundibulum is best seen in the parasternal long-axis view of the PA, which is obtained by medial and anterior angulation of the transducer from the parasternal long-axis view (Fig. 35–4). The pulmonary valve is also well seen with the infundibulum imaged proximal to the valve. M-mode of the pulmonary valve motion is of largely historical interest but is still occasionally performed. The pulmonary valve moves toward the PA with atrial systole and opens at the onset of RV contraction (see Fig. 35–4B). Loss of the A wave may occur with atrial fibrillation (AFib) and also in pulmonary hypertension (PH). Notching of the systolic motion may occur in PH but has also been described in PA dilatation with normal PA pressures.[21] Color Doppler will provide assessment of pulmonic regurgitation and turbulent flow associated with infundibular or pulmonic stenosis. Trace or mild pulmonic regurgitation is present in the majority of normal patients.[22] However, the jets are not parallel to the ultrasound (US) beam in this position and velocities are best measured in the parasternal short-axis view at the level of the aortic valve (Fig. 35–5). Both right-sided valves, the infundibulum and the RVOT are also well seen in this view.

The apical four-chamber view is most useful in demonstrating RV geometry (Fig. 35–6). The transducer must be properly positioned over the LV apex. Transducer positions medial to the correct on-axis view will visualize a greater portion of the RV free wall and cavity and may be misinterpreted as demonstrating RV enlargement. Common measurements of the right ventricle taken in the four-chamber view include the midventricular short axis (normal 3.5 ± 0.2 cm)[23] and a planed area of 18 ± 1.2 cm² in normal subjects. A general rule of thumb is that the area of a normal right ventricle is less than two thirds that of the left ventricle. This ratio increases in mild (0.6 to 1), moderate (1 to 1.5), and severe (>1.5) cases of RV dilatation. However, LV enlargement will obviously change this relationship. In the apical view, the moderator band transverses the RV cavity at midventricular level, connecting the free wall to the interventricular septum. The moderator band is present in approximately 75% of patients.[24] Furthermore, right atrial (RA) size may be planimetered in this view and the volume calculated using Simpson's rule and indexed to body surface area (BSA), similar to techniques for the left atrium. The peak velocity of TR is usually best measured in this view, with the US beam parallel to the jet.

The subcostal views may be useful for evaluation of the right ventricle particularly in patients with poor image quality of the apical four chamber (Fig. 35–7A). However, the difficulty in defining the anteroposterior plane of the four-chamber subcostal view makes assessment of the true RV size difficult. It is in this view, however, that the RV wall thickness is best measured because the US beam is perpendicular to the RV free wall and is not in the near field as in the parasternal views. While the normal RV free wall is 2 mm thick, a wall thickness of less than 5 mm is accepted as normal because of the difficulty in separating the RV free wall

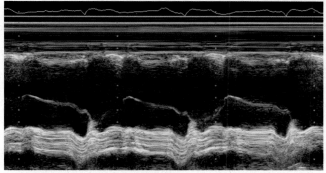

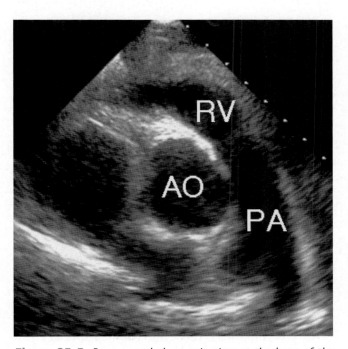

Figure 35–4. A, *Parasternal long axis of the pulmonary valve in systole and diastole. The right ventricular outflow tract (RV) is clearly imaged in this view. Although the details of the pulmonary valve are well seen, the pulmonary artery bifurcation is out of plane. B, M-mode of the pulmonary valve from the same view. The valve leaflets move towards the pulmonary artery with the atrial filling wave but do not open until the onset of right ventricular contraction. LV, left ventricle; PA, pulmonary artery.*

Figure 35–5. *Parasternal short-axis view at the base of the heart. The right ventricular outflow (RV) is imaged in the near field and the pulmonary artery bifurcation (PA) in the far field. The pulmonary artery flow is parallel to the ultrasound beam in this view. The right main pulmonary artery branch passes posterior to the ascending aorta (AO) and is partially imaged in this view.*

from the epicardium in some cases.[25,26] RV trabeculations should not be included in the measurement and cannot be reliably made from the standard apical four-chamber view. The subcostal short-axis view of the heart at the level of the aortic valve is ideal for demonstrating the pulmonic valve and PA and its bifurcation especially if the parasternal views are suboptimal (see Fig. 35–7B). The view is perpendicular to the interatrial septum facilitating the assessment of interatrial shunts. Remnant embryological structures, chiefly of importance in that they may be mistaken for pathology, such as Chiari network and Eustachian valve, may also be seen in this view.

Transesophageal Imaging

The right-sided structures should be systematically assessed in the standard transesophageal study. The initial view of the right ventricle is often the modified four-chamber view, obtained from the midesophagus in the transverse plane (imaging angle 0 degrees). This view of the right ventricle is foreshortened and does not necessarily represent true RV size or function. TR may be seen, but the jet is not parallel to the US beam and velocity measured in this view may be underestimated (Fig. 35–8). In the midesophageal longitudinal plane, (imaging angle 90 degrees) the probe may be rotated to assess the right atrium and superior vena cava (SVC) (Fig. 35–9). Patent foramen

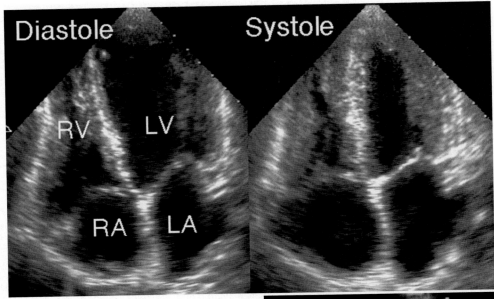

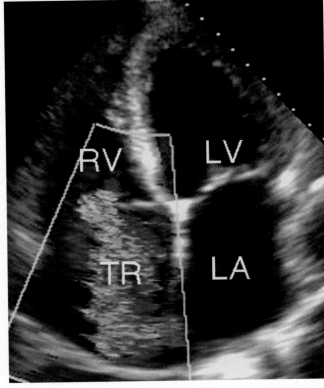

Figure 35–6. A, *Apical four-chamber view in diastole and systole. In diastole, the area of the right ventricle (RV) is less than two thirds of the area of the normal left ventricle (LV). Apical motion of the lateral tricuspid annulus is evident in systole. B, Color-Doppler imaging of the tricuspid regurgitant (TR) jet from the apical four-chamber view in systole in a different patient. The jet has a wide vena contracta, fills more than half of the right atrium, and extends to the back wall. These findings are consistent with moderately severe tricuspid regurgitation. LA, left atrium; RA, right atrium.*

ovale (PFO) are most reliably seen in this view with some rotation of the probe required to bring the junction of the primum and secundum septum into view. The RA appendage, broader based and triangular compared to the left atrial appendage, is seen in the far field in this view. An imaging plane of approximately 120 degrees with further rotation of the transducer will bring the TV into view. The TR jet is best measured in this view although the constraints of esophageal imaging may not allow the maximum ve-

locity to be obtained. An imaging angle of approximately 60 degrees with rotation toward the right will bring the pulmonary valve into view in the far field. These images are often suboptimal given the anterior location of the pulmonary valve and PA. Withdrawal of the transducer to the level of the aortic valve will bring the short axis of the superior vena cava into view. Further withdrawal in some patients allows visualization of the main PA to the right of the screen and the right main branch passing posteriorly to the

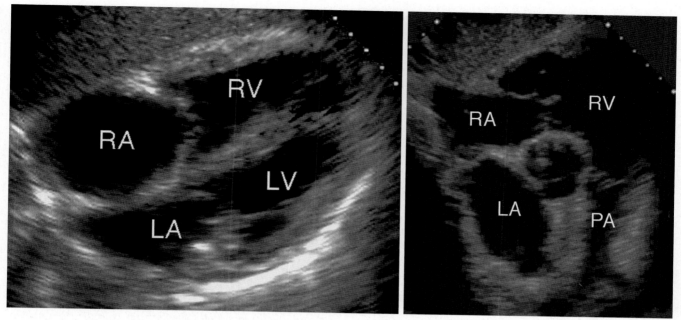

Figure 35-7. A, *Subcostal four-chamber view of the heart in systole. This view is coplanar with the apical four-chamber view. The right ventricular free wall is perpendicular to the ultrasound beam in this view, which is optimal for measurement of right ventricular wall thickness in diastole. B, Subcostal short axis of the heart at the base. The right atrium (RA), right ventricle (RV) and pulmonary artery (PA) are seen to surround the aortic root (unmarked) and the left atrium (LA). The bifurcation of the pulmonary artery is seen in the far field. The subcostal images may "save" the study if the other views are suboptimal. LV, left ventricle.*

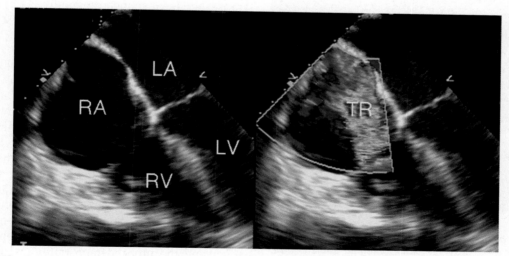

Figure 35-8. *Transesophageal echocardiographic modified four-chamber view in the mid-esophagus in the transverse plane (imaging angle is 0 degrees). The systolic view on the left demonstrates right atrial enlargement. Color-Doppler imaging shows a large jet of tricuspid regurgitation. The direction of the jet is nearly perpendicular to the ultrasound beam in this view and adequate assessment of tricuspid regurgitant jet velocity and pulmonary artery pressure is not possible. LA, left atrium; LV, left ventricle; RA, right atrium; RV, right ventricle.*

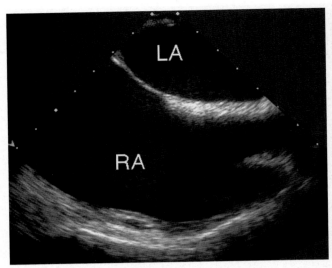

Figure 35–9. Transesophageal echocardiographic bicaval view of the interatrial septum from the mid-esophagus in the longitudinal plane (imaging angle is 90 degrees). The superior vena cava enters the right atrium (RA) to the right of the image and the broad based right atrial appendage is seen in the far field to the right below the junction of the superior vena cava. LA, left atrium.

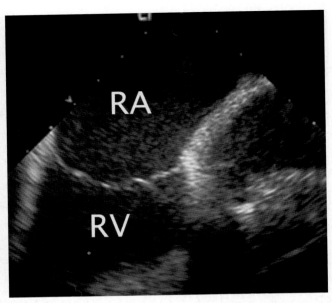

Figure 35–11. Intracardiac echocardiographic view of the tricuspid valve in systole. The catheter is in the right atrium and directed toward the right ventricle (RV). The tricuspid valve is closed in this systolic frame. The aortic root is imaged to the right of the screen.

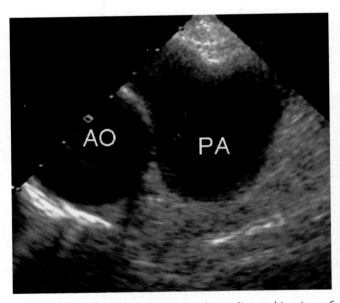

Figure 35–10. Transesophageal echocardiographic view of the pulmonary artery (PA) bifurcation from the high esophageal position in the transverse plane (imaging angle is 0 degrees). The main PA, to the right of the ascending aorta in this image is significantly enlarged. The right main branch of the PA passes posteriorly to the ascending aorta (AO). The proximal left branch is seen in the near field to the right of the screen.

aorta (Fig. 35–10). It is not possible to obtain reliable views of the left PA in most patients, although the actual bifurcation may be seen. In many patients, the carina passes between the esophagus and the great vessels, obscuring the high esophageal views. Trans-

gastric imaging provides a view similar to the short-axis transthoracic view although the inferior structures are portrayed at the top of the screen in the transesophageal echocardiography (TEE) views.

Intracardiac Imaging

Intracardiac echocardiography is usually performed with the transducer in the right atrium, having been introduced into the femoral vein and advanced through the IVC to the right atrium under fluoroscopy. The "home view" demonstrates the anterior and septal leaflets of the TV with the right ventricle in the far field[27] (Fig. 35–11). Clockwise rotation of the transducer brings the interatrial septum into view (Fig. 35–12). Posterior angulation of the transducer (achieved with the separate controls, which allow posteroanterior and right to left motion of the transducer tip) may be necessary for complete visualization of the septum. Further advancing the probe demonstrates the superior vena cava. Rotation at this level allows visualization of the RA appendage and the crista terminalis at the superior vena cava-RA junction.

In experienced hands, the probe may be advanced into the RV and the outflow tract to allow imaging of the left-sided structures and the infundibulum and pulmonary valve. The stiff catheter may provoke significant ventricular ectopy and right bundle branch block (RBBB). Perforation is also possible but has not been reported.

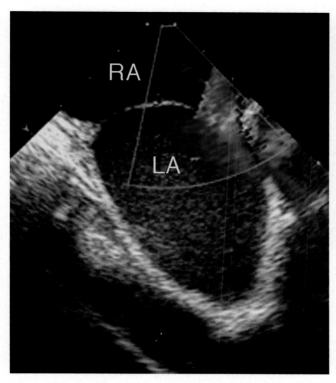

Figure 35-12. Intracardiac echocardiographic view of the interatrial septum. Clockwise rotation of the transducer from the "home view" with posterior angulation of the transducer within the right atrium (RA) allows assessment of the interatrial septum. There is a secundum atrial septal defect and color Doppler demonstrates a significant left to right shunt across the defect. LA, left atrium.

Doppler Assessment

Pulmonary Artery Outflow

The spectral envelope of the PA outflow is characteristically symmetric with a peak velocity of less than 0.8 m/s in adults.[28] An increase in velocity in the PA in the absence of pulmonary valve stenosis may occur with increased flow. High CO states, including pregnancy, anemia, and hepatic cirrhosis, may result in velocities that exceed 1.2 m/s but rarely significantly higher. In the absence of these conditions or pulmonary stenosis, an elevated PA velocity should precipitate the search for an intracardiac left-to-right shunt as the cause of the increased flow.

In the setting of PH, pulmonic valve opening is delayed as the right ventricle generates a higher pressure to open the valve. The acceleration time of the spectral envelope is decreased (Fig. 35–13) and correlates with the increase in PA pressure.[29] An acceleration time of less than 80 msec predicts an elevated mean pulmonary pressure greater than 20 mm Hg.[30] The acceleration time may also be indexed to the ejection time to correct for changes in heart rate.[31] However, these mea-

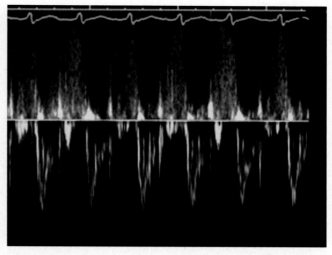

Figure 35-13. Pulsed-wave Doppler spectral display from the parasternal long-axis view of the pulmonary valve. Pulmonary outflow is seen below the baseline during systole. The acceleration time (from initiation of flow to peak velocity) is short, consistent with significant pulmonary hypertension.

surements are not routinely used in clinical studies as a result of their low sensitivity relative to changes in pulmonary vascular resistance (PVR).[32,33]

The cross-sectional area (CSA) of the pulmonary arterial system increases with the distance from the valve. This is in contradistinction to the systemic arterial circulation, a long tube with side branches. The normal pulmonary circulation operates as an open-ended reflector causing the reflected waves to be negative (or expansion) waves, further promoting forward flow of the ejected blood.[34] However, chronic PH causes stiffening of the pulmonary vessels and results in the reflected waves augmenting the pulmonary pressure similar to reflected waves within the aorta. The reflected wave occurs before valve closure, resulting in a premature partial closing of the valve and characteristic notching of the spectral envelope[35,36] (Fig. 35–14). The timing of the notch in the spectral Doppler envelope correlates with the M-mode timing of the notching of systolic motion of the pulmonary valve.

Measurement of Pulmonary Artery Pressure

During systole, the RV peak systolic pressure is equal to the peak pulmonary artery systolic pressure (PASP). This is readily calculated by applying the modified Bernoulli equation to the peak velocity of the TR jet.[37] Specifically,

$$PASP = 4v_{TR}^2 + RAP$$

in which *PASP* is the peak pulmonary artery systolic pressure (presumed to be equal to the RV peak systolic pressure), v_{TR} is the peak velocity of the TR jet

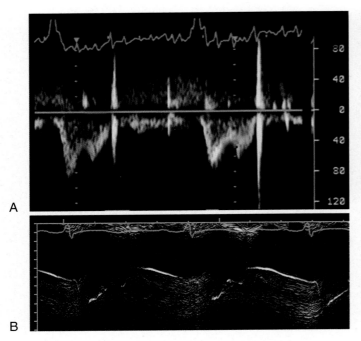

A

B

Figure 35–14. A, *Pulsed-wave Doppler from the parasternal long axis view of the pulmonary valve in a patient with severe pulmonary hypertension. The spectral envelope demonstrates systolic notching. B, M-mode of the pulmonary valve in the same patient. There is a loss of the normal A wave of the valve with atrial systole. There is partial closure of the valve in mid-systole (the "flying W" sign), which corresponds with the timing of systolic notching of the spectral Doppler envelope.*

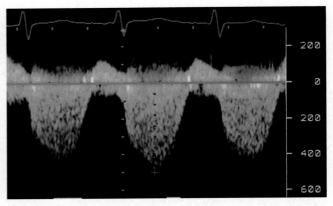

Figure 35–15. *Spectral display of continuous-wave Doppler from the apical four-chamber view across the tricuspid valve. The spectral envelope of the tricuspid regurgitant jet is seen in systole below the baseline. The peak velocity of the jet is 4.2 m/s, which predicts the systolic gradient between the right ventricle and right atrium is 71 mm Hg. The peak pulmonary artery pressure is 71 mm Hg plus the estimated right atrium pressure.*

obtained by continuous-wave Doppler, and *RAP* is the RA pressure (Fig. 35–15). When performed properly, this highly reproducible technique correlates closely with invasively derived PASP.[30,37-40] It is imperative to initially image the tricuspid regurgitant jet with color Doppler to align the continuous-wave US beam parallel to the regurgitant signal. Continuous-wave interrogation of the TR jet should be carried out in the RV inflow view, the short axis at the base, the apical four-chamber view, and the subcostal view. The highest velocity obtained should be used to calculate the peak RV systolic pressure. If pulmonic stenosis is present, the gradient across the pulmonic valve must be subtracted from the peak RV systolic pressure to obtain the peak PA pressure. In a technically limited study, agitated saline can be injected intravenously (IV) to enhance the TR jet signal and improve the measurement of the maximum TR jet velocity.[41]

The RA pressure can be measured directly by central line, but several methods have been described to assess RA pressure.[42] The scheme most commonly used in clinical practice assesses the diameter of the IVC while the patient performs a "sniff" (Fig. 35–16). Normally, the IVC collapses as the intrathoracic pressure de-

creases. However, with RA hypertension, IVC collapse is often less complete. To summarize:

IVC	RA Pressure (mm Hg)
Full collapse	5
>50% of initial diameter	10
<50% of initial diameter	15
No collapse	20

Positive pressure ventilation may abolish IVC collapse making this method unreliable in intubated patients.[43] If the IVC is poorly visualized and the RA size is normal, it can be assumed that the RA pressure is normal and 5 mm Hg should be used. Underestimation of the peak pressure will occur if the RA pressure is underestimated. This is of particular importance in the setting of "torrential" TR, in which RA pressure may exceed 20 mm Hg by a considerable amount, leading to an underestimate of PA pressure if 20 mm Hg is the maximum value used. Likewise, overestimation of PA pressure can occur as a result of an inappropriate right atrial pressure being added to the right ventricle-RA gradient. However, inaccurate measurement of a poorly seen spectral envelope may also lead to the inadvertent reporting of erroneous measurement.

It should be noted that newer hand held machines may not have the same Doppler capabilities as the standard machines and may miss significant PH.[44] This is of concern especially if the handheld systems are used by less experienced operators in intensive care unit (ICU) settings.

Pulmonary diastolic pressure may be measured by applying the modified Bernoulli equation to the pulmonary regurgitant jet velocity. The pulmonary regur-

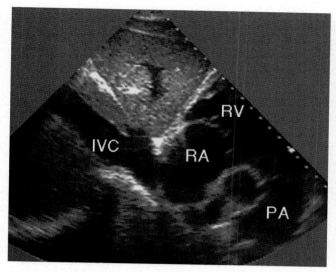

Figure 35–16. *Subcostal image of the inferior vena cava (IVC) as it enters the right atrium. With the transducer in this location, the patient is asked to sniff while the diameter of the IVC is monitored. PA, pulmonary artery; RA, right atrium; RV, right ventricle.*

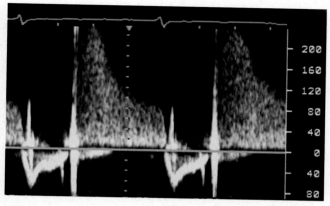

Figure 35–17. *Pulsed-wave Doppler of the pulmonary regurgitant jet from the parasternal short axis at the base. The velocity of the pulmonary regurgitant jet at end-diastole is 0.8 m/s, which is consistent with a normal pulmonary artery diastolic pressure.*

gitant jet velocity at end-diastole is used to estimate PA diastolic pressure (Fig. 35–17). The estimated RA pressure, assumed to be constant throughout the cardiac cycle, is added to the end-diastolic pulmonary regurgitant pressure gradient.[45] More controversial is the measurement of mean PA pressure, which has been shown to correlate with the early diastolic PR gradient.[46] However, the addition of estimated RA pressure to this value may worsen the correlation with invasively derived measurements.[47]

An alternate method to measure PA diastolic pressure is to measure the velocity of the TR jet velocity at the time of pulmonary valve opening. TR begins with isovolumic contraction, but the pulmonary valve does not open until RV pressure exceeds PA pressure. The TR jet velocity at this point in time can be used to calculate the PA diastolic pressure. Pulmonary valve opening is timed by measuring the interval between the beginning of the QRS to the onset of pulmonary systolic flow.[47,48]

Pulmonary Vascular Resistance

PVR is typically derived at right-sided heart catheterization and is equal to the transpulmonary gradient divided by the pulmonary flow Several authors have shown that the peak TR jet velocity divided by the velocity time integral (VTI) of the RVOT outflow spectral Doppler envelope is proportional to pulmonary resistance. Correlation with invasively measured pulmonary

resistance has shown that the resistance can be calculated from Doppler parameters using the equation:

$$PVR \text{ (Wood units)} = 10 \times TRV/VTI_{RVOT}$$

in which *TRV* is the peak TR velocity measured from the continuous-wave Doppler and *VTI*$_{RVOT}$ is the velocity time integral of the pulsed-wave Doppler spectral envelope in the *RVOT*. A *TRV/VTI*$_{RVOT}$ ratio of less than 0.2 is consistent with normal PVR.[49] Other groups have described methods for calculating pulmonary compliance and impedance noninvasively, but these parameters are not in standard clinical use.[50,51]

Quantitative Measurements

Right Ventricular Volume

The irregular shape of the RV cavity makes direct measurement of RV volume with two-dimensional echocardiography difficult. Much of the early work was based on comparison to angiographic models of RV geometry. The advent of magnetic resonance imaging (MRI) has rendered angiographic assessment obsolete and created a new gold standard for RV volume assessment. Simpson's rule has been applied to the right ventricle, but a true biplane Simpson's requires two orthogonal views with a common long axis. The apical four-chamber view is usually easily obtained. However, the subcostal four-chamber view, which is often used as the second view, is actually coplanar and not orthogonal to the apical view. Levine and colleagues demonstrated that RV volume could be approximated by the formula:

$$RV \text{ volume} = \tfrac{2}{3}A_1 \times L_2$$

in which A_1 is the area planimetered from the apical four-chamber view, and L is the length from the subcostal RVOT view.[52] This approach has the advantage of simplicity and takes the infundibulum into account in calculating the volume. Recently application of three-dimensional (3D) echocardiography to the right ventricle has yielded excellent correlation with in vitro models and magnetic resonance imaging volumes of the right ventricle.[53-55]

Right Ventricular Function

Most commonly, as with LV function, RV systolic function is assessed visually by the interpreting physician. However, the asymmetry of the RV contraction, its propensity to a more spherical geometry in response to overload, and the variable contribution of the infundibulum and septum to RV function make visual assessment fairly unreliable. Moreover, as mentioned previously, the right ventricle has a distinct pattern of contraction (longitudinal > transverse) as compared to the left ventricle, making simple visual assessment of RV free wall motion an incomplete surrogate for RV systolic function.

Volumetric assessments may be applied to systole and diastole to calculate RV EF. The simplicity of the area-length method makes it an attractive candidate for EF calculations[56]; however, the limitations inherent to the geometric assumptions of these methods have limited their application in clinical practice. Given the dramatic improvements in three-dimensional imaging, direct measurement of RV volume will no doubt replace previous two-dimensional methods for assessment of RV EF.[54] Currently however, three-dimensional estimates require offline analysis and remain cumbersome for the clinical laboratory.

Fractional area change ([RV end-diastolic area − RV end-systolic area/RV end-diastolic area] × 100), obtained in the apical four-chamber view, is an attractive alternative method for RV systolic function assessment because it does not require geometric assumptions and correlates well with RV EF.[57] However, measurement is often hampered by suboptimal endocardial definition and often high interobserver and intraobserver variability.

An alternative method involves measuring tricuspid annular plane systolic excursion (TAPSE). An M-mode cursor is placed through the lateral tricuspid annulus in the apical four-chamber view, and the absolute systolic displacement of the lateral tricuspid annulus is measured as the cardiac base contracts toward the apex[58] (Fig. 35–18). The advantages of TAPSE are that it is easy to perform, is highly reproducible, and correlates closely with RV EF and RV fractional area change in a variety of patient populations.[18,58-60] Moreover TAPSE does not require endocardial definition or geometric assumptions to quantify RV systolic function. The normal range for TAPSE has not been formally established,

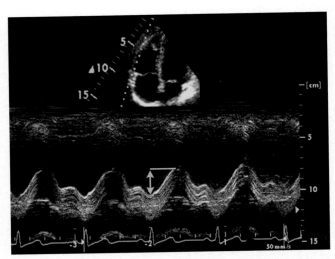

Figure 35–18. *M-mode of the lateral tricuspid annular plane systolic excursion (TAPSE). The maximum excursion from diastole to systole is measured in this frame. The TAPSE is 2.5 cm consistent with normal right ventricular systolic function.*

however, the average TAPSE for healthy subjects from several small studies is 2.5±0.5 cm,[61,62] with lesser values likely indicating mild (2 to 2.4 cm), moderate (1.5 to 1.9 cm) and severely (<1.5 cm) reduced RV function.[59,60]

Tissue Doppler imaging (TDI) can measure the velocity of the myocardium throughout the cardiac cycle. The RV free wall is most easily measured from the apical four-chamber view. The RV free wall has a higher systolic velocity in the longitudinal direction than the LV free wall. The systolic velocity correlates with TAPSE measurements and may be used to assess RV systolic function.[63] Others have applied myocardial strain (measure of deformation) and strain rate (rate of deformation) imaging to quantify LV systolic function.[64] However, their application to RV function is problematic because the RV free wall is too thin to allow for assessment of radial strain. Therefore, assessment has been thus far limited to longitudinal strain measured from the apical four-chamber view. Clinical application has been primarily in patients with congenital heart disease (CHD), particularly those with systemic right ventricles.[65,66] Proper acquisition is contingent on parallel alignment of the US beam with the RV free wall, which may require off-axis imaging with medial positioning of the transducer to bring the beam parallel to the RV free wall. Septal strain rate is influenced by both LV and RV function and may not be as useful as free wall assessments. Normal values have been established in children. In general the systolic strain in the midwall of the right ventricle is higher than either the basal or apical segments, and the right ventricle demonstrates higher strain and strain rates compared to the left ventricle.[67]

Similarly, the myocardial performance index (MPI; Tei index) has also been applied to RV function, which

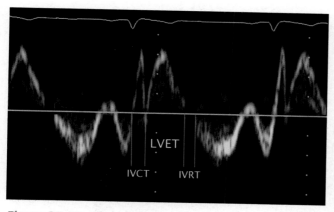

Figure 35–19. Tissue Doppler signal recorded from the right ventricular free wall. The components of the myocardial performance index (see text) are marked. IVCT, isovolumic contraction time; IVRT, isovolumic relaxation time; LVET, left ventricular ejection time.

is an integrative measure of both systolic and diastolic function, derived using the formula:

$$IVRT + IVCT/RVET$$

in which *IVRT* is the RV isovolumic relaxation time, *IVCT* is the isovolumic contraction time, and *RVET* is the RV ejection time. For the left ventricle, pulsed-wave Doppler can be used to measure the intervals because it is possible to position the sample volume to record both left ventricular outflow tract (LVOT) outflow and mitral inflow from a single location. However, this is not possible in the right ventricle, where the outflow tract is relatively distant and nonplanar with the tricuspid inflow. Therefore, tissue Doppler signals are typically used to measure the intervals (Fig. 35–19). Increasing values represent worsening function. In children, a mean value with normal RV function was 0.24.[68] The index has been applied to congenital heart disease and evaluation of systemic right ventricles[69-71] and in adults with pulmonary arterial hypertension (PAH; vida infra). MPI has also been used to identify patients with early RV dysfunction resulting from cardiac amyloidosis. In this study, nonsimultaneous recordings of PA outflow and TV inflow were used. The RV MPI in normal adult subjects was 0.28.[72] There is some concern that RV hypertrophy may shorten the IVRT leading to a paradoxically low MPI in the abnormal right ventricle with hypertrophy.[73] Moreover the derivation of the RV MPI is somewhat cumbersome, which has limited the applicability of this technique in clinical practice.

Pathophysiologic Response of the Right Ventricle

Pathophysiologically, RV dysfunction is classically divided into three categories: volume overload, pressure overload, and primary or inherent RV systolic dysfunc-

tion. As a result of its thin-walled and distensible design, the right ventricle is especially subject to changes in geometry when any one of these insults occur, and RV dysfunction typically manifests as a triad of RV dilatation (remodeling), right ventricle to left ventricle disproportion (with right to left septal shifting), with variable changes in RV systolic function.

Although lacking a reliable and clinically accessible gold standard for RV function, the integration of these stereotypical echocardiographic findings often provide a rationale basis for determining the cause of the underlying process. In addition, the treating physicians can be alerted to investigate relevant causes of dysfunction.

Volume Overload

In contrast to high-afterload states, isolated volume overload is better tolerated by the right ventricle. The most common causes of volume overload include TR or pulmonic regurgitation and congenital left-to-right shunt, such as atrial septal defect (ASD) or anomalous pulmonary drainage. Importantly, both TR and pulmonic regurgitation commonly occur secondary to PAH, in effect superimposing a volume load on a pressure-overloaded ventricle. Two-dimensional imaging of the valve is imperative, with findings, such as myxomatous degeneration, valve prolapse and dysplastic valve anatomy, identifying a primary valvular process. Regurgitation in the setting of a structurally normal valve suggests secondary dysfunction. In the later stages of large left-to-right cardiac shunts, severe pulmonary vascular disease can result, in which case the right-sided echocardiographic findings may be indistinguishable from other causes of pressure overload.

The hallmark of volume overload is RV, and often RA, dilatation. Naturally, there are limits imposed on the degree to which the right ventricle can dilate, largely dictated by pericardial constraint. Once the right-sided heart has dilated enough to occupy the potential pericardial space, any further increments in right-sided heart volume lead to reciprocal reductions in left-sided heart volumes, known as diastolic ventricular interdependence.[74] Echocardiographically, this manifests as interventricular (and interatrial) septal shifting from right to left, reduced septal to free wall LV dimensions, often with Doppler evidence of impaired early filling and diastolic function of the left ventricle[75-77] (Fig. 35–20). These findings, coupled with normal, or mildly elevated PA pressure by Doppler assessment implicate volume overload as the primary underlying process. An increase in the ratio of RV to LV end-diastolic area (or dimension) to greater than 1.5 indicates severe RV dilatation. In the early stages of volume overload, increased RV preload leads to increased RV systolic performance through increased sarcomere recruitment via the Frank-Starling mechanism. Thus the classic echocardiographic feature of a purely volume overloaded right ventricle is a dilated, hypercontractile right ventricle.[78] Over time, severe RV volume overload

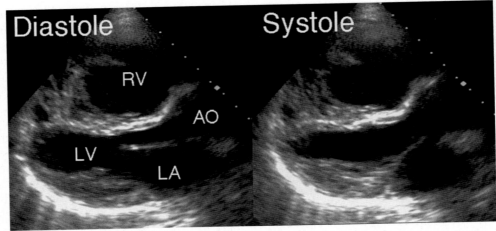

Figure 35–20. *Parasternal long-axis view in diastole and systole in a patient with severe right ventricular volume overload. The right ventricle (RV) is severely dilated. The septum deviates into the left ventricular cavity in diastole. In systole, there is paradoxical septal motion as the septum moves anteriorly toward the right ventricular free wall. Left ventricular function is impaired, but the interventricular septal motion aids in right ventricular ejection. AO, aorta; LA, left atrium; LV, left ventricle.*

may lead to RV systolic dysfunction, with the nearly invariable development of secondary TV regurgitation.

Isolated RV volume overload also leads to right-to-left interventricular septal flattening, imparting a D-shape to the left ventricle in diastole or frank bowing of the septum into the left ventricle in diastole.[79] The altered septal position leads to decreased left-sided heart filling, with decreased diastolic filling of the left ventricle resulting in a drop in LV SV and stroke work.[80] Conversely, in systole, the septum moves from left to right (paradoxical septal motion), restoring normal septal curvature and contributing to RV SV generation.[81] Paradoxical septal motion can be confused with dyskinetic anteroseptal wall motion resulting from ischemic heart disease. Attention to diastolic septal position and systolic thickening of the septal wall despite the overall motion will reliably distinguish these two processes and point toward RV volume overload as the primary hemodynamic disturbance.

Pressure Overload

The term *pressure overload* is used to encompass a variety of disease states that impose an increased afterload on the right ventricle, leading to RV dysfunction. PA pressure is often used synonymously with RV afterload, but strictly speaking this is incorrect and deserves clarification. PA pressure is the force that results from the interaction of pulmonary blood flow and the resistance and capacitive components of the pulmonary arterial circulation. It is the combination of PVR and proximal pulmonary arterial stiffness (which dictates the degree and timing of arterial wave reflection) that oppose ventricular ejection and comprise afterload. In many cases, RV pressure and RV afterload are collinear, which explains why the terms *pressure* and *afterload* have been used interchangeably. However, in a patient with a left-to-right shunt, such as an atrial septal de-

fect, pulmonary pressures may be significantly elevated as a result of a marked excess of pulmonary blood flow. In these patients, afterload is not increased despite the presence of PH because there is little to no opposition to ventricular ejection. Similarly, in a patient with a proximal pulmonary embolus, the estimated RV systolic pressure may be normal despite a massive increase in RV afterload with severe RV dysfunction.

The SV of the right ventricle, like the left ventricle, varies inversely with a rise in afterload. An increase in afterload will lead to decreased SV and increased end-systolic and end-diastolic volumes. As with volume overload, the right ventricle will dilate and assume a more spherical configuration. The consequent increase in chamber dimensions, along with increased intracavitary pressure leads to marked increases in RV wall tension, which the relatively nonmuscular right ventricle cannot overcome, and RV failure may ensue. The degree to which the right ventricle can tolerate an increase in afterload varies in direct proportion to baseline RV systolic function. In a patient with compromised RV function, a rise in RV afterload can be devastating. The rate at which the afterload stress is imposed is critically important. The more rapid the onset, the greater the impact is on RV function.[82,83] If the increase in afterload is chronic and progressive, RV remodeling allows the right ventricle to generate near-systemic, or at times, supra-systemic PA pressures.[84] The presence of RV hypertrophy, which is characterized by increased RV wall thickness (>5 mm; >10 mm when severe), marked intracavitary trabeculations, and thickening and prominence of the moderator band provides an important clue to longstanding RV pressure overload (Fig. 35–21). Interventricular septal motion also provides a clue to increased RV afterload; in this setting, the interventricular septum will often flatten or bow into the left ventricle during systole and will return to its normal configuration during diastole (Fig. 35–22). The degree of septal shift depends in part on the

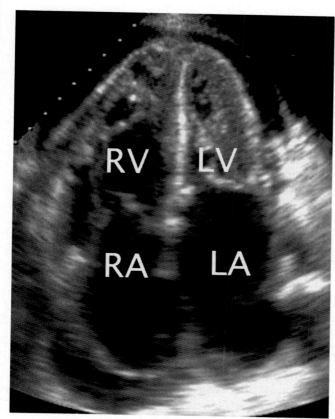

Figure 35–21. *Apical four-chamber view in a patient with severe pulmonary hypertension secondary to rheumatic mitral stenosis. Note the right ventricular enlargement and the trabeculations most prominent at the apex. The moderate band is also hypertrophied. Both atria are severely enlarged. The left ventricular cavity is small as a result of the mitral stenosis, but the left ventricular hypertrophy is a result of severe aortic stenosis, which is not shown in this image. LA, left atrium; LV, left ventricle; RA, right atrium; RV, right ventricle.*

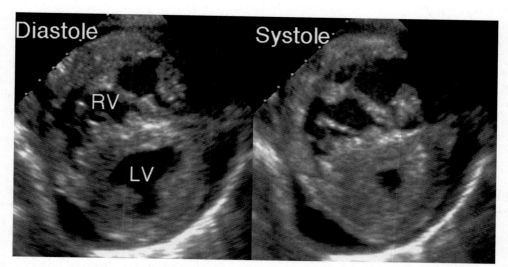

Figure 35–22. *Parasternal short axis at the level of the papillary muscles in diastole and systole. Severe right ventricular hypertrophy is demonstrated. The interventricular septum has a relatively normal configuration in diastole but flattens in systole ("D" sign). The right ventricular systolic pressures exceed left ventricular systolic pressures in this patient with severe pulmonary hypertension. In addition, there is a moderate pericardial effusion, which is a poor prognostic sign in pulmonary hypertension. LV, left ventricle; RV, right ventricle.*

relative distensibility of the interventricular septum. Septal hypertrophy attenuates septal shift and diastolic ventricular interaction in acute experimental models of RV pressure overload.[85,86] With further decompensation, typically characterized by the onset of TV regurgitation, there is an additional volume load imposed on the right ventricle, and the interventricular septum remains flat-tened or bowed into the left ventricle during systole and diastole. CS dilatation may also be seen in pressure overload. The CS is usually not visible in the parasternal long-axis view. In the absence of a persistent left superior vena cava, a dilated CS correlates with elevated RA pressure and RA size but not to the absolute level of PASP or to the presence of TR.[87]

Primary Right Ventricular Dysfunction

Primary RV dysfunction refers to impaired systolic function of the right ventricle that is load independent. The two most commonly encountered causes of primary RV dysfunction are acute RV ischemia and arrhythmogenic right ventricular dysplasia (ARVD). Acute RV ischemia almost invariably occurs in the setting of an acute inferior wall myocardial infarction (MI), typically when a coronary artery occlusion occurs proximal to the artery supplying the RV free wall. Thus echocardiographic examination often reveals severe RV systolic dysfunction often in conjunction with an inferior wall motion abnormality of the left ventricle.[5,88] MPI of the RV free wall has also been used to distinguish patients with RV infarction complicating an inferior myocardial infarction. An MPI greater than 0.7 was used as the cutoff value in one study of 60 patients.[89] ARVD is a rare condition, most typically occurring in young otherwise healthy patients who are diagnosed with a history of syncope and ventricular arrhythmias.[90] Echocardiographically, the right ventricle is often significantly dilated, with disproportion of right-sided to left-sided heart structures. Excessive endocardial trabeculations and a thickened and highly echogenic moderator band provide important clues to ARVD, at times with localized areas of akinesis or dyskinesis and aneurysms. Dilatation of the RVOT has been shown to be a distinguishing feature of ARVD.[91] There is often severe RV systolic dysfunction, with reductions in RV EF, RV fractional area change, and reduced tricuspid annular plane systolic excursion having been reported in these patients.[92] Importantly, in both ARVD and acute RV ischemia, PH is typically absent because inherent RV dysfunction often precludes generation high PA pressures.[5,90,93]

The Right-Sided Heart in Pulmonary Disease

Acute and chronic respiratory diseases can affect right-sided heart structure and function, a condition often referred to as cor pulmonale. Both pulmonary parenchymal and vascular diseases can lead to a reduction in the total pulmonary vascular surface area, which increases afterload. The degree of pulmonary vascular remodeling is typically far more severe in primary vascular disorders, resulting in much greater degrees of PH. An additional mechanism of increased PVR is hypoxic pulmonary vasoconstriction. Hypoxemia may, of course, occur with either entity.

Whatever the cause of the afterload stress, as discussed previously, RV dysfunction will typically manifest as a triad of RV systolic dysfunction, RV dilatation, and right ventricle to left ventricle disproportion. The tempo with which the afterload is imposed is critically important, relating to how conditioned the right ventricle is to accommodate such increases in load. As such, acute and chronic respiratory diseases often leave a distinct echocardiographic signature that can provide essential clues to the timing, severity, and nature of the underlying process (Table 35–1).

Acute Disease

Acute Pulmonary Embolism

Acute pulmonary embolism (PE) is the prototype for acute cor pulmonale. Acute obstruction of the pulmonary vasculature may lead to acute right-sided heart failure, and at times, total cardiovascular collapse. Obstruction of greater than 25% to 30% of the vascular bed is usually necessary to produce echocardiographic

TABLE 35–1. Echocardiographic Findings in Acute and Chronic Pulmonary Disease

	Acute	Chronic
RV enlargement	Yes—may demonstrate apical sharing	Yes—may demonstrate apical sharing
RVH	Absent	Present—moderator band may also show hypertrophy
TR	Present as a result of annular dilatation	Present as a result of annular dilatation
PR	Mild or less	Frequently moderate or severe
PHTN	Mean PA pressure <40 mm Hg	PASP may be suprasystemic
RV hypokinesis	May be severe Relative preservation of apical motion	RV dysfunction late finding
Septal shift	Present	Present but may be severe
PA dilation	Uncommon	Frequently present

PA, pulmonary artery; PASP, pulmonary artery systolic pressure; PHTN, pulmonary hypertension; RV, right ventricular; RVH, right ventricular hypertrophy; TR, tricuspid regurgitation.

findings. The severity of right-sided heart dysfunction is directly proportional to the degree of obstruction.[94,95] Thus a small subsegmental pulmonary embolus will typically not produce echocardiographic abnormalities. It is important to remember that a normal echocardiogram in the setting of a clinically suspected pulmonary embolus in no way rules out a PE, and further investigation is warranted.

RV dilatation is perhaps the most consistent echocardiographic finding in the setting of a large PE, relating to the natural tendency of the distensible right ventricle to dilate in response to a sudden increase in afterload.[96,97] Right-to-left septal shifting, often in both systole and diastole, may occur, compromising LV filling.[98] Thus there are limits to the efficacy of aggressive volume resuscitation in the setting of a massive PE with RV dysfunction because further RV distention via volume expansion may exacerbate ventricular interdependence, compromising LV filling and further decreasing CO.[99,100] Thus in the management of such patients, echocardiography is critical to document the relative position of the interventricular septum and the degree of right-sided to left-sided heart disproportion, which may help set limits on further volume resuscitation.

RV hypokinesis is also common in the setting of acute PE. The classic pattern of RV dysfunction in the setting of an acute PE includes mild to moderate hypokinesis of the basal and mid segments of the RV free wall, whereas the RV apex is "spared"—often referred to as the "McConnell" sign.[101] Visually, this is appreciated as hypokinesis from the base to the distal RV free wall, with a "buckling," or hinge point near the RV apex (Fig. 35–23). This contraction pattern is highly specific for a large pulmonary embolus. The mechanism may be the effect of the normally contracting LV apex on RV apical motion. A small series of regional strain analysis in acute pulmonary embolism has demonstrated midwall dysfunction with preserved basal and apical strain patterns.[102] Others have shown that the RV EF, tricuspid annular tissue Doppler velocity (longitudinal plane), and TAPSE are reduced in the setting of an acute PE.[103] RA hypertension is usually present. Subcostal imaging will demonstrate a dilated and noncollapsible IVC often accompanied by dilated hepatic veins.

The degree of PH is quite variable, again, depending on the ability of the right ventricle to maintain SV in the face of the vascular obstruction. In a previously healthy patient suffering from a large acute PE, it is uncommon for the right ventricle to generate a mean PA pressure greater than 40 mm Hg; thus a massive PE (30% to 40% vascular obstruction) can result in RV failure and cardiogenic shock with mean PA pressures of just 20 to 40 mm Hg.[98] The spectral envelope of the continuous-wave Doppler may also suggest systolic failure (Fig. 35–24). Conversely, patients with preexisting cardiopulmonary disease are able to generate higher pulmonary pressures acutely and may do so at a lesser degree of pulmonary vascular obstruction.[104] This is illustrated by the finding that the average transtricuspid flow velocity was significantly lower in patients with acute massive PE than in patients with subacute massive PE (3.0±0.4 m/s versus 4.2±0.6 m/s).[97] Increased PA impedance as a result of PE can also be inferred by Doppler examination because a shortened PA acceleration time (<60 to 100 ms), particularly in the presence of an RV systolic pressure less

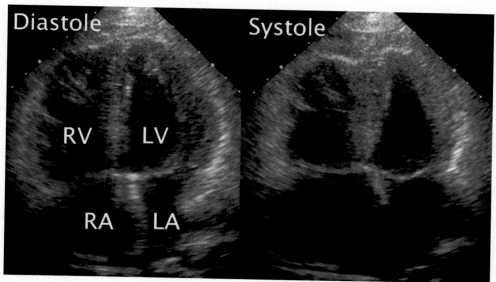

Figure 35–23. *Apical four-chamber view in diastole and systole in a patient with acute and massive pulmonary embolism. The right ventricle (RV) is severely diastolic image demonstrates severe dilatation. The interatrial septum deviates to the left consistent with right atrial hypertension. In systole, the RV does not appear to contract. However, there is motion at the right ventricular apex. This is a demonstration of "McConnell's sign" and should raise the suspicion of acute pulmonary embolism. LA, left atrium; LV, left ventricle; RA, right atrium.*

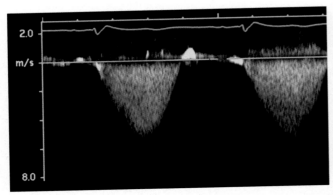

Figure 35-24. Spectral display of continuous-wave Doppler across the tricuspid valve in a patient with severe pulmonary hypertension and right ventricular systolic failure. The peak velocity is approximately 5 m/s, which predicts a pulmonary artery systolic pressure (PASP) of greater than 100 mm Hg. The tricuspid regurgitant jet velocity rises slowly, which demonstrates a decreased ability of the right ventricle to develop the necessary ejection pressure. The velocity falls off rapidly after the peak velocity is achieved. This pattern should raise the suspicion of right ventricular systolic failure.

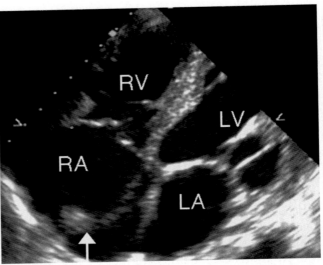

Figure 35-25. Off-axis four-chamber view. The right atrium (RA) and right ventricle (RV) are dilated. There is a mass in the RA (arrow), which represents a venous cast in transit. This cylindrical mass was highly mobile with the RA. There is right atrial hypertension as demonstrated by the shift of the interatrial septum to the left. The patient had already sustained a pulmonary embolism but was at risk for another and probably lethal event. The patient was taken to the operating room immediately after these images were obtained. LA, left atrium; LV, left ventricle.

than 60 mm Hg has been shown to be a specific indicator for acute PE.[105] These findings underscore the limitations of considering PA pressure and afterload as synonymous. In the setting of an acute massive PE, afterload may be critically increased, yet PASP is normal or only mildly increased. Thus it cannot be overemphasized that it is not the absolute magnitude of the rise in afterload but the relative impact of the afterload on ventricular function that dictates its hemodynamic significance. In the appropriate clinical setting, a dilated, hypokinetic right ventricle should dramatically increase the suspicion for an acute PE, regardless of the pulmonary pressures estimated by Doppler examination.

Right-sided heart thrombi or thrombi-in-transit occurred in 4% of 1135 patients with PE in the International Cooperative Pulmonary Embolism Registry[106] (Fig. 35-25). Thrombi may be visualized within the right atrium, ventricle, and occasionally, are seen straddling the interatrial septum. Characteristically, thrombi are highly mobile and change shape dynamically between systole (elongated) and diastole (spherical). Their presence is clearly a marker of high risk because these patients typically have suffered a massive PE and more often manifest overt RV dysfunction, greater hemodynamic compromise, and have a worse prognosis.[106] Although the optimal management strategy for these patients has not been established through large-scale prospective trials, the weight of the evidence suggests that in this setting, patients treated with heparin alone do poorly and that more aggressive therapy is indicated, such as thrombolysis or acute surgical or catheter-mediated intervention.[106,107]

The main PA and its bifurcation are well visualized by TEE. TEE has been shown to have comparable sensitivity (80% to 97%) and specificity (86% to 100%) as spiral computed tomography (CT) scan for the detection of central pulmonary emboli. Thus TEE may play a role in the diagnosis of central pulmonary emboli, perhaps best applied in the setting of clinical instability, in which bedside assessment and monitoring by TEE may be preferred over transporting the patient out of the intensive care unit (ICU) for spiral computed tomography examination. However, TEE may be problematic in the hypoxic but nonventilated patient, although no complications were reported in a series of 113 patients with acute PE undergoing TEE.

The primary value of echocardiography in acute PE is in the risk assessment of the individual patient. Echocardiographic evidence of RV hypokinesis predicts a twofold increase in mortality at 2 weeks and 3 months.[108-111] Even in hemodynamically stable patients, identification of RV dysfunction by echocardiography is an indication for thrombolytic therapy.[112] Echocardiography should be rapidly performed in every patient in whom the diagnosis of acute PE is made.[113] Likewise, patients with severe RV dysfunction in whom thrombolysis is contraindicated or those with severe RV dysfunction and shock may require more aggressive surgical or catheter-based therapies.[114,115] In addition, significant PH at the time of diagnosis (RV systolic pressure >50 mm Hg) predicts the presence of chronic thromboembolic PH at 1 year, and thus these patients should be referred to a PH center for monitoring and management following recovery from their acute event.[116]

Other Acute Respiratory Disease

Exacerbation of reactive airway disease, such as asthma and chronic obstructive pulmonary disease (COPD), has been associated with acute RV dysfunction. Small airway collapse leads to air trapping and alveolar distention, compressing small PAs and capillaries, and causes a rise in PVR. In the setting of acute bronchoconstriction, echocardiographic studies have shown acute RV dilatation during inspiration, with return of normal RV dimension during expiration, reflecting the effect of lung hyperinflation on impedance to RV ejection. Hypoxemia, hypercapnia, and acidosis further compound the rise in PVR and increased RV impedance. These same studies have also shown that as the right ventricle dilates during inspiration, LV cavity dimensions reciprocally diminish, reflecting the effects of right to left shifting of the interventricular septum, which may explain the frequent finding of pulsus paradoxus in patients with acute bronchoconstriction.[117,118]

Acute cor pulmonale can also be seen during other acute respiratory diseases, in particular, the acute respiratory distress syndrome (ARDS) and in patients with a significant pulmonary infection, such as community acquired pneumonia. Hypoxic vasoconstriction further increases PVR. Often these patients have a normal or increased CO, and PH is a common echocardiographic finding during the acute illness.[119] One study demonstrated a 25% incidence of acute cor pulmonale in patients with ARDS. Although patients with RV dysfunction required ventilation for longer periods, the outcome was not different from patients without evidence of RV failure.[120] Mechanical ventilation, and in particular positive end-expiratory pressure (PEEP), also impose an increased afterload on the right-sided heart through increased alveolar pressure, often while simultaneously decreasing venous return.[121-123] Based on the echocardiographic findings during their acute illness, patients are often labeled with the diagnosis of PH. However, these patients should have a repeat echocardiogram with Doppler estimation of pulmonary pressure once the acute illness and hypoxemia have resolved because correction of the acute hypoxemia will often result in normalization of PA pressure.

Chronic Respiratory Disease

The hallmark of chronic pulmonary disease leading to chronic cor pulmonale is PH. PH is defined as a mean PA pressure greater than 25 mm Hg at rest, or 30 mm Hg with exercise.[84] In chronic respiratory disease, PH may be secondary to diseases of the pulmonary vasculature or to various parenchymal lung disorders, often complicated by hypoxemia. The updated World Health Organization (WHO) classification system divides PH into five major categories, which provide a useful guide to the potential etiologies of PH.[124] This chapter focuses on WHO groups I (pulmonary arterial hypertension

[PAH]), III (PH associated with disorders of the respiratory system or hypoxemia), and IV (chronic thromboembolic disease). PH secondary to left-sided heart disease (WHO group II) will be discussed below (see Differentiation of Pulmonary Heart Disease from Primary Cardiac Disease), while PH related to uncommon causes such as compression of the pulmonary vasculature (group V) will not be discussed.

Fundamental to the evaluation of patients with chronic respiratory disease is the assessment of PA pressure, permitting both the diagnosis of PH and assessment of its severity. As discussed previously, continuous-wave Doppler interrogation of the tricuspid regurgitant jet is the most widely used method to assess RV systolic pressure, which reflects PASP assuming pulmonic stenosis is not present. Doppler consistently underestimated PA pressure compared with invasive pressure estimates by greater than 20 mm Hg in over 31% of patients with PH.[125] Overestimation of PA pressure, especially at the upper end of the normal range also occurs. Thus mildly elevated pulmonary pressures should be confirmed by right-sided heart catheterization before an extensive evaluation of PH.[126] Echocardiographic evidence of RV remodeling, right-sided to left-sided heart disproportion, septal shifting, and RV hypokinesis should greatly increase the clinical suspicion for significant acute or chronic respiratory disease.

Pulmonary Arterial Hypertension

PAH, defined as a mean pulmonary artery pressure greater than 25 mm Hg with a pulmonary capillary wedge pressure less than 15 mm Hg, results from disorders that localize to the distal pulmonary vasculature, and thus does not include patients with parenchymal lung disorders or thromboembolic disease. PAH is most commonly idiopathic (formerly referred to as primary PH). Other causes of PAH include collagen vascular disease, such as scleroderma, human immunodeficiency virus (HIV) infection, anorexigen use, and congenital left-to-right heart shunts. Common to all conditions listed under WHO group I are the pathologic findings within the small pulmonary vasculature of medial hypertrophy, intimal proliferation, and in advanced cases, obliteration of the distal vasculature. The reduction of the pulmonary vascular surface area leads to systemic or suprasystemic levels of PVR and pressure, RV decompensation, exercise intolerance, and in many cases, death.

Indices of right-sided heart size, ventricular interdependence, and depressed RV function have been correlated with disease severity and patient outcome in patients with PAH.[127,128] In addition, studies have consistently shown that the presence and severity of a pericardial effusion predicts poor outcome in patients with PAH.[129] Larger effusion size correlates with greater degrees of exercise intolerance, RA dilatation, greater interventricular septal displacement, and more severe

TR than patients without an effusion.[128,130,131] The exact mechanism of pericardial effusion in PAH is unclear. Effusion is typically found in patients with more globally decompensated right-sided heart function. Importantly, pericardiocentesis is not generally recommended in this setting because the pericardial effusion is a marker and not the cause of the right-sided heart decompensation. A disproportionate number of adverse events are reported in these patients at the time of the procedure.

Doppler echocardiography has also been used to quantify right-sided heart function in PAH. The severity of TR has been associated with poor outcome in PAH, likely reflecting the association between TR severity and RV dysfunction in these patients.[132,133] The RV MPI is significantly higher in patients with primary PH versus healthy control subjects (0.84±0.2 versus 0.28±0.04), with an increased MPI associated with reduced survival in patients with PAH.[133,134] Strain rate imaging also demonstrates moderate or severe RV abnormalities in all patients with significant PAH and improvement in these parameters after treatment with vasodilator therapy.[135]

In a recent prospective study in patients with PAH, a TAPSE less than 1.8 cm was strongly associated with impaired RV systolic function, greater degrees of right-sided heart remodeling, marked right-sided to left-sided heart disproportion, and a much higher incidence of significant pericardial effusion.[59] Patients with a TAPSE less than 1.8 cm also had smaller left-sided heart dimensions, more impaired LV filling, higher heart rates, and greater systemic vasoconstriction than patients with relative preservation of TAPSE. Survival estimates for patients with PAH with a TAPSE less than 1.8 cm were 60% and 50% at 1 and 2 years, respectively, versus 94% and 88% in patients with a TAPSE greater than or equal to 1.8 cm.

Serial echocardiography is useful to evaluate the efficacy of specific therapies in PAH. For example, 12-week infusion of prostacyclin has shown beneficial effects on RV size, curvature of the interventricular septum, and maximal tricuspid regurgitant jet velocity.[125] Similarly, 16 weeks of bosentan therapy has been shown to reduce RV end-systolic area, RV:LV diastolic area ratio, lessen interventricular septal shifting, improve LV early diastolic filling, and reduce the incidence of pericardial effusion in patients with PAH.[136] Future studies will need to focus on the clinical and prognostic impact of serial echocardiographic assessment of patients on specific therapies in PAH, and whether such information can be used to identify patients whom are responding favorably, versus those whom will require escalation of medical therapy, and/or referral for lung (heart/lung) transplantation.

Pulmonary Thromboembolic Disease

Chronic thrombotic occlusion of large PA segments is a rare complication of acute PE, resulting in chronic thromboembolic pulmonary hypertension (CTEPH) in

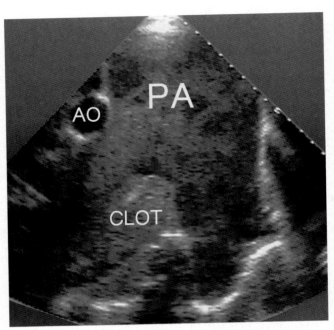

Figure 35-26. Parasternal short-axis view at the base of the heart in a patient with chronic thromboembolic pulmonary hypertension. The pulmonary artery (PA) is massively dilated and is many times the diameter of the aortic root (Ao), which is seen in cross section. There is spontaneous echocardiographic contrast within the main PA. There is a thrombus (CLOT) at the bifurcation of the main PA, which extends into the right main branch.

an estimated 0.1-0.5% of cases of acute PE[137-140] (Fig. 35-26). Progression of the disease likely results from a combination of narrowing of the proximal pulmonary vascular bed as a result of incompletely resolved thrombus, in situ thrombosis in areas of endothelial injury from prior acute embolic event, and the development of a distal arteriopathy in nonoccluded vascular segments that is similar to the small-vessel arteriopathy of idiopathic PAH.[141] The degree of elevation of PVR may be far greater than expected based on the angiographic level of pulmonary vascular obstruction, and a subset of patients may derive benefit from intravenous and inhaled prostacyclin analogues before and after pulmonary thromboendarterectomy.[142,143] Over time, progressive vascular obstruction and remodeling lead to marked increases in PVR, RV failure, and death if untreated. Because most patients are diagnosed late in their disease course, the manifestations of CTEPH are virtually indistinguishable from PAH or other forms of advanced PH, with the triad of RV enlargement, interventricular septal shifting, and RV systolic dysfunction being nearly universally present.[139] However, there are hemodynamic features that are unique to CTEPH that can be exploited both invasively and noninvasively that aid in distinguishing it from other forms of PAH, which may lead to a more rapid diagnosis.

The fundamental difference relates to the site of PVR. In CTEPH, vascular obstruction typically occurs in more proximal PA segments. The site of the pulmonary arterial wave reflection is closer to the pulmonic valve.[144,145] There is proportionally more reflection and the reflected waves arrive earlier during systole. Aside from the increased afterload imposed by this physiology, PA pulse pressure is often dramatically increased, particularly when referenced to mean PA pressure (so-called fractional pulse pressure).[146] The average fractional pulse pressure in CTEPH is 1.4 versus 0.8 in idiopathic PAH, with no overlap in these values between the two groups.[147] Using this noninvasive method, patients with CTEPH had a fractional pulse pressure was approximately 1.7, versus 0.9 in the idiopathic PAH group. Using a cutoff of 1.35, the sensitivity of fractional pulse pressure for CTEPH was 95% and the specificity was 100%.[147,148]

CTEPH is a potentially correctable form of PH, assuming timely and appropriate referral for pulmonary thromboendarterectomy. There is no upper limit of PVR or PA pressure that precludes surgical treatment.[149] Successful removal of clot burden can lead to rapid reversal of the pulmonary vascular obstruction, and dramatic improvement in right-sided heart function. This has been well illustrated in case series of severe CTEPH, where repeat echocardiography as early as 2 weeks, and as late as 1 year after pulmonary thromboendarterectomy showed significant reductions in RV systolic and diastolic area, decrease in TR, improvement in the RV fractional area change and decreased septal shifting with increases in LV size and marked improvements in early diastolic LV filling velocity.[150,151]

Secondary Pulmonary Hypertension

The chronic respiratory disorders associated with PH include COPD, interstitial lung disease (most commonly as a result of idiopathic pulmonary fibrosis), and disorders of alveolar hypoventilation, which include chronic neuromuscular disorders and sleep-disordered breathing. The pathogenesis of PH in COPD and interstitial lung disease relates in part to parenchymal lung destruction, which in essence, leads to collateral damage of the pulmonary vasculature and increased PVR. In addition, both acute hypoxic pulmonary vasoconstriction and the effects of chronic hypoxemia (and hypercapnia) on pulmonary vascular remodeling contribute to increased RV afterload in these conditions. The degree of elevation of PVR and PH in these patients is correlated to both the extent of parenchymal lung disease by radiography and pulmonary function testing and the severity of arterial hypoxemia. As a result, significant PH is uncommon in patients with COPD and interstitial lung disease whom have a forced expiratory volume (FEV1) greater than 1 L and a total lung capacity (TLC) greater than 50%.[152]

Alveolar hypoventilation also predisposes a patient to PH, via chronic hypoxemia, but intermittent hypoxemia is typically insufficient to result in chronic PH. Patients with obstructive sleep apnea who experience profound nocturnal oxygen desaturations do not usually develop PH, whereas PH is a common occurrence in subjects with the obesity-hypoventilation syndrome. The most significant predictors of PH in patients with sleep disordered breathing are daytime PO_2, PCO_2, FEV_1, and body mass index.[153] However, even in the absence of PH, obstructive sleep apnea is associated with RV dilatation and hypertrophy and decreases in RV systolic function as assessed by Doppler tissue imaging and tricuspid annular excursion.[154-156] Whether these changes are associated with the known LV diastolic dysfunction that accompanies sleep apnea is unclear.[157,158] The RV abnormalities have been shown to improve after successful continuous positive airway pressure (CPAP) therapy.[154]

A key differentiating feature of PH related to chronic respiratory disease is that it is relatively mild, with a mean PA pressure ranging between 20 and 35 mm Hg. Overt right-sided heart dysfunction is less common in these patients because they typically maintain a normal cardiac index and RA pressure until late stages of the respiratory disorder.[7] Nevertheless, subtle RV dysfunction may be observed with tissue Doppler imaging even in patients without PH.[159] The typical echocardiographic features of right-sided heart compromise will appear when the afterload becomes excessive.

Despite the lesser incidence and severity of PH in these patients, the presence of PH is a poor prognostic indicator in patients with COPD and interstitial lung disease, making its recognition of great clinical importance.[160,161] If RV function is preserved, PH may primarily be a marker of the severity of the underlying lung disease. However, the development of RV systolic failure may be a premorbid finding, reflecting an advanced stage of both cardiac and pulmonary disease.

Echocardiographic image quality tends to be suboptimal as a result of increased lung volumes, obesity, and pulmonary fibrosis, all of which can attenuate US penetration. Cardiac orientation is often abnormal, which may confound optimal Doppler alignment with the tricuspid regurgitant jet. These issues are well illustrated in a report of 374 patients with advanced lung disease who underwent right-sided heart catheterization and Doppler echocardiography less than 72 hours apart. Estimation of PASP was only possible in 44% of the population. There was only a modest overall correlation ($r = 0.69$) between invasively derived PASP and Doppler estimated pressure, with 52% of the patients having a pressure estimate that was greater than 10 mm Hg from the catheter-derived value.[162] The subcostal approach may confer additional diagnostic power in patients with hyperexpanded lungs.[163]

Systemic sclerosis and mixed connective tissue disease are associated with PH, detected by echocardiography in 13% to 28% of patients.[164,165] The PH may be isolated or associated with interstitial pulmonary fibrosis. Cor pulmonale with RV dilatation, hypertrophy and dysfunction will be detected on screening echocardiogram in a smaller number of patients.[166] Once again, early RV dysfunction, in the absence of PH may be detectable by tissue Doppler.[167] PH is discovered in fewer patients with sarcoidosis, approximately 5%. However, given the poor prognosis and the risk of cardiac involvement with sarcoid, these patients should also undergo routine screening echocardiography.[168-170]

Finally, refractory hypoxia in the setting of elevated right-sided pressures may be the result of right-to-left shunting through a stretched patent foramen ovale.[171-176] Injection of agitated saline will demonstrate prompt opacification of the left-sided heart demonstrating the cause of hypoxia. In some cases, percutaneous closure of the patent foramen ovale may dramatically improve the oxygenation.[173]

Pulmonary Venous Disease

Pulmonary veno-occlusive disease (PVOD) is a pattern of injury that may result from a variety of etiology factors. As a naturally occurring syndrome, it accounts for a small proportion of PH disease. Toxic exposures, infectious agents, including HIV and associations with autoimmune disease, have been described. Diagnosis by echocardiography has not been reported. The echocardiographic findings are essentially the same as in advanced PAH. However, acquired pulmonary vein stenosis may be detected echocardiographically. Pulmonary vein stenosis should be suspected when the inflow velocity is greater than 1.1 m/s and the flow is turbulent with little variation in velocity.[177] Clinically, this should be suspected in a patient following pulmonary vein isolation for ablation of atrial fibrillation.[178] Although the presentation may be acute and fulminant,

most commonly patients are diagnosed months after their procedure with a similar symptom complex as PVOD, including dyspnea, cough, fatigue, and hemoptysis.[179,180] Intracardiac echocardiography (ICE) guidance during the procedure may reduce the risk of injury.[181] MRI may be necessary to confirm the presence of pulmonary vein stenosis and to guide in stenting. Patients should be monitored by follow-up echocardiography after stenting as restenosis may occur.[182] The right superior pulmonary vein cannot be imaged by transthoracic echocardiography (TTE), and TEE or repeated MRI may be necessary for surveillance. Pulmonary vein thrombosis and occlusion has also been reported following heart and lung transplantation.[183,184] Intraoperative TEE may reduce the incidence of pulmonary venous complications and help with hemodynamic monitoring during these complicated surgeries.[185-187]

Differentiation of Pulmonary Heart Disease from Primary Cardiac Disease

Although this chapter has focused on the right ventricle and pulmonary arterial response to pulmonary disease, the most common cause of both PH and RV failure is left-sided heart disease.[188] In addition, patients with certain forms of cardiomyopathy that directly involve the RV are particularly intolerant to an increase in RV afterload. Distinction between primary left-sided heart disease and pulmonary disease should include a careful echocardiographic evaluation of the LV systolic and

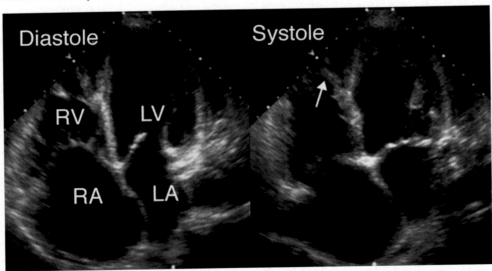

Figure 35–27. *Apical four-chamber view in diastole and systole in a patient with right ventricular failure resulting from longstanding LV failure. The left ventricular ejection fraction is markedly decreased as can be seen by comparison of the systolic and diastolic frames. The right ventricular function is also severely diminished. There was severe tricuspid regurgitation, which although not pictured, may be inferred by the systolic expansion of the right atrium (RA). LA, left atrium; LV, left ventricle; RV right ventricle.*

diastolic function, mitral inflow, pulmonary venous inflow patterns, and assessment of valvular function.

LV failure, whether systolic or diastolic, is characterized by a rise in LV end-diastolic pressure and subsequently in pulmonary capillary wedge pressure (PCWP). The development of PH is predicted more by the presence of a restrictive mitral inflow pattern and the degree of mitral regurgitation (MR) than the absolute degree of LV dysfunction measured by EF.[189] The development of RV dysfunction is a poor prognostic sign in patients with dilated cardiomyopathy[190,191] (Fig. 35–27). The development of significant TR or decreased tricuspid annular systolic excursion is particularly ominous.[192,193]

Mitral stenosis (MS) of any important degree, results in PH and RV remodeling.[194] Both PH and TR are likely to regress after successful treatment of mitral stenosis with valvuloplasty or surgical valve replacement.[195,196] In contrast, there was originally controversy as to whether isolated mitral regurgitation with normal LV systolic function could lead to PH.[197] It is now fully appreciated that subtle LV dysfunction may occur with severe mitral regurgitation before the development of overt failure. The development of PH at rest or on stress echocardiography is considered an indication for surgical repair.[198,199] In the setting of severe mitral regurgitation, preoperative PH predicts the development of postoperative LV dysfunction.[200]

KEY POINTS

- Complex RV geometry mandates assessment of anatomy and function from multiple echocardiographic views. Simple geometric assumptions cannot be used to model RV volumes.

- RV end-diastolic volume is 30% larger than LV end-diastolic volume, and RV EF is normally 35% to 45%. The mean systolic pressure and pulse pressure of the right ventricle are much lower than the left ventricle resulting in a lower stroke work.

- RV enlargement is manifest by RV end-diastolic diameter greater than 60% of LV end-diastolic diameter in the parasternal long axis and in the apical four-chamber view an area greater than two thirds of the LV area.

- PASP is calculated by the peak velocity of the TR jet with the formula: $PASP = 4v_{TR}^2 + RAP$. The RAP is calculated by the degree of collapse of the IVC with inspiration or sniff. The diastolic pressure can be calculated from the pulmonary regurgitant jet velocity.

- The right ventricle shortens more in the longitudinal plane than in the transverse plane. Tricuspid annular plane systolic excursion (TAPSE) correlates well with RV function because it is a measure of longitudinal shortening. Assessment of free wall motion is not reliable, in itself, as a measure of RV EF.

- Both severe TR and pulmonary regurgitation may cause volume overload of the right ventricle, but they are more likely to be secondary to severe PH or RV enlargement rather than as a result of primary valvular pathology. Careful echocardiographic assessment of valvular morphology will distinguish between primary and secondary valvular disease.

- Echocardiography in acute PE demonstrates RV enlargement, deviation of the interventricular and interatrial septum to the left side, and RV systolic failure with preservation of apical contraction. TR is invariably present, but the PASP is usually not severely elevated.

- Pulmonary arterial hypertension (PAH) can be distinguished by severe RV hypertrophy and PASP that may be near systemic. Compromise of LV filling and systolic function is the result of impingement on the LV cavity by the interventricular septum.

- Chronic thromboembolic pulmonary hypertension (CTEPH) will have similar echocardiographic features, but the PA pulse pressure is usually much greater than in other forms of PH.

- The most common cause of PH and RV dysfunction is left-sided dysfunction. Evidence of RV dysfunction mandates complete assessment of the valves and LV function to make this determination.

REFERENCES

1. Starr I, Jeffers W, Meade R: The absence of conspicuous increments of venous pressure after severe damage to the right ventricle of the dog, with a discussion of the relation between clinical congestive failure and heart disease. *Am Heart J* 26:291-301, 1943.
2. Wagner SRaD: By-passing the right ventricle. *Proceedings of the Society of Experimental Biology and Medicine* 71:69-71, 1948.
3. Donald DE, Essex HE: Pressure studies after inactivation of the major portion of the canine right ventricle. *Am J Physiol* 176:155-161, 1954.
4. Kagan A: Dynamic responses of the right ventricle following extensive damage by cauterization. *Circulation* 5:816-823, 1952.
5. Cohn JN, Guiha NH, Broder MI, Limas CJ: Right ventricular infarction. Clinical and hemodynamic features. *Am J Cardiol* 33:209-214, 1974.
6. Rich S, Levy PS: Characteristics of surviving and nonsurviving patients with primary pulmonary hypertension. *Am J Med* 76:573-578, 1984.
7. Schulman DS, Matthay RA: The right ventricle in pulmonary disease. *Cardiol Clin* 10:111-135, 1992.
8. Kussmaul WG, Noordergraaf A, Laskey WK: Right ventricular-pulmonary arterial interactions. *Ann Biomed Eng* 20:63-80, 1992.
9. Rushmer RF, Crystal DK, Wagner C: The functional anatomy of ventricular contraction. *Circ Res* 1:162-170, 1953.
10. Santamore WP, Dell'Italia LJ: Ventricular interdependence: significant left ventricular contributions to right ventricular systolic function. *Prog Cardiovasc Dis* 40:289-308, 1998.
11. Bakos A: The question of the function of the right ventricular myocardium: An experimental study. *Fed Proc* 7:724-732, 1948.
12. Hess DS, Bache RJ: Transmural right ventricular myocardial blood flow during systole in the awake dog. *Circ Res* 45:88-94, 1979.

13. Lowensohn HS, Khouri EM, Gregg DE, et al: Phasic right coronary artery blood flow in conscious dogs with normal and elevated right ventricular pressures. *Circ Res* 39:760-766, 1976.

14. Forman MB, Wilson BH, Sheller JR, et al: Right ventricular hypertrophy is an important determinant of right ventricular infarction complicating acute inferior left ventricular infarction. *J Am Coll Cardiol* 10:1180-1187, 1987.

15. Dell'Italia LJ, Santamore WP: Can indices of left ventricular function be applied to the right ventricle? *Prog Cardiovasc Dis* 40:309-324, 1998.

16. Maughan WL, Shoukas AA, Sagawa K, Weisfeldt ML: Instantaneous pressure-volume relationship of the canine right ventricle. *Circ Res* 44:309-315, 1979.

17. Geva T, Powell AJ, Crawford EC, et al: Evaluation of regional differences in right ventricular systolic function by acoustic quantification echocardiography and cine magnetic resonance imaging. *Circulation* 98:339-345, 1998.

18. Kaul S, Tei C, Hopkins JM, Shah PM: Assessment of right ventricular function using two-dimensional echocardiography. *Am Heart J* 107:526-531, 1984.

19. Leather, HA, et al: Longitudinal but not circumferential deformation reflects global contractile function in the right ventricle with open pericardium. *Am J Physiol Heart Circ Physiol* 290: H2369-H2375, 2006.

20. Clark TJ, Sheehan FH, Bolson EL: Characterizing the normal heart using quantitative three-dimensional echocardiography. *Physiol Meas* 27:467-508, 2006.

21. Bauman W, Wann LS, Childress R, et al: Mid systolic notching of the pulmonary valve in the absence of pulmonary hypertension. *Am J Cardiol* 43:1049-1052, 1979.

22. Maciel BC, Simpson IA, Valdes-Cruz LM, et al: Color flow Doppler mapping studies of "physiologic" pulmonary and tricuspid regurgitation: evidence for true regurgitation as opposed to a valve closing volume. *J Am Soc Echocardiogr* 4:589-597, 1991.

23. Bommer W, Weinert L, Neumann A, et al: Determination of right atrial and right ventricular size by two-dimensional echocardiography. *Circulation* 60:91-100, 1979.

24. Markiewicz W, Sechtem U, Higgins CB: Evaluation of the right ventricle by magnetic resonance imaging. *Am Heart J* 113:8-15, 1987.

25. Baker B, Scovil JA, Kane JJ, Murphy LL: Echocardiographic detection of right ventricular hypertrophy. *Am Heart J* 105:611-614, 1983.

26. Cacho A, Prakash R, Sarma R, Kaushik VS: Usefulness of two-dimensional echocardiography in diagnosing right ventricular hypertrophy. *Chest* 84:154-157, 1983.

27. Silvestry F, Wiegers S: *Intracardiac Echocardiography,* New York, Taylor and Francis, 2006, p. 120.

28. Gardin JM, Burns CS, Childs WJ, Henry WL: Evaluation of blood flow velocity in the ascending aorta and main pulmonary artery of normal subjects by Doppler echocardiography. *Am Heart J* 107:310-319, 1984.

29. Scapellato F, Temporelli PL, Eleuteri E, et al: Accurate noninvasive estimation of pulmonary vascular resistance by Doppler echocardiography in patients with chronic failure heart failure. *J Am Coll Cardiol* 37:1813-1819, 2001.

30. Stevenson JG: Comparison of several noninvasive methods for estimation of pulmonary artery pressure. *J Am Soc Echocardiogr* 2:157-171, 1989.

31. Beard JT 2nd, Newman JH, Loyd JE, Byrd BF 3rd: Doppler estimation of changes in pulmonary artery pressure during hypoxic breathing. *J Am Soc Echocardiogr* 4:121-130, 1991.

32. Vogel M, Weil J, Stern H, Buhlmeyer K: Responsiveness of raised pulmonary vascular resistance to oxygen assessed by pulsed Doppler echocardiography. *Br Heart J* 66:277-280, 1991.

33. Nanna M, Lin SL, Tak I, et al: Inaccuracy of Doppler estimates of pulmonary artery pressure using pulmonary flow acceleration time. *Can J Cardiol* 6:19-23, 1990.

34. Hollander, EH, et al: Negative wave reflections in pulmonary arteries. *Am J Physiol Heart Circ Physiol* 281:H895-H902, 2001.

35. Ha B, Lucas CL, Henry GW, et al: Effects of chronically elevated pulmonary arterial pressure and flow on right ventricular afterload. *Am J Physiol* 267(1 Pt 2):H155-H165, 1994.

36. Kitabatake A, et al: Noninvasive evaluation of pulmonary hypertension by a pulsed Doppler technique. *Circulation* 68:302-309, 1983.

37. Yock PG, Popp RL: Noninvasive estimation of right ventricular systolic pressure by Doppler ultrasound in patients with tricuspid regurgitation. *Circulation* 70:657-662, 1984.

38. Berger M, Haimowitz A, Van Tosh A, et al: Quantitative assessment of pulmonary hypertension in patients with tricuspid regurgitation using continuous wave Doppler ultrasound. *J Am Coll Cardiol* 6:359-365, 1985.

39. Chan KL, Currie PJ, Seward JB, et al: Comparison of three Doppler ultrasound methods in the prediction of pulmonary artery pressure. *J Am Coll Cardiol* 9:549-554, 1987.

40. Currie PJ, Seward JB, Chan KL, et al: Continuous wave Doppler determination of right ventricular pressure: a simultaneous Doppler-catheterization study in 127 patients. *J Am Coll Cardiol* 6:750-756, 1985.

41. Himelman RB, Stulbarg M, Kircher B, et al: Noninvasive evaluation of pulmonary artery pressure during exercise by saline-enhanced Doppler echocardiography in chronic pulmonary disease. *Circulation* 79:863-871, 1989.

42. Kircher BJ, Himelman RB, Schiller NB: Noninvasive estimation of right atrial pressure from the inspiratory collapse of the inferior vena cava. *Am J Cardiol* 66:493-496, 1990.

43. Marangoni S, Vitacca M, Quadri A, et al: Non-invasive haemodynamic effects of two nasal positive pressure ventilation modalities in stable chronic obstructive lung disease patients. *Respiration* 64:138-144, 1997.

44. Quiles J, Garcia-Fernandez MA, Almeida PB, et al: Portable spectral Doppler echocardiographic device: Overcoming limitations. *Heart* 89:1014-1018, 2003.

45. Masuyama T, Kodama K, Kitabatake A, et al: Continuous wave Doppler echocardiographic detection of pulmonary regurgitation and its application to noninvasive estimation of pulmonary artery pressure. *Circulation* 74:484-492, 1986.

46. Abbas AE, Fortuin FD, Schiller NB, et al: Echocardiographic determination of mean pulmonary artery pressure. *Am J Cardiol* 92:1373-1376, 2003.

47. Lanzarini L, Fontana A, Lucca E, et al: Noninvasive estimation of both systolic and diastolic pulmonary artery pressure from Doppler analysis of tricuspid regurgitant velocity spectrum in patients with chronic heart failure. *Am Heart J* 144:1087-1094, 2002.

48. Stephen B, Dalal P, Berger M, et al: Noninvasive estimation of pulmonary artery diastolic pressure in patients with tricuspid regurgitation by Doppler echocardiography [see comment]. *Chest* 116:73-77, 1999.

49. Abbas AE, Fortuin FD, Schiller NB, et al: A simple method for noninvasive estimation of pulmonary vascular resistance. *J Am Coll Cardiol* 41:1021-1027, 2003.

50. Huez S, Brimioulle S, Naije R, Vachiery JL: Feasibility of routine pulmonary arterial impedance measurements in pulmonary hypertension. *Chest* 125:2121-2128, 2004.

51. Dyer K, Lanning C, Das B, et al: Noninvasive Doppler tissue measurement of pulmonary artery compliance in children with pulmonary hypertension. *J Am Soc Echocardiogr* 19:403-412, 2006.

52. Levine R, Gibson TC, Aretz T, et al: Echocardiographic measurement of right ventricular volume. *Circulation* 69:497-505, 1984.

53. Shiota T, Jones M, Chikada M, et al: Real-time three-dimensional echocardiography for determining right ventricular stroke volume in an animal model of chronic right ventricular volume overload. *Circulation* 97:1897-1900, 1988.

54. Schindera ST, Mehwald PS, Sahn DJ, Kececioglu D: Accuracy of real-time three-dimensional echocardiography for quantifying right ventricular volume: Static and pulsatile flow studies in an anatomic in vitro model. *J Ultrasound Med* 21:1069-1075, 2002.

55. Sheehan FH, Bolson EL: Measurement of right ventricular volume from biplane contrast ventriculograms: Validation by cast and three-dimensional echo. *Catheter Cardiovasc Interv* 62:46-51, 2004.

56. Jiang L, Levine RA, Weyman AE: Echocardiographic assessment of right ventricular volume and function. *Echocardiography* 14:189-206, 1997.

57. Kovalova S, Necas J, Cerbak R, et al: Echocardiographic volumetry of the right ventricle. *Eur J Echocardiogr* 6:15-23, 2005.

58. Hammarstrom E, Wranne B, Pinto FJ, et al: Tricuspid annular motion. *J Am Soc Echocardiogr* 4:131-139, 1991.

59. Forfia PR, Fisher MR, Mathai SC, et al, Tricuspid annular displacement predicts survival in pulmonary hypertension. *Am J Respir Crit Care Med* 174:1034-1041, 2006.

60. Ghio S, Recusani F, Klersy C, et al: Prognostic usefulness of the tricuspid annular plane systolic excursion in patients with congestive heart failure secondary to idiopathic or ischemic dilated cardiomyopathy. *Am J Cardiol* 85:837-842, 2000.

61. Alam M, Wardell J, Andersson E, et al: Right ventricular function in patients with first inferior myocardial infarction: assessment by tricuspid annular motion and tricuspid annular velocity. *Am Heart J* 139:710-715, 2000.

62. Samad BA, Alam M, Jensen-Urstad K: Prognostic impact of right ventricular involvement as assessed by tricuspid annular motion in patients with acute myocardial infarction. *Am J Cardiol* 90:778-781, 2002.

63. Kukulski T, Hubbert L, Arnold M, et al: Normal regional right ventricular function and its change with age: A Doppler myocardial imaging study. *J Am Soc Echocardiogr* 13:194-204, 2000.

64. Marwick T: Measurement of strain and strain rate by echocardiography: Ready for prime time? *J Am Coll Cardiol* 47:1313-1327, 2006.

65. Frigiola A, Redington AN, Cullen S, Vogel M: Pulmonary regurgitation is an important determinant of right ventricular contractile dysfunction in patients with surgically repaired tetralogy of Fallot. *Circulation* 110(11 Suppl 1):II153-II157, 2004.

66. Weidemann F, Eyskens B, Mertens L, et al: Quantification of regional right and left ventricular function by ultrasonic strain rate and strain indexes after surgical repair of tetralogy of Fallot. *Am J Cardiol* 90:133-138, 2002.

67. Weidemann F, Eyskens B, Jamal F, et al: Quantification of regional left and right ventricular radial and longitudinal function in healthy children using ultrasound-based strain rate and strain imaging. *J Am Soc Echocardiogr* 15:20-28, 2002.

68. Ishii M, Eto G, Tei C, et al: Quantitation of the global right ventricular function in children with normal heart and congenital heart disease: A right ventricular myocardial performance index. *Pediatr Cardiol* 21:416-421, 2000.

69. Norozi K, Buchhorn R, Alpers V, et al: Relation of systemic ventricular function quantified by myocardial performance index (Tei) to cardiopulmonary exercise capacity in adults after Mustard procedure for transposition of the great arteries. *Am J Cardiol* 96:1721-1725, 2005.

70. Morhy SS, Andrade JL, Soares AM, et al: Non-invasive assessment of right ventricular function in the late follow-up of the Senning procedure. *Cardiol Young* 15:154-159, 2005.

71. Salehian O, Schwerzmann M, Merchant N, et al: Assessment of systemic right ventricular function in patients with transposition of the great arteries using the myocardial performance index: Comparison with cardiac magnetic resonance imaging. *Circulation* 110:3229-3233, 2004.

72. Kim W, Otsuji Y, Yuasa T, et al: Evaluation of right ventricular dysfunction in patients with cardiac amyloidosis using the Tei index. *J Am Soc Echocardiogr* 45-49, 2004.

73. Abd El Rahman MY, Abdul-Kahlig H, Vogel M, et al: Value of the new Doppler-derived myocardial performance index for the evaluation of right and left ventricular function following repair of tetralogy of Fallot. *Pediatr Cardiol* 23:502-507, 2002.

74. Belenkie I, Smith ER, Tyberg JV: Ventricular interaction: from bench to bedside. *Ann Med* 33:236-241, 2001.

75. Louie EK, Rich S, Brundage BH: Doppler echocardiographic assessment of impaired left ventricular filling in patients with right ventricular pressure overload due to primary pulmonary hypertension. *J Am Coll Cardiol* 1298-1306, 1986.

76. Mahmud E, Raisinghani A, Hassankhani A, et al: Correlation of left ventricular diastolic filling characteristics with right ventricular overload and pulmonary artery pressure in chronic thromboembolic pulmonary hypertension. *J Am Coll Cardiol* 40:318-324, 2002.

77. Marcus JT, Vonk Noordegraaf A, Roelveld RJ, et al: Impaired left ventricular filling due to right ventricular pressure overload in primary pulmonary hypertension: Noninvasive monitoring using MRI. *Chest* 119:1761-1765, 2001.

78. Arce OX, Knudson OA, Ellison MC, et al: Longitudinal motion of the atrioventricular annuli in children: Reference values, growth related changes, and effects of right ventricular volume and pressure overload. *J Am Soc Echocardiogr* 15:906-916, 2002.

79. St John Sutton MG, Takij AJ, Mercier LA, et al: Assessment of left ventricular function in secundum atrial septal defect by computer analysis of the M-mode echocardiogram. *Circulation* 60:1082-1090, 1979.

80. Popio KA, Gorlin R, Teichholz LE, et al: Abnormalities of left ventricular function and geometry in adults with an atrial septal defect. Ventriculographic, hemodynamic and echocardiographic studies. *Am J Cardiol* 36:302-308, 1975.

81. Bove AA, Santamore WP: Ventricular interdependence. *Prog Cardiovasc Dis* 23:365-388, 1981.

82. Guyton AC, Lindsey AW, Gilluly JJ: The limits of right ventricular compensation following acute increase in pulmonary circulatory resistance. *Circ Res* 2:326-332, 1954.

83. Wood KE: Major pulmonary embolism: Review of a pathophysiologic approach to the golden hour of hemodynamically significant pulmonary embolism. *Chest* 121:877-905, 2002.

84. Farber HW, Loscalzo J: Pulmonary arterial hypertension. *New Engl J Med* 351:1655-1665, 2004.

85. Little WC, Badke FR, O'Rourke RA: Effect of right ventricular pressure on the end-diastolic left ventricular pressure-volume relationship before and after chronic right ventricular pressure overload in dogs without pericardia. *Circ Res* 54:719-730, 1984.

86. Slinker BK, Chagas AC, Glantz SA: Chronic pressure overload hypertrophy decreases direct ventricular interaction. *Am J Physiol* 253(2 Pt 2):H347-H357, 1987.

87. Mahmud E, Raisinghani A, Kermati S, et al: Dilation of the coronary sinus on echocardiogram: Prevalence and significance in patients with chronic pulmonary hypertension. *J Am Soc Echocardiogr* 14:44-49, 2001.

88. Kinn JW, Aljuni SC, Samyn JG, et al: Rapid hemodynamic improvement after reperfusion during right ventricular infarction. *J Am Coll Cardiol* 26:1230-1234, 1995.

89. Ozdemir K, Alkuneser BB, Icli A, et al: New parameters in identification of right ventricular myocardial infarction and proximal right coronary artery lesion. *Chest* 124:219-226, 2003.

90. Fontaine G, Fontaliran F, Zenati O et al: Arrhythmogenic right ventricular dysplasia. *Annu Rev Med* 50:17-35, 1999.

91. Yoerger DM, Marcus F, Sherrill D, et al: Echocardiographic findings in patients meeting task force criteria for arrhythmogenic right ventricular dysplasia: new insights from the multidisciplinary study of right ventricular dysplasia. *J Am Coll Cardiol* 45:860-865, 2005.

92. Hebert JL, Chemla D, Gerard O, et al: Angiographic right and left ventricular function in arrhythmogenic right ventricular dysplasia. *Am J Cardiol* 93:728-733, 2004.

93. Faller M, Kessler R, Chaouat A, et al: Platypnea-orthodeoxia syndrome related to an aortic aneurysm combined with an aneurysm of the atrial septum. *Chest* 118:553-557, 2002.

94. McIntyre KM, Sasahara AA: The hemodynamic response to pulmonary embolism in patients without prior cardiopulmonary disease. *Am J Cardiol* 28:288-294, 1971.

95. Ribeiro A, Juhlin-Dannfelt A, Brodin LA, et al: Pulmonary embolism: Relation between the degree of right ventricle overload and the extent of perfusion defects. *Am Heart J* 135(5 Pt 1):868-874, 1998.

96. Come PC, Kim D, Parker JA, et al: Early reversal of right ventricular dysfunction in patients with acute pulmonary embolism after treatment with intravenous tissue plasminogen activator. *J Am Coll Cardiol* 10:971-978, 1987.

97. Kasper W, Geibel A, Tiede N, et al: Distinguishing between acute and subacute massive pulmonary embolism by conventional and Doppler echocardiography. *Br Heart J* 70:352-356, 1993.

98. Jardin F, Dubourg O, Gueret P, et al: Quantitative two-dimensional echocardiography in massive pulmonary embolism: Emphasis on ventricular interdependence and leftward septal displacement. *J Am Coll Cardiol* 10:1201-1206, 1987.

99. Belenkie I, Dani R, Smith ER, Tyberg JV: Ventricular interaction during experimental acute pulmonary embolism. *Circulation* 78:761-768, 1988.

100. Belenkie I, Dani R, Smith ER, Tyberg JV: Effects of volume loading during experimental acute pulmonary embolism. *Circulation* 80:178-188, 1989.

101. McConnell MV, Solomon SD, Rayan ME, et al: Regional right ventricular dysfunction detected by echocardiography in acute pulmonary embolism. *Am J Cardiol* 78:469-473, 1996.

102. Kjaergaard J, Sogaard P, Hassager C: Right ventricular strain in pulmonary embolism by Doppler tissue echocardiography. *J Am Soc Echocardiogr* 17:1210-1212, 2004.

103. Hsiao SH, Lee CY, Chang SM, et al: Pulmonary embolism and right heart function: Insights from myocardial Doppler tissue imaging. *J Am Soc Echocardiogr* 19:822-828, 2006.

104. McIntyre KM, Sasahara AA: Determinants of right ventricular function and hemodynamics after pulmonary embolism. *Chest* 65:534-543, 1974.

105. Kurzyna M, Torbicki A, Pruszczyk P, et al: Disturbed right ventricular ejection pattern as a new Doppler echocardiographic sign of acute pulmonary embolism. *Am J Cardiol* 90:507-511, 2002.

106. Torbicki A, Galie N, Covezzoli A, et al: Right heart thrombi in pulmonary embolism: Results from the International Cooperative Pulmonary Embolism Registry. *J Am Coll Cardiol* 41:2245-2251, 2003.

107. Pierre-Justin G, Pierard LA: Management of mobile right heart thrombi: A prospective series. *Int J Cardiol* 99:381-388, 2005.

108. Goldhaber SZ, Haire WD, Feldstein ML, et al: Alteplase versus heparin in acute pulmonary embolism: Randomized trial assessing right-ventricular function and pulmonary perfusion. *Lancet* 341:507-511, 1993.

109. Goldhaber SZ, Visani L, De Rosa M: Acute pulmonary embolism: Clinical outcomes in the International Cooperative Pulmonary Embolism Registry (ICOPER). *Lancet* 353:1386-1389, 1999.

110. Ribeiro A, Lindmarker P, Juhlin-Dannfelt A, et al: Echocardiography Doppler in pulmonary embolism: Right ventricular dysfunction as a predictor of mortality rate. *Am Heart J* 134:479-487, 1997.

111. Kucher N, Rossi E, De Rosa M, Goldhaber SZ: Prognostic role of echocardiography among patients with acute pulmonary embolism and a systolic arterial pressure of 90 mm Hg or higher. *Arch Intern Med* 165:1777-1781, 2005.

112. Konstantinides S, Geibel A, Heusel G, et al: Heparin plus alteplase compared with heparin alone in patients with submassive pulmonary embolism. *New Engl J Med* 347:1143-1150, 2002.

113. Goldhaber SZ: Thrombolysis for pulmonary embolism. *New Engl J Med* 347:1131-1132, 2002.

114. Sukhija R, Aronow WS, Lee J, et al: Association of right ventricular dysfunction with in-hospital mortality in patients with acute pulmonary embolism and reduction in mortality in patients with right ventricular dysfunction by pulmonary embolectomy. *Am J Cardiol* 95:695-696, 2005.

115. Leacche M, Unic D, Goldhaber SZ, et al: Modern surgical treatment of massive pulmonary embolism: results in 47 consecutive patients after rapid diagnosis and aggressive surgical approach [see comment]. *J Thorac Cardiovasc Surg* 129:1018-1023, 2005.

116. Ribeiro A, Lindmarker P, Johnsson H, et al: Pulmonary embolism: One-year follow-up with echocardiography Doppler and five-year survival analysis. *Circulation* 99:1325-1330, 1999.

117. Jardin F, Farcot JC, Boisante L, et al: Mechanism of paradoxic pulse in bronchial asthma. *Circulation* 66:887-894, 1982.

118. Settle HP Jr, Engel PJ, Fowler NO, et al: Echocardiographic study of the paradoxical arterial pulse in chronic obstructive lung disease. *Circulation* 62:1297-1307, 1980.

119. Ware LB, Matthay MA: The acute respiratory distress syndrome. *New Engl J Med* 342:1334-1349, 2000.

120. Vieillard-Baron A, Schmitt JM, Augarde R, et al: Acute cor pulmonale in acute respiratory distress syndrome submitted to protective ventilation: incidence, clinical implications, and prognosis. *Crit Care Med* 29:1551-1555, 2001. Erratum appears in *Crit Care Med* 30:26, 2002.

121. Jardin F, Vieillard-Baron A: Right ventricular function and positive pressure ventilation in clinical practice: from hemodynamic subsets to respirator settings. *Intensive Care Med* 29:1426-1434, 2003.

122. Jellinek H, Krenn H, Oczenski W, et al: Influence of positive airway pressure on the pressure gradient for venous return in humans. *J App Physiol* 88:926-932, 2000.

123. Piazza G, Goldhaber SZ: The acutely decompensated right ventricle: Pathways for diagnosis and management. *Chest* 1836-1852, 2005.

124. Simonneau G, Galie N, Rubin LJ, et al: Clinical classification of pulmonary hypertension. *J Am Coll Cardiol* 43(12 Suppl S):5S-12S, 2004.

125. Hinderliter AL, Willis PW 4th, Barst RJ, et al: Effects of long-term infusion of prostacyclin (epoprostenol) on echocardiographic measures of right ventricular structure and function in primary pulmonary hypertension. Primary Pulmonary Hypertension Study Group. *Circulation* 95:1479-1486, 1997.

126. Barst R, McGoon M, Torbicki A, et al: Diagnosis and differential assessment of pulmonary arterial hypertension. *J Am Coll Cardiol* 43:40S-47S, 2004.

127. McLaughlin VV, Presburg KW, Doyle RL, et al: Prognosis of pulmonary arterial hypertension: ACCP evidence-based clinical practice guidelines. *Chest* 126(1 Suppl):78S-92S, 2004.

128. Raymond RJ, Hinderliter AL, Willis PW, et al: Echocardiographic predictors of adverse outcomes in primary pulmonary hypertension. *J Am Coll Cardiol* 39:1214-1219, 2002.

129. Eysmann S, Palevsky HI, Reichek N, et al: Two-dimensional and Doppler echocardiographic and cardiac catheterization correlates of survival in primary pulmonary hypertension. *Circulation* 80:353-360, 1989.

130. Torbicki A, Kurzyna M: Pulmonary arterial hypertension: evaluation of the newly diagnosed patient. *Semin Respir Crit Care Med* 26:372-378, 2005.

131. Hinderliter AL, Willis PW 4th, Long W, et al: Frequency and prognostic significance of pericardial effusion in primary pulmonary hypertension. PPH Study Group. Primary pulmonary hypertension. *Am J Cardiol* 84:481-484, 1999.

132. Hinderliter AL, Willis PW 4th, Long WA, et al: Frequency and severity of tricuspid regurgitation determined by Doppler echo-

cardiography in primary pulmonary hypertension. *Am J Cardiol* 91:1033-1037, 2003.

133. Yeo TC, Dujardin KS, Tei C, et al: Value of a Doppler-derived index combining systolic and diastolic time intervals in predicting outcome in primary pulmonary hypertension. *Am J Cardiol* 81:1157-1161, 1998.

134. Tei C, Dujardin KS, Hodge DO, et al: Doppler echocardiographic index for assessment of global right ventricular function. *J Am Soc Echocardiogr* 9:838-847, 1996.

135. Borges A, Knebel F, Eddicks S, et al: Right ventricular function assessed by two-dimensional strain and tissue Doppler echocardiography in patients with pulmonary arterial hypertension and effect of vasodilator therapy. *Am J Cardiol* 98:530-534, 2006.

136. Galie N, Hinderliter AL, Torbicki A et al: Effects of the oral endothelin-receptor antagonist bosentan on echocardiographic and Doppler measures in patients with pulmonary arterial hypertension. *J Am Coll Cardiol* 41:1380-1386, 2003.

137. Cranshaw JH, Evans TW: Effect of lung injury on the pulmonary circulation. In Peacock AJ, Rubin LJ (eds): *Pulmonary circulation: Diseases and their treatment*, 2nd ed, New York, Oxford University Press, 2004, pp. 518-531.

138. Dartevelle P, Fadel E, Mussot S, et al: Chronic thromboembolic pulmonary hypertension. *Eur Respir J* 23:637-648, 2004.

139. Fedullo PF, Kerr KM, Auger WR, et al: Chronic thromboembolic pulmonary hypertension. *New Engl J Med* 345:1465-1472, 2001.

140. Auger W, Fedullo P, Jamieson S: Chronic thromboembolic pulmonary hypertension. In Peacock AJ, Rubin LJ (eds): *Pulmonary circulation: Diseases and their treatment*, 2nd ed, pp. 440-452.

141. Moser KM, Bloor CM: Pulmonary vascular lesions occurring in patients with chronic major vessel thromboembolic pulmonary hypertension. *Chest* 103:685-692, 1993.

142. Kramm T, Eberle B, Guth S, Mayer E: Inhaled iloprost to control residual pulmonary hypertension following pulmonary endarterectomy. *Eur J Cardiothorac Surg* 28:882-888, 2005.

143. Nagaya N, Sasaki N, Ando M, et al: Prostacyclin therapy before pulmonary thromboendarterectomy in patients with chronic thromboembolic pulmonary hypertension. *Chest* 123:338-343, 2003.

144. Castelain V, Herve P, Lecarpentier Y, et al: Pulmonary artery pulse pressure and wave reflection in chronic pulmonary thromboembolism and primary pulmonary hypertension. *J Am Coll Cardiol* 37:1085-1092, 2001.

145. Kim NH, Fesler P, Channick RN, et al: Preoperative partitioning of pulmonary vascular resistance correlates with early outcome after thromboendarterectomy for chronic thromboembolic pulmonary hypertension. *Circulation* 109:18-22, 2004.

146. Nakayama Y, Nakanishi N, Sugimachi M, et al: Characteristics of pulmonary artery pressure waveform for differential diagnosis of chronic pulmonary thromboembolism and primary pulmonary hypertension. *J Am Coll Cardiol* 29:1311-1316, 1997.

147. Tanabe N, Okada O, Abe Y, et al: The influence of fractional pulse pressure on the outcome of pulmonary thromboendarterectomy. *Eur Respir J* 17:653-659, 2001.

148. Nakayama Y, Sugimachi M, Nakanishi N, et al: Noninvasive differential diagnosis between chronic pulmonary thromboembolism and primary pulmonary hypertension by means of Doppler ultrasound measurement. *J Am Coll Cardiol* 31:1367-1371, 1998.

149. Jamieson SW, Kapelanski DP: Pulmonary endarterectomy. *Curr Probl Surg* 37:165-252, 2000.

150. Casaclang-Verzosa G, McCully RB, Oh JK, et al: Effects of pulmonary thromboendarterectomy on right-sided echocardiographic parameters in patients with chronic thromboembolic pulmonary hypertension. *Mayo Clin Proc* 81:777-782, 2006.

151. Menzel T, Kramm T, Wagner S, et al: Improvement of tricuspid regurgitation after pulmonary thromboendarterectomy. *Ann Thorac Surg* 73:756-761, 2002.

152. Strange C, Highland KB: Pulmonary hypertension in interstitial lung disease. *Curr Opin Pulmon Med* 11:452-455, 2005.

153. Bady E, Achkar A, Pascal S, et al: Pulmonary arterial hypertension in patients with sleep apnea syndrome. *Thorax* 55:934-939, 2000.

154. Shivalkar B, Van de Heyning C, Kerremans M, et al: Obstructive sleep apnea syndrome: more insights on structural and functional cardiac alterations, and the effects of treatment with continuous positive airway pressure. *J Am Coll Cardiol* 47:1433-1439, 2006.

155. Guidry UC, Mendes LA, Evans JC, et al: Echocardiographic features of the right heart in sleep-disordered breathing: The Framingham Heart Study. *Am J Respir Crit Care Med* 164:933-938, 2001.

156. Fishman AP: On keeping an eye on the right ventricle in sleep apnea. *Am J Respir Crit Care Med* 164:913-914, 2001.

157. Fung JW, Li TS, Choy DK, et al: Severe obstructive sleep apnea is associated with left ventricular diastolic dysfunction. *Chest* 121:422-429, 2002.

158. Niroumand M, Kuperstein R, Sasson Z, Hanly PJ, et al: Impact of obstructive sleep apnea on left ventricular mass and diastolic function. *Am J Respir Crit Care Med* 163:1632-1636, 2001.

159. Caso P, Galderisi M, Cicala S, et al: Association between myocardial right ventricular relaxation time and pulmonary arterial pressure in chronic obstructive lung disease: Analysis by pulsed Doppler tissue imaging. *J Am Soc Echocardiogr* 14:970-977, 2001.

160. Dallari R, Barozzi G, Pinelli G, et al: Predictors of survival in subjects with chronic obstructive pulmonary disease treated with long-term oxygen therapy. *Respiration* 61:8-13, 1994.

161. Nadrous HF, Pellikka PA, Krowka MJ, et al: Pulmonary hypertension in patients with idiopathic pulmonary fibrosis. *Chest* 128:2393-2399, 2005.

162. Arcasoy SM, Christie JD, Ferrari VA, et al: Echocardiographic assessment of pulmonary hypertension in patients with advanced lung disease. *Am J Respir Crit Care Med* 167:735-740, 2003.

163. Ferrazza A, Marino B, Giusti V, et al: Usefulness of left and right oblique subcostal view in the echo-Doppler investigation of pulmonary arterial blood flow in patients with chronic obstructive pulmonary disease. The subxiphoid view in the echo-Doppler evaluation of pulmonary blood flow. *Chest* 98:286-289, 1990.

164. Wigley FM, Lima JA, Mayes M, et al: The prevalence of undiagnosed pulmonary arterial hypertension in subjects with connective tissue disease at the secondary health care level of community-based rheumatologists (the UNCOVER study). *Arthritis Rheum* 52:2125-2132, 2005.

165. MacGregor AJ, Canavan R, Knight C, et al: Pulmonary hypertension in systemic sclerosis: Risk factors for progression and consequences for survival. *Rheumatology* 40:453-459, 2001.

166. de Azevedo AB, Sampio-Barras PD, Torres RM, Moreira C: Prevalence of pulmonary hypertension in systemic sclerosis. *Clin Exp Rheumatol* 23:447-454, 2005.

167. D'Andrea A, Stisi S, Bellissimo S, et al: Early impairment of myocardial function in systemic sclerosis: Non-invasive assessment by Doppler myocardial and strain rate imaging. *Eur J Echocardiogr* 6:407-418, 2005.

168. Sulica R, Teirstein AS, Kakarla S, et al: Distinctive clinical, radiographic, and functional characteristics of patients with sarcoidosis-related pulmonary hypertension. *Chest* 128:1483-1489, 2005.

169. Smedema J-P, Snoep G, van Kroonenburgh MP, et al: Cardiac involvement in patients with pulmonary sarcoidosis assessed at two university medical centers in the Netherlands. *Chest* 128:30-35, 2005.

170. Handa T, Nagai S, Miki S, et al: Incidence of pulmonary hypertension and its clinical relevance in patients with sarcoidosis. *Chest* 129:1246-1252, 2006.

171. Crawford LC, Panda M, Enjeti S: Refractory hypoxemia in right ventricular infarction: a case report. *South Med J* 99:79-81, 2006.

172. Shanoudy H, Soliman A, Raggi P, et al: Prevalence of patent foramen ovale and its contribution to hypoxemia in patients with obstructive sleep apnea. *Chest* 113:91-96, 1998.

173. Godart F, Porte HL, Rey C, et al: Postpneumonectomy interatrial right-to-left shunt: Successful percutaneous treatment. *Ann Thorac Surg* 64:834-836, 1997.

174. Zueger O, Soler M, Stulz P, et al: Dyspnea after pneumonectomy: The result of an atrial septal defect [see comment]. *Ann Thorac Surg* 63:1451-1452, 1997.

175. Estagnasie P, Djedaini K, LeBourdelles G, et al: Atrial septal aneurysm plus a patent foramen ovale. A predisposing factor for paradoxical embolism and refractory hypoxemia during pulmonary embolism. *Chest* 110:846-848, 1996.

176. Yun KL, Reichenspumer H, Schmoker J, et al: Heart transplantation complicated by a patent foramen ovale of the recipient atrial septum. *Ann Thorac Surg* 62:897-899, 1996.

177. Jander N, Minners J, Arentz T, et al: Transesophageal echocardiography in comparison with magnetic resonance imaging in the diagnosis of pulmonary vein stenosis after radiofrequency ablation therapy. *J Am Soc Echocardiogr* 18:654-659, 2005.

178. Packer DL, Keelan P, Munger TM, et al: Clinical presentation, investigation, and management of pulmonary vein stenosis complicating ablation for atrial fibrillation. *Circulation* 111:546-554, 2005.

179. Nilsson B, Chen X, Pehrson S, et al: Acute fatal pulmonary vein occlusion after catheter ablation of atrial fibrillation. *J Interv Card Electrophysiol* 11:127-130, 2004.

180. Arentz T, Jander N, von Rosenthal J, et al: Incidence of pulmonary vein stenosis 2 years after radiofrequency catheter ablation of refractory atrial fibrillation. *Eur Heart J* 24:963-969, 2003.

181. Marrouche NF, Martin DO, Wazni O, et al: Phased-array intracardiac echocardiography monitoring during pulmonary vein isolation in patients with atrial fibrillation: Impact on outcome and complications. *Circulation* 107:2710-2716, 2003.

182. Purerfellner H, Aichinger J, Martinek M, et al: Incidence, management, and outcome in significant pulmonary vein stenosis complicating ablation for atrial fibrillation. *Am J Cardiol* 93:1428-1431, 2004.

183. Bottio T, Angelini A, Testolin L, et al: How an undiscovered extensive peripheral pulmonary venous thrombosis destroyed a heart transplant: A case report. *Transplant Proc* 36:1551-1553, 2004.

184. Reilly MP, Plappert TJ, Wiegers SE: Cerebrovascular emboli related to pulmonary venous thrombosis after lung transplantation. *J Am Soc Echocardiogr* 11:299-302, 1998.

185. Ben-Dor I, Kramer MR, Raccah A, et al: Echocardiography versus right-sided heart catheterization among lung transplantation candidates. *Ann Thorac Surg* 81:1056-1060, 2006.

186. Hofer CK, Zollinger A, Rak M, et al: Therapeutic impact of intraoperative transesophageal echocardiography during noncardiac surgery. *Anaesthesia* 59:3-9, 2004.

187. Huang YC, Cheng YJ, Lin YH, et al: Graft failure caused by pulmonary venous obstruction diagnosed by intraoperative transesophageal echocardiography during lung transplantation. *Anesth Analg* 91:558-560, 2000.

188. Voelkel N, Quaife RA, Leinwand LA, et al: Right ventricular function and failure. *Circulation* 114:1883-1891, 2006.

189. Enriquez-Sarano M, Rossi A, Seward JB, et al: Determinants of pulmonary hypertension in left ventricular dysfunction. *J Am Coll Cardiol* 29:153-159, 1997.

190. Karatasakis GT, Karagounis LA, Kalyvas PA, et al: Prognostic significance of echocardiographically estimated right ventricular shortening in advanced heart failure. *Am J Cardiol* 82:329-334, 1998.

191. Di Salvo TG, Mathier M, Semigran MJ, Dec GW: Preserved right ventricular ejection fraction predicts exercise capacity and survival in advanced heart failure. *J Am Coll Cardiol* 25:1143-1153, 1995.

192. Faris R, Coats AJS, Henein MY: Echocardiography-derived variables predict outcome in patients with nonischemic dilated cardiomyopathy with or without a restrictive filling pattern. *Am Heart J* 144:343-350, 2002.

193. Hung J, Koelling T, Semigram MJ, et al: Usefulness of echocardiographic determined tricuspid regurgitation in predicting event-free survival in severe heart failure secondary to idiopathic-dilated cardiomyopathy or to ischemic cardiomyopathy. *Am J Cardiol* 82:1301-1303, 1998.

194. Sagie A, Freitas N, Paidal LR, et al: Doppler echocardiographic assessment of long-term progression of mitral stenosis in 103 patients: Valve area and right heart disease. *J Am Coll Cardiol* 28:472-479, 1996.

195. Fawzy ME, Hassan W, Stefadourous M, et al: Prevalence and fate of severe pulmonary hypertension in 559 consecutive patients with severe rheumatic mitral stenosis undergoing mitral balloon valvotomy. *J Heart Valve Dis* 13:942-947; discussion 947-948, 2004.

196. Hannoush H, Fawzy ME, Stefadourous M, et al: Regression of significant tricuspid regurgitation after mitral balloon valvotomy for severe mitral stenosis. *Am Heart J* 148:865-870, 2004.

197. Alexopoulos D, Lazzam C, Borrico S, et al: Isolated chronic mitral regurgitation with preserved systolic left ventricular function and severe pulmonary hypertension. *J Am Coll Cardiol* 14:319-322, 1989.

198. Rosenhek R, Radar F, Klaar U, et al: Outcome of watchful waiting in asymptomatic severe mitral regurgitation. *Circulation* 113:2238-2244, 2006.

199. Agricola E, Bombardini T, Oppizzi M, et al: Usefulness of latent left ventricular dysfunction assessed by Bowditch Treppe to predict stress-induced pulmonary hypertension in minimally symptomatic severe mitral regurgitation secondary to mitral valve prolapse. *Am J Cardiol* 95:414-417, 2005.

200. Yang H, Davidson WR Jr, Chambers CE, et al: Preoperative pulmonary hypertension is associated with postoperative left ventricular dysfunction in chronic organic mitral regurgitation: An echocardiographic and hemodymanic study. *J Am Soc Echocardiogr* 19:1051-1055, 2006.

Chapter 36

Echocardiographic Findings in Systemic Diseases Characterized by Immune-Mediated Injury

CARLOS A. ROLDAN, MD

The connective tissue diseases are chronic inflammatory states caused by autoimmunity. These diseases are more common in women than in men (with the exception of human leukocyte antigen B_{27}-related arthropathies), usually manifest from the second through the fifth decade, and cause significant morbidity and mortality.

Although the heart is not the principal target organ of these diseases, cardiovascular involvement is common and has serious consequences. The heart valves, pericardium, myocardium, coronary arteries, great vessels, and conduction system all may be involved. Estimates of the prevalence of cardiac involvement vary widely because of differences in study populations and methods of cardiac evaluation.

Echocardiography plays a major role in the better understanding of the prevalence, characteristics, severity, evolution, and response to therapy of the cardiovascular diseases associated with connective tissue diseases. The indications for echocardiography in patients with connective tissue diseases are similar to those of a general population. The increasing application of transesophageal, three-dimensional, intracardiac, tissue Doppler, myocardial strain, and contrast echocardiography will result in upward revision of current prevalence rates, characterization, prognosis, and therapy of heart disease in patients with connective tissue diseases. Echocardiography will play a major role in guiding and assessing the results of future percutaneous valve repair and replacement in these high-risk surgical candidates.

Systemic Lupus Erythematosus

Background

Systemic lupus erythematosus (SLE) is a chronic inflammatory disease that affects the musculoskeletal and mucocutaneous systems and frequently causes fatigue, myalgia, arthralgia or arthritis, photosensitivity, and serositis. Kidney, central nervous system (CNS), and cardiovascular disease are common and important causes of morbidity and mortality.

The most important forms of cardiac involvement in SLE are Libman-Sacks endocarditis, pericarditis, myocarditis, thrombosis or thromboembolism, coronary artery disease (CAD), and pulmonary hypertension.[1,2] Cardiovascular disease is the third most common cause of death of patients with SLE, after infections and renal disease.[3]

Associated Cardiovascular Involvement

Valve Disease

Valve disease in SLE is subdivided into Libman-Sacks (inflammatory) or thrombotic vegetations and leaflet thickening with or without fibrosis.[4,5] Mitral valve prolapse (MVP) is more prevalent (up to 22%) in lupus patients than in age-matched and gender-matched controls (5%).[6] About one third to one half of patients with SLE may have valve thickening or vegetations, but the degree of associated valve regurgitation is usually mild to moderate and therefore clinically silent.[4,5] However, subclinical disease may be complicated by cardioembolism or significant regurgitation as a result of recurrent immune-mediated valvulitis or infective endocarditis.[3,5,7]

The pathogenesis of valve disease in SLE includes an immune-complex mediated inflammation with subendothelial deposition of immunoglobulins and complement leading to an increased expression of $alpha_3$ $beta_1$ integrin on the endothelial cells; increased amount of collagen IV, laminin, and fibronectin; proliferation of blood vessels; inflammation, thrombus formation, and finally fibrosis.[8] The immune-complex mediated inflammation is exacerbated by a commonly associated increased systemic and local thrombogenesis mediated by antiphospholipid antibodies (aPL), which includes IgG or IgM anticardiolipin antibodies (aCL), lupus-anticoagulant (LA), or antibodies to plasma phospholipid-binding B_2-glycoprotein I. This constitutes the secondary antiphospholipid syndrome. The proposed mechanisms of valve damage by aPL include: (1) binding of aPL induces activation of endothelial cells and upregulation of the expression of adhesion molecules, secretion of cytokines, and abnormal metabolism of prostacyclins; (2) increased oxidized low-density lipoprotein (LDL) is taken up by macrophages, which leads to macrophage activation and further damage to endothelial cells; (3) aPL interfere with the regulatory functions of prothrombin, protein C, protein S, and tissue factor; and (4) a heparin-like induced thrombocytopenia.[9] However, the temporal association of valve disease with the duration, activity, and severity of SLE and the presence and levels of aPL is variable.[4,5,10-12] Libman-Sacks vegetations were originally described as cauliflower-like fibrous masses 2 to 4 mm in diameter that are located on any of the four cardiac valves. Active vegetations have central fibrinoid necrosis with fibroblastic proliferation and fibrosis surrounded by mononuclear and polymorphonuclear cellular infiltration, small hemorrhages, and platelet and fibrin thrombus.[2,4,5,13,14] Healed masses have central fibrosis, minimal or no inflammatory cell deposition, and no or hyalinized and endothelialized thrombus. Active, healed, and mixed masses can be seen in the same valve. Affected leaflets show replacement of the normal spongiosum and endothelial layers by postinflammatory fibrous tissue and infrequently by calcification. Almost all patients with Libman-Sacks vegetations have accompanying leaflet fibrosis, but fibrosis is more prevalent than Libman-Sacks vegetations among unselected patients with SLE.

Echocardiographic studies have shown that Libman-Sacks vegetations are usually less than 1 cm in diameter, vary in shape, have irregular borders, and have heterogeneous echo-density. The broad-based growths rarely move independently of the underlying valve structure. Lesions are more common on the mitral valve, can be attached to any portion of the mitral or aortic leaflets, and typically are seen on the atrial side of the mitral valve and on either side of the aortic cusps[4,5,7,15,16] (Figs. 36–1, 36–2, and 36–3). Lesions are rarely seen on right-sided heart valves. Echocardiographic studies estimate the prevalence of Libman-Sacks vegetations among patients with SLE as less than 10% by transthoracic echocardiography (TTE) and up to 35% by transesophageal echocardiography (TEE).[4,5,15,16]

Libman-Sacks vegetations and leaflet fibrosis are frequently accompanied by mild to moderate valve regurgitation but are otherwise usually clinically silent. Significant complications, such as cardioembolism and severe regurgitation resulting from recurrent or acute valvulitis, leaflet perforation including bioprosthetic leaflets, noninfective mitral valve chordal rupture, or infective endocarditis, occur in at least 20% of patients with valve disease.[5,17,18] Valve disease is more common in patients with focal ischemic brain injury on mag-

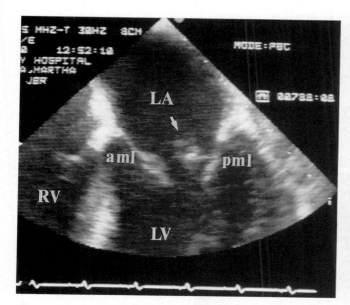

Figure 36–1. *Mitral valve Libman-Sacks vegetation and valve thickening in a patient with systemic lupus erythematosus. This transesophageal four-chamber view shows an irregular mass (arrow) of heterogeneous echo-density on the atrial side of the basal posterior mitral leaflet. Diffuse thickening predominantly of the middle and tip portions of the anterior (aml) and posterior (pml) mitral leaflets is also noted. Moderate mitral regurgitation was present. LA, left atrium; LV, left ventricle; RV, right ventricle. (From Roldan CA, Shively BK, Lau CC, et al: J Am Coll Cardiol 20:1127-1134, 1992.)*

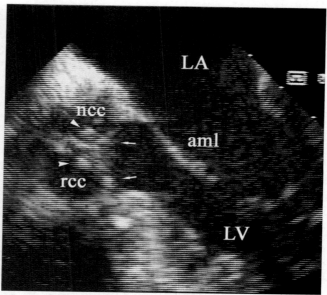

Figure 36–3. *Aortic valve Libman-Sacks vegetations and valve thickening in a patient with systemic lupus erythematosus. This transesophageal view longitudinal to the outflow tract demonstrates two well-defined small masses on the vessel side of the aortic right and noncoronary cusps (arrowheads). Mild localized thickening at the base of the right coronary cusp (rcc), the tip of the noncoronary cusp (ncc), and the tip of the anterior mitral leaflet (aml) is also noted (arrow). No aortic or mitral regurgitation was detected. LA, left atrium; LV, left ventricle; pml, posterior mitral leaflet.*

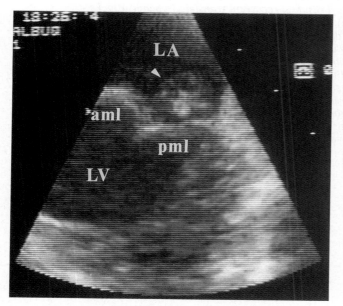

Figure 36–2. *Mitral valve Libman-Sacks vegetation and valve thickening in a patient with systemic lupus erythematosus. This transesophageal tangential portion of a four-chamber view shows a large mass (arrowhead) with heterogeneous echo-density on the atrial side of the basal posterior mitral leaflet. Associated diffuse thickening of both mitral leaflets is seen, and there was also mild mitral regurgitation. aml, anterior mitral leaflet; LA, left atrium; LV, left ventricle; pml, posterior mitral leaflet. (From Roldan CA, Shively BK, Lau CC, et al: J Am Coll Cardiol 20:1127-1134, 1992.)*

netic resonance imaging (MRI), in those with stroke or transient ischemic attack (TIA), and in those with non-focal neuropsychiatric manifestations of cognitive dysfunction, acute confusional state, seizures, or psychosis[7,19] (Figs. 36–4, 36–5, and 36–6). Transcranial Doppler studies also demonstrate a higher rates of microembolic events in patients with valve disease and neurologic events.[20-23] Infective endocarditis can mimic, accompany, or trigger a flare of SLE and can lead to severe valve dysfunction, heart failure (HF), and septic death. Similarly, a flare of SLE can mimic endocarditis (pseudoinfective endocarditis). A low white blood cell count, elevated aPL, and negative or low C-reactive protein may indicate pseudoinfective endocarditis.

The leaflet fibrosis (increased thickness and echo-reflectance) accompanying Libman-Sacks vegetations may cause reduced leaflet mobility, but valve stenosis is rare (<3%). In a TEE study, 48% of unselected patients with SLE who were younger than 60 years of age had abnormal leaflets, defined as leaflet thickness greater than 3 mm.[4,5,15] Because the decrease specificity of TTE for valve thickening, studies using this technique report highly variable but lower rates of valve thickening. Shadowing caused by leaflet scarring is observed in 12% of patients. Annular, subvalvular, and right-sided heart involvement is rare.

The natural history of SLE-associated valve disease appears to parallel that of the primary disease. Using

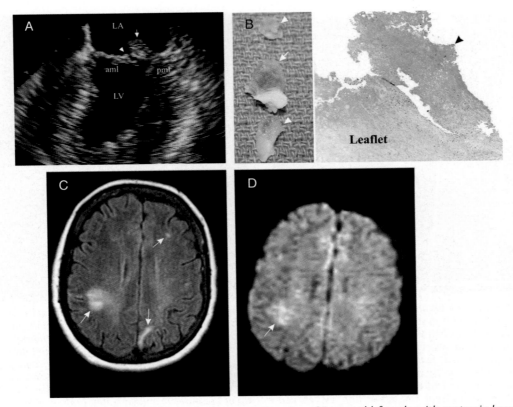

Figure 36–4. Mitral valve Libman-Sacks vegetations in a 31-year-old female with systemic lupus erythematosus and recurrent transient ischemic attacks. A, This transesophageal echocardiogram demonstrates a large vegetation on the atrial side and basal portion of the posterior mitral leaflet (pml) (arrow) and a small vegetation on the atrial side of the anterior mitral leaflet (aml) (arrowhead). Both leaflets had diffuse moderate thickening. Only mild mitral regurgitation was detected. The patient underwent mitral valve replacement as a result of recurrent transient ischemic attacks despite anticoagulation. B, Large vegetation (arrow) from the posterior leaflet and small vegetations (arrowheads) from the anterior leaflet. Histology of the leaflet revealed inflammation with mononuclear cells and fibrosis. Vegetations of predominant fibrinous material well adhered to the leaflet were demonstrated (arrowhead). C, This fluid attenuated inversion recovery magnetic resonance image demonstrates a recent cerebral infarct in the right occipitoparietal white matter (arrow on left). There are also left occipital and frontal lobe small cerebral infarcts (arrows on right). D, This diffusion-weighted image demonstrates a large area of hyperintensity (focally restricted diffusion) and confirms a recent infarct in the right occipitoparietal white matter (arrow). The cerebral infarcts in the left occipital and frontal hyperintense lesions are not visible by diffusion-weighted image indicating they are old infarcts. LA, left atrium; LV, left ventricle.

serial TEE, valve disease, especially valve vegetations, may appear de novo, resolve, change appearance, or progress independently of SLE disease duration, severity, activity, or therapy[5,15] (Fig. 36–7). The effect on valve masses of steroids or long-term anticoagulation has been variable.[24] Patients with valve vegetations or with moderate to severe valve dysfunction have a threefold to fourfold higher combined incidence of stroke, peripheral embolism, need for valve surgery, and death over a 2- to 8-year follow-up as compared to those without or mild valve disease.[5,7,17]

Rheumatic and SLE valve disease may have similar immunopathogenesis.[25] Except for elevation of antistreptolysin antibodies in rheumatic carditis, acute rheumatic and SLE endocarditis may have similar clinical, serologic, and echocardiographic findings. In their chronic states, the echocardiographic characteristics of these two conditions may overlap. In patients greater than 60 years of age, the pattern of valve scarring characteristic of SLE may be obscured by changes resulting from aging or atherosclerosis. The echocardiographic appearance of Libman-Sacks, thrombotic, and infective vegetations also overlap.[5,14,24,26,27]

Pericarditis

As many as 50% of patients with SLE suffer at least one episode of symptomatic pericarditis.[28,29] Most episodes are acute and are frequently associated with valvulitis, myocarditis, pleuritis, nephritis, and active

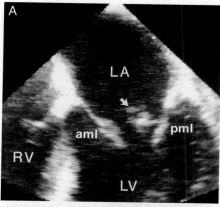

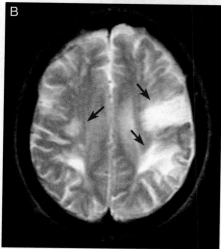

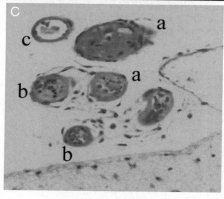

Figure 36-5. Mitral valve Libman-Sacks vegetation in a 47-year-old female with systemic lupus erythematosus and recurrent fatal stroke. A, This transesophageal echocardiogram demonstrates thickening of the mid and tip portions of the anterior (aml) and posterior (pml) mitral leaflets with a large vegetation on the midportion and atrial side of the posterior leaflet (arrow). B, This T2-weighted magnetic resonance imaging in this patient demonstrates generalized cortical atrophy, multiple areas of old cerebral infarcts characterized by loss of both gray and white matter (large areas of hyperintensity, arrows) in a cortical or subcortical pattern, and multiple areas of deep white matter abnormality consistent with widespread ischemic cerebrovascular disease. C, Histopathology of the brain demonstrated, cerebral vessels occlusion by fibrin thrombi (a); intimal hyperplasia, vessel wall thickening, and platelet thrombi (b); and an occasional patent blood vessel (c). LA, left atrium; LV, left ventricle; RV, right ventricle.

SLE.[29] Cardiac tamponade and constrictive pericarditis are uncommon (<2%).[28,29] Rarely, acute pericarditis and cardiac tamponade can be the initial manifestation of SLE. Because an effusion is not always present, the diagnosis of pericarditis rests on manifestations of the clinical syndrome not the echocardiogram. Because pericardial chest pain can be confounded or masked by musculoskeletal or pleural pain, echocardiography is of diagnostic value in these patients. Pericarditis typically yields serofibrinous, fibrinous, and rarely serosanguineous exudative fluid containing low complement level and antinuclear antibodies. By immunofluorescence, the pericardium shows granular deposition of immunoglobulins and C3 supporting an immune-complex–mediated injury.[30]

An effusion without accompanying signs and symptoms of pericarditis in a patient with SLE probably results from mild pericarditis or another process, such as nephrotic syndrome or uremia. Asymptomatic effusions are common incidental findings in patients with SLE, occurring in as many as 20% of those hospitalized with active disease.

Echocardiography is the standard method for the evaluation of suspected SLE pericarditis to assess the size of an effusion and look for signs of tamponade physiology, but findings are not specific for SLE disease. Tamponade is uncommon in SLE pericarditis, but the high morbidity rate of this complication and the potential for an atypical clinical presentation mandate careful evaluation.[28,29] As in tamponade from any cause, echocardiographic indicators of tamponade should prompt intensive monitoring or therapy. Echocardiographically guided pericardiocentesis has been successfully performed in series of patients with lupus with hemodynamically compromising pericardial effusions.[28] Also, serial echocardiography after fluid drainage or after antiinflammatory therapy help guide the need of other interventions.

Rarely, constrictive or infectious pericarditis may complicate SLE pericarditis.[31] Echocardiography is an effective screening method when constriction is under consideration. Echocardiography is insensitive for the detection of mild or moderate pericardial thickening. Cardiac magnetic resonance imaging or computed tomography (CT) are preferred methods for assessing pericardial thickness and are important confirmatory tests when the echocardiogram suggests constriction.

Myocardial Disease

Primary myocarditis is characterized by small foci of fibrinoid necrosis with infiltrates of plasma cells and lymphocytes, variable degrees of interstitial connective tissue, and focal myocardial scarring.[32,33] Immunofluorescence demonstrate granular immune-complexes and complement in the walls and perivascular tissues of

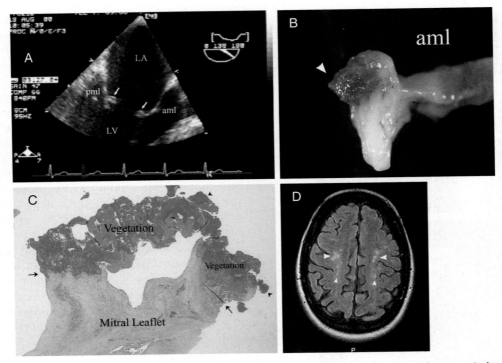

Figure 36–6. Mitral valve Libman-Sacks vegetations in a 28-year-old female with systemic lupus erythematosus and acute confusional state and cognitive dysfunction. A, This transesophageal echocardiographic view demonstrates small vegetations (arrows) on the atrial side and tip portions of the anterior (aml) and posterior mitral leaflets (pml) with associated leaflets' thickening and decreased mobility. Patient underwent valve replacement because associated symptomatic severe mitral regurgitation. B, Diffuse thickening with a Libman-Sacks vegetation on the atrial side and tip portion of the anterior leaflet is noted (arrowhead). C, Vegetation attached to the leaflets (arrows) demonstrated amorphous eosinophilic fibrinous to granular deposits admixed with histiocytes, inflammatory cells, and superficial microthrombi (arrowheads). The mitral leaflet demonstrated focal areas of myxoid degeneration and fibrinoid necrosis but no inflammation. D, This fluid attenuated inversion recovery image shows multifocal hyperintensities in the subcortical white matter typical of small infarcts (arrowheads). LA, left atrium; LV, left ventricle.

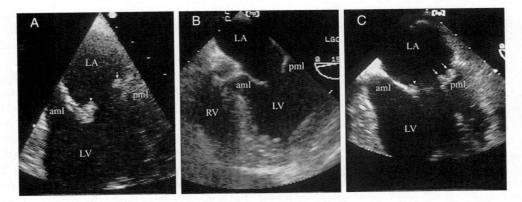

Figure 36–7. Resolution and reappearance of mitral valve Libman-Sacks vegetations in a 37-year-old female with systemic lupus erythematosus and a stroke. A, This initial transesophageal echocardiogram demonstrates two mitral valve vegetations: one on the atrial side of the tip of the anterior mitral leaflet (aml) (arrowhead) and another on the midportion of the posterior leaflet (pml) (arrow). Diffuse thickening of both mitral leaflets is also visible. Moderate mitral regurgitation was detected. B, Follow-up transesophageal echocardiogram obtained 2 months later shows resolution of both mitral valve vegetations and improvement in leaflet thickening. Mitral regurgitation was only mild. C, This transesophageal echocardiogram obtained 20 months later, when the patient had inactive systemic lupus erythematosus, shows reappearance of three mitral valve vegetations: one on the anterior mitral leaflet (arrowhead) and two on the posterior mitral leaflet (arrows). The thickening of both mitral leaflets also worsened. LA, left atrium; LV, left ventricle; RV, right ventricle.

myocardial blood vessels.[33] An association of cellular antigen Ro (SS-A) and La (SS-B) antibodies and myocarditis has been established, but their primary pathogenic role is still undefined.[34] Primary myocarditis with left ventricular (LV) diastolic and rarely global or regional systolic dysfunction occur in at least 10% of patients.[2,32,33] Rarely, acute lupus myocarditis manifested as clinical HF with global or segmental LV dysfunction may be the initial manifestation of active SLE.[33] Myocardial diastolic and less commonly systolic dysfunction in SLE result more often from endothelial dysfunction-mediated microvascular CAD. Rarely, small vessel vasculitis or epicardial coronary arteritis is a causal factor. Many Doppler echocardiography series including tissue Doppler in asymptomatic young patients without systemic or pulmonary hypertension and normal LV systolic function have demonstrated a high prevalence (15% to 35%) of subclinical myocardial disease manifested by variable degrees of LV and right ventricular (RV) diastolic dysfunction.[32,35-37] Parameters of impaired LV relaxation by mitral inflow, mitral annulus tissue Doppler, and color Doppler flow propagation velocities are predominant. In these studies, LV filling abnormalities occurred more frequently in patients with active SLE (64% versus 14%). Abnormal LV Doppler filling variables have been associated with reversible, fixed, and mixed myocardial perfusion defects in young patients with active SLE and normal coronary arteries.[38] As indicators of interstitial myocardial disease, echocardiographic tissue characterization demonstrates a decrease in the magnitude of cyclic variation of integrated backscatter.[37] These findings explain a greater than 20% prevalence of slow and disorganized myocardial conduction on signal average electrocardiography in unselected patients.[32] Also in unselected patients, the prevalence of a reduced resting LV ejection fraction (EF) is less than 20%.[4,5,8,32,35-37] Approximately one third of patients with SLE in a study demonstrated an exercise-induced fall or subnormal rise in EF.[39] Finally, a potentially reversible chloroquine sulfate-induced dilated or restrictive cardiomyopathy with marked myocardial cytoplasmic vacuolization and extensive myelin figures on histology has been recently reported.[40] Therefore, echocardiography may not separate active or past myocarditis from nontransmural ischemic myocardial injury in patients with active SLE. Coronary angiography and endomyocardial biopsy may be required to separate these conditions.

Thrombotic Diseases

Patients with SLE are subject to intracardiac thrombosis and cerebral or systemic thromboembolism resulting from underlying valve or myocardial disease independently of or exacerbated by aPL-induced thrombogenesis.[4,5,7,9,10,19] Substrates of high embolic potential are Libman-Sacks or thrombotic vegetations. Mitral valve vegetations are two to four times more common and strong independent predictors of focal ischemic brain injury on magnetic resonance imaging, stroke or transient ischemic attack, and nonfocal neuropsychiatric manifestations.[7,19] Also, a high prevalence of microembolic events using transcranial Doppler echocardiography has been demonstrated in patients with cerebral ischemic events.[22,23] Previous TTE and postmortem series of patients with SLE frequently identify Libman-Sacks vegetations as a probable cause of cardioembolism. Other substrates with high embolic potential are acute anterior myocardial infarction (MI), reduced LV EF (<35%), and atrial fibrillation (AFib). If substrates of high embolic potential are not identified on TTE, TEE is a reasonable next step to evaluate the presence of valve vegetations, atrial stasis or thrombi, aortic atheroma, and patent foramen ovale (PFO) or interatrial septal aneurysm.

Coronary Artery Disease

Autopsy studies show a 25% prevalence of epicardial coronary atherosclerosis in patients with SLE. Clinically evident disease is found in at least 10% of patients. After controlling for traditional risk factors for CAD, the risk of functional (abnormal vasodilation or microvascular disease) and atherosclerotic CAD in lupus patients is four to eight times higher than matched controls.[1,4,5] Chronic (>10 years) immune-mediated inflammation frequently exacerbated by aPL lead to CAD.[9,41-44] The following mechanisms have been proposed:

1. Activation of cellular and humoral immunity with activation of macrophages, CD4 T-cells and dendritic cells. The cytotoxicity of these cells to the endothelium and vascular wall results in increased vasoconstriction via decreased production of prostacyclin and prostaglandin I and increased thrombosis via release of platelet-derived growth factor and thromboxane A_2. The cytotoxic cells also produce interferon-γ, which destabilizes atherosclerotic plaques by suppressing synthesis of collagen, increase proliferation of smooth muscle cells, and activation of macrophages to release free radicals and matrix metalloproteinases.

2. Increased oxidation of low-density lipoprotein.

3. Increased production of inflammatory cytokines and chemokines such as heat shock proteins, C-reactive protein, rheumatoid factor, tumor necrosis factor-alpha (TNF-α), and interleukins. Interleukins are expressed on the endothelium of coronary arteries, recruit inflammatory cells, promote abnormal vascular smooth cell prolifera-

tion, induce oxidative stress, endothelial apoptosis, and up-regulation of adhesion molecules and chemokines).

4. Exacerbation of dyslipidemia, homocystinemia, and insulin resistance.

In patients with SLE, angina and MI may also result from coronary arteritis, in situ coronary thrombosis, or from embolization to a coronary artery from valve vegetations. Coronary arteritis should be suspected in a young patient with an acute coronary syndrome (ACS), especially if accompanied by active SLE and vasculitis affecting other organs. Coronary embolism or in situ thrombosis is rare but warrant consideration when MI occurs with no anginal prodrome or with a cardioembolic substrate or aPL.

In patients with or without chest pain syndrome and regional wall motion abnormalities on echocardiography, coronary angiography most commonly reveals normal coronaries or nonobstructive CAD.[12,45] Therefore, in these patients frequently unable to exercise, dobutamine stress echocardiography (DSE) yield low rate of abnormal results. Of uncertain significance, dobutamine echocardiography in patients with lupus has demonstrated up to 50% frequency of LV outflow tract gradient as compared to 20% reported in patients that do not have SLE.[45] Suspected CAD may warrant coronary angiography because of the confounding clinical and echocardiographic features of lupus myocarditis.

Pulmonary Hypertension

Pulmonary hypertension occurs in 5% to 14% of patients with SLE. The most common causes include interstitial lung disease, vasculitis, and thromboembolism.[46] Echocardiography is currently the technique most commonly used to diagnose and evaluate response to therapy of pulmonary hypertension in these patients. Myocardial and valve disease should also be considered as causes. Doppler echocardiography is valuable in the diagnosis, assessment of severity, and follow-up of SLE-associated pulmonary hypertension.

Primary Antiphospholipid Syndrome

Background

Primary antiphospholipid syndrome (PAPS) is defined by: (1) presence of aPL; (2) venous or arterial thrombosis or complicated pregnancy (fetal loss, preeclampsia, and eclampsia); and (3) lack of diagnostic criteria for other connective tissue disease. The diagnosis is established by one or more clinical criteria and one type of aPL on two or more occasions at least 6 weeks apart. The proposed pathogenesis of cardiovascular disease associated with PAPS is the result of aPL-induced functional and structural endothelial dysfunction, increased platelet aggregation, increased intrinsic and extrinsic coagulation pathways, and decreased fibrinolysis.[9,47,48] Cardiovascular disease occurs in 50% to 75% of patients with PAPS and manifest as valve disease, intracardiac thrombosis, pulmonary hypertension, nonobstructive coronary disease and myocardial disease.

Associated Cardiovascular Involvement

Valve Disease

Valve disease is the most common cardiac manifestation of PAPS. The prevalence, distribution, and characteristics of valve disease in PAPS mimic those of SLE.[49] Valve lesions are characterized by intravalvular thrombosis with focal necrosis and hemorrhage, vascular proliferation, histiocytic and fibroblastic infiltration, laminated and verrucous fibrin deposits, laminated or nodular fibrosis, and focal calcification.[14,50,51] Valve disease manifests as valve thickening, valve vegetations, and less commonly valve regurgitation. In controlled series using TTE, the prevalence of left-sided and predominantly of mitral valve disease ranges from 30% to 40% as compared to less than 5% in controls.[52] Using TEE, the prevalence of valve disease is higher (60% to 80%).[53] As in patients with SLE, valve lesions frequently persist unchanged (50% to 60%), appear de novo (20% to 30%), resolve (20%), and uncommonly progress (<20%) or need valve replacement (<10%) during a 1-year to 5-year follow-up.[54,55] Valve lesions have been associated with arterial thrombosis or thromboembolism to the brain (50%), coronary arteries (20% to 25%), and other arterial beds.[53,56] The effect of anticoagulation or antiinflammatory therapy on valve lesions has been variable, but no controlled longitudinal studies are available.[55,57,58]

Intracardiac Thrombosis

Patients with PAPS have an increased prevalence (15% to 20%) of right-sided and left-sided intracardiac thrombi.[59-61] Intracardiac thrombi include: (1) thrombotic valve vegetations consisting of platelet or fibrin thrombi formed on structurally abnormal or rarely normal valves, (2) left atrial appendage thrombi, (3) atrial or ventricular wall or free floating intracavitary thrombi, (4) obstructive thrombi creating a functional tricuspid or mitral stenosis,[62] and (5) atrial spontaneous echocardiographic contrast in patients in normal sinus rhythm. Right-sided heart thrombi are commonly associated with deep venous thrombosis

(DVT) or pulmonary embolism (PE) and rarely with intracardiac catheters. Intracardiac thrombi are best detected by TEE.

Pulmonary Hypertension

The prevalence of pulmonary hypertension on prospective echocardiographic series is at least 20% to 25% and is predominantly the result of chronic and recurrent pulmonary embolism and uncommonly to an abnormal vasospastic or in situ thrombotic vasculopathy.[55] Pulmonary hypertension is exacerbated by pregnancy and is one of the causes of death in these patients.[63]

Coronary Artery Disease

Hemostatic abnormalities and increased intake of oxidized low-density lipoprotein by activated macrophages in the coronary vessel wall cause endothelial damage and dysfunction, vasoconstriction, and thrombosis leading to functional or thrombotic microvascular disease and less often to atherosclerosis. A higher prevalence of increased intima-media thickness is common, but no plaques of the carotid arteries are reported in these patients.[64-67] A high prevalence (20% to 35%) of MI has been reported in patients with PAPS and results from microvascular disease, in situ coronary thrombosis, or coronary thromboembolism.[55,67-70] There are no series systematically using resting or stress echocardiography for detection of epicardial or microvascular CAD in these patients.

Myocardial Disease

In small controlled cross-sectional series using Doppler echocardiography in asymptomatic patients with PAPS, a high prevalence of LV diastolic dysfunction, predominantly of impaired relaxation, has been reported.[71,72] The mechanism of diastolic dysfunction includes primary myocardial disease, thrombotic microangiopathy, or decreased microvascular coronary vasodilation.[73] Rarely, catastrophic PAPS may manifest as dilated cardiomyopathy (DCM) with LV thrombus. RV diastolic dysfunction, predominantly impaired relaxation, is also common in patients with pulmonary hypertension.[36]

Rheumatoid Arthritis

Background

Rheumatoid arthritis is characterized by symmetric arthritis, potentially involving any synovial joint but usually affecting the metacarpophalangeal and proximal interphalangeal joints and wrists. In this disease, the patient's serum contains rheumatoid factor, a group of IgM or IgG antibodies directed against autologous IgG. No arthritic manifestations of rheumatoid arthritis include rheumatoid nodules, systemic vasculitis, glomerulonephritis, pulmonary fibrosis, and cardiovascular disease.[74,75] Clinically apparent heart disease occurs in as many as 25% to 40% of patients with rheumatoid arthritis and is more frequent in patients with long-standing disease; active extraarticular, erosive polyarticular, and nodular disease; systemic vasculitis; high serum titers of rheumatoid factor, an erythrocyte sedimentation rate greater than 55 mm per hour, and positive antinuclear antibodies. Heart disease is the third leading cause of death in patients with rheumatoid arthritis and account for nearly 40% of deaths in these patients.[76,77]

Associated Cardiovascular Involvement

Coronary Artery Disease

After controlling for traditional atherogenic risk factors, patients with rheumatoid arthritis have CAD two to three times more common than matched controls. Rheumatoid patients are often older than 50 years and more prone to atherosclerotic CAD. However, abnormal coronary artery vasodilation or microvascular disease is common. Coronary arteritis is rare. CAD accounts for 40% to 50% of the mortality of patients with rheumatoid arthritis.[74,78-80] The pathogenesis of their CAD is similar to that described for patients with SLE.[74,81-83] Patients with erythrocyte sedimentation rate (ESR) greater than 60 mm^3, higher levels of C-reactive protein, serum amyloid, soluble vascular adhesion molecule-1, and interferon-γ have reduced small and large arteries elasticity and have a twofold independent risk for MI, congestive heart failure (CHF), stroke, and cardiovascular mortality as compared to matched controls.[84-86] Patients with acute coronary syndromes have a higher recurrence rate of events and mortality than matched controls (58% versus 30% and 40% versus 15%, respectively).[87,88] A high prevalence (up to 61%) of subclinical CAD as determined by coronary artery calcification on electron-beam computed tomography is seen in patients with established disease as compared to those with recent onset of the disease (43%) and matched controls (38%).[89] Furthermore, cyclooxygenase-2 selective inhibitors, which inhibit prostaglandin I-2 (a vasodilator and inhibitor of platelet aggregation) and nonsteroidal antiinflammatory drugs (NSAIDs) increase the risk of acute coronary syndromes in patients with rheumatoid arthritis.[90] Amelioration of inflammation with low dose steroids, TNF-α blockers, or statins may decreased the effects of vascular inflammation and dysfunction and consequently of coronary events.[91-93] Coronary vasculitis is rare and affects small-sized or medium-sized intramyocardial arteries.[94]

As in the general population, resting and stress echocardiography are useful in the detection of wall motion abnormalities in those with obstructive CAD but have decreased sensitivity for microvascular disease. However, TTE can assess coronary flow reserve in those with microvascular disease.[95]

Pericarditis

Echocardiographic studies have shown pericardial effusions in as many as 50% of patients with rheumatoid arthritis, but symptomatic pericarditis is less common.[96] Pericarditis tends to occur in patients with active disease. Immunofluorescent staining of the pericardium reveals deposits of IgG, IgM, C3, and C1q, indicating autoimmune injury.[97] The pericardial effusion is exudative and bloody with a low glucose level, and it may contain rheumatoid factor. As with SLE pericarditis, tamponade and constriction are rarely reported. The role of echocardiography in the diagnosis and management of rheumatoid effusions parallels its role in SLE pericarditis.

Valve Disease

Estimates of the prevalence of valve disease in rheumatoid arthritis are highly variable. The reported prevalence rates of valve abnormalities is as low as 30% and usually occur in three forms, sometimes in four: (1) healed valvulitis with residual leaflet fibrosis and regurgitation and rarely stenosis, (2) valve nodules, (3) acute on chronic valvulitis, and rarely (4) acute valvulitis with variable degrees of regurgitation and with Libman-Sacks–like vegetations.[98-100] Acute and chronic valvulitis with resulting leaflet thickening and fibrosis is indistinguishable from that seen in SLE. In contrast, valve nodules appear to be unique to rheumatoid arthritis. These nodules can also be seen on valve rings, papillary muscle tips, and atrial or ventricular endocardium. Histologically, the valve nodules resemble subcutaneous nodules, containing a central portion of fibrinoid necrosis surrounded by a mononuclear infiltrate and sometimes by Langhans cells and giant cells. It is believed these nodules result from a process of focal vasculitis.

On echocardiography, rheumatoid valve nodules usually appear as small (<0.5 cm^2), spheroid masses with homogeneous reflectance, usually appearing singly and on any portion of the leaflet. The adjacent leaflet appears normal or shows mild sclerosis. This picture is unlike that of Libman-Sacks vegetations (compare Figs. 36–1 to 36–5 with Fig. 36–8). Acute valvulitis with superimposed valve masses mimics that of Libman-Sacks endocarditis (Fig. 36–9).

Rheumatoid valve disease is generally mild and asymptomatic, and it is less likely than SLE valve disease to result in clinically significant valve dysfunction. However, three uncommon manifestations

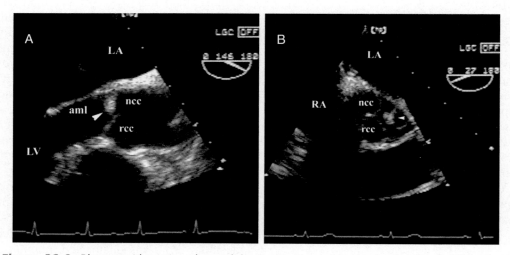

Figure 36–8. Rheumatoid aortic valve nodules in young asymptomatic patients. A, This transesophageal echocardiographic view longitudinal to the outflow tract in a 48-year-old woman with rheumatoid arthritis demonstrates an oval shape nodule with well defined borders and homogeneous soft tissue echo-reflectance within the midportion of the aortic noncoronary cusp (ncc) (arrowhead). The appearance of the right coronary cusps is normal. Aortic valve regurgitation was not demonstrated. B, This transesophageal echocardiographic short-axis view of the aortic valve in a 43-year-old man with rheumatoid arthritis demonstrates a well-defined nodule with homogeneously increased echo-reflectance within the tip and midportion of the left coronary cusp (arrowhead). Note the normal appearance of the uninvolved portions of the cusp and that of the ncc and right coronary cusps (rcc). Mild aortic valve regurgitation was detected. aml, anterior mitral leaflet; LA, left atrium; LV, left ventricle; RA, right atrium.

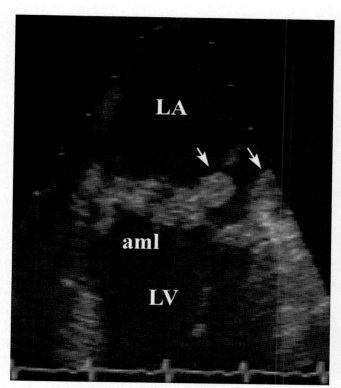

Figure 36–9. *Severe mitral valvulitis with Libman-Sacks–like vegetations in a 52-year-old female with severe rheumatoid arthritis and recurrent transient ischemic attacks. This close-up four chamber transesophageal echocardiographic view when patient presented with a transient ischemic attack demonstrates severe thickening with soft tissue echo-reflectance of the anterior and posterior mitral leaflets. Large, multi-lobed, with irregular borders, and with soft tissue echo-reflectant masses are noted on the atrial side of the anterior (aml) and posterior mitral leafets (arrows). LA, left atrium; LV, left ventricle.*

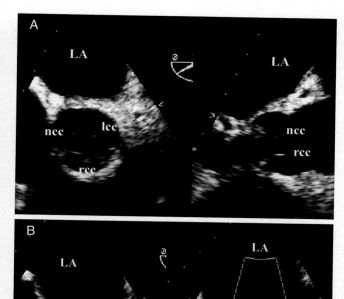

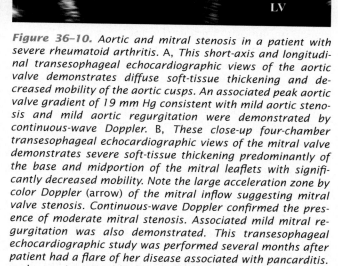

Figure 36–10. *Aortic and mitral stenosis in a patient with severe rheumatoid arthritis. A, This short-axis and longitudinal transesophageal echocardiographic views of the aortic valve demonstrates diffuse soft-tissue thickening and decreased mobility of the aortic cusps. An associated peak aortic valve gradient of 19 mm Hg consistent with mild aortic stenosis and mild aortic regurgitation were demonstrated by continuous-wave Doppler. B, These close-up four-chamber transesophageal echocardiographic views of the mitral valve demonstrates severe soft-tissue thickening predominantly of the base and midportion of the mitral leaflets with significantly decreased mobility. Note the large acceleration zone by color Doppler (arrow) of the mitral inflow suggesting mitral valve stenosis. Continuous-wave Doppler confirmed the presence of moderate mitral stenosis. Associated mild mitral regurgitation was also demonstrated. This transesophageal echocardiographic study was performed several months after patient had a flare of her disease associated with pancarditis. aml, anterior mitral leaflet; LA, left atrium; LV, left ventricle; lcc, left coronary cusp; ncc, noncoronary cusp; rcc, right coronary cusp.*

of the disease have been described: (1) valve thrombus overimposed on a valve nodule, Libman-Sacks–like vegetations, or valve strands complicated with systemic embolism[101,102]; (2) acute mitral or aortic valvulitis resulting in severe valve regurgitation and rarely stenosis[103] (Fig. 36–10); and (3) acute severe valve regurgitation from "rupture" of a nodule or a large nodule affecting leaflets coapation.[104,105]

Myocardial Disease

Some patients with rheumatoid arthritis have myocarditis, myocardial nodules, or cardiac amyloidosis. Evidence of present or past myocarditis is revealed at autopsy in as many as 30% of patients, but decreased LV systolic function by echocardiography is less common. Myocarditis has been associated with the presence of anti-SS-A/anti-SS-B autoantibod-

ies.[106] Recent controlled Doppler echocardiographic series using pulse and tissue Doppler, transmitral color flow propagation velocity, and myocardial performance index in young asymptomatic and patients who are not hypertensive have demonstrated a high prevalence of diastolic dysfunction, predominantly of impaired relaxation.[107,108] Also, large longitudinal series have demonstrated a high incidence (35% to 40%) of clinical diastolic HF independent of traditional cardiovascular risk factors for diastolic dysfunction.[109-111] The incidence of HF decreases with TNF-α blocker therapy.[112] As a result of residual interstitial myocardial fibrosis, patients with diastolic dysfunction have higher dispersion of repolarization as manifested by prolongation of the uncorrected and corrected QT dispersion.[113] Recently, a dilated or restrictive cardiomyopathy resulting from chloroquine therapy and characterized by myocyte enlargement resulting from perinuclear vacuolization and abundant myelinoid figures within myocytes has been reported.[114] The echocardiographic features of amyloidosis resulting from rheumatoid arthritis are nonspecific but may coexist or mimic rheumatoid constrictive pericarditis.

Pulmonary Hypertension

Pulmonary hypertension with normal pulmonary venous pressure may result from interstitial fibrosis, pulmonary vasculitis, or obliterative bronchiolitis. The prevalence of this disease is unknown but probably low. The mortality rate is high within 1 year of diagnosis. Prompt diagnosis is vital. Lung biopsy or bronchoalveolar lavage may confirm pulmonary vasculitis and bronchiolitis obliterans, both of which are frequently responsive to immunosuppressive therapy.

Pulmonary hypertension may not be accompanied by clinical or echocardiographic evidence of cor pulmonale, especially if the pulmonary artery (PA) pressure is less than 50 mm Hg. In controlled series of asymptomatic patients, the prevalence of pulmonary hypertension on echocardiography is five times higher in rheumatoid patients than in controls (21% versus 4%).[115]

If pulmonary hypertension is identified, echocardiography should also be used to rule out left atrial hypertension or a potential cause (e.g., LV dysfunction, mitral valve disease) and to follow the response to therapy.[116] In the absence of left-sided heart disease, the search for a treatable pulmonary cause should be pursued. When pulmonary hypertension is diagnosed with symptoms potentially caused by right-sided HF (e.g., exertional dyspnea, fatigue, peripheral edema), echocardiography is useful to assess the severity of RV dysfunction and tricuspid regurgitation and to estimate right atrial and pulmonary artery pressures.

Ankylosing Spondylitis

Background

Ankylosing spondylitis and other human leukocyte antigen-B$_{27}$-related (HLA-B$_{27}$-related) arthropathies are autoimmune diseases characterized by inflammation of the vertebral and sacroiliac joints. Arthritis of other joints, uveitis, and proximal aortitis and aortic valvulitis are common. Other complications are rare, and although arthritis may be disabling, the overall prognosis is good.

Associated Cardiovascular Involvement

Aortitis and Valve Disease

Among patients with ankylosing spondylitis, the prevalence rates of ascending aorta and aortic valve disease have varied widely, but aortitis and aortic regurgitation are commonly clinically important. Evidence of present or past inflammation is found in all layers of the aortic wall, and the process leads to dilation, fibrosis, and calcification.[117] The reason for selective injury of the proximal aorta is unknown. Aortic regurgitation (AR) is generally mild to moderate and results from the combination of dilation of the aortic root and annulus and thickening with retraction of the aortic cusps. Significant regurgitation is usually caused by acute valvulitis or supervening infective endocarditis.[118] The mitral valve may become abnormal when aortic root fibrosis extends downward into the anterior mitral leaflet. This often results in localized fibrotic thickening at the base of the anterior mitral leaflet, a condition called "subaortic bump."

In several echocardiographic studies, including a TEE series, aortic root thickening or sclerosis, increased stiffness, and dilation range from 20% to 60%, 60%, and 25% to 50% of patients, respectively.[119-121] Aortic valve thickening seen in 40% of patients manifested mainly as nodularities of the aortic cusps. Mitral valve thickening seen in one third of patients manifested predominantly as basal thickening of the anterior mitral leaflet, forming the characteristic subaortic bump. Valve regurgitation seen in almost half of patients was moderate in one third of them. Aortic root disease and valve disease were related to duration of the disease but not to its activity, severity, or therapy[119-122] (Figs. 36–11, 36–12, and 36–13). Mitral valve prolapse or myxomatous mitral leaflets with mild or moderate regurgitation is reported in 10% to 15% of patients.[121]

Conduction Abnormalities

Atrioventricular (AV) and intraventricular conduction blocks occur with a greater than expected frequency (>20%) in patients with ankylosing spondylitis.[123] Echocardiographic studies have demonstrated an association of conduction abnormalities with aortic root thickening and subaortic bump, "suggesting a role for extension of aortic root

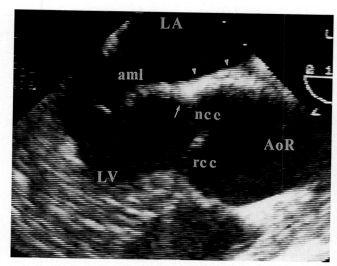

Figure 36–11. *Aortic root and aortic and mitral valve disease in a patient with ankylosing spondylitis. This transesophageal echocardiographic view longitudinal to the outflow tract in a 31-year-old man with progressive dyspnea of exertion and a diastolic murmur shows marked thickening of the posteromedial aortic root (arrowheads) extending to the basal portion of the noncoronary cusp (ncc) and into the base and midportions of the anterior mitral leaflet (subaortic bump, arrow). Mild thickening of the right coronary cusp (rcc) tip and mild aortic root dilation are also noted. Moderate to severe aortic regurgitation was demonstrated. Therefore, the patient underwent an uncomplicated aortic valve replacement. aml, anterior mitral leaflet; AoR, aortic root; LA, left atrium; LV, left ventricle.*

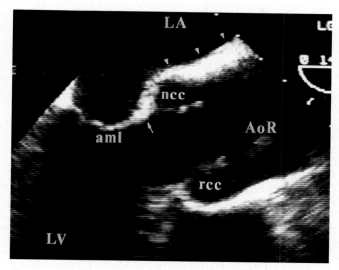

Figure 36–12. *Aortic root and aortic and mitral valve disease in a 43-year-old man with ankylosing spondylitis. This transesophageal echocardiographic view longitudinal to the outflow tract demonstrates severe sclerosis of the aortic root (AoR) predominantly of the posteromedial wall (arrowheads) extending to the base of the anterior mitral leaflet (aml) to form the subaortic bump (arrow). Moderate aortic root dilation is present. The noncoronary (ncc) and right coronary cusps (rcc) show mild localized thickening of their middle and tip portions. Moderate aortic regurgitation was demonstrated. LA, left atrium; LV, left ventricle.*

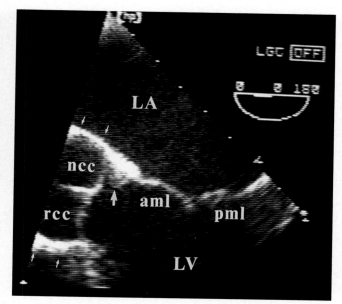

Figure 36–13. *Aortic root and mitral valve disease in a 41-year-old man with ankylosing spondylitis. This transesophageal echocardiographic view longitudinal to the outflow tract demonstrates sclerosis of the aortic root walls (small arrows) extending into the anterior mitral leaflet (aml) base and forming a large subaortic bump (large arrow). Decreased mobility of the anterior mitral leaflet was noted and mild mitral regurgitation was seen. The aortic valve cusps appear normal, and no aortic regurgitation was detected. LA, left atrium; LV, left ventricle; ncc, noncoronary cusp; pml, posterior mitral leaflet; rcc, right coronary cusp.*

fibrosis into the proximal septum and atrioventricular node.[117,119,123]

Myocardial and Pericardial Disease

The frequency of myocardial and pericardial disease in patients with ankylosing spondylitis may be higher than in the general population. The pathogenesis of myocardial disease may be related to increased connective tissue in the myocardium and/or microvascular disease.[124] Few controlled Doppler echocardiography series in young patients (<50 years old) with no clinical heart disease have uncommonly reported LV systolic dysfunction. In contrast, a 20% to 30% prevalence of diastolic dysfunction, predominantly impaired relaxation, has been reported.[121,122,125] In these studies, diastolic dysfunction was unrelated to age, disease duration, or disease activity. Rarely, cardiac amyloidosis with diastolic HF has been reported.[126]

The prevalence of pericardial disease in patients with ankylosing spondylitis is rare and probably similar to that of the general population (<2%). Echocardiographic studies report incidentally detected small pericardial effusions.

Scleroderma

Background

In scleroderma, excessive connective tissue overproduction and accumulation, structural and functional microvascular disease, and immune-complexes deposition affect the blood vessels, skin, joints, skeletal muscle, and multiple organs, including all structures of the heart. Thickening of the skin and Raynaud's phenomenon affect more than 90% of patients. In the diffuse type, there is symmetric fibrosis of the skin of the face, trunk, and extremities, with frequent involvement of internal organs. In the limited cutaneous type, the skin changes are limited to the extremities and face; internal organs are generally spared. This latter type is associated with the calcinosis, Raynaud's phenomenon, esophageal hypomotility, sclerodactyly, and telangiectasia (CREST) syndrome.

Cardiovascular disease occurs in as many as 50% of scleroderma patients.[127] CAD, myocarditis, pericarditis, and pulmonary and systemic hypertension-related heart disease occur. Arrhythmias and conduction abnormalities are less frequent. Overall, heart disease, pulmonary hypertension with or without cor pulmonale, and kidney disease are the leading causes of death in patients with scleroderma.

Associated Cardiovascular Involvement

Coronary Artery Disease

In scleroderma, the intramyocardial coronary arteries and arterioles are affected by two mechanisms: (1) abnormally increased vasoconstriction resulting from an immune-mediated inflammatory endothelial dysfunction or increased mast cell degranulation of vasoactive substances such as histamine, prostaglandin D_2, and leukotrienes C_4 and D_4. Intramyocardial coronary arterial spasm analogous to Raynaud's phenomenon occur.[128,129] Vasospasm of the epicardial coronary arteries is uncommon. (2) Obstructive microvascular disease resulting from intimal inflammation and fibrosis. The prevalence of epicardial atherosclerotic disease in patients with scleroderma is probably similar to that of a general population.

Because of predominant involvement of the intramyocardial coronary arteries, echocardiographic findings typical of transmural MI are uncommon. Using contrast-enhanced pulsed-wave (PW) Doppler TTE in a series of 27 patients without clinical evidence of ischemic heart disease, reduction in coronary flow reserve (<2.5) in the left anterior descending (LAD) coronary artery during adenosine infusion was detected in 52% of patients as compared to 4% of matched controls.[129] Severe reduction in coronary flow reserve (<2) was

seen in 19% of patients. Reduction in coronary flow reserve is more common in the diffuse form of scleroderma and is related to the duration and severity of the disease. As a result of functional and later on of obliterative microvascular disease, LV and RV diastolic and uncommonly systolic dysfunction can occur.[130,131] In contrast to typical atherosclerotic disease, areas of ischemic necrosis and fibrosis do not correspond to the regional distribution of a coronary artery, myocardial necrosis and fibrosis are predominantly subendocardial, and hemosiderin deposition is generally absent. Occasionally, a transmural MI resulting from epicardial coronary vasospasm can occur, and its echocardiographic diagnosis relies on the same findings as those of atherosclerotic disease. The cold pressor test with simultaneous myocardial perfusion scanning and echocardiography demonstrates transient wall motion abnormalities corresponding to as high as 70% frequency of reversible, fixed, or mixed perfusion abnormalities in patients with angiographically unremarkable epicardial coronary arteries.[127,132] Perfusion abnormalities improve with calcium channel blockers.

Myocardial Disease

Clinically apparent scleroderma-associated myocarditis is common but frequently unrecognized. Pathologic evidence of recent or past myocarditis is found in most patients.[133] Myocarditis is more common in patients with diffuse cutaneous involvement, anti-Scl70 antibodies, peripheral myopathy, and age older than 60 years. Patchy myocyte contraction band necrosis (typical of ischemia) with collagen replacement and myocardial fibrosis is characteristic of the disease and reported in up to 80% in postmortem series.

In echocardiographic studies, a reduced LV EF has been found in some asymptomatic patients, but it is more common in patients with clinical heart disease.[130,134-136] Associated RV dysfunction is reported commonly in patients with LV dysfunction. Reduced EF on echocardiography is associated with a high mortality rate (80% at 1 year) for those who develop clinical HF. In controlled cross-sectional and longitudinal studies using Doppler echocardiography, a high prevalence (30% to 50%) of parameters of abnormal LV relaxation and compliance is seen in unselected patients with either diffuse or limited cutaneous disease as compared to less than 10% in controls.[134,136] In a small series of 19 patients with scleroderma, impaired LV relaxation detected in 52% of patients was correlated with higher levels of soluble vascular cell adhesion molecules-1 and ESR and the duration and severity of Raynaud's. These data suggest that myocardial diastolic dysfunction result mainly from functional microvascular coronary disease.[135,137]

Myocardial ultrasonic videodensitometry in young patients with no diabetes or hypertension shows a high prevalence (30% to 90%) of decreased and heterogeneous integrated backscatter in the subendocardium of the septal and posterior walls.[124,138,139] Also, patients with scleroderma commonly have increased septal and posterior wall thickness. LV potentials on signal averaged electrocardiography, septal infarction pattern (Q waves in V_1 and V_2), ventricular arrhythmias, or conduction abnormalities on electrocardiography have also been noticed with increased frequency. Also, septal infarction patterns are associated with fixed septal or anteroseptal perfusion abnormalities. These findings suggest that myocardial dysfunction in patients with scleroderma is also related to increased interstitial collagen deposition and fibrosis.

Similarly, in controlled Doppler echocardiographic series, a high prevalence (40%) of RV diastolic dysfunction independently of pulmonary hypertension has been reported. These abnormalities include increased RV free wall thickness and right atrial systolic area, decrease in early filling velocity (E) and increased atrial filling velocity (A) tricuspid inflow velocities, decreased E/A ratio, increased global and regional isovolumic relaxation times (IVRTs), and reduce RV global filling.[140,141] In other series, RV diastolic dysfunction has been associated with LV diastolic dysfunction and pulmonary hypertension. In those with pulmonary hypertension, a higher prevalence and severity of RV diastolic dysfunction independently of age, heart rate, and LV mass has been reported.[142] A RV tissue Doppler E velocity of less than 0.11 m/s select patients with pulmonary artery pressure greater than 35 mm Hg, worse skin involvement, and positive anti-Scl-70 antibody. Finally, in patients with normal pulmonary artery pressure, a high prevalence (38%) of RV systolic dysfunction (EF < 35%) improve with nicardipine therapy.[131]

Pulmonary Hypertension and Cor Pulmonale

Interstitial lung disease and resultant pulmonary hypertension are a major feature of scleroderma.[143] Pulmonary fibrosis can occur in as many as 80% and pulmonary hypertension in as many as 35% to 50% of patients in series using Doppler echocardiography. Pulmonary hypertension secondary to inflammatory vasculopathy or pulmonary vasospasm is less common and is more commonly associated with the limited cutaneous type. Abnormal pulmonary function tests, abnormal lung uptake of gallium and technetium-99m Sestamibi, and radiographic abnormalities often precede cor pulmonale on echocardiography. Patients with pulmonary hypertension have a decreased survival of 81%, 63%, and 56% at 1, 2, and 3 years, respectively, from the diagnosis. In these patients,

decreased survival appears to be independent of the etiology of pulmonary hypertension.[144]

Pericarditis

Clinically evident or symptomatic pericardial disease occurs in 4% to 17% of patients with scleroderma and manifests as acute pericarditis and rarely as cardiac tamponade or pericardial constriction.[127,145,146] This low clinical prevalence contrast with that of postmortem and echocardiographic series, especially of asymptomatic pericardial effusions (30% to 50%). Symptomatic pericardial disease is two to four times more common in patients with the diffuse form than the limited cutaneous form of the disease[146] (Fig. 36-14). Pericardial disease is rarely the initial manifestation of scleroderma.[145] The pericardial effusion is usually an exudate, although without evidence of autoantibodies, immune complexes, or complement depletion.

Valve Disease

Published data suggest that scleroderma rarely cause valve disease. Unreplicated reports have described small masses similar to Libman-Sacks vegetations (one with probable embolization), aortitis and aortic regurgitation, and an unexplained increased frequency of mitral valve prolapse[147-149] (see Fig. 36-14). Finally, patients without hypertension with either diffuse or limited scleroderma have a decreased aortic distensibility as compared with controls.[150]

Polymyositis and Dermatomyositis

Background

Polymyositis and dermatomyositis are clinically similar diseases characterized by autoimmune-mediated skeletal muscle inflammation leading to symmetric proximal muscle weakness. Unlike polymyositis, dermatomyositis is accompanied by a rash on the face, neck, chest, and extensor surfaces of the extremities. Overlap syndromes frequently occur in which features of dermatomyositis or polymyositis are combined with those of SLE, rheumatoid arthritis, and scleroderma. Rarely, polymyositis or dermatomyositis can be associated with antiphospholipid antibody syndrome.

Myocarditis, pericarditis, and functional or structural microvascular CAD are the cardiac manifestations most commonly associated with polymyositis and dermatomyositis.[151,152] As a result of the lack of controlled cross-sectional and longitudinal studies, reported prevalence

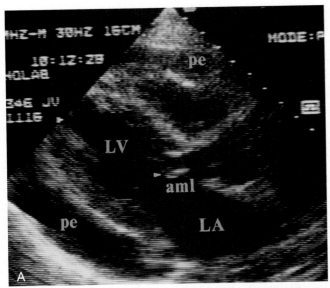

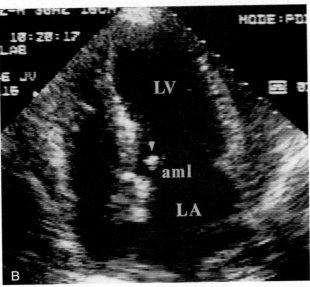

Figure 36-14. Mitral valve disease in a 72-year-old woman with scleroderma. Transthoracic long parasternal (A) and four-chamber (B) echocardiographic views show an irregular, highly reflectant nodularity in the midportion of the anterior mitral leaflet (aml) (arrowheads). Mild regurgitation was demonstrated. Despite the patient's age, no degenerative changes were detected in the mitral or aortic valve. Thus the valve abnormality is most likely related to scleroderma. Anterior and posterior pericardial effusion (pe) can be seen in the long parasternal view. LA, left atrium; LV, left ventricle. (From Roldan CA: In Braunwald E (ed): Atlas of Heart Diseases, vol 6., Philadelphia, 1996, Current Medicine, pp. 1-32.)

rates of cardiovascular disease are highly variable. Epicardial atherosclerotic CAD, conduction disorders, valve dysfunction, and pulmonary hypertension are uncommon. Although clinically manifested heart disease may occur in less than 25% of patients, it accounts for at least 10% mortality especially in those with myocarditis.

Associated Cardiovascular Involvement

Myocardial Disease

The pathogenesis of myocardial disease is either related to a direct myocardial inflammatory process and less likely to a functional microvascular disease.[153] In postmortem series, as many as 50% of patients with polymyositis or dermatomyositis show histologic evidence of active or healed myocarditis with variable degrees of mononuclear inflammation in the interstitium and perivascular areas, contraction band necrosis, and fibrosis. Approximately 10% to 20% of patients with myocarditis may develop cardiomyopathy.[154] The clinical prevalence of myocarditis is unknown. Patients with myocarditis frequently have active skeletal muscle myositis; as many as 50% of those with peripheral myositis, as indicated by uptake of technetium-99m pyrophosphate, also have myocardial uptake.[155,156] Rarely, a fulminant myocarditis with severe LV systolic dysfunction may be the initial manifestation of the disease.[157] Also, acute myocarditis can mimic clinically, electrocardiographically, and echocardiographically an acute MI.[158,159]

Limited prospective data, including two echocardiographic studies, suggest that few patients with polymyositis or dermatomyositis manifest wall motion abnormalities or a decreased LV EF during the course of their disease.[151-153,159] In noncontrolled small series, LV diastolic dysfunction as impaired relaxation has been reported in 12% to 40% of patients.[152]

An occasional patient with polymyositis or dermatomyositis develops findings of a hyperdynamic circulatory state accompanied by an elevated EF on echocardiography. The pathogenesis of this hyperkinetic heart syndrome is unknown, and patients are usually minimally symptomatic.

Pericarditis

The prevalence of clinically apparent pericardial disease in patients with polymyositis and dermatomyositis is low (≈10%). Pericarditis is more frequent in patients with the overlap syndrome and in children. Pericarditis and cardiac tamponade can rarely be the initial manifestation of the disease.[160] Echocardiographic series have shown an up to 25% prevalence of small and asymptomatic pericardial effusions. Cardiac tamponade and constriction are rare.

Coronary Artery Disease and Valve Disease

Epicardial CAD with angina has been reported in about 20% to 25% of patients. Microvascular disease is uncommon and coronary arteritis is rare.[153]

Noninfective valve vegetations similar to those seen in SLE have been reported.[161]

Mixed Connective Tissue Disease

Background

Mixed connective tissue disease is an overlap syndrome with features of SLE, rheumatoid arthritis (RA), scleroderma, and polymyositis. This disease is characterized by high titers of antibodies to nuclear ribonucleoprotein; patients also have speckled antinuclear antibodies and rheumatoid factor. Typical clinical features of this disease include Raynaud's phenomenon, hand edema, polyarthritis, sclerodactyly, interstitial pulmonary fibrosis, myositis, and esophageal hypomotility. As for polymyositis, the true prevalence of heart disease is unknown, but is highly variable (10% to 80%) with highest rates in echocardiographic series.[151] A correlation of heart disease with the severity and activity of the disease has not been clearly established.

Associated Cardiovascular Involvement

Pulmonary Hypertension

Pulmonary hypertension is a frequent and grave complication of mixed connective tissue disease, occurring in as many as 80% of patients. It most frequently affects patients with disease features of scleroderma. Proliferative vasculitis of the small and medium-sized pulmonary arteries and pulmonary fibrosis are the most common causes.[162] Pulmonary thromboembolism is rare.[163] Echocardiography is essential to the diagnosis and follow-up of these patients.

Pericarditis

Pericardial disease is common, but most patients have asymptomatic, small pericardial effusions on echocardiography. Clinical pericarditis has been reported in 25% to 30% of patients and rarely can be the initial manifestation of the disease.[151,164] Large pericardial effusion with tamponade rarely occurs and responds favorably to steroid therapy.[165,166] Nuclear ribonucleoprotein-immune complexes are found in the pericardial fluid.[164]

Valve Disease and Myocardial Disease

No data associating specific forms of valve disease with mixed connective disease have been reported. However, mitral valve prolapse has been reported in 20% to 25% of patients.[162,167,168] Myocarditis is characterized on histology by interstitial lymphocytic infiltrates and variable degrees of myocardial fibers necrosis and when acute and detected early can be reversible with steroids and intravenous pulse cyclophosphamide therapy.[169] On echocardiography, the spectrum of the diseases ranges from diastolic dysfunction to global or regional LV systolic dysfunction and HF.[170]

Coronary Artery Disease

As in other connective tissue diseases, CAD in patients with mixed connective tissue disease is related to functional microvascular disease. Acute MI or other acute coronary syndrome may result from small vessel disease, coronary vasospasm, in situ thrombosis, coronary embolism from a valve vegetation, and rarely arteritis.[171] Finally, acute myocarditis may mimic a MI (Table 36–1).

KEY POINTS

- Nonbacterial valve vegetations and leaflet fibrosis are seen in many patients with systemic lupus erythematosus (SLE), primary antiphospholipid syndrome (PAPS), and rheumatoid arthritis (RA).

- There is an increased prevalence of atherosclerotic coronary disease in patients with systemic inflammatory disorders, particularly SLE and RA independently of traditional atherogenic risk factors.

- Intracardiac thrombi are characteristic of PAPS.

- Pericarditis is common in patients with SLE, RA, polymyositis, dermatomyositis, and mixed connective tissue disease.

- LV diastolic dysfunction is the result of microvascular disease in patients in patients with SLE, PAPS, RA, scleroderma, and polymyositis or dermatomyositis.

- LV systolic dysfunction is uncommon and is the result of myocarditis in patients with SLE, PAPS, RA, scleroderma, and polymyositis or dermatomyositis.

- Pulmonary hypertension resulting from interstitial lung disease or vasculitis is seen in patients with SLE, scleroderma, and mixed connective tissue disorder.

- Proximal aortitis and valvulitis (with a characteristic subaortic bump) and conduction system disease are typical for ankylosing spondylitis (Table 36–2).

TABLE 36–1. Cardiovascular Involvement in Connective Tissue Diseases

Disease	Type of Involvement	Frequency (%)*	Key Characteristics
Systemic lupus erythematosus (SLE)	Libman-Sacks vegetations	10-35	Characteristic, but not exclusive of SLE. Can be inflammatory, thrombotic, or mixed vegetations. Vegetations frequently change in appearance, resolve, appear de novo, or reappear.
	Leaflet fibrosis	30-50	Frequently diffuse. Associated calcification is uncommon.
	Valve regurgitation (mild or worse)	30-50	Can be severe with acute valvulitis or with over imposed infection. Valve stenosis is rare (<3%).
	Pericarditis	10-50	Antinuclear antibodies in pericardial fluid are diagnostic but not always present. Tamponade or constriction is rare.
	Asymptomatic effusion	2-20	—
	Myocarditis/ cardiomyopathy	1-20	Primary myocarditis is associated with cellular antigen Ro (SS-A) and La (SS-B) antibody.
	Coronary disease		
	Atherosclerotic	10-30	Most commonly nonobstructive.
	Functional	25-30	Abnormal coronary vasodilation or microvascular disease. Microvascular thrombosis uncommon.
	Arteritis	Rare	Involves small and medium size vessels.
	Myocardial infarction	<10	A result of epicardial atherosclerosis, vasospasm, in situ thrombosis, or embolism. Arteritis is rare.
	Diastolic dysfunction†	15-35	Predominantly impaired left ventricular relaxation.
	Pulmonary hypertension	5-15	Caused by interstitial lung disease, vasculitis, and thromboembolism.
	Cardioembolism	15-20	More commonly to the brain (50%-80%).
Primary antiphospholipid syndrome (PAPS)	Valve vegetations	10-30	All valve abnormalities, especially valve vegetations, have similar characteristics and evolution as to those of SLE.
	Valve thickening	40-60	They are predominantly thrombotic but can be inflammatory or mixed. These vegetations also change in appearance over time, resolve, or reappear over time.
	Valve regurgitation	30-40	
	Intracardiac thrombosis	15-20	Includes thrombotic vegetations, adhered or free floating intracavitary thrombi, atrioventricular valves thrombi with inflow obstruction mimicking stenosis, and echocardiographic pseudocontrast.
	Pulmonary hypertension	20-25	More commonly secondary to pulmonary emboli, but pulmonary vasoconstriction or obstructive vasculopathy can occur.
	Coronary artery disease	20-30	Predominantly functional microvascular disease.
	Myocardial disease	15-30	Rarely primary inflammatory. Most commonly diastolic dysfunction due to microvascular coronary artery disease.
Rheumatoid arthritis (RA)	Coronary artery disease	40-65	Predominantly subclinical as detected by electron-beam CT.
	Atherosclerotic	>40	Two to four times higher than the general population, severe obstructive disease uncommon.
	Functional	>25	Abnormal coronary vasodilation or microvascular disease.
	Arteritis	Uncommon	Difficult to diagnose clinically.
	Myocardial infarction	10-15	Most commonly the result of epicardial atherosclerosis. Rarely, coronary vasospasm, in situ thrombosis, or embolism.
	Pericarditis	≤10	Occurs in patients with active disease, high rheumatoid factor level, and nodular disease; pericardial fluid can have rheumatoid factor.
	Asymptomatic effusion	30-50	—
	Leaflet fibrosis	>30	Leaflet fibrosis is indistinguishable from that of systemic lupus.
	Valve nodules	10-30	Characteristic of rheumatoid arthritis.

*Variability of rates is related to differences in patient population characteristics, study design, and diagnostic methods.
†Defined by Doppler echocardiographic criteria.

TABLE 36–1. Cardiovascular Involvement in Connective Tissue Diseases—cont'd

Disease	Type of Involvement	Frequency (%)*	Key Characteristics
Rheumatoid arthritis—cont'd	Valve regurgitation, ≥mild	>30	—
	Myocarditis/ cardiomyopathy	<10	Amyloid deposition is a rare cause.
	Diastolic dysfunction	30-40	Predominantly impaired left ventricular relaxation.
	Pulmonary hypertension	≈20	—
Ankylosing spondylitis	Proximal aortitis/valvulitis	20-60	Root sclerosis extending to base of anterior mitral leaflet and root dilatation are characteristic of the disease.
	Aortic regurgitation, ≥ mild	10-40	—
	Subaortic bump	10-40	Decreases anterior mitral leaflet mobility and causes regurgitation.
	Conduction system disease	>20	Extension of aortic root/annulus sclerosis into the proximal septum and atrioventricular node.
	Diastolic dysfunction	20-30	Predominantly impaired left ventricular relaxation.
	Pericarditis	<5	Primary immune mediated is uncommon.
	Asymptomatic effusion	<5	—
	Myocarditis/ cardiomyopathy	<5	Primary immune-mediated myocarditis is rare.
Scleroderma	Coronary disease		
	Atherosclerotic	<20	—
	Functional	≈50	Predominantly vasospastic or coronary Raynaud's.
	Myocarditis/ cardiomyopathy	10-50	Most commonly related to recurrent intramyocardial ischemia/ necrosis/fibrosis. Inflammatory uncommon.
	Diastolic dysfunction	30-50	Affects the left ventricle and right ventricle, and predominates as impaired relaxation.
	Pulmonary hypertension	35-50	Caused by pulmonary fibrosis, less commonly by vasculitis, vasospasm, or left heart disease.
	Pericarditis	5-20	—
	Asymptomatic effusion	30-40	—
	Valve disease	<10	Nonspecific. Mitral valve prolapse is common.
Polymyositis/ dermatomyositis	Myocarditis/ cardiomyopathy	>25	Primary myocarditis more common in patients with myositis. Diastolic dysfunction occurs in 10% to 40% of patients.
	Hyperkinetic heart syndrome	Rare	—
	Pericarditis	≈10	More frequent in children and in overlap syndrome.
	Asymptomatic effusion	5-25	—
	Coronary artery disease	≈20	Commonly nonobstructive atherosclerotic. Microvascular disease also common. Arteritis is rare.
	Valve disease	Unknown	Is nonspecific. Libman-Sacks–like vegetations are rare.
Mixed connective tissue disease	Pulmonary hypertension	≤80	More often resulting from proliferative vasculitis and pulmonary fibrosis.
	Pericarditis	5-30	—
	Asymptomatic effusion	Unknown	—
	Valve disease	Unknown	Nonspecific. High prevalence of mitral valve prolapse (20%-25%).
	Myocarditis/ cardiomyopathy	<5	—
	Coronary artery disease	Unknown	Predominantly microvascular disease.

TABLE 36–2. Key Echocardiographic Features of Valve Lesions in Selected Conditions

Disease	Affected Structures	Key Characteristics	Functional Sequelae
Systemic lupus erythematosus (SLE)	MV > AoV leaflets; rarely chordae, TV and PV; spares annuli.	Libman-Sacks vegetations: masses usually <1 cm in diameter, with heterogeneous echocardiographic reflectance (but not calcified) and with irregular borders; usually rounded shape. Attached to leaflet with a broad base. No independent motion. Lesions are located at any portion of leaflets, on atrial side of MV and aortic vessel or ventricular side of AoV. Diffuse leaflet thickening or sclerosis common; calcification uncommon and mild.	Mild to moderate MR or AR is common, but stenosis is rare. High potential embolic source.
Primary antiphospholipid syndrome	MV > AoV leaflets; rarely chordae, TV and PV; spares annuli.	Libman-Sacks–like vegetations with similar characteristic to those described for SLE.	Mild to moderate MR or AR are common. High potential embolic source.
Rheumatoid arthritis	MV, AoV leaflets, rarely annuli and chordae; spares TV and PV.	Rheumatoid nodules: masses usually <1 cm in diameter, with homogeneous soft-tissue echocardiographic reflectance and irregular border; usually rounded shape. Any location within the leaflet; leaflet thickening/sclerosis generally mild or absent. Libman-Sacks–like vegetations.	More than mild MR or AR is rare. Rupture of a nodule may lead to severe valve regurgitation. Rarely associated with cardioembolism. Associated with acute or recurrent valvulitis. Similar characteristics to those associated with SLE. High embolic potential. Postvalvulitis stenosis is rare.
Ankylosing spondylitis	Proximal aorta, annulus and AoV, base of anterior mitral leaflet; posterior MV leaflet, mitral annulus, and chordae spared.	Sclerosis, stiffness, and dilatation of Ao root extend to the annulus. AoV leaflet sclerosis is generally mild. Subaortic bump: a localized thickening of base of anterior mitral leaflet resulting from downward extension of Ao root and annular sclerosis.	Mild to moderate AR or MR are common. Stenosis not reported.
Rheumatic heart disease	90% involvement of MV and/or AoV; 10% TV and/or PV; annuli of valves and aortic root spared.	MV leaflet edges and chordae are most affected; with severe disease, sclerosis extends toward base of leaflet and may involve papillary muscles. Extensive calcification may occur. When localized, sclerosis may appear masslike, but very high echocardiographic reflectance is unlike other lesions, except degenerative. AoV cusp edges are affected in a similar pattern.	Leaflet edge fusion and chordal shortening produce a tethered mitral leaflet motion; analogous doming motion of the aortic cusps may be seen. If fusion predominates, stenosis results; if leaflet retraction predominates, regurgitation results.
Degenerative disorders	MV and AoV annuli and leaflets; uncommonly involves chordae and tip of papillary muscles.	Sclerosis is concentrated at base of leaflets and annulus, with progressive extension toward leaflet midportion, tip uncommonly involved. When localized, sclerosis may appear masslike or as nodules. Aortic valve nodules more commonly located at the base and commissural portions.	Annular calcification predominates for MV, with leaflet sclerosis less common and usually limited to posterior leaflet. MR rarely more than mild, and stenosis is rare and subclinical or mild. AoV leaflet sclerosis and fusion lead to stenosis, and leaflet distortion leads to AR, generally mild.

AR, aortic regurgitation; AoV, aortic valve; MR, mitral regurgitation; MV, mitral valve; PV, pulmonary valve; TEE, transesophageal echocardiography; TTE, transthoracic echocardiography; TV, tricuspid valve.

TABLE 36–2. Key Echocardiographic Features of Valve Lesions in Selected Conditions—cont'd

Disease	Affected Structures	Key Characteristics	Functional Sequelae
Infective endocarditis	Acute: mass with homogeneous soft-tissue reflectance and irregular borders; size and shape are highly variable, usually with narrow base, often pedunculated. Lesions almost always exhibit motion independent of underlying structure and almost always oscillatory. MV and TV lesions prolapse into atria in systole, AoV and PV lesions prolapse into outflow tracts in diastole. Lesions usually attached to distal third of leaflet. With AoV disease, additional vegetations may occur on anterior mitral leaflet and chordae. Chronic: localized thickening and/or increased reflectance of leaflet or chordae. Lesion is not necessarily distal on leaflet. Fibrous tissue reflectance and calcification are common.		Valve regurgitation is common and frequently severe; stenosis involving native valves is rare. Leaflet perforation or abscess formation occurs. Cardioembolism is common.
Valve or Lambl's excrescences[172]	Detected by TEE, rarely by TTE. Similarly high frequency (35%-40%) in healthy subjects, in patients with connective tissue diseases, and in patients with suspected cardioembolism. They are thin (0.6-2 mm in width), elongated (4-16 mm), hypermobile structures seen at or near the leaflets coaptation point, on the atrial side during systole for mitral and tricuspid valves and ventricular side during diastole for the aortic valve. Multivalvular involvement seen in 20%-25% of subjects.		Valve excrescences are not associated or cause valvular dysfunction, persist unchanged over time, and are not associated with aPL or with an increased risk of cardioembolism.

aPL, antiphospholipid antibodies.

REFERENCES

1. Doria A, Iaccarino L, Sarzi-Puttini P, et al: Cardiac involvement in systemic lupus erythematosus. *Lupus* 14:683-686, 2005.
2. Roberts WC, High ST: The heart in systemic lupus erythematosus. *Curr Probl Cardiol* 24:1-56, 1999.
3. Abu-Shakra M, Urowitz MB, Gladmann DD, et al: Mortality studies in systemic lupus erythematosus. Results from a single centre. I. Causes of death. *J Rheumatol* 22:1259-1264, 1995.
4. Roldan CA, Shively BK, Lau CC, et al: Systemic lupus erythematosus valve disease by transesophageal echocardiography and the role of antiphospholipid antibodies. *J Am Coll Cardiol* 20:1127-1134, 1992.
5. Roldan CA, Shively BK, Crawford MH: An echocardiographic study of valvular heart disease associated with systemic lupus erythematosus. *N Engl J Med* 335:1424-1430, 1996.
6. Evangelopoulos ME, Alevizaki M, Toumanidis S, et al: Mitral valve prolapse in systemic lupus erythematosus patients: clinical and immunological aspects. *Lupus* 12:308-311, 2003.
7. Roldan CA, Gelgand EA, Qualls CR, Sibbitt WL Jr: Valvular heart disease as a cause of cerebrovascular disease in patients with systemic lupus erythematosus. *Am J Cardiol* 95:1441-1447, 2005.
8. Afek A, Shoenfeld Y, Manor R, et al: Increased endothelial cell expression of alpha3beta1 integrin in cardiac valvulopathy in the primary (Hughes) and secondary antiphospholipid syndrome. *Lupus* 8:502-507, 1999.
9. Levine JS, Branch DW, Rauch J: The antiphospholipid syndrome. *N Engl J Med* 346:752-763, 2002.
10. Gleason CB, Stoddard MF, Wagner SG, et al: A comparison of cardiac valvular involvement in the primary antiphospholipid syndrome versus anticardiolipin-negative systemic lupus erythematosus. *Am Heart J* 125:1123-1129, 1993.
11. Leszczynski P, Straburzynska-Migaj E, Korczowska I, et al: Cardiac valvular disease in patients with systemic lupus erythematosus. Relationship with anticardiolipin antibodies. *Clin Rheumatol* 22:405-408, 2003.

12. Gentile R, Lagana B, Tubani L, et al: Assessment of echocardiographic abnormalities in patients with systemic lupus erythematosus: correlation with levels of antiphospholipid antibodies. *Ital Heart J* 1:487-492, 2000.

13. Libman E, Sacks B: A hitherto undescribed form of valvular and mural endocarditis. *Arch Intern Med* 33:701-737, 1924.

14. Eiken PW, Edwards WD, Tazelaar HD, et al: Surgical pathology of nonbacterial thrombotic endocarditis in 30 patients, 1985-2000. *Mayo Clin Proc* 76:1204-1212, 2001.

15. Omdal R, Lunde P, Rasmussen K, et al: Transesophageal and transthoracic echocardiography and Doppler-examinations in systemic lupus erythematosus. *Scand J Rheumatol* 30:275-281, 2001.

16. Kalke S, Balakrishanan C, Mangat G, et al: Echocardiography in systemic lupus erythematosus. *Lupus* 7:540-544, 1998.

17. Perez-Villa F, Font J, Azqueta M, Espinosa G, et al: Severe valvular regurgitation and antiphospholipid antibodies in systemic lupus erythematosus: a prospective, long-term, followup study. *Arthritis Rheum* 53:460-467, 2005.

18. Tikly M, Diese M, Zannettou N, et al: Gonococcal endocarditis in a patient with systemic lupus erythematosus. *Br J Rheumatol* 36:270-272, 1997.

19. Roldan CA, Gelgand EA, Qualls CR, Sibbitt WL Jr: Valvular heart disease is associated with nonfocal neuropsychiatric systemic lupus erythematosus. *J Clin Rheumatol* 12:3-10, 2006.

20. Morelli S, Bernardo ML, Viganego F, et al: Left-sided heart valve abnormalities and risk of ischemic cerebrovascular accidents in patients with systemic lupus erythematosus. *Lupus* 12:805-812, 2003.

21. Joven B, Mellor-Pita S, D'Cruz D, et al: Cerebral embolism complicating Libman-Sacks endocarditis-full recovery using tissue plasminogen activator. *J Rheumatol* 29:2022-2024, 2002.

22. Rademacher J, Sohngen D, Specker C, et al: Cerebral microembolism, a disease marker for ischemic cerebrovascular events in the antiphospholipid syndrome of systemic lupus erythematosus? *Acta Neurol Scand* 99:356-361, 1999.

23. Kumral E, Evyapan D, Keser G, et al: Detection of microemboli signals in patients with neuropsychiatric lupus erythematosus. *Eur Neurol* 47:131-135, 2002.

24. Espinola-Zavaleta N, Vargas-Barron J, Colmenares-Galvis T, et al: Echocardiographic evaluation of patients with primary antiphospholipid syndrome. *Am Heart J* 137:973-978, 1999.

25. Blank M, Aron-Maor A, Shoenfeld Y: From rheumatic fever to Libman-Sacks endocarditis: is there any possible pathogenetic link? *Lupus* 14:697-701, 2005.

26. Blanchard DG, Ross RS, Dittrich HC: Nonbacterial thrombotic endocarditis: Assessment by transesophageal echocardiography. *Chest* 102:954-956, 1992.

27. Shively BK, Gurule FT, Roldan CA, et al: Diagnostic value of transesophageal compared with transthoracic echocardiography in infective endocarditis. *J Am Coll Cardiol* 18:391-397, 1991.

28. Cauduro SA, Moder KG, Tsang TS, Seward JB: Clinical and echocardiographic characteristics of hemodynamically significant pericardial effusions in patients with systemic lupus erythematosus. *Am J Cardiol* 92:1370-1372, 2003.

29. Weich HS, Burgess LJ, Reuter H, et al: Large pericardial effusions due to systemic lupus erythematosus: a report of eight cases. *Lupus* 14:450-457, 2005.

30. Quismorio FP: Immune complexes in the pericardial fluid in systemic lupus erythematosus. *Arch Intern Med* 140:112-114, 1980.

31. Coe MD, Hamer DH, Levy CS, et al: Gonococcal pericarditis with tamponade in a patient with systemic lupus erythematosus. *Arthritis Rheum* 33:1438-1441, 1990.

32. Paradiso M, Gabrielli F, Masala C, et al: Evaluation of myocardial involvement in systemic lupus erythematosus by signal-averaged electrocardiography and echocardiography. *Acta Cardiol* 56:381-386, 2001.

33. Law WG, Thong BY, Lian TY, et al: Acute lupus myocarditis: clinical features and outcome of an oriental case series. *Lupus* 14:827-831, 2005.

34. Oshiro AC, Derbes SJ, Stopa AR, et al: Anti-Ro/SS-A and La/SS-B antibodies associated with cardiac involvement in childhood systemic lupus erythematosus. *Ann Rheum Dis* 56:272-274, 1997.

35. Cacciapuoti F, Galzerano D, Capogrosso P, et al: Impairment of left ventricular function in systemic lupus erythematosus evaluated by measuring myocardial performance index with tissue Doppler Echocardiography. *Echocardiography* 22:315-319, 2005.

36. Tektonidou MG, Ioannidis JP, Moyssakis I, et al: Right ventricular diastolic dysfunction in patients with anticardiolipin antibodies and antiphospholipid syndrome. *Ann Rheum Dis* 60:43-48, 2001.

37. Ueda T, Mizushige K, Aoyama T, et al: Echocardiographic observation of acute myocarditis with systemic lupus erythematosus. *Jpn Circ J* 64:144-146, 2000.

38. Lagana B, Schillaci O, Tubani L, et al: Lupus carditis: evaluation with technetium-99m MIBI SPECT and heart rate variability. *Myocard Angiol* 50:143-148, 1999.

39. Bahl VK: Myocardial systolic function in systemic lupus erythematosus: A study based on radionuclide ventriculography. *Cardiol Clin* 15:433-438, 1992.

40. Naqvi TZ, Luthringer D, Marchevsky A, et al: Chloroquine-induced cardiomyopathy-echocardiographic features. *J Am Soc Echocardiogr* 18:383-387, 2005.

41. Roman MJ, Shanker BA, Davies AB et al: Prevalence and correlates of accelerated atherosclerosis in systemic lupus erythematosus. *N Engl J Med* 349:2399-2406, 2003.

42. Rhaman P, Urowitz MB, Gladman DD, et al: Contribution of traditional risk factors to coronary artery disease in patients with systemic lupus erythematosus. *J Rheumatol* 26:2363-2368, 1999.

43. Borba EF, Bonfa E: Dyslipoproteinemia in systemic lupus erythematosus: Influence of disease activity and anticardiolipin antibodies. *Lupus* 6:533-539, 1997.

44. Dorai A, Schoenfeld Y, Pauletto P: Premature coronary disease in systemic lupus. *N Engl J Med* 350:1571-1575, 2004.

45. Codish S, Liel-Cohen N, Rovner M, et al: Dobutamine stress echocardiography in women with systemic lupus erythematosus: Increased occurrence of left ventricular outflow gradient. *Lupus* 13:101-104, 2004.

46. Galie N, Manes A, Farahani KV, et al: Pulmonary arterial hypertension associated to connective tissue diseases. *Lupus* 14:713-717, 2005.

47. Tenedios F, Erkan D, Lockshin MD: Cardiac involvement in the antiphospholipid syndrome. *Lupus* 14:691-696, 2005.

48. Lockshin MD, Tenedios F, Petri M, et al: Cardiac disease in antiphospholipid syndrome: Recommendations for treatment. Committee consensus report. *Lupus* 12:518-523, 2003.

49. Qaddoura F, Connolly H, Grogan M, et al: Valve morphology in the antiphospholipid syndrome: Echocardiographic features. *Echocardiography* 22:255-259, 2005.

50. Hojnik M, George J, Ziporen L, Shoenfeld Y: Heart valve involvement (Libman-Sacks endocarditis) in the antiphospholipid syndrome. *Circulation* 93:1579-1587, 1996.

51. Reisner SA, Brenner B, Haim N, et al: Echocardiography in nonbacterial thrombotic endocarditis: from autopsy to clinical entity. *J Am Soc Echocardiogr* 13:876-881, 2000.

52. Garcia-Torres R, Amigo MC, de la Rosa A, et al: Valvular heart disease in primary antiphospholipid syndrome (PAPS): Clinical and morphological findings. *Lupus* 5:56-61, 1996.

53. Turiel M, Muzzupappa S, Gottardi B, et al: Evaluation of cardiac abnormalities and embolic sources in primary antiphospholipid syndrome by transesophageal echocardiography. *Lupus* 9:406-412, 2000.

54. Turiel M, Sarzi-Puttinin P, Peretti A, et al: Five year follow-up by transesophageal echocardiographic studies in primary antiphospholipid syndrome. *Am J Cardiol* 96:574-579, 2005.

55. Espinola Zavaleta N, Montes RM, Soto ME, et al: Primary antiphospholipid syndrome: A 5-year transesophageal echocardiographic follow-up study. *J Rheumatol* 31:2402-2407, 2004.

56. Erdogan D, Goren MT, Diz-Kucukkaya R, Inanc M: Assessment of cardiac structure and left atrial appendage functions in primary antiphospholipid syndrome: A transesophageal echocardiographic study. *Stroke* 36:592-596, 2005.

57. Nesher G, Ilany J, Rosenmann D, Abraham AS: Valvular dysfunction in antiphospholipid syndrome: Prevalence, clinical features, and treatment. *Semin Arthritis Rheum* 27:27-35, 1997.

58. Shahian DM, Labib SB, Schneebaum AB: Etiology and management of chronic valve disease in antiphospholipid antibody syndrome and systemic lupus erythematosus. *J Card Surg* 10:133-139, 1995.

59. Yusuf S, Madden BP, Pumhrey CW: Left atrial thrombus caused by the primary antiphospholipid syndrome causing critical functional mitral stenosis. *Heart* 89:262, 2002.

60. Mottram PM, Gelman JS: Mitral valve thrombus mimicking a primary tumor in the antiphospholipid syndrome. *J Am Soc Echocardiogr* 15:746-748, 2002.

61. Ebato M, Kitai H, Kumakura H, et al: Thrombus on the tricuspid valve in a patient with primary antiphospholipid syndrome after implantation of an inferior vena cava filter. *Circ J* 66:425-427, 2002.

62. Mukhopadhyay S, Suryavanshi S, Yusu J, et al: Isolated thrombus producing tricuspid stenosis: an unusual presentation in primary antiphospholipid syndrome. *Indian Heart J* 56:61-63, 2004.

63. McMillan E, Martin WL, Waugh J, et al: Management of pregnancy in women with pulmonary hypertension secondary to SLE and antiphospholipid syndrome. *Lupus* 11:392-398, 2002.

64. Ames PRJ, Margarita A, Sokoll KB, et al: Premature atherosclerosis in primary antiphospholipid syndrome: preliminary data. *Ann Rheum Dis* 64:315-317, 2005.

65. Matsuura E, Lopez LR: Are oxidized LDL/b2-glycoprotein I complexes pathogenic antigens in autoimmune mediated atherosclerosis? *Clin Dev Immunol* 11:103-111, 2004.

66. Medina G, Casaos D, Jara LJ, et al: Increased carotid artery intima media thickness may be associated with stroke in primary antiphospholipid syndrome. *Ann Rheum Dis* 62:607-610, 2003.

67. Petri M: Detection of coronary artery disease and the role of traditional risk factors in the Hopkins Lupus Cohort. *Lupus* 9:170-175, 2000.

68. Cervera R: Coronary and valvular syndromes and antiphospholipid antibodies. *Thromb Res* 114:501-507, 2004.

69. Sletnes KE, Smith P, Abdelnoor M, et al: Antiphospholipid antibodies after myocardial infarction and their relation to mortality, reinfarction, and non-haemorrhagic stroke. *Lancet* 339:451-453, 1992.

70. Lagana B, Baratta L, Tubani L, et al: Myocardial infarction with normal coronary arteries in a patient with primary antiphospholipid syndrome—case report and literature review. *Angiology* 52:785-588, 2001.

71. Coudray N, de Zuttere D, Bletry O, et al: M mode and Doppler echocardiographic assessment of left ventricular diastolic function in primary antiphospholipid syndrome. *Br Heart J* 74:531-535, 1995.

72. Hasnie AM, Stoddard MF, Gleason CB, et al: Diastolic dysfunction is a feature of the antiphospholipid syndrome. *Am Heart J* 129:1009-1013, 1995.

73. Asherson RA, Cervera R, Piette JC, et al: Catastrophic antiphospholipid syndrome. Clinical and laboratory features of 50 patients. *Medicine (Baltimore)* 77:195-207, 1998.

74. Doria A, Sarzi-Puttini P, Shoenfeld Y: Second conference on heart, rheumatism and autoimmunity, Pescara, Italy, May 19-20, 2005. *Autoimmun Rev* 5:55-63, 2006.

75. Gerli R, Goodson NJ: Cardiovascular involvement in rheumatoid arthritis. *Lupus* 14:679-682, 2005.

76. Nicola PJ, Crowson CS, Maradit-Kremers H, et al: Contribution of congestive heart failure and ischemic heart disease to excess mortality in rheumatoid arthritis. *Arthritis Rheum* 54:60-67, 2006.

77. Gabriel SE, Crowson CS, Kremers HM, et al: Survival in rheumatoid arthritis: A population-based analysis of trends over 40 years. *Arthritis Rheum* 48:54-58, 2003.

78. Gonzalez-Gay MA, Gonzalez-Juanatey C, Martin J: Rheumatoid arthritis: A disease associated with accelerated atherogenesis. *Semin Arthritis Rheum* 35:8-17, 2005.

79. Sattar N, McInnes IB: Vascular comorbidity in rheumatoid arthritis: Potential mechanisms and solutions. *Curr Opin Rheumatol* 17:286-292, 2005.

80. Solomon DHM, Karlson EWM, Rimm EBS, et al: Cardiovascular morbidity and mortality in women diagnosed with rheumatoid arthritis. *Circulation* 107:1303-1307, 2003.

81. Gerli R, Schillaci G, Giordano A, et al: CD4 T lymphocytes contribute to early atherosclerotic damage in rheumatoid arthritis patients. *Circulation* 109:2744-2748, 2004.

82. Csiszar A, Ungvari Z: Synergistic effects of vascular IL-17 and TNF-alpha may promote coronary artery disease. *Med Hypotheses* 63:696-698, 2004.

83. Haskard DO: Accelerated atherosclerosis in inflammatory rheumatic diseases. *Scand J Rheumatol* 33:281-292, 2004.

84. Maradit-Kremers H, Crowson CS, Nicola PJ, et al: Increased unrecognized coronary heart disease and sudden deaths in rheumatoid arthritis: A population-based cohort study. *Arthritis Rheum* 52:402-411, 2005.

85. Wolfe F, Freundlich B, Straus WL: Increase in cardiovascular and cerebrovascular disease prevalence in rheumatoid arthritis. *J Rheumatol* 30:36-40, 2003.

86. Wong M, Toh L, Wilson A, et al: Reduced arterial elasticity in rheumatoid arthritis and the relationship to vascular disease risk factors and inflammation. *Arthritis Rheum* 48:81-89, 2003.

87. Douglas KM, Pace AV, Treharne GJ, et al: Excess recurrent cardiac events in rheumatoid arthritis patients with acute coronary syndrome. *Ann Rheum Dis* 65:348-353, 2006.

88. Wallberg-Johnson S, Cederfelt M, Rantapaa Dahlqvist S: Hemostatic factors and cardiovascular disease in active rheumatoid arthritis: An 8 year follow study. *J Rheumatol* 27:71-75, 2000.

89. Chung CP, Oeser A, Raggi P, et al: Increased coronary-artery atherosclerosis in rheumatoid arthritis: relationship to disease duration and cardiovascular risk factors. *Arthritis Rheum* 2005;52:3045-53.

90. Johnsen SP, Larson H, Tarone RE, et al: Risk of hospitalization for myocardial infarction among users of rofecoxib, celecoxib, and other NSAIDs: A population-based case-control study. *Arch Intern Med* 165:978-984, 2005.

91. Hurlimann D, Forster A, Noll G, et al: Anti-tumor necrosis factor-a treatment improves endothelial function in patients with rheumatoid arthritis. *Circulation* 106:2184-2187, 2002.

92. McCarey DW, McInnes IB, Madhok R, et al: Trial of atorvastatin in rheumatoid arthritis (TARA): Double-blind, randomized placebo controlled trial. *Lancet* 363:2015-2021, 2004.

93. Hermann F, Forster A, Chenevard R, et al: Simvastatin improves endothelial function in patients with rheumatoid arthritis. *J Am Coll Cardiol* 45:461-464, 2005.

94. Takayanagi M, Haraoka H, Kikuchi H, Hirohata S: Myocardial infarction caused by rheumatoid vasculitis: histological evidence of the involvement of T lymphocytes. *Rheumatol Int* 23:315-318, 2003.

95. Turiel M, Peretti R, Sarzi-Puttini P, et al: Cardiac imaging techniques in systemic autoimmune diseases. *Lupus* 14:727-731, 2005.

96. Wislowska M, Sypula S, Kowalik I: Echocardiographic findings and 24-h electrocardiographic Holter monitoring in patients

with nodular and non-nodular rheumatoid arthritis. *Rheumatol Int* 18:163-169, 1999.

97. Spalding DM, Haber P, Schrohenloher RE, Koopman WJ: Production of immunoglobulin and rheumatoid factor by lymphoid cells in rheumatoid pericardium. *Arthritis Rheum* 28:1071-1074, 1985.

98. Lee JS, Do IN, Kang DH, et al: Adult onset Still's disease as a cause of acute severe mitral and aortic regurgitation. *Korean J Intern Med* 20:264-267, 2005.

99. Anaya JM: Severe rheumatoid valvular heart disease. *Clin Rheumatol* 25:1-3, 2005.

100. Maksimowicz-McKinnon K, Mandell BF: Understanding valvular heart disease in patients with systemic autoimmune diseases. *Cleve Clin J Med* 71:881-885, 2004.

101. Kang H, Baron M: Embolic complications of a mitral valve rheumatoid nodule. *J Rheumatol* 31:1001-1003, 2004.

102. Gonzalez-Juanatey C, Garcia-Porrua C, Testa A, Gonzalez-Gay MA: Potential role of mitral valve strands on stroke recurrence in rheumatoid arthritis. *Arthritis Rheum* 49:866-867, 2003.

103. Mullins PA, Grace AA, Stewart SC, Shapiro LM: Rheumatoid heart disease presenting as acute mitral regurgitation. *Am Heart J* 122:242-245, 1991.

104. Arakawa K, Yamazawa M, Morita Y, et al: Giant rheumatoid nodule causing simultaneous complete atrioventricular block and severe mitral regurgitation: a case report. *J Cardiol* 46:77-83, 2005.

105. Howell A, Say J, Hedworth-Whitty: Rupture of the sinus of Valsalva due to severe rheumatoid heart disease. *Br Heart J* 34:537-540, 1972.

106. Lodde BM, Sankar V, Kok MR, et al: Adult heart block is associated with disease activity in primary Sjögren's syndrome. *Scand J Rheumatol* 34:383-386, 2005.

107. Levendoglu F, Temizhan A, Ugurlu H, et al: Ventricular function abnormalities in active rheumatoid arthritis: A Doppler echocardiographic study. *Rheumatol Int* 24:141-146, 2004.

108. Alpaslan M, Onrat E, Evcik D: Doppler echocardiographic evaluation of ventricular function in patients with rheumatoid arthritis. *Clin Rheumatol* 22:84-88, 2003.

109. Arslan S, Bozkurt E, Ali Sari R, Erol MK: Diastolic function abnormalities in active rheumatoid arthritis evaluation by conventional Doppler and tissue Doppler: Relation with duration of disease. *Clin Rheumatol* 25:294-299; Epub 2005 Oct 13.

110. Crowson CS, Nicola PJ, Kremers HM, et al: How much of the increased incidence of heart failure in rheumatoid arthritis is attributable to traditional cardiovascular risk factors and ischemic heart disease? *Arthritis Rheum* 52:3039-3044, 2000.

111. Nicola PJ, Maradit-Kremers H, Roger VL: The risk of congestive heart failure in rheumatoid arthritis: A population-based study over 46 years. *Arthritis Rheum* 52:412-420, 2005.

112. Wolfe F, Michaud K: Heart failure in rheumatoid arthritis: rates, predictors, and the effect of anti-tumor necrosis factor therapy. *Am J Med* 116:305-311, 2004.

113. Cindas A, Gokce-Kutsal Y, Tokgozoglu L, Karanfil A: QT dispersion and cardiac involvement in patients with rheumatoid arthritis. *Scand J Rheumatol* 31:22-26, 2002.

114. Roos JM, Aubry MC, Edwards WD: Chloroquine cardiotoxicity: Clinicopathologic features in three patients and comparison with three patients with Fabry disease. *Cardiovasc Pathol* 11:277-283, 2002.

115. Gonzalez-Juanatey C, Testa A, Garcia-Castelo A, et al: Echocardiographic and Doppler findings in long-term treated rheumatoid arthritis patients without clinically evident cardiovascular disease. *Semin Arthritis Rheum* 33:231-238, 2004.

116. Galie N, Manes A, Farahani KV, Pelino F, et al: Pulmonary arterial hypertension associated to connective tissue diseases. *Lupus* 9:713-717, 2005.

117. O'Neill TW: The heart in ankylosing spondylitis. *Ann Rheum Dis* 51:705-706, 1992.

118. Hoppmann RA, Wise CM, Challa R, Peacock J: Subacute bacterial endocarditis and ankylosing spondylitis. *Ann Rheum Dis* 47:423-427, 1988.

119. Roldan CA, Chavez J, Weist P, et al: Aortic root disease and valve disease associated with ankylosing spondylitis. *J Am Coll Cardiol* 32:1397-1404, 1998.

120. O'Neill TW, King G, Graham IH, Bresnihan B: Echocardiographic abnormalities in ankylosing spondylitis. *Ann Rheum Dis* 51:652-654, 1992.

121. Yildirir A, Aksoyek S, Calguneri M, et al: Echocardiographic evidence of cardiac involvement in ankylosing spondylitis. *Clin Rheumatol* 21:129-134, 2002.

122. Jimenez-Balderas FJ, Garcia-Rubi D, Perez-Hinojosa S, et al: Two-dimensional echo Doppler findings in juvenile and adult onset ankylosing spondylitis with long-term disease. *Angiology* 52:543-548, 2001.

123. Peters AJ, Wolde S, Sedney MI, et al: Heart conduction disturbance: An HLA-B27 associated disease. *Ann Rheum Dis* 50:348-350, 1991.

124. Brewerton DA, Gibson DG, Goddard DH, et al: The myocardium in ankylosing spondylitis: A clinical, echocardiographic and histopathological study. *Lancet* 1:995-998, 1987.

125. Crowley JJ, Donnelly SM, Tobin M, et al: Doppler echocardiographic evidence of left ventricular diastolic dysfunction in ankylosing spondylitis. *Am J Cardiol* 71:1337-1340, 1993.

126. Fujito T, Inoue T, Hoshi K, et al: Systemic amyloidosis following ankylosing spondylitis associated with congestive heart failure. A case report. *Jpn Heart J* 36:681-688, 1995.

127. Ferri C, Giuggioli M, Sebastian M, et al: Heart involvement in systemic sclerosis. *Lupus* 14:702-707, 2005.

128. Edwards JM, Porter JM: Raynaud's syndrome and small vessel arteriopathy. *Semin Vasc Surg* 6:56-65, 1993.

129. Montisci R, Vacca A, Garau P, et al: Detection of early impairment of coronary flow reserve in patients with systemic sclerosis. *Ann Rheum Dis* 62:890-893, 2003.

130. Aguglia G, Sgreccia A, Bernardo ML, et al: Left ventricular diastolic function in systemic sclerosis. *J Rheumatol* 28:1563-1567, 2001.

131. Meune C, Allanore Y, Devaux JY, et al: High prevalence of right ventricular systolic dysfunction in early systemic sclerosis. *J Rheumatol* 31:1941-1945, 2004.

132. Alexander EL, Firestein GS, Weiss JL, et al: Reversible cold-induced abnormalities in myocardial perfusion and function in systemic sclerosis. *Ann Intern Med* 105:661-668, 1986.

133. Banci M, Rinaldi E, Ierardi M, et al: 99mTc SESTAMIBI scintigraphic evaluation of skeletal muscle disease in patients with systemic sclerosis: diagnostic reliability and comparison with cardiac function and perfusion. *Angiology* 49:641-648, 1998.

134. Handa R, Gupta K, Malhotra A, et al: Cardiac involvement in limited systemic sclerosis: Non-invasive assessment in asymptomatic patients. *Clin Rheumatol* 18:136-139, 1999.

135. Armstrong GP, Whalley GA, Doughty RN, et al: Left ventricular function in scleroderma. *Br J Rheumatol* 35:983-988, 1996.

136. Maione S, Cuomo G, Giunta A, et al: Echocardiographic alterations in systemic sclerosis: A longitudinal study. *Semin Arthritis Rheum* 34:721-727, 2005.

137. Shahin AA, Anwar S, Elawar AH, et al: Circulating soluble adhesion molecules in patients with systemic sclerosis: Correlation between circulating soluble vascular cell adhesion molecule-1 (sVCAM-1) and impaired left ventricular diastolic function. *Rheumatol Int* 20:21-24, 2000.

138. Hirooka K, Naito J, Koretsune Y, et al: Analysis of transmural trends in myocardial integrated backscatter in patients with progressive systemic sclerosis. *J Am Soc Echocardiogr* 16:340-346, 2003.

139. Ferri C, Di Bello, Martini A, et al: Heart involvement in systemic sclerosis: An ultrasonic tissue characterization study. *Ann Rheum Dis* 57:296-302, 1998.

140. Lindqvist P, Caidahl K, Neuman-Andersen G, et al: Disturbed right ventricular diastolic function in patients with systemic sclerosis: a Doppler tissue imaging study. *Chest* 128:755-763, 2005.

141. Giunta A, Tirri E, Maione S, et al: Right ventricular diastolic abnormalities in systemic sclerosis. Relation to left ventricular involvement and pulmonary hypertension. *Ann Rheum Dis* 59:94-98, 2000.

142. D'Andrea A, Bellissimo S, Scotto di Uccio F, et al: Associations of right ventricular myocardial function with skin and pulmonary involvement in asymptomatic patients with systemic sclerosis. *Ital Heart J* 5:831-839, 2004.

143. Breit SN, Thornton SC, Penny R: Lung involvement in scleroderma. *Clin Dermatol* 12:243-252, 1994.

144. Mukerjee D, St George D, Coleiro B, et al: Prevalence and outcome in systemic sclerosis associated pulmonary arterial hypertension: Application of a registry approach. *Ann Rheum Dis* 62:1088-1093, 2003.

145. Gowda RM, Khan IA, Sacchi TJ, Vasavada BC: Scleroderma pericardial disease presented with a large pericardial effusion—a case report. *Angiology* 52:59-62, 2001.

146. Thompson AE, Pope JE: A study of the frequency of pericardial and pleural effusions in scleroderma. *Br J Rheumatol* 37:1320-1323, 1998.

147. Penmetcha M, Rosenbush SW, Harris CA: Cardiac valvular disease in scleroderma and systemic lupus erythematosus/scleroderma overlap associated with antiphospholipid antibodies. *J Rheumatol* 23:2171-2174, 1996.

148. Pullicino P, Borg R, Agius-Musccat H, Nadassy V: Systemic embolism from mitral vegetation in scleroderma. *J R Soc Med* 82:502-503, 1989.

149. Comens SM, Alpert MA, Sharp GC, et al: Frequency of mitral valve prolapse in systemic lupus erythematosus, progressive systemic sclerosis and mixed connective tissue disease. *Am J Cardiol* 63:369, 1989.

150. Moyssakis I, Gialafos E, Vassiliou V, et al: Aortic stiffness in systemic sclerosis is increased independently of the extent of skin involvement. *Rheumatology* 44:251-254, 2005.

151. Lundberg IE: Cardiac involvement in autoimmune myositis and mixed connective tissue disease. *Lupus* 14:708-712, 2005.

152. Gonzalez-Lopez L, Gamez-Nava JI, Sanchez L, et al: Cardiac manifestations in dermato-polymyositis. *Clin Exp Rheumatol* 14:373-379, 1996.

153. Riemekasten G, Opitz C, Audring H, et al: Beware of the heart: the multiple picture of cardiac involvement in myositis. *Rheumatology* 38:1153-1157, 1999.

154. Anders HJ, Wanders A, Rihl M, Kruger K: Myocardial fibrosis in polymyositis. *J Rheumatol* 26:1840-1842, 1999.

155. Buchpiguel CA, Roizenblatt S, Lucenn-Fernandez MF: Radioisotopic assessment of peripheral and cardiac muscle involvement and dysfunction in polymyositis/dermatomyositis. *J Rheumatol* 18:1359-1363, 1991.

156. Spiera R, Kagen L: Extramuscular manifestations in idiopathic inflammatory myopathies. *Curr Opin Rheumatol* 10:556-561, 1998.

157. Yukiiri K, Mizushige K, Ueda T, et al: Fulminant myocarditis in polymyositis. *Jpn Circ J* 65:991-993, 2001.

158. Morrison I, McEntegart A, Capell H: Polymyositis with cardiac manifestations and unexpected immunology. *Ann Rheum Dis* 61:1110-1111, 2002.

159. Tami LF, Bhasin S: Polymorphism of the cardiac manifestations in dermatomyositis. *Clin Cardiol* 16:260-264, 1993.

160. Martinez A, Vila LM, Rios-Olivares E: Predominance of CD4 T cells and Th2 cytokines in the pericardial fluid of a dermatomyositis patient with cardiac tamponade. *Clin Exp Rheumatol* 22:135, 2004.

161. Grillone P, Paolillo V, Presbitero P: Verrucous abacterial endocarditis and polymyositis. A possible association?. *G Ital Cardiol* 26:1303-1307, 1996.

162. Alpert MA, Goldberg SH, Singsen BH, et al: Cardiovascular manifestations of mixed connective tissue disease in adults. *Circulation* 68:1182-1193, 1983.

163. Ueda Y, Yamauchi Y, Makizumi K, et al: Successful treatment of acute right cardiac failure due to pulmonary thromboembolism in mixed connective tissue disease. *Jpn J Med* 30:568-572, 1991.

164. Beier JM, Nielsen HL, Nielsen D: Pleuritis-pericarditis: An unusual initial manifestation of mixed connective tissue disease. *Eur Heart J* 13:859-861, 1992.

165. Bezerra MC, Saraiva F Jr, Carvalho JF, et al: Cardiac tamponade due to massive pericardial effusion in mixed connective tissue disease: reversal with steroid therapy. *Lupus* 13:618-620, 2004.

166. Inoue T, Kamishirado E, Hayashi T, Morooka S: Fulminant hepatic failure due to cardiac tamponade associated with mixed connective tissue disease. *J Med* 28:129-135, 1997.

167. Leung W, Wong K, Lau C, et al: Echocardiographic identification of mitral valvular abnormalities in patients with mixed connective tissue disease. *J Rheumatol* 17:485-488, 1990.

168. Comens SM, Alpert MA, Sharp GC, et al: Frequency of mitral valve prolapse in systemic lupus erythematosus, progressive systemic sclerosis and mixed connective tissue disease. *Am J Cardiol* 63:369-370, 1989.

169. Hammann C, Genton CY, Delabays A, et al: Myocarditis of mixed connective tissue disease: favourable outcome after intravenous pulse cyclophosphamide. *Clin Rheumatol* 18:85-87, 1999.

170. Leung W, Wong K, Lau C, et al: Doppler-echo evaluation of left ventricular diastolic filling in patients with mixed connective tissue disease. *Cardiology* 77:93-100, 1990.

171. Jang JJ, Olin JW, Fuster V. A teenager with mixed connective tissue disease presenting with acute coronary syndrome. *Vasc Med* 9:31-34, 2004.

172. Roldan CA, Shively BKS, Crawford MH: Valve excrescences: Prevalence, evolution, and risk for cardioembolism. *J Am Coll Cardiol* 30:1308-1314, 1997.

Chapter 37

Echocardiography in the Evaluation of Cardiac Disease Resulting from Endocrinopathies, Renal Disease, Obesity, and Nutritional Deficiencies

MARCUS F. STODDARD, MD

A variety of endocrine disorders, renal diseases, nutritional deficiencies, and obesity may adversely alter cardiac function and structure and affect cardiovascular morbidity and mortality. These disorders may impair systolic and diastolic function, cause valvular regurgitation or stenosis, and lead to ventricular hypertrophy and dilation. These disorders may interact resulting in additive or synergistic adverse effects on cardiac function and structure. Although the cardiac manifestations of these disorders are nonspecific, their detection may have clinical relevance and a significant impact on patient management. Echocardiography plays an important role in the timely detection of cardiac abnormalities from these diverse disease entities, particularly in asymptomatic patients. In addition, echocardiography has been important in characterizing the frequency of and natural history of diet medication-related valvulopathy. If properly employed, echocardiography can play an important diagnostic role when anorexigen-induced valvulopathy is being considered.

Endocrinopathies and Heart Disease

Diabetic Heart Disease

Systolic Dysfunction in Diabetes

The presence of a dilated cardiomyopathy (DCM) specifically as a result of diabetes mellitus was first suggested by Rubler and colleagues[1] in 1972. At postmortem examination, cardiac enlargement, hypertrophy, and fibrosis were seen in four adult diabetic patients with histories of congestive heart failure (CHF) unexplained by coronary artery, hypertensive, valvular, congenital, or alcoholic heart disease. The existence of a diabetic DCM characterized by four-chamber enlargement and impaired systolic function was initially met with skepticism. Subsequent studies confirmed the existence of diabetic cardiomyopathy distinct from atherosclerotic or hypertensive heart disease.[2-4]

Systolic dysfunction in diabetic patients may consist of prolongation of the left ventricular (LV) preejection period, shortened LV ejection time, decreased ejection fraction (EF) and stroke volume (SV), and increased LV end-systolic volume.[5-7] As shown in recent studies, LV regional systolic myocardial performance is reduced in diabetes when assessed by strain, strain rate (SR), and myocardial tissue Doppler velocity.[8-10] Exercise may unmask potential abnormalities of systolic function unrelated to coronary artery disease (CAD) that were not apparent at rest in diabetes.[6] The factors accounting for diabetic cardiomyopathy are unknown and are likely multifactorial but may relate to diabetic microan-

giopathy of the coronary circulation, reduction in myocardial glucose supply and oxidation, impaired myocardial free fatty acid metabolism, abnormal regulation of intracellular calcium homeostasis, duration of diabetes, and type of diabetes.[11-14] The metabolic syndrome is a risk factor for adverse cardiovascular complications, such as heart failure (HF). Akin to diabetes mellitus, abnormalities of systolic function occur with the metabolic syndrome.[15]

Diastolic Dysfunction in Diabetes

Several studies confirm an association between diabetes mellitus and LV diastolic dysfunction. Compared with the impairment of LV systolic function, impairment of diastolic function appears to be an earlier sign of diabetic cardiomyopathy and can progress to symptomatic HF. Diastolic function is more likely to be impaired in diabetic patients with overt nephropathy, autonomic neuropathy, or retinopathy,[16-19] but diastolic dysfunction may occur in diabetic patients with uncomplicated disease.[20-22] In addition, diastolic dysfunction as determined by Doppler echocardiography may occur after only a few years of diabetes mellitus.[23] Recent studies using myocardial tissue Doppler imaging (TDI) have shown LV diastolic impairment at early stages in diabetes with a prevalence as high as 75%.[9,10,24-27] Similarly, right ventricular (RV) diastolic dysfunction is a feature of patients with diabetes but no overt heart disease.[28] Diastolic dysfunction in diabetes may consist of impaired LV relaxation, decreased compliance, or both conditions. Myocardial hypertrophy, interstitial collagen accumulation, and fibrosis occur in diabetic cardiomyopathy and may partially account for decreased ventricular compliance.[1,29]

Experiments implicate an abnormal reuptake of calcium into the sarcoplasmic reticulum in diabetes,[30] possibly accounting for impaired LV relaxation. Diastolic dysfunction in diabetes may manifest as prolongation of the isovolumetric relaxation time (IVRT), reduced early diastolic filling (E), increased atrial contribution to diastolic filling, and reduced diastolic myocardial ventricular tissue velocity or elastic recoil.[9,24-26,31,32] Importantly, LV diastolic dysfunction determined by pulsed Doppler echocardiography or tissue Doppler myocardial imaging in type II diabetic subjects adversely reduces maximal exercise capacity and tolerance.[33-35]

Echocardiographic Findings in Diabetes

The structural and functional cardiac abnormalities that may occur in persons with diabetes mellitus have been well characterized by means of echocardiography (Table 37-1). In people with diabetes, as compared with control subjects, conventional indexes de-

TABLE 37–1. Echocardiographic Findings in Diabetes Mellitus

Diastolic Dysfunction	Systolic Dysfunction	Structural Abnormalities
Spectral Doppler	*Spectral Doppler*	*M-Mode/Two-Dimensional*
↓Peak early filling velocity	↑LV preejection period	LV hypertrophy
↓E/A ratio	↓LV ejection time	LV enlargement
↑Percentage atrial contribution	*M-Mode/Two-Dimensional*	*Ultrasonic Integrated Backscatter*
↑Pressure half-time	↓Shortening fraction	Abnormal myocardial acoustics
↑Isovolumetric relaxation time	↓Velocity circumferential FS	↓Cyclic variation
↑Duration of rapid filling phase	↓Ejection fraction	
Color M-Mode	*Tissue Doppler Imaging*	
↓Inflow propagation rate	↓Peak systolic myocardial velocity	
Tissue Doppler Imaging		
↓Early diastolic myocardial peak velocity		
↓Early diastolic strain rate		

E/A, early to atrial velocity ratio; FS, fiber shortening; LV, left ventricular.

rived from pulsed Doppler echocardiography of mitral valve inflow have shown decreased peak early inflow velocity, decreased peak early to peak late filling velocity (E/A) ratio, increased pressure half-time (PHT), and increased atrial contribution to filling[9,20-22,36] (Fig. 37–1). Prolongation of the IVRT in diabetic patients has been demonstrated using continuous-wave (CW) Doppler echocardiography.[22] These abnormalities most likely reflect impairment in LV relaxation and occur in approximately 30% to 46% of asymptomatic young people with diabetes without ischemic, hypertensive, or valvular heart disease.[20,25] Abnormalities of diastolic filling can be further unmasked in patients with diabetes with normal diastolic filling at rest by performance of Valsalva maneuver or isometric handgrip exercise Doppler echocardiography.[25,37] Indexes of diastolic function derived by TDI are sensitive measures of abnormal diastolic function. Thus, it is not surprising that such indexes have been shown to be abnormal in diabetic subjects.[9,10,24-27,34] LV myocardial peak early diastolic velocity and strain are abnormally decreased. Importantly, the detection of diastolic dysfunction is enhanced by the addition of TDI parameters to that of conventional Doppler indexes (Fig. 37–2). Individual patients with diabetes may show an isolated abnormality in conventional or TDI indexes, which emphasizes the need for a comprehensive echocardiographic evaluation in the assessment of diastolic function (Fig. 37–3). Digitized M-mode echocardiography of the LV wall in diastole have shown prolongation of the rapid filling phase in more than 50% of young patients with diabetes who are insulin dependent.[38]

Several studies have demonstrated LV systolic dysfunction in patients with diabetes.[5-7,9,10,16,17,21,24] Peak LV myocardial systolic strain and peak systolic velocity may be reduced in patients with diabetes, representing an early stage of systolic dysfunction before abnormalities of more conventional echocardiographic indexes of systolic function.[8-10,24] In patients with dia-

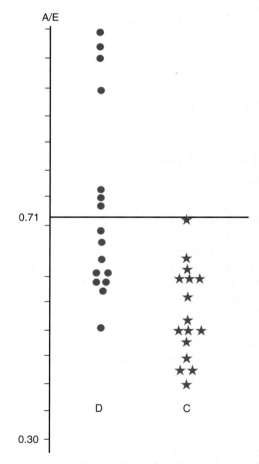

Figure 37–1. Individual values of peak atrial to peak early filling velocity (A/E) ratio of young insulin-dependent patients with diabetes (D) without retinopathy, nephropathy, or coronary artery disease are compared with those of normal control subjects (C). Abnormal filling is common in these young diabetic patients despite lack of other end-organ disease. (From Paillole C, Dahan M, Paycha F, et al: Am J Cardiol 64:1010-1016, 1989.)

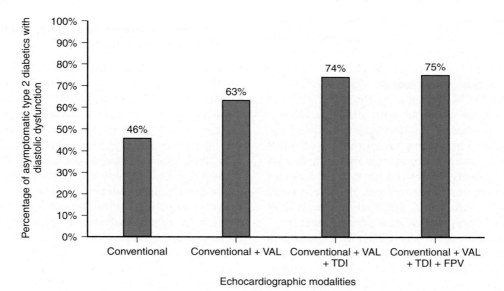

Figure 37–2. *Detection of left ventricular (LV) diastolic dysfunction in asymptomatic, normotensive patients with type 2 diabetes is enhanced by the addition of an abnormal Valsalva maneuver (VAL) response and/or abnormal tissue Doppler imaging (TDI) annular velocity to conventional Doppler indexes of diastolic filling. FPV, color M-mode derived LV inflow propagation rate. (From Boyer JK, Thanigaraj S, Schechtman KB, et al:* Am J Cardiol *93:870-875, 2004.)*

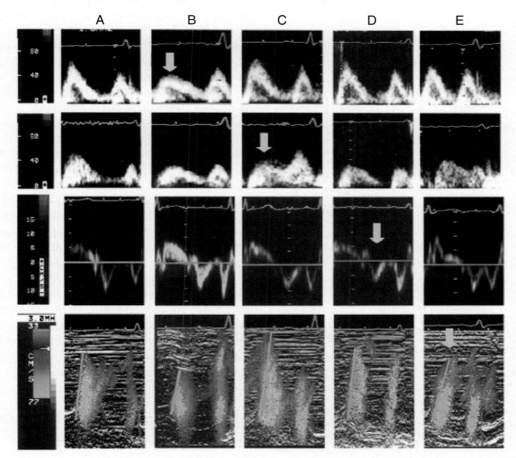

Figure 37–3. *Echocardiographic findings of diastolic function in five different patients with diabetes mellitus, designated as A, B, C, D, and E. Row 1, 2, 3, and 4 represent resting pulsed-Doppler mitral inflow, mitral inflow during the Valsalva maneuver, early diastolic tissue Doppler velocity, and color M-mode inflow propagation rate, respectively. Patient A shows no diastolic dysfunction abnormalities. In patients B through D, only one of the diastolic parameters (downward arrow) was abnormal when the remaining measurements were normal. (From Boyer JK, Thanigaraj S, Schechtman KB, et al:* Am J Cardiol *93:870-875, 2004.)*

betes with long-term, complicated disease, systolic time intervals are frequently abnormal and include prolongation of LV preejection period and shortening of ejection time.[5,7,22] Shortening fraction derived by M-mode echocardiography may be decreased in patients with diabetes with long-standing disease.[29,36] In young asymptomatic patients with diabetes, abnormalities of LV shortening fraction and velocity of circumferential fiber shortening measured by M-mode echocardiography may become evident immediately after exercise.[39] Divergent results have been reported in diabetic subjects on the response of peak systolic myocardial tissue velocity to dobutamine, with findings of a blunted increase[24] versus normal increase.[26]

Left ventricular hypertrophy (LVH) is a feature of diabetes mellitus and can be assessed by M-mode and two-dimensional (2D) echocardiography.[29,36] Abnormal myocardial acoustic properties characterized by a reduction in the cyclic variation of ultrasound-integrated backscatter can be detected in asymptomatic patients with diabetes and may reflect early subclinical cardiomyopathic changes attributable to collagen deposition in the heart[8,40] (Fig. 37–4).

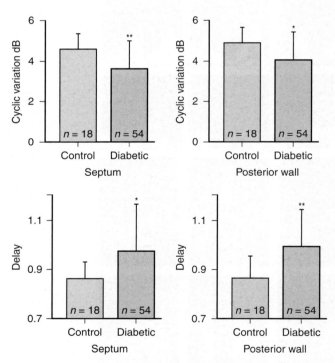

Figure 37–4. Comparison of myocardial acoustic properties from the left ventricular septum and posterior wall in control subjects and diabetic patients assessed by ultrasonic backscatter indexes (cyclic variation in decibels and delay). Patients with diabetes show an altered magnitude and delay of cyclic variation of backscatter consistent with a myopathic process despite the presence of normal ventricular size and function. **P < 0.01 and *P < 0.05 versus control subjects; error bars are standard deviation. (From Perez JE, McGill JB, Santiago JV, et al: J Am Coll Cardiol 19:1154-1162, 1992.)

Interaction of Diabetes with Hypertension, Renal Insufficiency, and Obesity

Diabetes and systemic hypertension are both independently associated with concentric LVH. The prevalence of concentric LVH and magnitude of relative wall thicknesses is greater in patients when these two diseases coexist as compared to when either are in isolation.[41] LV diastolic function is more impaired in patients with coexisting diabetes and hypertension as compared to those subjects with only one of these diseases.[9] LV diastolic dysfunction, independent of LVH, may markedly progress in patients with chronic renal failure and diabetes.[42] LV diastolic dysfunction is significantly more prevalent in obese patients with as compared to those without diabetes mellitus.[43] Lastly, in patients with diabetes the presence of obesity has a synergistic effect on the increase in LV mass corrected for height.[44]

Clinical Utility

Preventive cardiology depends on detection of disease in its earliest stages coupled with effective treatments. In people with diabetes mellitus, echocardiography may be useful in the early detection of LV diastolic dysfunction,[20-23,25] particularly with the emergence of TDI.[9,10,24-27,34] To appropriately apply Doppler echocardiography to assess LV diastolic function, a comprehensive approach must be employed and attention to detail is needed (see Chapter 11). Abnormal systolic function may be unmasked at an early stage in the disease by stress echocardiography (see Chapters 1 and 16).[37,40] Diastolic dysfunction correlates with worsening glycemic control.[45] Importantly, systolic and diastolic dysfunction in diabetes mellitus may be reversible or preventable with glycemic control[31,46] (Fig. 37–5). In patients with type 2 diabetes and hypertension, improved glycemic control promotes regression of LVH.[47] Echocardiographic screening of diabetic subjects, even if asymptomatic, for abnormalities in systolic and diastolic function or ventricular hypertrophy is advisable; particularly if there is the coexistence of diseases that potentiate the adverse effects of diabetes on cardiac structure and function, such as hypertension, renal failure, or obesity. The clinical utility of echocardiography in myocardial tissue characterization for fibrosis in the patient with diabetes is promising.[8,40]

Thyroid Disease and Heart Disease

Systolic Function and Thyroid Disease

Impairment of LV systolic function is a well-recognized feature of overt chronic hypothyroidism.[48-54] Myocardial contractility is depressed by hypothyroidism, possibly because of alterations in contractile protein isoforms. Animal models demonstrate that low thyroid

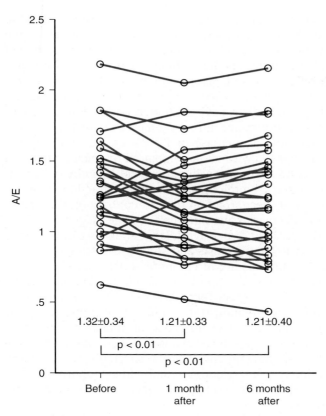

Figure 37–5. *Individual and mean data values of peak atrial to peak early filling velocity (A/E) ratio in non–insulin-dependent diabetic patients before and 1 and 6 months after glycemic control by insulin treatment. A significant reduction in A/E ratio occurs during treatment, consistent with improved diastolic filling. (From Hiramatsu K, Ohara N, Shigematsu S, et al: Am J Cardiol 70:1185-1189, 1992.)*

function induces cardiac atrophy and chamber dilatation from loss of arterioles, which impair myocardial blood flow.[55] These processes may lead to the development of DCM and CHF.[51] Subclinical or borderline hypothyroidism is a frequent and early form of thyroid failure, whereby circulating free thyroid hormone concentrations are normal, but thyroid stimulating hormone level is elevated. Recent echocardiographic studies using TDI have shown that systolic dysfunction may be evident in subclinical or borderline hypothyroidism during exercise but inconsistently present at rest.[56-59]

Hyperthyroidism has a multifaceted effect on the cardiovascular system. Enhanced resting LV contractile function is a consistent finding in overt hyperthyroidism.[53,60-63] During exercise, however, selected subjects with hyperthyroidism display a paradoxical decline or blunted increase in LVEF, SV, heart rate, and cardiac output (CO).[53,60,64] Kahaly and colleagues[65] demonstrated impaired cardiopulmonary exercise capacity in patients with overt hyperthyroidism, which was reversible in the euthyroid state. In addition, hyperthyroidism is associated with cardiomegaly and CHF. Importantly, a striking reversal of CHF and DCM resulting from hy-

perthyroidism may occur after induction of a euthyroid state.[61,66] For example, Umpierrez and colleagues[67] showed an increase in mean LV EF from 28% before to 55% after becoming euthyroid in patients with hyperthyroidism. Enhanced RV systolic function as assessed by myocardial peak systolic velocity derived from TDI is present in overt hyperthyroidism.[68] Subclinical hyperthyroidism is defined as a lower than normal thyroid stimulating hormone concentration in association with normal free thyroid hormone levels. It may be exogenous (i.e., induced by thyroid hormone treatment) or caused by endogenous thyroid disease. Several studies have shown subclinical hyperthyroidism, whether exogenous[69,70] or endogenous,[71] to increase LV systolic function while other researchers have reported no effect.[63,72-74]

Diastolic Function and Thyroid Disease

LV diastolic dysfunction is an associated feature of overt and subclinical hypothyroidism. M-mode and conventional Doppler echocardiographic indexes are consistent with impaired relaxation in overt hypothyroidism.[75] Subclinical hypothyroidism has been consistently shown to display diastolic dysfunction as evidenced by abnormalities in TDI-derived peak early diastolic myocardial velocity and relaxation time interval.[56-59] Importantly, impaired relaxation in overt and subclinical hypothyroidism may be reversed by thyroid hormone replacement.[56,75-77]

LV filling as assessed by Doppler echocardiography may be enhanced in untreated overt hyperthyroidism,[78,79] which may normalize after treatment induces a euthyroid state.[78] Exogenous subclinical hyperthyroidism is more consistently associated with diastolic dysfunction,[69,70,73,80] although others have failed to show diastolic dysfunction in this clinical setting.[72,74] Diastolic dysfunction when present in exogenous subclinical hyperthyroidism is partially reversible with achievement of a euthyroid state after medication titration.[80] Divergent results have been found in endogenous subclinical hyperthyroidism, with some investigators reporting associated diastolic dysfunction,[71] others noting no effect,[74] while still others finding an associated decrease in IVRT or potentially enhanced diastolic function.[63]

Structural, Valvular, and Pericardial Diseases

Pericardial effusion (PE) is a manifestation of overt hypothyroidism. The incidence of pericardial effusion in hypothyroidism varies with severity of disease and occurs in 30% to 80% of patients with advanced, severe disease[81-84] and in 3% to 6% of patients with mild disease.[85] Cardiac tamponade resulting from PE from hypothyroidism is rare.[86] Histological studies have demonstrated myofibril swelling and interstitial edema and fibrosis in the cardiac tissue of patients with hypothyroidism. Asymmetric septal hypertrophy may occur as a feature of overt hypothyroidism but appears to be rare.[87]

An association between Graves' disease and mitral valve prolapse (MVP) has been reported.[88,89] A prevalence as high as 16.5% to 25% of mitral valve prolapse in patients with Graves' disease has been found.[89,90] The basis for this association is unknown; however, prior studies suggest a possible autoimmune-mediated mechanism[91] or potential genetic linkage between Graves' hyperthyroidism and mitral valve prolapse.[92] In addition, mitral regurgitation (MR) has been seen in 71% of patients with Graves' disease, whereas tricuspid regurgitation (TR) may occur in 63% of such patients.[90] Importantly, moderate or severe tricuspid regurgitation can be seen in 29% of these patients and is associated with CHF.[90] Increased LV mass and prevalence of LVH is a feature of overt hyperthyroidism and endogenous or exogenous subclinical hyperthyroidism.[63,70,71,74,80] LV mass is substantially higher in patients with coexisting subclinical hyperthyroidism and hypertension, than when either disease is seen in isolation.[93]

Echocardiographic Findings in Thyroid Disease

M-mode, 2D, and Doppler echocardiography have been used to demonstrate impaired LV systolic function in patients with overt hypothyroidism (Tables 37–2 and 37–3). Several studies have shown prolongation of the LV preejection period and reduction of the shortening fraction, EF, velocity of circumferential fiber shortening, and systolic ejection force in overt hypothyroidism.[48-54] Although earlier studies failed to show systolic dysfunction via systolic intervals in patients with subclinical hypothyroidism, more recent studies differ and have shown increases in LV preejection period and preejection period to ejection time ratio in these subjects.[58,76,94] Patients with subclinical hypothyroidism have a blunted augmentation of cardiac performance during exercise as reflected by a less than normal increase in EF, SV or CO with stress.[95] TDI has likewise shown impaired regional myocardial systolic dysfunction in subclinical hypothyroidism as reflected by prolongation in precontraction time, increased precontraction time to contraction time ratio, and decreased annular peak systolic velocity[57,58] (Fig. 37–6). Overt hyperthyroidism enhances cardiac sensitivity to beta agonists and augments resting LV EF and rate, and velocity of circumferential fiber shortening, as assessed by 2D, Doppler, and M-mode echocardiography,[62-64] respectively. However, stress echocardiography may demonstrate a blunted response in LV EF, SV, and CO.[64] The influence of subclinical hypothyroidism on systolic function is variable with some studies showing enhanced LV shortening fraction and velocity of circumferential fiber shortening,[69-71] whereas others finding no effect on these parameters or EF.[63,72-74]

Impaired diastolic function of overt hypothyroid patients is manifested by prolongation in IVRT and reduction in early diastolic posterior wall thinning rate.[75,77] These abnormalities can be assessed by Doppler and M-mode echocardiography. In addition, myocardial performance index (i.e., isovolumetric contraction time + IVRT ÷ ejection time) may be prolonged in this

---

TABLE 37–2. Echocardiographic Findings in Hypothyroidism

Overt Hypothyroidism		
Systolic Dysfunction	**Diastolic Dysfunction**	**Structural Abnormalities**
M-Mode/Two-Dimensional	*M-Mode*	*M-Mode/Two-Dimensional*
↓Shortening fraction	↓Posterior wall thinning rate	LV enlargement
↓LV ejection fraction	*Spectral Doppler*	Pericardial effusion:
↓Velocity circumferential FS	↑Isovolumetric relaxation time	30%-80% (in advanced disease)
Spectral Doppler		3%-6% (in mild disease)
↑LV preejection period		
Subclinical Hypothyroidism		
Systolic Dysfunction	**Diastolic Dysfunction**	**Structural Abnormalities**
Tissue Doppler Imaging	*Tissue Doppler Imaging*	*M-Mode/Two-Dimensional*
↑Myocardial precontraction time	↑Myocardial relaxation time	LV hypertrophy
↓Annular peak systolic velocity	↓Annular peak early diastolic velocity	*Ultrasonic Integrated Backscatter*
Spectral Doppler	*Spectral Doppler*	↓Cyclic variation
↑LV preejection period	↑Isovolumetric relaxation time	
↑LV preejection period/	↓Peak early filling velocity	
LV ejection time	E/A ratio	

E/A, early to atrial velocity ratio; FS, fiber shortening; LV, left ventricular.

TABLE 37-3. Echocardiographic Findings in Hyperthyroidism

Overt Hyperthyroidism		
Enhanced Systolic Function	**Enhanced Diastolic Function**	**Structural Abnormalities**
M-Mode/Two-Dimensional ↑LV ejection rate ↑Velocity circumferential FS ↑LV ejection fraction	*Spectral Doppler* ↓Isovolumetric relaxation time ↓Early filling deceleration time ↑Early filling deceleration rate	*M-Mode/Two-Dimensional* LV enlargement ↑LV mass LV hypertrophy Mitral valve prolapse
Subclinical Hyperthyroidism		
Systolic Function	**Diastolic Function**	**Structural Abnormalities**
M-Mode/Two-Dimensional ↑or normal shortening fraction ↑or normal velocity circumferential FS Normal ejection fraction	*Spectral Doppler* ↑Isovolumetric relaxation time ↓or normal peak early filling velocity or normal E/A ratio	*M-Mode/Two-Dimensional* ↑LV mass

In overt hyperthyroidism stress echocardiography may demonstrate a blunted rise in left ventricular ejection fraction, stroke volume, and cardiac output, and dilated cardiomyopathy may occur.
FS, fiber shortening; LV, left ventricular.

disorder.[96] In subclinical hypothyroidism, LV diastolic dysfunction as evidenced by prolongation of IVRT derived from Doppler echocardiography has been consistently shown.[57,59,70,76,77,94] Lower peak early filling velocity or peak early to atrial velocity ratio may occur with this condition.[59] Lastly, TDI shows lower LV annular early diastolic velocity and prolonged myocardial relaxation time[58,59] (see Fig. 37–6).

Enhanced diastolic function of overt hyperthyroidism is manifested by a shortening of IVRT and deceleration time (DT) and an increase of early diastolic deceleration rate, as assessed by Doppler echocardiography.[78] Most studies have shown evidence of LV diastolic dysfunction in subclinical hyperthyroidism on the basis of conventional Doppler echocardiographic indexes, namely prolongation of IVRT and/or reduced E/A ratio.[69-71,73,80] However, other studies using the same indexes have shown no effect on diastolic function.[72,74]

2D echocardiography is an excellent technique to diagnose PE in overt hypothyroidism. The diagnosis of hypothyroidism can be easily missed in some medical conditions, such as Down's syndrome, and the finding of PE by echocardiography may lead to the correct diagnosis of thyroid dysfunction[97] (Fig. 37–7). Asymmetric hypertrophy, although rare in overt hypothyroidism, is clinically relevant and can be readily diagnosed with M-mode and 2D echocardiography.[87] In subclinical hypothyroidism, abnormalities of increased LV mass or myocardial texture can be diagnosed with 2D echocardiography[94] or ultrasonic tissue backscatter,[76] respectively. Increased LV mass and LVH, features of overt[63,70,98] and subclinical[71,74,80,93] hyperthyroidism can be diagnosed by M-mode and 2D echocardiography. Valvular

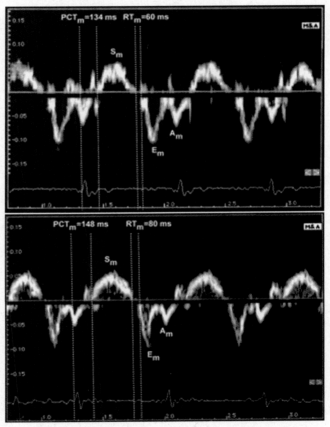

Figure 37–6. *Pulsed tissue Doppler pattern of posterior septum in a healthy subject* (upper panel) *and in a patient with subclinical hypothyroidism* (lower panel). *The peak myocardial early to atrial velocity (E_m/A_m) ratio is more than 1 in both cases, but myocardial precontraction time (PCT_m) and relaxation time (RT_m) are longer in the patient with subclinical hypothyroidism. (From Vitale G, Galderisi M, Lupoli GA, et al: J Clin Endocrinol Metab 87:4350-4355, 2002.)*

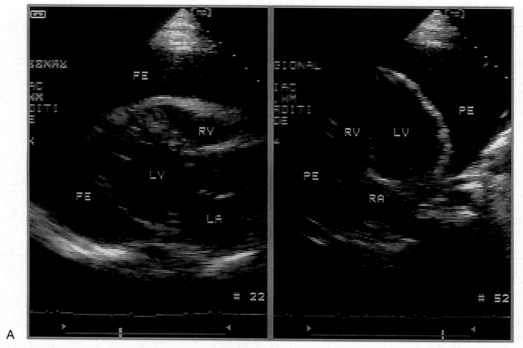

Figure 37–7. Transthoracic two-dimensional parasternal long-axis (A) and four-chamber (B) views demonstrating a large pericardial effusion (PE) with compression of the right ventricle (RV) and right atrium (RA) as a result of confirmed cardiac tamponade by invasive evaluation. This patient was a 26-year-old man with Down's syndrome who presented with dyspnea. Profound hypothyroidism was confirmed after the echocardiographic findings of pericardial effusion. LV, left ventricle; LA, left atrium.

heart disease, including mitral valve prolapse and hemodynamically significant mitral or tricuspid regurgitation, associated with overt hyperthyroidism can be assessed for clinical significance and progression with echocardiography.[89,90] Echocardiography has been used to demonstrate that pulmonary hypertension defined as peak pulmonary systolic pressure greater than 35 mm Hg may occur in as many as 41% of patients with overt hyperthyroidism.[99]

Clinical Utility

The cardiac abnormalities seen in patients with overt and subclinical hypothyroidism are potentially reversible.[76,77,100] M-mode, 2D, and Doppler echocardiography are useful for detecting and assessing the severity of cardiac abnormalities associated with hypothyroidism. TDI techniques have rapidly matured in the last few years and offer potential for a greater diagnostic yield for abnormalities of cardiac function, particularly diastolic dysfunction. An accurate diagnosis of HF in the setting of overt hypothyroidism may be problematic because of nonspecific symptoms. Echocardiographic findings of cardiac dysfunction and/or hemodynamically significant mitral or tricuspid regurgitation would support the diagnosis of HF and potentially affect the specific selection of medical therapy. Subclinical hypothyroidism adversely affects cardiac structure and func-

tion. Such findings are clinically relevant because they portend development of overt cardiac disease. Screening for cardiac disease in these patients should incorporate more sophisticated echocardiographic techniques, such as TDI. Otherwise, occult and reversible myocardial disease may go unrecognized. Pericardial tamponade in overt hypothyroidism is difficult to recognize and easily confused with HF.[86] Both may be diagnosed with dyspnea, tachycardia, jugular venous distention, enlarged cardiac silhouette, and peripheral edema. The diagnosis of cardiac tamponade is facilitated by the use of echocardiography. Adverse cardiac effects from overt or subclinical hyperthyroidism are potentially reversible with treatment once recognized.[70,71,80] In patients with overt hyperthyroidism, attributing exercise limitations to primary cardiac disease may be challenging on the basis of resting systolic function, which is typically enhanced. However, exercise echocardiography may be useful in unmasking a blunted improvement in systolic function with exercise and aid in treatment.[53,60,64] Studies addressing the potential clinical usefulness of TDI in this setting will further guide in the utility of echocardiography. Subclinical hyperthyroidism has a relevant clinical impact in that it adversely affects cardiac structure and function. Screening for these abnormalities with echocardiography, particularly using comprehensive measures of diastolic function, is advisable. Lastly, overt hyperthyroidism should be included in the differential diagnosis of pulmonary hypertension.

Acromegalic Heart Disease

Ventricular Hypertrophy in Acromegaly

Cardiovascular complications are a major cause of morbidity and mortality from acromegaly. LVH occurs in many patients with acromegaly and contributes to the morbidity and mortality from this disease.[101-112] The development of LVH in acromegaly is partially explained by the association of hypertension with this disease.[113,114] However, LVH may occur in a significant proportion of acromegalic patients in the absence of hypertension.[101-114] In addition, LV mass has been shown to increase with short-term growth hormone hypersecretion[115,116] and to regress after effective chronic pharmacologic therapy.[109-112,117-118] Pathologic studies on acromegalic hearts show extensive interstitial fibrosis. Ultrasonographic tissue characterization in uncomplicated acromegalic patients demonstrates an abnormal increase in echo-reflectivity,[111,119,120] which may revert to normal after cure or adequate control of the disease.[111,119] The type of LVH is typically concentric,[101,102,104] but eccentric hypertrophy whereby the increase in LV mass is predominantly on the basis of chamber dilation as compared to wall thickness has been reported.[119] Although asymmetric septal hypertrophy may develop in acromegaly, its reported prevalence among patients with this condition is highly variable.[101-105] Some studies have reported a rare association,[101,102,104] and others have described a frequent association[103,105] between asymmetric septal hypertrophy and acromegaly. In addition to concentric wall thickening, LV diastolic chamber enlargement develops in acromegaly and may occur in the absence of other associated diseases, such as hypertension, CAD, and diabetes mellitus.[101,102,104,105] The reported incidence of an increased LV mass in patients with acromegaly is 38% to 81%.[101-104,121] The development of RV hypertrophy in persons with acromegaly has also been described.[122]

Diastolic Dysfunction in Acromegaly

Given the frequent association of acromegaly with LVH, hypertension, premature CAD, and diabetes mellitus, it is not surprising that diastolic dysfunction often occurs in those with acromegaly.[107-112,121,122] Prolongation of IVRT and abnormal LV diastolic filling, characterized by reduction of early filling and augmentation of atrial contribution to filling, occur in most patients with acromegaly, even in the absence of hypertension, diabetes mellitus, or CAD.[121,122] Abnormalities of diastolic function often improve with treatment.[109,111,112,123] Disease duration and increased LV mass are important factors in the severity of impaired LV filling.[123] Abnor-

malities of RV filling similar to those of the left ventricle also occur.[116,122]

Systolic Function and Acromegaly

In the absence of long-standing, severe acromegaly complicated by hypertension, CAD, or diabetes mellitus, global LV systolic dysfunction in patients with acromegaly appears uncommon.[101-105,121,122] However, regional LV systolic dysfunction may be evident.[108,123] In patients with short-term acromegaly uncomplicated by hypertension, CAD, or diabetes mellitus, global LV systolic function, as assessed by shortening fraction, SV, and CO, typically is enhanced.[124] However, prolonged untreated acromegaly may lead to DCM and HF.[125,126] Acromegaly is characterized by excessive apoptosis of myocytes and nonmyocytes, which correlates with the extent of impairment in EF and disease duration, possibly explaining acromegalic cardiomyopathy.[125]

Valvular Heart Disease in Acromegaly

Acromegaly is associated with an increased prevalence of potentially significant aortic and MR.[127,128] Aortic regurgitation (AR) of a mild or greater severity reportedly occurs in 18% of patients with inactive acromegaly and increases to 31% if acromegaly is active (defined as elevated levels of growth hormone).[127] Severe MR has been noted in 5% of patients with acromegaly.[128] The prevalence of significant aortic or MR increases with duration of disease[128] (Fig. 37–8). Successful valvular surgery has been reported in these

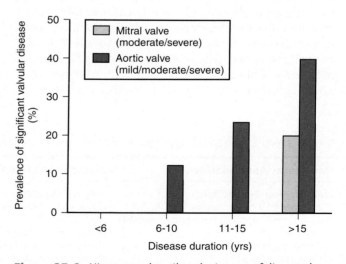

Figure 37–8. *Histogram describes the impact of disease duration on valvular disease (i.e., mild or greater aortic and moderate or greater mitral regurgitation) in patients with acromegaly. Binary logistic regression analysis showed a significant impact of disease duration on valvular disease with an odds ratio equal to 1.19; 95% confidence interval, 1.028-1.376 (i.e., every additional year of disease would result in a 19% increase in odds per year). (From Pereira AM, van Thiel SW, Lindner JR, et al: J Clin Endocrinol Metab 89:71-75, 2004.)*

patients,[128,129] with pathology findings of myxoid valvular degeneration.[128]

Echocardiographic Findings in Acromegaly

Echocardiography is well suited to delineate the protean cardiac manifestations of acromegaly (Table 37–4). M-mode and 2D echocardiographic findings include concentric LVH,[101,102,104,116] eccentric hypertrophy,[119] septal hypertrophy that may simulate hypertrophic cardiomyopathy (HCM),[103,105] RV hypertrophy,[122] and LV dilation.[101,102,104,106] In acromegaly, echocardiography is useful in diagnosing LVH and documenting its regression with therapy.[109-111,118,119] Pulsed Doppler echocardiography of transmitral valve velocities in these patients shows a reduction of peak early filling velocity and E/A ratio and an increase in peak atrial filling velocity and deceleration time of early filling.[109-111,116,122] Abnormalities of transtricuspid valve Doppler velocities similar to those of the mitral valve are a feature of acromegaly.[116,122] IVRT assessed by Doppler echocardiography is prolonged in acromegalic patients.[107-109,116,122] Pulsed Doppler echocardiography has shown abnormal superior vena cava (SVC) flow, characterized by a decrease in peak forward diastolic velocity and an increase in peak flow velocity reversal during atrial contraction.[122] These findings are consistent with biventricular diastolic dysfunction, possibly reflecting impaired ventricular relaxation. TDI of LV myocardium confirms regional diastolic dysfunction in patients with acromegaly as evidenced by a decrease in peak early diastolic myocardial velocity and peak early to atrial myocardial velocity ratio[112,123] (Fig. 37–9). Depending on duration of disease, EF by echocardiography at rest may be enhanced, normal, or reduced. Reduced peak myocardial systolic velocity by pulsed-wave TDI may be evident at rest with active acromegaly.[108] Exercise may show a blunted increase in EF, unmasking occult systolic dysfunction even when the disease is early in

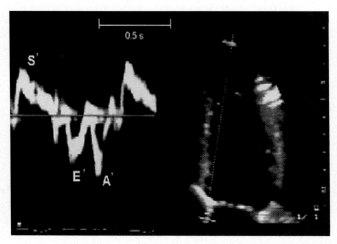

Figure 37–9. *Pulsed-wave Doppler tissue tracing of sepal mitral annulus in a patient with acromegaly. The peak annular early diastolic velocity (E') is reduced with resulting inversion of E' to peak atrial diastolic velocity (A') ratio (E'/A'). (From Bruch C, Herrmann B, Schmermund A, et al: Am Heart J 144:538-543, 2002.)*

its onset.[130] Ultrasonic integrated backscatter in patients with acromegaly shows reduced cyclic variation and increased derived collagen volume fraction, an index of myocardial fibrosis.[111,119]

Clinical Utility

Acromegaly frequently leads to heart disease, which may be asymptomatic. Clinical studies have demonstrated that suppression of growth hormone release by pharmacologic agents, such as octreotide acetate, a long-acting somatostatin synthetic peptide analog, in patients with acromegaly significantly reduces LVH and reduces abnormalities of IVRT and LV and RV filling.[109-111,118,131,132] The echocardiographic evaluation of cardiac size and function in patients with acromegaly is of value to assess ventricular hypertrophy and car-

TABLE 37–4. **Echocardiographic Findings in Acromegaly**

Structural Abnormalities	Diastolic Dysfunction (>50%)	Systolic Function
M-Mode/Two-Dimensional	*Spectral Doppler*	*M-Mode/Two-Dimensional*
Concentric LV hypertrophy (>50%)	↓Peak early filling velocity	*In short-term acromegaly*
Asymmetric septal hypertrophy (variable frequency)	↓E/A ratio	↑Ejection fraction
	↑Early filling deceleration time	↑Stroke volume
LV enlargement	↑Isovolumetric relaxation time	↑Cardiac output
↑LV mass (38%-81%)	Abnormal SVC flow	*In long-term acromegaly*
RV hypertrophy		Normal or ↓ejection fraction
Ultrasonic Integrated Backscatter	*Tissue Doppler Imaging*	*Tissue Doppler Imaging*
↓Cyclic variation	↓Early diastolic myocardial velocity	↓Peak myocardial systolic velocity
↑Derived collagen volume fraction	↓Early to atrial myocardial velocity ratio	

E/A, peak early to peak atrial velocity ratio; LV, left ventricular; RV, right ventricular; SVC, superior vena cava.

diac dysfunction. Prolongation of IVRT is the most sensitive conventional echocardiographic index of cardiac involvement in acromegaly and is useful in the evaluation in the subclinical stage of the disease.[107] Importantly, indexes derived from TDI appear more sensitive for myocardial involvement and should be useful in the serial evaluation of treated patients with acromegaly to detect cardiac involvement.[108,112] Ventricular hypertrophy and dysfunction are important indicators for aggressive treatment to control growth hormone levels as a means of improving heart disease in patients with excessive growth hormone.[117,124,131,132] The application of more sophisticated echocardiographic techniques, such as ultrasonic integrated backscatter to assess for myocardial fibrosis and collagen volume, await future investigations but are promising.[111,119] The echocardiographic manifestations of structural valvular disease in acromegaly have been described and include aortic and mitral valve fibrosis and calcification, and mitral annular calcification.[127] Significant MR and/or AR may ensue, occasionally progressing to the point of surgical intervention. Conventional color flow and spectral Doppler echocardiography should be used for the serial evaluation of patients with acromegaly and evidence of structural valvular disease, particularly if the disease has been long standing.[128]

Hyperparathyroidism and Heart Disease

Cardiac Calcification

The major cause of death in primary hyperparathyroidism patients is cardiovascular disease.[133-135] Hypercalcemia resulting from primary hyperparathyroidism may induce calcification of coronary arteries,[136] valves,[137-139] and myocardium.[137-140] Aortic valve calcification occurs in 46% to 63% of primary hyperparathyroidism patients, and mitral valve or submitral annulus calcification has been reported in 33% to 49% of these patients.[137-139] Aortic stenosis (AS) and mitral stenosis (MS) may result from primary hyperparathyroidism.[137,138] Myocardial calcific deposits have been re-

ported in 62% to 74% of patients with primary hyperparathyroidism.[137-139] Myocardial calcification mainly involves the interventricular septum and may result in third-degree heart block.[137,138]

Structure and Function in Hyperparathyroidism

LVH is a common feature of primary hyperparathyroidism and may be caused by an excessive serum concentration of parathyroid hormone or elevated extracellular calcium concentration.[138-143] Partial regression of LVH may occur 6 months to 1 year after parathyroidectomy in these patients.[138,139,141,142] Primary hyperparathyroidism is associated with hypercontractile function and may be a cause of HCM.[140] A reduced transmitral valve E/A ratio and prolonged IVRT by pulsed Doppler echocardiography has been reported in patients with primary hyperparathyroidism and suggests that LV diastolic dysfunction may be a feature of this disease.[143-146] Global LV systolic function appears little affected but may be slightly increased via ejection or shortening fraction.[146]

Echocardiographic Findings in Hyperparathyroidism

2D echocardiography is useful for determining the extent of myocardial and valvular calcification in patients with primary hyperparathyroidism (Table 37-5). The presence and severity of aortic or mitral stenosis can be assessed by Doppler echocardiography. M-mode and 2D echocardiographic methods are useful for evaluation of LVH and possible HCM.[140] Diastolic function can be assessed. Newer indexes of diastolic function, such as TDI, should be used to potentially detect myocardial disease at an early stage.

Clinical Utility

Echocardiography helps identify LVH and valvular stenosis in patients with primary hyperparathyroidism. Parathyroidectomy may promote regression of myocar-

TABLE 37-5. **Echocardiographic Findings in Primary Hyperparathyroidism**

Valvular Disease	Structural Abnormalities	Enhanced Systolic Function
M-Mode/Two-Dimensional/Doppler	*M-Mode/Two-Dimensional*	*Two-Dimensional*
Aortic valve calcification (46%-63%)	Myocardial calcification (62%-74%)	↑LV ejection fraction
Mitral valve/annulus calcification (33%-49%)	LV hypertrophy	
Aortic stenosis	Asymmetric septal hypertrophy	
Mitral stenosis		

LV, left ventricular.

dial hypertrophy and can be monitored by serial echocardiographic studies.[138,139,141,142]

Adrenal Diseases and Heart Disease

Cushing's Syndrome and Echocardiographic Features

Cushing's syndrome is associated with a fourfold increase in mortality rate as a result of cardiovascular complications.[147] Cushing's syndrome is caused by excessive secretion of adrenocortical hormones, which leads to hypertension, impaired glucose tolerance, diabetes, truncal obesity, hyperlipidemia, and a prothrombotic milieu. LVH frequently occurs in patients with this syndrome and is partially attributable to associated hypertension. An echocardiographic study showed LVH and asymmetric septal hypertrophy in 75% of patients with Cushing's syndrome.[148] Asymmetric septal hypertrophy in this syndrome is common and severe, with interventricular septal thickness ranging from 1.6 to 3.2 cm and the ratio of septal to posterior wall thickness ranging from 1.33 to 2.67.[148] Fallo and colleagues[149] noted LV concentric remodeling (i.e., high relative wall thickness without increased LV mass) in Cushing's syndrome that was independent of blood pressure. M-mode echocardiographically derived LV midwall fractional shortening may be decreased in Cushing's syndrome, consistent with systolic dysfunction.[150] Similarly, diastolic dysfunction consistent with impaired LV relaxation may be present as evidenced by a reduced transmitral peak early to atrial velocity ratio, and prolonged deceleration time.[150] The frequency of concentric remodeling and diastolic dysfunction increases with longer duration of disease. These abnormalities may contribute to the high cardiovascular morbidity seen in patients with Cushing's syndrome and suggest a role for echocardiography.

Primary Hyperaldosteronism and Echocardiographic Features

LV wall thickening without asymmetric septal hypertrophy is a feature of primary hyperaldosteronism.[151] Several investigators have reported concentric LVH in primary hyperaldosteronism,[152-154] evidence of diastolic dysfunction as reflected by reduced mitral valve peak early filling velocity and peak early to atrial velocity or integral ratio and increased atrial contribution to filling.[153-156] Not unexpectedly on the basis of prior findings of globally impaired diastolic function, regional myocardial diastolic function may be abnormal in primary hyperaldosteronism. For example, peak early diastolic myocardial velocity derived from TDI is decreased in this disease.[156] However, LV systolic function does not appear to be impaired as assessed by EF or regional

indexes, such as myocardial strain (i.e., percent deformation of myocardial segmental length) and peak systolic strain rate (i.e., peak rate of regional myocardial deformation).[156] In primary hyperaldosteronism, myocardial ultrasonic integrated backscatter demonstrate decreased cyclic variation, findings consistent with greater myocardial collagen content and fibrosis.[157,158] Experimental data support the concept that excessive aldosterone, independent of its hypertensive effect, may induce ventricular hypertrophy and fibrosis.[159] However, histological proof of myocardial fibrosis in humans from primary hyperaldosteronism remains to be shown.[159]

Clinical Utility

Regression of LVH in Cushing's syndrome after surgical treatment frequently occurs and may be dramatic.[148] Echocardiographic findings of severe LVH or HCM without obvious cause should raise the clinical suspicion of glucocorticoid excess, possibly from Cushing's syndrome. Regression of LVH may occur after surgical excision of an aldosterone-producing tumor in patients with primary hyperaldosteronism.[154] Pharmacologic agents, such as spironolactone, that antagonize mineralocorticoid receptors offer cardio protection and echocardiographic abnormalities of function or structure in these patients would suggest their need.

End-Stage Renal Disease and Heart Disease

Uremic Cardiomyopathy

CHF commonly occurs in patients with end-stage renal failure.[160] The pathogenesis of HF in uremic patients is complex and multifactorial and may include anemia, electrolyte and acid-base abnormalities, volume overload, hypertension, CAD, and uremic toxins. Although some studies have reported normal LV systolic function in patients with uremia,[161,162] many support the presence of a specific uremic cardiomyopathy.[163-167] The features of uremic cardiomyopathy include cardiac enlargement, impaired LV systolic function, and ventricular hypertrophy. In addition, after renal transplantation systolic function improves, LV volume decreases, and LVH regresses, independent of blood pressure control.[168] Secondary hyperparathyroidism resulting from uremia is a cause of LV systolic dysfunction.[166,169,170] Dilated nonischemic and nonvalvular cardiomyopathy associated with advanced secondary hyperparathyroidism in patients on chronic dialysis has been shown to considerably improve 6 months after parathyroidectomy, with mean LV EF and end-diastolic diameter practically normalizing.[169] LV systolic dysfunction is demonstrable in mild secondary hyperparathyroidism by the sensitive technique of TDI.[170]

Structural and Valvular Heart Disease in Renal Disease

Calcification of the myocardium, valves, or cardiac skeleton is found in most patients with end-stage renal disease and is caused by derangements in calcium and phosphorus metabolism.[171-177] Calcification of the aortic valve has been reported in 28% to 60% of patients with end-stage renal disease.[173-175,177] Mitral annular calcification has been described in 10% to 36% of patients on dialysis.[171,172] A study using transesophageal echocardiography (TEE), which offers enhanced 2D resolution as compared to transthoracic echocardiography (TTE) has shown that calcification may also occur in "atypical" areas, such as the base of both mitral leaflets and intervalvular fibrosa.[178]

Aortic valve regurgitation is a feature of renal failure and is explained by valvular calcification,[173,179] and it occurs in 13% of renal failure patients.[173] MR may occur in 38% of renal failure patients and may be caused by mitral annular calcification or LV dilation.[173] Tricuspid and pulmonic insufficiency occur with the same frequency as do MR and AR, respectively, in patients with chronic renal failure.[173,180] However, the mechanism of right-sided valvular regurgitation consists of increased pulmonary artery (PA) pressures as a consequence of hemodynamically significant MR as opposed to that of valvular calcification.[173,181]

Calcific aortic and mitral stenoses are important valvular abnormalities of renal failure. Occasionally, aortic and mitral stenoses may rapidly progress in patients with chronic renal failure, possibly because of associated secondary hyperparathyroidism.[177,182] Pericardial disease from renal failure may manifest as PE, pericardial thickening, or cardiac tamponade. Concentric LVH or asymmetric septal hypertrophy may be seen in renal failure patients with or without associated systemic hypertension.[183,184] In patients with renal failure with secondary hyperparathyroidism, eccentric LVH may occur, characterized by LV dilation and normal wall thickness.[185,186]

Diastolic Function and Renal Disease

LV diastolic dysfunction is associated with renal failure[170,187-189] and may persist after renal transplantation.[187,189] In renal failure, LVH is a common associated finding, but it is not a necessary feature to display diastolic dysfunction in this disease. The primary etiology of renal failure may likewise contribute to diastolic dysfunction, such as systemic hypertension or diabetes mellitus. The diastolic dysfunction is on the basis of impaired LV relaxation or ventricular noncompliance.

Echocardiographic Findings in Renal Disease

Structural or valvular abnormalities of the heart detectable by echocardiography occur in most patients with end-stage renal disease and may include atrial or ventricular dilation; concentric hypertrophy; asymmetric septal hypertrophy; mitral annulus calcification; aortic and mitral valve calcification; myocardial calcification; aortic, mitral, tricuspid, and pulmonic valvular regurgitation; aortic and mitral valve stenosis; and PE[163-167,171-173,175-183] (Figs. 37–10, 37–11, 37–12, and Table 37–6). Despite the many echocardiographic features of end-stage renal disease, none are diagnostic of a specific structural or valvular abnormality or of cardiomyopathy resulting from renal failure.

Hemodialysis is a commonly used treatment in patients with end-stage renal disease. An acute reduction in intravascular volume is associated with hemodialysis. It is not unanticipated that this treatment would significantly alter loading conditions. LV end-diastolic diameter derived by M-mode echocardiography may decrease on average by 4 mm after hemodialysis.[190] The decrease in LV end-diastolic diameter after hemodialysis results from a decrease in early filling without a compensatory increase in atrial contribution to filling as assessed by transmitral valve Doppler echocardiography.[190,191] Analogous to the effect of hemodialysis on conventional Doppler

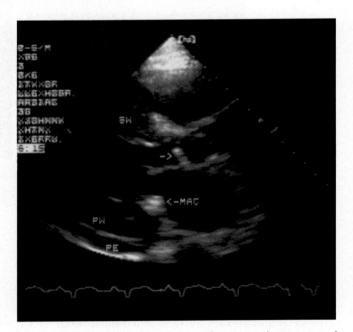

Figure 37–10. *Transthoracic two-dimensional parasternal long-axis view in a patient with chronic renal failure demonstrating associated mitral annular calcification (MAC), pericardial effusion (PE), a calcified aortic valve (arrow), and hypertrophy of the septal (SW) and posterior (PW) left ventricular walls.*

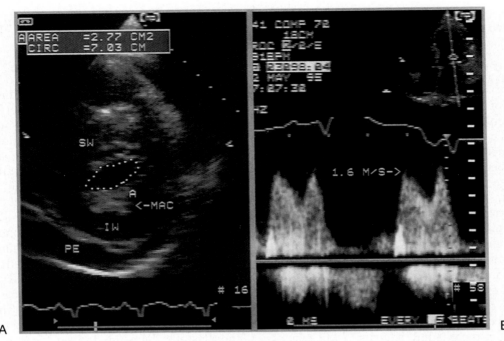

Figure 37–11. *Two-dimensional short-axis (A) and continuous-wave (B) Doppler echocardiography of the mitral valve in a patient with chronic renal failure demonstrating mitral stenosis from encroachment on the mitral orifice by mitral annular calcification (MAC). The planimetered mitral orifice area (A) was 2.77 cm², and the peak gradient by modified Bernoulli equation was 10 mm Hg. IW, inferoposterior wall; PE, pericardial effusion; SW, septal wall.*

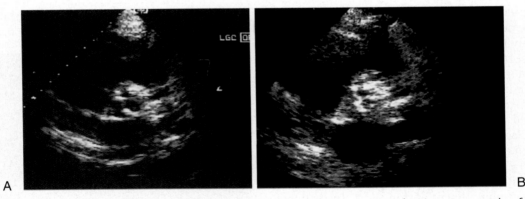

Figure 37–12. *Two-dimensional echocardiograms from short-axis view showing an example of mild aortic valve stenosis (A) that rapidly progressed to a severely stenotic and calcified aortic valve (B) in a chronic dialysis patient. (From Ohara T, Hashimoto Y, Matsumura A, et al: Circ J 69:1535-1539, 2005.)*

indexes of diastolic function, tissue Doppler echocardiographic indexes show a decrease in peak early diastolic annular and myocardial velocity but no change in late diastolic velocities.[192] Similarly, LV inflow propagation rate derived by color M-mode echocardiography decreases after hemodialysis in patients with EF greater than 50%.[193] Thus, the impact of preload reduction must be considered when diastolic function is being assessed in these patients after dialysis. The influence of hemodialysis on systolic function as assessed by M-mode or 2D echocardiog-

raphy is complex and may be influenced by dialysate composition,[194] dialysis-induced changes in serum electrolytes,[195] LV mass,[196] and previous treatment with a beta antagonist.[196] Systolic function after hemodialysis, as assessed by echocardiographically derived shortening fraction, LV EF, velocity of circumferential fiber shortening, or ratio of fractional shortening to end-systolic stress, may be enhanced,[197-200] depressed,[199,200] or unchanged.[190,194,198] Doppler echocardiographic findings of diastolic dysfunction in patients with renal failure include reduced transmitral

TABLE 37-6. Echocardiographic Findings in Renal Disease

Valvular Disease	Structural Abnormalities	Diastolic Dysfunction
M-Mode/Two-Dimensional/Doppler	*M-Mode/Two-Dimensional*	*Spectral Doppler*
Aortic valve calcification (28%-60%)	Concentric LV hypertrophy	↓Peak early filling velocity
Mitral annular calcification (10% to 36%)	Eccentric LV hypertrophy	↓E/A ratio
Aortic regurgitation (13%)	LV enlargement	↑Isovolumetric relaxation time
Mitral regurgitation (38%)	Asymmetric septal hypertrophy	*Tissue Doppler Imaging*
Aortic stenosis	Atrial enlargement	↓Early diastolic myocardial velocity
Mitral stenosis	Pericardial effusion	↓Annular peak early diastolic velocity
Tricuspid regurgitation	Pericardial thickening	*Systolic Dysfunction*
Pulmonic insufficiency	Myocardial calcification	*Two-dimensional*
	Ultrasonic Integrated Backscatter	↓LV ejection fraction
	↓Cyclic variation	
	↑Echoreflectivity	

E/A, peak early to peak atrial velocity ratio; LV, left ventricular.

peak early filling velocity and E/A ratio and prolonged IVRT.[187,188] In addition, TDI derived peak early diastolic annular and myocardial velocity is decreased.[170,189] Ultrasonic backscatter of myocardium in renal failure shows less homogeneity and greater reflectivity, reflecting cardiac calcification[199,200] and reduced cyclic variation[199,201] (Fig. 37–13).

Clinical Utility

Echocardiography is a useful noninvasive method of evaluating patients with end-stage renal disease who has cardiovascular symptoms. An accurate diagnosis of the cause of CHF in patients with renal failure on the basis of clinical assessment is challenging. CHF in

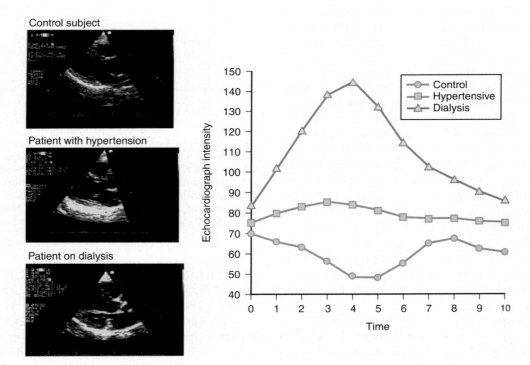

Figure 37–13. *Illustration of ultrasonographic videodensitometric analysis of myocardium in end-stage renal disease. Left panels show digitized two-dimensional echocardiographic images of the left ventricle (parasternal long-axis view) of a control subject, a hypertensive patient, and a dialysis patient. The graph on right demonstrates variation in echocardiographic intensity in the region of interest placed at the posterior wall level during one cardiac cycle divided into 12 frames for the control (red circle), hypertensive (purple square) and dialysis (blue triangle) groups. Time 0 is end-diastolic frame and time 4 is end-systolic frame. (From Di Bello V, Panichi V, Pedrinelli R, et al: Nephrol Dial Transplant 14:2184-2191, 1999.)*

patients with renal diseases frequently multifactorial and could be diagnosed on the basis of congestive cardiomyopathy, inadequate ventricular hypertrophy, valvular regurgitation, or stenosis. PE with secondary cardiac tamponade could simulate CHF. Conventional M-mode, 2D, and Doppler echocardiography are useful in the diagnosis of the many structural and valvular abnormalities that may cause HF in the patient with renal failure. In addition, newly emerging TDI and strain rate imaging offer to complement the conventional echocardiographic approaches in the comprehensive assessment of patients with renal failure for the elucidation of possible associated myocardial disease. Myocardial tissue characterization with ultrasonic integrated backscatter aids in the diagnosis of myocardial disease in patients with renal failure but has not been employed widely.

Echocardiography is useful for predicting survival in chronic dialysis patients.[202,203] Echocardiographic assessment of LV size and systolic function is a significantly better predictor of prognosis than clinical evaluation or electrocardiographic findings.[202] Patients on dialysis with abnormal LV systolic function and dilated LV cavities have a poor prognosis, with one study reporting a mean survival of 7.8 months in such patients.[202] A prospective study using serial echocardiography has shown that improvement in renal failure-related cardiac abnormalities (e.g., LVH and systolic dysfunction) 1 year after the patient starts dialysis is associated with an improved cardiac outcome over a mean follow-up period of 41 months.[204] Thus, serial echocardiography adds prognostic information beyond the initial study, an important application of echocardiography in the evaluation of patients with end-stage renal disease. LV diastolic dysfunction, independent of LVH, is markedly progressed in patients with chronic renal failure[205] and can play a dominant role in symptoms. Importantly, diastolic dysfunction manifest as pseudonormal or restrictive filling is a significant independent predictor of cardiac and overall mortality in these patients when on hemodialysis[203] (Fig. 37–14). LVH is a major risk factor for morbidity and mortality in patients with chronic renal failure. Its complete regression may occur with intense and multifaceted therapy,[206] making serial echocardiography useful in monitoring success of treatment.

Systemic hypotension induced by hemodialysis is occasionally serious or life threatening. In patients with dialysis-induced hypotension refractory to conventional therapy, echocardiography helps assess potential causes of hypotension after dialysis, such as intravascular volume depletion, impaired systolic function, or a hyperdynamic state with secondary intraventricular obstruction. Patients with impaired early LV filling and a short duration of early filling are

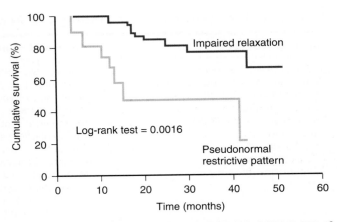

Figure 37–14. Kaplan-Meier estimates for the occurrence of death in patients with impaired relaxation (n = 49) and pseudonormal or restrictive pattern (n = 19) of diastolic dysfunction. (From Zaslavsky LMA, Pinotti AF, Gross JL: J Diabetes Complications 19:194-200, 2005.)

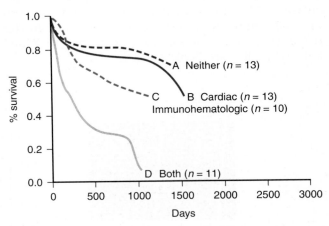

Figure 37–15. Survival curves for diabetic patients with immunohematologic and cardiac (i.e., left ventricular end-systolic diameter greater than 4 cm, shortening fraction less than 20%, and/or coronary artery disease) risk factors. Echocardiographic parameters are useful for prediction of reduced patient survival. (From Weinrauch LA, Delia JA, Monaco AP, et al: Am J Med 93:19-28, 1992.)

at higher risk for hemodynamic instability during hemodialysis and may be identified prospectively by Doppler echocardiography.[207]

In the preoperative evaluation for renal transplantation, echocardiography is useful for predicting patient and renal graft survival.[208] M-mode echocardiographically derived increased LV end-systolic diameter (=4 cm) and a decreased shortening fraction (<20%) are predictive of a reduced chance of patient survival[208] (Fig. 37–15). Decreased graft survival in patients who have had a renal transplant is predicted by elevated end-systolic diameter.[208]

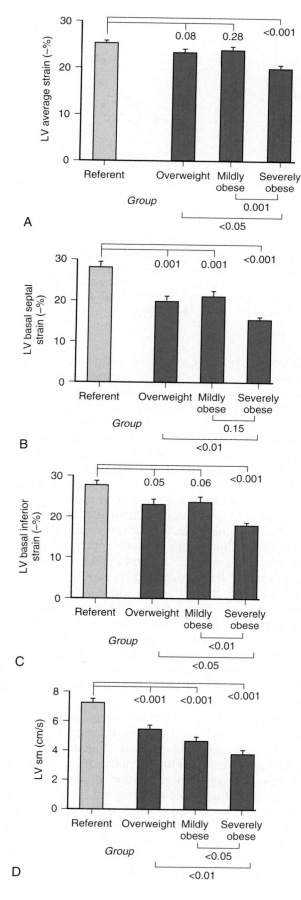

Obesity and Heart Disease

Systolic Function in Obesity

It has long been known that CHF is a frequent cause of death in morbidly overweight persons.[209,210] Long-standing obesity is associated with preclinical and clinical LVH, dilation,[211-216] and impaired LV systolic function.[214,217-222] These abnormalities of LV structure and function may occur in the absence of hypertension or CAD. These findings are consistent with the notion of an obesity cardiomyopathy.[215] However, recent investigators have reported in obese individuals an increase in EF as compared to control subjects[223-225] or no difference in EF.[226,227] It is suggested that global systolic function may be augmented in the early stages of obesity.[224] However, even in the face of normal global LV systolic function, abnormalities in regional myocardial function exist in people with obesity.[227] Wong and colleagues[227] have demonstrated in obese subjects with normal EF that regional indexes of systolic myocardial function are decreased in overweight, mildly obese, or severely obese subjects (Fig. 37–16).

Obesity is accompanied by increases in circulatory blood volume and CO, which are proportional to excess body weight.[216,218] The high-output state of morbid obesity occurs primarily from increases in adipose tissue blood flow. Resting heart rate is minimally affected, but SV is increased. Systolic function curves or indexes, such as the stroke work index to LV end-diastolic pressure or preejection period to LV ejection time ratio, however, may be reduced in patients who are obese, consistent with depressed myocardial systolic function.[219,221]

Reduced LV EF and attenuation of the normal increase in EF with exercise may occur in morbidly obese people.[221] In such individuals, increased LV mass is associated with an attenuation of the normal increase in LV EF during exercise[221] (Fig. 37–17). Weight reduction in subjects with obesity is associated with improvement in systolic function.[214,222,228,229] RV systolic function may be impaired due to obesity.

Diastolic Function in Obesity

Abnormalities of LV filling have been reported in asymptomatic, otherwise healthy obese people.[223,225,226,230,231] Prolongation of IVRT occurs in obesity.[223,225-227,229,232] Regional myocardial diastolic function as assessed by TDI shows impairment in people

Figure 37–16. *Relation of body mass index (BMI) with systolic measures of myocardial average strain (A), basal septal strain (B), basal inferior strain (C), and average systolic velocity (D). LV, left ventricular. (From Wong CY, O'Moore-Sullivan T, Leano R, et al:* Circulation *110:3081-3087, 2004.)*

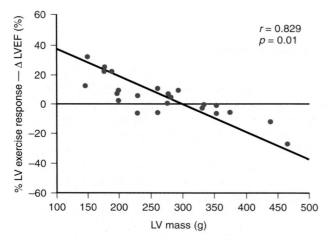

Figure 37–17. *Correlation of left ventricular (LV) mass versus change in LV ejection fraction (LVEF) during exercise (i.e., LV exercise response) in morbidly obese subjects. Increasing LV mass is associated with a decreasing LV exercise response. LV, left ventricular; LVEF, left ventricular ejection fraction. (From Alpert MA, Singh A, Terry BE, et al: Am J Cardiol 63:1478-1482, 1989.)*

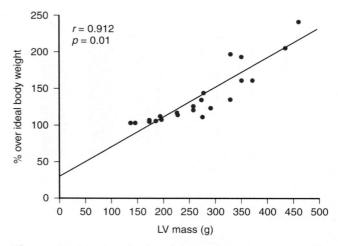

Figure 37–18. *Correlation of left ventricular mass versus percentage over ideal body weight in morbidly obese subjects. Increasing severity of obesity is associated with greater left ventricular mass. (From Alpert MA, Singh A, Terry BE, et al: Am J Cardiol 63:1478-1482, 1989.)*

who are obese.[227,233] These global and regional findings may be noted in the absence of systolic dysfunction and are consistent with LV diastolic dysfunction. Impaired LV relaxation, compliance, or both occur in patients who are obese because of the associated LVH. Weight reduction is associated with improvement in LV diastolic filling and isovolumetric relaxation,[222,228,234] and tissue Doppler indexes of regional diastolic function.[235]

Structural Abnormalities in Obesity

Compared with control subjects of normal weight with similar blood pressure, patients who are obese show an increase in left atrial diameter and area, aortic root diameter, LV end-diastolic diameter, septal and posterior wall thickness, and LV mass.[213,226,227] Obesity causes eccentric hypertrophy (i.e., LV dilation and normal or mildly increased wall thickness). The eccentric hypertrophy in obesity is accounted for by chronic increased intravascular volume.[213] This partially explains the association between increasing LV mass and severity of obesity[220] (Fig. 37–18). Inadequate hypertrophy of the LV wall to normalize wall stress in the face of a dilated cavity occurs in some people who are obese and may account for impaired myocardial systolic function.[215] Weight loss induces significant reductions in LV end-diastolic diameter, end-systolic wall stress, and LV mass.[230,231,236,237]

Anorexigen Use, Valvulopathy, and Pulmonary Hypertension in Obesity

Obesity is associated with serious cardiovascular health risks, such as heart disease, stroke, and systemic hypertension. Appetite-suppressant medications or anorexi-

gens with diverse mechanisms of action are used in the treatment of obese subjects to promote weight reduction. Much has been learned about the prevalence and natural history of valvulopathy from anorexigens since the original report by Connolly and colleagues[238] noting the association of valvular heart disease and the use of specific anorexigens, which alter serotonin metabolism. In 1997 Connolly and colleagues[238] reported 24 obese individuals with echocardiographic findings of pathologic MR or AR who had been treated with fenfluramine and phentermine. Structural abnormalities by echocardiography in these cases included aortic or mitral leaflet thickening, diastolic doming of the anterior mitral leaflet and immobility of the posterior mitral leaflet, shortening and thickening of chordae tendineae, and retraction of aortic valve leaflets.[238] Furthermore, histopathologic and gross pathological findings available for three of these subjects included fibrotic endocardial changes of valve leaflets and chordae tendineae with a "stuck on plaque" appearance and white glistening valves, which were indistinguishable from the features of carcinoid or ergotamine valvulopathy.[238,239]

Based on pooled data from five echocardiographic surveys, the Food and Drug Administration (FDA) reported a prevalence of 33% of at least mild AR or "moderate" (i.e., cases interpreted as mild to moderate MR were analyzed as moderate in severity) MR in subjects after the use of anorexigens, namely fenfluramine or dexfenfluramine with or without phentermine.[240] A nonrandomized echocardiographic study noted a frequency of mild or greater AR, and/or moderate or greater MR in 22.7% of patients receiving dexfenfluramine or fenfluramine, higher than that of controls which was 1.3%.[241] However, subsequent studies employing matched control subjects and blinding of echocardiographic interpretations have shown a considerably lower prevalence from 6.3% to 11.3% (unadjusted for background rates) of aortic valvular regurgitation in association with the use of anorexigens when the FDA criteria (i.e., mild or greater AR) were met.[242-244] Part of this variance may relate to duration of use and dose of anorexigens or echocardiographic methods and study design. Studies have shown no association between anorexigen use and valvular heart disease when duration of treatment was less than 3 months.[245,246] No single study has shown a statistically significant association between moderate or severe MR and the use of diet medications. However, metaanalysis of four studies showed a statistically significant increase of moderate or greater MR in patients treated for greater than 90 days with fenfluramine or dexfenfluramine as compared to controls (i.e., 3.5% versus 1.8%).[247] In addition, case reports of significant MR in users of anorexigens have been reported.[248-251] The natural history of valvulopathy from fenfluramine derivatives has been better clarified. Aortic or mitral valvular regurgitation that meets the FDA criteria in severity when present appears far more likely to remain stable or to regress than to progress in obese subjects after cessation of the use of fenfluramine or dexfenfluramine.[252-260] Ideally, quantitative measures, such as effective regurgitant orifice area (EROA), volume and flow rate by proximal isovelocity surface area (PISA), vena contracta (VC), regurgitant fraction, jet height relative to the outflow tract in the case of AR, or jet area relative to left atrial area for MR, should be employed to assess regurgitation severity.[261,262] The need for valve surgery from anorexigen-valvulopathy has been reported,[238,249-251,263-266] but in the context of the millions of individuals who have been treated with diet medications, this is a rare outcome.[251,267,268] Lastly, valve surgery when needed has arisen while diet medications are being used or in proximity to their discontinuation but not many years after cessation of anorexigens.

A prospective epidemiologic study has shown a significantly greater risk for primary pulmonary hypertension in obese subjects treated with anorexigens as compared with control subjects.[269] The use of appetite suppressants, including dexfenfluramine or fenfluramine, for longer than 3 months showed an odds ratio of 23 (95% confidence interval [CI], 6.9 to 77) for primary pulmonary hypertension in obese individuals.[269] Echocardiography is a useful modality to estimate peak PA systolic pressure and should play an important role in the noninvasive estimation of PA pressure in obese subjects when pulmonary hypertension on the basis of anorexigen use is suspected. However, Weyman and colleagues[270] have shown that peak pulmonary systolic pressure, estimated by echocardiography, is greater than 35 mm Hg in nearly one third of otherwise normal obese individuals. The prevalence of elevated pulmonary pressures in morbidly obese individuals living at moderate altitude may be in excess of 96%.[271] These data suggest caution when ascribing mild elevation of PA systolic pressure to anorexigen use in obese subjects.

Echocardiographic Findings in Obesity

The M-mode and 2D echocardiographic features of chronic obesity consist of aortic root, left atrial, and LV enlargement and eccentric hypertrophy[213,231,226] (Table 37-7). Gender differences may play a role in the structural response to obesity. Obesity in young otherwise healthy women is associated with concentric LV remodeling (i.e., an increase in the relative wall thickness but not LV mass).[272] Although SV, as assessed by pulsed Doppler and 2D echocardiography, is increased in people who are obese, this change is accounted for by LV dilation.[232] M-mode echocardiographically derived LV shortening fraction and 2D-determined EF may be reduced in morbid obesity[214,217-222,228,234] (Fig. 37-19). However, global systolic function may be augmented in the early stages of obesity with an increase in EF.[224] Abnormalities in regional myocardial systolic function exist in people with obesity,[227,272] namely

TABLE 37-7. Echocardiographic Findings in Obesity

Structural Abnormalities	Systolic Dysfunction	Diastolic Dysfunction
M-Mode/Two-Dimensiona	*M-Mode/Two-Dimensional*	*Spectral Doppler*
Eccentric LV hypertrophy	↓LV ejection fraction	↑Isovolumetric relaxation time
LV enlargement	↓Shortening fraction	↓E/A ratio
↑LV mass	*Spectral Doppler*	*Tissue Doppler Imaging*
↑Left atrial size	↓PEP/LVET ratio	↓Early diastolic myocardial velocity
↑Aortic root diameter	*Tissue Doppler Imaging*	↓Annular peak early diastolic velocity
Ultrasonic Integrated Backscatter	↓Peak myocardial systolic velocity	
Cyclic variation		

E/A, early to atrial velocity ratio; LV, left ventricular; PEP/LVET, preejection to left ventricular ejection time.

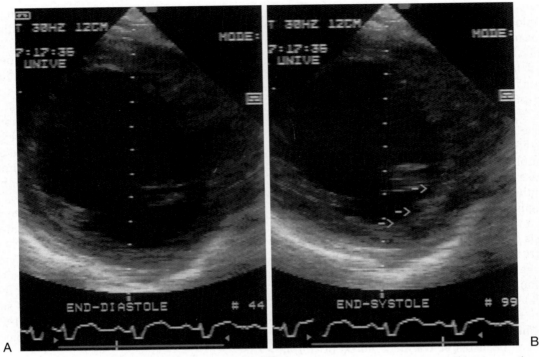

Figure 37–19. Transesophageal two-dimensional short-axis view of the left ventricle at the papillary muscle level in a patient with obesity cardiomyopathy. A, Eccentric hypertrophy. B, Reduced systolic function. The anterolateral wall was the best-contracting segment (arrows).

myocardial peak strain and peak systolic velocity measured from basilar LV segments are decreased in overweight, mildly obese, or severely obese subjects. The Doppler echocardiographically derived preejection period to LV ejection time ratio is increased in obesity.[232] The pulsed Doppler-derived IVRT may be prolonged in obesity.[229,232] Transmitral valve Doppler indexes of diastolic filling may be abnormal for these patients and show decreased peak early filling velocity,[230] increased peak atrial filling velocity,[229,230] reduced E/A ratio,[223-231] increased atrial contribution to filling,[228] and reduced deceleration rate of early filling.[228-230] These findings may be more commonly seen if obesity is morbid, of long duration, and associated with eccentric hypertrophy[230,231,234] (Fig. 37–20). In addition, recent studies have shown decreased LV diastolic function with tissue Doppler-derived early diastolic annular velocity.[233] RV systolic and diastolic dysfunction is present in obese people as demonstrated by tissue Doppler-derived measures of RV peak systolic and diastolic myocardial velocity, respectively.[273] Ultrasonic myocardial tissue characterization in obese subjects demonstrates increased myocardial reflectivity with reduced cyclic variation.[227] Obesity is associated with numerous comorbid conditions, such as diabetes mellitus, hypertension, obstructive sleep apnea, and metabolic syndrome, which interact to effect cardiac structure and function.[274-277] Moderate or severe LV diastolic dysfunction

is more prevalent when obesity is complicated by diabetes[274] or obstructive sleep apnea.[275] Similarly, obese subjects have disproportionately more LV mass and LVH when the condition is associated with systemic hypertension[276] or metabolic syndrome.[277]

Clinical Utility

The echocardiographic findings of obesity are nonspecific. However, echocardiography is useful in the assessment of obese patients with CHF. Appraisal of LV systolic function, diastolic filling, chamber size, and hypertrophy, and RV function may help guide medical therapy. Substantial weight reduction by the morbidly obese may improve LV and RV systolic and diastolic function, decrease LV chamber size, and reduce LV mass.[214,228,235-237]

Echocardiography may be of benefit in obese subjects with suspected aortic or mitral valvulopathy on the basis of anorexigen use. However, attempting to apply the FDA criteria for valvulopathy, which are based solely on the presence of at least mild AR or MR, is simplistic and not clinically helpful. Isolated AR or MR in the presence of an otherwise structurally normal valve as assessed by echocardiography may well be a normal variant. In addition, preexisting conditions, such as rheumatic disease, before to the use of anorexigens may also explain valvulopathy and should be

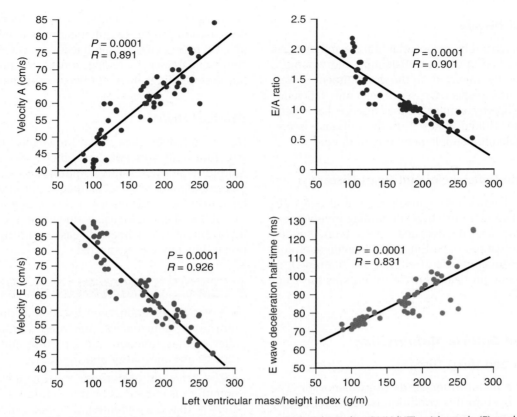

Figure 37–20. *Correlation of left ventricular mass to height index (LVM/HT) with peak (E) and peak atrial filling (A) wave velocities, peak early filling velocity to peak atrial filling velocity (E/) ratio, and E wave deceleration half-time. All indexes of diastolic function become increasingly impaired as LVM/HT increases. (From Alpert MA, Lambert CR, Boyd TE, et al:* Am Heart J *130:1068-1073, 1995.)*

considered.[278] The presence of aortic or mitral valvular thickening unexplained by other causes in combination with at least mild AR or at least greater than mild MR, respectively, should be present before a diagnosis of anorexigen-induced valvulopathy can be entertained. In addition, data from Weyman and colleagues[270] suggest caution when attributing mild elevation of PA systolic pressure as estimated by echocardiography to anorexigen use in obese subjects.

Technical issues in the performance and interpretation of echocardiography in obese subjects are important. Body habitus in these patients may make acquisition of adequate transthoracic views challenging. Subcostal views complement standard approaches and should be employed. Transesophageal echocardiography should be considered whenever necessary to circumvent limitations of transthoracic echocardiography. Lastly, several quantitative measures should be employed to assess changes in severity of regurgitation over time[261,262] because reliance on qualitative assessments or any single method is unreliable and may lead to erroneous conclusions on the clinically relevant question of progression, stability, or regression in valvular heart disease.[279]

Nutritional Deficiencies and Heart Disease

Vitamin and Trace Element Deficiencies and Heart Disease

Beriberi Heart Disease

Severe thiamine deficiency persisting for at least 3 months is the cause of a clinical syndrome called beriberi. Heart disease in patients with beriberi is characterized by biventricular failure and marked edema[280-282] associated with a high CO and arteriolar vasodilation. RV failure may predominate, but significant elevation of LV end-diastolic and pulmonary capillary wedge pressures (PCWPs) may occur. The disease has been virtually eliminated in the United States, but it can be seen in alcoholic people who become thiamine deficient. The hemodynamic abnormalities are reversible with thiamine therapy but may not respond to inotropic agents or diuretics. The possibility of thiamine deficiency and beriberi heart disease should be considered in cases of refractory CHF presumed to result from alcoholic cardiomyopathy.

Keshan Heart Disease

A DCM characterized by myocardial fibrosis and necrosis has been described in China.[283] Selenium and vitamin E deficiency may be important in the development of Keshan heart disease. Suspected cases of selenium deficiency and cardiomyopathy similar to this disease have been reported in the United States.[284] Keshan disease is preventable by selenium supplementation in the diet.

Other Vitamin Deficiencies and Heart Disease

Vitamin C deficiency may cause scurvy and heart abnormalities. The manifestations of cardiac involvement in scurvy may include dyspnea, chest pain, sudden death, PR interval prolongation, and ST-segment abnormalities. The direct effects of vitamin A, vitamin D, or niacin deficiency on heart muscle in humans have not been established.

Protein and Calorie Malnutrition

Kwashiorkor and Heart Disease

Protein-calorie malnutrition leads to kwashiorkor. The heart disease seen in this condition is characterized by atrophy of cardiac muscle fibers, interstitial edema, vacuolization of myocardial fibers, and low-output CHF. Although the condition is rare in developed nations, it may contribute to heart disease in patients with chronic illnesses or anorexia nervosa.

Echocardiography and Nutritional Deficiencies

Few studies of the echocardiographic features of heart disease resulting from nutritional deficiencies have been reported and the findings tend to be nonspecific. Echocardiographic features of beriberi cardiomyopathy or selenium deficiency cardiomyopathy include LV enlargement and decreased indexes of systolic function (Table 37–8). In children, LV diameter and mass, as assessed by M-mode echocardiography, are decreased in protein-calorie malnutrition proportional to the reduction in body size.[285] In children, LV systolic function may be decreased in protein-calorie malnutrition and manifested by a decrease in shortening fraction, mean velocity of circumferential fiber shortening, and systolic time interval,[286] but these findings have not been consistently shown.[285]

Clinical Utility

Nutritional deficiencies may adversely affect cardiac structure and function and increase cardiovascular morbidity and mortality. Appropriate nutritional replacement may reverse cardiac abnormalities caused by nutritional deficiencies. Echocardiography may be useful for the noninvasive documentation of cardiac involvement when heart disease resulting from nutritional deficiency is suspected.

KEY POINTS

■ A variety of endocrine disorders, renal diseases, nutritional deficiencies, and obesity may adversely alter cardiac function and structure and affect cardiovascular morbidity and mortality.

■ The detection of diastolic dysfunction in endocrinopathies is enhanced by the addition of TDI parameters to that of conventional Doppler indexes.

■ PE may be seen in overt hypothyroidism or may be the first indication of thyroid dysfunction.

■ HF resulting from hypothyroidism is accurately diagnosed by echocardiography.

■ In patients with acromegaly, echocardiographic findings include concentric LVH, eccentric hypertrophy, septal hypertrophy that may simulate HCM, RV hypertrophy, and LV dilation.

■ Aortic valve calcification occurs in 46% to 63% of primary hyperparathyroidism patients, and mitral valve or submitral annulus calcification has been reported in 33% to 49% of these patients.

■ Echocardiographic findings of severe LVH or HCM without obvious cause should raise the clinical suspicion of glucocorticoid excess, possibly from Cushing's syndrome.

TABLE 37–8. Echocardiographic Findings in Nutritional Deficiencies

Beriberi Heart Disease (Thiamine Deficiency)	Keshan Heart Disease (Selenium Deficiency)	Kwashiorkor (Protein-Calorie Malnutrition)
LV enlargement	LV enlargement	↓LV mass
↓LV ejection fraction	↓LV ejection fraction	↓LV end-diastolic diameter
RV enlargement	Segmental LV WMA	↓Shortening fraction
		↓Velocity circumferential FS

FS, fiber shortening; LV, left ventricular; RV, right ventricular; WMA, wall motion abnormality

■ In patients with end-stage renal disease, findings include atrial or ventricular dilation; concentric hypertrophy; asymmetric septal hypertrophy; mitral annulus calcification; aortic and mitral valve calcification; myocardial calcification; aortic, mitral, tricuspid, and pulmonic regurgitation; aortic and mitral valve stenosis; and PE.

■ The natural history of valvulopathy from fenfluramine derivatives has been better clarified. Aortic or mitral valvular regurgitation that meets the FDA criteria in severity when present appears far more likely to remain stable and/or to regress than to progress in obese subjects after cessation of the use of fenfluramine or dexfenfluramine.

REFERENCES

1. Rubler S, Dlugash J, Yucheoglu YZ, et al: New type of cardiomyopathy associated with diabetic glomerulosclerosis. *Am J Cardiol* 30:595-602, 1972.
2. Hamby RI, Zoneraich S, Sherman L: Diabetic cardiomyopathy. *J Am Med Assoc* 229:1749-1754, 1974.
3. Zarich SW, Nesto RW: Diabetic cardiomyopathy. *Am Heart J* 118:1000-1012, 1989.
4. Uuisturpa MIJ, Mustonen JN, Airaksinen KEJ: Diabetic heart muscle disease. *Ann Med* 22:377-386, 1990.
5. Ahmed SS, Jaferi GA, Narang RM, Regan TJ: Preclinical abnormality of left ventricular function in diabetes mellitus. *Am Heart J* 89:153-158, 1975.
6. Vered Z, Battler A, Segal P, et al: Exercise-induced left ventricular dysfunction in young men with asymptomatic diabetes mellitus (diabetic cardiomyopathy). *Am J Cardiol* 54:633-637, 1984.
7. Senevirathe BIB: Diabetic cardiomyopathy: The preclinical phase. *Br Med J* 1:1444-1446, 1977.
8. Fang ZY, Yuda S, Anderson V, et al: Echocardiographic detection of early diabetic myocardial disease. *J Am Coll Cardiol* 41:611-617, 2003.
9. Kosmala W, Kucharski W, Przewlocka-Kosmala M, Mazurek W: Comparison of left ventricular function by tissue Doppler imaging in patients with diabetes mellitus without systemic hypertension versus diabetes mellitus with systemic hypertension. *Am J Cardiol* 94:395-399, 2004.
10. Fang ZY, Schull-Meade R, Downey M, et al: Determinants of subclinical diabetic heart disease. *Diabetologia* 48:394-402, 2005.
11. Zoneraich S, Silverman G, Zoneraich O: Primary myocardial disease, diabetes mellitus, and small vessel disease. *Am Heart J* 5:754-755,1980.
12. Nitenberg A, Valensi P, Sachs R, et al: Impairment of coronary vascular reserve and ACh-induced coronary vasodilation in diabetic patients with angiographically normal coronary arteries and normal left ventricular systolic function. *Diabetes* 42:1017-1025, 1993.
13. Ohtake T, Yokayama I, Watanabe T, et al: Myocardial glucose metabolism in noninsulin-dependent diabetes mellitus patients evaluated by FDG-PET. *J Nucl Med* 36:456-463, 1995.
14. Malhotra A, Sanghi V: Regulation of contractile proteins in diabetic heart. *Cardiovasc Res* 34:34-40, 1997.
15. Wong CY, O-Moore-Sullivan T, Fang ZY, et al: Myocardial and vascular dysfunction and exercise capacity in the metabolic syndrome. *Am J Cardiol* 96:1686-1691, 2005.
16. Shapiro LM, Leatherdale BA, Mackinnon J, Fletcher RF: Left ventricular function in diabetes mellitus II: Relation between clinical features and left ventricular function. *Br Heart J* 45:129-132, 1981.
17. Sanderson JE, Brown DJ, Rivellese A, Kohner E: Diabetic cardiomyopathy? An echocardiographic study of young diabetics. *Br Med J* 1:404-407, 1978.
18. Sampson MJ, Chambers JB, Sprigings DC, Drury PL: Abnormal diastolic function in patients with type I diabetes and early nephropathy. *Br Heart J* 64:266-274, 1990.
19. Poirier P, Bogaty P, Philippon F, et al: Preclinical diabetic cardiomyopathy: Relation of left ventricular diastolic dysfunction to cardiac autonomic neuropathy in men with uncomplicated well-controlled type 2 diabetes. *Metabolism* 52:1056-1061, 2003.
20. Zarich SW, Arbuckle BE, Cohen LR, et al: Diastolic abnormalities in young asymptomatic diabetic patients assessed by pulsed Doppler echocardiography. *J Am Coll Cardiol* 12:114-120, 1988.
21. Takenaka K, Sakanioto T, Amarro K: Left ventricular filling determined by Doppler echocardiography in diabetes mellitus. *Am J Cardiol* 61:1140-1143, 1988.
22. Paillole C, Dahan M, Paycha F, et al: Prevalence and significance of left ventricular filling abnormalities determined by Doppler echocardiography in young type I (insulin-dependent) diabetic patients. *Am J Cardiol* 64:1010-1016, 1989.
23. Di Bonito P, Cuomo S, Moio N, et al: Diastolic dysfunction in patients with non-insulin-dependent diabetes mellitus of short duration. *Diabet Med* 13:321-324, 1996.
24. Fang ZY, Najos-Valencia O, Leano R, Marwick TH: Patients with early diabetic heart disease demonstrate a normal myocardial response to dobutamine. *J Am Coll Cardiol* 42:446-453, 2003.
25. Boyer JK, Thanigaraj S, Schechtman KB, Perez JE: Prevalence of ventricular diastolic dysfunction in asymptomatic, normotensive patients with diabetes mellitus. *Am J Cardiol* 93:870-875, 2004.
26. Von Bibra H, Thrainsdottir IS, Hansen A, et al: Tissue Doppler imaging for the detection and quantitation of myocardial dysfunction in patients with type 2 diabetes mellitus. *Diab Vasc Dis Res* 2:24-30, 2005.
27. Di Bonito P, Moio N, Cavuto L, et al: Early detection of diabetic cardiomyopathy: Usefulness of tissue Doppler imaging. *Diabet Med* 22:1720-1725, 2005.
28. Kosmala W, Colonna P, Przewlocka-Kosmala M, Mazurek W: Right ventricular dysfunction in asymptomatic diabetic patients. *Diabetes Care* 27:2736-2738, 2004.
29. Galderisi M, Anderson KM, Wilson PWF, Levy D: Echocardiographic evidence for the existence of a distinct diabetic cardiomyopathy (the Framingham Heart Study). *Am J Cardiol* 68:85-89, 1991.
30. Ganguly PK, Pierce GN, Dhalla KS, Dhalla NS: Defective sarcoplasmic reticular calcium transport in diabetic cardiomyopathy. *Am J Physiol* 224:E528-E535, 1983.
31. Hiramatsu K, Ohara N, Shigematsu S, et al: Left ventricular filling abnormalities in non-insulin-dependent diabetes mellitus and improvement by a short-term glycemic control. *Am J Cardiol* 70:1185-1189, 1992.
32. Diamant M, Lamb HJ, Groeneveld Y, et al: Diastolic dysfunction is associated with altered myocardial metabolism in asymptomatic normotensive patients with well-controlled type 2 diabetes mellitus. *J Am Coll Cardiol* 42:328-335, 2003.
33. Poirier P, Garneau C, Bogaty P, et al: Impact of left ventricular diastolic dysfunction on maximal treadmill performance in normotensive subjects with well-controlled type 2 diabetes mellitus. *Am J Cardiol* 85:473-477, 2000.
34. Saraiva RM, Duarte DM, Duarte MP, et al: Tissue Doppler imaging identifies asymptomatic normotensive diabetes with dia-

stolic dysfunction and reduced exercise tolerance. *Echocardiography* 22:561-570, 2005.

35. Fang ZY, Sharman J, Prins JB, Marwick TH: Determinants of exercise capacity in patients with type 2 diabetes. *Diabetes Care* 28:1643-1648, 2005.

36. Devereux RB, Roman MJ, Paranicas M, et al: Impact of diabetes on cardiac structure and function: The strong heart study. *Circulation* 101:2271-2276, 2000.

37. Tarumi N, Iwasaka T, Takahashi N, et al: Left ventricular diastolic filling properties in diabetic patients during isometric exercise. *Cardiology* 83:316-323, 1993.

38. Airaksinen J, Ikaheimo M, Kaila J, et al: Impaired left ventricular filling in young female diabetics. *Acta Med Scand* 216:509-516, 1984.

39. Baum VC, Levitsky LL, Englander RM: Abnormal cardiac function after exercise in insulin-dependent diabetic children and adolescents. *Diabetes Care* 10:319-323, 1987.

40. Perez JE, McGill JB, Santiago JV, et al: Abnormal myocardial acoustic properties in diabetic patients and their correlation with the severity of disease. *J Am Coll Cardiol* 19:1154-1162, 1992.

41. Eguchi K, Kario K, Hoshide S, et al: Type 2 diabetes is associated with left ventricular concentric remodeling in hypertensive patients. *Am J Hypertens* 18:23-29, 2005.

42. Miyazato J, Horio T, Takiuchi S, et al: Left ventricular diastolic dysfunction in patients with chronic renal failure: impact of diabetes mellitus. *Diabet Med* 22:730-736, 2005.

43. Di Stante B, Galandauer I, Aronow WS, et al: Prevalence of left ventricular diastolic dysfunction in obese persons with and without diabetes mellitus. *Am J Cardiol* 95:1527-1528, 2005.

44. Kuperstein R, Hanly P, Niroumand M, Sasson Z: The importance of age and obesity on the relation between diabetes and left ventricular mass. *J Am Coll Cardiol* 37:1957-1962, 2001.

45. Shishehbor MH, Hoogwerf BJ, Schoenhagen P, et al: Relation of hemoglobin A1c to left ventricular relaxation in patients with type 1 diabetes mellitus and without overt heart disease. *Am J Cardiol* 91:1514-1517, A9, 2003.

46. Grandi AM, Piantanida E, Franzetti I, et al: Effect of glycemic control on left ventricular diastolic function in type 1 diabetes mellitus. *Am J Cardiol* 97:71-76, 2006.

47. Felicio JS, Ferreira SR, Plavnik FL, et al: Effect of blood glucose on left ventricular mass in patients with hypertension and type 2 diabetes mellitus. *Am J Hypertens* 13:1149-1154, 2000.

48. Buccino RA, Spann JF Jr, Pool PE, et al: Influence of the thyroid state on the intrinsic contractile properties and energy stores of the myocardium. *J Clin Invest* 46:1669-1682, 1967.

49. Amidi M, Leon DF, DeGroot WJ, et al: Effect of the thyroid state on myocardial contractility and ventricular ejection rate in man. *Circulation* 38:229-239, 1968.

50. Crowley WF Jr, Ridgway EC, Bough EW, et al: Noninvasive evaluation of cardiac function in hypothyroidism: Response to gradual thyroxine replacement. *N Engl J Med* 296:1-6, 1977.

51. Santos AD, Miller RP, Mathew PK, et al: Echocardiographic characterization of the reversible cardiomyopathy of hypothyroidism. *Am J Med* 68:675-682, 1980.

52. Forfar J, Muir A, Toft A: Left ventricular function in hypothyroidism. *Br Heart J* 48:278-284, 1982.

53. Smallridge RC, Goldman MH, Raines K, et al: Rest and exercise left ventricular ejection fraction before and after therapy in young adults with hyperthyroidism and hypothyroidism. *Am J Cardiol* 60:929-931, 1987.

54. Lee RT, Plappert M, St John Sutton MG: Depressed left ventricular systolic ejection force in hypothyroidism. *Am J Cardiol* 65:526-527, 1990.

55. Tang YD, Kuzman JA, Said S, et al: Low thyroid function leads to cardiac atrophy with chamber dilatation, impaired myocardial blood flow, loss of arterioles, and severe systolic dysfunction. *Circulation* 112:3122-3130, 2005.

56. Arinc H, Gunduz H, Tamer A, et al: Tissue Doppler echocardiography in evaluation of cardiac effects of subclinical hypothyroidism. *Int J Cardiovasc Imaging,* Epub 2005 Nov 2.

57. Zoncu S, Pigliaru F, Putzu C, et al: Cardiac function in borderline hypothyroidism: A study by pulsed wave tissue Doppler imaging. *Eur J Endocrinol* 152:527-533, 2005.

58. Vitale G, Galderisi M, Lupoli GA, et al: Left ventricular myocardial impairment in subclinical hypothyroidism assessed by a new ultrasound tool: pulsed tissue Doppler. *J Clin Endocrinol Metab* 87:4350-4355, 2002.

59. Kosar F, Sahin I, Turan N, et al: Evaluation of right and left ventricular function using pulsed-wave tissue Doppler echocardiography in patients with subclinical hypothyroidism. *J Endocrinol Invest* 28:704-710, 2005.

60. Forfar JC, Muir AL, Sawers SA, Toft AD: Abnormal left ventricular function in hyperthyroidism: Evidence for a possible reversible cardiomyopathy. *N Engl J Med* 307:1165-1170, 1982.

61. Iskandrian AS, Rose L, Hakki A, et al: Cardiac performance in thyrotoxicosis: Analysis of 10 untreated patients. *Am J Cardiol* 51:349-352, 1983.

62. Martin WH, Spina RJ, Korte E: Effect of hyperthyroidism of short duration on cardiac sensitivity to beta-adrenergic stimulation. *J Am Coll Cardiol* 19:1185-1191, 1992.

63. Petretta M, Bonaduce D, Spinelli L, et al: Cardiovascular haemodynamics and cardiac autonomic control in patients with subclinical and overt hyperthyroidism. *Eur J Endocrinol* 145:691-696, 2001.

64. Kahaly GJ, Wagner S, Nieswandi J, et al: Stress echocardiography in hyperthyroidism. *J Clin Endocrinol Metab* 84:2308-2313, 1999.

65. Kahaly G, Hellermann J, Mohr-Kahaly S, et al: Impaired cardiopulmonary exercise capacity in patients with hyperthyroidism. *Chest* 109:57-61, 1996.

66. Pereira N, Parisi A, Dec GW, et al: Myocardial stunning in hyperthyroidism. *Clin Cardiol* 23:298-300, 2000.

67. Umpierrez GE, Challapalli S, Patterson C: Congestive heart failure due to reversible cardiomyopathy in patients with hyperthyroidism. *Am J Med Sci* 310:99-102, 1995.

68. Arinc H, Gunduz H, Tamer A, et al: Evaluation of right ventricular function in patients with thyroid dysfunction. *Cardiology* 105:89-94, 2006.

69. Biondi B, Fazio S, Palmieri EA, et al: Left ventricular diastolic dysfunction in patients with subclinical hyperthyroidism. *J Clin Endocrinol Metab* 84:2064-2067, 1999.

70. Fazio S, Biondi B, Carella C, et al: Diastolic dysfunction in patients on thyroid-stimulating hormone suppressive therapy with levothyroxine: beneficial effect of beta-blockade. *J Clin Endocrinol Metab* 80:2222-2226, 1995.

71. Biondi B, Palmieri EA, Fazio S, et al: Endogenous subclinical hyperthyroidism affects quality of life and cardiac morphology and function in young and middle-aged patients. *J Clin Endocrinol Metab* 85:4701-4705, 2000.

72. Shapiro LE, Sievert R, Ong L, et al: Minimal cardiac effects in asymptomatic athyreotic patients chronically treated with thyrotropin-suppressive doses of L-thyroxine. *J Clin Endocrinol Metab* 83:2607-2608, 1997.

73. Mercuro G, Panzuto MG, Bina A, et al: Cardiac function, physical exercise capacity, and quality of life during long-term thyrotropin-suppressive therapy with levothyroxine: effect of individual dose tailoring. *J Clin Endocrinol Metab* 85:159-164, 2000.

74. Sgarbi JA, Villaca FG, Garbeline B, et al: The effects of early antithyroid therapy for endogenous subclinical hyperthyroidism in clinical and heart abnormalities. *J Clin Endocrinol Metab* 88:1672-1677, 2003.

75. Vora J, O'Malley BP, Petersen S, et al: Reversible abnormalities of myocardial relaxation in hypothyroidism. *J Clin Endocrinol Metab* 61:269-272, 1985.

76. Monzani F, Di Bello V, Caraccio N, et al: Effect of levothyroxine on cardiac function and structure in subclinical hypothyroidism: A double blind, placebo-controlled study. *J Clin Endocrinol Metab* 86:1110-1115, 2001.

77. Virtanen VK, Saha HH, Groundstroem KW, et al: Thyroid hormone substitution therapy rapidly enhances left-ventricular diastolic function in hypothyroid patients. *Cardiology* 96:59-64, 2001.

78. Mintz G, Pizzarello R, Klein I: Enhanced left ventricular diastolic function in hyperthyroidism: Noninvasive assessment and response to treatment. *J Clin Endocrinol Metab* 73:146-150, 1991.

79. Thomas MR, McGregor AM, Jewitt DE: Left ventricle filling abnormalities prior to and following treatment of thyrotoxicosis-is diastolic dysfunction implicated in thyrotoxic cardiomyopathy? *Eur Heart J* 14:662-668, 1993.

80. Smit JW, Eustatia-Rutten CF, Corssmit EP, et al: Reversible diastolic dysfunction after long-term exogenous subclinical hyperthyroidism: A randomized, placebo-controlled study. *J Clin Endocrinol Metab* 90:6041-6047, 2005.

81. Kerber RE, Sherman B: Echocardiographic evaluation of pericardial effusion in myxedema: Incidence and biochemical and clinical correlations. *Circulation* 52:823-827, 1975.

82. Hardisty CA, Naik DR, Munro DS: Pericardial effusion in hypothyroidism. *Clin Endocrinol* 13:349-354, 1980.

83. Hradec J: The advantage of the use of echocardiographic evaluation in hypothyroid patients. *Endokrinologie* 75:187-196, 1980.

84. Khaleeli AA, Memon N: Factors affecting resolution of pericardial effusions in primary hypothyroidism: A clinical, biochemical and echocardiographic study. *Postgrad Med J* 58:473-476, 1982.

85. Kabadi UM, Kumar SP: Pericardial effusion in primary hypothyroidism. *Am Heart J* 120:1393-1395, 1990.

86. Manolis AS, Varriale P, Ostrowski RM: Hypothyroid cardiac tamponade. *Arch Intern Med* 147:1167-1169, 1987.

87. Altman DI, Murray J, Milner S, et al: Asymmetric septal hypertrophy and hypothyroidism in children. *Br Heart J* 54:533-538, 1985.

88. Channick BJ, Adlin EV, Marks AD: Hyperthyroidism and mitral-valve prolapse. *N Engl J Med* 305:497-500, 1981.

89. Brauman A, Algom M, Gliboa Y, et al: Mitral valve prolapse in hyperthyroidism of two different origins. *Br Heart J* 53:374-377, 1985.

90. Kage K, Kira Y, Sekine I, et al: High incidence of mitral and tricuspid regurgitation in patients with Graves' disease detected by two-dimensional color Doppler echocardiography. *Intern Med* 32:374-376, 1993.

91. Evangelopoulou ME, Alevizaki M, Toumanidis S, et al: Mitral valve prolapse in autoimmune thyroid disease: An index of cystemic autoimmunity? *Thyroid* 9:973-977, 1999.

92. Kontopoulos A, Harsoulis P, Adam K, et al: Frequency of HLA antigens in Graves' hyperthyroidism and mitral valve prolapse. *J Heart Valve Dis* 5:543-547, 1996.

93. Tamer I, Sargin M, Sargin H, et al: The evaluation of left ventricular hypertrophy in hypertensive patients with subclinical hyperthyroidism. *Endocr J* 52:421-425, 2005.

94. Di Bello V, Monzani F, Giorgi D, et al: Ultrasonic myocardial textural analysis in subclinical hypothyroidism. *J Am Soc Echocardiogr* 13:832-840, 2000.

95. Kahaly GJ: Cardiovascular and atherogenic aspects of subclinical hypothyroidism. *Thyroid* 10:665-679, 2000.

96. Doin FL, Borges Mda R, Campos O, et al: Effect of central hypothyroidism on Doppler-derived myocardial performance index. *J Am Soc Echocardiogr* 17:622-629, 2004.

97. Werder EA, Torresani T, Navratil F, et al: Pericardial effusion as a sign of acquired hypothyroidism in children with Down syndrome. *Eur J Pediatr* 152:397-398, 1993.

98. Dorr M, Wolff B, Robinson DM, et al: The association of thyroid function with cardiac mass and left ventricular hypertrophy. *J Clin Endocrinol Metab* 90:673-677, 2005. Epub 2004 Nov 2.

99. Merce J, Ferras S, Oltra C, et al: Cardiovascular abnormalities in hyperthyroidism: A prospective Doppler echocardiographic study. *Am J Med* 118:126-131, 2005.

100. Ciulla MM, Paliotti R, Cortelazzi D, et al: Effects of thyroid hormones on cardiac structure: A tissue characterization study in patients with thyroid disorders before and after treatment. *Thyroid* 11:613-619, 2001.

101. Martins JB, Kerber RE, Sherman BM, et al: Cardiac size and function in acromegaly. *Circulation* 56:863-869, 1977.

102. Savage DD, Henry WL, Eastman RC, et al: Echocardiographic assessment of cardiac anatomy and function in acromegalic patients. *Am J Med* 67:823-829, 1979.

103. Smallridge RC, Rajfer S, Davia J, Schaaf M: Acromegaly and the heart: An echocardiographic study. *Am J Med* 66:22-27, 1979.

104. Mather HM, Boyd MJ, Jenkins JS: Heart size and function in acromegaly. *Br Heart J* 41:697-701, 1979.

105. Morvan D, Komajda M, Grimaldi A, et al: Cardiac hypertrophy and function in asymptomatic acromegaly. *Eur Heart J* 12:666-672, 1991.

106. Hradec J, Marek J, Kral J, et al: Long-term echocardiographic follow-up of acromegalic heart disease. *Am J Cardiol* 72:205-210, 1993.

107. Ozbey N, Oncul A, Bugra Z, et al: Acromegalic cardiomyopathy: Evaluation of the left ventricular diastolic function in the subclinical stage. *J Endocrinol Invest* 20:305-311, 1997.

108. Mercuro G, Zoncu S, Colonna P, et al: Cardiac dysfunction in acromegaly: Evidence by pulsed wave tissue Doppler imaging. *Eur J Endocrinol* 143:363-369, 2000.

109. Vianna CB, Vieira ML, Mady C, et al: Treatment of acromegaly improves myocardial abnormalities. *Am Heart J* 143:873-876, 2002.

110. Lombardi G, Colao A, Marzullo P, et al: Improvement of left ventricular hypertrophy and arrhythmias after lanreotide-induced GH and IGF-I decrease in acromegaly. A prospective multi-center study. *J Endocrinol Invest* 25:971-976, 2002.

111. Bogazzi F, Di Bello V, Palagi C, et al: Improvement of intrinsic myocardial contractility and cardiac fibrosis degree in acromegalic patients treated with somatostatin analogues: A prospective study. *Clin Endocrinol (Oxf)* 62:590-596, 2005.

112. van Thiel SW, Bax JJ, Biermasz NR, et al: Persistent diastolic dysfunction despite successful long-term octreotide treatment in acromegaly. *Eur J Endocrinol* 153:231-238, 2005.

113. Colao A, Baldelli R, Marzullo P, et al: Systemic hypertension and impaired glucose inherance are independently correlated to the severity of the acromegalic cardiomyopathy. *J Clin Endocrinol Metab* 85:193-199, 2000.

114. Lopez-Velasco R, Escobar-Morreale HF, Vega B, et al: Cardiac involvement in acromegaly: Specific myocardiopathy or consequence of systemic hypertension? *J Endocrinol Metab* 82:1047-1053, 1997.

115. Fazio S, Cittadini A, Biondi B, et al: Cardiovascular effects of short-term growth hormone hypersecretion. *J Clin Endocrinol Metab* 85:179-182, 2000.

116. Minniti G, Jaffrain-Rea ML, Maroni C, et al: Echocardiographic evidence for a direct effect of GH/IGF-I hypersecretion on cardiac mass and function in young acromegalics. *Clin Endocrinol (Oxf)* 49:101-106, 1998.

117. Lombardi G, Colao A, Ferone D, et al: Cardiovascular aspects in acromegaly: Effects of treatment. *Metabolism* 45:1157-1160, 1996.

118. Colao A, Marzullo P, Ferone D, et al: Cardiovascular effects of depot long-acting somatostatin analog Sandostatin LAR in acromegaly. *J Clin Endocrinol Metab* 85:3132-3140, 2000.

119. Ciulla MM, Epaminonda P, Paliotti R, et al: Evaluation of cardiac structure by echoreflectivity analysis in acromegaly: Effects of treatment. *Eur J Endocrinol* 151:179-186, 2004.

120. Ciulla M, Arosio M, Barelli MV, et al: Blood pressure-independent cardiac hypertrophy in acromegalic patients. *J Hypertens* 17:1965-1969, 1999.

121. Rodrigues IA, Caruana MP, Lahiri A, et al: Subclinical cardiac dysfunction in acromegaly: Evidence for a specific disease of heart muscle. *Br Heart J* 62:185-194, 1989.

122. Fazio S, Cittadini A, Sabatini D, et al: Evidence for biventricular involvement in acromegaly: A Doppler echocardiographic study. *Eur Heart J* 14:26-33, 1993.

123. Bruch C, Herrmann B, Schmermund A, et al: Impact of disease activity on left ventricular performance in patients with acromegaly. *Am Heart J* 144:538-543, 2002.

124. Thuesen L, Christensen SE, Weeke J, et al: A hyperkinetic heart in uncomplicated active acromegaly: Explanation of hypertension in acromegalic patients? *Acta Med Scand* 223:337-343, 1988.

125. Frustaci A, Chimenti C, Setoguchi M, et al: Cell death in acromegalic cardiomyopathy. *Circulation* 23:1426-1434, 1999.

126. Bihan H, Espinosa C, Valdes-Socin H, et al: Long-term outcome of patients with acromegaly and congestive heart failure. *J Clin Endocrinol Metab* 89:5308-5313, 2004.

127. Colao A, Spinelli L, Marzullo P, et al: High prevalence of cardiac valve disease in acromegaly: an observational, analytical, case-control study. *J Clin Endocrinol Metab* 88:3196-3201, 2003.

128. Pereira AM, van Thiel SW, Lindner JR, et al: Increased prevalence of regurgitant valvular heart disease in acromegaly. *J Clin Endocrinol Metab* 89:71-75, 2004.

129. Cable DG, Dearani JA, O'Brien T, et al: Surgical treatment of valvular heart disease in patients with acromegaly. *J Heart Valve Dis* 9:828-831, 2000.

130. Colao A, Spinelli L, Cuocolo A, et al: Cardiovascular consequences of early-onset growth hormone excess. *J Clin Endocrinol Metab* 87:3097-3104, 2002.

131. Lim MJ, Barkan AL, Buda AJ: Rapid reduction of left ventricular hypertrophy in acromegaly after suppression of growth hormone hypersecretion. *Ann Intern Med* 117:719-726, 1992.

132. Merola B, Cittadini A, Colao A, et al: Chronic treatment with the somatostatin analog octreotide improves cardiac abnormalities in acromegaly. *J Clin Endocrinol Metab* 77:790-793, 1993.

133. Ronni-Sivula H: Causes of death in patients previously operated on for primary hyperparathyroidism. *Ann Chir Gynaecol* 74:13-18, 1974.

134. Palmer M, Adami HO, Bergstrom R, et al: Mortality after surgery for primary hyperparathyroidism: A follow-up of 441 patients operated on from 1956 to 1979. *Surgery* 102:1-7, 1987.

135. Niederle B, Roka R, Wolosyczrek W, et al: Successful parathyroidectomy in primary hyperparathyroidism: A clinical follow-up study of 212 consecutive patients. *Surgery* 102:903-909, 1987.

136. Herrman G, Hehrmann R, Scholz HC, et al: Parathyroid hormone in coronary artery disease: Results of a prospective study. *J Endocrinol Invest* 9:256-271, 1986.

137. Niederle B, Stefenelli T, Glogar D, et al: Cardiac calcific deposits in patients with primary hyperparathyroidism: Preliminary results of a prospective echocardiographic study. *Surgery* 108:1052-1057, 1990.

138. Stefenelli T, Mayr H, Bergler-Klein J, et al: Primary hyperparathyroidism: Incidence of cardiac abnormalities and partial reversibility after successful parathyroidectomy. *Am J Med* 95:197-202, 1993.

139. Stefenelli T, Abela C, Frank H, et al: Cardiac abnormalities in patients with primary hyperparathyroidism: Implications for follow-up. *J Clin Endocrinol Metab* 82:106-112, 1997.

140. Symons C, Fortune F, Greenbaum RA, Dandona P: Cardiac hypertrophy, hypertrophic cardiomyopathy, and hyperparathyroidism: An association. *Br Heart J* 54:539-542, 1985.

141. Stefenelli T, Abela C, Frank H, et al: Time course of regression of left ventricular hypertrophy after successful parathyroidectomy. *Surgery* 12:157-161, 1997.

142. Piovesan A, Molineri N, Casasso F, et al: Left ventricular hypertrophy in primary hyperparathyroidism: Effects of successful parathyroidectomy. *Clin Endocrinol (Oxf)* 50:321-328, 1999.

143. Nappi S, Saha H, Virtanen V, et al: Left ventricular structure and function in primary hyperparathyroidism before and after parathyroidectomy. *Cardiology* 93:229-233, 2000.

144. Dalberg K, Brodin LA, Jublin-Dannfelt A, et al: Cardiac function in primary hyperparathyroidism before and after operation: An echocardiographic study. *Eur J Surg* 162:171-176, 1996.

145. Ohara N, Hiramatsu K, Shigematsu S, et al: Effect of parathyroid hormone on left ventricular diastolic function in patients with primary hyperparathyroidism. *Miner Electrolyte Metab* 21:63-66, 1995.

146. Nilsson IL, Aberg J, Rastad J, Lind L: Left ventricular systolic and diastolic function and exercise testing in primary hyperparathyroidism-effects of parathyroidectomy. *Surgery* 128:895-902, 2000.

147. Boscaro M, Barzon L, Fallo F, Sonino N: Cushing's syndrome. *Lancet* 357:783-791, 2001.

148. Sugihara N, Shimizu M, Kita Y, et al: Cardiac characteristics and postoperative courses in Cushing's syndrome. *Am J Cardiol* 69:1475-1480, 1992.

149. Fallo F, Budano S, Sonino N, et al: Left ventricular structural characteristics in Cushing's syndrome. *J Hum Hypertens* 8:509-513, 1994.

150. Muiesan ML, Lupia M, Salvetti M, et al: Left ventricular structural and functional characteristics in Cushing's syndrome. *J Am Coll Cardiol* 41:2275-2279, 2003.

151. Suzuki T, Abe H, Nagata S, et al: Left ventricular structural characteristics in unilateral renovascular hypertension and primary aldosteronism. *Am J Cardiol* 1:1224-1227, 1988.

152. Tanabe A, Naruse M, Naruse K, et al: Left ventricular hypertrophy is more prominent in patients with primary aldosteronism than in patients with other types of secondary hypertension. *Hypertens Res* 20:85-90, 1997.

153. Rossi GP, Sacchetto A, Pavan E, et al: Remodeling of the left ventricle in primary aldosteronism due to Conn's adenoma. *Circulation* 9568:675-682, 1997.

154. Rossi GP, Sacchetto A, Visentin F, et al: Changes in left ventricular anatomy and function in hypertension and primary aldosteronism. *Hypertension* 27:1039-1045, 1996.

155. Rossi GP, Sacchetto A, Pavan E, et al: Left ventricular systolic function in primary aldosteronism and hypertension. *J Hypertens* 16:2075-2077, 1998.

156. Stowasser M, Sharman J, Leano R, et al: Evidence for abnormal left ventricular structure and function in normotensive individuals with familial hyperaldosteronism type I. *J Clin Endocrinol Metab* 90:5070-5076, 2005.

157. Rossi GP, Di Bello V, Ganzaroli C, et al: Excess idosterone is associated with alterations of myocardial texture in primary aldosteronism. *Hypertension* 40:23-27, 2002.

158. Kozáková M, Buralli S, Palombo C, et al: Myocardial ultrasonic backscatter in hypertension: relation to aldosterone and endothelin. *Hypertension* 41:230-236, 2003.

159. Schmidt BM, Schmeider RE: Aldosterone-induced cardiac damage: Focus on blood pressure independent effects. *Am J Hypertens* 16:80-86, 2003.

160. Capelli JP, Kasparian H: Cardiac work demands and left ventricular function in end-stage renal disease. *Ann Intern Med* 86:261-267, 1977.

161. Gueron M, Berlyne GM, Nord E, Ben Ari J: The case against the existence of a specific uremic myocardiopathy. *Nephron* 15:2-4, 1975.

162. Lewis BS, Milne FJ, Goldberg B: Left ventricular function in chronic renal failure. *Br Heart J* 38:1229-1239, 1976.

163. Ianhez LE, Lowen J, Sabbaga E: Uremic myocardiopathy. *Nephron* 15:17-28, 1975.

164. Prosser D, Parsons V: The case for a specific uraemic myocardiopathy. *Nephron* 15:4-7, 1975.

165. Drueke T, Le Pailleur C, Meilhac B, et al: Congestive cardiomyopathy in uraemic patients on long-term haemodialysis. *Br Med J* 1:350-353, 1977.

166. Lai KN, Whitford J, Buttfield I, et al: Left ventricular function in uremia: Echocardiographic and radionuclide assessment in patients on maintenance hemodialysis. *Clin Nephrol* 23:125-133, 1985.

167. London GM, Fabiani F, Marchais SJ, et al: Uremic cardiomyopathy: An inadequate left ventricular hypertrophy. *Kidney Int* 31:973-980, 1987.

168. Parfrey PS, Harnett JD, Foley RN, et al: Impact of renal transplantation on uremic cardiomyopathy. *Transplantation* 60:908-914, 1995.

169. Goto N, Tominaga Y, Matsuoka S, et al: Cardiovascular complications caused by advanced secondary hyperparathyroidism in chronic dialysis patients; special focus on dilated cardiomyopathy. *Clin Exp Nephrol* 9:138-141, 2005.

170. Iqbal A, Jorde R, Lunde P, et al: Left ventricular dysfunction in subjects with mild secondary hyperparathyroidism detected with pulsed wave tissue Doppler echocardiography. *Cardiology* 105:1-8, 2006.

171. Nestico PF, DePace NL, Kotler MN, et al: Calcium phosphorus metabolism in dialysis patients with and without mitral annular calcium: Analysis of 30 patients. *Am J Cardiol* 51:497-500, 1983.

172. Maher ER, Young G, Smyth-Walsh B, et al: Aortic and mitral valve calcification in patients with end-stage renal disease. *Lancet* 2:875-877, 1987.

173. Bryg RJ, Gordon PR, Migdal SD: Doppler-detected tricuspid, mitral or aortic regurgitation in end-stage renal disease. *Am J Cardiol* 63:750-752, 1989.

174. Schonenberger A, Winkelspecht B, Kohler H, et al: High prevalence of aortic valve alterations in haemodialysis patients is associated with signs of chronic inflammation. *Nephron Clin Pract* 96:c48-c55, 2004.

175. Panuccio V, Tripepi R, Tripepi G, et al: Heart valve calcifications, survival, and cardiovascular risk in hemodialysis patients. *Am J Kidney Dis* 43:479-484, 2004.

176. Ohara T, Hashimoto Y, Matsumura A, et al: Accelerated progression and morbidity in patients with aortic stenosis on chronic dialysis. *Circ J* 69:1535-1539, 2005.

177. Strozecki P, Odrowaz-Sypniewska G, Manitius J: Cardiac valve calcifications and left ventricular hypertrophy in hemodialysis patients. *Ren Fail* 27:733-738, 2005.

178. Madu EC, D'Cruz IA, Wall B, et al: Transesophageal echocardiographic spectrum of calcific mitral abnormalities in patients with end-stage renal disease. *Echocardiography* 17:29-35, 2000.

179. Matalon R, Moussalli ARJ, Nidus BD, et al: Functional aortic insufficiency: A feature of renal failure. *N Engl J Med* 285:1522-1523, 1971.

180. Perez JE, Smith CA, Meltzer VN: Pulmonic valve insufficiency: A common cause of transient diastolic murmurs in renal failure. *Ann Intern Med* 103:497-502, 1985.

181. Depace NL, Ross J, Iskandrian AS, et al: Tricuspid regurgitation: Noninvasive techniques for determining causes and severity. *J Am Coll Cardiol* 3:1540-1550, 1984.

182. Fujise K, Amerling R, Sherman W: Rapid progression of mitral and aortic stenosis in a patient with secondary hyperparathyroidism. *Br Heart J* 70:282-284, 1993.

183. Bernardi D, Bernice L, Cini G, et al: Asymmetric septal hypertrophy in uremic-normotensive patients on regular hemodialysis: An M-mode and two-dimensional echocardiographic study. *Nephron* 39:30-35, 1985.

184. Straumann E, Bertel O, Meyer B, et al: Symmetric and asymmetric left ventricular hypertrophy in patients with end-stage renal failure on long-term hemodialysis. *Clin Cardiol* 21:672-678, 1998.

185. Zoccali C, Benedetto FA, Mallamaci F, et al: Left ventricular mass monitoring in the follow-up of dialysis patients: Prognostic value of left ventricular hypertrophy progression. *Kidney Int* 65:1492-1498, 2004.

186. London GM, DeVernejoul MC, Fabiani F, et al: Secondary hyperparathyroidism and cardiac hypertrophy in hemodialysis patients. *Kidney Int* 32:900-907, 1987.

187. Huting J: Diastolic left ventricular function after renal transplantation in patients with normal and hypertrophied myocardium. *Clin Cardiol* 15:845-850, 1992.

188. Bardaji A, Vea AM, Gutierrez C, Ridao C, et al: Left ventricular mass and diastolic function in normotensive young adults with autosomal dominant polycystic kidney disease. *Am J Kidney Dis* 32:970-975, 1998.

189. Hayashi SY, Rohani M, Lindholm B, et al: Left ventricular function in patients with chronic kidney disease evaluated by colour tissue Doppler velocity imaging. *Nephrol Dial Transplant* 21:125-132, 2006.

190. Sztajzel J, Ruedin P, Monin C, et al: Effect of altered loading conditions during haemodialysis on left ventricular filling pattern. *Eur Heart J* 14:655-661, 1993.

191. Hung KC, Huang HL, Chu CM, et al: Effects of altered volume loading on left ventricular hemodynamics and diastolic filling during hemodialysis. *Ren Fail* 26:141-147, 2004.

192. Oguzhan A, Arinc H, Abaci A, et al: Preload dependence of Doppler tissue imaging derived indexes of left ventricular diastolic function. *Echocardiography* 22:320-325, 2005.

193. Lin SK, Hsiao SH, Lee TY, et al: Color M-mode flow propagation velocity: is it really preload independent? *Echocardiography* 22:636-641, 2005.

194. Sztajzel J, Ruedin P, Stoermann C, et al: Effects of dialysate composition during hemodialysis on left ventricular function. *Kidney Int* 41:S60-S66, 1993.

195. Wizemann V, Soetanto R, Thormann J, et al: Effects of acetate on left ventricular function in hemodialysis patients. *Nephron* 64:101-105, 1993.

196. Artis AK, Alpert MA, Van Stone J, et al: Effect of hemodialysis on left ventricular systolic function in the presence and absence of beta-blockade: Influence of left ventricular mass. *Am J Nephrol* 11:289-294, 1991.

197. DiBello V, Bianchi AM, Caputo MT, et al: Fractional shortening/end-systolic stress correlation in the evaluation of left ventricular contractility in patients treated by acetate dialysis and lactate haemofiltration. *Nephrol Dial Transplant* 5:115-118, 1990.

198. Gupta S, Dev V, Kumar MV, Dash SC: Left ventricular diastolic function in end-stage renal disease and the impact of hemodialysis. *Am J Cardiol* 71:1427-1430, 1993.

199. Di Bello V, Panichi V, Pedrinelli R, et al: Ultrasonic videodensitometric analysis of myocardium in end-stage renal disease treated with haemodialysis. *Nephrol Dial Transplant* 14:2184-2191, 1999.

200. Pizzarelli F, Dattolo P, Ferdeghini EM, Morales MA: Parameters derived by ultrasonic myocardial characterization in dialysis patients are associated with mortality. *Kidney Int* 68:1320-1325, 2005.

201. Fatema K, Hirono O, Masakane I, et al: Dynamic assessment of myocardial involvement in patients with end-stage renal disease by ultrasonic tissue characterization and serum markers of collagen metabolism. *Clin Cardiol* 27:228-234, 2004.

202. Weinrauch LA, D'Elia JA, Gleason RE, et al: Usefulness of left ventricular size and function in predicting survival in chronic dialysis patients with diabetes mellitus. *Am J Cardiol* 70:300-303, 1992.

203. Zaslavsky L, Pinotti A, Gross J: Diastolic dysfunction and mortality in diabetic patients on hemodialysis: A 4.25-year controlled prospective study. *J Diabetes Complications* 19:194-200, 2005.

204. Foley RN, Parfrey PS, Kent GM, et al: Serial change in echocardiographic parameters and cardiac failure in end-stage renal disease. *J Am Soc Nephrol* 11:912-916, 2000.

205. Miyazato J, Horio T, Takiuchi S, et al: Left ventricular diastolic dysfunction in patients with chronic renal failure: impact of diabetes mellitus. *Diabet Med* 22:730-736, 2005.

206. Hampl H, Sternberg C, Berweck S, et al: Regression of left ventricular hypertrophy in hemodialysis patients is possible. *Clin Nephrol* 58(Suppl 1):S73-S96, 2002.

207. Rozich JD, Smith B, Thomas JD, et al: Dialysis-induced alterations in left ventricular filling: mechanisms and significance. *Am J Kidney Dis* 17:277-285, 1991.

208. Weinrauch LA, D'Elia JA, Monaco AP, et al: Preoperative evaluation for diabetic renal transplantation: Impact of clinical, laboratory, and echocardiographic parameters on patient and allograft survival. *Am J Med* 93:19-28, 1992.

209. Counihan TB: Heart failure due to extreme obesity. *Br Heart J* 18:425-426, 1956.

210. Alexander JK, Pettigrove JR: Obesity and congestive heart failure. *Geriatrics* 22:101-108, 1967.

211. Alexander JK: Obesity and the heart. *Curr Probl Cardiol* 5:6-41, 1980.

212. Messerli FH: Cardiovascular effects of obesity and hypertension. *Lancet* 1:165-168, 1982.

213. Messerli FH, Sundgaard-Riise K, Reisin ED, et al: Dimorphic cardiac adaption to obesity and arterial hypertension. *Ann Intern Med* 99:757-761, 1983.

214. Alpert MA, Terry BE, Kelly DL: Effect of weight loss on cardiac chamber size, wall thickness and left ventricular function in morbid obesity. *Am J Cardiol* 55:783-786, 1985.

215. Alexander JK: The cardiomyopathy of obesity. *Prog Cardiovasc Dis* 27:325-333, 1985.

216. Nakajima T, Fujioka S, Tokunaga K, et al: Noninvasive study of left ventricular performance in obese patients: Influence of duration of obesity. *Circulation* 71:481-486, 1985.

217. Nakajima T, Fujioka S, Tokunaga K, et al: Correlation of intraabdominal fat accumulation and left ventricular performance in obesity. *Am J Cardiol* 64:235-239, 1989.

218. Garcia LC, Laredo C, Arriaga J, Barnanco JG: Echocardiographic findings in obesity. *Rev Invest Clin* 34:235-239, 1982.

219. Romano M, Carella G, Cotecchia MR, et al: Abnormal systolic time intervals in obesity. *Am Heart J* 112:356-360, 1986.

220. Alpert MA, Singh A, Terry BE, et al: Effect of exercise on left ventricular systolic function and reserve in morbid obesity. *Am J Cardiol* 63:1478-1482, 1989.

221. DeDivitiis O, Fazio S, Petitto M, et al: Obesity and cardiac function. *Circulation* 64:477-482, 1981.

222. Karason K, Wallentin I, Larsson B, et al: Effects of obesity and weight loss on cardiac function and valvular performance. *Obes Res* 6:422-429, 1998.

223. Iacobellis G, Ribaudo MC, Leto G, et al: Influence of excess fat on cardiac morphology and function: study in uncomplicated obesity. *Obes Res* 10:767-773, 2002.

224. Pascual M, Pascual DA, Soria F, et al: Effects of isolated obesity on systolic and diastolic left ventricular function. *Heart* 89:1152-1156, 2003.

225. Iacobellis G, Ribaudo MC, Zapputerreno A, et al: Adapted changes in left ventricular structure and function in severe uncomplicated obesity. *Obes Res* 12:1616-1621, 2004.

226. Morricone L, Malavazos AE, Coman C, et al: Echocardiographic abnormalities in normotensive obese patients: relationship with visceral fat. *Obes Res* 10:489-498, 2002.

227. Wong CY, O'Moore-Sullivan, T, Leano R, et al: Alterations of left ventricular myocardial characteristics associated with obesity. *Circulation* 110:3081-3087, 2004.

228. Alpert MA, Terry BE, Mulekar M, et al: Cardiac morphology and left ventricular function in normotensive morbidly obese patients with and without congestive heart failure, and effect of weight loss. *Am J Cardiol* 80:736-740, 1997.

229. Mureddu GF, de Simone G, Greco R, et al: Left ventricular filling pattern in uncomplicated obesity. *Am J Cardiol* 77:509-514, 1996.

230. Zarich SW, Kowalchuk GJ, McGuire MP, et al: Left ventricular filling abnormalities in asymptomatic morbid obesity. *Am J Cardiol* 68:377-381, 1991.

231. Chakko S, Mayor M, Allison MD, et al: Abnormal left ventricular diastolic filling in eccentric left ventricular hypertrophy of obesity. *Am J Cardiol* 68:95-98, 1991.

232. Stoddard MF, Tseuda K, Thomas M, et al: The influence of obesity on left ventricular filling and systolic function. *Am Heart J* 124:694-699, 1992.

233. Willens HJ, Chakko SS, Lowery MH, et al: Tissue Doppler imaging of the right and left ventricle in severe obesity (body mass index >35kg/m²). *Am J Cardiol* 94:1087-1090, 2004.

234. Alpert MA, Lambert CR, Terry BE, et al: Influence of left ventricular mass on left ventricular diastolic filling in normotensive morbid obesity. *Am Heart J* 130:1068-1073, 1995.

235. Willens HJ, Chakko SC, Byers P, et al: Effects of weight loss after gastric bypass on right and left ventricular function assessed by tissue Doppler imaging. *Am J Cardiol* 95:1521-1524, 2005.

236. Alpert MA, Lambert CR, Panayiotou H, et al: Relation of duration of morbid obesity to left ventricular mass, systolic function, and diastolic filling, and effect of weight loss. *Am J Cardiol* 76:1194-1197, 1995.

237. Himeno E, Nishino K, Nakashima Y, et al: Weight reduction regresses left ventricular mass regardless of blood pressure level in obese subjects. *Am Heart J* 131:313-319, 1996.

238. Connolly HM, Crary JL, McGoon MD, et al: Valvular heart disease associated with fenfluramine-phentermine. *N Engl J Med* 337:581-588, 1997.

239. Redfield MM, Nicholson WJ, Edwards WD, et al: Valve disease associated with ergot alkaloid use: echocardiographic and pathologic correlations. *Ann Intern Med* 117:50-52, 1992.

240. Centers for Disease Control and Prevention: Cardiac valvulopathy associated with exposure to fenfluramine or dexfenfluramine: US Department of Health and Human Services interim public health recommendations, November 1997. *J Am Med Assoc* 278:1729-1731, 1997.

241. Khan MA, Herzog CA, St. Peter JV, et al: The prevalence of cardiac valvular insufficiency assessed by transthoracic echocardiography in obese patients treated with appetite-suppressant drugs. *N Engl J Med* 339:713-718, 1998.

242. Shively BK, Roldan CA, Gill EA, et al: Prevalence and determinants of valvulopathy in patients treated with dexfenfluramine. *Circulation* 100:2161-2167, 1999.

243. Gardin JM, Schumacher D, Constantine G, et al: Valvular abnormalities and cardiovascular status following exposure to dexfenfluramine or phentermine/fenfluramine. *J Am Med Assoc* 283:1703-1709, 2000.

244. Jollis JG, Landolfo CK, Kisslo J, et al: Fenfluramine and phentermine and cardiovascular findings effect of treatment duration on prevalence of valve abnormalities. *Circulation* 101:2071-2077, 2000.

245. Weissman NJ, Tighe JF Jr, Gottdiener JS, et al: An assessment of heart valve abnormalities in obese patients taking dexfenfluramine, sustained-release dexfenfluramine, or placebo. *N Engl J Med* 339:725-732, 1998.

246. Burger AJ, Sherman HB, Charlamb MJ, et al: Low prevalence of valvular heart disease in 226 phentermine-fenfluramine protocol subjects prospectively followed for up to 30 months. *J Am Coll Cardiol* 34:1153-1158, 1999.

247. Sachdev M, Miller, WC, Ryan, T, et al: Effect of fenfluramine-derived diet pills on cardic valves: a meta-analysis of observational studies. *Am Heart J* 144:1065-1073, 2002.

248. Vagelos R, Jacobs M, Popp RL, et al: Reversal of phen-fen associated valvular regurgitation documented by serial echocardiography. *J Am Soc Echocardiogr* 15:653-657, 2002.

249. Aurigemma GP, Ronen A, Cuenoud H, et al: Severe mitral valve regurgitation associated with dexfenfluramine use. *Cardiology* 98:215-217, 2002.

250. Biswas SS, Donovan CL, Forbess JM, et al: Valve replacement for appetite suppressant-induced valvular heart disease. *Ann Thorac Surg* 67:1819-1822, 1999.

251. Caccitolo JA, Connolly HM, Rubenson DS, et al: Operation for anorexigen-associated valvular heart disease. *J Thorac Cardiovasc Surg* 122:656-664, 2001.

252. Hensrud DD, Connolly HM, Grogan M, et al: Echocardiographic improvement over time after cessation of use of fenfluramine and phentermine. *Mayo Clin Proc* 74:1191-1197, 1999.

253. Weissman NJ, Tighe JF, Gottdiener JS, et al: Prevalence of valvular regurgitation associated with dexfenfluramine three to five months after discontinuation of treatment. *J Am Coll Cardiol* 34:2088-2095, 1999.

254. Gardin JM, Weissman NJ, Leung C, et al: One year echocardiographic follow-up on patients treated with anorexigens. *Int J Obesity* 24:S188, 2000.

255. Khan MA, St. Peter JV, Herzog CA, et al: Does the severity of appetite suppressant-related aortic valve insufficiency change over time after stopping exposure to drug? *Circulation* 102:II-369, 2000.

256. Mast ST, Jollis JG, Ryan T, et al: The progression of fenfluramine-associated valvular heart disease assessed by echocardiography. *Ann Intern Med* 134:261-266, 2001.

257. Davidoff R, McTiernan A, Constantine G, et al: Echocardiographic examination of women previously treated with fenfluramine: long-term follow-up of a randomized, double-blind, placebo-controlled trial. *Arch Intern Med* 161:1429-1436, 2001.

258. Gardin JM, Weissman NJ, Leung C, et al: Clinical and echocardiographic follow-up of patients previously treated with dexfenfluramine or phentermine/fenfluramine. *J Am Med Assoc* 286:2011-2014, 2001.

259. Weissman NJ, Panza JA, Tighe JF, et al: Natural history of valvular regurgitation 1 year after discontinuation of dexfenfluramine therapy: A randomized, double-blind, placebo-controlled trial. *Ann Intern Med* 134:267-273, 2001.

260. Klein AL, Griffin BP, Grimm RA, et al: Natural history of valvular regurgitation using side-by-side echocardiographic analysis in anorexigen-treated subjects. *Am J Cardiol* 96:1711-1717, 2005.

261. Quiñones MA, Otto CM, Stoddard M, et al: Recommendations for quantification of Doppler echocardiography: A report from the Doppler quantification task force of the nomenclature and standards committee of the American Society of Echocardiography. *J Am Soc Echocardiogr* 15:167-184, 2002.

262. Zoghbi WA, Enriquez-Sarano M, Foster E, et al: Recommendations for evaluation of the severity of native valvular regurgitation with two-dimensional and Doppler echocardiography. *J Am Soc Echocardiogr* 16:777-802, 2003.

263. Steffee CH, Singh HK, Chitwood WR: Histologic changes in three explanted native cardiac valves following use of fenfluramines. *Cardiovasc Pathol* 8:245-253, 1999.

264. Doty JR, Bull DA, Flores JH, et al: Valve repair and replacement for valvular heart disease secondary to phetermine-fenfluramine use. *Circulation* 104:II-685, 2001.

265. McDonald PC, Wilson JE, Gao M, et al: Quantitative analysis of human heart valves: does anorexigen exposure produce a distinctive morphological lesion? *Cardiovasc Path* 11:251-262, 2002.

266. Volmar KE, Hutchins GM: Aortic and mitral fenfluramine-phentermine valvulopathy in 64 patients treated with anorectic agents. *Arch Pathol Lab Med* 125:1555-1561, 2001.

267. Jick H, Vasilakis C, Weinrauch LA, et al: A population-based study of appetite-suppressant drugs and the risk of cardiac-valve regurgitation. *N Engl J Med* 339:719-724, 1998.

268. Eichelberger JP, Pearson TA, Gajary E, et al: 15 year outcome data on patients treated with fenfluramine/phentermine combination. *J Am Soc Echocardiogr* 12:355, 1999.

269. Abenheim L, Moride Y, Brenot F, et al: Appetite suppressant drugs and the risk of primary pulmonary hypertension. *N Engl J Med* 335:609-616, 1996.

270. Weyman AE, Davidoff R, Gardin J, et al: Echocardiographic evaluation of pulmonary artery pressure with clinical correlates in predominantly obese adults. *J Am Soc Echocardiogr* 15:454-462, 2002.

271. Valencia-Flores M, Rebollar V, Santiago V, et al: Prevalence of pulmonary hypertension and its association with respiratory disturbances in obese patients living at moderately high altitude. *Int J Obes Relat Metab Disord* 28:1174-1180, 2004.

272. Peterson LR, Waggoner AD, Schechtman KB, et al: Alterations in left ventricular structure and function in young healthy obese women: Assessment by echocardiography and tissue Doppler imaging. *J Am Coll Cardiol* 43:1399-1404, 2004.

273. Wong CY, O'Moore-Sullivan T, Leano R, et al: Association of subclinical right ventricular dysfunction with obesity. *J Am Coll Cardiol* 47:611-616, 2006.

274. Di Stante B, Galandauer I, Aronow WS, et al: Prevalence of left ventricular diastolic dysfunction in obese persons with and without diabetes mellitus. *Am J Cardiol* 95:1527-1528, 2005.

275. Sidana J, Aronow WS, Ravipati G, et al: Prevalence of moderate or severe left ventricular diastolic dysfunction in obese persons with obstructive sleep apnea. *Cardiology* 104:107-109, 2005.

276. Kuch B, Muscholl M, Luchner A, et al: Gender specific differences in left ventricular adaptation to obesity and hypertension. *J Hum Hypertens* 12:685-691, 1998.

277. de Simone G, Palmieri V, Bella JN, et al: Association of left ventricular hypertrophy with metabolic risk factors: the HyperGEN study. *J Hypertens* 20:323-331, 2002.

278. Kimmel SE, Keane MG, Crary JL, et al: Detailed examination of flenfluramine-phentermine users with valve abnormalities identified in Fargo, North Dakota. *Am J Cardiol* 84:304-308, 1999.

279. Gottdiener JS, Panza JA, St John Sutton M, et al: Testing the test: the reliability of echocardiography in the sequential assessment of valvular regurgitation. *Am Heart J* 144:115-121, 2002.

280. Ayzenberg O, Silber MH, Bortz D: Beriberi heart disease: A case report describing the hemodynamic features. *S Afr Med J* 68:263, 1985.

281. Akram H, Maslowski AH, Smith BL, Nichols MG: The haemodynamic, histopathological and hormonal features of alcoholic beriberi. *Q J Med* 50:359, 1981.

282. Carson P: Alcoholic cardiac beriberi. *Br Med J* 284:1817, 1982.

283. Tang SC, Liu YX, Jin ZH, et al: M-mode echocardiographic features of children with Keshan disease. A preliminary observation of 106 cases. *Chin Med J* 97:795-800, 1984.

284. Fleming CR, Lie JT, McCall JT, et al: Selenium deficiency and fatal cardiomyopathy in a patient on home parenteral nutrition. *Gastroenterology* 83:689-693, 1982.

285. Ocal B, Unal S, Zorlu P, et al: Echocardiographic evaluation of cardiac functions and left ventricular mass in children with malnutrition. *J Paediatr Child Health* 37:14-17, 2001.

286. Phornphatkul C, Pongprot Y, Suskind R, et al: Cardiac function in malnourished children. *Clin Pediatr* 33:147-154, 1994.

Chapter 38

Echocardiography in Patients with Inherited Connective Tissue Disorders

MARK LEWIN, MD

Forms of Connective Tissue Disorders

Whereas connective tissue disorders affect multiple organs, the impact on the cardiovascular system is considered the most dangerous. These disorders are known to cause progressive degeneration of the integument, joints, pleura, and eyes. Although there is potential for both left-sided and right-sided heart involvement, clinically important pathology is typically confined to the mitral valve, aortic valve, and the aorta itself.

As opposed to other forms of cardiovascular disease, many patients come to medical attention not because of symptoms referable to the cardiovascular system but rather because of findings associated with one of the noncardiac organ systems noted previously. Additionally, identification of cardiovascular pathology may be noted on screening cardiac assessment as the result of the presence of a defined or suspected connective tissue disorder in another family member. Echocardiography is the mainstay of cardiac screening for the cardiac manifestations of connective tissue disorders. As in many other cardiac disorders, transesophageal imaging complements transthoracic in developing a thorough set of data. In addition, other noninvasive imaging modalities (i.e., computed tomography [CT] and magnetic resonance imaging [MRI]) contribute to diagnosis in selected circumstances. Although Marfan syndrome is the most common connective tissue disorder leading to cardiovascular compromise, a number of other inherited and congenital conditions are known to affect the cardiac structures in similar ways (Table 38–1). These conditions will be elucidated in this chapter. In addition, the spectrum of disease and the methods of assessment will be highlighted.

Marfan Syndrome

Marfan syndrome is a well-described heritable disorder of connective tissue with a broad phenotypic spectrum. Major clinical manifestations include the cardiovascular, ocular, and skeletal systems. Diagnosis is almost exclusively based on clinical criteria (Table 38–2) as put forth by the Ghent nosology.[1] Myopia and lens dislocation are common findings of the ocular system. Skeletal system involvement is characterized by bone overgrowth and joint laxity. Cardiovascular manifestations include dilatation of the aorta (typically at the level of the sinus of Valsalva), a predisposition for aortic dissection, mitral valve prolapse (MVP) with or without regurgitation, tricuspid valve prolapse, and enlargement of the main pulmonary artery (PA). The Ghent criteria are divided into those termed *major* and those termed *minor*. The major criteria include those that carry high diagnostic specificity (because they are relatively uncommon in other conditions and in the general population). In the absence of a family history, or a fibrillin 1 *(FBN1)* mutation, the diagnosis of Marfan syndrome requires the presence of major criteria in two organ systems and involvement within a third system. In the presence of a family history or a known *FBN1* mutation, one major and one minor criterion are

required for diagnosis. In younger children who do not fulfill sufficient criteria to confirm a diagnosis, serial evaluations are recommended as a result of the potential for evolving clinical conditions that could progress such that a diagnosis is eventually achieved.

Marfan syndrome is inherited in an autosomal dominant manner with 25% of patients representing sporadic, new mutations without a family history.[2] Once an individual is diagnosed with Marfan syndrome, first-degree relatives should be screened for the condition (by physical examination, accompanied by ophthalmologic assessment and echocardiography when felt to be clinically appropriate). The age related penetrance is high and both interfamilial and intrafamilial variability are well described. Molecular genetic testing of the *FBN1* gene (locus 15q21.1) reveals a causative mutation in approximately 70% to 90% of individuals fulfilling the clinical diagnostic criteria for Marfan syndrome.[3]

Although there has been considerable effort invested in defining genotype-phenotype correlations for Marfan syndrome, few if any definitive correlations have emerged. Thus far none have been shown specific enough to influence clinical management. Of those that have emerged, the patients with the most severe form of Marfan syndrome (also termed the *infantile Marfan syndrome*) and an identifiable *FBN1* mutation tend to harbor mutations in the central portion of the gene, between exons 24 to 32.[4-6] Interestingly, mutations have been also found in this region in other patients with classic, atypically severe, and milder forms of Marfan syndrome and other fibrillinopathies.[6-8] By way of contrast, mutations in FBN1 resulting in milder forms of a type 1 fibrillinopathy have also been described. These include mutations in the C-terminus region of FBN1 resulting in only the skeletal manifestations of Marfan syndrome.[9] Mutations in exons 59 to 65 of *FBN1*[10] and exons 1 to 10[11] have been associated with phenotypes lacking significant aortic involvement or with only late onset and relatively mild cardiovascular features.

In an effort to identify other genetic modifiers of the wide variability inherent in Marfan syndrome, Giusti and colleagues[12] investigated the possible role of hyperhomocysteinemia and specifically the C677T methylenetetrahydrofolate reductase (MTHFR) polymorphism as a factor influencing the severity of cardiovascular manifestations in Marfan syndrome. Patients were subdivided based on the degree of cardiac involvement and total homocysteine, cysteine, folate, and B_{12} levels were measured together with C677T MTHFR genotyping. The prevalence of homozygotes for the C677T polymorphism was significantly higher in patients with aortic dissection than in patients without dissection, patients with mild cardiac involvement, and in control subjects. However, further analysis indicated that it was total homocysteine that remained associated with the severe cardio-

TABLE 38–1. Inherited and Congenital Disorders Associated with Aortic Dilation and/or Mitral Valve Prolapse

Marfan syndrome
Ehlers-Danlos syndrome
Homocystinuria
Thoracic aortic aneurysm and dissection syndrome (TAADS)
Familial thoracic aortic aneurysm
MASS phenotype
Bicuspid aortic valve
Coarctation of the aorta
Mitral calve prolapse syndrome
Turner syndrome
Osteogenesis imperfecta

TABLE 38–2. **Features of Marfan Syndrome**

	Major Criteria	Minor Criteria
Skeletal	*At least four of the following:* Pectus deformity requiring surgery Reduced upper-to-lower segment ratio for age Wrist and thumb signs Scoliosis Reduced elbow extension Pes planus Protrusio acetabulare (abnormally deep acetabulum with accelerated erosion)	*Two major components or one major component and at least two of the following:* Moderate pectus excavatum Joint hypermobility High arched palate with dental crowding Malar hypoplasia, or retrognathia, or down-slanting palpebral fissures
Integument	—	*At least one of the following:* Striae atrophicae without obvious cause Recurrent or incisional hernia
Cardiovascular	*At least one of the following:* Dilatation of the ascending aorta involving the sinuses of Valsalva Dissection of the ascending aorta	*At least one of the following:* Mitral valve prolapse Idiopathic main pulmonary artery dilatation Descending thoracic or abdominal aorta dilatation before the age of 50 years
Ocular	Ectopia lentis	*At least two of the following:* Abnormally flat cornea Increased axial length of the globe Myopia
Family/genetic history	*At least one of the following:* First-degree relative with Marfan syndrome Presence of a mutation in *FBN1* known to cause Marfan syndrome	—
Other	Dural ectasia Spontaneous pneumothorax	—

Requirements for diagnosis: In the absence of an unequivocally affected first-degree relative, one should require involvement of the skeleton and at least two other systems with a minimum of one major manifestation (ectopia lentis, aortic dilatation or aortic dissection, or dural ectasia). In the presence of an unequivocally affected first-degree relative, one requires only that two organ systems be involved.
FBN1, fibrillin 1.

vascular phenotype in their study group rather than the C677T MTHFR genotype. The authors conclude that this association suggests a role for hyperhomocysteinemia and the MTHFR genotype in the phenotypic variability of the cardiovascular manifestations seen in Marfan syndrome. In due course, other genetic modifiers of Marfan syndrome and the cardiovascular phenotype will likely be identified.

Ehlers-Danlos

There are multiple forms of Ehlers-Danlos syndrome, each manifested by particular phenotypic features. The most common forms are type III, otherwise termed *benign hypermobility syndrome,* and the classic form, previously designated as types I and II but now recognized as forming a clinical continuum (involving hyperextensibility, fragile "cigarette paper" skin which heals poorly, scoliosis, and hernias). The classic form of Ehlers-Danlos is uncommonly associated with cardiac features of MVP, aortic root dila-

tion, and an increased susceptibility to dissecting aortic aneurysm.[13] Cardiovascular surgery is not tolerated well as a result of the friable nature of the tissues resulting in disruption of vascular integrity. Types I and III are inherited in an autosomal dominant fashion and are caused by a disorder in synthesis of collagen.

Type IV is also termed the *malignant* form of Ehlers-Danlos syndrome in that there is an increased susceptibility to spontaneous vascular dissection. These large vessel dissections can involve the aorta, but the cerebral and abdominal large arteries are also at risk.[14,15] The sites of arterial rupture are the thorax and abdomen (50%), head and neck (25%), and extremities (25%). Although uncommon, the vascular type of Ehlers-Danlos syndrome is a cause of stroke in young adults. The mean age of intracranial aneurysmal rupture, spontaneous carotid-cavernous sinus fistula, and cervical artery aneurysm is 28 years.[16] Hyperelastic tissues and hyperextensible joints are less frequent manifestations, but easy bruising and poor wound healing are commonly seen. Inheritance is autosomal dominant with the defect occurring in the type 3 collagen gene located on chromosome 2.[17]

All patients with Ehlers-Danlos syndrome (irrespective of particular type) should undergo screening echocardiographic assessment. Patients with types I, II, and IV (more commonly associated with cardiovascular manifestations) should be evaluated annually by echocardiography to develop a serial assessment of aortic dilation and mitral valve disease. Aortic insufficiency may develop. The indications for surgical repair are similar to Marfan syndrome with the caveat being that the fragile nature of the large vessels in type IV results in a more complex surgical patient and associated higher surgical morbidity and mortality as a result of the loss of vascular integrity.

Homocystinuria

This disorder is defined as the presence of excessive homocystine in the urine. The most common form of homocystinuria is caused by a metabolic disorder in which a deficiency of cystathionine β-synthase results in an elevation of blood methionine and subsequent deposition of its precursor homocysteine in the urine. The inheritance occurs in an autosomal recessive pattern with variable phenotypic expression even within the same family. Clinical findings can include mental retardation or developmental delay, ectopia lentis, coagulopathies, and many of the same skeletal features present in Marfan syndrome including scoliosis, arachnodactyly, tall stature, and pectus deformities. As opposed to the aortic dilation seen in patients with Marfan syndrome, this entity is not generally present in homocystinuria. From a cardiovascular standpoint, these patients can develop arterial and venous thromboses, which can lead to peripheral or cerebral vascular disease in both children and adults.[18] This is complicated by vascular injury including medial degeneration of the aorta and large arteries, with intimal hyperplasia and fibrosis. There is resultant pulmonary embolism with associated right ventricular (RV) hypertension and ischemic coronary disease with the potential for myocardial infarction.

Other Fibrillinopathies

FBN1 mutations have also been reported in distinct phenotypes that have overlap with Marfan syndrome, including MVP syndrome, the MASS phenotype (Myopia, MVP, mild Aortic enlargement, nonspecific Skin/Skeletal signs), apparently isolated ectopia lentis, predominant or isolated skeletal features of Marfan syndrome and familial aortic aneurysm or dissection.[3] Together, Marfan syndrome and the Marfan-related phenotypes have been termed the type 1 fibrillinopathies.

Congenital contractural arachnodactyly (CCA), another connective tissue disorder similar to Marfan syndrome, is caused by fibrillin-2 (FBN2) mutations. It can be difficult to differentiate between these two syndromes because of the similar skeletal complications including arachnodactyly, pectus deformities, and scoliosis. However, CCA usually presents with multiple joint contractures and crumpled ear helices. There is the occasional finding of aortic root dilation, and in addition eye involvement can be seen.[19]

Another disease locus has been mapped to 16p12-13 and causes mutations in the smooth muscle myosin heavy chain (MYH11) gene. These individuals have been shown to have thoracic aortic aneurysm and dissection, marked aortic stiffness, and in addition a predilection for persistent patency of the ductus arteriosus.[20] Individuals with this mutation have decreased aortic compliance and a higher pulse wave velocity. Young asymptomatic carriers frequently already have indices of aortic stiffness similar to older symptomatic patients. Histologic examination shows large areas of medial degeneration with little smooth muscle content. Thus the MYH11 mutation is felt to confer early and severe reduction in the elasticity of the aortic wall. From a physiologic perspective, this would be consistent with the role of smooth muscle cells in maintaining appropriate mechanical properties to the thoracic aorta.[21]

Transforming Growth Factor-Beta Receptor Mutations

The most recent exciting breakthrough in the understanding of the etiology of connective tissue disorders involves the transforming growth factor, TGF-β. In 1993, a large family with features suggestive of Marfan syndrome was reported to lack a mutation in the Marfan loci within the fibrillin gene.[22] This family was shown to have a mutation mapped to the 3p24 loci; this was subsequently termed Marfan type II (MFS2).[23] The MFS2 gene has been shown to encode TGF-β, yielding the first evidence that there is a direct link between abnormal TGF-β signaling and connective tissue disorders. Further clarity to this relationship occurred with the identification that mutations in the transforming growth factor-β receptor type-2 gene (TGFBR2) have been found to be associated with the Marfan phenotype, further expanding our understanding of Marfan type II. The features of Marfan type II typically include skeletal, cardiac, and (typically mild) ocular findings.[24] Recent data suggest a functional relationship between FBN1 and TGF-β signaling, suggesting a link between these two abnormal proteins of the extracellular connective tissue matrix and the development of the pathologic features of Marfan syndrome.[25]

Mutations in TGFBR and TGFBR2 have been found in association with a recently described connective tissue disorder termed *Loeys-Dietz syndrome*.[26] This syndrome is characterized by a bifid uvula, hypertelorism, cleft palate, and generalized arterial tortuosity with ascending aortic aneurysm. Although the phenotype is variable, in general it is felt that these individuals have a worse cardiovascular risk profile (including aortic dissection at a younger age, and at a smaller aortic diameter) than is the case for Marfan syndrome. Other features may include craniosynostosis, brain malformations, mental retardation, and aneurysms or dissection throughout the arterial tree. The *TGFBR's* regulate multiple cellular functions including cell proliferation, differentiation, and organization. The extent of clinical overlap between Marfan syndrome, Loeys-Dietz syndrome, and other mutations of the *TGFBR* family remain unclear. In a study by Mizuguchi and colleagues, four out of five *TGFBR2* mutations were found in patients fulfilling diagnostic criteria for Marfan syndrome based upon the revised Ghent criteria.[24] In a study of 41 unrelated patients who fulfilled the Marfan syndrome clinical criteria, two patients were found to have *TGFBR1* mutations and five patients were found to have *TGFBR2* mutations,[27] again suggesting the extensive clinical overlap between patients with Marfan syndrome and those with *TGFBR* mutations.

Thoracic Aortic Aneurysm and Dissection

Thoracic aortic aneurysm and dissection (TAAD) is a severe and well-described feature of many inherited connective tissue disorders including Marfan's and Ehlers-Danlos syndrome. However familial clustering of TAAD is more complex and heterogeneous. Twenty percent of patients with TAAD who do not have Marfan syndrome are found to have a first-degree relative with the disease.[28] Although fibrillin mutations have been found in some families with aortic aneurysms along with features suggestive of a connective tissue disorder but inadequate criteria to warrant the diagnosis of Marfan syndrome,[3] in some families TAAD segregates as an isolated finding. Studies have mapped loci for nonsyndromic familial TAAD to three loci: 5q13-15 *(TAAD1)*, 3p24-25 *(TAAD2)*, and 11q23.2-q24 *(FAA1)*.[22,29,30] The *TAAD2* locus overlaps the second locus for Marfan syndrome *(MFS2)*[12,23,31] on the *TGFBR2* gene and may be the etiology of 5% of familial TAAD cases.[32]

Histopathology

The fibrous structures of the heart are composed primarily of connective tissue proteins. These serve as a framework whereby the contractile myocardial tissue is structurally supported. Connective tissue also supports the underlying structure of the large blood vessels and valves. Collagen and elastin fibrils underlie the endocardial cells of the heart and blood vessels. Type I collagen fiber bundles make up the support structure for the atrioventricular valves and constitute the primary elements of the valvar fibrous rings. The major structural support of the large blood vessels is elastin and collagen types I and III; lesser amounts of types IV, V, and VI collagen also contribute to vessel wall integrity.

The aorta is comprised of three layers, the intima, media, and adventitia. The medial layer consists of concentric layers of smooth muscle cells, collagen, and elastin with extracellular matrix proteoglycans. In connective tissue disorders, dilation of the aortic root is caused by degenerative changes as a result of loss of smooth muscle cells, fragmentation of elastic fibers, increase in collagen, replacement of this degenerated tissue with "cysts."[33] This degenerative process is therefore termed *cystic medial necrosis* and is seen not only in the case of patients with Marfan syndrome[34] but also in biopsy or autopsy aortic specimens from patients with a range of disease processes, including the dilated aortic root associated with a bicuspid aortic valve, familial thoracic aortic aneurysms,[11] Turner syndrome,[35] Ehlers-Danlos syndrome type IV,[36] coarctation of the aorta and other congenital heart defects,[37,38] and in association with adult polycystic kidney disease.[39] In addition, pathology of the medial layer seen with cystic medial necrosis has been described as part of the degenerative cardiovascular changes of aging and is exacerbated in the presence of systemic hypertension.[40]

Spectrum of Disease: Echocardiographic Findings

Aortic Dilation

The aortic root is comprised of the aortic valve annulus, the sinus of Valsalva, the sinotubular junction, and the ascending aorta. By convention, echocardiographic measurements of these regions are performed from the parasternal long-axis view at early systole (Fig. 38–1). The regions of the aortic arch are best viewed from the suprasternal notch (Fig. 38–2). Additionally, the aortic valve and ascending aorta may be imaged in children from the subcostal imaging plane (Figs. 38–3, 38–4, and 38–5). In the presence of a connective tissue disorder, dilation may occur at any position along the aortic root and throughout the descending thoracic and abdominal aorta. However, the most typical sites of dilation encompass the sinus of Valsalva, sinotubular junction, and proximal ascending aorta. These sites develop the most significant pathology in that their position

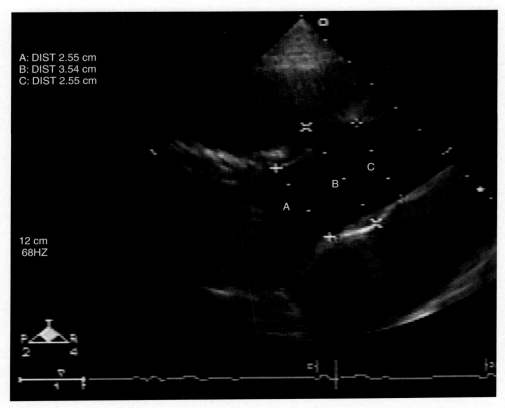

A: DIST 2.55 cm
B: DIST 3.54 cm
C: DIST 2.55 cm

12 cm
68HZ

Figure 38–1. Fourteen-year-old with Marfan syndrome; imaging performed in the parasternal long-axis plane. Moderate dilation of the aortic valve (A): 26 mm; 4 z-scores. Sinus of Valsalva (B): 38 mm; 4.3 z-scores. Mild sinotubular junction dilation (C): 28 mm; 2.7 z-scores. (Z-score is equivalent to standard deviation.)

subjects them to the highest sheer stresses as a result of pulsatile expansion during systole.[41] Effacement of the sinotubular junction is a common finding, in which the sinotubular junction and proximal ascending aorta develop a "flattened" appearance and have essentially the same diameter as the sinus of Valsalva (Fig. 38–6). The term *effacement* is qualitative and is not associated with defined measurements. In fact, effacement encompasses a spectrum of findings, initially manifest subtle changes in the natural tendency for the sinotubular junction to abruptly change direction and caliber at the onset of the proximal ascending aorta. As the severity of effacement progresses, there is a progressive transition to a morphologic pattern characterized by a constant caliber of vessel from the sinus of Valsalva through the proximal ascending aorta.

In addition, as the severity of aortic root dilation worsens, aortic insufficiency can develop. This is a result of either asymmetric dilation of one or more cusps or generalized dilation at the aortic valve annulus. Either mechanism has the potential to alter the geometry of the aorta in such a manner that insufficiency will develop (Figs. 38–7 and 38–8).

In those situations in which the thoracic aorta can not be imaged completely using transthoracic echo-

cardiography (TTE), transesophageal echocardiography (TEE) should be employed. Studies suggest that TEE is comparable to CT scan in defining thoracic aortic aneurysms.

The normal adult abdominal aorta measures 2 cm at the level of the celiac trunk and 1.8 cm just below the renal arteries. Tapering occurs as the aorta approaches the level of the iliac arteries. Most abdominal aortic aneurysms form between the renal and iliac arteries. Clinically significant abdominal aortic aneurysms measure greater than 4 cm in diameter. High degrees of sensitivity and specificity should be expected from abdominal ultrasound (US) or echocardiography, but excessive body habitus can occasional hamper complete visualization. In these cases abdominal aortic angiography, CT scan, or aortic MRI should provide data with which to achieve a definitive diagnosis.

Aortic aneurysms are classified as either true or false (pseudoaneurysm). A true aneurysm involves weakening and dilation of the entire vessel wall. A pseudoaneurysm occurs when a full thickness defect in the aortic wall allows blood to circulate out of the confines of the artery. The circulating blood is contained by the surrounding soft tissues. The most common etiologies for a true aneurysm include atherosclerosis, medial

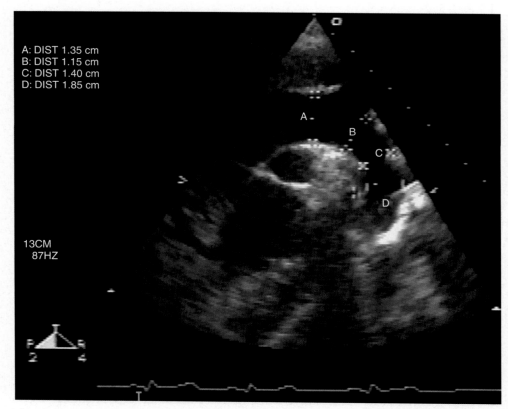

A: DIST 1.35 cm
B: DIST 1.15 cm
C: DIST 1.40 cm
D: DIST 1.85 cm

13CM
87HZ

Figure 38–2. Aortic arch imaging from the suprasternal long-axis imaging plane at end-systole demonstrating the appropriate locations to measure the distal ascending aorta (A) just before the innominate artery, the transverse aorta (B) between the innominate artery and the left carotid artery, the aortic isthmus (C) just before the left subclavian artery, and the proximal descending aorta (D) just beyond the left subclavian artery.

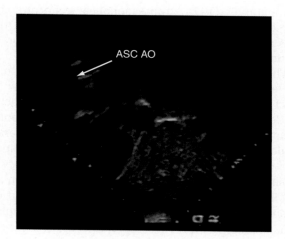

Figure 38–3. Three-year-old with a TGF-β mutation; subcostal short-axis imaging allows visualization of the left ventricular outflow tract through the ascending aorta (Asc Ao).

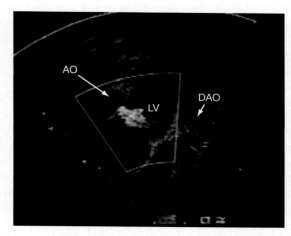

Figure 38–4. Three-year-old with a TGF-β mutation; subcostal short-axis imaging identifies moderate aortic regurgitation resulting from dilation of the aortic root (AO). DAO, descending thoracic aorta; LV, left ventricle.

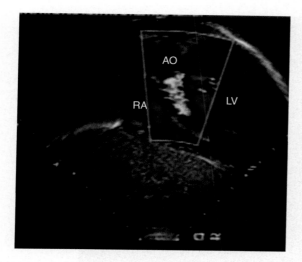

Figure 38–5. Three-year-old with a TGF-β mutation; subcostal long-axis imaging of moderate aortic regurgitation. AO, aortic root; LV, left ventricle; RA, right atrium.

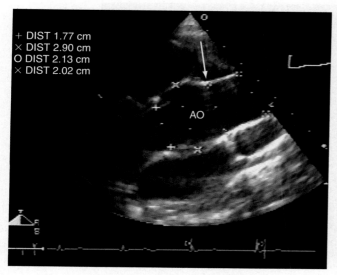

Figure 38–6. Parasternal long-axis view demonstrating dilation of the aortic root (AO) resulting in effacement of the sinotubular junction (arrow).

degeneration, and aortic dissection. Pseudoaneurysms are often the result of trauma or infection (e.g., endocarditis). Sinus of Valsalva aneurysm is associated with a number of secondary phenomena. The expansion of the aneurysm typically takes the path of least resistance into the right-sided heart structures. Affected sites can include aortic valve leaflet distortion and aortic regurgitation (AR), coronary artery occlusion, right ventricular outflow tract (RVOT) obstruction, tricuspid regurgitation (TR), obstruction of the right PA,

and descending aortic obstruction.[42,43] By using two-dimensional (2D) echocardiography, the dilated sinus can be elucidated.

Aortic Dissection

Patients with acute aortic dissection require emergent assessment and therapy. Prompt diagnosis is crucial to differentiate these patients from those with worrisome symptoms as a result of more benign conditions. Mortality is estimated at approximately 1% per hour in the first 48 hours for those patients who survive to reach an acute care setting.[44] In addition to providing a diagnosis, the details of anatomy and physiology are vital to care. These include classification of the dissection, definition of the site of rupture, detection of extravasation, assessment of aortic regurgitation, and assessment of side-branch involvement.[45] TTE provides a rapid and readily accessible diagnostic tool and in many cases can answer all of the above questions. TTE is frequently diagnostic in the detection of proximal aortic root dissection by revealing a progressively enlarging aortic root. In addition, the presence of a dissecting hematoma is oftentimes identified.[46]

However often further imaging is required, and TEE serves as a valuable next-line imaging modality. In experienced hands, TEE should detect virtually all cases of descending aortic dissection. One large multicenter study reported a sensitivity and specificity of 99% and 98%, respectively, in the diagnosis of aortic dissection by transesophageal imaging.[47] Combining 2D, color and pulsed Doppler modalities during the transesophageal study should allow for the detection of sites of communication between true and false lumen, site of rupture, presence of hematoma, presence of valve involvement, and the identification of aortic ulceration. Merging transesophageal data with that obtained via transthoracic imaging of the transverse arch should allow for complete delineation of the thoracic aorta. Sinus of Valsalva dissection can be accompanied by rupture of an aneurysm into adjoining cardiac structures.[48] Pulsed and color Doppler interrogation can detect the associated findings that occur in this situation. A complete discussion of aortic dissection can be found in Chapter 33.

Other Aortic Arch Manifestations

In addition to the natural history of aortic dilation and dissection that occurs in a subset of patients with connective tissue disorders, pathologic dilation can occur after aortic root surgery. In a study of patients with Marfan syndrome, a retrospective analysis was performed based on presence or absence of prior elective aortic root surgery.[49] Multivariate analysis showed that a previous elective aortic root surgery was associ-

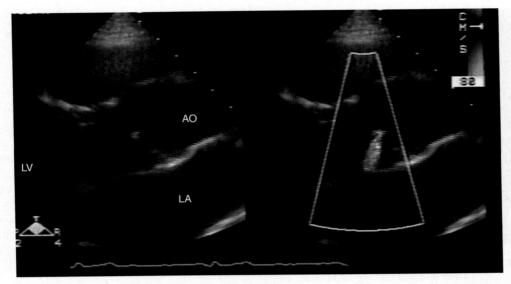

Figure 38–7. Parasternal long-axis view (color compare) *demonstrating mild aortic regurgitation with an eccentric jet directed towards the mitral valve anterior leaflet. AO, aortic root; LA, left atrium; LV, left ventricle.*

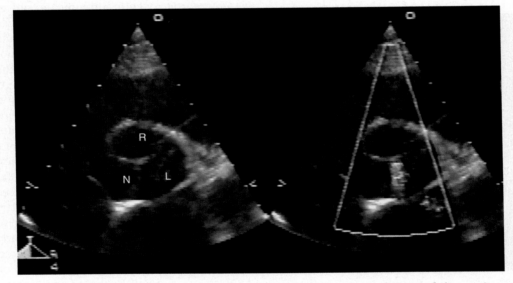

Figure 38–8. Parasternal short-axis view demonstration asymmetric dilation of the aortic root causing more pronounced dilation of the right aortic cusp (R) and a resultant jet of eccentric aortic insufficiency. L, left aortic cusp, N, noncoronary cusp.

ated with a fourfold increased risk of subsequent dilation of the descending aorta. In addition, an increased descending aortic diameter was associated with a higher risk of aortic root dissection, independent of the diameter of the aortic root itself. The authors raised a cautionary flag in that only 37% of their patient population had complete measurements obtained at all aortic levels, suggesting the possibility that a large number of patients with a dangerous degree of aortic dilation are going undetected even when imaging studies are performed.

The dogma has been that males with Marfan syndrome are at higher risk than females for the development of premature death as a result of aortic root dissection. A prospective evaluation of aortic root growth by serial echocardiography in 113 men and 108 women with Marfan syndrome demonstrated that at baseline, women had a 5-mm smaller aortic root diameter adjusted for age than men.[50] Average aortic root growth was similar in men and women. Men and women were divided into subgroups: fast and slow aortic root growers. One in seven men (1.5 mm/year) and one in nine women (1.8 mm/year) had fast-growing aortic root diameters. In both men and women, more aortic root dissections (25% versus 4%; $p < 0.001$) were observed in fast growers than in slow growers (four men versus nine women). The authors propose a reduction in the cut-off value for elective aortic root replacement in women by 5 mm, thus substantially reducing the development of aortic root dissections.

Mitral Valve Prolapse

MVP is defined as the displacement of abnormally thickened and redundant mitral valve leaflets into the left atrium during systole (Figs. 38–9 and 38–10). This geometric change in the integrity of the valve can result in poor coaptation and resultant mitral regurgitation (MR). MR will eventually lead to left atrial and subsequently left ventricular (LV) dilation, which in-and-of itself will worsen the degree of regurgitation. Echocardiography is the current gold standard for the diagnosis and evaluation of MVP. Echocardiographic criteria have been established for the detailed assessment of the mitral valve; MVP is now defined as displacement of one or both leaflets by greater than 2 mm above the mitral annulus in the parasternal long-axis or apical long-axis view. It is optimal to diagnose MVP only from the parasternal views, with apical imaging providing only confirmatory information. MVP is further divided into classic and nonclassic forms: classic is defined as leaflet thickness greater than 5 mm; in the nonclassic form the leaflets are less than 5 mm. Complications of endocarditis or the development of severe MR are more typically seen in the classic form of the disease.[51] The connective tissue disorders are more commonly associated with redundancy of the mitral valve leaflets resulting in MVP. This is in distinction to MVP in the adult population caused by calcific disease in which the leaflets are less redundant but more thickened.

Evaluation of the valve has been greatly enhanced since the introduction of three-dimensional (3D) imaging. Although MVP is typically sporadic, it is also associated with disorders of connective tissues including Marfan syndrome, Ehlers-Danlos syndrome, osteogenesis imperfecta, and the MASS phenotype (defined earlier). As the association of Marfan syndrome and MVP is common, the suspicion arose that isolated MVP might be the result of a mutation of *FBN1*.[52] However this association has never been established.

MVP is the most prevalent valve abnormality in Marfan syndrome with a reported prevalence of greater than 35%.[53] It is important to recognize that surgical repair of MR can exacerbate aortic dilation postoperatively as a result of the increased hemodynamic stresses on the aorta.

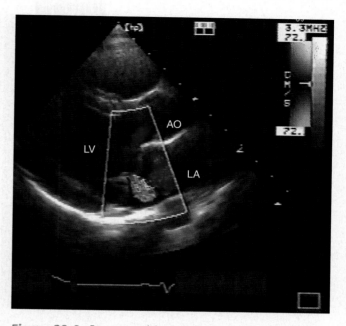

Figure 38–9. *Parasternal long-axis view of the mitral valve during systole demonstrating redundant chordae, buckling of the anterior and posterior mitral valve leaflets, and resultant mitral valve prolapse and mitral regurgitation. The mitral valve leaflets are displaced in a postero-superior direction into the left atrium (LA). AO, aortic root; LV, left ventricle.*

Bicuspid Aortic Valve

Familial recurrence of a bicuspid aortic valve has been well described, validating the inherited basis of this condition.[54,55] Patients with a bicuspid aortic valve are at increased risk of aortic aneurysm and dissection (Fig. 38–11). This appears to be secondary to pathologic changes in the aortic wall including cystic medial necrosis, loss of elastic fibers, increased apoptosis, and altered smooth muscle cell alignment.[56] Patients with a bicuspid valve have larger aortic root dimensions and an increased rate of aortic dilation over time (Fig. 38–12). Up to 15% of aortic dissections may occur in individuals with a bicuspid aortic valve.[57] The term *poststenotic dilation* was previously used as a hemodynamic explanation for the finding of aortic root dilation in the presence of a bicuspid aortic valve. However, it is now understood that this relationship is in fact the result of aortic pathology, which is independent of the aortic valve disease itself.[58,59] The increased risk of aortic dissection in patients with a bicuspid valve is limited to a small group of the overall population of patients with a bicuspid valve.[60,61] Even after valve replacement, surgery for a bicuspid valve is a strong risk factor for subsequent aortic dissection. It is probable that the concomitant finding of a bicuspid aortic valve and aortic aneurysm and dissection is a manifestation of what is the general class of systemic connective tissue disorders.[62]

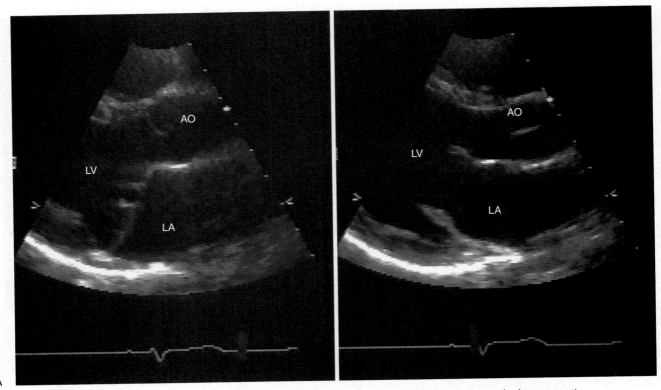

Figure 38–10. *A, Parasternal long-axis view of the mitral valve during end-systole demonstrating, buckling of the anterior and posterior mitral valve leaflets and resultant mitral valve prolapse. B, Parasternal long-axis view of the mitral valve at end-diastole demonstrating, thickening of the anterior and posterior mitral valve leaflet tips. AO, aortic root; LA, left atrium; LV, left ventricle.*

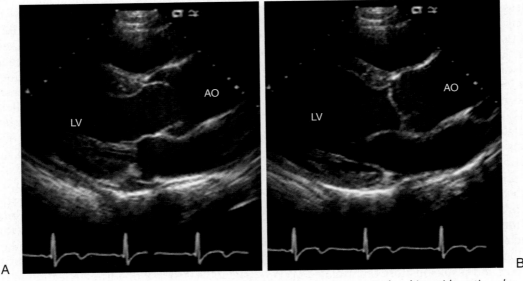

Figure 38–11. *A, Parasternal long-axis view during systole. Patient with a bicuspid aortic valve, doming of the aortic valve leaflets, effacement of the sinotubular junction, and dilation of the aortic root (AO). B, Parasternal long-axis view during diastole. Bicuspid aortic valve demonstrating eccentric valve leaflet closure and dilation of the sinus of Valsalva. LV, left ventricle.*

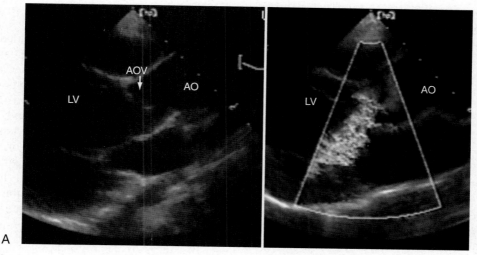

Figure 38–12. A, *Ten-year-old with Loeys-Dietz syndrome and severe aortic insufficiency secondary to a bicuspid aortic valve and severe aortic root dilation. Parasternal long-axis view of the thickened aortic valve leaflets (AOV), dilated left ventricle (LV), and aneurysm of the aortic root (AO).* B, *Parasternal long-axis view of the severe jet of aortic regurgitation resulting from the combined aortic valve and aortic root pathologic processes.*

Although multiple factors have been implicated in aortic dissection,[63] little is known of why or how a bicuspid aortic valve predisposes to aneurysm formation and dissection. In an attempt to address this question, Schaefer and colleagues[64] describe differences in aortic dimensions and elasticity between different phenotypes. Subjects with type 1 bicuspid aortic valve (anterior-posterior leaflet orientation with or without a raphe in the position demarcated by the left and right coronary cusps) have a larger dimension and increased wall stiffness at the sinuses of Valsalva (Fig. 38–13) than those with type 2 bicuspid aortic valve (right-left leaflet orientation with or without a raphe in the position demarcated by the right coronary and noncoronary cusps). The mechanism for these differences may be that the composition and elastic properties of the aortic wall are genetically related to aortic valve morphology. Hemodynamic differences may also contribute, with genetic upregulation altered by flow and force exerted on the aortic wall dependent on aortic valve morphology.

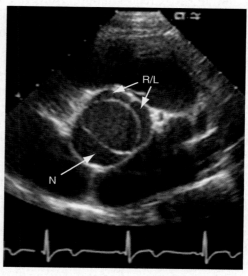

Figure 38–13. Parasternal short-axis view of a patient with a dilated aortic root and associated bicuspid aortic valve. The valve pathology is the result of fusion of the left (L) and right (R) coronary cusps. A raphe is noted between the left and right cusps. N, noncoronary cusp.

Left Ventricle

Although aortic arch and mitral valve disease are most commonly seen in the presence of connective tissue disorders, abnormalities of LV systolic and diastolic function are beginning to be elucidated.

Diastolic Function. Using both cardiac MRI and echocardiography, LV diastolic function has been evaluated in a number of small studies. Impaired LV diastolic function has been demonstrated with echocardiographic identification of an increase in deceleration time (DT) and an increase in isovolumic relaxation time (IVRT); these findings were attributed to impaired elastic recoil.[65] An unusual pattern of transmitral flow in which decreased ventricular compliance (decreased deceleration time) and reduced myocardial relaxation both occur.[66] Using tissue Doppler, a prolongation of the early filling phase with reduced velocities at the mitral annulus (Ea) has been demonstrated; this would suggest that myocardial tissue relaxation is impaired.[67]

Echocardiographic data obtained in children as young as 3 years of age with Marfan syndrome demonstrate early LV diastolic function (relaxation) impairment.[65] More recently, in a study of 40 children and young adults with Marfan syndrome, when compared to normal age-matched controls echocardiographic indices of LV diastolic function (including prolonged deceleration time and isovolumic relaxation time, and decreased mitral E/A ratio) also suggested impaired relaxation.[68] The presence early in life of increased myocardial stiffness, followed later in life by the development of aortic wall stiffness as the aorta distends,[69] may together contribute to the development of LV systolic and diastolic dysfunction.

Systolic Function. Reduced systolic contractility in Marfan syndrome has been thought to be solely a secondary phenomenon as a result associated aortic and/or mitral valve regurgitation. However, it has been suggested that in the absence of valvular heart disease subtle findings would suggest that LV systolic contractility is adversely affected. A small series from the Mayo clinic demonstrated no significant deterioration in ejection fraction (EF), LV end-systolic, end-diastolic dimensions; in addition this study followed these parameters serially over a 10-year period without obvious changes developing longitudinally.[70] However, these findings differed from a more recent large-scale study of 234 adults with Marfan syndrome. Although none of the patients met criteria for dilated cardiomyopathy (DCM), a small subset of the patients did show increased LV end-systolic and end-diastolic dimensions, with an associated mild deterioration in ejection fraction.[71] In additional meridional wall stress was similar between patients and controls suggesting that as opposed to an alteration in afterload causing LV impairment, more likely the observed differences were the result of primary LV contractile dysfunction.

The pathogenesis of LV systolic and diastolic dysfunction in patients with Marfan syndrome is incompletely understood but is likely the result of the primary structural and functional disorder in the *FBN1* protein. Microfibrils, which act as scaffolding for the formation of elastic fibers and contribute to their function, play an important role in mediating elastic recoil. These microfibrils contain the protein *FBN1* as one of their primary components. In that mutations in *FBN1* interfere with microfibril function, this in turn would be predicted to lead to impairment of LV diastolic elastic recoil.

Pulmonary Artery

As opposed to the well-defined left-sided heart pathology, abnormalities of the right-sided heart are less well recognized. Dilation of the main PA does occur, and serial echocardiographic measurements should be obtained. In the adult population, good correlation has been demonstrated between progressive dilation of the aortic root and main PA.[72] However, dangerous PA pathology as a result of PA aneurysm or dissection has not been reported, and the clinical significance of this finding requires further clarification. The population with associated pulmonary hypertension may be at risk given the expected abnormal increase in tensile stress thus placed on the PA.

Natural History

The majority of patients with Marfan syndrome present with ascending aortic dilation or dissection. Rarely does a patient have a type B dissection of the descending thoracic aorta. However, there is evidence that identification of progressive descending aortic dilation will predict the eventual development of dissection in this region.[49] For this reason, even in the absence of significant ascending aortic dilation, recommendations have been made that serial assessment include careful monitoring of the entire aorta (from the level of the aortic valve to the abdominal aorta).

A distinct (and typically severe form) of Marfan syndrome can be seen early in life termed *infantile Marfan syndrome.* Multivalvular disease is common, most often resulting in MVP with associated marked MR and severe skeletal and pulmonary emphysematous changes. Congestive heart failure (CHF) and respiratory compromise often lead to early demise.[73]

The pregnant woman with Marfan syndrome is at increased risk for aortic dissection, although the risk is low when the aorta is less than 4 cm.[74] Echocardiograms should be performed serially throughout the pregnancy, especially during the third trimester when growth acceleration can occur.

In general, TTE assessment is performed annually in patients with mild to moderate aortic dilation so long as these findings have been stable. In young children and in those who have severe disease, echocardiograms typically are performed on a 6-month basis. Conversely, individuals without aortic dilation but with other features suggestive of a connective tissue disorder or a strong family history, echocardiograms are generally performed every few years until adulthood. In patients who manifest rapidly progressive disease and are thus approaching criteria for surgical intervention, reevaluation at a minimum of every 6 months is recommended. Rapid progres-

TABLE 38–3. Summary of Clinical and Echocardiographic Findings for the Most Common Forms of Connective Tissue Disorders

	Affected Cardiac Structures	Characteristic Findings	Functional Sequelae	Prevalence
Marfan	MV Aortic root Ascending aorta	MVP TV prolapse Dilation of the aortic root	Mitral regurgitation Aortic regurgitation Susceptibility to dissecting aortic aneurysm	3:10,000
Ehlers-Danlos Type IV	Aortic root Large and small arteries	Large and small arterial aneurysm Arteriovenous fistulae	Aortic regurgitation Susceptibility to dissecting aortic aneurysm Dissection often spontaneous	≈1:250,000
Bicuspid aortic valve	Aortic valve Ascending aorta	Aortic valve dysfunction Dilation of the ascending aorta	Aortic regurgitation Aortic stenosis Ascending aortic dissection	≈1:100
TGF-β mutations	Aortic arch	Arterial tortuosity	Aortic dissection (possibly at a smaller aortic diameter than Marfan syndrome)	Unknown
TAAD	Thoracic aorta	Dilation of the aortic root Aneurysm of the thoracic aorta	Ascending aortic dissection Descending thoracic aortic dissection	Unknown: Aortic aneurysms result in 15,000 U.S. deaths per year

MV, mitral valve; MVP, mitral valve prolapse; TAAD, thoracic aortic aneurysm and dissection; TGF, transforming growth factor; TV, tricuspid valve.

sion generally is defined as growth approaching 5 mm every 6 months. Table 38–3 summarizes the clinical cardiac and echocardiographic features found in the most common connective tissue disorders. In addition, the prevalence of these connective tissue conditions in the general population is reviewed.

Methods of Assessment

Standard 2D echocardiography remains the screening tool for the assessment of valve morphology and for the measurement of aortic dimensions. The precision of this assessment is operator dependent and is also mitigated by image quality (primarily due to issues of patient body habitus). Oblique measurements of the aorta can overestimate actual dimensions as will occur for an aortic diameter that is not drawn perpendicular to the aortic flow center line. These measurements are typically acquired from the parasternal long-axis view, the long axis of the suprasternal notch, and the subcostal plane. Some labs will measure the sinus of Valsalva using M-mode. Although this can provide reproducible and accurate measurement data, we typically make all measurements from 2D echocardiography with data

acquired at early systole. The aortic valve annulus, sinus of Valsalva, and sinotubular junction (and the proximal aspect of the ascending aorta) are obtained from the parasternal long-axis view (Fig. 38–14). The distal ascending aorta (just before the takeoff of the innominate artery), the transverse aortic arch, the aortic isthmus are measured from the suprasternal notch (Fig. 38–15). In some individuals, the proximal descending aorta can be imaged from the parasternal window. In the pediatric population it is common to obtain suitable images to visualize the distal thoracic aorta and abdominal aorta from the subcostal imaging plane (Figs. 38–16 and 38–17). There should be a consistent attempt to obtain images and make measurements of each of these areas in every patient who comes through the echocardiography laboratory.

Imaging of the valves can be enhanced by the acquisition of 3D data. With the availability of live 3D, one can now obtain valve structure and function information in such a manner that immediate decisions can be made regarding the nature of the pathologic process. In addition, live 3D color Doppler can now be achieving with some systems, and this further enhances are understanding of valve pathophysiology. Although 3D can

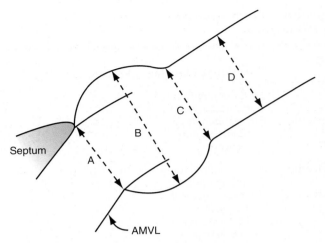

Figure 38–14. Schematic representation of the aortic root from the echocardiographic parasternal long-axis view demonstrating the aortic valve annulus (A), sinus of Valsalva (B), sinotubular junction (C), and proximal ascending aorta (D). Measurements are obtained at early systole.

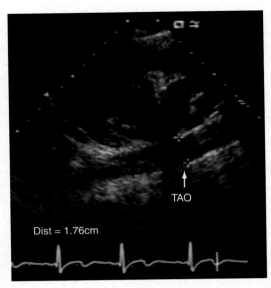

Figure 38–16. Subcostal long-axis image demonstrating the preferred location at which to measure the distal descending thoracic aorta (TAO). Dist, distance.

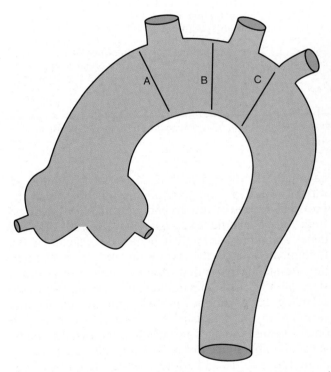

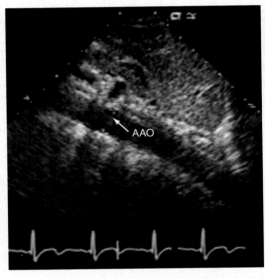

Figure 38–17. Subcostal long-axis image demonstrating the preferred location at which to measure the abdominal aorta (AAO) inferior to the diaphragm.

Figure 38–15. Schematic representation of the suprasternal long-axis imaging plane. From this echocardiographic view measurements are obtained of the distal ascending aorta (A) just before the innominate artery, transverse arch (B), between the innominate artery and the left carotid artery, and the aortic isthmus (C) just before the left subclavian artery.

also be used for the acquisition of aortic arch images, this requires unique operator skills. Therefore many labs obtain valve data by 3D on a relatively frequent basis, but acquisition of 3D volume rendered images of the aortic arch is less common.

Normalization of aortic measurements is an important aspect surrounding accurate data interpretation. Dependence on the accuracy of these normalized data is particularly acute in the pediatric population, in which rapid changes occur during growth. Because of the prognostic significance of aortic measurements in patients with connective tissue disorders, aortic dimensions have been extensively studied with 2D echocardiography. Normal values have been reported for children and adults based on a range of indices including age, body surface area (BSA), and height.[75-80]

In a study of 52 normal infants and children (aged 1 month to 15 years) and 135 normal adults (aged 20 to 74 years), the aorta was measured at end-diastole in the parasternal long-axis view at four levels: aortic annulus, sinus of Valsalva, sinotubular junction, and proximal ascending aorta at its maximal dimension. Of note, in this study 2D measurements at the sinus of Valsalva were larger than those obtained by M-mode. These larger 2D values, normalized using M-mode nomograms, falsely diagnosed aortic dilation in 40% of normal children and adults.[77]

Rigorous decisions are critical regarding which set of data will be used as the standard in any individual echocardiography laboratory. Once a published data set has been agreed on and implemented, all subsequent patient studies should be normalized using the same criteria. In the situation in which patients are plotted against differing normal data sets, wide variation in divergence from the norm can occur. As opposed to the use of published data sets, some groups have relied upon either internally derived normal controls or unpublished data obtained from large institutional studies.[81]

The pediatric patient with marked aortic dilation often presents a difficult clinical dilemma. Although the aorta may be 50% to 75% larger than predicted when normalized for body surface area, little data is available to assign a definitive risk for the short-term development of aortic dissection. Medical centers approach this problem in different ways, with no universally accepted algorithm. In an attempt to better predict pediatric risk for aortic dissection, noninvasive assessment of aortic wall dysfunction has been undertaken. In 19 pediatric patients with Marfan syndrome, transthoracic M-mode tracings were used to calculate aortic elastic properties.[82] Significant differences from control patients were seen; patients with Marfan syndrome demonstrated decreased aortic distensibility, increased aortic wall stiffness indices, decreased systolic diameter increase, and decreased maximum systolic area increase. Although this study did not attempt to predict future risk, further work of this type may allow use to provide better prognostic data for the pediatric population with connective tissue disorders.

Limitations of Assessment

Although transthoracic 2D and M-mode assessment are the most common methods of assessing the mitral valve and aorta in patients with connective tissue disorders, there are a number of limitations associated with these methods. Data acquisition is equipment and operator dependent. Measurements of aortic dimensions are affected by patient body habitus, and significant overestimation can be introduced into these measurements if oblique measurements are obtained.

TEE is a value tool in assessing the aorta in those patients with difficult transthoracic acoustic images. In addition to the routine use as a tool to obtain accurate measurements of the aortic root, TEE can also be used to evaluate properties of aortic distensibility. Measurement of aortic distensibility, stiffness index, and pulsed-wave velocity can be obtained using M-mode data from the transesophageal short-axis view. Tissue Doppler imaging (TDI) has been applied to the evaluation of thoracic aortic elasticity in patients with Marfan syndrome. Acceleration time, maximum wall expansion velocity, and wall strain were calculated from tissue Doppler imaging tracings in 31 patients with Marfan syndrome. Data derived from transesophageal imaging found that tissue Doppler imaging data was complementary to M-mode, together serving as a significant predictor of progressive aortic dilation and eventual dissection.[83]

Therapeutic Strategies

Pharmacologic

For the past 2 decades, the standard of care in the treatment of patients with Marfan syndrome with associated aortic dilation has been beta-adrenergic blockade. The validation for this approach is based on data on longitudinal follow-up data assessing the progression of aortic dilation with and without beta-blocker therapy demonstrating a beneficial response in a subset of these patients.[84] Treated patients showed slower aortic root growth, less risk of the development of aortic dissection, less common need for aortic surgery, and less mortality. This therapeutic strategy has been demonstrated in adults and children.[85] Although therapy does not necessarily result in avoidance of aortic surgery altogether, in general surgical intervention is forestalled. In addition, the presence of significant aortic dilation has been shown to be less amenable to beta-blocker therapy than is the case for the earlier treatment of the patient with milder aortic dilation.[84] Some studies have demonstrated improved ascending aortic stiffness associated with beta-blocker therapy in patients with Marfan syndrome,[86,87] whereas others have shown no effect or worsening of indices of aortic stiffness.[88] The initiation of beta-blocker therapy is typically based on a confirmed clinical diagnosis of Marfan syndrome (based upon the modified Ghent criteria) and the attainment of quantitative aortic root dilation. This is generally defined as the presence of aortic root dimensions as measured by echocardiography or MRI greater than 2 z-scores from the mean for body surface area. (Z-score is equivalent to standard deviation.)

In patients intolerant of beta-blocker therapy, either because of associated reactive airways disease or other side effects (e.g., fatigue or dizziness secondary to hypotension), other pharmacologic strategies have been employed to delay progressive aortic dilation. These include calcium channel blockers[85] and angiotensin-converting enzyme (ACE) inhibitors. In a 3-year longitudinal study of patients with Marfan syndrome, comparing therapy with beta-blockers versus ACE inhibitors, patients treated with the later were shown to have less aortic dilation.[89] In addition, using echocardiographic measurements both aortic stiffness index and aortic distensibility improved with ACE inhibitor therapy.

Recent data has suggested a role for the angiotensin-1 receptor antagonist, losartan. Studies have shown that myxomatous mitral valve disease, aortic dilation, and impaired pulmonary alveolar septation, all features of the murine model of Marfan syndrome are mediated by excessive TGF-β signaling. It has been hypothesized that losartan may delay aortic dilation as a result of its effect in inhibiting TGF-β signaling in the aortic wall. Treatment with losartan in a mouse model of Marfan syndrome that carries a *FBN1* mutation demonstrated histological improvement in aortic wall elastic matrix architecture. In addition, there was echocardiographic evidence of reduced aortic growth in the losartan-treated group.[90] This therapy suggests an exciting new line of investigation in that it employs a strategy, which is directed at disease pathogenesis, and may be the first step toward actual disease prevention.

Surgical

In adults with Marfan syndrome or one of the other connective tissue disorders, the threshold for consideration of aortic root replacement occurs when the diameter reaches 5 cm.[91,92] A clearly established risk exists when the aortic dimension exceeds 6 cm, with a four-fold increase in the cumulative risk of aortic dissection or rupture.[91] Factors that are used to modify these parameters downward include rapid aortic growth (>1 cm per year), a family history of premature aortic dissection (at <5 cm) and the associated finding of moderate or severe aortic regurgitation (AR). However some patients (even in the absence of factors which would place them at higher risk) develop aortic dissection at a diameter less than 5 cm.[92] For this reason, patient education regarding the symptoms of aortic dissection is crucial.

In the younger pediatric population with Marfan syndrome (before adolescence), it is relatively uncommon to identify aortic pathology of such severity that surgical intervention must be considered. However when this situation does exist, decisions surrounding timing of aortic surgery are complicated by the lack of adequate data to predict when the risk of aortic dissection has reached unacceptable levels. At my institution, the preadolescent child with a connective tissue disorder would be a candidate for surgery under the following conditions:

1. Maximum normalized aortic dimension greater than 8 to 10 standard deviations above the mean for body surface area

2. Accelerating aortic growth (>5 mm per 6 months)
3. Family history of aortic dissection
4. Additional pathologic lesion requiring intervention (i.e., aortic regurgitation, MR secondary to MVP)

The actual decision to procedure with aortic surgery in the pediatric population is frequently based on less well-defined theoretical concerns. Oftentimes a maximum aortic dimension greater than 8 to 10 standard deviations from the mean (as listed previously) is accepted.

Surgical intervention for aortic dilation typically takes the form of either a composite graft and associated valve replacement (Bentall technique)[93] or procedures performed when the aortic valve remains competent and therefore the valve is "spared."[94,95] The results of aortic replacement in adults are encouraging. In a report by Gott and colleagues[92] on 675 Marfan patients who underwent aortic replacement, a 1.5% operative mortality was seen in elective cases as compared to 11.7% for emergency surgeries. Five-year and ten-year survival was 84% and 75%, respectively.

Although the success of aortic surgery has improved dramatically, postoperative complications remain. Pseudoaneurysm at the graft site or graft dehiscence is frequently difficult to detect by transthoracic imaging. In these situations TEE has been clearly demonstrated to provide additional diagnostic data.[96,97]

Alternate Diagnostic Approaches

MRI and cardiac CT can be used in patients who have limited acoustic images or require detailed assessment in the situation in which ambiguous data is present. This might include the patient with unusual tortuosity of the aortic arch, the question of dilation extending into the carotid arteries or circle of Willis or when an aortic dissection cannot be entirely excluded. However, it must be kept in mind that just as is the case with echocardiographic assessment, the accuracy of CT and MRI evaluation are reliant on availability of appropriate equipment and are operator dependent.

Advances in MRI have allowed for the evaluation of aortic elasticity in patients with Marfan syndrome. The elasticity of the aorta has been found to be reduced in these patients. MRI velocity mapping of the aorta demonstrates reduced aortic distensibility during systole and increased pulse wave propagation.[98] Use of MRI velocity encoding demonstrates a positive response to beta-blocker therapy with a reduction in pulsed-wave propagation after beta-blocker treatment. These techniques not only yield important information regarding the biophysical properties of the aorta in patients with connective tissue disorders but may also provide data in order to predict individual patient risk.[98]

KEY POINTS

■ A variety of disorders can lead to connective tissue abnormalities, with many of these conditions manifesting similar cardiac features of aortic dilation and dissection, and MVP.

■ Although Marfan syndrome remains a clinical diagnosis, primarily based on defined cardiac, skeletal, ocular findings, refinement in genetic testing has improved diagnostic rates to close to 90%.

■ In addition to the well-described fibrillin mutations associated with connective tissue disease, the role of TGF-β as a cause of these conditions is increasingly evident.

■ In connective tissue disorders, dilation of the aortic root is caused by degenerative changes of smooth muscle cells, elastic fibers, and collagen, resulting in cystic changes termed *cystic medial necrosis*.

■ Changes in mitral and aortic valve fibrous ring integrity, combined with dilation of the surrounding tissues causing alteration in valve geometry, result in the hemodynamic disturbances seen in the connective tissue disorders (predominantly regurgitation).

■ In virtually all children and most adults TTE is highly predictive of the pathologic changes in the mitral valve, aortic valve and aortic arch associated with the connective tissue disorders.

■ TEE and other imaging modalities (3D echocardiography, MRI, and CT) serve as adjunct modalities to diagnosis.

■ In addition to valve and large vessel disease, the connective tissue disorders may also affect systolic and diastolic LV function.

■ When surgical intervention is contemplated for a bicuspid aortic valve in children and young adults in which the aorta is dilated, careful consideration should be given to possible connective tissue conditions that might complicate the procedure and recuperation.

■ In the growing child and teen, quantitative assessment of the aortic arch must incorporate the use of a well-validated nomogram to ensure clear understanding of the severity of dilation and rate of growth.

REFERENCES

1. De Paepe A, Devereux RB, Dietz HC, et al: Revised diagnostic criteria for the Marfan syndrome. *Am J Med Genet* 62:417-426, 1996.
2. Gray JR, Bridges AB, Faed MJ, et al: Ascertainment and severity of Marfan syndrome in a Scottish population. *J Med Genet* 31:51-54, 1994.
3. Judge DP, Dietz HC: Marfin syndrome. *Lancet* 366:1965-1976, 2005.
4. Dietz H, Francke U, Furthmayr H, et al: The question of heterogeneity in Marfan syndrome. *Nat Genet* 9:228-231, 1995.
5. Schrijver I et al: Cysteine substitutions in epidermal growth factor-like domains of fibrillin-1: distinct effects on biochemical and clinical phenotypes. *Am J Hum Genet* 65(4):1007-1020, 1999.
6. Wang M, Price C, Han J, et al: Recurrent mis-splicing of fibrillin exon 32 in two patients with neonatal Marfan syndrome. *Hum Mol Genet* 4:607-613, 1995.
7. Dietz HC, Pyeritz RE: Mutations in the human gene for fibrillin-1 (FBN1) in the Marfan syndrome and related disorders. *Hum Mol Genet* 4:1799-1809, 1995.
8. Nijbroek G, Sood S, McIntosh I, et al: Fifteen novel FBN1 mutations causing Marfan syndrome detected by heteroduplex analysis of genomic amplicons. *Am J Hum Genet* 57:8-21, 1995.
9. Milewicz DM, Grossfield J, Cao SN, et al: A mutation in FBN1 disrupts profibrillin processing and results in isolated skeletal features of the Marfan syndrome. *J Clin Invest* 95:2373-2378, 1995.
10. Palz M, Tiecke F, Booms P, et al: Clustering of mutations associated with mild Marfan-like phenotypes in the 3' region of FBN1 suggests a potential genotype-phenotype correlation. *Am J Med Genet* 91:212-221, 2000.
11. Guo D, Hasham S, Kuang SQ, et al: Familial thoracic aortic aneurysms and dissections: genetic heterogeneity with a major locus mapping to 5q13-14. *Circulation* 103:2461-2468, 2001.
12. Giusti B, Porciani MC, Brunelli T, et al: Phenotypic variability of cardiovascular manifestations in Marfan syndrome. Possible role of hyperhomocysteinemia and C677T MTHFR gene polymorphism. *Eur Heart J* 24:2038-2045, 2003.
13. Leier CV, Call TD, Fulkerson PK, Wooley CF: The spectrum of cardiac defects in the Ehlers-Danlos syndrome, types I and III. *Ann Intern Med* 92:171-178, 1980.
14. Pope FM, Kendall BE, Slapak GI, et al: Type III collagen mutations cause fragile cerebral arteries. *Br J Neurosurg* 5:551-574, 1991.
15. Bellenot F, Boisgard S, Kantelip B, et al: Type IV Ehlers-Danlos syndrome with isolated arterial involvement. *Ann Vasc Surg* 4:15-19, 1990.
16. North KN, Whiteman DA, Pepin MG, Byers PH: Cerebrovascular complications in Ehlers-Danlos syndrome type IV. *Ann Neurol* 38:960-964, 1995.
17. Emanuel BS, Cannizzaro LA, Seyer JM, Myers JC: Human alpha 1(III) and alpha 2(V) procollagen genes are located on the long arm of chromosome 2. *Proc Natl Acad Sci U S A* 82:3385-3389, 1985.
18. Mudd SH, Skovby F, Levy HL, et al: The natural history of homocystinuria due to cystathionine beta-synthase deficiency. *Am J Hum Genet* 37:1-31, 1985.
19. Gupta PA, Wallis DD, Chin TO, et al: FBN2 mutation associated with manifestations of Marfan syndrome and congenital contractural arachnodactyly. *J Med Genet* 41:e56, 2004.
20. Zhu L, Vranckx R, Khau Van Kien P, et al: Mutations in myosin heavy chain 11 cause a syndrome associating thoracic aortic aneurysm/aortic dissection and patent ductus arteriosus. *Nat Genet* 38:343-349, 2006.
21. Laurent S, Boutouyrie P, Lacolley P: Structural and genetic bases of arterial stiffness. *Hypertension* 45:1050-1055, 2005.
22. Boileau C, Jondeau G, Babron MC, et al: Autosomal dominant Marfan-like connective-tissue disorder with aortic dilation and skeletal anomalies not linked to the fibrillin genes. *Am J Hum Genet* 53:46-54, 1993.
23. Collod G, Babron MC, Jondeau G, et al: A second locus for Marfan syndrome maps to chromosome 3p24.2-p25. *Nat Genet* 8:264-268, 1994.
24. Mizuguchi T, Collod-Beroud G, Akiyama T, et al: Heterozygous TGFBR2 mutations in Marfan syndrome. *Nat Genet* 36:855-860, 2004.

25. Boileau C, Jondeau G, Mizuguhi T, Matsumoto N: Molecular genetics of Marfan syndrome. *Curr Opin Cardiol* 20:194-200, 2005.

26. Loeys BL, Chen J, Neptune ER, et al: A syndrome of altered cardiovascular, craniofacial, neurocognitive and skeletal development caused by mutations in TGFBR1 or TGFBR2. *Nat Genet* 37:275-281, 2005.

27. Singh KK, Rommel K, Mishra A, et al: TGFBR1 and TGFBR2 mutations in patients with features of Marfan syndrome and Loeys-Dietz syndrome. *Hum Mutat* 27:770-777, 2006.

28. Coady MA, Davies RR, Roberts M, et al: Familial patterns of thoracic aortic aneurysms. *Arch Surg* 134:361-367, 1999.

29. Hasham SN, Willing MC, Guo DC, et al: Mapping a locus for familial thoracic aortic aneurysms and dissections (TAAD2) to 3p24-25. *Circulation* 107:3184-3190, 2003.

30. Vaughan CJ, Casey M, He J, et al: Identification of a chromosome 11q23.2-q24 locus for familial aortic aneurysm disease, a genetically heterogeneous disorder. *Circulation* 103:2469-2475, 2001.

31. Gilchrist DM: Marfan syndrome or Marfan-like connective-tissue disorder. *Am J Hum Genet* 54:553-554, 1994.

32. Pannu H, Fadulu VT, Chang J, et al: Mutations in transforming growth factor-β receptor type II cause familial thoracic aortic aneurysms and dissections. *Circulation* 112:513-520, 2005.

33. Roberts WC, Honig HS: The spectrum of cardiovascular disease in the Marfan syndrome: a clinico-morphologic study of 18 necropsy patients and comparison to 151 previously reported necropsy patients. *Am Heart J* 104:115-135, 1982.

34. McKusick VA: The cardiovascular aspects of Marfan's syndrome: a heritable disorder of connective tissue. *Circulation* 11:321-342, 1955.

35. Lin AE, Lippe B, Rosenfeld RG: Further delineation of aortic dilation, dissection, and rupture in patients with Turner syndrome. *Pediatrics* 102(1): e12,1998.

36. Pepin M, Schwarze U, Superti-Furga A, Byers PH: Clinical and genetic features of Ehlers-Danlos syndrome type IV, the vascular type. *N Engl J Med* 342:673-680, 2000.

37. Lindsay J Jr: Coarctation of the aorta, bicuspid aortic valve and abnormal ascending aortic wall. *Am J Cardiol* 61:182-184, 1988.

38. Niwa K, Perloff JK, Bhuta SM, et al: Structural abnormalities of great arterial walls in congenital heart disease: Light and electron microscopic analyses. *Circulation* 103:393-400, 2001.

39. Leier CV, Baker PB, Kilman JW, Wooley CF: Cardiovascular abnormalities associated with adult polycystic kidney disease. *Ann Intern Med* 100:683-688, 1984.

40. Schlatmann TJ, Becker AE: Histologic changes in the normal aging aorta: Implications for dissecting aortic aneurysm. *Am J Cardiol* 39:13-20, 1977.

41. Robicsek F, Thubrikar MJ: Hemodynamic considerations regarding the mechanism and prevention of aortic dissection. *Ann Thorac Surg* 58:1247-1253, 1994.

42. Engel PJ, Held JS, van der Bel-Kahn J, Spitz H: Echocardiographic diagnosis of congenital sinus of Valsalva aneurysm with dissection of the interventricular septum. *Circulation* 63:705-711, 1981.

43. Shaffer EM, Snider AR, Beekham RH, et al: Sinus of Valsalva aneurysm complicating bacterial endocarditis in an infant: diagnosis with two-dimensional and Doppler echocardiography. *J Am Coll Cardiol* 9:588-591, 1987.

44. Khan IA, Nair CK: Clinical, diagnostic, and management perspectives of aortic dissection. *Chest* 122:311-328, 2002.

45. Erbel R, Alfonso F, Boileau C, et al: Diagnosis and management of aortic dissection. *Eur Heart J* 22:1642-1681, 2001.

46. Granato JE, Dee P, Gibson RS: Utility of two-dimensional echocardiography in suspected ascending aortic dissection. *Am J Cardiol* 56:123-129, 1985.

47. Erbel R, Engberding R, Daniel W, et al: Echocardiography in diagnosis of aortic dissection. *Lancet* 1:457-461, 1989.

48. Yokoi K, Kambe T, Ichimaya S, et al: Ruptured aneurysm of the right sinus of Valsalva: Two pulsed Doppler echocardiographic studies. *J Clin Ultrasound* 9:505-510, 1981.

49. Engelfriet PM, Boersma E, Tijssen JG, et al: Beyond the root: Dilatation of the distal aorta in the Marfan syndrome. *Heart* 92(9):1238-1243, 2006.

50. Meijboom LJ, Timmermans J, Zwinderman AH, et al: Aortic root growth in men and women with the Marfan's syndrome. *Am J Cardiol* 96:1441-1444, 2005.

51. Marks AR, Choong CY, Sanflippo AJ, et al: Identification of high-risk and low-risk subgroups of patients with mitral-valve prolapse. *N Engl J Med* 320:1031-1036, 1989.

52. Dietz HC, Cutting GR, Pyeritz RE, et al: Marfan syndrome caused by a recurrent de novo missense mutation in the fibrillin gene. *Nature* 352:337-339, 1991.

53. van Karnebeek CD, Naeff MS, Mulder BJ, et al: Natural history of cardiovascular manifestations in Marfan syndrome. *Arch Dis Child* 84:129-137, 2001.

54. Huntington K, Hunter AG, Chan KL: A prospective study to assess the frequency of familial clustering of congenital bicuspid aortic valve. *J Am Coll Cardiol* 30:1809-1812, 1997.

55. Clementi M, Notari L, Borghi A, Tenconi R: Familial congenital bicuspid aortic valve: a disorder of uncertain inheritance. *Am J Med Genet* 62:336-338, 1996.

56. Fedak PW, Verma S, Weisel RD, et al: Clinical and pathophysiological implications of a bicuspid aortic valve. *Circulation* 106:900-904, 2002.

57. Ward C: Clinical significance of the bicuspid aortic valve. *Heart* 83:81-85, 2000.

58. Keane MG, et al: Bicuspid aortic valves are associated with aortic dilatation out of proportion to coexistent valvular lesions. *Circulation* 102:III35-III39, 2000.

59. Ferencik M, Pape LA: Changes in size of ascending aorta and aortic valve function with time in patients with congenitally bicuspid aortic valves. *Am J Cardiol* 92:43-46, 2003.

60. Roberts CS, Roberts WC: Dissection of the aorta associated with congenital malformation of the aortic valve. *J Am Coll Cardiol* 17:712-716, 1991.

61. Nistri S, Sorbo MD, Marin M, et al: Aortic root dilatation in young men with normally functioning bicuspid aortic valves. *Heart* 82:19-22, 1999.

62. Lewin MB, Otto CM: The bicuspid aortic valve: adverse outcomes from infancy to old age. *Circulation* 111:832-844, 2005.

63. Nienaber CA, Eagle KA: Aortic dissection: new frontiers in diagnosis and management: Part I: from etiology to diagnostic strategies. *Circulation* 108:628-635, 2003.

64. Schaefer BM, Lewin MB, Stout KK, Byers PH, Otto CM: Usefulness of bicuspid aortic valve phenotype to predict elastic properties of the ascending aorta. *Am J Cardiol* 99:686-690, 2007.

65. Savolainen A, Nisula L, Keto P, et al: Left ventricular function in children with the Marfan syndrome. *Eur Heart J* 15:625-630, 1994.

66. Porciani MC, Giurlani L, Chelucci A, et al: Diastolic subclinical primary alterations in Marfan syndrome and Marfan-related disorders. *Clin Cardiol* 25:416-420, 2002.

67. De Backer JF, Devos D, Segers P, et al: Primary impairment of left ventricular function in Marfan syndrome. *Int J Cardiol* 112:353-358, 2005.

68. Das BB, Taylor AL, Yetman AT: Left ventricular diastolic dysfunction in children and young adults with Marfan syndrome. *Pediatr Cardiol* 27:256-258, 2006.

69. Hirata K, Triposkiadis F, Sparks E, et al: The Marfan syndrome: Abnormal aortic elastic properties. *J Am Coll Cardiol* 18:57-63, 1991.

70. Chatrath R, Beauschesne LM, Connolly HM, et al: Left ventricular function in the Marfan syndrome without significant valvular regurgitation. *Am J Cardiol* 91:914-916, 2003.

71. Meijboom LJ, Timmermans J, van Tintelen JP, et al: Evaluation of left ventricular dimensions and function in Marfan's syndrome without significant valvular regurgitation. *Am J Cardiol* 95:795-797, 2005.

72. Nollen GJ, van Schijndel KE, Timmermans J, et al: Pulmonary artery root dilatation in Marfan syndrome: quantitative assessment of an unknown criterion. *Heart* 87:470-471, 2002.

73. Gross DM, Robinson LK, Smith LT, et al: Severe perinatal Marfan syndrome. *Pediatrics* 84:83-99, 1989.

74. Lind J, Wallenburg HC: The Marfan syndrome and pregnancy: a retrospective study in a Dutch population. *Eur J Obstet Gynecol Reprod Biol* 98:28-35, 2001.

75. Tacy TA, Vermilion RP, Ludomirsky A: Range of normal valve annulus size in neonates. *Am J Cardiol* 75:541-543, 1995.

76. Roge CL, Silverman NH, Hart PA, Ray RM: Cardiac structure growth pattern determined by echocardiography. *Circulation* 57:285-290, 1978.

77. Roman MJ, Devereux RB, Kramer-Fox R, O'Loughlin J: Two-dimensional echocardiographic aortic root dimensions in normal children and adults. *Am J Cardiol* 64:507-512, 1989.

78. Nidorf SM, Picard MH, Triulzi MO, et al: New perspectives in the assessment of cardiac chamber dimensions during development and adulthood. *J Am Coll Cardiol* 19:983-988, 1992.

79. Sheil ML, Jenkins O, Sholler GF: Echocardiographic assessment of aortic root dimensions in normal children based on measurement of a new ratio of aortic size independent of growth. *Am J Cardiol* 75:711-715, 1995.

80. Daubeney PE, Blackstone EH, Weintraub RG, et al: Relationship of the dimension of cardiac structures to body size: an echocardiographic study in normal infants and children. *Cardiol Young* 9:402-410, 1999.

81. Colan S: Normal echocardiographic values in infants and children (Boston Children's Hospital; unpublished data).

82. Baumgartner D, Baumgartner C, Matyas G, et al: Diagnostic power of aortic elastic properties in young patients with Marfan syndrome. *J Thorac Cardiovasc Surg* 129:730-739, 2005.

83. Vitarelli A, Conde Y, Cimino E, et al: Aortic wall mechanics in the Marfan syndrome assessed by transesophageal tissue Doppler echocardiography. *Am J Cardiol* 97:571-577, 2006.

84. Shores J, Berger KR, Murphy EA, Pyeritz RE: Progression of aortic dilatation and the benefit of long-term beta-adrenergic blockade in Marfan's syndrome. *N Engl J Med* 330:1335-1341, 1994.

85. Rossi-Foulkes R, Roman MJ, Rosen SE, et al: Phenotypic features and impact of beta blocker or calcium antagonist therapy on aortic lumen size in the Marfan syndrome. *Am J Cardiol* 83:1364-1368, 1999.

86. Groenink M, de Roos A, Mulder BJ, et al: Changes in aortic distensibility and pulse wave velocity assessed with magnetic resonance imaging following beta-blocker therapy in the Marfan syndrome. *Am J Cardiol* 82:203-208, 1998.

87. Yin FC, Brin KP, Ting CT, Pyeritz RE: Arterial hemodynamic indexes in Marfan's syndrome. *Circulation* 79:854-862, 1989.

88. Haouzi A, Berglund H, Pelikan PC, et al: Heterogeneous aortic response to acute beta-adrenergic blockade in Marfan syndrome. *Am Heart J* 133:60-63, 1997.

89. Yetman AT, Bornemeier RA, McCrindle BW: Usefulness of enalapril versus propranolol or atenolol for prevention of aortic dilation in patients with the Marfan syndrome. *Am J Cardiol* 95:1125-1127, 2005.

90. Habashi JP, Judge DP, Holm TM, et al: Losartan, an AT1 antagonist, prevents aortic aneurysm in a mouse model of Marfan syndrome. *Science* 312:117-121, 2006.

91. Davies RR, Goldstein LJ, Coady MA, et al: Yearly rupture or dissection rates for thoracic aortic aneurysms: simple prediction based on size. *Ann Thorac Surg* 73:17-27; discussion 27-28, 2002.

92. Gott VL, Greene PS, Alejo DE, et al: Replacement of the aortic root in patients with Marfan's syndrome. *N Engl J Med* 340:1307-1313, 1999.

93. Bentall H, De Bono A: A technique for complete replacement of the ascending aorta. *Thorax* 23:338-339, 1968.

94. Miller DC: Valve-sparing aortic root replacement in patients with the Marfan syndrome. *J Thorac Cardiovasc Surg* 125:773-778, 2003.

95. Sarsam MA, Yacoub M: Remodeling of the aortic valve anulus. *J Thorac Cardiovasc Surg* 105:435-438, 1993.

96. Yasuda H, Sakagoshi N, Lim YJ, Mishima M, et al: Pseudoaneurysm after Bentall operation diagnosed by transesophageal echocardiography. *Ann Thorac Surg* 78:1478, 2004.

97. Ballal RS, Gatewood RP, Nanda NC, et al: Usefulness of transesophageal echocardiography in the assessment of aortic graft dehiscence. *Am J Cardiol* 80:372-376, 1997.

98. Groenink M, de Roos A, Mulder BJ, et al: Biophysical properties of the normal-sized aorta in patients with Marfan syndrome: Evaluation with MR flow mapping. *Radiology* 219:535-540, 2001.

Chapter 39

Aging Changes Seen on Echocardiography

MICHAEL A. CHEN, MD, PhD

Background and Importance

By 2030, in the United States, an estimated 71.5 million people will be age 65 or older (35 million in 2000), with 9.6 million of them over the age of 85 (4.2 million in 2000).[1] Cardiovascular disease is the leading cause of death and disability, and advanced age is a major risk factor. Normal aging results in pervasive changes in cardiovascular structure and function and alterations in other organ systems. Many normal age-related changes in cardiovascular structure and function are readily identifiable on echocardiography. This is also true of conditions that are pathologic but common in the elderly.

Basic Principles and Echocardiographic Approach

The echocardiographic techniques used to acquire images and other data are the same for the elderly as for younger people.

Normal Changes in Cardiac Structure

Left Ventricular Wall Thickness and Chamber Dimensions

Multiple studies have demonstrated increases in left ventricular (LV) wall thickness with age in patients without a history of hypertension, valvular or other cardiovascular disease[2-5] (Fig. 39-1). These cross-sectional studies involved from 53 to 136 normal healthy subjects, and documented mild increases in LV wall thickness. For example, in a study by Gardin and colleagues, 136 adults (78 men and 58 women aged 20 to 97 years) without

The author acknowledges Kiran B. Sagar, MD, and Abraham C. Parail, MD, the previous authors of this chapter in *The Practice of Clinical Echocardiography*, second edition.

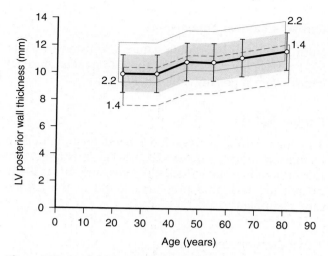

Figure 39–1. *Plot of left ventricular posterior wall thickness in late diastole in millimeters versus age in years. For each age group the mean (circle) and 95% prediction interval (blue shaded) for normal values are depicted for a body surface area (BSA) of 1.8 m². The 95% prediction intervals are also shown for subjects with BSA values of 1.4 m² (dashed lines) and 2.2 m² (solid lines). LV, left ventricular. (From Gardin JM, Henry WL, Savage DD, et al: J Clin Ultrasound 7:439-447, 1979. Copyright © 1979, John Wiley & Sons. Reprinted by permission of John Wiley & Sons, Inc.)*

evidence of cardiovascular disease were studied.[2] The patients were stratified into six age groups and significant increases in wall thickness with age were found. Comparing the youngest group (21 to 30 years), with the oldest group (>70 years), the mean septal wall thickness increased from 9.8 mm to 11.8 mm, and the mean posterior wall thickness increased from 10.1 mm to 11.8 mm. This represented increases of 20% and 18%, respectively.

Left Ventricular Mass

Based on data documenting increased wall thickness with increasing age, a number of prior echocardiographic studies have suggested that there is an age-related increase in LV mass (sometimes indexed for weight or height).[6,7] The formula for LV mass that is commonly used was derived by Devereux and colleagues.[8] The formula is as follows:

$$LV\ mass\ (g) = 0.80 \times 1.04([VST_d + LVID_d + PWT_d]^3 - [LVID_d]^3) = 0.6$$

in which VST_d is ventricular septal thickness at end-diastole, $LVID_d$ is LV internal dimension at end-diastole, and PWT_d is LV posterior wall thickness at end-diastole.

In contrast to these findings, a recent study (part of the Baltimore Longitudinal Study of Aging), which used volunteers without cardiovascular disease (136 men, 200 women), using magnetic resonance imaging (MRI) showed that wall thickness increased with age and short-axis diastolic dimension did not change with age (similar to prior echocardiographic data). On the other

hand, LV length declined in both sexes over time. The resulting estimate of LV mass revealed no age relationship in women, although there was an age-related decline in men (resulting from a smaller increase in wall thickness). This suggests that with time, the left ventricle becomes thicker and more spherical.[9]

The reason for the discrepancy in the findings between M-mode and two-dimensional (2D) echocardiographic data and magnetic resonance imaging data lies in the algorithms used to calculate LV mass in the former techniques. These algorithms, such as the formula derived by Devereux and colleagues,[8] assume an ellipsoid shaped cavity and do not take into account changes in cavity shape. Thus, the calculations will be less accurate with cavities that are, for example, more spherical. Three-dimensional (3D) echocardiography has been shown to be a more accurate technique than two-dimensional (2D) echocardiography in estimating LV mass in studies comparing the two techniques against weighing of the left ventricle in both human and animal studies.[10-12] 3D echocardiography derived LV mass estimates have also been shown to correlate well with those estimates derived from MRI.[13,14]

Aortic Root Diameter

There is a mild increase in the aortic root diameter seen with age (Fig. 39–2). There is an approximately 6% increase in a normal population between the fourth and eighth decades.[3] A study of serial chest X-rays (CXRs) taken over 17 years noted an increase from 3.4 to 3.8 cm.[15] This enlargement may present an extra stimulus to the left ventricle to hypertrophy because it represents a larger blood volume that must be pushed forward.

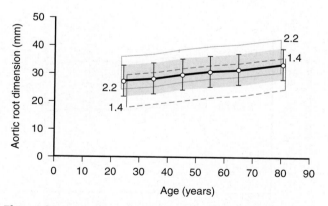

Figure 39–2. *Aortic root dimension in late diastole is plotted in millimeters versus age in years. The mean value for each age group is depicted by a circle plotted at the mean age in the age group. The bracket and shaded area on either side of the circle represents the interval for normal values for a subject with a body surface area of 1.8 m². The 95% prediction intervals are also shown for subjects with body surface area values of 1.4 m² (dashed lines) and 2.2 m² (solid lines). (From Gardin JM, Henry WL, Savage DD, et al: J Clin Ultrasound 7:439-447, 1979. Copyright © 1979, John Wiley & Sons. Reprinted by permission of John Wiley & Sons, Inc.)*

Left Atrial Size

There is a significant increase in size of the left atrium with age (Fig. 39–3).

Left Ventricular Dimensions

In the studies that have documented increases in LV wall thickness, measurements of LV end-diastolic and end-systolic dimensions showed either a slight decrease to no change with age[2,3,6] (Fig. 39–4 and Table 39–1). Because LV stroke volume (SV) is the difference of LV end-diastolic and end-systolic volumes, supine resting LV stroke volume is also assumed to be unrelated to age.

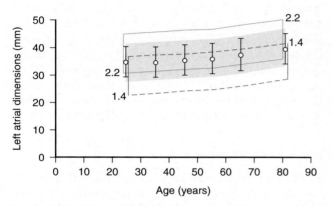

Figure 39–3. *Left atrial dimension in late diastole in millimeters versus age in years. For each age group the mean and 95% prediction intervals for normal values are depicted. The solid and dashed lines as per Figure 39–2. (From Gardin JM, Henry WL, Savage DD, et al: J Clin Ultrasound 7:439-447, 1979. Copyright © 1979, John Wiley & Sons. Reprinted by permission of John Wiley & Sons, Inc.)*

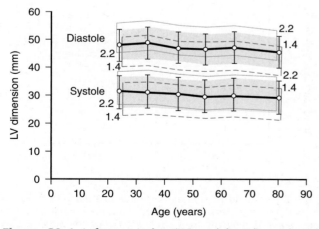

Figure 39–4. *Left ventricular (LV) end-diastolic and end-systolic dimensions in millimeters versus age in years. For each age group the mean and 95% prediction intervals for normal values are depicted. The solid and dashed lines as per Figure 39–2. (From Gardin JM, Henry WL, Savage DD, et al: J Clin Ultrasound 7:439-447, 1979. Copyright © 1979, John Wiley & Sons. Reprinted by permission of John Wiley & Sons, Inc.)*

Cardiac Chamber Dimensions

Normal echocardiographic values are listed in Table 39–1. These normal changes should be taken into account when reporting abnormalities.

Cardiac Valves

The four cardiac valves have been documented to change in morphology with age. These changes are most notable in the left-sided valves, and this is likely related to the higher pressures found in the associated chambers.

Valve Circumference

Valve circumference has been found to increase with age.[16] In one study of 765 patients, the mean valve circumference, when indexed for body surface area (BSA), progressively rose through adult life, a trend that was greater for the semilunar than for the atrioventricular valves. Krovetz[17] reanalyzed data regarding aortic valve size and found that after approximately 18 to 21 years of age the size of the aortic annulus increases in a near linear fashion (Fig. 39–5).

Valve Thickness

One autopsy study of 200 disease-free hearts demonstrated significant increases in mean thickness of the aortic and mitral valves with increasing age. This study showed that compared with subjects who were less than 20 years of age, those who were older than 60 years had valves that were twice as thick (Table 39–2).[18]

Valvular Calcification

Aging is associated with thickening and calcification of the aortic valve cusps also called aortic valve sclerosis and the mitral and aortic valve annuli (termed *mitral annular calcification* (MAC) and *aortic annular calcification*, respectively) (Figs. 39–6 and 39–7). Calcium is found at the bases of the aortic cusps and at the annulus and at the margins of closure of the mitral leaflets on the atrial side and in the mitral valve annulus. The term *senile calcification syndrome* was coined to describe patients with aortic valve sclerosis, MAC, and calcification of the epicardial coronary arteries.[19]

Various studies in elderly subjects have identified prevalence as high as approximately 50% for each of these lesions.[20-24] Although aortic valve sclerosis is equally common in men and women, MAC is more frequently seen in women. The prevalence by age of MAC in one study is listed in Table 39–3.

TABLE 39-1. Mean Values of Echocardiographic Parameters for Three Age Groups

Parameter	Group I (25-44 Years)	Group II (45-64 Years)	Group III (65-84 Years)
Mitral valve E-F slope (mm/s)	102.3±3.7 (52)	79.0±3.8 (35)*	67.1±5.2 (18)†
Aortic root, diastole (mm)	30.9±0.6 (45)	32.0±0.6 (34)	32.9±0.8 (17)‡
LV Wall Thickness (mm)			
Systolic	15.4±0.5 (33)	17.6±0.7 (15)	18.8±0.6 (12)*
Diastolic	8.7±0.3 (33)	9.8±0.5 (16)	10.7±0.5 (13)*
Systolic/m^2	7.6±0.3 (33)	9.2±0.3 (15)†	10.0±0.4 (12)†
Diastolic/m^2	4.3±0.1 (33)	5.0±0.2 (16)*	5.7±0.2 (13)†§
LV Dimension (mm)			
Systolic	34.4±1.1 (37)	32.1±0.89 (17)	32.1±1.4 (11)
Diastolic	51.8±1.03 (37)	50.8±1.3 (17)	51.2±1.4 (11)
Systolic/m^2	17.3±0.5 (37)	16.7±0.5 (17)	16.8±0.6 (11)
Diastolic/m^2	26.0±0.5 (37)	26.4±0.6 (17)	27.0±0.7 (11)
Fractional shortening of the minor semi–axis	0.34±0.01 (37)	0.36±0.01 (17)	0.37±0.02 (11)
Vcf (circ/s)	1.17±0.04 (37)	1.23±0.04 (17)	1.30±0.08 (11)

The number of subjects is given in parentheses next to the mean and standard error of the mean.
*$p < 0.01$ as compared with group I.
†$p < 0.001$ as compared with group I.
‡$p < 0.05$ as compared with group I.
§$p < 0.05$ as compared with group II.
LV, left ventricular; Vcf, velocity of circumferential fiber shortening.
Adapted from Gerstenblith G, Frederiksen J, Yin FCP: *Circulation* 56:273–277, 1977. Reproduced with permission. Copyright 1977 American Heart Association.

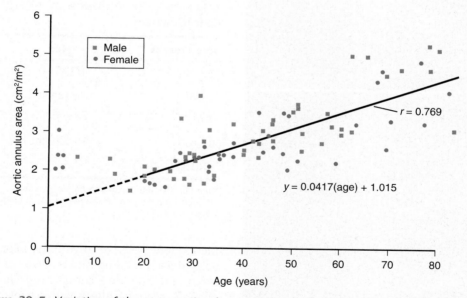

Figure 39–5. *Variation of the cross-sectional area of the aorta at the valve level with age. The regression line shown is for patients over 20 years of age. Patients under 20 years of age, in general, have higher aortic annulus areas per square meter than predicted by the regression equation. (From Krovetz LJ: Am Heart J 90:569-574, 1975.)*

Normal Changes in Cardiac Function

Left Ventricular Systolic Function

Resting ejection fraction (EF), percent fractional shortening, and cardiac output (CO) by echocardiography and by radionuclide ventriculography are unaffected by age in healthy normotensive people.[25-27] To maintain a normal ejection time in the setting of late systolic augmentation of aortic impedance, there is a prolonged contractile activation of the LV wall in the elderly.[27] This prolonged contractile activation means that when mitral valve opens, myocardial relaxation is

TABLE 39–2. Aortic Valve Thickness by Age Range in 200 Normal Hearts*

Age (Years)	Range (mm)	Mean ± SD (mm)
<20	0.35-1.55	0.67±0.21
20-59	0.40-2.10	0.87±0.27
≥60	0.55-3.50	1.42±0.51

*Thicknesses of all three cusps were combined, and the mean (±SD) was calculated.
SD, standard deviation.
Adapted from Sahasakul Y, Edwards WD, Naessens JM, et al: *Am J Cardiol* 62:424-430, 1988. Reproduced with permission.

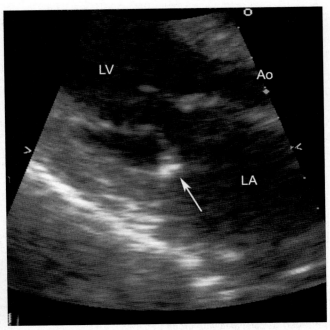

Figure 39–7. Mitral annular calcification. Note the nodule of calcium on the posterior annulus of the mitral valve (arrow) in this parasternal long-axis view. Ao, aorta; LA, left atrium; LV, left atrium.

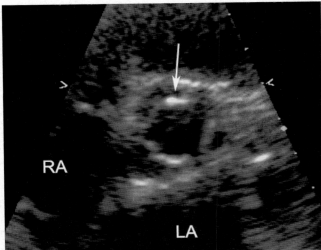

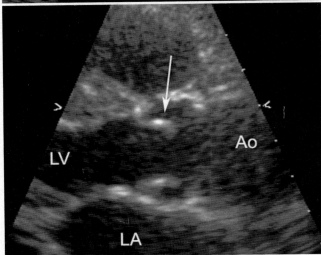

Figure 39–6. Aortic sclerosis. Note the bright nodularity present on the leaflets (arrows) in both short-axis (A) and long-axis (B) views of the aortic valve in systole. Ao, aorta; LA, left atrium; RA, right atrium.

TABLE 39–3. Prevalence of Mitral Annular Calcification

Age (Years)	Men	Women
62-70	4/22 (18)*	7/35 (20)*
71-80	13/42 (31)	40/110 (34)
81-90	44/75 (59)	146/226 (65)
91-100	19/22 (86)	56/96 (89)
101-103		3/3 (100)

*Number affected per total number (percent).
Adapted from Aronow WS, Schwartz KS, Koenigsberg M: *Am J Cardiol* 59:1213-1214, 1987.

incomplete (relative to younger people) and thus, the early diastolic filling rate is lower in the elderly. Studies of rat and dog cardiac muscle have shown no change in contractile function (resting tension, peak isometric tension, maximal rate of tension development) with age.[27,28]

Left Ventricular Diastolic Function

Although LV systolic performance in the aged is preserved, LV diastolic function changes markedly with age. Seminal work in this area showed a reduction in mitral valve E-F closure slope on M-mode echocardiography.[2,3] Later work using pulsed Doppler examination confirmed that there was a reduction in early diastolic peak filling rate (peak E-wave velocity) of approximately 50% between 20 and 80 years of age. There is a concomitant increase with age in peak A-wave velocity, representing late LV filling resulting from atrial contraction. This atrial "kick" is powered by a modest age-related increase in left atrial size. It is reasonable to consider the augmented atrial contribution to LV filling to be a successful compensatory mechanism to the reduced early diastolic filling rate into the thicker, presumably less compliant ventricle.

There have been a number of mechanisms proposed to explain the changes in diastolic function that occur with aging, and likely all play some role. These mechanisms include a lower rate of calcium accumulation by the sarcoplasmic reticulum.[29] Studies of whole animal hearts and isolated cardiac muscle have documented prolong isovolumic relaxation and increased myocardial diastolic stiffness.[30] Sclerosis of the mitral leaflets with resultant prolonged diastolic filling time (late closure) has also been proposed as a possible mechanism, as has an increase in afterload.

Data from the Framingham Heart Study was used to establish reference values for various Doppler parameters for elderly patients and is depicted in Table 39–4.[31] These data were obtained by studying 114 men and women aged 70 to 87 years of age who were screened and found to be free of cardiovascular disease. Notably, the vast majority (87%) of these subjects had peak E/A velocity ratios less than 1, 75% had values less than 0.86, and 25% had values less than 0.62. Because normal young subjects have E/A velocities greater than 1, it may be inappropriate to use this as the normal standard against which to compare the diastolic function of an elderly person (Fig. 39–8; see Chapter 11).

Cardiac Response to Pressor Stress

The usual response of increases in blood pressure and heart rate (HR) in response to sustained, isometric handgrip is altered in healthy elderly as opposed to young people. HR does not increase as much in the older group, but blood pressure is increased more than in the young. Accompanying these changes are mild increases in echocardiographically measured LV diastolic and systolic dimensions that occur in the aged.[32,33] Similar changes in LV cavity size and blunted HR increase has been seen in response to phenylephrine infusion in healthy older versus younger volunteers.[34] It therefore appears that results from reduced contractile reserve in the aged heart in response to increased afterload, overall systolic performance is maintained by cavity enlargement (i.e., the Frank-Starling mechanism).

Cardiac Response to Exercise Stress

Multiple studies have shown that VO$_2$max declines with age. This findings is likely multifactorial and involves changes in cardiac output, pulmonary function, muscle function, among other factors. There has also been a documented age associated decline in maximum exercise cardiac output, which is a result of the aforementioned blunted HR response to exercise. With exercise, stroke volume is maintained with aging. The mechanism by which this occurs is that larger LV end diastolic volumes are achieved with exercise, which offsets the blunted capacity of the aging heart to reduce end-systolic volume. The larger LV end-diastolic volume is achieved to some degree as a result of the slower HR (longer diastolic filling time) and the larger end-systolic volume.[35]

TABLE 39–4. Mean and Percentile Values of Doppler Diastolic Filling Indices for 114 Study Subjects over 70 Years of Age

Diastolic Indices	Mean	Lower Percentiles		Median Percentiles		Upper Percentiles	
		5%	10%	50%	75%	90%	95%
E-velocity (m/s)	0.44	0.25	0.26	0.41	0.51	0.69	0.76
A-velocity (m/s)	0.59	0.38	0.43	0.56	0.68	0.80	0.84
E/A (ratio)	0.76	0.48	0.52	0.70	0.86	1.05	1.21
E/A TVI (ratio)	1.36	0.79	0.90	1.33	1.57	1.76	1.94
AFF (ratio)	0.40	0.29	0.32	0.40	0.44	0.49	0.52
AT (s)	0.06	0.02	0.03	0.05	0.07	0.08	0.09
DT (s)	0.14	0.09	0.10	0.14	0.16	0.19	0.23

AFF, atrial filling fraction; AT, acceleration time; DT, deceleration time; A-velocity, peak velocity A; E-velocity, peak velocity E; E/A, ratio of early to late peak velocities; E/A TVI, ratio of early to late time velocity integrals.
Modified from Sagie A, Benjamin EJ, Golderisi M, et al: *J Am Soc Echocardiogr* 6:570-576, 1993.

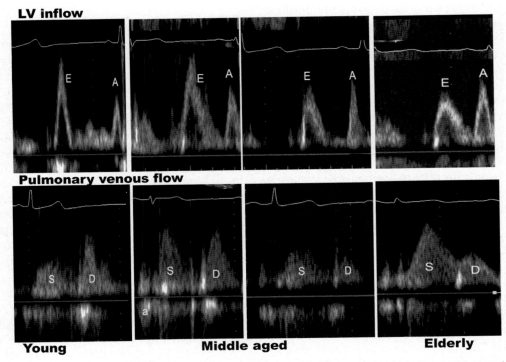

Figure 39–8. Example mitral inflow (upper panels) *and pulmonary vein* (lower panels) *Doppler tracings from normal young, middle aged, and elderly individuals. Showing the normal progression of changes in left ventricular filling. A, pulmonary vein atrial reversal; D, diastolic pulmonary vein flow; E, peak early filling velocity; LV, left ventricle; S, systolic pulmonary vein flow.*

Ejection fraction, however, does not increase as much in older healthy individuals as in younger ones, and they do not reach the same peak as in younger people.[35] This results from a decreased ability to reduce their end systolic volumes. These findings likely result from multiple mechanisms. These include reduced myocardial contractility, increased vascular afterload, diminished autonomic modulation of LV contractility and arterial afterload, and arterial-ventricular load mismatching.[36]

Clinical Utility and Outcome Data

Valvular Heart Disease

Aortic Valve Sclerosis

Aortic valve sclerosis is one end of the spectrum of calcific aortic valvular disease. Aortic sclerosis is characterized by mild leaflet thickening without restriction of outflow, and at the other end of the spectrum is severe calcification that may progress to aortic stenosis (AS) with restricted leaflet motion and obstruction to LV outflow. The lesions of aortic sclerosis are complex focal subendothelial plaquelike lesions located on the aortic side of the valve leaflet that extend to the fibrosa layer. These lesions are probably reactions to increased mechanical or decreased shear stresses. Mechanical stresses are greatest on the aortic side near the attach-

ments of the leaflets to the aortic root. Shear stress across the noncoronary cusp is lowest because of a lack of diastolic coronary blood flow, which probably explains why the noncoronary cusp is usually the first affected.[37] Patients with AS who have bicuspid valves tend to present 20 years younger than patients with trileaflet valves, which supports the concept that mechanical stress (bileaflet valves are subject to a greater amount of such stress) is important in the pathogenesis of the disease.[37] The lesions of aortic valve sclerosis are active, with evidence of an accumulation of an inflammatory cell infiltrate, microscopic calcification, an accumulation of low-density lipoproteins (LDLs) and lipoprotein(a), and evidence of low-density lipoprotein oxidation.[38-41] As the process continues, calcification increases, and there is active bone formation.[42] Ultimately, leaflet calcification can become so severe that opening of the valve is impaired and hemodynamically significant AS results.

In longitudinal studies documenting progression from aortic valve sclerosis to AS, moderate stenosis (jet velocity 3 to 4 m/s) was found in 3% of patients in one study and 5% in a second, and severe stenosis (jet velocity >4 m/s) in 2.5% of patients in both studies.[43,44] Although the vast majority of patients will not progress to significant AS, given the high prevalence of aortic valve sclerosis in the aging population, the sheer number of people who could be affected is high, and thus its identification is important (see also Chapter 23).

Mitral Annular Calcification

MAC is characterized by calcification at the leaflet base and in the annulus. It has been classified by its anatomic position. Most cases of MAC involve the posterior annulus with bright echos seen at the basal posterior wall, at the junction with the posterior mitral leaflet. Anterior MAC is defined by bright echoes located at the base of the anterior mitral valve leaflet and may extend from the annulus throughout the base of the heart into the mitral and aortic valves.[45] Although many echocardiographers use personal subjective criteria to grade the severity of MAC, a more systematic approach has also been used.[46] Mild MAC can be defined as involving less than one third of the annular circumference (<3 mm in thickness) and are usually restricted to the angle between the posterior leaflet of the mitral valve and the LV posterior wall. Moderate MAC involves less than two thirds of the annular circumference (3 to 5 mm in thickness). In severe MAC more than two thirds of the circumference is affected (>5 mm in thickness), usually extending beneath the entire posterior mitral leaflet and may make a complete circle.

MAC and Valvular Dysfunction. There is a wide spectrum of calcification in MAC and is probably progressive (Fig. 39–9). It usually begins with a small amount of calcium deposition at the basal insertion of the posterior mitral leaflet. Calcification of the annular connective tissue ensues and may form a ridge or ring that encircles the leaflets. As it progresses further, it may bulge into the LV cavity below the posterior leaflet and lift the leaflets toward the left atrium.[47,48] A larger extent of involvement may render the base of the posterior leaflet immobile and result in varying amounts of valvular regurgitation.[49] Actual leaflet calcification, however, is rare. The severity of MAC seems to be correlated with the severity of associated mitral regurgitation when it is present.[50-52]

Mitral stenosis (MS) as a result of MAC has also been described. In contrast to rheumatic mitral stenosis in which there is commissural fusion, in MAC associated mitral stenosis, the leaflets are not fused and the leaflet tips are thin, but the increased flow velocities are a result of the decreased mitral annular excursion resulting from calcification.[53]

MAC and Other Pathology. MAC is associated with left atrial well as LV enlargement.[46,54-56] In a prospective study of 976 elderly patients with and without MAC, left atrial enlargement was 2.4 times more prevalent in patients with MAC than in those without MAC.[54]

MAC and Conduction Abnormalities. Likely secondary to concomitant calcification within the conduction system (which may be contiguous because calcium extends from the annulus into the interventricular septum), MAC is associated with conduction abnormalities, such as atrioventricular (AV) block, sinoatrial node disease, bundle branch block, left anterior fascicular block, and nonspecific intraventricular conduction delay.[46,57,58]

MAC and Atrial Fibrillation. Likely owing to the associated left atrial enlargement, atrial fibrillation (AFib) is more common in patients with MAC than without it. In various studies, the relative risk was increased from 2.8 to 12 times.[46,55-59]

MAC and Thromboembolism. MAC is associated with a number of conditions that predispose to thromboembolic stroke, including AFib, mitral regurgitation and stenosis, left atrial enlargement, and congestive heart failure (CHF). In addition, MAC has been associated with aortic atheromata,[60] complex aortic debris,[61] and calcification of the thoracic aorta,[62] all of which could be sources of thromboembolic. On the other hand, there is reason to suspect that MAC itself may be involved in providing a source for thromboemboli. Although the calcification in MAC is usually covered by

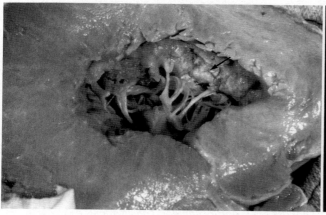
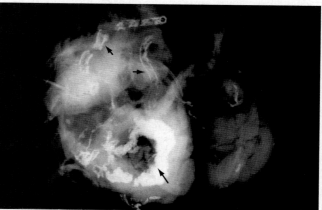

A   B

Figure 39–9. A, *Ventricular aspect of the mitral valve shows nodules of calcium deposited at the annulus adherent to the valve leaflet and chordae* (arrow). B, *Postmortem radiograph shows nearly O-shaped mitral annular calcification* (large arrow) *and calcified coronary arteries* (small arrows).

a layer of endothelium, ulceration of the lining may expose the calcium and serve as a starting point for fibrin-platelet clot, which may embolize.[54,58] A number of studies that tried to control for other factors have revealed an association of MAC with cerebral embolization, with relative risks of 1.5 to 5.[46,54,59,63-66]

Studies have found MAC to be an independent risk factor for stroke in patients who were in AFib and those who were in sinus rhythm.[59] This has led to some advocating prophylactic anticoagulation in patients with MAC, regardless of rhythm.[67]

MAC and Endocarditis. The abnormal valve morphology, hemodynamics, and endothelium have been implicated as predisposing the valve to infection (endocarditis).[54,58] In particular, patients with MAC and chronic renal failure, seem to be at especially high risk.[68] Treatment of patients with antibiotics may also be less effective because the avascular nature of the mitral annulus predisposes to periannular abscesses, and therefore some advocate antibiotic prophylaxis for patients with MAC undergoing invasive procedures. The American Heart Association guidelines do not recommend endocarditis prophylaxis for native valvular heart disease, including MAC.[69,70]

Aortic Valve Sclerosis and MAC and Outcome

Several studies have found a strong association between MAC and aortic valve sclerosis with adverse cardiovascular outcomes and mortality.[24,71-74] Otto and colleagues found that in 5621 men and women 65 years of age or older who were participants in the Cardiovascular Health Study that aortic sclerosis (without hemodynamically significant outflow obstruction) was associated with an approximately 50% increase risk of death from cardiovascular causes and a 40% increase in the risk of myocardial infarction (MI).[24] In another study of 2358 elderly patients, those with aortic valve sclerosis had a risk of developing a new coronary event that was 1.8 times higher than those without it.[75] Lending support to the concept that calcific aortic valve disease and atherosclerotic vascular disease have a shared pathogenesis is data from Otto and colleagues' study that older age, male gender, smoking, hypertension, and hyperlipidemia were associated with aortic sclerosis.

In a recent study, Barasch and colleagues investigated the prevalence and clinical outcomes of MAC, aortic valve sclerosis, and aortic annular calcification.[76] Again using data from the Cardiovascular Health Study, 3929 subjects with a mean age of 76 years, 60% of whom were women, MAC was seen in 42% of subjects, aortic annular calcification in 44%, and aortic valve sclerosis in 54%. The rate of all three conditions being found in a single subject was 17%. Subjects with these conditions tended to be older, and those with mitral annular calcification had worse risk profiles (e.g., left ventricular hypertrophy (LVH), increased left atrial size, abnormal

ejection fraction, increased carotid intimal media thickness, dyslipidemia, elevated C-reactive protein) than those with aortic valve sclerosis and aortic annular calcification. In addition, this study showed that the severity of MAC (estimated from 2-D echocardiography, semiquantitatively) was associated with a higher prevalence of atherosclerotic vascular disease, independent of other risk factors. These conditions were associated with a significantly elevated risk of cardiovascular disease endpoints, and the strongest association was with the combined group (MAC and aortic annular calcification and aortic valve sclerosis) with CHF (odds ratio [OR] 2.04, 95% confidence interval [CI] 1.34 to 3.09). (Figs. 39–10 and 39–11 and Table 39–5).

Although not definitively proven, a good deal of research has strongly suggested a relationship between calcification of the fibrous skeleton of the heart and aortic valve cusps and advanced atherosclerosis.[77-80] Inflammation and abnormalities of lipid metabolism have both been implicated in the development of both atherosclerosis and aortic valve calcification.[81-84] Other data has failed to support the association of inflammatory markers with calcific aortic valvular disease however.[85]

Left Ventricular Hypertrophy

Data from both the Framingham study and the Cardiovascular Health Study confirm that LVH is a potent predictor of morbidity and mortality from coronary heart disease, CHF, and stroke.[86-88]

The relationship between age and LVH is complex. Evaluation of data from the Framingham Heart Study

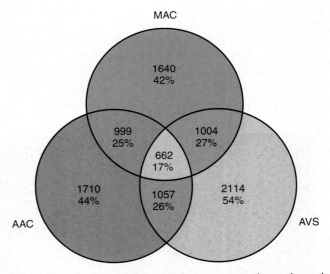

Figure 39–10. *The relationship between mitral annular calcification, aortic annular calcification, and aortic valve sclerosis in 3929 participants in the Cardiovascular Health Study. Numbers are total numbers of patients, and percentages refer to the percent of the total population of 3929 study participants. AAC, aortic annular calcification; AVS, aortic valve sclerosis, MAC, mitral annular calcification. (From Barasch E, Gottdiener JS, Marino-Larsen EK, et al: Am Heart J 151:39-47, 2006. Reprinted with permission.)*

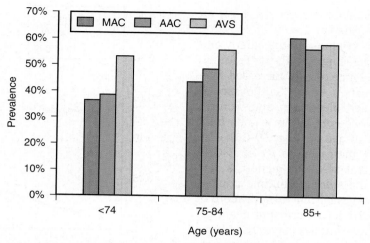

Figure 39–11. *The distribution of mitral annular calcification, aortic annular calcification, and aortic valve sclerosis in the three age groups of the 3929 participants enrolled in the Cardiovascular Health Study. MAC: P less than 0.001; AAC: P less than 0.001; AVS: P equal to 0.055. AAC, aortic annular calcification; AVS, aortic valve sclerosis, MAC, mitral annular calcification. (From Barasch E, Gottdiener JS, Marino-Larsen EK, et al: Am Heart J 151:39-47, 2006. Reprinted with permission.)*

TABLE 39–5. Odds Ratios (95% Confidence Interval) for the Association of Cardiac Calcification with Cardiovascular Events

Calcification Category	MI, OR (95% CI)	Stroke, OR (95% CI)	Angina Pectoris, OR (95% CI)	CHF, OR (95% CI)	Revascularization, OR (95% CI)
MAC	1.70 (1.38-2.09)	1.84 (1.40-2.41)	1.29 (1.11-1.51)	1.69 (1.31-2.17)	1.50 (1.18-1.91)
AAC	1.17 (0.95-1.54)	1.13 (0.86-1.48)	1.21 (1.03-1.42)	1.75 (1.34-2.27)	1.33 (1.04-1.71)
AVS	1.27 (1.03-1.57)	1.16 (0.88-1.53)	1.24 (1.06-1.45)	1.02 (0.79-1.31)	1.07 (0.84-1.37)
MAC + AAC + AVS	1.86 (1.32-2.62)	1.95 (1.26-3.03)	1.60 (1.24-2.07)	2.04 (1.34-3.09)	1.85 (1.21-2.84)

The study involved the 3929 participants enrolled in the Cardiovascular Health Study.
AAC, aortic annular calcification; AVS, aortic valve sclerosis; CHF, congestive heart failure; CI, confidence interval; MAC, mitral annular calcification; MI, myocardial infarction; OR, odds ratio.
From Barasch E, Gottdiener JS, Marino-Larsen EK, et al: *Am Heart J* 151:39-47, 2006. Reprinted with permission.

revealed that age, height, systolic blood pressure, and body mass index (BMI) were significant and independent predictors of LV mass in 4972 people aged 17 to 90 years. However, when people were screened out of the analysis who met one of the following conditions: evidence of cardiovascular disease on history, physical examination, electrocardiogram (ECG), chest X-ray or echocardiography, had blood pressure greater than or equal to 140/90, were on medications for cardiopulmonary disease, or were greater than or equal to 20% above or below recommended weight for height, age was no longer a significant correlate of LV mass.[89] Thus, it seems that the increases in LV mass that are seen with age are often confounded by coexisting cardiopulmonary disease.

Left Atrial Size and Outcomes

Elevated left atrial size has been shown to be a marker of cardiovascular risk. Largely from studies carried out in elderly populations, an enlarged left atrium is associated with an increased risk of AFib, stroke, and death

(including post-myocardial infarction and in patients with dilated cardiomyopathies).[90-94] Using data from the Strong Heart Study, Kizer and colleagues showed that left atrial diameter (normal defined as <3.8 cm for women, <4.2 cm for men) was an independent predictor of incident cardiovascular events after adjustment for other factors (clinical, echocardiographic, inflammatory).[95] See Table 39–6 and Figure 39–12. The relative utility of various measures of left atrial size, including volume, area, and diameter, is an area of active research, with some data indicating that left atrial volume is the more robust marker for cardiovascular events.[96]

Congestive Heart Failure

The reversal of early and late diastolic filling with age results in preserved end-diastolic and stroke volume (and therefore cardiac output), but a reduction in LV compliance may cause an elevated LV end-diastolic pressure in the elderly, especially with tachycardia. This would be expected to cause dyspnea to be more easily provoked and presumably forms the basis of CHF in some patients (see Chapter 29).

The syndrome of CHF is common in the elderly and is more prevalent with increasing age. In the Framingham Heart Study, the incidence of CHF increased five-fold from age 40 to 70 years.[97] In the Cardiovascular Health Study, which studied older men and women, found an increased prevalence of CHF in women from 4.1% at age 70 to 14.3% at age 85 (Fig. 39–13). The figures for men were 7.8% increasing to 18.4%.[98] CHF with normal or near-normal systolic function is also particularly prevalent in the elderly. Multiple population-based studies have suggested that 50% or more of the elderly patients with CHF have normal or near-normal systolic function. These studies have also documented that CHF with preserved systolic function is more common in women than in men.[99-101] Because women outnumber men in the older age group, the problem is even more prevalent with advancing age.

There are multiple etiologies of CHF with preserved systolic function and several are listed in Table 39–7.[102] Evaluation of patients with CHF by echocardiography can lead to a diagnosis of the etiology of CHF and as such can lead to more appropriate evaluation and treatment of the condition. It is important to recognize how prevalent CHF is in the elderly and the fact that patients with heart failure and preserved systolic function also have impaired survival (although in some studies not to the same degree).[103-105] Furthermore, it has been shown that patients who do not have the syndrome of CHF but who have been found to have diastolic dysfunction also have higher mortality than those with normal diastolic function.[106]

Coronary Artery Disease and Stress Testing

The identification of findings supportive of a diagnosis of coronary artery disease (CAD) is common in the elderly because age is a major risk factor for coronary

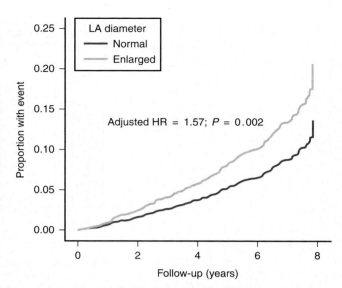

Figure 39–12. *Incidence of cardiovascular events by left atrial diameter in the Strong Heart Study, a study of 2084 middle-aged and elderly persons. Adjusted Kaplan-Meier curves of first cardiovascular events according to presence or absence of left atrial enlargement. HR, heart rate; LA, left atrium. (Adapted from Kizer JR, Bella JN, Palmieri V, et al: Am Heart J 151:412-418, 2006. Reprinted with permission.)*

disease. Wall motion abnormalities, wall thinning, and aneurysm formation from prior myocardial infarction may be seen (see Chapters 15 and 16).

Stress echocardiography (exercise or pharmacologic) is a modality commonly used to evaluate for coronary artery disease and sometimes to evaluate myocardial viability. The techniques used are the same for the elderly as for the younger patient. Age-adjusted normative values for target HR and exercise time are widely available. In addition, treadmill protocols that have a more gentle increase in speed or incline are common (e.g., Modified Bruce, Naughton, Balke protocols). Because many elderly have comorbid conditions that make exercise stress testing unattractive or impossible (e.g., chronic

TABLE 39–6. Cardiovascular Endpoints by Left Atrial Size

Clinical Outcome	Enlarged Left Atrium (*n* = 461)		Normal Left Atrium (*n* = 2343)		*p-value*
	N	*%*	*N*	*%*	
First cardiovascular event	86	18.7	282	12.0	<0.001
Fatal and nonfatal CHD*	52	11.2	169	7.2	0.003
Fatal and nonfatal stroke	15	3.3	51	2.2	0.186
Fatal and nonfatal CHF	19	4.1	62	2.6	0.084
Any cardiovascular death	23	5.0	67	2.9	0.018

*Includes fatal and nonfatal myocardial infarction, sudden cardiac death, and other fatal and nonfatal coronary heart disease.
CHD, coronary heart disease; CHF, congestive heart failure.
Data from the 2084 middle-aged and elderly participants in the Strong Heart Study. Adapted from Kizer JR, Bella JN, Palmieri V, et al: *Am Heart J* 151:412-418, 2006. Reprinted with permission.

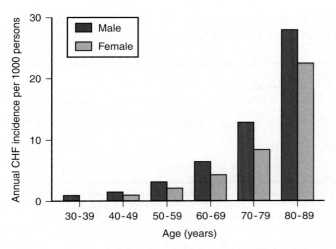

Figure 39-13. The relationship between age and heart failure in the Cardiovascular Health Study. CHF, congestive heart failure. (From Kitzman DW, Gardin JM, Gottdiener JS, et al: Am J Cardiol 87:413-419, 2001.)

TABLE 39-7. Heart Failure with Normal Left Ventricular Systolic Function

Diastolic Heart Failure
Hypertension
Restrictive cardiomyopathy
Infiltrative cardiomyopathy
Hypertrophic cardiomyopathy
Noncompaction cardiomyopathy

Right-Sided Heart Failure
Severe pulmonary hypertension
Right ventricular infarction
Arrhythmogenic right ventricular dysplasia
Atrial septal defect

Valvular Heart Diseases
Severe valvular stenosis
Severe valvular regurgitation

Pericardial Disease
Cardiac tamponade
Constrictive pericarditis

Intracardiac Mass
Atrial myxoma
Apical eosinophilic thrombus

Pulmonary Vein Stenosis

Congenital Heart Diseases

Adapted from Oh JK, Hatle L, Tajik AJ, et al: *J Am Coll Cardiol* 47:500-506, 2006. Reprinted with permission.

obstructive pulmonary disease [COPD], orthopedic or arthritic conditions, neuromuscular disorders, peripheral vascular disease), the use of pharmacologic stress increases the number of patients eligible for stress testing in this age group. Vasodilators, such as adenosine or dipyridamole and catecholamines (dobutamine) as pharmacologic stress agents, are used in this population.

Studies in elderly patients referred for stress testing on clinical grounds and in the post-myocardial infarction population have demonstrated the value of exercise, adenosine, dipyridamole, and dobutamine echocardiography in predicting clinical outcomes.[107-111]

There is some data that suggests that dobutamine stress echocardiography (DSE) is more sensitive and accurate but equally as specific as adenosine stress echocardiography (Table 39-8).

Safety

The safety profile of these various types of stress testing in the elderly is good. Exercise echocardiography is similar to standard exercise testing with regard to safety, although some caution is needed as patients are guided back to the scanning bed from the treadmill. In one study of 454 patients, half were 70 years of age or older and half were younger than 70 years of age, dobutamine stress echocardiography was associated with higher rates in the elderly versus younger patients of asymptomatic hypotension (defined as a drop in systolic blood pressure of >20 mm Hg) of 37% versus 12%. There were also significantly higher rates of supraventricular tachycardia (7% versus 1%) and of premature ventricular contractions (74% versus 32%). There was a nonsignificant trend toward more frequent ventricular tachycardia (5% versus 2%) and of AFib (3% versus 0.4%). The authors report that all arrhythmias resolved with either dobutamine infusion cessation or with administration of metoprolol.[112] Similar results were reported by Hiro and colleagues[113]

Dipyridamole and adenosine can cause bronchospasm, hypotension, and arrhythmias, and for the most part these effects do not seem to be age related.[114,115] However, elderly patients undergoing adenosine stress tests may be more likely to experience transient atrioventricular block. In one study of 120 patients who were 70 years old or older this occurred in 6% of tests.[116] In another study it occurred in 18% of patients who were 75 years of age or older versus 8% in those younger than 75 years of age.[117]

Cardiogenic Thromboembolism

Cardiac sources of embolism are thought to be responsible for ischemic strokes in as many as 20% of cases.[118] Embolization of the components of MAC and of atherosclerotic intraaortic debris are more common in elderly patients. See Figures 39-7, 39-9, and 39-14. Not all studies have found an association between mitral annular calcification and stroke, however.[88,119] Aortic sclerosis has also been associated with the risk of stroke, but an independent association between aortic valve calcification and cerebral infarcts has only been demonstrated in the presence of AS.[24,119,120] As with

TABLE 39–8. Sensitivity, Specificity, and Accuracy of Dobutamine and Adenosine Stress Echocardiography in the Detection of Coronary Artery Disease in Older Adults

	Sensitivity				Specificity	Accuracy
	Overall	**1VD**	**2VD**	**3VD**		
Dobutamine	86.5% (77/89)	74% (14/19)	88% (22/25)	91% (41/45)	84% (26/31)	86% (103/120)
Adenosine	66.3% (59/89)	42% (8/19)	76% (19/25)	71% (32/45)	90% (28/31)	72.5% (87/120)
P value	<0.001	0.227	0.124	<0.01	<0.001	<0.001

Data in parentheses indicate number of patients. This study enrolled 120 patients 70 years old or older with chest pain and known or suspected coronary artery disease who underwent both dobutamine and adenosine stress echocardiography, as well as coronary angiography.
1VD, one-vessel coronary artery disease; 2VD, two-vessel coronary artery disease; 3VD, three-vessel coronary artery disease.
From Anthopoulos LP, Bonou MS, Kardaras FG, et al: *J Am Coll Cardiol* 28(1):52-59, 1996. Reprinted with permission.

younger patients, LV thrombus (usually associated with LV dysfunction), left atrial thrombus (usually associated with AFib and flutter), vegetations, paradoxic emboli (across a patent foramen ovale [PFO]), and myxoma are no more prevalent in the elderly. Many studies have demonstrated the higher sensitivity of transesophageal echocardiography (TEE) to detect potential sources of embolism, including in the elderly population[121,122] (see Chapter 40).

Cardiac Amyloidosis

Amyloid infiltration of the heart in the elderly has been described for decades and has been variously termed *senile amyloidosis of the heart* or *amyloidosis localized to the heart*[123,124] (see Chapter 29). However, a more appropriate term is probably *systemic senile amyloidosis* because evidence of small amyloid deposits have been found in the aorta, lung, gastrointestinal (GI) tract, liver, and kidney.[125,126] In addition to systemic senile amyloidosis, amyloid infiltration of the heart occurs in primary amyloidosis, amyloidosis associated with multiple myeloma and secondary amyloidosis, which is associated with chronic inflammation. In one autopsy study of 244 patients who were older than 60 years of age, amyloid was found in the heart in 50% of patients.[127] Although it infrequently causes clinical symptoms or signs,[128,129] it has been associated with AFib (particularly when found in the ventricular myocardium), ventricular arrhythmias, and with CHF (usually when there is a large burden of involvement).[130,131] The protein of senile amyloidosis is different from primary amyloidosis and it portends a much better prognosis.[132] Studies have shown a male predominance in primary systemic but an even greater predominance in the senile type.[131,132] In a study by Smith and colleagues that compared patients with senile and primary amyloidosis, the male to female ratio was 5.5:1 for the senile group, and 1.6:1 for

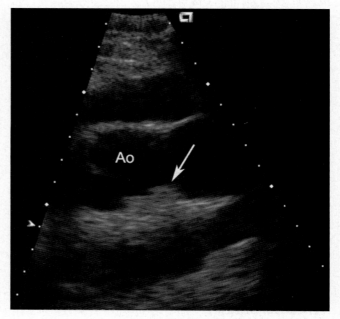

Figure 39–14. *Atherosclerotic plaque in the aortic root* (arrow). *Long-axis view of the aortic valve and ascending aorta. Ao, aorta.*

the primary group.[131] The patients with senile amyloidosis were older with a mean age of 83 years, whereas only 4 of the 21 patients with primary amyloidosis were over 70 years old. Amyloid deposits can be found in the ventricular myocardium and in the atrial mural endocardium. Less common sites of deposition in the senile type include the valves, epicardium, and intramyocardial blood vessels.[133] Echocardiographic evidence of cardiac amyloidosis includes increased myocardial echo-genicity with a "speckle" pattern, increased interatrial septal thickness, and valve thickening, the latter two characteristics are common in other conditions. Finding LVH on echocardiography along with a low-voltage pattern on an electrocardiogram is suggestive of an infiltrative cardiomyopathy.

Clinical Recommendations

1. Norms for chamber dimensions should be adjusted based on age.

2. Although valvular calcification is common (aortic valve sclerosis, aortic annular calcification. and mitral annular calcification) because its presence is associated with adverse outcomes, it should not be considered normal. Instead it should be viewed as important risk markers.

3. Diastolic filling parameters commonly change with age in a generally predictable manner but do predispose patients to having adverse events or outcomes (e.g., AFib, CHF). Thus, they should not be considered normal, but rather, the specific physiologic abnormalities should be described (e.g., impaired relaxation).

4. Although stress testing is generally safe to perform in the elderly population, practitioners should be aware that these patients are more likely than younger patients to experience supraventricular tachycardia, premature ventricular contractions, and asymptomatic hypotension with dobutamine and transient atrioventricular block with adenosine.

KEY POINTS

- Age is a major risk factor for cardiovascular disease, and many normal and pathologic changes that are common with age are readily detected on echocardiography.

- There are changes in cardiac structure affecting the left ventricle, left atrium, and valves.

- There are predictable changes in LV performance with age, particularly changes in diastolic function.

- Valvular calcification (including aortic valve sclerosis, aortic annular calcification, and mitral annular calcification) is common and is associated with adverse outcomes in the elderly.

- Pharmacologic stress testing is common in the elderly, and a heightened awareness of possible complications is advisable.

- LVH, elevated cardiac mass, and increased left atrial size are associated with adverse outcomes.

- CHF, and in particular diastolic heart failure, are common in the elderly.

REFERENCES

1. Federal Interagency Forum on Aging-Related Statistics: *Older Americans 2004: Key Indicators of Well-Being*, Washington, DC, Government Printing Office, 2004, p. 68.

2. Gardin JM, Henry WL, Savage DD, et al: Echocardiographic measurements in normal subjects. Evaluation of an adult population without clinically apparent heart disease. *J Clin Ultrasound* 7:439-447, 1979.

3. Gerstenblith G, Fredreriksen J, Yin FCP: Echocardiographic assessment of a normal adult aging population. *Circulation* 56:273-277, 1977.

4. Pearson AC, Grudipath CV, Labovitz AJ: Effects of aging left ventricular structure and function. *Am Heart J* 121:871-873, 1991.

5. Henry WL, Gardin JM, Ware JH: Echocardiographic measurement in normal subjects from infancy to old age. *Circulation* 62:1054-1061, 1980.

6. Dannenberg AL, Levy D, Garrison RJ: Impact of age on echocardiographic left ventricular mass in healthy population. The Framingham Study. *Am J Cardiol* 64:1066-1068, 1989.

7. Shub C, Klein AL, Zachariah PK, et al: Determination of left ventricular mass by echocardiography in a normal population: effect of age and sex in addition to body size. *Mayo Clin Proc* 69:205-221, 1994.

8. Devereux RB, Alonso DR, Lutas EM: Echocardiographic assessment of left ventricular hypertrophy: Comparison with necropsy findings. *Am J Cardiol* 57:450-458, 1986.

9. Hees PS, Fleg JL, Lakatta EG: Left ventricular remodeling with age in normal men versus women: Novel insights using three-dimensional magnetic resonance imaging. *Am J Cardiol* 90:1231-1236, 2002.

10. Sapin PM, Gopal AS, Clarke GB: Three-dimensional echocardiography compared to two dimensional echocardiography for measurement of left ventricular mass anatomic validation in an open chest canine model. *Am J Hypertens* 9:467-474, 1996.

11. Gopal AS, Keller AM, Shen Z: Three-dimensional echocardiography: in vitro and in vivo validation of left ventricular mass and comparison with conventional echocardiographic methods. *J Am Coll Cardiol* 24:504-513, 1994.

12. Hubka M, Bolson EL, McDonald JA: Three-dimensional echocardiographic measurement of left and right ventricular mass and volume: in vitro validation. *Int J Cardiovasc Imaging* 18:111-118, 2002.

13. Gopal AS, Schnellbaecher MJ, Shen Z: Freehand three-dimensional echocardiography for determination of left ventricular volume and mass in patients with abnormal ventricles: comparison with magnetic resonance imaging. *J Am Soc Echocardiogr* 10:853-861, 1997.

14. Mor-Avi V, Sugeng L, Winert L: Fast measurement of left ventricular mass with real-time three-dimensional echocardiography: Comparison with magnetic resonance imaging. *Circulation* 110:1814-1818, 2004.

15. Ensor RE, Fleg JL, Kim YC: Longitudinal chest x-ray changes in normal men. *J Gerontol* 38:307-314, 1983.

16. Kitzman DW, Sihloz DH, Hagen PT: Age-related changes in normal human hearts during the first 10 decades of life. Part II (maturity): A quantitative anatomic study of 765 specimens from subjects 20-99 years old. *Mayo Clin Proc* 63:137-146, 1988.

17. Krovetz LJ: Age-related changes in the size of the aortic valve annulus in man. *Am Heart J* 90:569-574, 1975.

18. Sahasakul Y, Edwards WD, Naessens JM, et al: Age-related changes in aortic and mitral valve thickness. Implication for two-dimensional echocardiography based on autopsy study of 200 normal hearts. *Am J Cardiol* 62:424-430, 1988.

19. Roberts WC: The senile cardiac calcification syndrome. *Am J Cardiol* 58:572-574, 1986.

20. Boon A, Lodder J, Cheriex E, Kessels F: Mitral annulus calcification is not an independent risk factor for stroke: A cohort study of 657 patients. *J Neurol* 244:535-541, 1997.

21. Aronow WS, Schwartz KS, Konigsberg M: Correlation of serum lipids calcium and phosphorus, diabetes mellitus, aortic valve stenosis and history of systemic hypertension with presence or absence of mitral annular calcification in persons older than 62 years in a long-term health care facility. *Am J Cardiol* 59:381-382, 1987.

22. Aronow WS, Ahn C, Shirani J, et al: Comparison of frequency of new coronary events in older subjects with and without valvular aortic sclerosis. *Am J Cardiol* 83:599-600, A8, 1999.

23. Tolstrup K, Roldan CA, Qualls CR, et al: Aortic valve sclerosis, mitral annular calcium, and aortic root sclerosis as markers of atherosclerosis in men. *Am J Cardiol* 89:1030-1034, 2002.

24. Otto CM, Lind BK, Kitzman DW: Association of aortic-valve sclerosis with cardiovascular mortality and morbidity in the elderly. *N Eng J Med* 341:142-147, 1999.

25. Port S, Cobb FR, Coleman RE: Effect of age on the response of the left ventricular ejection fraction to exercise. *N Engl J Med* 303:1133-1137, 1980.

26. Rodeheffer RJ, Gerstenbligh G, Becker LC: Exercise cardiac output is maintained with advancing age in healthy human subjects. *Circulation* 69:203-213, 1984.

27. Laktta EG, Gerstenblith G, Angell CS, et al: Prolonged contraction duration in aged myocardium. *J Clin Invest* 55:61-68, 1975.

28. Yin FCP, Weisfeldt ML, Milnor WR: Role of aortic input impedance in the decreased cardiovascular response to exercise with aging in dogs. *J Clin Invest* 68:28-38, 1981.

29. Froelich JP, Lakatta EG, Beard E, et al: Studies of sarcoplasmic reticulum function and contraction duration in young and aged rat myocardium. *J Mol Cell Cardiol* 10:427-438, 1978.

30. Wei JY, Spurgeon HA, Lakatta EG: Excitation-contradiction in rat myocardium: alterations with adult aging. *Am J Physiol* 246:H784-H791, 1984.

31. Sagie A, Benjamin EJ, Golderisi M, et al: Reference values for Doppler indexes of left ventricular diastolic filling in the elderly. *J Am Soc Echocardiogr* 6:570-576, 1993.

32. Petrofsky JS, Burse RL, Lind AR: Comparison of physiologic responses of men and women to isometric exercise. *J Appl Physiol* 38:863-868, 1975.

33. Swinne CJ, Shapiro EP, Lima SD, et al: Age-associated changes in cardiac performance during isometric exercise in normal subjects. *Am J Cardiol* 69:823-826, 1992.

34. Yin FC, Raizes GS, Guarnieri T, et al: Age-associated decrease in ventricular response to haemodynamic stress during beta-adrenergic blockade. *Br Heart J* 40:1349-1355, 1978.

35. Fleg JL, O'Connor FC, Gerstenblith G, et al: Impact of age on the cardiovascular response to dynamic upright exercise in healthy men and women. *J Appl Physiol* 78:890-900, 1995.

36. Fleg L, Lakatta EG: Normal aging of the cardiovascular system. In Aronow WS, Fleg JL (eds): *Cardiovascular Disease in the Elderly,* New York, Marcel Dekker, 2004.

37. Freeman, RV, Otto CM: Spectrum of calcific aortic valve disease: Pathogenesis, disease progression, and treatment strategies. *Circulation* 111:3316-3326, 2004.

38. Otto CM, Kuusisto J, Reichenbach DD, et al: Characterization of the early lesion in "degernarative" valvular aortic stenosis: histological and immunohistochemical studies. *Circulation* 90:844-853, 1994.

39. Olsson M, Dalsgaard CJ, Haegerstrand A, et al: Accumulation of T lymphocytes and expression of interleukin-2 receptors in nonrheumatic stenotic aortic valves. *J Am Coll Cardiol* 23:1162-1170, 1994.

40. O'Brien KD, Reichenbach DD, Marcovina SM, et al: Apoliopoproteins B, (a) and E accumulate in the morphologically early lesion of "degenerative" valvular aortic stenosis. *Arterioscler Thromb Vasc Biol* 16:523-532, 1996.

41. Olsson M, Thyberg J, Nilsson J: Presence of oxidized low density lipoprotein in nonrheumatic stenotic aortic valves. *Arterioscler Thromb Vasc Biol* 19:1218-1222, 1999.

42. Mohler ER, Gannon F, Reynolds C, et al: Bone formation and inflammation in cardiac valves. *Circulation* 103:1522-1528, 2001.

43. Cosmi JE, Kort S, Tunick PA, et al: The risk of the development of aortic stenosis in patients with "benign" aortic valve thickening. *Arch Intern Med* 162:2345-2347, 2002.

44. Faggiano P, Antonini-Canterin F: Progression of aortic valve sclerosis to aortic stenosis. *Am J Cardiol* 91:99-101, 2003.

45. Nair CK, Aronow WS, Sketch MH, et al: Clinical and echocardiographic characteristics of patients with mitral annular calcification: comparison with age- and sex-matched control subjects. *Am J Cardiol* 51:992-995, 1983.

46. Nair CK, Thomson W, Ryschon K, et al: Long-term follow-up of patients with echocardiographically detected mitral annular calcium and comparison with age- and sex-matched control subjects. *Am J Cardiol* 63:465-470, 1989.

47. Fulkerson PK, Beaver BM, Anseon JL: Calcification of the mitral annulus. Etology, clinical associations, complications, and therapy. *Am J Med* 66:967-977, 1979.

48. Roberts WC, Perloff JK: Mitral valvular disease. A clinicopathologic survey of the conditions causing the mitral valve to function normally. *Ann Intern Med* 77:939-975, 1972.

49. Karl S, Pearlman SD, Touchstone DA, et al: Prevalence and mechanism of mitral regurgitation in the absence of intrinsic abnormalities of mitral leaflets. *Am Heart J* 118:963-972, 1989.

50. Aronow WS, Kronzon I: Correlation of prevalence and severity of mitral regurgitation and mitral stenosis determined by Doppler echocardiography with physical signs of mitral regurgitation and mitral stenosis in 100 patients aged 62 to 100 years with mitral annular calcium. *Am J Cardiol* 60:1189-1190, 1997.

51. Pearlman JD, Touchstone DA, Esquival L: Prevalence and mechanisms of mitral regurgitation in the absence of intrinsic abnormalities of the mitral leaflets. *Am Heart J* 118:963-972, 1989.

52. Labovitz AJ, Nelson JG, Windhorst DM, et al: Frequency of mitral valve dysfunction from mitral annular calcium as detected by Doppler echocardiography. *Am J Cardiol* 55:133-137, 1985.

53. Osterberger LE, Goldstein S, Khaja F, et al: Functional mitral stenosis in patients with massive annular calcification. *Circulation* 64:472-476, 1981.

54. Aronow WS, Koenigsberg, Kronzon I, et al: Association of mitral annular calcium with new thromboembolic stroke and cardiac events at 39-month follow-up in elderly patients. *Am J Cardiol* 65:1511-1512, 1990.

55. Savage DD, Garrison RJ, Castelli WP: Prevalence of submitral (annular) calcium and its correlates in a general population-based sample (the Framingham Study). *Am J Cardiol* 51:1375-1378, 1983.

56. Nair CK, Sudhakaran C, Aronow WS, et al: Clinical characteristics of patients younger than 60 years with mitral annular calcium: Comparison with age- and sex-matched control subjects. *Am J Cardiol* 54:1286-1287, 1984.

57. Nair CK, Sketch MH, Desai R, et al: High prevalence of symptomatic bradyarrhythmias due to atrioventricular node-fascicul *Am Heart J* 103:226-229, 1982.

58. Fulkerson PK, Beaver BM, Auseon JC, Graber HL: Calcification of the mitral annulus:etiology, clinical associations, complications and therapy. *Am J Med* 66:967-977, 1979.

59. Aronow WS, Ahn C, Kronzon I, et al: Association of mitral annular calcium with new thromboembolic stroke at 44-month follow-up of 2,148 persons, mean age 81 years. *Am J Cardiol* 81:105-106, 1998.

60. Tolstrup K, Roldan CA, Qualls CR, et al: Aortic valve sclerosis, mitral annular calcium, and aortic root sclerosis as markers of atherosclerosis in men. *Am J Cardiol* 89:1030-1034, 2002.

61. Rubin DC, Hawke MW, Plotnick GD: Relation between mitral annular calcium and complex intraaortic debris. *Am J Cardiol* 71:1251-1252, 1993.

62. Adler Y, Motro M, Shemesh J, et al: Association of mitral annular calcium on spiral computed tomography (dual-slice mode) with thoracic aorta calcium in patients with systemic hypertension. *Am J Cardiol* 89:1420-1422, 2002.

63. Boston Area Anticoagulation Trial for Atrial Fibrillation Investigators: The effect of low-dose warfarin on the risk of stroke in patients with nonrheumatic atrial fibrillation. *N Engl J Med* 323:1505-1511, 1990.

64. Stein JH, Soble JS: Thrombus associated with mitral valve calcification. A possible mechanism for embolic stroke. *Stroke* 26:1697-1699, 1995.

65. Lin C-S, Schwartz IS, Champman I: Calcification of the mitral annulus fibrosus with systemic embolization. *Arch Pathol Lab Med* 111:411, 1987.

66. Aronow WS, Koenigsberg M, Kronzon J, et al: Association of mitral annular calcium with new thromboembolic stroke and cardiac events at 39-month follow-up in elderly patients. *Am J Cardiol* 59:181-182, 1987.

67. Cheitlin MD, Aronow WS: Mitral regurgitation, stenosis, and annular calcification. In Aronow WS, Fleg JL (eds): *Cardiovascular Disease in the Elderly,* New York, Marcel Dekker, 2004.

68. Schott CR, Kotler MN, Parry WR, et al: Mitral annular calcification: Clinical and echocardiographic correlations. *Arch Intern Med* 137:1143-1150, 1977.

69. Burnside JW, DeSanctis RW: Bacterial endocarditis on calcification of the mitral annulus fibrosus. *Ann Intern Med* 76:615-618, 1972.

70. Dajani AS, Taubert KA, Wilson W, et al: Prevention of bacterial endocarditis. Recommendations by the American Heart Association. *Circulation* 96:358-366, 1997.

71. Aronow WS, Ahn C, Shirani J, et al: Comparison of frequency of new coronary events in older subjects with and without valvular aortic sclerosis. *Am J Cardiol* 83:599-600, A8, 1999.

72. Fox CS, Vasan RS, Parise H, et al: Framingham Heart Study. Mitral annular calcification predicts cardiovascular morbidity and mortality: the Framingham Heart Study. *Circulation* 107:1492-1496, 2003.

73. Benjamin EJ, Plehn JF, D'Agostino RB, et al: Mitral annular calcification and the risk of stroke in an elderly cohort. *N Engl J Med* 327:374-379, 1992.

74. Olsen MH, Wachtell K, Bella JN, et al: Aortic valve sclerosis relates to cardiovascular events in patients with hypertension (a LIFE substudy). *Am J Cardiol* 95:132-136, 2005.

75. Aronow WS, Ahn C, Shirani J, et al: Comparison of frequency of new coronary events in older subjects with and without valvular aortic sclerosis. *Am J Cardiol* 83:599-600, 1999.

76. Barasch E, Gottdiener JS, Marino-Larsen EK, et al: Clinical significance of calcification of the fibrous skeleton of the heart and aortosclerosis in community dwelling elderly. The Cardiovascular Health Study (CHS). *Am Heart J* 151:39-47, 2006.

77. Benjamin 1992, Boon, 1997, Cao JJ, et al: C-Reactive protein, carotid intima-media thickness, and incidence of ischemic stroke in the elderly: The Cardiovascular Health Study. *Circulation* 108:166-170, 2003.

78. Adler Y, Levinger U, Koren A, et al: Association between mitral annulus calcification and peripheral arterial atherosclerotic disease. *Angiology* 51:639-646, 2000.

79. Adler Y, Koren A, Fink N, et al: Association between mitral annulus calcification and carotid atherosclerotic disease. *Stroke* 29:1833-1837, 1998.

80. Nair CK, Aronow WS, Sketch MH: Clinical and echocardiographic characteristics of patients with mitral annular calcification comparison with sex-matched control subjects. *Am J Cardiol* 51:1373-1378, 1983.

81. Ross R: Atherosclerosis: an inflammatory disease. *N Engl J Med* 340:115-126, 1999.

82. Mohler III ER, Gannon F, Reynolds C, et al: Bone formation and inflammation in cardiac valves. *Circulation* 103:1522-1528, 2001.

83. O'Brien KD, Shavelle DM, Caulfield MT, et al: Association of angiotensin-converting enzyme with low-density lipoprotein in aortic valvular lesions and in human plasma. *Circulation* 106:2224-2230, 2002.

84. Novaro GM, Sachar R, Pearce GL, et al: Assocation between apolipoprotein E alleles and calcific valvular heart disease. *Circulation* 108:1804-1808, 2003.

85. Agmon Y, Khandheria BK, Jamil Tajik A, et al: Inflammation, infection and aortic valve sclerosis: Insights from the Olmstead County (Minnesota) population. *Atherosclerosis* 174:337-342, 2004.

86. Levy D, Garrison RJ, Savage DD, et al: Prognostic implications of echocardiographically determined left ventricular mass in the Framingham Heart Study. *N Engl J Med* 1990:322:1561-1566.

87. Levy D, Garrison RJ, Savage DD, et al: Left ventricular mass and incidence of coronary heart disease in an elderly cohort: The Framingham Heart Study. *Ann Intern Med* 110:101-107, 1989.

88. Gardin JM, McClelland R, Kitzman D, et al: M-mode echocardiographic predictors of six- to seven-year incidence of coronary heart disease, stroke, congestive heart failure, and mortality in an elderly cohort (the Cardiovascular Health Study). *Am J Cardiol* 87:1051-1057, 2001.

89. Savage DD, Levy D, Dannenberg AL, et al: Association of echocardiographic left ventricular mass with body size, blood pressure and physical activity (the Framingham Study). *Am J Cardiol* 65:371-376, 1990.

90. Tsang T, Barnes M, Bailey K, et al: Left atrial volume: important risk marker of incident atrial fibrillation in 1655 older men and women. *Mayo Clin Proc* 76:467-475, 2001.

91. Barnes ME, Miyasaka Y, Seward JB, et al: Left atrial volume in the prediction of first ischemic stroke in an elderly cohort without atrial fibrillation. *Mayo Clin Proc* 79:1008-1014, 2004.

92. Tsang TS, Barnes ME, Gersh BJ, et al: Prediction of risk for first age-related cardiovascular events in an elderly population: the incremental value of echocardiography. *J Am Coll Cardiol* 42:1199-1205, 2003.

93. Moller J, Hillis G, Oh J, et al: Left atrial volume: a powerful predictor of survival after acute myocardial infarction. *Circulation* 107:2207-2212, 2003.

94. Rossi A, Cicoira M, Zanolla L, et al: Determinants and prognostic value of left atrial volume in patients with dilated cardiomyopathy. *J Am Coll Cardiol* 40:1425-1430, 2002.

95. Kizer JR, Bella JN, Palmieri V, et al: Left atrial diameter as an independent predictor of first clinical cardiovascular events in middle-aged and elderly adults: The Strong Heart Study (SHS). *Am Heart J* 151:412-418, 2006.

96. Tsang, TSM, Abhayaratna WP, Barnes ME, et al: Prediction of cardiovascular outcomes with left atrial size: Is volume superior to area or diameter? *J Am Coll Cardiol* 47:1018-1023, 2006.

97. Kannel WB: Epidemiological aspects of heart failure. *Cardiol Clin* 7:1-9, 1989.

98. Kitzman DW, Gardin JM, Gottdiener JS, et al: Importance of heart failure with preserved systolic function in patients = 65 years of age. CHS Research Group. Cardiovascular Health Study. *Am J Cardiol* 87:413-419, 2001.

99. Gottdiener JS, Arnold AM, Aurigemma GP, et al: Predictors of congestive heart failure in the elderly: The Cardiovascular Health Study. *J Am Coll Cardiol* 35:1628-1637, 2000.

100. Senni M, Tribouilloy CM, Rodeheffer RJ, et al: Congestive heart failure in the community: A study of all incident cases in Olmsted County, Minnesota, in 1991. *Circulation* 98:2282-2289, 1998.

101. Vasan RS, Larson MG, Benjamin EJ, et al: Congestive heart failure in subjects with normal versus reduced left ventricular ejection fraction: Prevalence and mortality in a population-based cohort. *J Am Coll Cardiol* 33:1948-1955, 1999.

102. Oh JK, Hatle L, Tajik, AJ, et al: Diastolic heart failure can be diagnosed by comprehensive two-dimensional and Doppler echocardiography. *J Am Coll Cardiol* 47:500-506, 2006.

103. Badano, LP, Albanese, MC, DeBiaggio PD, et al: Prevalence, clinical characteristics, quality of life, and prognosis of patients with congestive heart failure ad isolated left ventricular diastolic dysfunction. *J Am Soc Echocardiogr* 17:253-261, 2004.

104. Philbin, EF, Rocco TA Jr, Lindenmuth NW, et al: Systolic versus diastolic heart failure in community practice: Clinical features, outcomes, and the use of angiotensin-converting enzyme inhibitors. *Am J Med* 109:605-613, 2000.

105. Tsutsui, H, Tsuchihashi M, Takeshita A, et al: Mortality and readmission of hospitalized patients with congestive heart failure and preserved versus depressed systolic function. *Am J Cardiol* 88:530-533, 2001.

106. Redfield, MM, Jacobsen SJ, Burnett, et al: Burden of systolic and diastolic ventricular dysfunction in the community: appreciating the scope of the heart failure epidemic. *J Am Med Assoc* 289:194-202, 2003.

107. Arruda AM, Das MK, Roger VL, et al: Prognostic value of exercise echocardiography in 2632 patients ≥65 years of age. *J Am Coll Cardiol* 37:1036-1041, 2001.

108. Smart S, Sagar K, Tresch D: Age-related determinants of outcome after acute myocardial infarction: a dobutamine-atropine stress echocardiographic study. *J Am Geriatr Soc* 50:1176-1185, 2002.

109. Anthopoulos LP, Bonou MS, Kardaras FG, et al: Stress echocardiography in elderly patients with coronary artery disease: Applicability, safety and prognostic value of dobutamine and adenosine echocardiography in elderly patients. *J Am Coll Cardiol* 28:52-59, 1996.

110. Camerieri A, Picano E, Landi P, et al: Prognostic value of dipyridamole echocardiography early after myocardial infarction in elderly patients. Echo Persantine Italian Cooperative (EPIC) Study Group. *J Am Coll Cardiol* 22:1809-1815, 1993.

111. Sicari R, Pasanisi E, Venneri L, et al: Echo Persantine International Cooperative (EPIC) Study Group; Echo Dobutamine International Cooperative (EDIC) Study Group. Stress echo results predict mortality: a large-scale multicenter prospective international study. *J Am Coll Cardiol* 41:589-595, 2003.

112. Elhendy A, van Domburg RT, Bax JJ, et al: Safety, hemodynamic profile, and feasibility of dobutamine stress technetium myocardial perfusion single-photon emission CT imaging for evaluation of coronary artery disease in the elderly. *Chest* 117:649-656, 2000.

113. Hiro J, Hiro T, Reid CL, et al: Safety and results of dobutamine stress echocardiography in women versus men and in patients older and younger than 75 years of age. *Am J Cardiol* 80:1014-1020, 1997.

114. Ranhosky A, Kempthorne-Rawson J: The safety of intravenous dipyridamole thallium myocardial perfusion imaging. Intravenous Dipyridamole Thallium Imaging Study Group. *Circulation* 81:1205-1209, 1990.

115. Lam JY, Chaitman BR, Glaenzer M, et al: Safety and diagnostic accuracy of dipyridamole-thallium imaging in the elderly. *J Am Coll Cardiol* 11:585-589, 1988.

116. Anthopoulos LP, Bonou MS, Kardaras FG, et al: Stress echocardiography in elderly patients with coronary artery disease: applicability, safety and prognostic value of dobutamine and adenosine echocardiography in elderly patients. *J Am Coll Cardiol* 28:52-59, 1996.

117. Hashimoto A, Palmer EL, Scott JA: Complications of exercise and pharmacologic stress tests: Differences in younger and elderly patients. *J Nucl Cardiol* 6:612-619, 1999.

118. Sherman DG, Dyken ML, Fisher M, et al: Antithrombotic therapy for cerebrovascular disorders. *Chest* 95:140S-155S, 1989.

119. Boon A, Lodder J, Cheriex E, Kessels F: Risk of stroke in a cohort of 815 patients with calcification of the aortic valve with or without stenosis. *Stroke* 27:847-851, 1996.

120. Petty GW, Khanderia BK, Whisnant JP, et al: Predictors of cerebrovascular events and death among patients with valvular heart disease. A population-based study. *Stroke* 31:2628-2635, 2000.

121. Blum A, Reisner S, Farbstein Y: Transesophageal echocardiography (TEE) vs. transthoracic echocardiography (TTE) in assessing cardiovascular sources of emboli in patients with acute ischemic stroke. *Med Sci Monit* 10:CR521-CR523, 2004.

122. Gambini C, Paciaroni E: The role of transesophageal echocardiography in the diagnosis of ischemic stroke in the elderly. *Arch Gerontol Geriatr* 20:37-42, 1995.

123. Josselson AJ, Pruitt RD, Edwards JE: Amyloid disease of the heart. *Med Clin North Am* 34:1137, 1950.

124. Pomerance A: The pathology of senile cardiac amyloidosis. *Br J Pathol Bacteriol* 91:357, 1966.

125. Pitkänen P, Westermark P, Cornwell GC III: Senile systemic amyloidosis. *Am J Pathol* 117:391-399, 1984.

126. Cornwell GG III, Murdoch WL, Kyle RA, et al: Frequency and distribution of senile cardiovascular amyloid. A clinicopathologic correlation. *Am J Med* 75:618-623, 1983.

127. Hodkinson HM, Pomerance A: The clinical significance of senile cardiac amylodosis: a prospective clinico-pathologic study. *Q J Med* 46:381-387, 1977.

128. Wright JR, Calkins E: Amyloid in the aged heart: frequency and clinical significance. *J Am Geriatr Soc* 23:97-103, 1975.

129. Shah PM, Abelmann WH, Gersh BJ: Cardiomyopathies in the elderly. *J Am Coll Cardiol* 10(suppl A):77A-79A, 1987.

130. Johansson B, Westermark P: Senile systemic amyloidosis: A clinico-pathological study of twelve patients with massive amyloid infiltration. *Int J Cardiol* 32:83-92, 1991.

131. Smith TJ, Kyle RA, Lie JT: Clinical significance of histopathologic patterns of cardiac amyloidosis. *Mayo Clin Proc* 59:547, 1984.

132. Kyle RA, Spittell PC, Gertz MA, et al: The premortem recognition of systemic senile amyloidosis with cardiac involvement. *Am J Med* 171:395-400, 1996.

133. Lie JT, Hammond PI: Pathology of the senescent heart: Anatomic observations on 237 autopsy studies of patients 90-105 years old. *Mayo Clin Proc* 63:552, 1988.

Chapter 40

Echocardiographic Evaluation of the Patient with a Systemic Embolic Event

EDMOND W. CHEN, MD • RITA F. REDBERG, MD, MSc

Cerebrovascular Ischemia

Stroke, a sudden development of a focal neurologic deficit, remains the third leading cause of death in the United States, accounting for about 1 out of every 15 deaths and the second leading cause of death globally.[1,2] In the United States, in 2003 alone, there were 700,000 strokes that contributed to 273,000 deaths and about one million hospitalizations. With stroke prevalence now at 5.5 million individuals (using 2003 data), total cost (direct and indirect economic burden) is estimated to have reached $57.9 billion in 2006.[2]

Approximately 10% of all diagnosed strokes occur in patients younger than 45 years of age, with variable prevalence reported across different racial and ethnic groups.[3-7] Up to 40% of strokes occur in patients without occlusive cerebrovascular disease; and it is estimated that the source is of cardiac origin in 15% to 20% of the cases.[8,9] Another 30% to 40% (100,000 to 200,000 per year) are in the category of stroke of undetermined cause, also known as cryptogenic stroke, defined by the Trial of ORG 10172 in Acute Stroke Treatment (TOAST) classification as brain infarction that is not attributable to a source of definite cardioembolism, large artery atherosclerosis, or small artery disease despite extensive vascular, cardiac, and serologic evaluation.[9-16]

Because diagnostic imaging modalities have become more routine and widely available, an increasing num-

TABLE 40–1. Stroke Occurrence by Type

Type of Stroke	Occurrence (%)
Atherosclerotic thrombosis	20
Lacunae	5-10
Embolism	20
Hemorrhage	10-20
Vascular	5
Indeterminate	35-40

ber of findings have been observed in these subjects with embolic and cryptogenic stroke and have been suggested as potential origin of these cerebrovascular events (Table 40–1). Although for most of these conditions, a definitive causal relationship is yet to be proven, promising research especially in the therapeutic front is underway.

Cardiac tumors can be a source of emboli, but the most commonly implicated sources are thrombi from the left atrial appendage or left ventricle, left atrial spontaneous contrast, atrial septal aneurysm associated with a patent foramen ovale (PFO), thrombi traversing a PFO (i.e., paradoxical emboli), valve vegetations (infected or sterile), fibrinous mitral valve strands, protruding aortic atheroma of the aortic arch and ascending aorta, and emboli associated with mitral and aortic prostheses.

Echocardiography has proven to be invaluable in defining the cause of cerebrovascular ischemia in patients without occlusive cerebrovascular disease or where additional diagnostic information can influence the choice of therapeutic options, such as anticoagulation.[17-21] This chapter discusses indications for, clinical value of, and the limitations of transthoracic echocardiography (TTE), transesophageal echocardiography (TEE), and contrast echocardiography in this setting; particular emphasis is placed on the utility and insights provided by TEE in cases of stroke and the impact of echocardiography on patient management.

Transthoracic Echocardiography

Indications

As with many diagnostic challenges, the workup for an embolic event includes taking a comprehensive patient history, performing a complete physical examination, relevant laboratory evaluation, and obtaining an electrocardiogram (ECG), often followed by a carotid duplex ultrasound (US). If significant carotid stenosis is identified, some centers proceed with surgical endarterectomy, preceded often with magnetic resonance angi-

ography or less routinely performed today, cerebral angiography. In recent years, especially in those with increased perioperative risks, carotid angioplasty has become increasingly popular.[22,23]

In the search for a cardiac source of emboli, if there is no evidence of cardiac disease indicated by the history, physical examination, or electrocardiogram, the yield of findings from a TTE for the identification of a source of lesions usually is less than 1%.[24-28] A pooled analysis of 13 studies found that TTE yielded a source incidence of 0.7% in patients with no cardiac history; in patients with clinical cardiac abnormalities, the yield increased to 13%.[29] In a review of 280 patients between 19 and 96 years of age who underwent TTE for assessing suspected systemic emboli, Come and colleagues[24] found a 35% incidence of abnormalities that might have predisposed patients to systemic embolism and a 4% incidence of lesions that were possibly or probably responsible for emboli. Among patients who had known cardiovascular disease, 47% of them had associated abnormalities that might have predisposed to systemic embolism and 4% had lesions possibly or probably responsible for emboli. In contrast, the group without cardiovascular disease, the rates were 14% and 0%, respectively.

In another study of 138 patients with one or more recent episodes of focal cerebral ischemia, in whom a cardiac mechanism was suspected or no probable mechanism of ischemia was identified, intracardiac thrombus was found in 9 patients (6.5%); 32 patients (23.2%) had other cardiac disorders, possibly related to the ischemic event; and the remaining 97 patients (70.3%) had study results that were normal or added nothing to the clinical findings. Two-dimensional (2D) echocardiography was of limited value in assessing patients with no clinical cardiac disease or hypertension only; it was more valuable for patients known to have cardiac disease, especially atrial fibrillation (AFib).[26]

Routine echocardiography can be considered in the evaluation of patients suspected of cerebral embolism, although the yield is low.[29-32] In particular, routine echocardiography is now recommended for young patients especially those 45 years of age or younger who have experienced an embolic event.[32,33] This is partly due to a higher likelihood that the identifiable abnormality may be an attributable source of cerebral embolism as opposed to concurrent cerebrovascular disease associated with the degenerative process of aging in the elderly.[32] Many of the findings associated with cerebrovascular ischemia in this age group, such as PFO, spontaneous echocardiographic contrast (SEC), and atrial septal aneurysm, are best seen by TEE. However, the utility of TEE has not yet been established, and it is not clear whether any of these findings are actually a cause of embolism or whether these findings mandate specific treatment (Table 40–2). For older patients (>65 years), a growing body of data implicates atheromas in the

TABLE 40–2. Echocardiographic Evaluation of Cardiac Source of Embolus

	H&P Factors That Increase the Likelihood of This Finding	Age Group	Best Diagnostic Test
Probable Source of Embolus			
Left atrial thrombus	Mitral valve disease, atrial fibrillation	Any age	TEE
LV thrombus	CAD, history of myocardial infarction	>50 years	TTE
Vegetation, mitral or aortic (>10 mm)	Fever, weight loss, changing murmurs	Any age	TEE (preferred)/TTE
Myxoma	Systemic symptoms	Any age	TTE/TEE
Possible Source of Embolus			
PFO	No specific	<55 years	TTE with contrast
Atrial septal aneurysm	No specific	<55 years	TEE
Left atrial size >4 cm	Mitral value disease, decreased LV compliance	Any age	TTE
Aortic atheroma	CAD, advanced age	>60 years	TEE
Prostheses, mitral or aortic	Varied	Any age	TEE
Rheumatic mitral valve disease	History of rheumatic fever	Any age	TTE
Mitral annular calcification	Advanced age	>55 years	TTE
Atrial septal defect	No specific or decreased exercise tolerance	<40 years	TEE (preferred)/TTE
Fibrinous valve strands	No specific	Any age	TEE
Mitral valve prolapse	Atypical CP, early systolic murmur	Any age	TTE
Vegetation (<10 mm)	Fever	Any age	TEE (preferred)/TTE
LV aneurysm	CAD	>50 years	TTE
Dilated cardiomyopathy	Fatigue, reduced exercise tolerance	Any age	TTE

Ao, aorta; ASA, atrial septal aneurysm; CAD, coronary artery disease; CP, chest pain; H&P, history and physical; LA, left atrium; LAA, left atrial appendage; LV, left ventricular; MAC, mitral annular calcification; MV, mitral valve; MVP, mitral valve prolapse; PFO, patent foramen ovale; SEC, spontaneous echo contrast; TEE, transesophageal echocardiography; TTE, transthoracic echocardiography; –, patients without cardiovascular disease; +, patients with cardiovascular disease.

aorta as a source of embolic events, which may increase the yield of TEE findings in this group as well.

Findings and Techniques

Left Atrial Size

TTE is an excellent method to evaluate left atrial size. The left atrial diameter can be measured in the parasternal long-axis and short-axis views by M-mode or directly from the 2D image (online or offline). Normally, the left atrial diameter is less than 4 cm. Measurements of left atrial diameter should be made at end-systole, from leading edge to leading edge. M-mode echocardiography has been shown to predict angiographic left atrial area,[34] but it has limitations that compromise accurate volume estimates. 2D volumetric measurement is generally preferred and correlates well with cine-computed tomographic measurements of atrial volume.[35-38]

The left atrium is best imaged in the two-chamber and four-chamber apical views, with the patient in steep left recumbency and with suspended respiration. Atrial volume can then be calculated by a single-plane area-length method from each view or by using the biplane method of discs. Normal left atrial volume is approximately 36 mL or 20 mL/m^2. This volume is increased in athletes.[39]

The atrial appendage, especially in enlarged atria, can sometimes be visualized in the apical views. Occasionally, a particularly large thrombus can be seen in the enlarged left atrium by TTE (Fig. 40–1). The sensitivity of TTE for the detection of left atrial thrombus is 25% to 57% overall and 63% to 83% for left atrial cavity thrombus. Specificity is 94% to 99%, as confirmed at surgery. Most thrombi occur, however, in the left

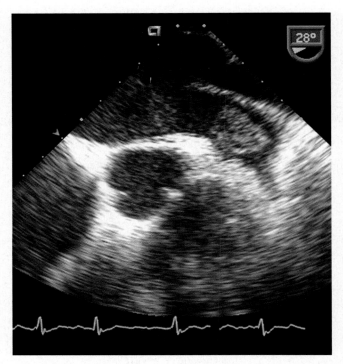

Figure 40–1. Left atrial thrombus seen on transesophageal echocardiography. This 75-year-old woman had congestive heart failure with enlarged left atrium and was in atrial fibrillation. There was no intrinsic mitral valve disease. (Courtesy of Bill PC Hsieh, MD.)

atrial appendage, which is a posterior structure, and the sensitivity of TTE for detecting left atrial appendage thrombi drops to 0% to 16%.[40-42] An enlarged left atrium, particularly in a patient with AFib, may have an intraatrial thrombus, suggesting the need for TEE to better visualize left atrial appendage thrombus or the need for presumptive anticoagulation.

Mitral Annular Calcification

Despite a number of studies that have suggested an association between mitral annular calcification and stroke,[26,28,43-48] the role of mitral annular calcification in stroke remains unclear. In an analysis of M-mode echocardiograms in 1159 members of the Framingham study, Benjamin and colleagues[49] contended that mitral annular calcification was an independent risk factor for stroke, especially embolic stroke. This association was maintained in subjects without AFib, congestive heart failure (CHF), or clinically apparent coronary artery disease (CAD). These authors postulated that the mechanism may be calcific emboli or that the mitral annular calcification may serve as a nidus for thrombus.[49] In another prospective study of 2148 subjects, patients with mitral annular calcification were more likely to suffer a cerebrovascular event, with a risk ratio of 2.6 ($P = 0.001$). This risk was further increased in the presence of mitral stenosis (MS) and AFib;[47] however, the Stroke Preven-

tion in Atrial Fibrillation-II (SPAF-II) trial of 568 patients failed to find such an association.[50] A prospective cohort study of 657 patients with mitral annular calcification identified by 2D echocardiography showed no increased incidence of stroke.[51]

Mitral annular calcification is easily detected by TTE. Using 2D criteria, it is best identified in the same views in which the mitral valve is seen: the parasternal long-axis and short-axis views, and the two-chamber and four-chamber apical views. Mitral annular calcification is visually defined as increased echo-density in the mitral annulus, which is a C-shaped structure and distinct from the mitral valve. Annular calcification occurs posteriorly, may extend toward the base of the heart, and can appear to infiltrate the myocardium. Extensive mitral annular calcification can obscure visualization of the thin mitral valve leaflets and can cause decreased mitral valve excursion, although usually not severe MS.

Mitral annular calcification can be graded as mild, moderate, or severe. Autopsy studies reveal this condition in approximately 10% of patients.[52,53] It is associated with obesity, elevated systolic blood pressure, aging, aortic stenosis (AS), coronary artery disease, and hypertrophic obstructive cardiomyopathy. It is found predominantly in elderly women, with an incidence of 12% in women over 70.[52] Mitral annular calcification occurs earlier in patients who are undergoing renal dialysis, and it may be associated with the presence of aortic atheroma as well.[54,55] Perhaps because mitral annular calcification is often a marker atherosclerotic disease, patients with mitral annular calcification often have an increased risk of both cardiovascular and cerebrovascular events.[48,56-59]

Left Ventricular Wall Motion and Thrombus

TTE is an excellent method for evaluating left ventricular (LV) wall motion abnormalities and thrombus in most patients. The identification of wall motion abnormalities, particularly of an aneurysm, greatly increases the likelihood of finding an associated LV thrombus.

These masses generally are seen in the setting of wall motion abnormalities, particularly anterior and apical, or cardiomyopathy (Fig. 40–2). Thrombi are visually defined as a distinct mass of echoes in the LV cavity that are seen clearly throughout the cardiac cycle in at least two different echocardiographic views. They appear as irregular sessile or mobile structures that are contiguous with the endocardium in an area of abnormal wall motion, such as ischemic or infarcted myocardium.

Thrombi are best seen in the four-chamber apical view by TTE because the transducer is closest to the cardiac apex in this view. Identification of thrombi can be made more certain by using off-axis views that are directed toward or across the apex. In some cases, the transducer may be directed inferiorly or caudally across

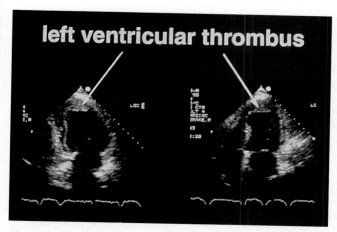

left ventricular thrombus

Figure 40–2. Left ventricular apical thrombus seen in the two-chamber (left) and four-chamber (right) views in transthoracic echocardiography from a 56-year-old man with ischemic cardiomyopathy. The thrombus appears as a cap adherent to the apex. (Courtesy of Ray Stainback, MD.)

the apical impulse location, the "back-handed" apical view. In this process, it is best to use a high-frequency transducer (3.5 or 5 MHz). This view combined with the use of a higher-frequency transducer increase the examiner's ability to detect apical thrombus. Rarely, thrombi may form in the left ventricle, in the setting of transient ischemia or coronary spasm, with normal wall motion seen by echocardiography. Thrombi also are seen in patients with dilated cardiomyopathies (DCMs) secondary to ischemic or nonischemic causes. In difficult cases, especially with TTE images, intravenous (IV) contrast agent can be used to better delineate the endocardial border thereby, augmenting the image and potentially enhancing the quality of more subtle changes.

The incidence of embolization from ventricular thrombus in dilated cardiomyopathy is approximately 1% to 4% per year.[9,60-65] The independent risk factors for stroke are low ejection fraction (EF), older age, and the absence of aspirin or anticoagulation therapy. Thrombi that are protruding and mobile are most likely to embolize.[66] Echocardiography is useful in this setting to identify thrombi and to target patients who may benefit from anticoagulation.[9,43,62,66,67] Patients known to be at high risk for embolization, such as those in AFib or those with a history of previous embolization, may be considered for anticoagulation therapy with proper weighing of individual risks and benefits.

In cases of anterior myocardial infarction (MI), embolic risk is greatest in the first 3 months after the infarction.[67-72] After that period, the clot has organized and is less of an embolic risk, and 40% of clots resolve spontaneously.[73] More recent data suggest an increased incidence of stroke long after the initial infarction. In the Survival and Ventricular Enlargement (SAVE) trial, 2231 patients with LV dysfunction following an episode of MI were prospectively followed for a mean of 42 months. During the study, 4.6% of these patients experienced strokes, with an estimated 5-year rate of stroke of 8.1%.[74] Presently, anticoagulation therapy is recommended following MI in patients unable to take aspirin, patients with persistent AFib, and patients with LV thrombus. The American College of Cardiology and American Heart Association (ACC/AHA) Task Force on acute MI considers anticoagulation therapy a class I indication for patients with LV thrombus (for at least 3 months and indefinitely in patients without an increased risk of bleeding) and class II indication in patients requiring secondary prevention, having LV dysfunction and extensive regional wall motion abnormalities, and having severe LV dysfunction, with or without CHF.[75]

Transesophageal Echocardiography

Indications

TEE offers higher resolution imaging than TTE because the adjacent, airless imaging pathway allows the use of 5-MHz to 7.5-MHz probes. This advantage becomes particularly evident when studying structures close to the probe, such as the left atrium (and left atrial appendage) and thoracic aorta. All series that compare TTE with TEE show that the latter is superior for identifying potential sources of arterial emboli.[27,33,76-81]

The data for the effect of age on the usefulness of TEE in evaluating emboli are evolving. As stated previously, patients with no cardiac disease have an extremely low likelihood of positive findings on TTE, generally less than 1%. Even though TEE is superior to TTE in identifying potential sources of emboli in patients without known cardiac disease, overall yield is increased to only 1.6% in a pooled analysis.[29] Thus, patients with a history of ischemic stroke and who are under 45 to 55 years of age tend to have a low overall yield as well. Although some authorities recommend TEE evaluation of embolic events as the initial diagnostic test for patients younger than 45 to 55 years of age with no other heart disease,[32] others do not recommend such an approach.[29] In any case, this age group is less likely to have occlusive cerebrovascular disease. Findings best visualized by TEE, such as PFO, atrial septal aneurysm, atrial septal defect (ASD), and SEC, have been associated with embolic events in this group of patients. All comparative studies show a higher yield of diagnostic findings by TEE; what remains unclear is whether these possible and probable sources of embolism are truly responsible for ischemic events. This enigma is complicated by studies that have found occlusive cerebrovascular disease and probable or possible cardiac sources of emboli in the same patients.

Even in patients already on anticoagulation, findings from TEE may have incremental value and impact to the care of these patients. TEE-guided cardioversion is now a common practice, with reasonable safety profile.[82,83] In the original Assessment of Cardioversion Using Transesophageal Echocardiography (ACUTE) trial, one of the underlying assumptions was that the presence of thrombus is associated with an increased risk of thromboembolism associated with cardioversion. Of the 571 patients who underwent TEE, 6 patients (1.1%) had embolism and 79 (13.8%) had TEE-identified thrombus. Interestingly, for patients who had embolic events, none had a TEE-identified thrombus. Instead five of the six patients (83.3%) had one or more abnormal TEE findings of SEC, aortic atheroma, PFO, atrial septal aneurysm, and mitral valve strands. In fact, these TEE risk factors were more predictive of thromboembolic risk and provided statistically significant incremental value (chi-square 38.0; $p < 0.001$) for identification of risk. This underscored the importance of these potential risk factors and argues for perhaps for aggressive risk factor modification or more intense or prolonged anticoagulation even in patients who are already on oral anticoagulation.[84]

Findings and Techniques

Left Atrial Appendage Thrombus

Left atrial appendage evaluation is now an integral part of a complete TEE, especially in patients suspected of cardioembolic event.[85,86] Most left atrial thrombi occur in the left atrial appendage. Because the left atrium and its appendage are posterior structures lying in the far field of the image, the appendage is poorly visualized on TEE, so that TEE is necessary to look for a left atrial appendage thrombus. TEE has the advantages of higher frequency transducers and closer proximity to the left atrium. The sensitivity for detection of left atrial cavity and appendage thrombi by TEE is 90% to 95%, with a specificity of 95% to 100%.[41,42]

The left atrial appendage can be visualized in the basal transverse and longitudinal planes. Multiplane imaging optimizes views of the left atrial appendage. One is often able to see this structure most clearly at 30-degree rotation of the image plane. The appendage is easily recognized by its characteristic triangular structure (Fig. 40-3). It is important to be familiar with the appearance of a normal left atrial appendage because the appendage is traversed by pectinate muscles along its length. When one is familiar with the normal ridgelike appearance of the left atrial appendage, a thrombus is more easily recognized. Thrombus may be recognized by identifying a mobile or sessile, irregularly shaped, gray, textured density that is clearly separate from the lining of the atrial appendage (Fig. 40-4).

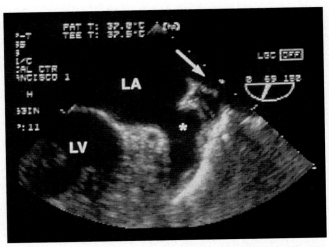

Figure 40-3. *Normal left atrial appendage (LAA) (asterisk) seen in a multiplane basal short-axis transesophageal echocardiographic view. Note the typical crescentic structure of the LAA and its normal ridged lining. The* arrow *identifies the left superior pulmonary vein (LSPV). There is a normal fibrous structure that separates the LAA and LSPV, which is nicknamed the "warfarin ridge" because it can be mistaken for a left atrial clot. LA, left atrium; LV, left ventricle.*

It is a clearly defined echo-dense intracavitary mass, acoustically distinct from the endocardium. Commonly associated echocardiographic features are increased left atrial size and SEC.

Left atrial appendage thrombi occur most often in patients who are in AFib, although 5% to 10% of left atrial thrombi are seen in patients who are in normal sinus rhythm and are without mitral valve disease. The incidence of left atrial thrombus identified by TEE in patients with systemic emboli ranges from 5% to 17% in reported series, with the incidence increasing in series in which a higher percentage of the patients studied had MS or AFib.

Left atrial appendage function predicts formation of spontaneous contrast and subsequent clot and should be an integral part of a TEE examination, especially in patients with concomitant AFib.[42,87-96] A complete evaluation of the left atrial appendage also includes evaluation of its velocity and flow pattern (see Chapter 41; Fig. 41-5). This can be done by placing a pulsed-Doppler sample volume in the left atrial appendage approximately 1 cm from the orifice, where normal left atrial appendage flow has been characterized. In a TEE study of left atrial flow in 109 patients, the forward left atrial appendage contraction wave was measured as 46±18 cm/s, followed by a retrograde filling wave of 46±17 cm/s in sinus rhythm. In 40% of patients in sinus rhythm, additional forward and retrograde velocities of 23±10 and 22±11 cm/s, respectively, were seen. In contrast, AFib was associated with reduced forward and retrograde flows in an irregular pattern.[97]

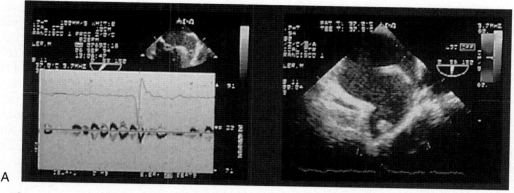

Figure 40–4. *A 47-year-old woman with atrial fibrillation who underwent transesophageal echocardiography before planned cardioversion. A, Pulsed Doppler sampling in the left atrial appendage shows a low-velocity fibrillatory pattern associated with stasis and thrombi. B, Transesophageal echocardiographic view of the left atrium showing chamber enlargement, spontaneous contrast, and left atrial appendage thrombus. (Courtesy of Ray Stainback, MD.)*

Reduced antegrade appendage flow velocity is associated with a higher incidence of left atrial thrombus. Mugge and colleagues[98] pointed out the usefulness of left atrial appendage function in assessing embolic risk. The association between atrial appendage thrombus in this structure and embolic stroke has been established, as has the association between appendage dysfunction and the tendency to form thrombus. The study demonstrated a strong association between atrial appendage thrombus and SEC in the atrial cavity and with embolic events if the appendage flow velocity fails to exceed 25 cm/s.[98] In the SPAF-III TEE substudy, 37% of the 382 patients showed flow velocity reduced to 20 cm/s or less, which was associated with a higher incidence of left atrial thrombus (17% compared with 5% in patients with higher velocity, $P < 0.001$).[99] Subsequent analysis of TEE findings of 721 patients in the SPAF-III study supported that finding. Multivariate analysis found antegrade flow velocity of less than 20 cm/s (relative risk 2.6; $P = 0.02$) to be associated with left atrial appendage thrombus.[100]

If left atrial appendage thrombus is seen by TEE, the patient should undergo anticoagulation therapy. Any correctable causes of left atrial dysfunction should be evaluated following satisfactory treatment and resolution of the thrombus. For example, if the patient is in AFib, cardioversion should be considered, as discussed in Chapter 41. If the patient has mitral valve disease, consideration of treatment—mitral valvuloplasty or surgery—is warranted (see Chapter 21).

Spontaneous Echocardiographic Contrast

SEC in the left atrium is a dramatic finding on echocardiography. It is defined as the presence of dynamic, smoke-like, swirling echoes.[101] To optimize detection of SEC, a high-frequency transducer (=5 MHz) should be used, and the entire left atrial cavity and appendage should be carefully imaged in a basal short-axis view and a four-chamber view. The gain and compression settings need to be optimized to avoid missing low-amplitude echoes. Spontaneous echocardiographic contrast is seen best with higher gains and can be differentiated from white-noise artifact by the characteristic swirling motion (Fig. 40–5). To maximize detection of intermittent left atrial SEC, sufficient time should be allowed for imaging. Because it depends on transducer frequency and gain settings of the instrument, SEC is difficult to quantitate. If frequencies higher than 5 MHz are used, low-intensity contrast can be seen in normal subjects without mitral regurgitation (MR) who have normal or slightly reduced cardiac output. If gain settings are too low or if there is bright light in the ex-

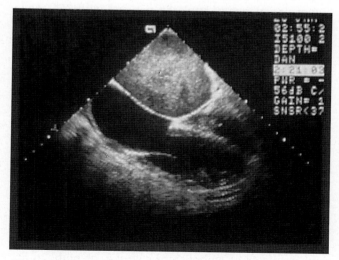

Figure 40–5. *Transesophageal echocardiography, four-chamber view, showing spontaneous contrast filling the dilated left atrium of this 70-year-old woman with rheumatic mitral stenosis. (Courtesy of Ray Stainback, MD.)*

amination setting (e.g., in the operating room [OR]), spontaneous contrast can be missed. This finding is best seen using a 5-MHz or greater frequency transducer, with the gain set high enough to create uniform low-level background noise throughout the atrium.

SEC can be seen by TTE[102] but is more frequently identified by TEE, reported in up to 20% of patients undergoing TEE in some centers.[103] This increased detection of SEC by TEE was confirmed in a larger study of 400 consecutive TEE patients, in whom SEC in the left atrium was seen in 19%. SEC was not seen in any patient by TTE in this study.[104]

SEC can be found in the left atrial appendage, right atrium, left ventricle, or descending aorta. In all these sites, SEC generally is associated with a low-flow state and increased thrombotic risk, although there are rare reports of SEC in patients with no significant cardiac abnormalities.[103-109] SEC is thought to represent increased echo-genicity because of the aggregation of blood cells at low shear rates. A number of reports correlated local coagulation or systemic hematologic abnormalities, or both, such as anticardiolipin antibody, sedimentation rate, and fibrinogen levels, with an increased incidence of SEC.[109-113] In the SPAF-III study, plasma fibrinogen greater than 35 mg/dL ($P < 0.001$) was associated with the identification of any SEC; however, dense SEC was associated only with age in the multivariate model.[109]

Furthermore, SEC can be found in the left atrium in conditions associated with stasis of blood in the left atrium, such as AFib, left atrial thrombus, and enlarged left atrium secondary to MS. Its incidence is increased in the setting of acute MI even with normal sinus rhythm.[114] In one report of TEE studies of 1288 patients in normal sinus rhythm, SEC was seen in 2% of the patients. The presence of SEC was associated with a higher prevalence of stroke in patients with SEC when compared with controls, (83% versus 56%; $P = 0.02$).[115] Abnormal left atrial appendage function is an important predictor of SEC formation and is frequently associated with AFib. Thus, reduced appendage function should prompt search or attention to possible SEC.[87-96]

SEC is also associated with age and MR.[101] However, SEC is not seen in patients with severe MR (unless the left atrium is large) probably because the mitral regurgitant jet agitates the left atrial blood pool. The absence of SEC in MR appears to be associated with decreased embolic risk.[116,117] In a large TEE study, MR was an independent predictor of the absence of SEC.[101] In this study of 400 patients, Black and colleagues[101] found SEC in 19%, 95% of whom showed AFib or MS. In MS and in nonvalvular AFib, SEC was the only independent predictor of embolism, or stroke, or both. In another study, SEC was found to carry a relative risk ratio of 10.6 for patients with MS in AFib compared to those without SEC. In a study of 47 patients with MS in sinus rhythm, Bernstein and colleagues[118] found that SEC did

not predict clinical events but was a predictor of more severe stenosis (i.e., it was a marker of stasis).

Even in the absence of AFib or mitral valve disorder, SEC may be more frequently observed in those with more severe LV dysfunction.[96] In a study of 500 consecutive patients with stroke, 10 out of 45 patients with sinus rhythm and depressed LV ejection fraction of 45% or lower had evidence of SEC. In multivariate analysis, ejection fraction of 35% or less and a left atrial appendage flow velocity of 55 cm/s or less were independent predictors of SEC or thrombus ($p < 0.05$).

Right atrial SEC is seen in conditions that promote stasis of right atrial blood, including AFib and an enlarged right atrium, as in cor pulmonale. It is less likely to be seen in patients with severe tricuspid regurgitation (TR). LV SEC is seen in states of low flow, such as cardiomyopathy and LV aneurysm.[66]

Descending aortic SEC has been associated with severe LV dysfunction leading to reduced cardiac output and low flow in the descending aorta. It also may be seen in the false lumen of patients with aortic dissection.[119,120]

Atrial Septum

Structures and findings in the atrial septum generally are better identified and characterized better by TEE than by other methods.

Atrial Septal Aneurysm. Atrial septal aneurysm has been identified in 1% of all patients in a large autopsy study;[121] it is seen in 0.2% of all TTE readings[122] and in 3% to 8% of all TEE readings.[79,123,124] In a population-based sample of 363 subjects in Olmsted County, Minnesota, the prevalence of atrial septal aneurysm found on TEE was 2.2%.[124] An atrial septal aneurysm appears as a redundant, highly mobile membranous portion of the atrial septum and is defined as a billowing or localized outpouching greater than 11 mm from the plane of the septum with a base of 1.5 cm.[125] It is associated with ASDs or PFO in up to 77% of cases.[78,124,126] The speculation is that atrial septal aneurysm may be a remnant, perhaps, of a healed ASD. It has been suggested that the presence of right-to-left shunt (which occurs up to 78% of the patients with atrial septal aneurysm), may be the underlying mechanism by which systemic embolism may occur.[79,124,127-130]

The best view for identifying an atrial septal aneurysm by TTE is the parasternal short-axis view at the level of the atria. It also may be visualized in the four-chamber apical view or in the subcostal view. However, for definitive diagnosis, TEE is superior to TTE. In a review of 195 cases, only 53% of cases of TEE-identified atrial septal aneurysms were diagnosed with TTE.[129] The best view for identifying an atrial septal aneurysm by TEE is the basal longitudinal view at the level of the atrial septum or the four-chamber view using the transverse plane at the level of the midesophagus. To define an atrial septal aneurysm, measurements of the total excursion of the localized bulging of the septum primum should be made. If the bulging occurs consistently into either atrium, excursion should be measured from the maximal point of the bulging to an imaginary line connecting the nonaneurysmal segments of the septum primum at the base of the aneurysm. The distance between the maximal extent of aneurysmal bulging and this imaginary line is considered the excursion distance. If there is cardiorespiratory variation in the excursion of the aneurysm, the maximal distance of excursion into either atrium should be added to determine the total phasic excursion. Atrial septal aneurysm can be classified according to its intrusion into the left or right atrium and to its motion during respiratory cycle.[79] One group recently proposed a classification scheme based on the direction of bulging. They suggested that each subtype may have different clinical correlates;[131] however, this scheme awaits further validation. Alternatively, atrial septal aneurysm can also be classified based on its association with PFO or perforation(s) and has suggested utility in transcatheter correction.[132]

The association of atrial septal aneurysm with stroke remains unclear. Recently, in the Stroke Prevention Assessment of Risk in a Community (SPARC) study of 363 subjects with a history of cerebral embolism, atrial septal aneurysm was more frequently identified (7.9% versus 2.2% of controls, odds ratio 3.65; $P = 0.002$); and, in 86% of the patients with atrial septal aneurysm, TEE failed to identify other potential causes.[124] In a prospective study of 42 patients with a history of atrial septal aneurysm, however, who were identified from 846 patients who had undergone cardiac surgery, no association was shown between stroke and atrial septal aneurysm. During the mean follow-up of 69.5 months, no patient demonstrated any cerebrovascular or embolic event.[133] Similarly in a study of 581 patients with an ischemic stroke of unknown origin who received aspirin, no recurrence was observed in those with isolated atrial septal aneurysm. However, the presence of both atrial septal aneurysm and PFO was associated with a significant risk of recurrent stroke (hazard ratio [HR], 4.17; 95% confidence interval [CI], 1.47 to 11.84).[134,135] Like PFO, transcutaneous and surgical correction techniques are available; however, their utility has not been proven. Likewise, medical therapy has yet to be defined. In the 630 patient Patent Foramen Ovale in Cryptogenic Stroke (PICSS) study, the presence of atrial septal aneurysm (11.5%, 69 out of 600 patients with interpretable TEEs) did not modify the risk of recurrent stroke or death associated with PFO, and no difference in outcome between aspirin and warfarin therapy was observed among patients with both an atrial septal aneurysm and a PFO.[136]

Lipomatous Hypertrophy. It may be difficult to appreciate lipomatous hypertrophy by TTE because the atrial septum sits in the far field of the image, where beam-spread artifact often obscures the details of the septum. On TEE, the entity appears as a characteristic dumbbell-shaped interatrial septum that involves the septum primum and venous portions but always spares the PFO (Fig. 40-6). In some cases, this entity can be mistaken for a tumor, but its sessile behavior, location, and fatty nature identify it as benign. It is more common with aging and may be associated with diabetes. There is no specific treatment indicated (except to avoid surgery for tumor).

Lipomatous hypertrophy of the interatrial septum has been suggested to be associated with arterial embolization and pulmonary emboli[137] and with arrhythmias and sudden death.[138] However, in the TEE in SPARC thickness of interatrial septum (IAS) was carefully measured ($n = 384$) and found to be related to the aging process and not correlated with atherosclerotic risk factors.[139]

Contrast Technique. Agitated saline contrast study is useful for identifying a PFO or ASD but must be undertaken meticulously.[140] The saline contrast technique requires a three-way stopcock and sterile normal saline. A syringe containing 3 mL of normal saline and 0.1 mL of air is attached to one part of the stopcock, and an empty syringe is attached to the other stopcock; the third port is attached to a catheter (e.g., Intracath) placed in the antecubital vein. Contrast is then agitated by passing it forcefully between the two syringes until it has an opalescent appearance (Fig. 40-7). A vigorous

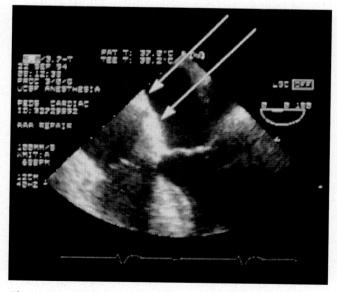

Figure 40-6. *Lipomatous septal hypertrophy* (arrows) *seen in a horizontal plane four-chamber transesophageal echocardiographic view of the atrial septum. Note the dumbbell-shaped appearance of the septum with the thin portion of the fossa ovalis separating the two lipomatous areas of septum, an incidental finding in a 68-year-old man undergoing vascular surgery.*

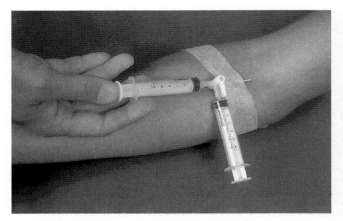

Figure 40–7. *Set-up for a saline contrast injection. A three-way stopcock is attached to a 20-gauge intracatheter in the patient's antecubital vein with two syringes attached. A saline and air mixture is then added, agitated until milky white, and vigorously injected during echocardiographic imaging.*

bolus injection is made into the antecubital vein while the atrial septum is being visualized. Massaging and elevating the upper arm can facilitate arrival of the bolus of contrast medium into the heart, as can the use of at least a 20-gauge catheter. Increased quantities of saline (up to 10 mL) can be used if the contrast effect is inadequate, particularly in larger patients. Contrast is seen passing from the right to the left atrium if there is a patent communication and right atrial pressure exceeds left atrial pressure.

Atrial Septal Defect. ASDs can be a route for paradoxical emboli. Defects are identified on 2D echocardiography using the same views as previously described for identifying atrial septal aneurysm. As with other findings in the atrial septum, identifying ASDs is readily increased by the use of TEE[141,142] and is particularly applicable for detecting sinus venosus defects.[143] ASDs may be suspected or identified using 2D echocardiography and should be confirmed by Doppler echocardiography (Fig. 40–8) and by the use of contrast. An ASD is identified by a negative contrast effect (Fig. 40–9), the lack of contrast resulting from blood flow across the ASD, thus "washing out" the contrast from the right atrium. Although there may be a transient rise in right atrial pressure during early systole, the contrast injection can be reliably performed during the resting state and during provocative maneuvers that transiently raise right atrial pressure above left atrial pressure, such as Valsalva's maneuver or a cough.

The appearance of contrast in the left atrium provides only a qualitative assessment of interatrial shunting; the actual shunt fraction cannot be measured by this technique. Other echocardiographic indicators, however, such as right-chamber enlargement, suggest a hemodynamically significant left-to-right shunt.

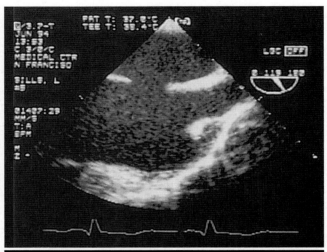

A

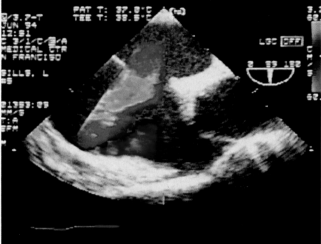

B

Figure 40–8. *This 44-year-old woman was evaluated for decreasing exercise tolerance and a murmur. Transthoracic echocardiograph showed right-sided chamber enlargement. A, Biatrial multiplane transesophageal echocardiography view at 119 degrees shows dropout of the atrial septum and an enlarged right atrium. B, Color-flow Doppler in longitudinal view confirms the flow across the secundum atrial septal defect.*

Patent Foramen Ovale. PFO has been associated with cryptogenic stroke. It occurs in approximately 25% of all adult hearts as a consequence of the failure of the septum secundum to fuse to the septum primum over the foramen ovale. The foramen ovale is a one-way valve allowing flow from the right to the left atrium. In fetal life, the foramen ovale serves as a conduit for high-oxygen, high-glucose blood to reach the fetal heart and brain and usually closes within several hours of birth because of increased pulmonary resistance.

Visualization of the foramen ovale requires imaging directly over the interatrial septal foraminal area. The foramen lies within the thin portion of the fossa ovalis. Agitated saline contrast or color Doppler allows identification of a PFO. The atrial septum should be visualized and carefully aligned in the four-chamber apical

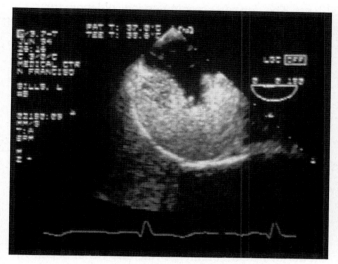

Figure 40–9. *Saline contrast injection in the patient seen in Figure 40–8 shows a negative contrast effect secondary to left-to-right flow across the atrial septal defect.*

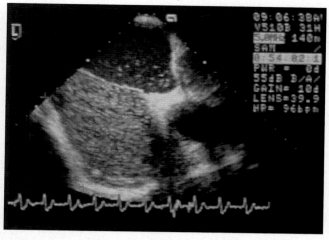

Figure 40–10. *This 48-year-old man had a history of transient ischemic attacks. Longitudinal plane transesophageal echocardiography biatrial view saline contrast injection shows opacification of the right atrium and multiple microbubbles passing into the left atrium, consistent with a patent foramen ovale.*

view. After contrast is injected, the echocardiogram should be closely observed for opacification of the right atrium with contrast and then for passage of microbubbles from the right atrium into the left atrium. A PFO is defined as the passage of more than three microbubbles from the right atrium to the left atrium within the first three cardiac cycles after opacification of the right atrium with contrast (Fig. 40–10).

If no bubbles pass with spontaneous respiration, during which there is reversal of atrial pressure gradient in early systole, the injections should be repeated while the patient is asked to perform Valsalva's maneuver. The patient should be asked to release the Valsalva strain as the right atrium begins to opacify. With a successful Valsalva maneuver, the atrial septum can be seen to bow transiently from right to left, indicating raised right atrial pressure. Inspiration during this maneuver may cause increased impedance secondary to lung expansion and thereby decrease the echocardiographic image quality or ever alter the imaging plane, and the echocardiographer should be prepared for this. If patients cannot perform Valsalva's maneuver, they may be asked to cough. The agitated saline contrast study, especially when combined with TEE and Valsalva maneuver is now widely regarded as the most sensitive test for detection of a PFO.[140,144] There are alternative techniques that may improve the sensitivity of PFO detection, especially when TTE is the imaging modality employed.[145,146] However, in cases in which definitive identification is important, again TEE is probably the test of choice.

TEE has increased the detection rate for PFO.[27] In a study of 238 patients that compared the value of transthoracic and transesophageal color Doppler and contrast echocardiography for detecting a PFO, a PFO was detected by contrast TEE in 22%, whereas only 8% were detected by contrast TTE. A PFO was detected in 50% of patients younger than 40 years of age and with otherwise unexplained ischemic stroke. A higher sensitivity is exhibited by TEE than for TTE for detecting PFO, and PFOs are observed in significant numbers in younger patients with embolic events.[77]

There have been numerous studies linking the presence of PFO with stroke, particularly in younger patients, defined as younger than 40 years,[147] 45 years,[148] or 55 years of age,[149] and in patients who have had cryptogenic stroke.[150] Lechat and colleagues[149] found the prevalence of PFO to be significantly higher in a group of patients under 55 years of age with stroke (40%) than in an age-matched control group (10%). The prevalence of PFO in this younger stroke group is as high as 40% to 74% in reported series.[151-153]

Because PFOs are a common finding and their size and permeability vary greatly, as presumably would their embolic risk, several studies have sought to define echocardiographically characteristics of "high-risk" PFO. Characteristics include larger PFOs and right-to-left shunting.[154-158] One study of PFO in patients with cerebral ischemia showed increased separation between the septum primum and septum secundum, increased mobility of the foramen ovale membrane and defects of larger size (2.8 versus 0.7 cm) than in patients without ischemia. Patients with these findings had a 12.5% recurrence rate of cerebral ischemia at 24 months ($P = 0.05$).[156] The same group later reported that in 101 patients with a PFO and a history of stroke, those who had PFO at rest and membrane mobility greater than 6.5 mm had a recurrent stroke rate of 16.3% compared to those with PFO only with maneuvers and mobility less than

6.5 mm (4.3%; $P = 0.05$).[158] In another contrast TEE study of 74 consecutive patients referred for ischemic stroke, 23 patients had PFO. Separating patients into those with strokes of determined origin versus cryptogenic strokes showed that the PFO dimension was significantly larger in patients with cryptogenic stroke than in those with an identifiable cause of stroke (2.1 to 1.7 versus 0.57 ± 0.78 mm; $P < 0.01$). The number of microbubbles crossing the interatrial septum was also greater in patients with cryptogenic stroke than in those with an identifiable cause of stroke (13.9 ± 10.7 versus 1.6 ± 0.8; $P < 0.0005$). The authors concluded that patients with cryptogenic stroke have larger PFOs with more extensive right-to-left interatrial shunting than patients with stroke of determined cause and that TEE is useful for identifying these characteristics.[155] When magnetic resonance imaging (MRI) and computed tomography (CT) imaging data of 95 patients with a history of ischemic stroke, who had undergone TEE, were analyzed, one study found that patients with larger PFOs had more abnormal findings. For example, superficial infarcts occurred more frequently in patients, who had PFOs 2 mm or longer, than in patients with no PFO or PFOs 2 mm or shorter (50% versus 21%; $P = 0.02$).[159]

Because approximately 25% to 30% of the normal population have PFO, other investigators have suggested caution in interpreting this finding as a cause of cerebral ischemia.[33,160-163] There are several reasons for the difficulties in extrapolating from the finding of a PFO by echocardiography or autopsy to the likelihood that this entity is responsible for a stroke. A PFO is a one-way valve that opens when right atrial pressure exceeds left atrial pressure, either transiently, such as during a Valsalva maneuver, coughing, or sneezing, or in conditions that cause chronically elevated right atrial pressure. For a stroke to occur, there must be a thrombus on the right side of the heart, presumably originating from a deep venous thrombosis (DVT), which happens to be passing through the heart at the same time that right atrial pressure is elevated. If there is not chronic right-sided pressure elevation, the investigator must postulate that the patient had a transient right-sided pressure elevation at the exact time of transit of the thrombus. Further complicating the interpretation of this echocardiographic finding, echocardiography detects a PFO of only 5 to 15 μm, the size of the microbubbles injected as contrast media, but a thrombus must be approximately 1 mm to cause a clinical event. A number of studies, however, found an association with deep venous thromboses and with embolic events in patients with PFO, providing a potential source for paradoxical embolism.[164,165] In a study of 227 patients, 56 were noted to have interatrial shunting. Fifty-three of the 56 patients underwent venography of the lower limbs. Five (9.5%) patients were noted to have acute deep venous thrombosis, of which four were clinically

silent. The authors recommended phlebography for patients with PFO and embolic event.[165]

If a PFO is identified in a patient with cerebrovascular ischemia, anticoagulation therapy with warfarin or aspirin has been suggested.[166] Unfortunately, existing data are largely derived from small retrospective series and heterogeneous populations. Because of the common occurrence of PFO in the population, causal relationship is difficult to establish. The true recurrence rate is unknown at this time, and as such, effects of potential therapeutic benefits from drugs, devices, or surgery are difficult to measure. In the Lausanne Stroke Study, 140 consecutive patients with clinical evidence of cerebral embolism and PFO were followed for a mean period of 3 years.[113] Only eight patients had a recurrent infarct (1.9% per year). In the French Study Group on Patent Foramen Ovale and Atrial Septal Aneurysm of 132 patients with PFO or atrial septal aneurysm, with mean follow-up of 22.6 months, only 8 patients had a stroke, yielding an actuarial risk of 2.3% at 2 years.[114] Using decision analysis, Nendaz and colleagues found that even when modeling the recurrence rate at 0.8% per year based on reported rates in the community, any therapeutic option may be potentially beneficial.[115] The presence of PFO was not associated with an increased risk of stroke in a prospective review of the 585 patients age 45 years or older in the SPARC study.[162] Similarly in a case-control study of 1072 residents in the Olmsted County, Minnesota, presence of PFO was not associated with an increased risk of stroke.[163] Interestingly, the French PFO-ASA study found that although isolated PFO or atrial septal aneurysm was each associated with a low recurrent rate, 2.3% and 0% over a 4-year period, the combination of PFO and atrial septal aneurysm was associated with excess recurrent stroke at 15.2% and was independent risk factor of recurrent stroke.[134]

In the PICSS, a substudy of the original Warfarin-Aspirin Recurrent Stroke Study (WARSS) study, PICSS randomized 630 patients with a history of recent ischemic stroke who underwent TEE to adjusted dose warfarin (target INR 1.4 to 2.8) or aspirin (at 325 mg/day). PFO was present in 204 patients (33.8%). There was no significant difference in the time to primary endpoints of recurrent ischemic stroke or death (HR, 1.17; 95% CI 0.60 to 2.37; 2-year event rates 14.3% versus 12.7%; $P = 0.84$). Size of PFO or the presence of atrial septal aneurysm did not modify outcome.[136] Obviously the role of medical therapy, especially which therapy (antiplatelet versus anticoagulation) remains undefined. Interestingly, in a retrospective review of 100 patients, 50% of whom had TEE-diagnosed PFO, the main effect of that diagnosis was the institution of warfarin and a trend toward aspirin discontinuation.[167]

Although surgical closure has demonstrated some success,[168,169] it is unclear when a surgical approach may be indicated. In a review of 5 studies of total of 161 patients, the annual rate of stroke 0.34% (95% CI, 0.01 to 1.89) and of stroke or death is 0.85% (95% CI, 0.10 to 3.07).[170] Despite high success rate, at least one report suggested that residual shunting may remain in a patients who underwent surgical closure of PFO and that surgical treatment of PFO cannot be considered gold standard for definitive therapy.[171] Recently transcatheter closure devices have become popular largely based on nonrandomized data. In a largest review of transcatheter closure device use in 403 patients from 1998 to 2004, namely the Cardia PFO occluder, newer generations of devices are associated with a lower annual thromboembolic event rate of two percent.[172] As suggested, given the uncertainties concerning indications for PFO closure for cryptogenic stroke, risk associated with any therapy or device (pharmacological or otherwise) must by necessity be low.[173,174] This cannot be overemphasized especially because there is increasing interest in exploring PFO closure for nonlethal conditions, such as migraine.[175-177] As the American Academy of Neurology concludes, there is insufficient evidence to recommend routine closure of PFOs in patients with cryptogenic stroke.[178] Until data from randomized controlled studies are available, careful assessment of risks and benefits is essential in determining the merits of antiplatelet, anticoagulation, transcatheter closure devices, or surgical correction for each individual. Given the uncertainties of cause and effect and lack of compelling evidence for any therapy, no specific recommendation can be made. However, specific echocardiographic findings, such as size and degree of shunt, may help identify patients at highest risk of recurrence where benefits may outweigh risks.

Chiari's Network

Chiari's remnant is a remnant of the right venous valve from fetal life. It runs from the inferolateral part of the right atrium and extends onto the atrial septum in the region of the lower portion of the limbus of the fossa ovalis. Also known as Chiari's network, it is a fenestrated, filamentous structure that typically has an undulating appearance in real-time imaging (Fig. 40–11). When not fenestrated, it is known as the eustachian valve or valve of the inferior vena cava, a normal structure. This structure can be seen in the right atrium by TTE in the four-chamber apical view and is even better visualized by TEE. It is easily identified in the bicaval (90-degree) view of the right atrium and can also be seen by looking at the basal short-axis view in the horizontal plane.

These structures are normal variants and should be differentiated from right atrial clots. Chiari's networks may retain their role from fetal life, when they facilitated flow from the inferior vena cava across the PFO. Data on Chiari's network is limited, but in one study of 1436 patients who underwent TEE, Chiari's network was

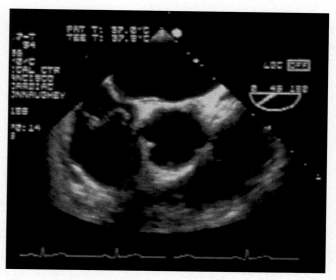

Figure 40–11. *Basal transesophageal echocardiographic view at 45 degrees showing the filamentous Chiari's network in the right atrium.*

present in 2% of the patients. It was more frequently associated with PFO (83% versus 28% control; $P < 0.001$) and atrial septal aneurysm (24%). Chiari's network was significantly more common in patients with unexplained embolic events than in patients evaluated for other indications (4.6% versus 0.5%; $P < 0.001$).[179]

Mitral Valve Strands

Several TEE studies have identified mitral valve strands in a high proportion of patients with a history of systemic embolism. The reported prevalence ranges widely, from 2% to 41%.[180-186] In a cohort of 1475 randomly selected subjects in Olmsted County, Minnesota, mitral valve strands were identified in 47% of patients, of whom 98% had no prior history of stroke.[187] The true prevalence, however, remains unknown.

Mitral valve strands appear as small, fine threadlike material arising from the atrial surface of the mitral valve and have motion independent of the valve. In the literature, the term *valve strand* is often used interchangeably with Lambl's excrescence or valve excrescence. Unfortunately, there is no uniform definition of this entity. Valve strands are more commonly associated with the mitral valve but can occur on the atrial side of the tricuspid valve and on the ventricular side of the aortic valve. They have also been identified on prosthetic valves.[127] The histology of mitral valve strands is unknown. They may represent degenerative changes of the leaflet because they are associated with calcified or thickened mitral valves. They may also represent thrombi, fibrin strands, torn chordae, or redundant leaflets. Gross examination of a mitral valve that had filamentous strands seen by TEE revealed the strands to be consistent with a Lambl's excrescence.

The role of mitral valve strands in cerebral embolism remains in question. A number of retrospective studies suggested a potential association with embolic events.[163,180-184] In one study, 9% of patients 50 years of age or younger had mitral valve strands as the only identified cardiac abnormality; however, aortic atheroma were not routinely investigated.[183] In the French Study of Aortic Plaques in Stroke, 284 patients with a history of stroke were prospectively followed for 2 to 4 years. Mitral valve strands were found in 22.5% of the 284 case patients compared with 12.1% of the controls. The presence of mitral valve strands was associated with an increased risk of stroke, with an odds ratio of 2.2 ($P = 0.005$). Further analysis, however, showed a lack of increase in recurrence of stroke.[184] In another prospective TEE study, patients with mitral valve strands were prospectively followed clinically and with repeat TEE. The prevalence of valve strands appeared similar in the both normal subjects and patients with a history of stroke, with a reported prevalence of up to 47% of the subjects. Not only was there no association with future embolic events, TEE findings of valve strands persisted unchanged over time.[185] Thus, the contribution of mitral valve strands in embolic stroke is likely small.

Intracardiac Tumors

Cardiac tumors are rare, with an incidence of 0.001% to 0.28% in autopsy series.[188] They can, however, be a source of embolus. Although stroke is not an uncommon complication of patients with malignancies, tumor embolization as a cause of stroke in these patients is exceedingly rare.[189] Cardiac metastases occur in 2% to 20% of patients with malignancies, most commonly lung or breast cancer. The most common primary cardiac tumors are myxomas, 80% of which occur in the left atrium, attached to the fossa ovale by a stalk. They can usually be recognized with TTE by their typical location and appearance (Fig. 40–12). Myxomas often contain cysts and may have dermal elements such as

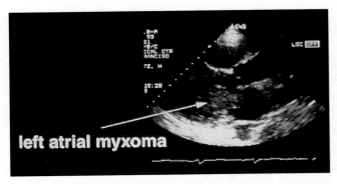

Figure 40–12. This patient is a 62-year-old woman with symptoms of weight loss and syncope. Transthoracic echocardiographic showed large left atrial myxoma that prolapsed through mitral valve in the parasternal long-axis view.

bone, giving them a calcified appearance. TEE, however, has the advantages of better localizing the stalk, more clearly defining the characteristic heterogeneous appearance and mobility, and identifying any involvement of or any damage to the mitral valve[190,191] (Fig. 40–13). These advantages are invaluable in planning the surgical approach because these tumors, once identified, should always be removed in view of their embolic potential-highly mobile tumors with broad bases of attachment have much higher embolic potential than the well-encapsulated variety.[192]

Lambl's Excrescences and Papillary Fibroelastomas

Myxomas also occur on valves, but valve tumors are most often fibroelastomas.[193,194] Papillary fibroelastomas are rare, accounting for 7% to 8% of nonmalignant cardiac tumors. They usually are discovered at autopsy, with an autopsy incidence of 0.002% to 0.33%, although the detection rate in their premorbid stage is higher with increasing use of echocardiography. They have a characteristic appearance on echocardiography and are commonly attached to a left-sided valve. They are usually found in older patients (>60 years), although they have been reported in patients ranging from 3 to 86 years of age.

The literature is confusing because of a profusion of names for the same entity; *cardiac papilloma, papillary fibroma, giant Lambl's excrescence,* and *papillary endocardial tumor* have all been used to describe what is properly called a *papillary fibroelastoma.* Some reports differentiate Lambl's excrescences from papillary fibroelastomas by composition and location; Lambl's excrescences lack the rich acid mucopolysaccharide matrix and smooth muscle cells that are found in papillary fibroelastomas, which occur along the line of valve closure at contact points and are more likely to occur in multiples (Fig. 40–14).

Papillary fibroelastomas have multiple papillary fronds and can appear like a sea anemone attached to the endocardial surface of the valves by a small pedicle. They rarely exceed 1 cm in diameter. Lambl first described them in 1856 as small filiform projections on the cusps of aortic valves. These tumors can form a nidus for platelet and fibrin aggregation and lead to systemic or neurologic emboli.

They are most commonly identified on the valves as left-sided valvular structures much more commonly than as right-sided structures. They have also been found on the chordae and papillary apparatus, LV septum, left ventricular outflow tract (LVOT), LV free wall, and the left atrium.[195,196] Clinical manifestations include such conditions as cerebral embolism,[197] MI,[198] sudden death,[199] pulmonary embolism (PE),[200] and syncope.[201] In one striking case, a 3.5-year-old child was diagnosed with acute embolic stroke. Evaluation,

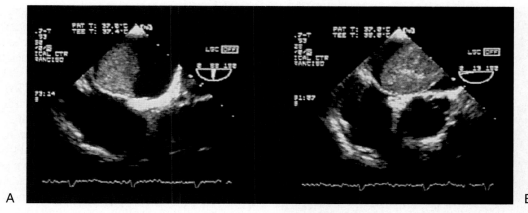

Figure 40–13. *A 30-year-old woman whose physical examination was remarkable for a diastolic rumble and tumor plop. She underwent transesophageal echocardiography before myxoma resection. Biatrial longitudinal view (A) and biatrial horizontal view (B) show left atrial myxoma with a heterogeneous appearance; it is attached to the interatrial septum. (Courtesy of Ray Stainback, MD.)*

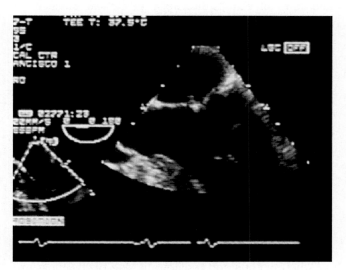

Figure 40–14. *Small mass seen attached to the mitral valve consistent with Lambl's excrescence.*

which included echocardiography, revealed papillary fibroelastoma as the only potential source.[202]

A review of echocardiograms at the Mayo Clinic from 1980 to 1995 found 54 patients with an echocardiographic diagnosis of papillary fibroelastomas; 17 of these patients were confirmed by pathologic diagnosis. They represented 0.019% of all patients who underwent echocardiographic evaluation during this period of time. TEE was more helpful in identifying the condition than was TTE. Most of the tumors (81.5%) were found on the valvular endocardium, usually on the left side. Despite the association with valvular surfaces, valvular dysfunction is uncommon. The echocardiographic finding included small pedunculated tumors (usually <1.5 cm), with a refractive appearance and intratumoral echolucency. Embolic events were observed in 20% of these patients. Surgical resection in

this study was curative, with no new embolic events occurring at follow-up.[195] Rarely, papillary fibroelastoma can be multiple affecting different areas of the heart.[203,204]

In general surgical resection is preferred in symptomatic patients, especially if valvular integrity can be preserved.[205,206] Anticoagulation therapy has been recommended when asymptomatic papillary fibroelastomas are identified or in nonsurgical candidates; surgical excision is recommended for patients with a history of embolic events. These recommendations are based on anecdotal observations and not on data from clinical trials.

Valvular Vegetation

Acute bacterial endocarditis with deposition of vegetative material on one of the cardiac valves is another possible source of cardiac embolus (see Chapter 22). Systemic embolization is observed in about one third of cases, with up to 65% of these events involving the central nervous system (CNS).[207-211] Most embolic events are observed during the first 2 weeks of therapy.[212]

Echocardiography is useful for identifying vegetations. Localization of vegetations to the precise cusp of attachment is possible by M-mode echocardiography, but only masses larger than 5 mm in diameter can be detected by M-mode methods.[213] Even when 2D imaging supplanted M-mode echocardiography as the imaging mode of choice, sensitivity for vegetation detection remained suboptimal.[214] This sensitivity was improved when TEE was used in the study of endocarditis[215] (Fig. 40–15).

In the early 1990s, several studies examined the difference in sensitivity between TTE and TEE.[216-220] Although specificity for both TTE and TEE is high (98% to 100%), the sensitivity of TTE is 44% to 60% for vegetation, and the sensitivity of TEE is 88% to 100%.[32,221]

In a study of TTE for the diagnosis of endocarditis, a group at Duke University[222] looked at the site, size, mo-

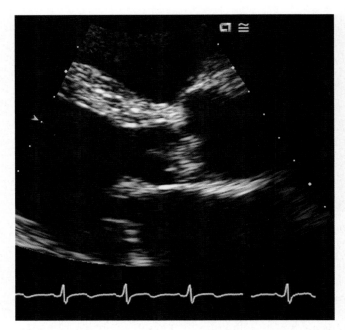

Figure 40-15. This 64-year-old man who presented with fever and cerebral and peripheral emboli underwent aortic valve replacement. Transthoracic echocardiographic long-axis view showing aortic vegetation. (Courtesy of Elizabeth Ryan, MD.)

bility, shape, and attachment of vegetations. There was high interobserver agreement on the presence and location of vegetations but less agreement on the size, mobility, and shape. Vegetation size was helpful in predicting emboli, with vegetations larger than 10 mm more likely to embolize (>50% versus 42%). Generally, findings from TTE were not helpful in predicting complications. In one study in which 57 patients with acute infective endocarditis underwent both TTE and TEE, neither modality helped predict embolic complications.[210]

In a similar study using TEE, Mugge and colleagues[223] also found that the only echocardiographic finding predictive of embolic events was the size of the vegetation mass. They found a stronger association between vegetation size and embolic events than in the Duke study. This association was particularly true for mitral valve vegetations, perhaps owing to the increased sensitivity of transesophageal imaging (Fig. 40-16). In this study, vegetations larger than 10 mm were more likely to embolize (46% versus 20%; $P < 0.001$). Other researchers also have found that the size of the vegetation is related to the chance of embolization.[222,224-226] Vegetations on the mitral valve are thought to have the highest embolic risk for cerebrovascular events.[227,228]

In a recent prospective multicenter study, 384 consecutive patients with definite diagnosis of infective endocarditis by Duke criteria underwent TEE. Echocardiographic findings of maximal vegetation length greater than 10 mm (odds ratio 9; $P = 0.004$) and severe vegetation mobility defined as prolapsing vegetation that

crosses the cooptation plane of the leaflets during cardiac cycle (odds ratio 2.4; $P = 0.04$) independently predicted risk of new embolic events. In particular, vegetation length of 15 mm or greater was associated with an 80% increased risk of death in 1 year ($P = 0.02$).

The American Heart Association (AHA) consensus panel now recommends routine echocardiography in patients suspected of infective endocarditis. In particular, TEE is central to the diagnosis of infective endocarditis and is indicated especially in patients with moderate to high clinical suspicion for infective endocarditis and in endocarditis with high risk features, such as large or mobile vegetations, valvular insufficiency, suggestion of perivalvular extension, or secondary valvular dysfunction, or if the patients are difficult to image with TTE.[32,229] Repeat or follow-up TEE is also of significant value.[229] Despite the compelling value, diagnostically and prognostically,[221,230] confusion regarding indications and roles of echocardiography in clinical practice remains common, leading to potential misuse.[231,232]

Intraoperative Transesophageal Echocardiography

Neurologic sequelae from cardiopulmonary bypass surgery are increasingly recognized as common. In particular, stroke is a reported complication that occurs in 2% to 6% of procedures.[233,234] Interestingly, the prevalence of neurological complications in some series is on the rise, perhaps a reflection of the change in recipients of cardiopulmonary bypass surgery (i.e., patients undergoing such surgery today are higher risks with more comorbidities than in previous decades). There are several insights from TEE studies that show promise for reducing this serious complication.

Atheromatous aortic plaque is one of the most important risk factors for embolic events during cardiac surgery. One possible explanation could be that placement of the aortic cannula may dislodge the plaque; this is especially likely for a mobile and protruding atheroma. Other maneuvers that may dislodge the aortic atheroma during cardiopulmonary bypass surgery are overaggressive palpation, aortic cross-clamping, anastomosis of proximal vein grafts to the ascending aorta, and the "sandblast" effect of high-pressure cannula flow against the aortic wall. Intraoperative TEE monitoring allows identification of plaque location, and the anesthesiologist or cardiologist can guide the surgeon in placement of the aortic cannula to avoid plaque. Guidance of cannula placement by TEE has been more accurate than direct palpation in identification of aortic atheroma in the operating room.[18,235,236] There is evidence that intraoperative TEE guidance to avoid atheroma during cannula placement can decrease the risk of stroke.[237-239] Katz and colleagues[237] reported a case of intraoperative TEE monitoring dur-

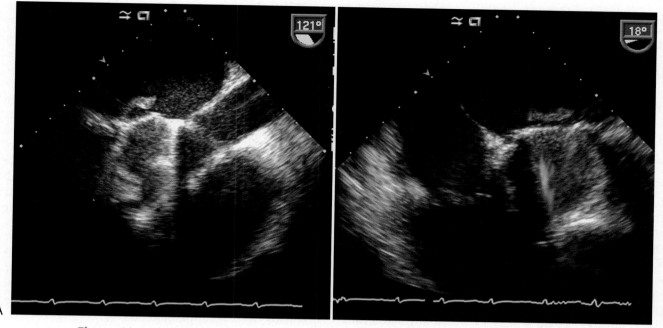

Figure 40–16. *This 68-year-old woman presented with fevers 1-year post–mitral valve replacement. A, Transesophageal echocardiographic view shows mechanical mitral prosthesis with a vegetation protruding into the left atrium. Shadowing from mitral prosthesis is noted. B, Four-chamber transesophageal echocardiographic view of the same vegetation. (Courtesy of Bill PC Hsieh, MD.)*

ing cardiopulmonary bypass in which a mobile atheroma was seen to disappear as the cannula was inserted into the arch in the region of the atheroma. The patient awoke with a neurologic deficit.

Other techniques that have been used in an attempt to reduce embolic events during cardiopulmonary bypass surgery include hypothermic circulatory arrests, a long aortic cannula, and aortic arch débridement in patients at high risk for emboli, as determined by TEE.[235,240] Aortic arch endarterectomy, however, has been found to be associated with a higher risk of intraoperative stroke.[241] Epiaortic surface imaging may be even more accurate than TEE in identifying aortic plaque[241] because it allows the most precise localization of plaque and avoids the shadowing that can obscure imaging in the anterior portion of the aorta, particularly if multiplane TEE is not available.

Thoracic Aortic Atheroma

Atheromatous changes in the thoracic aorta are now recognized as an important risk factor for embolic events. Because of their location, TEE is by far the imaging modality of choice.[242-244] To image the descending aorta, it is best to start from the transgastric view. The TEE probe should be rotated 180 degrees from the transgastric view and withdrawn slowly into the esophagus. The depth of field can be adjusted to 4 to 6 cm because the descending aorta is quite close to the esophagus. This magnifies the image and facilitates identifying intimal thickening and plaque. The distance of the probe tip from the incisors should be annotated every 5 cm and at any point where there is an abnormality. Biplane or multiplane probes should be used for imaging, whenever possible. A systematic approach including frequent fine manipulation and magnification is essential, especially to characterize the location and features of the atheromatous plaques. Meticulous attention to optimal contrast gain is also important. Often a reduction of contrast and change in harmonic setting can help prevent overlooking more subtle abnormalities.

To examine the aortic arch, the probe should be rotated anteriorly at approximately 20 cm from the incisors. This structure is best imaged with biplane or multiplane technology. Further manipulation can help identify atherosclerotic changes near the innominate arteries as well. It is best to image the arch at the conclusion of the TEE examination because many patients experience reflex gagging at this insertion level, and the probe can then be withdrawn after completion of aortic arch imaging. Atherosclerotic plaque often involves the arch and descending thoracic aorta. The atherosclerotic changes are commonly graded from I to IV (Table 40–3).

Atherosclerotic changes in the aorta are common in the general population. In an autopsy series of 500 consecutive patients, ulcerated plaques were detected in 5% of the patients with no history of cerebrovascular disease. In patients with a history of stroke, however, the prevalence of plaque at this site was 26%.

TABLE 40–3. Grading of Aortic Plaques

Class	Characteristics
I	Normal intimal
II	Minimal intimal thickening
III	Raised irregular plaque <5 mm
IV	Complex protruding plaque with ≥5 mm thickness, ulceration, or calcified density

In patients who had cerebral infarcts without hemorrhage, the prevalence was 28%.[245] In a prospective study of 120 autopsies, aortic arch atheroma was associated with increased risk of stroke (HR, 5.8; 95% CI, 1.1 to 31.7).[246] In case-control studies of patients with a history of stroke who underwent TEE, the prevalence ranges from 14% to 33%. On the other hand, ulcerated plaques are only seen in 5% of the control patients in these studies.[247-256] In studies in which any significant aortic atheroma in patients with a history of ischemic stroke is considered, the prevalence is approximately 27%.[249-257] The prevalence of significant aortic arch disease is approximately 14%.[248,258]

Since the embolic potential of aortic atheromas was first described by Tunick and Kronzon[247] in 1990, numerous papers have documented an association between atheromatous changes in the aorta and systemic emboli.[247-255] Atheromas at highest risk for embolization are those that protrude 4 mm or more into the aortic lumen or are pedunculated and have freely mobile components (Fig. 40–17). Amarenco and colleagues[248] using TEE in a prospective case-control study of 250 patients over 60 years of age, discovered a higher incidence of plaque 4 mm or thicker in the ascending aorta and proximal arch in patients with no known explanation for stroke, compared with a control group of cerebrovascular-accident patients with known or possible causes of stroke (28% versus 8%). After adjustment for atherosclerotic risk factors, the odds ratio for ischemic stroke among patients with such plaques was 9.1. Plaques 4 mm or thicker in the aortic arch were not associated with AFib or stenosis of the extracranial internal carotid artery. In contrast, plaques that were 1 to 3.9 mm thick were frequently associated with carotid stenosis of 70% or greater. These results confirm a strong, independent association between atherosclerotic disease of the aortic arch and the risk of ischemic stroke, especially for thick plaques.[248] More recently, Tanaka and colleagues noted that more moderate atheroma of 3.5 mm or greater was frequently observed in patients with undetermined cause of stroke and an independent predictor of subsequent cardiovascular event.[259]

Not only does aortic plaque pose an apparent risk factor for the first stroke, but also thoracic aortic atheroma 4 mm or thicker predicts recurrent events. In a follow-up study of 331 patients admitted for stroke, originally described by Amarenco and colleagues[248] the incidence of recurrent stroke was 11.9 per 100 person-years in patients with atheroma 4 mm or thicker compared with those whose aortic-wall thickness was 1 to 3.9 mm and less than 1 mm (P < 0.001). After adjusting for other potential risk factors for stroke, the presence of aortic plaques 4 mm or thicker was found to be an independent predictor of recurrent stroke.[258] In a smaller study, Dressler and colleagues also noted a high recurrent stroke rate of 38% in 1 year.[260] Interestingly, in the SPAF-III substudy, complex aortic atheroma independently predicted increased risk of stroke.[261] Complex aortic atheroma independently predicted risk of recurrence, also at 12% per year.[99]

In addition, patients with complex aortic atheroma are at risk for vascular embolic events. In a prospective TEE study of the risk of vascular events in patients with protruding aortic atheromas, 42 of 521 patients had protruding atheromas and no other source of emboli. They

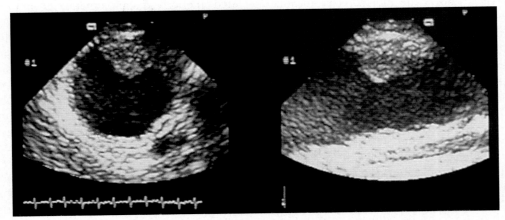

Figure 40–17. This 70-year-old man was undergoing coronary artery bypass grafting. A, Horizontal plane transesophageal echocardiographic view of the descending aorta shows a large aortic atheroma protruding into the aortic lumen. Intimal thickening and irregularity are also noted. B, Longitudinal transesophageal echocardiographic view of the same plaque.

were followed for up to 2 years and compared with a control group without atheromas, matched for age, gender, and hypertension. In 42 patients with atheromas, 14 (33%) had 19 vascular events (five brain, two eye, four kidney, one bowel, seven lower extremity) during follow-up; in 42 control patients, 3 (7%) had vascular events (two brain and one eye). Univariate analysis identified only protruding atheromas as significantly correlating with events, and multivariate analysis showed that only protruding atheromas independently predicted events.[262] In the French Study of Aortic Plaques in Stroke, the incidence of vascular events was 26 per 100 person-years of follow-up.[99] In a follow-up study of echocardiographic correlates of vascular events, the same group noted with interest that ulceration did not increase the risk of vascular events. The lack of calcification markedly increased the risk of subsequent vascular events (relative risk of 10.3, $P < 0.001$). The authors postulated that the lack of calcification may be associated with more vulnerable plaques.[263]

In contrast, an analysis from the SPARC study found that aortic plaque 4 mm or thicker was not associated with a significant increase in risk of neurological events.[264] Similarly, a recent population-based case-control study based in Olmstead County failed to demonstrate a significant association between complex aortic atheroma and the incidence of neurological events.[265] However, given the small number of patients with such aortic lesions, these studies may be underpowered to show any discernable difference.

Pathophysiologically, limited evidence suggests embolic strokes probably result from thromboembolic occlusion by the mobile elements in these complex aortic plaques. In a pathologic and TEE study, the mobile elements seen on TEE intraoperatively appeared on pathologic examination to be thrombi. For identification of thrombus, TEE had a sensitivity of 91% and a specificity of 90%.[266] In a separate pathologic and TEE study, again the mobile elements seen intraoperatively in the aorta were associated with thrombosis that was confirmed pathologically.[267] In 1998, Freedberg and colleagues described a case report of a patient with protruding atheroma who died of an embolic phenomenon. For the first time, emboli from these atheroma were visualized in transit on TEE.[268] Together these studies provide a plausible pathologic basis for thromboembolism in patients with aortic atheromas.

A high risk of embolic events related to invasive procedures also has been shown in patients with aortic atherosclerosis, particularly those patients with pedunculated aortic plaques.[269-271] In one study of patients with aortic arch disease and atheroma 5 mm or thicker, 17% of the 59 patients suffered an embolic event following cardiac catheterization through the femoral approach compared with 3% of controls ($P = 0.01$). Similarly, 5 of 10 patients who underwent placement of intraaortic balloon pump experienced an embolic event

compared with zero events in 12 controls ($P = 0.02$).[270] If possible, TEE examination of the thoracic aorta in selected patients should be performed before invasive aortic procedures such as left-sided heart catheterization and intraaortic balloon pulsation. If pedunculated plaque or mobile thrombus is identified, invasive aortic procedures should be undertaken only with the understanding of an increased embolic risk in these patients. Some operators prefer to perform left-sided heart catheterization from the arm, using the Sones technique in these high-risk patients-for whom TEE is key in identification-if angiography is indicated. Because aortic atherosclerosis seen by TEE is a marker for coronary artery disease,[259,272,273] patients at high risk for emboli often are the ones who need invasive procedures.

The treatment of atheromatous plaque is not well defined. Earlier reports of peripheral embolization in patients on warfarin raised concerns about the safety of anticoagulation in these patients.[274] The increasing use of warfarin in clinical practice, however, has thus far been found to be safe. Perhaps the largest controlled experience with warfarin is in the area of AFib. In SPAF-III, as discussed previously, patients with complex aortic plaques in the setting of AFib have a fourfold increased rate of stroke ($P = 0.005$). The use of warfarin decreased the risk by as much as 75% ($P = 0.02$).[99] A number of uncontrolled studies have all found a lower incidence of stroke with the use of warfarin.[252,260,275] The lack of randomized controlled data makes rational treatment challenging.

Interestingly, atheromatous lesions may be dynamic in nature. Montgomery and colleagues[276] performed serial TEE examinations in patients with significant atheromatous disease of the aorta. No intervention was prescribed. During a 20-month period, 7 of the 10 patients with severe atherosclerotic aortic disease developed a new mobile lesion. The same number of patients showed resolution of a previously documented mobile lesion. Of note, only one clinical embolic event was documented in these patients.[276] Tunick and colleagues examined 519 patients with severe aortic plaques retrospectively.[277] The use of antiplatelet or warfarin was not associated with a reduction of new embolic events. The need for better clinical data is clear.

In the Detection and Management of Associated Atherothrombotic Locations in Patients with a Recent Atherothrombotic Ischemic Stroke (DETECT) survey, Leys and colleagues evaluated 753 patients with ischemic stroke and identified 47.5% of the patients with associated atherosclerosis of coronary artery disease, aortic atheroma, or peripheral arterial disease. In particular, aortic atheroma was noted in 17% of the patients, underscoring the high probability of concomitant atherosclerotic disease, and regardless of the need for potential anticoagulation, the need for aggressive risk factor modification is clear.[278] In another study of 245 consecutive patients who underwent TEE for stroke of undetermined origin, long-term survival was assessed. In a mean follow-up period of 3 (1.4 to 4.8) years, death occurred in 19.2% of patients. TEE findings included PFO (18.8%), left atrium or left ventricle thrombus (2.4%), spontaneous echo contrast (3.7%), atrial septal aneurysm (3.3%), valve vegetation, mass, or tumor (7.8%), complex aortic atheroma (14.7%), and composite of any cardiac source of embolus (39.2%). Complex aortic atheroma was the only independent predictor of death (HR, 2.7; 95% CI, 1.4 to 5.3). This suggests further evaluation, potential treatment, and risk factor modification in these patients may be of benefit.[279]

Until outcome data are available, the use of antiplatelet or anticoagulation therapy should be reserved for patients with a history of otherwise unexplained embolic event and high-risk echocardiographic features, such as severe aortic atheroma.[280] This is an area of continued and active study (Table 40-4).

Percutaneous Valvuloplasty

An embolic rate of approximately 4% is associated with percutaneous balloon mitral valvuloplasty (see Chapter 21). The embolic event can occur during the procedure or in the first few days following the initial procedure and is often associated with a highly calcified valve. This feature can be identified echocardiographically and echocardiography may serve to influence the occurrence or course of the procedure.[281-283]

Mitral Valve Prolapse

Mitral valve prolapse (MVP) is another common finding that is purportedly associated with emboli in some studies. It is defined echocardiographically if two of the following four criteria are present: (1) superior displacement of any part of the mitral leaflets above the annulus 2 mm or more in the parasternal long-axis view; (2) marked superior displacement (>3 mm) of the bellies of the anterior and posterior mitral leaflets above the annulus, with the coaptation point at or above the annular plane in the four-chamber apical view; (3) increased mitral leaflet thickness (>5 mm); and (4) pathologic MR.

Ischemic neurologic events were previously thought to be highly correlated with MVP, especially in patients under 45 years of age.[284,285] Some of these studies, however, were done using M-mode criteria for MVP. By

TABLE 40-4. Studies in Progress

Names	Description	Primary Endpoint
ARCH	An international randomized controlled trial comparing the efficacy of warfarin (target INR 2-3) with that of aspirin (at 75-325 mg/day) plus clopidogrel (at 75 mg/day) in patients with a history of ischemic stroke within 6 months and an aortic arch atheroma that is either mobile or 4 mm or thicker. The target enrollment is 1500 patients, enrollment period of 3 years, and total study duration of 5 years.	Composite of recurrent stroke, acute myocardial infarction, peripheral embolism, and vascular death.
CLOSURE 1	The Evaluation of the STARflex Septal Closure System in Patients with a Stroke or Transient Ischemic Attack as a result of Presumed Paradoxical Embolism through CLOSURE 1 study is randomized controlled trial to evaluate the safety and efficacy of the STARFlex septal closure system versus best medical therapy in patients with a stroke or transient ischemic attack as a result of presumed paradoxical embolism through a patent foramen ovale. The study began in 2003, with a target enrollment of 1600 patients.	Two-year incidence of stroke or transient ischemic attack.
CODICIA	A multicenter study based in Spain with target enrollment of 500 patients within 30 days of cryptogenic stroke. The objective is to compare the risk of recurrent stroke in cryptogenic stroke patients who have a patent foramen ovale with right-to-left shunting with the risk of recurrence in cryptogenic stroke patients with normal cardiac anatomy. Eligible patients will undergo contrast transcranial Doppler ultrasonography with saline solution infusion. Subsequently, patients with massive right-to-left shunting will receive contrast TEE, while those without right-to-left shunting will receive either contrast TEE or TTE. The study began in year 2000 and is due to conclude.	The incidence of transient ischemic attack and recurrent stroke.
WARCEF	A randomized, double-blind, multicenter study, funded by the National Institutes of Health, with a target enrollment of 2860 and follow-up of 3-5 years. Patients with left ventricular ejection of 35% or less in the absence of atrial fibrillation or mechanical prosthetic heart valves are randomized to warfarin (INR 2.5-3) or aspirin (at 325 mg/day).	Event free survival in 3-5 years for composite of death or stroke (ischemic or hemorrhagic).

ARCH, aortic arch related cerebral hazard study; CODICIA, Recurrent Crytopgenic Stroke and Right to Left Shunt: A 5-year Follow-Up Study; INR, International Normalized Ratio; TEE, transesophageal echocardiography; TTE, transthoracic echocardiography; WARCEF, warfarin-aspirin reduced cardiac ejection fraction study.

these criteria, 7% to 21% of a healthy population was defined as having MVP. Since then, there has been more accurate definition of MVP using 2D criteria.

Using the currently accepted criteria for MVP, the association between MVP and ischemic neurologic events is no longer observed. Earlier studies found MVP in up to 40% of younger patients with stroke or transient ischemic attack, but Gilon and colleagues found MVP in only 1.9% to 2.7% of younger patients, using accepted 2D criteria. Furthermore, this case-control study of 213 patients 45 years of age or younger suggested that MVP was not associated with an increased incidence of stroke.[286] In a population-based cohort study of 1079 residents of Olmsted County, Minnesota, patients with echocardiographic diagnosis of MVP between 1975 and 1989, without prior stroke or transient ischemic attack (TIA), were followed until the development of their first stroke. Patients with MVP had a twofold increase of incidence of stroke (standardized morbidity ratio, 2.1; 95% CI, 1.3 to 3.2). After adjustment of risk factors, such as age, diabetes, congestive heart failure, AFib, and mitral valve replacement, however, no association between MVP and stroke was seen. Of note, the mean age at initial stroke was 78 years of age.[287] In a subsequent follow-up of 49 patients with MVP and a history of ischemic stroke, no increased incidence of recurrent stroke was identified.[288] In the offsprings of the Framingham Heart Study, MVP was seen in 2.4% of 3491 subjects. The natural history, as in other studies, was benign, with no increase in ischemic stroke risks.[289] The increased risk observed in some studies may be explained in part by MR that can be associated with MVP, as evidenced in another longer-term follow-up study (up to 10 years) again in the Olmsted County. In this study, individuals with MVP were observed to have increased risk of neurological events (risk ratio 2.2; 95% CI, 1.5 to 3.2; $P < 0.001$); this increased risk was, however, associated with age and clinically significant mitral valve regurgitation and had increased risk of neurological events.[290]

Attribution of Embolic Events to a Cardiac Source

Approximately 20% of strokes are thought to result from a cardiac source of embolism, and 40% are of undetermined origin, but an increasing number in the latter category have been associated with the various echocardiographic findings discussed in this chapter. Despite the strong association between echocardiographic findings of a source of embolus and stroke, it remains difficult to show a true cause-and-effect association.

What is the best course when a possible or probable source of systemic embolism is discovered? Recent data from large trials have actually made therapeutic decision even more challenging. In particular, role of warfarin in the treatment of stroke remains controversial. WARSS compared the efficacy of adjusted-dose warfarin (international normalized ratio [INR] 1.4 to 2.8) to aspirin (325 mg/day) in 2206 patients with a history of ischemic stroke for recurrent stroke or death with 2 years. No treatment effects between warfarin and aspirin were noted.[291] Interestingly, in the post-hoc analyses of the cryptogenic subgroup, warfarin was associated with worse outcome in those with moderate stroke severity.[292] Similarly, The Warfarin-Aspirin Symptomatic Intracranial Disease (WASID) trial compared the efficacy of warfarin (INR 2 to 3) to aspirin (1300 mg/day) in 569 patients with know intracranial arterial stenosis and found no benefits of warfarin over aspirin. Enrollment into the study was in fact terminated early because of excess death and major hemorrhage in the warfarin arm.[293] On the other hand, dual antiplatelet therapy with aspirin and clopidogrel appeared not to be superior to aspirin alone in the multicenter 15,603 patients Clopidogrel for High Atherothrombotic Risk and Ischemic Stablization, Management, and Avoidance (CHARISMA) study.[294] In the multicenter 7599 patients Management of Atherothrombois with Clopidogrel in High-Risk Patients with Recent Transient Ischemic Attack or Ischemic Stroke (MATCH) study, dual antiplatelet therapy was not superior to clopidogrel and with excess bleeding in the combination arm.[295] In contrast, combined analyses of 40,000 randomized patients from International Stroke Trial (IST)[296] and Chinese Acute Stroke Trial (CAST)[297] showed that early use of aspirin is associated with a significant reduction of recurrent ischemic stroke (1.6% versus 2.3%, $P < 0.001$).[298] Clearly, in the absence of compelling data, individualized treatment tailored to patient's need with proper weighing of risks and benefits is important in the management of this challenging problem.

Influence of Echocardiographic Evaluation on Patient Management

Several studies have examined how echocardiographic evaluation of patients with embolic events influences patient management. In the Significance of Transesophageal Echocardiography in the Prevention of Recurrent Stroke (STEPS) study, 242 patients with unexplained cerebral ischemia underwent TEE and were followed for 1 year. Recurrent stroke occurred in 17 of 132 (13%) of the patients in the aspirin group versus 5 of 110 (5%) of the patients receiving warfarin ($P < 0.02$). The TEE findings again played a major role in determining the pharmacological therapy.[275]

Dawn and colleagues evaluated the relative impact of TEE on management of 234 patients who presented with stroke, transient ischemic attack, or peripheral embolism. Findings observed on TEE diagnosed 59% of the patients, resulted in a change in medical or surgical treatment in 30% of the patients, and influenced initiation of oral anticoagulation in 12% of the patients.[299] The authors concluded that TEE had a significant impact in defining care of patients with unexplained thromboembolism. In another study of 503 consecutive patients with stroke by Harloff and colleagues TEE identified high risk and potential sources of stroke in 8% and 22.6% of 212 potential candidates for oral anticoagulation, who were then prescribed oral anticoagulation. High-risk sources were defined as aortic plaques 4 mm or greater, left atrial or left atrial appendage thrombi, SEC, and left atrial flow less than 30 cm/s. Potential sources were defined as PFO, atrial septal aneurysm, and aortic plaques less than 4 mm. The remaining 147 patients were treated with antiplatelet agents or statin. The authors concluded that TEE was indispensable in guiding appropriate anticoagulation therapy.[19] Of course, until outcome of these patients is known, or if clear benefits of associated therapy have been defined, the true appropriateness of TEE-guided therapy cannot be assessed.

In support of the above findings, McNamara and colleagues performed a cost-effectiveness analysis on the value of echocardiography in the clinical management of stroke. In their analysis, the indication for anticoagulation therapy was limited to only left atrial or left atrial appendage thrombus. Interestingly, they found that TTE alone or in sequence with TEE was not cost-effective compared with TEE alone. Because of their findings, they recommended TEE in all patients with new stroke.[300] Because a diagnostic test in this case is most useful when a clear decision or outcome can be readily defined (i.e., a defined change in therapy), it is little wonder TEE may not influence therapeutic choices in smaller strokes, such as small cortical strokes.[301] Until optimal treatment paradigm is defined for each associated disorder, it remains a challenge to define appropriateness of TEE. This question is now being addressed in several clinical trials, of which the results will be available in the next few years.

Summary

Common sense and good medical judgment based on best available evidence should guide the work-up and management of systemic embolism. We have outlined a simple approach to the echocardiographic evaluation of patients with a suspected embolic event (Fig. 40–18). Echocardiography is often recommended in patients suspected of a cardioembolic stroke. This recommendation is particularly strong for groups that have a possible contraindication to anticoagulation and if it is important to define precisely the risks and benefits of anticoagulation. Conversely, the recommendation for echocardiography is weakened for patients who would be anticoagulated regardless of echocardiographic findings. Both the AHA Echocardiography Task Force and the Canadian Task Force on Preventive Health Care considered echocardiography to be not useful in cases where findings of the echocardiogram do not alter management, particu-

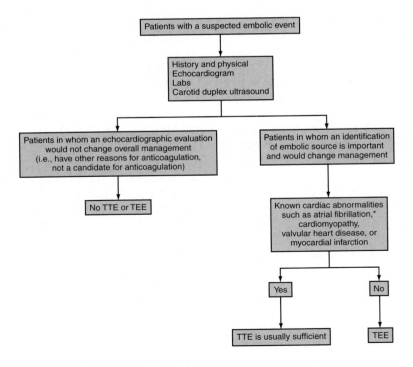

*In general, patients with atrial fibrillation and a stroke should be anticoagulated.

Figure 40–18. Echocardiographic evaluation of patients with a systemic embolic event. TEE, transesophageal echocardiography; TTE, transthoracic echocardiography.

larly in anticoagulation.[29,32] At this time, anticoagulation for many of the associated echocardiographic findings are not supported by clear clinical data.[278] Extreme care should be exercised in using echocardiographic findings to direct care of patients with suspected systemic embolic, until cause and effect for any potential etiology has been firmly established and risk and benefits of various therapeutic alternatives have been defined. The results of randomized clinical trials will help further refine the management and work-up of patients with embolic events.

KEY POINTS

■ Up to 40% of strokes occur in patients without occlusive cerebrovascular disease, and 15% to 20% of the cases are estimated to be of cardiac origin.

■ If there is no clinical evidence of cardiac disease, the yield of transthoracic echocardiography (TTE) for the identification of a source of embolus usually is less than 1%.

■ Echocardiography is recommended in patients 45 years of age or younger who have experienced an embolic event.

■ TEE is superior to TTE for identifying potential sources of cerebral emboli such as aortic atheroma, atrial septal aneurysm, atrial septal defect, left atrial appendage thrombus, PFO, and spontaneous contrast.

■ TEE has increased the detection rate for PFO. However, given the uncertainties concerning indications for PFO closure for cryptogenic stroke, one must balance risk and benefits before considering any definitive therapy.

■ Although stroke is not an uncommon complication of patients with malignancies, tumor embolization as a cause of stroke in these patients is exceedingly rare.

■ Aortic atheroma is a common and dynamic pathological process in patients with suspected stroke, especially among patients with concomitant cardiovascular or vascular disease.

■ Because a diagnostic test in this case is most useful when a clear decision and/or outcome can be readily defined (i.e., a defined change in therapy), use of echocardiography must be balanced by thoughtful medical deduction with attention to its potential influence on choice of therapy.

REFERENCES

1. Feigin VL, Lawes CM, Bennett DA, Anderson CS: Stroke epidemiology: a review of population-based studies of incidence, prevalence, and case-fatality in the late 20th century. *Lancet Neurol* 2:43-53, 2003.

2. Thom T, Haase N, Rosamond W, et al: Heart disease and stroke statistics—2006 update: a report from the American Heart Association Statistics Committee and Stroke Statistics Subcommittee. *Circulation* 113:e85-e151, 2006.

3. Gandolfo C, Conti M: Stroke in young adults: epidemiology. *Neurol Sci* 24(Suppl 1):S1-S3, 2003.

4. Bendixen BH, Posner J, Lango R: Stroke in young adults and children. *Curr Neurol Neurosci Rep* 1:54-66, 2001.

5. Bogousslavsky J, Pierre P: Ischemic stroke in patients under age 45. *Neurol Clin* 10:113-124, 1992.

6. Chong JY, Sacco RL: Epidemiology of stroke in young adults: race/ethnic differences. *J Thromb Thrombolysis* 20:77-83, 2005.

7. Kittner SJ, Stern BJ, Wozniak M, et al: Cerebral infarction in young adults: The Baltimore-Washington Cooperative Young Stroke Study. *Neurology* 50:890-894, 1998.

8. Ferro JM: Cardioembolic stroke: an update. *Lancet Neurol* 2:177-188, 2003.

9. Cardiogenic brain embolism. The second report of the Cerebral Embolism Task Force. *Arch Neurol* 46:727-743, 1989.

10. Sacco RL, Ellenberg JH, Mohr JP, et al: Infarcts of undetermined cause: The NINCDS Stroke Data Bank. *Ann Neurol* 25:382-390, 1989.

11. Bogousslavsky J, Van Melle G, Regli F: The Lausanne Stroke Registry: analysis of 1,000 consecutive patients with first stroke. *Stroke* 19:1083-1092, 1988.

12. Petty GW, Brown RD Jr, Whisnant JP, et al: Ischemic stroke subtypes: A population-based study of incidence and risk factors. *Stroke* 30:2513-2516, 1999.

13. Kolominsky-Rabas PL, Weber M, Gefeller O, et al: Epidemiology of ischemic stroke subtypes according to TOAST criteria: incidence, recurrence, and long-term survival in ischemic stroke subtypes: A population-based study. *Stroke* 32:2735-2740, 2001.

14. Schulz UG, Rothwell PM: Differences in vascular risk factors between etiological subtypes of ischemic stroke: importance of population-based studies. *Stroke* 34:2050-2059, 2003.

15. Schneider AT, Kissela B, Woo D, et al: Ischemic stroke subtypes: a population-based study of incidence rates among blacks and whites. *Stroke* 35:1552-1556, 2004.

16. Lee BI, Nam HS, Heo JH, Kim DI: Yonsei Stroke Registry. Analysis of 1,000 patients with acute cerebral infarctions. *Cerebrovasc Dis* 12:145-151, 2001.

17. Flachskampf FA, Decoodt P, Fraser AG, et al: Guidelines from the Working Group. Recommendations for performing transesophageal echocardiography. *Eur J Echocardiogr* 2:8-21, 2001.

18. Kuhl HP, Hanrath P: The impact of transesophageal echocardiography on daily clinical practice. *Eur J Echocardiogr* 5:455-468, 2004.

19. Harloff A, Handke M, Reinhard M, et al: Therapeutic strategies after examination by transesophageal echocardiography in 503 patients with ischemic stroke. *Stroke* 37:859-864, 2006.

20. Beaulieu Y, Marik PE. Bedside ultrasonography in the ICU: Part 2. *Chest* 128:1766-1781, 2005.

21. Beaulieu Y, Marik PE: Bedside ultrasonography in the ICU: Part 1. *Chest* 128:881-895, 2005.

22. Nowygrod R, Egorova N, Greco G, et al: Trends, complications, and mortality in peripheral vascular surgery. *J Vasc Surg* 43:205-216, 2006.

23. Meyers PM, Schumacher HC, Higashida RT, et al: Use of stents to treat extracranial cerebrovascular disease. *Annu Rev Med* 57:437-454, 2006.

24. Come PC, Riley MF, Bivas NK: Roles of echocardiography and arrhythmia monitoring in the evaluation of patients with suspected systemic embolism. *Ann Neurol* 13:527-531, 1983.

25. Greenland P, Knopman DS, Mikell FL, et al: Echocardiography in diagnostic assessment of stroke. *Ann Intern Med* 95:51-53, 1981.

26. Lovett JL, Sandok BA, Giuliani ER, Nasser FN: Two-dimensional echocardiography in patients with focal cerebral ischemia. *Ann Intern Med* 95:1-4, 1981.

27. Pearson AC, Labovitz AJ, Tatineni S, Gomez CR: Superiority of transesophageal echocardiography in detecting cardiac source of embolism in patients with cerebral ischemia of uncertain etiology. *J Am Coll Cardiol* 17:66-72, 1991.

28. Robbins JA, Sagar KB, French M, Smith PJ: Influence of echocardiography on management of patients with systemic emboli. *Stroke* 14:546-549, 1983.

29. Kapral MK, Silver FL: Preventive health care, 1999 update: 2. Echocardiography for the detection of a cardiac source of embolus in patients with stroke. Canadian Task Force on Preventive Health Care. *CMAJ* 161:989-996, 1999.

30. Nicholson WJ, Triantafyllou A, Helmy T, Lerakis S: Part 2: use of echocardiography in the evaluation of patients with suspected cardioembolic stroke. *Am J Med Sci* 330:243-246, 2005.

31. Lerakis S, Nicholson WJ: Part I: use of echocardiography in the evaluation of patients with suspected cardioembolic stroke. *Am J Med Sci* 329:310-316, 2005.

32. Cheitlin MD, Armstrong WF, Aurigemma GP, et al: ACC/AHA/ASE 2003 guideline update for the clinical application of echocardiography—summary article: a report of the American College of Cardiology/American Heart Association Task Force on Practice Guidelines (ACC/AHA/ASE Committee to Update the 1997 Guidelines for the Clinical Application of Echocardiography). *J Am Coll Cardiol* 42:954-970, 2003.

33. DeRook FA, Comess KA, Albers GW, Popp RL: Transesophageal echocardiography in the evaluation of stroke. *Ann Intern Med* 117:922-932, 1992.

34. Hirata T, Wolfe SB, Popp RL, et al: Estimation of left atrial size using ultrasound. *Am Heart J* 78:43-52, 1969.

35. Lang RM, Bierig M, Devereux RB, et al: Recommendations for chamber quantification. *Eur J Echocardiogr* 7:79-108, 2006.

36. Lang RM, Bierig M, Devereux RB, et al: Recommendations for chamber quantification: a report from the American Society of Echocardiography's Guidelines and Standards Committee and the Chamber Quantification Writing Group, developed in conjunction with the European Association of Echocardiography, a branch of the European Society of Cardiology. *J Am Soc Echocardiogr* 18:1440-1463, 2005.

37. Kircher B, Abbott JA, Pau S, et al: Left atrial volume determination by biplane two-dimensional echocardiography: Validation by cine computed tomography. *Am Heart J* 121:864-871, 1991.

38. Vandenberg BF, Weiss RM, Kinzey J, et al: Comparison of left atrial volume by two-dimensional echocardiography and cine-computed tomography. *Am J Cardiol* 75:754-757, 1995.

39. Wang Y, Gutman JM, Heilbron D, et al: Atrial volume in a normal adult population by two-dimensional echocardiography. *Chest* 86:595-601, 1984.

40. Manning WJ, Silverman DI, Waksmonski CA, et al: Prevalence of residual left atrial thrombi among patients with acute thromboembolism and newly recognized atrial fibrillation. *Arch Intern Med* 155:2193-2198, 1995.

41. Manning WJ, Weintraub RM, Waksmonski CA, et al: Accuracy of transesophageal echocardiography for identifying left atrial thrombi. A prospective, intraoperative study. *Ann Intern Med* 123:817-822, 1995.

42. Agmon Y, Khandheria BK, Gentile F, Seward JB: Echocardiographic assessment of the left atrial appendage. *J Am Coll Cardiol* 34:1867-1877, 1999.

43. Nishide M, Irino T, Gotoh M, et al: Cardiac abnormalities in ischemic cerebrovascular disease studied by two-dimensional echocardiography. *Stroke* 14:541-545, 1983.

44. Bogousslavsky J, Hachinski VC, Boughner DR, et al: Cardiac and arterial lesions in carotid transient ischemic attacks. *Arch Neurol* 43:223-228, 1986.

45. Rem JA, Hachinski VC, Boughner DR, Barnett HJ: Value of cardiac monitoring and echocardiography in TIA and stroke patients. *Stroke* 16:950-966, 1985.

46. Good DC, Frank S, Verhulst S, Sharma B: Cardiac abnormalities in stroke patients with negative arteriograms. *Stroke* 17:6-11, 1986.

47. Aronow WS, Koenigsberg M, Kronzon I, Gutstein H: Association of mitral anular calcium with new thromboembolic stroke and cardiac events at 39-month follow-up in elderly patients. *Am J Cardiol* 65:1511-1512, 1990.

48. Kizer JR, Wiebers DO, Whisnant JP, et al: Mitral annular calcification, aortic valve sclerosis, and incident stroke in adults free of clinical cardiovascular disease: The Strong Heart Study. *Stroke* 36:2533-2537, 2005.

49. Benjamin EJ, Plehn JF, D'Agostino RB, et al: Mitral annular calcification and the risk of stroke in an elderly cohort. *N Engl J Med* 327:374-379, 1992.

50. Predictors of thromboembolism in atrial fibrillation: II. Echocardiographic features of patients at risk. The Stroke Prevention in Atrial Fibrillation Investigators. *Ann Intern Med* 116:6-12, 1992.

51. Boon A, Lodder J, Cheriex E, Kessels F: Mitral annulus calcification is not an independent risk factor for stroke: a cohort study of 657 patients. *J Neurol* 244:535-541, 1997.

52. Savage DD, Garrison RJ, Castelli WP, et al: Prevalence of submitral (anular) calcium and its correlates in a general population-based sample (the Framingham Study). *Am J Cardiol* 51:1375-1378, 1983.

53. Pomerance A: Pathological and clinical study of calcification of the mitral valve ring. *J Clin Pathol* 23:354-361, 1970.

54. Adler Y, Koren A, Fink N, et al: Association between mitral annulus calcification and carotid atherosclerotic disease. *Stroke* 29:1833-1837, 1998.

55. Adler Y, Vaturi M, Fink N, et al: Association between mitral annulus calcification and aortic atheroma: a prospective transesophageal echocardiographic study. *Atherosclerosis* 152:451-456, 2000.

56. Tunca A, Karanfil A, Koktener A, et al: Association between mitral annular calcification and stroke. *Jpn Heart J* 45:999-1005, 2004.

57. Fox CS, Vasan RS, Parise H, et al: Mitral annular calcification predicts cardiovascular morbidity and mortality: The Framingham Heart Study. *Circulation* 107:1492-1496, 2003.

58. Soylu M, Demir AD, Arda K, et al: Association between mitral annular calcification and carotid atheroma. *Angiology* 52:201-204, 2001.

59. Kamensky G, Lisy L, Polak E, et al: Mitral annular calcifications and aortic plaques as predictors of increased cardiovascular mortality. *J Cardiol* 37(Suppl 1):21-26, 2001.

60. Fuster V, Gersh BJ, Giuliani ER, Tajik AJ, Brandenburg RO, Frye RL: The natural history of idiopathic dilated cardiomyopathy. *Am J Cardiol* 47:525-531, 1981.

61. Meltzer RS, Visser CA, Fuster V: Intracardiac thrombi and systemic embolization. *Ann Intern Med* 104:689-698, 1986.

62. Baker DW, Wright RF: Management of heart failure. IV. Anticoagulation for patients with heart failure due to left ventricular systolic dysfunction. *J Am Med Assoc* 272:1614-1618, 1994.

63. Crawford TC, Smith WTT, Velazquez EJ, et al: Prognostic usefulness of left ventricular thrombus by echocardiography in dilated cardiomyopathy in predicting stroke, transient ischemic attack, and death. *Am J Cardiol* 93:500-503, 2004.

64. Sharma ND, McCullough PA, Philbin EF, Weaver WD: Left ventricular thrombus and subsequent thromboembolism in patients with severe systolic dysfunction. *Chest* 117:314-320, 2000.

65. Stokman PJ, Nandra CS, Asinger RW: Left ventricular thrombus. *Curr Treat Options Cardiovasc Med* 3:515-521, 2001.

66. Mikell FL, Asinger RW, Elsperger KJ, et al: Regional stasis of blood in the dysfunctional left ventricle: echocardiographic detection and differentiation from early thrombosis. *Circulation* 66:755-763, 1982.

67. Chesebro JH, Ezekowitz M, Badimon L, Fuster V: Intracardiac thrombi and systemic thromboembolism: detection, incidence, and treatment. *Annu Rev Med* 36:579-605, 1985.

68. Dexter DD Jr, Whisnant JP, Connolly DC, O'Fallon WM: The association of stroke and coronary heart disease: a population study. *Mayo Clin Proc* 62:1077-1083, 1987.

69. Haugland JM, Asinger RW, Mikell FL, Elsperger J, Hodges M. Embolic potential of left ventricular thrombi detected by two-dimensional echocardiography. Circulation. 1984 Oct;70(4):588-98.

70. Johannessen KA, Nordrehaug JE, von der Lippe G, Vollset SE: Risk factors for embolisation in patients with left ventricular thrombi and acute myocardial infarction. *Br Heart J* 60(2):104-110, 1998.

71. Kupper AJ, Verheugt FW, Peels CH, et al: Left ventricular thrombus incidence and behavior studied by serial two-dimensional echocardiography in acute anterior myocardial infarction: left ventricular wall motion, systemic embolism and oral anticoagulation. *J Am Coll Cardiol* 13:1514-1520, 1989.

72. Arvan S, Boscha K: Prophylactic anticoagulation for left ventricular thrombi after acute myocardial infarction: A prospective randomized trial. *Am Heart J* 113:688-693, 1987.

73. Stratton JR, Nemanich JW, Johannessen KA, Resnick AD: Fate of left ventricular thrombi in patients with remote myocardial infarction or idiopathic cardiomyopathy. *Circulation* 78:1388-1393, 1988.

74. Loh E, Sutton MS, Wun CC, et al: Ventricular dysfunction and the risk of stroke after myocardial infarction. *N Engl J Med* 336:251-257, 1997.

75. Antman EM, Anbe DT, Armstrong PW, et al: ACC/AHA guidelines for the management of patients with ST-elevation myocardial infarction; A report of the American College of Cardiology/American Heart Association Task Force on Practice Guidelines (Committee to Revise the 1999 Guidelines for the Management of patients with acute myocardial infarction). *J Am Coll Cardiol* 44:E1-E211, 2004.

76. Cujec B, Polasek P, Voll C, Shuaib A: Transesophageal echocardiography in the detection of potential cardiac source of embolism in stroke patients. *Stroke* 22:727-733, 1991.

77. Hausmann D, Mugge A, Becht I, Daniel WG: Diagnosis of patent foramen ovale by transesophageal echocardiography and association with cerebral and peripheral embolic events. *Am J Cardiol* 70:668-672, 1992.

78. Lee RJ, Bartzokis T, Yeoh TK, et al: Enhanced detection of intracardiac sources of cerebral emboli by transesophageal echocardiography. *Stroke* 22:734-739, 1991.

79. Pearson AC, Nagelhout D, Castello R, et al: Atrial septal aneurysm and stroke: A transesophageal echocardiographic study. *J Am Coll Cardiol* 18:1223-1229, 1991.

80. Pop G, Sutherland GR, Koudstaal PJ, et al: Transesophageal echocardiography in the detection of intracardiac embolic sources in patients with transient ischemic attacks. *Stroke* 21:560-565, 1990.

81. Labovitz AJ, Camp A, Castello R, et al: Usefulness of transesophageal echocardiography in unexplained cerebral ischemia. *Am J Cardiol* 72:1448-1452, 1993.

82. Klein AL, Grimm RA, Murray RD, et al: Use of transesophageal echocardiography to guide cardioversion in patients with atrial fibrillation. *N Engl J Med* 344:1411-1420, 2001.

83. Klein AL, Grimm RA, Jasper SE, et al: Efficacy of transesophageal echocardiography-guided cardioversion of patients with atrial fibrillation at 6 months: a randomized controlled trial. *Am Heart J* 151:380-389, 2006.

84. Thambidorai SK, Murray RD, Parakh K, et al: Utility of transesophageal echocardiography in identification of thrombogenic milieu in patients with atrial fibrillation (an ACUTE ancillary study). *Am J Cardiol* 96:935-941, 2005.

85. Flachskampf FA: The standard TEE examination: procedure, safety, typical cross-sections and anatomic correlations, and systematic analysis. *Semin Cardiothorac Vasc Anesth* 10:49-56, 2006.

86. Donal E, Yamada H, Leclercq C, Herpin D: The left atrial appendage, a small, blind-ended structure: A review of its echocardiographic evaluation and its clinical role. *Chest* 128:1853-1862, 2005.

87. Kamalesh M, Copeland TB, Sawada S: Severely reduced left atrial appendage function: a cause of embolic stroke in patients in sinus rhythm? *J Am Soc Echocardiogr* 11:902-904, 1998.

88. Panagiotopoulos K, Toumanidis S, Saridakis N, et al: Left atrial and left atrial appendage functional abnormalities in patients with cardioembolic stroke in sinus rhythm and idiopathic atrial fibrillation. *J Am Soc Echocardiogr* 11:711-719, 1998.

89. Omran H, Jung W, Rabahieh R, et al: Imaging of thrombi and assessment of left atrial appendage function: A prospective study comparing transthoracic and transesophageal echocardiography. *Heart* 81:192-198, 1999.

90. Bilge M, Eryonucu B, Guler N, et al: Transesophageal echocardiography assessment of left atrial appendage function in untreated systemic hypertensive patients in sinus rhythm. *J Am Soc Echocardiogr* 13:271-276, 2000.

91. Ozer N, Tokgozoglu L, Ovunc K, et al: Left atrial appendage function in patients with cardioembolic stroke in sinus rhythm and atrial fibrillation. *J Am Soc Echocardiogr* 13:661-665, 2000.

92. Antonielli E, Pizzuti A, Palinkas A, et al: Clinical value of left atrial appendage flow for prediction of long-term sinus rhythm maintenance in patients with nonvalvular atrial fibrillation. *J Am Coll Cardiol* 39:1443-1449, 2002.

93. Alessandri N, Mariani S, Ciccaglioni A, et al: Thrombus formation in the left atrial appendage in the course of atrial fibrillation. *Eur Rev Med Pharmacol Sci* 7:65-73, 2003.

94. Illien S, Maroto-Jarvinen S, von der Recke G, et al: Atrial fibrillation: relation between clinical risk factors and transesophageal echocardiographic risk factors for thromboembolism. *Heart* 89:165-168, 2003.

95. Handke M, Harloff A, Hetzel A, et al: Left atrial appendage flow velocity as a quantitative surrogate parameter for thromboembolic risk: determinants and relationship to spontaneous echocontrast and thrombus formation—a transesophageal echocardiographic study in 500 patients with cerebral ischemia. *J Am Soc Echocardiogr* 18:1366-1372, 2005.

96. Handke M, Harloff A, Hetzel A, et al: Predictors of left atrial spontaneous echocardiographic contrast or thrombus formation in stroke patients with sinus rhythm and reduced left ventricular function. *Am J Cardiol* 96:1342-1344, 2005.

97. Jue J, Winslow T, Fazio G, et al: Pulsed Doppler characterization of left atrial appendage flow. *J Am Soc Echocardiogr* 6:237-244, 1993.

98. Mugge A, Kuhn H, Nikutta P, et al: Assessment of left atrial appendage function by biplane transesophageal echocardiography in patients with nonrheumatic atrial fibrillation: Identification of a subgroup of patients at increased embolic risk. *J Am Coll Cardiol* 23:599-607, 1994.

99. Transesophageal echocardiographic correlates of thromboembolism in high-risk patients with nonvalvular atrial fibrillation. The Stroke Prevention in Atrial Fibrillation Investigators Committee on Echocardiography. *Ann Intern Med* 128:639-647, 1998.

100. Goldman ME, Pearce LA, Hart RG, et al: Pathophysiologic correlates of thromboembolism in nonvalvular atrial fibrillation: I. Reduced flow velocity in the left atrial appendage (The Stroke Prevention in Atrial Fibrillation [SPAF-III] study). *J Am Soc Echocardiogr* 12:1080-1087, 1999.

101. Black IW, Hopkins AP, Lee LC, Walsh WF: Left atrial spontaneous echo contrast: a clinical and echocardiographic analysis. *J Am Coll Cardiol* 18:398-404, 1991.

102. Iliceto S, Antonelli G, Sorino M, et al: Dynamic intracavitary left atrial echoes in mitral stenosis. *Am J Cardiol* 55:603-606, 1985.

103. Castello R, Pearson AC, Labovitz AJ: Prevalence and clinical implications of atrial spontaneous contrast in patients undergoing transesophageal echocardiography. *Am J Cardiol* 65:1149-1153, 1990.

104. Daniel WG, Nellessen U, Schroder E, et al: Left atrial spontaneous echo contrast in mitral valve disease: an indicator for an increased thromboembolic risk. *J Am Coll Cardiol* 11:1204-1211, 1988.

105. Chimowitz MI, DeGeorgia MA, Poole RM, et al: Left atrial spontaneous echo contrast is highly associated with previous stroke in patients with atrial fibrillation or mitral stenosis. *Stroke* 24:1015-1019, 1993.

106. Leung DY, Black IW, Cranney GB, et al: Prognostic implications of left atrial spontaneous echo contrast in nonvalvular atrial fibrillation. *J Am Coll Cardiol* 24:755-762, 1994.

107. Brown J, Sadler DB. Left atrial thrombi in non-rheumatic atrial fibrillation: assessment of prevalence by transesophageal echocardiography. *Int J Cardiovasc Imaging* 9:65-72, 1993.

108. Jones EF, Calafiore P, McNeil JJ, et al: Atrial fibrillation with left atrial spontaneous contrast detected by transesophageal echocardiography is a potent risk factor for stroke. *Am J Cardiol* 78:425-429, 1996.

109. Asinger RW, Koehler J, Pearce LA, et al: Pathophysiologic correlates of thromboembolism in nonvalvular atrial fibrillation: II. Dense spontaneous echocardiographic contrast (The Stroke Prevention in Atrial Fibrillation [SPAF-III] study). *J Am Soc Echocardiogr* 12:1088-1096, 1999.

110. Fatkin D, Loupas T, Low J, Feneley M: Inhibition of red cell aggregation prevents spontaneous echocardiographic contrast formation in human blood. *Circulation* 96:889-896, 1997.

111. Fatkin D, Herbert E, Feneley MP: Hematologic correlates of spontaneous echo contrast in patients with atrial fibrillation and implications for thromboembolic risk. *Am J Cardiol* 73:672-676, 1994.

112. Peverill RE, Harper RW, Gelman J, et al: Determinants of increased regional left atrial coagulation activity in patients with mitral stenosis. *Circulation* 94:331-339, 1996.

113. Heppell RM, Berkin KE, McLenachan JM, Davies JA: Haemostatic and haemodynamic abnormalities associated with left atrial thrombosis in non-rheumatic atrial fibrillation. *Heart* 77:407-411, 1997.

114. Bilge M, Guler N, Eryonucu B, Asker M: Frequency of left atrial thrombus and spontaneous echocardiographic contrast in acute myocardial infarction. *Am J Cardiol* 84:847-849, A8, 1999.

115. Nendaz M, Sarasin F, Boyousslavsky J: How to prevent stroke recurrence in patients with patent foramen ovale: anticoagulants, antiaggregants, foramen closure, or nothing? *Eur Neurol* 37(4):199-204, 1997.

116. Blackshear JL, Pearce LA, Asinger RW, et al: Mitral regurgitation associated with reduced thromboembolic events in high-risk patients with nonrheumatic atrial fibrillation. Stroke Prevention in Atrial Fibrillation Investigators. *Am J Cardiol* 72:840-843, 1993.

117. Fatkin D, Kelly RP, Feneley MP: Relations between left atrial appendage blood flow velocity, spontaneous echocardiographic contrast and thromboembolic risk in vivo. *J Am Coll Cardiol* 23:961-969, 1994.

118. Bernstein NE, Demopoulos LA, Tunick PA, et al: Correlates of spontaneous echo contrast in patients with mitral stenosis and normal sinus rhythm. *Am Heart J* 128:287-292, 1994.

119. Velho FJ, Dotta F, Scherer L, et al: Association between the effect of spontaneous contrast in the thoracic aorta and recent ischemic stroke determined by transesophageal echocardiography. *Arq Bras Cardiol* 82:52-56, 47-51, 2004.

120. Panidis IP, Kotler MN, Mintz GS, et al: Right ventricular function in coronary artery disease as assessed by two-dimensional echocardiography. *Am Heart J* 107:1187-1194, 1984.

121. Silver MD, Dorsey JS: Aneurysms of the septum primum in adults. *Arch Pathol Lab Med* 102:62-65, 1978.

122. Hanley PC, Tajik AJ, Hynes JK, et al: Diagnosis and classification of atrial septal aneurysm by two-dimensional echocardiography: report of 80 consecutive cases. *J Am Coll Cardiol* 6:1370-1382, 1985.

123. Schneider B, Hofmann T, Meinertz T, Hanrath P: Diagnostic value of transesophageal echocardiography in atrial septal aneurysm. *Int J Cardiovasc Imaging* 8:143-152, 1992.

124. Agmon Y, Khandheria BK, Meissner I, et al: Frequency of atrial septal aneurysms in patients with cerebral ischemic events. *Circulation* 99:1942-1944, 1999.

125. Schneider B, Hanrath P, Vogel P, Meinertz T: Improved morphologic characterization of atrial septal aneurysm by transesophageal echocardiography: Relation to cerebrovascular events. *J Am Coll Cardiol* 16:1000-1009, 1990.

126. Lucas C, Goullard L, Marchau M Jr, et al: Higher prevalence of atrial septal aneurysms in patients with ischemic stroke of unknown cause. *Acta Neurol Scand* 89:210-213, 1994.

127. Belkin RN, Kisslo J: Atrial septal aneurysm: recognition and clinical relevance. *Am Heart J* 120:948-957, 1990.

128. Cabanes L, Mas JL, Cohen A, et al: Atrial septal aneurysm and patent foramen ovale as risk factors for cryptogenic stroke in patients less than 55 years of age. A study using transesophageal echocardiography. *Stroke* 24:1865-1873, 1993.

129. Mugge A, Daniel WG, Angermann C, et al: Atrial septal aneurysm in adult patients. A multicenter study using transthoracic and transesophageal echocardiography. *Circulation* 91:2785-2792, 1995.

130. Mattioli AV, Aquilina M, Oldani A, Longhini C, Mattioli G: Atrial septal aneurysm as a cardioembolic source in adult patients with stroke and normal carotid arteries. A multicentre study. *Eur Heart J* 22:261-268, 2001.

131. Olivares-Reyes A, Chan S, Lazar EJ, et al: Atrial septal aneurysm: a new classification in two hundred five adults. *J Am Soc Echocardiogr* 10:644-656, 1997.

132. Ewert P, Berger F, Vogel M, et al: Morphology of perforated atrial septal aneurysm suitable for closure by transcatheter device placement. *Heart* 84:327-331, 2000.

133. Burger AJ, Jadhav P, Kamalesh M: Low incidence of cerebrovascular events in patients with incidental atrial septal aneurysm. *Echocardiography* 14:589-596, 1997.

134. Mas JL, Arquizan C, Lamy C, et al: Recurrent cerebrovascular events associated with patent foramen ovale, atrial septal aneurysm, or both. *N Engl J Med* 345:1740-1746, 2001.

135. Lamy C, Giannesini C, Zuber M, et al: Clinical and imaging findings in cryptogenic stroke patients with and without patent foramen ovale: The PFO-ASA Study. Atrial Septal Aneurysm. *Stroke* 33:706-711, 2002.

136. Homma S, Sacco RL, Di Tullio MR, et al: Effect of medical treatment in stroke patients with patent foramen ovale: Patent foramen ovale in Cryptogenic Stroke Study. *Circulation* 105:2625-2631, 2002.

137. Abboud H, Brochet E, Amarenco P: Lipomatous hypertrophy of the inter-atrial septum and stroke. *Cerebrovasc Dis* 18:178, 2004.

138. Zarauza MJ, Alonso F, Hidalgo M, et al: [Lipomatous hypertrophy of the interatrial septum simulating an atrial mass in a patient with a pulmonary embolism: its diagnosis by transesophageal echocardiography and percutaneous biopsy]. *Rev Esp Cardiol* 46:761-764, 1993.

139. Agmon Y, Meissner I, Tajik AJ, et al: Clinical, laboratory, and transesophageal echocardiographic correlates of interatrial septal thickness: a population-based transesophageal echocardiographic study. *J Am Soc Echocardiogr* 18:175-182, 2005.

140. Gill EA Jr, Quaife RA: The echocardiographer and the diagnosis of patent foramen ovale. *Cardiol Clin* 23:47-52, 2005.

141. Konstantinides S, Kasper W, Geibel A, et al: Detection of left-to-right shunt in atrial septal defect by negative contrast echocardiography: a comparison of transthoracic and transesophageal approach. *Am Heart J* 126:909-917, 1993.

142. Hausmann D, Daniel WG, Mugge A, et al: Value of transesophageal color Doppler echocardiography for detection of different types of atrial septal defect in adults. *J Am Soc Echocardiogr* 5:481-488, 1992.

143. Kronzon I, Tunick PA, Freedberg RS, et al: Transesophageal echocardiography is superior to transthoracic echocardiography in the diagnosis of sinus venosus atrial septal defect. *J Am Coll Cardiol* 17:537-542, 1991.

144. Woods TD, Patel A: A critical review of patent foramen ovale detection using saline contrast echocardiography: When bubbles lie. *J Am Soc Echocardiogr* 19:215-222, 2006.

145. Lindeboom JE, van Deudekom MJ, Visser CA: Traditional contrast echocardiography may fail to demonstrate a patent foramen ovale: Negative contrast in the right atrium may be a clue. *Eur J Echocardiogr* 6:75-78, 2005.

146. Cerrato P, Grasso M, Imperiale D, et al: Stroke in young patients: enteropathogenesis and risk factors in different age classes. *Cerebrovasc Dis* 18:154-159, 2004.

147. Webster MW, Chancellor AM, Smith HJ, et al: Patent foramen ovale in young stroke patients. *Lancet* 2:11-12, 1988.

148. Jeanrenaud X, Bogousslavsky J, Payot M, et al: [Patent foramen ovale and cerebral infarct in young patients]. *Schweiz Med Wochenschr* 120:823-829, 1990.

149. Lechat P, Mas JL, Lascault G, et al: Prevalence of patent foramen ovale in patients with stroke. *N Engl J Med* 318:1148-1152, 1988.

150. Di Tullio M, Sacco RL, Gopal A, et al: Patent foramen ovale as a risk factor for cryptogenic stroke. *Ann Intern Med* 117:461-465, 1992.

151. de Belder MA, Tourikis L, Leech G, Camm AJ: Risk of patent foramen ovale for thromboembolic events in all age groups. *Am J Cardiol* 69:1316-1320, 1992.

152. Klotzsch C, Janssen G, Berlit P: Transesophageal echocardiography and contrast-TCD in the detection of a patent foramen ovale: experiences with 111 patients. *Neurology* 44:1603-1606, 1994.

153. Kizer JR, Devereux RB: Clinical practice. Patent foramen ovale in young adults with unexplained stroke. *N Engl J Med* 353:2361-2372, 2005.

154. Kerut EK, Norfleet WT, Plotnick GD, Giles TD: Patent foramen ovale: a review of associated conditions and the impact of physiological size. *J Am Coll Cardiol* 38:613-623, 2001.

155. De Castro S, Cartoni D, Fiorelli M, et al: Morphological and functional characteristics of patent foramen ovale and their embolic implications. *Stroke* 31:2407-2413, 2000.

156. De Castro S, Cartoni D, Fiorelli M, et al: Patent foramen ovale and its embolic implications. *Am J Cardiol* 86:51G-52G, 2000.

157. Homma S, Di Tullio MR, Sacco RL, et al: Characteristics of patent foramen ovale associated with cryptogenic stroke. A biplane transesophageal echocardiographic study. *Stroke* 25:582-586, 1994.

158. Hausmann D, Mugge A, Daniel WG: Identification of patent foramen ovale permitting paradoxic embolism. *J Am Coll Cardiol* 26:1030-1038, 1995.

159. Steiner MM, Di Tullio MR, Rundek T, et al: Patent foramen ovale size and embolic brain imaging findings among patients with ischemic stroke. *Stroke* 29:944-948, 1998.

160. Falk RH: PFO or UFO? The role of a patent foramen ovale in cryptogenic stroke. *Am Heart J* 121:1264-1266, 1991.

161. Konstadt SN, Louie EK: Echocardiographic diagnosis of paradoxical embolism and the potential for right to left shunting. *Am J Cardiovasc Imaging* 8:28-38, 1994.

162. Meissner I, Khandheria BK, Heit JA, et al: Patent foramen ovale: innocent or guilty? Evidence from a prospective population-based study. *J Am Coll Cardiol* 47:440-445, 2006.

163. Petty GW, Khandheria BK, Meissner I, et al: Population-based study of the relationship between patent foramen ovale and cerebrovascular ischemic events. *Mayo Clin Proc* 81:602-608, 2006.

164. Stollberger C, Slany J, Schuster I, et al: The prevalence of deep venous thrombosis in patients with suspected paradoxical embolism. *Ann Intern Med* 119:461-465, 1993.

165. Lethen H, Flachskampf FA, Schneider R, et al: Frequency of deep vein thrombosis in patients with patent foramen ovale and ischemic stroke or transient ischemic attack. *Am J Cardiol* 80:1066-1069, 1997.

166. Bogousslavsky J, Devuyst G, Nendaz M, et al: Prevention of stroke recurrence with presumed paradoxical embolism. *J Neurol* 244:71-75, 1997.

167. Boddicker KA, Kerber RE: Does transesophageal echocardiographic demonstration of a patent foramen ovale in patients with a recent cerebral ischemic event change anticoagulation therapy? *J Am Soc Echocardiogr* 18:357-361, 2005.

168. Homma S, Di Tullio MR, Sacco RL, et al: Surgical closure of patent foramen ovale in cryptogenic stroke patients. *Stroke* 28:2376-2381, 1997.

169. Dearani JA, Ugurlu BS, Danielson GK, et al: Surgical patent foramen ovale closure for prevention of paradoxical embolism-related cerebrovascular ischemic events. *Circulation* 100(19 Suppl):II171-II175, 1999.

170. Homma S, Sacco RL: Patent foramen ovale and stroke. *Circulation* 112:1063-1072, 2005.

171. Schneider B, Bauer R: Is surgical closure of patent foramen ovale the gold standard for treating interatrial shunts? An echocardiographic follow-up study. *J Am Soc Echocardiogr* 18:1385-1391, 2005.

172. Spies C, Strasheim R, Timmermanns I, Schraeder R: Patent foramen ovale closure in patients with cryptogenic thrombo-embolic events using the Cardia PFO occluder. *Eur Heart J* 27:365-371, 2006.

173. Maisel WH, Laskey WK: Patent foramen ovale closure devices: moving beyond equipoise. *J Am Med Assoc* 294:366-369, 2005.

174. Thomson JD: Percutaneous PFO closure, further data but many unanswered questions. *Eur Heart J* 27:258-259, 2006.

175. Diener HC, Weimar C, Katsarava Z: Patent foramen ovale: paradoxical connection to migraine and stroke. *Curr Opin Neurol* 18:299-304, 2005.

176. Schwerzmann M, Nedeltchev K, Lagger F, et al: Prevalence and size of directly detected patent foramen ovale in migraine with aura. *Neurology* 65:1415-1418, 2005.

177. Giardini A, Donti A, Formigari R, et al: Transcatheter patent foramen ovale closure mitigates aura migraine headaches abolishing spontaneous right-to-left shunting. *Am Heart J* 151:922 e1-e5, 2006.

178. Messe SR, Silverman IE, Kizer JR, et al: Practice parameter: recurrent stroke with patent foramen ovale and atrial septal aneurysm: report of the Quality Standards Subcommittee of the American Academy of Neurology. *Neurology* 62:1042-1050, 2004.

179. Schneider B, Hofmann T, Justen MH, Meinertz T: Chiari's network: normal anatomic variant or risk factor for arterial embolic events? *J Am Coll Cardiol* 26:203-210, 1995.

180. Leung DY, Black IW, Cranney GB, et al: Selection of patients for transesophageal echocardiography after stroke and systemic embolic events. Role of transthoracic echocardiography. *Stroke* 26:1820-1824, 1995.

181. Freedberg RS, Goodkin GM, Perez JL, et al: Valve strands are strongly associated with systemic embolization: a transesophageal echocardiographic study. *J Am Coll Cardiol* 26:1709-1712, 1995.

182. Roberts JK, Omarali I, Di Tullio MR, et al: Valvular strands and cerebral ischemia. Effect of demographics and strand characteristics. *Stroke* 28:2185-2188, 1997.

183. Tice FD, Slivka AP, Walz ET, et al: Mitral valve strands in patients with focal cerebral ischemia. *Stroke* 27:1183-1186, 1996.

184. Cohen A, Tzourio C, Chauvel C, et al: Mitral valve strands and the risk of ischemic stroke in elderly patients. The French Study

of Aortic Plaques in Stroke (FAPS) Investigators. *Stroke* 28:1574-1578, 1997.

185. Roldan CA, Shively BK, Crawford MH: Valve excrescences: prevalence, evolution and risk for cardioembolism. *J Am Coll Cardiol* 30:1308-1314, 1997.

186. Nighoghossian N, Derex L, Perinetti M, et al: Course of valvular strands in patients with stroke: cooperative study with transesophageal echocardiography. *Am Heart J* 136:1065-1069, 1998.

187. Meissner I, Whisnant JP, Khandheria BK, et al: Prevalence of potential risk factors for stroke assessed by transesophageal echocardiography and carotid ultrasonography: The SPARC study. Stroke Prevention: Assessment of Risk in a Community. *Mayo Clin Proc* 74:862-869, 1999.

188. McAllister HA, Jr, Hall RJ, Cooley DA: Tumors of the heart and pericardium. *Curr Probl Cardiol* 24:57-116, 1999.

189. Rogers LR: Cerebrovascular complications in patients with cancer. *Semin Neurol* 24:453-460, 2004.

190. Alam M, Sun I: Transesophageal echocardiographic evaluation of left atrial mass lesions. *J Am Soc Echocardiogr* 4:323-330, 1991.

191. Shyu KG, Chen JJ, Cheng JJ, et al: Comparison of transthoracic and transesophageal echocardiography in the diagnosis of intracardiac tumors in adults. *J Clin Ultrasound* 22:381-389, 1994.

192. Pinede L, Duhaut P, Loire R: Clinical presentation of left atrial cardiac myxoma. A series of 112 consecutive cases. *Medicine (Baltimore)* 80:159-172, 2001.

193. Narang J, Neustein S, Israel D: The role of transesophageal echocardiography in the diagnosis and excision of a tumor of the aortic valve. *J Cardiothorac Vasc Anesth* 6:68-69, 1992.

194. Thomas MR, Jayakrishnan AG, Desai J, et al: Transesophageal echocardiography in the detection and surgical management of a papillary fibroelastoma of the mitral valve causing partial mitral valve obstruction. *J Am Soc Echocardiogr* 6:83-86, 1993.

195. Klarich KW, Enriquez-Sarano M, Gura GM, et al: Papillary fibroelastoma: echocardiographic characteristics for diagnosis and pathologic correlation. *J Am Coll Cardiol* 30:784-790, 1997.

196. Yee HC, Nwosu JE, Lii AD, et al: Echocardographic features of papillary fibroelastoma and their consequences and management. *Am J Cardiol* 80:811-814, 1997.

197. Sastre-Garriga J, Molina C, Montaner J, et al: Mitral papillary fibroelastoma as a cause of cardiogenic embolic stroke: Report of two cases and review of the literature. *Eur J Neurol* 7:449-453, 2000.

198. Deodhar AP, Tometzki AJ, Hudson IN, Mankad PS: Aortic valve tumor causing acute myocardial infarction in a child. *Ann Thorac Surg* 64:1482-1484, 1997.

199. Prahlow JA, Barnard JJ: Sudden death due to obstruction of coronary artery ostium by aortic valve papillary fibroelastoma. *Am J Forensic Med Pathol* 19(2):162-165, 1998.

200. Rubin MA, Snell JA, Tazelaar HD, et al: Cardiac papillary fibroelastoma: an immunohistochemical investigation and unusual clinical manifestations. *Mod Pathol* 8:402-407, 1995.

201. Ganjoo AK, Johnson WD, Gordon RT, et al: Tricuspid papillary fibroelastoma causing syncopal episodes. *J Thorac Cardiovasc Surg* 112:551-553, 1996.

202. de Menezes IC, Fragata J, Martins FM: Papillary fibroelastoma of the mitral valve in a 3-year-old child: case report. *Pediatr Cardiol* 17:194-195, 1996.

203. Kanarek SE, Wright P, Liu J, et al: Multiple fibroelastomas: a case report and review of the literature. *J Am Soc Echocardiogr* 16:373-376, 2003.

204. Eslami-Varzaneh F, Brun EA, Sears-Rogan P: An unusual case of multiple papillary fibroelastoma, review of literature. *Cardiovasc Pathol* 12:170-173, 2003.

205. Gowda RM, Khan IA, Nair CK, et al: Cardiac papillary fibroelastoma: a comprehensive analysis of 725 cases. *Am Heart J* 146:404-410, 2003.

206. Georghiou GP, Shapira Y, Stamler A, et al: Surgical excision of papillary fibroelastoma for known or potential embolization. *J Heart Valve Dis* 14:843-847, 2005.

207. Hill EE, Herijgers P, Herregods MC, Peetermans WE: Evolving trends in infective endocarditis. *Clin Microbiol Infect* 12:5-12, 2006.

208. Di Salvo G, Habib G, Pergola V, et al: Echocardiography predicts embolic events in infective endocarditis. *J Am Coll Cardiol* 37:1069-1076, 2001.

209. Steckelberg JM, Murphy JG, Ballard D, Bailey K, Tajik AJ, Taliercio CP, et al: Emboli in infective endocarditis: the prognostic value of echocardiography. *Ann Intern Med* 114:635-640, 1991.

210. De Castro S, Magni G, Beni S, et al: Role of transthoracic and transesophageal echocardiography in predicting embolic events in patients with active infective endocarditis involving native cardiac valves. *Am J Cardiol* 80:1030-1034, 1997.

211. Bayer AS, Bolger AF, Taubert KA, et al: Diagnosis and management of infective endocarditis and its complications. *Circulation* 98:2936-2948, 1998.

212. Mylonakis E, Calderwood SB: Infective endocarditis in adults. *N Engl J Med* 345:1318-1330, 2001.

213. Hirschfeld DS, Schiller N: Localization of aortic valve vegetations by echocardiography. *Circulation* 53:280-285, 1976.

214. Peterson SP, Schiller N, Stricker RB: Failure of two-dimensional echocardiography to detect aspergillus endocarditis. *Chest* 85:291-294, 1984.

215. Habib G: Embolic risk in subacute bacterial endocarditis: Determinants and role of transesophageal echocardiography. *Curr Infect Dis Rep* 7:264-271, 2005.

216. Birmingham GD, Rahko PS, Ballantyne F 3rd: Improved detection of infective endocarditis with transesophageal echocardiography. *Am Heart J* 123:774-781, 1992.

217. Pedersen WR, Walker M, Olson JD, et al: Value of transesophageal echocardiography as an adjunct to transthoracic echocardiography in evaluation of native and prosthetic valve endocarditis. *Chest* 100:351-356, 1991.

218. Shively BK, Gurule FT, Roldan CA, et al: Diagnostic value of transesophageal compared with transthoracic echocardiography in infective endocarditis. *J Am Coll Cardiol* 18:391-397, 1991.

219. Sochowski RA, Chan KL: Implication of negative results on a monoplane transesophageal echocardiographic study in patients with suspected infective endocarditis. *J Am Coll Cardiol* 21:216-221, 1993.

220. Shapiro SM, Young E, De Guzman S, et al: Transesophageal echocardiography in diagnosis of infective endocarditis. *Chest* 105:377-382, 1994.

221. Evangelista A, Gonzalez-Alujas MT: Echocardiography in infective endocarditis. *Heart* 90:614-617, 2004.

222. Heinle S, Wilderman N, Harrison JK, et al: Value of transthoracic echocardiography in predicting embolic events in active infective endocarditis. Duke Endocarditis Service. *Am J Cardiol* 74:799-801, 1994.

223. Mugge A, Daniel WG, Haverich A, Lichtlen PR: Diagnosis of noninfective cardiac mass lesions by two-dimensional echocardiography. Comparison of the transthoracic and transesophageal approaches. *Circulation* 83:70-78, 1991.

224. Rohmann S, Erbel R, Darius H, et al: Prediction of rapid versus prolonged healing of infective endocarditis by monitoring vegetation size. *J Am Soc Echocardiogr* 4:465-474, 1991.

225. Mugge A, Daniel WG, Frank G, Lichtlen PR: Echocardiography in infective endocarditis: reassessment of prognostic implications of vegetation size determined by the transthoracic and the transesophageal approach. *J Am Coll Cardiol* 14:631-638, 1989.

226. Thuny F, Di Salvo G, Belliard O, et al: Risk of embolism and death in infective endocarditis: prognostic value of echocardiography: a prospective multicenter study. *Circulation* 112:69-75, 2005.

227. Rohmann S, Erbel R, Gorge G, et al: Clinical relevance of vegetation localization by transoesophageal echocardiography in infective endocarditis. *Eur Heart J* 13:446-452, 1992.

228. Cabell CH, Pond KK, Peterson GE, et al: The risk of stroke and death in patients with aortic and mitral valve endocarditis. *Am Heart J* 142:75-80, 2001.

229. Baddour LM, Wilson WR, Bayer AS, et al: Infective endocarditis: diagnosis, antimicrobial therapy, and management of complications: A statement for healthcare professionals from the Committee on Rheumatic Fever, Endocarditis, and Kawasaki Disease, Council on Cardiovascular Disease in the Young, and the Councils on Clinical Cardiology, Stroke, and Cardiovascular Surgery and Anesthesia, American Heart Association: endorsed by the Infectious Diseases Society of America. *Circulation* 111: e394-e434, 2005.

230. Rosen AB, Fowler VG Jr, Corey GR, et al: Cost-effectiveness of transesophageal echocardiography to determine the duration of therapy for intravascular catheter-associated Staphylococcus aureus bacteremia. *Ann Intern Med* 130:810-820, 1999.

231. Thangaroopan M, Choy JB: Is transesophageal echocardiography overused in the diagnosis of infective endocarditis? *Am J Cardiol* 95:295-297, 2005.

232. Kuruppu JC, Corretti M, Mackowiak P, Roghmann MC: Overuse of transthoracic echocardiography in the diagnosis of native valve endocarditis. *Arch Intern Med* 162:1715-1720, 2002.

233. McKhann GM, Grega MA, Borowicz LM Jr, et al: Stroke and encephalopathy after cardiac surgery: An update. *Stroke* 37:562-571, 2006.

234. Hogue CW Jr, Barzilai B, Pieper KS, et al: Sex differences in neurological outcomes and mortality after cardiac surgery: a society of thoracic surgery national database report. *Circulation* 103:2133-2137, 2001.

235. Ribakove GH, Katz ES, Galloway AC, et al: Surgical implications of transesophageal echocardiography to grade the atheromatous aortic arch. *Ann Thorac Surg* 53:758-761; discussion 62-63, 1992.

236. Iglesias I, Bainbridge D, Murkin J: Intraoperative echocardiography: Support for decision making in cardiac surgery. *Semin Cardiothorac Vasc Anesth* 8:25-35, 2004.

237. Katz ES, Tunick PA, Rusinek H, et al: Protruding aortic atheromas predict stroke in elderly patients undergoing cardiopulmonary bypass: experience with intraoperative transesophageal echocardiography. *J Am Coll Cardiol* 20:70-77, 1992.

238. Grossi EA, Bizekis CS, Sharony R, et al: Routine intraoperative transesophageal echocardiography identifies patients with atheromatous aortas: impact on "off-pump" coronary artery bypass and perioperative stroke. *J Am Soc Echocardiogr* 16:751-755, 2003.

239. Katsnelson Y, Raman J, Katsnelson F, et al: Current state of intraoperative echocardiography. *Echocardiography* 20:771-780, 2003.

240. Grossi EA, Kanchuger MS, Schwartz DS, et al: Effect of cannula length on aortic arch flow: protection of the atheromatous aortic arch. *Ann Thorac Surg* 59:710-712, 1995.

241. Stern A, Tunick PA, Culliford AT, et al: Protruding aortic arch atheromas: risk of stroke during heart surgery with and without aortic arch endarterectomy. *Am Heart J* 138:746-752, 1999.

242. Macleod MR, Amarenco P, Davis SM, Donnan GA: Atheroma of the aortic arch: an important and poorly recognized factor in the etiology of stroke. *Lancet Neurol* 3:408-414, 2004.

243. Macleod MR, Donnan GA: Atheroma of the aortic arch: the missing link in the secondary prevention of stroke? *Expert Rev Cardiovasc Ther* 1:487-489, 2003.

244. Amarenco P: Cryptogenic stroke, aortic arch atheroma, patent foramen ovale, and the risk of stroke. *Cerebrovasc Dis* 20(Suppl 2):68-74, 2005.

245. Amarenco P, Duyckaerts C, Tzourio C, et al: The prevalence of ulcerated plaques in the aortic arch in patients with stroke. *N Engl J Med* 326:221-225, 1992.

246. Khatibzadeh M, Mitusch R, Stierle U, et al: Aortic atherosclerotic plaques as a source of systemic embolism. *J Am Coll Cardiol* 27:664-669, 1996.

247. Tunick PA, Kronzon I: Protruding atherosclerotic plaque in the aortic arch of patients with systemic embolization: A new finding seen by transesophageal echocardiography. *Am Heart J* 120:658-660, 1990.

248. Amarenco P, Cohen A, Tzourio C, et al: Atherosclerotic disease of the aortic arch and the risk of ischemic stroke. *N Engl J Med* 331:1474-1479, 1994.

249. Jones EF, Kalman JM, Calafiore P, et al: Proximal aortic atheroma. An independent risk factor for cerebral ischemia. *Stroke* 26:218-224, 1995.

250. Stone DA, Hawke MW, LaMonte M, et al: Ulcerated atherosclerotic plaques in the thoracic aorta are associated with cryptogenic stroke: A multiplane transesophageal echocardiographic study. *Am Heart J* 130:105-108, 1995.

251. Di Tullio MR, Sacco RL, Gersony D, et al: Aortic atheromas and acute ischemic stroke: a transesophageal echocardiographic study in an ethnically mixed population. *Neurology* 46:1560-1566, 1996.

252. Ferrari E, Vidal R, Chevallier T, Baudouy M: Atherosclerosis of the thoracic aorta and aortic debris as a marker of poor prognosis: benefit of oral anticoagulants. *J Am Coll Cardiol* 33:1317-1322, 1999.

253. Matsumura Y, Osaki Y, Fukui T, et al: Protruding atherosclerotic aortic plaques and dyslipidemia: correlation to subtypes of ischemic stroke. *Eur J Echocardiogr* 3:8-12, 2002.

254. Di Tullio MR, Sacco RL, Savoia MT, et al: Aortic atheroma morphology and the risk of ischemic stroke in a multiethnic population. *Am Heart J* 139:329-336, 2000.

255. Kazui S, Levi CR, Jones EF, et al: Risk factors for lacunar stroke: A case-control transesophageal echocardiographic study. *Neurology* 54:1385-1387, 2000.

256. Yahia AM, Kirmani JF, Xavier AR, et al: Characteristics and predictors of aortic plaques in patients with transient ischemic attacks and strokes. *J Neuroimaging* 14:16-22, 2004.

257. Tunick PA, Perez JL, Kronzon I: Protruding atheromas in the thoracic aorta and systemic embolization. *Ann Intern Med* 115:423-427, 1991.

258. Atherosclerotic disease of the aortic arch as a risk factor for recurrent ischemic stroke. The French Study of Aortic Plaques in Stroke Group. *N Engl J Med* 334:1216-1221, 1996.

259. Tanaka M, Yasaka M, Nagano K, et al: Moderate atheroma of the aortic arch and the risk of stroke. *Cerebrovasc Dis* 21:26-31, 2006.

260. Dressler FA, Craig WR, Castello R, Labovitz AJ: Mobile aortic atheroma and systemic emboli: efficacy of anticoagulation and influence of plaque morphology on recurrent stroke. *J Am Coll Cardiol* 31:134-138, 1998.

261. Zabalgoitia M, Halperin JL, Pearce LA, et al: Transesophageal echocardiographic correlates of clinical risk of thromboembolism in nonvalvular atrial fibrillation. Stroke Prevention in Atrial Fibrillation III Investigators. *J Am Coll Cardiol* 31:1622-1626, 1998.

262. Tunick PA, Rosenzweig BP, Katz ES, et al: High risk for vascular events in patients with protruding aortic atheromas: a prospective study. *J Am Coll Cardiol* 23(5):1085-1090, 1994.

263. Cohen A, Tzourio C, Bertrand B, et al: Aortic plaque morphology and vascular events: A follow-up study in patients with ischemic stroke. FAPS Investigators. French Study of Aortic Plaques in Stroke. *Circulation* 96:3838-3841, 1997.

264. Meissner I, Khandheria BK, Sheps SG, et al: Atherosclerosis of the aorta: risk factor, risk marker, or innocent bystander? A prospective population-based transesophageal echocardiography study. *J Am Coll Cardiol* 44:1018-1024, 2004.

265. Petty GW, Khandheria BK, Meissner I, et al: Population-based study of the relationship between atherosclerotic aortic debris and cerebrovascular ischemic events. *Mayo Clin Proc* 81:609-614, 2006.

266. Vaduganathan P, Ewton A, Nagueh SF, et al: Pathologic correlates of aortic plaques, thrombi and mobile "aortic debris" imaged in vivo with transesophageal echocardiography. *J Am Coll Cardiol* 30:357-363, 1997.

267. Laperche T, Laurian C, Roudaut R, Steg PG: Mobile thromboses of the aortic arch without aortic debris. A transesophageal echocardiographic finding associated with unexplained arterial embolism. The Filiale Echocardiographie de la Societe Francaise de Cardiologie. *Circulation* 96:288-294, 1997.

268. Freedberg RS, Tunick PA, Kronzon I: Emboli in transit: the missing link. *J Am Soc Echocardiogr* 11:826-828, 1998.

269. Karalis DG, Chandrasekaran K, Victor MF, et al: Recognition and embolic potential of intraaortic atherosclerotic debris. *J Am Coll Cardiol* 17:73-78, 1991.

270. Karalis DG, Quinn V, Victor MF, et al: Risk of catheter-related emboli in patients with atherosclerotic debris in the thoracic aorta. *Am Heart J* 131:1149-1155, 1996.

271. Keeley EC, Grines CL: Scraping of aortic debris by coronary guiding catheters: a prospective evaluation of 1000 cases. *J Am Coll Cardiol* 32:1861-1865, 1998.

272. Sen S, Wu K, McNamara R, et al: Distribution, severity and risk factors for aortic atherosclerosis in cerebral ischemia. *Cerebrovasc Dis* 10:102-109, 2000.

273. Acarturk E, Demir M, Kanadasi M: Aortic atherosclerosis is a marker for significant coronary artery disease. *Jpn Heart J* 40:775-781, 1999.

274. Hilton TC, Menke D, Blackshear JL: Variable effect of anticoagulation in the treatment of severe protruding atherosclerotic aortic debris. *Am Heart J* 127:1645-1647, 1994.

275. Labovitz AJ: Transesophageal echocardiography and unexplained cerebral ischemia: A multicenter follow-up study. The STEPS Investigators. Significance of transesophageal echocardiography in the prevention of recurrent stroke. *Am Heart J* 137:1082-1087, 1999.

276. Montgomery DH, Ververis JJ, McGorisk G, et al: Natural history of severe atheromatous disease of the thoracic aorta: A transesophageal echocardiographic study. *J Am Coll Cardiol* 27:95-101, 1996.

277. Tunick PA, Nayar AC, Goodkin GM, et al: Effect of treatment on the incidence of stroke and other emboli in 519 patients with severe thoracic aortic plaque. *Am J Cardiol* 90(12):1320-1325, 2002.

278. Leys D, Woimant F, Ferrieres J, et al: Detection and management of associated atherothrombotic locations in patients with a recent atherothrombotic ischemic stroke: Results of the DETECT survey. *Cerebrovasc Dis* 21:60-66, 2006.

279. Ward RP, Don CW, Furlong KT, Lang RM: Predictors of long-term mortality in patients with ischemic stroke referred for transesophageal echocardiography. *Stroke* 37:204-208, 2006.

280. Albers GW, Amarenco P, Easton JD, et al: Antithrombotic and thrombolytic therapy for ischemic stroke: the Seventh ACCP Conference on Antithrombotic and Thrombolytic Therapy. *Chest* 126(3 Suppl):483S-512S, 2004.

281. Drobinski G, Montalescot G, Evans J, et al: Systemic embolism as a complication of percutaneous mitral valvuloplasty. *Cathet Cardiovasc Diagn* 25:327-330, 1992.

282. Demirtas M, Usal A, Birand A, et al: A serious complication of percutaneous mitral valvuloplasty: systemic embolism. How can we decrease it? Case history. *Angiology* 47:285-289, 1996.

283. Liu TJ, Lai HC, Lee WL, et al: Immediate and late outcomes of patients undergoing transseptal left-sided heart catheterization for symptomatic valvular and arrhythmic diseases. *Am Heart J* 151:235-241, 2006.

284. Barnett HJ, Boughner DR, Taylor DW, et al: Further evidence relating mitral-valve prolapse to cerebral ischemic events. *N Engl J Med* 302:139-144, 1980.

285. Nishimura RA, McGoon MD, Shub C, et al: Echocardiographically documented mitral-valve prolapse. Long-term follow-up of 237 patients. *N Engl J Med* 313:1305-1309, 1985.

286. Gilon D, Buonanno FS, Joffe MM, et al: Lack of evidence of an association between mitral-valve prolapse and stroke in young patients. *N Engl J Med* 341:8-13, 1999.

287. Orencia AJ, Petty GW, Khandheria BK, et al: Risk of stroke with mitral valve prolapse in population-based cohort study. *Stroke* 26:7-13, 1995.

288. Orencia AJ, Petty GW, Khandheria BK, et al: Mitral valve prolapse and the risk of stroke after initial cerebral ischemia. *Neurology* 45:1083-1086, 1995.

289. Freed LA, Levy D, Levine RA, et al: Prevalence and clinical outcome of mitral-valve prolapse. *N Engl J Med* 341:1-7, 1999.

290. Avierinos JF, Brown RD, Foley DA, et al: Cerebral ischemic events after diagnosis of mitral valve prolapse: a community-based study of incidence and predictive factors. *Stroke* 34:1339-1344, 2003.

291. Mohr JP, Thompson JL, Lazar RM, et al: A comparison of warfarin and aspirin for the prevention of recurrent ischemic stroke. *N Engl J Med* 345:1444-1451, 2001.

292. Sacco RL, Prabhakaran S, Thompson JL, et al: Comparison of warfarin versus aspirin for the prevention of recurrent stroke or death: Subgroup analyses from the warfarin-aspirin recurrent stroke study. *Cerebrovasc Dis* 22:4-12, 2006.

293. Chimowitz MI, Lynn MJ, Howlett-Smith H, et al: Comparison of warfarin and aspirin for symptomatic intracranial arterial stenosis. *N Engl J Med* 352:1305-1316, 2005.

294. Bhatt DL, Fox KA, Hacke W, et al: Clopidogrel and aspirin versus aspirin alone for the prevention of atherothrombotic events. *N Engl J Med* 354:1706-1717, 2006.

295. Diener HC, Bogousslavsky J, Brass LM, et al: Aspirin and clopidogrel compared with clopidogrel alone after recent ischemic stroke or transient ischemic attack in high-risk patients (MATCH): randomized, double-blind, placebo-controlled trial. *Lancet* 364:331-337, 2004.

296. The International Stroke Trial (IST): A randomized trial of aspirin, subcutaneous heparin, both, or neither among 19,435 patients with acute ischemic stroke. International Stroke Trial Collaborative Group. *Lancet* 349:1569-1581, 1997.

297. CAST: Randomized placebo-controlled trial of early aspirin use in 20,000 patients with acute ischemic stroke. CAST (Chinese Acute Stroke Trial) Collaborative Group. *Lancet* 349:1641-1649, 1997.

298. Chen ZM, Sandercock P, Pan HC, et al: Indications for early aspirin use in acute ischemic stroke: A combined analysis of 40,000 randomized patients from the Chinese acute stroke trial and the international stroke trial. On behalf of the CAST and IST collaborative groups. *Stroke* 31:1240-1249, 2000.

299. Dawn B, Hasnie AM, Calzada N, et al: Transesophageal echocardiography impacts management and evaluation of patients with stroke, transient ischemic attack, or peripheral embolism. *Echocardiography* 23:202-207, 2006.

300. McNamara RL, Lima JA, Whelton PK, Powe NR: Echocardiographic identification of cardiovascular sources of emboli to guide clinical management of stroke: a cost-effectiveness analysis. *Ann Intern Med* 127:775-787, 1997.

301. Rabinstein AA, Chirinos JA, Fernandez FR, et al: Is TEE useful in patients with small subcortical strokes? *Eur J Neurol* 13:522-527, 2006.

Chapter 41

The Role of Echocardiography in Atrial Fibrillation and Flutter

WARREN J. MANNING, MD

Technologic advances in two-dimensional (2D) and Doppler ultrasonography have led to the emergence of echocardiography as an integral tool in the evaluation and management of patients with cardiac rhythm disturbances. Transthoracic echocardiography (TTE) and transesophageal echocardiography (TEE) provide detailed information about cardiac anatomy and function. Patients with ventricular tachyarrhythmias are routinely referred for echocardiographic examination for identification of suspected structural heart disease. Echocardiography may also play a role in the localization of bypass tracts in Wolff-Parkinson-White syndrome[1] and in the choice of optimal pacemaker type, lead position, and settings in patients with hemodynamic compromise related to rhythm disturbances[2] and characterization of ventricular dyssynchrony and respondents to cardiac resynchronization therapy (CRT).[3,4]

In addition to ventricular arrhythmias, both TTE and TEE provides useful information in the evaluation and management of patients with atrial arrhythmias, particularly atrial fibrillation (AFib). In this chapter, we review the detailed structural and functional information derived from TTE and TEE and how these data assist in the evaluation and management of patients with AFib and atrial flutter.

Echocardiographic Assessment of Atrial Anatomy and Function

Left Atrial Anatomy

TTE has long been recognized as a reliable and reproducible method to assess the anatomy of the body of the left atrium. M-mode echocardiography[5-7] allows for the measurement of left atrial dimension in the parasternal long-axis or short-axis orientations. Overall, this unidimensional index correlates well with angiographically derived left atrial area and volume[6,7] but may be disproportionately erroneous in common disease states associated with asymmetric atrial dilation, such as mitral valve disease.[8]

Two-dimensional TTE provides more accurate assessment of atrial anatomy. The left atrium is well seen from both the parasternal and the apical windows. In many laboratories, left atrial anatomy is characterized by the M-mode or 2D dimension from the parasternal long-axis or short-axis and the left atrial length from the apical four-chamber view. Because the left atrium is not spherically shaped and asymmetric enlargement may occur, 2D derived left atrial volume provides a more accurate measure of left atrial size[9] and is advocated by the American Society of Echocardiography[10] and more favorably compares with volumetric methods, such as cardiovascular magnetic resonance imaging (MRI) and computed tomography (CT).[11,12] With the biplane method,[13] maximum left atrial area and length are measured in the apical four-chamber (A_{4C}, L_{4C}) and two-chamber (A_{2C}, L_{2C}) orientations with volume derived as:

$$\text{Left Atrial Volume} = \frac{1.7\ (A_{4C})\ (A_{2C})}{L_{4C} + L_{2C}}$$

Population-based studies suggest left atrial volumes of 41.9 ± 11.9 ml or when normalized for body surface area, 22 ± 5 ml/m^2.[14] Increasing left atrial volume has been shown to predict development of AFib in the general population[15] and patients postcardiac surgery[16] and hypertrophic cardiomyopathy (HCM).[17,18] Biplane and Simpson's methods compare closely.[13] In situations in which there is focal atrial asymmetry, such as distortion of the left atrium from an extrinsic structure (e.g., mediastinal tumor, hiatal hernia, or descending thoracic aortic aneurysm), accurate calculation of left atrial volume may be improved by using a Simpson approach.

TEE is a well tolerated but moderately invasive diagnostic imaging technique that allows for superior visualization of posterior structures, such as the left atrium and atrial appendage. Although TEE may be used to assess the body of the left atrium from orientations analogous to transthoracic imaging,[19] its greatest advantage is in evaluation of the anatomy and function of the left and right atrial appendages.

Identification of Left Atrial Thrombi

Anatomic imaging of the body of the left atrium may be readily obtained from 2D TTE, but identification or exclusion of left atrial and left atrial appendage thrombi are best reserved for TEE. The sensitivity of TTE for the detection of left atrial thrombi (Fig. 41–1) has been estimated at only 39% to 63%,[20-22] with limited success for identifying thrombi in the left atrial appendage. Even with modified views,[23] visualization of the left atrial appendage may be accomplished in less than 20% of patients.[24] Though identification of atrial appendage thrombi using more modern TTE equipment has been described,[25] this has not been confirmed by larger series or other groups.

Imaging of the left atrial appendage is readily accomplished with multiplane TEE (Fig. 41–2). The normal length and neck width of the adult left atrial appendage in the horizontal and vertical imaging planes are 28 ± 5 mm and 16 ± 5 mm, respectively.[26] Left atrial appendage anatomic indexes are dependent on imaging plane, with greater neck width and cross-sectional area (CSA) when observed at a 135-degree imaging plane as compared with a 45-degree or 90-degree plane,[27] consistent with its shape idealized as a special ungula of a right circular cylinder.[27] Multiple lobes and trabeculations are common (see Fig. 41–2).

The accuracy of TEE for the identification of left atrial thrombi has been reported by several investigators. Aschenberg and colleagues[24] were among the first to report on preoperative monoplane TEE for atrial thrombi. Among 21 consecutive patients presenting for routine mitral valve replacement, 6 patients had TEE evidence of left atrial thrombi. All six thrombi were

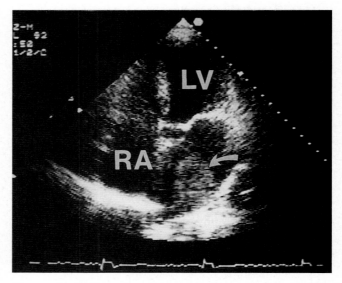

Figure 41–1. Transthoracic echocardiographic image taken from the apical four-chamber view obtained with a 5 MHz imaging transducer. Note the thrombus (arrow) along the posterior wall of the left atrium in this patient with rheumatic mitral stenosis. LV, left ventricle; RA, right atrium.

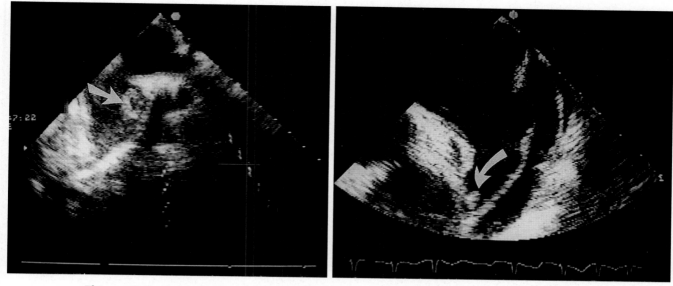

Figure 41-2. *Transesophageal echocardiographic image taken in the horizontal plane using a 5 MHz imaging transducer.* A, *15-mm thrombus (arrow) near the mouth of the left atrial appendage;* B, *4-mm thrombus (arrow) at the tip of the left atrial appendage. (From Manning WJ, Reis GJ, Douglas PS: Br Heart J 67:171, 1992.)*

confirmed at surgery and no additional thrombi were seen on direct inspection. Mügge and colleagues[28] subsequently reported on 12 patients with atrial thrombi detected by monoplane TEE who were referred for cardiac surgery. All thrombi were confirmed on direct inspection. Similarly, Olson and colleagues[29] performed monoplane TEE in 20 patients immediately before mitral valve replacement or mitral valve repair. They prospectively identified all three atrial thrombi seen at surgery, including two in the left atrium and one in the right atrium. Finally, in the largest monoplane TEE series, Hwang and colleagues[30] reported on more than 200 patients with rheumatic mitral valve disease undergoing TEE within 3 days of valve surgery. Sensitivity and specificity for detection of atrial thrombus were 93% and 100%, respectively.

Over the past decade, multiplane TEE technology has become the standard with superior visualization of the left atrial appendage. In my experience of nearly 200 consecutive patients undergoing monoplane, biplane, or multiplane intraoperative TEE immediately before mitral valve surgery, TEE sensitivity and specificity for left atrial thrombi were 100% and 99%, respectively.[31] I have found the 0-degree, 90-degree, and 135-degree imaging planes particularly advantageous for assessing the left atrial appendage.

Right Atrial Anatomy

The right atrium has not been as well studied by either TTE or TEE. As is the case with the left atrium, 2D TTE provides a reasonably comprehensive assessment of right atrial volume. The primary transthoracic window is the apical four-chamber view, with right atrial area

estimated using a length-diameter ellipsoid formula. Parasternal short-axis and subxiphoid windows provide complementary data. The right atrial appendage is rarely appreciated from TTE, but TEE at 90-degree (Fig. 41–3) and 135-degree imaging orientations readily allow for visualization of this structure.[32] Right atrial appendage area and length are independent of transducer orientation with areas of 5.4 ± 2.4 cm[2] and lengths of 4.0 ± 0.9 cm reported for those in sinus rhythm.[32] Care must be taken to avoid mistaking normal structures (such as the Eustachian valve or Chiari network) for thrombi.[32,33]

TTE and TEE sensitivity and specificity data for identification of right atrial thrombi are relatively sparse. Schwartzbard and colleagues[34] reported on 20 patients with TEE evidence of right atrial thrombus, including 7 confirmed at surgery. TTE identified thrombus in only six patients (30%). All right atrial appendage thrombi were missed by TTE.

Atrial Mechanical Function

In addition to providing information about atrial anatomy, echocardiography is a powerful tool for evaluation of atrial systolic performance. The atria are traditionally believed to have two primary functions: as passive conduits or reservoirs for oxygenated blood passing from the vena cava or lungs to the ventricles and as booster pumps to augment passive diastolic ventricular filling.

Before the advent of echocardiography, assessment of atrial mechanical function had been limited to invasive catheter-based techniques,[35] which are impractical for serial assessments. M-mode echocardiographic as-

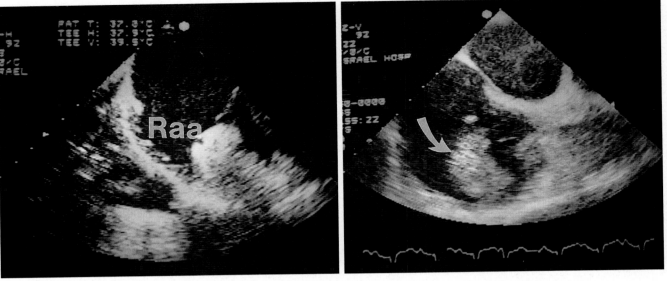

Figure 41–3. *Transesophageal echocardiographic image depicting normal right atrial appendage (RAA) in the horizontal imaging plane* (A) *and another patient with a right atrial thrombus* (arrow) *in the vertical plane* (B).

sessment of mitral valve motion can be used in patients with cardiac arrhythmias and was first described by Gabor and Winsberg.[36] Normal anterior mitral leaflet excursion is 13 mm,[36,37] with depressed excursion seen with mitral stenosis (MS), low cardiac output (CO), and in association with atrial mechanical dysfunction.

With the development of 2D-guided pulsed Doppler technology, transmitral Doppler spectra have become recognized as an accurate technique for quantifying atrial mechanical function. In the absence of aortic insufficiency, left ventricular (LV) filling may be divided into passive and active phases. The initial (early, or E) wave in the transmitral Doppler flow profile represents passive ventricular filling, and the final (atrial, or A) wave represents active filling during atrial systole (Fig. 41–4). This transmitral Doppler flow profile can be influenced by a number of factors, including heart rate (HR), loading conditions, and sample volume position. The most common indexes of interest include peak A wave velocity, percentage of A wave filling, and peak and percentage E/A ratios. Peak E and A wave velocities vary considerably with sample position. In my laboratory, I generally assess the transmitral profile at its maximum (between the tips of the mitral leaflets).

In addition to the previously described quantitative indexes of transmitral Doppler data, the transmitral Doppler profile may also be used to calculate atrial ejection force, defined as that force that the atrium exerts to propel blood into the left ventricle.[38] The atrial ejection force is based on Newtonian mechanics and is proportional to the mitral orifice area and the square of the peak A wave velocity. As with more traditional E wave and A wave indexes, atrial ejection force may be dependent on loading parameters, although this subject remains to be more completely

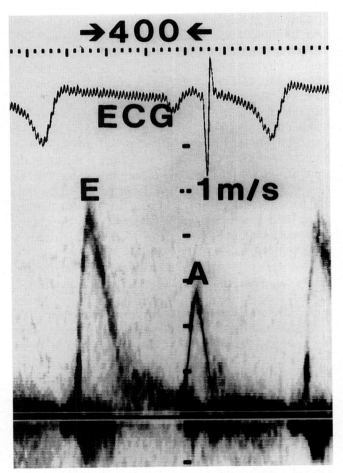

Figure 41–4. *Spectral display of transmitral pulsed Doppler echocardiographic flow velocity. The time scale (top) is measured in milliseconds. A, atrial filling wave; E, early filling wave; ECG, electrocardiogram. (From Manning WJ, Silverman DI, Katz SE, et al: J Am Coll Cardiol 22:222, 1993. With permission from the American College of Cardiology.)*

studied. If calculation of atrial ejection force is desired, a pulsed Doppler sample position at the level of the mitral annulus would be geometrically more appropriate.

Left Atrial Appendage Function

Because the left atrial appendage is a "blind pouch," volumetric ejection must equal inflow during each cardiac cycle. Pollick and Taylor[39] noted that patients with sinus rhythm who were free of atrial thrombus had a characteristic contractile left atrial appendage apex and a noncontractile base. 2D TEE-guided pulsed Doppler has allowed for further characterization of left atrial appendage systolic performance. The pulsed Doppler profile taken at the mouth of the left atrial appendage displayed characterizing ejection and filling phases (Fig. 41–5A). In a healthy adult population, peak left atrial appendage ejection and filling velocities are 46±18 cm/s and 46±17 cm/s, respectively.[40] Investigators have subsequently characterized left atrial appendage flow patterns as having four distinct morphologic types (see Fig. 41–5): type I, sinus; type II, flutter (regularized saw-tooth); type III, fibrillatory (irregular saw-tooth) with ejection velocity greater than 0.2 m/s; and type IV, stagnant/absent flow with peak ejection velocity of 0.2 m/s or less. In rare instances, there may be a discontinuity between the body of the atrium and appendage[41,42] with sinus pattern on transmitral flow but a fibrillatory pattern in the appendage. As compared with anatomic indexes, which appear to be dependent on imaging plane, Doppler indexes of atrial appendage ejection and inflow are independent of imaging plane.[27] Spontaneous echocardiographic contrast (SEC), a marker for stasis, is typically seen with type III or IV appendage flow, whereas left atrial appendage thrombi are most commonly seen with type IV flow.[43,44] As with transmitral Doppler data, left atrial appendage flow velocities are dependent on Doppler sample position and loading conditions.[45]

Right atrial appendage function has not been as well studied. One report indicated normal right atrial appendage ejection velocity of 40 + 16 cm/s, significantly lower than left atrial appendage ejection velocity.[32]

Echocardiography and Atrial Fibrillation

Prevalence of Atrial Fibrillation

AFib is a common arrhythmia, with an overall prevalence of 0.4% in the United States[46] and is responsible for more than 180,000 hospital admissions annually.[46] Its prevalence increases sharply with increasing age and is found in up to 4% of people over 60 years of

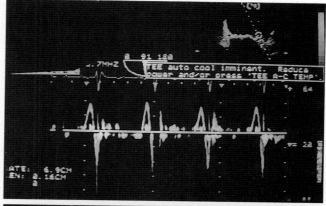

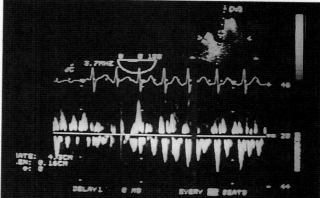

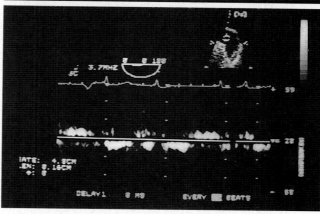

Figure 41–5. Spectral display of pulsed Doppler echocardiographic flow velocity with the sample volume at the mouth of the left atrial appendage. A, Patient in sinus rhythm. B, Patient with atrial fibrillation with active appendage ejection. C, Patient with atrial fibrillation with minimal atrial appendage mechanical function. The vertical calibration markings for each represent 0.2 m/s intervals.

age.[47] Data from the Framingham Heart Study suggest that an increased E/A ratio was associated with an increased risk for the subsequent development of AFib.[48] In an earlier Framingham Heart Study, the presence of chronic AFib was associated with a near doubling of both overall and cardiovascular mortality.[49] Atrial flutter is a far less common sustained arrhythmia. Analogous detailed epidemiologic studies are not available.

Symptoms and Clinical Impact

AFib is characterized by a lack of organized atrial mechanical and electrical activity. This condition promotes stasis of blood within the atria and increases the risk of thrombus formation. Thromboembolism associated with AFib is believed to account for nearly half of all cardiac sources of emboli. In addition to the risk of thrombus formation, loss of organized atrial mechanical activity impairs the atrium's ability to act as a "booster" pump and thus impairs ventricular filling (and consequently cardiac output).[50] The mechanical function of the atria appears to be less severely impaired in atrial flutter, but thrombus formation remains a concern, particularly among patients with alternating AFib and flutter or flutter in the setting of MS or LV systolic dysfunction.

Important clinical issues related to AFib include the following:

1. Thromboembolism, including cerebral and other systemic emboli and pulmonary emboli. These events are likely the result of the migration of thrombi formed within the atria during the period of AFib or may relate to new thrombus formation during the periconversion period. Among patients with nonvalvular AFib, the vast majority (>90%) of atrial thrombi reside in the left atrial appendage (a structure best visualized by TEE). TEE evidence of SEC and depressed atrial appendage ejection velocity (<0.2 m/s) are markers for increased risk for both thrombus formation and for clinical thromboembolism.[44,51-53]

2. Hemodynamic decompensation, which may include depressed cardiac output, congestive heart failure (CHF), fatigue, and pulmonary edema. Decompensation is particularly common among patients with a noncompliant ventricle. Such a situation may occur with normal aging and with left ventricular hypertrophy (LVH) related to systemic hypertension or aortic stenosis (AS). This hemodynamic deterioration is particularly common in the setting of a rapid ventricular rate, during which the diastolic filling period is preferentially shortened.

3. Palpitations, most commonly associated with AFib with a rapid (>100 per minute) ventricular response. Patients with controlled ventricular rates (<100 per minute) are often asymptomatic.

4. Tachycardia-induced cardiomyopathy, which may occur in patients with poorly controlled, rapid ventricular rates.

Atrial Size and Atrial Fibrillation

Left atrial enlargement is common among patients with AFib, particularly those with mitral valve disease or systemic hypertension. Data suggest that left atrial enlarge-

ment decreases the likelihood that long-term maintenance of sinus rhythm will be maintained.[54,55] Aronow and colleagues[56] studied 588 patients and found that an enlarged left atrium was present in 57% of patients with chronic AFib as compared with only 8% of those with sinus rhythm. Data from the Framingham Heart Study suggest that among those without a history of AFib, left atrial enlargement is among the strongest predictors for the subsequent development of nonvalvular AFib.[49] Several groups have reported that left atrial size increases with progressive duration of AFib.[57-59]

Although AFib promotes further left atrial enlargement, there are data suggesting that cardioversion and maintenance of sinus rhythm may reverse this process. Using M-mode techniques, DeMaria and colleagues[37] reported a decrease in left atrial size within 1 hour of cardioversion. I studied a group of 21 patients with AFib of 5 months' duration.[60] Patients with persistent sinus rhythm had significantly smaller left atria 3 months after cardioversion as compared with precardioversion data. In contrast, the group of patients who reverted to AFib had no change in left atrial size. Similarly, Gosselink and colleagues[61] reported on atrial size in 41 patients with chronic AFib undergoing precardioversion and 6-month postcardioversion TTE. Both left and right atrial volumes decreased among patients with persistent sinus rhythm, with no change in the group who reverted to AFib. Van Gelder and colleagues[62] reported on 120 patients with chronic AFib who were cardioverted and remained in sinus rhythm for at least 6 months. Significant regression of both left and right atrial size was documented (except in patients with MS). Similar results have also been seen 1 year after pulmonary vein ablation.[63] These data strongly suggest that restoration of sinus rhythm may reverse the process of progressive left and right atrial enlargement.

Because atrial enlargement may be deleterious and cardioversion to sinus rhythm may prevent or reverse such dilation, I believe that avoidance of cardioversion should not be based on an absolute left atrial size. Patients with chronic (>1 year) AFib, rheumatic mitral valve disease, and prominent left atrial enlargement (>6 cm), however, are far less likely to be maintained in sinus rhythm after conversion.[64]

Detection of Atrial Thrombi in Atrial Fibrillation

AFib is believed to be responsible for almost half of cardiogenic thromboembolism. Several large, multicenter, prospective randomized studies have now confirmed the beneficial effect of chronic anticoagulation (International Normalized Ratio [INR] 2 to 3) in patients with AFib[65-69] for clinical stroke prevention, with one retrospective study suggesting an INR of greater than 2.5 immediately before cardioversion to be particularly beneficial.[70] Because TTE is so limited for the assessment of atrial thrombi,[20-22] data on the prevalence of left atrial thrombi was not available until the introduction of TEE. Among patients presenting with AFib of greater than 2 days' or of unknown duration, I found atrial thrombi in 13%,[71,72] of which more than 92% were left atrial thrombi and nearly all of these involved the left atrial appendage. These data are similar to those reported by others[73-78] but higher than the approximately 6% incidence of clinical thromboembolism following cardioversion without anticoagulation.[79-82] This apparent discrepancy can be explained by the fact that some thrombi may not migrate, and some embolic events may be clinically silent.[83,84] Patients at particularly high risk for atrial thrombi (Table 41-1) included those with rheumatic mitral valve disease, depressed LV systolic function, recent thromboembolism,[85] and TEE evidence of severe left atrial SEC and complex aortic debris.[53,84] Duration of AFib and left atrial dimension are not predictive of left atrial thrombi.[71,72]

In contrast to data suggesting that moderate or worse mitral regurgitation (MR) is protective against clinical thromboembolism,[86,87] researchers have found that mitral regurgitation is not protective against left atrial thrombi (see Table 41-1) among those with new onset AFib.[71]

Immediate cardioversion is generally advocated for patients with AFib of less than 24 hours' duration,[88] under the assumption that the prevalence of atrial thrombi in this group was low. This common teaching was challenged when Stoddard and colleagues[89] reported a 14% prevalence of atrial thrombi among patients with AFib of less than 3 days' duration and a prevalence of 27% in those with a duration of 3 days or more in a predominantly male population. In contrast, I found an incidence of clinical thromboembolism following cardioversion (without antecedent TEE or prolonged warfarin anticoagulation) of less than 1% among patients with AFib of less than 2 days' duration.[90] Thus, prolonged warfarin or screening TEE are likely not needed in this group (unless they have a history of thromboembolism, severe LV dysfunction, or MS). Although I perform cardioversion of AFib of less than 48 hours' duration without prolonged warfarin or screening TEE, I do initiate therapeutic anticoagulation at presentation (rather than delaying anticoagulation until the patient has been in AFib for 48 hours).

As might be expected, atrial thrombi are more common among patients with AFib with acute thromboembolism. In my experience, residual left atrial thrombi are found in more than 40% of these patients.[91] Because this group represents a high clinical risk for whom chronic warfarin is indicated, I do not routinely perform TEE to search for thrombi in this group but do so if cardioversion is desired.

Right atrial thrombi appear to be far less common among patients with AFib and represent less than 5% of all atrial thrombi.[71,72,92] Right atrial SEC is distinctly unusual. It is seen in only 10% of patients with AFib[71] but is highly predictive for right atrial thrombi.

Chronic Atrial Fibrillation and Predictors of Thromboembolism

Compared with patients with new-onset AFib and undergo TEE before cardioversion, risk factors of thromboembolism differ in patients with chronic AFib. Prior

---

TABLE 41-1. Characteristics of Patients at Risk for Atrial Thrombi

	Entire Group	Left Atrial Thrombus	No Left Atrial Thrombus	*p* Value
Total number	533*	70	463	—
Age (year)	71.6±13	70.7±14	71.7±13.2	0.55
Gender (% female)	45.9	54.3	44.4	0.16
First episode of AF (%)	60	64.3	59.1	0.49
Duration of AF (weeks)	4.4±9.3	5.8±15.4	3.9±8	0.18
History of thromboembolism (%)	8.3	28.9	7.3	0.003
Left atrial SEC (%)	48	85.5	36.9	0.0001
Left atrial dimension (cm)	4.6±0.7	4.7±0.7	4.6±0.7	0.29
Mitral regurgitation (0-3+)	1.3±0.9	1.2±0.6	1.3±0.9	0.35
Left ventricular dysfunction (%)	40.9	60.7	38.1	0.002

Data presented are mean value ±SD.
*TEE could not be completed in six patients. Data for these six are excluded.
AF, atrial fibrillation; SD, standard deviation; SEC, spontaneous echocardiographic contrast.
Adapted from The Stroke Prevention in Atrial Fibrillation Investigators: *Ann Intern Med* 116:6-12, 1992.

thromboembolism and LV systolic dysfunction are among the strongest independent predictors of thromboembolism in patients with chronic AFib.[93] The TEE substudies of the Stroke Prevention in Atrial Fibrillation Investigators Committee (SPAF) III study[53] have extended echocardiographic indexes known to be associated with thromboembolism to include dense SEC, depressed (<20 cm/s) left atrial appendage ejection velocity, left atrial thrombus, and complex aortic plaque. Importantly, the SPAF-III data suggest that these TEE indexes may identify high-risk and low-risk subgroups from among clinically high-risk patients (age, female gender, systemic hypertension, LV dysfunction, or prior thromboembolism).[53]

Guidance of Early Cardioversion

Cardioversion of AFib is performed in an effort to improve cardiac function, relieve symptoms, and decrease the risk of thrombus formation. Data from several large prospective studies now indicate no mortality or thromboembolic advantage to aggressive cardioversion and maintenance of sinus rhythm (versus chronic anticoagulation and rate control).[94-96] However, for symptomatic patients who are difficult to rate control, cardioversion is still advocated. Unfortunately, successful cardioversion is associated with an approximately 6% incidence of clinical thromboembolism among patients who are not systematically anticoagulated for several weeks prior to cardioversion.[79-82] Because atrial thrombi are poorly detected by TTE, conventional care of patients with AFib of unknown or prolonged (>2 days') duration had demanded that these patients receive several weeks of anticoagulation before cardioversion, followed by several weeks of anticoagulation after cardioversion while atrial mechanical function recovers.[97] Although no randomized and only two prospective studies[73,76] have been reported, 3 to 4 weeks of warfarin therapy appears to decrease the risk of an embolic event following cardioversion to less than 1.6%.[70,73,76,81,82] The majority of these clinical embolic events occur within the first 10 days after cardioversion.[98] Use of warfarin, however, carries a risk of major (2%) and minor (10% to 20%) hemorrhagic complications.[73,76,99] In addition, many patients develop a subtherapeutic INR during the month leading to cardioversion. For these individuals, the warfarin dose is increased and the "1-month clock" restarted, an approach supported by TEE studies demonstrating left atrial appendage thrombi in these patients.[100,101] Finally, conventional therapy leads to a delay in cardioversion for the large majority of patients who do not have an atrial thrombus, and a second hospitalization is needed later for cardioversion.

Rationale and Advantages

The risks and benefits of a TEE-guided approach to cardioversion are summarized in Table 41–2. A TEE-guided approach to early and safe cardioversion has

TABLE 41–2. Benefits and Risks of Transesophageal Echocardiography–Guided Cardioversion

Benefits

Shorter initial duration of atrial fibrillation (AFib)
  Enhanced recovery of atrial mechanical function
  More rapid resolution of symptoms of congestive heart failure (CGF)
  Increased likelihood that sinus rhythm will be maintained
No need to return for elective cardioversion after 1 month of warfarin anticoagulation
Shorter total duration of AFib
  Fewer hemorrhagic complications
  Lower cost for warfarin medication and monitoring
Fewer thromboembolic events than conventional therapy (?)
More cost-effective than conventional therapy
Identify high-risk population that requires lifelong warfarin regardless of clinical risk factors (?)

Risks

Transesophageal echocardiography (TEE) "misses" clinically relevant thrombi that subsequently migrate and cause stroke or thromboembolism
Morbidity associated with TEE
Cost of TEE

several advantages over traditional strategies for hospitalized patients with AFib. Currently, up to 8 weeks of oral anticoagulation are recommended with cardioversion,[88,102,103] including 3 to 4 weeks before and after cardioversion. This period of anticoagulation exposes patients to a significant risk of a hemorrhagic complication[73,76,99] by doubling the exposure of systemic anticoagulation. For unclear reasons, the AFib population appears to be at increased risk of hemorrhagic complications during the second month of anticoagulation.[73]

Early cardioversion offers physiologic advantages over traditional therapy. A shorter duration of AFib before cardioversion is among the strongest predictors for long-term maintenance of sinus rhythm.[55] Almost 60% of patients hospitalized for AFib at my hospital[71,72] have been in AFib for less than 1 month. For these individuals, traditional treatment of 3 to 4 weeks of anticoagulation before cardioversion serves to more than double the total period of AFib before cardioversion. The TEE-guided approach has been shown to be associated with fewer recurrences of AFib[72] and to increased prevalence of sinus rhythm at 6 months postcardioversion.[104]

Early cardioversion may also lead to a more rapid return to normal atrial function. The time required for return of atrial mechanical function is directly related to the duration of AFib before cardioversion.[97,105] Patients with AFib less than 2 weeks before cardioversion appear to have complete return of atrial mechanical function within 24 hours of cardioversion, whereas those with AFib of 2 to 6 weeks require a week, and those with AFib for more than 6 weeks require up to 3 weeks.[97] With elimination of a TTE, a TEE approach to guide early cardioversion also appears to have cost savings.[106,107] Finally, a TEE approach may also reduce the incidence of thromboembolism after cardioversion. The costs of the TEE approach include the morbidity of TEE, cost of TEE, and risk that TEE will not be adequate to identify atrial thrombi, which subsequently migrate and cause clinical events.

Current Data

I reported on my experience with a TEE-guided approach (Fig. 41–6) to early cardioversion among 533 patients with AFib of unknown or prolonged duration who underwent precardioversion TEE in the absence of prolonged chronic anticoagulation.[71,72,92] Seventy-six atrial thrombi were identified in 70 patients (13%). Of the 463 without TEE evidence of thrombi, 413 (89%) were successfully cardioverted to sinus rhythm, all without prolonged anticoagulation, and 1 (0.2%; 95% confidence interval [CI], 0 to 0.8%) experienced a clinical thromboembolic event. The one adverse event occurred in an elderly woman with mild MS who was diagnosed 1 week after cardioversion with a brachial artery embolus. She had been therapeutically anticoagulated between TEE and diagnosis with the adverse event.[72] None of the 70 patients with atrial thrombi were cardioverted, but 5 (7%) died during the index hospitalization. Repeat TEE to document resolution of atrial thrombi was recommended for all with atrial thrombi, with cardioversion only after documentation of thrombus resolution.

Other prospective studies using a similar anticoagulation regimen have shown similar results. Stoddard and colleagues[75] reported on 82 patients scheduled for elective cardioversion of AFib. Atrial thrombi were identified in 13% of patients. Sixty-six of 71 patients without atrial thrombi underwent successful cardioversion, and no patient experienced a clinical embolic event. The pilot study data from the Assessment of Cardioversion Using Transesophageal Echocardiography (ACUTE) trial reported no thromboembolic complications among 47 patients treated with an anticoagulation strategy similar to mine.[73] Finally, data from the 1222-patient, multicenter, randomized ACUTE trial,[76] which directly compared conventional therapy of

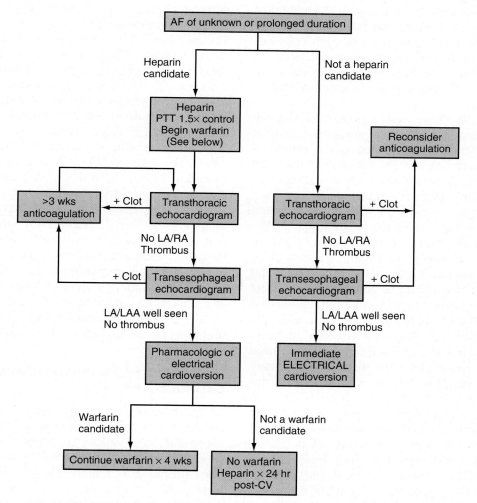

Figure 41–6. Schematic of the transesophageal echocardiographic protocol. *AF, atrial fibrillation; CV, cardioversion; LA, left atrium; LAA, left atrial appendage; PTT, partial thromboplastin time. (From Manning WJ, Silverman DI, Keighley CS, et al:* J Am Coll Cardiol 25:1356, 1995.)

4 weeks of precardioversion warfarin with a strategy of therapeutic anticoagulation followed by TEE and early cardioversion if no atrial thrombi are seen. Equivalence was found for both approaches, though with 0.5% thromboembolic events in the conventional arm and 0.8% in the TEE arm. Of note, nearly all of the adverse events in the ACUTE TEE arm occurred while the patient had a subtherapeutic (<2) INR or was in AFib, while the adverse events in the conventional therapy arm occurred in patients in sinus rhythm and with therapeutic INR. These data highlighted the importance of therapeutic postcardioversion anticoagulation. Interestingly, the absence of an atrial thrombus on a prior TEE does not appear to preclude the need for a TEE if a patient returns with AFib in the absence of chronic anticoagulation.[108]

Although these reports are encouraging, several adverse events have occurred among patients with a "negative" TEE for atrial thrombi who have undergone early cardioversion using monoplane TEE or in the absence of systemic anticoagulation.[109] Many underwent electrical cardioversion several days or weeks following TEE with no anticoagulation during this interval. For these patients, it is impossible to exclude the possibility that atrial thrombi may have formed either between the TEE and cardioversion or even after cardioversion. Impaired atrial mechanical function,[97,110] impaired atrial appendage function,[111,112] or new spontaneous contrast[75,112] have all been documented following cardioversion.

Although no data have been reported for conventional cardioversion approaches, a prospective study of 127 patients undergoing TEE-guided cardioversion reported no clinical embolic events, but cerebral magnetic resonance imaging demonstrated 4.7% of patients had new embolic lesions suggestive of embolic lesions.[113]

As in my original report,[92] I strongly recommend that all patients being considered for multiplane TEE-guided early cardioversion be therapeutically anticoagulated with intravenous (IV) heparin or warfarin at the time of TEE, continuing through cardioversion, and that warfarin anticoagulation be continued for at least 1 month after cardioversion. TEE should be performed (without preceding TTE to reduce costs[106]) immediately before cardioversion to adequately visualize the atria and appendages and to exclude the presence of atrial thrombi. Heightened vigilance for thrombi is necessary if there is prominent SEC or poor (<0.2 m/s) atrial appendage ejection velocity. If a thrombus is seen on TEE, cardioversion should be deferred and the patient maintained on warfarin for 4 weeks followed by repeat TEE to document thrombus resolution before cardioversion.[114] Patients with right atrial appendage thrombi should be treated in a similar manner. If the atrial appendage cannot be adequately "cleared" of thrombus, the patient should be treated conservatively with 3 to 4 weeks of therapeutic warfarin before cardioversion.

The use of low molecular weight precardioversion anticoagulation or as a bridge to therapeutic warfarin to expedite patient discharge has been less extensively studied but appears to be a reasonable option with regards to safety and shortens hospitalization.[11,115,116]

Although not directly supported by prospective clinical trials, it is my clinical practice to treat patients with AFib who have TEE evidence of atrial thrombi with "life-long" warfarin (INR, 2 to 3) even after resolution of thrombus has been documented and cardioversion to sinus rhythm has been achieved. I believe such an approach is prudent given that the overall recurrence rate of AFib is high, and these patients have already selected themselves as being at increased risk for atrial thrombus formation.[53] One prospective study with serial cranial magnetic resonance imaging scans reported that over half of patients with left atrial appendage thrombi on TEE suffered cerebral embolism or death during the succeeding 3 years.[117]

Resolution of Atrial Thrombi

The use of several weeks of anticoagulation before cardioversion results in a reduction of cardioversion-related thromboembolism from 6% to less than 1%. The mechanism by which warfarin conveys this beneficial effect had been presumed to be thrombus organization and adherence to the atrial endocardium, thus reducing the likelihood of postcardioversion migration.[118] Consistent with this hypothesis, several investigators have reported that atrial thrombi in patients with rheumatic mitral valve disease may not resolve even after several months of warfarin.[119-120] In nonrheumatic, new-onset AFib, a different mechanism appears responsible. I have found that after 4 weeks of warfarin, almost 85% of atrial thrombi have completely resolved[113] (Fig. 41–7). Similar data have been reported by others.[74,78,121,122] These data support the hypothesis that the mechanism of warfarin's benefit is related to thrombus resolution or silent migration and prevention of new thrombus formation (rather than thrombus organization). Although randomized data are not available, I interpret these data as supportive of the need for follow-up TEE examination for documentation of thrombus resolution before cardioversion.[114]

Mechanism of Thromboembolism after Cardioversion

Although usually occurring within 72 hours, thromboembolism has been reported up to 10 days following successful cardioversion in patients with maintained sinus rhythm.[98] Such adverse events have classically been attributed to migration of left atrial thrombi that were present at the time of cardioversion.[88] TEE has documented the new appearance of, or more pronounced, spontaneous left atrial contrast following

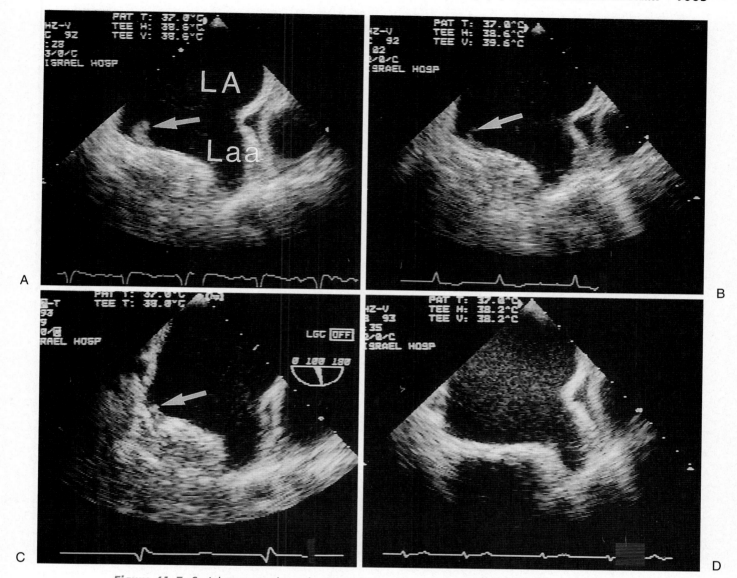

Figure 41–7. Serial transesophageal echocardiographic studies showing the left atrium and left atrial appendage viewed in the vertical plane with a 5 MHz biplane probe. The thrombus (arrow) is in the body of the left atrium, closely associated with the mitral annulus in the posterior portion of the left atrium. A, Initial study demonstrating a mobile 12-mm thrombus. B, Thrombus persists but is smaller after 1 week of warfarin therapy. C, After 3 weeks of warfarin, the thrombus continues to be seen (arrow). D, Complete resolution of thrombus is seen after 5.5 weeks of warfarin. LA, left atrium; LAA, left atrial appendage. (From Collins LJ, Silverman DI, Douglas PS, Manning WJ: Circulation 93:162, 1995, with permission. Copyright 1995 American Heart Association.)

electrical cardioversion.[75,112] In addition, more depressed left atrial appendage ejection velocity is common after spontaneous or electrical cardioversion.[111,112] These findings have led to the hypothesis that atrial thrombi may form after cardioversion resulting from atrial injury or stunning. Indeed, LV "stunning" as a result of electrical cardioversion has been previously described,[123,124] and relatively impaired atrial mechanical function has been seen after electrical (as compared with pharmacologic) cardioversion.[105,125] Finally, in rare instances, there may be a discontinuity between the body of the atrium and the appendage[41,42] with a sinus pattern on the surface electrocardiogram and transmitral Doppler echocardiogram but a fibrillatory pattern in the appendage. Premature discontinuation of warfarin may thereby lead to new thrombus formation. These data all emphasize the importance of therapeutic (INR 2 to 3) warfarin anticoagulation during the pericardioversion period. For patients who are not considered candidates for out-of-hospital warfarin, I recommend therapeutic anticoagulation with heparin for at least 24 hours after cardioversion.

Assessment of Return of Atrial Mechanical Function after Cardioversion

The noninvasive nature of echocardiography makes it the ideal modality for the serial assessment of atrial function after cardioversion. DeMaria and colleagues[37] reported serial M-mode data of anterior mitral leaflet excursion before and after cardioversion among 35 patients with AFib of 14 months' duration. One hour after cardioversion, prominent mitral A waves were found in 94% of their study group, although anterior leaflet excursion was less than that seen in normal subjects (7.5 mm versus 13 mm). These early data suggested that atrial mechanical contraction was reduced after cardioversion despite normal atrial depolarizations on electrocardiography. Two patients had no discernible atrial anterior mitral leaflet motion, and both of these patients reverted to AFib within 1 week. These investigators also found an increased LV end-diastolic dimension, with unchanged end-systolic dimension, consistent with an improvement in LV ejection fraction (EF). Orlando and colleagues[126] also used M-mode echocardiography to evaluate atrial function after cardioversion. Five hours after cardioversion, 4 of their 15 patients (27%) had no mitral A wave. In their experience, neither the presence of an A wave nor its amplitude correlated with long-term maintenance of sinus rhythm.

Pulsed Doppler echocardiography permits serial noninvasive evaluation of flow across the mitral valve and is thus ideally suited to assess atrial systolic function. Transmitral Doppler spectra accurately reflect the left atrial contribution to total LV filling. As reported by Van Gelder and colleagues[127] and Viswanathan and colleagues,[128] these temporal changes in transmitral Doppler spectra parallel improvements in LV ejection fraction[128] and peak oxygen consumption.[127]

Shapiro and colleagues[110] reported transmitral Doppler data from a group of patients with AFib of 2 days' duration or less. Peak A wave velocities immediately after cardioversion were similar to those in a control (sinus) population. In contrast, patients with a duration of AFib of greater than 1 year before cardioversion had significantly smaller A wave amplitude after cardioversion. I performed serial transmitral pulsed Doppler examination in 21 patients undergoing elective cardioversion, with a duration of AFib of 5 months.[56] Over 3 months of follow-up, there were significant increases in both peak A wave velocity and percent atrial contribution to total LV filling (Fig. 41–8). Neither index returned to normal until 3 weeks after cardioversion. Additional studies have confirmed that transmitral Doppler data are not predictive of the long-term maintenance of sinus rhythm.[126,129] Thus, it appears that return of atrial mechanical function is not sufficient to allow for premature discontinuation of postcardioversion anticoagulation.

Atrial compartment surgery, or the maze procedure, has received considerable interest as an approach to prevent recurrent AFib. Shyu and colleagues[130] studied 22 patients with chronic AFib who underwent atrial compartment operations. Over 70% of their group had no transmitral A wave 1 week after surgery, despite sinus rhythm on the surface electrocardiogram. Even after 2 months, 40% of their patients had not regained evidence of A waves. Of note, right atrial mechanical function appeared to recover more rapidly than left atrial mechanical function. Though less well studied, recovery of atrial mechanical function has also been demonstrated after pulmonary vein isolation.[131]

Studies of atrial mechanical function in patients with AFib of an intermediate (3-day to 4-week) duration had been previously limited by the relative scarcity of such patients. This was as a result of the recommendation that patients with AFib of more than 2 days' duration receive anticoagulation for 3 to 4 weeks before cardioversion. My TEE cardioversion trial allowed me to evaluate atrial function among patients with this intermediate duration of AFib. I found that both the immediate peak A velocity and the percentage A wave filling were significantly lower (Fig. 41–9) in the groups with AFib of moderate (>2 up to 6 weeks) and prolonged (>6 weeks) duration as compared with the patients with AFib of only brief (=2 weeks) duration.[97] This depression in peak A velocity persisted until at least 1 week following cardioversion. In addition, 1 week after cardioversion, both peak A velocity and percentage A wave filling were depressed in the group with AFib of prolonged duration as compared with the group with AFib of moderate duration. As compared with 3-month postcardioversion data, full recovery of atrial mechanical function was achieved within 24 hours for patients with brief (<2 weeks) duration, within 1 week for patients with moderate (2 to 6 weeks) duration, and within 1 month for patients with prolonged (>6 weeks) duration of AFib. Twenty-seven patients (45%) reverted to AFib during follow-up. Those reverting to AFib had a longer duration prior to cardioversion (10.2 versus 5.3 weeks; $P = 0.04$). There were no differences in left atrial dimension, patient age, mode of cardioversion, peak A wave velocity, or percentage of A wave filling among patients who reverted to AFib compared with those with sustained sinus rhythm.

Evidence of Electrical Injury to the Atria

LV myocardial injury as a result of electrical cardioversion has been previously described.[123,124] TEE data acquired with electrical cardioversion have shown new or more pronounced spontaneous left atrial contrast following electrical cardioversion[75,112] and depressed left atrial appendage ejection velocity.[111] I reported on transmitral Doppler data from 33 patients with AFib

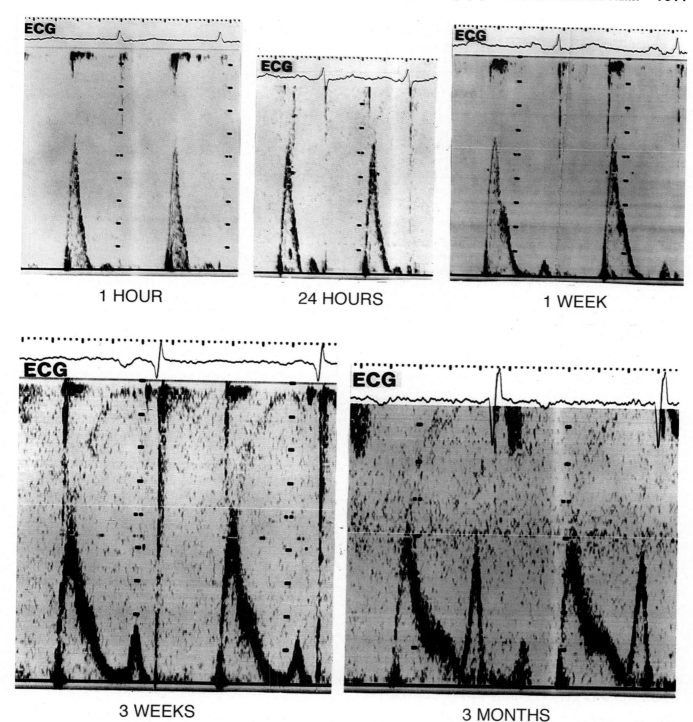

Figure 41–8. *Serial transmitral pulsed Doppler inflow velocity profiles from an individual patient. Note the progressive increase in peak atrial filling wave wave velocity during the observation period. For each spectrum, the vertical calibration markings indicate 0.2 m per second flow velocity. ECG, electrocardiogram. (From Manning WJ, Leeman DE, Gotch PJ, Come PC: J Am Coll Cardiol 13:620, 1989. Reprinted with permission from the American College of Cardiology.)*

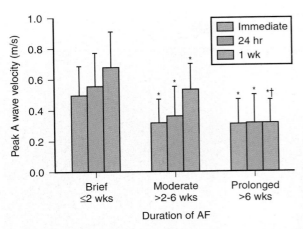

Figure 41–9. Comparison of transmitral pulsed Doppler peak atrial filling (A) wave velocity among patients with brief (≤2 weeks), moderate (2 to 6 weeks), and prolonged (>6 weeks) atrial fibrillation immediately after, at 24 hours, and at 1 week after cardioversion. *P < 0.05 versus brief duration. †P < 0.05 versus moderate duration. AF, atrial fibrillation. (From Manning WJ, Silverman DI, Katz SE, et al: J Am Coll Cardiol 23:1537, 1994.)

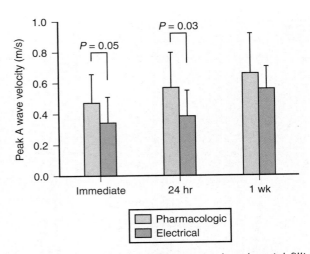

Figure 41–10. Comparison of transmitral peak atrial filling (A) wave velocity among patients who underwent pharmacologic and electrical cardioversion. (From Manning WJ, Silverman DI, Katz SE, et al: Am J Cardiol 75:626, 1995. With permission from Excerpta Medica Inc.)

of less than 5 weeks' duration following elective electrical or pharmacologic (primarily quinidine or procainamide) cardioversion using transmitral Doppler examination.[125] Immediately following cardioversion, patients who underwent electrical cardioversion demonstrated lower peak A wave velocity as compared with those who were cardioverted pharmacologically (Fig. 41–10). This depression in atrial systolic function was also present at the 24-hour study but had resolved at 1 week. Similarly, Mattiolo and colleagues[132] randomized 64 patients with AFib (duration 1 day to 6 months) to either direct-current shock or pharmacologic cardioversion. They found that the recovery of atrial mechanical function occurred sooner with pharmacologic cardioversion. Finally, Pollak and Falk[133] performed electrical cardioversion in 37 patients receiving sotalol or placebo. They found relatively depressed atrial function among the group receiving sotalol as compared with those receiving placebo.

Spontaneous Echocardiographic Contrast

SEC, or "smoke," refers to the presence of dynamic smokelike echoes in a cardiac cavity and is occasionally seen by TTE in the left atrium in patients with MS and AFib. More commonly, SEC is identified on TTE of the LV apex with a high-frequency transducer in patients with an apical aneurysm. SEC likely represents stasis of blood within the cavity, but it may also reflect alterations in blood components, such as platelets, red cells, and fibrinogen. Black and colleagues[134] found an association between SEC and erythrocyte aggregation in low shear rate conditions. Aspirin and warfarin

therapy do not appear to affect the presence of left atrial spontaneous echo contrast.[134] At least mild SEC may be seen in over half of patients with AFib[53,71,92] and in over 80% of patients with AFib and left atrial appendage thrombi.[71] Among patients with nonvalvular AFib, Chimowitz and colleagues[135] found that left atrial SEC was associated with an increased risk of stroke, a finding also confirmed by Bernhardt and colleagues[84] for both clinical and silent strokes. Black and colleagues[134] found that SEC by TEE was an independent predictor of left atrial thrombus among patients with suspected cardioembolism. Although unproved, it seems likely that recovery of atrial mechanical function would decrease or abolish SEC. SPAF-III TEE data[53] suggest that warfarin anticoagulation decreases the risk of thromboembolism in patients with SEC.

Echocardiography and Atrial Flutter

Sustained atrial flutter is far less common then AFib. As a result, there are fewer data regarding atrial function at baseline and following cardioversion. It has generally been accepted that the relatively preserved atrial mechanical function (Fig. 41–11) with atrial flutter results in a lower risk of thromboembolism (as compared with AFib). In a retrospective review, Arnold and colleagues[82] reported on 122 patients with atrial flutter at the time of cardioversion, including 74% who were not receiving anticoagulation. No patient experienced a clinical thromboembolic event. These data

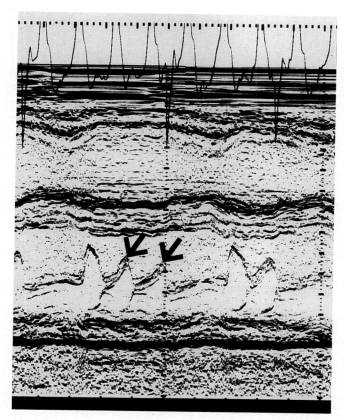

Figure 41–11. M-mode echocardiographic image depicting motion of the anterior mitral leaflet (arrows) *corresponding to flutter waves on the electrocardiogram in a patient with atrial flutter.*

would support the concept that patients with atrial flutter do not require anticoagulation before cardioversion. However, there have been reports of atrial thrombus identified during TEE study among patients with atrial flutter[78,136,137] and postcardioversion thromboembolism. A limitation of interpreting the literature on atrial flutter is the definition of the arrhythmia. For many studies, a patient is defined as having atrial flutter if it is the rhythm during the intervention or period of observation (e.g., at the time of TEE or cardioversion). Many patients may have alternating periods of AFib and flutter, making clinical distinction of pure atrial flutter difficult. Irani and colleagues[138] performed TEE in 47 consecutive patients with atrial flutter (and without AFib by history or Holter monitoring). They found that 11% of patients had left atrial thrombus, and 31% had SEC, values similar to those found in patients with AFib. Similar to my findings for AFib, moderate or severe mitral regurgitation was not protective against thrombus formation for this group.

Jordaens and colleagues[139] studied 22 patients with atrial flutter with serial transmitral Doppler echocardiography after cardioversion. Analogous to data on AFib, they found that 20% of patients had Doppler evidence of atrial standstill immediately after cardio-

version. There was a progressive increase in peak A wave velocity and percentage of A wave filling over a 6-week period. Based on these data, my recommendation is to treat patients with atrial flutter who have periods of AFib ("atrial flutter-fibrillation") in the same manner as those with isolated AFib. When it is certain that a patient has sustained atrial flutter, particularly for a short period of time, it may be reasonable to cardiovert without anticoagulation, although individualized risk-benefit considerations are most appropriate. I would generally treat conservatively patients who had atrial flutter in the setting of rheumatic mitral valve disease, a history of thromboembolism, or LV systolic dysfunction, with short-term anticoagulation and screening TEE or 1 month of anticoagulation prior to elective cardioversion.

Current and Future Areas of Investigation

As the ability of echocardiography to provide detailed structural and functional information about the heart continues to grow, so likely will its role in the evaluation and optimal management of patients with AFib. Among the areas of current and future investigation are:

1. Improved methods of assessment of atrial mechanical function with applications of tissue Doppler imaging.

2. Randomized prospective studies to further define the safety of TEE to guide early cardioversion among patients with AFib as in the ACUTE Trial.

3. Prospective studies examining the frequency of silent cerebral embolism among patients treated with conventional therapy.

4. Assistance in localization of structural abnormalities and foci of abnormal electrical activity, including assistance in radiofrequency ablation of arrhythmic foci.

5. Identification of clinical or echocardiographic indexes that predict recurrence of AFib or identify a group at low risk for thromboembolism so as to minimize postcardioversion anticoagulation.

Summary

Echocardiography provides a valuable tool for the evaluation and management of patients with AFib or atrial flutter. Continued technologic advances and investigation will likely lead to an expanding role for echocardiography in this growing patient population.

KEY POINTS

■ Left atrial volume (normalized for body surface area) is preferred for characterization of atrial size.

■ Increased left atrial size is a risk factor for the development of AFib.

■ TEE is highly accurate for identification of atrial thrombi and superior to TTE.

■ For patients with AFib, TEE risk factors for clinical thromboembolism include left atrial appendage thrombus, severe SEC, depressed (<0.2 m/s) atrial appendage ejection velocity and complex aortic plaque.

■ TEE will identify atrial thrombi in approximately 13% of patients presenting with new-onset AFib of greater than 2 days duration. The vast majority of thrombi is within or involves the left atrial appendage.

■ In concert with precardioversion therapeutic anticoagulation with unfractioned heparin, low molecular weight heparin, or warfarin, a TEE-guided strategy of early cardioversion is comparable to 1 month of precardioversion warfarin with a risk of clinical thromboembolism of less than 1%.

■ After cardioversion, left atrial and left atrial appendage mechanical function remains depressed, emphasizing the need for therapeutic warfarin for at least 1 month after cardioversion.

■ For patients with new onset, nonvalvular AFib who have TEE evidence of atrial thrombi, greater than 75% of the thrombi will resolve after 1 month of therapeutic warfarin.

■ Recovery of atrial mechanical function after cardioversion is related to the duration of AFib.

■ Data for atrial flutter suggest that the incidences of atrial thrombi and thromboembolism are slightly reduced compared with AFib, but that these patients should likely be treated with AFib guidelines.

REFERENCES

1. Okumura M, Okajiha S, Sotobata I, et al: Non-invasive localization of the pre-excitation site in patients with the Wolff-Parkinson-White syndrome. *Jpn Heart J* 21:157, 1980.
2. Iwase M, Sotobata I, Yokata M, et al: Evaluation by pulsed Doppler echocardiography of the atrial contribution to left ventricular filling in patients with DDD pacemakers. *Am J Cardiol* 58:104, 1986.
3. Gorcsan III J, Kanzake H, Bazaz R, et al: Usefulness of echocardiographic tissue synchronization imaging to predict acute response to cardiac resynchronization therapy. *Am J Cardiol* 93:1178-1181, 2004.
4. Bax JJ, Bleeker GB, Marwick TH, et al: Left ventricular dyssynchrony predicts response and prognosis after cardiac resynchronization therapy. *J Am Coll Cardiol* 44:1834-1840, 2004.
5. Hirata T, Wolfe SB, Popp RL, et al: Estimation of left atrial size using ultrasound. *Am Heart J* 78:43, 1969.
6. Ten Cate FJ, Kloster FE, van Dorp WG, et al: Dimensions and volumes of the left atrium and ventricle determined by single beam echocardiography. *Br Heart J* 1974;36:737-746, 1974.
7. Yabek SM, Isabel-Jones J, Bhatt DR, et al: Echocardiographic determination of left atrial volumes in children with congenital heart disease. *Circulation* 53:268, 1976.
8. Loperfido F, Pennestri F, Digaetano A, et al: Assessment of left atrial dimensions by cross-sectional echocardiography in patients with mitral valve disease. *Br Heart J* 50:570, 1983.
9. Lester SJ, Ryan EW, Schiller NB, Foster E: Best method in clinical practice and in research studies to determine left atrial size. *Am J Cardiol* 84:929-932, 1999.
10. Lang RM, Bierig M, Devereux RB, et al: Recommendations for chamber quantification: a report from the American Society of Echocardiography's Guidelines and Standards Committee and the Chamber Quantification Writing Group, developed in conjunction with the European Association of Echocardiogrpahy, a branch of the European Society of Cardiology. *J Am Soc Echocardiogr* 18:1440-1463, 2005.
11. Rodevan O, Bjornerheim R, Ljosland M, et al: Left atrial volumes assessed by three- and two-dimensional echocardiography compared with MRI estimates. *Int J Cardiovasc Imaging* 15:397-410, 1999.
12. Vandenberg BF, Weiss RM, Kinzey J, et al: Comparison of left atrial volume by two-dimensional echocardiography and cine-computed tomography. *Am J Cardiol* 75:754-757, 1995.
13. Ujino K, Barnes ME, Cha SS, et al: Two-dimensional echocardiographic methods for assessment of left atrial volume. *Am J Cardiol* 98:1185-1188, 2006.
14. Pritchett AM, Jacobsen SJ, Mahoney DW, et al: Left atrial volume as an index of left atrial size: population based study. *J Am Coll Cardiol* 41:1036-1043, 2003.
15. Tsang TS, Barnes ME, Bailey KR, et al: Left atrial volume: important risk marker of incident atrial fibrillation in 1655 older men and women. *Mayo Clin Proc* 76:467-475, 2001.
16. Osranek M, Fatema K, Qaddoura F, et al: Left atrial volume predicts the risk of atrial fibrillation after cardiac surgery: A prospective study. *J Am Coll Cardiol* 48:779-786, 2006.
17. Tani T, Tanabe K, Ono M, et al: Left atrial volume and risk of paroxysmal atrial fibrillation in patients with hypertrophic cardiomyopathy. *J Am Soc Echocardiogr* 17:644-648, 2004.
18. Losi MA, Betocchi S, Aversa M, et al: Determinants of atrial fibrillation development in patients with hypertrophic cardiomyopathy. *Am J Cardiol* 94:895-900, 2004.
19. Drexler M, Erbel R, Müller U, et al: Measurement of intracardiac dimensions and structures in normal young adult subjects by transesophageal echocardiography. *Am J Cardiol* 65:1491, 1990.
20. Schweizer P, Bardos P, Erbel R, et al: Detection of left atrial thrombi by echocardiography. *Br Heart J* 45:148, 1981.
21. DePace NL, Soulen RL, Kotler MN, et al: Two-dimensional echocardiographic detection of intraatrial masses. *Am J Cardiol* 48:954, 1981.
22. Shrestha NK, Moreno FL, Narciso FV, et al: Two-dimensional echocardiographic diagnosis of left atrial thrombus in rheumatic heart disease: A clinicopathologic study. *Circulation* 67:341, 1983.
23. Herzog CA, Bass D, Kane M, et al: Two-dimensional echocardiographic imaging of left atrial appendage thrombi. *J Am Coll Cardiol* 3:1340, 1984.
24. Aschenberg W, Schlüter M, Kremer P, et al: Transesophageal two-dimensional echocardiography for the detection of left atrial appendage thrombus. *J Am Coll Cardiol* 7:163, 1986.
25. Omran H, Jung W, Rabahieh R, et al: Imaging of thrombi and assessment of left atrial appendage function: A prospective

study comparing transthoracic and transesophageal echocardiography. *Heart* 81:192, 1999.

26. Cohen GI, White M, Sochowski RA, et al: Reference values for normal adult transesophageal echocardiographic measurements. *J Am Soc Echocardiogr* 8:221-230, 1995.

27. Chan SK, Kannam JP, Douglas PS, Manning WJ: Multiplane transesophageal echocardiographic assessment of left atrial appendage anatomy and function. *Am J Cardiol* 76:528, 1995.

28. Mügge A, Daniel WG, Hausmann D, et al: Diagnosis of left atrial appendage thrombi by transesophageal echocardiography: Clinical implications and follow-up. *Am J Cardiac Imag* 4:173, 1990.

29. Olson JD, Goldenberg IF, Pedersen W, et al: Exclusion of atrial thrombus by transesophageal echocardiography. *J Am Soc Echocardiogr* 5:52, 1992.

30. Hwang JJ, Chen JJ, Lin SC, et al: Diagnostic accuracy of transesophageal echocardiography for detecting left atrial thrombi in patients with rheumatic heart disease having undergone mitral valve operations. *Am J Cardiol* 72:677, 1993.

31. Manning WJ, Weintraub RM, Waksmonski CA, et al: Accuracy of transesophageal echocardiography for identifying left atrial thrombi: A prospective, intraoperative study. *Ann Intern Med* 123:817, 1995.

32. Subramaniam B, Riley MF, Panzica, PJ, Manning WJ: Transesophageal echocardiographic assessment of right atrial appendage anatomy and function: comparison with the left atrial appendage and implications for local thrombus formation. *J Am Soc Echocardiogr* 47:612-618, 2006.

33. Katz ES, Freedberg RS, Rutkovsky L, et al: Identification of an unusual right atrial mass as a Chiari Network by biplane transesophageal echocardiography. *Echocardiogr* 9:273, 1992.

34. Schwartzbard AZ, Tunick PA, Rosenzweig BP, et al: The role of transesophageal echocardiography in the diagnosis and treatment of right atrial thrombi. *J Am Soc Echocardiogr* 12:64, 1999.

35. Rowlands DJ, Logan WF, Howitt G: Atrial function after cardioversion. *Am Heart J* 74:149, 1967.

36. Gabor GE, Winsberg F: Motion of the mitral valves in cardiac arrhythmias: Ultrasonic cardiographic study. *Invest Radiol* 5:355, 1970.

37. DeMaria AN, Lies JE, King JF, et al: Echographic assessment of atrial transport, mitral movement and ventricular performance following electroversion of supraventricular arrhythmias. *Circulation* 51:273, 1975.

38. Manning WJ, Silverman DI, Katz SE, et al: Atrial ejection force: A new method for the assessment of atrial systolic function. *J Am Coll Cardiol* 22:221, 1993.

39. Pollick C, Taylor D: Assessment of left atrial appendage function by transesophageal echocardiography: Implications for the development of thrombus. *Circulation* 84:223, 1991.

40. Jue J, Winslow T, Fazio G, et al: Pulsed Doppler characterization of left atrial appendage flow. *J Am Soc Echocardiogr* 6:237, 1993.

41. Seto TB, Buchholz A, Douglas PS, Manning WJ: When the body and appendage of the left atrium disagree: "Focal" atrial fibrillation-implications for atrial thrombus formation and risk of thromboembolism. *J Am Soc Echocardiogr* 12:1097, 1999.

42. Bellotti P, Spirito P, Lupi G, Vecchio C: Left atrial appendage function assessed by transesophageal echocardiography before and on the day after elective cardioversion for nonvalvular atrial fibrillation. *Am J Cardiol* 81:1199, 1998.

43. Rubin DN, Katz SE, Riley MF, et al: Evaluation of left atrial appendage anatomy and function in recent onset atrial fibrillation by transesophageal echocardiography. *Am J Cardiol* 78:774, 1996.

44. Fatkin D, Kelly RP, Feneley MP: Relations between left atrial appendage blood flow velocity, spontaneous echocardiographic contrast and thromboembolic risk in vivo. *J Am Coll Cardiol* 23:961, 1994.

45. Hoit BD, Shao Y, Gabel M: Influence of acutely altered loading conditions on left atrial appendage flow velocities. *J Am Coll Cardiol* 24:1117, 1994.

46. Thom T, Haase N, Rosamond W, et al: AHA Statistical Update. Heart Disease and Stroke Statistics - 2006 Update. A report from the American Heart Association Statistics Committee and Stroke Statistics Subcommittee. *Circulation* 113:e85-e151, 2006.

47. Lloyd-Jones DM, Wang TJ, Leip EP, et al: Lifetime risk for development of atrial fibrillation: the Framingham Heart Study. *Circulation* 110:1042-1046, 2004.

48. Vasan RS, Larson MG, Levy D, et al: Doppler transmitral flow indexes and risk of atrial fibrillation (the Framingham Heart Study). *Am J Cardiol* 91:1079-1083, 2003.

49. Vaziri SM, Larson MG, Benjamin EJ, Levy D: Echocardiographic predictors of nonrheumatic atrial fibrillation. The Framingham Heart Study. *Circulation* 89:724, 1984.

50. Morris JJ, Entman M, North WC, et al: The changes in cardiac output with reversion of atrial fibrillation to sinus rhythm. *Circulation* 31:670, 1965.

51. Zabalgoitia M, Halperin JL, Pearce LA, et al. for the Stroke Prevention in Atrial Fibrillation III Investigators: Transesophageal echocardiographic correlates of clinical risk of thromboembolism in nonvalvular atrial rfibrilaltion. *J Am Coll Cardiol* 31:1622, 1998.

52. Black IW, Hopkins AP, Lee LC et al: Left atrial spontaneous echo contrast: A clinical and echocardiographic analysis. *J Am Coll Cardiol* 18:398, 1991.

53. The Stroke Prevention in Atrial Fibrillation Investigators Committee: Transesophageal echocardiographic correlates of thromboembolism in high-risk patients with nonvalvular atrial fibrillation. *Ann Intern Med* 128:639, 1998.

54. Hoglund C, Rosenhame G: Echocardiographic left atrial dimension as a predictor of maintaining sinus rhythm after conversion of atrial fibrillation. *Acta Med Scand* 217:411, 1985.

55. Dittrich HC, Erickson JS, Schneiderman T, et al: Echocardiographic and clinical predictors for outcome of elective cardioversion of atrial fibrillation. *Am J Cardiol* 63:193, 1989.

56. Aronow WS, Schwartz KS, Koenigsberg M: Prevalence of enlarged left atrial dimension by echocardiography and its correlation with atrial fibrillation and an abnormal P terminal force in lead V1 of the electrocardiogram in 588 elderly persons. *Am J Cardiol* 59:1003, 1987.

57. Petersen P, Kastrup J, Brinch K, et al: Relation between left atrial dimension and duration of atrial fibrillation. *Am J Cardiol* 60:382, 1987.

58. Sanfillippo AJ, Abascal VM, Sheehan M, et al: Atrial enlargement as a consequence of atrial fibrillation: A prospective echocardiographic study. *Circulation* 82:792, 1990.

59. Suarez GS, Lampert S, Ravid S, et al: Changes in left atrial size in patients with lone atrial fibrillation. *Clin Cardiol* 14:652, 1991.

60. Manning WJ, Leeman DE, Gotch PJ, et al: Pulsed Doppler evaluation of atrial mechanical function after electrical cardioversion of atrial fibrillation. *J Am Coll Cardiol* 13:617, 1989.

61. Gosselink ATM, Crijns HJGM, Hamer HPM, et al: Changes in left and right atrial size after cardioversion of atrial fibrillation: Role of mitral valve disease. *J Am Coll Cardiol* 22:1666, 1993.

62. Van Gelder IC, Crijns HJ, Van Gilst WH, et al: Decrease of right and left atrial sizes after direct current electrical cardioversion in chronic atrial fibrillation. *Am J Cardiol* 167:93, 1991.

63. Reant P, Lafitte S, Jais P, et al: Reverse remodeling of the left cardiac chambers after catheter ablation after 1 year in a series

of patients with isolated atrial fibrillation. *Circulation* 112:2896-2903, 2005.

64. Brodsky MA, Allen BJ, Capparelli EV, et al: Factors determining maintenance of sinus rhythm after chronic atrial fibrillation with left atrial dilatation. *Am J Cardiol* 63:1065, 1989.

65. The Boston Area Anticoagulation Trial for Atrial Fibrillation Investigators: The effect of low-dose warfarin on the risk of stroke in patients with non-rheumatic atrial fibrillaton. *N Engl J Med* 323:1505, 1990.

66. Petersen P, Godrfredsen J, Boysen GK, et al: Placebo-controlled, randomised trial of warfarin and aspirin for prevention of thromboembolic complications in chronic atrial fibrillation: the Copenhagen AFASAK study. *Lancet* 1:175, 1989.

67. Stroke Prevention in Atrial Fibrillation Study Group Investigators: Stroke Prevention in Atrial Fibrillation Study: Final results. *Circulation* 84:527, 1991.

68. Connolly SJ, Laupacis A, Gent M, et al: Canadian atrial fibrillation (CAFA) study. *J Am Coll Cardiol* 18:349, 1991.

69. Ezekowitz MD, Bridgers SL, James KE, et al: Warfarin in the prevention of stroke associated with nonrheumatic atrial fibrillation. Veterans Affairs Stroke Prevention in Nonrheumatic Atrial Fribrillation Investigators. *N Engl J Med* 327:1406, 1993.

70. Gallagher MM, Hennessy BJ, Edwardsson N, et al: Embolic complications of direct current cardioversion of atrial arrhythmias: Association with low intensity of anticoagulation at the time of cardioversion. *J Am Coll Cardiol* 40:926-933, 2002.

71. Manning WJ, Silverman DI, Keighley CS, et al: Transesophageal echocardiographically facilitated early cardioversion from atrial fibrillation using short-term anticoagulation: Final results of a prospective 4.5 year study. *J Am Coll Cardiol* 25:1354, 1995.

72. Weigner MJ, Thomas LR, Patel U, et al: Transesophageal echocardiography facilitated early cardioversion from atrial fibrillation: Short-term safety and impact on maintenance of sinus rhythm at 1 year. *Am J Med* 110:694, 2001.

73. Klein AL, Grimm RA, Black IW, et al: Cardioversion guided by transesophageal echocardiography: The ACUTE Pilot Study. A randomized control trial. Assessment of cardioversion using tranesophageal echocardiography. *Ann Intern Med* 126:200, 1997.

74. Corrado G, Tadeo G, Beretta S, et al: Atrial thrombi resolution after prolonged anticoagulation in patients with atrial fibrillation: A transesophageal echocardiography study. *Chest* 115:140, 1999.

75. Stoddard MF, Dawkins P, Prince CR, Longaker RA: Transesophageal echocardiographic guidance of cardioversion in patients with atrial fibrillation. *Am Heart J* 129:1204, 1995.

76. Klein AL, Grimm RA, Murray RD, et al: Use of transesophageal echocardiography to guide cardioversion in patients with atrial fibrillation. *N Engl J Med* 344:1411, 2001.

77. Wu LA, Chandrasekaran K, Friedman PA, et al: Safety of expedited anticoagulation in patients undergoing transesophageal echocardiographic-guided cardioversion. *Am J Med* 119:142, 2006.

78. Corrado G, Santarone M, Beretta S, et al: Early cardioversion of atrial fibrillation and atiral flutter guided by transesophageal echocardiography. A single centre 8.5-year experience. *Europace* 2:119-126, 2000.

79. Resnekov L, McDonald L: Complications in 220 patients with cardiac dysrhythmias treated by phased direct current shock, and indications for electroversion. *Br Heart J* 29:926, 1967.

80. Lown B, Perlroth MG, Kaiddbey S, et al: "Cardioversion" of atrial fibrillation: A report on the treatment of 65 episodes in 50 patients. *N Engl J Med* 269:325, 1963.

81. Bjerkelund C, Ornig OM: The efficacy of anticoagulant therapy in preventing embolism related to D.C. electrical conversion of atrial fibrillation. *Am J Cardiol* 23:208, 1969.

82. Arnold AZ, Mick MJ, Mazurek RP, et al: Role of prophylactic anticoagulation for direct current cardioversion in patients with atrial fibrillation or atrial flutter. *J Am Coll Cardiol* 19:851, 1992.

83. Ezekowitz MD, James KE, Nazarian SM, et al: Silent cerebral infarction in patients with nonrheumatic atrial fibrillation. The Veterans Affairs Stroke Prevention in Nonrheumatic Atrial Fibrillation Investigators. *Circulation* 92:2178, 1995.

84. Bernhardt P, Schmidt H, Hammerstingl C, et al: Patients with atrial fibrillation and dense spontaneous echo contrast at high risk. A prospective and serial follow-up over 12 months with transesophgeal echocardiography and cerebral magnetic resonance imaging. *J Am Coll Cardiol* 45:1807-1812, 2005.

85. The Stroke Prevention in Atrial Fibrillation Investigators: Predictors of thromboembolism in atrial fibrillation: II. Echocardiographic features of patients at risk. *Ann Intern Med* 116:6-12, 1992.

86. Blackshear JL, Pearce LA, Asinger RW, et al: Mitral regurgitation associated with reduced thromboembolic events in high-risk patients with nonrheumatic atrial fibrillation. *Am J Cardiol* 72:840, 1993.

87. Nakagami H, Yamamoto K, Ikeda U, et al: Mitral regurgitation reduces the risk of stroke in patients with nonrheumatic atrial fibrillation. *Am Heart J* 136:528, 1998.

88. Pritchett ELC: Management of atrial fibrillation. *N Engl J Med* 326:1264, 1992.

89. Stoddard MF, Dawkins PR, Prince CR, et al: Left atrial appendage thrombus is not uncommon in patients with acute atrial fibrillation and a recent embolic event: A transesophageal echocardiographic study. *J Am Coll Cardiol* 25:452, 1995.

90. Weigner MJ, Caulfield TA, Danias PG, et al: Risk for clinical thromboembolism associated with conversion to sinus rhythm in patients with atrial fibrillation lasting less than 48 hours. *Ann Intern Med* 126:615, 1997.

91. Manning WJ, Silverman DI, Waksmonski CA, et al: Prevalence of residual left atrial thrombi among patients presenting with thromboembolism and newly recognized atrial fibrillation. *Arch Intern Med* 155:2193, 1995.

92. Manning WJ, Silverman DI, Gordon SPF, et al: Cardioversion from atrial fibrillation without prolonged anticoagulation with use of transesophageal echocardiography to exclude the presence of atrial thrombi. *N Engl J Med* 328:750, 1993.

93. Gage BF, Waterman AD, Shannon W, et al: Validation of clinical classification schemes for predicting stroke: results from the National Registry of Atrial Fibrillation. *J Am Med Assoc* 285:2864, 2001.

94. Wyse DG, Waldo AL, DiMarco JP, et al: A comparison of rate control and rhythm control in patients with atrial fibrillation. The atrial fibrillation follow-up investigation of rhythm management (AFIRM) investigators. *N Engl J Med* 347:1825, 2002.

95. Van Gelder IC, Hagens VE, Bosker HA, et al: A comparison of rate control and rhythm control in patients with recurrent persistent atrial fibrillation. *N Engl J Med* 347:1834, 2002.

96. Carlsson J, Miketic S, Windeler J, et al: Randomized trial of rate-control versus rhythm-control in persistent atrial fibrillation: The Strategies of Treatment of Atrial Fibrillation (STAF) study. *J Am Coll Cardiol* 41:1690, 2003.

97. Manning WJ, Silverman DI, Katz SE, et al: Impaired left atrial mechanical function after cardioversion: Relationship to the duration of atrial fibrillation. *J Am Coll Cardiol* 23:1535, 1994.

98. Berger M, Schweitzer P: Timing of thromboembolic events after electrical cardioversion of atrial fibrillation or flutter: A retrospective analysis. *Am J Cardiol* 82:1545, 1998.

99. Weinberg DM, Mancini GBJ: Anticoagulation for cardioversion of atrial fibrillation. *Am J Cardiol* 63:745, 1989.

100. Shen X, Li H, Rovang K, et al: Prevalence of intra-atrial thrombi in atrial fibrillation patients with subtherapeutic international normalized ratios while taking conventional anticoagulation. *Am J Cardiol* 90:660, 2002.

101. Corrado G, Beretta S, Sormani L, et al: Prevalence of atrial thrombi in patients with atrial fibrillation/flutter and subtherapeutic anticoagulation prior to cardioversion. *Eur J Echocardiogr* 2004;5:257-261, 2004.

102. Fuster V, Ryden LE, Cannom DS, et al: ACC/AHA/ESC 2006 Guidelines for the management of patients with atrial fibrillation - Executive summary. A report of the American College of Cardiology/American Heart Association Task Force on Practice Guidelines and the European Society of Cardiology Committee for Practice Guidelines (Writing Committee to Revise the 2001 Guidelines for the Management of Patients with Atrial Fibrillation). *Circulation* 114:700-752, 2006.

103. Singer DE, Albers GW, Dalen JE, et al: 7th ACCP Consensus Conference on Antithrombotic Therapy: Antithrombotic therapy in atrial fibrillation. *Chest* 126:429S-456S, 2004.

104. Klein AL, Grimm RA, Jasper SE, et al: Efficacy of transesophageal echocardiography-guided cardioversion of patients with atrial fibrillation at 6 months: A randomized controlled trial. *Am Heart J* 151:380-389, 2006.

105. Harjai KJ, Mobarek SK, Cheirif J, et al: Clinical variables affecting recovery of left atrial mechanical function after cardioversion from atrial fibrillation. *J Am Coll Cardiol* 30:481, 1997.

106. Seto TB, Taira DA, Tsevat J, et al: Cost-effectiveness of transesophageal echocardiographic-guided cardioversion: A decision analytic model for patients admitted to the hospital with atrial fibrillation. *J Am Coll Cardiol* 29:122, 1997.

107. Klein AL, Murray RD, Becker ER, et al: Economic analysis of a transesophageal echocardiography-guided approach to cardioversion of patients with atrial fibrillation: the ACUTE economic data at eight weeks. *J Am Coll Cardiol* 43:1217-1224, 2004.

108. Shen X, Li H, Rovang K, et al: Transesophageal echocardiography before cardioversion of recurrent atrial fibrillation: does absence of previous atrial thrombi preclude the need of a repeat test? *Am Heart J* 146:741-745, 2003.

109. Black IW, Fatkin D, Sagar KB, et al: Exclusion of atrial thrombus by transesophageal echocardiography does not preclude embolism after cardioversion of atrial fibrillation: A multicenter study. *Circulation* 89:2509, 1994.

110. Shapiro EP, Effron MB, Lima S, et al: Transient atrial dysfunction after conversion of chronic atrial fibrillation to sinus rhythm. *Am J Cardiol* 62:1202, 1988.

111. Grimm RA, Stewart WJ, Maloney JD, et al: Impact of electrical cardioversion for atrial fibrillation on left atrial appendage function and spontaneous echo contrast: Characterization by simultaneous transesophageal echocardiography. *J Am Coll Cardiol* 22:1359, 1993.

112. Fatkin D, Kuchar DL, Thorburn CW, et al: Transesophageal echocardiography before and during direct current cardioversion of atrial fibrillation: Evidence for atrial stunning as a mechanism of thromboembolic complications. *J Am Coll Cardiol* 23:307, 1994.

113. Bernhardt P, Schmidt H, Hammerstingl C, et al: Incidence of cerebral embolism after cardioversion of atrial fibrillation: A prospective study with transesophageal echocardiography and cerebral magnetic resonance imaging. *J Am Soc Echocardiogr* 18:649-653, 2005.

114. Seto TB, Taira DA, Manning WJ: Cardioversion in patients with atrial fibrillation and left atrial thrombi on initial transesophageal echocardiography: Should transesophageal echocardiography be repeated before elective cardioversion? A cost effectiveness analysis. *J Am Soc Echocardiogr* 12:508, 1999.

115. deLuca I, Sorino M, De Luca L, et al: Pre and post-cardioversion transesophageal echocardiography for brief anticoagulation therapy with enoxaparin in atrial fibrillation patients: A prospective study with a 1-year follow-up. *Int J Cardiol* 102:447-454, 2005.

116. Klein AL, Jasper SE, Katz WE, et al: The use of enoxaparin compared to unfractionated heparin for short-term antithrombotic therapy in atrial fibrillation patients undergoing TEE-guided cardioversion: Assessment of cardioversion using transesophageal echocardiography (ACUTE) II randomized multicenter pilot study. *Eur Heart J* 27:2858-2865, 2006.

117. Bernhardt P, Schmidt H, Hammerstingl C, et al: Atrial thrombi— a prospective follow-up study over 3 years with transesophageal echocardiography and cranial magnetic resonance imaging. *Echocardiography* 23:388-394, 2006.

118. Goldman MJ: The management of chronic atrial fibrillation: Indications for and method of conversion to sinus rhythm. *Prog Cardiovasc Dis* 3:465, 1960.

119. Tsai LM, Hung JS, Chen JH, et al: Resolution of left atrial appendage thrombus in mitral stenosis after warfarin therapy. *Am Heart J* 121:1232, 1991.

120. Pytlewski G, Panidis IP, Combs W, et al: Resolution of left atrial thrombus with warfarin by transesophageal echocardiography before percutaneous commisurotomy in mitral stenosis. *Am Heart J* 128:843, 1994.

121. Collins LJ, Silverman DI, Douglas PS, Manning WJ: Cardioversion of non-rheumatic atrial fibrillation: Reduced thromboembolic complications with 4 weeks of pre-cardioversion anticoagulation are related to atrial thrombus resolution. *Circulation* 92:160, 1995.

122. Jaber WA, Prior DL, Thamilarasan M, et al: Efficacy of anticoagulation in resolving left atrial and left atrial appendage thrombi: A transesophageal echocardiographic study. *Am Heart J* 140:150-156, 2000.

123. Ehsani A, Ewy GA, Sobel BE: Effects of electrical countershock on serum creatine phosphokinase (CPK) isoenzyme activity. *Am J Cardiol* 37:12, 1976.

124. Yarbrough R, Ussery G, Whitley J: A comparison of the effects of A.C. and D.C. countershock on ventricular function in thoracotomized dogs. *Am J Cardiol* 14:504, 1964.

125. Manning WJ, Silverman DI, Katz SE, et al: Temporal dependence of the return of atrial mechanical function on the mode of cardioversion of atrial fibrillation to sinus rhythm. *Am J Cardiol* 75:624, 1995.

126. Orlando JR, van Herick R, Aronow WS, et al: Hemodynamics and echocardiograms before and after cardioversion of atrial fibrillation to normal sinus rhythm. *Chest* 76:521, 1979.

127. Van Gelder IC, Crijns HJGM, Blanksma PK, et al: Time course of hemodynamic changes and improvement of exercise tolerance after cardioversion of chronic atrial fibrillation unassociated with cardiac valve disease. *Am J Cardiol* 72:560, 1993.

128. Viswanathan K, Daniak S, Salomone K, et al: Effect of atrial fibrillation on improvement in left ventricular performance. *Am J Cardiol* 88:439-441, 2001.

129. Dethy M, Chassat C, Roy D, Mercier LA: Doppler echocardiographic predictors of recurrence of atrial fibrillation after cardioversion. *Am J Cardiol* 62:723, 1988.

130. Shyu KG, Cheng JJ, Chen JJ, et al: Recovery of atrial function after atrial compartment operation for chronic atrial fibrillation in mitral valve disease. *J Am Coll Cardiol* 24:392, 1994.

131. Donal E, Grimm RA, Yamada H, et al: Usefulness of Doppler assessment of pulmonary vein and left atrial appendage flow following pulmonary vein isolation of chronic atrial fibrillation in predicting recovery of left atrial function. *Am J Cardiol* 95:941, 2005.

132. Mattiolo AV, Castelli A, Andria A, et al: Clinical and echocardiographic features influencing recovery of atrial function after cardioversion of atrial fibrillation. *Am J Cardiol* 82:1368, 1998.

133. Pollak A, Falk RH: Aggravation of postcardioversion atrial dysfunction by sotalol. *J Am Coll Cardiol* 25:665, 1995.

134. Black IW, Hopkins AP, Lee LC, et al: Left atrial spontaneous echo contrast: A clinical and echocardiographic analysis. *J Am Coll Cardiol* 18:398, 1991.

135. Chimowitz MI, DeGeorgia MA, Poole RM, et al: Left atrial spontaneous echo contrast is highly associated with previous stroke in patients with atrial fibrillation or mitral stenosis. *Stroke* 24:1015, 1993.

136. Orsinelli DA, Pearson AC: Usefulness of transesophageal echocardiography to screen for left atrial thrombus before elective cardioversion for atrial fibrillation. *Am J Cardiol* 72:1337, 1993.

137. Bikkina M, Alpert MA, Mulekar M, et al: Prevalence of intraatrial thrombus in patients with atrial flutter. *Am J Cardiol* 76:186-189, 1995.

138. Irani WN, Grayburn PA, Afridi I: Prevalence of thrombus, spontaneous echo contrast, and atrial stunning in patients undergoing cardioversion of atrial flutter. *Circulation* 95:962-966, 1997.

139. Jordaens L, Missault L, Germonpré E, et al: Delayed restoration of atrial function after conversion of atrial flutter by pacing or electrical cardioversion. *Am J Cardiol* 71:63, 1993.

Part Eight

Adult Congenital Heart Disease and Cardiac Tumors

General Echocardiographic Approach to the Adult with Suspected Congenital Heart Disease

MICHELLE GURVITZ, MD

The author acknowledges A. Rebecca Snider, MD, the previous author of this chapter in *The Practice of Clinical Echocardiography*, second edition.

The population of adults with congenital heart disease (CHD) is growing rapidly in the United States.[1-3] Adult patients with CHD have a variety of heart conditions, from simple "holes in the heart" to complex single ventricle anatomy. Some have undergone palliation or complete surgical repair whereas others remain with their native heart condition or present de novo in adulthood. Many childhood patients will have a long lapse in medical follow-up and then are diagnosed later in adulthood with complications of the underlying condition.[4-7] In all of these situations, echocardiography remains the mainstay of diagnosis for patients with CHD.[8-10] There are many approaches to echocardiographic imaging for adult patients with CHD; one of these methods is discussed in this chapter.

First, the positioning of the heart within the chest is addressed, followed by the definition and morphology of the cardiac chambers, valves, and great vessels. Further analysis is based on the segmental approach, which describes the alignments and relationships of the atria, ventricles, and great arteries. These fundamentals are necessary for recognition of the different morphologic cardiac components in either the usual or unusual anatomic arrangements. Next, the chapter reviews the more common anatomic arrangements that create normal hearts and congenital heart anomalies. This is followed by a review of issues surrounding the assessment of the univentricular heart. Finally, there is a brief discussion on the use of color and spectral Doppler to identify shunts and valvular lesions in CHD. Regardless of the specific disease, repair, technology, or technique at hand, there are certain general principles to keep in mind when imaging patients with CHD:

- First, the presence of one congenital abnormality often means that there may be more. It is crucial to complete a comprehensive two-dimensional (2D) and Doppler evaluation in view of the possibility that there will be more than one anomaly.

- Second, there may be exceptions to the "rules" of CHD and cardiac development. Thus, the physician must always describe what is present, even if that information seems inconsistent with what is known about conventional CHD lesions.

- Third, no physician or sonographer should hesitate to get a second opinion. Even the best congenital echocardiographers need assistance at times.

- Fourth, the larger body habitus of adults makes echocardiography more difficult than in children. Often, imaging requires other strategies to complement the echocardiography. These often include transesophageal echocardiography (TEE), magnetic resonance imaging (MRI), computed tomography (CT) scanning, or cardiac catheterization.[11-15]

Basic Principles

The cardiologist should expect that adult patients with CHD often will not know specific information regarding their heart disease. Many of the patients are not familiar with the name of their heart condition or the particular aspects of surgical or catheter-based interventions. Some may understand it was a hole in the heart or a "narrow valve" or a "single pumping chamber," but many will not be able to describe it in any detail.[16,17] The clinician, however, can derive a number of clues from basic patient information, and that information will help guide the physician and sonographer. This includes:

1. Has the patient had surgery?
2. If so, how many? Were they sternotomies, thoracotomies, or both?
3. Is the patient cyanotic?
4. Has the patient had any catheter-based interventional procedures?

For example, if the patient reports a narrow valve, had no surgeries but a catheter-based procedure, and is acyanotic, one might expect aortic stenosis (AS) or pulmonary stenosis with a small chance of mitral valve disease. Of course, even with this information the clinician has to keep an open mind when diagnosing CHD because patients with CHD may have more than one condition. The echocardiography lab needs to be familiar with anatomic variations of CHD. However, even though most congenital heart anomalies are well described in the pediatric cardiology literature, the nomenclature for some complex anatomic lesions remains disputed. For example, the segmental relationships of the cardiac structures have been variously classified from an embryologic perspective, a physiologic perspective, and even a surgical or interventional perspective.[18-21] In some cases, there is no universal agreement as to the definition of a ventricle let alone complete segmental anatomy of certain conditions. Some of these controversies are discussed further in this chapter. With these terminology disagreements in mind, this text focuses on identifying and describing the cardiac chambers and great vessels, their anatomic alignment, and the position of the heart relative to the systemic venous system and other organs.

Cardiac Position

The heart is normally positioned in the left chest with the apex pointing leftward. Depending on cardiac rotation in development, the heart may take other positions (or malpositions) including location in the mid-chest, the right chest, or even outside the chest (ectopia cordis).[22,23] The spatial position of a particular structure or organ in the body is known as the situs. The condition in which the heart and the other body organs are found in a usual arrangement is termed situs solitus. This includes a left-sided heart, left-sided stomach and spleen, and a right-sided liver. Departures from this normal organ arrangement are specially defined. For example, a complete inversion of the thoracic and abdominal viscera, resulting in a heart positioned in the right side of the thoracic cavity with a rightward-pointing apex, and inversion of the abdominal organs and lungs, is called situs inverse totalis[18,20,21] (Fig. 42–1). Several other combinations can and do occur. For example, patients might have the heart positioned in the right chest but situs solitus of other organs or the heart positioned in the left chest with situs inversus of the other organs. Both of these situations are more often associated with a structurally abnormal heart.[24] A small percentage of patients have an unusual and inconsistent arrangement of the viscera, with the heart positioned in either the mid-chest or right or left thorax. This is often referred to as heterotaxy syndrome or asplenia and polysplenia syndromes.[25]

The Left-Sided Heart

The normal position of the heart is in the left chest with a leftward-pointing apex. In certain cases, resulting from anatomic abnormalities, such as hypoplasia of the left lung, the heart may be located in the extreme left chest. This condition is called levoposition. In this situation, however, the heart usually maintains normal segmentation and connections. In some cases of het-

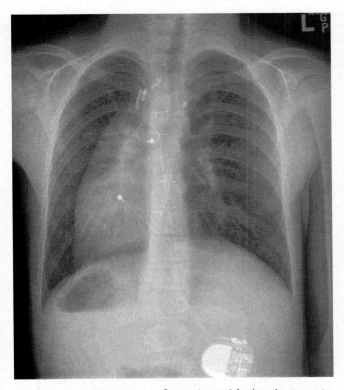

Figure 42–1. Chest X-ray of a patient with situs inversus totalis: The cardiac apex points rightward. The air bubble of the stomach is visualized in the upper right abdomen. The bronchi are also reversed with a trilobed lung on the left and a bilobed lung on the right. A pacemaker is seen in the abdomen with leads to the atrium and ventricle. Of note, there are also vascular coils noted in the right upper chest.

erotaxy abnormalities, the heart remains positioned in the left side of the chest but is commonly associated with congenital heart defects.[24,25]

The Right-Sided Heart

Anatomy

A right-sided heart is known as dextrocardia with three basic types: dextroposition, mirror-image dextrocardia, and dextroversion[22,26] (Fig. 42–2).

Dextroposition occurs when mechanical considerations, such as right lung hypoplasia or severe scoliosis, displace the heart to the right side of the thorax. In these cases, the heart retains a leftward-pointing apex and normal arterial and venous connections. The visceral and atrial positioning is most often situs solitus, and the condition is usually not associated with intracardiac CHD. Mirror-image dextrocardia may be seen with complete situs inversus. In this condition the heart is positioned in the right thorax with a rightward-pointing apex. The chamber and vessel relationships within the heart are usually normal, but the relative positions of the anatomic components are reversed or mirror-image in relation to the normal left-sided heart. A heart with mirror-image dextrocardia often has a right aortic arch and descending thoracic aorta.[23,27] Dextroversion describes a heart that has not rotated the cardiac apex to the left during embryologic development, resulting in a rightward-apex with situs solitus of the other organs or with other unusual arrangements of the viscera. As with a leftward heart with situs inversus, these cases have an increased rate of intracardiac congenital heart defects. In some studies that correlation reaches a majority of patients with dextroversion having associated congenital heart defects.[25,28]

Imaging Approach

When imaging the patient with suspected dextrocardia or cardiac malposition, the first step is determining abdominal situs and cardiac positioning. This is best done by starting with the subcostal view. In the normal subcostal short-axis view, the spine is positioned in the middle with the pulsatile aorta in cross section to the patient's left, just anterior to the spine. The collapsible inferior vena cava (IVC) is seen in cross section to the patient's right and further anterior of the spine (Fig. 42–3). Ideally, before referral for an echocardiogram for suspected CHD, the patient has had a chest X-ray (CXR) showing the lung anatomy, liver, stomach bubble, and the positioning of the heart within the thorax. In dextroposition, the heart and its segmental connections usually remain normally related—albeit located to the right of the midline. The usual echocardiographic views can be employed, but they should be adjusted for the rightward positioning

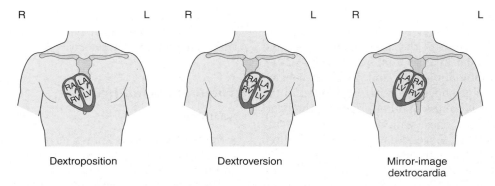

Dextroposition   Dextroversion   Mirror-image dextrocardia

Figure 42–2. *Diagrammatic representation of the types of dextrocardia. In dextroposition (in situs solitus), the entire heart is shifted to the right chest, either because of a space-occupying mass in the left chest or because of absence of the normal lung volume filling the right chest. Usually, the alignment of the major axis of the heart is normal (pointed toward the left) or rotated slightly vertically; however, the entire heart is shifted to the right of midline or to the retrosternal area. The parasternal long-axis and short-axis views are obtained with the usual orientation of the plane of sound but with the transducer positioned just to the right of the sternum. The apical views are also obtained with the usual orientation of the plane of sound but with the transducer positioned just to the right of the lower sternal border. In dextroversion (in situs solitus), there is failure of apical pivoting. The cardiac apex is to the right of midline and the atria are usually in their normal positions or shifted slightly to the right. The major axis of the heart is aligned from the left shoulder toward the right hip. The parasternal long-axis view is obtained with the plane of sound oriented in the mirror-image direction of normal. Because the atria are usually normally positioned and the great arteries arise normally from the ventricles, the parasternal short-axis view is obtained with a normal orientation of the plane of sound. In mirror-image dextrocardia (situs inversus totalis) the heart is located in the mirror-image position of normal. Both atria are usually entirely to the right of the sternum, and the cardiac apex is usually in the right fifth or sixth intercostal space at the anterior axillary line; hence, the major axis of the heart is aligned between the left shoulder and right hip. The parasternal long-axis view is obtained from the right second or third intercostal space with the plane of sound oriented in a mirror-image direction of normal (from left shoulder to right hip). The parasternal short-axis view is obtained from the same transducer location with the plane of sound also oriented in the mirror-image direction of normal (from right shoulder to left hip). The apical views are obtained with the transducer positioned in the right fifth or sixth intercostal space in the anterior axillary line and with the plane of sound oriented in a mirror-image direction of normal. LA, left atrium; LV, left ventricle; RA, right atrium; RV, right ventricle.*

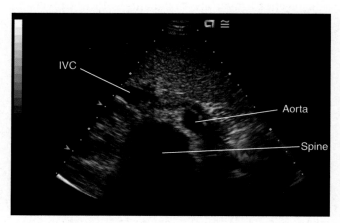

Figure 42–3. *Subcostal short-axis view in a patient with abdominal and atrial situs solitus. The aorta is leftward and anterior of the spine. The inferior vena cava (IVC) is rightward and slightly more anterior.*

and are frequently displaced to the right of the sternum.[23] In mirror-image dextrocardia with visceral situs inversus, the apex of the heart points toward the right leg, and the long-axis of the heart is oriented from left shoulder to right leg. The intracardiac connections are

often normally related, however, the morphologic right atrium and ventricle are positioned leftward of the morphologic left atrium and ventricle. The apex of the heart is usually positioned as inverted from normal and can be found in the right fifth or sixth intercostal space in the anterior axillary line. Although further cardiac imaging in this condition can be confusing, the result is that the images either appear normal or are the mirror image of a normally positioned heart. For example, the parasternal long-axis view is obtained with the transducer oriented along the long axis of the heart from left shoulder toward right leg. Once recorded, the images look like those obtained in the usual parasternal long-axis view because there is no right-left orientation, only superior-inferior and anterior-posterior. The parasternal short-axis views are obtained in the orthogonal plane. In the short-axis view, right-left and anterior-posterior orientation is obtained so the image in a patient with dextrocardia looks like the "usual" view, only backwards or right-left inverted. The images obtained in the apical four-chamber view are "backward appearing," similar to the parasternal short axis, and they are obtained with the transducer positioned at the apex of the heart. The sonographer or physician should be careful not to invert the image so that it appears normal: This will be confusing on later review of the study and misleading regarding the relationship of the heart within the thorax. The imaging positions for dextroversion are similar to that for mirror-image dextrocardia. Often, however, the heart is often not positioned as far rightward in the chest; moreover, this condition carries a much higher incidence of intracardiac congenital heart abnormalities (Fig. 42–4).

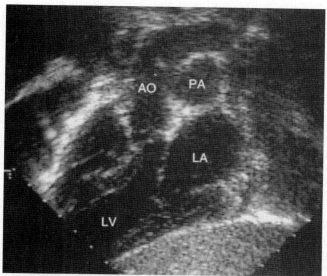

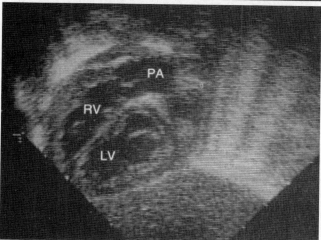

Figure 42–4. Subcostal four-chamber views from a patient with dextroversion of the cardiac apex. A, The left-sided ventricle has a smooth septal surface and is therefore the morphologic left ventricle (LV). The LV gives rise to a vessel that arches and is therefore the aorta (AO). B, The plane of sound has been tilted far anteriorly. The right-sided ventricle has a prominent moderator band in its apical portion and is therefore a morphologic right ventricle (RV). The RV gives rise to a vessel that dives posteriorly and is therefore a pulmonary artery (PA). Other echocardiographic views showed that this patient had atrial situs solitus; therefore, the atrioventricular and ventriculoarterial connections are normal. The only abnormality in this heart is failure of pivoting of the cardiac apex to the left. LA, left atrium.

In any patient with dextrocardia, views of the aortic arch are obtained in the usual fashion in the suprasternal notch. In these conditions it is important to identify the presence of a right-sided or left-sided arch, descending aorta, and the branching pattern of the head and neck vessels.

Cardiac Morphology

General

The heart's anatomic position and function do not always reflect the morphology of a chamber. For example, a left-sided ventricular chamber connected to an aortic outflow is not always a morphologic left ventricle. In certain congenital heart defects there are absent or atretic valves, chambers, or great vessels. In these cases, identifying the morphology of each chamber becomes more challenging. However, once familiar with the usual morphologic landmarks of the cardiac chambers and great arteries, the abnormal anatomic variants and unusual anatomic relationships found in many CHDs become easier to differentiate and recognize (Table 42–1).

TABLE 42–1. Morphologic Characteristics of Cardiac Chambers, Valves, and Great Arteries

Morphologic Chamber	Identifying Features
Right atrium	Receives IVC and has Eustachian valve Broad-based and trabecular appendage
Left atrium	Receives pulmonary veins (usually) Long and finger-like appendage
Tricuspid valve and right ventricle	AV valve is trileaflet and has septal attachments Heavily trabeculated chamber with moderator band Discrete inflow and outflow portions
Mitral valve and left ventricle	AV valve is bileaflet and attaches to papillary muscles, not septum Chamber is smooth walled
Aorta and aortic valve	Trileaflet semilunar valve Gives rise to coronaries and head and neck vessels
Pulmonary artery and pulmonary valve	Trileaflet semilunar valve Vessel bifurcates early into right and left branches

AV, atrioventricular; IVC, inferior vena cava.

Atria

The right atrium is most easily characterized by its appendage. This is a broad-based and triangular structure that lies anterior to the chamber. Often there is a visible Eustachian valve arising from the orifice of the IVC, directed toward the mid-portion of the interatrial septum. More specifically, the tissue of the valve runs along the inferior portion of the atrium and is directed toward the limbus or the inferior portion of the fossa ovalis (Fig. 42–5).

The right atrium is also identified by connections with the suprahepatic portion of the IVC. Even when there are abnormal connections of the superior vena cava (SVC), the suprahepatic portion of the IVC rarely connects anywhere except the morphologic right atrium.[29,30] Finally, the abdominal situs may also help identify atrial anatomy. The atrial situs usually follows the abdominal situs; in situs solitus—with the liver on the right and the stomach on the left—one would expect a right-sided morphologic right atrium.[25,28] The left atrium is also best characterized by its appendage. This is a narrow and finger-like or windsock structure that lies anterior to the left atrium. The flap-valve of the foramen ovale, if present, should be found on the left surface of the interatrial septum and is a useful landmark. Finally, the practitioner should look for the connections of at least three individual pulmonary veins—with a minimum of at least one each from the right and left sides—entering an atrial chamber. This finding most always indicates a left atrium.[29,30] However, if the pulmonary veins come to a confluence and empty into an accessory vertical vein before entering an atrial chamber, that chamber is not necessarily a morphologic left atrium.

Atrioventricular Valves and Ventricles

When there are two atrioventricular (AV) valves and two ventricular chambers, the valves travel with the morphologically appropriate ventricle. Thus, identifying a tricuspid valve also identifies the right ventricle; identifying a right ventricle signals an associated tricuspid valve. The mitral valve likewise associates with the left ventricle (Fig. 42–6).

The tricuspid valve has three leaflets positioned as anterior, posterior, and septal. The leaflets are attached to a network of small papillary muscles on the right ventricular free wall and the interventricular septum. Papillary muscles arising from the septal surface are distinctive of the right ventricle. As a result, papillary septal attachments are unique to the tricuspid valve and right ventricle. If two distinct AV valves are present in the heart, then the tricuspid valve is usually the one more apically displaced.[29,30] The right ventricle is also identified by its coarse trabeculations. There are a number of muscular bands within the chamber that cross from the septal to the parietal surface. The most prominent of these is the moderator band, situated in the mid-cavitary portion of the ventricle (see Fig. 42–6). The relationship of inflow and outflow portions also differentiates the right ventricle from the left ventricle. The right ventricle has a distinct outflow portion consisting of infundibular or conal muscular tissue. Consequently, the outflow semilunar valve and great artery are displaced from the inflow valve, unlike the morphologic left ventricle. The mitral valve is the AV valve associated with the morphologic left ventricle. The valve has two leaflets, one each in the anterior and posterior positions. Typically, little or no conal tissue separates the left ventricular inflow and outflow, allowing for fibrous continu-

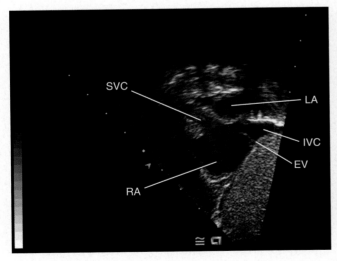

Figure 42–5. Subcostal saggital view in a patient with normal return of the superior vena cava (SVC) and inferior vena cava (IVC) to the right atrium. The eustachian valve (EV) is visualized near the origin of the IVC. The left atrium is also shown. LA, left atrium; RA, right atrium.

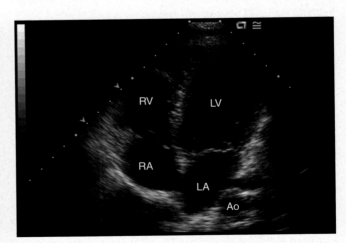

Figure 42–6. Apical four-chamber view showing the normal relationships of the atria and ventricles. The moderator band is well seen toward the apex of the trabeculated right ventricle (RV). The tricuspid valve is shown with one leaflet aimed toward the septum and is slightly apically displaced from the mitral valve. The left ventricle (LV) is smooth walled. At least two pulmonary veins can be seen entering the left atrium (LA). Ao, aorta; RA, right atrium.

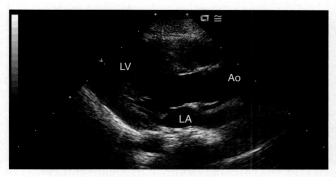

Figure 42–7. *Parasternal long-axis view showing the mitral valve apparatus attaching to papillary muscles away from the interventricular septum. The mitral annulus is shown in continuity with the aortic valve. Ao, aorta; LA, left atrium; LV, left ventricle.*

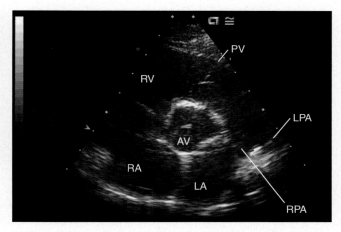

Figure 42–8. *Parasternal short-axis view showing the pulmonary valve anterior and slightly leftward of the aortic valve. The main pulmonary artery is shown bifurcating into right and left branch pulmonary arteries (RPA and LPA). AV, aortic valve; LA, left atrium; PV, pulmonary valve; RA, right atrium; RV, right ventricle.*

ity of the mitral and left ventricular outflow valve. The mitral valve apparatus is attached to two dominant papillary muscles, the superiorly positioned anterolateral and the more inferior posteromedial papillary muscles. Unlike the situation with the tricuspid valve, neither of the papillary muscles arises from the interventricular septum. The left ventricular chamber itself is smoothed walled and bullet shaped in comparison to the trabeculated and somewhat triangular right ventricle. There is no separation of inflow and outflow, so there is usually continuity between the mitral valve and the left ventricular outflow valve[29,30] (Fig. 42–7).

Semilunar Valves and Great Arteries

The pulmonary valve is a trileaflet semilunar valve associated with a pulmonary artery (PA). The PA is identified as the great artery arising from the heart that bifurcates early into right and left branches headed toward the lungs (Fig. 42–8). In the normal heart, the PA is found anterior to the aorta as it arises from the heart. But in CHD, this is not always the case. Thus, the best identification is usually a morphologic description of bifurcation of the vessel. Be aware, however, that there are exceptions. For example, conditions of isolated branch PA atresia are rare but do exist. The aortic valve is a semilunar, three-leaflet valve associated with the aorta and aortic arch. The aorta gives rise to the origins of the right and left coronary arteries. The cusps or leaflets of the aortic valve are named right, left, and non-coronary: the right and left cusps are associated with the origins, respectively, of the right and left coronary arteries. About 1% to 2% of people in the United States are thought to have a bicuspid, or two-leaflet, aortic valve.[31] The aorta itself is identified as the great vessel that does not bifurcate early and from which the coronary arteries and head and neck arteries originate (Fig. 42–9). It is a rare case where the coronary arteries do not arise from the aorta. Although the aortic arch normally arises leftward, it also can be

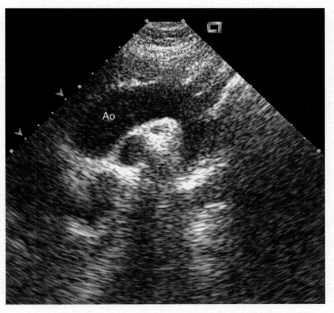

Figure 42–9. *Aortic arch visualized from the suprasternal notch view. The head and neck vessels are shown arising from the transverse arch. Ao, aorta.*

rightward. When the aortic arch arises rightward, it can be associated with mirror-image branching of the head and neck vessels. The sidedness of the arch is most easily identified by evaluating the direction of the first bifurcating head and neck vessel. If this first artery bifurcates rightward, then the aortic arch is usually leftward; and if the first artery goes leftward, then the aortic arch is most commonly a right arch. If there is no bifurcation of the first head and neck vessel, more involved abnormalities, such as aberrant subclavian arteries arising from the more distal aorta and vascular rings, should be sought.[32-34] There can be a number of variations on the positioning of the head and neck vessels; they are best defined by tracing each as far as possible in the suprasternal long-axis and short-axis views.

Cardiac Anatomy

General Segmental Approach

The heart is anatomically described by the relationships of the atria, ventricles, great arteries, and the relationship of these to the systemic and pulmonary venous connections. Clinically, the segmental approach defines the heart by identifying these relationships within the patient (Table 42–2).

Generally, the easiest way to determine chamber and great vessel alignment is to follow the flow of blood through the heart. In the complete examination, three segments of the heart require description: the atria, the ventricles, and the great vessels. In the normal heart, the concordant arrangement has a right atrium aligned with a right ventricle, the ventricle further aligned with a PA; and a left atrium aligned with left ventricle, further aligned with the aorta. Any other alignment or arrangement between segments is considered discordant.[18,20,21,35]

In the segmental approach, the atria can take three possible configurations. Atrial situs solitus has normal position, with a morphologic right atrium on the anatomic right side. Atrial situs inversus has reverse positioning, with a morphologic right atrium on the anatomic left side. Atrial situs ambiguous has atrial morphology too difficult to determine, leaving the sidedness unclear. Often this will involve what appears to be two right or two left atria. The atrial situs and abdominal visceral situs are usually similar.[20,21,35] The ventricular segmental arrangement occurs in one of two positions determined embryologically by the bulboventricular looping of the heart. The first and normal orientation is the dextro-looped, or d-looped, ventricles. In this case, the morphologic right ventricle is located more anteriorly and on the anatomic right side. The second possibility is levo-looped or l-looped where the morphologic right ventricle is on the anatomic left side.[20,21,35]

The ventricles give rise to the outflows and great arteries. The description and segmentation of the great artery anatomy is the most confusing and somewhat controversial part of the segmental approach. The usual alignment of the great arteries has the aorta arising from the morphologic left ventricle and the PA arising from the morphologic right ventricle. In that arrangement, the aortic valve is aligned posterior and rightward of the pulmonary valve. In abnormal relations of the great vessels, the aorta arises from a morphologic right ventricle and the PA arises from a morphologic left ventricle; both great vessels arise from a single ventricular chamber; or there is only a single outflow present (truncus arteriosus or atresia of one of the great arteries).[20,21,35] Some definitions of abnormally related or 'transposed' great vessels rely on the orientation of the vessels in relation to each other—noting that transposition occurs when the aorta is anterior to the PA. Other accepted definitions describe transposition as an abnormal alignment of the great vessel with the ventricle. In this definition, vessels are considered transposed if the aorta arises from the morphologic right ventricle and the PA from the left ventricle. Any other relationships of the great vessels to the ventricles, such as double-outlet ventricles, are considered malposed.[20,21,35] Because the morphology may depart in many ways from the normal arrangement, it is crucial that the clinician describe the anatomy found in the patient, including the relationship of the great arteries to the ventricles and to each other.

TABLE 42–2. General Echocardiographic Approach

Abdominal situs	Solitus (liver on right, stomach on left) Inversus (liver on left/transverse, stomach on the right)
Atrial anatomy and systemic venous connections	Solitus (right atrium on right side) Inversus (right atrium on left side) Ambiguous or indeterminate
Atrioventricular connection	Two AV valves Common AV valve AV valve atresia Straddling or overriding AV valve
Ventricular morphology and relationships	d-loop (right ventricle on right side) l-loop (right ventricle on left side) Univentricular heart
Semilunar valves	Two semilunar valves Common semilunar valve (truncus) Semilunar valve atresia
Great artery relationships and connections	Concordant Discordant Double outlet (left or right ventricle) Common outlet (truncus arteriosus) Single outlet (great artery atresia)

AV, atrioventricular.

Concordant and Discordant Arrangements

There are four possible AV and ventriculoarterial anatomic or segmental relationships (Table 42–3). Concordance refers to the normal alignments, and discordance refers to abnormal alignments. First, there is normal cardiac alignment with AV and ventriculoarterial concordance. Second, there is AV concordance and ventriculoarterial discordance, or d-transposition of the great arteries (d-TGA) (Fig. 42–10). Third, one can also have AV discordance with ventriculoarterial discordance. This is known as congenitally corrected transposition of the great arteries (CCTGA) or l-transposition of the great arteries (l-TGA) (Fig. 42–11). Fourth, there is AV discordance with ventriculoarterial concordance. This arrangement is rare and can occur with different great artery arrangements and includes isolated ventricular inversion, isolated atrial noninversion, or anatomically corrected malposition of the great vessels. As

one example, in isolated ventricular inversion, the morphologic right atrium is aligned with a morphologic left ventricle, which is aligned with an aorta. Physiologically it is similar to d-TGA.[18,21,36]

Other Nonsegmental Abnormalities

Apart from the segmental alignment of the heart, two areas of connections between these segments can also contribute to congenital abnormalities. The first is the AV connection, consisting of the AV valves and inlet portion of the interventricular septum. The second is the ventriculoarterial connection, consisting of the semilunar valves and outflow portion of the ventricular septum. Abnormalities in the valves or the inlet and outflow regions of the heart require appropriate descriptions along with the segmental anatomy. For example, in common congenital heart anomalies, such as a complete AV canal defect or tetralogy of Fallot, there is usually normal or concordant segmental alignments but there are inlet or outflow abnormalities. General guidelines regarding such abnormal segmental alignments and segment connections are discussed here.

TABLE 42–3. Anatomic Alignments and Relationships

Atrioventricular Connection	Ventriculoarterial Connection	Congenital Heart Defect
Concordant	Concordant	Normal heart
Concordant	Discordant	d-TGA
Discordant	Discordant	Congenitally corrected TGA
Discordant	Concordant	Isolated ventricular inversion or anatomically corrected malposition

TGA, transposition of the great arteries.

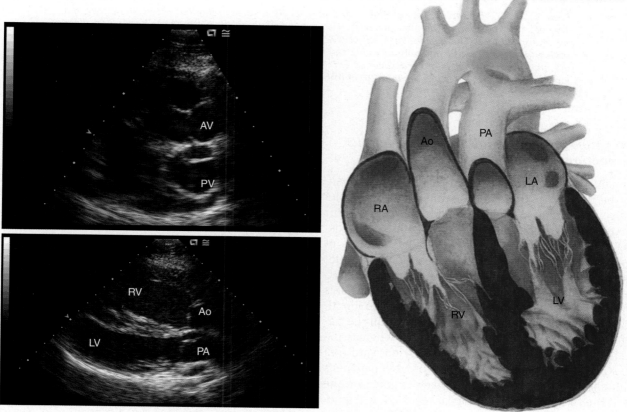

Figure 42–10. *The parasternal long-axis and short-axis views show the great arterial relationships in d-transposition of the great arteries. The pulmonary artery (PA) and pulmonary valve (PV) are shown posterior to the aorta (Ao) and aortic valve (AV). The great vessels are shown as side-by-side, which is a common finding in d-TGA. LA, left atrium; LV, left ventricle; RA, right atrium; RV, right ventricle.*

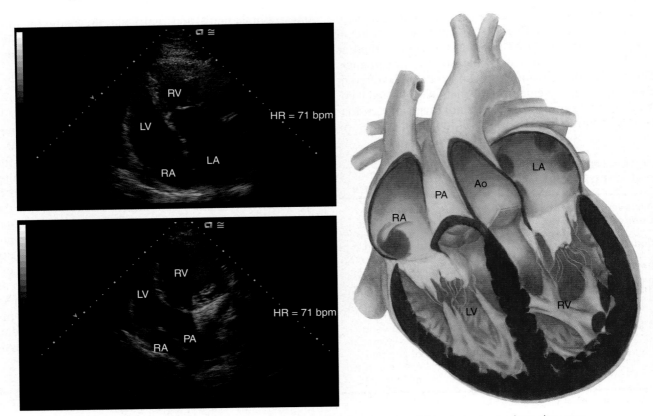

Figure 42–11. The apical four-chamber and off-axis parasternal long-axis views show the anatomy of l-transposition of the great arteries. There is atrioventricular discordance and ventriculoarterial discordance. The morphologic left ventricle is on the anatomic right side and gives rise to a pulmonary artery that is in continuity with the mitral valve. The tricuspid valve has a mild Ebsteinoid malformation that is often associated with l-TGA. HR, heart rate; LA, left atrium; LV, morphologic left ventricle; RA, right atrium; RV, morphologic right ventricle.

Determination of Atrial Situs and Venous Connections

In many patients with CHD, the segmental anatomy may be unclear or the diagnosis unknown. If so, the cardiac positioning in the thorax and the orientation of the apex are best analyzed beginning with the subcostal view. That view also helps determine the situs of the liver, the position of the IVC and abdominal aorta, and the relationship of the hepatic portion of the IVC drainage to the right atrium. In the subcostal short-axis view, the spine, liver, aorta, and IVC should be identified. In the usual arrangement, the aorta is on the patients's left and just anterior to the spine, whereas the IVC is noted even further anteriorly and rightward (see Fig. 42–3). The liver is visualized on the patients's right, and often the air of the stomach is noted on the left. If the stomach and liver appear reversed, a diagnosis of complete situs inversus or heterotaxy syndrome should be considered. If the IVC is not present, an azygous or hemiazygos vein, positioned posteriorly along the spine and just to the right or left of the aorta respectively, should be sought. Be aware that in certain cases

the aorta may descend on the right side of the spine.[37] The connection of the IVC to the atrial chamber is often visible when sweeping anteriorly in the subcostal short-axis view. When the hepatic portion of the IVC is present, the chamber will almost always be a morphologic right atrium.[18,20,21] Visualization of the right atrial appendage in the subcostal short-axis view can also help confirm the anatomy, but the appendage may be difficult to see in adults with larger body habitus. The SVC will usually be visualized draining into a morphologic right atrium after rotating the transducer into the subcostal sagittal view. Oftentimes, the right-sided SVC and IVC are seen in the same plane entering the right-sided atrium (see Fig. 42–5). This view may be difficult to obtain in some adults. The right-sided SVC may also be seen in the suprasternal short-axis view aiming rightward of the aorta (Fig. 42–12). If the SVC is not seen in these views, appears small, or an innominate vein is absent, consider the diagnosis of a persistent embryologic left-sided SVC. If the right SVC is not visualized in any view entering the right atrium and the patient has had heart surgery, it is possible that the SVC has been attached directly to the right PA (Glenn

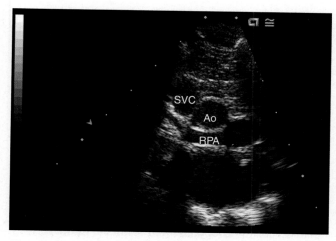

Figure 42-12. The superior vena cava is well seen to the right of the aorta in the suprasternal short-axis view angled rightward. The right pulmonary artery (RPA) is also visualized. Ao, aorta; SVC, superior vena cava.

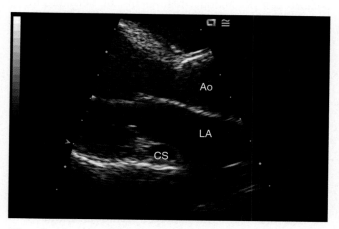

Figure 42-13. Parasternal long-axis view showing a prominent coronary sinus (CS). The most common association with this finding is a persistent left superior vena cava. Ao, aorta; LA, left atrium.

shunt). In some cases, particularly in patients with heterotaxy syndrome, both right and left SVCs may be present.[25,28] A persistent left SVC will be seen when there is failure of the embryologic left SVC to regress. This has been reported to occur in 0.3% to 0.5% in the general population and up to 4% to 5% of those with CHD.[24,38,39] A left SVC often explains a coronary sinus (CS) that appears prominent in the apical view or is easily visualized in the parasternal long-axis view posterior to the left atrium (Fig. 42-13). (If no left SVC is present, the dilated coronary sinus may also be explained by anomalous pulmonary venous drainage or a fistula to the CS.) Although the left SVC typically drains to the CS, it occasionally drains directly to the left atrium. The subcostal saggital view aiming leftward or the parasternal short-axis view often best show the left SVC draining into the CS near the level of the mitral annulus. In addition, the suprasternal short-axis view

aimed to the left of the aorta, following inferiorly toward the CS, is also useful. Dual SVCs can be seen in the subcostal saggital view or the suprasternal short-axis view.[38,39] Drainage of all four individual pulmonary veins should be defined as well as possible. This allows the clinician to evaluate a diagnosis of total or partial anomalous pulmonary venous return and helps determine the morphologic left atrium. It would be unusual to see unrepaired total anomalous pulmonary venous return in an adult or older teen as this almost always must be diagnosed and fixed in childhood. However, other abnormalities of the pulmonary veins might be diagnosed in adulthood including partial anomalous venous return (one or two pulmonary veins returning to the systemic venous system or right atrium directly) and cor triatriatum.[40]

Identification of all four pulmonary veins on transthoracic imaging often is not possible in adults; typically transesophageal imaging or another imaging modality is needed. In infants and children, the individual drainage of the pulmonary veins is best seen in the subcostal four-chamber view, the parasternal short-axis view, or a lower window in the suprasternal short-axis view. Color Doppler is helpful in identifying the orifice of the individual veins. If drainage of the individual pulmonary veins into the left atrium is not identified and a right-to-left shunt is identified at the atrial level, a pulmonary venous confluence with a vertical vein connection to the systemic venous system should be sought. In this case of total anomalous pulmonary venous return, the confluence most often lies posterior to the left atrium, and is visible in the parasternal long-axis, suprasternal, or subcostal views depending if the drainage is intracardiac, supracardiac, or infracardiac, respectively. Pulmonary veins can also have mixed drainage, with individual veins seen draining to the left atrium, directly to the right atrium or the CS. In partial anomalous pulmonary venous return, usually two or three veins are seen entering the left atrium. The other veins, most commonly from the right side, often enter the SVC or the right atrium directly. This often occurs in association with an atrial septal defect (ASD), particularly of the sinus venosus type. However, the partial anomalous pulmonary venous return is an isolated finding in approximately 20% of cases.[40-42] Patients with partial anomalous pulmonary venous return will often have right atrial and ventricular enlargement of uncertain etiology.

In rare cases, the pulmonary veins can drain to the left atrium but have incomplete integration with it. This condition is known as cor triatriatum and occurs when a membrane is present in the left atrium that separates and prevents some or all of the pulmonary veins from draining through the corresponding AV valve. Physiologically, this condition can be asymptomatic until adulthood if mild. However, the condition may mimic mitral stenosis (MS) and may show up in childhood if severe.[43,44]

One further distinction regarding atrial anatomy should be mentioned. In rare conditions known as heterotaxy syndromes, the atrial and visceral situs are unusual and may be difficult to define. In some of these cases, the morphology of the two atria may look similar, and the two chambers may resemble dual right or dual left atria. These findings are often associated with abnormal visceral anatomy. If dual atria are identified, investigation for other anomalies is important. Abnormalities of the systemic and pulmonary veins, and inflow and outflow anomalies, such as AV canal defects or double outlet right ventricles, are commonly associated with heterotaxy syndromes.[25,28]

Determination of Atrioventricular Valves and Ventricles

Once the atrial arrangement has been identified, the alignment with the ventricle or ventricles is next to be defined. This is simplest when there are two ventricular chambers and two AV valves. As mentioned, the AV valve follows the chamber morphology. If there are two well-formed ventricular chambers, attempts are then made to morphologically distinguish a right from a left ventricle. In identifying ventricles, the evaluation for shape, trabeculations, and a moderator band is best done in the apical four-chamber view, further using the parasternal long-axis and short-axis views (see Fig. 42–6). If there are well-formed AV valves and interventricular septum, then the valve attachments to the interventricular septum may also help differentiate the morphology of the chambers. Only a morphologic right ventricle will have an AV valve with septal attachments. A single dominant ventricle or a univentricular heart pose further difficulties and will be covered in more detail later in the chapter.

The AV valves require description and interrogation in their own right, not just in relation to the ventricles. The valves may be morphologically abnormal or abnormally positioned even though the segments are concordant. The valve arrangements and attachments are well seen in the apical four-chamber, parasternal long-axis and short-axis, and subcostal sagittal views. Several arrangements or abnormalities of the AV valves can occur without corresponding abnormalities of segmentation or other chamber alignments. For example, there may be imperfect closure of the leaflets or abnormalities in the chordal apparatus of one of the two valves. On the mitral side, this can result in clefts, parachute, and arcade valves. A cleft is a separation in the valve leaflet that does not allow for full coaptation and results in mitral regurgitation (Fig. 42–14). A parachute mitral valve involves a single dominant or asymmetric papillary muscle. An arcade mitral valve is attached by short chords to multiple diminutive papillary muscle heads. The parachutes and arcades can be stenotic, regurgitant, or normally functioning.[45] On the tricuspid valve side, apical displacement and tethering of the septal and posterior leaflets results in Ebstein's anomaly[46] (Fig. 42–15).

Another AV valve abnormality occurs when the patient has a common AV valve in place of two separate valves, as seen with AV septal defects. In that case, there will be a primum atrial septal defect, an inlet ventricular septal defect, and a single AV valve with usually five leaflets that separates the atria from the respective ventricles. The most common leaflet arrangements of the single AV valve are anterior and posterior bridging leaflets, right and left lateral leaflets, and a right accessory leaflet. As a result of the common AV valve, the right and left sides are notably situated at the same level in the inlet; this differs from the usual

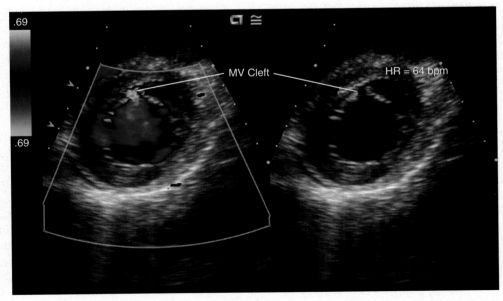

Figure 42–14. *Parasternal short-axis view at the level of the mitral valve shows a small cleft in the anterior leaflet. BPM, beats per minute; HR, heart rate; MV, mitral valve.*

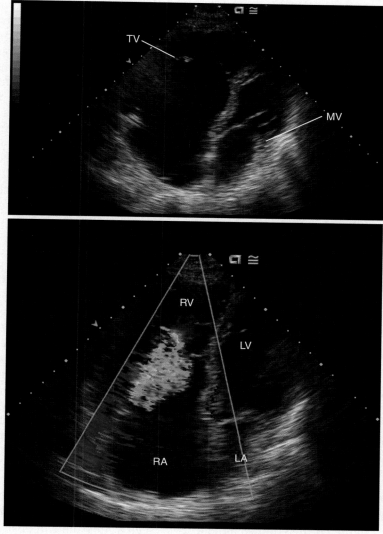

Figure 42–15. *Apical four-chamber view with and without color Doppler shows a patient with severe Ebstein's anomaly of the tricuspid valve. There is apical displacement of the tricuspid valve and severe tricuspid regurgitation. LA, left atrium; LV, left ventricle; MV, mitral valve; RA, right atrium; RV, right ventricle; TV, tricuspid valve.*

position of mild apical displacement of the tricuspid valve relative to the mitral. The common valve may have attachments at the crest of the septum, or there may be no septal attachments at all.[47] In the adult, even if the AV septal defect has been repaired, the left and right AV valves will remain at the same level. A partial AV canal defect, consisting of a primum atrial septal defect and cleft mitral valve, can show up as unrepaired in adults.[48] The cleft can be best visualized when interrogating the mitral valve in the parasternal short-axis view. Subaortic obstruction resulting from the typical gooseneck deformity of the left ventricular outflow tract or resulting from accessory septal attachments should be considered in both repaired and unrepaired AV canal defects. Other confusing AV alignments are presented by straddling, overriding, or atretic AV

valves. With straddle or override, the affected AV valve is at least partially committed to the opposite ventricular chamber—either by the direction of the inflow (straddling) or the alignment of the valve annulus (overriding).[49-50] When only one AV valve is present and it is not a common AV valve, the other valve is probably atretic or not fully formed. The most common form of this is atresia of the tricuspid valve with a resultant hypoplastic right ventricle, usually known solely as "tricuspid atresia." Congenital heart anomalies with atresia of one AV valve usually involve complex anatomy and often a heart with a single dominant ventricular chamber. With a rare abnormality of crisscross AV valves the systemic and pulmonary venous flows cross to opposite ventricles in the unoperated heart or the right-sided atrium flows into the left-sided ventricle (and vice-versa) without mixing oxygenated and de-oxygenated blood. This is an embryologic rotational defect and can occur with AV and ventriculoarterial concordance or discordance. This defect is suspected when there are two AV valves that cannot be visualized in parallel in any of the routine views.[51-53]

Determination of Semilunar Valves and Great Arteries

The relationship of the ventricles to the outflow valve and arteries is most easily described when there are two distinct ventricular chambers and two distinct arterial outflow vessels. In the normally positioned heart, the aortic valve and origin of the aorta arise from the left ventricle and are posterior and slightly rightward of the pulmonary valve and PA origin arising from the right ventricular outflow tract. The relationship of the great arteries to the ventricular chambers is well seen in the parasternal long-axis and short-axis views and the apical four-chamber view (see Figs. 42–7 and 42–8).

From the parasternal long-axis view, the posterior vessel arising from the posterior ventricle is followed to determine if it gives rise to an aorta with head and neck vessels or a PA that turns further posteriorly and bifurcates early. These relationships can also be evaluated when sweeping anteriorly from the AV valves in the apical four-chamber view. The first vessel to come into view is the posterior great vessel; again, one can determine if it is an aorta or PA based on the early bifurcation or the presence of coronary and head and neck arteries. A great artery is considered aligned with a ventricular chamber if half or more of that artery orifice is committed to the chamber. The alignment with the ventricular chamber can then be determined as concordant (e.g., aorta with left ventricle) or discordant (e.g., PA with left ventricle). The distinction between concordance and discordance becomes difficult when both great arteries arise from one chamber or there is only a single outflow. As with the AV valves, this anatomy still requires description. In some of the more recent classifications, these types of great artery relationships are termed malposed rather than transposed. In the double-outlet ventricle, both great arteries arise from a single ventricular chamber that is usually a morphologic right ventricle. In a rare instance, the arteries will arise from a morphologic left ventricle. There are many definitions and multiple anatomic variations comprising a diagnosis of double-outlet ventricles. In one definition, each great artery has some subarterial conal tissue, and thus, neither will be in fibrous continuity with the mitral valve. In the simpler definition of the double-outlet right ventricle, the anterior vessel arises completely from the right ventricle, and the posterior vessel may override the septum but will be more than 50% committed from the right ventricle.[53] Truncus arteriosus is another outflow tract abnormality. In this diagnosis, instead of two outflows from one ventricle, there is a single outflow acting for both ventricles. The single outflow divides into both the aorta and either a main PA or individual branch PAs. As before, this is best diagnosed by following the outflow vessel in the apical four-chamber or parasternal long-axis and short-axis views to determine the branching patterns. In most cases, by the time a patient has reached adulthood, the truncus arteriosus either will have been repaired in childhood or the patient will have severe cyanosis and have developed Eisenmenger physiology. Once the individual great arteries have been identified, it is important to trace them distally as far as possible to examine for additional extracardiac congenital malformations. The imaging of the bifurcation of the normally positioned branch PAs is best performed in the parasternal short-axis view. The pulmonary valve is seen giving rise to a main PA and the bifurcation of the right and left branches (see Fig. 42–8). The individual branches can also be visualized in the suprasternal notch views with the right PA best seen in the suprasternal short-axis view (see Fig. 42–12), whereas the left pulmonary artery can be seen by angling slightly leftward of the standard suprasternal long-axis view. The PAs should be interrogated for absence or stenosis of a branch PA or other abnormalities, such as a patent ductus arteriosus or aortopulmonary window. The aorta is visualized in multiple views to investigate as many of its segments as possible. The aortic valve and proximal ascending aorta are well seen in the usual parasternal long-axis view. The more distal aortic arch is best visualized from the suprasternal notch long-axis view. Often the entire transverse aortic arch and proximal portion of the descending thoracic aorta can be seen at this angle. It is an excellent view to interrogate for coarctation of the aorta or patent ductus arteriosus. When possible, the descending aorta should also be imaged from the subcostal views in both the short axis and long axis. Examining abdominal aortic pulsatility can be helpful in determining a distal coarctation or the severity of a more proximal coarctation.[54] Other extracardiac congenital abnormalities can be seen when imaging the aorta and branch PAs, including a patent ductus arteriosus or an aortopulmonary window. A patent ductus arteriosus is seen as a vascular connection arising from the aorta, near the typical origin of a left subclavian artery and entering the left PA. If the ductus is small, it may be difficult to see in two-dimensional imaging but will be visible as continuous left-to-right shunting from the aorta to the PA with color Doppler imaging. If the ductus is large and not discovered until adulthood, it is likely the patient will have elevated pulmonary vascular resistance or Eisenmenger physiology and there may be little residual shunting. An aortopulmonary window is usually seen as a connection between the main PA and the ascending aorta. It is best visualized in the parasternal short-axis view, but may be difficult to discern in two-dimensional images; often color and spectral Doppler are required. As with a large ductus arteriosus, an aortopulmonary window may be hard to diagnose even with Doppler in adulthood because the unrepaired patients will have elevated PA pressures and have developed Eisenmenger physiology.

Univentricular Heart

General

As with some congenital malformations previously discussed, the univentricular heart engenders its own debate over nomenclature.[18-21,29] Different terms are employed to describe these hearts, including primitive ventricles, univentricular hearts, and univentricular AV connections. Morphologically, the potential rudimentary chambers associated with a single dominant ventricular chamber include those associated with an outflow vessel (outflow chamber) and those associated with neither an inflow nor outflow (trabecular chamber). Some pathologists prefer to call these types of rudimentary chambers "ventricles" and describe the anatomy from an embryologic perspective. Others define a ventricle as a chamber that receives 50% of an inflow valve.[18] Still others describe the anatomy and morphology as it is found in the heart, such as double-inlet left ventricle or unbalanced AV canal with hypoplastic left ventricle. For purposes of this section, the univentricular heart refers to a heart in which the AV connection is predominantly related to a single ventricular chamber that is either morphologically right or left in origin. Occasionally the morphology of the chamber cannot be determined; these instances are referred to as univentricular heart of indeterminate type.[56,57] In the adult, the patient with a univentricular heart may show up to the echocardiography lab as either unrepaired or with a palliative or reparative surgery. Unless familiar with the different nomenclatures, it is often the best practice simply to describe the chambers present and the relationships to the valves and great vessels. Determining the morphology of the dominant ventricular chamber focuses on the anatomic landmarks, the AV connections, and the ventriculoarterial connections. Although there may be two AV valves entering a common chamber, such as in double-inlet left ventricle, there can also be atresia of one of the valves or a common AV valve.[56-60] In the univentricular heart, the AV valves are often malformed in some way and may not carry the normal morphologic conditions of a mitral and tricuspid valve. These are more appropriately identified as right and left AV valves. Moreover, the ventriculoarterial connections can take any arrangement, including normally related, transposed, double outlet, or atresia of one of the vessels.[56-60]

Left Ventricular Type

The morphologic left ventricular type univentricular heart is the more common form of single ventricular chamber found in adults (Fig. 42–16). The rudimentary chamber is usually located at the base, anterior and superior to the ventricle, and often gives rise to the aortic outflow. The orientation of the chambers is most often l-looped, with the morphologic left ventricle somewhat rightward and the rudimentary chamber to the left; d-looping, however, also exists.[56-60] The connection between the ventricle and the rudimentary chamber, often called the bulboventricular foramen, is best seen in the subcostal and parasternal long-axis and short-axis views. In the long-axis view, the open-

SINGLE VENTRICLE OF LV TYPE:

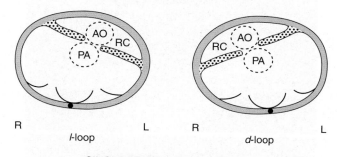

SINGLE VENTRICLE OF RV TYPE:

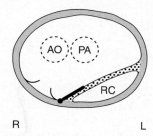

Figure 42–16. *Diagrammatic representation of the anatomic features used to diagnose the type of univentricular heart on two-dimensional echocardiography. The drawings represent parasternal short-axis projections. In single ventricle of the left ventricular (LV) type, the trabecular septum (stippled) and rudimentary chamber (RC) are anterior to the atrioventricular valves. The trabecular septum runs to the acute or obtuse margin of the heart and not to the crux of the heart (black circle). Thus, there is no intervening septum at the crux of the heart between the atrioventricular valves. Most often, the RC is at the left basal aspect of the heart (l-loop); however, it can also be located less frequently at the right basal aspect of the heart (d-loop). Most commonly, the ventriculoarterial connections are discordant with the aorta (AO) arising from the RC and the pulmonary artery (PA) arising from the main ventricle (depicted in the diagram); however, any ventriculoarterial connection is possible. In single ventricle of the right ventricular (RV) type, the RC and trabecular septum are posterior to the atrioventricular valves. The trabecular septum courses to the crux of the heart, and there is usually left atrioventricular valve atresia (shown). Most commonly, the ventriculoarterial connections are double outlet from the main ventricle (shown); however, any ventriculoarterial connection is possible.*

ing to the anterior rudimentary chamber is seen leading to an outflow vessel. In the coronal view, both the right and left AV valves can be seen opening into the posterior ventricle, whereas the rudimentary chamber is visualized anteriorly (Fig. 42–17).

The AV valves can also be seen in the apical four-chamber view entering into a common chamber with no intervening inlet septum.[56,57,61] Although there are usually two separate AV valves, stenosis or atresia of one of the valves can occur as can entry of a common

valve. In a majority of these patients, the great arteries are transposed and the aorta will arise from the rudimentary chamber, whereas the PA will arise from the morphologic left ventricle.[56,57,61]

Right Ventricular Type

In adulthood, the less commonly seen condition is the single ventricular chamber of the right ventricular type (see Fig. 42–16). In this case, the rudimentary chamber is located posterior and inferior to the morphologic right ventricle.[56-62] This chamber may be located to the right (l-loop) or to the left (d-loop) of the dominant right ventricle. In patients with a univentricular heart of the right ventricular type and a common inlet, some may exhibit other features consistent with heterotaxy syndromes.

The AV valves may be a common inlet, single inlet with atresia of one valve, or a double inlet.[25] The AV valve communications and the rudimentary chamber are best seen in the apical and subcostal four-chamber views because the valves lie more anteriorly and the rudimentary chamber lies more posteriorly. The rudimentary chamber usually does not give rise to any of the outflow vessels. Most often the patient will have a form of double-outlet right ventricle, with both great arteries arising from the right ventricle or a single aorta with pulmonary atresia.

Other Univentricular Physiology Hearts

Special mention should be made of some subtle differences and difficulties in describing a few of the univentricular lesions. For example, there are differences in describing a double-inlet left ventricle with right AV valve atresia, as opposed to diagnosing tricuspid atresia or, similarly, the differences between a univentricular heart of the right ventricular type with absent left AV valve, as opposed to a hypoplastic left heart with mitral atresia. Although there are physiologic similarities, there are anatomic and embryologic differences in the development of these conditions. Visually, however, the differences may be difficult to determine. One echocardiographic distinction can be found in the positioning of the atria and the interventricular septum. In the cases of tricuspid atresia and hypoplastic left heart syndrome, the atria often lie over the associated ventricular chamber and the ventricular septum can be visualized up to the crux of the heart in the inlet septum. In the other cases of the univentricular hearts, the inlet portion of the septum is often missing and the atria will be seen over the dominant chamber not the rudimentary chambers. However, in the adult who has often had multiple surgeries, these distinctions may be quite difficult.

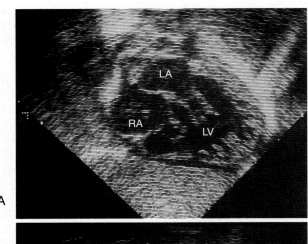

A

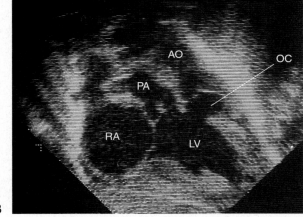

B

Figure 42–17. Subcostal coronal views from a patient with univentricular heart of the left ventricular type and discordant ventriculoarterial connections. A, The transducer has been tilted posteriorly to image the inlets of the heart. This view is a posterior plane passing through both atrioventricular valve inlets and the crux of the heart; therefore, this plane lies posterior to the trabecular septum and rudimentary chamber. Note the "kissing" atrioventricular valve with no intervening ventricular septum oriented to the crux of the heart. Both atrioventricular valves empty into the large posterior left ventricle (LV). B, The transducer has been tilted anteriorly to image the outflow tracts. The LV is connected to a posterior pulmonary artery (PA). A small rightward and anterior outlet chamber (OC) gives rise to an anterior and rightward aorta (Ao). Note that many of the echocardiographic features of transposition of the great vessels are seen. The great vessels are aligned parallel and the posterior PA has a posterior sweep. LA, left atrium; RA, right atrium.

Color and Spectral Doppler

General

Anatomy is obviously crucial, but it is only one part of the CHD evaluation. Color and spectral Doppler imaging are both critical tools in any comprehensive investigation of congenital heart lesions. In particular, Doppler imaging plays an important role in identifying intracardiac shunt lesions, such as ventricular septal defects (VSDs), valve abnormalities, such as pulmonary stenosis, and residual embryologic vascular connections, such as a left SVC to the CS. Similarly, the Doppler techniques help identify the direction of flow. These techniques also quantify flow in intracardiac shunting and valvular abnormalities.

Intracardiac Shunts

Once the anatomy and relationships of the chambers and great artery and venous connections have been determined, abnormalities between those chambers require investigation:

- The interatrial and interventricular septa are closely examined for intracardiac shunting; and
- The AV and semilunar valves are interrogated for stenosis and regurgitation, regardless of the positioning within the heart.

Moreover, with univentricular hearts or single ventricles it is crucial to determine any connection be-tween the ventricular chamber and rudimentary outflow chamber. It is important to determine if there is obstruction in this region. Finally, the aorta and PAs are interrogated for stenosis at any point along the anatomic course. Atrial shunts are sought by examining the interatrial septum in multiple views. These views include the apical four-chamber, parasternal short-axis and subcostal sagittal planes (Fig. 42–18). The subcostal view is often helpful as it shows the secundum septum and the venosus septa of the IVC and SVC. However, in many adults, the subcostal images may not be clear. If an interatrial shunt is identified, the direction and velocity of flow between the interatrial chambers is reported. The degree of shunting can be estimated by the degree of right ventricular enlargement. Alternatively, it can be determined quantitatively by calculating a pulmonary to systemic flow ratio, using the flow across the pulmonary valve (Qp) and flow across the aortic valve (Qs) in an otherwise structurally normal heart.[55]

The interrogation for interatrial defects requires careful attention. With other signs of an intracardiac shunting, such as unexplained right ventricular enlargement, the interrogation needs to include the venosus and primum portions of the septum. If the images are limited by body habitus, a bubble contrast study may be required. Like the interatrial septum, the interventricular septum is interrogated in multiple views. These include the apical four-chamber, and parasternal long-axis and short-axis views (Fig. 42–19). For each view, it is important to image from the apex to the base

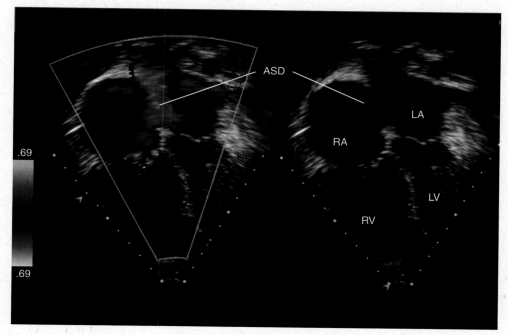

Figure 42–18. *Apical four-chamber view showing large secundum atrial septal defect (ASD). There is also significant right atrial (RA) and right ventricular (RV) enlargement. LA, left atrium; LV, left ventricle.*

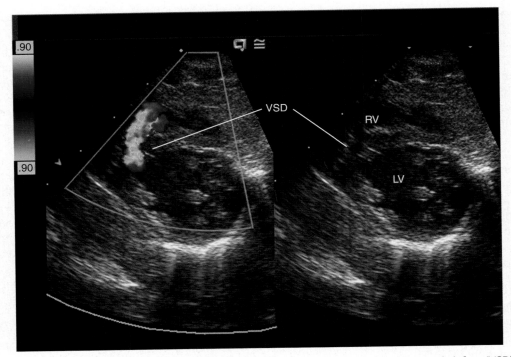

Figure 42–19. Parasternal short-axis view showing a muscular ventricular septal defect (VSD). The defect is difficult to appreciate in the two-dimensional view, however, the left-to-right shunt is easily seen with color Doppler. LV, left ventricle; RV, right ventricle.

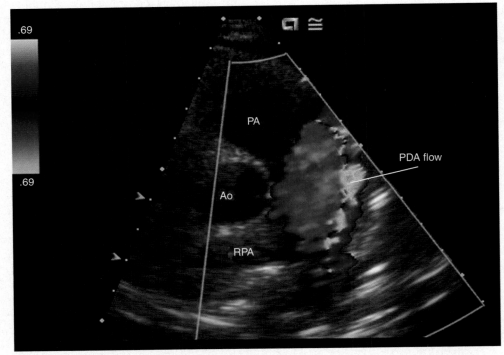

Figure 42–20. Parasternal short-axis view with color Doppler shows the left-to-right shunt (red flow) of the patent ductus arteriosus (PDA) into the main pulmonary artery (PA). Ao, aorta; RPA, right branch pulmonary artery.

of the septum. In the apical four-chamber and parasternal long-axis views, aim the transducer anteriorly and posteriorly to interrogate the outflow and inflow portions of the septum respectively. The sector width should be narrow, and the color gain decreased, to identify smaller shunts. As with atrial level shunting, the direction and velocity of flow can be estimated using both color and spectral Doppler. Note that with some serpiginous, or small, muscular defects, velocity interrogation may be inaccurate.

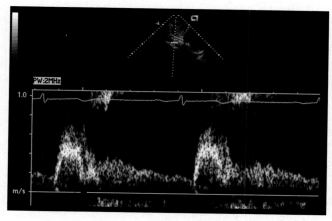

Figure 42-21. Spectral Doppler profile of the descending aortic flow with an antegrade run-off into diastole.

Great Artery Abnormalities

As with the normal heart, complete evaluation for valvar stenosis and regurgitation using color and spectral Doppler is important. In CHD, several anomalies, discussed in relation to the aortic arch and PA, are better defined using Doppler interrogation. The aortic arch is best visualized in the suprasternal views. Color and spectral Doppler interrogation are used to investigate for flow acceleration, particularly in the area of the isthmus just at—or distal to—the left subclavian artery origin. Turbulence in this area suggests a coarctation or a patent ductus arteriosus. The small ductus is identified as having continuous left-to-right shunting from the aorta into the PA (Fig. 42-20), whereas the larger ductus may have low velocity or bidirectional shunting if the patient has developed Eisenmenger physiology. In the case of a coarctation, there is increased velocity of flow across the narrowed area with persistent antegrade diastolic run-off. The downstream and abdominal aortic flow is also interrogated in the subcostal view to evaluate for blunting of pulsatile flow and/or persistent diastolic run-off (Fig. 42-21).

The branch PAs are best interrogated by Doppler in the parasternal short-axis and suprasternal views for stenosis and other flow abnormalities. If a patent ductus arteriosus is suspected, the diastolic flow into the PA from the aorta is often seen with color in these views. The PA branches can also be interrogated in the subcostal sagittal view if the patient has good subcostal images.

KEY POINTS

■ The segmental approach begins with the identification of the atrial and abdominal situs and continues with the identification of ventricular and arterial relationships. The atria are defined by the appendages and by the systemic and pulmonary venous connections. The right atrium has a broad appendage and is associated with the suprahepatic IVC. The left atrium has a narrow appendage and is associated with the pulmonary venous return.

■ The right ventricle is recognized by the presence of a moderator band and association with a tricuspid valve, whereas the left ventricle is bullet shaped and is associated with a mitral valve. The tricuspid valve has three leaflets and attachments to the interventricular septum. The mitral valve has two leaflets attached to papillary muscles opposite the interventricular septum. In the normal heart, the tricuspid valve is more apically displaced.

■ The great arteries are denoted by the bifurcation patterns as they exit the heart. Either vessel can be anterior or posterior or either can be right or left. The aorta bifurcates more distally and gives rise to the coronary arteries and head and neck vessels. The PA bifurcates early into the right and left PA branches.

■ Normal segmental alignment is when the right atrium is associated with the right ventricle and pulmonary artery and the left atrium with the left ventricle and the aorta.

■ The most common abnormalities with discordant relationships are (1) d-transposition of the great arteries with AV concordance and ventriculoarterial discordance and (2) l-transposition of the great arteries or congenitally corrected transposition of the great arteries with AV discordance and ventriculoarterial discordance.

■ Abnormalities of the AV and semilunar valves are common, even with normal segmentation. Some of the more frequent findings include bicuspid aortic and pulmonary valves, Ebsteinoid tricuspid valves, and cleft mitral valves. Abnormalities can also include common, atretic, straddling, and overriding atrioventricular valves, as well as common, overriding, or atretic semilunar valves.

■ The univentricular heart refers to a heart in which the AV connection is predominantly related to a single ventricular chamber that is either morphologically right or left in origin. In the left ventricular type, the rudimentary chamber is usually anterior and superior and gives rise to the aorta. In the right ventricular type, the rudimentary chamber is usually inferior and posterior and is not associated with an outflow vessel.

■ Full functional assessment with color and spectral Doppler is required for:

–all intracardiac valves to assess stenosis and regurgitation,

–the atrial and interventricular septa for evidence of shunting, and

–the aorta and PAs for evidence of flow abnormalities and shunts

REFERENCES

1. Warnes CA, Liberthson R, Danielson GK, et al: The 32nd Bethesda Conference Task Force 1: The changing profile of congenital heart disease in adult life. *J Am Coll Cardiol* 37:1170-1175, 2001.

2. Hoffman JI, Kaplan S, Liberthson RR: Prevalence of congenital heart disease. *Am Heart J* 147:425-439, 2004.

3. Niwa K, Perloff JK, Webb GD, et al: Survey of specialized tertiary care facilities for adults with congenital heart disease. *Int J Cardiol* 96:211-216, 2004.

4. Child JS, Collins-Nakai RL, Alpert JS, et al: Task force 3: Workforce description and educational requirements for the care of adults with congenital heart disease. *J Am Coll Cardiol* 37:1183-1187, 2001.

5. Gurvitz MZ, Chang RK, Ramos FJ, et al: Variations in adult congenital heart disease training in adult and pediatric cardiology fellowship programs. *J Am Coll Cardiol* 46:893-898, 2005.

6. Reid GJ, Irvine MJ, McCrindle BW, et al: Prevalence and correlates of successful transfer from pediatric to adult health care among a cohort of young adults with complex congenital heart defects. *Pediatrics* 113:e197-e205, 2004.

7. Wacker A, Kaemmerer H, Hollweck R, et al: Outcome of operated and unoperated adults with congenital cardiac disease lost to follow-up for more than five years. *Am J Cardiol* 95:776-779, 2005.

8. Kaemmerer H, Stern H, Fratz S, et al: Imaging in adults with congenital cardiac disease (ACCD). *Semin Thorac Cardiovasc Surg* 48:328-335, 2000.

9. Child JS: Echo-Doppler and color-flow imaging in congenital heart disease. *Cardiol Clin* 8:289-313, 1990.

10. Moodie DS: Diagnosis and management of congenital heart disease in the adult. *Cardiol Rev* 9:276-281, 2001.

11. Goo HW, Park IS, Ko JK, et al: Computed tomography for the diagnosis of congenital heart disease in pediatric and adult patients. *Int J Cardiovasc Imaging* 21:347-365, 2005.

12. Boxt LM: Magnetic resonance and computed tomographic evaluation of congenital heart disease. *J Magn Reson Imaging* 19:827-847, 2004.

13. Okuda S, Kikinis R, Geva T, et al: 3D-shaded surface rendering of gadolinium-enhanced MR angiography in congenital heart disease. *Pediatr Radiol* 30:540-545, 2000.

14. Hartnell GG, Cohen MC, Meier RA, Finn JP: Magnetic resonance angiography demonstration of congenital heart disease in adults. *Clin Radiol* 51:851-857, 1996.

15. Hirsch R, Kilner PJ, Connelly MS, et al: Diagnosis in adolescents and adults with congenital heart disease. Prospective assessment of individual and combined roles of magnetic resonance imaging and transesophageal echocardiography. *Circulation* 90:2937-2951, 1994.

16. Chessa M, De Rosa G, Pardeo M, et al: Illness understanding in adults with congenital heart disease. *Ital Heart J* 6:895-899, 2005.

17. Dore A, de Guise P, Mercier LA: Transition of care to adult congenital heart centres: what do patients know about their heart condition? *Can J Cardiol* 18:141-146, 2002.

18. Tynan MJ, Becker AE, Macartney FJ, et al: Nomenclature and classification of congenital heart disease. *Br Heart J* 41:544-553, 1979.

19. Jacobs ML, Mayer JE Jr: Congenital Heart Surgery Nomenclature and Database Project: single ventricle. *Ann Thorac Surg* 69(4 suppl):s197-s204, 2000.

20. Van Praagh R: Terminology of congenital heart disease: glossary and commentary. *Circulation* 56:139-143, 1977.

21. Van Praagh R: Segmental approach to diagnosis. In Fyler D (ed): *Nadas' Pediatric Cardiology*. Philadelphia, Hanley and Belfus, 1992, pp. 27-36.

22. Huhta JC, Hagler DJ, Seward JB, Tajik AJ, Julsrud PR, Ritter DG. Two-dimensional echocardiographic assessment of dextrocardia: A segmental approach. *Am J Cardiol* 50:1351-1360, 1982.

23. Snider AR, Serwer GA, Ritter SB: *Echocardiography in Pediatric Heart Disease*, 2nd ed. St. Louis, Mosby-Year Book, 1997, pp. 560-562.

24. Perloff JK: *The Clinical Recognition of Congenital Heart Disease*, 4th ed. Philadelphia, WB Saunders, 1994.

25. Van Praagh S, Santini F, Sanders S: Cardiac malpositions with special emphasis on visceral heterotaxy. In Fyler D (ed): *Nadas' Pediatric Cardiology*. Philadelphia, Hanley and Belfus, 1992, pp. 589-608.

26. Van Praagh R, Van Praagh S, Vlad P, et al: Anatomic types of congenital dextrocardia: diagnostic and embryologic implications. *Am J Cardiol* 13:510-531, 1964.

27. Garg N, Agarwal BL, Modi N, et al: Dextrocardia: an analysis of cardiac structures in 125 patients. *Int J Cardiol* 88:143-155, 2003.

28. Stanger P, Rudolph AM, Edwards JE: Cardiac malpositions: An overview based on study of sixty-five necropsy specimens. *Circulation* 56:159-172, 1977.

29. Van Praagh R, Van Praagh S: Morphologic anatomy. In Fyler D (ed): *Nadas' Pediatric Cardiology*. Philadelphia, Hanley and Belfus, 1992, pp. 27-36.

30. Shinebourne EA, Macartney FJ, Anderson RH: Sequential chamber localization—logical approach to diagnosis in congenital heart disease. *Br Heart J* 38:327-340, 1976.

31. Roberts WC: The congenitally bicuspid aortic valve—a study of 85 autopsy cases. *Am J Cardiol* 26:72, 1970.

32. Celano V, Pieroni DR, Gingell RL, Roland JM: Two-dimensional echocardiographic recognition of the right aortic arch. *Am J Cardiol* 51:1507-1512, 1983.

33. Shrivastava S, Berry JM, Einzig S, Bass JL: Parasternal cross-sectional echocardiographic determination of aortic arch situs: A new approach. *Am J Cardiol* 55:1236-1238, 1985.

34. Snider AR, Serwer GA, Ritter SB: *Echocardiography in Pediatric Heart Disease*, 2nd ed. St. Louis, Mosby-Year Book, 1997, pp. 476-478.

35. Van Praagh R: The importance of segmental situs in the diagnosis of congenital heart disease. *Semin Roentgenol* 20:254-271, 1985.

36. Van Praagh R, Durnin R, Jockin H, et al: Anatomically corrected malposition of the great arteries (S, D, L). *Circulation* 51:20-31, 1975.

37. Snider AR, Serwer GA, Ritter SB: *Echocardiography in Pediatric Heart Disease*, 2nd ed. St. Louis, Mosby-Year Book, 1997, pp. 558-560.

38. Tak T, Crouch E, Drake GB: Persistent left superior vena cava: Incidence, significance and clinical correlates. *Int J Cardiol* 82:91-93, 2002.

39. Buirski G, Jordan SC, Joffe HS, Wilde P: Superior vena caval abnormalities: Their occurrence rate, associated cardiac abnormalities and angiographic classification in a paediatric population with congenital heart disease. *Clin Radiol* 37:131-138, 1986.

40. Gustafson RA, Warden HE, Murray GF, Hill RC, Rozar GE: Partial anomalous pulmonary venous connection to the right side of the heart. *J Thorac Cardiovasc Surg* 98:861-868, 1989.

41. Wong ML, McCrindle BW, Mota C, Smallhorn JF: Echocardiographic evaluation of partial anomalous pulmonary venous drainage. *J Am Coll Cardiol* 26:503-507, 1995.

42. Snider AR, Serwer GA, Ritter SB: *Echocardiography in Pediatric Heart Disease*, 2nd ed. St. Louis, Mosby-Year Book, 1997, pp. 474-475.

43. Alphonso N, Norgaard MA, Newcomb A, et al: Cor triatriatum: presentation, diagnosis and long-term surgical results. *Ann Thorac Surg* 80:1666-1671, 2005.

44. Slight RD, Nzewi OC, Buell R, Mankad PS: Cor-triatriatum sinister presenting in the adult as mitral stenosis: an analysis of factors which may be relevant in late presentation. *Heart Lung Circ* 14:8-12, 2005.

45. Grenadier E, Sahn DJ, Valdes-Cruz LM, et al: Two-dimensional echo Doppler study of congenital disorders of the mitral valve. *Am Heart J* 107:319-325, 1984.

46. Anderson KR, Zuberbuhler JR, Anderson RH, et al: Morphologic spectrum of Ebstein's anomaly of the heart: a review. *Mayo Clin Proc* 54:174-180, 1979.

47. Anderson RH, Ho SY, Falcao S, et al: The diagnostic features of atrioventricular septal defect with common atrioventricular junction. *Cardiol Young* 8:33-49, 1998.

48. Gatzoulis MA, Hechter S, Webb GD, Williams WG: Surgery for partial atrioventricular septal defect in the adult. *Ann Thorac Surg* 67:504-510, 1999.

49. Pessotto R, Padalino M, Rubino M, et al: Straddling tricuspid valve as a sign of ventriculoatrial malalignment: A morphometric study of 19 postmortem cases. *Am Heart J* 138:1184-1195, 1999.

50. Rice MJ, Seward JB, Edwards WD, et al: Straddling atrioventricular valve: Two-dimensional echocardiographic diagnosis, classification and surgical implications. *Am J Cardiol* 55:505-513, 1985.

51. Anderson KR, Lie JT, Sieg K, et al: A criss-cross heart. Detailed anatomic description and discussion of morphogenesis. *Mayo Clin Proc* 52:569-575, 1977.

52. Hery E, Jimenez M, Didier D, et al: Echocardiographic and angiographic findings in superior-inferior cardiac ventricles. *Am J Cardiol* 63:1385-1389, 1989.

53. de la Cruz MV, Cayre R, Arista-Salado Martinez O, et al: The infundibular interrelationships and the ventriculoarterial connection in double outlet right ventricle. Clinical and surgical implications. *Int J Cardiol* 35:153-164, 1992.

54. Shaddy RE, Snider AR, Silverman NH, Lutin W: Pulsed Doppler findings in patients with coarctation of the aorta. *Circulation* 73:82-88, 1986.

55. Snider AR, Serwer GA, Ritter SB: *Echocardiography in Pediatric Heart Disease,* 2nd ed. St. Louis, Mosby-Year Book, 1997, p. 191.

56. Rigby ML, Anderson RH, Gibson D, et al: Two dimensional echocardiographic categorisation of the univentricular heart. Ventricular morphology, type, and mode of atrioventricular connection. *Br Heart J* 46:603-612, 1981.

57. Huhta JC, Seward JB, Tajik AJ, et al: Two-dimensional echocardiographic spectrum of univentricular atrioventricular connection. *J Am Coll Cardiol* 5:149-157, 1985.

58. Beardshaw JA, Gibson DG, Pearson MC, et al: Echocardiographic diagnosis of primitive ventricle with two atrioventricular valves. *Br Heart J* 39:266-275, 1977.

59. Soto B, Pacifico AD, Di Sciascio G: Univentricular heart: an angiographic study. *Am J Cardiol* 49:787-794, 1982.

60. Ho SY, Zuberbuhler JR, Anderson RH: Pathology of hearts with a univentricular atrioventricular connection. *Perspect Pediatr Pathol* 12:69-99, 1988.

61. Snider AR, Serwer GA, Ritter SB: *Echocardiography in Pediatric Heart Disease,* 2nd ed. St. Louis, Mosby-Year Book, 1997, pp. 343-351.

62. Shinebourne EA, Lau KC, Calcaterra G, Anderson RH: Univentricular heart of right ventricular type: clinical, angiographic and electocardiographic features. *Am J Cardiol* 46:439-445, 1980.

Chapter 43

Echocardiographic Evaluation of the Adult with Unoperated Congenital Heart Disease

MARY ETTA E. KING, MD

Caring for adults with congenital heart disease (CHD) who have not had prior surgical intervention is a fascinating lesson in the natural history of congenital anomalies of the heart. It can also be a remarkable tribute to the tolerance, adaptation, and perseverance of the patient in the face of long-standing cardiac disability. In managing adults with unoperated CHD, three clinical subgroups emerge: patients with mild or slowly progressive defects who do not require intervention; patients who have eluded previous diagnosis and are still amenable to surgical correction or transcatheter intervention; and patients with abnormalities that are deemed inoperable. It is the task of the cardiologist to evaluate each patient thoroughly to determine optimal management.

Echocardiography has been a major advance for cardiologists in diagnosing and evaluating the anatomic and physiologic status of the adult with CHD. The technique is not without challenge or difficulty, however. Cardiac enlargement and hypertrophy and associated scoliosis cause chest wall deformities that limit transthoracic ultrasound (US) access. Congenital or acquired pulmonary disease and cardiac malpositions lend additional impediment to surface echocardiographic imag-

TABLE 43-1. Congenital Heart Defects in the Unoperated Adult

Most Common	Less Common	Rare
Bicuspid aortic valve	Ventricular septal defect	Double-outlet right ventricle
Pulmonic stenosis	Discrete subaortic stenosis	Complete transposition
Coarctation of the aorta	Patent ductus arteriosus	Truncus arteriosus
Atrial septal defect	Ebstein's anomaly	Tricuspid atresia
	Tetralogy of Fallot	Univentricular heart
	Coronary arteriovenous fistula	
	Sinus of Valsalva aneurysm	
	Corrected transposition	

ing. Transesophageal echocardiography (TEE) is useful in circumventing some of these difficulties and plays a major adjunctive role in evaluating and managing the adult with CHD.[1,2] Increasingly, alternate imaging modalities, such as magnetic resonance imaging (MRI) and computed tomography (CT), are playing important complementary roles in the complete evaluation of the adult with CHD.[3,4] It has been said that "chance favors the prepared mind." Thus, the likelihood of an accurate diagnosis with any of these technologies requires a clear understanding of congenital heart defects and the expected sequelae and complications.

This chapter includes the clinical features and echocardiographic evaluation and management of congenital heart defects that are encountered in the adult patient without the benefit of previous surgical intervention. Discussion includes valvular abnormalities, disorders affecting the left ventricular outflow tract (LVOT) and aorta, septal defects and shunt lesions, and the complex congenital abnormalities most frequently encountered. The relative frequency of these anomalies in the unoperated adult is shown in Table 43-1. (Additional discussion of complex congenital lesions can be found in Chapter 42.)

Valvular Abnormalities

Bicuspid Aortic Valve

The congenitally bicuspid aortic valve is the most frequent of all congenital heart defects, occurring in approximately 1% to 2% of the U.S. population.[5] There are a number of factors that suggest a genetic basis for this common defect. Familial studies indicate an autosomal dominant transmission with variable penetrance, but the genetic locus or loci are as yet undetermined.[5] Morphologically, the bicuspid valve may have two

equal cusps with a single central commissure, or the cusps may be disparate in size, with an eccentric commissure and the larger cusp containing a raphe.

Functionally, a bicuspid valve may be nonstenotic and nonregurgitant, which is especially true in the adolescent and young adult, of whom as many as one third have no significant functional impairment. Progression of stenosis is common, however, even in valves with mild dysfunction. By the age of 60 years, 53% of bicuspid valves are stenotic, and by the age of 70 years, 73% become significantly stenotic. Of individuals older than 40 years who require aortic valve replacements, about 30% have a congenitally abnormal aortic valve.[6] The mechanism of progressive valvular dysfunction appears to be a "wear-and-tear" process leading to fibrosis and calcification.

Congenitally bicuspid aortic valves have a known association with abnormalities of the aorta (see Chapter 33). Aortic coarctation occurs in a small percentage of patients with bicuspid aortic valves. Aortic dissection is another abnormality recognized for its association with a bicuspid aortic valve (Fig. 43-1). Reported studies have shown that 5% to 9% of patients with dissecting aneurysms of the aorta also have a bicuspid aortic valve. Pathologic study of the aorta in these patients revealed changes consistent with cystic medial necrosis.[7,8] Poststenotic dilation of the ascending aorta has long been recognized in congenital aortic stenosis (AS) and has traditionally been attributed to mechanical impingement of a jet lesion eccentrically directed by the domed leaflets. However, the ascending aorta may be dilated even in functionally normal bicuspid valves, raising the possibility that aortic dilation may be caused by a developmental defect affecting both the valve and the aortic root.[9] Recent reports have shown an increase in vascular smooth muscle cell apoptosis and increased metalloproteinase activity in the aortic wall of patients with bicuspid aortic valves, suggesting a genetic abnormality of the aortic wall.[10-12] Periodic echocardiographic assessment of the ascending aorta is therefore indicated in all patients with a bicuspid aortic valve regardless of the functional status of the valve itself.

Another group of malformations associated with a bicuspid aortic valve is Shone's complex. This complex comprises several levels of inflow or outflow obstruction to the left heart: supramitral ring, congenital mitral stenosis (MS), discrete subaortic membrane, bicuspid aortic valve, and coarctation. Whereas most patients with this "left heart blight" have received evaluation and treatment as children, milder forms may be seen in the adult population, prompting careful assessment of the mitral valve structure, subaortic region, and aortic arch in the adult with a bicuspid aortic valve.

Infectious endocarditis is a significant problem for patients with congenital AS. Unfortunately, it may be the first mode of presentation for a patient with a previ-

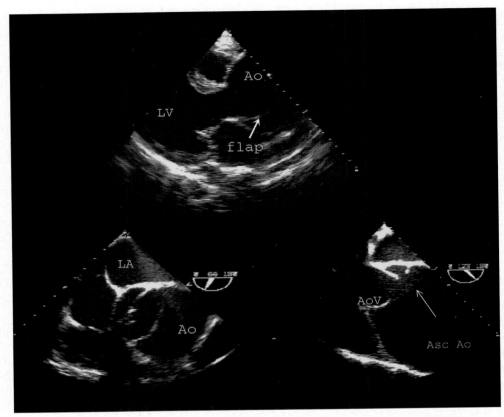

Figure 43–1. Echocardiographic views from a patient with a bicuspid aortic valve and a chronic aortic dissection. The parasternal long-axis view (top) demonstrates the markedly dilated proximal ascending aorta with a suggestion of an intimal flap (arrow). At surgical repair, the transesophageal echocardiography showed a bicuspid aortic valve (bottom left) and confirmed an intimal tag in the dilated aortic root (bottom right). Ao, aorta; AoV, aortic valve; Asc Ao, ascending aorta; LA, left atrium; LV, left ventricle.

ously undiagnosed bicuspid aortic valve. Natural history studies of young adults with congenital AS found a 35-fold higher incidence of endocarditis in that group than in the general population.[13,14] A slightly higher incidence was seen in those patients with aortic regurgitation (AR). Progression of valvular infection to the surrounding aortic root may occur if there is a delay in diagnosis and treatment or in the presence of a particularly invasive microorganism.

Echocardiographic Evaluation

The distinctive echocardiographic features of the congenitally bicuspid aortic valve include systolic doming in the parasternal long-axis views and the demonstration of a single commissural line with two functional valve cusps in the parasternal short-axis views. Particular care must be taken to assess the valve in systole and in diastole. In patients with asymmetric leaflets and a prominent raphe, the valve may appear tricuspid in diastole; however, the elliptical "football" shape of the systolic orifice indicates that the raphe is not a functional commissure. The valve leaflets often are thick-

ened and fibrotic, more so with increasing age. When extensive calcification occurs, doming may no longer be noted and the morphology of the cusps in the short-axis views may be difficult to distinguish from calcific stenosis of a tricuspid aortic valve.

Valvular stenosis should be evaluated with pulsed-wave (PW) and continuous-wave (CW) Doppler imaging exactly as one would a stenotic trileaflet aortic valve. Because of the eccentric nature of the stenotic jet in congenital AS, Doppler sampling from the right parasternal window may detect the highest systolic velocities and should always be attempted in addition to the usual apical and suprasternal notch sampling. In ongoing follow-up, serial aortic valve areas should be routinely calculated by the continuity equation in addition to peak and mean gradients. The development of left ventricular (LV) dysfunction may mask progression of stenosis if valve gradients alone are used to assess the severity of stenosis.[15]

Valvular regurgitation is frequently present and may be the predominant functional abnormality in the adolescent and young adult. Careful echocardiographic inspection of the valve leaflets may give an indication of whether regurgitation is caused by fibrosis and retraction of the commissural margins of the leaflets, cusp prolapse, aneurysmal enlargement of the root and valve annulus, or valvular destruction secondary to endocarditis. Doppler color flow imaging readily detects the regurgitant flow and can be used to semiquantitate the degree of aortic regurgitation. Serial assessment of the effect of regurgitation on ventricular size and function should be performed just as described for a regurgitant trileaflet aortic valve.

The subvalvular LVOT and the mitral valve should be carefully investigated for congenital anomalies. Associated coarctation must be excluded, and the size and shape of the ascending aorta should be serially followed.

TEE may be useful if valve morphology is difficult to determine transthoracically and if such information would guide a surgical attempt at valve repair (Fig. 43–2). Additionally, more accurate aortic and pulmonary annular dimensions can be measured if a pulmonary autograft (Ross procedure) is planned or to guide the choice of a mechanical valve. Evaluation of endocarditis and aortic root abscess are also indications for a transesophageal study. Quantitative functional assessment of the valve usually is more accurate from the transthoracic approach, although transgastric views usually allow adequate Doppler alignment for valve gradients.

Management

Confirmation of the presence of a bicuspid aortic valve and echocardiographic-Doppler determination of the severity of stenosis and regurgitation assist in clinical management decisions. Patients with mild to moderate degrees of stenosis or regurgitation require more regular surveillance. Periodic cardiologic follow-up is important given the progression of valve dysfunction with age and the associated aortic root pathology. The adolescent and young adult with a bicuspid aortic valve should have echocardiographic-Doppler study every year if the mean gradient is greater than 30 mm Hg, peak gradient greater than 50 mm Hg, or if the aortic root or ascending aorta measures greater than 5 cm, or if root enlargement is progressing greater than or equal to 0.5 cm/year.[16]

Development of chest pain, syncope, congestive heart failure (CHF), left ventricular hypertrophy (LVH)

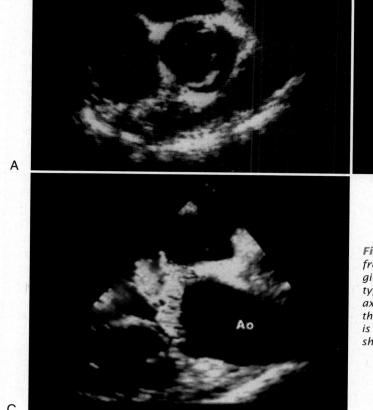

A

B

C

Figure 43–2. Transesophageal echocardiographic images from a patient with a bicuspid valve and severe aortic regurgitation. A, An aortic valve in cross section demonstrates the typical elliptic orifice of a bicuspid valve in systole. B, A long-axis view of the left ventricular outflow tract (LVOT) shows that prolapse and malcoaptation of the right coronary leaflet is the cause of the patient's significant aortic regurgitation, shown in C. Ao, aorta.

with strain, significant arrhythmia, or a mean Doppler gradient of greater than 50 mm Hg are indications for further investigation and possible intervention. In the young adult with supple valve leaflets, balloon valvuloplasty has shown success in relieving significant AS and is probably the method of choice.[16,17] Aortic regurgitation, however, generally increases by at least one grade after percutaneous balloon dilation, limiting the usefulness of this procedure in a patient with combined stenosis and more than mild regurgitation.[18] Indications for aortic balloon valvuloplasty include the lack of significant valve calcification and a peak-to-peak aortic gradient of greater than 50 mm Hg in a symptomatic patient or greater than 60 mm Hg in an asymptomatic patient. Intervention in an asymptomatic patient may be indicated for a lower gradient of greater than 50 mm Hg if the patient wishes to participate in competitive athletics or become pregnant.[16]

With newer expertise in surgical aortic valve repair, current indications for surgical intervention in the adolescent and young adult with a bicuspid aortic valve may undergo closer scrutiny. Concerns about valve replacement and anticoagulation in young adults may be unnecessary if initial enthusiasm for aortic valve repair or the Ross procedure is maintained.[19-21] The Ross procedure involves translocation of the patient's native pulmonary valve into the aortic position and replacement of the pulmonary valve with an aortic homograft. The premature calcification and degeneration that have plagued the homograft and heterologous bioprosthetic aortic valves are not a problem when the patient's own pulmonary valve is used in the aortic position. Some enlargement of the neoaortic sinuses has been observed in the immediate postoperative period, which does not appear to progress with longer follow-up.[20,21] The long-term outcome of an aortic homograft in the place of the translocated pulmonary valve is uncertain, but intermediate follow-up has shown reasonable durability, with a 9% failure rate and a 12% incidence of dysfunction in a large series of patients. The rate of freedom from dysfunction for older children and adults was 87% at 8 years. Use of a pulmonary homograft was associated with lower rates of failure and dysfunction.[22]

Pulmonary Stenosis

Congenital valvular pulmonary stenosis is a common anomaly that has a slightly higher prevalence in women. This anomaly generally follows a benign course with increasing age. Children and adolescents with mild pulmonary stenosis (peak gradient < 25 mm Hg) have less than a 5% chance of requiring valvotomy during childhood and essentially no need for intervention in adulthood. Those with more moderate degrees of stenosis (peak gradient of 25 to 50 mm Hg) have only a 20% likelihood of requiring intervention.[23]

Pulmonary valve morphology in the adult usually involves a supple but thickened valve with commissural fusion or a bicuspid valve. Calcification is rarely seen even in older patients. Poststenotic dilation of the main and left pulmonary arteries (PAs) is common. Pulmonary regurgitation is frequently present, but it is usually mild. Valvular stenosis is usually an isolated finding; however, acquired infundibular stenosis, supravalvular stenosis, branch pulmonary stenoses, and atrial septal defect (ASD) are occasionally associated. Abnormalities of the pulmonary valve and PA are part of several genetic syndromes, such as Noonan's syndrome, William's syndrome, Trisomy 13 through 15 and 18, and congenital rubella. Because of the benign nature of this lesion, patients with pulmonary stenosis are likely to escape detection during childhood and first come to medical attention during their adult years.

Echocardiographic Evaluation

Recording diagnostic two-dimensional (2D) images of the pulmonary valve in adults can be difficult because of the frequent interference of overlying lung tissue. Positioning the patient in a high left lateral decubitus position and imaging during held expiration, however, may improve the ability to visualize the valve leaflets and the PA. Apical or subcostal views of the right ventricular outflow tract (RVOT) also are useful in assessing the adult with pulmonary stenosis. Leaflet thickening may actually enhance echocardiographic visualization of the valve, and the presence of poststenotic dilation of the mid-portion or distal portion of the main PA often is a clue to previously unsuspected valvular pathology. Classic valvular stenosis causes systolic doming of the leaflets (Fig. 43–3). PW Doppler demonstrates an increase in systolic velocity that begins at the valvular level, and CW Doppler allows estimation of the peak and mean transvalvular gradient. Color flow mapping distinctly delineates the turbulent jet of high-velocity flow into the main PA. Because of the horizontal substernal course of the RVOT, accurate peak Doppler flow velocities sometimes are difficult to obtain from the parasternal approach. Sampling of the highest peak systolic velocity may be more accurate from the apical or subxiphoid approach. In older patients, long-standing valvular obstruction leads to significant right ventricular (RV) hypertrophy including the infundibular portion of the ventricle. Dynamic infundibular obstruction thus adds to the right ventricle-PA gradient over time. Doppler flow patterns from sampling within the infundibulum typically demonstrate the dagger-shaped, late-peaking systolic signal characteristic of dynamic obstructions.[24]

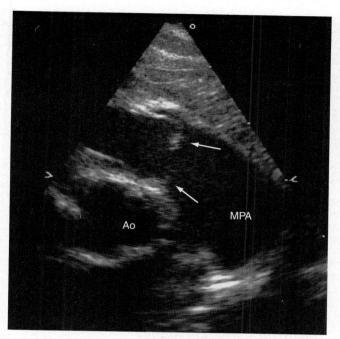

Figure 43–3. Parasternal long-axis echocardiographic view of the right ventricular outflow tract in a patient with valvular pulmonary stenosis. The valve leaflets are thickened and dome into the pulmonary artery in systole (arrows). There is poststenotic dilation of the main pulmonary artery. Ao, aorta; MPA, main pulmonary artery.

Management

In general, the adult with mild valvular pulmonary stenosis (peak systolic gradient < 30 mm Hg) requires no specific intervention. Decisions regarding intervention in patients with mild-to-moderate stenosis should be individualized, but intervention is recommended for symptomatic patients with a peak-to-peak gradient greater than 30 mm Hg and in asymptomatic patients with a peak-to-peak gradient greater than 40 mm Hg.[16] Balloon valvotomy has become the treatment of choice for this group of patients.[26] Echocardiographic evaluation is quite helpful, both for determining which patient is most likely to respond favorably and to follow the results of the dilation. A small pulmonary annulus and markedly thickened, cartilaginous leaflets predict a poor response to dilation. In addition, the patient who has acquired significant infundibular hypertrophy may demonstrate a high postprocedural gradient. Regression of hypertrophy, however, occurs in a large percentage of patients after removal of the valvular component of obstruction and thus does not constitute a contraindication to balloon valvuloplasty.[27] In such cases with apparent residual obstruction, reassessment of Doppler gradients is recommended over the following 6 months before proceeding to a second valvuloplasty or surgical valvotomy.

Mitral Valve Anomalies

Adults with congenital anomalies of the mitral valve usually present with the clinical findings of mitral regurgitation. Thus, when patients are referred for echocardiographic evaluation of the severity of mitral regurgitation (MR) and suitability for mitral valve repair, one of several congenital problems in mitral valve structure may be found. A cleft in the anterior leaflet occurs either as an isolated abnormality or as part of a complex involving defects in the atrioventricular (AV) septum. A double-orifice mitral valve results from abnormal fusion of the embryonic endocardial cushions. Patients with this anomaly may have two equal orifices or one large mitral orifice and a smaller vestigial one. Functionally, the double-orifice mitral valve can be stenotic or regurgitant. A parachute mitral valve has abnormal attachments of the valve leaflets to the papillary muscles. Classically, one large centrally placed papillary muscle is present with all chordae from both leaflets converging on this muscle; however, a variation of this pattern occurs in which two papillary muscles are present but with all or most of the chordal attachments devoted to one papillary muscle. Although this arrangement often creates significant inflow obstruction in infancy and childhood, the coexistence of redundant leaflet tissue and chordae and strategically placed commissures and clefts may produce a valve that functions with minimal obstruction. A variety of other minor aberrant arrangements of the papillary muscles may be noted echocardiographically in adults that contribute to inadequate coaptation of the mitral leaflets during systole. For example, it is common to find an additional posterior papillary muscle with chordal attachments creating a bifid appearance of the posterior leaflet. A papillary muscle on the high lateral or anterolateral wall (the papillary muscle of Moulaert) may have chordal attachments from the anterior leaflet, resulting in a triangular mitral valve orifice.[28]

Echocardiographic Evaluation

Echocardiographic assessment of congenital mitral anomalies uses all the usual windows for evaluating the mitral valve. The parasternal short-axis view defines the number of leaflets, a single or double orifice, the presence of a cleft, and the number and location of the papillary muscles (Fig. 43–4). The orientation of the anterior leaflet cleft is toward the anterior septum in cases of isolated mitral valve cleft and toward the mid or inferior septum in patients with an associated AV septal defect. Long-axis or off-axis views may be needed to follow the chordal attachments to their respective papillary muscles. PW, CW, and color Doppler all are important to assess the functional significance of these structural anomalies. Doppler quantification of

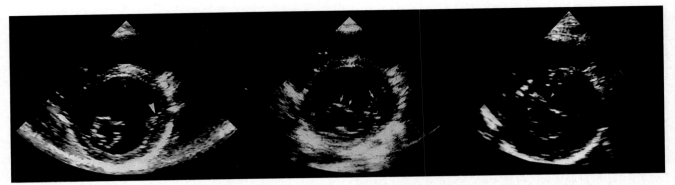

Figure 43–4. *Parasternal short-axis echocardiographic views of the left ventricle at the mitral valve level. Left, Parachute mitral valve with anterior and posterior leaflets inserting on the posteromedial papillary muscle. A small anterolateral papillary muscle is present* (arrowhead) *but does not receive any valvular attachments. Center, Double-orifice mitral valve. There is a discrepancy in orifice size, with the medial orifice* (double arrows) *being larger than the lateral* (single arrow) *orifice. Right, Cleft anterior leaflet from a patient with a partial atrioventricular canal defect. The two portions of the anterior leaflet* (arrowheads) *are attached to the interventricular septum.*

the severity of MS and mitral regurgitation is discussed in Chapters 18 and 21. Abnormal flow patterns created by any of the congenital mitral valve lesions predispose to the development of infectious endocarditis. Mitral anomalies are sometimes first detected when the adolescent or young adult is referred for an echocardiographic search for valvular vegetations in the setting of clinical endocarditis.

Management

Management of congenital MS or mitral regurgitation in the adolescent and adult follows similar clinical guidelines as that in acquired mitral valve disease. Intervention for congenital MS is indicated for symptomatic patients with a mean mitral gradient of 10 mm Hg and for asymptomatic patients with pulmonary hypertension and a mean gradient of 10 mm Hg.[16] Balloon mitral valvuloplasty has been attempted in congenital MS but carries a significant risk of valve disruption and should only be attempted in selected cases by centers with experience with this lesion.[29] Intervention for patients with congenital mitral regurgitation should be reserved for those patients with symptomatic severe mitral regurgitation or asymptomatic patients with severe mitral regurgitation and LV dysfunction.[16] With the increasing success of mitral valve repair, delaying surgical treatment to avoid a prosthetic valve has become less imperative.[30,31] Preoperative or intraoperative TEE determination of exact leaflet anatomy and the mechanism of valve dysfunction has been a vital factor in predicting successful plastic repair.[32] TEE features of interest include the presence and degree of calcification or fibrosis, adequacy and mobility of individual leaflets, site and direction of the regurgitant jet, and presence of leaflet clefts and papillary muscle anomalies.

Tricuspid Valve Anomalies

There are several congenital abnormalities that affect the tricuspid valve. The dysplastic tricuspid valve with inflow obstruction and regurgitation is part of the spectrum of hypoplastic right heart. Another congenital abnormality of the tricuspid valve occurs from involvement of the tricuspid leaflets in the septal aneurysm which forms around a membranous ventricular septal defect (VSD), resulting in tricuspid regurgitation (TR). The most widely recognized congenital abnormality of the tricuspid valve, however, is Ebstein's anomaly. The malformation described by Ebstein consists of apical displacement of the septal and posterior tricuspid leaflets associated with an enlarged anterior leaflet that is variably bound to the RV free wall. The septal or posterior leaflet may be rudimentary or dysplastic. Downward displacement of the functional valve orifice creates an enlarged right atrium and an atrialized portion of the right ventricle. The true right ventricle is frequently hypoplastic and functionally impaired. The infundibular portion of the right ventricle and the PA may be mildly underdeveloped. An ASD or patent foramen ovale (PFO) is present in the majority of patients.[33] The clinical presentation of this anomaly is quite variable, ranging from severe cyanosis in the newborn to mild tricuspid regurgitation or arrhythmia in the adult. The latter finding may be secondary to marked right atrial enlargement or to tachyarrhythmias in conjunction with Wolff-Parkinson-White syndrome, which is found in 10% to 15% of patients with Ebstein's anomaly.[34] The Ebstein's valve can be functionally obstructive and is variably regurgitant. Diagnosis in the adolescent or adult is commonly made during echocardiographic evaluation of clicks and murmurs heard on auscultation or as a part of clinical investigations for the cause of tachyarrhythmias. Occasionally, a patient with unexplained cyanosis or paradoxical embolization is found to have Ebstein's anomaly.

Echocardiographic Evaluation

Echocardiography is ideally suited for the anatomic delineation of the tricuspid valve leaflets. The parasternal inflow view of the right heart, when properly aligned, demonstrates the apical displacement of the posterior leaflet and the elongated sail-like anterior leaflet arising normally from the tricuspid annulus. The apical four-chamber plane is optimal for defining the origin of the septal leaflet, the degree of adherence of the anterior leaflet to the free wall, and the size of the true right ventricle (Fig. 43–5). It should be noted that apical displacement of the coaptation point alone can be seen in conditions which dilate the tricuspid annulus and create incomplete closure of the leaflets, such as an ASD with RV volume overload. These conditions differ from Ebstein's anomaly in that the tricuspid leaflets all arise normally from the annular plane. To classify a displaced septal leaflet as diagnostic of Ebstein's anomaly, the measured distance between the mitral leaflet insertion

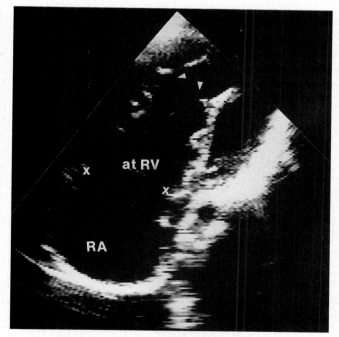

Figure 43–5. Apical four-chamber echocardiographic view in a patient with Ebstein's malformation of the tricuspid valve. The view has been modified to best demonstrate the tricuspid leaflets in diastole. There is marked enlargement of the right atrium (RA) and atrialized right ventricle (at RV), with the true right ventricle composed only of the area between the valve leaflets and the apex. The tricuspid annulus is shown (x), and the origin of the septal leaflet is displaced apically (arrowheads). The anterior leaflet is elongated but not tightly bound to the right ventricular free wall. RA, right atrium.

and the origin of the tricuspid septal leaflet in the apical view should be greater than 8 mm/m^2.[35]

Echocardiographic evaluation of Ebstein's anomaly should also note the relative sizes and contractility of the atrialized and the true right ventricle. Color flow Doppler detects tricuspid regurgitation, which may be severe or can be present as multiple eccentric regurgitant jets through commissures in the funnel-like valve orifice. Inflow obstruction is rarely manifested as an elevated transvalvular gradient; instead, the displaced valve leaflets provide a resistance to forward flow that elevates systemic venous pressure and drives flow right to left across the atrial communication. Careful 2D imaging of the interatrial septum and color Doppler interrogation should demonstrate an atrial septal communication in most patients. Agitated saline contrast injection may be useful if imaging is suboptimal or the shunt is not apparent by color Doppler. TEE provides additional information about leaflet origins and chordal attachments and better direct imaging of the interatrial septum in adults with difficult transthoracic studies.

In some individuals with Ebstein's malformation, late development of clinical heart failure occurs as a result of LV dysfunction.[36] This may be due to LV noncompaction in some instances.[37] In others, compression of the LV by the massive right heart enlargement impairs diastolic filling. With significant distortion of the LV cavity by the enlarged right heart chambers, calculation of LV volumes and ejection fraction (EF) by the simpler echocardiographic methods is difficult. Qualitative estimation of LV function and measures of diastolic function, however, can provide useful clinical information regarding LV performance. Use of nongeometic indices of ventricular function, such as the myocardial performance index (MPI), has also been useful in this patient group.[38]

Management

Patients with Ebstein's malformation frequently remain asymptomatic, leading full and active lives despite marked structural abnormality of the tricuspid valve and right atrial enlargement. Although some centers have suggested that tricuspid valve repair should be recommended in the asymptomatic patient if the cardiothoracic ratio is greater than 65%, many centers would restrict intervention to those with progressive cyanosis, severe tricuspid regurgitaion, LV or RV failure, paradoxical embolization, or intractable arrhythmias. Surgical repair of the abnormal tricuspid valve is preferred to valve replacement if the anatomy is favorable. Good results have been reported[39] when there is sufficient size and mobility of the anterior leaflet to permit it to serve as a monocusp valve after plication of the right atrium and atrialized right ventricle and with a bileaflet repair if the posterior leaflet is large enough to contribute to valve coaptation.[40,41] Echocardiographic assessment of the size and mobility of the leaflets, the degree of displacement, and the function of the right ventricle is critical for the selection of patients most suitable for valve repair. Several scoring systems have been proposed for categorizing the severity of the Ebstein's malformation (Fig. 43–6). One method simply assigns three categories based on the ratio of septal leaflet displacement to overall septal length (septal leaflet attachment ratio [SLAr]): SLAr less than 0.45 is mild, SLAr 0.45 to 0.60 is moderate, and SLAr greater than 0.60 is severe).[42] Another measure of the severity of valve displacement uses a ratio of the area of the right atrium and atrialized right ventricle to that of the combined area of the true right ventricle, left atrium and left ventricle as measured in an apical four-chamber view: ratio less than 0.5 is grade 1, ratio 0.5 to 0.99 is grade 2, ratio 1 to 1.49 is grade 3, and ratio greater than or equal to 1.5 is grade 4.[36] A third method incorporates the degree of anterior leaflet tethering, degree of septal and posterior leaflet displacement, and size and function of the atrialized right ventricle in a classification from A to D.[43] These indices have been correlated with long-term clinical outcome or success with valve repair, with increasing grades of severity having higher morbidity and mortality and less successful surgical results.

Left Ventricular Outflow Tract and Aorta

Subaortic Stenosis

Subaortic obstruction in the adult occurs in several forms. A discrete form, the subaortic membrane, is a developmental anomaly that is rarely seen in neonates but appears in older children and young adults. It has been postulated that turbulent flow in the LVOT stimulates the growth of "rest" tissue in the region of the membranous septum, creating the discrete outflow obstruction.[44] Discrete subaortic stenosis is usually formed by a thin fibrous membrane attached circumferentially or along a portion of the circumference of the LVOT. It may lie immediately adjacent to the base of the aortic leaflets or be attached more distally near the junction of the muscular and membranous portion of the interventricular septum. Occasionally the entire circumferential structure is composed of muscle, creating a muscular subaortic collar. In older patients, what began as a discrete membrane may be complicated by the development of muscular subaortic hypertrophy. The muscular hypertrophy obscures the thinner membrane, thus masking the true pathophysiology of the obstructive process. Long-segment tubular narrowing of the LVOT is seen more commonly in children, usually requiring surgical attention before the adult years.

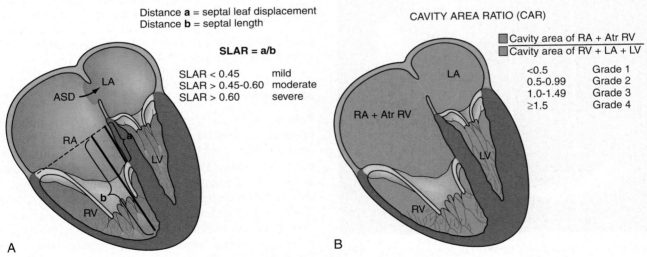

Figure 43–6. Diagrammatic representations of two scoring systems for the severity of the valvular abnormality in Ebstein's anomaly. A, A ratio of the displacement distance of the septal tricuspid leaflet (a) to the length of the septum (b) gives a quantitative measure that can be used to indicate mild, moderate or severe displacement.[42] B, The cavity area of the right atrium and atrialized right ventricle is compared to the sum of the cavity areas of the true right ventricle, the left atrium and left ventricle with quantitative classification into Grades 1 through 4.[36] ASD, atrial septal defect; Atr RV, atrialized right ventricle; LA, left atrium; LV, left ventricle; RA, right atrium; RV, right ventricle; SLAR, septal leaflet attachment ratio. (Modified with permission from Mayo Foundation for Medical Information and Research.)

As previously mentioned, discrete subaortic stenosis may occur in association with other obstructive lesions affecting the left heart-supramitral ring, bicuspid aortic valve, and coarctation. In addition, aortic valve endocarditis may occur because of the abnormal flow patterns created by the subaortic narrowing. Subaortic membranes also are found as part of a complex that includes a perimembranous VSD and an obstructive muscle bundle in the right ventricle.[45] With increasing age, the VSD may close spontaneously, leaving the patient with a discrete obstruction of the LVOT and a muscular collar in the right ventricle. Late development of discrete subaortic stenosis has been described in patients with complete or partial AV canal defects, especially after surgical repair.[46]

Echocardiographic Evaluation

Echocardiographic detection of a subaortic membrane is typically made in the parasternal long-axis views of the LVOT in which a linear structure protrudes from the left surface of the interventricular septum and the base of the anterior mitral leaflet is tented up by the tension of the circumferential membrane (Fig. 43–7). In some cases, the membrane is difficult to visualize unless the US beam is directly incident to the plane of the obstructing membrane. Low parasternal or apical long-axis views are thus more likely to detect the fine linear structure. When the membrane originates immediately beneath the aortic valve, its detection requires appreciation of subtle abnormality in the excursion of the aortic cusps and observation of a persistent echo in systole when the aortic cusp opens into the sinus of Valsalva. Unexplained turbulence and increased flow velocities by Doppler across an apparently normal aortic valve also are a clue to the presence of a high dis-

crete subaortic membrane. Systolic flow acceleration by PW or color Doppler occurs proximal to the aortic valve. Aortic regurgitation is commonly found in these patients as a result of long-standing subaortic flow disturbance or from infectious endocarditis. Initial and serial assessment of outflow tract pressure gradients by Doppler is important because progression of both the severity of obstruction and the degree of aortic regurgitation is well described in younger patients.[47] As with other lesions, TEE may be helpful in the patient with limited transthoracic access to delineate the exact nature of LV obstruction. This approach is particularly useful in cases with mixed or multiple-level obstruction. Both midesophageal views of the subaortic area and transgastric images of the LVOT are useful for obtaining diagnostic information.

Management

Surgical excision of the circumferential membrane is recommended for patients with symptoms, LVH with strain, or a significant outflow gradient. Controversy still exists regarding surgical intervention in the asymptomatic patient with lower gradients. Some have argued that resection of the membrane preserves the aortic valve from further trauma and reduces or prevents progressive aortic regurgitation.[48] Others have found that subaortic stenosis follows a less predictable course, with stenosis and regurgitation remaining trivial over many years.[49-51] The frequent need for reoperation and the development of aortic regurgitation despite surgical excision indicate caution in recommending surgical intervention in the asymptomatic patient with only a mild hemodynamic abnormality. Close clinical and echocardiographic follow-up is warranted, and endocarditis prophylaxis should be con-

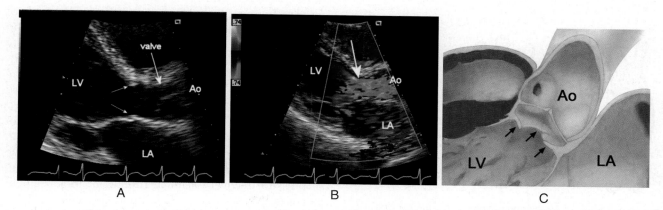

Figure 43–7. A, *Parasternal long-axis echocardiographic view of the left ventricle (LV) from a patient with discrete subaortic stenosis. The discrete subaortic membrane is shown as a linear density protruding from the upper left septal surface and anterior mitral valve leaflet (arrows). The anterior aortic sinus is distorted and has prolapsed into the perimembranous ventricular septal defect immediately below it (arrowhead). B, Color flow Doppler shows acceleration of blood flow proximal to the aortic valve. C, Illustration of the anatomy of a discrete membranous subaortic membrane. Ao, aorta; LA, left atrium; LV, left ventricle.*

sidered. When surgical excision is indicated, intraoperative TEE can be helpful to monitor the success of membrane removal and detect complications, such as mitral valve perforation or iatrogenic creation of a VSD.

Percutaneous balloon dilation has been attempted in patients with discrete fibrous membranes.[52,53] Selection criteria for optimal success include a thin discrete membrane less than 3 mm in width, a sufficient distance between the membrane and aortic valve to permit a subaortic chamber, and the absence of more than grade 2 aortic regurgitation. Intermediate followup has shown a substantial reduction in gradient that persists over 5 years in 48% of patients, with no significant change in the degree of aortic regurgitation.[53] In one series, patients older than 13 years of age had the lowest rate of recurrent stenosis after balloon dilation; however, potential damage to the mitral and aortic valves and incomplete relief of obstruction dictates a cautious approach in applying this technique. Certainly in adults with acquired secondary muscular outflow obstruction, percutaneous dilation is unlikely to produce the desired results.

Supravalvular Aortic Stenosis

Supravalvular AS is an uncommon lesion that occurs as either a discrete membrane at the sinotubular junction, an "hourglass" deformity, or a diffuse hypoplasia of the entire ascending aorta (Fig. 43–8). The hourglass deformity is encountered most frequently, constituting 66% of cases of supravalvular obstruction, whereas diffuse hypoplasia (20%) and discrete membranous stenosis (10%) are less common.[54] Obstruction at the supravalvular level occurs as an isolated abnormality or part of an inherited syndrome. William's syndrome is one such inherited abnormality associated with mild mental retardation, failure to thrive, characteristic "elfin" facies, and multiple peripheral pulmonary stenoses. A familial autosomal dominant form of supravalvular AS also occurs unassociated with mental retardation.[55] Recent genetic studies have suggested that the underlying cause of supravalvar AS is a mutation of the elastin gene on chromosome 7q11.23, which leads to an arteriopathy of varying severity but most uniformly expressed in the supravalvar aorta.[56]

Functionally, supravalvular stenosis may occur as an incidental finding associated with a systolic murmur and no gradient. In other cases, the lesion is progressively obstructive or part of a diffuse process affecting the aorta, coronary ostia, brachiocephalic origins, and pulmonary arterial tree. The aortic valve leaflets are often normal; however, in some patients the cusps are distorted by the supravalvar constriction or incorporated into the stenosing ring. When progressive obstruction and failure of normal aortic growth occurs, LVH and the typical symptoms of AS appear.

Echocardiographic Evaluation

Echocardiographic detection of supravalvular stenosis relies on careful inspection of the sinotubular junction and proximal ascending aorta, which is possible with cranial angulation in right or left parasternal windows, or from suprasternal notch views. The diameter of the normal aorta at the sinotubular junction equals or slightly exceeds that of the aortic annulus. The tubular portion of the ascending aorta should never be smaller than the aortic annulus.[57]

Echocardiographic-Doppler study should determine the type of supravalvular lesion and the severity of stenosis. Although routine echocardiographic study in adults now more often includes views of the ascending aorta above the sinuses of Valsalva, this portion of the aorta is frequently not imaged and thus a diagnosis of supravalvar stenosis is easily missed. The impetus to look specifically for this lesion may be a high-velocity turbulent flow detected by CW Doppler across an otherwise normal aortic valve. Accurate assessment of the supravalvular gradient by Doppler is best determined from the right parasternal or suprasternal window rather than from the cardiac apex. Doppler estimates of the severity of stenosis correlate poorly, however, with catheter-obtained gradients and often overestimate the true degree of obstruction because of the phenomenon of pressure recovery seen in tubular or long-segment stenoses.[58]

Imaging of the proximal branch pulmonary arteries should be attempted in patients with William's syndrome, although associated branch stenoses of the PAs may be too distal for echocardiographic detection. An alternate imaging modality, such as CT or MRI, is a

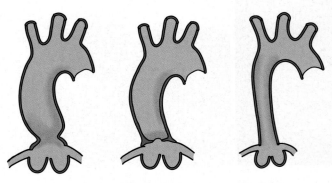

Hour-glass type   Membranous type   Tubular type

Figure 43–8. *The three major types of supravalvular aortic stenosis. Left, Discrete infolding of the aorta at the sinotubular junction produces an hour-glass deformity. Center, Membranous weblike obstruction. Right, Diffuse tubular hypoplasia of the ascending aorta.*

useful adjunct to evaluate more extensive extracardiac involvement of the aorta and PAs.

Management

The decision for surgical intervention for supravalvular AS is made according to the same indications as for valvular obstruction—significant outflow gradient with LVH or symptoms. The morphology of the supravalvular narrowing dictates the type of repair required, varying from patch aortoplasty to partial root replacement. A good relief of obstruction for this lesion should be possible with low mortality and without a need for reoperation.[59,60] Abnormalities of the aortic valve leaflets may persist after repair of the root and merit clinical and echocardiographic surveillance. Associated branch pulmonary stenoses may require balloon dilation or surgical arterioplasty.

Sinus of Valsalva Aneurysms

Congenital aneurysms of the aortic sinuses of Valsalva are thought to result from a weakness in the aortic media at its junction with the annulus fibrosus. A small diverticulum or finger-like protrusion extends most commonly from the right or noncoronary sinus. Because the aortic sinuses are almost entirely intracardiac, the aneurysms extend into regions of the heart that lie adjacent to the affected aortic sinus. The right ventricle and right atrium are common termination sites for aneurysms of the right aortic sinus. Aneurysms of the noncoronary sinus usually enter the right atrium.[61] Over time, the aneurysm may enlarge to become a "windsock," potentially causing obstructive problems in the RVOT or tricuspid valve. Rarely, sinus of Valsalva aneurysms burrow into the interventricular septum, causing AV conduction defects.[62] Protrusion into the LVOT may create outflow tract obstruction.[63]

Congenital sinus of Valsalva aneurysms come to clinical attention most typically in adolescence and young adulthood when the protruding structure ruptures into the receiving chamber. Acute rupture of a large aneurysm causes retrosternal or epigastric pain and severe dyspnea from CHF. By contrast, perforation of a small aneurysm may go unnoticed until a continuous murmur is heard by auscultation or chronic CHF from the long-standing volume overload brings the patient to medical attention. Coronary artery compression by a sinus of Valsalva aneurysm is an interesting though unusual mode of presentation.[64]

Echocardiographic Evaluation

Sinus of Valsalva aneurysms may be an incidental finding on echocardiographic study, but they are discovered more often during echocardiographic-Doppler evaluation of a continuous murmur with the suspected diagnosis of patent ductus arteriosus (PDA) or coronary artery fistula.[65,66] Parasternal long-axis and short-axis views of the aortic sinuses demonstrate the finger-like windsock extending from the base of the sinus toward the site of termination (Fig. 43–9). The originating sinus may be somewhat enlarged, but the native morphology of the root and valve is usually not significantly distorted. It is important to determine that the aneurysm originates from the aortic sinus above the plane of the aortic valve to distinguish this lesion from the more common aneurysm of the membranous interventricular septum. Delineation of a normal coronary artery origin and lumen size distinguishes the sinus of Valsalva aneurysm from a coronary artery fistula. Acquired aortic fistulas after endocarditis can be differentiated because they lack the extended aneurysmal channel seen with a congenital sinus of Valsalva aneurysm. Color flow Doppler demonstrates continuous turbulent flow within the aneurysm and into the receiving chamber. In patients with a significant left-to-right shunt, left atrial and LV enlargement reflect the size of the volume overload, and right heart chamber enlargement occurs when the aneurysm communicates with the right atrium. Mild aortic regurgitation is expected from distortion of the aortic cusp, and root enlargement is a result of long-standing volume overload. Severe aortic regurgitation should raise the suspicion of aneurysm rupture into the LVOT or secondary endocarditis affecting the aortic valve leaflets.

Management

Small unruptured aneurysms found incidentally can be followed expectantly. Larger aneurysms or those that are adversely affecting surrounding structures should be electively excised. Ruptured sinus of Valsalva aneurysms require surgical closure to prevent late congestive symptoms caused by volume overload and to decrease the susceptibility to infectious endocarditis.

Coarctation of the Aorta

Coarctation of the aorta in the adolescent and adult is most often discovered during investigation of hypertension found in the course of routine physical examination. Weak or absent femoral pulses, LVH on the electrocardiogram (ECG), or a systolic murmur in the back or through collaterals in conjunction with the hypertension results in a referral to the echocardiographic laboratory or cardiologist's office for definitive diagnosis.

The anatomic lesion found most commonly in adults is a discrete ridge or diaphragm narrowing the aortic

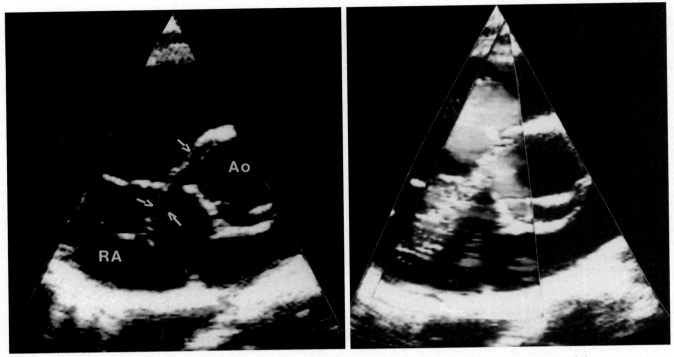

Figure 43–9. *Parasternal short-axis echocardiographic images of the aorta (Ao) at the base of the heart. A, Aneurysm of the right coronary sinus of Valsalva shown as a narrow "windsock" protruding into the right atrium (RA) (arrows). B, Color flow Doppler image demonstrates turbulent flow filling the narrow channel and creating a shunt from the aorta into the right atrium.*

lumen just below the left subclavian artery and opposite the ductus arteriosus or ligamentum arteriosum. Poststenotic enlargement of the descending thoracic aorta is usually present. Rarely, the coarctation lies more distally in the thoracic or abdominal aorta. Functionally, patients seen as adults are usually asymptomatic because the degree of obstruction created by the coarctation is mild or moderate, or collateral vessels bypass a more severe stenosis.

About 50% of patients with adult coarctation have a bicuspid aortic valve.[67] Other structural defects of the left heart, such as discrete subaortic membranes or mitral valve anomalies occasionally are present, and a small VSD or residual patency of the ductus arteriosus may coexist. The natural history of adult coarctation of the aorta is complicated by cerebrovascular accidents from ruptured berry aneurysms, aortic dissection, and endocarditis or endarteritis. Up to 20% of patients with Turner's syndrome may have coarctation and nearly 50% have a bicuspid aortic valve, prompting the need for echocardiographic assessment and follow-up of these patients into adulthood.[68]

Echocardiographic Evaluation

Echocardiographic diagnosis of coarctation relies on 2D visualization of the anatomy of the aortic arch and Doppler detection of flow disturbance in the descend-

ing aorta (Fig. 43–10). Although the aorta can be imaged in part from a variety of parasternal views, suprasternal notch or right parasternal windows provide the best access to the region of interest. Because the site of coarctation can be difficult to visualize, patient positioning maneuvers that optimize the suprasternal view are important. In the long-axis view of the aortic arch, the brachiocephalic vessels should be identified and traced distally if possible. Just beyond the left subclavian artery, a shelf of infolded tissue narrows the aortic lumen. The thoracic aorta distal to the coarctation is often dilated from the systolic jet through the stenotic area.

Color flow Doppler detects a narrowed flow stream at the point of coarctation and systolic flow acceleration, with continuation of flow into diastole in cases of significant obstruction. In fact, when 2D imaging is indistinct, the color flow turbulence may alert the sonographer to the site of obstruction. CW Doppler in patients with discrete obstruction shows a typical pattern of increased systolic flow velocity and a continued gradient in diastole. Doppler gradients *(ΔP)* estimated from the peak systolic velocity (V_2) of the CW Doppler signal usually overestimate the catheter-measured gradient. Better correlations have been shown when the velocity proximal to the coarctation (V_1) is included in the Bernoulli equation [$\Delta P = 4(V_2^2 - V_1^2)$] or when both the peak systolic velocity and pressure half-time

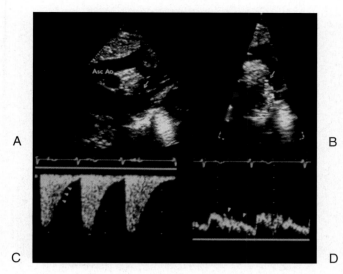

Figure 43–10. A, *Suprasternal long-axis echocardiographic view of the aortic arch depicts tubular narrowing of the transverse arch with discrete coarctation at the isthmus* (arrow). B, *Doppler color flow mapping shows aliasing and turbulence beginning at the site of discrete obstruction* (arrow). C, *Continuous-wave Doppler signal was obtained in the descending thoracic aorta and illustrates a high peak velocity in systole (3 m/s) with a gradient that persists during early diastole* (arrowheads). D, *Pulsed-wave Doppler signal obtained from the descending abdominal aorta. There is blunting of the systolic upstroke and turbulent continuous flow during diastole* (arrowheads) *indicative of significant obstruction to flow located more proximally in the aorta. Asc Ao, ascending aorta.*

(PHT) of the diastolic gradient are considered.[69,70] Long-segment narrowing of the aorta without discrete obstruction causes acceleration of flow, giving high peak velocities by CW Doppler. Conversion of these velocities into systolic gradients mistakenly predicts significant coarctation. The lack of a diastolic gradient helps to distinguish flow acceleration from true obstruction. Doppler flow patterns in the descending abdominal aorta are extremely useful in detecting upstream obstruction.[71] Patients with tubular narrowing but without a discrete obstruction demonstrate a normal pattern of abdominal aortic flow-rapid systolic upstroke, relatively laminar flow signal, and no continuation of flow into diastole. With coarctation, the flow profile has a delay in the systolic upstroke, turbulence in systole, and variable degrees of diastolic antegrade flow (see Fig. 43–10). Routinely including the Doppler profile of abdominal aortic flow in the clinical examination is an excellent method to screen for unsuspected coarctation. Adults with coarctation may have considerable tortuosity of the transverse arch, making both visualization and alignment for accurate Doppler detection of gradient impossible. In such cases, a high degree of suspicion is generated by abnormal flow in the abdominal aorta, directing a more dili-

gent search from off-axis views or with a stand-alone CW Doppler probe.

Although Doppler flow patterns are relatively easy to obtain in most adults with coarctation, direct imaging of the anatomy of the arch and descending aorta is frequently limited. Alternative imaging modalities often are necessary to further define the exact details of the obstruction and to guide decisions for management. TEE can detect the site and configuration of the obstruction. Long-axis views allow quantitation of luminal narrowing; however, Doppler gradients are difficult to obtain because the affected region of the aorta generally lies perpendicular to the interrogating Doppler beam.[72] Visualization of branch vessels and collaterals are limited with TEE, thus making other imaging techniques more useful in defining the coarctation and pertinent arch anatomy. MRI is an accurate noninvasive imaging tool for displaying complete arch anatomy, and newer applications allow velocity mapping as well. Spiral CT with contrast and three-dimensional (3D) reconstruction also provides an exquisite noninvasive rendering of the arch anatomy, branch vessels, and collaterals.[73,74] Angiography may still be required in the older adult to assess the degree of collateral development and coronary anatomy if surgical repair is planned.

Management

Indications for intervention in the adult with coarctation include hypertension, a significant pressure gradient between the upper and lower extremities, and a reduction in luminal diameter of greater than 50%. Some centers recommend percutaneous balloon dilation for discrete lesions in adolescents and young adults, finding good relief of the gradient, improvement in hypertension, and a low rate of restenosis.[75] Small saccular aneurysms may occur at the dilation site either acutely or on later follow-up. Although some of these aneurysms have been surgically repaired, serial follow-up of others has shown no progression in size and no rupture or dissection. The long-term outcome of these iatrogenic aneurysms is uncertain, however. Intravascular echocardiography performed immediately after dilation can demonstrate the intimal tear that routinely occurs during balloon angioplasty.[76] Transthoracic echocardiographic (TTE) evaluation after angioplasty is helpful in assessing residual gradient and restenosis, but it cannot reliably detect the presence of small aneurysms. Repeat MRI or angiography is needed for follow-up evaluation of this complication.

The use of balloon-expandable intravascular stents is now routinely applied in the treatment of aortic coarctation. Early and intermediate follow-up suggests excellent relief of stenosis without a significant incidence of stent migration, fracture, restenosis, or thromboembolic complications, leading some centers to consider stent placement as the procedure of choice for uncomplicated adult coarctation.[77,78]

Surgical repair of coarctation in the adult can be accomplished with low operative mortality and good intermediate outcome.[79] Attention to the degree of collateral formation is important to ensure adequate perfusion during cross-clamping and to prevent spinal cord injury. Prosthetic bypass grafts or other alternatives to mobilization and end-to-end anastomosis may be required in adults with less elastic tissue or with unfavorable anatomy such as hypoplasia of the transverse arch or coarctation adjacent to brachiocephalic vessels. Residual hypertension is common after late repair of coarctation.

Septal Defects and Shunt Lesions

Atrial Septal Defects

After the bicuspid aortic valve, ASDs are the most common congenital lesion found in adolescents and adults, constituting nearly 22% of adult congenital heart defects. The ostium secundum defect is the most frequent (75%) followed by the ostium primum type (15% to 20%) and the sinus venosus defect (5%).[80] A rare form of atrial septal communication is the coronary sinus (CS) septal defect in which the roof of the CS is partially or completely absent, allowing left-to-right shunt from the left atrium into the CS and thence into the right atrium (Fig. 43–11).

A PFO, the fetal communication between the overlapping layers of the primum and secundum portions of the atrial septum, persists in 10% to 18% of adults as determined by echocardiographic contrast injection and as many as 25% to 30% of patients in autopsy series.[81,82] Because of failure of fusion of the two septal layers, the flap of septum primum covering the fossa ovalis may open transiently with changes in the transatrial pressure gradient, allowing the passage of flow in either direction. Additionally, this thin membranous layer may have multiple small perforations or develop into a septal aneurysm with or without an atrial shunt. Improved detection of atrial defects and more aggressive investigation in patients with cerebrovascular events has generated great interest regarding the association of PFO, atrial septal aneurysm, and cryptogenic stroke.[83-85] Although there is still no consensus as to the risk of stroke implied by the presence of a PFO, it is clear, that the potential for a right-to-left embolus exists when there is any form of communication in the interatrial septum.

Patients with shunting at the atrial level are usually asymptomatic until middle to late adult years. If their atrial defect has not been diagnosed during childhood

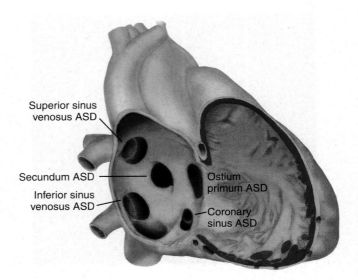

Figure 43–11. *Diagrammatic representation of the interatrial septum as viewed from a cutaway view of the right heart to demonstrate atrial septal defect location. The superior and inferior sinus venosus atrial septal defects (ASD) are shown near the entry of the superior vena cava (SVC) and inferior vena cava (IVC), respectively. The secundum ASD is centrally positioned, the primum ASD inferiorly located near the atrioventricular valves, and the coronary sinus septal defect drains through the mouth of the coronary sinus.*

by the physical findings of a widely split second heart sound and pulmonic flow murmur, detection may occur by routine chest X-ray findings of cardiomegaly and pulmonary plethora. Beginning in the fourth or fifth decades of life, symptoms of fatigue, dyspnea on exertion, and atrial arrhythmia develop. RV failure and paradoxical embolization also may be the mode of presentation in older patients with ASDs. Endocarditis is quite rare, most often seen in patients with accompanying mitral valve anomalies.

Echocardiographic Evaluation

Patients with ASDs require echocardiographic assessment of the anatomic abnormality of the atrial septum, the hemodynamic effect of shunt flow, and the presence of any associated defects (Table 43–2). Imaging of the interatrial septum is best performed with subxiphoid views when these are available. The true apical four-chamber view is unreliable because false-positive septal dropout often occurs in the midatrial septum. An off-axis four-chamber view obtained by sliding midway between the apical and subxiphoid views, however, yields a more perpendicular interface between the interrogating US beam and the interatrial septum. Parasternal short-axis and right parasternal views are supplemental windows for imaging the atrial septum. The septum primum covering the fossa ovalis is thinner than either the superior portions of the septum or the

TABLE 43-2. Atrial Septal Defect: Associated Lesions

Type of Atrial Septal Defect	Associated Lesion
Secundum ASD	MVP, PS, PAPVR
Primum ASD	Cleft MV, inlet VSD, or septal aneurysm
Sinus venosus ASD	PAPVR—right PVs, overriding SVC
Coronary sinus septal defect	Unroofed CS, L-SVC, PAPVR, or TAPVR

ASD, atrial septal defect; CS, coronary sinus; L-SVC, left superior vena cava; MV, mitral valve; MVP, mitral valve prolapse; PAPVR, partial anomalous pulmonary venous return; PS, pulmonic stenosis; SVC, superior vena cava; TAPVR, total anomalous pulmonary venous return; VSD, ventricular septal defect.

region near the crux of the heart. Mobility of the septum primum or aneurysmal deformity (>1 cm deviation from the plane of the basal septum) raises the suspicion of a PFO. True ASDs should have a distinct edge visible at the blood-tissue interface. All aspects of the atrial septum should be inspected, including the superior rim, with visualization of the superior vena caval entry. Right parasternal views are especially helpful for imaging this area. When the atrial defect can be imaged directly, measurement of its dimensions in orthogonal planes, the septal rims, and its size relative to the entire atrial septal length should be made.

PW and color flow Doppler add additional diagnostic power to the transthoracic examination. In any of the views mentioned previously, the passage of flow across an apparent atrial defect further confirms the presence of an interatrial communication (Fig. 43–12). When right heart pressures are normal, a clear stream of flow occurs in late systole with accentuation in diastole. Elevation of right heart pressures decreases the transseptal pressure gradient, and shunt flow then may be difficult to distinguish from other low-velocity atrial flows.

Contrast echocardiography plays an important diagnostic role in cases in which the imaging and Doppler findings are equivocal. With rapid intravenous (IV) injection of 5 ml of agitated saline (or saline mixed with a small amount of the patient's blood), highly reflective microbubbles appear in the right atrium and right ventricle. Contrast passes into the left atrium and left ventricle within three to five cardiac cycles in the presence of an interatrial communication (see Fig. 43–12). Even when left-to-right shunting is predominant, there is a period of transient right-to-left shunting during which contrast can pass into the left atrium. The right-to-left pressure gradient can be augmented by having the patient cough or perform a Valsalva ma-

neuver. A negative contrast effect occurs with left-to-right shunts when unopacified blood enters the densely opacified right atrium. Negative contrast is a less reliable diagnostic feature, however, because flow from the inferior vena cava (IVC) or CS may create the same appearance. Sensitivities of 92% to 100% have been reported for detection of ASDs by transthoracic contrast echocardiography.[86,87] It has been suggested that injection from the leg may improve the sensitivity of the contrast technique because the eustachian valve tends to direct inferior vena caval flow across the fossa ovalis.[88]

TTE study also helps to define the hemodynamic effects of shunt flow. Right atrial and RV enlargement and dilation of the main PA are expected with shunts of 1.5:1 or greater. The pulmonary veins are prominent, but the left atrium is usually normal in size unless there is associated mitral regurgitation or LV failure. The interventricular septum in the cross-sectional views of the left ventricle is flattened in diastole and moves paradoxically toward the right ventricle in systole.

Specific quantification of shunt volume by echocardiographic-Doppler techniques has been attempted by several methods, all of which remain semi-quantitative in clinical use. PW Doppler determination of cardiac output (CO) has been validated with a high degree of accuracy in the experimental setting.[89] The ratio of PW Doppler-determined cardiac output across the pulmonary and aortic valves gives an estimate of the pulmonary-to-systemic flow ratio (Q_p/Q_s). This technique is not accurate if the flow across either valve is influenced by something other than the intracardiac shunt, such as valvular stenosis, subvalvular obstruction, or significant valvular regurgitation. Application of this method to the clinical arena has been less successful, partly because of the difficulty of obtaining accurate dimensions of the pulmonary annulus in adults.

When color flow mapping became a part of the echocardiographic diagnostic armamentarium, there was initial enthusiasm for its quantitative potential. Planimetry of the area of the flow stream within the right atrium has been compared with shunt volumes but with poor correlations.[90] Better correlation has been shown when the diameter of the color flow stream at the atrial defect is compared with shunt ratios,[91] but this remains semi-quantitative with considerable overlap between patients with small, moderate, and large shunts. This result might be expected because the color flow diameter simply reflects the anatomic dimension of the atrial defect, and although it bears a gross relationship to the size of the shunt, factors such as RV compliance and PA pressures cause variation in the volume of shunt for a given ASD size.

Estimation of PA pressure is an important part of the echocardiographic assessment of atrial shunts. The PA

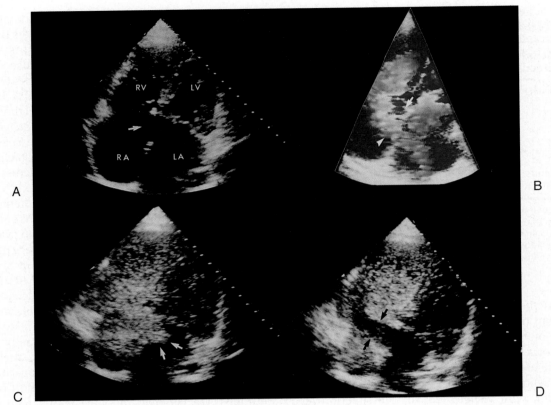

Figure 43–12. *Series of apical four-chamber echocardiographic views from a patient with a large ostium primum atrial septal defect. A, Large defect in the inferior portion of the atrial septum (arrow). B, Doppler color flow mapping readily detects the passage of flow through the defect (arrow, arrowhead). C, After intravenous injection of agitated saline, a positive contrast effect is observed as opacified blood from the right atrium (RA) crosses from right to left (arrows). D, Shunting of unopacified blood from the left atrium (LA) creates a negative contrast effect in the right atrium (arrows). LV, left ventricle; RV, right ventricle. (From Levine RA, et al: Echocardiography: Principles and clinical application. In Eagle KA, Haber E, DeSanctis RW, Austen WG [eds]:* The Practice of Cardiology. *Boston, Little, Brown and Company, 1989, p 1555.)*

pressure is easily and reliably determined by applying the simplified Bernoulli equation to the peak velocity of the tricuspid regurgitation jet to obtain the pressure gradient between right ventricle and right atrium.[92] If the patient does not have tricuspid regurgitation, other subjective signs of pulmonary hypertension may be present. For example, the interventricular septum is flattened in systole if RV systolic pressure is greater than half the systemic pressure. Systolic notching on the pulmonic valve M-mode or the PA Doppler flow profile also indicates significant elevation of PA pressure. Applying the modified Bernoulli equation to the end-diastolic velocity of the pulmonary regurgitation jet provides quantitative information about PA diastolic pressure as well.

Associated abnormalities should be sought as part of the complete transthoracic examination (see Table 43–2). Mitral valve prolapse (MVP) occurs with large RV volume overload, usually from geometric distortion of the left ventricle but occasionally from a myxomatous mitral valve. A cleft in the anterior mitral leaflet is usually present with ostium primum ASDs. Significant mitral regur-

gitation occurs with increasing age.[93] Valvular pulmonic stenosis is present in a small number of patients, and when it is significant it can promote right-to-left shunting across the ASD with resultant cyanosis.

The drainage of all four pulmonary veins should be established if possible in any patient with an ASD. Anomalous return of the right upper and middle lobe veins is found in the majority of patients with superior sinus venosus ASDs and in a small percentage of patients with ostium secundum ASDs. The right veins drain to the superior vena cava (SVC) either at the junction with the right atrium or more distally along the course of the SVC. Echocardiographic-Doppler detection of this anomaly is difficult in adults, but it can be attempted with long-axis and short-axis right parasternal views of the SVC and occasionally can be appreciated in subcostal views of the SVC. A turbulent flow stream entering the SVC laterally and posteriorly represents the pulmonary vein inflow. Anomalous drainage of the right lower vein to the inferior vena cava occurs with the "scimitar syndrome" in association with an inferior sinus venosus ASD. Right parasternal views that focus on the inferior vena caval entry to the right atrium are most useful to search for the anomalous pulmonary venous inflow.

TEE has proved to be superior to transthoracic study in adult patients for detecting patency of the foramen ovale, small secundum ASDs, sinus venosus defects, and anomalous pulmonary venous return.[94-96] Although the presence of an interatrial shunt and an estimate of its hemodynamic significance can be determined adequately by TTE, defect sizing and specific anatomic detail are much more accurately obtained from the transesophageal approach (Fig. 43–13).

The interatrial septum is easily imaged with the probe in the midesophageal position. At zero degrees, the crux of the heart is well seen, and ostium primum or secundum atrial defects are most apparent. From the 90-degree bicaval view, the superior vena caval entry to the right atrium is clearly defined and superior sinus venosus defects with anomalous pulmonary venous entry can be detected. The flaplike opening of the PFO also can be appreciated in this view. Color flow mapping confirms the presence of shunting, and saline contrast injection may be useful if proof of right-to-left shunting is needed. ASDs vary in shape, making measurements of the defect in two orthogonal views important. The pulmonary veins can be identified from both the transverse and the longitudinal planes.

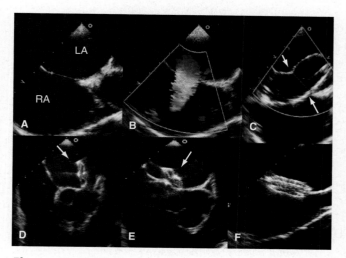

Figure 43–13. Transesophageal echocardiographic images of the interatrial septum in a patient with a secundum atrial septal defect undergoing transcatheter device closure with an Amplatz septal occluder. A, Measurement of defect size. B, The left-to-right shunt across the defect is apparent by color flow Doppler. C, Balloon sizing is performed by measuring the diameter at the waist of an inflated balloon (arrows). D, The Amplatz device is demonstrated (arrow) being deployed in the left atrium. E, The left atrial portion of the Amplatz device (arrow) is fully deployed along the left atrial septal surface. F, The Amplatz device is fully deployed and well aligned with the septum. LA, left atrium; RA, right atrium.

Management

Patients with an isolated ASD and a significant left-to-right shunt should have elective closure of the defect because of the possibility of progressive pulmonary hypertension and the late development of RV failure and atrial arrhythmias. Closure may be appropriate even for patients with smaller shunts because of the tendency for shunt size to increase with age resulting from alterations in LV compliance, and because of the ever-present risk of paradoxical embolization. Surgical mortality for this lesion is quite low, and long-term follow-up shows improvement in symptoms, decrease or stabilization of pulmonary hypertension, and near-normal long-term survival rates in patients repaired before the age of 25 years.[97-99] Patients with elevation of pulmonary arteriolar resistance greater than 15 U/m^2 are not good surgical candidates and are better managed medically.[100]

There is some divergence of opinion regarding closure of atrial defects in the older adult. One natural history study[101] found no difference in survival or symptoms and no difference in the incidence of new arrhythmias, stroke, emboli, cardiac failure, or progressive pulmonary hypertension between medically and surgically managed patients over the age of 25 years. A subsequent large series of adults over the age of 40 years, however, demonstrated a significant reduction in mortality and dramatic improvement in functional class after ASD closure compared with a similar group managed medically. The risk of atrial arrhythmias and attendant embolic complications was not altered by ASD closure.[102] Thus, with low surgical morbidity and mortality and with the availability of transcatheter closure devices, closure of ASDs with a significant shunt without severe pulmonary hypertension is recommended regardless of age.[103]

At the present time, patients with an incidentally detected PFO do not require intervention. The occurrence of an embolic stroke or peripheral embolus in the patient with a PFO and no other obvious embolic source can be considered justification for anticoagulation or for surgical or device closure, particularly in the younger adult. Current Food and Drug Administration (FDA) guidelines indicate that device closure may be pursued if a patient has a recurrent event while on anticoagulation or has a contraindication to warfarin.[104] The results of several ongoing clinical trials are needed to determine if anticoagulation or antiplatelet agents alone are equally effective to PFO closure in preventing recurrent embolic events.[105,106]

Percutaneous closure of ASDs is rapidly becoming the treatment modality of choice. Several different transcatheter closure devices have been designed for this purpose. The Amplatz Septal Occluder (AGA Medical, Golden Valley, Minn.), the Helex ASD device (W. L. Gore, Flagstaff,

Ariz.) and the Amplatzer Cribriform device (AGA Medical Corp., Golden Valley, Minn.) are the only devices fully approved for clinical use for ASD closure, but several other devices are in the investigative stages in the United States and may be approved in the near future.[107,108] The basic device is a flexible wire framework covered with fabric or filled with foam, that folds inside a catheter delivery system. One portion of the device is extruded on the left atrial side of the ASD, the delivery sheath is withdrawn across the defect, and the other portion of the device is deployed along the right atrial side. Newer generation devices have a thick central core that allows the device to be self-centering within the defect (Fig. 43–14). This characteristic provides better immediate closure rates and permits closure of larger atrial defects because less overlap is required to ensure that the device remains well seated. For any of the current devices, the best results are achieved when the atrial defect is centrally located in the interatrial septum

because extension of the device beyond the edges of the defect may impinge on the AV valves or extend into the SVC, right upper pulmonary vein, or CS. Thus, sinus venosus and ostium primum ASDs would be excluded from consideration for device closure.

Echocardiography plays an essential role in the selection of patients most suitable for device closure. Assessment of the defect size, the overall length of the interatrial septum, the amount of septal rim around the defect, and the degree of mobility or aneurysm of the septum primum are all important in evaluating a patient for device closure. Although TTE can provide some of this information, TEE generally is more accurate in adults. Because some traction is applied to the atrial septum in the process of placing the occluding device, the balloon-stretched diameter is the measurement that is most reliable in selecting a device that will not slip through the ASD. Thus in clinical practice, TTE is used to diagnose the shunt at the atrial level, catego-

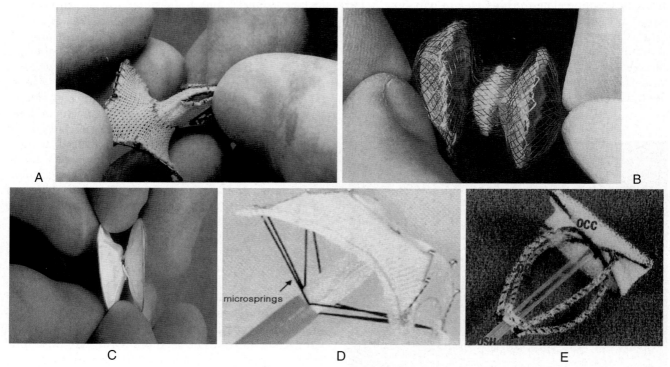

Figure 43–14. *Transcatheter closure devices for atrial septal defects. A, The Das self-centering device. The edges of the left atrial disc are retracted to show the central collar, which promotes centering of this device within the septal defect. B, The Amplatzer septal occluder is a double-disc device with a nitinol wire frame and a broad waist that centers the device. C, The Gore Helex device, which is extruded as a single helical disc with a narrow waist. D, The STARFlex version of the CardioSEAL septal occluder. Hinges midway along each leg promote retroflexion of the legs toward the septum. Microsprings assist in centering the device in the defect. E, The Sideris button device modified with centering wires attached to the occluder (OCC), which is introduced with a pushing catheter (PUSH). (A, From Das GS, Voss G, Jarvis G, et al: Circulation 88(part I):1756, 1993. B, From Sharafuddin MJ, Gu X, Titus JL, et al: Circulation 95:2162, 1997. Reproduced with permission. Copyright American Heart Association. C, Courtesy of N. Wilson, MD. D, From Hausdorf G, Kaulitz R, Paul T, et al: Am J Cardiol 84:1113, 1999. Reproduced with permission. Copyright Elsevier, Ltd. E, From Sideris EB, Sideris SE, Fowlkes JP, et al: Circulation 81:314, 1990.)*

rize the location of the atrial defect and its approximate size, determine the shunt size, and detect any associated defects. If device closure is considered, TEE before or during catheterization can further define the anatomy, and the balloon-stretched diameter can be measured. Transesophageal guidance in the catheterization laboratory has greatly facilitated the optimal placement of the closure device parallel to the plane of the interatrial septum and centered across the defect. Additionally, deployment in the atrial appendage or within the mitral valve orifice can be avoided under direct observation by TEE. The fully deployed device can then be observed for a period of time before the procedure is completed to ensure that it remains in a good position. Color flow Doppler and contrast echocardiography determine residual patency immediately after deployment (see Fig. 43–13). Some centers prefer the use of intracardiac echocardiography (ICE) to monitor device placement. The US-tipped catheter can be inserted intravenously with local anesthesia and manipulated by the interventionalist, avoiding the need for anesthesia and a separate TEE procedural staff. In experienced hands, intracardiac echocardiography monitoring has been shown to be equally reliable for delineating the ASD or PFO, and for assessing device deployment.[109]

Follow-up studies of device closure of ASDs have shown a high rate of successful placement. Residual patency rates are small, with a continued decrease in shunting over time. Although a number of complications have been described (device embolization, malposition, device erosion through the atrial wall or aorta, endocarditis, and thrombotic emboli), the complication rate is low.[107,110] Endothelialization of the device is thought to occur within 6 months when properly aligned flush with the native septum.[111]

Anomalous Pulmonary Venous Return

Connection of some or all of the pulmonary veins to the systemic venous circulation results in a left-to-right shunt and RV volume overload. Embryologically these anomalies are a result of persistence of early fetal connections between the developing lung buds and the systemic venous pathways, with subsequent failure of incorporation of the common pulmonary venous confluence with the left atrium.[112] Total anomalous pulmonary venous return (TAPVR) is a distinct rarity in the adult because the degree of hemodynamic derangement usually brings the patient to medical attention during infancy or early childhood. Therefore, the patients most frequently encountered with abnormal pulmonary venous connection in the adult years are those with partial anomalous pulmonary venous return (PAPVR). Although there are a myriad of possible anomalous connections (Fig. 43–15), the right pulmonary veins are more often involved than the left

veins.[113] Commonly the right pulmonary veins enter the SVC, the SVC-right atrial junction, or directly to the right atrium, with or without an associated sinus venosus ASD. When the right pulmonary veins connect to the inferior vena cava, often associated with an inferior sinus venosus ASD, the term "scimitar syndrome" has been applied, referring to the curvilinear shadow noted on chest X-ray from the enlarged venous channel. Anomalous drainage of the left pulmonary veins usually terminates via an ascending vertical vein into the innominate vein, but occasionally one or both left pulmonary veins connect to the CS.

The clinical presentation of this anomaly is similar to that of an ASD, with a pulmonic flow murmur, RV volume overload, dyspnea, and exercise intolerance. In theory the amount of left-to-right shunt with PAPVR should be small because each pulmonary vein carries only 25% of the total pulmonary blood flow. However the lower resistance encountered in the right atrium causes preferential shunting of flow to the pulmonary segments that are draining anomalously, thereby creating a more significant left-to-right shunt.

Echocardiographic Evaluation

As mentioned previously, PAPVR should be suspected whenever a sinus venosus ASD is present and should be considered carefully in patients with a secundum ASD as well. The presence of right heart enlargement without an atrial shunt or other obvious cause of an RV volume overload is also a signal to inspect the pulmonary venous return carefully. Pulmonary venous entry to the left atrium should be sought in the parasternal short-axis views of the left atrium, the apical four-chamber view, the subxyphoid views of the left atrium, and the suprasternal "crab view" of the left atrium using color flow Doppler to demonstrate the venous inflow streams. If some of the pulmonary veins do not appear to clearly enter the left atrium, attention should be directed to the known systemic venous entry points. Suprasternal or right parasternal views of the SVC and innominate vein may demonstrate enlargement and more vigorous flow if this is the pathway for the anomalous drainage. Alternatively, the inferior vena cava or the CS may be dilated if pulmonary venous flow is diverted into these systemic venous channels. Direct visualization of the pulmonary vein entry is often difficult in the adult patient by TTE but is occasionally possible when the potential sites of entry are carefully inspected using color Doppler. In experienced hands, TEE is accurate in diagnosing PAPVR and delineating the sites of anomalous entry.[113] MRI and spiral CT are excellent adjuncts to echocardiography for diagnosing PAPVR.[114,115] Cardiac catheterization and angiography still play a role in adults who may need concomitant assessment of coronary artery disease.

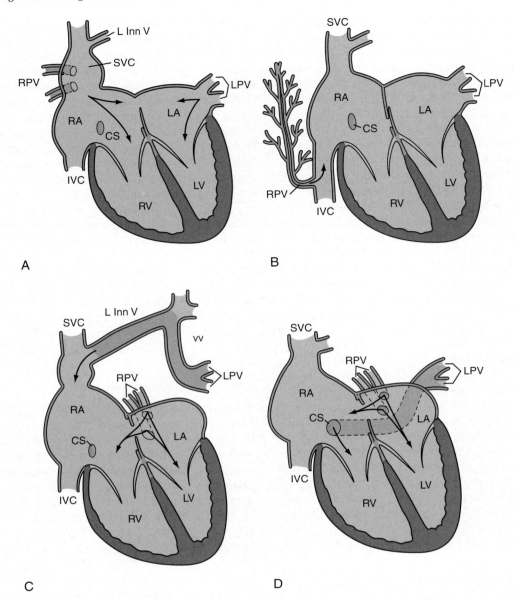

Figure 43–15. *Diagrammatic depiction of several different types of partial anomalous pulmonary venous return. A, The right pulmonary veins drain to the superior vena cava. B, The right pulmonary veins drain to the inferior vena cava. C, Anomalous drainage of the left pulmonary veins via an ascending vertical vein to the left innominate vein. D, Depicts drainage of the left pulmonary veins to the coronary sinus. CS, coronary sinus; IVC, inferior vena cava; LA, left atrium; L Inn V, left innominate vein; LPV, left pulmonary veins; LV, left ventricle; RA, right atrium; RPV, right pulmonary veins; RV, right ventricle; SVC, superior vena cava; vv, vertical vein. (Reproduced by permission from Adams, Emmanouilides, Riemenschneider: Heart Disease in Infants, Children, and Adolescents, 4th ed., Williams & Wilkins, Baltimore, 1989, p 583.)*

Management

Partial anomalous drainage of a single pulmonary vein usually does not create a significant hemodynamic disturbance and requires no intervention. PAPVR, which causes an RV volume overload or which occurs in association with an ASD, should undergo surgical correction. The surgical repair is individualized for the type of abnormal drainage, but whenever possible, the anomalous veins are redirected to the left atrium via a baffle with closure of any associated ASD.[116]

Ventricular Septal Defects

VSDs are the most common congenital anomaly recognized at birth, but they account for only about 10% of cases of CHD in the adult. This decrement in prevalence is in part the result of a high rate of spontaneous closure during the first few years of life. In addition, moderate and large lesions generally cause symptoms of CHF, dyspnea, and failure to thrive in childhood, requiring medical and surgical intervention long before adulthood. The VSDs that persist in adult years, therefore, are either small defects, larger defects that have diminished in size by one of several natural processes, or large defects with irreversible pulmonary vascular disease. Spontaneous closure does occur in later years but is uncommon. The incidence of infectious endocarditis for patients with VSDs is low in the current antibiotic era; however, the risk is higher for adults than children, and it is higher for patients with associated aortic regurgitation.[117]

The most common location for adult VSDs is the membranous ventricular septum (see Fig. 43–16 for VSD locations). Shunt flow passes from the LVOT to the right ventricle just beneath the septal leaflet of the tricuspid valve. Membranous septal aneurysm formation may occur by fibrous tissue proliferation and incorporation of the septal tricuspid valve leaflet. The aneurysm limits shunt flow and occasionally closes the defect entirely. Aneurysms may become quite large and have been noted to cause turbulence and obstruction in the RVOT (Fig. 43–17). Distortion of the septal leaflet from incorporation into the septal aneurysm may create a communication from the LVOT into the right

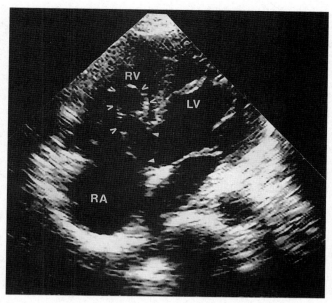

Figure 43–17. Apical four-chamber echocardiographic image from a patient with a perimembranous ventricular septal defect (closed arrowheads) and a large membranous septal aneurysm (open arrowheads). The aneurysm protrudes into the right ventricle (RV) and has incorporated tricuspid septal leaflet tissue. LV, left ventricle; RA, right atrium.

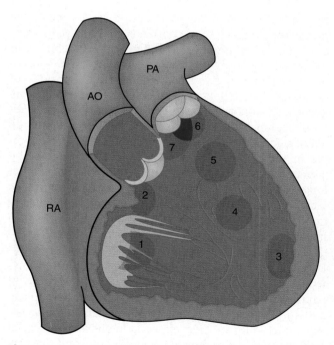

Figure 43–16. Diagrammatic representation of the interventricular septum as viewed from the right ventricular surface with the location of typical ventricular septal defects shown by number: 1, Inlet or canal-type ventricular septal defect; 2, membranous ventricular septal defect; 3, 4, and 5, muscular ventricular septal defects; 6 and 7, subarterial or supracristal ventricular septal defects. Ao, aorta; PA, pulmonary artery; RA, right atrium. (Reproduced with permission from King ME, De Moor M: Current Science, Inc 1:312, 1999.)

atrium, a Gerbode defect. Over time, this defect leads to a RV volume overload, right atrial enlargement, and atrial arrhythmias. In some membranous VSDs, the support of the right aortic cusp is undermined, leading to prolapse of this cusp into the defect. Progressive aortic regurgitation often becomes a more important hemodynamic issue than the ventricular shunt. Subaortic membranes also may develop in association with membranous VSDs during adolescence or early adulthood. Another important associated finding in patients with membranous VSDs is the so-called double-chambered right ventricle. A low-lying obstructive muscle bundle develops between the inlet and outlet portions of the right ventricle and may lie either proximal or distal to the VSD. This RV outflow obstruction results in RV hypertension, which may be mistaken for pulmonary hypertension from the VSD shunt if the muscle bundle is not detected (Table 43–3).

Muscular VSDs are the next most common type of septal defect. Because smaller defects of this type often close spontaneously, the ones that persist in adulthood are generally quite large, sometimes multiple, and associated with pulmonary vascular obstructive disease (Eisenmenger's syndrome). These patients may present with cyanosis from reversal of shunt flow. Pulmonary hypertension is avoided in a few individuals by the development of muscular hypertrophy of the RVOT, a sort of natural pulmonary banding referred to as the Gasul phenomenon.[118] Hypertrophy of the moderator

TABLE 43–3. Ventricular Septal Defect: Associated Lesions

Type of Ventricular Septal Defect	Associated Lesion
Membranous VSD	Septal aneurysm, DSAS, DCRV, AoV prolapse
Supracristal or subarterial VSD	AoV prolapse
Inlet VSD	Cleft MV or TV, primum ASD, straddling AV valve

AoV, aortic valve; ASD, atrial septal defect; AV, atrioventricular; DCRV, double chambered right ventricle; DSAS, discrete subaortic stenosis; MV, mitral valve; TV, tricuspid valve; VSD, ventricular septal defect.

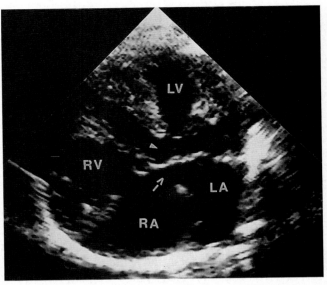

Figure 43–18. Apical four-chamber echocardiographic image of a type C complete atrioventricular canal defect. The large-inlet ventricular septal defect (arrowhead) *and primum atrial septal defect* (arrow) *are crossed by a central bridging leaflet that has no chordal attachments to the crest of the interventricular septum. LA, left atrium; LV, left ventricle; RA, right atrium; RV, right ventricle.*

band also can restrict shunt flow across sizable apical muscular defects, and when this occurs, the LV and the RV apex become one chamber, giving the cardiac apex an aneurysmal appearance.

Defects of the supracristal or subpulmonary septum are found more commonly in patients of Asian descent and are associated with a high incidence of aortic regurgitation.[119] Prolapse of the right or left coronary cusp into the VSD actually may decrease the VSD shunt while creating more severe aortic regurgitation. Occasionally the aortic sinus is extruded through the defect and ruptures, causing a fistula from the aorta to RVOT.

Defects in the inlet septum are usually the result of a defect in the formation of the AV septum. Because the formation of this portion of the septum is intimately associated with the development of the AV valves and the crux of the heart, associated AV valve anomalies and a primum ASD are common (Fig. 43–18). Clefts in either the mitral or tricuspid valves or a common AV valve may occur. The tricuspid valve occasionally straddles the inlet VSD, with chordal insertions that cross the defect into the left ventricle. When the VSD is small, dense chordal tissue crossing the defect may effectively obstruct flow, limiting the shunt size. Fibrous aneurysms also occur with AV septal defects, decreasing or closing the ventricular septal communication. In most cases, however, an inlet VSD is large and rarely closes spontaneously. Adults with this lesion develop pulmonary vascular obstructive disease early in life. AV septal defects are frequently seen in adults with Down syndrome, in whom surgery may have been declined because of the patient's neurologic and functional limitations.

Echocardiographic Evaluation

The interventricular septum is a complex fibrous and muscular structure requiring careful interrogation of all aspects by 2D imaging and color Doppler to detect VSDs

(Fig. 43–19). Membranous VSDs are best seen in the parasternal long-axis and short-axis views as echo dropout beneath the aortic valve and near the attachment of the septal leaflet of the tricuspid valve. Apical or subcostal five-chamber views also demonstrate the position of the defect in relation to the LVOT and tricuspid valve. Associated abnormalities of the right aortic cusp, subaortic region, and septal aneurysm formation should be delineated. The presence of an obstructive muscle bundle in the right ventricle should also be sought. The supracristal VSD can be appreciated in the parasternal long-axis view of the RVOT or the parasternal short-axis view at the base of the heart, located immediately proximal to the pulmonic valve. If the right aortic cusp has become distorted and prolapses into the VSD, the defect itself may not be detectable without color or PW Doppler. Muscular septal defects may be located anywhere within the trabecular septum. Careful scrutiny of parasternal short-axis sweeps and apical, off-axis apical, and subcostal views is required to detect muscular defects. Inlet VSDs are most apparent in apical or subcostal four-chamber views directed posteriorly toward the crux of the heart. Associated abnormalities of the atrial septum and the AV valves also can be appreciated from this vantage point.

Assessment of left atrial and LV chamber size and LV function is important. Long-standing volume overload is associated with enlargement of left heart structures and may cause LV failure in the adult. In the clinical

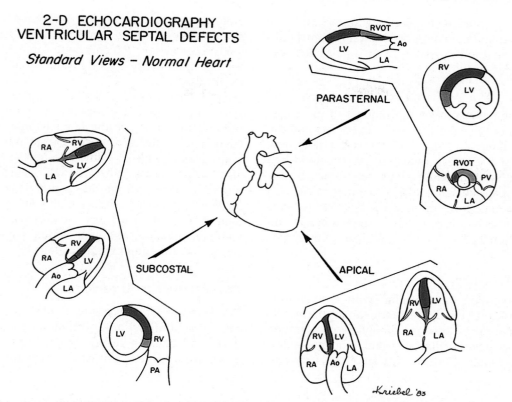

Figure 43–19. *Standard two-dimensional echocardiographic views with color coding of the location of the common types of ventricular septal defects. The membranous septum is coded in red, the supracristal or infundibular septum in orange, the inlet septum in green and the muscular septum in blue. Ao, aorta; LA, left atrium; LV, left ventricle; PA, pulmonary artery; PV, pulmonary valve; RA, right atrium; RV, right ventricle; RVOT, right ventricular outflow tract. (From Levine RA, et al: In Eagle KA, Haber E, DeSanctis RW, Austen WG [eds]: The Practice of Cardiology. Boston, Little, Brown and Company, 1989, p 1554.)*

setting of endocarditis, vegetations can be detected on the aortic valve, the membranous septal aneurysm, or the tricuspid septal leaflet. Endarteritis at the site of the jet lesion within the right ventricle or RVOT is usually not detectable by 2D imaging unless vegetations are extensive.

Color flow mapping greatly enhances the sensitivity of detection of all forms of VSDs. Left-to-right shunts are readily detected as turbulent jets crossing the septum into the right ventricle when the pulmonary pressures are normal. Ambiguity may occur when there is little difference between left and right heart pressures because shunt flow is low in velocity and difficult to distinguish from other low-velocity flow within the right heart. PW and CW Doppler studies are helpful to confirm the timing and velocity of shunt flow. With small membranous and supracristal VSDs, low-velocity diastolic shunt flow may precede the high-velocity systolic jet, presumably owing to slight differences in late diastolic pressures between left and right ventricles. This diastolic flow is sometimes mistaken clinically for aortic regurgitation or

another aortic runoff lesion such as a sinus of Valsalva fistula or coronary artery fistula.

CW Doppler measurement of the VSD peak jet velocity allows estimation of RV systolic pressures, and consequently PA systolic pressures. By applying the modified Bernoulli equation, one can calculate the pressure gradient between the left and the right ventricle from the VSD peak velocity. Subtracting this gradient from the cuff systolic blood pressure yields the RV systolic pressure (Fig. 43–20). Alignment as parallel as possible to the direction of the VSD jet prevents underestimation of the gradient between the ventricles. Sampling from multiple windows or off-axis views may be required to achieve the best alignment.

Shunt quantification by PW Doppler can be performed in the same way as with ASDs. Measurement of cardiac output across pulmonic and aortic valves is made, and the pulmonic-to-systemic flow ratio (Q_p/Q_s) is computed. The turbulence created in the PA by shunt flow from nearby membranous and supracristal defects may make measurement of the pulmonary flow velocity integral inaccurate.

An alternative method for deriving shunt ratios involves calculating the volumetric shunt flow across the VSD and adding it to the systemic cardiac output to get pulmonary flow:

$$Q_p = Q_s + VSD\ shunt$$

The VSD shunt volume is the product of the cross-sectional area of the color flow jet at the defect and the flow velocity integral of the CW Doppler systolic flow signal (see Fig. 43–20). In one study, this method had better correlation with shunt ratios determined by the Fick method than the standard PW Doppler calculation of Q_p/Q_s.[120] It may prove particularly useful in patients with pulmonary stenosis or in whom the pulmonary annulus or pulmonary flow profile is difficult to measure.

Management

Surgical intervention for the adult with a small VSD with no significant LV volume overload and normal PA pressures is not necessary. Periodic follow-up is important, to reassess ventricular size and function and to follow PA pressures. Closure of a small VSD may be indicated when intervention is needed for associated abnormalities, such as significant aortic regurgitation or RVOT obstruction. Patients with large VSDs and irreversible pulmonary hypertension should be managed medically.

Device closure of VSDs has been accomplished in selected cases, and it is approved by the Food and Drug Administration for specific clinical applications.[121] Muscular defects are most easily closed but perimembranous defects with or without septal aneurysms have also been successfully treated with device closure. Appropriate placement requires a sufficient distance from the aortic valve (>3 mm) or the AV valves to avoid damaging these structures. Acquired heart block, device embolization, and endocarditis have all been described as infrequent complications.[122]

Patent Ductus Arteriosus

The PDA is a fetal necessity to allow diversion of flow from the nonfunctioning pulmonary circuit into the aorta and back to the placenta. The ductal channel arises from the PA bifurcation near the origin of the

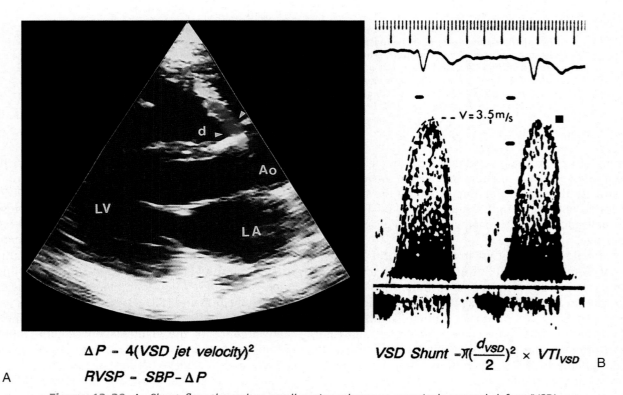

$$\Delta P = 4(VSD\ jet\ velocity)^2$$

A

$$RVSP = SBP - \Delta P$$

$$VSD\ Shunt = \pi\left(\frac{d_{VSD}}{2}\right)^2 \times VTI_{VSD}$$

B

Figure 43–20. *A, Shunt flow through a small perimembranous ventricular septal defect (VSD). B, Continuous-wave Doppler spectral tracing of the VSD shunt flow. The peak systolic velocity is 3.5 m/s. Dotted lines trace the flow velocity integral of the shunt flow. Estimation of right ventricular systolic pressure (RVSP) can be made by the formula on the* lower left, *using four times the square of the peak velocity. Calculation of the VSD shunt is possible using the formula on the* lower right, *including the diameter of the VSD and the flow velocity integral of the continuous-wave Doppler tracing. Ao, aorta; d, diameter of the flow stream at the septal surface; LA, left atrium; LV, left ventricle; P, pressure; SBP, systolic blood pressure; VTI, velocity time integral.*

left PA and passes to the lesser curvature of the aorta just opposite the left subclavian artery. Ductal shape is quite variable, sometimes being a long, tortuous channel or a conical connection or even a short window-like communication (Fig. 43–21). The ductus arteriosus normally closes spontaneously within the first 24 to 48 hours of life. Persistence beyond the neonatal period is abnormal, and spontaneous closure after the first year of life is distinctly uncommon. This lesion is found in only about 2% of adults with CHD. It is usually an isolated anomaly, but it can occur in association with complex lesions, VSD, or coarctation. After 30 years of age, the ductal tissue becomes calcified and more friable. Aneurysms of the ductus arteriosus or the closed ductal diverticulum also occur and may rupture. Infectious endocarditis is more common in the second and third decades of life, affecting the pulmonary end of the ductal channel.

The clinical presentation of an adult with a PDA depends on the size of the shunt. Trivial shunts may be clinically silent, detected by an echocardiographic-Doppler study that was requested for an unrelated lesion. Small ductal shunts produce a continuous murmur at the upper left sternal border, which can be confused with the murmur of a coronary artery fistula, combined AS and regurgitation, or a VSD with aortic regurgitation. Patients with moderate or large shunts develop CHF and atrial arrhythmias from the long-standing LV volume overload. With the onset of pulmonary hypertension and reversal of the shunt, the murmur decreases in intensity or disappears and differential cyanosis of the lower extremities may be noticed.

Echocardiographic Evaluation

2D imaging of the ductus arteriosus is accomplished with ease in the neonate and young child, but it becomes progressively more difficult in adolescents and adults. The direct view of the ductal channel is best obtained in a high left parasternal window at the PA bifurcation where the left PA crosses the descending thoracic aorta. The main PA appears to "trifurcate," with the third channel being the ductus. Visualization is possible also in suprasternal notch views of the aorta focused on the lesser curvature opposite the left subclavian artery. Diagnosis of a PDA in the adult usually is made with color flow Doppler imaging rather than direct 2D imaging. The left-to-right flow stream appears as a red jet in diastole entering the main PA near the left PA origin (Fig. 43–22). Although PDA shunt flow is continuous, the systolic component is usually washed along with systolic flow in the main PA. If flow can be visualized within the ductus itself, however, a continuous Doppler signal is present. As the PA pressures rise, the velocity of the PDA shunt decreases and it becomes more difficult to distinguish a discrete PDA jet from other low-velocity flows within the dilated pulmonary vessel. Adults with a dilated main PA often have a low-velocity retrograde flow in late systole from swirling of flow within the enlarged vessel. PW Doppler can distinguish this from ductal flow by the difference in timing. Continuous flow into the PA also is seen with coronary artery fistulas and with an aortopulmonary window. Demonstration of the color Doppler flow stream emanating from the bifurcation and originating within the descending thoracic aorta should confirm that the shunt comes from a PDA.

CW Doppler sampling of ductal shunt flow is important for estimation of PA pressure. When the US beam is aligned from the high left parasternal window directly into the mouth of the PDA, systolic and diastolic flow velocity can be recorded. Applying the modified Bernoulli equation, the peak systolic velocity of the PDA jet can be used to calculate the systolic gradient between the aorta and PA. Subtracting this gradient from the cuff systolic aortic blood pressure yields the PA systolic pressure.

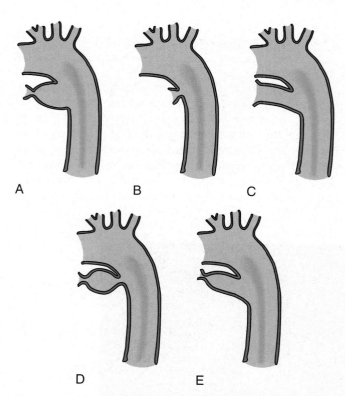

Figure 43–21. *The various shapes of a patent ductus arteriosus as seen angiographically. The ductus is shown arising from the lesser curvature of the aortic arch. Its configuration varies from a window-like communication to a long tortuous channel (A to E). Knowledge of the ductal shape is important in choosing the best method of transcatheter closure. (Modified from Krichenko A, et al: Am J Cardiol 63:878, 1989. Reprinted by permission of the publisher. Copyright 1989 by Excerpta Medica Inc.)*

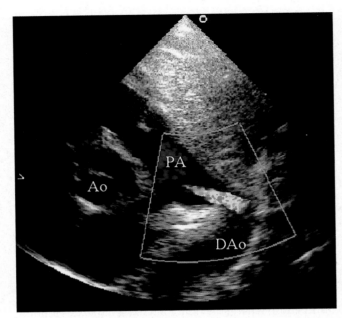

Figure 43–22. *Parasternal short-axis echocardiographic view of the heart at the base, demonstrating a small patent ductus arteriosus. The stream of left-to-right shunt flow is shown in color as it passes from the descending thoracic aorta (DAo) to the pulmonary artery (PA). Ao, aorta.*

Management

Closure of a PDA is recommended for all but the clinically silent or the severely hypertensive ductus. Angiographic, MRI, or CT delineation of the ductal shape is still recommended for surgical planning and for decisions regarding device closure in the adult. Surgical mortality in repairing this lesion is low, but calcification of the ductus or a short, wide ductal shape complicates the procedure. Transcatheter closure of the ductus arteriosus is now the treatment of choice for children and adults. Several types of devices are currently in use, including a pluglike occluder within the ductus, umbrella devices that occlude the orifices at each end of the ductus, and coils that are extruded within the ductus and thrombose the channel.[123] TEE guidance of device placement has not played as critical a role for the ductus arteriosus as for ASDs. The difficulty in imaging the anatomic details of the ductus arteriosus by TEE limits the usefulness of the modality, and fluoroscopic monitoring alone is sufficient for accurate placement.

TTE Doppler assessment after device closure is quite helpful to ensure appropriate device position and assess residual shunting. The highly reflective device can be appreciated by 2D imaging at the pulmonary bifurcation and along the lesser curvature of the aorta. Malpositioning of the PDA devices can result in protrusion of a portion of the occluder into the aortic lumen or into the main PA[124] (Fig. 43–23). Feasibility and efficacy of device or coil occlusion of the PDA are excellent with 98% occlusion at 6 and 12 months. Complication rates are low, but include device or coil embolization, hemolysis, and left PA stenosis.[123]

Coronary Fistulas

A coronary artery fistula is an abnormal communication of a coronary artery with a cardiac chamber, great vessel, or other vascular structure without passing through the myocardial capillary bed. Most coronary fistulas are congenital, resulting either from persistence of embryonic channels between the cardiac chambers and the developing coronary circulation or from aberrant connection of some of the coalescing coronary

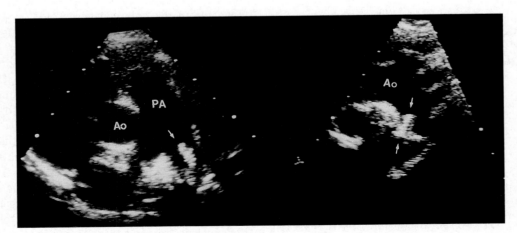

Figure 43–23. *Echocardiographic images from a patient after patent ductus arteriosus closure with a Sideris device. Left, In the parasternal short-axis view the counteroccluder (arrow) is seen near the origin of the left pulmonary artery (PA). Right, The occluder protrudes into the aortic lumen (double arrows) in the suprasternal notch view. Ao, aorta.*

channels to the PA. Coronary fistulas have been reported in 0.2% of coronary angiograms, usually as incidental findings.[125] The clinical presentation depends on the site of termination of the fistula and the degree of shunting. Over 90% of fistulas terminate in the right heart—right ventricle, right atrium, PA, CS, or SVC. A continuous murmur is caused by shunting from the aorta to the right heart. When the fistula communicates with the left ventricle, the murmur is audible only in diastole. Shunting is usually modest (Q_p/Q_s < 1.5:1), but it may progress over time by gradual enlargement of the fistulous tract or from the development of systemic hypertension. Signs of RV volume overload and CHF may appear later in life from the long-standing left-to-right shunt. The shunt is rarely large enough to cause severe pulmonary hypertension. Angina, and rarely myocardial infarction, occurs in a small percentage of patients from "coronary steal" as the fistula diverts flow from the normal coronary circulation.[126]

Echocardiographic Evaluation

Echocardiographic-Doppler diagnosis of coronary artery fistulas begins with the detection of enlargement of the proximal coronary artery involved in the abnormal communication. The affected coronary vessel is diffusely enlarged (>0.6 cm) and can often be traced to the site of termination with knowledge of the expected coronary course and the usual sites of fistulous communication. Aneurysmal lakes may develop near the communication with the receiving chamber or vessel, appearing as large sonolucent regions (Fig. 43–24). Enlargement of the right or left heart chambers gives an indication of the significance of left-to-right shunting.

Color flow Doppler demonstrates continuous flow within the involved coronary artery and helps to localize the exit site.[127,128] When a small fistula from the left coronary artery to the PA is present, a tiny stream of continuous flow may be found incidentally in the proximal main PA. Larger fistulas are diagnosed by scanning the right atrium, right ventricle, and left ventricle for a continuous turbulent flow signal (Fig. 43–25).

TEE also can detect coronary enlargement and visualize the enlarged and aneurysmal channels of the fistula. It is particularly helpful intraoperatively to assess residual fistulous flow and segmental wall motion after ligation of the feeding coronary vessel.[129]

Contrast echocardiography has been used in conjunction with angiography to detect fistulous communication when there are multiple entry sites of a coronary fistula.[130] If the fistula terminates in both the right and the left ventricles, angiographic contrast may stream preferentially to the lower-pressure chamber. Faint opacification of the left ventricle easily may be overlooked. With injection of agitated saline into the arterial catheter, however, even a trace appearance of contrast in the left ventricle is obvious echocardiographically.

Management

Small, clinically silent coronary fistulas do not require closure. Patients with fistulas that are large enough to cause coronary dilation should be followed clinically for the development of symptoms of coronary regurgitation or significant right or LV volume overload. Coronary angiography is generally necessary to completely evaluate the coronary circulation for coexistent athero-

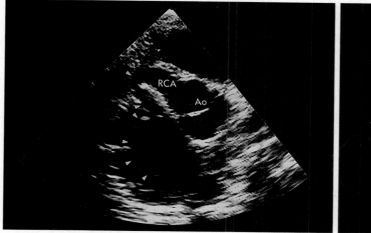
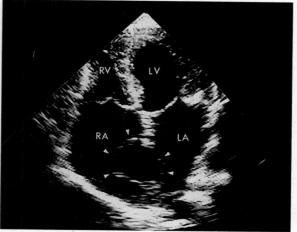

A

B

Figure 43–24. Echocardiographic images from a patient with a coronary artery fistula from right coronary artery (RCA) to right atrium (RA). A, In the parasternal short-axis view the RCA is markedly dilated and tortuous, feeding a large venous lake adjacent to the interatrial septum (arrowheads). B, Apical four-chamber view demonstrates the venous lake along the right atrial septal surface (arrowheads). Ao, aorta; LA, left atrium; LV, left ventricle; RV, right ventricle.

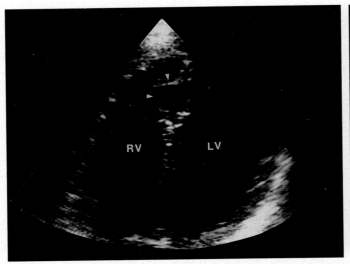

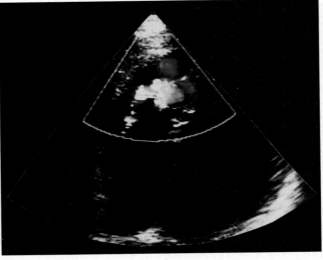

Figure 43-25. *Apical echocardiographic images from a patient with a coronary artery fistula terminating in the right ventricular apex. A, A small venous lake (arrowheads) is apparent along the right septal surface. B, Entry of flow into the right ventricle from the fistula is clearly demonstrated by color flow Doppler. LV, left ventricle; RV, right ventricle.*

sclerotic disease and for complete anatomic delineation of the fistula. Closure of large fistulas may be approached surgically or with transcatheter coil occlusion or devices, depending on the specific anatomy of the lesion.[131,132]

Complex Congenital Heart Disease

Adults who survive with complex congenital heart defects represent a small but intriguing fraction of an adult cardiology practice. In the current surgical era, most patients with complex lesions have had the benefit of either palliative or corrective surgery during childhood (see Chapter 44). The occasional patient reaches adulthood without prior intervention and seeks medical attention for symptoms which may be typical of acquired heart disease—congestive failure, angina, valvular disease, arrhythmia, endocarditis—only to be found to have complex CHD when an echocardiographic study is performed. A brief consideration is given here to some of the complex lesions that permit natural survival into adulthood.

Tetralogy of Fallot

The tetralogy originally described by Fallot in 1888 consisted of a large VSD, an overriding aorta, pulmonary stenosis, and RV hypertrophy (Fig. 43-26). About 15% of patients have an atrial septal communication (pentalogy of Fallot), and 25% have a right aortic arch.

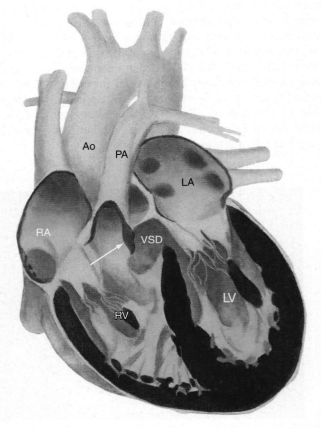

Figure 43-26. *Diagrammatic representation of tetralogy of Fallot which shows the large subaortic ventricular septal defect (VSD), the aorta (Ao) straddling the ventricular defect, and the deviation of the conal septum (arrow) into the right ventricular outflow tract creating subpulmonary stenosis.*

Anomalous origin of the left anterior descending (LAD) coronary artery from the right coronary artery or bilateral left anterior descending vessels occurs in 5% to 9% of patients, complicating patch repair of the RVOT because the anomalous vessel passes over the RVOT.[133,134]

Physiologically, the clinical picture with tetralogy of Fallot (TOF) is that of a VSD with RV outflow obstruction of variable severity. Most patients develop severe cyanosis either at birth or within the first year of life, requiring surgical palliation or correction. Only 11% of patients survive to 20 years of age without intervention.[135] With only a modest degree of pulmonary stenosis, patients can survive with few symptoms into adult years. Paradoxically, the other group of late survivors without surgery includes patients with complete obstruction to RV outflow. This subgroup—having pulmonary atresia with VSD—has multiple congenital aortic-to-pulmonary collaterals capable of supplying the pulmonary circulation so as to produce only modest clinical desaturation. Cerebrovascular accidents or brain abscess, complications of polycythemia and cyanosis, bacterial endocarditis, acquired aortic valve disease, and arrhythmias account for much of the morbidity and mortality in the adult with uncorrected TOF.

Echocardiographic Evaluation

Echocardiographic-Doppler evaluation can accurately define the characteristic features of TOF. The malalignment VSD usually is large and lies immediately beneath the dilated overriding aortic root (Fig. 43–27). In parasternal views of the left ventricle, the size of the VSD can be appreciated. The direction and velocity of shunt flow across the defect are easily determined in these planes by color flow and PW Doppler imaging. Unless the VSD has become restrictive over time, the shunt is low velocity and predominantly right to left. Parasternal short-axis views of the RVOT and aorta demonstrate the typical anterior deviation of the conal septum, narrowing the RVOT (see Fig. 43–27). A small pulmonary annulus, valvular pulmonary stenosis, and hypoplasia of the main and branch pulmonary arteries also are visible in this view. The systolic gradient across the stenotic outflow tract should be measured by CW Doppler imaging. In patients with native or acquired pulmonary atresia, the RVOT is filled with muscle and ends blindly with no visible pulmonary valve leaflets and no detectible flow by PW Doppler. When the parasternal views are not able to visualize the PA because of chest wall or lung interference, scanning from the suprasternal notch or high left subclavicular area may provide the necessary access to the branch pulmonary arteries. The proximal right PA is measurable in nearly all patients with confluent pulmonary arteries. Suprasternal or high parasternal views of the ascending aorta are most accurate for measuring the right PA, which passes behind the aorta as a small cross-sectional lumen in the long-axis plane, or a small linear vessel in the short-axis plane. Aortopulmonary collaterals can be detected, but they often are not fully delineated by either MRI or 2D echocardiography.[136,137] Apical and subcostal five-chamber views depict the large subaortic VSD and the overriding aorta. Acquired aortic valve stenosis and regurgitation also can be further evaluated at this point in the examination. Moving the

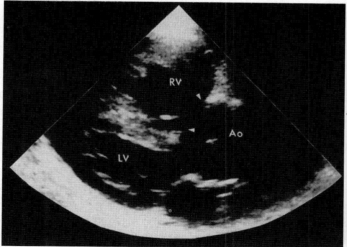
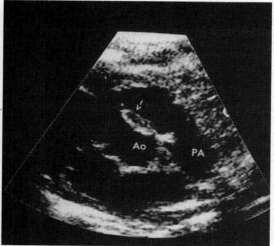

A   B

Figure 43–27. Echocardiographic images from a patient with tetralogy of Fallot. A, Parasternal long-axis view of the left ventricle (LV) illustrates a large malalignment ventricular septal defect with aortic overriding of the interventricular septum (arrowheads). B, Anterior deviation of the parietal band (arrow) is apparent in the parasternal short-axis image, creating obstruction in the right ventricular outflow tract. Ao, aorta; PA, pulmonary artery; RV, right ventricle.

scan plane even more anteriorly from the five-chamber view brings the RVOT into view. This approach may provide better alignment of the Doppler cursor for sampling the RVOT gradient.

In the cross-sectional views of the aortic root at the base of the heart, attempts should be made to visualize the coronary arteries. Enlargement of the right coronary orifice hints at a larger blood supply through this vessel, perhaps caused by the anomalous origin of the left anterior descending coronary artery. Careful attention should be directed to cross-sectional lumina seen anterior to the RVOT in high parasternal views and to anteriorly coursing vessels arising from the proximal right coronary artery. Although some success has been reported with transthoracic study of the coronary arteries in adults with TOF,[138] coronary arteriography or an alternate imaging modality is still needed as part of the preoperative assessment in the adult.

Transesophageal imaging in TOF can provide nearly all the important diagnostic information. Malalignment of the conal septum is apparent in midesophageal longitudinal views of the RVOT or from the transgastric approach. The pulmonary valve anatomy and the size of the main and right PA can be determined from transverse views in the midesophagus or high esophagus. The left PA is often more difficult to image. The VSD and overriding aorta can be appreciated in transverse views from the midesophagus and from transgastric views.

Management

The majority of adults with TOF should be candidates for complete repair. Surgery for this lesion can be accomplished in the adult with acceptable mortality and with gratifying relief of cyanosis and improvement in functional class (see Chapter 44).[139,140] In the subgroup with pulmonary atresia, decisions regarding surgical correction are based on the confluence and size of the PAs and the size and distribution of aortopulmonary collaterals.

Congenitally Corrected Transposition

Congenitally corrected transposition is a malformation in which the great arteries are transposed but the ventricles are inverted and discordant relative to the atria, resulting in a "double switch" that physiologically corrects the circulation. In the absence of associated lesions, corrected transposition may go clinically unnoticed and is entirely compatible with a normal lifespan.[141] VSD, pulmonary outflow obstruction, and an Ebstein-like malformation of the left-sided tricuspid valve, however, are frequently present (Fig. 43–28). Complete heart block is commonly seen because of the abnormal pathway of the conduction system.

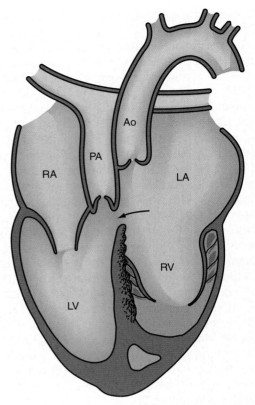

Figure 43–28. *Anatomic features of congenitally corrected transposition. The aorta (Ao) lies anterior and to the left of the pulmonary artery (PA). It arises from the morphologic right ventricle (RV), which is left sided. The most commonly associated lesions include pulmonary stenosis, ventricular septal defect* (arrow), *and an Ebstein-like malformation of the left-sided tricuspid valve. LA, left atrium; LV, left ventricle; RA, right atrium. (From King ME: In Weyman AE [ed]:* Principles and Practice of Echocardiography. *Philadelphia, Lea & Febiger, 1994, p 1038, with permission.)*

Even with associated lesions, corrected transposition is quite compatible with survival into adult years. The limiting feature in many patients is the function of the systemic right ventricle. The anatomic right ventricle may not be functionally suited to carry the long-term burden of systemic afterload, particularly with additional volume loading from ventricular shunts or AV valve regurgitation.[142]

The anatomic features and echocardiographic diagnosis of this complex are reviewed in Chapter 42. Clinical echocardiographic-Doppler follow-up in patients with congenitally corrected transposition is directed primarily toward monitoring systemic RV function and systemic AV valve regurgitation. Ventricular shunting and pulmonary outflow obstruction also require serial assessment. Standard geometric models for assessing LV volumes and ejection fraction do not accurately model the unusual shape of the systemic right ventricle; therefore, the Simpson's rule method using two orthogonal apical planes may be a more accurate echocardiographic method for calculating systemic ventricular volume and function in this group. As three-dimensional echocardiography becomes more clinically applicable, it may be the optimal method for determining ventricular volumes because it does not require geometric assumptions. Radionuclide rest and exercise ejection fractions and MRI also are useful for following systemic RV function.[143] An alternative nongeometric means of serially following systemic ventricular function is this group of patients is the myocardial performance index, which uses Doppler measures of isovolumic time intervals and ejection time.[144]

The asymptomatic patient with corrected transposition requires no intervention. Both patient and physician need to be aware of the propensity to develop complete heart block, and invasive cardiac procedures should be avoided unless they contribute to clinical management. Also, because of ventricular inversion, the electrocardiogram in corrected transposition shows deep Q waves in the right precordial leads that can be mistaken for an ischemic injury. RV failure frequently develops with increasing age and medical therapy with afterload reduction is indicated.[142]

Patients with associated VSD and pulmonic stenosis should be managed in similar fashion to those with normal ventricular connections. Endocarditis prophylaxis is generally recommended. If pulmonary outflow obstruction is severe enough to require operative correction or if significant regurgitation of the systemic tricuspid valve requires surgical attention, the options for repair are either physiologic or anatomic. Physiologic repair would entail simply repairing or replacing the tricuspid valve, closing the VSD, or bypassing the pulmonary stenosis with a left ventricle-PA conduit. This, however, leaves the anatomic right ventricle as the systemic ventricle, which is problematic for long-term survival. Anatomic repair requires a double switch, with either an atrial or arterial switch and a Rastelli procedure to connect the left ventricle to the aorta with a right ventricle-PA conduit. Although the anatomic approach entails more extensive surgery, the result is an anatomic left ventricle as the systemic ventricle and an unloading of the right ventricle with its abnormal tricuspid valve. The choice of surgical approach must be individualized to the patient's anatomy and physiology.[145,146]

Double-Outlet Right Ventricle

As its name implies, double-outlet right ventricle is a condition in which both great arteries arise entirely or mostly from the right ventricle. A VSD is present to allow the left ventricle to eject into the right-sided aorta and PA. The great arteries are separated from the ventricles by bilateral subarterial conus and arise in parallel from the heart, often lying side by side. The location of the VSD relative to the aorta or PA and the presence or absence of pulmonary stenosis determines the hemodynamic picture of the patient with double-outlet right ventricle (Fig. 43–29). If the VSD is subpulmonary, the physiology is similar to that of complete transposition. A subaortic VSD with pulmonary stenosis is physiologically indistinguishable from TOF. Survival to adolescence and adulthood is possible when the ventricular septal shunt is restricted by pulmonary stenosis of moderate degree. The patient is obligatorily cyanotic, but the degree of cyanosis is influenced by streaming across the VSD and by the severity of pulmonary obstruction.

Echocardiographic diagnosis of double-outlet right ventricle is made by demonstrating the origin of both great arteries primarily from the right ventricle

DOUBLE OUTLET RV

Subpulmonic VSD — Subaortic VSD — Doubly committed VSD — Uncommitted VSD

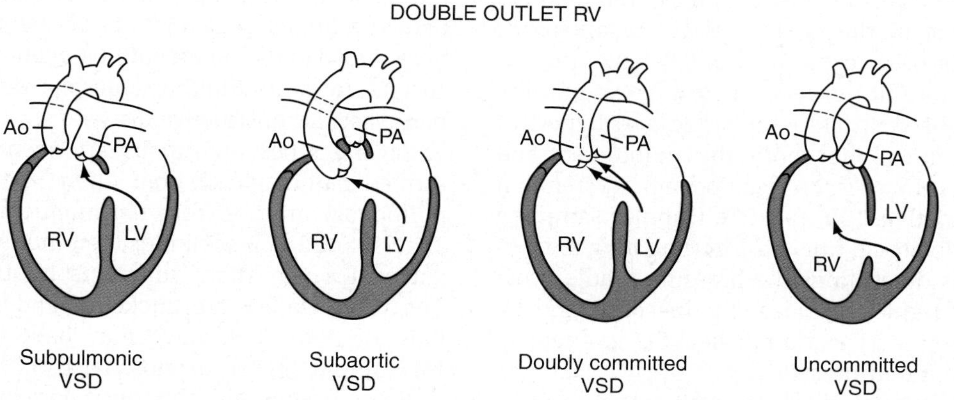

Figure 43–29. Subtypes of double-outlet right ventricle (RV) based on the position of the ventricular septal defect (VSD). The VSD may lie immediately beneath the pulmonary artery (PA) (far left), predominantly below the aorta (Ao) with or without pulmonary stenosis (left center), or beneath both great vessels (right center) or may be unrelated to either great artery. LV, left ventricle. (From King ME: In Weyman AE [ed]: Principles and Practice of Echocardiography. Philadelphia, Lea & Febiger, 1994, p 1042, with permission.)

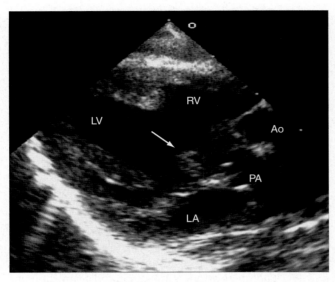

Figure 43–30. Parasternal long-axis echocardiographic view from a patient with double-outlet right ventricle. The view has been oriented to display the parallel origin of the great arteries from the anterior ventricle. The arrow points to the subpulmonary conal muscle which separates the pulmonary valve from the mitral valve. Ao, aorta; LA, left atrium; LV, left ventricle; PA, pulmonary artery; RV, right ventricle.

(Fig. 43–30). In many instances, the posterior great vessel overrides the interventricular septum similar to the anatomy of TOF or complete transposition with VSD. The key distinguishing feature of double-outlet right ventricle is the lack of fibrous continuity between the mitral valve and its nearest semilunar valve. In the parasternal long-axis plane, this feature is apparent as a muscular separation between the base of the anterior mitral leaflet and whichever semilunar valve is more posterior. Doming of the pulmonary valve and the presence of subpulmonary stenosis can also be demonstrated in this view.

In the parasternal short-axis planes, the relative position and size of the great vessels are apparent. Sweeps from the base to the ventricular level demonstrate the anterior and rightward origin of the outflow vessels. The right ventricle is enlarged and hypertrophied because it supplies both the pulmonary and systemic circuits. LV pressure may be suprasystemic if the VSD is restrictive. PW and CW Doppler sampling of the VSD velocity in the parasternal long-axis or short-axis views determines the pressure gradient between left and right ventricles. In this case, the LV pressure is estimated by adding the VSD gradient to the cuff systolic blood pressure.

Apical and subcostal views are well suited to demonstrate the ventriculoarterial relationship and to establish the position of the VSD relative to the great arteries. Delineation of the degree of override of the posterior great vessel can be demonstrated from these planes; however, variations in angulation can create marked variations in the apparent origin of the vessel

in question. The parasternal long-axis view is more accurate to assess the degree to which the posterior vessel arises from the right ventricle. Inspection of the VSD for tricuspid valve chordal apparatus is important because the tricuspid valve may have chordal attachments to the crest of the septal defect or to the conal septum. This scenario would make intracardiac repair of the VSD more difficult and thus influences surgical planning. Finally, Doppler assessment of the transpulmonary gradient should be made from the apical or subcostal approach.

Management

Adults with double-outlet right ventricle who have a protected pulmonary bed and preserved ventricular function should be considered for complete repair to remove the complications of cyanosis, to remove the risk of cerebral embolus or brain abscess, and to prevent eventual RV failure. Surgical correction ideally attempts to connect the left ventricle to the aorta, close the VSD, and relieve pulmonary stenosis. These goals are achieved in different ways depending on the size and location of the VSD (see Chapter 44).[147]

Truncus Arteriosus

Persistent truncus arteriosus is a rare malformation in which a single arterial trunk arising from the heart supplies the coronary, pulmonary, and systemic circulation. A large VSD is invariably present. Embryologically, this anomaly has been attributed to improper septation of the primitive arterial trunk, although another hypothesis attributes this malformation to infundibular and pulmonary atresia with subsequent failure of truncal septation, making persistent truncus arteriosus a close relative of TOF.[148] Survival beyond 1 year of age without surgical intervention is rare; however, adult survival is possible if branch pulmonary stenoses or severe truncal valve stenosis protects the pulmonary circulation. Some patients survive to early adulthood despite developing pulmonary vascular obstructive disease.

Several types of truncus arteriosus have been described pathologically that differ in the origin of the pulmonary arteries from the main trunk (Fig. 43–31). Types I and II are seen most commonly. The semilunar valve of a persistent truncus is frequently abnormal. The valve leaflets are thickened and stenotic, regurgitant, or both. The valve may have two (8%), three (61%), four (31%), or more cusps.[149]

Echocardiographically, this anomaly must be distinguished from TOF with pulmonary atresia. Both demonstrate a large central arterial vessel overriding the septum above a large malalignment VSD. The aortic valve in truncus arteriosus is commonly abnormal in structure and function, whereas that in TOF is usually normal. There is no semblance of a RVOT with a per-

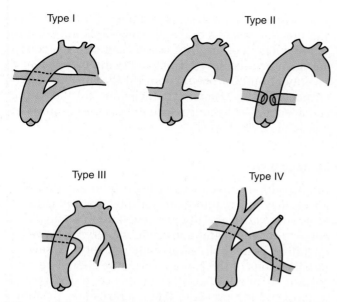

Type I   Type II

Type III   Type IV

Figure 43–31. Subtypes of persistent truncus arteriosus. Most commonly, the main pulmonary artery arises from the posterolateral border of the truncus (type I) or the branches arise independently from the proximal vessel (type II). Rarely, the right pulmonary artery arises from the truncus and the left lung is supplied by collaterals from the descending aorta (type III). Another unusual variant includes hypoplasia of the ascending trunk with interrupted aortic arch. The pulmonary arteries arise from the proximal portion of the truncus arteriosus, and a large patent ductus arteriosus supplies the descending aorta (type IV). (From King ME: In Weyman AE [ed]: Principles and Practice of Echocardiography. Philadelphia, Lea & Febiger, 1994, p 1045, with permission.)

sistent truncus arteriosus, whereas in TOF the outflow tract occupies its usual position but is small and filled with muscle. In the types of truncus arteriosus encountered most frequently, the main PA or its branches arise directly from the ascending trunk, whereas in TOF, the small PA or branches cannot be shown to have direct communication with the ascending aorta. Both of these malformations have a right aortic arch in about one third of cases.

High right and left parasternal views are the most useful in detecting the origins of the pulmonary arteries. Evaluation of the truncal valve is made in the same way one would assess a native aortic valve, inspecting the number of cusps in the parasternal short-axis views and the degree of stenosis and regurgitation by Doppler from the apex. Concentric hypertrophy of both left and right ventricles would be expected in the adult with truncus arteriosus, and ventricular function may be impaired.

Patients with a protected pulmonary vascular bed are amenable to surgical correction with closure of the VSD and a conduit from the right ventricle to the PA. If the pulmonary arteries arise separately, some form of arterioplasty is required to unify the pulmonary arteries. Truncal valve replacement may also be needed.

Tricuspid Atresia

Tricuspid atresia constitutes 1% to 3% of all congenital heart defects, and fewer than 10% of patients survive beyond childhood without surgery.[150] In this malformation, the atrioventricular valve of the morphologic right ventricle is absent or imperforate. The right ventricle is variably underdeveloped and the left heart is compensatorily enlarged. An atrial septal communication is present to allow egress of blood from the blind right atrium, and a VSD of variable size is usually present. The great vessels may be normally related (60% to 70%) or transposed, with or without obstruction to pulmonary blood flow. The physiology in the adult is that of a central mixing lesion creating cyanosis, with VSD and pulmonic stenosis, or VSD and pulmonary vascular disease. The adult with uncorrected tricuspid atresia is susceptible to the usual complications of this physiologic state, namely endocarditis, brain abscess, and right-to-left embolic events.

Echocardiographic Evaluation

In the place of the tricuspid valve, a thick band of fibromuscular tissue is recognized by 2D imaging (Fig. 43–32). No evidence of flow can be demonstrated by color or PW Doppler. The right atrium is enlarged, often with a prominent eustachian valve. The size of the right ventricle is related to the size of the VSD during fetal development. It may be vestigial and slitlike with a small VSD or nearly normal in size with a large VSD. Progressive restriction of the VSD may occur.[151] When the great vessels are normally

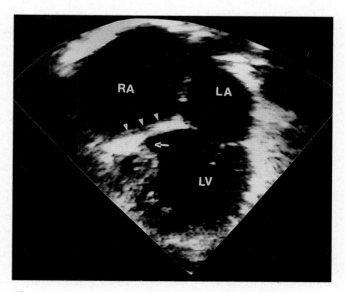

Figure 43–32. Transesophageal echocardiographic view of a patient with tricuspid atresia. The atretic tricuspid valve is shown as a thick, fibrous ridge (arrowheads) at the base of the enlarged right atrium (RA). A ventricular septal defect is present (arrow) leading into a tiny right ventricular chamber. LA, left atrium; LV, left ventricle.

related, progressive VSD closure creates further obstruction to pulmonary blood flow. In patients with transposed great arteries, the systemic blood flow is jeopardized. Thus, serial determination of the VSD size by 2D imaging and VSD gradient by Doppler is an important part of echocardiographic evaluation.

The left ventricle in this anomaly is enlarged, and systolic function may be impaired from long-standing volume overload. Quantitative assessment of ventricular function is performed by the usual echocardiographic methods and is an important factor in determining surgical options.

Echocardiographic study in the patient with tricuspid atresia also must focus on the presence, size, and origin of the aorta and PA. The orientation and relative size of the great arteries and associated abnormalities of the valvular and subvalvular region all can be appreciated from parasternal windows. Apical and subcostal images are particularly useful in establishing ventriculoarterial relationships and measuring gradients across the semilunar valves and outflow tracts.

The interatrial septum in the adult with uncorrected tricuspid atresia generally has a large, unrestricted atrial defect in the form of a stretched PFO or secundum ASD. Apical, subcostal, or right parasternal windows optimally should delineate the atrial septum and demonstrate right-to-left shunt by PW and color Doppler.

Management

Patients with tricuspid atresia and restricted pulmonary blood flow may be candidates for a Fontan procedure, which diverts systemic venous return directly to the PA. The optimal candidate must have good LV function, no significant mitral regurgitation, and normal branch PA anatomy and pulmonary resistance. Natural survivors with tricuspid atresia and pulmonary vascular disease are not currently amenable to surgical correction but may be considered for heart-lung transplantation.[152]

Univentricular Heart

The basic element of the univentricular heart is communication of both atria or a common atrium with a single main ventricular chamber. Natural survival of adolescents and adults with this complex congenital anomaly depends on fortuitous streaming of oxygenated and unoxygenated blood and protection of the pulmonary circulation by an optimal degree of pulmonary stenosis. Ventricular failure develops with increasing age.

The important aspects to ascertain echocardiographically in patients with this anomaly are (1) the presence and location of an accessory chamber; (2) the number and functional status of the AV valves; (3) the number and orientation of the great vessels and their relation to the main or accessory chamber; (4) the presence and severity of outflow obstruction; (5) the functional performance of the systemic ventricle; and (6) the nature and adequacy of venous return in the case of atresia of one of the AV valves.

Management

Adults with a univentricular heart who are well balanced may not require surgical intervention as long-term survival in the unoperated state in some cases equals that following corrective surgery.[153] However operative correction employing one of the several modifications of the Fontan procedure should be considered to provide relief from the complications of cyanosis and prevent late ventricular dysfunction.[154,155] Patient eligibility requires adequate PA size and confluence, low PA resistance, competent systemic AV valves, good ventricular function with low ventricular end-diastolic pressure, and no obstruction to ventricular outflow. If the patient does not meet these eligibility criteria, palliative surgery with either a cavopulmonary or aortopulmonary shunt is a low risk alternative with reasonable long-term outcome.[156]

KEY POINTS

■ Adults with CHD may escape detection during childhood because their lesion is mild or slowly progressive because their physiology is well balanced or protective, or because of poor access to medical care.

■ The mode of presentation of the adult with unoperated CHD is often similar to adults with acquired heart disease—CHF, arrhythmia, murmur, hypertension, endocarditis.

■ Bicuspid aortic valve is the most common form of CHD in the adult and requires continued follow-up for progressive stenosis or regurgitation, aortic coarctation, and aortic root dilatation.

■ Despite marked structural abnormality, patients with Ebstein's anomaly are often able to lead full and active lives but may experience adverse events such as tachyarrhythmias, paradoxical emboli, progressive disability from tricuspid regurgitation, or left heart failure.

■ Discrete subaortic stenosis may be masked by development of septal hypertrophy, requiring careful TTE and TEE studies to elicit the correct pathophysiology.

■ Aortic coarctation is easily missed by transthoracic imaging, but PW Doppler sampling in the abdominal aorta may alert the examiner to the flow disturbance more proximal in the aorta.

■ Doppler gradients in supravalvar AS and long-segment aortic coarctation often overestimate the true gradient due to flow acceleration in a tubular vessel with pressure recovery.

■ Sinus venosus ASDs are the most frequently missed atrial defect by TTE resulting from incomplete imaging of the most superior aspect of the septum; TEE is usually required to detect the defect and evaluate partial anomalous pulmonary venous drainage.

■ In the cyanotic adult with unoperated CHD, detecting the presence of pulmonary stenosis at any level may convert the clinical status from inoperable to surgically treatable.

■ Alternative imaging modalities, such as MRI and CT, are important adjuncts to echocardiography in the complete assessment of adult CHD.

REFERENCES

1. Sreeram N, Sutherland GR, Geuskens R, et al: The role of transoesophageal echocardiography in adolescents and adults with congenital heart defects. *Eur Heart J* 12:231, 1991.
2. Marelli AJ, Child JS, Perloff JK: Transesophageal echocardiography in congenital heart disease in the adult. *Cardiol Clin* 3:505, 1993.
3. Samyn MM: A review of the complementary information available with cardiac magnetic resonance imaging and multi-slice computed tomography (CT) during the study of congenital heart disease. *Int J Cardiovasc Imaging* 20:569-578, 2004.
4. Boxt LM: Magnetic resonance and computed tomographic evaluation of congenital heart disease. *J Magn Reson Imaging* 19:827-847, 2004.
5. Huntington K, Hunter AG, Chan KL: A prospective study to assess the frequency of familial clustering of congenital bicuspid aortic valve. *J Am Coll Cardiol* 30:1809-1812, 1997.
6. Fenoglio JJ, McAllister HA Jr, DeCastro CM, et al: Congenital bicuspid aortic valve after age 20. *Am J Cardiol* 39:164, 1977.
7. Sabet HY, Edwards WD, Tazelaar HD, et al: Congenitally bicuspid aortic valves: A surgical pathology study of 542 cases (1991 through 1996) and a literature review of 2715 additional cases. *Mayo Clin Proc* 74:14, 1999.
8. Roberts CS, Roberts WC: Dissection of the aorta associated with congenital malformation of the aortic valve. *J Am Coll Cardiol* 17:712, 1991.
9. Keane MG, Wiegers SE, Plappert T, et al: Bicuspid aortic valves are associated with aortic dilatation out of proportion to coexistent valvular lesions. *Circulation* 102(suppl 3):III35-III39, 2000.
10. Bonderman D, Gharehbaghi-Schnell E, Wollenek G, et al: Mechanism underlying aortic dilatation in congenital aortic valve malformation. *Circulation* 99:2138, 1999.
11. Niwa K, Perloff JK, Bhuta SM, et al: Structural abnormalities of great arterial walls in congenital heart disease: light and electron microscopic analyses. *Circulation* 103:393-400, 2001.
12. Nataatmadja M, West M, West J, et al: Abnormal extracellular matrix protein transport associated with increased apoptosis of vascular smooth muscle cells in Marfan syndrome and bicuspid aortic valve thoracic aortic aneurysm. *Circulation* 108(Suppl 1): II329-II334, 2003.
13. Gersony WM, Hayes CJ, Driscoll DJ, et al: Bacterial endocarditis in patients with aortic stenosis, pulmonary stenosis, or ventricular septal defect. *Circulation* 87(suppl I):I-121, 1993.
14. Griffin MR, Wilson WR, Edwards WD, et al: Infective endocarditis: Olmsted County, Minnesota, 1950 through 1981. *J Am Med Assoc* 254:1199, 1985.
15. Otto CM, Pearlman AS, Gardner CL: Hemodynamic progression of aortic stenosis in adults using Doppler echocardiography. *J Am Coll Cardiol* 7:509, 1986.
16. ACC/AHA 2006 Guidelines for the management of patients with valvular heart disease: executive summary: A Report of the American College of Cardiology/American Heart Association Task Force on Practice Guidelines. *Circulation* 114:450-527, 2006.
17. Rosenfeld HM, Landzberg MJ, Perry SB, et al: Balloon aortic valvuloplasty in the young adult with congenital aortic stenosis. *Am J Cardiol* 73:1112, 1994.
18. Justo RN, McCrindle BW, Benson LN, et al: Aortic valve regurgitation after surgical versus percutaneous balloon valvotomy for congenital aortic valve stenosis. *Am J Cardiol* 77:1332, 1996.
19. Ross D, Jackson M, Davies J: The pulmonary autograft-A permanent aortic valve. *Eur J Cardiothorac Surg* 6:113, 1992.
20. Savoye C, Auffray J-L, Hubert E, et al: Echocardiographic follow-up after Ross Procedure in 100 patients. *Am J Cardiol* 85:854, 2000.
21. Kouchoukos NT, Masetti P, Nickerson NJ, et al: The Ross procedure: long-term clinical and echocardiographic follow-up. *Ann Thorac Surg* 78:773-781, 2004.
22. Niwaya K, Knott-Craig CJ, Lane M, et al: Cryopreserved homograft valve in the pulmonary position: Risk analysis for intermediate-term failure. *J Thorac Cardiovasc Surg* 117:141, 1999.
23. Hayes CJ, Gersony WM, Driscoll DJ, et al: Second natural history study of congenital heart defects: Results of treatment of patients with pulmonary valvar stenosis. *Circulation* 87(suppl I):I-28, 1993.
24. Nishimura RA, Pieroni DR, Bierman FZ, et al: Second natural history study of congenital heart defect. Pulmonary stenosis: Echocardiography. *Circulation* 87(suppl I):I-73, 1993.
25. Dajani AS, Taubert KA, Wilson W, et al: Prevention of bacterial endocarditis: Recommendations by the American Heart Association. *J Am Med Assoc* 277:1794-1801, 1997.
26. Teupe CH, Burger W, Schrader R, Zeiher AM: Late (five to nine years) follow-up after balloon dilation of valvular pulmonary stenosis in adults. *Am J Cardiol* 80:240-242, 1997.
27. McCrindle BW: Independent predictors of long-term results after balloon pulmonary valvuloplasty. *Circulation* 89:1751, 1994.
28. Moulaert AJ, Oppenheimer-Dekker A: Anterolateral muscle bundle of the left ventricle, bulboventricular flange and subaortic stenosis. *Am J Cardiol* 37:78, 1976.
29. Moore P, Adatia I, Spevak PJ, et al: Severe congenital mitral stenosis in infants. *Circulation* 89:2099-2106, 1994.
30. Chauvaud S, Fuzellier JF, Houel R, et al: Reconstructive surgery in congenital mitral valve insufficiency (Carpentier's techniques): long-term results. *J Thorac Cardiovasc Surg* 115:84-93, 1998.
31. McCarthy JF, Neligan MC, Wood AE: Ten year's experience of an aggressive reparative approach to congenital mitral valve anomalies. *Eur J Cardiothorac Surg* 10:534-539, 1996.
32. Marwick TH, Stewart WJ, Currie PJ, et al: Mechanisms of failure of mitral valve repair: An echocardiographic study. *Am Heart J* 122:149, 1991.
33. Anderson KR, Zuberbuhler JR, Anderson RH, et al: Morphologic spectrum of Ebstein's anomaly of the heart: A review. *Mayo Clin Proc* 54:174, 1979.

34. Watson H: Natural history of Ebstein's anomaly of tricuspid valve in childhood and adolescence: An international cooperative study of 505 cases. *Br Heart J* 36:417, 1974.

35. Seward JB: Ebstein's anomaly: Ultrasound imaging and hemodynamic evaluation. *Echocardiography* 10:641-664, 1993.

36. Celermajer DS, Bull C, Till JA, et al: Ebstein's anomaly: Presentation and outcome from fetus to adult. *J Am Coll Cardiol* 23:170, 1994.

37. Attenhofer Jost CH, Connolly HM, O'Leary PW, et al: Left heart lesions in patients with Ebstein anomaly. *Mayo Clin Proc* 80:361-368, 2005.

38. Eidem BW, Tei C, O'Leary PW, et al: Nongeometric quantitative assessment of right and left ventricular function: myocardial performance index in normal children and patients with Ebstein anomaly. *J Am Soc Echocardiogr* 11:849-856, 1998.

39. Danielson GK, Driscoll DJ, Mair DD, et al: Operative treatment of Ebstein's anomaly. *J Thorac Cardiovasc Surg* 104:1195, 1992.

40. Hetzer R, Nagdyman N, Ewert P, et al: A modified repair technique for tricuspid incompetence in Ebstein's anomaly. *J Thorac Cardiovasc Surg* 115:857-868, 1998.

41. Quaegebeur JM, Sreeram N, Fraser AG, et al: Surgery for Ebstein's anomaly: the clinical and echocardiographic evaluation of a new technique. *J Am Coll Cardiol* 17:722-728, 1991.

42. Attie F, Rosas M, Rijlaarsdam M, et al: The adult patient with Ebstein anomaly. Outcome in 72 unoperated patients. *Medicine* 79:27-36, 2000.

43. Carpentier A, Chauvaud S, Mace L, et al: A new reconstructive operation for Ebstein's anomaly of the tricuspid valve. *J Thorac Cardiovasc Surg* 96:91, 1988.

44. Gewillig M, Daenen W, Dumoulin M, et al: Rheologic genesis of discrete subvalvular aortic stenosis: A Doppler echocardiographic study. *J Am Coll Cardiol* 19:818, 1992.

45. Ward CJB, Culham JAG, Patterson MWH, et al: The trilogy of double-chambered right ventricle, perimembranous ventricular septal defect and subaortic narrowing—a more common association than previously recognized. *Cardiol Young* 5:140-146, 1995.

46. Ben-Shachar G, Moller JH, Castaneda-Zuniga W, et al: Signs of membranous subaortic stenosis appearing after correction of persistent common atrioventricular canal. *Am J Cardiol* 48:340, 1981.

47. Shem-Tov A, Schneeweiss A, Motro M, et al: Clinical presentation and natural history of mild discrete subaortic stenosis: Follow-up of 1-17 years. *Circulation* 66:509, 1982.

48. Douville EC, Sade RM, Crawford FA, et al: Subvalvular aortic stenosis: Timing of operation. *Ann Thorac Surg* 50:29, 1990.

49. Rohlicek CV, del Pino SF, Hosking M, et al: Natural history and surgical outcomes for isolated discrete subaortic stenosis in children. *Heart* 82:708-713, 1999.

50. DeVries AR, Hess J, Witsenburg M, et al: Management of fixed subaortic stenosis: A retrospective study of 57 cases. *J Am Coll Cardiol* 19:1013, 1992.

51. Oliver JM, Gonzalez A, Gallego P, et al: Discrete subaortic stenosis in adults: increased prevalence and slow rate of progression of the obstruction and aortic regurgitation. *J Am Coll Cardiol* 38:835-842, 2001.

52. Rao PS: Balloon angioplasty of fixed subaortic stenosis. *J Invasive Cardiol* 11:197-199, 1999.

53. Suarez de Lezo J, Pan M, Medina A, et al: Immediate and follow-up results of transluminal balloon dilation for discrete subaortic stenosis. *J Am Coll Cardiol* 18:1309, 1991.

54. Morrow AG, Waldhauser JA, Peters RL, et al: Supravalvular aortic stenosis. *Circulation* 20:1003, 1959.

55. Logan WGWE, Wyn JE, Walker E, et al: Familial supravalvular aortic stenosis. *Br Heart J* 27:547, 1965.

56. Stamm C, Friehs I, Ho SY, et al: Congenital supravalvar aortic stenosis: A simple lesion? *Eur J Cardiothorac Surg* 19:195-202, 2001.

57. Weyman AE, Caldwell RL, Hurwitz RA, et al: Cross-sectional echocardiographic characterization of aortic obstruction. I: Supravalvular aortic stenosis and aortic hypoplasia. *Circulation* 57:491, 1978.

58. Tani LY, Minich LL, Pagotto LT, Shaddy RE: Usefulness of Doppler echocardiography to determine the timing of surgery for supravalvar aortic stenosis. *Am J Cardiol* 86:114-116, 2000.

59. Flaker G, Teske D, Kilman J, et al: Supravalvular aortic stenosis: A 20-year clinical perspective and experience with patch aortoplasty. *Am J Cardiol* 51:256, 1983.

60. Myers JL, Waldhausen JA, Cyran SE, et al: Results of surgical repair of congenital supravalvular aortic stenosis. *J Thorac Cardiovasc Surg* 105:281-287, 1993.

61. Sakakibara S, Konno S: Congenital aneurysm of the sinus of Valsalva: Anatomy and classification. *Am Heart J* 63:405, 1962.

62. Segab C, Davy JM, Scheuble C, et al: Atrioventricular block disclosing an isolated congenital aneurysm of the sinus of Valsalva, extending into the septum and not ruptured. *Arch Mal Coeur Vaiss* 74:1233, 1981.

63. Rothbaum DA, Dillon JC, Chang S, et al: Echocardiographic manifestations of right sinus of Valsalva aneurysm. *Circulation* 49:768, 1974.

64. Hiyamuta K, Ohtsuki T, Shimamatsu M, et al: Aneurysm of the left aortic sinus causing acute myocardial infarction. *Circulation* 67:1151, 1983.

65. Desai AG, Sharma S, Kumar A, et al: Echocardiographic diagnosis of unruptured aneurysm of right sinus of Valsalva. *Am Heart J* 109:363, 1985.

66. Matsumoto M, Matsui H, Beppu S, et al: Echocardiographic diagnosis of ruptured aneurysm of sinus of Valsalva. *Circulation* 53:382, 1976.

67. Liberthson RR, Pennington DG, Jacobs ML, et al: Coarctation of the aorta: Review of 234 patients and clarification of management problems. *Am J Cardiol* 43:835, 1979.

68. Saenger P: Turner's syndrome. *N Engl J Med* 335:1749-1754, 1996.

69. Marx GR, Allen HD: Accuracy and pitfalls of Doppler evaluation of the pressure gradient in aortic coarctation. *J Am Coll Cardiol* 7:1379, 1986.

70. Carvalho JS, Redington AN, Shinebourne EA, et al: Continuous wave Doppler echocardiography and coarctation of the aorta: Gradients and flow patterns in the assessment of severity. *Br Heart J* 64:133, 1990.

71. Sanders SP, MacPherson D, Yeager SB: Temporal flow velocity profile in the descending aorta in coarcation. *J Am Coll Cardiol* 7:603, 1986.

72. Ryan K, Sanyal RS, Pinheiro L, et al: Assessment of aortic coarctation and collateral circulation by biplane transesophageal echocardiography. *Echocardiography* 9:277, 1992.

73. Becker C, Soppa C, Fink U, et al: Spiral CT angiography and 3D reconstruction in patients with aortic coarctation. *Eur Radiol* 7:1473-1477, 1997.

74. Mohiaddin RH, Kilner PJ, Rees S, et al: Magnetic resonance volume flow and jet velocity mapping in aortic coarctation. *J Am Coll Cardiol* 22:1515, 1993.

75. Rao PS: Coarctation of the aorta. *Curr Cardiol Reports* 7:425-434, 2005.

76. Harrison JK, Sheikh KH, Davidson CJ, et al: Balloon angioplasty of coarctation of the aorta evaluated with intravascular ultrasound imaging. *J Am Coll Cardiol* 15:906, 1990.

77. Ebeid MR, Prieto LR, Latson LA: Use of balloon-expandable stents for coarctation of the aorta: initial results and intermediate-term follow-up. *J Am Coll Cardiol* 30:1847-1852, 1997.

78. Hornung TS, Benson LN, McLaughlin PR: Interventions for aortic coarctation. *Cardiol Rev* 10:139-148, 2002.

79. Kirklin JW, Barrett-Boyes BG (eds): Coarctation of the aorta and interrupted aortic arch. In *Cardiac Surgery*, 2nd ed. New York, Churchill Livingstone, 1993, pp. 1263-1326.

80. Moodie DS: Diagnosis and management of congenital heart disease in the adult. *Cardiol Rev* 9:276-281, 2001.

81. Hagen PT, Scholz DG, Edwards WD: Incidence and size of patent foramen ovale during the first 10 decades of life: An autopsy study of 965 normal hearts. *Mayo Clin Proc* 59:17, 1984.

82. Lynch JJ, Schuchard GH, Gross CM, et al: Prevalence of right-to-left atrial shunting in a healthy population: Detection by Valsalva maneuver contrast echocardiography. *Am J Cardiol* 53:1478, 1984.

83. Cabanes L, Mas JL, Cohen A, et al: Atrial septal aneurysm and patent foramen ovale as risk factors for cryptogenic stroke in patients less than 55 years of age: A study using transesophageal echocardiography. *Stroke* 24:1865, 1993.

84. Kizer JR, Devereux RB: Clinical practice. Patent foramen ovale in young adults with unexplained stroke. *New Engl J Med* 353:2361-2372, 2005.

85. Mugge A, Daniel WG, Angermann C: Atrial septal aneurysm in adult patients. A multicenter study using transthoracic and transesophageal echocardiography. *Circulation* 91:2785, 1995.

86. Fraker TD Jr, Harris PJ, Behar VS, et al: Detection and exclusion of interatrial shunts by two-dimensional echocardiography and peripheral venous injection. *Circulation* 59:379, 1979.

87. Grenadier E, Alpan G, Keidar S, et al: M-mode and two-dimensional contrast echocardiography in adult patients with atrial septal defects. *Clin Cardiol* 6:588, 1983.

88. Seward JB, Tajik AJ, Sungler JG, et al: Echocardiographic contrast studies: Initial experience. *Mayo Clin Proc* 40:163, 1975.

89. Stewart WJ, Jiang L, Mich R, et al: Variable effects of changes in flow rate through the aortic, pulmonic and mitral valves on valve area and flow velocity: Impact on quantitative Doppler flow calculations. *J Am Coll Cardiol* 6:653, 1985.

90. Sherman FS, Sahn DJ, Valdes-Cruz LM, et al: Two-dimensional Doppler color flow mapping for detecting atrial and ventricular septal defects. Studies in an animal model and in the clinical setting. *Herz* 12:212, 1985.

91. Pollick C, Sullivan H, Cujec B, et al: Doppler color-flow mapping assessment of shunt size in atrial septal defect. *Circulation* 78:522, 1988.

92. Yock PG, Popp RL: Noninvasive estimation of right ventricular systolic pressure by Doppler ultrasound in patients with tricuspid regurgitation. *Circulation* 70:657, 1984.

93. Liberthson RR, Boucher CA, Fallot JT, et al: Severe mitral regurgitation: A common occurrence in the aging patient with secundum atrial septal defect. *Clin Cardiol* 4:229, 1981.

94. Hausmann D, Daniel WG, Mugge A, et al: Value of transesophageal color Doppler echocardiography for detection of different types of atrial septal defect in adults. *J Am Soc Echocardiogr* 5:481, 1992.

95. Kronzon I, Tunick PA, Freedberg RS, et al: Transesophageal echocardiography is superior to transthoracic echocardiography in the diagnosis of sinus venosus atrial septal defect. *J Am Coll Cardiol* 17:537, 1991.

96. Belkin RN, Pollack BD, Ruggiero ML, et al: Comparison of transesophageal and transthoracic echocardiography with contrast and color flow Doppler in the detection of patent foramen ovale. *Am Heart J* 128:520, 1994.

97. Murphy JG, Gersh BJ, McGoon MD, et al: Long-term outcome after surgical repair of isolated atrial septal defect: Follow-up at 27 to 32 years. *N Engl J Med* 323:1645, 1990.

98. Horvath KA, Burke RP, Collins JJ, et al: Surgical treatment of adult atrial septal defect: Early and long-term results. *J Am Coll Cardiol* 20:1156, 1992.

99. Liberthson RR, Boucher CA, Strauss HW, et al: Right ventricular function in adult atrial septal defect. *J Am Coll Cardiol* 47:56, 1981.

100. Steele PM, Fuster V, Cohen M, et al: Isolated atrial septal defect with pulmonary vascular obstructive disease-long-term follow-up and prediction of outcome after surgical correction. *Circulation* 76:1037, 1987.

101. Shah D, Azhar M, Oakley CM, et al: Natural history of secundum atrial septal defect in adults after medical or surgical treatment: A historical prospective study. *Br Heart J* 71:224, 1994.

102. Konstantinides S, Geibel A, Olschewski M, et al: A comparison of surgical and medical therapy for atrial septal defect in adults. *N Engl J Med* 333:469, 1995.

103. Gatzoulis MA, Redington AN, Somerville J, Shore DF: Should atrial septal defects in adults be closed? *Ann Thorac Surg* 61:657-659, 1996.

104. Homma S, Sacco RL: Patent foramen ovale and stroke. *Circulation* 112:1063-1072, 2005.

105. Messe SR, Silverman IE, Kizer JR, et al: Practice parameter: recurrent stroke with patent foramen ovale and atrial septal aneurysm: report of the Quality Standards Subcommittee of the American Academy of Neurology. *Neurology* 62:1042-1050, 2004.

106. Messe SR, Cucchiara B, Luciano J, Kasner: SEPFO management: neurologists vs cardiologists. *Neurology* 65:172-173, 2005.

107. Rao PS: Catheter closure of atrial septal defects. *J Invasive Cardiol* 15:398-400, 2003.

108. Pedra CAC, Pihkala J, Lee K-J et al: Transcatheter closure of atrial septal defects using the Cardio-seal implant. *Heart* 84:320, 2000.

109. Boccalandro F, Baptista E, Muench A, et al: Comparison of intracardiac echocardiography versus transesophageal echocardiography guidance for percutaneous transcatheter closure of atrial septal defect. *Am J Cardiol* 93:437-440, 2004.

110. Hein R, Buscheck F, Fischer E, et al: Atrial and ventricular septal defects can safely be closed by percutaneous intervention. *J Intervent Cardiol* 18:515-522, 2005.

111. Kreutzer J, Ryan CA, Gauvreau K, et al: Healing response to the clamshell device for closure of intracardiac defects in humans. *Catheter Cardiovasc Interv* 54:101-111, 2001.

112. Kraybill KA, Lucas RV: Abnormal pulmonary venous connections. In Emmanoulides GC, Riemenschneider TA, Allen HD, Gutgesell H (eds): *Heart Disease in infants, children, and adolescents including the fetus and young adult.* Baltimore, Williams & Wilkins, 1995, pp. 838-874.

113. Ammash NM, Seward JB, Warnes CA, et al: Partial anomalous pulmonary venous connection: Diagnosis by transesophageal echocardiography. *J Am Coll Cardiol* 29:1351-1358, 1997.

114. Masui T, Seelos KC, Kersting-Sommerhoff BA, Higgins CB: Abnormalities of the pulmonary veins: evaluation with MR imaging and comparison with cardiac angiography and echocardiography. *Radiology* 181:645-649, 1991.

115. Remy-Jardin M, Remy J: Spiral CT angiography of the pulmonary circulation. *Radiology* 212:615-636, 1999.

116. Atrial septal defect and partial anomalous pulmonary venous connection. In Kirklin JW, Barrett-Boyes BG (eds): *Cardiac Surgery*, 2nd ed, New York, Churchill Livingstone, 1993.

117. Gersony WM, Hayes CJ, Driscoll DJ, et al: Bacterial endocarditis in patients with aortic stenosis, pulmonary stenosis, or ventricular septal defect. *Circulation* 87(suppl I): I-121-I-126, 1993.

118. Gasul BM, Dillon RJ, Vela V: The natural transformation of ventricular septal defects into ventricular septal defects with pulmonary stenosis. *Am J Dis Child* 94:424, 1957.

119. Tohyama K, Satomi G, Momma K: Aortic valve prolapse and aortic regurgitation associated with subpulmonic ventricular septal defect. *Am J Cardiol* 79:1285, 1997.

120. Sabry AF, Reller MD, Silberbach M, et al: Comparison of four Doppler echocardiographic methods for calculating pulmonary-to-systemic shunt flow ratios in patients with ventricular septal defect. *Am J Cardiol* 75:611, 1995.

121. Holzer R, Balzer D, Cao QL, et al: Device closure of muscular ventricular septal defects using the Amplatzer muscular ven-

tricular septal defect occluder: immediate and mid-term results of a U.S. registry. *J Am Coll Cardiol* 43:1257-1263, 2004.

122. Hijazi ZM: Device closure of ventricular septal defects. *Catheter Cardiovasc Interv* 60:107-114, 2003.

123. Moore JW, Levi DS, Moore SD, et al: Interventional treatment of patent ductus arteriosus in 2004. *Catheter Cardiovasc Interv* 64:91-101, 2005.

124. Ottenkamp J, Hess J, Talsma MD, Buis-Liem TN: Protrusion of the device: A complication of catheter closure of patent ductus arteriosus. *Br Heart J* 68:301, 1992.

125. Hobbs RE, Mullit HD, Raghavan PV, et al: Coronary artery fistulae: A 10-year review. *Cleve Clin Q* 49:191, 1982.

126. Cottier C, Kiowski W, von Bertrab R, et al: Multiple coronary arteriocameral fistulas as a cause of myocardial ischemia. *Am Heart J* 115:181, 1988.

127. Sanders SP, Parness IA, Colan SD: Recognition of abnormal connections of coronary arteries with the use of Doppler color flow mapping. *J Am Coll Cardiol* 13:922, 1989.

128. Shakudo M, Yoshikawa J, Yoshida K, et al: Noninvasive diagnosis of coronary artery fistula by Doppler color flow mapping. *J Am Coll Cardiol* 13:1572, 1989.

129. Reeder GS, Tajik AJ, Smith HC: Visualization of coronary artery fistula by two-dimensional echocardiography. *Mayo Clin Proc* 55:185, 1980.

130. Cooper MJ, Bernstein D, Silverman NH: Recognition of left coronary artery fistula to the left and right ventricles by contrast echocardiography. *J Am Coll Cardiol* 6:923, 1985.

131. Okubo M, Nykanen D, Benson LN: Outcomes of transcatheter embolization in the treatment of coronary artery fistulas. *Catheter Cardiovasc Interv* 52:510-517, 2001.

132. Armsby LR, Keane JF, Sherwood MC, et al: Management of coronary artery fistulae. Patient selection and results of transcatheter closure. *J Am Coll Cardiol* 39:1026-1032, 2002.

133. Dabizzi RP, Caprioli G, Aiazzi L, et al: Distribution and anomalies of coronary arteries in tetralogy of Fallot. *Circulation* 61:95, 1980.

134. Fellows KE, Smith J, Keane JF: Preoperative angiography in infants with tetrad of Fallot. *Am J Cardiol* 47:1279, 1981.

135. Bertranou EG, Blackstone EH, Hazelrig JB, et al: Life expectancy without surgery in tetralogy of Fallot. *Am J Cardiol* 42:458-466, 1978.

136. Huhta JC, Piehler JM, Tajik AJ, et al: Two-dimensional echocardiographic detection and measurement of the right pulmonary artery-ventricular septal defect: Angiographic and surgical correlation. *Am J Cardiol* 49:1235, 1982.

137. Gomes AS, Lois JF, Williams RG: Pulmonary arteries: MR imaging in patients with congenital obstruction of the right ventricular outflow tract. *Radiology* 174:51, 1990.

138. Berry JM, Einzig S, Krabill K, et al: Evaluation of coronary artery anatomy in patients with tetralogy of Fallot by two-dimensional echocardiography. *Circulation* 78:149, 1988.

139. Hu DC, Seward JB, Puga FJ, et al: Total correction of tetralogy of Fallot at age 40 years and older: Long-term follow-up. *J Am Coll Cardiol* 5:40, 1985.

140. Nollert GD, Fischlein T, Bouterwek S, et al: Long-term results of total repair of tetralogy of Fallot in adulthood 35 years follow-up

in 104 patients corrected at the age of 18 or older. *Thorac Cardiovasc Surg* 45:178-181, 1997.

141. Lieberson AD, Schumacher RR, Childress RH, et al: Corrected transposition of the great vessels in a 73-year-old man. *Circulation* 39:96, 1969.

142. Graham TP, Bernard YD, Mellen BG, et al: Long-term outcome in congenitally corrected transposition of the great arteries: A multi-institutional study. *J Am Coll Cardiol* 36:255, 2000.

143. Benson LN, Burns R, Schwaiger M, et al: Radionuclide angiographic evaluation of ventricular function in isolated congenitally corrected transposition of the great arteries. *Am J Cardiol* 58:319, 1986.

144. Eidem BW, O'Leary PW, Tei C, Seward JB: Usefulness of the myocardial performance index for assessing right ventricular function in congenital heart disease. *Am J Coll Cardiol* 86:654-658, 2000.

145. Mavroudis C, Backer CL: Physiologic versus anatomic repair of congenitally corrected transposition of the great arteries. *Semin Thorac Cardiovasc Surg Pediatr Card Surg Annu* 6:16-26, 2003.

146. Alghamdi AA, McCrindle BW, Van Arsdell GS: Physiologic versus anatomic repair of congenitally corrected transposition of the great arteries: Meta-analysis of individual patient data. *Ann Thorac Surg* 81:1529-1535, 2006.

147. Kleinert S, Sano T, Weintraub RG, et al: Anatomic features and surgical strategies in double-outlet right ventricle. *Circulation* 96:1233-1239, 1997.

148. VanPraagh R, VanPraagh S: The anatomy of common aortico-pulmonary trunk (truncus arteriosus communis) and its embryologic implications. *Am J Cardiol* 166:406, 1965.

149. Calder L, VanPraagh R, VanPraagh S, et al: Truncus arteriosus communis: Clinical, angiocardiographic, and pathologic findings in 100 patients. *Am Heart J* 92:23, 1976.

150. Dick M, Fyler DC, Nadas AS: Tricuspid atresia: Clinical course in 101 patients. *Am J Cardiol* 36:327, 1975.

151. Rao PS: Further observations on the spontaneous closure of physiologically advantageous ventricular septal defects in tricuspid atresia: Surgical implications. *Ann Thorac Surg* 35:121, 1983.

152. Pigula FA, Gandhi SK, Ristich J, et al: Cardiopulmonary transplantation for congenital heart disease in the adult. *J Heart Lung Transplant* 20:297-303, 2001.

153. Hager A, Kaemmerer H, Eicken A, et al: Long-term survival of patients with univentricular heart not treated surgically. *J Thorac Cardiovasc Surg* 123:1214-1217, 2002.

154. van Doorn CA, de Leval MR: The Fontan operation in clinical practice: indications and controversies. *Nat Clin Pract Cardiovasc Med* 2:116-117, 2005.

155. DeLeval MR, Kimes P, Gewillig M, et al: Total cavopulmonary connection: A logical alternative to atriopulmonary connection for complex Fontan operations. *J Thorac Cardiovasc Surg* 96:682, 1988.

156. Gatzoulis MA, Munk MD, Williams WG, Webb GD: Definitive palliation with cavopulmonary or aortopulmonary shunts for adults with single ventricle physiology. *Heart* 83:51-57, 2000.

Chapter 44

Echocardiographic Evaluation of the Adult with Postoperative Congenital Heart Disease

JOHN S. CHILD, MD

■ General Postoperative Congenital Heart Disease Issues
  Atrial and Ventricular Incisions
  Anatomic and Valvular Residua and Sequelae
  Ventricular Function
  Conduits, Patches, and Prosthetic Materials

■ Palliative Procedures
  Pulmonary Artery Banding
  Palliative Aortopulmonary Shunts
  Glenn Shunts

■ Corrective Procedures for Simple Lesions
  Atrial Septal Defects
  Ventricular Septal Defects
  Patent Ductus Arteriosus
  Bicuspid Aortic Valve
  Subaortic Stenosis
  Coarctation of the Aorta
  Ebstein Anomaly
  Pulmonic Stenosis
  Anomalies of the Coronary Arteries

■ Repair of Complex Malformations
  Atrial Switch Surgery
  Arterial Switch Surgery
  Total Anomalous Pulmonary Venous Connection
  Fontan Atrial Surgery
  Atrioventricular Septal Defects
  Biventricular Repairs
  Tetralogy of Fallot
  Common Transposition of the Great Arteries
  Congenitally Corrected Transposition of the Great Arteries
  Double-Outlet Right Ventricle

The incidence of moderate and severe forms of congenital heart disease (CHD) is approximately 6 per 1000 live births (19 per 1000 if a bicuspid aortic valve [BAV] is included).[1] In the last 60 years, advances in diagnosis and in catheter and surgical treatment resulted in nearly 1 million adult survivors with CHD in the United States.[2-6] There are now more adults than children with CHD.[7] Some surgical techniques, nonexistent 3 decades ago, are now used in adolescents and adults whose physiology and anatomic substrate allowed survival either without surgery or with palliative procedures. Other operations rarely performed today exist in many adult survivors of their childhood CHD surgeries. Familiarity with previous and current procedures is needed because surgical and catheter techniques continue to evolve.[8] Except for perhaps ligation or device closure of patent ductus arteriosus (PDA) or suture closure of a simple secundum atrial septal defect (ASD), there a few cures; most surgically modified CHD leave behind (residua) or cause (sequelae) problems ranging from trivial to serious.[6,8]

Adults with CHD may be seen in adult echocardiographic laboratories accustomed to evaluating acquired cardiac diseases and possibly simple CHD. Complex palliative or corrective procedures are not well known by most medical cardiologists without special training.[9] The evaluation and management of adult CHD requires detailed knowledge of the (1) original anatomy and physiology; (2) dynamic changes in anatomy and physiology that occur with time; (3) effects of adult diseases (e.g., systemic arterial hypertension, coronary artery disease [CAD]) or conditions (e.g., pregnancy) on that physiology; (4) types of operative repair (both past and present) for each complex of lesions; (5) presence and extent of possible postoperative residua, sequelae, and complications; and (6) proper selection, performance, and interpretation of modalities required for anatomic imaging and hemodynamic assessment.[10]

It is impractical to repetitively catheterize these individuals; combined two-dimensional (2D) and Doppler echocardiography are often more useful than angiography in providing details of valvular anatomy and in visualizing patches and ventricular wall thickness.[10] Echocardiography is nearly equivalent to angiography in displaying the connections of the pulmonary and systemic veins to the atria, intraatrial anatomy, and the connections of the atria or ventricles to the great arteries.[10-13] Where questions remain, magnetic resonance imaging (MRI) or computed tomographic (CT) imaging are of great value.[13] Interpretation is best done using the segmental approach with identification of atrial, ventricular, and arterial segments and determination of (1) atrial and ventricular situs, (2) connections of the atria to the ventricles and ventricles to the great arteries, and (3) relationships of the ventricles and great arteries.[10-12,14] Spectral and color flow Doppler permit localization and quantitation of stenosis and regurgitation, extracardiac and intracardiac conduit stenosis, pulmonary and systemic venous obstruction, septal or patch shunts; and intracardiac hemodynamics.[2] Conduit course and obstruction, pulmonary artery (PA)

branches, or aortopulmonary collaterals may also require angiography or magnetic resonance imaging for full delineation but in such instances can be applied selectively.[13]

Many adults with CHD have "geometrically–challenged" ventricles (e.g., the systemic right ventricle in congenitally corrected transposition or d-transposition of the great arteries, the incised or patched right ventricle in tetralogy of Fallot [TOF], or even a single ventricle) and standard measures of ventricular function may be less reliable.[7] The ventricular myocardial performance index (MPI) is a useful nongeometric measure that examines systole (ejection time) and the isovolumic contraction and relaxation times (technically not isovolumic if regurgitation is present).[15-20] Doppler evaluation of diastolic function and Doppler tissue and strain rate (SR) imaging are now being used to evaluate global and regional ventricular function in CHD.[21-25]

Transesophageal echocardiography (TEE) images areas often not seen on transthoracic echocardiography (TTE; e.g., coarctation, sinus venosus ASDs, pulmonary venous connections) and provides more complete depiction of complex anatomy.[10-12] TEE evaluation must be thorough because unsuspected lesions may be found (e.g., ASDs, anomalous pulmonary venous connections, muscular ventricular septal defects [VSDs]) that may need repair at the time of surgery. TEE allows good visualization of the origins of the coronary arteries, main PA branches, and entire aorta. TEE is the standard for intraoperative and postoperative evaluation of complex CHD surgery.[10-12] Before cardiopulmonary bypass (CPB), TEE refines anatomic diagnosis and detects unsuspected defects that may require modification of the operative approach. After discontinuation of cardiopulmonary bypass and resumption of normal cardiac activity, adequacy of repair is evaluated and additional repair directed when the initial result is unsatisfactory. Any residua and surgical sequelae are documented. TEE in the postoperative care unit elucidates causes of general complications (e.g., hypotension, tamponade, ventricular dysfunction), or, complications of specific CHD surgeries, such as the Fontan procedure (e.g., lateral tunnel thrombus).

General Postoperative Congenital Heart Disease Issues

Atrial and Ventricular Incisions

Electric instability may occur after atrial or ventricular incisional scars or aneurysms or after insertion of intracardiac patches or conduits with possible disruption of the conduction system[6-8,26] (Table 44–1). Patients with intraatrial baffles or conduits (e.g., Mustard and Fontan

TABLE 44–1. General Postoperative Issues in Congenital Heart Disease

Postoperative Issue	Examples
Electric instability	Atrial arrhythmias after intraatrial baffle procedures Ventricular arrhythmias after ventriculotomy
Residual anatomic defects	Bicuspid aortic valve in patient with aortic coarctation Residual mitral regurgitation after cleft leaflet or primum atrial septal defect repair Pulmonic regurgitation after tetralogy of Fallot repair Dilated aortic root Missed muscular ventricular septal defect
Impaired ventricular function	Chronic volume overload resulting from valve regurgitation Anatomic right ventricle functioning as the systemic ventricle Single functioning ventricle
Prosthetic materials	Degeneration of septal patches, intracardiac and extracardiac conduits Prosthetic valve dysfunction Thrombus formation Risk of infective endocarditis Obstruction or leaking of conduits

procedures) frequently suffer atrial arrhythmias; superimposed pressure overload on a ventriculotomy site may cause ventricular arrhythmias[8] (Fig. 44–1). Because certain subgroups of postoperative CHD often require pacemaker therapy, there are concerns about diminished ventricular contractility over the long term with pacing via one ventricle (usually the right).[27,28] As such, ventricular resynchronization by biventricular or multisite pacing may be of value and is amenable to evaluation by echocardiographic-Doppler.[29,30]

Anatomic and Valvular Residua and Sequelae

Postoperative anatomic and valvular sequelae and residua must be sought.[6,8] BAVs, common with aortic coarctation, continue to pose risks of progressive stenosis, regurgitation, and endocarditis despite coarctation repair. Variations on a parachute mitral valve, also associated with coarctation and other stenoses in sequence on the left-sided circulation, are detected by imaging a decreased interpapillary muscle distance and Doppler evidence of inflow obstruction. Repair of an ostium primum ASD with cleft mitral leaflet may leave residual mitral regurgitation (MR) or the sequel of mitral stenosis (MS); subaortic stenosis as a result of anomalous chordal attachments should be sought. In repaired Fallot's tetralogy, pulmonary regurgitation (PR) is a sequel to valvulotomy or transannular incision and patch. Mild-moderate low-pressure pulmonic regurgitation is common and well tolerated; severe pulmonic regurgitation may cause right ventricular (RV) dilatation and tricuspid regurgitation (TR), particularly if there is residual RV outflow obstruction. Muscular

VSDs may have been missed and should be sought by color flow imaging (Fig. 44–2). A dilated aortic root or trunk may occur TOF, transposition of the great arteries, or single ventricle in association with pulmonic stenosis, and late aortic regurgitation (AR) is common in adults (Fig. 44–3). Atrioventricular (AV) valve regurgitation, common preoperatively in Fontan patients, may progress postoperatively.

Ventricular Function

Valvular lesions pose a risk for endocarditis and, if severe, affect long-term ventricular performance.[31] Operative myocardial preservation often was faulty in previous decades. The later in life the patient is operated, the less the regression of ventricular hypertrophy. Long term, a subaortic right ventricle operating at systemic pressures or a single functioning ventricle in a univentricular heart—even after a Fontan—may have an irreversible decline in contractility. Ventricular function may suffer if a prosthetic patch or conduit origin is large, if an incisional aneurysm acts as a "windkessel," or if valvular or conduit obstruction and regurgitation or large shunt overloads the heart.

Conduits, Patches, and Prosthetic Materials

Septal patches, prosthetic valves, and conduits may degenerate.[8,10] Foreign bodies, such as pacer wires or mechanical valvular prostheses, risk thrombus formation or endocarditis (Fig. 44–4). Bioprosthetic valves and conduits often develop obstruction or regurgitation resulting from degenerative changes and

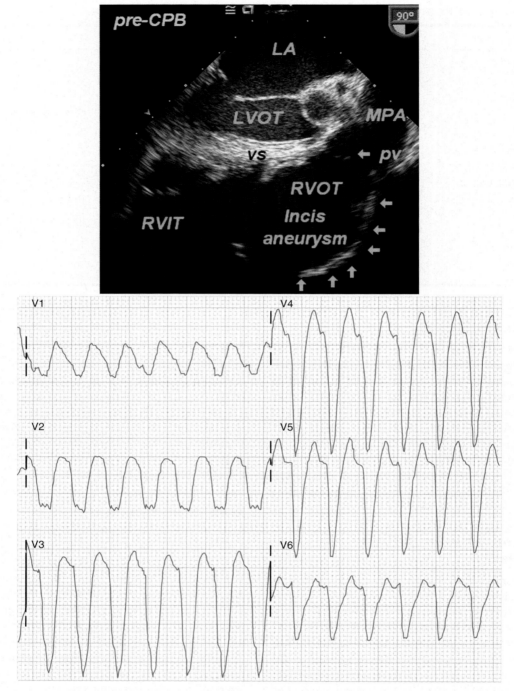

Figure 44–1. *Tetralogy of Fallot. Intraoperative pre-cardiopulmonary bypass (pre-CPB) transesophageal echocardiography shows right ventricular outflow tract (RVOT) incisional (incis) dyskinetic aneurysm and scar, which was then revised and a pulmonary valve inserted for severe pulmonary regurgitation. Patient showed up at the emergency department with palpitations, and the electrocardiogram showed ventricular tachycardia (precordial leads are shown here). LA, left atrium; LVOT, left ventricular outflow tract; MPA, main pulmonary artery; PV, pulmonary valve; RVIT, right ventricular inflow tract.*

calcification or by intimal ingrowth, particularly in adolescents and young adults. External conduits may be kinked by compression between the heart and sternum. Obstruction can occur at the exit from the ventricle, at a bioprosthetic valve, or at the distal insertion site. An internal conduit may develop leaks, internal obstruction, or kinking or may partially obstruct the chamber within which it sits. Some conduits have unusual courses resulting from altered great artery relationships; therefore, multiple precor-

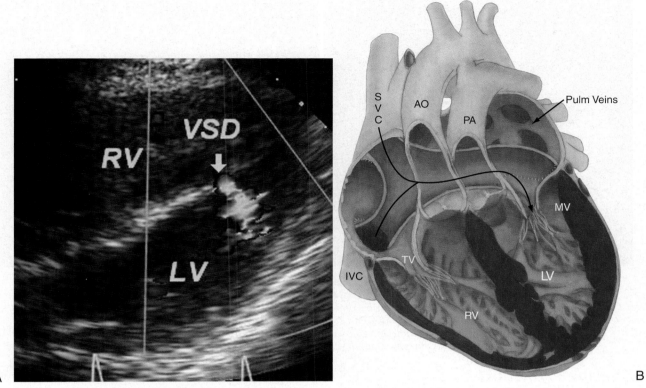

A

B

Figure 44-2. *D-transposition of the great arteries (DTGA) late after intraatrial baffle surgery (Mustard) with residual unrecognized apical muscular ventricular septal defect (VSD) in a modified transthoracic apical view. A small right ventricle (RV) to left ventricle (LV) shunt is seen as a small color flow jet (arrow), which represents a left-to-right shunt given the RV is the subaortic ventricle, and the LV is the subpulmonic ventricle. B, Geometry of Mustard baffle repair. The atrial baffle causes systemic venous blood to course anteriorly and leftward from the rightward cavae to the mitral valve and LV; this results in the posterior pulmonary veins coursing rightward and then anterior to the tricuspid valve and RV.*

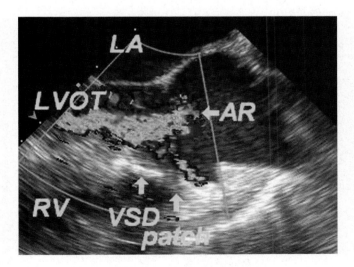

Figure 44-3. *Intraoperative transesophageal echocardiography reveals baseline images prior to aortic valve replacement and aortic root repair for severe aortic regurgitation (AR) and dilated aortic root (measured 52 mm at sinuses) late after previously repaired tetralogy of Fallot. The old ventricular septal defect (VSD) patch is well seen. LA, left atrium; LVOT, left ventricular outflow tract; RV, right ventricle; RVOT, right ventricular outflow tract.*

dial and subcostal transducer positions or multiplane TEE may be required for an adequate anatomic-hemodynamic evaluation. Continuous-wave (CW) Doppler is directed into the conduit from multiple angles to predict the pressure gradient; most conduits curve and the proper angle to record the true peak velocity may be difficult to obtain.[10] CW Doppler of AV valve regurgitation quantitates ventricular systolic pressure and estimates significant conduit stenosis.

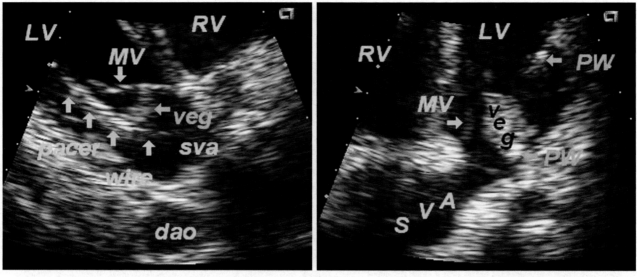

Figure 44–4. *D-transposition of the great arteries late post Mustard with pacemaker previously inserted for sick sinus syndrome. The patient had fevers and bacteremia. Transthoracic echocardiographic views: modified parasternal long-axis view (A) and zoomed portion of four-chamber apical view (B) reveal a vegetation (veg) on the pacer wire (PW), which passes via the systemic venous atrium (SVA) from the superior vena cava to the left ventricle (LV). The vegetation resolved after 6 weeks of antibiotic therapy. Dao, descending aorta; MV, mitral valve; RV, right ventricle.*

Palliative Procedures

Pulmonary Artery Banding

PA banding may be used to decrease the volume and pressure effects of a large shunt at the ventricular level to avoid heart failure or pulmonary hypertension (Table 44–2 and Fig. 44–5). The band site is evaluated by echocardiographic anatomic imaging, the best band placement being the mid-portion of the PA; a band that is too close to the valve may interfere with

valve function, a band that has slipped onto the bifurcation may cause branch artery stenosis. Inadequate banding allows pulmonary hypertension. Band stenosis gradient is quantitated by aligning the CW Doppler beam with the color flow jet via the iatrogenic stenosis (see Fig. 44–5). Because most lesions that require banding have large VSDs, PA systolic pressure can be estimated as systolic systemic blood pressure minus the peak pressure gradient across the band (provided that there is no left ventricular outflow tract [LVOT] obstruction).

TABLE 44–2. Palliative Procedures for Congenital Heart Disease

Name of Procedure	Description	Complications
Pulmonary artery banding	Constriction of main pulmonary artery	Inadequate band with consequent pulmonary vascular disease Branch pulmonary artery stenosis Pulmonic valve dysfunction
Waterston shunt	Ascending aorta to right pulmonary artery	Pulmonary hypertension resulting from too large a shunt
Potts shunt	Descending aorta to left pulmonary artery	Kinking of branch pulmonary arteries
Blalock-Taussig shunt	Subclavian artery to branch pulmonary artery	Inadequate shunt to maintain pulmonary blood flow
Modified Blalock-Taussig shunt	Gore-Tex graft from subclavian artery to pulmonary artery	Excessive shunt resulting in pulmonary hypertension
Glenn shunt	Superior vena cava to right pulmonary artery with division of main pulmonary artery	Postoperative cyanosis resulting from increased collaterals from superior to inferior vena cava or pulmonary arteriovenous fistulas
Bidirectional Glenn shunt	Superior vena cava to both (undivided) pulmonary arteries	Postoperative cyanosis resulting from increased collaterals from superior to inferior vena cava or pulmonary arteriovenous fistulas

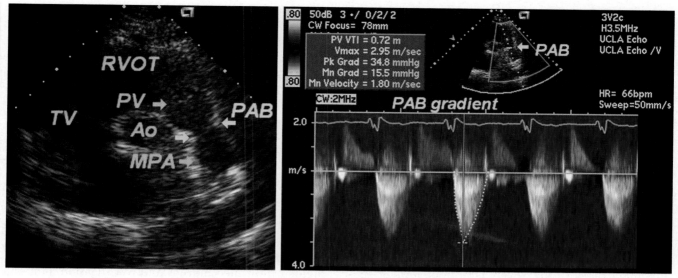

Figure 44–5. This patient had a previous pulmonary artery band (PAB) as a neonate before subsequent repair of an atrioventricular septal defect as an infant. The parasternal long-axis transthoracic echocardiographic view shows that the pulmonary artery band (PAN) was not completely removed. The accompanying continuous-wave Doppler study reveals residual stenosis with a mean systolic gradient of 15.5 mm Hg. Ao, aorta; MPA, main pulmonary artery; PV, pulmonary valve; RVOT, right ventricular outflow tract; TV, tricuspid valve.

Palliative Aortopulmonary Shunts

Palliative systemic arterial to pulmonary arterial shunts are performed for CHD characterized by decreased pulmonary arterial flow (e.g., TOF) (Fig. 44–6). The shunts from the high-pressure aorta to the low-pressure PA can be evaluated for patency by CW Doppler, which should reveal nonlaminar flow in both systole and diastole toward the PA in the absence of pulmonary hypertension.

The Waterston (ascending aorta to right PA) and Potts (descending aorta to left PA) shunts are discrete side-to-

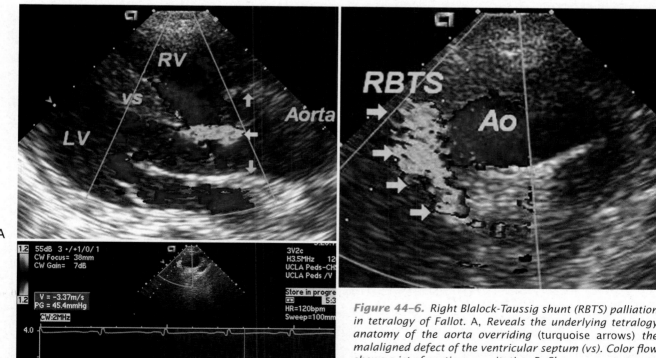

Figure 44–6. Right Blalock-Taussig shunt (RBTS) palliation in tetralogy of Fallot. A, Reveals the underlying tetralogy anatomy of the aorta overriding (turquoise arrows) the malaligned defect of the ventricular septum (vs). Color flow shows a jet of aortic regurgitation. B, Shows a suprasternal notch view of the RBTS descending (yellow arrows) rightward along the transverse aorta (Ao). C, Shows the continuous-wave Doppler of the RBTS with continuous high-velocity flow with peaking in systole (sys) but persisting throughout diastole (diast) indicating low pulmonary vascular resistance. LV, left ventricle; RV, right ventricle.

side connections. Potts and Waterston anastomoses are now rarely performed because of problems with precise control of size and possible pulmonary hypertension or kinking of branch PAs, which may complicate further repair. TTE imaging of these anastomoses is often difficult in adults and may require TEE in which proper Doppler alignment with color flow imaging makes it possible to calculate the Bernoulli equation gradient. PA systolic pressure is estimated by subtracting the peak systolic pressure gradient from the brachial artery systolic peak pressure. As PA pressures rise, diastolic flow decreases more than systolic flow; diminutive diastolic flow indicates increased diastolic pulmonary pressure.

A classic Blalock-Taussig shunt is a direct end-to-side anastomosis between a subclavian artery and a branch PA, usually on the side opposite the aortic arch (see Fig. 44–6). A modified Blalock-Taussig shunt uses a 4-mm to 5-mm Gore-Tex tube or vein graft from aorta or subclavian artery to the PA. Imaging of a Blalock-Taussig shunt uses suprasternal and supraclavicular views augmented by color flow imaging. Estimation of PA pressure may be unreliable in a long curving connection; a low gradient may be seen in the presence of adequate

flow and normal PA pressures. The flow should be virtually continuous; as such, it must be distinguished from a patent ductus (see Fig. 44–6). If the shunt is small or occluded, flow decreases or is lost. Doppler is helpful in the early postoperative period in a patient who continues to have cyanosis to assess adequacy of the shunt versus other causes of postoperative cyanosis (e.g., atelectasis). If the shunt is too large and results in pulmonary hypertension (fortunately an uncommon event), the diastolic flow decreases first, with decreased systolic flow later as pulmonary vascular resistance rises to equal systemic resistance.

Glenn Shunts

A classic Glenn shunt is anastomosis of the end of the superior vena cava (SVC) to the side of the right PA divided from the main PA and SVC ligation as it enters the right atrium. A bidirectional Glenn allows SVC flow to both PAs, causing improved systemic oxygen saturation without ventricular volume overload, useful as definitive palliation or as a staging for subsequent Fontan procedures in complex congenital

TABLE 44–3. Corrective Procedures for "Simple" Congenital Heart Lesions

Lesion	Corrective Procedure	Complications and Residual Abnormalities
Atrial septal defect	Suture repair, patch closure, or transcatheter closure	Residual shunting Associated mitral valve abnormalities Persistent pulmonary hypertension Right-sided heart chamber enlargement
Ventricular septal defect	Surgical repair (via right transatrial approach)	Residual patch leak Arrhythmias if ventricular incision needed
Patent ductus arteriosus	Surgical ligation or catheter device closure	Residual shunting (more likely if calcified)
Bicuspid aortic valve	Surgical or balloon valvuloplasty Pulmonic autograft Valve replacement	Associated lesions (ventricular septal defect, coarctation) Restenosis Prosthetic valve dysfunction
Subaortic stenosis	Excision of membrane or fibromuscular ridge	Aortic regurgitation Iatrogenic ventricular septal defect Mitral valve injury Recurrent stenosis
Coarctation of aorta	Multiple repair procedures	Residual or recurrent coarctation Left ventricular hypertrophy Associated lesions (e.g., bicuspid aortic valve, supramitral ring)
Ebstein anomaly	Surgical repair	Residual tricuspid regurgitation Associated lesions (patent foramen ovale, atrial septal defects, pulmonic stenosis, ventricular septal defects)
Pulmonic stenosis	Balloon dilation Surgical repair	Residual stenosis Pulmonic regurgitation Dynamic right ventricular outflow obstruction (early postoperative)
Coronary artery anomalies	Various repair procedures	Left ventricular dysfunction Mitral regurgitation

heart disease not amenable to biventricular repair. Echocardiographic imaging from right supraclavicular or suprasternal notch windows can show the course of the SVC and the size of the connection to the right pulmonary artery. TEE imaging at 90 to 110 degrees alignment identifies the right atrium and upper stump of the SVC and then, with rotation of the probe rightward, the SVC-right PA connection. Combined color flow and spectral Doppler evaluate anastomosis patency.[10-12]

Recurrent late postoperative cyanosis may be via collateral venous flow from the SVC to the inferior vena cava (IVC) or from pulmonary arteriovenous fistulae. Echocardiographic contrast detects these extracardiac shunts; after injection into an arm vein, late flow into the left atrium identifies pulmonary arteriovenous fistulae, whereas prompt appearance in the right atrium reveals azygous-venous collaterals to the IVC.[2] Fistulae and venous collaterals are amenable to catheter directed coil embolization.

Corrective Procedures for Simple Lesions

Simple lesions are isolated shunts, obstructive malformations, or regurgitant lesions (Table 44–3). Complex malformations have two or more simple lesions, often with malpositions of veins, chambers, or great arteries and associated cyanosis.[10]

Atrial Septal Defects

ASDs are among the most common unoperated and postoperative congenital heart defects. A secundum ASD, the most common, has conventionally been closed by direct surgical repair with good results even in adults older than 40 years of age.[32-34] Recently, transcatheter device closure for secundum defects of appropriate size and rim for current devices has been successful with a low rate of complications.[35-39] Both TEE and intracardiac echocardiography (ICE) are valuable in guiding proper insertion of ASD closure devices.[40,41] Echocardiographic examination after ASD closure searches for residual shunting, associated mitral abnormalities, pulmonary hypertension, and degree of resolution of right-sided heart chamber enlargement.[10,42] Patch leaks are infrequently seen, provided that severe pulmonary hypertension was not present. A previously sizable shunt will have a decrease in but not necessarily normalization of RV size and increased left ventricular (LV) size plus improved RV and LV myocardial performance index.[42]

Sinus venosus ASD, often associated with anomalous pulmonary venous connections to the SVC, often requires TEE for precise diagnosis (Figs. 44–7 and 44–8). Repair requires patching of the defect with autologous pericardium so as to also baffle the anomalous pulmo-

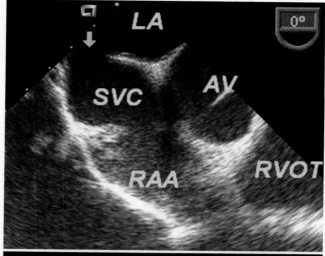

A

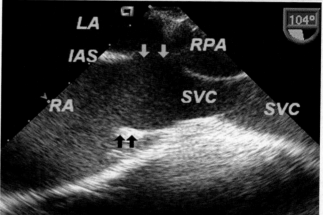

B

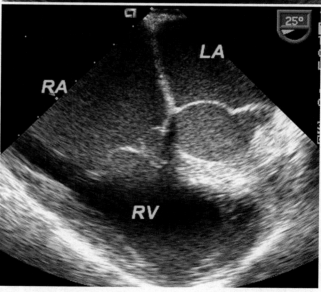

C

Figure 44–7. *Sinus venosus atrial septal defect on preoperative multiplane transesophageal echocardiography that shows a horizontal plane* (A) *and vertical plane* (B) *of the defect* (turquoise arrows) *between the left atrium (LA) and superior vena cava (SVC); the mouth of the SVC to the right atrium (RA) is seen on the vertical plane with the crista terminalis depicted by the black arrows. C, Shows a dilated RA and right ventricle (RV). AV, aortic valve; IAS, interatrial septum; LV, left ventricle; RAA, right atrial appendage; RPA, right pulmonary artery; RVOT, right ventricular outflow tract.*

nary venous drainage to the left atrium via the ASD. TEE is valuable to evaluate the adequacy of patch closure of the defect with attention to possible SVC or pulmonary venous obstruction (Fig. 44–9).

AV canal-type ASD will be considered in the section on complex repairs. A coronary sinus (CS) ASD, the rar-

est form, consists of partial or complete absence of the coronary sinus with connection of the left atrium to the right atrium via the usual location of the coronary sinus ostium, usually with a persistent left SVC that joins the roof of the left atrium.[24] A coronary sinus ASD may be associated with complete AV septal defects or tricuspid atresia (and may first be detected after a Fontan repair).

Ventricular Septal Defects

VSD, a common congenital lesion alone or in combination with other anomalies, may occur anywhere in the ventricular septum. VSD may be classified as membranous, muscular, inlet, outlet, or malalignment. VSD may be characterized as restrictive or nonrestrictive according to whether there is a pressure gradient from left to right ventricle. In adults, substantial left-to-right shunt resulting from a nonrestrictive VSD is rarely a result of pulmonary vascular disease (Eisenmenger's syndrome). Spontaneous closure of perimembranous VSD occurs frequently, mainly by adherence of septal tricuspid leaflet tissue but occasionally by prolapse of an aortic cusp into the defect. TR may develop. AR (especially with outlet supracristal defects) may occur; operative closure of the VSD usually prevents progression. Small defects risk infective endocarditis; once endocarditis occurs, it may be argued that closure of the VSD will diminish subsequent risk. Nine of 296 patients who underwent closure of isolated VSD developed endocarditis; three of the nine had no known residual shunt.[43]

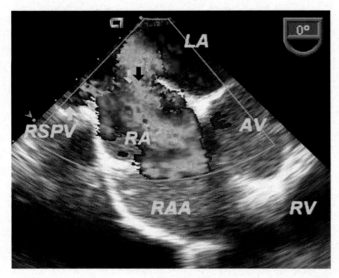

Figure 44-8. *Sinus venosus atrial septal defect (patient in Fig. 44–7) with transesophageal echocardiography color flow imaging showing the shunt from left atrium (LA) into the superior vena cava (SVC) and right atrium (RA) plus shows the entrance partial anomalous pulmonary venous connection of the right superior pulmonary vein (RSPV) into the RA rather than to the LA. AV, aortic valve; RAA, right atrial appendage; RV, right ventricle.*

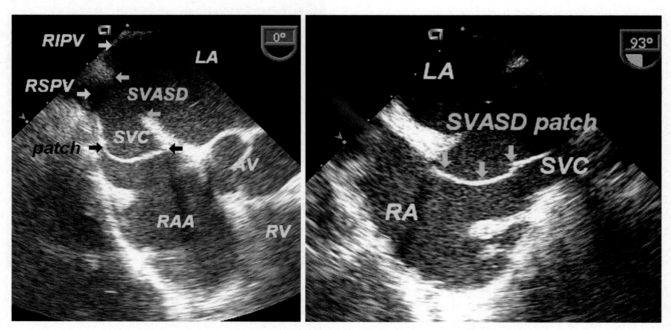

Figure 44-9. *Sinus venosus atrial septal defect with partial anomalous pulmonary venous connection. Intraoperative transesophageal echocardiography in the patient from Figures 44–7 and 44–8 after patch repair (SVASD patch) of the defect where the patch redirects the right superior pulmonary vein (RSPV) flow to the left atrium (LA) via the defect, which is left open. The superior vena cava (SVC) is mildly narrowed but patent. The right inferior pulmonary vein (RIPV) is seen to enter the LA normally. AV, aortic valve; RA, right atrium; RAA, right atrial appendage; RV, right ventricle.*

A simple VSD is closed by right transatrial approach to avoid electrical and mechanical consequences of ventricular incisions. Multiple muscular VSDs may require left ventriculotomy for visualization with the risks of ventricular arrhythmia and ventricular dysfunction. Investigation for patch leaks is imperative, preferably in the operating room (OR) at the time of closure to allow re-repair at that time. Color flow imaging after closure of a large VSD may show previously undetected smaller defects. Transcatheter device closure has been helpful for multiple muscular VSDs, for persistent postoperative VSD in complex conotruncal malformations, acquired postinfarction VSD, and recently is being applied to perimembranous VSD.[44] TEE or intracardiac echocardiography during the procedure decreases fluoroscopy time, determines the device position relative to the defect and adjacent valves and detects residual shunting.

Patent Ductus Arteriosus

PDA is ordinarily detected in childhood, but undiagnosed cases are seen each year during routine echocardiography for other reasons. Operative closure of PDA in the young leaves few residua; in adults, calcification is common and can tear during ligation. Catheter device closure is effective provided the size is less than 7 mm and previous endarteritis at the site has not occurred, which could weaken the vessel wall. TEE is useful in verifying complete uncomplicated closure. Color flow imaging search for residual shunting is essential to confirm success or the need for further device closure and for advice on antiinfective endocarditis prophylaxis.

Bicuspid Aortic Valve

BAV, the most common congenital cardiac malformation, may initially be functionally normal but with time most develop significant stenosis or regurgitation.[45,46] Associated lesions (e.g., VSD, aortic coarctation) should be sought. There is an associated tissue defect of the aortic wall with a tendency to aneurysm and ascending aortic dissection.[47]

Surgical or balloon catheter valvuloplasty can palliate young adults but may cause AR. Most patients ultimately require valve replacement with a mechanical or bioprosthetic valve (homograft or heterograft or Ross procedure) or repair. The Ross procedure (pulmonary autograft to the aortic position, heterograft or homograft to the pulmonary position, with or without reimplantation of the coronary arteries) reduces bioprosthetic degeneration in the aortic position, decreases the reoperation rate, and avoids long-term anticoagulation. Bioprosthetic pulmonary valve degeneration is often well tolerated but late reoperation is likely.

Concerns about pulmonary root autografts in the aortic position include potential for dilation of the wall of the PA with continued exposure to systemic arterial pressure and the development of progressive neoaortic valvular regurgitation. Because cardiopulmonary bypass time is longer than for simple valve replacement, meticulous attention to myocardial preservation and to the technique of coronary reimplantation is required. Precise measurement of the pulmonary and aortic annuli to ensure parity and demonstration of only mild or no pulmonary regurgitation are helpful in deciding on the Ross procedure. Intraoperative TEE achieves these goals and verifies valvular and myocardial function and normal flow at coronary reimplantation sites.

Subaortic Stenosis

Subaortic stenosis, most commonly resulting from a discrete fibromuscular ridge, may be isolated or may complicate perimembranous VSDs before or after closure.[48-50] Aortic valve regurgitation is more likely the closer the membrane is to the aortic valve. Excision of the membrane or fibromuscular ridge in association with focal septal myomectomy is the treatment of choice to reduce the likelihood of recurrence. If associated AR is moderate or less, surgical repair may avoid replacement. Intraoperative TEE verifies relief of obstruction, lack of mitral injury, absence of iatrogenic VSD, and only mild or absent AR.[10] Surveillance for recurrence with stenosis and development or progression of AR is mandatory.

Coarctation of the Aorta

Many survivors of coarctation surgical repair exist; those treated with catheter balloon dilatation or stenting are steadily increasing[51,52] (Figs. 44–10 and 44–11). Residua, sequelae, or complications are frequent and require lifelong follow-up.[6,53-57] BAV, aortic medial defects, abnormal medium sized arterial reactivity, and intracranial aneurysms are commonly associated with coarctation suggesting a common developmental abnormality with diffuse arteriopathy.[6,58-62] Repairs include resection of coarctation with end-to-end anastomosis, patch or subclavian flap aortoplasty, or interposition conduit (see Fig. 44–10). If the condition is symptomatic, repair is best done in infancy; otherwise, timing is elective, but the later in life repair is performed, the more likely persistent hypertension and accelerated coronary artery disease. Suprasternal notch echocardiographic views are useful for imaging of residual or recurrent coarctation narrowing or aneurysm formation. Color flow imaging shows the narrowed site with proximal acceleration; CW Doppler is necessary to show the systolic gradient.[10] Continued diastolic forward flow through the zone of narrowing denotes significant obstruction (see Fig. 44–10). Exercise echocardiographic-Doppler is useful for follow-up of repaired coarctation to detect exercise-related hypertension and coarctation gradients. TEE is more effective than surface echo in evaluating the extent and degree of coarctation. Doppler peak systolic velocity

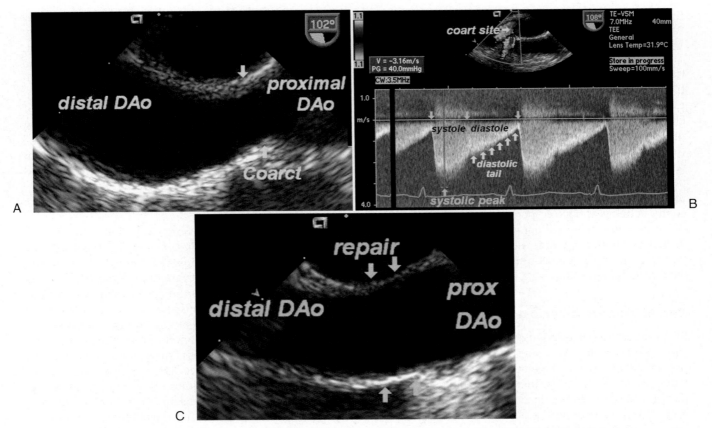

Figure 44–10. *A, Shows the prerepair aortic coarctation anatomy (coarct) with dilatation of the distal portion of the descending aorta (DAo) that was nonpulsatile in contrast to the excessively pulsatile proximal DAo. B, The continuous-wave Doppler, which is not able to be precisely aligned with true angle of the coarctation, as such the peak recorded velocity of 3.16 m/s is an underestimate of the true peak instantaneous systolic gradient; regardless, the continued diastolic tail reveals that this is a significantly obstructive coarctation. C, Shows the postoperative repair with no residual anatomic coarctation.*

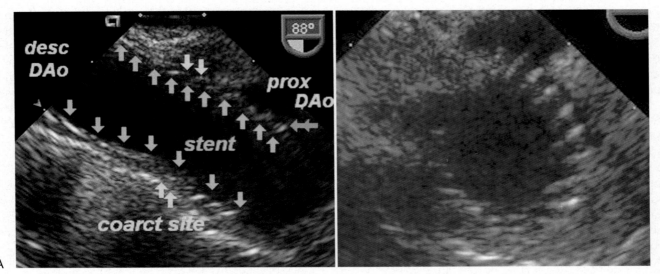

Figure 44–11. *A, A long-axis transesophageal echocardiographic image of the proximal and distal descending aorta (Dao) with only minimal residual narrowing at the coarctation (coarct) site. B, A short-axis image through the upper stent.*

in the descending aorta correlates better with residual narrowing of the aortic isthmus or distal aortic arch than does the systolic blood pressure gradient between the upper and lower limbs; peak velocities greater than 2.5 m/s effectively detect greater than 25% narrowing. Prolongation of anterograde flow during diastole indicates a significant morphologic abnormality (e.g., restenosis or aneurysmal dilation).

Left ventricular hypertrophy (LVH) and LV function should be quantified; associated left-sided obstructive lesions (e.g., BAV, supramitral ring) must be sought. Postoperative endarteritis is rare but can result in a pseudoaneurysm. Balloon catheter dilation and stenting is often applied to recurrent or residual postoperative coarctation but is effective and safe in native coarctation.[51] Intravascular or TEE during balloon dilation or stenting and intraoperatively is useful to show a good result and detect tear or dissection[10] (see Fig. 44–11).

Ebstein Anomaly

Ebstein anomaly has significant morbidity resulting from arrhythmias and right-sided heart failure and even sudden death, possibly as a result of ventricular arrhythmias arising in the pathology of the atrialized right ventricle.[21,63-65] It is characterized by apical displacement of the septal tricuspid leaflet with adherence of the septal and posterior tricuspid leaflets to the underlying myocardium, resulting in downward displacement of the functional annulus and an atrialized RV chamber in its inflow portion. The anterior leaflet is redundant and may have abnormal fenestrations or tethering to ventricular myocardium. The true tricuspid annulus is dilated; TR is usual. Comprehensive echocardiographic definition of the tricuspid anatomy is usually adequate for diagnosis and prediction of suitability for repair and avoids the need for preoperative catheterization.[10,11,66,67] Associated anomalies include patent foramen ovale (PFO), ASD, pulmonary valve stenosis or atresia, VSDs, and TOF. LV function can be decreased.[68] Tricuspid valve repair and annuloplasty with RV plication and right atrial reduction are preferable to valve replacement.[8,69-76] An anterior leaflet that is elongated, untethered, and freely mobile is necessary for best repair; a dysplastic, tethered, or fenestrated valve is undesirable. Intraoperative TEE verifies satisfactory reduction in TR without stenosis, repair of associated defects, and adequacy of myocardial preservation.

Pulmonic Stenosis

Pulmonic stenosis may be subvalvular, valvular, or supravalvular. Management requires elucidation of severity and site of stenosis and of associated abnormalities (e.g., VSD or ASD). Some adults are still seen with previous surgical valvuloplasty for isolated valvular pulmonic stenosis, but balloon catheter dilatation is now usual except in dysplastic valves.[8] Immediately after valvuloplasty the severely hypertrophied right ventricular outflow tract (RVOT) may develop dynamic subpulmonic stenosis manifest by late-peaking high velocities, which typically regress over time. Follow-up of residual stenosis or sequelae of pulmonary regurgitation is required.

Double-chambered right ventricle, a variation of subpulmonic stenosis, resulting from aberrant muscle bundles at the junction of the inlet and outlet portions of the right ventricle proximal to the infundibulum, is often associated with VSD and occasionally subaortic stenosis.[10] Only the inlet right ventricle is under pressure from the pulmonic stenosis and, despite hypertrophy of that portion, the electrocardiogram (ECG) shows remarkably low-voltage RV forces. Resection of the obstructing muscle bundles is indicated when there is more than mild stenosis.

Anomalies of the Coronary Arteries

Coronary artery anomalies include abnormal origin of the right, left main, or left coronary artery branches from one coronary cusp or the other, associated abnormal courses of the anomalous artery, and abnormal connections to other vessels or chambers (e.g., coronary arteriovenous fistula, anomalous origin of the left coronary artery from the PA).[8,10,11] Some are benign; others may result in myocardial ischemia, ventricular dysfunction, arrhythmias, and sudden death. Abnormalities of the course of the coronary arteries seen in TOF or transposition complexes are important in relation to the technique of surgical repair. Echocardiography, particularly TEE, has had success in identifying coronary abnormalities.

Anomalous origin of the left coronary artery from the PA is often associated with myocardial ischemia, congestive heart failure (CHF), MR, and arrhythmias. Surgical approaches include simple ligation of the left coronary artery at its attachment to the pulmonary trunk, saphenous vein or internal mammary artery bypass grafting, direct reimplantation of the coronary to the aorta, and (via a surgically created aortopulmonary window) fashioning of a tunnel that directs blood flow from the aorta to the left coronary ostium. Postoperative imaging of this connection in the operating room is necessary. Long-term echocardiographic evaluation includes quantitation of global and regional LV function and degree of MR.

Repair of Complex Malformations

Atrial Switch Surgery

Atrial switch surgery (e.g., Mustard and Senning) is the reason most people born with complete transposition of the great arteries are adolescents and young adults today[8] (Table 44-4). A combination of atrial septal tissue, pericardium, or synthetic material is used to fash-

TABLE 44-4. Corrective Procedures for "Complex" Malformations

Lesion	Corrective Procedure	Complications and Residual Abnormalities
TGA	Atrial switch surgery (Mustard procedure)	Rhythm and conduction disturbances Baffle leaks and obstruction Vena caval and pulmonary venous obstruction Tricuspid regurgitation Right ventricular dysfunction
TGA	Arterial switch procedure	Supravalvular pulmonic stenosis Supravalvular aortic stenosis (less common) Regional wall motion abnormalities of the left ventricle
Tricuspid atresia or double-inlet single ventricle	Fontan repair (right atrium to pulmonary artery or right ventricle)	Cavoatrial shunting, atrial septal shunting, thrombus, right atrial to pulmonary artery obstruction
Atrioventricular canal defects	Patching of ASD or VSD combined with valve repair	Residual mitral regurgitation Iatrogenic mitral stenosis Subaortic stenosis Patch leaks
Tetralogy of Fallot	VSD patch and relief of infundibular pulmonic stenosis	Pulmonic regurgitation Right ventricular aneurysms (with older repairs) Residual right ventricular outflow obstruction Ventricular septal patch leaks
TGA with VSD and pulmonic stenosis	Rastelli repair (conduit from right ventricle to pulmonary artery with VSD patch directing subaortic flow)	VSD patch leak, subaortic obstruction Prosthetic valve dysfunction
TGA with VSD and subaortic stenosis	Damus-Kaye-Stansel procedure	VSD patch leak Pulmonic regurgitation
Congenitally corrected TGA	Various repairs, depending on associated defects	Left-sided atrioventricular valve regurgitation Heart block Systemic (anatomic right) ventricular systolic dysfunction
Double-outlet right ventricle	Rastelli repair	Obstruction of left ventricular to aortic baffle Residual VSDs Obstruction in right-sided conduit

ASD, atrial septal defect; TGA, transposition of great arteries; VSD, ventricular septal defect.

ion a baffle that reroutes systemic venous return to the subpulmonary morphologic left ventricle and pulmonary venous return to the subaortic morphologic right ventricle (Figs. 44-4, 44-12, and 44-13). The atrial cavity is therefore divided into two portions: an anterior chamber receiving the systemic venous return and a posterior chamber receiving the pulmonary venous return. Sequelae and complications include dysrhythmias (sinus node dysfunction and atrial arrhythmias are frequent) and conduction disturbances, baffle leaks or obstruction, vena caval and pulmonary venous obstruction, TR, dysfunction of the right ventricle and even sudden death.[6,7,77-82] RV dysfunction may be the result of ischemia or fibrosis.[83-85] Residual defects may include pulmonic stenosis, LVOT obstruction, VSD patch leaks, and pulmonary hypertension.

TTE Doppler from multiple windows routinely allows imaging of the intraatrial pulmonary venous and systemic venous portions of the atrial switch[10] (see Figs.

44-4, 44-12, and 44-13). Presystolic flow reversal with atrial contraction into the hepatic venous confluence and SVC provides indirect evidence of caval anastomotic patency. If echocardiographic contrast injected into a peripheral arm vein promptly enters the systemic venous atrium, the superior vena caval anastomosis is patent. In obstruction at the superior vena caval connection, azygous or other venous collaterals to the IVC will cause contrast to first enter the IVC and then the systemic venous atrium. TR may occur with or without diminished RV function. Long-term performance of the systemic right ventricle is often abnormal, especially in the VSD repair subgroup. In addition to evaluating RV size and ejection fraction (EF), measuring RV myocardial performance index is useful.[10,18] TEE may be needed for accurate imaging of the entrance site of all four pulmonary veins and for imaging of the caval junctions with the systemic venous baffle.[11,12] Peripheral venous contrast injections help detect baffle leaks. With

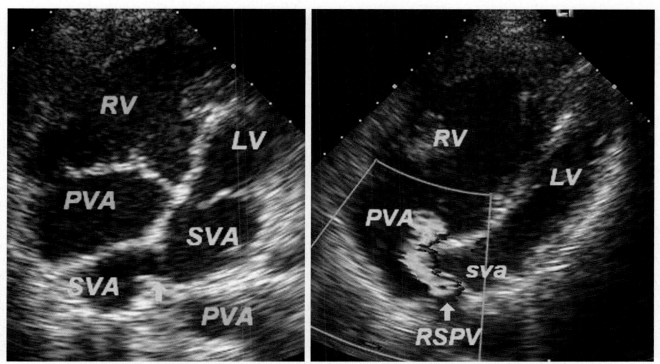

Figure 44–12. *Transthoracic echo of apical views in dextro-transposition of the great arteries (DTGA) late status post-Mustard procedure. A, The alignment with the systemic venous atrium (SVA) with minimal narrowing in the mid-portion (arrow); the pulmonary venous atrium (PVA) wraps around the SVA and thus is seen only in two parts. The SVA connects the vena cavae with the left ventricle (LV) via a portion of the previous left atrium, and the PVA connects the posterior left atrium and pulmonary veins to the right ventricle (RV) via a portion of the previous right atrium. B, The alignment of the image plane with the PVA and demonstrates color flow acceleration at a narrowing of the origin of the right superior pulmonary vein (RSPV). The PVA now courses obliquely across the SVA, which is only incompletely seen. In both images, the subaortic systemic RV is dilated.*

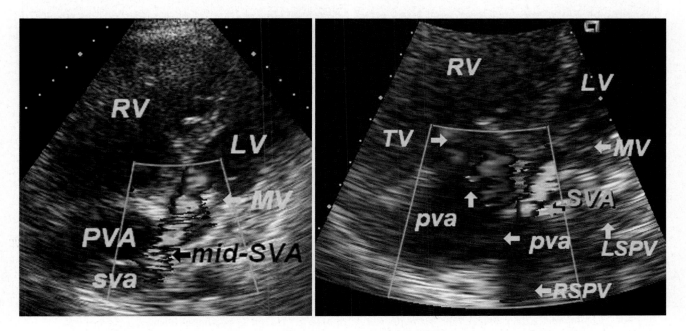

Figure 44–13. *Transthoracic echocardiographic of apical views in dextro-transposition of the great arteries (DTGA) late status post-Mustard procedure show a patent pulmonary venous atrium (PVA) with color flow acceleration of a significantly narrowed mid-portion of the systemic venous atrium (SVA) baffle. LSPV, left superior pulmonary vein; LV, left ventricle; MV, mitral valve; RSPV, right superior pulmonary vein; RV, right ventricle; TV, tricuspid valve.*

TEE, obstructed caval-baffle, mid-baffle, or pulmonary venous baffle sites are diagnosed by an increased peak velocity of continuous systolic and diastolic flow in combination with documented turbulent flow.

Arterial Switch Surgery

Because of late problems after atrial switch surgery, the arterial switch operation (ASO) is preferred when possible. Issues include supravalvular aortic or PA stenosis at the anastomoses and abnormalities of the proximal coronary arterial anastomoses and kinking and of the adequacy of the coronary microcirculation.[86-90] Postoperative echocardiography plays an important role in evaluating the arterial anastomoses. Supravalvular pulmonary stenosis is the most frequent complication of ASO. Neoaortic root dilatation and adequacy of the neoaortic (anatomic pulmonary) valve is a long-term concern. Proximal coronary artery patency can be confirmed by intraoperative echocardiography. Myocardial perfusion defects are relatively common after ASO; coronary events after ASO are not uncommon, usually occur early, and may be a cause of sudden death.[89,91] Regional wall motion abnormalities have been seen after two-stage repairs and correlate with myocardial perfusion defects.[92]

Total Anomalous Pulmonary Venous Connection

Total anomalous pulmonary venous connection (TAPVC) is the result of lack of development of communication of the common pulmonary vein and the left atrium. Most adults arrive already diagnosed and corrected with connection of the common pulmonary vein to the left atrium and closure of the obligatory ASD. After repair of TAPVC, color flow and pulsed-wave (PW) Doppler provide useful information regarding the presence of pulmonary venous obstruction.

Fontan Atrial Surgery

Fontan-type atrial surgery, used when biventricular repair is not possible (e.g., tricuspid atresia or double-inlet single ventricle or complex straddling of AV valves, or crisscross relationships and superior-inferior ventricles—where two functioning ventricles cannot be established) has frequent short-term and long-term morbidity and mortality.[93-96] The several variants of the Fontan repair all result in complete or near-complete (hemi-Fontan) separation of the pulmonary and systemic circulations. The right atrium was an integral part of the original Fontan anatomy. Many adults still

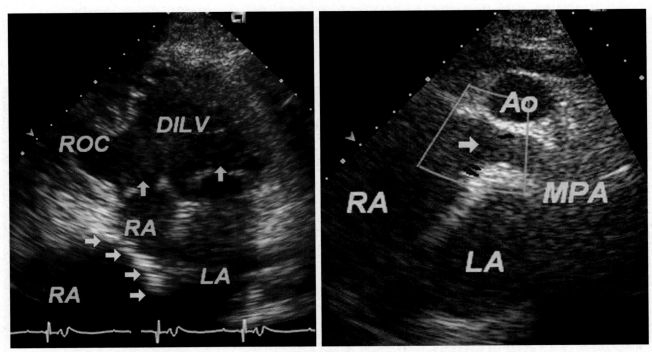

Figure 44–14. *Univentricular atrioventricular connection with double-inlet single left ventricle (DILV) with small residual right outlet chamber (ROC) status postclassic Fontan with right atrial to pulmonary artery connection. The malposed great arteries are not shown here—aorta arises from ROC, pulmonary trunk (now oversewn) from the DILV. A, The patch exclusion* (multiple arrows) *of a portion of the right atrium (RA) that will be part of the Fontan connection. B, A suprasternal view of the RA to pulmonary artery (MPA) pathway. Ao, aortic arch; LA, left atrium; MPA, main pulmonary artery.*

exist that had the old style direct right atrial-PA anastomosis or the modified right atrial RV connection[94] (Figs. 44–14 and 44–15). In high-risk Fontan patients, an adjustable ASD or fenestration may be performed.[97,98] In double-inlet single ventricle, a direct atriopulmonary connection with patch exclusion of the right AV valve was a common modification of the Fontan procedure. Current total cavopulmonary connection (TCPC) is more hemodynamically efficient[99] (Fig. 44–16). The TCPC is either an extracardiac tube connecting IVC to

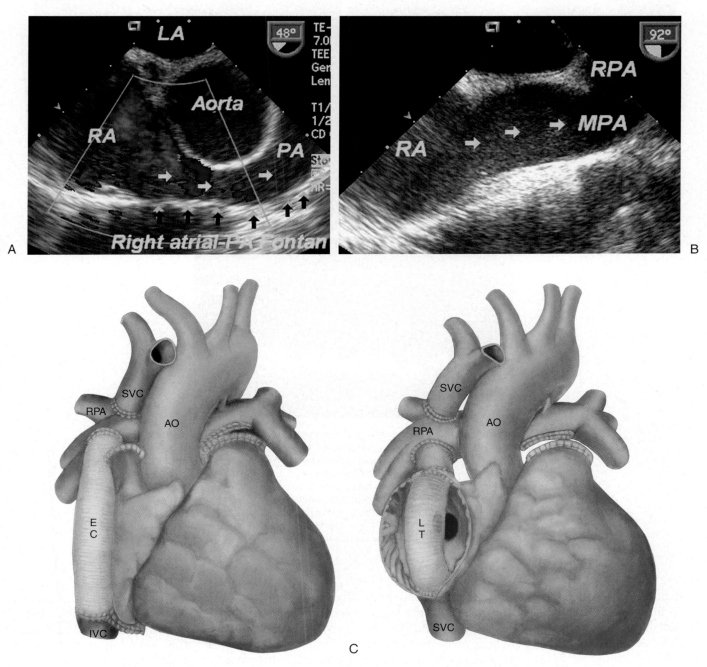

Figure 44–15. A, *Right atrium (RA) to pulmonary artery (PA) Fontan in tricuspid atresia. Transesophageal echocardiography in a horizontal* (A) *and vertical* (B) *plane shows a widely patent connection.* C, *Two variations on Total Cavopulmonary Connection "Fontan" repair procedures with external conduit (EC) type* (right), *internal lateral tunnel (LT)* (left), *with each type of connection draining inferior vena cava (IVC) blood and the reattached superior vena cava (SVC) blood to the RPA. AO, aorta; LA, left atrium; MPA, main pulmonary artery; RPA, right pulmonary artery.*

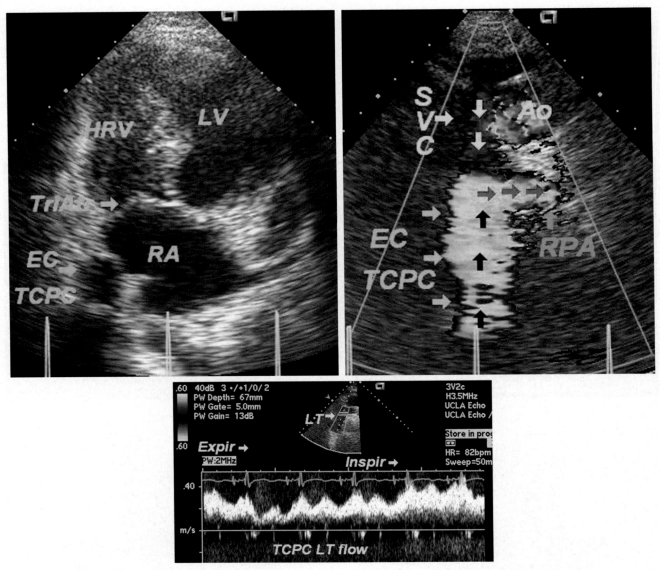

Figure 44–16. *Total cavopulmonary connection (TCPC) using an extracardiac (EC) tube from the inferior vena cava plus a superior vena cava (SVC) anastomosis to the right pulmonary artery (RPA) in a hypoplastic right ventricle (HRV) with tricuspid atresia (TriAtr) in which a biventricular repair was not possible. The four-chamber equivalent transthoracic imaging shows the HRV, TriAtr, the right atrium (RA), and left ventricle (LV). Because of the image plane required to image the EC TCPC, the left atrium is not well seen. The suprasternal notch imaging with color flow shows the flow in the EC TCPC up toward the RPA and the SVC flow rightward of the aortic arch (Ao) down to the RPA. Pulsed-wave Doppler sampling of the ETCPC flow shows normal continuous biphasic flow toward the RPA with respiratory variation. expir, expiration; inspir, inspiration; LT, lateral tunnel.*

right PA plus connection of SVC to pulmonary artery or an intracardiac tube or lateral tunnel using the lateral wall of the right atrium to bring IVC to PA with the SVC attached to right PA.[99-103] In adults whose Fontan circulation is failing or atrial arrhythmias are difficult to control, conversion to either a modern TCPC often with a modified maze procedure with right atrial size reduction is considered. Patch exclusion of the right atrium may result in right AV valve regurgitation. Postoperative subaortic stenosis (dynamic or fixed—at the bulboventricular foramen in single ventricle, at the subaortic

conus in tricuspid atresia with transposed great arteries) must be sought[10-12,104] (Fig. 44–17). The most common complications in the atrial portion of the Fontan circulation include cavoatrial shunting, atrial septal shunting, thrombus, and right atrium to PA obstruction; atrial arrhythmias are frequent.[93,94,96,102,103] Surgical sequelae purposely left behind in high-risk patients include atrial fenestrations and adjustable ASDs.[98]

In adults, right atrial-RV conduits are occasionally seen by TTE examination but right atrial-pulmonary connections can be difficult to visualize[10-12] (see Figs. 44–14

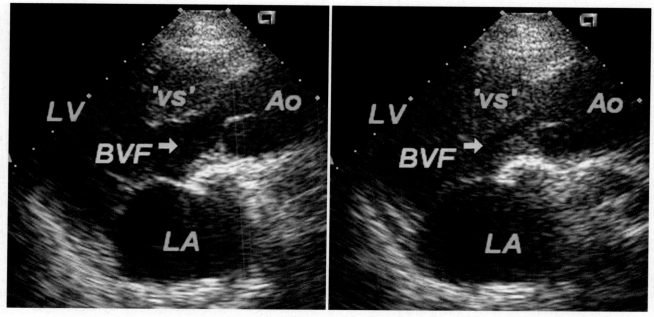

Figure 44–17. Fontan patient with single left ventricle (LV) with the aorta (Ao) arising from a small outlet chamber. End-diastolic (A) and end-systolic (B) frames of the bulboventricular foramen show a mildly narrowed bulboventricular foramen (BVF) in diastole relative to the size of the proximal aorta (AO) with near obliteration of the BVF during systole causing dynamic subaortic stenosis. Note that the aortic valve appears closed in both frames—this was a result of marked systolic flutter with premature closure of the aortic valve resulting from the dynamic BVF obstruction. "Vs" indicates the "ventricular septum," which is a misnomer in that there are not two well-formed ventricles. LA, left atrium.

and 44–15). Evaluation of ventricular hypertrophy and systolic and diastolic function is important as they are determinants of long-term outcome.[105,106] Multiplane TEE consistently images the Fontan anastomosis, although not always with the necessary alignment to allow accurate spectral Doppler assessment of peak velocity profiles[10-12] (see Fig. 44–15).

In the Fontan patient, an important determinant of outcome is the systolic and diastolic function of the systemic ventricle and its AV valve, both of which are readily evaluated by TTE Doppler studies.[104-107] TEE is useful when directed at suspected complications or known residua of the Fontan atrial anatomy (baffle shunts, thrombi, stenotic connections) (see Fig. 44–15).

With no functioning subpulmonary right ventricle in most with the Fontan repair, PA flow shows a biphasic or triphasic pattern with diastolic velocities equal to or greater than systolic, with accentuation of diastolic velocity at the time of right atrial contraction[108] (see Fig. 44–16). Inspiration augments PA flow velocities, and pulmonary and systemic venous flow profiles remain relatively normal in patients with normal left (or single) ventricular function (see Fig. 44–16). Abnormal systemic ventricular performance is reflected in a reduced pulmonary arterial flow pattern velocity with decreased change on inspiration and a predominantly systolic profile.

Intraoperative TEE ensures patent connections and helps size any surgical ASD or fenestration. Postoperative TEE may be required in the intensive care unit (ICU) in Fontan patients to search for known complica-

tions (e.g., increasing PA pressures with decreased cardiac output [CO] and right-sided heart failure resulting from lateral tunnel Fontan thrombus embolization). TEE can also be used in the interventional catheterization laboratory to guide postoperative closure of surgical ASDs or fenestration.

Atrioventricular Septal Defects

Atrioventricular septal defects (AVSDs), also known as AV canal defects, are a group of anomalies that share a defect at the site of the AV septum and abnormalities of the AV valves.[10-12,14] They are considered complex lesions because of the usual association of two or more abnormalities. These defects may be partial (partial endocardial cushion or primum ASDs, cleft mitral leaflet, or inlet VSD) or complete and will usually have been corrected in childhood or adolescence. The usual partial AVSD in adults is a primum ASD plus an anterior mitral leaflet cleft with abnormal chordal attachments to the LVOT and variable degrees of MR. Repair requires primum ASD patching and mitral valve repair. Complete AVSD, rarely first diagnosed in adults, are seen in patients surviving to adulthood after childhood repair. Complete AVSD has a large septal defect with interatrial and interventricular components plus a common AV valve that connects both atria and both ventricles.

Follow-up imaging examines adequacy of mitral repair and amount of regurgitation and presence of iatrogenic mitral stenosis or subaortic stenosis. Subaortic stenosis may be the result of a discrete fibromuscular narrowing or abnormal LVOT attachments of anomalous chords and leaflet tissue or may develop postoperatively because of reduction of LV outflow size as the cleft in the mitral leaflet is apposed.[10] Owing to combined preoperative right and LV volume overload, the size and function of both ventricles must be quantified postoperatively. Occasionally, TR can be substantial and tricuspid valvular repair requires postoperative evaluation. In addition, in complete AVSD repairs, the VSD patch must be evaluated. Some patients, especially those with Down syndrome, can have pulmonary vascular disease; tricuspid and pulmonary regurgitant jets should quantify PA pressure. To minimize significant residual defects (e.g., valvular regurgitation, patch leaks), intraoperative TEE should be used.[10-12]

Biventricular Repairs

Biventricular repairs result in two well-formed functional ventricles with a subpulmonic ventricle and a subaortic ventricle that are able to provide a circulation in series without an admixture of venous and systemic blood. Most complex congenital cardiac malformations amenable to biventricular repair are cyanotic and consist of a mixture of septal defects; obstructive and regurgitant valvular, subvalvular, or supravalvular lesions; and malpositions of the cardiac chambers and great arteries.[8] Anatomic substrates that are typical candidates include TOF, pulmonary atresia with VSD, transposition complexes of the great arteries, and double-outlet ventricles.[8,10] The basic theme includes patch closure of a VSD and reconstitution of ventricular to pulmonary arterial blood flow. If pulmonic stenosis cannot be directly repaired for anatomic or conduction system reasons, the PA must be ligated or the valve oversewn and a conduit placed from the ventricle to PA. Long-term postoperative survival is affected by age at operation, degree of relief of the loading conditions imposed on the ventricular myocardium, myocardial protection during operation, electrophysiologic sequelae, and the durability of prosthetic materials, especially valved or nonvalved conduits.

Tetralogy of Fallot

TOF is the most common complex congenital malformation with cyanosis at birth in which patients live to adulthood because of the length of time that palliative (see Fig. 44–6) and corrective procedures have been available[8] (Figs. 44–1, 44–3, and 44–18 to 44–21). TOF is the result of anterior deviation of the outlet septum with infundibular narrowing and a malaligned VSD. Echocardiography shows the malaligned VSD with aortic override plus a spectrum of RVOT and PA obstructive lesions from mild to complete pulmonary atresia[10-12,14] (see Fig. 44–6). Numerous associated defects

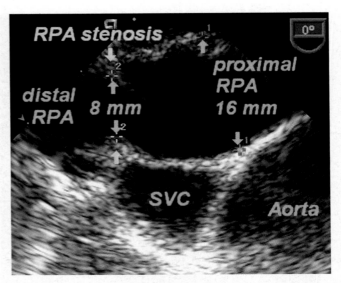

Figure 44–18. Previously repaired tetralogy of Fallot after initial palliation with a right Blalock-Taussig shunt. During pre-cardiopulmonary intraoperative transesophageal echocardiography before pulmonary valve replacement for severe pulmonary valve regurgitation, right pulmonary artery (RPA) stenosis—probably a consequence of the previous Blalock-Taussig shunt—was found, which also underwent repair. SVC, superior vena cava.

must be identified for proper surgical and postoperative management (e.g., ASDs, endocardial cushion abnormalities, Ebstein malformation, muscular VSDs, absent pulmonic valve or left PA, abnormal origin of one PA from the aorta, systemic and pulmonary venous anomalies, discrete subaortic stenosis, right-sided aortic arch, aortopulmonary window, aortopulmonary collaterals, and coronary artery anomalies).[10]

TOF repair includes patch closure of the VSD and usually a RVOT incision to relieve infundibular stenosis (see Figs. 44–1, 44–3, 44–19 and 44–20). The RV incision at times must extend through the pulmonary annulus plus a transannular patch. Pulmonary valve, trunk, or branch artery stenosis should be relieved (see Fig. 44–18). If there is extreme pulmonic stenosis or pulmonary atresia, a valved conduit connects the right ventricle to PA. After TOF repair, long-term concerns focus on the right ventricle and its outflow tract, the pulmonic valve and PA, the left ventricle, the aortic valve and ascending aorta, and electrophysiologic residua and sequelae[6,8,15,26,109-144] (see Figs. 44–1, 44–3, and 44–18 to 44–20).

When repaired in the first 5 years of life, late RV function remains normal in the absence of significant RV outflow obstruction provided low-pressure pulmonic valve regurgitation is only mild to moderate. Severe pulmonic regurgitation causes RV enlargement and failure, and TR, particularly if there is any residual RVOT, pulmonary valve, or pulmonary artery (e.g., branch stenosis) obstruction (see Figs. 44–18 to

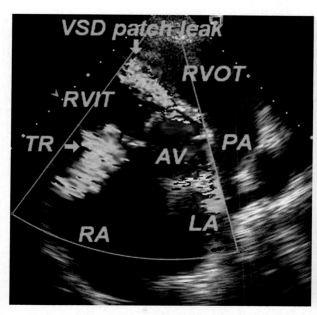

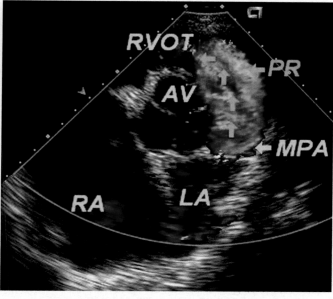

Figure 44-19. *Tetralogy of Fallot late after prior intracardiac repair. Transthoracic echocardiographic parasternal short-axis images. A, Shows residual ventricular septal defect (VSD) patch leak and tricuspid regurgitation (TR). B, Severe pulmonary regurgitation (PR)—the color-flow imaging is shown in diastole with marked wide open laminar diastolic flow from the main pulmonary artery (MPA) back toward the right ventricular outflow tract (RVOT). AV, aortic valve; LA, left atrium; PA, pulmonary artery; RA, right atrium; RVIT, right ventricular inflow tract.*

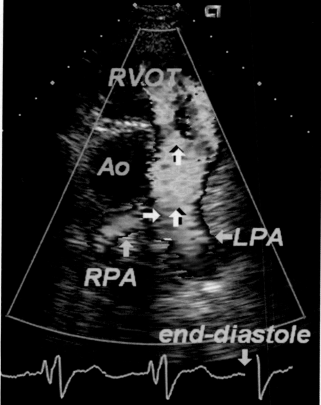

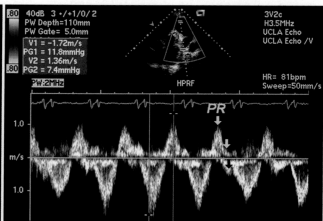

Figure 44-20. *Tetralogy of Fallot late after prior intracardiac repair. A, The short-axis images of severe pulmonary regurgitation with retrograde diastolic flow from the right and left pulmonary artery branches (RPA and LPA, respectively) back toward the right ventricular outflow tract (RVOT). B, The pulsed-wave Doppler sample in the RVOT, which reveals that there is termination of the pulmonary regurgitation (PR) velocity late in diastole with subsequent presystolic reversal consistent with right ventricular restrictive physiology. Ao, aorta.*

44–20). Postoperative RVOT scars and aneurysms may be present and risk ventricular arrhythmias and sudden death (see Fig. 44–1). Two-dimensional echocardiography with color flow and spectral Doppler examine the RV outflow and PA anatomy for obstruction or regurgitation (see Figs. 44–19 and 44–20); CW Doppler tricuspid regurgitant jet velocities reflect RV systolic pressure.[10] VSD leaks, usually eccentric, may occur anywhere along the patch and require color flow imaging for detection (see Fig. 44–19). RV restrictive physiology late after repair of tetralogy is common as detected by Doppler hemodynamics; the atrial filling pressure wave (A wave) contributes to forward pulmonary flow and shortens the duration of pulmonary regurgitation resulting in less RV enlargement and better exercise tolerance[10,106,120,125,145] (see Fig. 44–20). When severe pulmonary regurgitation results in impaired exercise performance, increasing RV size with decreasing RV systolic function and increasing TR, pulmonary valve replacement is necessary. Aerobic capacity has been shown to improve after pulmonary valve replacement for severe pulmonary regurgitation after previous TOF repair even if the RV size and function does not.

Late postoperative LV function in TOF is related to age at the time of repair and to previous volume overload from palliative shunt procedures. Patients with severe cyanotic TOF have decreased left-sided heart volumes and decreased LV ejection fractions related to the reduced pulmonary arterial blood flow. Repair in the first 2 years of life allows LV mass and volume to normalize; with repair after 2 years of age, left-sided heart volumes increase, but LV function remains subnormal. Medial aortic disease can cause a dilated aortic root or trunk (see Fig. 44–3); AR is common and at times has resulted in biventricular failure.[47] Any combination of persistent VSD patch leaks, ventricular to pulmonary outflow obstruction, and significant valvular regurgitation may cause serious ventricular overload. Inadequate operative myocardial preservation or the preexistence of volume overload (as with large palliative shunts before more complete hemodynamic repair) may cause ventricular failure over the long term.[8]

Common Transposition of the Great Arteries

Transposition complexes have each great artery arising from the wrong ventricle (ventriculoarterial discordance). This definition is independent of the spatial relationships of the great arteries and the presence or absence of a subaortic infundibulum. In d-transposition of the great arteries (DTGA), each atrium connects to its anatomically appropriate ventricle (AV concordance), but that ventricle gives rise to an anatomically inappropriate great artery (ventriculoarterial discordance). The aorta arises from the right ventricle (with aortic-mitral discontinuity) and usually sits right of and anterior to the PA, which emerges from the left ventricle. This results in two separate and parallel circulations, and some communication between the two circulations must exist or be made iatrogenically after birth to sustain life.[8]

Echocardiographic imaging must define the course of each of the great arteries and (1) identify the size and location of a VSD, (2) confirm the presence and severity of pulmonic stenosis, (3) detect other shunts, and (4) evaluate the presence and severity of valvular regurgitation.[10-12] Dynamic subvalvular pulmonic stenosis can be the result of systolic anterior mitral motion into the LVOT or dynamic subpulmonic septal contraction with obstruction versus fixed subvalvular stenosis. The pulmonary valve may be the site of obstruction. The location of the obstruction affects surgical planning; if not addressed, these problems contribute to postoperative morbidity and mortality.

Long-term outcome of surgical intervention for DTGA, with or without VSD and pulmonic stenosis depends on the type of repair.[4-6] In the past, most underwent intraatrial baffle procedures (e.g., Mustard or Senning), causing persistence of a systemic subaortic right ventricle and tricuspid valve (see Figs. 44–2, 44–12, and 44–13); in contrast, the ASO is now used and the left ventricle is the systemic ventricle. Rastelli repair (Fig. 44–21), whether for TGA or for double-outlet right ventricle (DORV) with VSD and pulmonary stenosis, uses an external conduit from right ventricle to PA and an intraventricular tunnel via the VSD from left ventricle to

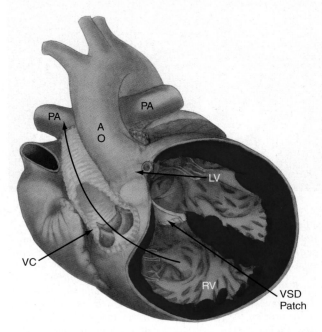

Figure 44–21. Great arteries in Rastelli repair with left ventricle (LV) baffled to aorta (AO) by VSD patch, and right ventricle (RV) baffled to pulmonary artery (PA) by valved conduit (VC).

aorta. An internal tunnel may develop a patch leak or obstruction resulting from kinking or may partially obstruct the chamber through which it transits. Long-term concerns include durability of a bioprosthesis, patency of conduits, VSD patch leaks, and postoperative electrophysiologic residua and sequelae.[8]

The Damus-Kaye-Stansel (DKS) procedure, as applied to DTGA with a VSD without pulmonic stenosis but with subaortic stenosis, consists of end-to-side anastomosis of the proximal PA to aorta, oversewing of the aortic valve or proximal aorta and a VSD patch. The right ventricle is connected to the distal main PA, now separated from the proximal main PA, by a valved conduit. A variation of the DKS is used in single ventricle with transposition of great arteries and subaortic stenosis (bulboventricular foramen obstruction). Imaging of the pulmonary arterial to aortic anastomosis establishes lack of obstruction, pulmonary regurgitation, conduit patency, or VSD patch leaks.

Congenitally Corrected Transposition of the Great Arteries

Congenitally corrected transposition of the great arteries (CCTGA) consists of discordant AV and ventriculoarterial connections with ventricular inversion (right atrium enters the left ventricle via a mitral valve, left atrium enters the right ventricle via a tricuspid valve; left ventricle gives rise to the PA, right ventricle gives rise to the aorta). The AV valves follow their ventricles, revealing the left-sided systemic ventricle as the anatomic right ventricle and vice versa. Echocardiographic crux anatomy shows the left atrioventricular valve (AVV) more apically placed than the right AVV, identifying tricuspid and mitral valves, respectively. The aorta leaves the right ventricle leftward and anterior and left ventricle connects to a rightward and posterior pulmonary trunk, well shown on short-axis parasternal views or angulated apical or subcostal views.[8,10] Associated anomalies include ASD, Ebstein-like abnormality of the left-sided tricuspid valve and TR (physiologically equivalent to MR), VSD, and subvalvar (fixed or dynamic) or valvar pulmonic stenosis. A large VSD with significant pulmonic stenosis or severe systemic AVV regurgitation prompts consideration of surgery. A Rastelli procedure may be used in CCTGA with a VSD and subvalvular pulmonary stenosis. The left ventricle may be connected to the PA via a valved conduit, whereas the right ventricle supplies the aorta once the VSD is patched. The subpulmonary stenosis is often not resected because of the high incidence of complete heart block.

Three issues materially influence long-term postoperative survival: (1) progressive TR, (2) high incidence of heart block often caused by operation, and (3) progressive decrease systemic subaortic morphologic right ventricle function.[6,8,146,147] AVV regurgitation is common preoperatively, is difficult to repair (often requiring replacement instead), may progress postoperatively, poses a continuing risk of endocarditis, and may affect long-term ventricular performance.

Double-Outlet Right Ventricle

DORV, a heterogeneous category, has both great arteries committed to the right ventricle; the VSD may be committed to the aorta (subaortic, infracristal), to the PA (subpulmonic, supracristal), to both (doubly committed, subarterial), or to neither. The VSD location affects the streaming characteristics of blood and degree of cyanosis, and the capacity for and type of repair.[8] The presence or absence of pulmonary stenosis or increased pulmonary vascular resistance is a determinant of outcome. DORV with a subpulmonary VSD and a RV or biventricular pulmonary trunk (Taussig-Bing anomaly) may clinically resemble complete transposition of great arteries with a nonrestrictive VSD. Cyanosis is usually mild initially but progresses as pulmonary vascular resistance rises. Favorable regulation of pulmonary blood flow occasionally establishes adequate, but not excessive, flow, with consequent amelioration of LV volume overload.

Echocardiography must address the spatial relationships between the great arteries, the outflow tract for each artery, the location and type of VSD, and the relationship of the VSD to the aorta. Associated anomalies must be sought (e.g., malpositions, AV canal or septal defects, etc.).

Rastelli repair for DORV with subaortic VSD and pulmonic stenosis consists of an external right ventricle to PA conduit and an intraventricular left ventricle to the aorta via the VSD tunnel. The intraventricular course of the LV to the aortic baffle can be long and kinking may occur; this is best evaluated intraoperatively with TEE. A right ventricle to PA valved conduit can develop obstruction. In DORV of a TOF type with normally related great arteries and a subaortic VSD, the repair may use a septal patch and primary repair of the site of pulmonic stenosis without resort to a conduit. Residual defects in the native ventricular septum or around the patch may be more frequent in repair of DORV than in TOF, presumably because the distance from the VSD to the aorta is greater and more complex as a result of both the proximity of tricuspid valve tissue and anomalies of the ventricular septal musculature. Intramural residual interventricular defects seen after repair of conotruncal malformations, most commonly DORV, are found around the anterior portion of the patch between the neosystemic outflow tract and right ventricle and require careful color flow imaging to detect. In such cases, device occluder placement has reduced the shunt; successful surgical closure may require removal and reattachment of the anterior portion of the patch.

KEY POINTS

- Advances in surgical and catheter treatments have resulted in more adults with CHD than children with CHD in the United States.

- Many adult echocardiographic laboratories are unprepared for the full range of previously operated or complex CHD. Study of these patients should be done where expertise is best, whether in an adult or pediatric laboratory.

- Combined echocardiographic imaging with color flow imaging and spectral Doppler recordings of postoperative CHD provide comprehensive anatomic, functional, and hemodynamic details.

- For best results, imaging and hemodynamic study requires detailed knowledge of (1) the anatomic and hemodynamic faults of the original defect; (2) the types of operative repairs (both past and present) available for each complex of lesions; and, (3) the potential residua, sequelae, and complications of the old and new repairs.

- It is imperative that complementary imaging and hemodynamic modalities (echocardiogram with Doppler and echo-contrast versus magnetic resonance imaging or computed tomography versus cardiac catheterization) be integrated for the most useful elucidation of the specific operated CHD substrate.

REFERENCES

1. Hoffman JI, Kaplan S: The incidence of congenital heart disease. *J Am Coll Cardiol* 39:1890-1900, 2002.
2. Hoffman JI, Kaplan S, Liberthson RR: Prevalence of congenital heart disease. *Am Heart J* 147:425-439, 2004.
3. Warnes CA, Liberthson R, Danielson GK, et al: Task force 1: the changing profile of congenital heart disease in adult life. Care of the adult with congenital heart disease. Presented at the 32nd Bethesda Conference, Bethesda, Maryland, October 2-3, 2000. *J Am Coll Cardiol* 37:1170-1175, 2001.
4. Graham TP Jr: The year in congenital heart disease. *J Am Coll Cardiol* 45:1887-1899, 2005.
5. Graham TP: Jr. The year in congenital heart disease. *J Am Coll Cardiol* 43:2132-2141, 2004.
6. Warnes CA: The adult with congenital heart disease: born to be bad? *J Am Coll Cardiol* 46:1-8, 2005.
7. Williams RG, Pearson GD, Barst RJ, et al: Report of the National Heart, Lung, and Blood Institute Working Group on research in adult congenital heart disease. *J Am Coll Cardiol* 47:701-707, 2006.
8. Perloff JK, Child JS: *Congenital Heart Disease in Adults*, 2nd ed. Philadelphia, WB Saunders, 1998.
9. Child JS, Collins-Nakai RL, Alpert JS, et al: Task force 3: Workforce description and educational requirements for the care of adults with congenital heart disease. Care of the adult with congenital heart disease. Presented at the 32nd Bethesda Conference, Bethesda, Maryland, October 2-3, 2000. *J Am Coll Cardiol* 37:1183-1187, 2001.
10. Child JS: Transthoracic and transesophageal echocardiographic imaging: Anatomic and hemodynamic assessment. In Perloff JK CJ (ed): *Congenital Heart Disease in Adults*, 2nd ed. Philadelphia, WB Saunders, 1998, pp. 91-128.
11. Child JS: Congenital heart disease. In Roelandt JRTC, Pandian NG (eds): *Multiplane Transesophageal Echocardiography*. New York, Churchill Livingstone, 1996, pp. 173-198.
12. Child JS: Atria and related structures. In Roelandt JRTC, Pandian NG (eds): *Multiplane Transesophageal Echocardiography*. New York, Churchill Livingstone, 1996, pp. 139-154.
13. Sahn DJ, Vick GW 3rd: Review of new techniques in echocardiography and magnetic resonance imaging as applied to patients with congenital heart disease. *Heart* 86(Suppl 2):II41-II53, 2001.
14. Child JS: Echo-Doppler and color-flow imaging in congenital heart disease. *Cardiol Clin* 8:289-313, 1990.
15. Eidem BW, O'Leary PW, Tei C, et al: Usefulness of the myocardial performance index for assessing right ventricular function in congenital heart disease. *Am J Cardiol* 86:654-658, 2000.
16. Eidem BW, Tei C, O'Leary PW, et al: Nongeometric quantitative assessment of right and left ventricular function: Myocardial performance index in normal children and patients with Ebstein anomaly. *J Am Soc Echocardiogr* 11:849-856, 1998.
17. Williams RV, Ritter S, Tani LY, et al: Quantitative assessment of ventricular function in children with single ventricles using the Doppler myocardial performance index. *Am J Cardiol* 86:1106-1110, 2000.
18. Salehian O, Schwerzmann M, Merchant N, et al: Assessment of systemic right ventricular function in patients with transposition of the great arteries using the myocardial performance index: Comparison with cardiac magnetic resonance imaging. *Circulation* 110:3229-3233, 2004.
19. Tei C, Dujardin KS, Hodge DO, et al: Doppler echocardiographic index for assessment of global right ventricular function. *J Am Soc Echocardiogr* 9:838-847, 1996.
20. Tei C, Nishimura RA, Seward JB, et al: Noninvasive Doppler-derived myocardial performance index: Correlation with simultaneous measurements of cardiac catheterization measurements. *J Am Soc Echocardiogr* 10:169-178, 1997.
21. Tede NH, Shivkumar K, Perloff JK, et al: Signal-averaged electrocardiogram in Ebstein's anomaly. *Am J Cardiol* 93:432-436, 2004.
22. Vogel M, Derrick G, White PA, et al: Systemic ventricular function in patients with transposition of the great arteries after atrial repair: a tissue Doppler and conductance catheter study. *J Am Coll Cardiol* 43:100-106, 2004.
23. Jamal F, Bergerot C, Argaud L, et al: Longitudinal strain quantitates regional right ventricular contractile function. *Am J Physiol Heart Circ Physiol* 285:H2842-H2847, 2003.
24. Chaliki HP, Mohty D, Avierinos J-F, et al: Outcomes after aortic valve replacement in patients with severe aortic regurgitation and markedly reduced left ventricular function. *Circulation* 106:2687-2693, 2002.
25. Cheung MM, Smallhorn JF, McCrindle BW, et al: Non-invasive assessment of ventricular force-frequency relations in the univentricular circulation by tissue Doppler echocardiography: A novel method of assessing myocardial performance in congenital heart disease. *Heart* 91:1338-1342, 2005.
26. Perloff JK, Natterson PD: Atrial arrhythmias in adults after repair of tetralogy of Fallot. *Circulation* 91:2118-2119, 1995.
27. Nahlawi M, Waligora M, Spies SM, et al: Left ventricular function during and after right ventricular pacing. *J Am Coll Cardiol* 44:1883-1888, 2004.
28. Barber BJ, Batra AS, Burch GH, et al: Acute hemodynamic effects of pacing in patients with Fontan physiology: A prospective study. *J Am Coll Cardiol* 46:1937-1942, 2005.
29. Bacha EA, Zimmerman FJ, Mor-Avi V, et al: Ventricular resynchronization by multisite pacing improves myocardial performance in the postoperative single-ventricle patient. *Ann Thorac Surg* 78:1678-1683, 2004.

30. Janousek J, Tomek V, Chaloupecky VA, et al: Cardiac resynchronization therapy: A novel adjunct to the treatment and prevention of systemic right ventricular failure. *J Am Coll Cardiol* 44:1927-1931, 2004.

31. Child JS, Perloff JK, Kubak B: Infective endocarditis: risks and prophylaxis. In Perloff JK, Child JS (eds): *Congenital Heart Disease in Adults*, 2nd ed. Philadelphia, WB Saunders, 1998, pp. 129-143.

32. Konstantinides S, Geibel A, Olschewski M, et al: A comparison of surgical and medical therapy for atrial septal defect in adults. *N Engl J Med* 333:469-473, 1995.

33. Attie F, Rosas M, Granados N, et al: Surgical treatment for secundum atrial septal defects in patients >40 years old. A randomized clinical trial. *J Am Coll Cardiol* 38:2035-2042, 2001.

34. Attenhofer Jost CH, Connolly HM, Danielson GK, et al: Sinus venosus atrial septal defect: long-term postoperative outcome for 115 patients. *Circulation* 112:1953-1958, 2005.

35. Krumsdorf U, Ostermayer S, Billinger K, et al: Incidence and clinical course of thrombus formation on atrial septal defect and patient foramen ovale closure devices in 1,000 consecutive patients. *J Am Coll Cardiol* 43:302-309, 2004.

36. Chessa M, Carminati M, Butera G, et al: Early and late complications associated with transcatheter occlusion of secundum atrial septal defect. *J Am Coll Cardiol* 39:1061-1065, 2002.

37. Du ZD, Hijazi ZM, Kleinman CS, et al: Comparison between transcatheter and surgical closure of secundum atrial septal defect in children and adults: results of a multicenter nonrandomized trial. *J Am Coll Cardiol* 39:1836-1844, 2002.

38. Masura J, Gavora P, Podnar T: Long-term outcome of transcatheter secundum-type atrial septal defect closure using Amplatzer septal occluders. *J Am Coll Cardiol* 45:505-507, 2005.

39. Vida VL, Barnoya J, O'Connell M, et al: Surgical versus percutaneous occlusion of ostium secundum atrial septal defects: results and cost-effective considerations in a low-income country. *J Am Coll Cardiol* 47:326-331, 2006.

40. Hijazi ZM, Cao Q, Patel HT, et al: Transesophageal echocardiographic results of catheter closure of atrial septal defect in children and adults using the Amplatzer device. *Am J Cardiol* 85:1387-1390, 2000.

41. Mullen MJ, Dias BF, Walker F, et al: Intracardiac echocardiography guided device closure of atrial septal defects. *J Am Coll Cardiol* 41:285-292, 2003.

42. Salehian O, Horlick E, Schwerzmann M, et al: Improvements in cardiac form and function after transcatheter closure of secundum atrial septal defects. *J Am Coll Cardiol* 45:499-504, 2005.

43. Moller JH, Patton C, Varco RL, et al: Late results (30 to 35 years) after operative closure of isolated ventricular septal defect from 1954 to 1960. *Am J Cardiol* 68:1491-1497, 1991.

44. Fu YC, Bass J, Amin Z, et al: Transcatheter closure of perimembranous ventricular septal defects using the new Amplatzer membranous VSD occluder: Results of the U.S. phase I trial. *J Am Coll Cardiol* 47:319-325, 2006.

45. Fedak PWM, Verma S, David TE, et al: Clinical and pathophysiological implications of a bicuspid aortic valve. *Circulation* 106:900-904, 2002.

46. Lewin MB, Otto CM: The bicuspid aortic valve: adverse outcomes from infancy to old age. *Circulation* 111:832-834, 2005.

47. Niwa K, Perloff JK, Bhuta SM, et al: Structural abnormalities of great arterial walls in congenital heart disease: Light and electron microscopic analyses. *Circulation* 103:393-400, 2001.

48. Gersony WM: Natural history of discrete subvalvar aortic stenosis: Management implications. *J Am Coll Cardiol* 38:843-845, 2001.

49. Van Arsdell G, Tsoi K: Subaortic stenosis: at risk substrates and treatment strategies. *Cardiol Clin* 20:421-429, 2002.

50. Oliver JM, Gonzalez A, Gallego P, et al: Discrete subaortic stenosis in adults: Increased prevalence and slow rate of progression of the obstruction and aortic regurgitation. *J Am Coll Cardiol* 38:835-842, 2001.

51. Carr JA: The results of catheter-based therapy compared with surgical repair of adult aortic coarctation. *J Am Coll Cardiol* 47:1101-1107, 2006.

52. Carr JA, Amato JJ, Higgins RS: Long-term results of surgical coarctectomy in the adolescent and young adult with 18-year follow-up. *Ann Thorac Surg* 79:1950-1955; discussion 1955-1956, 2005.

53. Vriend JW, Mulder BJ: Late complications in patients after repair of aortic coarctation: Implications for management. *Int J Cardiol* 101:399-406, 2005.

54. Vriend JW, Zwinderman AH, de Groot E, et al: Predictive value of mild, residual descending aortic narrowing for blood pressure and vascular damage in patients after repair of aortic coarctation. *Eur Heart J* 26:84-90, 2005.

55. Toro-Salazar OH, Steinberger J, Thomas W, et al: Long-term follow-up of patients after coarctation of the aorta repair. *Am J Cardiol* 89:541-547, 2002.

56. Stewart AB, Ahmed R, Travill CM, et al: Coarctation of the aorta life and health 20-44 years after surgical repair. *Br Heart J* 69:65-70, 1993.

57. Cohen M, Fuster V, Steele PM, et al: Coarctation of the aorta. Long-term follow-up and prediction of outcome after surgical correction. *Circulation* 80:840-845, 1989.

58. Warnes CA: Bicuspid aortic valve and coarctation: Two villains part of a diffuse problem. *Heart* 89:965-966, 2003.

59. Boyum J, Fellinger EK, Schmoker JD, et al: Matrix metalloproteinase activity in thoracic aortic aneurysms associated with bicuspid and tricuspid aortic valves. *J Thorac Cardiovasc Surg* 127:686-691, 2004.

60. Celermajer DS, Greaves K: Survivors of coarctation repair: fixed but not cured. *Heart* 88:113-114, 2002.

61. von Kodolitsch Y, Aydin MA, Koschyk DH, et al: Predictors of aneurysmal formation after surgical correction of aortic coarctation. *J Am Coll Cardiol* 39:617-624, 2002.

62. Vriend JW, de Groot E, Mulder BJ: Limited effect of early repair on carotid arterial wall stiffness in adult post-coarctectomy patients: In response to the article by Heger M, Willfort A, Neunteufl T, Rosenhek R, Gabriel H, Wollenek G, Wimmer M, Maurer G, Baumgartner H. Vascular dysfunction after coarctation repair is related to the age at surgery. *Int J Cardiol* 100:335-336, 2005.

63. Attie F, Rosas M, Rijlaarsdam M, et al: The adult patient with Ebstein anomaly. Outcome in 72 unoperated patients. *Medicine (Baltimore)* 79:27-36, 2000.

64. Celermajer DS, Bull C, Till JA, et al: Ebstein's anomaly: presentation and outcome from fetus to adult. *J Am Coll Cardiol* 23:170-176, 1994.

65. Zuberbuhler JR, Allwork SP, Anderson RH: The spectrum of Ebstein's anomaly of the tricuspid valve. *J Thorac Cardiovasc Surg* 77:202-211, 1979.

66. Shiina A, Seward JB, Edwards WD, et al: Two-dimensional echocardiographic spectrum of Ebstein's anomaly: Detailed anatomic assessment. *J Am Coll Cardiol* 3:356-370, 1984.

67. Shiina A, Seward JB, Tajik AJ, et al: Two-dimensional echocardiographic—surgical correlation in Ebstein's anomaly: Preoperative determination of patients requiring tricuspid valve plication vs replacement. *Circulation* 68:534-544, 1983.

68. Benson LN, Child JS, Schwaiger M, et al: Left ventricular geometry and function in adults with Ebstein's anomaly of the tricuspid valve. *Circulation* 75:353-359, 1987.

69. Chauvaud S: Ebstein's malformation. Surgical treatment and results. *Thorac Cardiovasc Surg* 48:220-223, 2000.

70. Augustin N, Schmidt-Habelmann P, Wottke M, et al: Results after surgical repair of Ebstein's anomaly. *Ann Thorac Surg* 63:1650-1656, 1997.

71. Augustin N, Schreiber C, Lunge R: Valve preserving treatment of Ebstein's anomaly: Perioperative and follow-up results. *Thorac Cardiovasc Surg* 48:316, 2000.

72. Knott-Craig CJ, Overholt ED, Ward KE, et al: Neonatal repair of Ebstein's anomaly: Indications, surgical technique, and medium-term follow-up. *Ann Thorac Surg* 69:1505-1510, 2000.

73. Knott-Craig CJ, Overholt ED, Ward KE, et al: Repair of Ebstein's anomaly in the symptomatic neonate: An evolution of technique with 7-year follow-up. *Ann Thorac Surg* 73:1786-1792; discussion 1792-1783, 2002.

74. Mair DD, Seward JB, Driscoll DJ, et al: Surgical repair of Ebstein's anomaly: Selection of patients and early and late operative results. *Circulation* 72:II70-II76, 1985.

75. Quaegebeur JM, Sreeram N, Fraser AG, et al: Surgery for Ebstein's anomaly: the clinical and echocardiographic evaluation of a new technique. *J Am Coll Cardiol* 17:722-728, 1991.

76. Pressley JC, Wharton JM, Tang AS, et al: Effect of Ebstein's anomaly on short- and long-term outcome of surgically treated patients with Wolff-Parkinson-White syndrome. *Circulation* 86:1147-1155, 1992.

77. Kammeraad JA, van Deurzen CH, Sreeram N, et al: Predictors of sudden cardiac death after Mustard or Senning repair for transposition of the great arteries. *J Am Coll Cardiol* 44:1095-1102, 2004.

78. Sarkar D, Bull C, Yates R, et al: Comparison of long-term outcomes of atrial repair of simple transposition with implications for a late arterial switch strategy. *Circulation* 100(19 suppl): II176-II181, 1999.

79. Wilson NJ, Clarkson PM, Barratt-Boyes BG, et al: Long-term outcome after the mustard repair for simple transposition of the great arteries. 28-year follow-up. *J Am Coll Cardiol* 32:758-765, 1998.

80. Puley G, Siu S, Connelly M, et al: Arrhythmia and survival in patients >18 years of age after the mustard procedure for complete transposition of the great arteries. *Am J Cardiol* 83:1080-1084, 1999.

81. Gelatt M, Hamilton RM, McCrindle BW, et al: Arrhythmia and mortality after the Mustard procedure: a 30-year single-center experience. *J Am Coll Cardiol* 29:194-201, 1997.

82. Gatzoulis MA, Walters J, McLaughlin PR, et al: Late arrhythmia in adults with the mustard procedure for transposition of great arteries: a surrogate marker for right ventricular dysfunction? *Heart* 84:409-415, 2000.

83. Babu-Narayan SV, Goktekin O, Moon JC, et al: Late gadolinium enhancement cardiovascular magnetic resonance of the systemic right ventricle in adults with previous atrial redirection surgery for transposition of the great arteries. *Circulation* 111:2091-2098, 2005.

84. Millane T, Bernard EJ, Jaeggi E, et al: Role of ischemia and infarction in late right ventricular dysfunction after atrial repair of transposition of the great arteries. *J Am Coll Cardiol* 35:1661-1668, 2000.

85. Lubiszewska B, Gosiewska E, Hoffman P, et al: Myocardial perfusion and function of the systemic right ventricle in patients after atrial switch procedure for complete transposition: Long-term follow-up. *J Am Coll Cardiol* 36:1365-1370, 2000.

86. Losay J, Hougen TJ: Treatment of transposition of the great arteries. *Curr Opin Cardiol* 12:84-90, 1997.

87. Losay J, Touchot A, Serraf A, et al: Late outcome after arterial switch operation for transposition of the great arteries. *Circulation* 104(suppl 1):I121-I126, 2001.

88. Schwartz ML, Gauvreau K, del Nido P, et al: Long-term predictors of aortic root dilation and aortic regurgitation after arterial switch operation. *Circulation* 110(suppl 1):II128-II132, 2004.

89. Legendre A, Losay J, Touchot-Kone A, et al: Coronary events after arterial switch operation for transposition of the great arteries. *Circulation* 108(suppl 1):II186-II190, 2003.

90. Oskarsson G, Pesonen E, Munkhammar P, et al: Normal coronary flow reserve after arterial switch operation for transposition of the great arteries: An intracoronary Doppler guidewire study. *Circulation* 106:1696-1702, 2002.

91. Rickers C, Sasse K, Buchert R, et al: Myocardial viability assessed by positron emission tomography in infants and children after the arterial switch operation and suspected infarction. *J Am Coll Cardiol* 36:1676-1683, 2000.

92. De Caro E, Ussia GP, Marasini M, et al: Transoesophageal atrial pacing combined with transthoracic two dimensional echocardiography: Experience in patients operated on with arterial switch operation for transposition of the great arteries. *Heart* 89:91-95, 2003.

93. van den Bosch AE, Roos-Hesselink JW, Van Domburg R, et al: Long-term outcome and quality of life in adult patients after the Fontan operation. *Am J Cardiol* 93:1141-1145, 2004.

94. Gates RN, Laks H, Drinkwater DC Jr, et al: The Fontan procedure in adults. *Ann Thorac Surg* 63:1085-1090, 1997.

95. Gersony DR, Gersony WM: Management of the postoperative Fontan patient. *Prog Pediatr Cardiol* 17:73-79, 2003.

96. Veldtman GR, Nishimoto A, Siu S, et al: The Fontan procedure in adults. *Heart* 86:330-335, 2001.

97. Thompson LD, Petrossian E, McElhinney DB, et al: Is it necessary to routinely fenestrate an extracardiac fontan? *J Am Coll Cardiol* 34:539-544, 1999.

98. Laks H, Pearl JM, Haas GS, et al: Partial Fontan: advantages of an adjustable interatrial communication. *Ann Thorac Surg* 52:1084-1094; discussion 1094-1085, 1991.

99. de Zelicourt DA, Pekkan K, Wills L, et al: In vitro flow analysis of a patient-specific intraatrial total cavopulmonary connection. *Ann Thorac Surg* 79:2094-2102, 2005.

100. Pearl JM, Laks H, Stein DG, et al: Total cavopulmonary anastomosis versus conventional modified Fontan procedure. *Ann Thorac Surg* 52:189-196, 1991.

101. Kuroczynski W, Kampmann C, Choi YH, et al: The Fontan-operation: from intra- to extracardiac procedure. *Cardiovasc Surg* 11:70-74, 2003.

102. Azakie A, McCrindle BW, Van Arsdell G, et al: Extracardiac conduit versus lateral tunnel cavopulmonary connections at a single institution: Impact on outcomes. *J Thorac Cardiovasc Surg* 122:1219-1228, 2001.

103. Mavroudis C, Backer CL, Deal BJ, et al: Total cavopulmonary conversion and maze procedure for patients with failure of the Fontan operation. *J Thorac Cardiovasc Surg* 122:863-871, 2001.

104. Lan YT, Chang RK, Laks H: Outcome of patients with double-inlet left ventricle or tricuspid atresia with transposed great arteries. *J Am Coll Cardiol* 43:113-119, 2004.

105. Border WL, Syed AU, Michelfelder EC, et al: Impaired systemic ventricular relaxation affects postoperative short-term outcome in Fontan patients. *J Thorac Cardiovasc Surg* 126:1760-1764, 2003.

106. Tede NH, Child JS: Diastolic dysfunction in patients with congenital heart disease. *Cardiol Clin* 18:491-499, 2000.

107. Cheung YF, Penny DJ, Redington AN: Serial assessment of left ventricular diastolic function after Fontan procedure. *Heart* 83:420-424, 2000.

108. Di Sessa TG, Child JS, Perloff J, et al: Systemic venous and pulmonary arterial flow patterns after Fontan's procedure for tricuspid atresia or single ventricle. *Circulation* 70:989-902, 1984.

109. Niwa K, Siu SC, Webb GD, et al: Progressive aortic root dilation in adults late after repair of tetralogy of Fallot. *Circulation* 106:1374-1378, 2002.

110. Warnes CA, Child JS: Aortic root dilatation after repair of tetralogy of Fallot: Pathology from the past? *Circulation* 106:1310-1311, 2002.

111. Roest AAW, de Roos A, Lamb HJ, et al: Tetralogy of Fallot: Postoperative delayed recovery of left ventricular stroke volume after physical exercise—Assessment with fast MR imaging. *Radiology* 226:278-284, 2003.

112. Roos-Hesselink J, Perlroth MG, McGhie J, et al: Atrial arrhythmias in adults after repair of tetralogy of Fallot. Correlations

with clinical, exercise, and echocardiographic findings. *Circulation* 91:2214-2219, 1995.

113. Murphy JG, Gersh BJ, Mair DD, et al: Long-term outcome in patients undergoing surgical repair of tetralogy of Fallot. *N Engl J Med* 329:593-599, 1993.

114. Mahle WT, Parks WJ, Fyfe DA, et al: Tricuspid regurgitation in patients with repaired Tetralogy of Fallot and its relation to right ventricular dilatation. *Am J Cardiol* 92:643-645, 2003.

115. Lucron H, Marcon F, Bosser G, et al: Induction of sustained ventricular tachycardia after surgical repair of tetralogy of Fallot. *Am J Cardiol* 83:1369-1373, 1999.

116. Khairy P, Landzberg MJ, Gatzoulis MA, et al: Value of programmed ventricular stimulation after tetralogy of Fallot repair: A multicenter study. *Circulation* 109:1994-2000, 2004.

117. Joffe H, Georgakopoulos D, Celermajer DS, et al: Late ventricular arrhythmia is rare after early repair of tetralogy of Fallot. *J Am Coll Cardiol* 23:1146-1150, 1994.

118. Helbing WA, Roest AA, Niezen RA, et al: ECG predictors of ventricular arrhythmias and biventricular size and wall mass in tetralogy of Fallot with pulmonary regurgitation. *Heart* 88:515-519, 2002.

119. Hokanson JS, Moller JH: Significance of early transient complete heart block as a predictor of sudden death late after operative correction of tetralogy of Fallot. *Am J Cardiol* 87:1271-1277, 2001.

120. Helbing WA, Niezen RA, Le Cessie S, et al: Right ventricular diastolic function in children with pulmonary regurgitation after repair of tetralogy of Fallot: Volumetric evaluation by magnetic resonance velocity mapping. *J Am Coll Cardiol* 28:1827-1835, 1996.

121. Hazekamp MG, Kurvers MMJ, Schoof PH, et al: Pulmonary valve insertion late after repair of Fallot's tetralogy. *Eur J Cardiothorac Surg* 19:667-670, 2001.

122. Harrison DA, Siu SC, Hussain F, et al: Sustained atrial arrhythmias in adults late after repair of tetralogy of Fallot. *Am J Cardiol* 87:584-588, 2001.

123. Gatzoulis MA: Tetralogy of Fallot. In Gatzoulis MA, Webb GD, Daubeney PEF (eds): *Diagnosis and Management of Adult Congenital Heart Disease.* St. Louis, Churchill Livingstone, 2003, pp. 315-326.

124. Gatzoulis MA, Balaji S, Webber SA, et al: Risk factors for arrhythmia and sudden cardiac death late after repair of tetralogy of Fallot: A multicentre study. *Lancet* 356:975-981, 2000.

125. Gatzoulis MA, Clark AL, Cullen S, et al: Right ventricular diastolic function 15 to 35 years after repair of tetralogy of Fallot. Restrictive physiology predicts superior exercise performance. *Circulation* 91:1775-1781, 1995.

126. El Rahman MYA, Abdul-Khaliq H, Vogel M, et al: Relation between right ventricular enlargement, QRS duration, and right ventricular function in patients with tetralogy of Fallot and pulmonary regurgitation after surgical repair. *Heart* 84:416-420, 2000.

127. Dittrich S, Vogel M, Dahnert I, et al: Surgical repair of tetralogy of Fallot in adults today. *Clin Cardiol* 22:460-464, 1999.

128. Dodds GA, III, Warnes CA, Danielson GK: Aortic valve replacement after repair of pulmonary atresia and ventricular septal defect or tetralogy of Fallot. *J Thorac Cardiovasc Surg* 113:736-741, 1997.

129. Discigil B, Dearani JA, Puga FJ, et al: Late pulmonary valve replacement after repair of tetralogy of Fallot. *J Thorac Cardiovasc Surg* 121:344-351, 2001.

130. Daliento L, Folino AF, Menti L, et al: Adrenergic nervous activity in patients after surgical correction of tetralogy of Fallot. *J Am Coll Cardiol* 38:2043-2047, 2001.

131. Chandar JS, Wolff GS, Garson A Jr, et al: Ventricular arrhythmias in postoperative tetralogy of Fallot. *Am J Cardiol* 65:655-661, 1990.

132. Chaturvedi RR, Shore DF, Lincoln C, et al: Acute right ventricular restrictive physiology after repair of tetralogy of Fallot: Association with myocardial injury and oxidative stress. *Circulation* 100:1540-1547, 1999.

133. Bricker JT: Sudden death and tetralogy of Fallot. Risks, markers, and causes. *Circulation* 92:158-159, 1995.

134. Bacha EA, Scheule AM, Zurakowski D, et al: Long-term results after early primary repair of tetralogy of Fallot. *J Thorac Cardiovasc Surg* 122:154-161, 2001.

135. Ghai A, Silversides C, Harris L, et al: Left ventricular dysfunction is a risk factor for sudden cardiac death in adults late after repair of tetralogy of Fallot. *J Am Coll Cardiol* 40:1675-1680, 2002.

136. Geva T, Sandweiss BM, Gauvreau K, et al: Factors associated with impaired clinical status in long-term survivors of tetralogy of Fallot repair evaluated by magnetic resonance imaging. *J Am Coll Cardiol* 43:1068-1074, 2004.

137. Abd El Rahman MY, Hui W, Yigitbasi M, et al: Detection of left ventricular asynchrony in patients with right bundle branch block after repair of tetralogy of Fallot using tissue-Doppler imaging-derived strain. *J Am Coll Cardiol* 45:915-921, 2005.

138. Davlouros PA, Kilner PJ, Hornung TS, et al: Right ventricular function in adults with repaired tetralogy of Fallot assessed with cardiovascular magnetic resonance imaging: detrimental role of right ventricular outflow aneurysms or akinesia and adverse right-to-left ventricular interaction. *J Am Coll Cardiol* 40:2044-2052, 2002.

139. Davos CH, Davlouros PA, Wensel R, et al: Global impairment of cardiac autonomic nervous activity late after repair of tetralogy of Fallot. *Circulation* 106(suppl 1):I69-I75, 2002.

140. Frigiola A, Redington AN, Cullen S, et al: Pulmonary regurgitation is an important determinant of right ventricular contractile dysfunction in patients with surgically repaired tetralogy of Fallot. *Circulation* 110(suppl 1):II153-II157, 2004.

141. Tulevski, II, Hirsch A, Dodge-Khatami A, et al: Effect of pulmonary valve regurgitation on right ventricular function in patients with chronic right ventricular pressure overload. *Am J Cardiol* 92:113-116, 2003.

142. Vliegen HW, van Straten A, de Roos A, et al: Magnetic resonance imaging to assess the hemodynamic effects of pulmonary valve replacement in adults late after repair of tetralogy of Fallot. *Circulation* 106:1703-1707, 2002.

143. Babu-Narayan SV, Kilner PJ, Li W, et al: Ventricular fibrosis suggested by cardiovascular magnetic resonance in adults with repaired tetralogy of Fallot and its relationship to adverse markers of clinical outcome. *Circulation* 113:405-413, 2006.

144. Giannopoulos NM, Chatzis AC, Bobos DP, et al: Tetralogy of Fallot: influence of right ventricular outflow tract reconstruction on late outcome. *Int J Cardiol* 97(suppl 1):87-90, 2004.

145. van Straten A, Vliegen HW, Lamb HJ, et al: Time course of diastolic and systolic function improvement after pulmonary valve replacement in adult patients with tetralogy of Fallot. *J Am Coll Cardiol* 46:1559-1564, 2005.

146. Graham TP, Jr., Bernard YD, Mellen BG, et al: Long-term outcome in congenitally corrected transposition of the great arteries: a multi-institutional study. *J Am Coll Cardiol* 36:255-261, 2000.

147. Beauchesne LM, Warnes CA, Connolly HM, et al: Outcome of the unoperated adult who presents with congenitally corrected transposition of the great arteries. *J Am Coll Cardiol* 40:285-290, 2002.

Chapter 45

Cardiac Tumors

CHARLES J. BRUCE, MD, MBChB

The author thanks Bridgette A. Wagner for her assistance with this chapter.

Background

Although cardiac tumors are rare with an autopsy frequency of only 0.001% to 0.03%,[1,2] they represent an important group of cardiovascular abnormalities because an early and accurate diagnosis may permit a curative procedure or in some circumstances, may even avoid unnecessary surgery.[3-5] Before the introduction of two-dimensional (2D) echocardiography in the 1970s, antemortem diagnosis of cardiac tumors was exceptionally unusual.[6] However, with the advent of 2D transthoracic echocardiography (TTE), the ability to identify cardiac tumors antemortem has been possible. Moreover, antemortem diagnosis of cardiac masses and tumors has steadily increased. This has been brought about by improvements in imaging technology including higher frequency transthoracic imaging transducers, harmonic imaging, and refinements in transesophageal echocardiography (TEE), including multiplane TEE and three-dimensional (3D) imaging.[7,8] Echocardiography is well suited as the initial imaging modality in patients suspected of having a cardiac tumor because it is a simple noninvasive technique with widespread availability and relatively low cost (Table 45–1). Nevertheless, other imaging modalities including computed tomography (CT) and magnetic resonance imaging (MRI) do provide additional diagnostic information and should be seen as ancillary complementary techniques[9] because they can provide information for staging and treatment planning, particularly when surgical resection is being considered.[10]

Patients with cardiac tumors may be diagnosed with cardiovascular related or constitutional symptoms. However, more often than not, a cardiac mass is discovered incidentally during an echocardiographic examination performed for an unrelated indication. These incidental masses usually represent thrombi or vegetations; often occurring in a particular clinical milieu with associated unique concomitant echocardiographic abnormalities.[5] If a mass is indeed a tumor, it is most likely malignant secondary to a known malignant process elsewhere, usually from the breast, lung, or malignant melanoma. Much less likely, the mass represents a primary cardiac tumor. In this case it is most likely benign, with a nearly 50% likelihood of being a myxoma. Malignant primary cardiac tumors are rare and represent only approximately one quarter of primary cardiac tumors. These are most often a variety of sarcoma.

TABLE 45–1. Echocardiography in the Evaluation, Diagnosis, and Treatment of Cardiac Tumors

A. Evaluation of Cardiac Masses
Normal variant anatomy
Nontumor masses and disorders mimicking tumors
  Thrombi
  Vegetation
  Infiltrative disorder
  Device hardware

B. Diagnosis of Tumor
Morphology
  Location
  Attachment site
  Mobility
  Size
  Shape
Hemodynamic impact

C. Guiding Interventions
Percutaneous biopsy
Pericardiocentesis
Intraoperative assessment pre-CPB and post-CPB

CPB, cardiopulmonary bypass.

Clinical symptoms and signs are often determined by location of the tumor rather than its histologic type.[11,12] Thus, the clinical significance of a benign tumor may be just as important as a malignant type. Benign tumors may be locally invasive impairing myocardial contractility or causing valve dysfunction presenting with heart failure or resulting in systemic or pulmonary embolism, conduction system disease, or fatal arrhythmias. Often, tumors are diagnosed with pericardial effusions with or without tamponade, others may be diagnosed with constitutional or systemic symptoms.

The benefit of echocardiography lies in its ability to demonstrate precise anatomic details and pathology. It delineates the morphologic appearance, location and motion of tumors, and determines the hemodynamic consequences of the tumor, if any.[13] The sensitivity of echocardiography is greatest for endocardial lesions where the contrast between the tumor and the echolucent chamber is greatest, permitting accurate characterization of the size and mobility of the mass. Intramyocardial lesions are less well appreciated, whereas pericardial tumors are the most difficult to detect, mainly because of the increased pericardial echodensity and its far-field position. MRI and/or CT offer benefits over echocardiography in defining lesions in these locations[14] and are also helpful in staging tumors, assessing degree of mural infiltration, detecting pericardial involvement, and presence of tumor extension or metastases (Table 45–2).

TTE and TEE have unique attributes and limitations when evaluating cardiac tumors. Although the availability of TTE is widespread and is simpler to perform, multiplane TEE generates higher resolution images of structures, particularly near the esophagus. It is thus not only better suited to detect tumors in the superior vena cava (SVC), right atrium, pulmonary arteries (PAs), left atrium, and descending thoracic aorta but is also helpful to distinguish these masses from thrombi and vegetations.[15,16] Overall, TEE has better sensitivity and specificity than TTE, especially when identifying smaller tumors.[17] It is also particularly useful in distinguishing true pathology from normal or normal-variant cardiac anatomy, for example, a prominent crista terminalis or lipomatous hypertrophy of the interatrial septum.[4] However, TEE is not as good at identifying left ventricular (LV) apical masses and if this is a clinical concern, TTE should be performed.[15,18]

The following discussion reviews the clinical scope of cardiac tumors and their incidence. A clinical classification is presented and the echocardiographic and pathologic correlation of the most common individual tumors is addressed in descending order of their prevalence. Alternative or complementary imaging techniques are also briefly discussed. Finally, conditions mimicking cardiac tumors and newer, emerging echocardiographic technologies with potential to better evaluate cardiac tumors are also discussed.

TABLE 45-2. Diagnostic Techniques for the Diagnosis of Cardiac Tumors

	Radiography	CT	Angiography	MRI	Echocardiography
Primary Benign					
Myxoma	+	++	+++	++++	+++++
Pericardial cyst	++	+++	0	+++++	+
Lipoma	+	+++	+	+++++	+++
Fibroelastoma	0	0	0	+++	+++++
Rhabdomyoma	0	+	+	++++	+++++
Fibroma	0	+	+	++++	++++
Primary Malignant					
Sarcomas	+	++	++	+++++	+++
Mesotheliomas	+	+++	+	+++++	++
Lymphomas	++	+++	+	+++++	++
Secondary Tumors					
Direct extension	+	+++	++	+++++	+++
Venous extension	0	+	+++	++++	++++
Metastatic spread	+	++	+	++++	++

0, of no use; +, of limited use; ++, may be of use; +++, useful; ++++, very useful; +++++, preferred diagnostic tool.
Adapted from Salcedo EE, Cohen GI, White RD, Davison MB: *Curr Probl Cardiol* 17:73-137, 1992.

Cardiac Tumors: Scope of the Problem

Primary cardiac tumors are rare entities with an autopsy frequency ranging from 0.001% to 0.03%.[19] Three quarters of these tumors are benign with nearly half the benign tumors representing myxomas.[20-24] The remaining benign tumors in descending order of frequency include lipomas, papillary fibroelastomas, and rhabdomyomas.[19] Traditionally, papillary fibroelastomas have been considered less frequent than myxoma and lipomas, but it is increasingly recognized in the literature, and in my experience, that papillary fibroelastoma may in fact now represent the most common form of benign cardiac tumor.[25] This fact underscores the increasing antemortem diagnosis of cardiac masses as a result of the ever-increasing use of echocardiography and the enhanced images newer echocardiographic technology affords. Furthermore the incidence of cardiac tumors does vary with age, with rhabdomyomas and fibromas being the most common benign cardiac tumors in children. Therefore, age at diagnosis should be considered as it may as it may aid in the differential diagnosis.

About one quarter of primary cardiac tumors are malignant, 95% of which are sarcomas, the remaining 5% are by lymphomas.[18,26,27] Of the sarcoma group, the most common in reported series are undifferentiated, followed by angiosarcomas, leiomyosarcomas, and rhabdomyosarcomas.

Secondary malignant disease of the heart and pericardium are considerably more common than primary cardiac malignancy, some estimates 30 to 1000 times more common.[27,28] In random autopsy series, the frequency of metastatic involvement is 0.4%; and in patients with diagnosed cancer cardiac involvement is as high as 20%.[16,29-31] Spread to the heart is generally via direct tumor extension, venous/lymphatic spread, or arterial metastasis. The most common underlying malignancies with secondary cardiac involvement include carcinoma of the lung, breast, esophagus, stomach, kidneys, melanoma, lymphoma, and leukemia.

TABLE 45-3. Approximate Incidence of Benign Tumors of the Heart in Adults and Children

	Incidence (%)	
	Adults	**Children**
Myxoma	45	15
Lipoma	20	—
Papillary fibroelastoma	15	—
Angioma	5	5
Fibroma	3	15
Hemangioma	5	5
Rhabdomyoma	1	45
Teratoma	<1	15

Adapted from Shapiro LM: *Heart* 85:218-222, 2001.

Classification of Cardiac Tumors

A proposed classification is considered in Figure 45–1. An additional classification considers a pediatric versus adult population. There is s significant difference in tumor type in the pediatric versus adult population (Table 45–3). Tumors may also be characterized by the locations in which they are most commonly found (Table 45–4 and Fig. 45–2).

CLASSIFICATION OF PRIMARY AND SECONDARY CARDIAC TUMORS

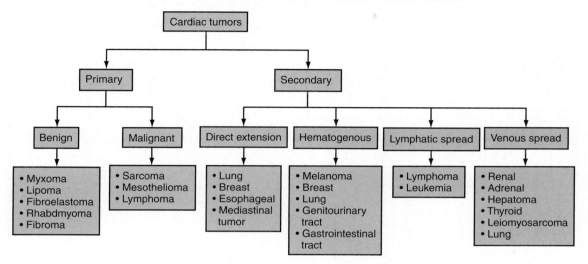

Figure 45–1. Classification of primary and secondary cardiac tumors. (Adapted from Salcedo EE, Cohen GI, White RD, Davison MB: Curr Probl Cardiol *17:73-137, 1992.*)

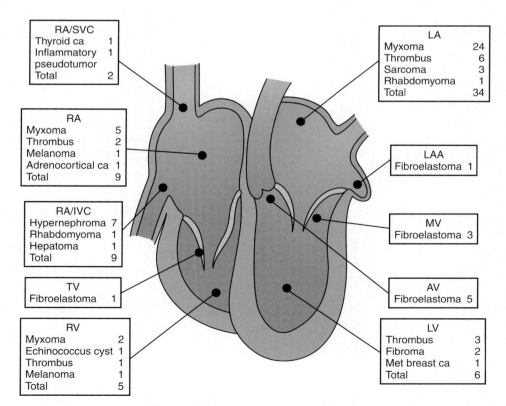

Figure 45–2. Diagram illustrating the distribution and pathologic characteristics of the masses according to intracardiac attachment site. AV, aortic valve; ca, carcinoma; IVC, inferior vena cava; LA, left atrium; LAA, left atrial appendage; LV, left ventricle; met, metastatic; MV, mitral valve; RA, right atrium; RV, right ventricle; SVC, superior vena cava; TV, tricuspid valve. (From Dujardin KS, Click RL, Oh JK: J Am Soc Echocardiogr *13:1080-1083, 2000.*)

TABLE 45-4. Features of Benign Primary Cardiac Tumors

Type of Tumor (Prevalence)	Patient Age When Diagnosed	Associated Syndromes	Most Common Location	Typical Morphologic Characteristics	Echocardiographic Features	CT Features	MRI Features*
Myxoma (50% of all primary cardiac neoplasms)	30-60 (younger if associated with Carney complex)	Carney complex	Interatrial septum at fossa ovalis, left atrium more common than right	Gelatinous, attached to stalk; calcification common; hemorrhage or necrosis common	Mobile tumor, narrow stalk	Heterogeneous, low attenuation	Heterogeneous, bright on T2WI; heterogeneous enhancement
Lipoma (approximately 60 cases)	Variable	A few cases associated with tuberous sclerosis	Pericardial space or any cardiac chamber	Large, broad-based; no calcification, hemorrhage, or necrosis	Usually hypoechoic in the pericardial space, echogenic in a cardiac chamber	Homogeneous fat attenuation (low attenuation)	Homogeneous fat signal intensity (increased T1); no enhancement
Papillary fibroelastoma (uncertain)	Middle-aged, elderly	None	Cardiac valves	Small (<1 cm), frond-like, narrow stalk; calcification rare (n = 2); no hemorrhage or necrosis	"Shimmering" edges	Usually not seen	Usually not seen
Rhabdomyoma	Infants, children <4 years	Tuberous sclerosis	Left ventricle, right ventricle in walls on aortic valves outflow tract	Mural pedunculated *multiple*, variable size, spontaneous regression	Brighter than surrounding myocardium	Hypodense on contrast CT	Isointense to myocardium T2WI; hyperintense to myocardium T2WI
Fibroma (100 cases since 1976)	Infants, children, young adults	Gorlin syndrome	Ventricles	Large, intramural; calcification common; no hemorrhage or necrosis	Intramural, calcified	Low attenuation, calcified	Isointense on T1WI; dark on T2WI; usually little to no enhancement
Hemangioma	All ages mean 4th decade	None	Anywhere; one third in right ventricle, one third in left ventricle; one fourth in right atrium	Multilobulated, unilocular, cystic, <1-8 cm	"Solid" echo-dense	Intense central contrast enhancement	Rapid enhancement increased T2WI signal
Paraganglioma (<50 cases)	Young adults	Many possible but almost always sporadic	Left atrium, coronary arteries, aortic root	Broad-based, infiltrative or circumscribed; calcification rare (n = 1); hemorrhage or necrosis common	Echogenic, relatively immobile	Low attenuation	Typically isointense or heterogeneous on T1WI, bright on T2WI; marked enhancement

*T1WI, T1-weighted images, T2Wi, T2-weighted images.
CT, computed tomography; MRI, magnetic resonance imaging.
Adapted from Araoz PA, Mulvagh SL, Tazelaar HD, et al: *Radiographics* 20:1303-1319, 2000.

Primary Benign Cardiac Tumors

Cardiac Myxomas

Three quarters of all primary cardiac tumors are benign, and nearly half of these are myxomas. Myxomas occur in all age groups, most frequently between the third and sixth decades of life (with an approximate incidence of 45% in adults and 15% in children).[32] Women are more commonly affected.[33-38] Although myxomas usually occur sporadically as an isolated tumor in the left atrium, familial myxomas have been reported (accounting for 7% of myxomas).[39-42] The familial myxomas occur as an inherited, autosomal dominant disorder, in combination with two or more of the following conditions: skin myxomas (single or multiple), cutaneous lentiginosis, myxoid fibroadenomas of the breast, pituitary adenomas, primary adrenocortical micronodular dysplasia with Cushing's syndrome, and testicular tumors (characteristically large cell calcifying Sertoli cell tumors). These syndromes are grouped under the Carney complex, named after the physician who first described the familial nature of the disorder.[26] These patients tend to be younger and may have the germline mutation PRKAR1A.[43] They are also more likely to have multiple myxomas and have an increased risk of recurrence after resection.[33]

Clinical Setting

The clinical features of myxomas, like most cardiac tumors, are determined by their location, size, and mobility. These characteristics are easily addressed by echocar-

diography. Most patients are diagnosed with one or more features of the triad of embolism, intracardiac obstruction, and constitutional symptoms. Dyspnea may occur secondary to atrioventricular (AV) valve obstruction. Occasionally, there are no symptoms, particularly with small tumors. There is a risk of recurrence after resection (5%), more commonly with familial myxomas.[44] Thus, semiannual surveillance echocardiographic follow-up has been recommended following surgery.[32,45]

Location

Cardiac myxomas usually develop in the atria, 75% originating in the left atrium and 15% to 20% in the right atrium. They characteristically arise from or near the interatrial septum at the border of the fossa ovalis membrane.[11,34-36,46] Occasionally they may grow through the fossa ovalis and into both atria. Myxomas may also originate (in descending order of frequency) from the posterior atrial wall, anterior atrial wall, and atrial appendage. Three percent to four percent of myxomas originate in the left ventricle and three percent to four percent in the right.[32,46] Tumors are usually solitary. Multiple tumors or atypical locations suggest familial myxoma. Myxomas of the heart valves have been reported but are extremely rare (Figs. 45–3 and 45–4).

Gross Appearance

The gross appearance of cardiac myxomas is variable. The tumors range in size from 1 to 15 cm in diameter but most frequently measure 5 to 6 cm in diameter.[32] Myxo-

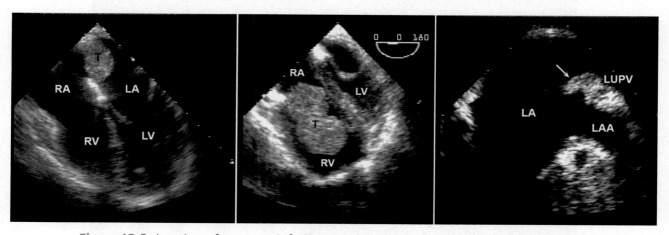

Figure 45–3. *Locations of myxomas.* Left, *Transesophageal echocardiographic four-chamber view demonstrating a 3.5-cm lobulated left atrial myxoma (T) arising from the fossa ovalis membrane. A mass at this location typically represents an atrial myxoma. At surgery, several "streamers" were attached to the tumor, not seen on echocardiography. Middle, A transesophageal echocardiographic four-chamber view demonstrates a right ventricular myxoma (T) measuring 7 by 4 cm that arises from the anterior tricuspid valve leaflet. This tumor extended through the right ventricular outflow tract and pulmonary valve (not shown). Myxomas arising from unusual locations or from multiple sites should raise suspicion of Carney complex (see Fig. 45–2). Right, Transesophageal echocardiograph in a 70-year-old woman with a stroke. An 8-mm left atrial myxoma (arrow) is seen attached to the "Q tip" (junction of the left upper pulmonary vein [LUPV] and left atrial appendage orifice [LAA]). A lesion at this location may be confused with a thrombus. The mass did not resolve with anticoagulation. At surgery, an additional smaller friable lesion was identified inferior to the primary lesion shown. LA, left atrium; LV, left ventricle; RV, right ventricle; RA, right atrium.*

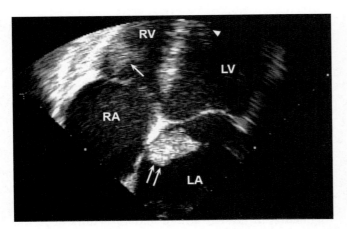

Figure 45–4. *A 19-year-old woman with a stroke. On examination there were cutaneous myxomas and lentigines of the lips. A transesophageal echocardiogram demonstrates multiple intracardiac myxomas. Tumors are seen in the left atrium near the fossa ovalis (double arrows) and related to the anterior tricuspid valve leaflet (single arrow). A left ventricular myxoma attached to the anterior septum is also present but is poorly seen in this still frame image (arrowhead). At surgery, an additional small right ventricular apical myxoma was also identified using a thoracoscope. This was not appreciated on preoperative or intraoperative echocardiography. This patient was diagnosed with Carney complex. A repeat echocardiogram 4 years after tumor excision demonstrated no recurrence. This case also stresses the importance of carefully looking for additional lesions. LA, left atrium; LV, left ventricle; RV, right ventricle; RA, right atrium.*

mas are generally polypoid, often pedunculated, frequently arising from a narrow stalk, and are rarely sessile. They are usually round or ovoid in shape with a smooth or gently lobulated surface (Fig. 45–5). The mobility of the tumor depends on its consistency, which varies in part depending on the extent of attachment and the length of its stalk. Polypoid myxomas are usually compact and show little tendency toward spontaneous fragmentation. The less common villous or papillary myxomas have a surface consisting of multiple fine villous extensions that are fragile and tend to break off. The risk of embolization is greatest with these tumors[19,47-49] (Table 45–5). Adding to their embolic potential, they frequently have organized thrombi on their surface. Internally, myxomas often contain cysts and areas of necrosis and hemorrhage. Calcification has been observed but is rare and is found only in 10% to 20% of cases.[20,32] Occasionally myxomas may become infected.[50-53]

Echocardiographic Features

Echocardiography can define the location, size, shape, attachment, and mobility of the myxoma.[19,32] Multiple myxomas may be missed, particularly if the imager is distracted by finding the index tumor. Careful evaluation of all cardiac chambers is necessary to exclude multiple tumors. The characteristic narrow stalk is the most important distinguishing feature followed by tumor mobil-

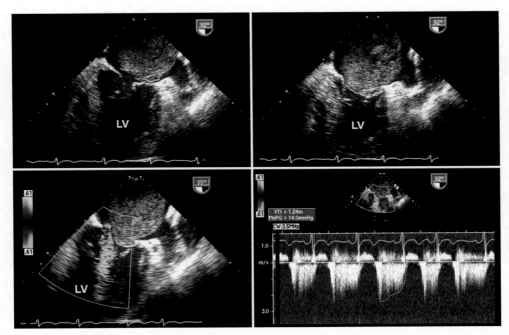

Figure 45–5. *A 64-year-old woman complained of exertional and resting chest heaviness and shortness of breath for 3 months. The transesophageal echocardiogram demonstrates the typical echocardiographic appearance of a large left atrial myxoma. Top left panel, A systolic frame demonstrating a large 5-by-7-cm ovoid mass in the left atrium arising from a narrow stalk attached to the fossa ovalis (not shown). Top right panel, A diastolic frame demonstrating the myxoma prolapsing through the mitral valve resulting in functional mitral valve stenosis (bottom left and bottom right panels). The mean gradient across the mitral valve is 14 mm Hg. LV, left ventricle.*

TABLE 45-5. Morphologic Features of Myxomas Related to Embolism

Morphologic Features	Emboli		
	Yes (*n* = 10)	No (*n* = 27)	*P* Value
Villous surface	90	37	0.007
Diameter, mm	48±17	62±26	0.132
Gross calcifications	0	15	0.557

Values given as percentage or mean plus or minus standard deviation, unless otherwise specified.
Adapted from Acebo E, Val-Bernal JF, Gomez-Roman JJ, Reveulta JM: *Chest* 123:1379-1385, 2003.

ity and distensibility.[9] When these features of a left atrial mass are seen, a diagnosis of cardiac myxoma can be made with a high degree of confidence,[54] especially if the stalk originates from the atrial septum. The internal echocardiographic appearance may be homogeneous or have central areas of hyperlucency representing necrotic foci and hemorrhage.[55,56] Internal areas of calcification may be present. Depending on their size and mobility, myxomas may result in left or right ventricular inflow obstruction, the degree of obstruction sometimes varying with body position (see Fig. 45-5). TEE may provide additional important information detecting the precise site of insertion and morphologic features of atrial and ventricular myxomas. It is also more sensitive for identifying small tumors (1 to 3 mm in diameter) and satellite tumors.[15,17,54,57-59]

Other Imaging Modalities

Tumor mobility, tumor distensibility and the thin delicate stalk are not as well demonstrated by CT or MRI.[9] However, unlike echocardiography, CT and MRI can differentiate tissue composition, better identifying solid, liquid, hemorrhagic, and fatty space-occupying tumors. CT and MRI findings of cardiac myxomas are variable, usually reflecting their gross pathologic features. Because of their gelatinous consistency, they have heterogeneous low attenuation at CT and calcification, if present, is also seen. They have markedly increased signal intensity on T2-weighted magnetic resonant images.[60,61] Presence of calcification or hemosiderin may result in areas of decreased signal intensity. Contrast enhancement is usually heterogeneous reflecting the presence of necrotic areas.[9,62]

Differential Diagnosis

Differentiation of cardiac myxoma from vegetations or thrombi is important. Usually the echocardiographic appearance of a cardiac myxoma is quite distinctive. Sometimes, however, the diagnosis may be less certain,

particularly when the myxoma has an unusual location or attachment, such as the left atrial appendage. In these instances the clinical scenario (atrial fibrillation [AFib]), associated echocardiographic findings (impaired ventricular function, left atrial enlargement and spontaneous echocardiographic contrast [SEC]) and CT or MRI findings are helpful in distinguishing thrombus from tumor. Sometimes, if the mass is small, a diagnostic trial of anticoagulation can be attempted and imaging repeated to confirm resolution.

Papillary Fibroelastoma

The true prevalence of papillary fibroelastomas is unknown. The reported prevalence of papillary fibroelastoma varies and is likely underreported because they are asymptomatic and thus underrepresented in surgical series, sometimes not appearing at all.[63] However, in a surgical series from the Mayo Clinic[20] and the Armed Forces Institute of Pathology (AFIP),[63] they accounted for 10% of primary cardiac tumors and were thus the second most common primary cardiac tumor.[5] Also, with the advent of echocardiography and improving imaging techniques, cardiac papillary fibroelastoma is being detected earlier and increasingly reported.[6] These benign endocardial papillomas predominantly affect the cardiac valves accounting for three quarters of all cardiac valvular tumors.[5] Patients with papillary fibroelastomas are often asymptomatic (30%) and diagnosed incidentally.[5,64] However, the clinical consequences of papillary fibroelastomas are significant and have been increasingly recognized as causes of stroke, transient ischemic attack (TIA), systemic embolism, and sudden cardiac death.[5,64]

Clinical Setting

Cardiac papillary fibroelastomas occur in all age groups but are predominantly identified in adulthood, particularly between the fourth and eighth decades of life.[5,64] The mean age of detection is approximately 60 years and may reflect the increased use of echocardiography in older patients. Men and women are equally affected. The natural history of these tumors has not been characterized because serial studies using echocardiography have not been performed. They are considered generally slow-growing tumors but are clinically important because they may serve as a nidus for thrombus formation and potential thromboembolism.

Gross Pathology

Grossly, papillary fibroelastomas are small (usually less than 1 cm in diameter [mean 9 mm] but can be as large as 7 cm).[5] When these tumors occur in the cardiac chambers, they are larger than those found on the aortic and mitral valves.[64] These tumors have a characteristic flower-like appearance with multiple papillary fronds attached to the endocardium by a short pedicle and when immersed in saline, they exhibit the typical "sea anemone" appearance.[64,65] The papillary fronds are narrow, elongated, and branching and merge imperceptibly into the substance of the valve. Sometimes, the gross appearance of the characteristic papillary structure may be obscured by attached thrombi.[66,67] Calcification rarely occurs, having been reported in only two cases.[66]

Location

Papillary fibroelastomas usually develop on cardiac valves (75% to 90%) but may arise anywhere in the heart, originating from the left ventricle, ostium of the right and left coronary arteries, left atrial appendage, atrial and ventricular septum, right atrium, left ventricular outflow tract [LVOT], Eustachian valve, and Chiari network. They have also been found in the right atrial appendage, and right ventricular outflow tract (RVOT) (Fig. 45–6).

Left-sided valves are affected 95% of the time, with aortic valve involvement slightly more common than the mitral valve.[5,64] Valvular papillary fibroelastomas usually arise from the mid-portion of the valve rather than the free edge (a distinguishing characteristic from Lambl's excrescences). Those that originate from the semilunar valves most often project into the arterial lumen but sometimes project into the ventricular cavity or even prolapse across the valve in diastole. Those originating on the AV valves project into the atria. Rarely, they may arise from the subvalvular apparatus of the mitral and tricuspid valves.[68,69] Papillary fibroelastomas are usually solitary but can occur at multiple sites (9%).[5,64]

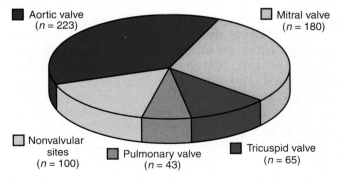

■ Aortic valve (n = 223)
□ Mitral valve (n = 180)
□ Nonvalvular sites (n = 100)
▨ Pulmonary valve (n = 43)
■ Tricuspid valve (n = 65)

Location of cardiac papillary fibroelastoma (n = 611 patients).

Figure 45–6. Location of cardiac papillary fibroelastoma. (From Gowda RM, Khan IA, Nair CK, et al: Am Heart J 146:404-410, 2003.)

Clinical Manifestations

Most papillary fibroelastomas are discovered incidentally while undergoing echocardiography for unrelated reasons or during evaluation of a cardiac source of embolism.[5] Like most cardiac tumors, their clinical presentation depends on many factors including tumor location, size, growth rate, and tendency for embolization. The most common clinical presentations include cerebral and systemic embolization and coronary artery occlusion. Patients may also be diagnosed with heart failure and sudden cardiac death. Embolism is thought to occur from superimposed thrombi or fragmentation of the papillary fronds themselves (sometimes both) as, on occasion, confirmed tumor fragments have been isolated in embolic material.[5,64]

Echocardiographic Diagnosis

Papillary fibroelastomas are easily detected by echocardiography. Although TTE can readily detect these tumors, the superior resolution of TEE makes this the definitive imaging modality to confirm the characteristic appearance of these usually small, highly mobile tumors and plays a central role in the search for multiple lesions.[5,70,71]

On 2D echocardiography, papillary fibroelastomas are characterized by a small, mobile, pedunculated valvular or less commonly, endocardial mass, which on many occasions, flutters or prolapses into the cardiac chamber during systole or diastole (Fig. 45–7). Usually they have a well-defined "head," but they may appear as elongated strand-like projections. Characteristically, they have a stippled edge with a "shimmer" or "vibration" at the interface of the tumor with the surrounding blood, a finding that may distinguish them from thrombi.[5,72] Rather than being pedunculated and mobile, the tumors may be sessile. Sometimes the tumor may be missed because they are small, the examination is not performed carefully enough because the clinical index of suspicion is low or because they are masked by an associated lesion or degenerative valvular disease.[64] If a papillary fibroelastoma is suspected as a source of embolism, a transesophageal echocardiogram should be performed. A proposed treatment algorithm based on imaging characteristics is presented in Figure 45–8.

Other Imaging Modalities

CT and MRI are inferior to echocardiography because they do not allow real-time imaging, and the temporal resolution is inadequate because most of these tumors are small and attached to moving valves. The main disadvantage of MRI is susceptibility to motion artifact.[5,9]

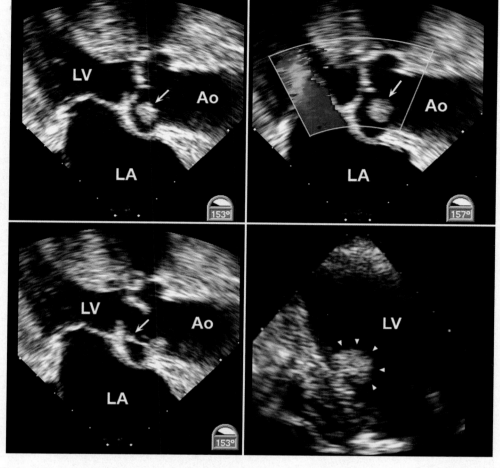

Figure 45–7. An incidental mass was identified in an 80-year-old woman undergoing a routine transthoracic echocardiogram. The transesophageal echocardiogram demonstrates a 14-by-10-mm globular mass with an irregular border (arrow, top panels) attached to the aortic surface of the aortic valve noncoronary cusp by a thin stalk (arrow, left bottom panel). Apart from aortic valve sclerosis, there were no associated valvular abnormalities or evidence of valvular destruction. Right bottom panel, Multiple papillary fibroelastomas were seen on transthoracic echocardiography in a 33-year-old woman with Hodgkin's lymphoma and radiation-induced heart disease. In this zoomed apical two-chamber view image, one papillary fibroelastoma is seen attached to the endocardial surface of the midinferior left ventricular wall. The fimbriated surface can be appreciated (arrowheads). Although papillary fibroelastomas are most commonly found on valves, they may arise anywhere in the heart. Ao, aorta; LA, left atrium; LV, left ventricle.

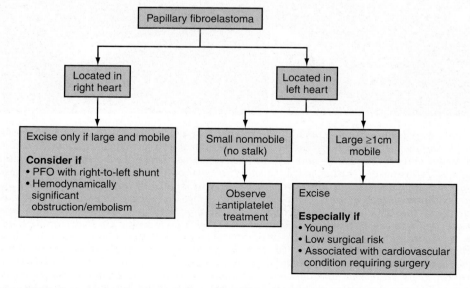

Figure 45–8. Proposed management of papillary fibroelastomas based on echocardiographic findings. PFO, patent foramen ovale.

Differential Diagnosis

Again, the differential diagnosis includes thrombi, vegetations, other heart tumors, degenerative valvular calcification, and Lambl's excrescences (Fig. 45–9). Lambl's excrescences may be difficult to distinguish from papillary fibroelastomas.[73] These filiform fronds, first described by Lambl in 1856,[74] occur by definition at the sites of valve closure and are thought be the result of wear-and-tear lesions that originate as small thrombi on the endocardium of the contact margins of the valves at the site of minor endothelial damage, akin to the frayed edges of an old shirt cuff. In AV valves, Lambl's excrescences are found at the site of valve closure on the atrial surface, but on semilunar valves, they can occur anywhere on the valve. Unlike papillary fibroelastomas, they usually do not occur on the arterial side of the semilunar valves or on the mural endocardium.[5] Unlike papillary fibroelastomas, Lambl's excrescences are much more common, reported in up to 85% of adults with multiple tumors present in more than 90% of cases. Papillary fibroelastomas, in contrast, are typically larger and more gelatinous and are present on valves away from the valvular lines of closure. They may also be found on endo-

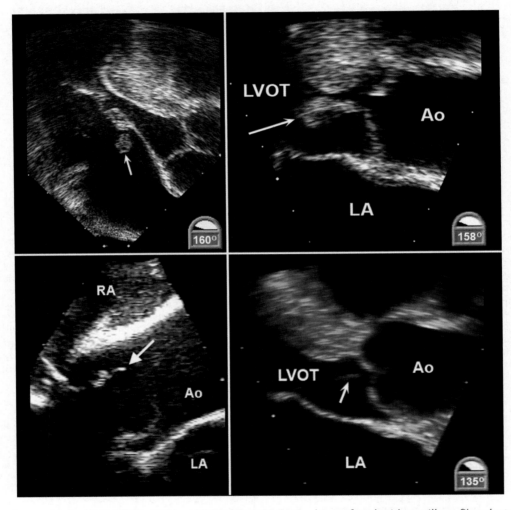

Figure 45–9. Vegetations and Lambl's excrescences may be confused with papillary fibroelastomas. The top panels demonstrate vegetations of the mitral (top left panel) and aortic (top right panel) valves in two patients with culture positive enterococcal faecalis endocarditis. The vegetation on the aortic valve (arrow) is attached to the left ventricular outflow tract aspect of the aortic valve. It is highly mobile and like the mitral vegetation, is associated with valve destruction and severe aortic regurgitation (not shown). Unlike papillary fibroelastomas, these vegetations do not have a characteristic thin stalk and "fimbriated" shimmering edge. Papillary fibroelastomas are usually not associated with valve destruction. Examples of a Lambl's excrescence are shown attached to the aortic valve (arrows) in systole, in the (left bottom panel) and diastole (right bottom panel). This fine filamentous highly mobile strand-like structure prolapses through the valve into the left ventricular outflow tract in diastole. Unlike a papillary fibroelastoma, there is no globular "head" component at its distal end, and unlike a vegetation, apart from associated degenerative valve disease, overt valve destruction is unusual. Ao, aorta; LA, left atrium; LVOT, left ventricular outflow tract; RA, right atrium.

cardial surfaces of the atria and ventricles.[31,75-78] Despite these reported differences, it can sometimes be difficult to distinguish these two abnormalities noninvasively.

Other Benign Cardiac Tumors

Lipoma and Lipomatous Hypertrophy

Lipomatous hypertrophy of the atrial septum is a benign condition and is not a true tumor. It is discussed here because it is often confused with a lipoma. Lipomatous hypertrophy is defined as "any deposit of fat in the atrial septum at the level of the fossa ovalis that exceeds 2 cm in transverse dimension."[63] Lipomatous hypertrophy involves the interatrial septum, sparing the fossa ovalis membrane,[63] resulting in a characteristic dumbbell shape (Fig. 45–10). It results from adipose cell hyperplasia and is associated with increasing age and obesity.[79,80] It is a nonneoplastic condition and may be associated with atrial arrhythmias. It may rarely result in superior vena cava obstruction.[81] Echocardiographically, the atrial septum may measure up to 3 cm in thickness and appears hyperechoic. Unlike lipomatous hypertrophy, lipomas are much less common. Unfortunately the number of reported cases is not clear from the literature because some series do not

differentiate between lipomas and lipomatous hypertrophy.[63] These homogeneous fatty encapsulated tumors usually arise from the epicardial surface, most often from a broad pedicle, and grow into the pericardial space.[9] Subendocardial lipomas are often small and sessile, whereas subepicardial lipomas tend to be larger. Subendocardial lipomas may also grow as broad-based pedunculated masses protruding into the cardiac chambers. Lipomas are usually asymptomatic but may cause symptoms due to local compression (rarely lipomas become quite large weighing as much as 4.8 kg)[82] or cause arrhythmias, and occasionally may arise from the interatrial septum and extend into the left atrial cavity mimicking a cardiac myxoma. Lipomas, unlike myxomas however, have a broad base of attachment and are not as mobile as myxomas.[83,84] An unusual observation is that the echocardiographic appearance of lipomas varies depending on their particular location. In the pericardial space they may appear echogenic, entirely hypoechoic, or have hypoechoic regions.[85-87] Intracavitary lipomas on the other hand are homogeneous and hyperechoic.[84,88] The reason for this difference is not known[9] (Fig. 45–11).

If diagnostic uncertainty exists, with respect to identifying lipomatous hypertrophy or lipoma, CT and MRI are diagnostic as a result of their high specificity in identifying fat.[9,89-91] In fact because the dumbbell appearance

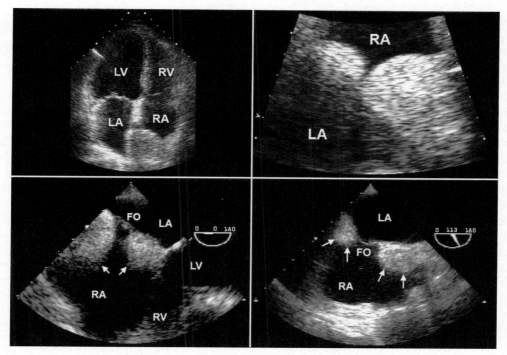

Figure 45-10. These panels demonstrate the typical appearance of exuberant lipomatous hypertrophy of the atrial septum. Top left panel, *Transthoracic echocardiogram, apical four-chamber view, demonstrating a dumb-bell shaped mass in relation to the interatrial septum. The fossa ovalis membrane, which is characteristically spared in this condition, is thin, with most of the hypertrophy involving the superior limbus resulting in a masslike lesion in the roof of the right atrium.* Top right panel, *A zoomed image from a subcostal transthoracic echocardiographic view in the same patient.* Bottom, *Transesophageal echocardiographic views of lipomatous hypertrophy (arrows). Again, characteristically, the fossa ovalis membrane is spared. FO, fossa ovalis membrane; LA, left atrium; LV, left ventricle; RA, right atrium; RV, right ventricle.*

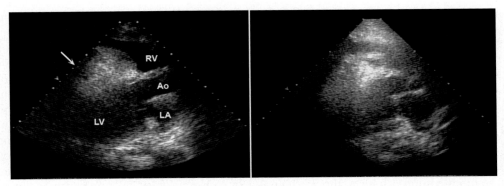

Figure 45–11. Parasternal long-axis view images from a transthoracic echocardiogram in a 40-year-old woman with syncope and ventricular tachycardia are shown. A large poorly defined hyperechoic homogeneous intracardiac mass (arrow) involving the anterior interventricular septum is present. This mass also involved the anterior wall and extended to the apex. The size of the mass could not be accurately assessed because of acoustic shadowing, typical for a lipoma in this location, (right panel). There was no evidence of significant outflow tract or valvular obstruction. Magnetic resonance imaging of the heart was diagnostic demonstrating the typical appearance of a lipoma. Ao, aorta; LA, left atrium; LV, left ventricle; RV, right ventricle.

is so characteristic for lipomatous hypertrophy and non-invasive imaging is so specific for fat, a percutaneous tissue biopsy or surgical biopsy is unnecessary.[92]

Hemangioma

Hemangiomas are benign vascular tumors that represent only 2.8% to 10% of primary cardiac tumors.[93,94] They can arise anywhere in the heart and have been found in both ventricles, both atria, on the epicardial surface, and in the pericardium.[95-99] These tumors are seen more frequently in males than females, at all ages, with a mean age at diagnosis of 43 years.[100] These tumors are usually asymptomatic and are discovered incidentally by echocardiography, CT, MRI, or at autopsy.[101] Symptoms depend on anatomic location and size of the tumor. They may cause arrhythmias, pericardial effusions, congestive heart failure (CHF), right ventricular outflow tract obstruction, coronary insufficiency, and sudden cardiac death.[96] From a review of 56 reported cases, the localization of these tumors is approximately one third in the right ventricle, one third in the left ventricle, and one quarter in the right atrium. Other locations include the interatrial septum and interventricular septum and left atrium in 10% of cases. In one third of cases, multiple extensive tumors are present. The size of cardiac hemangiomas ranges from less than 1 cm to more than 8 cm.[96] Morphologically, the tumors have been variably described as a solid echodense bulge of the interventricular septum, a large multilobulated mass or a unilocular mass with a cystic structure.[98] Although echocardiography can detect the tumor and its location, there are unfortunately no uniform diagnostic echocardiographic criteria[98] (Fig. 45–12). TEE provides incremental information regarding the accurate localization of the tumor and estimation of intracardiac and extracardiac extension and determining the attachment site. It is also useful to assess whether there is extension of right atrial tumors into the great veins.[16] Cardiac catheterization and MRI are considered superior complementary diagnostic techniques. Cardiac catheterization reveals a characteristic "tumor blush" resulting from the tumor vascularity, and MRI can demonstrate the increased vascularity of the hemangioma with rapid enhancement during first pass gadolinium contrast infusion.[102-105]

The natural history of cardiac hemangiomas is poorly documented. Nevertheless, as the hemodynamic consequences of the tumor cannot be predicted, resection is recommended when feasible.

Rhabdomyoma

This intramyocardial tumor is the most frequent cardiac neoplasm of childhood representing 60% of pediatric cardiac tumors[14] and is often diagnosed in the first year of life, increasingly in utero with the use of fetal echocardiography[93,95,96,99,106,107] (Fig. 45–13). There is a well-described and common association with rhabdomyoma and tuberous sclerosis, an autosomal dominant syndrome characterized by hamartomas in several organs, epilepsy, mental deficiency, and characteristic skin lesions. In fact, nearly 50% of infants with tuberous sclerosis are reported to have a rhabdomyoma.[108-110]

These tumors are almost always multiple and occur with equal frequency in the left and right ventricles growing in the ventricular walls or on the AV valves. They vary in size from a few millimeters to a few centimeters and may be pedunculated often obstructing ventricular inflow or outflow. Hemorrhage and calcification are uncommon.[111] Echocardiographically, they appear well circumscribed and slightly brighter than the surrounding normal myocardium[14] (Fig. 45–14).

Rhabdomyomas appear hypodense on contrast CT, isointense to myocardium on T1-weighted images and hyperintense on T2-weighted images.[112] In contrast, fi-

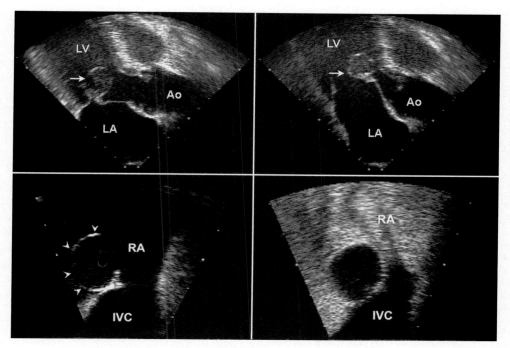

Figure 45–12. Top panels, *An incidental finding noted on transthoracic echocardiography in a 53-year-old man with ischemic heart disease led to this transesophageal echocardiogram. A 2-cm thin walled echo-lucent mass (arrow) consistent with a hemangioma is seen attached to the ventricular aspect of the anterior mitral valve leaflet. Echocardiographic contrast administered intravenously is seen within the tumor confirming its vascular nature. Bottom panels, Another example of a hemangioma measuring 1.7 by 1.5 cm involving the Eustachian valve at the inferior vena cava–right atrial junction. The outline of the hemangioma is clearly demarcated by administration of agitated saline contrast injection via an antecubital vein. Ao, aorta; IVC, inferior vena cava; LA, left atrium; LV, left ventricle; RA, right atrium.*

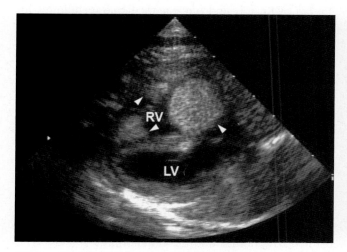

Figure 45–13. *This fetal echocardiogram, longitudinal axis view, demonstrates multiple well-circumscribed large and small tumors (arrowheads), typical for rhabdomyomas. These masses result in near obliteration of the right ventricular cavity. LV, left ventricle; RV, right ventricle.*

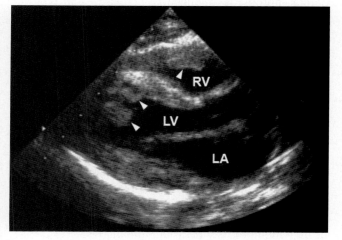

Figure 45–14. *A transthoracic echocardiogram, parasternal long-axis view, in a 9-month-old child with tuberous sclerosis demonstrates multiple intracardiac tumors (arrowheads) in both the left and right ventricles. These lesions in this clinical setting are typical for rhabdomyomas and their size can be expected to regress with time. LA, left atrium; LV, left ventricle; RV, right ventricle.*

bromas (also a common childhood cardiac tumor) appear as dark solitary masses often with calcification on T2-weighted images.[113]

A characteristic and peculiar feature of rhabdomyomas is spontaneous regression (Fig. 45–15). The tumors usually regress in size or number or both in most patients less than 4 years of age. This phenomenon oc-

curs less so in older patients probably accounting for their higher incidence in children, and why, if found in adults, they are usually smaller than those typically seen in children.[110] These tumors are associated with a higher incidence of ventricular preexcitation and Wolff-

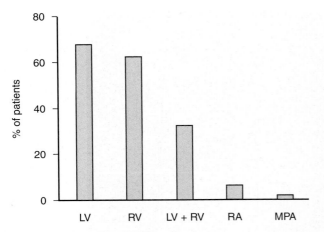

Figure 45–15. *Echocardiographic location of cardiac rhabdomyoma in the various cardiac chambers in 47 patients with tuberous sclerosis. Some patients had tumors in more than one cardiac chamber. LV, left ventricle; MPA, main pulmonary artery; RA, right atrium; RV, right ventricle. (From Nir A, Tajik AJ, Freeman WK, et al: Am J Cardiol 76:419-421, 1995.)*

Parkinson-White syndrome and may increase the risk of arrhythmia.[110] Because spontaneous tumor resolution is common, management is expectant in asymptomatic patients. Occasionally, surgical resection is necessary if the tumors are large resulting in structural or hemodynamic complications.[114-118]

Cardiac Fibroma

Cardiac fibroma is a congenital neoplasm that typically affects children, one third of whom are younger than 1 year when diagnosed. Like rhabdomyomas, they may also be detected in utero. It is the most common resected cardiac neoplasm in children and second most common benign primary cardiac tumor in children found at autopsy.[63,119] Fibromas have been rarely reported in adults.[120] Males and females are equally affected with a mean age of diagnosis of 13 years. There is an increased prevalence of cardiac fibromas in Gorlin syndrome, an autosomal dominant condition associated with multiple basal cell carcinomas, jaw cysts, skeletal anomalies and tendency to develop neoplasms in several organ systems.[121-123] Patients with fibromas usually present with arrhythmias, heart failure, cyanosis, syncope, chest pain, or sudden death. One third may be asymptomatic.[63,119]

Cardiac fibromas are usually located in the ventricles most often involving the left ventricular free wall, the intraventricular septum, the right ventricle, and rarely the atria.[124,125] The tumors are characteristically solitary (unlike rhabdomyoma), circumscribed, and often centrally calcified without cystic change, necrosis, or hemorrhage (although this may be present in large tumors).[20,63,126-128] The typical echocardiographic appearance is of a discreet often obstructive, echogenic, noncontractile mass ranging in size from 1 to 10 cm in diameter (mean 5 cm) in a ventricular wall.[63] The tumor may be nodular and discreet and may even mimic

hypertrophic cardiomyopathy or ventricular septal hypertrophy[124,128-130] (Fig. 45–16).

On CT, fibromas appear as homogenous masses with soft tissue attenuation that may be either infiltrative or sharply marginated. Calcification is often seen. On MRI, they are homogeneous and hypointense on T2-weighted images and iso-intense relative to muscle on T1-weighted images. They demonstrate little or no contrast material enhancement.[9,127] MRI also demonstrates the extent of myocardial infiltration, which can guide tumor resection.[131]

Surgery appears to be the optimal treatment in patients with symptomatic resectable tumors. The role of surgery in patient with asymptomatic tumors is less clear because cardiac fibromas can remain dormant for many years and even regress.[127] However, because of fatal arrhythmias, surgery is often recommended despite absence of symptoms. Transplantation is considered for large and unresectable tumors.

Cardiac Paraganglioma

This is an exceedingly rare tumor with only 30 cases reported before 1992 and 20 cases in the subsequent 10 years. Patients may present with symptoms of catecholamine excess or resulting from compression of adjacent structures. Echocardiography, particularly TEE, identifies ovoid, well-demarcated tumors characteristically within the AV groove adjacent to the epicardial arteries near the tricuspid and mitral annuli[132] (Fig. 45–17). MRI, CT, and nuclear medicine techniques for localizing extra adrenal paragangliomas are also useful in detecting and characterizing these tumors.

Malignant Primary Cardiac Tumors

Malignant primary tumors are rare. Metastatic disease or secondary cardiac malignancy on the other hand is 30 times more common. Only approximately 15% of primary cardiac tumors are malignant. The vast majority (95%) of these primary malignant tumors is sarcomas, and the remaining 5% is made up of primary cardiac lymphomas and mesotheliomas.[27]

Sarcoma

Sarcomas are most frequently diagnosed between the third and fifth decades of life and are found equally in men and women. They can arise at any part of the heart.[133] The clinical course is dismal, rapidly progressive with death occurring as a result of widespread local infiltration, intracavitary obstruction, or metastases, often already present at the time of initial diagnosis. Although sarcomas can be differentiated histologically, their echocardiographic characteristics are not signifi-

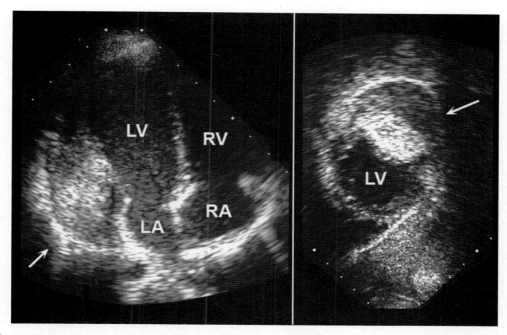

Figure 45–16. An apical four-chamber view (left) and parasternal short-axis view (right), from a transthoracic echocardiogram in a 5-year-old girl, demonstrate a solitary circumscribed 4-by-5-cm noncontractile left ventricular fibroma (arrow) involving the free wall and occupying a significant portion of the left ventricular cavity, interfering with left ventricular filling. The central portion appears bright consistent with calcification. LA, left atrium; LV, left ventricle; RA, right atrium; RV, right ventricle.

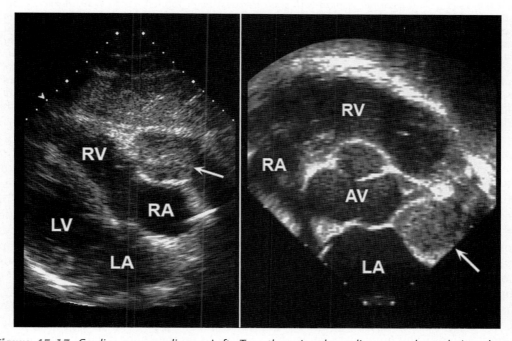

Figure 45–17. Cardiac paragangliomas. Left, Transthoracic echocardiogram, subcostal view, demonstrates an echogenic, ovoid well demarcated intrapericardial 6-by-5-cm mass in the right atrioventricular groove producing mass effect but without invading the right atrial wall (arrow). There is no associated pericardial effusion. Right, Transthoracic echocardiogram in a different patient, parasternal short-axis view, demonstrates a mass (arrow) adjacent to the aortic valve, immediately beneath the aortic arch and adherent to the left pulmonary artery. Masses in these locations (left and right) are characteristic of this rare tumor. AV, aortic valve; LA, left atrium; LV, left ventricle; RA, right atrium; RV, right ventricle.

cantly unique to permit a reliable noninvasive histologic distinction (Figs. 45-18 and 45–19).

Angiosarcomas are most common with a male to female ratio of about two to one. They usually arise in the right atrium or pericardium. The presenting signs and symptoms are nonspecific and may include right-sided heart failure, symptoms of pericardial involvement, or vena caval obstruction.[18,25,134] Echocardiography usually

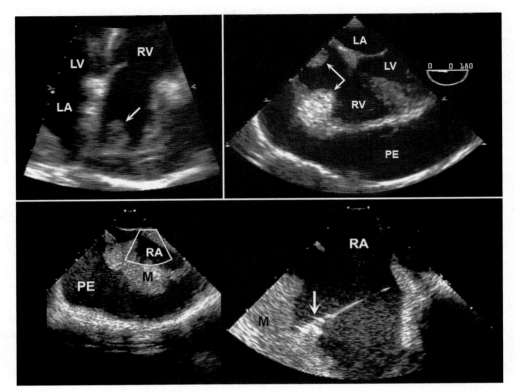

Figure 45–18. *A 33-year-old woman with pleuritic chest pain.* Top left panel, *Transthoracic echocardiogram, apical four-chamber zoomed view, demonstrates an irregular mass in the right atrium* (arrow) *with an associated posterior pericardial effusion predominantly located around the right ventricle. Top right panel, A transesophageal echocardiographic image demonstrates the same right atrial mass (arrows). Associated abnormal thickening of the right atrial wall and atrioventricular groove is appreciated. Bottom panel, Intracardiac ultrasound imaging guides percutaneous pericardial effusion drainage and biopsy of the tumor. The intracardiac ultrasound probe tip is located within the body of the right atrium. The bioptome (arrow) is seen facilitating biopsy of tumor tissue and avoiding the uninvolved thin right atrial wall. Pathology confirmed angiosarcoma. LA, left atrium; LV, left ventricle; M, mass; PE, pericardial effusion; RA, right atrium; RV, right ventricle.*

demonstrates a broad-based right atrial mass near the inferior vena cava (IVC). Epicardial, endocardial, and intracavitary extension is common. At surgery, local spread of the tumor to the pleural mediastinum is often found. Pulmonary metastases are frequent, and survival after diagnosis rarely exceeds 6 months.

Rhabdomyosarcomas account for 20% of sarcomas.[135] Multiple sites of myocardial involvement are common without predilection to any particular cardiac location.[26] Fibrosarcomas, histiosarcomas, and osteosarcomas constitute the remaining histological subtypes of sarcomas. Osteosarcomas characteristically develop near the junction of the pulmonary veins and can extend into these vessels, a feature readily appreciated with TEE.[4]

Primary Cardiac Lymphoma

The diagnosis of primary cardiac lymphoma requires (1) absence of lymphoma outside the pericardial sac (after a complete autopsy examination) and (2) the bulk of the tumor resides within the pericardium or cardiac symptoms arise from lymphomatous cardiac

infiltration at the time of initial diagnosis. Although the incidence is exceedingly rare (1% of primary cardiac tumors in the AFIP Series report),[136] the incidence of cardiac lymphoma is increasing because of lymphoproliferative disorders related to viral infections (Epstein-Barr virus and human immunodeficiency virus [HIV]) and immunocompromised transplanted patients.[137-143] They usually present during the fourth decade with a slight predominance in men. All areas of the heart can be involved including the pericardium. The lymphoma may become intracavitary and produce obstruction. The lesions appear as nodules and rarely as polypoid growths on the endocardial surface. Although echocardiography is a sensitive imaging technique, a definitive tissue diagnosis is still required.[144]

Mesotheliomas

Pericardial mesotheliomas are malignant tumors of the pericardium, which present clinically either as pericarditis, a pericardial effusion, or both. Some may present with features of constrictive pericarditis and signs of right-sided heart failure[14] (Fig. 45–20). These tumors are more

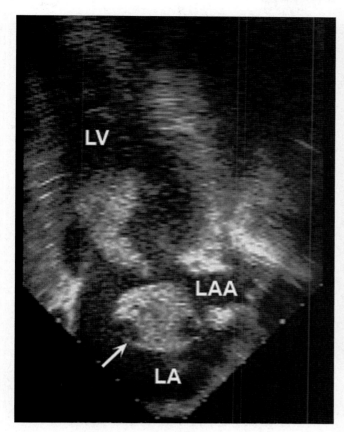

Figure 45–19. This transesophageal echocardiogram, in a 46-year-old man with a prior history of right axillary malignant schwannoma demonstrates a large heterogenous appearing left atrial tumor (arrow). Two hypoechoic lesions are consistent with necrotic foci. A serpiginous component is seen prolapsing through the open mitral valve into the left ventricular cavity in diastole. The tumor, a metastatic neurofibrosarcoma, arose from the right upper pulmonary vein (not shown). LA, left atrium; LAA, left atrial appendage; LV, left ventricle.

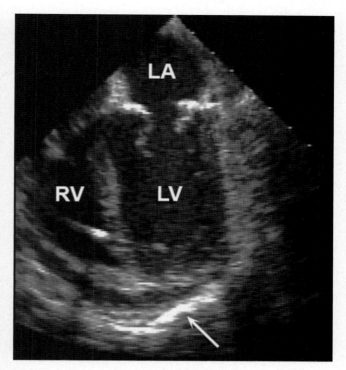

Figure 45–20. A transesophageal echocardiogram, four-chamber view, in a 47-year-old man with Hodgkin's disease treated with radiation and chemotherapy presenting with a clinical diagnosis of constrictive pericarditis is shown. The pericardium is thickened (arrow), and there is a small associated pericardial effusion. The visceral pericardium also appears thick. At surgery, the pericardium was thick and friable. Histology confirmed pericardial mesothelioma. LA, left atrium; LV, left ventricle; RV, right ventricle.

common in adults. Unlike pleural mesotheliomas, there is no association with asbestosis. Although solitary pericardial mesotheliomas occur, more frequently they cover most of the parietal and visceral surface of the pericardium encasing the heart. In contrast to sarcomas, invasion into the myocardium is only superficial. CT and MRI define tumor extent and degree of myocardial invasion.

Secondary or Metastatic Malignant Tumors of the Heart

Whereas primary tumors of the heart are rare, secondary tumors are common. Among unselected autopsies the incidence is about 4% and may be as high as 20% in patients dying from malignancy.[29,145] Malignant tumors spread to the heart by direct extension, usually from mediastinal tumors, hematogenous spread, lymphatic spread, or intraluminal extension from the IVC.[146] Metastatic involvement can be either localized or dif-

fuse. The nodules may be found in discreet locations or encase the epicardial surface. Pericardial effusion or cardiac tamponade may often be the initial presentation of secondary cardiac involvement. The noninvasive imaging appearance of metastatic deposits seldom distinguishes the tumor type. Rather, a careful evaluation looking for the primary tumor or a detailed history of prior malignancy provides the strongest clue.[25]

Direct Extension

Most secondary tumors of the heart arise contiguously from tumors in the chest cavity, most commonly breast, lung, or esophageal carcinoma. The initial clinical manifestation of these tumors is usually the result of pericardial involvement, and consequently, the most common echocardiographic finding in these patients is a pericardial effusion with or without cardiac tamponade.[14]

Hematogenous Spread

Metastatic spread to the heart is usually hematogenous with right-sided and left-sided metastases equally reported.[14] Ninety percent of metastases are clinically silent.[26]

Malignant melanoma, although a less common tumor than lung or breast carcinoma, is well recognized as having the highest rate of cardiac metastasis of any tumor,[147] with as many as 50% of all autopsy cases having cardiac involvement.[147] Moreover, more cases of cardiac involvement are being diagnosed as a result of rising melanoma incidence and increasing survival. Melanoma can involve any cardiac chamber and any cardiac structure, but most metastases are located in the myocardium and valvular involvement is rare (Fig. 45–21). Glancy and colleagues found cardiac involvement in 45 of 70 cases of metastatic melanoma.[148] Most had multiple small metastases throughout the heart with the right atrium most commonly involved. Intracavitary metastases from malignant melanoma make up the majority of published cases and are usually discovered incidentally.[147] In patients with a history of melanoma who have cardiac symptoms, cardiac involvement can be ascertained using either TTE or TEE, although TEE is better suited to identify smaller lesions and to define mobility and attachment.[15,149,150] MRI also demonstrates site of mural attachment but defines extension of tumor into adjacent mediastinal structures better than TEE.[147] It also produces a characteristic hyperintense signal on T1-weighted images as a result of paramagnetic scavenging by melanin.[147]

Malignant carcinoid heart disease, usually manifesting with characteristic valvular abnormalities, may rarely be diagnosed with metastatic cardiac disease typified by intramyocardial masses. These usually occur in the setting of known carcinoid syndrome[151] (Fig. 45–22).

Lymphatic Spread

Most patients with cardiac metastases from lymphomas or leukemias have concomitant involvement of their mediastinal lymph nodes. Stagnated lymph flow allows for retrograde extension of the tumor. Lymphomas form discreet endomyocardial masses, which are usually clinical silent.

Intraluminal Venous Extension

Tumors may propagate within blood vessels returning to the heart, most commonly originating from abdominal tumors via the IVC to the right-sided heart. Renal cell carcinoma, adrenal carcinoma, hepatocellular carcinoma, and uterine leiomyosarcoma are the most common tumors that reach the heart in this manner.[14] Of these, renal cell carcinoma is most common. These tumors usually appear as large elongated masses inside and emanating from the IVC and entering the right atrium, sometimes extending into the right ventricle[4,152] (Fig. 45–23). These intraluminal tumors may be distinguished from simple thrombi because they have a rather more "masslike" appearance, unlike thrombi, which usually appear as long, thin elongated venous casts.[153]

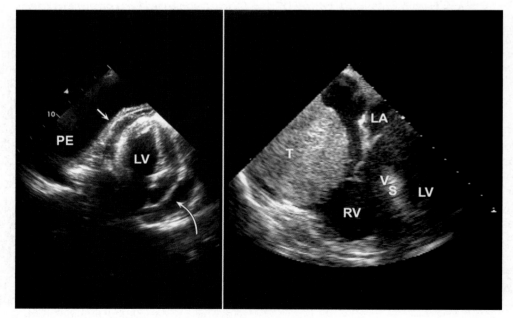

Figure 45–21. A transthoracic echocardiogram, four-chamber apical view, demonstrates metastatic melanoma to the pericardium (left). The pericardium around the left ventricle is thickened with an irregular surface and texture (arrow). There is a moderate to large pericardial effusion around the right ventricle and right atrium (curved arrow) and large pleural effusion. Right, A transesophageal echocardiogram in a 72-year-old man with a history of melanoma presenting with fatigue demonstrates a 4-by-6-cm polypoid tumor arising from the right atrium and prolapsing into the right ventricle. Importantly, the tumor does not arise from the atrial septum, a factor potentially distinguishing it from a myxoma. It did not arise from the inferior vena cava (not shown). At surgery, the tumor was black in color, and pathology confirmed metastatic melanoma. LA, left atrium; LV, left ventricle; PE, pericardial effusion; RV, right ventricle; T, tumor; VS, ventricular septum.

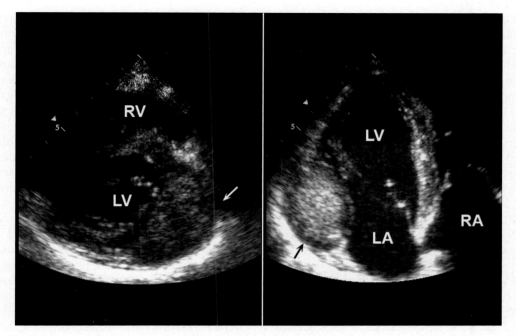

Figure 45–22. The transthoracic echocardiographic images demonstrate unusual cardiac involvement with metastatic carcinoid tumor. Left, Parasternal short-axis image at the basal left ventricular level demonstrates the large metastatic tumor located in the lateral wall (arrow). Right, Apical four-chamber view demonstrates the relationship of the tumor to the atrioventricular groove, distorting the mitral annulus and mitral leaflet (arrow). A 3D echocardiogram demonstrating the same tumor and its relationship to the mitral valve apparatus is shown in Figure 45–26. LA, left atrium; LV, left ventricle; RA, right atrium; RV, right ventricle.

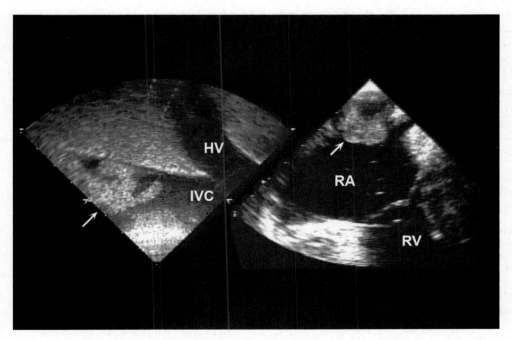

Figure 45–23. These transesophageal echocardiographic images from different patients demonstrate classic venous extension of tumor thrombus from the kidney into the inferior vena cava characteristic for hypernephroma (renal cell carcinoma). A complex tumor thrombus is seen within the lumen of the inferior vena cava (arrow). The most distal extent of the tumor is 2 cm proximal to the origin of the hepatic vein. No intracardiac tumor was present in this patient. The right image demonstrates tumor extension from the inferior vena cava into the right atrium (arrow). Both these tumors were successfully removed via a cavotomy under intraoperative transesophageal echocardiography guidance. Transesophageal imaging confirmed complete removal of the tumor thrombus without embolization. HV, hepatic vein; IVC, inferior vena cava; RA, right atrium; RV, right ventricle.

Diagnostically, TEE is useful because it provides excellent visualization of venous inflow to the heart. It can also guide complete en-bloc resection of the abdominal and intraluminal tumor and enable real-time monitoring of tumor embolization[4,154-156] (see Fig. 45–23). On occasion, these tumors may also cross a patent foramen ovale (PFO), appearing as a thrombus-in-transit. In cases of intraluminal leiomyosarcoma, multiple points of attachment in the IVC may help distinguish these tumors from renal cell carcinoma or hepatoma. Thyroid carcinoma has been described growing along the superior vena cava into the right atrium[157] and carcinoma of the lung may also extend into the left atrium intraluminally directly from the pulmonary veins.[14,153,158]

The Differential Diagnosis of Cardiac Tumors, Masses, and Normal and Normal-Variant Cardiac Structures

When confronted with a suspected mass, as always, it is important to integrate all the clinical information, for example, age and prior history of malignancy, with all the echocardiographic information. The most likely etiology of an intracardiac mass is a thrombus, followed by a vegetation. Primary cardiac tumors are rare, with metastatic involvement of the heart more frequent and usually occurring in the setting of previously diagnosed malignancy. Often, a cardiac mass is diagnosed when in fact the mass really represents an unusual tomographic plane of a normal cardiac structure or normal variant of cardiac anatomy. It is important to distinguish these findings from cardiac tumors. Table 45–6 includes the most common normal or variants of normal cardiac anatomy that are often confused with abnormal masses or tumors. Apart from the clinical history, associated echocardiographic findings also provide important clues as to the etiology of the mass. For example, thrombi and vegetations have characteristic echocardiographic features but in addition, they can often be distinguished from one another and from other cardiac masses by their particular intracardiac location (e.g., left atrial appendage or ventricular apex versus valve leaflets) and the "company they keep" (e.g., atrial fibrillation, left atrial enlargement, mitral valve disease, valvular destruction, and bacteremia). Thrombi seldom occur as an isolated finding. Ventricular thrombi usually occur in the setting of coronary artery disease (CAD) with associated akinetic or dyskinetic myocardial segments, most commonly an aneurysmal left ventricular apex with concomitant left ventricular dysfunction. Atrial thrombi usually occur within the left atrial appendage in patients with atrial fibrillation, mitral valve disease, and left atrial enlargement. Ancillary features of sluggish blood flow, such as spontaneous echocardiographic contrast (SEC) and reduced left atrial appendage emptying velocities, may be present. Another useful clinical strategy to determine whether a mass is a thrombus or a tumor is to perform a serial echocardiographic evaluation following a period of systemic anticoagulation. Thrombi usually resolve after 4 weeks of anticoagulation, whereas tumors will either increase in size or remain unchanged despite anticoagulation (Fig. 45–24).

TABLE 45–6. Normal or Normal-Variant Cardiac Structures, Noncardiac Tumor Pathology, and Intracardiac Hardware That May Be Confused with Cardiac Tumors

Normal or Normal-Variant Cardiac Structures	Myocardium
Right atrium	Asymmetric ventricular hypertrophy
Crista terminalis	Noncompaction of the left ventricle
Eustachian valve	Hypereosinophilic syndrome
Chiari network	Atrial septum
Left atrium	Lipomatous hypertrophy
Floor of left upper pulmonary vein adjacent to the left	Atrial septum aneurysm
atrial appendage ("Q-tip")	Extracardiac
Right ventricle	Compression of left atrium by aorta
Moderator band	Coronary aneurysm or fistula
Left ventricle	Potential space of the transverse sinus
Papillary muscles	Left lower lobe atelectasis
Noncardiac Tumor Pathology	Hematoma
Intracardiac	Hiatal hernia
Thrombi	Pericardial fat infiltration
Valves	Mediastinal tumor
Vegetations (infective and marantic)	***Intracardiac Hardware***
Lambl's excrescence	Pacing leads
Flail or prolapsing leaflet	Swan-Ganz catheter
Severed mitral valve apparatus after mitral valve	Central line catheter
replacement	
Fatty tricuspid valve annulus	
Mitral annular calcification	

Vegetations may be confused with cardiac tumors (Fig. 45–25). However, apart from papillary fibroelastomas, primary tumors of the cardiac valves are exceedingly rare. Vegetations appear as mobile echogenic masses attached to valves and are usually diagnosed in the setting of known or suspected valve disease and bacteremia. Occasionally, when vegetations are seen in the absence of a bacteremia, other clinical features, such as rheumatologic disease or underlying malignancy, may signify Libman-Sacks endocarditis. Valvular vegetations in the setting of infective endocarditis are also usually accompanied by features of valvular

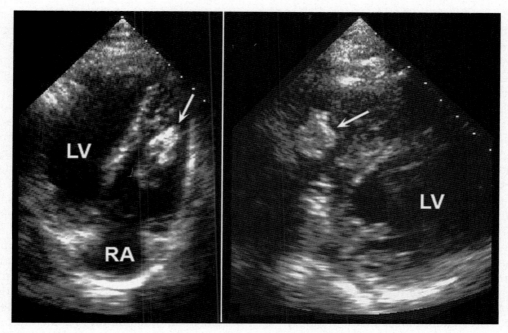

Figure 45–24. A transthoracic echocardiogram (right, apical four-chamber view; left, parasternal short-axis view) in a 20-year-old with pulmonary embolism shows a calcified thrombus in the right ventricular apex (arrow). The etiology of the mass was indeterminate and did not resolve after a month of systemic anticoagulation. Surgical excision was advised. Histology demonstrated a calcified amorphous tumor (CAT) or thrombus with a mixed inflammatory infiltrate and associated calcification. LV, left ventricle; RA, right atrium.

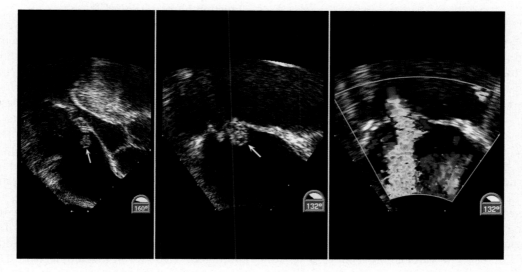

Figure 45–25. Vegetations may be confused with papillary fibroelastomas. These transesophageal echocardiographic images demonstrate distinguishing characteristics of endocarditis. A mobile 6-by-7-mm globular vegetation (arrow) is attached to the atrial aspect of the anterior mitral valve leaflet tip, seen in diastole (left) and systole (middle). Color flow imaging of the mitral valve (right) demonstrates severe mitral regurgitation secondary to destruction of the mitral valve as a result of a perforation of the anterior leaflet. This characteristic mass lesion, associated with valvular destruction and positive blood cultures, is consistent with a diagnosis of a vegetation and thus infective endocarditis.

destruction and consequent regurgitation. Nonvalvular vegetations occur at sites of turbulence and may be attached to the ventricular endocardial surface in patients with hypertrophic obstructive cardiomyopathy and in patients with septal defects.

Infiltrative disorders involving the heart may mimic cardiac tumors. These include cardiac involvement by sarcoidosis,[159] Wegener's granulomatosis,[160] hypereosinophilic syndrome,[161] and tuberculosis. Also, specific pathologic cardiac disorders reported to have been confused with cardiac tumors[162] include cardiac varices,[163] coronary artery fistula,[164] coronary artery aneurysm,[164,165] atrial septal aneurysm,[166,167] intramyocardial hematoma following percutaneous intervention,[168] blood cysts,[169] and pericardial cysts.[170]

Normal cardiac structures potentially confused with tumors include the Eustachian valve, Chiari network, lipomatous hypertrophy of the atrial septum, and the ridge of tissue seen between the left superior pulmonary vein and left atrial appendage on TEE commonly referred to as the "Q-tip." Even a diaphragmatic hernia may be confused with a cardiac tumor. This can be readily identified by having the patient drink a carbonated beverage while being imaged and confirming the presence of gas bubbles in the stomach. Knowledge of these normal cardiac structures and normal variants of cardiac anatomy is important to avoid unnecessary additional evaluation, biopsy, or operation (see Table 45–6).

Role of Newer Echocardiographic Techniques in the Imaging of Cardiac Tumors

Although TTE is an excellent screening tool, as a result of the limited image frequency of the transducer, detection of small tumors is insensitive. Transthoracic imaging has improved with the advent of tissue harmonic imaging, particularly in obese patients or those with chronic lung disease, and this has probably contributed to the increasing diagnosis of cardiac tumors antemortem. Nevertheless, TEE is more sensitive than TTE in diagnosing small tumors, particularly papillary fibroelastomas. The reported diagnostic sensitivity for detecting mass lesions by TTE and TEE is 93% and 97%, respectively.[171] TEE is also more sensitive in detecting abnormalities involving the posterior cardiac structures, particularly the atria, interatrial septum, and pulmonary veins. Intracardiac ultrasound (US), using a variable frequency (5 to 10 MHz) phased array transducer affixed to the end of a deflectable catheter has been recently introduced. These transducers provide high-resolution images of intracardiac structures and have been used to guide intracardiac tumor biopsy (see Fig. 45–22). However, because this is an invasive technique more widespread application for cardiac tumor diagnosis is limited.[172,173]

From both a diagnostic and therapeutic standpoint, echocardiography not only has an important and established role in invasive procedures related to diagnostic biopsy of cardiac masses but also in the therapeutic or diagnostic drainage of suspected malignant pericardial effusions. Open thoracotomy, cardiopulmonary bypass and resection, or open biopsy remains the diagnostic standard.[173-178] However, in patients with right-sided lesions (most commonly malignant) who may be too ill, have unresectable disease or only need a diagnostic tissue biopsy before chemotherapy, TEE or intracardiac echocardiography can be especially useful to guide percutaneous biopsy. Real-time visualization of the procedure enhances safety, minimizing risk of inadvertent damage to delicate surrounding structures, and increasing diagnostic yield by directing the bioptome to the tumor tissue directly, as compared with using fluoroscopy alone. For pericardial effusions, concomitant TTE complements percutaneous pericardiocentesis. This approach has been well described and not only enhances safety of the procedure but also permits immediate hemodynamic assessment following pericardiocentesis and serial assessment following ongoing pericardial drainage.

Intraoperative TEE is also an important tool in guiding surgical intervention. In a report from the Mayo Clinic on patients undergoing cardiac surgery primarily for resection of mass lesions, intraoperative TEE added diagnostic information that resulted in modification of the surgical procedure, both before and after cardiopulmonary bypass in 16% of cases. In fact, this study and others have documented the importance of confirming that the mass is indeed present immediately before the skin incision to avoid unnecessary surgery for tumors that may have embolized in the period between initial detection and surgery.[179,180]

In recent years, 3D TTE and TEE have evolved into a new clinical diagnostic tool in cardiac imaging.[181-184] Using this technique, anatomy and pathology can be appreciated without having to perform "mental reconstruction" of the problem permitting morphologic, volume, and spatial assessment of masses and tumors in vivo[185] (Fig. 45–26). It also permits noninvasive "sectioning" of the mass to better evaluate its morphologic and spatial characteristics thereby reportedly helping guide preoperative decision making.[181,185] Unlike CT or MRI, a hemodynamic assessment can be performed at the same time.

Although 3D reconstruction can be derived from both TTE and TEE studies, transthoracic imaging yields poor quality images if poor acoustic windows are encountered. This can be overcome with TEE, provided the probe is stabilized and the study is gated to respiration and heart rate.[186] 3D TEE also permits volume quantification of intracardiac mass lesions. These volume assessments have been shown to correlate well with in vitro measured volumes of surgical specimens.[30] Currently transthoracic image resolution and quality is suboptimal for detection of small tumors.

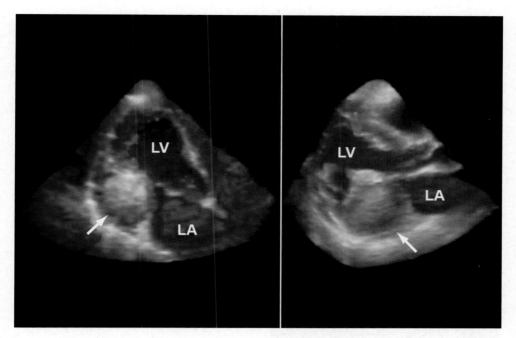

Figure 45–26. *3D echocardiography applied to cardiac tumor diagnosis. A full volume 3D echocardiogram, apical four-chamber (left) and modified parasternal long-axis view (right) shows an intracardiac carcinoid tumor (arrow) in the left atrioventricular groove and its relationship to the mitral valve. These images are complimentary to the standard 2D images from the same patient in Figure 45–22. LA, left atrium; LV, left ventricle.*

Therefore, standard 2D imaging techniques should still be used to identify cardiac tumors.

Analysis of myocardial motion using tissue Doppler imaging (TDI) has also been used to characterize differences in tissue velocity of tumors versus normal myocardial tissue. Strain imaging, derived from either tissue velocity data or speckle tracking algorithms, is less susceptible to translational motion. It identifies contracting from noncontracting tissue and thus may be potentially helpful in distinguishing noncontractile tumors and thrombi from normal contracting myocardium. This concept has already been explored to identify and distinguish fibromas and rhabdomyomas.[187,188] Fibromas are composed of fibroblasts and collagen, and rhabdomyomas are composed of altered myocytes. Consequently the fibroma has less deformability than the rhabdomyoma or the surrounding normal myocardium. Echocardiographic derived strain data can identify this deformation or lack thereof, providing additional diagnostic information to identify and distinguish these tumors (Fig. 45–27). This technique can also be employed using tagged MRI, but it is labor intensive.[189]

Although the concept that unique ultrasound-tissue interaction holds potential in distinguishing abnormal from normal cardiac tissue, and despite being extensively explored in carefully controlled experiments, ultrasound-based tissue characterization has not proved practical or robust enough to be useful clinically.[190-192]

Echocardiographic contrast imaging may be useful in evaluating cardiac tumors by enhancing border defini-tion, better outlining tumor location and site of attachment and also by distinguishing vascular from avascular structures (e.g., thrombi by assessment of myocardial perfusion).[193] Perfusion imaging has improved significantly with advances in second-generation contrast agents and new imaging techniques, such as power modulation.[194-196] Both qualitative and quantitative differences in gray scale have been reported in various cardiac masses using this technique.[195] Malignant and highly vascular tumors demonstrated greater enhancement than adjacent myocardium, whereas myxomas demonstrated partial perfusion and quantitatively less enhancement than surrounding myocardium. Thrombi demonstrated no perfusion. In this study perfusion imaging also identified pericardial malignancy—an area less well appreciated using standard noncontrast imaging. Although promising, a limitation of this method in clinical practice is that it is time consuming, requiring off-line analysis of time intensity curves. Also, the technique requires skill and experience in contrast administration and image acquisition.

Targeted microbubble delivery represents an exciting frontier. Echocardiographic contrast bubbles are being engineered to target tumors to "unmask" them, making them easier to identify and characterize and also potentially to serve as vehicles for targeted therapy delivery. A recent study in a tumor-bearing mouse model has evaluated the use of contrast microbubbles targeted to tumor vasculature via conjugation with the tumor-binding peptide arginine-arginine-leucine. Using this technique the investigators were able to distinguish

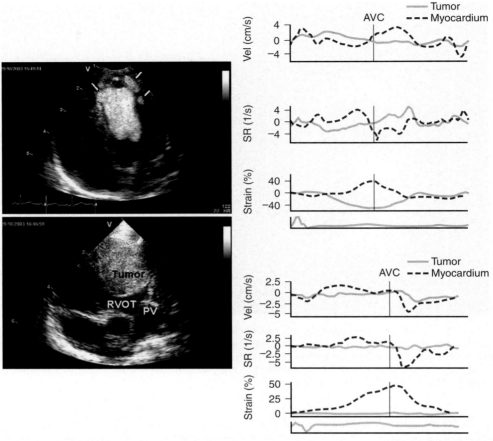

Figure 45–27. *Newer echocardiographic-based strain analysis applied to cardiac tumor diagnosis. Top, An apical four-chamber view shows three cardiac tumors in the left ventricle (arrows) consistent with rhabdomyomas. Corresponding longitudinal color Doppler myocardial imaging curves are shown recorded from the tumor and adjacent interventricular septum. The upper, mid and lower curves demonstrate myocardial velocity, strain rate and strain, respectively. In early systole, the tumor moves and deforms in the same direction as the surrounding myocardium. Later in systole, the myocardium squeezes the soft mass in the opposite direction. Bottom, Parasternal short-axis shows a fibroma attached to the right ventricular free wall extending toward the right ventricular outflow tract. In this case the fibroma neither moves nor deforms. These tissue Doppler characteristics may potentially be used to differentiate the rhabdomyoma from fibroma. AVC, aortic valve closure; PV, pulmonary valve; RVOT, right ventricular outflow tract; SR, strain rate; Vel, velocity. (From Ganame J, D'Hooge J, Mertens L: Eur J Echocardiogr 6:461-464, 2005, with permission.)*

normal tissue and tumor tissue in vivo. This pioneering work may open the possibility of ultrasonic molecular imaging of tumor angiogenesis in the clinical setting, thereby permitting improved noninvasive identification of tumors, assessment of malignant potential, and monitoring of tumor response.[197]

Summary

Echocardiography remains a vital noninvasive method of detecting and diagnosing cardiac tumors. Although cardiac tumors are rare, they are increasingly recognized antemortem, permitting earlier diagnosis and curative therapy. Echocardiography provides precise anatomic location and hemodynamic impact of most cardiac tumors. It is less sensitive in detecting intramyocardial and pericardial lesions. Other modalities, such as CT and MRI, are often better suited for tumor or metastases in these locations and should be seen as complementary imaging techniques. Moreover, these techniques are also helpful to determine extra cardiac spread. Echocardiography, particularly TEE and on occasion intracardiac ultrasound, provide echocardiographic guidance for percutaneous biopsy and diagnosis of cardiac masses. Also, echocardiography significantly aids and improves safety of percutaneous pericardiocentesis. Newer echocardiography techniques including contrast, tissue Doppler imaging, and speckle tracking do provide additional information and hold promise in refining the echocardiographic diagnosis of cardiac tumors. As always, when using echocardiography to assess cardiac tumors, all available clinical information should be integrated to maximize its diagnostic potential.

KEY POINTS

■ Cardiac tumors are rare. Incidental cardiac masses usually represent thrombi or vegetations. Three quarters of primary cardiac tumors are benign.

■ Myxomas are the most common benign primary cardiac tumor occurring sporadically as an isolated tumor in the left atrium usually attached to the fossa ovalis by a thin stalk. Multiple tumors or atypical locations suggest familial myxoma.

■ Papillary fibroelastomas, characterized by a small, mobile pedunculated anemone-like mass with a stippled edge, are the most common valvular tumors.

■ Lipomatous hypertrophy of the atrial septum may be confused with an intracardiac tumor. It results in a dumbbell-shaped intraatrial septum with characteristic sparing of the fossa ovalis membrane. The diagnosis can be confirmed by MRI or CT.

■ Rhabdomyomas are the most frequent cardiac neoplasm in childhood. They are almost always multiple, occurring in both left and right ventricles and can be expected to spontaneously regress in size in most patients less than 4 years of age. They are seen in 50% of infants with tuberous sclerosis.

■ Cardiac fibromas are the most common resected cardiac tumor in childhood. These characteristically solitary circumscribed tumors are usually located in the ventricles.

■ Only 15% of primary cardiac tumors are malignant, the vast majority of which (95%) are sarcomas. Sarcomas do not have a characteristic echocardiographic appearance. They are most commonly found in the right atrium. Widespread local infiltration is usually present and the clinical course is dismal.

■ Secondary cardiac malignancy or metastatic disease is 30 times more common than primary cardiac tumors. Malignant tumors spread to the heart by direct extension, hematogenous, lymphatic and intraluminal spread. Malignant melanoma has the highest rate of cardiac metastasis of any tumor. Renal cell carcinoma is the most common tumor to spread to the heart by the IVC.

■ Multiple tumors may be missed, particularly if the imager is distracted by finding the index tumor. Careful evaluation of all cardiac chambers is necessary to exclude multiple tumors.

■ When confronted with a suspected mass, it is important to integrate all the clinical information to make the most accurate noninvasive diagnosis.

REFERENCES

1. Reynen K: Frequency of primary tumors of the heart. *Am J Cardiol* 77:107, 1996.
2. Lam KY, Dickens P, Chan AC: Tumors of the heart. A 20-year experience with a review of 12,485 consecutive autopsies. *Arch Pathol Lab Med* 117:1027-1031, 1993.
3. Piazza N, Chughai T, Toledano K, et al: Primary cardiac tumors: Eighteen years of surgical experience on 21 patients. *Can J Cardiol* 20:1443-1448, 2004.
4. Goldman JH, Foster E: Transesophageal echocardiographic (TEE) evaluation of intracardiac and pericardial masses. *Cardiol Clin* 18:849-860, 2000.
5. Gowda RM, Khan AI, Nair CK, et al: Cardiac papillary fibroelastoma: A comprehensive analysis of 725 cases. *Am Heart J* 146:404-410, 2003.
6. Howard RA, Aldea GS, Shapira OM, et al: Papillary fibroelastoma: Increasing recognition of a surgical disease. *Ann Thorac Surg* 68:1881-1885, 1999.
7. Fyke FE 3rd, Segard JB, Edwards WD, et al: Primary cardiac tumors: Experience with 30 consecutive patients since the introduction of two-dimensional echocardiography. *J Am Coll Cardiol* 5:1465-1473, 1985.
8. Endo A, Ohtahara A, Kinugawa T, et al: Characteristics of 161 patients with cardiac tumors diagnosed during 1993 and 1994 in Japan. *Am J Cardiol* 79:1708-1711, 1997.
9. Araoz PA, Mulvagh SL, Tazelaar HD, et al: CT and MR imaging of benign primary cardiac neoplasms with echocardiographic correlation. *Radiographics* 20:1303-1319, 2000.
10. Tatli S, Lipton MJ: CT for intracardiac thrombi and tumors. *Int J Cardiovasc Imaging* 21:115-131, 2005.
11. Vander Salm TJ: Unusual primary tumors of the heart. *Semin Thorac Cardiovasc Surg* 12:89-100, 2000.
12. Colucci WS: Primary tumors of the heart. In Braunwald E, Zipes DP, Libby P (eds): *Heart Disease*, 6th ed. Philadelphia, WB Saunders, 2001.
13. Parissis JT, Zezas S, Sfiras N, Kastellanos S: An atypical left atrial myxoma causing intracavitary pressure gradient and typical diastolic transmitral flow of severe mitral stenosis. *Int J Cardiol* 102:165-167, 2005.
14. Salcedo EE, Cohen GI, White RD, Davison MB: Cardiac tumors: Diagnosis and management. *Curr Probl Cardiol* 17:73-137, 1992.
15. Mugge A, Daniel WG, Haverich A, Litchlen PR: Diagnosis of noninfective cardiac mass lesions by two-dimensional echocardiography. Comparison of the transthoracic and transesophageal approaches. *Circulation* 83:70-78, 1991.
16. Leibowitz G, Keller MM, Daniel WG, et al: Transesophageal versus transthoracic echocardiography in the evaluation of right atrial tumors. *Am Heart J* 130:1224-1227, 1995.
17. Samdarshi TE, Mahan EF 3rd, Nanda NC, et al: Transesophageal echocardiographic diagnosis of multicentric left ventricular myxomas mimicking a left atrial tumor. *J Thorac Cardiovasc Surg* 103:471-474, 1992.
18. Herrmann MA, et al: Primary cardiac angiosarcoma: A clinicopathologic study of six cases. *J Thorac Cardiovasc Surg* 103:655-664, 1992.
19. Acebo E, Val-Bernal JF, Gomez-Roman JJ, Reveulta JM: Clinicopathologic study and DNA analysis of 37 cardiac myxomas: A 28-year experience. *Chest* 123:1379-1385, 2003.
20. Tazelaar HD, Locke TJ, McGregor CG: Pathology of surgically excised primary cardiac tumors. *Mayo Clin Proc* 67:957-965, 1992.
21. Molina JE, Edwards JE, Ward HB: Primary cardiac tumors: experience at the University of Minnesota. *Thorac Cardiovasc Surg* 38(Suppl 2):183-191, 1990.
22. Larrieu AJ, Jamieson WR, Tyers GF, et al: Primary cardiac tumors: Experience with 25 cases. *J Thorac Cardiovasc Surg* 83:339-348, 1982.

23. Odim J, Reehal V, Laks H, et al: Surgical pathology of cardiac tumors. Two decades at an urban institution. *Cardiovasc Pathol* 12:267-270, 2003.

24. Kamiya H, Yasuda T, Nagamine H, et al: Surgical treatment of primary cardiac tumors: 28 years' experience in Kanazawa University Hospital. *Jpn Circ J* 65:315-319, 2001.

25. Butany J, Nair V, Naseemuddin A, Nair GM, et al: Cardiac tumors: Diagnosis and management. *Lancet Oncol* 6:219-228, 2005.

26. Shapiro LM: Cardiac tumors: Diagnosis and management. *Heart* 85:218-222, 2001.

27. Roberts WC: Primary and secondary neoplasms of the heart. *Am J Cardiol* 80:671-682, 1997.

28. Chiles C, Woodward PK, Gutierrez FR, Link KM: Metastatic involvement of the heart and pericardium: CT and MR imaging. *Radiographics* 21:439-449, 2001.

29. Cohen GU, Perry TM, Evans JM: Neoplastic invasion of the heart and pericardium. *Ann Intern Med* 42:1238-1245, 1955.

30. Ahmed S, Nanda NC, Miller AP, et al: Volume quantification of intracardiac mass lesions by transesophageal three-dimensional echocardiography. *Ultrasound Med Biol* 28:1389-1393, 2002.

31. McAllister HA Jr: Papillary fibroelastoma: Tumors of the cardiovascular system. *AFIB Atlas of Tumor Pathology* 15:20-25, 1978.

32. Reynen K: Cardiac myxomas. *N Engl J Med* 333:1610-1617, 1995.

33. Pinede L, Duhaut P, Loire R: Clinical presentation of left atrial cardiac myxoma. A series of 112 consecutive cases. *Medicine (Baltimore)* 80:159-172, 2001.

34. Kuon E, Kreplin M, Weiss W, Dahm JB: The challenge presented by right atrial myxoma. *Herz* 29:702-709, 2004.

35. Keeling IM, Oberwalder P, Anelli-Monti M, et al: Cardiac myxomas: 24 years of experience in 49 patients. *Eur J Cardiothorac Surg* 22:971-977, 2002.

36. Jelic J, Milicic D, Alfirevic I, et al: Cardiac myxoma: Diagnostic approach, surgical treatment and follow-up. A twenty years experience. *J Cardiovasc Surg (Torino)* 37(suppl 1):113-117, 1996.

37. Centofanti P, Di Rosa E, Deorsola L, et al: Primary cardiac tumors: Early and late results of surgical treatment in 91 patients. *Ann Thorac Surg* 68:1236-1241, 1999.

38. Selkane C, Amahzoune B, Chavanis N, et al: Changing management of cardiac myxoma based on a series of 40 cases with long-term follow-up. *Ann Thorac Surg* 76:1935-1938, 2003.

39. Akbarzadeh Z, Esmailzadeh M, Yousefi A, et al: Multicentric familial cardiac myxoma. *Eur J Echocardiogr* 6:148-150, 2005.

40. Carney JA, Gordon H, Carpenter PC, et al: The complex of myxomas, spotty pigmentation, and endocrine overactivity. *Medicine (Baltimore)* 64:270-283, 1985.

41. Vidaillet HJ Jr, Seward JB, Fyke FE 3rd, et al: "Syndrome myxoma": A subset of patients with cardiac myxoma associated with pigmented skin lesions and peripheral and endocrine neoplasms. *Br Heart J* 57:247-255, 1987.

42. Edwards A, Bermudez C, Piwonka G, et al: Carney's syndrome: Complex myxomas. Report of four cases and review of the literature. *Cardiovasc Surg* 10:264-275, 2002.

43. Szucs RA, Rehr RB, Yanovich S, Tatum JL: Magnetic resonance imaging of cardiac rhabdomyosarcoma. Quantifying the response to chemotherapy. *Cancer* 67:2066-2070, 1991.

44. Bhan A, Mehrotra R, Choudhary SK, et al: Surgical experience with intracardiac myxomas: Long-term follow-up. *Ann Thorac Surg* 66:810-813, 1998.

45. Hermans K, Jaarsma W, Plokker HW, et al: Four cardiac myxomas diagnosed three times in one patient. *Eur J Echocardiogr* 4:336-338, 2003.

46. Percell RL Jr, Henning RJ, Siddique Patel M: Atrial myxoma: case report and a review of the literature. *Heart Dis* 5:224-230, 2003.

47. Heath D: Pathology of cardiac tumors. *Am J Cardiol* 21:315-327, 1968.

48. Schanz U, Schneider J: [Endocardial myxoma. Current aspects of its histopathogenesis]. *Schweiz Med Wochenschr* 114:850-857, 1984.

49. Prichard RW: Tumors of the heart; review of the subject and report of 150 cases. *AMA Arch Pathol* 51:98-128, 1951.

50. Schweiger MJ, Hafer JG Jr, Brown R, Gianelly RE: Spontaneous cure of infected left atrial myxoma following embolization. *Am Heart J* 99:630-634, 1980.

51. Graham HV, von Hartitzsch B, Medina JR: Infected atrial myxoma. *Am J Cardiol* 38:658-661, 1976.

52. Joseph P, Himmelstein DU, Mahowald JM, Stullman WS, et al: Atrial myxoma infected with Candida: First survival. *Chest* 78:340-343, 1980.

53. Quinn TJ, Codini MA, Harris AA: Infected cardiac myxoma. *Am J Cardiol* 53:381-382, 1984.

54. Obeid AI, Marvasti M, Parker F, Rosenberg J: Comparison of transthoracic and transesophageal echocardiography in diagnosis of left atrial myxoma. *Am J Cardiol* 63:1006-1008, 1989.

55. Thier W, Schluter M, Krebber HJ, et al: Cysts in left atrial myxomas identified by transesophageal cross-sectional echocardiography. *Am J Cardiol* 51:1793-1795, 1983.

56. Rahilly GT Jr, Nanda NC: Two-dimensional echographic identification of tumor hemorrhages in atrial myxomas. *Am Heart J* 101:237-239, 1981.

57. Dittmann H, Voelker W, Karsch KR, Seipel L: Bilateral atrial myxomas detected by transesophageal two-dimensional echocardiography. *Am Heart J* 118:172-173, 1989.

58. Engberding R, Daniel WG, Erbel R, et al: Diagnosis of heart tumors by transesophageal echocardiography: A multicentre study in 154 patients. European Cooperative Study Group. *Eur Heart J* 14:1223-1228, 1993.

59. Perez de Isla L, de Castro R, Zamoran JL, et al: Diagnosis and treatment of cardiac myxomas by transesophageal echocardiography. *Am J Cardiol* 90:1419-1421, 2002.

60. Masui T, Takahashi M, Miura K, et al: Cardiac myxoma: Identification of intratumoral hemorrhage and calcification on MR images. *AJR Am J Roentgenol* 164:850-852, 1995.

61. Lie JT: Petrified cardiac myxoma masquerading as organized atrial mural thrombus. *Arch Pathol Lab Med* 113:742-745, 1989.

62. Restrepo CS, Largoza A, Lemos DF, et al: CT and MR imaging findings of malignant cardiac tumors. *Curr Probl Diagn Radiol* 34:1-11, 2005.

63. Burke A: Tumors of the heart and great vessels. In *Atlas of Tumor Pathology*. Washington, DC, Armed Forces Institute of Pathology, 1996, pp. 1-98.

64. Sun JP, Asher CR, Yang XS, et al: Clinical and echocardiographic characteristics of papillary fibroelastomas: A retrospective and prospective study in 162 patients. *Circulation* 103:2687-2693, 2001.

65. Burn CG, Bishop MB, Davies JN: A stalked papillary tumor of the mural endocardium. *Am J Clin Pathol* 51:344-346, 1969.

66. Paelinck B, Vermeersch P, Kockx M: Calcified papillary fibroelastoma of the tricuspid valve. *Acta Cardiol* 53:165-167, 1998.

67. Burke A: Papillary fibroelastomas: Tumors of the heart and great vessels. *AFIB Atlas of Tumor Pathology* 16:47-54, 1996.

68. Bottio T, Basso C, Rizzoli G, et al: Case report: Fibroelastoma of the papillary muscle of the mitral valve. Diagnostic implications and review of the literature. *J Heart Valve Dis* 11:288-291, 2002.

69. Fabricius AM, Heidrich L, Gutz U, Mohr FW: Papillary fibroelastoma of the tricuspid valve chordae with a review of the literature. *Cardiovasc J S Afr* 13:122-124, 2002.

70. Brown RD Jr, Khandheria BK, Edwards WD: Cardiac papillary fibroelastoma: A treatable cause of transient ischemic attack and ischemic stroke detected by transesophageal echocardiography. *Mayo Clin Proc* 70:863-868, 1995.

71. Kanarek SE, Wright P, Liu J, et al: Multiple fibroelastomas: A case report and review of the literature. *J Am Soc Echocardiogr* 16:373-376, 2003.

72. Klarich KW, Enriquez-Sarano M, Gura GM et al: Papillary fibroelastoma: Ehocardiographic characteristics for diagnosis and pathologic correlation. *J Am Coll Cardiol* 30:784-790, 1997.

73. Daveron E, Jain M, Kelley GP et al: Papillary fibroelastoma and Lambl's excrescences: echocardiographic diagnosis and differential diagnosis. *Echocardiography* 22:461-463, 2005.

74. Lambl V: Papillare excrescenzen an der semilunar-klappe der aorta. *Wien Med Wochenschr* 6:244-247, 1856.

75. Boone SA, Campagna M, Walley VM: Lambl's excrescences and papillary fibroelastomas: are they different? *Can J Cardiol* 8:372-376, 1992.

76. Paraf F, Berrebi A, Chauvaud S, et al: [Mitral papillary fibroelastoma in a HIV infected patient]. *Presse Med* 28:962-964, 1999.

77. Shirani J, Metveyeva P, et al: Transient loss of vision as the presenting symptom of papillary fibroelastoma of aortic valve. *Cardiovasc Pathol* 6:237-240, 1997.

78. Okada K, Sueda T, Orihashi K, et al: Cardiac papillary fibroelastoma on the pulmonary valve: A rare cardiac tumor. *Ann Thorac Surg* 71:1677-1679, 2001.

79. Basu S, Folliguet T, Anselmo M, et al: Lipomatous hypertrophy of the interatrial septum. *Cardiovasc Surg* 2:229-231, 1994.

80. Zeebregts CJ, Hensens AG, Timmermans J, et al: Lipomatous hypertrophy of the interatrial septum: Indication for surgery? *Eur J Cardiothorac Surg* 11:785-787, 1997.

81. Breuer M, Wipperman J, Franke U, Wahlers T: Lipomatous hypertrophy of the interatrial septum and upper right atrial inflow obstruction. *Eur J Cardiothorac Surg* 22:1023-1025, 2002.

82. Lang-Lazdunski L, Oroudji M, Pansard Y, et al: Successful resection of giant intrapericardial lipoma. *Ann Thorac Surg* 58:238-240; discussion 240-241, 1994.

83. Vanderheyden M, De Sutter J, Wellens F, Andries E: Left atrial lipoma: Case report and review of the literature. *Acta Cardiol* 53:31-32, 1998.

84. Mousseaux E, Idy-Peretti I, Bittoun J, et al: MR tissue characterization of a right atrial mass: Diagnosis of a lipoma. *J Comput Assist Tomogr* 16:148-151, 1992.

85. Mullen, JC, et al: Right atrial lipoma. *Ann Thorac Surg* 59(5):1239-1241, 1995.

86. King SJ, Smallhorn JF, Burrows PE: Epicardial lipoma: Imaging findings. *AJR Am J Roentgenol* 160:261-262, 1993.

87. Doshi S, Halim M, Singh H, Patel R: Massive intrapericardial lipoma, a rare cause of breathlessness. Investigations and management. *Int J Cardiol* 66:211-215, 1998.

88. Kamiya H, Ohno M, Iwata H, et al: Cardiac lipoma in the interventricular septum: Evaluation by computed tomography and magnetic resonance imaging. *Am Heart J* 119:1215-1217, 1990.

89. Kozelj M, Angelski R, Pavcnik D: Lipomatous hypertrophy of the interatrial septum: Diagnosis by echocardiography and magnetic resonance imaging. A case report. *Angiology* 46:863-866, 1995.

90. Restrepo CS, Largoza A, Lemos DF, et al: CT and MR imaging findings of benign cardiac tumors. *Curr Probl Diagn Radiol* 34:12-21, 2005.

91. Tuna IC, Julsrud PR, Click RL, et al: Tissue characterization of an unusual right atrial mass by magnetic resonance imaging. *Mayo Clin Proc* 66:498-501, 1991.

92. Nadra I, Dawson D, Schmitz SA, et al: Lipomatous hypertrophy of the interatrial septum: A commonly misdiagnosed mass often leading to unnecessary cardiac surgery. *Heart* 90:e66, 2004.

93. McAllister HA Jr: Tumors of the cardiovascular system. In *Atlas of Tumor Pathology*. Washington DC, Armed Forces Institute of Pathology, 1978, pp. 46-52.

94. Alsaileek A, Tepe SM, Alveraz L, et al: Diagnostic features of cardiac hemangioma on cardiovascular magnetic resonance, a case report. *Int J Cardiovasc Imaging* 22:699-702, 2006.

95. Lapenna E, De Bonis M, Torracca L, et al: Cavernous hemangioma of the tricuspid valve: Minimally invasive surgical resection. *Ann Thorac Surg* 76:2097-2099, 2003.

96. Kojima S, Sumiyoshi M, Suwa S, et al: Cardiac hemangioma: A report of two cases and review of the literature. *Heart Vessels* 18:153-156, 2003.

97. Matsumoto Y, Watanabe G, Endo M, Sasaki H: Surgical treatment of a cavernous hemangioma of the left atrial roof. *Eur J Cardiothorac Surg* 20:633-635, 2001.

98. Landolphi DR, Belkin RN, Hjemdahl-Monsen CE, LaFaro RJ: Cardiac cavernous hemangioma mimicking pericardial cyst: Atypical echocardiographic appearance of a rare cardiac tumor. *J Am Soc Echocardiogr* 10:579-581, 1991.

99. Hangler HB, Vorderwinkler KP, Fend F, Dapunt OE: Intramural right atrial myocardial hemangioma treated by emergency surgery. *Eur J Cardiothorac Surg* 11:782-784, 1997.

100. Sarjeant JM, Butany J, Cusimano RJ: Cancer of the heart: Epidemiology and management of primary tumors and metastases. *Am J Cardiovasc Drugs* 3:407-421, 2003.

101. Perk G, Yim J, Varkey M, et al: Cardiac cavernous hemangioma. *J Am Soc Echocardiogr* 18:979, 2005.

102. Fukuzawa S, Yamamoto T, Shimada K, et al: Hemangioma of the left ventricular cavity: Presumptive diagnosis by magnetic resonance imaging. *Heart Vessels* 8:211-214, 1993.

103. Moniotte S, Geva T, Perez-Atayde A, et al: Images in cardiovascular medicine. Cardiac hemangioma. *Circulation* 112:e103-e104, 2005.

104. Brizard C, Latremouille C, Jebara VA, et al: Cardiac hemangiomas. *Ann Thorac Surg* 56:390-394, 1993.

105. Broadwater B, McAdams HP, Dodd L: Case report: Pericardial hemangioma. *J Comput Assist Tomogr* 20:954-956, 1996.

106. Freedom RM, Lee KJ, MacDonald C, Taylor G: Selected aspects of cardiac tumors in infancy and childhood. *Pediatr Cardiol* 21:299-316, 2000.

107. Kagan KO, Schmidt M, Kuhn U, Kimmig R: Ventricular outflow obstruction, valve aplasia, bradyarrhythmia, pulmonary hypoplasia and non-immune fetal hydrops because of a large rhabdomyoma in a case of unknown tuberous sclerosis: A prenatal diagnosed cardiac rhabdomyoma with multiple symptoms. *BJOG* 111:1478-1480, 2004.

108. Bass JL, Breningstall GN, Swaiman KF: Echocardiographic incidence of cardiac rhabdomyoma in tuberous sclerosis. *Am J Cardiol* 55:1379-1382, 1985.

109. Smith HC, Watson GH, Patel RG, Super M: Cardiac rhabdomyomata in tuberous sclerosis: Their course and diagnostic value. *Arch Dis Child* 64:196-200, 1989.

110. Nir A, Tajik AJ, Freeman WK, et al: Tuberous sclerosis and cardiac rhabdomyoma. *Am J Cardiol* 76:419-421, 1995.

111. Burke A: *Atlas of Tumor Pathology*, 16th ed. Washington DC, Armed Forces Institute of Pathology, 1996, pp. 1-11, 55-67, 69-78, 79-85.

112. Fujita N, Caputo GR, Higgins CB: Diagnosis and characterization of intracardiac masses by magnetic resonance imaging. *Am J Cardiovasc Imaging* 8:69-80, 1994.

113. Grebenc ML, Rosado de Christenson ML, Burke AP, et al: Primary cardiac and pericardial neoplasms: Radiologic-pathologic correlation. *Radiographics* 20:1073-1103; quiz 1110-1111, 1112, 2000.

114. Bosi G, Lintermans JP, Pellegrino PA, et al: The natural history of cardiac rhabdomyoma with and without tuberous sclerosis. *Acta Paediatr* 85:928-931, 1996.

115. Smythe JF, Dyck JD, Smallhorn JF, Freedom RM: Natural history of cardiac rhabdomyoma in infancy and childhood. *Am J Cardiol* 66:1247-1249, 1990.

116. Becker AE: Primary heart tumors in the pediatric age group: A review of salient pathologic features relevant for clinicians. *Pediatr Cardiol* 21:317-323, 2000.

117. Jacobs JP, Konstantakos AK, Holland FW 2nd, et al: Surgical treatment for cardiac rhabdomyomas in children. *Ann Thorac Surg* 58:1552-1555, 1994.

118. Jozwiak S, Kawalec W, Dluzewska J, et al: Cardiac tumors in tuberous sclerosis: Their incidence and course. *Eur J Pediatr* 153:155-157, 1994.

119. Beghetti M, Gow RM, Haney I, et al: Pediatric primary benign cardiac tumors: A 15-year review. *Am Heart J* 134:1107-1114, 1997.

120. Kanemoto N, Usui K, Fusegawa Y: An adult case of cardiac fibroma. *Intern Med* 33:10-12, 1004.

121. Coffin CM: Congenital cardiac fibroma associated with Gorlin syndrome. *Pediatr Pathol* 12:255-262, 1992.

122. Herman TE, Siegel MJ, McAlister WH: Cardiac tumor in Gorlin syndrome. Nevoid basal cell carcinoma syndrome. *Pediatr Radiol* 21:234-235, 1991.

123. Gorlin RJ: Nevoid basal-cell carcinoma syndrome. *Medicine (Baltimore)* 66:98-113, 1987.

124. Parmley LF, Salley RK, Williams JP, Head GB 3rd: The clinical spectrum of cardiac fibroma with diagnostic and surgical considerations: Noninvasive imaging enhances management. *Ann Thorac Surg* 45:455-465, 1988.

125. de Ruiz M, Potter JL, Stavinoha J, et al: Real-time ultrasound diagnosis of cardiac fibroma in a neonate. *J Ultrasound Med* 4:367-369, 1985.

126. Ferguson HL, Hawkins EP, Cooley LD: Infant cardiac fibroma with clonal t(1;9)(q32;q22) and review of benign fibrous tissue cytogenetics. *Cancer Genet Cytogenet* 87:34-37, 1996.

127. Burke AP, Rosado de Christenson M, Templeton PA, Virmani R: Cardiac fibroma: Clinicopathologic correlates and surgical treatment. *J Thorac Cardiovasc Surg* 108:862-870, 1994.

128. Basso C, Valente M, Poletti A, et al: Surgical pathology of primary cardiac and pericardial tumors. *Eur J Cardiothorac Surg* 12:730-737; discussion 737-738, 1997.

129. Veinot JP, O'Murchu B, Tazelaar HD, et al: Cardiac fibroma mimicking apical hypertrophic cardiomyopathy: A case report and differential diagnosis. *J Am Soc Echocardiogr* 9:94-99, 1996.

130. Grinda JM, Mace L, Dervanian P, Neveux JY: Obstructive right ventricular cardiac fibroma in an adult. *Eur J Cardiothorac Surg* 13:319-321, 1998.

131. Gutberlet M, Abdul-Khaliq H, Stiller B, et al: Giant fibroma in the left ventricle of an infant: Imaging findings in magnetic resonance imaging, echocardiography and angiography. *Eur Radiol* 12(suppl 3):S143-S148, 2002.

132. Osranek M, Bursi F, Gura GM, et al: Echocardiographic features of pheochromocytoma of the heart. *Am J Cardiol* 91:640-643, 2003.

133. Donsbeck AV, Ranchere D, Coindre JM, et al: Primary cardiac sarcomas: An immunohistochemical and grading study with long-term follow-up of 24 cases. *Histopathology* 34:295-304, 1999.

134. Janigan DT, Husain A, Robinson NA: Cardiac angiosarcomas. A review and a case report. *Cancer* 57:852-859, 1986.

135. Castorino F, Masiello P, Quattrocchi E, Di Bendentto G: Primary cardiac rhabdomyosarcoma of the left atrium: An unusual presentation. *Tex Heart Inst J* 27:206-208, 2000.

136. McAllister HA Jr: Primary tumors and cysts of the heart and pericardium. *Curr Probl Cardiol* 4:1-51, 1979.

137. Holladay AO, Siegel RJ, Schwartz DA: Cardiac malignant lymphoma in acquired immune deficiency syndrome. *Cancer* 70:2203-2207, 1992.

138. Burtin P, Guerci A, Boman F, et al: Malignant lymphoma in the donor heart after heart transplantation. *Eur Heart J* 14:1143-1145, 1993.

139. Kelsey RC, Saker A, Morgan M: Cardiac lymphoma in a patient with AIDS. *Ann Intern Med* 115:370-371, 1991.

140. Pousset F, Le Heuzey JY, Pialoux G, et al: Cardiac lymphoma presenting as atrial flutter in an AIDS patient. *Eur Heart J* 15:862-864, 1994.

141. Le Heuzey JY, Pousset F, Pialoux G: Letter to the editor. *Arch Mal Coeur Vaiss* 89:269, 1996.

142. Denis J, Hery B, Crepin V, et al: Malignant tumoral lymphoma of the heart in human immunodeficiency virus infection: Diagnosis by echocardiography. *Arch Mal Coeur Vaiss* 88:507-510, 1995.

143. Pettelot G, Gibelin P, Blanc P, et al: Complete regression of cardiac non-Hodgkin's lymphoma after 23 months with chemotherapy. *Arch Mal Coeur Vaiss* 89:379-381, 1996.

144. Tighe DA, Hochman A, Levij IS, Stern S: Primary cardiac lymphoma. *Echocardiography* 17:345-347, 2000.

145. Brian S, et al: Clinical diagnosis of secondary tumors of the heart and pericardium. *Dis Chest* 55:202, 1959.

146. Longo R, Mocini D, Santini M, et al: Unusual sites of metastatic malignancy: case 1. Cardiac metastasis in hepatocellular carcinoma. *J Clin Oncol* 22:5012-5014, 2004.

147. Gibbs P, Cebon JS, Calafiore P, Robinson WA: Cardiac metastases from malignant melanoma. *Cancer* 85:78-84, 1999.

148. Glancy DL, Roberts WC: The heart in malignant melanoma. A study of 70 autopsy cases. *Am J Cardiol* 21:555-571, 1968.

149. Obeid AI, al Mudamgha A, Smulyan H: Diagnosis of right atrial mass lesions by transesophageal and transthoracic echocardiography. *Chest* 103:1447-1451, 1993.

150. Reeder GS, Khandheria BK, Seward JB, Tajik AJ: Transesophageal echocardiography and cardiac masses. *Mayo Clin Proc* 66:1101-1109, 1991.

151. Pandya UH, Pellikka PA, Enriquez-Sarano M, et al: Metastatic carcinoid tumor to the heart: Echocardiographic-pathologic study of 11 patients. *J Am Coll Cardiol* 40:1328-1332, 2002.

152. Lee TM, Chen MF, Liau CS, Lee YT: Role of transesophageal echocardiography in the management of metastatic tumors invading the left atrium. *Cardiology* 88:214-217, 1997.

153. Kullo IJ, Oh JK, Keeney GL, et al: Intracardiac leiomyomatosis: Echocardiographic features. *Chest* 115:587-591, 1991.

154. Swenson JD, Hullander RM, Nolan JE, York JK: Renal cell carcinoma in the inferior vena cava demonstrated by transesophageal echocardiography. *J Cardiothorac Vasc Anesth* 7:335-336, 1993.

155. Singh I, Jacobs LE, Kotler MN, Ioli A: The utility of transesophageal echocardiography in the management of renal cell carcinoma with intracardiac extension. *J Am Soc Echocardiogr* 8:245-250, 1995.

156. Hasnain JU, Watson RJ: Transesophageal echocardiography during resection of renal cell carcinoma involving the inferior vena cava. *South Med J* 87:273-275, 1994.

157. Kim RH, Mautner L, Henning J, Volpe R: An unusual case of thyroid carcinoma with direct extension to great veins, right heart, and pulmonary arteries. *Can Med Assoc J* 94:238-243, 1966.

158. Podolsky LA, Jacobs LE, Ioli A, Kotler MN: TEE in the diagnosis of intravenous leiomyomatosis extending into the right atrium. *Am Heart J* 125:1462-1464, 1993.

159. Joffe II, Lampert C, Jacobs LE, et al: Cardiac sarcoidosis masquerading as a metastatic tumor: The role of transthoracic and transesophageal echocardiography. *J Am Soc Echocardiogr* 8:933-937, 1995.

160. Herbst A, Padilla MT, Prasad AR, et al: Cardiac Wegener's granulomatosis masquerading as left atrial myxoma. *Ann Thorac Surg* 75:1321-1323, 2003.

161. Eroglu E, Di Salvo G, Herbots L, et al: Restrictive left ventricular filling in hypereosinophilic syndrome as a result of partial cavity obliteration by an apical mass: A strain/strain rate study. *J Am Soc Echocardiogr* 16:1088-1090, 2003.

162. Ker J, Van Beljon J: Diaphragmatic hernia mimicking an atrial mass: A two-dimensional echocardiographic pitfall and a cause of postprandial syncope. *Cardiovasc J S Afr* 15:182-183, 2004.

163. Harrity PJ, Tazelaar HD, Edwards WD, et al: Intracardiac varices of the right atrium: a case report and review of the literature. *Int J Cardiol* 48:177-181, 1995.

164. Choi BJ, Chang HJ, Choi SY, et al: A coronary artery fistula with saccular aneurysm mimicking a right atrial cystic mass. *Jpn Heart J* 45:697-702, 2004.

165. Anfinsen OG, Aaberge L, Geiran O, et al: Coronary artery aneurysms mimicking cardiac tumor. *Eur J Echocardiogr* 5:308-312, 2004.

166. Malaterre HR, Cohen F, Kallee K, et al: Giant interatrial septal aneurysm mimicking a right atrial tumor. *Int J Cardiovasc Imaging* 14:163-166, 1998.

167. Pappas KD, Arnaoutoglou E, Papadopoulos G: Giant atrial septal aneurysm simulating a right atrial tumor. *Heart* 90:493, 2004.

168. Cheng HW, Hung KC, Lin FC, Wu D: Spontaneous intramyocardial hematoma mimicking a cardiac tumor of the right ventricle. *J Am Soc Echocardiogr* 17:394-396, 2004.

169. Timperley J, Mitchell AR, Becher H: Primary cardiac lymphoma. *Eur J Echocardiogr* 4:327-330, 2003.

170. Padder FA, Conrad AR, Manzar JK, et al: Echocardiographic diagnosis of pericardial cyst. *Am J Med Sci* 313:191-192, 1997.

171. Meng Q, Lai H, Lima J, et al: Echocardiographic and pathologic characteristics of primary cardiac tumors: A study of 149 cases. *Int J Cardiol* 84:69-75, 2002.

172. Bruce CJ, Packer DL, Seward JB: Intracardiac Doppler hemodynamics and flow: New vector, phased-array ultrasound-tipped catheter. *Am J Cardiol* 83:1509-1512, A9, 1999.

173. Bruce CJ, Nishimura RA, Rihals CS, et al: Intracardiac echocardiography in the interventional catheterization laboratory: Preliminary experience with a novel, phased-array transducer. *Am J Cardiol* 89:635-640, 2002.

174. Segar DS, Bourdillon PD, Elsner G, et al: Intracardiac echocardiography-guided biopsy of intracardiac masses. *J Am Soc Echocardiogr* 8:927-929, 1995.

175. Malouf JF, Thompson RC, Maples WJ, Wolfe JT: Diagnosis of right atrial metastatic melanoma by transesophageal echocardiographic-guided transvenous biopsy. *Mayo Clin Proc* 71:1167-1170, 1996.

176. Lynch M, Clements SD, Shanewise JS, et al: Right-sided cardiac tumors detected by transesophageal echocardiography and its usefulness in differentiating the benign from the malignant ones. *Am J Cardiol* 79:781-784, 1997.

177. Burling F, Devlin G, Heald S: Primary cardiac lymphoma diagnosed with transesophageal echocardiography-guided endomyocardial biopsy. *Circulation* 101:E179-E181, 2000.

178. Jurkovich D, de Marchena E, Bilsker M, et al: Primary cardiac lymphoma diagnosed by percutaneous intracardiac biopsy with combined fluoroscopic and transesophageal echocardiographic imaging. *Catheter Cardiovasc Interv* 50:226-233, 2000.

179. Dujardin KS, Click RL, Oh JK: The role of intraoperative transesophageal echocardiography in patients undergoing cardiac mass removal. *J Am Soc Echocardiogr* 13:1080-1083, 2000.

180. Ofori CS, Sharma BN, Moore LC, et al: Disappearing cardiac masses—the importance of intraoperative transesophageal echocardiography. *J Heart Valve Dis* 3:688-689, 1994.

181. Borges AC, Witt C, Bartel T, et al: Preoperative two- and three-dimensional transesophageal echocardiographic assessment of heart tumors. *Ann Thorac Surg* 61:1163-1167, 1996.

182. Espinola-Zavaleta N, Morales GH, Vargas-Barron K, et al: Three-dimensional transesophageal echocardiography in tumors of the heart. *J Am Soc Echocardiogr* 15:972-979, 2002.

183. Lokhandwala J, Lui Z, Jundi M, et al: Three-dimensional echocardiography of intracardiac masses. *Echocardiography* 21:159-163, 2004.

184. Mehmood F, Nanda NC, Vengala S, et al: Live three-dimensional transthoracic echocardiographic assessment of left atrial tumors. *Echocardiography* 22:137-143, 2005.

185. Handke M, Schocholin A, Schafer DM, et al: Myxoma of the mitral valve: Diagnosis by 2-dimensional and 3-dimensional echocardiography. *J Am Soc Echocardiogr* 12:773-776, 1999.

186. Veiga Mde F, Lopes MG, Pinto FJ: Dynamic three-dimensional reconstruction of the heart by transesophageal echocardiography. *Arq Bras Cardiol* 72:559-568, 1999.

187. Ganame J, D'Hooge J, Mertens L: Different deformation patterns in intracardiac tumors. *Eur J Echocardiogr* 6:461-464, 2005.

188. Pauliks LB, Miller S, Banerjee A: Intracardiac fibroma in nevoid-basal cell carcinoma (gorlin) syndrome: Tissue characterization by strain rate imaging. *Echocardiography* 23:79-80 2006.

189. Bouton S, Yang A, McCrindle BW, et al: Differentiation of tumor from viable myocardium using cardiac tagging with MR imaging. *J Comput Assist Tomogr* 15:676-678, 1991.

190. Green SE, Joynt LF, Fitzgerald PJ, et al: In vivo ultrasonic tissue characterization of human intracardiac masses. *Am J Cardiol* 51:231-236, 1983.

191. Xiao G, Brady M, Noble JA, Zhang Y: Segmentation of ultrasound B-mode images with intensity inhomogeneity correction. *IEEE Trans Med Imaging* 21:48-57, 2002.

192. Hao X, Bruce CJ, Pislaru C, Greenleaf JF: Characterization of reperfused infarcted myocardium from high-frequency intracardiac ultrasound imaging using homodyned K distribution. *IEEE Trans Ultrason Ferroelectr Freq Control* 49:1530-1542, 2002.

193. Lepper W, Shivalkar B, Rinkevich D, et al: Assessment of the vascularity of a left ventricular mass using myocardial contrast echocardiography. *J Am Soc Cardiogr* 15:1419-1422, 2002.

194. Campani R, Calliadi F, Bottinelli F, et al: Contrast enhancing agents in ultrasonography: Clinical applications. *Eur J Radiol* 27(suppl 2):S161-S170, 1998.

195. Kirkpatrick JN, Wong T, Bednarz JE, et al: Differential diagnosis of cardiac masses using contrast echocardiographic perfusion imaging. *J Am Coll Cardiol* 43:1412-1419, 2004.

196. Tousek P, Orban M, Schomig A, Firschke C: Images in cardiovascular medicine. Real-time perfusion echocardiography of an intracardiac mass. *Circulation* 107:2390, 2003.

197. Weller GE, Wong MK, Modzelewski RA, et al: Ultrasonic imaging of tumor angiogenesis using contrast microbubbles targeted via the tumor-binding peptide arginine-arginine-leucine. *Cancer Res* 65:533-539, 2005.

Index

A

Note: Page numbers followed by the letter f refer to figures and those followed by t refer to tables.